WALKER'S
PEDIATRIC
GASTROINTESTINAL
DISEASE

PHYSIOLOGY • DIAGNOSIS • MANAGEMENT

VOLUME ONE

5

EDITORS

RONALD E. KLEINMAN, MD
Charles Wilder Professor of Pediatrics
Harvard Medical School
Physician-in-Chief and Chair, Department of Pediatrics
Massachusetts General Hospital for Children
Boston, Massachusetts

OLIVIER J. GOULET, MD, PhD
Chief, In-Patient Gastroenterology Unit
Necker-Enfants Malades Hôpital
Professor of Pediatrics
Faculty of Medicine Necker
University of Paris V
Paris, France

GIORGINA MIELI-VERGANI, MD, PhD, FRCPCH
Alex Mowat Professor of Pediatric Hepatology
Department of Liver Studies and Transplantation
Guy's, King's, and St. Thomas' School of Medicine
London, UK

IAN R. SANDERSON, MSc, MD, FRCP, FRCPCH
Professor of Paediatric Gastroenterology
Head, Centre for Gastroenterology
Centre for Digestive Disease
Blizard Institute of Cell & Molecular Science
London, UK

PHILIP M. SHERMAN, MD, FRCPC
Professor of Paediatrics, Microbiology, and Dentistry
Hospital for Sick Children
University of Toronto
Canada Research Chair in Gastrointestinal Disease
Toronto, Ontario, Canada

BENJAMIN L. SHNEIDER, MD
Professor of Pediatrics
Department of Pediatrics
University of Pittsburgh School of Medicine
Pittsburgh, Pennsylvania

Walker's

Pediatric Gastrointestinal Disease

5

Physiology • Diagnosis • Management

VOLUME ONE

2008
People's Medical Publishing House—USA
Shelton, CT

People's Medical Publishing House—USA
2 Enterprise Drive, Suite 509
Shelton, CT 06484
Tel: 203-402-0646
Fax:203-402-0854
E-mail: info@pmph-usa.com

PMPH-USA

08 09 10 11 12 / IPP / 9 8 7 6 5 4 3 2 1

ISBN 978-1-55009-364-3
Printed in China
Managing Editor: Patricia Binder: Production Editor: Catherine Travelle; Typesetter: Aptara; Cover Designer: Alex Wheldon

Sales and Distribution

United States
BC Decker Inc
P.O. Box 785
Lewiston, NY 14092-0785
Tel: 905-522-7017; 800-568-7281
Fax: 905-522-7839; 888-311-4987
E-mail: info@bcdecker.com
www.bcdecker.com

UK, Europe, Middle East
McGraw-Hill Education
Shoppenhangers Road
Maidenhead
Berkshire, England SL6 2QL
Tel: 44-0-1628-502500
Fax: 44-0-1628-635895
www.mcgraw-hill.co.uk

Mexico and Central America
ETM SA de CV
Calle de Tula 59
Colonia Condesa
06140 Mexico DF, Mexico
Tel: 52-5-5553-6657
Fax: 52-5-5211-8468
E-mail: editoresdetextosmex@prodigy.net.mx

Canada
McGraw-Hill Ryerson Education
Customer Care
300 Water Street
Whitby, Ontario, L1N 9B6
Tel: 1-800-565-5758
Fax: 1-800-463-5885

Singapore, Malaysia,Thailand, Philippines, Indonesia, Vietnam, Pacific Rim, Korea
McGraw-Hill Education
60 Tuas Basin Link
Singapore 638775
Tel: 65-6863-1580
Fax: 65-6862-3354

Brazil
Tecmedd Importadora E Distribuidora De Livros Ltda.
Avenida Maurílio Biagi, 2850
City Ribeirão, Ribeirão Preto – SP – Brasil
CEP: 14021-000
Tel: 0800 992236
Fax: (16) 3993-9000
E-mail: tecmedd@tecmedd.com.br

Foreign Rights
John Scott & Company
International Publishers' Agency
P.O. Box 878
Kimberton, PA 19442
Tel: 610-827-1640
Fax: 610-827-1671
E-mail: jsco@voicenet.com

Australia, New Zealand
McGraw-Hill Australia
Pyt LtdLevel 2, 82 Waterloo Road North Ryde, NSW, 2113 Australia
Customer Service Australia
Phone: +61 (2) 9900 1800
Fax: +61 (2) 9900 1980
E-mail: cservice_sydney@mcgraw-hill.com

Customer Service New Zealand
Phone (Free Phone): +64 (0) 800 449 312
Fax: (Free Phone): +64 (0) 800 449 318
Email: cservice@mcgraw-hill.co.nz

India, Bangladesh, Pakistan, Sri Lanka
CBS Publishers & Distributors
4596/1A-11, Darya Ganj
New Delhi-2, India
Tel: 232 71632
Fax: 232 76712
E-mail: cbspubs@vsnl.com

Japan
United Publishers Services Limited
1-32-5 Higashi-Shinagawa
Shinagawa-Ku, Tokyo 140-0002
Tel: 03 5479 7251
Fax: 03 5479 7307

PREFACE TO THE FIFTH EDITION

The fifth edition of this textbook is being published in advance of World Congress-3 of Pediatric Gastroenterology, Hepatology, and Nutrition to be held in Igaussu Falls, Brazil, in August 2008. This timeline has been developed to provide a timely and comprehensive update to health care providers worldwide, who have the privilege of caring for children with gastrointestinal and liver disorders. To provide harmony and reduce unnecessary duplication, this textbook was developed in concert with the latest edition of the *Nutrition in Pediatrics* edited by Drs. Christopher Duggan, John Watkins and Allan Walker.

This new edition marks the end of an era: Professor Allan Walker has stepped down from his leadership position, having turned over the management and responsibility for this edition over to Ron Kleinman, and his co editors. The team of editors wishes to thank Allan publicly for his sage guidance and leadership over many years, and to acknowledge that we continue to rely on his input and feedback in formulating what is now referred to as *Walker's Pediatric Gastrointestinal Disease*. We also enthusiastically welcome the addition of Professor Giorgina Mieli-Vegani from London to the group of editors who are responsible for this edition of the Walker textbook.

The intent of this edition of the textbook is to provide a comprehensive overview of the most recent advances in our subspecialty. A cadre of leading experts from all around the world has been assembled as authors of the various chapters, so as to provide an international perspective for a rapidly evolving and increasingly technical subspecialty. The chapters included in this edition of the Walker textbook are intended to provide the most current concepts regarding the pathophysiologic basis of gastrointestinal and hepatologic disorders affecting newborns, children and adolescents, a consideration of the differential diagnosis, and evidence-based approaches to the diagnosis and treatment of these conditions.

The editors have greatly enjoyed having a leadership role in developing the 5th edition of this textbook. We trust that the content provided herein will assist in the continuing medical education of those who are involved in providing the best available health care to our most precious resource, children.

Ronald E. Kleinman
Olivier J. Goulet
Giorgina Mieli-Vergani
Ian R. Sanderson
Philip M. Sherman
Benjamin L. Shneider
September 2007

DEDICATIONS

With deepest gratitude to Martha, Adam, Emily, Scott and Avery Isabel for their love and support.

Ronald E. Kleinman, MD

With my deep appreciation to Professor Allan Walker who invited me to join the editorship of this book; to my senior colleagues, Professors Jean Rey, Claude Ricour and Jacques Schmitz, who encouraged me to enter pediatric gastroenterology and nutrition; and to my wife, Véronique, and our children, Pierre-Arthur, Charles, Alix and Marine, who have supported me in my work for so many years.

Olivier J. Goulet, MD, PhD

To Bill Rizzo

Ian R. Sanderson, MD

This book is dedicated to trainees—past, current, and future—who make the journey through life in academic medicine so interesting, meaningful, and rewarding.

Philip M. Sherman, MD

To my wife, Abigail, and my daughters, Elizabeth and Caitlin, for their tremendous love, support, and sacrifices without which this and my other professional accomplishments would not be possible. I would also like to acknowledge my colleague and friend, Sukru Emre, for all of his insights into pediatric hepatology.

Benjamin L. Shneider, MD

CONTENTS

CONTRIBUTORS

NADEEM AHMAD AFZAL, MBBS, MRCPCH, MRCP (UK)
Specialist Registrar
Center for Pediatric Gastroenterology
Royal Free Hampstead National Health Service Trust
London, England
Interventional Endoscopy: Recent Innovations

STEPHEN JOHN ALLEN, MBChB, MRCP (UK) PAEDS, DTM&H, MD
Reader in Paediatrics
The School of Medicine
University of Wales Swansea
Swansea, Wales, United Kingdom
Malnutrition

BEATRICE C. AMADI, MD, MMED, DIPLOMA IN PAED.
   GASTROENTEROLOGY
University of Zambia
School of Medicine
Department of Paediatrics and Child Health
University Teaching Hospital
Lusaka, Zambia
Parasitic and Fungal Infections

PAUL ASHLEY, BDS, PhD, FDS, PAED DENT
Senior Lecturer Paediatric Dentistry
Division of Paediatric Dentistry
University College London
London, England
Disorders of the Oral Cavity

KAMRAM BADIZADEGAN, MD
Assistant Professor of Pathology & Health Science and Technology
Harvard Medical School
Massachusetts General Hospital
Boston, Massachusetts
Other Neoplasms

WILLIAM F. BALISTRERI, MD
Dorothy M.M. Kersten Professor of Pediatrics
Department of Pediatrics
University of Cincinnati College of Medicine
Cincinnati, Ohio
Approach to Neonatal Cholestasis

COLIN BALL, MD
Consultant Paediatrician
Department of Paediatrics
King's College Hospital
Denmark Hill
London, England
Immune Deficiency and the Liver

SANJAY BANSAL, MD, MRCP
Senior Registrar
Department of Paediatric Hepatology
King's College Hospital
London, England
Acute Liver Failure

DORSEY M. BASS, MD
Associate Professor of Pediatrics
Department of Pediatrics
Stanford University
Palo Alto, California
Viral Infections of the Intestinal Tract

DOMINIQUE C. BELLI, MD
Pediatric Gastroenterology Unit
Children's Hospital of Geneva
Geneva, Switzerland
Upper Gastrointestinal Endoscopy

SUZANNE BENDER, MD
Clinical Instructor
Department of Psychiatry
Harvard University Medical School
Boston, Massachusetts
Management of Surgical Patients

KEITH J. BENKOV, MD
Associate Professor
Department of Pediatrics
Mount Sinai School of Medicine
New York, New York
*Ultrasonography, Computed Tomography,
Magnetic Resonance Imaging*

MARC A. BENNINGA, MD, PhD
Head of the Department of Pediatric
Gastroenterology and Nutrition
Department of Pediatric GI and Nutrition
Emma Children's Hospital/AMC
Amsterdam, The Netherlands
*Chronic Abdominal Pain Including Functional
Abdominal Pain, Irritable Bowel Syndrome and
Abdominal Migraine*

MARK J. BERGERON, MD
Department of Pediatrics
University of Minnesota
Minneapolis, Minnesota
Bilirubin Metabolism

JORGE A. BEZERRA, MD
Professor of Pediatrics
Department of Pediatrics
University of Cincinnati
Cincinnati, Ohio
Biliary Atresia

JULIE E. BINES, MD, FRACP
Victor and Loti Smorgon Professor of Paediatrics
Department of Paediatrics
University of Melbourne
Parkville, Australia
Intestine Failure–Associated Liver Disease

THOMAS BLANCHARD, PhD
Assistant Professor
Department of Biological Sciences
University of Tennessee at Martin
Martin, Tennessee
Immune and Inflammatory Disorders: Inflammation

GABRIELLA BOCCIA, MD
Assistant Professor
Department of Pediatrics
University of Naples Federico II
Naples, Italy
*Normal Motility and Development of the Intestinal
Neuroenteric System*

OSVALDO BORELLI, MD, PhD
Reader
Department of Pediatrics
University of Rome "La Sapienza"
Rome, Italy
*Normal Motility and Development of the Esophageal
Neuroenteric System*

KEVIN E. BOVE, MD
Professor
Department of Pediatrics
University of Cincinnati College of Medicine
Cincinnati, Ohio
Bile Acid Synthesis and Metabolism
*Lysosomal Acid Lipase Deficiencies, Wolman's Disease
    and Cholesteryl Ester Storage Disease*

ANNAMARIE BRODERICK, MB, BCH, BAO, MMEDSC, DCH, MRCPI
Department of Pediatrics
University College Dublin
Children's Research Centre, Our Lady's Hospital for Sick Children
Dublin, Ireland
Gallbladder Disease

BILLY BOURKE, MD, FRCPI
Research Strand, Inflammation, Infection & Immunity
Department of Pediatrics
University College Dublin
Dublin, Ireland
Helicobacter Pylori and Peptic Ulcer Disease

NICOLE BROUSSE, MD, PhD
Professor of Pathology
Hôpital Necker-Enfants Malades
Paris V-Université René Descartes
Paris, France
Autoimmune Enteropathy and IPEX Syndrome

LAURA BULL, PhD
Associate Professor of Medicine
Department of Biopharmacology Science
University of California at San Francisco
San Francisco, California
Disorders of Biliary Transport

TARIQ BURKI, MBBS, FCPS, FRCS
Department of Paediatric Surgery
The Royal Hospital London
London, England
Pediatric Ostomy

BRENDA BURSCH, PhD
Professor
Division of Child Psychiatry
David Geffen School of Medicine at UCLA
Los Angeles, California
Gastrointestinal Features of Pediatric Illness Falsification

ROSS N. BUTLER, MSc, PhD
Professor
Department of Physiology
University of Adelaide
Adelaide, Australia
Breath Analysis

ASSAD M. BUTT, MBBS(LONDON), DCH(LONDON), FRCPCH
Honorary Consultant
Department of Paediatrics
Brighton & Sussex University Medical School
Brighton, England
The Pancreas: Tumors

ANNE MARIE CAHILL
Chief, Interventional Radiology Division
Children's Hospital of Philadelphia
University of Pennsylvania
School of Medicine
Philadelphia, Pennsylvania
Interventional Radiology in the GI Tract in Children

MICHAEL S. CAPLAN, MD
Associate Professor of Pediatrics
Department of Pediatrics
Northwestern University, Feinberg School of Medicine
Evanston, Illinois
Necrotizing Enterocolitis

HELEN CARTY, FRCR, FRCPI, FRCP, FRCPCH, FFRRCSI(HON)
Professor of Paediatric Radiology
Department of Medical Imaging
University of Liverpool
Liverpool, England
Plain Radiographs and Contrast Studies

DAVID CASSON, BA, MBBS, MRCPI
Honorary Lecturer
Department of Medicine
University of Liverpool
Liverpool, England
Radionuclide Diagnosis

JEAN PIERRE CÉZARD, MD, PhD
Professeur
Department of Gastroenterology
Paris VII
Paris, France
Normal Physiology of Intestinal Digestion and Absorption

MEI-HWEI CHANG, MD
Professor
Department of Pediatrics
National Taiwan University
College of Medicine
Taipei, Taiwan
Hepatitis B Virus

ERIKA C. CLAUD, MD
Assistant Professor
Department of Pediatrics
Division of Neonatology
University of Chicago
Chicago, Illinois
Necrotizing Enterocolitis

GEOFFREY CLEGHORN, MBBS, FRACP, FACG, FQA
Associate Professor and Head
Department of Pediatrics and Child Health
University of Queensland
Brisbane, Australia
Pharmacological Therapy of Exocine Pancreatic Insufficiency

ANDREW B. COOPER, PhD
Research Assistant Professor
Department of Natural Resources/EOS
University of New Hampshire
Durham, New Hampshire
*Methodology: Statistical Analysis, Test Interpretation, Basic
Principles of Screening with Application for Clinical Study*

CATHERINE CORD-UDY, MBBS, FRACS(PAED SURG)
Consultant Paediatric Surgeon
Department of Paediatric Surgery
The Royal Hospital London
London, England
Pediatric Ostomy

RICHARD T. LEE COUPER, MD
Department of Paediatrics
University of Adelaide
Adelaide, Australia
Pancreatic Function Tests

NICHOLAS M. CROFT, MBBS, PhD, FRCPCH
Senior Lecturer
Department of Paediatric Gastroenterology
Barts and The London, Queen Mary's School
of Medicine and Dentistry
London, England
Ulcerative and Indeterminate Colitis

SALVATORE CUCCIARA, MD, PhD
Professor
Department of Pediatrics
University of Rome "La Sapienza"
Rome, Italy
*Normal Motility and Development of the Esophageal
Neuroenteric System*

CARLA D. CUTHBERT, PhD
Fellow, Clinical-Biochemical Genetics
Department of Laboratory Medicine and Pathology
Mayo Medical School
Rochester, Minnesota
Inherited Abnormalities in Mitochondrial Fatty Acid Oxidation

STEVEN J. CZINN, MD
Professor
Departments of Pediatrics and Pathology
Case Western Reserve University School of Medicine
Cleveland, Ohio
Immune and Inflammatory Disorders: Inflammation

ALAN DANEMAN, MD
Department of Diagnostic Imaging
Hospital for Sick Children
Toronto, Ontario, Canada
Plain Radiographs and Contrast Studies

MARK DAVENPORT, ChM FRCS (PAEDS)
Reader in Paediatric Surgery
Department of Paediatric Surgery
Kings College, London
London, England
The Liver: Anatomy and Embryology

GEOFFREY P. DAVIDSON, MBBS, MD, FRACP
Professor
Department of Pediatrics
University of Adelaide
Adelaide, Australia
Breath Analysis

ANDREW S. DAY, MB, CHB, MD, FRACP
Senior Lecturer
Division of Paediatrics
University of New South Wales
School of Women's and Children's Health
Sydney, Australia
Other Causes of Gastritis

GIULIO DE MARCO, MD
Doctor
Department of Pediatrics
University of Naples Federico II
Naples, Italy
Persistent Diarrhea

LEE A. DENSON, MD
Assistant Professor
Department of Pediatrics
University of Cincinnati College of Medicine
Cincinnati, Ohio
Other Viral Infections

GUSTAVO ANDRADE DE PAULO, MD, MSc, PhD
Department of Gastroenterology
Universidade Federal de São Paulo
São Paulo, Brazil
Endoscopic Retrograde Cholangiopancreatography

PASCAL DE SANTA BARBARA, PhD
Department of Muscle and Pathologies
University of Montpellier
Montpellier, France
The Intestine: Anatomy and Embryology

ANIL DHAWAN, MD, FRCPCH
Honorary Senior Lecturer
Department of Paediatrics
Guy's, King's and St. Thomas School of Medicine
London, England
Acute Liver Failure

CARLO DI LORENZO, MD
Professor
Department of Pediatrics
University of Pittsburgh School of Medicine
Pittsburgh, Pennsylvania
Motility Disorders
Normal Motility and Development of the Gastric Neuroenteric System

GIOVANNI DI NARDO, MD
Clinical and Research Fellow
Department of Pediatrics
University of Rome "La Sapienza"
Rome, Italy
Normal Motility and Development of the Esophageal Neuroenteric System

BRENDAN DRUMM, MD, FRCPC, FRCPI
Professor
Department of Pediatrics
University College of Dublin
Dublin, Ireland
Helicobacter pylori and Peptic Ulcer Disease

HONG DU, PhD
Associate Professor
Department of Pediatrics
University of Cincinnati College of Medicine
Cincinnati, Ohio
*Lysosomal Acid Lipase Deficiencies: Wolman's
Disease and Cholesteryl Ester Storage Disease*

PETER R. DURIE, MD, FRCPC
Professor
Department of Pediatrics
University of Toronto
Toronto, Ontario, Canada
Shwachman-Diamond Syndrome

MOUNIF EL-YOUSSEF, MD
Associate Professor
Department of Pediatrics
Mayo Medical School
Rochester, Minnesota
Systemic Conditions Affecting the Liver

MICHAEL J. G. FARTHING, DSc(MED), MD, FRCP, FMEDSCI
Professor of Medicine
St. Georges Hospital Medical School
University of London
London, England
Parasitic and Fungal Infections

ALESSIO FASANO, MD
Professor and Director
Mucosal Biology Research Center
University of Maryland School of Medicine
Baltimore, Maryland
Bacterial Infections

MILTON J. FINEGOLD, MD
Professor of Pathology and Pediatrics
Department of Pathology
Baylor College of Medicine
Houston, Texas
Liver Tumors

YIGAEL FINKEL, MD, PhD
Department of Pediatric Gastroenterology and Nutrition
Astrid Lindgren Children's Hospital
Stockholm, Sweden
Short Bowel Syndrome

CLAUDIO FIOCCHI, MD
Professor
Departments of Medicine, Pathology and Pediatrics
Case Western Reserve University School of Medicine
Cleveland, Ohio
Immune and Inflammatory Disorders: Inflammation

THOMAS M. FISHBEIN, MD
Director
Small Bowel Transplantation
Transplant Institute
Georgetown University
Washington, District of Columbia
Small Intestinal Transplantation

ROBERT E. FLEMING, MD
Associate Professor of Pediatrics
Department of Pediatrics/Newborn Medicine
Saint Louis University
St. Louis, Missouri
Hemochromatosis

VICTOR L. FOX, MD
Assistant Professor
Department of Pediatrics
Harvard Medical School
Boston, Massachusetts
*Gastrointestinal Endoscopy: Patient Preparation and
General Considerations
Gastrointestinal Endosonography*

JULIANA C. FREM, MD
Fellow
Department of Pediatrics
Emory University School of Medicine
Atlanta, Georgia
Other Neuromuscular Disorders

DEBORAH K. FREESE, MD
Associate Professor
Department of Pediatrics
Mayo Medical School
Rochester, Minnesota
Systemic Conditions Affecting the Liver

GLENN T. FURUTA, MD
Assistant Professor
Department of Gastroenterology and Nutrition
The Children's Hospital
Boston, Massachusetts
Eosinophilic Gastrointestinal Disease

NARMER F. GALEANO, MD
Attending Physician
Division of Pediatric Gastroenterology
Maimonides Infants and Children's Hospital of Brooklyn
New York, New York
Mitochondrial Function and Dysfunction

CHERYL E. GARIEPY, MD, FAAP
Assistant Professor
Department of Pediatrics and Communicable Diseases
University of Michigan
Ann Arbor, Michigan
Hirschsprung's Disease

KEVIN J. GASKIN, MD, FRACP
James Fairfax Professor of Paediatric Nutrition
Discipline of Paediatrics & Child Health
University of Sydney
Sydney, Australia
Cystic Fibrosis

MARK A. GILGER, MD
Professor of Pediatrics
Department of Pediatrics
Baylor College of Medicine
Houston, Texas
Gastrointestinal Bleeding
Upper Gastrointestinal Bleeding

RANJANA GOKHALE, MD
University of Chicago Comer Children's Hospital
University of Chicago Pediatric Specialists
Chicago, Illinois
Atypical Colitis and Other Inflammatory Diseases

BENJAMIN D. GOLD, MD
Associate Professor of Pediatrics and Microbiology
Department of Pediatrics
Emory University School of Medicine
Atlanta, Georgia
Other Neuromuscular Disorders

REGINO P. GONZÁLEZ-PERALTA, MD
Associate Professor and Director
Department of Pediatrics
Pediatric Hepatology and Liver Transplantation
University of Florida College of Medicine
Gainesville, Florida
Hepatitis C Virus

FRÉDÉRIC GOTTRAND, MD, PhD
Professor
Faculté de Medecine
Université de Lille 2
Lille, France
Acid Peptic Disease

OLIVIER J. GOULET, MD, PhD
Chief, In-Patient Gastroenterology Unit
Necker-Enfants Malades Hôpital
Professor of Pediatrics
Faculty of Medicine Necker
University of Paris V
Paris, France
Autoimmune Enteropathy and IPEX Syndrome
Congenital Enteropathies
Gastrointestinal Manifestations of Primary
Immunodeficiency Diseases
Short Bowel Syndrome

GLENN R. GOURLEY, MD, AGAF
Professor of Pediatrics
Research Director, Pediatric Gastroenterology
Department of Pediatrics
University of Minnesota
Minneapolis, Minnesota
Bilirubin Metabolism

GREGORY A. GRABOWSKI, MD, FACMG
Professor
Department of Pediatrics
University of Cincinnati College of Medicine
Cincinnati, Ohio
Lysosomal Acid Lipase Deficiencies: Wolman
Disease and Cholesteryl Ester Storage Disease

FIONA GRAEME-COOK, MB, FRCP
Assistant Professor
Department of Pathology
Harvard Medical School
Boston, Massachusetts
Tumors of the Pediatric Esophagus and Stomach

BRUNO GRIDELLI, MD
Professor of Surgery
Department of Surgery
University of Pittsburgh School of Medicine
Pittsburgh, Pennsylvania
Liver Transplantation

ANNE M. GRIFFITHS, MD, FRCP (C)
Professor of Paediatrics
Department of Paediatrics
University of Toronto
Toronto, Ontario, Canada
Crohn's Disease

STEFANO GUANDALINI, MD
Professor
Department of Pediatrics
University of Chicago
Chicago, Illinois
Acute Diarrhea

ALFREDO GUARINO, MD
Professor
Department of Pediatrics
University of Naples Federico II
Naples, Italy
Persistent Diarrhea

DAVID J. HACKAM, MD, PhD
Roberta Simmons Assistant Professor
Division of Pediatric Surgery
University of Pittsburgh
School of Medicine
Pittsburgh, Pennsylvania
Peritonitus and Intra-abdominal Abscesses

NEDIM HADZIC, MD
Professor, Honorary Senior Lecturer Paediatric Hepatology
Department of Child Health, Institute of Liver Studies
King's College Hospital
Denmark Hill
London, England
Immune Deficiency and the Liver

ERIC HASSALL, MBCHB, FRCPC, FACG
Professor
Department of Pediatrics
University of British Columbia
Vancouver, British Columbia, Canada
Gastroesophageal Reflux

JAMES E. HEUBI, MD
Professor of Pediatrics
Division of Pediatric Gastroenterology, Hepatology & Nutrition
Cincinnati Children's Hospital
Cincinnati, Ohio
Bile Acid Synthesis and Metabolism

PATRICIA L. HIBBERD, MD, PhD
Director, Center for Global Health Research
Department of Public Health and Family Medicine
Tufts University School of Medicine
Boston, Massachusetts
Methodology: Statistical Analysis, Test Interpretation, Basic Principles of Screening with Application for Clinical Study

SIMON HORSLEN, MB, CHB, MRCP(UK), FRCPCH
Professor of Pediatrics
Department of Pediatrics
University of Washington
Seattle, Washington
Disorders of Carbohydrate Metabolism

SARAH HOTCHIN, RN
Specialist Sister, Paediatric Surgery and Stoma Care
The Royal London Hospital
London, England
Pediatric Ostomy

JEAN-PIERRE HUGOT, MD, PhD
Professor
Faculté de Médicine Bichat
Université Paris VII
Paris, France
Crohn's Disease

PAUL E. HYMAN, MD
Department of Pediatric Gastroenterology
University of Kansas
Kansas City, Kansas
Gastrointestinal Features of Pediatric Illness Falsification

ESSAM IMSEIS, MD
Fellow, Division of Gastroenterology and Nutrition
C. S. Mott Children's Hospital
Department of Pediatrics and Communicable Diseases
University of Michigan School of Medicine
Ann Arbor, Michigan
Hirschsprung's Disease

MIHO INOUE, MD
Clinical Fellow
Department of Pediatrics
University of Toronto
Division of Clinical Pharmacology and Toxicology
Toronto, Ontario, Canada
Drug-Induced Bowel Injury

ERIKA ISOLAURI, MD, PhD
Department of Pediatrics
Professor of Pediatrics
University of Turku
Turku, Finland
Probiotics

SHINYA ITO, MD, FRCPC
Professor
Department of Pediatrics
University of Toronto
Division of Clinical Pharmacology and Toxicology
Toronto, Ontario, Canada
Drug-Induced Bowel Injury

TOM JAKSIC, MD, PhD
Associate Professor
Department of Surgery
Harvard University
Children's Hospital
Boston, Massachusetts
Benign Perianal Lesions

DOMINIQUE M. JAN, MD
Visiting Professor
Department of Surgery
Columbia University
New York, New York
The Pancreas: Congenital Anomalies

SIDNEY JOHNSON, MD
Chief Surgical Resident
Department of Surgery
Children's Hospital Boston
Harvard Medical School
Boston, Massachusetts
Benign Perianal Lesions

CHRISTOPHER D. JOLLEY, MD
Associate Professor and Chief
Department of Pediatrics
University of Florida College of Medicine
Gainesville, Florida
Hepatitis C Virus

NICOLA L. JONES, MD, FRCPC, PhD
Associate Professor
Department of Paediatrics and Physiology
University of Toronto
Toronto, Ontario, Canada
Microbial Interactions with Gut Epithelium

STACY A. KAHN, MD
Fellow
University of Chicago
Department of Pediatrics
Comer Children's Hospital
Chicago, Illinois
Acute Diarrhea

SAUL J. KARPEN, MD, PhD
Associate Professor
Departments of Pediatrics and Molecular and Celluar Biology
Baylor College of Medicine
Houston, Texas
The Liver: Bile Formation and Cholestasis

STUART S. KAUFMAN, MD
Associate Professor of Pediatrics and Surgery
Georgetown University School of Medicine
Georgetown, District of Columbia
Small Intestinal Transplantation

ROBIN KAYE, MD
Associate Professor of Radiology
School of Medicine
University of Pennsylvania
Philadelphia, Pennsylvania
Interventional Radiology in the GI Tract in Children

PAUL KELLY, MA, MD, FRCP
Reader
Institute of Cell and Molecular Science
Barts and the London School of Medicine
London, England
HIV and Other Secondary Immunodeficiencies
Parasitic and Fungal Infections

SIMON E. KENNY, BSc(HONS), MBCHB(HONS), MD,
    FRCS(PAED SURG), FAAP
Honorary Senior Lecturer in Child Health
Department of Child Health
University of Liverpool
Liverpool, England
The Intestine: Congenital Anomalies Including Hernias

BARBARA S. KIRSCHNER, MD, FAAP
Professor of Pediatrics
Department of Pediatrics
The Pritzker School of Medicine
University of Chicago
Chicago, Illinois
Atypical Colitis and Other Inflammatory Diseases

RONALD E. KLEINMAN, MD
Charles Wilder Professor of Pediatrics
Harvard Medical School
Physician-in-Chief and Chair, Department of Pediatrics
Massachusetts General Hospital for Children
Boston, Massachusetts

A.S. KNISELY, MD
Consultant Histopathologist
Institute of Liver Studies
King's College Hospital
London, England
Liver Biopsy Interpretation

SIBYLLE KOLETZKO, MD
Professor
Department of Pediatrics
Ludwig Maximilians University
Munich, Germany
Other Dysmotilities Including Chronic Intestinal Pseudo-Obstruction
    Syndrome

AMETHYST C. KURBEGOV, MD, MPH
Clinical Fellow
Department of Pediatrics
Baylor College of Medicine
Houston, Texas
Bile Formation and Cholestasis

JACOB C. LANGER, MD, FRCS(C)
Professor
Department of Surgery
University of Toronto
Toronto, Ontario, Canada
Surgical Aspects of Inflammatory Bowel Disease in Children

MONICA LANGER, MD
Resident, General Surgery
Department of Surgery
University of British Columbia
Vancouver, British Columbia, Canada
Benign Perianal Lesions

GREGORY Y. LAUWERS, MD
Associate Professor
Department of Pathology
Harvard Medical School
Boston, Massachusetts
Tumors of the Pediatric Esophagus and Stomach

DANIEL AVI LEMBERG, BSc (MED), MBBS, DIPPAED, FRACP
Lecturer
Department of Paediatric Gastroenterology
University of New South Wales
School of Women's and Children's Health
Sydney, Australia
Other Causes of Gastritis

B U.K. LI, MD
Professor of Pediatrics
Department of Pediatrics
Medical College of Wisconsin
Milwaukee, Wisconsin
Nausea, Vomiting, and Pyloric Stenosis

CHRIS A. LIACOURAS, MD
Professor of Pediatrics
University of Pennsylvania
School of Medicine
Philadelphia, Pennsylvania
Eosinophilic Gastrointestinal Disease

STEVEN N. LICHTMAN, MD, FRCPC
Professor
Department of Pediatrics
University of North Carolina at Chapel Hill
School of Medicine
Chapel Hill, North Carolina
Small Bowel Bacterial Overgrowth

JENIFER R. LIGHTDALE, MD, MPH
Assistant in Pediatrics
Department of Pediatrics
Harvard Medical School
Boston, Massachusetts
Outcomes Research in Pediatric Gastroenterology

CLAUDE LIGUORY, MD
Medical Doctor
Endoscopy Unit
Alma Clinic
Paris, France
Endoscopic Retrograde Cholangiopancreatography

DAVID ALLDEN LLOYD, MCHIR, FRCS, FCS(SA),
    FRCSC(PED SURG), FACS
Emeritus Professor
Department of Child Health
University of Liverpool
Liverpool, England
The Intestine: Congenital Anomalies Including Hernias

DOLORES LÓPEZ-TERADA, MD, PHD
Assistant Professor
Department of Pathology
Baylor College of Medicine
Houston, Texas
Liver Tumors

MARK E. LOWE, MD, PHD
Professor of Pediatrics
Department of Pediatrics
University of Pittsburgh
Pittsburgh, Pennsylvania
Acute and Chronic Pancreatitis
Pancreatic Function and Dysfunction

DENNIS P. LUND, MD
Associate Professor
Department of Surgery
University of Wisconsin School of Medicine
Madison, Wisconsin
Appendicitis

WALLACE K. MACNAUGHTON, PHD
Professor
Department of Physiology and Biophysics
University of Calgary
Calgary, Alberta, Canada
Radiation Induced Bowel Injury

GIUSEPPE MAGGIORE, MD
Associate Professor of Pediatrics
Department of Pediatrics
University of Pisa
Pisa, Italy
Liver Transplantation

MARKKU MÄKI, MD, PHD
Professor
Department of Pediatrics
University of Tampere Medical School
Tampere, Finland
Celiac Disease

MARTIN G. MARTIN, MD, MPP
Professor of Pediatrics
Department of Pediatrics
University of California at Los Angeles
Los Angeles, California
Congenital Intestinal Transport Defects

EMMANUAL MAS, MD, MSc
Doctor
Department of Pediatrics
Children's Hospital, University of Toulouse
Toulouse, France
Toxic and Traumatic Injury of the Esophagus

DIETRICH MATERN, MD
Assistant Professor
Department of Laboratory Medicine and Pathology
Mayo Clinic College of Medicine
Rochester, Minnesota
Inherited Abnormalities in Mitochondrial Fatty Acid Oxidation

CAL S. MATSUMOTO, MD, FACS
Assistant Professor of Surgery
Department of Pediatric Liver and Intestinal Transplantation
Georgetown University Hospital
Washington, District of Columbia
Small Intestinal Transplantation

SUZANNE V. MCDIARMID, MB, CHB
Professor
David Geffen School of Medicine
University of California at Los Angeles
Los Angeles, California
End-Stage Liver Disease

LAURENT MICHAUD, MD
Medical Doctor
Division of Gastroenterology, Hepatology and Nutrition
Hôpital Jeanne de Flandre
Faculty of Medicine and Children's Hospital
Lille, France
Lower Gastrointestinal Bleeding

GIORGINA MIELI-VERGANI, MD, PHD, FRCPCH
Alex Mowat Professor of Pediatric Hepatology
Department of Liver Studies and Transplantation
Guy's, King's, and St. Thomas' School of Medicine
London, England
Autoimmune Liver Disease

ALEXANDER G. MIETHKE, MD
Fellow
Pediatric Gastroenterology, Hepatology and Nutrition
Cincinnati Children's Hospital
Cincinnati, Ohio
Approach to Neonatal Cholestasis

MICHAEL R. MILLAR, MB, CHB, MD, FRCPATH
Honorary Senior Lecturer
Centre for Infectious Diseases
Barts and the London School of Medicine and Dentistry,
Queen Mary College, University of London
London, England
Antimicrobials

BIREN P. MODI, MD
Research Fellow
Department of Surgery
Harvard University
Children's Hospital
Boston, Massachusetts
Benign Perianal Lesions

V. MOHAN, MD, FRCP(UK), FRCP(GLASGOW), PHD, DSC, FNASC
Chairman and Chief Diabetologist
Dr. Mohan's Diabetes Specialties Center and Madras
Diabetes Research Foundation
Chennai, India
Juvenile Tropical Pancreatitis

JEAN-FRANÇOIS MOUGENOT, MD
Pediatric Gastroenterologist
Director of Pediatric Digestive Endoscopic Units
Hôpital Robert Debré and Hôpital Necker-Enfants Malades
Paris, France
Endoscopic Retrograde Cholangiopancreatography
Intestinal Polyps and Polyposis
Upper Gastrointestinal Endoscopy

M. SUSAN MOYER, MD
Professor of Pediatrics
Medical Director
Schubert-Martin IBD Center
Cincinnati Children's Hospital
Cincinnati, Ohio
Intestinal Obstruction

SIMON MURCH, BSC, PHD, FRCP, FRCPCH
Senior Lecturer
Centre for Paediatric Gastroenterology
Royal Free and University College School of Medicine
London, England
Food Allergic Enteropathy

KAREN F. MURRAY, MD
Professor of Pediatrics
Department of Pediatrics
University of Washington
Seattle, Washington
Disorders of Amino Acid Metabolism

HASSAN Y. NAIM, PHD
Professor and Chairman of Biochemistry
Department of Physiological Chemistry
School of Veterinary Medicine, Hanover
Hanover, Germany
Genetically Determined Disaccharidase Deficiency

KAREN NORTON, MD
Associate Professor
Department of Radiology and Pediatrics
Mount Sinai School of Medicine
New York, New York
Ultrasonography, Computed Tomography,
Magnetic Resonance Imaging

SAMUEL NURKO, MD, MPH
Assistant Professor
Department of Pediatrics
Harvard Medical School
Boston, Massachusetts
Gastrointestinal Manometry: Methodology and Indications

MARK R. OLIVER, MBBS, MD, FRACP
Senior Fellow
Department of Paediatrics
University of Melbourne
Melbourne, Australia
Pancreatic Function Tests

JEAN-PIERRE OLIVES, MD
Professor of Pediatrics
Department of Pediatrics
Université de Toulouse
Toulouse, France
Toxic and Traumatic Injury of the Esophagus

SYLVIANE OLSCHWANG, MD, PHD
Researcher
Institut Paoli-Calmettes
Marseille, France
Intestinal Polyps and Polyposis

CHEE YEE OOI (KEITH), MB, BS, DIPPAED
Conjoint Associate Lecturer
Faculty of Medicine
University of New South Wales
Randwick, Australia
Other Causes of Gastritis

P. PEARL O'ROURKE, MD
Associate Professor, Pediatrics
Department of Pediatrics
Harvard Medical School
Harvard University
Boston, Massachusetts
Ethics and Regulatory Issues

DINESH S. PASHANKAR, MD, MRCP
Associate Professor
Department of Pediatrics
Yale University School of Medicine
New Haven, Connecticut
Bacterial, Parasitic and Other Infections

PRUE M. PEREIRA-FANTINI, PHD
Research Officer
Department of Infection, Immunity and Environment
Murdoch Children's Research Institute
Parkville, Australia
Intestine Failure – Associated Liver Disease

DAVID H. PERLMUTTER, MD
Vira I. Heinz Professor and Chair
Professor of Cell Biology and Physiology
Department of Pediatrics
University of Pittsburgh School of Medicine
Pittsburgh, Pennsylvania
α1-Antitrypsin Deficiency

MICHEL PEUCHMAUR, MD, PHD
Chief of Pathology Department
Robert Debré Hospital
Paris, France
Intestinal Polyps and Polyposi

ALAN DAVID PHILLIPS, BA, PhD, FRCPCH
Honorary Reader
Department of Pediatrics and Child Health
Royal Free and University College Medical School
University College London
London, England
Congenital Enteropathies
Genetically Determined Disaccharidase Deficiency
Intestinal Biopsy

C. S. PITCHUMONI, MD, FRCP(C), FACP, MPH, MACG
Clinical Professor of Medicine
Department of Medicine
Robert Wood Johnson School of Medicine and Drexel University
New Brunswick, New Jersey
Juvenile Tropical Pancreatitis

STEPHEN R. PORTER, MD, PhD, FDS, RCS, RCSE
Associate Dean and Professor, Head of Oral Medicine
Department of Oral Medicine
Eastman Dental Institute for Oral Health Care Sciences
London, England
Disorders of the Oral Cavity

RIAD RAHHAL, MD
Clinical Assistant Professor
Department of Pediatrics
University of Iowa
Iowa City, Iowa
Functional Constipation

GRANT A. RAMM, PhD
Head, Hepatic Fibrosis Group
The Queensland Institute of Medical Research
Royal Brisbane Hospital
Brisbane, Australia
Fibrogenesis and Cirrhosis

GERALD V. RAYMOND, MD
Associate Professor of Neurology
Johns Hopkins University School of Medicine
Baltimore, Maryland
Zellweger Syndrome and Other Disorders of Peroxisomal Metabolism

PIERO RINALDO, MD, PhD
Professor
Department of Laboratory Medicine and Pathology
Mayo Clinic College of Medicine
Rochester, Minnesota
Inherited Abnormalities in Mitochondrial Fatty Acid Oxidation

SILVIA RIVA, MD
Attending Pediatrician
Department of Medicine
ISMETT Hospital
Palermo, Italy
Liver Transplantation

DRUCILLA J. ROBERTS, MD
Department of Pathology
Massachusetts General Hospital
Boston, Massachusetts
The Stomach and Duodenum: Anatomy, Embryology, and Congenital Anomalies

EVE A. ROBERTS, MD, FRCPC (C)
Professor
Department of Pediatrics, Medicine, and Pharmacology
University of Toronto School of Medicine
Toronto, Ontario, Canada
Drug-Induced Hepatotoxicity in Children

PHILIP ROSENTHAL, MD
Professor of Pediatrics and Surgery
Department of Pediatrics
University of California, San Francisco
San Francisco, California
Disorders of the Biliary Tract: Other Disorders

ORI D. ROTSTEIN, MD, MSC, FRCSC, FACS
Senior Scientist
Division of Cellular & Molecular Biology
Toronto General Research Institute (TGRI)
Toronto, Ontario, Canada
Peritonitis and Intra-abdominal Abscesses

MARION ROWLAND, MB, PhD
Research Assistant
Department of Pediatrics
University College Dublin
Dublin, Ireland
Helicobacter Pylori and Peptic Ulcer Disease

COLIN D. RUDOLPH, MD, PhD
Professor of Pediatrics
Department of Pediatric Gastroenterology & Nutrition
Medical College of Wisconsin
Milwaukee, Wisconsin
Gastroesophageal Reflux

FRANK M. RUEMMELE, MD, PhD
Department of Pediatrics
Hôpital Necker-Enfants Malades
Faculty of Medicine
Paris V – Descartes
Paris, France
Autoimmune Enteropathy and IPEX Syndrome

SEPPO SALMINEN, PhD
Professor, Director
Functional Foods Forum, Health Biosciences Program
University of Turku
Turku, Finland
Probiotics

MARIANNE SAMYN, MD, FRCPCH
Consultant Paediatric Hepatologist
Paediatric Liver Centre
King's College Hospital
London, England
Autoimmune Liver Disease

IAN R. SANDERSON, MSc, MD, FRCP, FRCPCH
Professor of Paediatric Gastroenterology
Head, Centre for Gastroenterology
Centre for Digestive Disease
Blizard Institute of Cell & Molecular Science
London, UK

MIGUEL SAPS, MD
Assistant Professor of Pediatrics
Feinberg School of Medicine
Northwestern University
Chicago, Illinois
Motility Disorders
Normal Motility and Development of the Gastric Neuroenteric System

GHISLAINE SAYER, MRCP, DMRD, FRCR
Doctor
Department of Medical Imaging
University of Liverpool School of Medicine
Liverpool, England
Plain Radiographs and Contrast Studies

MICHELA G. SCHÄPPI, MD
Registrar
Division of Gastroenterology
Department of Pediatrics
Hôpital des Enfants Malades
University of Geneva
Geneva, Switzerland
Upper Gastrointestinal Endoscopy

STEVEN C. SCHOLZMAN, MD
Clinical Instructor in Psychiatry, Lecturer in Education
Department of Psychiatry
Harvard Medical School, Harvard Graduate School of Education
Boston, Massachusetts
Management of Surgical Patients

RICHARD A. SCHREIBER, MDCM, FRCP (C)
Clinical Professor
Department of Pediatrics
University of British Columbia
Vancouver, British Columbia, Canada
Bacterial, Parasitic and Other Infections

ANDREA SCHWARZER, MD
Division of Pediatric Gastroenterology and Hepatology
Ludwig-Maximilians University Medical School
Munich, Germany
Other Dysmotilities Including Chronic Intestinal Pseudo-Obstruction Syndrome

ERNEST G. SEIDMAN, MD, FRCPC, FACG
Professor
Department of Pediatrics
University of Montreal
Montreal, Quebec, Canada
Gastrointestinal Manifestations of Primary Immunodeficiency Diseases

KENNETH D. R. SETCHELL, PhD
Professor of Pediatrics
School of Medicine
University of Cincinnati
Cincinnati, Ohio
Bile Acid Synthesis and Metabolism

RAANAN SHAMIR, MD
Associate Professor
Department of Medicine
Ruth and Bruce Rappaport Faculty of Medicine
Technion, Institute of Technology
Haifa, Israel
Prebiotics, Synbiotics and Fermented Products

EYAL SHEMESH, MD
Assistant Professor
Department of Psychiatry
University of Pennsylvania
Philadelphia, Pennsylvania
Adherence to Medical Regimens

ROSS W. SHEPHERD, MD, FRACP, FRCP
Professor
Department of Pediatrics
Washington University School of Medicine
St. Louis, Missouri
Fibrogenesis and Cirrhosis

PHILIP M. SHERMAN, MD, FRCPC
Professor of Paediatrics, Microbiology and Dentistry
Hospital for Sick Children
University of Toronto
Canada Research Chair in Gastrointestinal Disease
Toronto, Ontario, Canada

DELANE SHINGADIA, FRCPCH, MPH
Doctor
Department of Child Health
Barts and The London School of Medicine and Dentistry
Queen Mary College, University of London
London, England
HIV and Other Secondary Immunodeficiencies

BENJAMIN L. SHNEIDER, MD
Professor of Pediatrics
Department of Pediatrics
University of Pittsburgh School of Medicine
Pittsburgh, Pennsylvania
Disorders of Biliary Transport

VIRPI V. SMITH, PhD
Honorary Lecturer
Gastroenterology Unit
Institute of Child Health
University College London
London, England
Intestinal Biopsy

MARCO SPADA, MD, PhD
Associate Professor of Surgery
Department of Surgery
University of Pittsburgh
Pittsburgh, Pennsylvania
Liver Transplantation

ROBERT H. SQUIRES JR., MD
Professor of Pediatrics
University of Pittsburgh School of Medicine
Pittsburgh, Pennsylvania
Ultrasonography, Computed Tomography, Magnetic Resonance Imaging

ANNAMARIA STAIANO, MD
Associate Professor
Department of Pediatrics
University of Naples Federico II
Naples, Italy
Normal Motility and Development of the Intestinal Neuroenteric System

STEVEN J. STEINBERG, PhD
Assistant Professor
Department of Neurology
Johns Hopkins University School of Medicine
Baltimore, Maryland
Zellweger Syndrome and Other Disorders of Peroxisomal Metabolism

JENNIFER P. STEVENS, MS
Medical Student
Harvard Medical School
Boston, Massachusetts
Ethics and Regulatory Issues

EKKEHARD STURM, MD, PhD
Doctor
University of Tuebingen
University Hospital
Tuebingen, Germany
Disorders of the Intrahepatic Bile Ducts

HANIA SZAJEWSKA, MD
Professor of Pediatrics
Department of Pediatrics
The Medical University of Warsaw
Warsaw, Poland
Prebiotics, Synbiotics and Fermented Products

STUART TANNER, CBE, FRCP, FRCPCH
Emeritus Professor of Paediatrics
Academic Unit of Child Health
University of Sheffield
Sheffield, England
Wilson's Disease

JONATHAN E. TEITELBAUM, MD, FAAP
Assistant Professor
Department of Pediatrics
Drexel University School of Medicine
Philadelphia, Pennsylvania
The Gastrointestinal System in Systemic Endocrinopathies
Mouth and Esophagus: Congenital Anomalies

MAURICIO R. TEREBIZNIK, PhD
Assistant Professor
Department of Cell and Systems Biology
University of Toronto
Toronto, Ontario, Canada
Microbial Interactions with Gut Epithelium

NIKHIL THAPAR, BSc(HONS), BM(HONS), MRCP(UK), MRCPCH
Research Fellow
Department of Enteric Neurodevelopment
National Institute for Medical Research
London, England
Stomach and Duodenum: Anatomy, Embryology and Congenital Anomalies

ERICA THOMAS, RGN, RSCN, DPNS, BSc (HONS)
Senior Sister Paediatric Surgery
Department of Paediatric Nursing
The Royal London Hospital
City University London
London, England
Pediatric Ostomy

MIKE THOMSON, MBChB, DCH, FCRP, FRCPCH
Senior Lecturer
Centre for Paediatric Gastroenterology
Sheffield Medical School
Sheffield, England
Esophagitis
Ileocolonoscopy and Enteroscopy
Interventional Endoscopy: Recent Innovations

FRANCO TORRENTE, MD
Clinical Assistant
Department of Pediatric Gastroenterology
G. Gaslini Institute
Genoa, Italy
Food Allergic Enteropathy

SILVIA TORTORELLI, MD, PhD
Fellow, Clinical Biochemical Genetics
Department of Laboratory Medicine and Pathology
Mayo Clinic College of Medicine
Rochester, Minnesota
Inherited Abnormalities in Mitochondrial Fatty Acid Oxidation

DAVID N. TUCHMAN, MD
Assistant Professor of Pediatrics
Department of Pediatrics
Johns Hopkins University
Baltimore, Maryland
Disorders of Deglutition

DOMINIQUE TURCK, MD
Professor of Pediatrics
Faculty of Medicine
University of Lille
Lille, France
Lower Gastrointestinal Bleeding

ALIYE UC, MD
Assistant Professor of Pediatrics
Department of Pediatrics
University of Iowa
Iowa City, Iowa
Functional Constipation

YVAN VANDENPLAS, MD, PhD
Staff Gastroenterologist
Department of Pediatrics
Academisch Zeikenhuis-Vrye Universiteit Brussel
Brussels, Belgium
pH and Impendance Measurements in Infants and Children

DIEGO VERGANI, MD, PhD, FRCP
Professor of Liver Immunopathology
Department of Liver Studies and Transplantation
Guy's, King's, and St. Thomas' School of Medicine
London, England
Autoimmune Liver Disease

HENKJAN J. VERKADE, MD, PhD
Professor of Pediatrics
Department of Pediatrics
University of Groningen Medical Center
Groningen, The Netherlands
Disorders of the Intrahepatic Bile Ducts

ARINE M. VLIEGER, MD
Pediatrician
Department of Pediatrics
St. Antonius Hospital
Nieuwegein, The Netherlands
Chronic Abdominal Pain Including Functional Abdominal Pain, Irritable Bowel Syndrome and Abdominal Migraine

PIERRE-YVES VON DER WEID, PhD
Associate Professor
Department of Pharmacology & Therapeutics,
Physiology & Biophysics
University of Calgary Faculty of Medicine
Calgary, Alberta, Canada
Lymphatic Disorders

W. ALLAN WALKER, MD
Conrad Taff Professor of Nutrition and Pediatrics
Department of Pediatrics
Harvard Medical School; Harvard School of Public Health
Boston, Massachusetts
Pediatric Gastroenterology, A Historical Perspective

JOHN WALKER-SMITH, MD, FRCP, FRACP, FRCPCH
Department of Paediatric Gastroenterology
Royal Free Hospital
University College Medical School
London, England
Pediatric Gastroenterology: A Historical Perspective

MU WANG, MD
Assistant Professor
Adjunct Professor of Informatics
Department of Biochemistry and Molecular Biology
Indiana University School of Medicine
Indianapolis, Indiana
Systemic Conditions Affecting the Liver

BRAD W. WARNER, MD
Professor of Surgery
Program Director, Pediatric Surgery Residency
Cincinnati Children's Hospital
Cincinnati, Ohio
Intestinal Obstruction

PAUL A. WATKINS, MD, PhD
Professor
Department of Neurology
Johns Hopkins University School of Medicine
Kennedy Krieger Institute
Baltimore, Maryland
Zellweger Syndrome and Other Disorders of Peroxisomal Metabolism

DAVID C. WHITCOMB, MD, PhD
Professor of Medicine
Department of Medicine
University of Pittsburgh
Pittsburgh, Pennsylvania
Pancreatitis: Acute and Chronic Pancreatic Function and Dysfunction

K. LYNETTE WHITFIELD, MD
Fellow
Department of Pediatrics
Baylor College of Medicine
Houston, Texas
Upper Gastrointestinal Bleeding

PETER F. WHITINGTON, MD
Professor of Pediatrics and Medicine
Northwestern University
Feinberg School of Medicine
Chicago, Illinois
Hemochromatosis

HELEN J. WILLIAMS, MB, CHB, MRCPCH, FRCR
Honorary Senior Clinical Lecturer
Department of Paediatrics
University of Birmingham
Birmingham, England
Radionuclide Diagnosis

MARK WILKS, BSc DIP BACTERIAL, PhD
Honorary Senior Lecturer
Centre for Infectious Diseases
Barts and the London School of Medicine and Dentistry
Queen Mary College, University of London
London, England
Antimicrobials

MICHAEL WILSCHANSKI, MBBS
Senior Lecturer
Department of Pediatrics
Hebrew University
Jerusalem, Israel
Other Hereditary and Acquired Pancreatic Disorders

EYTAN WINE, MD
PhD Candidate
The Hospital for Sick Children
Sherman Laboratory
Cell Biology Research Program
Toronto, Ontario, Canada
Microbial Interactions with Gut Epithelium

ERNST M. WRIGHT, PhD, DSc, FRS
Professor of Physiology
Department of Physiology
University of California at Los Angeles
Los Angeles, California
Congenital Intestinal Transport Defects

KLAUS-PETER ZIMMER, MD
Professor
Division of Gastroenterology
Westfalische Wilhelms Universitat
Munster, Germany
Genetically Determined Disaccharidase Deficiency

Introduction

Pediatric Gastroenterology: A Historical Perspective

W. Allan Walker, MD

John Walker-Smith, MD

The rise of pediatrics as a specialty was a natural outcome of the foundation of hospitals specifically for children in the nineteenth century. By the end of the century, chairs of pediatrics had been created. It was also at that time that gastroenterology emerged as a specialty of general medicine. However, it was not until the 1960s that pediatric gastroenterology began to emerge as a subspecialty within pediatrics. The reason for its emergence related naturally to the clinical need of a significant body of child patients. However, its development was catalyzed by the development of specialized techniques, which resulted in a significant improvement in accurate diagnosis. These improvements in large measure centered upon the ability to safely, and with minimal distress to the child, biopsy the gastrointestinal tract and the liver. Pari passu with this advance in accuracy of diagnosis based chiefly upon tissue diagnosis, the tissue provided, enabled a greater understanding of the pathology and pathophysiology of disease. It was a classical example of service and research proceeding side by side for the child's benefit. From the beginning, pediatric gastroenterology has been rooted in clinical science. So, scientific advances in nutrition, immunology, and related disciplines have been rapidly applied to clinical practice. Advances in surgery have also had considerable impact on pediatric gastroenterology practice, perhaps most notably the development of liver and more recently small intestinal transplantation.

In this introductory chapter of the fifth edition of this textbook, we attempt to summarize the historical evolution of our field, highlighting some of those disorders that have their onset during infancy or childhood or are unique to that age period and that have spurred the development of the discipline. We also review the defining events in the establishment of the subspecialty and speculate on the directions it may follow into the new millennium. All of these serve as a preface to a significantly expanded fifth edition of this textbook. All chapters have been revised and updated to reflect the advances in science and clinical practice that have occurred since the publication of the fourth edition. The textbook has also been significantly expanded to reflect the extraordinary advances in our understanding of the development and pathophysiology of the gastrointestinal tract at the cellular and molecular levels.

ONTOGENY OF PEDIATRIC GASTROENTEROLOGY

The concept of organ-specific subspecialties in medicine began at the end of the nineteenth century. For example, the American Gastroenterological Association was established in 1897 in Philadelphia.[1] It took almost another century before such subspecialties of pediatrics were established. The European and North American societies of pediatric gastroenterology were incorporated in 1968 and 1973, respectively, and, more recently, the Latin American (1974) and the Asian Pan Pacific (1993) societies formally organized. A major impediment to the development of this field was a notion among pediatricians that gastrointestinal conditions could be fully addressed within the purview of general pediatrics. Although this undoubtedly is true for common acute gastrointestinal conditions (eg, neonatal regurgitation and rotavirus gastroenteritis), it quickly became clear that the diagnosis and treatment of chronic, complex, and often debilitating conditions affecting the liver, pancreas, gastrointestinal tract as well as the nutritional status of pediatric patients required a specific knowledge and experience acquired only through specialized training. Heretofore, this need had been filled by gastroenterologists in internal medicine. In general, this approach was acceptable as long as it involved an older child or adolescent. However, these internists had little or no expertise in managing young patients with gastrointestinal problems unique to pediatrics, (eg, inborn errors in bilirubin metabolism, congenital intestinal absorptive defects and other metabolic diseases (α_1-antitrypsin disease [α_1-AT]), and congenital malformations of the liver and gastrointestinal tract. As we have acquired a better understanding of the phenotypic expression of disease, we now recognize that later childhood or adult onset of disease may have its pathophysiologic origin in utero or in early infancy. This is illustrated by the "Barker hypothesis" (eg, intrauterine programming)[2] as the basis for adult-onset type II diabetes or obesity and the importance of early appropriate bacterial colonization of the gut in the prevention of immune-mediated diseases such as allergy (asthma) or autoimmune diseases (Crohn's disease).[3] To better diagnose and manage these patients, pediatricians left pediatrics to train in adult gastroenterology and adapted this training to the care of infants and children. In the early 1970s, small selective divisions of pediatric gastroenterology and nutrition were established in North America and Europe by pediatricians trained in adult gastroenterology programs. These divisions became nascent training centers for future pediatric gastroenterologists. In three short decades, the field has evolved to become an established pediatric subspecialty worldwide.

DEVELOPMENT OF DIAGNOSTIC AND THERAPEUTIC APPROACHES TO GASTROINTESTINAL DISEASE STATES IN CHILDREN

Table 1 is adapted from a recent comprehensive review of the history of pediatric gastroenterology, hepatology, and nutrition[4] including a list of diagnostic techniques and therapeutic approaches that have helped shape the unique expertise of the pediatric gastroenterologist. We highlight a few representative conditions from this list below. A complete discussion of each disorder is found in subsequent chapters in the book.

Celiac Disease

Celiac disease is a unique genetically predisposed condition that, although lifelong, often presents in infancy and childhood. In postwar Holland, Dicke

---

Table 1 Medical Events Leading to the Emergence of Pediatric Gastroenterology

Small intestinal biopsy
Parenteral nutrition
Safe pediatric ileocolonoscopy
Percutaneous liver biopsy
Pathophysiology of hereditary disorders of absorption
Rise of gut immunology and food allergy research
Oral rehydration
Advances in pediatric surgery
   Portoenterostomy (Kasai) procedure for biliary atresia
   Organ transplant
   Liver
   Small bowel
Pathophysiology of metabolic liver disease
   (eg, α_1-antitrypsin genetic defect)
Genetic basis for disease
   Cystic fibrosis
   α_1-Antitrypsin disease
   Crohn's disease

Adapted from Walker-Smith, Walker.[4]

demonstrated that this chronic, malabsorptive condition associated with severe "failure to thrive" was caused by intolerance to gluten, a major constituent of several grains, particularly wheat.[5] This observation that a common condition in infants and children was not an infectious gastroenteritis but instead a food intolerance launched pediatric gastroenterology as a subspecialty of pediatrics in Europe. In 1957, Dr Jack Sakula, a pediatrician, and Dr Margot Shiner, a gastroenterologist, published a diagnostic technique that could be used to diagnose celiac disease.[6]

More recently, celiac disease has been linked to specific human leukocyte antigen (HLA) loci (DQ2 and DQ8), suggesting a genetically based underlying immunologic defect.[7] Currently, it is considered to be an autoimmune disease, with transglutaminase as the putative autoantigen.[8] With modern infant feeding guidelines, including exclusive breast-feeding for four or more months, the classic presentation of celiac disease in early infancy (chronic diarrhea or malabsorption associated with severe failure to thrive) is much less common today. In fact, as the condition presents in a less classical fashion in later childhood and in adults, it becomes part of a differential diagnosis for irritable bowel syndrome and inflammatory bowel disease.[9] Furthermore, it has been associated with other autoimmune diseases such as type I diabetes, hypothyroidism, so on, which can also confuse the diagnosis.[10] As serologic tests with high sensitivity and specificity for celiac disease have come into routine use (IgA antiendomysial and tissue transglutaminase antibodies), subclinical celiac disease and atypical presentations of the disorder have been recognized, and the true prevalence of this disorder has significantly increased.[11] These advances in noninvasive diagnostic tests, along with a better understanding of the pathogenesis of the disease, have allowed the pediatric gastroenterologist to manage the disease and its complications more efficiently (see Chapter 16.1, "Celiac Disease").

α1-Antitrypsin Deficiency Disease

In 1969, Sharp and colleagues reported that the inherited disorder α_1-AT deficiency was associated with neonatal hepatitis syndrome, leading to cirrhosis.[12] Subsequently, when the percutaneous liver biopsy technique was adapted for use in infants and children,[13] this condition could be distinguished from other neonatal hepatic conditions, such as biliary atresia. In follow-up studies by Sharp and others, a mutant form of α_1-AT (PiZZ) was identified as a sequestered protein in the endoplasmic reticulum of hepatocytes, and this histopathologic feature became diagnostic of the disease.[14,15] Initially, α_1-AT–associated hepatitis was thought to be due to a failure of its release into the hepatic interstitium to neutralize proteases in the portal circulation that could cause hepatocellular damage.[16] More recently, the hepatic lesion has been ascribed to hepatocyte toxicity caused by the retained mutant form of α_1-AT in hepatocytes.[17] However, using sophisticated "cutting edge" cell biologic techniques,

Perlmutter and colleagues[18] and others[19] have suggested that the process is much more complex and involves not only accumulation of misfolded mutant forms of α_1-AT in hepatocyte endoplasmic reticulum but also disruption of other subcellular functions leading to liver damage. They also suggest that genetic variants of α_1-AT can define phenotypic hepatic disease expression.[20] This common metabolic liver disease can now be distinguished from other liver conditions (eg, tyrosinemia, biliary atresia) and managed in an appropriate prospective manner. Of interest, α_1-AT-deficient liver disease is a common cause of liver transplant in pediatric patients (see Chapter 35.4, "α_1-Antitrypsin Deficiency").[21]

Cystic Fibrosis

It is now generally recognized that cystic fibrosis is a genetically determined condition that often presents with pancreatic insufficiency, malabsorption, progressive, obstructive lung disease, and progressive biliary cirrhosis. Initially, with an incomplete understanding of the pathogenesis of this condition, patients died in childhood from severe lung failure.[22] However, the recent discovery that a cellular membrane transporter for chloride is defective in patients with cystic fibrosis, as well as the cloning of this transporter for the cystic fibrosis transmembrane conductance regulator (CFTR)[23] promises more effective approaches to management of the pulmonary and gastrointestinal complication of this disorder. The association of genotypes with phenotypes in patients with cystic fibrosis has the potential to facilitate the diagnosis and management of patients with cystic fibrosis.[24] The obvious extension of having cloned the gene is the potential for gene therapy to prevent the severe disease complications. Until this is established, however, some patients with progressive disease leading to lung and liver failure may undergo combined lung and liver transplant as the ultimate "rescue" therapy. In addition, new therapeutic approaches to enhancing membrane chloride transport and to the prevention of *Pseudomonas* and other infections of the lung have met with some success.[25] This condition is also an example of a unique pancreatic disorder that presents in infancy and childhood. A complete discussion of the molecular biology of this disorder, its diagnosis, and approaches to treatment is found in Chapter 45.1, "Cystic Fibrosis."

Intrahepatic Cholestasis

Major advances have occurred in our understanding of the molecular mechanisms responsible for the formation and transport of bile in the liver and biliary tract. These are fully described in Chapter 28.1, "Bile Formation and Cholestasis," and Chapter 35.9, "Biliary Transport." The recent discovery that the hydrolysis of adenosine triphosphate (ATP) is necessary for canalicular transport of bile salts has led to the finding that bile acid transporters are members of the ATP-binding cassette transporter superfamily of proteins. Many of these proteins, such as the bile salt export pump, have now been identified. Disorders such as

Byler disease can now be renamed according to the defects in transport proteins that are responsible for them. This elucidation of the molecular and physiologic process of bile formation sets the stage for extraordinary advances in the diagnosis and treatment of these inherited disorders, as well as a host of disorders characterized by cholestasis found in both children and adults. New observations are discussed in this edition.

ADVANCES IN DIAGNOSTIC TECHNOLOGY

A major factor in the rise of pediatric gastroenterology has been the technological advance in diagnosis. Tissue diagnosis is at the heart of much investigation of gastrointestinal and liver disease in children. A portion of this textbook is dedicated to a description of techniques used in determining a tissue diagnosis as well as the major advances that have occurred in understanding the disorders themselves.

It was the development of small intestinal biopsy and liver biopsy in children that were the most significant advances that played the chief roles in the development of the specialty. The observation by Sakula and Shiner in 1957[6] that there was a flat small intestinal mucosa in children with celiac disease followed by the observation by Anderson in 1960[26] that this abnormality responded to a gluten-free diet transformed the practical management of children with celiac disease. From this came the concept that permanent gluten-sensitive enteropathy was the basic pathology of celiac disease. The principle that diagnosis of celiac disease required intestinal tissue obtained from a small intestinal biopsy during elimination and later challenge with gluten first arose in Europe, but then became accepted internationally.[27]

Shiner used a cumbersome rigid tube biopsy technique. It was the subsequent advent of the Crosby capsule and its modification as a pediatric biopsy capsule which made this diagnostic technique popular, practical, and safe. The early days of biopsy in children were overshadowed by occurrences of bowel perforation. This did not occur once it was understood that the pediatric capsule should have a porthole diameter of 2.5 mm rather than the adult diameter of 5 mm to avoid this mishap.[28]

Access to small intestinal mucosa enabled the disaccharidase assay to be performed on the tissue obtained by biopsy. This also permitted a classification of sugar malabsorption disorders.[29] It soon became clear that secondary disaccharidase deficiency was a very common problem in infants with chronic diarrhea. Breath hydrogen testing for carbohydrate malabsorption came to be used as a less invasive way to make the diagnosis, especially in older children.

The development of the technique of total parenteral nutrition by Wilmore and Dudrick[30] in 1968 was of pivotal importance for the establishment of pediatric gastroenterology. Children with intractable diarrhea and other disorders that previously would have died from starvation now survived. Thus, the ability to safely biopsy the small intestine provided research, diagnostic, and potential therapeutic opportunities for a whole range of "new" disorders such as familial enteropathy, microvillous atrophy, tufting enteropathy, and autoimmune enteropathy.

The development of fiberoptic endoscopy with flexible instruments has further changed the scene. Increasingly, both upper and lower endoscopy with multiple biopsies has become the diagnostic norm with the Crosby capsule passing out of clinical use in most centers. This technique has transformed the accurate diagnosis of chronic inflammatory bowel disease where ileocolonoscopy with multiple biopsies has become central to the modern diagnostic approach.[31]

However, as Hamilton[32] has stated in the first edition, the newer diagnostic techniques including biopsy, imaging, and endoscopy are often invasive and unpleasant for the child patient. Yet trainees want to perform a large number of procedures, manufacturers want to sell equipment, and parents want action taken. Hamilton emphasized the need for sound compassionate wisdom to be applied by the clinicians who are caring for children with gastroenterological problems. A theme of the book has been to provide the latest information concerning diagnostic advances, particularly those that employ minimally invasive or noninvasive methods, so that sound clinical decisions concerning diagnosis and management of these children may be made earlier in the course of the illness and be based upon accurate data, acquired within a compassionate framework.

ADVANCES IN MANAGEMENT

Advances in management, both medical and surgical, have been a feature of the development of our subspecialty. Such advances have included the use of oral rehydration therapy and enteral nutrition. New medication options, such as therapeutic monoclonal antibodies, have made a major difference in the lives of children with liver and gastrointestinal disorders. With a better understanding of the molecular mechanisms of disease and developmental pharmacology, drugs can be designed to treat a condition and, in particular, a specific patient while minimizing the risks of adverse side effects. Thus, major advances in diagnosis, management, and treatment of gastrointestinal disorders in pediatric patients have come about as a result of the remarkable expansion in our understanding of the development and pathophysiology of the gastrointestinal tract at the cellular and genetic/molecular levels. Just one example is the recognition of *CARD 15/NOD2* mutations in Crohn's disease.[33]

MAJOR DEFINING EVENTS IN THE SUBSPECIALTY CENTERS OF EXCELLENCE

In the early 1960s, small pediatric-based centers of excellence in the care of children with gastrointestinal disorders formed and focused on common gastrointestinal problems unique to the referral region. For example, several centers in Europe and the United Kingdom specialized in the care of patients with celiac disease, whereas others in France and the United Kingdom began to attract infants with chronic, life-threatening liver diseases. Ultimately, these centers began to provide care for a broader-based spectrum of gastrointestinal disorders. With increasing interest in pediatric gastroenterology among academic pediatric centers, small "splinter groups" (eg, the "Pediatric Gut Club") began to have organized symposia at national pediatric meetings or as satellite symposia at meetings of adult gastroenterologists. As interest in this pediatric subspecialty grew, the need for formally organized societies emerged.

PEDIATRIC GASTROENTEROLOGY SOCIETIES

The natural evolution of the increasing interest in pediatric gastroenterology was the establishment of formal societies in the late 1960s or early 1970s. The European Society for Paediatric Gastroenterology was established in 1968 and held its first independent meeting in Paris in 1968 with representatives from the Netherlands, Sweden, France, Italy, and the United Kingdom.[34] This society grew steadily over the next three decades into the European Society for Paediatric Gastroenterology, Hepatology, and Nutrition (ESPGHAN) which exists today (currently with almost 600 members). The formal organization of a society has been a catalyst for increased numbers of European and United Kingdom pediatricians choosing to exclusively practice or conduct research in gastrointestinal diseases. Among other benefits, it has also led to the establishment of guidelines for the diagnosis and management of several common pediatric gastrointestinal diseases (eg, celiac disease, gastrointestinal allergy, neonatal hyperbilirubinemia).

The North American Society of Pediatric Gastroenterology, Hepatology and Nutrition (NASPGHAN) was established in 1973 as an extension of the informal Pediatric Gut Club. It sponsored an evening symposium at the annual meeting of the Society for Pediatric Research and American Pediatric Society. As additional physicians with an interest in pediatric gastroenterology or with formal gastrointestinal training joined the Society, the venue for its annual symposium moved to the American Gastroenterological Association's (AGA's) national meeting. Finally, in 1984, the Society established its own independent annual meeting, which has occurred yearly since then, either separately or in conjunction with the ESPGHAN and more recently with LASPGN, ASPSPGAN, CAPGAN (World Congress). The establishment of a formal society for pediatric gastroenterology in North America has led to subspecialty boards and multiple formally constituted and recognized training programs (3 years' duration) approved by the Accreditation Council on Graduate Medical Education (ACGME). NASPGHAN now has over 1,000 members. In the last two decades, additional international societies have been established in other parts of the world. In 1974, the Latin Society for Paediatric Gastroenterology and Nutrition (LASPGAN) was founded to formalize interaction among pediatric gastroenterologists in countries in South and Central America and to establish exchanges with NASPGHAN.

In like manner, in 1993, the Asian Pan Pacific Society of Paediatric Gastroenterology (APPSPGN) was established as an extension of a group of pediatricians interested in gastroenterology in Asia who had been informally meeting since the 1960s. This society began holding large meetings every other year in venues throughout Asia. In 1994, the Commonwealth Association of Paediatric Gastroenterology and Nutrition (CAPGAN) was founded to include both developing and industrialized countries that are or were part of the British Commonwealth. With the recognition that these new societies represented almost 3,000 physicians worldwide, the decision was made to hold a world congress every 4 years. This began with a highly successful first world congress held in Boston, Massachusetts, in 2000, which had over 3,000 attendees. The second world congress was held in Paris, France, in 2004 and had even more attendees. A third world congress is planned for 2008 in Brazil. These meetings resulted in position papers defining and outlining management of several gastrointestinal conditions that are accepted as standard practice guidelines worldwide.[35] In addition, a Federation of Societies of Pediatric Gastroenterology, Hepatology and Nutrition was formed to coordinate the relationships and joint activities of the four major regional societies. A major benefit of these newly organized relationships has been the fostering of collaborative studies and exchange training programs, as well as greater awareness of major gastrointestinal health problems in developing countries. Recently, the National Institutes of Health (NIH) has made substantial efforts to foster collaborative studies of pediatric gastrointestinal and liver disorders as well. This includes multicenter programs to study acute liver failure, biliary atresia, nonalcoholic fatty liver disease, and small intestinal failure. These NIH-sponsored programs represent a major milestone in the development of pediatric gastroenterology.

JOURNAL OF PEDIATRIC GASTROENTEROLOGY AND NUTRITION

In 1982, the *Journal of Pediatric Gastroenterology and Nutrition* was first published as a private journal. In 1991, the journal became the official journal of ESPGHAN and NASPGHAN, and, in 1995, the other two regional societies, LASPGN and APPSPGN, became affiliates with representation on the editorial board. This journal has expanded and now receives manuscripts from clinical and basic research physician scientists worldwide. Through this journal, societies can publish position papers, supplements from major meetings, abstracts from national meetings, and medical opinions from leaders in the field. It has also helped to establish the field of pediatric gastroenterology in the eyes of the medical community worldwide.

ROLE OF TEXTBOOKS

It was natural that once a body of clinical and scientific knowledge developed, textbooks of pediatric gastroenterology should appear. The first texts to appear in English were published at the beginning of the 1970s (Silverman et al 1971,[36] Anderson and Burke 1975,[37] Walker-Smith 1975,[38] Gryboski 1975[39]).

In 1991, the first edition of *Pediatric Gastrointestinal Disease* was published.[40] The subtitle *Pathophysiology Diagnosis and Management* was of key importance. A major aim of the text was to deal extensively with the pathophysiologic basis of gastrointestinal and hepatic diseases and how this related to modern diagnosis and management. The conception of this book had its origins in a collaborative publication by three of the editors JA Walker-Smith, JR Hamilton, and WA Walker who had coedited a small book, *Practical Pediatric Gastroenterology*, in 1983.[41] The editors interacted well and WA Walker took the initiative to edit a comprehensive text.[40] The text also aimed to provide a comprehensive and complete account of gastrointestinal, pancreatic, and liver disorders of children as a reference text for pediatricians, pediatric gastroenterologists, and gastroenterologists alike. These were ambitious aims and the resulting book appeared in two volumes with a total of 1,785 pages. In fact, this first edition symbolized the coming of age of the discipline of pediatric gastroenterology as a fullfledged subspecialty of pediatrics. The amount of information and expanding literature in this field is accumulating at such a pace that the editors have decided to update the textbook with each world congress in an effort to provide a current and comprehensive reference for physicians caring for children with gastrointestinal problems. After the third edition, a change in editorship began and a European editor was added. With the fifth edition, an entirely new editorship has been established as the mantel is passed to new leaders in the field, including the addition of the first female editor. Thus, the fifth edition symbolizes the maturity of the discipline worldwide.

THE DEVELOPING CHILD: A UNIQUE CHALLENGE TO THE PEDIATRIC GASTROENTEROLOGIST

In the introductory chapter to the third edition of this textbook, Dick Hamilton emphasized that the pediatric gastroenterologist must have an in-depth knowledge of the morphologic and functional development of the gastrointestinal tract to understand and manage gastrointestinal symptoms and disorders in pediatric patients.[32] For example, many infants may have regurgitation during early feeding in infancy.[42] This condition is usually not pathologic and improves with time as the gastrointestinal tract matures. At a later stage in life, however, the same persistent symptoms might portend serious disease such as obstruction or inflammation.[43] Without a complete knowledge of developing gut function in infancy, inappropriate diagnostic interventions could be instituted and unnecessary invasive therapy undertaken.

In contrast, a missed diagnosis of a serious gastrointestinal condition that affects gastrointestinal function could lead to severe "failure to thrive" and, if a chronic condition ensues, to growth retardation. Microvillus inclusion disease, Hirschsprung disease, and other congenital disorders of gut and liver function are examples of disorders that have been identified as a result of an expanding understanding of gut morphogenesis. Furthermore, a chronic condition such as inflammatory bowel disease that interferes with the child's emotional and physical development during the vulnerable period of adolescence might have a lifelong impact on adult stature and psychosocial stability if not treated properly. These problems need a specialized knowledge of the normal expected pattern of physical and psychological development in the pediatric patient and an appreciation for the impact of chronic or serious illness on the child's quality of life. The pediatric gastroenterologist therefore needs to understand his or her patient population, know the unique age-related conditions that can affect the gastrointestinal tract, and be able to distinguish symptoms and signs that are related to gut development from that of serious disease. Said in another way, certain gastrointestinal signs occurring during different periods of life (infancy, childhood, and adolescence) often evoke a very different differential diagnosis and approach. Two examples may underscore the uniqueness of caring for pediatric patients with gastrointestinal problems. A major diagnostic problem occurring during childhood that requires careful evaluation by the pediatric gastroenterologist is the child with recurrent abdominal pain (RAP). In most instances, RAP is not due to a serious "organic" gastrointestinal condition but instead may relate to stresses in the child's life, such as school adjustment problems, learning difficulties, a dysfunctional family situation, or a low pain threshold, all manifesting themselves as recurrent gastrointestinal symptoms (eg, pain, diarrhea, constipation).[44]

The pediatric gastroenterologist (like his or her counterparts in internal medicine) must be able to separate complaints that originate from a serious physical gastrointestinal disorder (eg, early inflammatory bowel disease, *Helicobacter pylori* gastritis) from functional, often agerelated, complaints. He or she must carefully decide on appropriate diagnostic tests without being too invasive or "feeding" into the child or parent's fear of serious illness. If the symptoms of abdominal pain are diagnosed as functional RAP, the pediatric gastroenterologist must reassure the patient and parents without offending them and prepare an acceptable approach to management. The thoughtful consideration of RAP in this textbook provides a major insight into the diagnosis and management of this condition (see Chapter 24.3, "Chronic Abdominal Pain").

Another condition unique to pediatric gastroenterology is "breast milk colitis."[45] This condition presents with bloody diarrhea in infancy in young infants who are exclusively breastfed. Parents anxious about caring for a vulnerable newborn may overreact, fearing the worst for their baby. As pediatric gastroenterologists, we know that the immaturely developed mucosal immune system in neonates, activated by foreign proteins (cow milk proteins) present in breast milk from the maternal diet and breast milk cytokines and other active immune factors, can temporarily cause sigmoid-rectal inflammation and blood in the stools. The condition is transient and requires either limiting the maternal diet or temporarily taking the infant off breast milk. Over time, the condition clears, and no residual intestinal problems persist. Our expanding understanding of the maturation and physiology of the gut immune system and the presence and function of biologically active factors in breast milk are areas of unique interest and importance to the pediatric gastroenterologist. With this knowledge and experience, infants with this and other immune-related inflammatory conditions can be spared unnecessary investigation and treatments. What we have just briefly described are but a few examples that underscore the need for subspecialists with formal credentials in pediatric gastroenterology and nutrition. A more detailed account of the emergence of pediatric gastroenterology and hepatology has been published with contributions from some of those who were pioneers in the discipline.[46]

FUTURE OF THE SUBSPECIALTY: PEDIATRIC GASTROENTEROLOGY IN THE TWENTY-FIRST CENTURY

Having provided historical evidence for our specialty's evolution as an established component of pediatric medicine, let us speculate about the future of our field during the twenty-first century. Advances in medicine and science will make the future practice of pediatric gastroenterology an exciting and fulfilling professional experience. In the last few years, the Human Genome Project has been completed. With this database, we can systematically begin to identify genes that are responsible for organ development, as well as those that cause or influence the development of complex gastrointestinal conditions (eg, *CARD15/NOD2* mutations and Crohn's disease). Because so many of the disorders seen by pediatric gastroenterologists have an inherited basis, they serve as biologic examples that lead to significant discoveries regarding the mechanisms of disorders that spread well beyond the sphere of pediatric gastroenterology. Table 2 depicts some scientific, diagnostic, and therapeutic breakthroughs that will shape the specialty of pediatric gastroenterology in the twenty-first century.

Table 2 Approaches That Will Enhance the Future Practice of Pediatric Gastroenterology in the Twenty-First Century

DNA microarrays
Single nucleotide polymorphisms (SNPs)
Proteomics
Genomics
RNAai knockdown
Stem cells
Nutrient–gene interaction
MRI
Targeted therapy

As a result of the advances in molecular genetics, we will also be in a better position to make earlier diagnoses of chronic debilitating conditions (eg, cystic fibrosis, inflammatory bowel disease, celiac disease) before they cause irreversible damage to the pediatric patient. This is particularly true in the identification of single nucleotide polymorphisms (SNPs) that render signaling pathways or enzymatic function inoperative and may either contribute to the pathogenesis of disease or facilitate environmental factors causing disease or at best act as a biomarker for the prediction of disease. Examples of SNPs identified in pediatric gastrointestinal diseases are the NOD2/CARD15 polymorphism is Crohn's disease[47] and a TLR-2 SNP in allergic disease states.[48] By providing genotype–phenotype associations with genetically determined diseases, we can modify the patient's environment to minimize the severity of disease expression. Patients can also be tested for genetically determined responses to therapeutic interventions (eg, use of 6-mercaptopurine in inflammatory bowel disease patients). Effective gene therapy is clearly within sight. Using molecular and cellular biologic techniques, we can define the precise cellular mechanism of disease and ultimately develop genetic profiles that will allow patients to be identified before expression of the disease phenotypic and its consequences occur. The challenge, of course, will be to identify only those who would actually develop disease and not to mislabel the otherwise healthy carrier of "disease-related" genes.

We have now begun to understand how microorganisms and their molecular patterns mediate health and disease in the gastrointestinal tract.[49] Several years ago, a molecular pattern recognition receptor for endotoxin (lipopolysaccharide [LPS]) was identified on intestinal lymphoid cells. This receptor was termed the Toll-like receptor (TLR) because of its conserved structure similar to the Toll receptor in *Drosophila melanogaster*, which determines organism orientation and innate immunity. This receptor was noted to have an intracellular signal transduction schema similar to the interleukin-1β receptor. Interaction with LPS resulted in an upregulation of nuclear factor κB, an inflammatory cytokine transcription factor, which generated the inflammatory response to endotoxin. This discovery has led to a better understanding of the mechanism of endotoxin-induced shock and new approaches to

its prevention. The TLR that principally interacts with LPS is termed TLR4. In addition to this receptor, which has been cloned, nine other TLRs have been identified and cloned, and other molecular patterns of both gram-positive and gram-negative bacteria, as well as viruses, have been identified as their ligands.[50] This genomic/molecular biologic discovery has opened up the field of innate immunity and has identified the role of the gut epithelium in its effector response. Since the last edition, this field of research has exploded. We now know that initial microbial colonization and the interaction of colonizing commensal bacteria with TLRs on developing enterocytes and intestinal dendritic cells/lymphocytes can provide the basis for development of a normal mucosal immune system and lower the risk of developing immune-mediated disease states (eg, allergy and autoimmune disease). This concept has been depicted as the "hygiene hypothesis."[3,51] As a result of this knowledge, a new form of therapy for these conditions is emerging (eg, probiotics) to provide surrogate colonization under conditions when inadequate or potentially harmful initial colonization occurs (eg, Cesarean section or excessive use of perinatal antibiotics).[52] Thus, our understanding of how intestinal pathogens and commensal organisms communicate with the gut through the epithelial surface lining or underlying lymphoid elements is expanding rapidly, with very important future health care implications.

The role of nutrition and nutritional status in the development of disease later in life is another area of investigation that may provide important therapeutic benefits. The observations made by David Baker and colleagues[2] that nutrition during pregnancy may affect the expression of chronic diseases, such as obesity, coronary vascular disease, and hypertension in adulthood, serves as the basis for much of the work taking place now on this topic. These are but a few of the many examples to be found in the following chapters of this textbook of areas of research and investigation that will influence the direction of care of pediatric patients with gastrointestinal, liver, pancreatic, and nutritional disorders over the coming years.

SUMMARY AND CONCLUSIONS

The growth of pediatric gastroenterology has been extraordinary to be beheld. It has been a pleasure for the authors to observe and be part of this remarkable development, which has benefited so many children with hitherto debilitating and sometimes fatal disorders. Many of these children can lead normal and fulfilling lives.

The pediatric gastroenterologist must have a complete understanding of pediatric development and gastrointestinal diseases unique to specific age groups, not only to optimally diagnose and manage symptoms and disorders but also to enhance the quality of life for children and adolescents.

The current state of the art in understanding and management of gastrointestinal disorders in child patients is set forth in this new edition of this textbook. We look forward to future editions with much enthusiasm as there is still much to be done for those children where cure is not yet possible. We have unbounded enthusiasm for future developments.

REFERENCES

1. Kirsner JB. The Development of American Gastroenterology. New York: Raven Press; 1990.
2. Gillman MW. Epidemiological challenges in studying the fetal origins of adult chronic disease. Int J Epidemiol 2003;3:294–9.
3. Guarner F, Bourdet-Sicard R, Brandtzaeg P, et al. Mechanisms of disease: The hygiene hypothesis revisited. Nat Clin Pract 2006;3:275–84.
4. Walker Smith J, Walker WA. The development of pediatric gastroenterology. A historical overview. Pediatr Res 2003;53:706–15.
5. Dicke WK. Celiac disease [thesis]. Utrecht: University of Utrecht; 1950.
6. Sakula J, Shiner M. Celiac disease with atrophy of the small intestinal mucosa. Lancet 1957;ii:876–7.
7. Kagnoff MF. Celiac disease pathogenesis: The plot thickens. Gastroenterology 2002;123:939–41.
8. Godkin A, Jewell D. The pathogenesis of celiac disease. Gastroenterology 1998;115:206–10.
9. Hill ID, Dirks MH, Liptak GS, et al. Guideline for the diagnosis and treatment of celiac disease in children: Recommendations of the North American Society for pediatric gastroenterology, hepatology and nutrition. J Pediatr Gastroenterol Nutr 2005;40:1–19.
10. Farrell RJ, Kelly CP. Current concepts. N Engl J Med 2002;346:180–8.
11. Farrell RJ, Kelly CP. Diagnosis of celiac sprue. Am J Gastroenterol 2001;96:3237–46.
12. Sharp HL, Bridges PA, Krivit W, Freier EF. Cirrhosis associated with alpha-1-antitrypsin deficiency: A previously unrecognized inherited disorder. J Lab Clin Med 1969;73:934–9.
13. Sharp H. Liver biopsy. In: Walker-Smith J, Walker WA, editors. A Concise History of Paediatric Gastroenterology, 2004. p. 29–37.
14. Sharp HL. Alpha-1-antitrypsin deficiency. Hosp Pract 1971; 6:83–96.
15. Sveger T, Eriksson S. The liver in adolescents with alpha-1-antitrypsin deficiency. Hepatology 1995;22:514–7.
16. Wu Y. A lag in intracellular degradation of mutant α-1-antitrypsin correlates with the liver disease phenotype in homozygous PIZZ-α₁ antitrypsin deficiency. Proc Natl Acad Sci U S A 1994;91:9014–8.
17. McCracken AA, Kruse BK, Brown JL. Molecular basis for defective secretion of variants having altered potential for salt bridge formation between amino acids 240 and 242. Mol Cell Biol 1989;9:1408–14.
18. Perlmutter DH, Travis J, Punsal PI. Elastase regulates the synthesis of its inhibitors, α₁-proteinase inhibitor, and exaggerates the defect in homozygous PIZZ α₁-proteinase inhibitor deficiency. J Clin Invest 1988;81:1774–8.
19. McCracken AA, Brodsky JL. Assembly of ER-associated protein degradation in vitro: Dependence on cytoso, calnexin and ATP. J Cell Biol 1996;132:291–8.
20. Qu D, Teckman JH, Omura S, Perlmutter DH. Degradation of mutant secretory protein, α₁-proteinase Z, in the endoplasmic reticulum requires proteasome activity. J Biol Chem 1996; 271:22791–5.
21. Adrian-Casavilla F, Reyes J, Tzakis A, et al. Liver transplantation for neonatal hepatitis as compared to the other two leading indications for liver transplantation in children. J Hepatol 1994;21:1035–9.
22. Davis PB. Clinical pathophysiology and manifestations of lung disease. In: Yankaskas JR, Knowles, MR, editors. Cystic Fibrosis in Adults. Philadelphia: Lippincott-Raven; 1999. p. 45–67.
23. Riordan JR, Rommens JM, Karem B, et al. Identification of the cystic fibrosis gene: Cloning and characterization of complementary DNA. Science 1989;245:1066–72.
24. Durno C, Corey M, Zielenski J, et al. Genotype and phenotype correlations in patients with cystic fibrosis and pancreatitis. Gastroenterology 2002;123:1857–64.
25. Davis PB, Byard PJ, Konstan MW. Identifying treatments that halt progression of pulmonary disease in cystic fibrosis. Pediatr Res 1997;41:161–5.

26. Anderson CM. Histological changes in the duodenal mucosa in celiac disease. Arch Dis Child 1960;419–523.

27. Meeuwisse GW. Diagnostic criteria in coeliac disease. Acta Paediatr 1970;59:461–7.

28. Partin JC, Schubert WK. Precautionary note on the use of the intestinal biopsy capsule in infants and emaciated children. N Engl J Med 1966;274:94–5.

29. Weijers HA, van de Kamer JH, Dicke WK, Ijsseling J. Diarrhoea caused by deficiency of sugar splitting enzymes. Acta Paediatr (Uppsala) 1961;50:55–9.

30. Wilmore DW, Dudrick SJ. Growth and development of an infant receiving all nutrients exclusively via a vein. JAMA 1968;20:860–4.

31. Gleason WA, Tedesco FJ, Keating JP, Goldstein PD. Fibreoptic gastrointestinal endoscopy in infants and children. J Pediatr 1974;85:810–2.

32. Hamilton JR. The pediatric patient: Early development and the digestive system. In: Walker WA, Durie P, Hamilton JR, et al, editors. Pediatric Gastrointestinal Disease, 3rd edition. Hamilton, ON: BC Decker; 2000. p. 1–11.

33. Ferraris A, Torres B, Knafelz D, et al. Relationship between *CARD15*, *SLC22A4/5*, and *DLG5* polymorphisms and early-onset inflammatory bowel diseases: An Italian multicentric study. Inflamm Bowel Dis 2006;12:355–61.

34. Strandvik B. ESPGAN: The European Society for Pediatric Gastroenterology and Nutrition 25 years' memories 1968–1992. J Pediatr Gastroenterol Nutr 1993;21:11–9.

35. Booth I, Cunha Ferriera R, Desjeux J-F. Recommendations for composition of oral rehydration solutions for the children of Europe. J Pediatr Gastroenterol Nutr 1972;14:113–5.

36. Roy C, Silverman A, Cozzetto FJ. Pediatric Clinical Gastroenterology, 1st edition. St. Louis: CV Mosby; 1971.

37. Anderson CM, Burke V. Pediatric Gastroenterology, 1st edition. Oxford: Blackwell Scientific; 1975.

38. Walker-Smith JA. Diseases of the Small Intestine in Childhood, 1st edition. Turnbridge Wells, UK: Pitman Medical; 1975.

39. Gryboski J. Gastrointestinal problems in the infant. In: Major Problems in Clinical Pediatrics, Volume XIII, 1st edition. Philadelphia: WB Saunders; 1975.

40. Walker WA, Durie P, Hamilton JR, et al. Pediatric Gastrointestinal Disease: Pathophysiology Diagnosis Management. Hamilton, ON: BC Decker; 1991.

41. Walker-Smith J, Hamilton R, Walker WA, editors. Practical Pediatric Gastroenterology, 2nd edition. Hamilton, ON: BC Decker; 1996.

42. Dumont RC, Rudolph CD. Development of gastrointestinal motility in the infant and child. Gastroenterol Clin North Am 1994;23:655–71.

43. Bourke B, Jones N, Sherman P. *Helicobacter pylori* infection and peptic ulcer disease in children. Pediatr Infect Dis J 1996;15:1–13.

44. Jeffrey RB, Federle MP, Tolentino CS. Periappendiceal inflammatory masses: CT-directed management and clinical outcome in 70 patients. Radiology 1988;167:13–9.

45. Xanthou M, Bines J, Walker WA. Human milk and intestinal host defense in newborns. An update. Adv Pediatr 1995;42:171–208.

46. Walker-Smith JA, Walker WA. A Concise History of Paediatric Gastroenterology. Bladon Medical Publishing.

47. Russell RK, Drummond HE, Nimmo EE, et al. Genotype-phenotype analysis in childhood-onset Crohn's disease: *NOD2/CARD15* variants consistently predict phenotypic characteristics of severe disease. Inflamm Bowel Dis 2005; 11:955–64.

48. Eder W, Klimecki W, Yu L, et al. Toll-like receptor 2 as a major gene for asthma in children of European farmers. J Allergy Clin Immunol 2004;113:482–8.

49. Aderem A, Ulevitch RJ. Toll-like receptors in the induction of the innate immune response. Nature 2000;406:782–7.

50. Lasker MV, Nair SK. Intracellular TLR signaling: A structural perspective on human disease. J Immunol 2006; 177:11–6.

51. Bach JF. The effect of infections on susceptibility to autoimmune and allergic disease. N Engl J Med 2002;347: 911–20.

52. DiGiacinto C. Probiotics ameliorate recurrent Th-1 mediated murine colitis by inducing Il-10 and IL-10-dependent TFG (β) bearing regulating cells. J Immunol 2005;174: 3237–46.

I | MOUTH AND ESOPHAGUS

1

Congenital Anomalies

Jonathan E. Teitelbaum, MD, FAACP

Congenital anomalies of the mouth and esophagus are relatively common. The majority of these anomalies are readily apparent at birth or, in many cases, can be appreciated on prenatal ultrasonography. Increasing knowledge of the embryologic events that result in the normal development of these structures has led to the identification of various genes and gene products that help to orchestrate these events. With that, there has been a rapid advancement in identifying various genetic mutations that result in abnormalities of development and subsequent syndromic and nonsyndromic presentations.

These malformations are associated with various clinical presentations. Whereas some allow patients to be asymptomatic, others can cause difficulties in feeding or articulation or life-threatening respiratory difficulties. More complex malformations often require multidisciplinary teams, including surgeons (general, otolaryngologic, and orthodontic), gastroenterologists, speech pathologists, and geneticists.

FACIAL CLEFTS (CLEFT LIPS AND PALATES)

Oral clefts are among the most common of all birth defects, second only to clubfoot. Cleft lip with or without cleft palate (CL[P]) occurs with an incidence of 1 in 500 to 1 in 2,500 in different populations based on ethnic group, geographic location, and socioeconomic conditions.[1] The highest incidence is among native Americans (3.6 in 1,000 live births), whereas among Blacks, it is less (0.3 in 1,000 live births). Whites have an incidence of 1 in 1,000 live births. Defects are unilateral in 80%.[2]

Isolated cleft palate (CP) occurs in approximately 1 in 2,000 live births, and there is little to no racial preponderance.[2] CL(P) is more common in boys, whereas CP is seen more commonly in girls. The cause is likely multifactorial disruption of embryologic morphogenesis.[2]

Higher birth order may also be a risk factor for CL(P) and CP. However, studies are not conclusive and may be confounded by other factors, such as advanced maternal or paternal age or increased exposure to teratogens, which, in themselves, may be the risk factors.[3] While nonsyndromic clefts are generally thought to be relatively benign conditions, a study reveals that the perinatal mortality rate for babies with isolated facial clefts was significantly higher than the background population (odds ratio 3.3).[4]

The risk of having subsequent children with clefts is different for those with CL(P) from those with CP. When both parents are unaffected and have an affected child, the risk of recurrence is 4.4% for CL(P) and 2.5% for CP. If one parent is affected, the risk is increased to 15.8% for CL(P) and 14.9% for CP. If two children are affected and the parents are unaffected, the risk for a third child is 9% for CL(P) and 1% for CP.[2] Concordance among monozygotic twins ranges between 40 and 60%, whereas it is 5% among dizygotic twins. The lack of 100% concordance rates among monozygotic twins argues against genetic events alone being responsible for the clefting phenotype.[5]

Cleft lip is a unilateral or bilateral gap in the upper lip and jaw, which is formed during the third to seventh week of embryologic development.[1] The incisive foramen divides the hard palate into a primary and secondary palate. The primary palate lies anterior to the incisive foramen and includes the bony premaxilla, mucoperiostal covering, and incisor teeth. The secondary palate is posterior to the incisive foramen and is composed of the horizontal plates of the maxilla and palatine bone. The remaining dentition arrives from the secondary palate. Primary palate formation begins at 4 to 5 weeks gestation with the fusion of the paired median nasal prominences. This marks the separation of the oral and nasal cavities. Ultimately, the median nasal prominences give rise to dental arch, incisor teeth, and philtrum of the upper lip. Formation of the secondary palate

(hard and soft) begins at approximately the seventh week of gestation. The posterior maxillary prominences form palatal shelves, which rotate inferiorly and medially to fuse with the vomer in the midline. Anterior to posterior palatal closure occurs in a zipper-like fashion. At 9 weeks gestation, the hard palate fuses with the septum to complete the separation of the oral and nasal cavities. The soft palate is composed of five paired muscles: tensor veli palatini, levator veli palatini, palatoglossus, palatopharyngeus, and musculus uvulae. Midline approximation of the soft palatal musculature marks the completion of palatogenesis at approximately 12 weeks gestation.[2]

The multifactorial inheritance model is currently the most widely accepted theory of nonsyndromic clefts. In this model the risk of developing a given anomaly is determined by the presence of either genetic or environmental liabilities. Each liability occurs in a normal distribution within the population. The accumulation of multiple small liabilities eventually reaches a threshold, beyond which a defect occurs. Variable penetrance of the phenotype for many genes results in non-Mendelian inheritance patterns. Ongoing research is investigating the role that associated features play in the familial transmission patterns of nonsyndromic clefts. Associated features include fluctuating and directional asymmetry, non-right-handedness, dermatoglyphic patterns, craniofacial morphology, orbicularis oris muscle defects, structural brain and vertebral anomalies, minor physical anomalies, and velopharyngeal incompetence.[6]

An estimated 300 syndromes include CL(P) in their phenotype; however, syndromic clefts account for only 30% of CL(P).[1] The proportion of patients with CP who are syndromic versus nonsyndromic remains unresolved, with estimates varying widely, between 15 and 80%.[1] Approximately 25% of syndromic clefts are associated with Stickler syndrome, whereas another 15% are associated with velocardiofacial syndrome.[2] The most common malformations in association with clefts are found in the central nervous system and the skeletal system, followed by the urogenital and cardiovascular systems.[7] Various syndromes associated with CP (Table 1) and CL(P) (Table 2) have been described.

Defects in the *PVRL1* gene (chromosome 11q23) result in abnormal formation of nectin 1, a cell–cell adhesion molecule expressed in the developing face and palate that is essential for fusion of the medial edge epithelia. A 50% reduction in the amount of nectin 1 appears to be a risk factor for nonsyndromic CL(P) in patients on Margarita Island and Venezuela.[1] A similar gene, *OFC3* (19q13, MIM#600757), has also been implicated in nonsyndromic CL(P) based on genetic linkage studies. Other candidate genes include *OFC1* (6p24.3, MIM#119530), *OFC2* (2p13, MIM#602966), *OFC4* (1q, MIM#608371), *OFC5* (MSX1, *4p16.1*, MIM #608874), *OFC6* (MIM#608864), *TP63* (3q27), *TGFA* (2p13), *TBX22*,1 *PGD1* (1p36), 6 methylenetetrahydrofolate reductase (1q36),[8–9] transcobalbumin 2,[10] and TGFalpha (2p13).[8] A defect in the *CDH1/* E-cadherin gene (MIM#192090) has been associated with CL(P) and hereditary diffuse gastric cancer.[11]

The role of teratogens in the formation of clefts has been supported by studies suggesting causation associated with maternal exposure to corticosteroids, phenytoin, valproic acid,[5] thalidomide,[5] alcohol,[5] cigarettes,[5] dioxin,[5] or retinoic acid; maternal diabetes mellitus; maternal

Table 1 Cleft Palate or Bifid Uvula without Cleft Lip

Syndrome	Omim Number*
Catel-Manzke	302380
Cerebrocostomandibular	117650
Deletion 4q	
Dubowitz	223370
Duplication 3q	
Duplication 10q	
Escobar	265000
Femoral hypoplasia–unusual facies	134780
Fibrochondrogenesis	228520
Hay-Wells syndrome of ectodermal dysplasia	106260
Hydrolethalus	236680
Kabuki make-up	147920
Kniest dysplasia	156550
Marden-Walker	248700
Meckel-Gruber	249000
Nager	154400
Orofaciodigital	311200
Otopalatodigital, type I	311300
Otopalatodigital, type II	304120
Popliteal pterygium	119500
Retinoic acid embryopathy	243440
Short-rib polydactyly, type II	263520
Velocardiofacial	192430
Spondyloepiphyseal dysplasia congenita	183900
Stickler	108300
Treacher Collins	154500
Van der Woude	119300

Adapted from Jones.[90]
*Searching the OMIM (Online Mendelian Inheritance in Man) can be done at <http://www.ncbi.nlm.nih.gov/omim./>

Table 2 Syndromes with Cleft Lip with or without Cleft Palate

Syndrome	OMIM Number*
Deletion 4p	
Ectrodactyly-ectodermal dysplasia clefting	604292
Fryns	229850
Hay-Wells syndrome of ectodermal dysplasia	106260
Holoprosencephaly sequence	157170
Miller	247200
Mohr	252100
Orofaciodigital	311200
Popliteal pterygium	119500
Rapp-Hodgkin ectodermal dysplasia	129400
Roberts	268300
Short-rib polydactyly, type II	263520
Trisomy 13	
Van der Woude	119300

Adapted from Jones.[90]
*Searching the OMIM (Online Mendelian Inheritance in Man) can be done at <http://www.ncbi.nlm.nih.gov/omim/>.

hormone imbalance; and maternal vitamin and nutrient deficiency.[12] While there is no consensus that any particular teratogen or environmental factor is implicated in most clefts,[1] some suggest that the risk may be increased with exposure to oxygenated (odds ratio 1.8), chlorinated (odds ratio 9.4), and petroleum (odds ratio 3.6) solvents.[13] Folic acid may have a protective effect to reduce the risk of clefting, although this is controversial.[8,14] Studies also suggest that maternal zinc deficiency may be associated with nonsyndromic clefting.[15–16]

Prenatal diagnosis allows for early parental counseling. Current technology can detect CL(P) at gestational week 15 because the soft tissues of the fetal face become distinct to transabdominal ultrasonography.[7] During the second trimester, ultrasonography detects less than 20% of cases of isolated CL(P) and far fewer cases of isolated CP.[7] However, syndromic CL(P) is detected at 38%, perhaps because a more detailed scan is undertaken given the associated anomalies, or because these clefts are larger and more readily visualized. Optimum timing for diagnosis is regarded as 20 to 22 weeks gestation. The ability to see the defect is influenced by the position of the fetus, position of an overlying hand or umbilical cord, maternal obesity, multiple pregnancies, oligohydramnios, and the experience of the technician. The use of transvaginal ultrasonography and three-dimensional ultrasonography also increases the sensitivity and specificity of the test.[2] Recently, real-time magnetic resonance imaging has also been proven useful in prenatal diagnosis of CP.[17] A delay of greater than 24 hours in diagnosis of nonsyndromic cleft palate without cleft lip in the newborn can occur in as much as 37%.[18] Those with a delay in diagnosis often had feeding problems or nasal regurgitation. The authors suggest that all newborns should undergo visual inspection of the palate as palpation alone is inadequate.

Initial evaluation of a patient with CP should include prenatal care, birth history, teratogen exposure, and a family history of clefting or syndromes. A multidisciplinary team is often helpful in assessing the family's medical and psychosocial needs. The cleft team should consist of a surgeon, otologist, audiologist, dentist (orthodontist or oral surgeon), social worker, geneticist, pediatrician, nutritionist, and speech pathologist. Breastfeeding is possible in some patients with a short or narrow cleft.[19] Infants with larger clefts can rarely generate adequate suction for traditional breast or bottle-feeding. Various specialized nipples have been created to facilitate feeding. Feeding typically takes longer, and frequent burping may be required in these infants because they often swallow large amounts of air. Infants should be weighed on a weekly basis initially to ensure adequate intake.[2] Evidence suggests that children with CL have a lesser degree of weight and length impairment in the first few years of life as compared to those children with cleft lip and palate or CP.[20]

Palatal clefting disrupts all layers of the normal palate architecture, including mucosa, muscle, and bone. The muscles of the soft palate must wrap anteriorly and insert on the cleft margin or the posterior palate. Aberrant tensor veli palatini insertion results in eustachian tube dysfunction, so nearly all CP patients will have chronic otitis media requiring myringotomy tube placement. Abnormal insertion of the levator veli palatini results in loss of normal velopharyngeal competence.[2]

CP may be classified as primary or secondary, complete or incomplete, unilateral or bilateral, or submucous. Primary CP results in incomplete closure of the hard palate anterior to the incisive foramen, whereas secondary CP results in a midline defect posterior to the incisive foramen. Secondary clefts appear to be distinct genetic entities, unrelated to cleft lip but often associated with Pierre Robin sequence (PRS). Complete CP involves the primary, secondary, and soft palate and is usually associated with cleft lip. Submucous CP results from inadequate development of the muscles of the soft palate without disruption of the mucosa. They can characteristically include a bifid uvula, dehiscence of the central palatal musculature (may be palpable or result in bluish discoloration in the midline, termed a zona pellucida), and loss of the posterior nasal spine.[2]

Presurgical orthopedic techniques are used to modify the shape of the cleft deformity before definitive cleft repair. These increase the ease of the primary repair, normalize facial growth, and prevent alveolar collapse. Active techniques include finger massage, lip taping and strapping, and oral prosthetics. Passive techniques are aimed at inhibiting tongue protrusion between the palatal shelves by using oral obturators. Although these techniques have been shown to effectively narrow the distance between alveolar segments, no differences in esthetic outcome, need for revision surgery, or improvement in feeding have been prospectively demonstrated.[2]

Palatoplasty aims to separate the oral and nasal cavities and restore velopharyngeal competence. An aggressive approach must be balanced with the risk of maxillary growth disturbance.[2]

Although 90% of patients with a cleft lip have repair between 3 and 6 months of age,[21] the timing of CP repair is controversial. Proponents of early CP repair (3 to 6 months) believe that early velopharyngeal competence is critical to normal speech development. Proponents of late palatal repair (2 to15 years) believe that the risk of iatrogenic disruption of palatal growth and midfacial hypoplasia outweighs the risk of speech abnormalities. Clefts delayed for more than 2 years generally require obturation to overcome velopharyngeal incompetence and allow normal speech development. Oral obturators placed prior to 2 years are often poorly tolerated. The lack of clear evidence supporting early versus late repair has led to a compromise in which most surgeons perform repair from 12 to 24 months.[2] Experience with neonatal cleft lip and palate repair has been described as safe, although long-term follow-up is not yet available.[22] Recently, fetal surgery for CL(P) has also been described.[23] The risks of repair include bleeding, infection, wound breakdown, palatal fistula, inhibition of maxillary growth, and velopharyngeal incompetence.[2] A description of the various surgical techniques used in palatal repair is beyond the scope of this chapter.

The emergence of the deciduous teeth is disrupted by the clefting process. The mean emergence age of the cleft side upper deciduous lateral incisor is delayed by 8 months when an alveolar cleft is present and by 13 months when an alveolar and palatal cleft is present. However, if early orthopedic plates are used, the lower incisors emerge earlier than normal. The emergence of the deciduous primary molar is also delayed in patients with clefts.[21] Also, children with cleft lip and/or palate were found to be at risk for dental caries, with the highest incidence found in the teeth adjacent to the oral cleft.

Special consideration should be given to advising the parent to provide breast milk to infants with CP. This is based on a study by Paradise and colleagues, who evaluated 315 infants with CP. Freedom from effusion in one or both ears at one or more visits was found in 2.7% of those fed cow's milk or soy formula exclusively and 32% of those fed with breast milk exclusively or in part for varying periods.[24] General growth patterns of children with clefts do not differ significantly from those without clefts.[21]

PIERRE ROBIN SEQUENCE

Pierre Robin, a French stomatologist, described the association of micrognathia and glossoptosis (posterior displacement of the tongue into the pharynx) in 1923 and added CP in a 1934 report. This triad is now known as the Pierre Robin sequence (MIM#261800), with the word "sequence" being used to reflect the series of events leading to the

clinical phenotype. The significant respiratory symptoms associated with PRS distinguish it from simple CP. An estimate on the incidence varies from 1 in 2,000 to 1 in 30,000.[25] Mortality ranges from 2.2 to 26%, with the cause of death typically related to obstructive apnea and failure to thrive.[26]

The initiating event appears to be mandibular deficiency. In early development, the retroposition of the mandible results in maintaining the tongue in a high position within the nasopharynx. Tongue position prevents the medial growth and fusion of the palatal shelves, and a resultant U-shaped cleft occurs.[25] The degree of the defects results in marked clinical heterogeneity.

The nature of the mandibular hypoplasia is heterogeneous and includes positional malformations in which the mandible has normal growth potential, but external factors, such as oligohydramnios, multiple births, or uterine anomalies, prevent full development; intrinsic mandibular hypoplasia in which there is reduced growth potential, such as is seen with genetic syndromes; neurologic or neuromuscular abnormalities in which abnormal mandibular movement prevents tongue descent, as seen with myotonic dystrophy and arthrogryposis; and connective tissue disorders.[25]

Approximately 20 to 40% of affected individuals are classified as having nonsyndromic PRS. These patients have normal growth potential and development if airway and feeding problems are prevented.[25] Some potential candidate genes have been identified including *GAD67* (2q31), *PVRL1* (11q23-q24), and *SOX9* (17q24.3-q25.1).[27] The majority of PRS cases are associated with various recognized syndromes (Table 3), the most common of which include Stickler syndrome (34%), velocardiofacial syndrome (11%), fetal alcohol syndrome (10%), and Treacher Collins syndrome (5%).[28]

At birth, patients with PRS have marked anteroposterior mandibular deficiency. The base of the nose is often flattened, and a palatal cleft is present. The possibility for mandibular catch-up

Table 3 Syndromes Associated with Pierre Robin Sequence

Syndrome	OMIM Number*
Beckwith-Wiedemann	130650
Cerebrocostomandibular	117650
Distal arthrogryposis	301830
Femoral-facial syndrome (bilateral femoral dysgenesis)	134780
Fetal alcohol	
Larsen	150250
Miller-Dieker lissencephaly	247200
Spondyloepiphyseal dysplasia congenita	183900
Stickler syndrome	108300
Treacher Collins	154500
Trisomy 18	
Velocardiofacial	192430

Adapted from St-Hilaire.[25]

*Searching the OMIM (Online Mendelian Inheritance in Man) can be done at <http://www.ncbi.nlm.nih.gov/omim/>.

growth is related to the etiology of the PRS. When mandibular deficiency is due to positioning, the micrognathia will likely self-correct. However, syndromic PRS often involves altered mandibular growth potential, and correction is less likely.[25] Hearing levels in patients with PRS revealed 83% to have bilateral conductive hearing loss, whereas 60% of CP patients (with or without cleft lip) had hearing loss. All patients with hearing loss had middle ear effusion.[29]

Airway obstruction is multifactorial, involving both anatomic and neuromuscular components. Neuromuscular impairment of the genioglossus and other pharyngeal muscles predisposes PRS patients to airway collapse. Mechanical obstruction is the result of the retroposition of the mandible and diminished anterior traction on the tongue. The airway obstruction may lead to associated cor pulmonale, failure to thrive, and cerebral impairment owing to hypoxia.[25] A study by Sher and colleagues using nasopharyngoscopy found that 59% of the obstruction was the result of posterior movement of the tongue contacting the posterior pharyngeal wall.[30]

If the airway compromise is due to glossoptosis, then positioning has been the mainstay of treatment. Patients are placed in the prone position so as to rely on gravity to displace the tongue anteriorly. However, this maneuver does not allow for easy observation of signs of respiratory distress should airway obstruction occur. For this reason, some have advocated the use of a weighted wire to bring the tongue forward.[25]

The use of a nasopharygeal airway has been described, with good results. The tube should have an internal diameter of 3.0 to 3.5 mm and can be advanced to 8 mm until good air movement is observed. Typically, a single tube is sufficient. Gavage feedings through a nasogastric tube are recommended when this tube is in place.[25] A study of 22 neonates treated with nasopharyngeal airway and nasogastric feeding demonstrated this approach to be safe and allowed for improved growth, development, and parental bonding.[31]

The use of a tongue to lip adhesion or glossopexy was also designed to relieve abnormal tongue positioning. In this procedure, the tongue is sutured in place in a more anterior position. Although this can alleviate upper airway obstruction, there is a significant failure rate and a large percentage will require additional interventions for feeding or airway issues.[32] In addition, complications include tongue laceration, wound infection, dehiscence, injury to the Wharton duct, and scar formation of the lip, chin, and mouth.[25] A study by LeBlanc and colleagues suggests that this procedure does not adversely affect speech when compared with affected patients who did not undergo glossopexy.[33]

The use of mandibular distraction osteogenesis has been described as a definitive structural resolution of the micrognathia with correction of the hard and soft tissues. The technique is technically demanding and requires good compliance from the parents.[34] Tracheostomy would be a final alternative for those patients who do not respond to nonsurgical measures. Other procedures described include subperiosteal release of the floor of the mouth and hyomandibulopexy.[25] Recently, the use of a molded dental appliance, termed a modified nutrition plate, in a newborn with PRS was described which forced the tongue to displace anteriorly to its normal position relieving airway obstruction and allowed for normal feeding.[35]

Feeding difficulties have been reported to be due to poor tongue mobility or poor muscle coordination during swallowing. This leads to poor suck and poor bolus propagation. A recent study revealed over 50% of patients to have temporary feeding problems that resolved by 1 year of life, whereas almost 25% have chronic feeding problems. Overall, 40% required some form of enteral tube feeding.[26] Electromyography during bottle-feeding revealed incoordination between oral and pharyngeal phases of swallowing. Esophageal motility studies revealed increased lower esophageal sphincter mean resting pressure and incomplete or asynchronous lower esophageal sphincter relaxation; simultaneous contractions, multipe-aked waves, and very high amplitude waves along the esophageal body; and increased mean upper esophageal sphincter resting pressure and asynchronous upper esophageal sphincter relaxation.[36] Various feeding-facilitating techniques including pacifier, massage to relax and anteriorizer the tongue, long and soft bottle nipple, global symmetric position, and insertion of the nipple on the tongue have been shown to foster oral feeding in this population.[37]

A study by Abadie and colleagues evaluated 66 neonates with isolated PRS. These authors hypothesized that PRS is the result of brainstem dysfunction that causes poor mandibular growth owing to impaired oral motility in utero. They evaluated the patients with esophageal manometry, laryngoscopy, and Holter-electrocardiography recording. They also graded the degree of clefting, glossoptosis, and retrognathia. They found that 98% had feeding difficulty within the first week of life and 81% had problems for the first 3 months of life. Transient solid food dysphagia was present in 18 to 60%, depending on the severity of their PRS. Manometric abnormalities were present, as previously described. Acute life-threatening events were present in 30% overall, with higher proportions seen in more severely affected individuals. Vagal overactivity was demonstrated in 59%.[38]

Early failure to thrive is seen relatively commonly and is often multifactorial. Factors implicated in poor weight gain include feeding difficulties, syndrome-related hypoxemia, respiratory insufficiency, increased caloric demand, prematurity, and related operations. In addition, gastroesophageal reflux and respiratory infections may contribute. Full catch-up growth in height and weight typically occurs during early childhood.[26]

A mild variant of the PRS has been described in which there is mild retrognathia and a high arched palate. These patients were noted to share manometric abnormalities with classic PRS and presented with early feeding resistance.[39]

PSEUDOPALATAL CLEFTS

Some patients have marked lateral hard palate swellings. These are typically associated with a high arched palate and median furrow. Careful examination reveals an intact palate despite the misleading appearance of a cleft. Such pseudopalatal clefts are common in patients with Apert syndrome (MIM#101200) and have been described in Crouzon disease (MIM#123500) as well. No treatment is indicated.[40]

EPULIS (GINGIVAL GRANULAR CELL TUMOR OF THE NEWBORN)

The first case of congenital epulis was reported in 1871. This rare benign soft tissue tumor occurs more frequently in females than males. No links to genetic defects or teratogens have been identified. The tumor is most commonly at the lateral alveolar ridge, where the lateral incisor or canine teeth erupt. The lesions are firm and smooth with a fleshy pink color and often pedunculated. The tumors range in size from 1 mm to 9 cm and are multiple in 10%. The histogenesis remains controversial, with proposed origins as odontogenic, fibroblastic, histiocytic, myogenic, and neurogenic.[41] Congenital lesions can present as masses protruding from the mouth and can prevent nutrition and partially restrict respiration. Clinically, one may see occasional spontaneous regression and lack of postnatal tumor growth. Treatment is typically with simple excision.[41–42] The lesion should be differentiated from granular cell myoblastoma. There have been no documented recurrences or malignant transformation of an epulis.

EPIGNATHUS TERATOMAS

Epignathus teratomas are rare congenital malformations giving rise to oropharyngeal tumors. They are classified as mature teratoma. The estimated incidence for all mature teratomas is 1 in 4,000 live births, and at least 2% are oropharyngeal. The lesions do not appear to be familial in nature; however, there is a female predominance of 3:1 over males.[43] Epignathus teratomas occur more frequently in children of young mothers and can be associated with polyhydramnios owing to swallowing difficulty. Prenatal detection of these tumors has rarely been reported.[43] Placental edema owing to fetal cardiac decompensation based on the vascular nature of the tumors has been described as pre-eclampsia.[44]

The clinical presentation is based on the size and location of the tumor. Large tumors can result in early neonatal asphyxia. Computed tomography (CT) and magnetic resonance imaging (MRI) allow preoperative assessment of the tumor. Intracranial extension should be suspected in the event of sphenoid dehiscence.[44]

Histologically, they are composed of various tissues of ecto-, endo-, and mesodermal origin. The site of origin appears to be the craniopharyngeal canal. The implantation of the base can be single or multiple. The majority of these tumors have their point of attachment at the base of the skull in the posterior region of the nasopharynx. The tumors can be multiple and are associated with other malformations in 6% of cases. CP is the most common associated anomaly; however, bifid tongues and noses have been described. Differential diagnosis usually includes rhabdomyosarcoma of the tongue, retinoblastoma, nasal glioma, heterotopic thyroid, cystic lymphangioma, nasoethmoid meningoencephalocele, sphenoid meningoencephalocele, and giant epulis.[44]

Treatment consists of early and total surgical resection using an oral approach. Malignant degeneration has never been described in association with epignathus teratomas. Recurrence has not been reported.[44]

RANULA

A cyst-like swelling in the mouth floor, ranula, has been described since the days of Hippocrates. They are unilateral and unilocular and confined to the sublingual space, causing no discomfort. Their origin is typically due to mucus extravasation from the sublingual salivary gland that results in a pseudocyst. This condition is rare in the neonatal period but has been detected antenatally on ultrasonography.[45]

The ranula is characterized by a translucent blue color reflecting the viscous mucus contained within and the vascular congestion of the overlying mucosa. They are typically soft and slow to enlarge. Traumatic rupture is common, but with healing of the roofing mucosa, recurrences develop. Larger cysts may cause tongue displacement and result in difficulty with mastication, swallowing, and speech. Treatment initially can involve marsupialization and packing of the cystic lumen with gauze. Maintaining the packing for at least 10 days promotes fibrosis and sealing of the leaking salivary duct. Alternatively, the use of injecting the lesion with a sclerosing agent (eg, OK-432) has been described in children and adults,[46] and the use of a water-based laser system (eg, Er, Cr:YSGG laser) has been reported as well.[47] Recurrences can be treated with a more extensive intraoral excision of the culpable sublingual salivary gland[48.]

NATAL AND NEONATAL TEETH

Natal teeth are those observable in the oral cavity at birth, whereas neonatal teeth are those that erupt during the first month of life. The reported incidence is somewhat varied, but among larger studies, the range is between 1 in 1,118 and 1 in 30,000. Overall, there does not appear to be a gender predilection, although some studies suggest that the incidence may be slightly higher among females.[49]

The etiology of early eruption is unknown, although it has been related to several factors, including superficial position of the germ, infection or malnutrition, febrile states, eruption accelerated by febrile incidents or hormonal stimulation, hereditary transmission of an autosomal dominant gene, osteoblastic activity within the germ area related to the remodeling phenomenon, and hypovitaminosis. At times, premature eruption is described in which an immature rootless tooth exfoliates within a short time. This phenomenon, in distinction to early eruption, has been designated "expulsive Capdepont follicle," may result from trauma to the alveolar margin at delivery, and is associated with gingival inflammation. Natal and neonatal teeth owing to early eruption have been related to various syndromes, including Hallermann-Streiff (MIM#234100), Ellis-van Creveld (MIM#225500), craniofacial dysostosis, multiple steatocystoma (MIM#184510), congenital pachyonychia (MIM167200), and Sotos (MIM#117550).[49]

Clinically, the teeth may be conical or may be normal in size and shape and opaque yellow-brown in color. They can be classified as mature or immature based on their structure and development. Histologically, most of the crowns are covered with hypoplastic enamel of varying degree and severity. In addition, they often have absence of root formation, ample and vascularized pulp, and irregular dentin formation and lack of cementum formation. These teeth can be differentiated from cysts of the dental lamina and Bohn nodules by radiographic examination.[49]

Radiographic verification of the relationship of the tooth and adjacent structures, nearby teeth, and the presence or absence of a germ in the primary tooth area allows one to determine if the tooth belongs to the normal dentition. Indeed, most natal and neonatal teeth are primary teeth of the normal dentition (95%) and not supernumerary teeth. The teeth are usually in the region of the lower incisors (85%) and double in 61% of the cases.[49]

Treatment depends in part on the tooth's implantation, degree of mobility, difficulty sucking or breastfeeding, possibility of traumatic injury, and whether the tooth is part of the normal dentition or supernumerary. If the tooth is part of the normal dentition and well implanted, it should be left in the arch to avoid loss of space and collapse of the developing mandibular arch, which could lead to future malocclusion. Removal should be considered only if there is difficulty in feeding or they are highly mobile, with risk of aspiration. However, it should be noted that, to date, there are no reports of aspiration of a natal or neonatal tooth. If indicated, extraction is relatively easy and can be accomplished with forceps or even the fingers; however, some experts caution that they should not be removed prior to day 10 of life owing to risk of hemorrhage. This risk, however, is lessened if vitamin K is administered prior to extraction, as is typically performed as part of immediate neonatal care.[49]

TONGUE LESIONS

Tongue development begins at 3 to 4 weeks gestation from the first three to four brachial arches.[50] Specifically, the tongue arises from four swellings (median tongue bud, two lateral tongue buds, and hypobranchial eminence), which merge to form the tongue.[50] Pediatric tongue lesions represent 2.4% of all pediatric oral and maxillofacial tumors. Most lesions are benign and include various local neoplastic solid tumors, cysts, polyps, benign neoplasms, and diffuse hypertrophy. Anterior lesions do not typically obstruct the aerodigestive tract and are typically asymptomatic. Posterior lesions may present with acute respiratory distress or dysphagia. Excision of these lesions may hamper function owing to injury to superficial lingual nerves. Diffuse lesions can present with chronic protrusion, respiratory distress, dysphagia, dysarthria, or salivation. Surgical repair aims at preserving motility, taste, and cosmetic appearance.[51]

Osseous christmas are lesions composed of normal bone mass within the soft tissue. When present in the tongue, they are typically posterior near the foramen cecum. Patients' ages range between 5 and 73 years, with an increased frequency in the third and fourth decades. A female predominance has been observed. The origin is thought to be ossified remnants of brachial arches. They may appear as densely calcified masses on plain film and noncontrast CT. Differential diagnosis includes extraskeletal osteosarcoma and chondrosarcoma, which are both less likely in a pediatric population. Treatment is via surgical excision. No recurrences or malignant transformations have been reported.[51]

Hamartomas represent benign tumor-like proliferation of a tissue in its usual anatomic location. Fewer than 15 cases of lingual hamartomas have been reported, although some may have been mischaracterized as mesenchymomas. Lingual hamartomas occur in more than 50% of the orofaciodigital syndromes.[51] Airway obstruction can be a problem with large lesions. Treatment is local resection.

Lingual teratomas occur at the foramen cecum, where the embryologic tongue buds converge. Grossly, they are typically encapsulated, cystic, solid, or multiloculated masses that may contain hair, skin, cartilage, or mucous membrane tissue. The cause is unknown but thought to be secondary to entrapment of embryologic epithelial cells along the lines of closure for the first and second branchial arch or the differentiation of multipotential cells sequestered during closure of the anterior neuropore.[51]

Aglossia is likely due to a lack of development of the lateral lingual swellings of the mandibular arch. This is an extremely rare anomaly, with only a few reports existing among living children.[50] This typically occurs in association with other malformations and has been associated with aglossia-adactylia syndrome (Hanhart syndrome, MIM#103300) and Goldenhar syndrome (MIM#164210), in which one can see partial aglossia. In surviving patients, swallowing may improve after several months.[50] A recent report of a girl with aglossia proposed that micrognathia, microsomia, congenital absence of mandibular incisors, and collapse of the mandibular arch were the result of abnormal tongue development. This same girl had subclinical hypothyroidism.[52]

Microglossia is a not so rare malformation, often associated with other congenital syndromes (Table 4).[50] Clinical difficulties depend on the degree of microglossia and associated findings. Patients may have some difficulty with articulation.

Tongue hemihypertrophy or hemiatrophy is usually associated with auricular, mandibular, and maxillary hypoplasia. Affected patients have less developed musculature of the soft palate and tongue on the affected side. Parotic gland aplasia or hypoplasia may also be an associated anomaly. Parry-Romberg syndrome (MIM#141300) and congenital hemifacial hyperplasia are syndromes associated with this anomaly.[50]

Macroglossia is defined as a resting tongue that protrudes beyond the teeth or alveolar ridge. Sequelae owing to macroglossia include articulation errors, particularly in pronouncing consonants requiring the tongue tip to approximate the alveolar ridge or roof of the mouth (ie, s, z, sh, t, d, n). One may also develop an anterior open bite, prognathism, increased ramus to body angle, and flattening of the alveolar ridge. Deglutition issues may also arise and result in failure to thrive owing to inadequate intake. Airway obstruction may be a further complication and may lead to pulmonary hypertension and cor pulmonale. Acute respiratory distress owing to sudden respiratory obstruction has also been described.[53]

Lymphangioma is the most common etiology of macroglossia in children. It can be apparent at birth 60% of the time, with 95% becoming symptomatic by 2 years of life. The lymphangioma shares a common embryologic origin with cystic hygroma because both arise from lymphatic tissue rests derived from the primitive jugular sac.

Table 4 Syndromes Associated with Microglossia	
Syndrome	OMIM Number*
Aglossia-adactylia (oromandibular limb hypogenesis)	103300
Distal arthrogryposis, type II (Freeman-Sheldon)	193700
Faciocardiomelic dysplasia	227270
Hydrolethalus	236680
Myopathy, congenital nonprogressive, with Möbius sequence and Robin sequence	254940
Pierre Robin sequence	261800

Adapted from Hazelbaker.[58]
*Searching the OMIM (Online Mendelian Inheritance in Man) can be done at <http://www.ncbi.nlm.nih.gov/omim/>.

They typically involve the anterior two-thirds of the tongue. There is a coincident cystic hygroma in 7%. Grossly, it appears as a nodular swelling on the dorsum of the tongue or a water-filled blister. Discoloration of the tongue is due to blue-red vascular blebs deep within the vesicles. Increasing size can result from inflammation or trauma with hemorrhage into the lymphatic spaces. Recurrence after resection is common and arises from residual unremoved tissue.[53]

There are multiple syndromes associated with macroglossia (Table 5). Neonatal hypothyroidism, cretinism, has been associated with macroglossia. Here the tongue is enlarged owing to myocyte hypertrophy and myxedematous tissue deposition. The tongue is smooth and symmetrically enlarged. Treatment involves controlling the underlying endocrine condition, typically by the use of exogenous thyroid hormone.[53]

Beckwith-Wiedemann syndrome (MIM# 130650), described in 1964, also causes macroglossia. Possible patterns of inheritance include autosomal dominant inheritance with variable expressivity, contiguous gene duplication at 11p15, and genomic imprinting resulting from a defective or absent copy of the maternally derived gene. The incidence is estimated at 1 in 13,500 live births.[54] Associated features include exomphalos, gigantism, facial flame nevus, ear lobe anomalies, mild microcephaly, prominent occiput, maxillary hypoplasia, and short orbital floor. Macroglossia is present in 95% of affected individuals. Hypoglycemia is also a prominent feature owing to pancreatic cell hyperplasia.

Hemangiomas, congenital vascular malformations, may present as macroglossia. Histologically, one sees endothelium-lined vascular spaces. Therapy includes systemic and intralesional steroids and laser excision.[53] Rhabdomyosarcoma of the tongue causes macroglossia and accounts for 20% of head and neck rhabdomyosarcomas. Chemotherapy affords a 70% 3-year survival rate.[53] Neurofibromatosis may be associated with macroglossia when affected individuals develop neurofibromas in the tongue. They are typically unilateral and slow growing. Early surgical excision is recommended

Table 5 Syndromes Associated with Macroglossia

Syndrome	OMIM Number*
4p+	
Beckwith-Wiedemann	130650
Generalized gangliosidosis (GM1)	230500
Mannosidosis, αB	248500
Mucopolysaccharidosis I (Hurler)	252800
Mucopolysaccharidosis II (Hunter)	309900
Mucopolysaccharidosis VI, A and B	253200
Neurofibromatosis	162200
Pycnodysostosis or osteopetrosis	265800
Simpson-Golabi-Behmel	312870
X-linked α-thalassemia/mental retardation	301040

Adapted from Weiss, White.[53]
*Searching the OMIM (Online Mendelian Inheritance in Man) can be done at <http://www.ncbi.nlm.nih.gov/omim/>.

prior to spread to the floor of the mouth, thus allowing for total excision.[53] Pseudomacroglossia can be seen in those instances in which there is a small mandible (eg, Down syndrome, PRS).[53]

Treatment of macroglossia with surgical excision is based on the effects on feeding, dentition, speech, and airway compromise. Initially, the patient may achieve benefit from nursing in the prone position or feeding through a nasogastric tube. Management involves a multidisciplinary team of an otolaryngologist, a speech therapist, and an orthodontist. Goals include the restoration of the size and shape of the tongue, preservation of function, and correction of dental arch anomalies. Typically, surgery is performed by 4 to 7 months to avoid maxillofacial deformities and speech defects.[53]

Long tongue has rarely been described in which affected persons have an extremely lengthy tongue with extreme mobility. This has been documented in Ehlers-Danlos syndrome.[50] There do not appear to be any clinical manifestations.

Accessory tongue is a very rare malformation in which the tongue is attached to the tonsil or a process arising from one side of the base of the tongue.[50]

Cleft of bifid tongue has been described with Goldenhar syndrome, orofaciodigital syndrome types I (MIM#311200) and II (MIM#252100), CP lateral synechia syndrome (MIM#119550), and focal dermal hypoplasia (MIM#305600).[50]

Lingual thyroid occurs when thyroid gland elements persist in the area of the foramen cecum. This is typically along the midline, immediately posterior to the foramen cecum and resting on a broad base. The color varies from red to purple.[50] The lingual thyroid mass usually increases in size as the child ages owing to the effect of thyroid-stimulating hormone on this marginally functioning thyroid. Common presenting symptoms are dysphagia, dysphonia, dyspnea, and, occasionally, pain. Rarely the lesion can obstruct the airway, and a CO_2 laser has been reported as being a useful tool in helping to remove a portion of the lesion so that the airway can be secured.[55] A thyroid scan is required to determine the amount of active thyroid tissue because this may be the patient's only functioning thyroid tissue. Management considerations include functional, metabolic, and cosmetic factors. Euthyroid, asymptomatic patients can be followed carefully over time. Patients with abnormalities in their thyroid function can be managed with hormone therapy; otherwise, surgical resection is warranted. There is an increased frequency of thyroid carcinoma in lingual thyroid tissue.[40]

Other syndromes with associated tongue anomalies include Melkersson-Rosenthal syndrome (MIM#155900), in which one-third of affected individuals have a folded tongue; Coffin-Lowry syndrome (MIM#303600), in which patients have been observed to have a deep central lingual groove and thickened lips; Riley-Day syndrome (MM#223900), in which one observes decreased numbers of fungiform and circumvallate papillae; and Klippel-Trenaunay-Weber

syndrome (MIM#149000), in which there may be angiomatosis of the tongue.[50]

Ankyloglossia, tongue-tie, is a congenital anomaly characterized by an abnormally short lingual frenulum, which may restrict tongue tip mobility. Incidence figures reported in the literature vary from 0.02 to 4.8%, and there is a male-to-female ratio of 3 to 1.[56] Ankyloglossia occurs most frequently as an isolated anatomic variation. An increased prevalence has been noted among children of mothers who abused cocaine.[56] It may also be associated with various syndromes, including Opitz syndrome (MIM#300000), orofaciodigital syndrome, and X-linked CP (MIM#303400). The long-term outcome of ankyloglossia is unknown because there are no long-term studies; however, some authors postulate that the short frenulum can elongate spontaneously, with progressive stretching and thinning with use.[56] This might account for the perception that this disorder is more common among children than adults. Sequelae from ankyloglossia are debated; some feel that it is rarely symptomatic, whereas others state that it results in infant feeding difficulties, speech disorders, and mechanical and social difficulties.[56] Surveys report that the majority of lactation consultants feel that ankyloglossia can hamper breastfeeding and result in sore nipples, poor latching on and sucking mechanics, poor infant weight gain, and early weaning.[56] This is, in part, supported by a recent prospective study in which 36 infants with ankyloglossia were compared with normal controls. Although both groups were able to successfully breastfeed for at least 2 months, the affected group reported more frequent nipple pain and difficulty latching on (25 vs 3% for controls).[57] There does not appear to be a problem with affected infants ability to bottle-feed, although this should not be used as an argument to avoid breastfeeding attempts.[56]

Speech sounds that may be affected by tongue tip mobility include lingual sounds and sibilants such as t, d, z, s, th, n, l. Although ankyloglossia can be a cause of articulation problems and effortful speech, it is not a cause of speech delay.[56]

Additional problems reported by older children and adults include difficulty in intraoral toilet (lip licking and sweeping away oral debris), cuts under the tongue, creation of a diasthesis between the lower central incisors, and poorly fitting dentures. Social difficulties may also occur, including playing a wind instrument, licking ice cream, and "French kissing."[56]

Diagnosis is based on physical examination in which the frenulum is abnormally short and inserts onto the tongue at or near the tongue tip. The tongue may appear notched or heart shaped on protrusion. Protrusion is limited and may not extend beyond the lower lip. Hazelbaker, a lactation consultant, devised an assessment tool for lingual frenulum function to be used on neonates. Based on a scoring of seven lingual movements from 0 to 2, low scorers are recommended to undergo frenotomy.[58] However, despite this and other more complex measuring scales, there appears to be no way to predict, based on examination, those children who are likely to have problems related to ankyloglossia.[56]

The timing of surgical correction is controversial. Some feel that given the rare incidence of complications, it is warranted to wait until such complications develop, whereas others feel that prophylactic treatment is warranted, especially in light of the minimal surgical risks.[56] Additional considerations with respect to timing include the fact that delayed repair beyond 1 year of age often requires general surgery, whereas younger children tolerate the procedure in a clinic setting. Frenotomy, clipping of the frenulum, is rapid and easy and is best suited for infants. The discomfort is brief and minor and may not warrant anesthesia. In children over age 1 year, frenuloplasty is preferred. Here the frenulum is released via sequential cuts, as is done with frenotomy, and then the resultant wound is closed with a suture. As with frenotomy, antibiotics are not required, and rare postoperative pain can be managed with acetaminophen. Improvements in breastfeeding are often immediate, given that that was the source of the feeding problem. Similarly, articulation improves in 75% of patients postoperatively among patients with ankyloglossia-related problems. Complications of repair include infection, excessive bleeding, recurrent ankyloglossia owing to scarring, new speech disorder, and glossoptosis.[56]

CYSTIC HYGROMA

Cystic hygromas are congenital malformations of the lymphatic system. They are characterized by single or multiple fluid-filled lesions occurring at sites of lymphatic-venous connections. They typically develop between the late first trimester and early second trimester. The incidence of cystic hygroma is unknown; however, rates as high as 1 in 100 have been reported.[59]

The lymphatic system develops at the end of the fifth week as endothelium grows out from the venous system. Six lymphatic sacs, two jugular sacs draining the head, neck, and arms; two iliac sacs draining the legs and lower trunk; and two sacs draining the gut (the retroperitoneal sac and the cisterna chili), develop in close proximity to the body's large veins. Through centrifugal extension and branching, the lymphatic vessels arise from these sacs. The right and left thoracic ducts connect with the venous system at the junction of the internal jugular and subclavian veins at the end of the sixth week of gestation.[59]

The anatomic distribution and severity of lymphatic vessel anomalies vary with the underlying disorder. They range in size from that of a small pouch to giant extensions along the length of the body. They tend to infiltrate tissue planes, including the tongue and the floor of the mouth. This can lead to life-threatening airway compromise. Owing to their large size and tissue involvement, endotracheal intubation may be difficult, and tracheotomy is necessary to secure the airway. They are either smooth or irregular in contour, the latter suggesting a multilocular fluid collection. Hygroma spaces are lined by endothelial cells and contain serous lymphatic fluid. They are typically located in the posterior neck. Numerous syndromes have been associated with cystic hygromas (Table 6), as well as exposure to alcohol, aminopterin, and trimethadone.[59]

In the multicenter first and second trimester evaluation of risk (FASTER) trial, cystic hygroma was identified in 134 among 38,167 screened cases (1 in 285). Chromosomal abnormalities including trisomy 21, Turner syndrome, trisomy 18 were found in 51%. Major structural fetal malformations, mainly cardiac and skeletal, were diagnosed in 34%. Overall survival with normal pediatric outcome was detected in only 17%. Thus, the finding of a cystic hygroma in the first trimester is the strongest prenatal association with aneuploidy and should prompt further diagnostic evaluation and counseling.[60]

Prenatal diagnosis can ensure that the appropriate surgical personnel are in the delivery room and thus offer the best chance for a good outcome.[61] Indeed, operating while the patient remains on placental support and ex utero intrapartum treatment have been described.[62–63] Before excision is attempted, the extent of the lesion and its relationship to surrounding structures must be considered. For superficial lesions, ultrasonography with or without Doppler may help to define the lesion. For more complex lesions, CT and MRI have proven useful. Complete excision is the treatment of choice. However, because their extension can be marked and their involvement of vital structures and nerves is common, removal may not be possible. Postoperative complications of recurrence, wound seroma, infection, and nerve damage occur in 30% or more of cases. If the lesion is only partially resected, recurrence rates approach 100%.[59] Nonsurgical treatment with either bleomycin or OK-432 (lyophilized incubation mixture of group A *Streptococcus pyogenes*) has shown some efficacy.[59]

ESOPHAGEAL DUPLICATION

Congenital duplications may arise along the length of the gastrointestinal system. Although midgut duplications are the most common, foregut duplications (esophagus, stomach, and parts 1 and 2 of the duodenum) account for approximately one-third.[64] Among the foregut duplications, esophageal duplications are the most common. The duplications may appear as cysts, diverticulae, and tubular malformations, all of which are thought to have a similar embryologic origin. Gastric mucosa is frequently observed within the wall of the duplication irrespective of their site of origin.[65]

Esophageal duplications are often identified on chest radiograph and barium esophagogram as posterior mediastinal masses.[65] Duplication cysts may be difficult to distinguish from bronchogenic cysts, which can also cause external compression of the esophagus. Vertebral anomalies are concomitantly found in approximately 50% of cases.[64] Many of these are associated with intraspinal abnormalities. This association is best explained embryologically by the split notochord syndrome. The notochord, present from the third week of gestation, may split, allowing endodermal gut to herniate through the gap, resulting in a cyst or fistula. The cyst may interfere with anterior fusion of the vertebral mesoderm, accounting for the vertebral anomalies.[64]

The most common presenting symptom of an esophageal duplication cyst within neonates is respiratory distress owing to the enlarging cyst pressing on the adjacent lungs and airways. Among older children, dysphagia is a more common complaint. Smaller cysts may remain asymptomatic for years and be noted incidentally on chest radiography. Older children may develop massive gastrointestinal or bronchial hemorrhage and spinal meningitis because the wall of the duplication erodes owing to production of acid from the gastric lining of the duplication.

Diagnosis is usually accomplished radiographically as a mass on a chest radiograph or as a compressing mass on contrast esophagogram. Communicating lesions can also be noted to fill with contrast. Chest CT or MRI is helpful in further defining the lesion. Prenatal ultrasonographic visualization has been described.[66]

Management is best accomplished via surgical excision of the duplication. However, excision is not always possible, particularly if the esophagus and duplication share a common wall

Table 6 Syndromes Associated with Cystic Hygroma

Syndrome	OMIM Number*
Achondrogenesis type II	200610
Achondroplasia	100800
Beckwith-Wiedemann	130650
Cornelia de Lange	122470
Cowden disease	158350
Cumming	211890
Districhiasis-lymphedema	153400
Fraser	219000
Fryns	229850
Hereditary lymphedema	153100
Multiple pterygium	253290
Noonan	163950
Oculodental digital dysplasia	164200
Opitz-Frias	145410
Pena-Shokeir	208150
Polysplenia	208530
Proteus	176920
Roberts	268300
Thrombocytopenia absent radii	274000
Trisomy 13	
Trisomy 18	
Trisomy 21	
Turner	
Williams	194050
Zellweger	214100

Adapted from Gallagher.[59]

*Searching the OMIM (Online Mendelian Inheritance in Man) can be done at <http://www.ncbi.nlm.nih.gov/omim/>.

for any distance. Excision of the bulk of the duplication with stripping of the mucosa on the esophageal wall is an option for those cysts that are unresectable. Resection via minimal access thoracocsopic surgery has been described,[67] as well as endoscopic resection.[68]

ESOPHAGEAL STENOSIS

Congenital esophageal stenosis is defined as an intrinsic stenosis caused by a congenital malformation of the esophageal wall that is not necessarily present at birth. The etiology is classified as tracheobronchial rest (TBR), membranous diaphragm (MD), and segmental hypertrophy of the muscularis and diffuse fibrosis of the submucosa. The stenosis owing to TBR is the most common and MD is the least common.[69] The overall incidence of esophageal stenosis is estimated at 1 in 25,000 to 50,000 live births, with the incidence of other congenital anomalies associated with congenital esophageal stenosis ranging from 17 to 33%.[70] Symptoms vary with the location and severity of the stenosis. High esophageal lesions typically present with respiratory symptoms, whereas lower lesions present with vomiting. The majority present with the introduction of solids and signs and symptoms of dysphagia.[69]

Esophagograms are helpful in making the diagnosis, and confirmation by endoscopy is diagnostic. When strictures are identified, congenital lesions must be differentiated from acid-related strictures and from compression of the esophagus from external structures such as vascular rings. The majority of cases attributable to TBR are in the distal portions of the esophagus, whereas fibromuscular stenosis (FMS) and MD occur more commonly in the middle third. The FMS is classically 1 to 4 cm in length, has a smooth wall with an hourglass configuration, is located at the junction of the middle and lower thirds of the esophagus, and results in only partial obstruction of the esophageal lumen. TBR is typically found within 3 cm of the gastric cardia and often results in high-grade obstruction. MD is more common in the midesophagus.[69] Endoscopic ultrasound has been shown to be helpful in differentiating FMS from TBR as the later contains hyperechoic lesions consistent with cartilage.[71]

Segmental stenosis attributable to TBR and FMS can be associated with esophageal atresia and tracheoesophageal fistula (TEF) and accounts for up to one-third of reported cases. TBR, like esophageal atresia, is due to abnormal separation of the foregut into the trachea and esophagus, which occurs at day 25 of gestation. This accounts for their frequent association. MD is likely a form of "partial" esophageal atresia,[69] although case reports of complete obstruction of the esophagus by an intraluminal mucosal diaphragm have been described.[72]

Treatment of congenital esophageal stenosis is typically via excision with end-to-end reanastomosis. If this is in proximity to the lower esophageal sphincter, an accompanying fundoplication

should be performed. Some controversy, however, exists as to whether some of these lesions, particularly those with FMS, can be treated by dilatation. Dilatations are not always successful, and there is a risk of perforation. Esophageal webs (MD) may be more amenable to simple dilatation.[69] There have also been reports of treatment of MD with endoscopic laser division.[73] In case of short segmental stenosis owing to TBR, circular myomectomy has been described.[74]

ESOPHAGEAL ATRESIA

The first reported case of esophageal atresia was an autopsy finding by Durston in 1670. Shortly thereafter, in 1697, Thomas Gibson provided the first clinical description of a TEF.[75] The first successful staged repair was reported in 1939 by Laven and Ladd.[75] Haight reported the first successful primary anastomosis with fistula ligation in 1941.[75] Prior to these reports, esophageal atresia was a uniformly fatal congenital anomaly.

The exact cause remains unknown. Normal development of the foregut begins during the fourth week of embryonic life as the foregut endoderm differentiates into a ventral respiratory part and a dorsal esophageal part.[76] Traditionally, scientists speculated that the ventral and dorsal parts achieve separation by week 7 of embryonic life after formation of lateral longitudinal tracheoesophageal folds which fuse in the midline as a septum. Incomplete fusion was thought to result in TEF.[76] Kluth, in his study on chick embryos, hypothesized that it is excessive ventral invagination of the ventral pharyngoesophageal fold that results in TEF.[77] A study of

the Adriamycin rat model suggests that the initial event is esophageal atresia, and it is the lung bud that forms the stomach accounting for the fistula.[78] Developmental disorders of circulation have also been proposed. Genes of the retinoic acid receptor, HOXD group, sonic hedgehog, Gli family, Foxf1, thyroid transcription factor, and Tbx4 misexpression have been linked to these malformations.[75–76]

Overall, the incidence of esophageal atresia is 1 in 3,000 to 1 in 4,000 live births, with the highest rate among Whites.[79] There is a 0.5 to 2% risk of recurrence among siblings of an affected child. Prolonged maternal use of contraceptive pills and exposure to progesterone and estrogen during pregnancy have been implicated as teratogens. Esophageal atresia with TEF takes a number of forms (Figure 1); the most common anomaly, accounting for 85% of cases, comprises a blind-ending esophageal pouch with a fistula from the trachea to the distal esophagus.

Approximately 50 to 70% cases have associated anomalies, including cardiac (11 to 49%), genitourinary (24%), gastrointestinal (24%), and skeletal (13%). Approximately 10% of patients are classified within the VACTERL (MIM#192350) association in which three or more of the following anomalies are found: vertebral, anorectal, cardiac, TEF, and renal and radial limb anomalies. Driver and colleagues reported the associated anomalies in 134 patents with esophageal atresia with or without TEF. Of these, 31 had gastrointestinal anomalies, including anorectal malformation (52%), duodenal atresia (19%), malrotation (13%), jejunoileal atresia (10%), duplication (3%), and hiatal hernia (3%).[80] Mee and colleagues identified 119 infants with con-

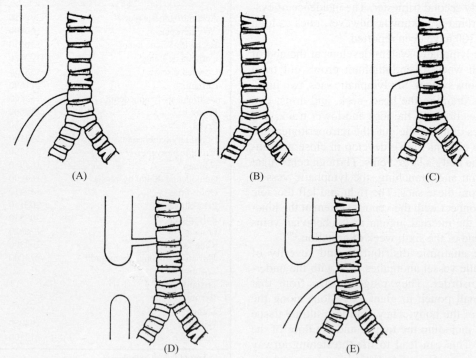

Figure 1 Types of esophageal atresia with or without fistula. The incidence of each is as follows: (A) esophageal atresia (EA) with distal tracheoesophageal fistula (TEF), 85%; (B) EA without TEF, 8%; (C) isolated TEF, 4%; (D) EA with proximal TEF, 2%; (E) EA with distal and proximal TEF, <1%>. (By Jean Hyslop, Medical Artist, Royal Hospital for Sick Children, Yorkhill, Glasgow, UK.)

genital cardiac anomalies of 554 patients with esophageal atresia. The most common included atrial septal defect (ASD) (8%), ventricular septal defect (VSD) (28%), tetralogy of Fallot (13%), and patent ductus arteriosus (PDA) (13%).[81] Other associations have been noted.[75] Syndromes associated with esophageal atresia and TEF are listed in Table 7.

The proximal blind esophageal pouch is typically hypertrophied and has a good blood supply. It is adherent to the trachea, which often has more muscle than cartilage, and thus results in tracheomalacia. The distal pouch is narrow and small; fistulae typically open into the trachea near the carina. The gastroesophageal sphincter is typically incompetent, and the vagus nerve is often defective, accounting for improper peristalsis.[75]

The diagnosis is suspected if there is evidence of polyhydramnios and a smaller than usual gastric bubble. Together these findings have a positive predictive value of 56%.[82] Prenatal ultrasonography may also demonstrate an anechoic structure in the fetal neck, representing the upper pouch. After birth, newborns are typically mucusy and require frequent suctioning. With feeding, there may be coughing, vomiting, and cyanosis. If a distal fistula is present, one may see progressive abdominal distention because the stomach and intestines fill with air introduced from the trachea. With a delay in diagnosis, the patients may develop pneumonitis.

The diagnosis is facilitated by the attempted introduction of a nasogastric tube that meets resistance prior to entering the stomach as it coils in the esophagus. A radiograph with the tube in place reveals the coiled esophageal tube. The presence of a TEF is recognized by the presence of intestinal air. The introduction of contrast into the proximal pouch is hazardous owing to the aspiration risk and is typically not warranted. Preoperative bronchoscopy is recommended by some to localize the fistula, exclude an upper pouch fistula, and identify a right-sided aortic arch. Echocardiography is also typically performed preoperatively to assess for associated cardiac defects and determine the laterality of the aortic arch, and thus allow for decision making as to the surgical approach.[75] A right-sided arch occurs in less than 2% of the cases.

The rare H-type TEF (4%) can be more difficult to diagnose because patients may not be as symptomatic in the immediate newborn period. Patients often present with a history of choking and respiratory difficulty with feeds. They may also have a history of recurrent pneumonia or asthma. Routine esophagography may fail to demonstrate the fistulous connection; therefore, if there is a high index of suspicion, the study should be performed via a nasogastric tube that is slowly withdrawn into the esophagus so that better visualization of the esophageal mucosa can be obtained. Esophagogastroscopy similarly may not be able to visualize the fistula, whereas bronchoscopy is typically the test of choice. H-type TEF has been successfully closed endoscopically with electrocautery and histoacryl glue.[83]

If possible, endotracheal intubation prior to surgery should be avoided because air introduced into the bowel via the TEF can cause abdominal distention and potential perforation.[84] The surgical approach is via a standard extrapleural thoracotomy with division of the fistula and single-layer end-to-end anastomosis using polyglycolic acid sutures. The two ends of the esophagus are typically within 2 cm, allowing anastomosis. Long gap atresias of greater than 2.5 cm pose special problems and may necessitate colonic interposition or pulling the stomach proximately into the chest to allow continuity. Surgical repair utilizing minimal access thoracoscopic surgery has been described.[85] The use of drainage tubes or gastrostomy has been abandoned, and early alimentation is practiced.[86] In long gap esophageal atresia with or without TEF in which anastomosis cannot be accomplished despite lengthening myotomies, ligation of the fistula, if present, and gastrostomy with delayed primary repair have been advocated, particularly in small for date or preterm infants. Suctioning of secretions from the proximal pouch or creation of a "spit fistula" is required until subsequent reanastomosis.

Postoperatively, there is a risk of anastomotic leak (10 to 17%),[86] leading to formation of a salivary fistula, pneumonitis, and/or mediastinitis. Salivary fistula may respond to prolonged parenteral nutrition, ventilatory support, and antibiotics. After the immediate postoperative period, patients are at risk for anastomotic strictures, which may require dilatation, or reanastomosis. If the stricture is resistant to dilatation, it is likely due to concomitant gastroesophageal reflux disease, with acid-related inflammation.

Gastroesophageal reflux is a common problem owing to the impaired esophageal peristalsis. Clinically, the incidence is thought to be between 25 and 40%; however, when pH monitoring is performed, the incidence rises to 70%.[86] Poorly controlled reflux can result in acid-related strictures or life-threatening aspiration pneumonia. Antireflux surgery is considered for those patients with persistent difficulties despite medical therapy. However, fundoplication carries a

25% risk of recurrent reflux, and in these patients with poor esophageal motility difficulty, postoperative dysphagia and food impaction have been observed.[84]

Tracheomalacia or other structural tracheal anomalies can occur in up to 75% of patients.[86] Some may have severe manifestations and require either tracheostomy or aortopexy. Other, less affected individuals have noisy breathing, stridor, or a "barky" cough. Tracheal anomalies appear to occur only in the presence of a TEF and are not seen in isolated esophageal atresia.[86]

Poor outcome is still seen in children with low birth weight (<1,500 g) and major cardiac anomalies. These risk factors are reflected in the Waterston (Table 8) and Spitz (Table 9) classification schemes for prediction of outcomes in children with esophageal atresia and TEF. Among the infants in the original Waterston report, group A had a 95% survival, group B had a 68% survival, and group C had a 6% survival.[87] With advances in neonatology, reclassification does not include respiratory illness as a separate risk factor. According to the Spitz classification, in the absence of low birth weight and cardiac anomalies (group I), there is a 97% survival, 57% if one risk factor is present (group II), and 22% if both are present (group III).[75] The question as to whether patients who underwent TEF repair during infancy are at risk for esophageal adenocarcinoma has been raised.[88]

CONGENITAL LARYNGOTRACHEOESOPHAGEAL CLEFT

The first laryngotracheoesophageal cleft was described by Richter in 1792, who palpated a common cavity at the level of the larynx and hypopharynx in a newborn with feeding difficulties.[89]

The respiratory system develops as a foregut outpouching starting at day 20 of gestation.

Table 7 Syndromes Associated with Esophageal Atresia and Tracheoesophageal Fistula

Syndrome	OMIM Number*
CHARGE	214800
Fanconi syndrome	227650
McKusick-Kaufman syndrome	236700
Trisomy 21	
VACTERL	192350

Adapted from Banerjee.[75]
CHARGE = coloboma of the eye, heart anomaly, choanal atresia, retardation, and genital and ear anomalies; VACTERL = vertebral, anal, cardiac, tracheal, esophageal, renal, and limb anomalies.
*Searching the OMIM (Online Mendelian Inheritance in Man) can be done at <http://www.ncbi.nlm.nih.gov/omim/>.

Table 8 Waterston Classification of Infants with Esophagel Atresia with Tracheoesophageal Fistula

A	Birth weight over 5.5 pounds and well
B	Birth weight between 4 and 5.5 pounds and well, or higher birth weight with moderate pneumonia and other congenital anomalies
C	Birth weight under 5 pounds or higher birth weight but severe pneumonia and severe congenital anomalies

Adapted from Waterston.[87]

Table 9 Spitz Classification of Infants with Esophageal Atresia with Tracheoesophageal Fistula

I	Birth weight greater than or equal to 1.5 kg and no congenital heart disease
II	Birth weight less than 1.5 kg or congenital heart disease
III	Birth weight less than 1.5 kg and congenital heart disease

Adapted from Banerjee.[75]

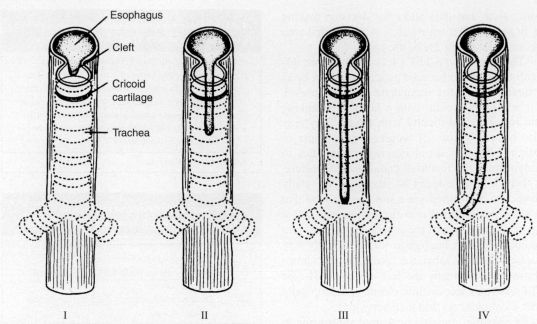

Figure 2   Types of laryngotracheoesophageal clefts. (By Jean Hyslop, Medical Artist, Royal Hospital for Sick Children, Yorkhill, Glasgow, UK.)

An abnormality in tracheoesophageal septum formation or progression accounts for a laryngotracheoesophageal cleft involving the tracheal rings. Failure of cricoid fusion may occur following failure of the septum to reach the appropriate level. Absence of cricoid fusion in isolation results in a laryngeal cleft.[89]

Numerous classification schemes have been devised. The most commonly quoted is that devised by Ryan in which type I is a cleft above the cricoid, type II is beyond the cricoid lamina, type III is up to the carina, and type IV is into the mainstem bronchi (Figure 2).[89]

Most cases appear to be sporadic; however, a mouse model exists in which a laryngotracheoesophageal cleft is inherited as an autosomal recessive mutation. Laryngotracheoesophageal clefts are seen in up to 50% of patients with Opitz (BBB/G) syndrome (MIM#145410). They also are seen with other anomalies, including TEF, anal atresia, malrotation, microgastria, and bronchobiliary fistula. Cardiac anomalies occur in up to one-third of cases and include VSD, PDA, coarctation of the aorta, and transposition of the great vessels. Associations with hypospadia, unilateral lung hypoplasia, and renal agenesis have also been reported.[89]

Neonatal symptoms may be subtle or obvious, with respiratory distress owing to recurrent aspiration pneumonia. One may also see cyanosis, coughing, choking, stridor exacerbated by feeds, sialorrhea, or a weak, toneless, or hoarse cry.

Chest radiography may reveal an aspiration pneumonia, persistent esophageal air, and distended bowel. Nasogastric tubes may be noted to be displaced along the anteroposterior plane on lateral radiography. CT and bronchoscopy can help to define the extent of the laryngotracheoesophageal cleft. The presence of an intact arytenoid fold excludes the diagnosis of a cleft. Swallowing studies with small volumes show simultaneous filling of the esophagus and trachea.[89]

Surgical repair is the definitive treatment. The most common approach is a lateral pharyngotomy through a vertical lateral cervical incision. Care must be taken not to damage the recurrent larygeal nerve on the side opposite the approach. All but the smallest clefts will require tracheostomy, and specialized tubes have been developed to prevent pressure on the posterior wall. Postoperative complications include fistulization, granulation tissue at the repair site, esophageal and subglottic stenosis, nerve injury, and aspiration.[89]

After repair, esophageal dysmotility still places the patient at risk for aspiration. Gastric division with a draining gastrostomy in the proximal segment and a feeding gastrostomy in the distal segment is widely used to protect the esophageal anastomosis. Alternatively, fundoplication with feeding gastrostomy or jejunostomy may suffice. After healing, feeding therapy is often required.[89]

REFERENCES

1. Spritz R. The genetics and epigenetics of orofacial clefts. Curr Opin Pediatr 2001;13:556–60.
2. Strong E, Buckmiller L. Management of cleft palate. Fac Plast Surg Clin North Am 2001;9:15–25.
3. Vieira A, Orioli I. Birth order and oal clefts: A meta analysis. Teratology 2002;66:209–16.
4. Ngai CW, Martin WL, Tonks A, et al. Are isolated facial cleft lip and palate associated with increased perinatal mortality? A cohort study from the West Midlands Region 1995-1997. J Matern Fetal Neonatal Med 2005;17: 203–6.
5. Murray J. Gene/environment causes of cleft lip and/or palate. Clin Genet 2002;61:248–56.
6. Weinberg SM, Neiswanger K, Martin RA, et al. The Pittsburgh oral-facial cleft study: Expanding the cleft phenotype. Background and justification. Cleft Palate Craniofac J 2006;43:7–20.
7. Johnson N, Sandy J. Prenatal diagnosis of cleft lip and palate. Cleft Palate Craniofac J 2003;40:186–9.
8. Carinci F, Pezzetti F, Scapoli L, et al. Recent developments in orofacial cleft genetics. J Craniofac Surg 2003;14:130–43.
9. Mostowska A, Hozyasz K, Jagodzinski P. Maternal MTR genotype contributes to the risk of nonsyndromic cleft lip and palate in the Polish population. Clin Genet 2006;69:512–7.
10. Martinelli M, Scapoli L, Palmieri A, et al. Study of four genes belonging to the folate pathway: Transcobalamin 2 is involved in the onset of nonsyndromic cleft lip with or without cleft palate. Hum Mutat 2006;27:294 .
11. Frebourg T, Oliveira C, Hochain P, et al. Cleft lip/palate and CDH1/E-cadherin mutations in families with hereditary diffuse gastric cancer. J Med Genet 2006;43:138–42.
12. Krapes IP, van Rooij IA, Ocke MC, et al. Maternal nutritional status and the risk for orofacial cleft offspring in humans. J Nutr 2004;134:3106–13.
13. Chevrier C, Dananche B, Bahuau M, et al. Occupational exposure to organic solvent mixtures during pregnancy and the risk of nonsyndromic oral clefts. Occup Environ Med 2006;27:Epub.
14. Shaw GM, Carmichael SL, Laurent C, Rasmussen SA. Maternal nutrient intakes and risk of orofacial clefts. Epidemiology 2006;17:285–91.
15. Krapels IP, Rooij IA, Wevers RA, et al. Myo-inositol, glucose and zinc status as risk factors for nonsyndromic cleft lip with or without cleft palate in offspring: A case control study. BJOG 2004;111:661–8.
16. Tamura T, Munger RG, Corcoran C, et al. Plasma zinc concentrations of mothers and the risk of nonsyndromic oral clefts in their children: A case control study in the Philippines. Birth Defects Res A Clin Mol Teratol 2005;73: 612–6.
17. Kazan-Tannus JF, Levine D, McKenzie C, et al. Real-time magnetic resonance imaging aids prenatal diagnosis of isolated cleft palate. J Ultrasound Med 2005;24:1533–40.
18. Habel A, Elhadi N, Sommerlad B, Powell J. Delayed detection of cleft palate: An audit of newborn examination. Arch Dis Child 2006;91:238–40.
19. Garcez LW, Giugliani ER. Population-based study on the practice of breastfeeding in children born with cleft lip and palate. Cleft Palate Craniofac 2005;42:687–93.
20. Montagnoli LC, Barbieri MA, Bettiol H, et al. Growth impairment of children with different types of lip and palate clefts in the first 2 years of life: A crosssectional study. J Pediatr (Rio J) 2005;81:461–5.
21. Prahl-Andersen B. Dental treatment of predental and infant patients with clefts and craniofacial anomalies. Cleft Palate Craniofac J 2000;37:528–32.
22. Sandberg D, Magee W, Denk M. Neonatal cleft lip and palate repair. AORN J 2002;75:490–8.
23. Papadopulos NA, Papadopoulos MA, Kovacs L, et al. Foetal surgery and cleft lip and palate: Current status and new perspectives. Br J Plast Surg 2005;58:593–607.
24. Paradise J, Elster B, Tan L. Evidence in infants with cleft palate that breast milk protects against otitis media. Pediatrics 1994;94:853–60.
25. St-Hilaire H, Buchbinder D. Maxilofacial pathology and management of Pierre Robin sequence. Otolaryngol Clin North Am 2000;33:1241–56.
26. Vanden Elzen AP, Semmekrot B, Bongers E, et al. Diagnosis and treatment of the Pierre Robin sequence: Results of a retrospective clinical study and review of the literature. Eur J Pediatr 2001;160:47–53.
27. Jakobsen LP, Knudsen MA, Lespinasse J, et al. The genetic basis of the Pierre Robin Sequence. Cleft Palate Craniofac J 2006;43:1555–9.
28. Shprintzen R. The implications of the diagnosis of Robin sequence. Cleft Palate Craniofac J 1992;29:205–9.
29. Handzic J, Bagatin M, Subotic R, Cuk V. Hearing levels in Pierre Robin syndrome. Cleft Palate Craniofac J 1995;32:30–6.
30. Sher A, Sphrintzen R, Thorpy M. Endoscopic observations of obstructive sleep apnea in children with anomalous upper airways: Predictive and therapeutic value. Int J Pediatr Otorhinolaryngol 1986;11:135–46.
31. Wagener S, Rayatt S, Tatman A, et al. Management of infants with Pierre Robin sequence. Cleft Palate Craniofac J 2003;40:180–5.
32. Denny AD, Amm CA, Schaefer RB. Outcomes of tongue-lip adhesion for neonatal respiratory distress caused by Pierre Robin sequence. J Craniofac Surg 2004;15: 819–23.
33. LeBlanc SM, Golding-Kushner KJ. Effect of glossopexy on speech sound production in Robin sequence. Cleft Palate Craniofac J 1992;29:239–45.
34. Denny A, Amm C. New technique for airway correction in neonates with severe Pierre Robin sequence. J Pediatr 2005;147:97–101.
35. Oktay H, Baydas B, Ersoz M. Using a modified nutrition plate for early intervention in a newborn infant with Pierre Robin sequence: A case report. Cleft Palate Craniofac J 2006;43:370–3.
36. Baudon J, Renault F, Goutet J, et al. Motor dysfunction of the upper digestive tract in Pierre Robin sequence as assessed by sucking-swallowing electromyography and esophageal manometry. J Pediatr 2002;140:719–23.

37. Nassar E, Marques IL, Trindade AS, Jr, Bettiol H. Feeding-facilitating techniques for the nursing infant with Robin sequence. Cleft Palate Craniofac J 2006;43:55–60.

38. Abadie V, Morisseau-Durand M, Beyler C, et al. Brainstem dysfunction: A possible neuroembryological pathogenesis of isolated Pierre Robin sequence. Eur J Pediatr 2002; 161:275–80.

39. Abadie V, Andre A, Zaouche A, et al. Early feeding resistance: A possible consequence of neonatal oro-oesophageal dyskinesia. Acta Paediatr 2001;90:738–45.

40. Gray S, Parkin J. Congenital malformations of the mouth and pharynx. In: Bluestone C, Stool S, Kenna M, editors. Pediatric Otolaryngology, Vol. 2. Philadelphia: WB Saunders; 1996. p. 985–98.

41. Ugras S, Demirtas I, Bekerecioglu M, et al. Immunohistochemical study on histogenesis of congenital epulis and review of the literature. Pathol Int 1997;47:627–32.

42. Olsen JL, Marcus JR, Zuker RM. Congenital eppulis. J Craniofac Surg 2005;16:161–4.

43. Gull I, Wolman I, Har-Toov J, et al. Antenatal sonographic diagnosis of epignathus at 15 weeks of pregnancy. Ultrasound Obstet Gynecol 1999;13:271–3.

44. Vandenhaute B, Leteurtre E, Lecomte-Houcke M, et al. Epignathus teratoma: Report of three cases with a review of the literature. Cleft Palate Craniofac J 2000;37:83–91.

45. Moya JF, Sulzberger SC, Recasens JD, et al. Antenatal diagnosis and management of a ranula. Ultrasound Obstet Gynecol 1998;11:147–8.

46. Rho MH, Kim DW, Kwon JS, et al. OK-432 sclerotherapy of plunging ranula in 21 patients: It can be a substitute for surgery. AJNR Am J Neuroradiol 2006;27:1090–5.

47. Zola M, Rosenberg D, Anakwa K. Treatment of a ranula using an Er,Cr:YSGG laser. J Oral Maxillofac Surg 2006;64:823–7.

48. Mandel L. Ranula, or, what's in a name? N Y State Dent J 1996;62:37–9.

49. Cunha R, Boer F, Torriani D, Frossard W. Natal and neonatal teeth: Review of the literature. Pediatr Dent 2001;23: 158–62.

50. Emmanouil-Nikoloussi E, Kerameos-Foroglou C. Developmental malformations of human tongue and associated syndromes [review]. Bull Group Int Rech Sci Stomatol Odontol 1992;35:5–12.

51. Horn C, Thaker H, Tampakopoulou D, et al. Tongue lesions in the pediatric population. Otolaryngol Head Neck Surg 2001;124:164–9.

52. Kantaputra P, Tanpaiboon P. Thyroid dysfunction in a patient with aglossia. Am J Med Genet A 2003;122:274–7.

53. Weiss L, White J. Macroglossia: A review. J La State Med Soc 1990;142:13–6.

54. Thorburn MJ, Wright ES, Miller CG, Smith-Read EHM. Exomphalos-macroglossia-gigantism syndrome in Jamaican infants. Am J Dis Child 1970;119:316–21.

55. Hafidh Ma, Sheahan P, Khan NA, et al. Role of CO_2 laser in the management of obstructive ectopic lingual thyroids. J Laryngol Otol 2004;118:807–9.

56. Lalakea M, Messner A. Ankyloglossia: Does it matter? Pediatr Clin North Am 2003;50:381–97.

57. Messner A, Lalakea M, Aby J, et al. Ankyloglossia: Incidence and associated feeding difficulties. Arch Otolaryngol Head Neck Surg 2000;126:36–9.

58. Hazelbaker A. The assessment tool for lingual frenulum function [master's thesis]. Pasadena, CA: Pacific Oaks College; 1993.

59. Gallagher P, Mahoney M, Gosche J. Cystic hygroma in the fetus and newborn. Semin Perinatol 1999;23:341–56.

60. Malone FD, Ball RH, Nyberg DA, et al. First-trimester septated cystic hygroma: Prevalence, natural history, and pediatric outcome. Obstet Gynecol 2005;106:288–94.

61. Suzuki N, Tsuchida Y, Takahashi A, et al. Prenatally diagnosed cystic lymphangioma in infants. J Pediatr Surg 1998;33:1599–604.

62. Skarsgard E, Chitkara U, Krane E, et al. The OOPS procedure (operation on placental support): In utero airway management of the fetus with prenatally diagnosed tracheal obstruction. J Pediatr Surgery 1996;31:826–8.

63. Mychaliska G, Bealer J, Graf J, et al. Operating on placental support: The ex utero intrapartum treatment procedure. J Pediatr Surg 1997;32:230–1.

64. Carachi R, Azmy A. Foregut duplications. Pediatr Surg Int 2002;18:371–4.

65. Bajpai M, Mathur M. Duplications of the alimentary tract: Clues to the missing links. J Pediatr Surg 1994;29:1361–5.

66. Gul A, Tekoglu G, Aslan H, et al. Prenatal sonographic features of esophageal and ileal duplications at 18 weeks of gestation. Prenat Diagn 2004;24:969–71.

67. Merry C, Spurbeck W, Lobe T. Resection of foregut-derived duplications by minimal-access surgery. Pediatr Surg Int 1999;15:224–6.

68. Will U, Meyer F, Bosseckert H. Successful endoscopic treatment of an esophageal duplication cyst. Scand J Gastroenterol 2005;40:995–9.

69. Ramesh J, Ramanujam T, Jayaram G. Congenital esophageal tenosis: Report of three cases, literature review, and proposed classification. Pediatr Surg Int 2001;17:188–92.

70. Vasudevan S, Kerendi F, Lee H, Ricketts R. Management of congenital esophageal stenosis. J Pediatr Surg 2002;37:1024–6.

71. Usui N, Kamata S, Kawahara H, et al. Usefulness of endoscopic ultrasonography in the diagnosis of congenital esophageal stenosis. J Pediatr Surg 2002;37:1744–6.

72. Sharma A, Sharma K, Sharma C, et al. Congenital esophageal bstruction by intraluminal mucosal diaphragm. J Pediatr Surg 1991;26:213–5.

73. Roy G, Cohen R, Williams S. Endoscopic laser division of an sophageal web in a child. J Pediatr Surg 1996;31:439–40.

74. Maeda K, Hisamatsu C, Hasegawa T, et al. Circular myotomy for the treatment of congenital esophageal stenosis owing to tracheobronchial remnant. J Pediatr Surg 2004;39:1765–8.

75. Banerjee S. Oesophageal atresia—the touch stone of pediatric surgery. J Indian Med Assoc 1999;97:432–5.

76. Felix JF, Keijzer R, van Dooren MF, et al. Genetics and developmental biology of oesophageal atresia and tracheo-oesophageal fistula: Lessons learned from mice relevant for pediatric surgeons. Pediatr Surg Int 2004;20:731–6.

77. Kluth D, Steding G, Seidl W. The embryology of foregut malformations. J Pediatr Surg 1987;22:389–93.

78. Diez-Pardo JA, Baoquan Q, Navarro C, et al. A new rodent experimental model of esophageal atresia and tracheoesophageal fistula: Preliminary report. J Pediatr Surg 1996;31:498–502.

79. Sparey C, Jawaheer G, Barrett A, Robson S. Esophageal atresia in the Northern Region Congenital Anomaly Survey, 1985-1997: Prenatal diagnosis and outcome. Am J Obstet Gynecol 2000;182:427–31.

80. Driver C, Shankar K, Jones M, et al. Phenotypic presentation and outcome of esophageal atresia in the era of the Spitz classification. J Pediatr Surg 2001;35:1419–21.

81. Mee R, Beasley S, Auldist A, Myers N. Influence of congenital heart disease on management of oesophageal atresia. Pediatr Surg Int 1992;7:90–3.

82. Stringer MD, McKenna KM, Goldstein RB, et al. Prenatal diagnosis of esophageal atresia. J Pediatr Surg 1995; 30:1258–63.

83. Tzifa KT, Maxwell EL, Chait P, et al. Endoscopic treatment of congenital H-type and recurrent tracheoesophageal fistula with electrocautery and histoacryl glue. Int J Pediatr Otorhinolaryngol 2006;70:925–30.

84. Maoate K, Myers N, Beasley S. Gastric perforation in infants with oesophageal atresia and distal tracheo-oesophageal fistula. Pediatr Surg Int 1999;15:24–7.

85. Allal H, Kalfa N, Lopez M, et al. Benefits of the thoracoscopic approach for short- or long-gap esophageal atreia. J Laparoendosc Adv Surg tech A 2005;15:673–7.

86. Spitz L. Esophageal atresia and tracheoesophageal fistula in children. Curr Opin Pediatr 1993;5:347–52.

87. Waterston D, Carter RB, Aberdeen E. Oesophageal atresia: Tracheo-oesophageal fistula. A study of survival in 218 infants. Lancet 1962;i:819–22.

88. Alfaro L, Bermas H, Fenoglio M, et al. Are patients who had a tracheoesophageal fistula repair during infancy at risk for esophageal adenocarcinoma during adulthood? J Pediatr Surg 2005;40:719–20.

89. Carr M, Clarke K, Webber E, Giacomantonio M. Congenital laryngotracheoesophageal cleft. J Otolaryngol 1999;28: 112–7.

90. Jones K. Smith's Recognizable Patterns of Human Malformation. Philadelphia: WB Saunders; 1997.

2

Disorders of the Oral Cavity

Stephen Porter, MD, PhD, FDS, RCS, RCSE
Paul Ashley, BDS, PhD, FDS Paed Dent

The oral cavity is the most accessible part of the gastrointestinal tract. Signs or symptoms of disease in the oral cavity may reflect disease restricted to the mouth (eg, dental caries): however, they may also be diagnostic of other conditions affecting the gastrointestinal tract (eg, oral lesions of Crohn's disease) or indicate disease occurring in other systems (eg, mucosal ulceration in cyclic neutropenia). While not quite a "window to the soul," the appearance of the hard and soft tissues of the mouth can give us useful clues as to the condition of the gastrointestinal tract and the body as a whole. This chapter describes the more common disorders that arise in the mouths of children and discusses the impact of gastrointestinal disease on the mouth.

DISORDERS OF TEETH

Teeth start to develop 5 weeks after commencement of embryogenesis; this process continues until the third permanent molars are complete at age 20 years. They begin from a thickening of the stomodeal epithelium, and development is regulated by interactions between neural crest-derived mesenchymal cells and the oral environment. (Precise mechanisms are still unclear, although over 200 genes are implicated.[1]) Disturbance of this process (either as a result of genetic mutation or environmental factors) can give rise to defects of tooth number, shape/size, structure, or eruption—dependent on the type of disturbance and at which point in the tooth development sequence that occurs. Genetic defects causing abnormalities of number, shape, or size are associated with mechanisms regulating tooth morphogenesis, those causing abnormalities of structure being defects of connective tissue (eg, type 1 collagen) or other components of the extracellular matrix. Enamel and dentine are not remodeled once formed; hence, defects may be the result of disease processes or other environmental insults that happened several years earlier. Some of the more common disorders are described below.

DISORDERS OF TOOTH NUMBER

These can be classified as hypodontia (missing teeth) or supernumerary teeth (extra teeth).

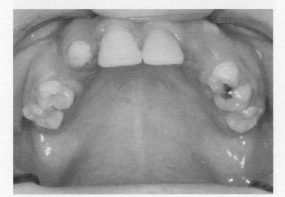

Figure 1 Hypodontia.

Hypodontia

Hypodontia is one of the most common dental anomalies, affecting up to 20% of the population.[2-4] One or more teeth may be affected, and the permanent teeth are more commonly affected than the primary teeth (primary dentition, 0.5 to 0.9%; permanent dentition, 1.6 to 9.6%, excluding third molars[2]) (Figure 1). The most commonly missing teeth are third molars, followed by maxillary lateral incisors and mandibular second premolars. Population studies have shown that tooth agenesis can be manifested as an isolated finding (either sporadic or familial) or part of a syndrome (see Table 1). One of the more common genetically determined disorders that can cause hypodontia is ectodermal dysplasia.

Ectodermal Dysplasias

The ectodermal dysplasias (EDs) comprise a large group of genetically determined disorders, clinically characterized by alterations of two or more ectodermally derived structures, giving rise to a wide variety of defects of the skin, nail, hair, or sweat glands.[5]

There are multiple congenitally missing primary teeth, coronoid primary incisors, with moderately to severely taurodontic second primary molars. Supernumerary cusps may also occur. The permanent teeth are always reduced in number and the crown shape of any present teeth is usually abnormal; in particular, the permanent incisal crowns are often conical or pointed, whereas the permanent molar crowns have a reduced diameter. The absence of teeth results in an underdevelopment of the alveolar processes

Table 1 Dental Anomalies in Childhood
Anomalies of tooth number
Hypodontia
Ectodermal dysplasia
Idiopathic hypodontia
Others (in chondroectodermal dysplasia, achondroplasia, Rieger syndrome, incontinentia pigmenti [Bloch-Sulzberger syndrome], Seckel syndrome)
Supernumerary teeth
Supplemental teeth
Others (supernumerary teeth in Apert syndrome, Gardner syndrome, cleidocranial dysplasia, Down syndrome, Crouzon anemia, orofaciodigital syndrome, Hallerman-Streiff syndrome)
Anomalies of tooth size
Microdontia
Macrodontia
Connation (fusion or germination)
Anomalies of tooth shape
Dilaceration
Dens in dente
Dens evaginatus
Taurodontism
Anomalies of eruption (see Table 3)
Anomalies of tooth color (see Table 4)

and hence a reduction in the lower third of the face height and lip protuberance, the latter causing dry, cracked, and fissured lips.[5-8]

ED typically encompasses a spectrum of ectodermal abnormalities. Individuals with anhidrotic forms may be liable to heat intolerance, which may give rise to episodes of hyperthermia, eventually leading to cerebral damage. Sparse blonde hair, including a reduced density of eyebrow and eyelash hair, is common in ED. The nails may appear dystrophic and brittle. The periocular skin may show a fine wrinkling with hyperpigmentation. As the salivary glands are ectodermally derived, patients may have varying degrees of salivary gland aplasia, xerostomia, and an increased liability to dental caries.[9]

Early dental intervention affords the child the opportunity to develop normal forms of speech, chewing, and swallowing; normal facial support; improved temporomandibular joint function; and improved self-esteem.[10-11] When a child with ED reaches his or her early teens, orthodontic treatment may be indicated, together with definitive restorative dental care possibly including endosseous implants.[12]

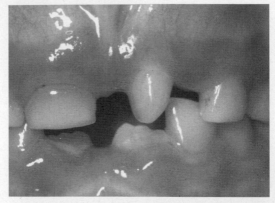

Figure 2 Supernumery tooth in site of upper central incisor.

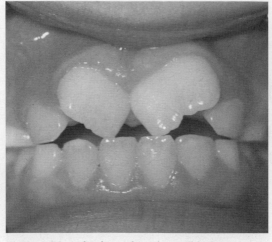

Figure 3 Macrodontia—enlarged central incisors.

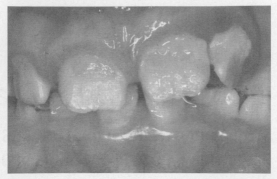

Figure 4 Amelogenesis imperfecta—gross loss of normal anatomy of the permanent dentition.

Supernumerary Teeth

Supernumerary teeth occur more commonly in the permanent dentition than the primary dentition (prevalence in the primary dentition, 0.3 to 0.8%: permanent dentition, 0.1 to 3.8%.[13]) and are more common in males than in females (permanent dentition only, ratio of 2:1). Supernumerary teeth may occur singly or in multiples (although this is rare) in either the maxilla or mandible (Figure 2). In the primary dentition, they are usually normal or conical in form. In the permanent dentition, the teeth may be conical, supplemental (normal form), tuberculate (barrel shaped), or odontomatous (hamartomatous malformation composed of more than one type of tissue).[14] The conical supernumerary is the most common defect seen and usually occurs in the palate between the central incisors where it is referred to as a mesiodens. The etiology is not understood but is probably multifactorial with both genetic and environmental factors having an input. As with hypodontia supernumerary teeth can be manifested as an isolated finding (either sporadic or familial) or as part of a syndrome (see Table 1), the most common of which is probably

cleidocranial dysplasia. Of relevance to gastrointestinal disease, supernumery teeth and odontomes may be a feature of Gardner's syndrome.

Both supernumerary and supplemental teeth can cause delayed or failed eruption of adjacent teeth and, when unerupted, may cause resorption of adjacent roots and/or dentigerous cyst formation. Management is usually by extraction.

DISORDERS OF TOOTH SIZE/SHAPE

Teeth may be increased (macrodontia) (Figure 3) or decreased (microdontia) in size or exhibit malformation of the crown. Macrodontia and microdontia are both rare; microdontia may be associated with hypodontia. Abnormalities of shape are more common and come in a wide variety of forms. These include abnormalities of cusp formation, such as invaginations where an ingrowth of enamel epithelium results in a pit or invagination within the tooth. Other abnormalities of form include additional cusps or fusion of teeth together to form the so called "double teeth." Other defects of tooth size and shape are detailed in Table 2 and in the relevant sections of this chapter.

DISORDERS OF TOOTH STRUCTURE

Primary Disorders of Enamel Formation

Amelogenesis Imperfecta. Amelogenesis imperfecta comprises a group of disorders with genetic heterogeneity characterized by defects of enamel. Classification schemes of amelogenesis imperfecta vary with a combination of phenotype (hypoplastic, hypocalcified, and hypomature) and mode of inheritance (autosomal dominant or recessive and sex-linked dominant or recessive) most commonly being employed. Reported prevalence varies widely (1:4,000 to 1:14,000), the autosomal dominant types being the most common (85%).[15–16]

The clinical appearance of affected teeth varies widely from a pitted appearance of the enamel seen in some hypoplastic types to the yellow/brown enamel and excessive wear observed in hypomaturation or hypocalcified types (Figure 4). The clinical features of amelogenesis imperfecta may have a similar appearance to fluoro-

sis or molar-incisal hypomineralization (MIH). Children with amelogenesis imperfecta require evaluation and management by specialists in pediatric dentistry, together with other relevant specialists (eg, clinical genetics).[17] Treatment aims are to preserve the existing structures and improve esthetics.

Primary Disorders of Dentine Formation

There are two main type of dentine disorder, dentine dysplasia and dentinogenesis imperfecta both of which have an autosomal dominant mode of inheritance.[15,18]

Dentine Dysplasia. This uncommon condition is characterized by normal-shaped crowns of the primary and/or permanent teeth but with an amber or opalescent appearance owing to abnormal structure of the underlying dentine. In dentine dysplasia type I (radicular dentine dysplasia), there is obliteration of the pulp chambers, short or absent roots, and resultant tooth mobility and migration. In type II disease (coronal dentine dysplasia and pulpal dysplasia), the clinical consequences are not as severe as that of type I, tends to affect the deciduous dentition more than the permanent dentition, and the root structure may be unaffected.[18]

Dentinogenesis Imperfecta. This is probably the most well known of the primary dentinal disorders, presumably as a consequence of its potentially profound clinical presentation. At least three types of disease are known[19] with a reported prevalence (USA) of type II of 1:8,000.[20] Features of the disease are broadly common across all groups, the teeth having a gray/blue/amber appearance and the enamel shearing off the underlying dentine leading to rapid wear (Figure 5). The crowns are bulbous and have a pronounced cervical constriction. The roots are short and rounded, and the pulp chambers may become rapidly obliterated. The three types of dentinogenesis imperfecta can be differentiated:

Type I: Associated with osteogenesis imperfecta types IB, IIIB, or IVB. Also associated with Ehlers-Danlos syndrome type II, Goldblatt's syndrome, Schimke immuno-osseous dysplasia, and skeletal dysplasia.[21] Typically the primary teeth are affected more severely than the permanent teeth.

Type II: "Classic" dentinogenesis imperfecta sometimes referred to as hereditary opalescent

Table 2 Disorders of Tooth Shape and Size	
Disorder	Comments
Dilaceration	A bend in the root or crown of a tooth. Usually affects the permanent incisors. Arises as a consequence of childhood trauma to teeth.
Connation (double teeth)	Teeth joined together. More common in the deciduous than in permanent dentition. May represent fusion or partial development (germination) of teeth.
Macrodontia	Abnormally enlarged teeth. Uncommon but usually affects all of the dentition.
Microdontia	Abnormally small teeth. Uncommon.
Taurodontism	Not a true defect of tooth shape. A radiologic feature characterized by an enlarged pulp chamber, long crown, and short roots.
Prominent tubercles or cusps	A variety of defects may occur.
Enamel cleft	Small cleft in the enamel crown in the cervical region.

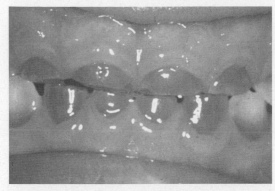

Figure 5 Dentinogenesis imperfecta—note the discoloration and excess wear (attrition) of the teeth.

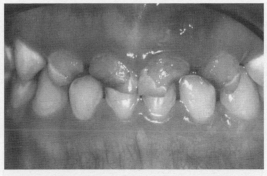

Figure 6 Dental decay (caries). Early decay causes decalcification (white patches), while later disease causes tooth tissue loss.

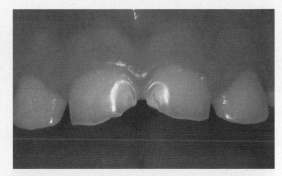

Figure 7 Erosion of the smooth surfaces of teeth.

dentine. This can be distinguished from type I by the fact that both primary and permanent teeth are affected with equal severity.

Type III: Sometimes termed the Brandywine variant (after the residents of an area of southern Maryland, in whom it was first observed). This is clinically similar to types I and II, but there are also "shell teeth," characterized by an abnormally large pulp chamber.

ACQUIRED DISORDERS OF TOOTH STRUCTURE

Dental Caries (Decay) and Sequelae

Dental caries is probably the most common of all human diseases and is caused by the demineralization of the dental hard tissues by metabolic acids of the dental plaque biofilm.[22] There is constant ionic exchange between the plaque biofilm and the tooth surface; dental caries occurs if this equilibrium is disturbed. This may be due to changes in available carbohydrates, the microbial composition of the plaque biofilm, or other factors such as the ability of the saliva to act as a pH buffer. Of greatest clinical significance, dietary sucrose is the most likely underlying cause of caries. There has been a decline in carious experience among the children of industrialized nations since the 1960s; however, it is now largely concentrated in children from deprived backgrounds.[23]

Caries initially manifests as areas of white decalcification of the enamel, with later destruction of the enamel and dentine (Figure 6). Early decay is asymptomatic, although later disease, when there is involvement of the dentine, gives rise to short-term localized pain in response to hot, cold, and sweet foods. Unchecked decay eventually results in severe pulpal inflammation and death, and possibly inflammation of the apical areas of the periodontium (periapical periodontitis).

Periapical periodontitis will give rise to local long-standing pain, usually in response to hot and cold foods and particularly with occlusal pressure. The affected tooth may be slightly elevated, and there may be formation of a sinus that drains from the gingivae at the level of the apex of the tooth. Periapical infection can give rise to periapical abscess formation ("gum boil") and cellulitis, the latter occasionally causing pyrexia and

malaise, as well as facial swelling. Other possible sequelae of a periapical abscess include periapical (radicular) cyst formation or, rarely, discharge of a sinus onto the skin. Rarely the cellulitis can be so severe as to compromise the airway, and infection may even give rise to necrotizing fasciitis.

Dental caries is typically due to a diet high in fermentable carbohydrates and tends to occur in the fissures of premolars and molars, although it can arise interdentally between any tooth. In addition, xerostomia owing to salivary gland disease or local radiotherapy greatly increases the risk of caries development. Caries in under 5-year olds is classified as early childhood caries (ECC) and is characterized by poor feeding practices (including use of a bottle containing sugary drinks or sweetened milk or soy-based milk preparations high in carbohydrate) and rapid disease progression, teeth appearing to break down upon eruption. Bovine milk will not cause caries. Prolonged (over the age of 1 year) on demand breastfeeding has been associated with caries development, however, this is controversial.[24]

TOOTH SURFACE LOSS

Generalized loss of tooth surface may be due to attrition, abrasion, erosion, or some combination of these.

Dental Erosion

Dental erosion is the consequence of acids of nonbacterial origin destroying the enamel. It is commonly associated with excessive consumption of low-pH beverages but is also associated with any condition where chronic vomiting or reflux may occur. This will include gastro-esophageal reflux disease (GORD),[25] bulimia, or anorexia nervosa. Other conditions that may predispose to erosion include use of acidic medicaments (acetylsalicylic acid, ascorbic acid, liquid hydrochloric acid, iron tonics, and acidic saliva stimulants/substitutes) and individuals on a lactovegetarian diet where the combined effect of associated hyposalivation, high consumption of low-pH foodstuffs, and the abrasive effect of the coarse fresh food can promote erosion.[26]

Dental erosion is increasingly common, especially in the developed world. Depending on the method of classification, teeth examined,

and city of study, 11.6 to 48% of examined 12- to 14-year-old children may have some degree of dental erosion.[27]

Almost any tooth surface can be affected, but, typically, the palatal aspects of the upper anterior teeth become thinned and smooth (Figure 7). Management of erosion begins with elimination of the causative agent, though this may be difficult (eg, GORD). Teeth can then be restored as required to improve esthetics and function as required.

Attrition and Abrasion

Attrition is the loss of dental hard tissues as a consequence of mastication. Attrition is a normal feature of the late deciduous dentition and is particularly noticeable on the incisors and canines. Severe attrition of the permanent dentition in childhood is uncommon but may arise with severe malocclusion and may be a feature of Rett syndrome.[28]

Abrasion is the loss of dental hard tissues owing to frictional damage by foreign hard substances, typically a toothbrush. It is uncommon in children. Abrasion typically gives rise to concavities within the dentine (and to a lesser extent the enamel) of the cervical margins of teeth.

DEVELOPMENTAL DENTAL DEFECTS

Genetic causes of enamel defects have been previously detailed; however, there are environmental insults that can disturb the development of enamel to produce a similar outcome. Possibly the most well known of these is fluorosis.

Fluorosis

Excess fluoride intake, either as a consequence of drinking water with a naturally high-fluoride concentration or following excess ingestion of fluoride supplements (eg, in toothpaste or fluoride tablets), will cause a mineralization defect of enamel if taken during enamel development. Mild fluorosis presents as chalky white patches of the enamel of otherwise normal teeth; more severe disease manifests with intrinsic brown staining of the enamel; and severe fluorosis gives rise to brown pitting, mottling, and brittleness of the enamel (Figure 8). As expected, the enamel associated with fluorosis is less liable to dental caries than normal enamel, although in severe fluorosis, the pitting and mottling can lead to

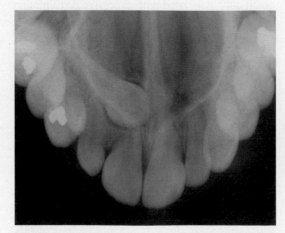

Figure 8 Gross fluorosis of the teeth.

unusual patterns of dental decay, for example, on the smooth surfaces of teeth which can present as a papery white appearance of the tooth if mild, through to severe hypoplasia.[29] Fluorosis most commonly affects the permanent dentition; although in areas where there is endemic fluorosis, the deciduous teeth will also be affected.

Other Developmental Defects

A variety of other developmental defects of teeth can arise, depending on the features of which the nature of the insult. Transient insults can give rise to a line in the crown enamel corresponding to the chronology of the insults. Alternatively, if the insult is more prolonged, then there may be generalized enamel defects (as seen in low-birth-weight children), inadequate root formation, or even agenesis of the tooth. A specific clinical entity has recently been observed hypoplasia of the first permanent molar teeth with or without discoloration of the molar incisor hypomineralisation (MIH). The etiology of MIH is not fully understood, but it is thought to be some unspecified environmental insult (eg, viral infection) in the first year of life.[30]

DISORDERS OF ERUPTION/ EXFOLIATION

Disorders of eruption or exfoliation (tooth loss) encompass early or late eruption/exfoliation of primary or permanent teeth and also anomalies of position (Table 2).[31] Diagnosis may be difficult due to a variation in eruption times, particularly in the primary dentition.

Early Eruption

Conditions that may be associated with generalized early eruption of teeth include hyperpituitarism and other endocrine disorders, Proteus syndrome, and Soto's syndrome. In newborn children, natal or neonatal teeth sometimes occur. These are primary teeth in 90% of cases and should be left. The 10% of cases that are supplemental/supernumerary teeth are often mobile and are usually removed.

Early Exfoliation

Early loss of primary teeth is associated with periodontal disease in the infant or child. This is

Table 3 Defects of Dental Eruption
Neonatal teeth
Ellis-van Creveld syndrome
Hallerman-Streiff syndrome
Pachyonychia congenita
Premature eruption
Precocious puberty
Hyperthyroidism
Hemifacial hypertrophy
Sotos syndrome
Sturge-Weber syndrome
Delayed eruption
Local causes
Hyperdontia
Small skeletal base
Ankylosis of deciduous teeth
Systemic causes
Albright hereditary osteodystrophy
Cleidocranial dysplasia
Down syndrome
Hypothyroidism
Hypopituitarism
Gardner syndrome
Goltz syndrome
Incontinentia pigmenti

usually part of a more serious systemic condition such as Papillon-Lefevre syndrome (due to a deficiency of cathepsin C) or congential neutropenias. Other metabolic conditions that may cause early exfoliation include hypophosphatasia or acrodynia (mercury poisoning).[32]

Delayed Eruption

As with early eruption, a generalized delay in eruption may be caused by endocrine disorders, in this case disorders such as hypothyroidism. Local causes of delayed eruption might be supernumerary tooth, dilacerated root, or impactions (Figure 9).

Delayed Exfoliation

Generalized delay of exfoliation of primary teeth is uncommon, and it can be seen in hereditary gingivofibromatosis or where there are no permanent teeth. Localized delays in exfoliation may be a result of ankylosis.

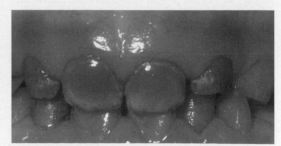

Figure 9 Delayed eruption of an upper permanent canine—there is no obvious cause for this.

Table 4 Abnormal Tooth Color
Extrinsic discoloration
Food stuffs
Drugs (eg, chlorhexidine)
Poor plaque control
Intrinsic discoloration
Caries
Trauma
Restorative materials
Internal resorption
Fluorosis
Tetracyclines
Congenital disorders of dentine and enamel structure
Erythropoietic porphyria
Severe neonatal (or early childhood) jaundice

DENTAL DISCOLORATION AND STAINING

The teeth can be extrinsically or, more rarely, intrinsically stained (Table 4).

Most discoloration of teeth in childhood is due to dental caries. Enamel decalcified by dental decay can become stained with foodstuffs, and caries that arrests takes on a black appearance. Teeth that become nonvital, typically owing to trauma, may take on a darkened color because of the pigments associated with pulpal necrosis, whereas internal resorption of the dentine can produce pink spots on the crowns of affected teeth.[3]

Systemic tetracycline therapy in the years of crown development can give rise to gray, yellow, or brown pigmentation of the teeth. The degree and color of tooth discoloration will depend upon the dose, duration, and type of tetracycline prescribed. Fluorosis causes variable degrees of tooth discoloration, which have already been described. Other, albeit uncommon, causes of intrinsic pigmentation of the teeth include congenital erythropoietic porphyria (Figure 10),[33] hemolytic disease of the newborn, and hyperbilirubinemia owing to rare disease such as biliary atresia. Chlorhexidine gluconate mouthrinse and gel cause brown extrinsic staining of the teeth. The stain can be easily removed by professional dental cleaning and can be prevented by application of chlorhexidine immediately following regular tooth cleaning, because the chlorhexidine stains the pellicle that forms on teeth within a few minutes after tooth cleaning.[34]

Figure 10 Intrinsic staining of the primary dentition secondary to porphyria.

GINGIVAL AND PERIODONTAL DISEASE IN CHILDHOOD

Most gingival disease in childhood is plaque-related gingival inflammation (gingivitis); however, a wide range of congenital disorders can give rise to gingival and periodontal manifestations. Gingival and periodontal disease in childhood most commonly manifests as swelling (Table 5), accelerated periodontal destruction (Table 6), and/or ulceration (Table 7).

Non-specific Gingivitis

Acute. Acute non-specific gingivitis is due to inflammation secondary to local accumulation of plaque. Signs of acute gingivitis develop within 7 to 10 days of plaque accumulation and initially arise on the interdental papillae before spreading to the adjacent free gingival margins. Rarely, there may be involvement of the attached gingivae. Acute gingivitis initially manifests as redness and swell-

Table 5 Causes of Gingival Swelling in Childhood

Local causes of generalized enlargement
  Chronic gingivitis
  Hyperplastic gingivitis owing to mouth breathing

Local causes of localized enlargement
  Abscesses
  Fibrous epulides
  Exostoses
  Eruption cysts

Systemic causes of generalized enlargement
  Congenital disease
    Hereditary gingival fibromatosis
    Mucopolysaccharidoses
    Mucolipidoses
    Hypoplasminogenemia
    Lipoid proteinosis
    Infantile systemic hyalinosis
  Acquired disease
    Drugs
      Phenytoin
      Cyclosporine
      Amlodipine
      Diltiazem
      Felodipine
      Isradipine
      Lacidipine
      Lercanidipine
      Nicardipine
      Nifedipine
      Nimodipine
      Nisoldipine
      Verapamil
      Others
    Crohn's disease
    Leukemia (acute myeloid)
    Scurvy

Systemic causes of localized enlargement
  Heck disease
  Tuberous sclerosis
  Cowden disease
  Fibrous epulis
  Giant cell epulis
  Pyogenic granuloma
  Papilloma
  Crohn's disease, orofacial granulomatosis and
    related conditions
  Kaposi sarcoma and other (rare) neoplasms

Table 6 Systemic Causes of Enhanced Gingival/Periodontal Destruction

Primary immunodeficiencies
  Reduced neutrophil number
    Cyclic neutropenia
    Benign familial neutropenia
    Other primary neutropenias
  Defective neutrophil function
    Hyperimmunoglobulinemia E
    Kartagener syndrome
    Chronic granulomatous disease
    Chédiak-Higashi syndrome
    Acatalasia
    Leukocyte adhesion deficiency
    Actin dysfunction syndrome
  Other immunodeficiencies
    Fanconi anemia
    Down syndrome
    Severe combined immunodeficiency

Other congenital disorders
  Hypophosphatasia
  Ehlers-Danlos syndrome type III, IV and VIII
  Acro-osteolysis (Hajdu-Cheney syndrome)
  Type Ib glycogen storage disease
  Oxalosis
  Dyskeratosis benigna intraepithelialis mucosae et
    cutis hereditara
  Familial dysautonomia (Riley-Day syndrome)
  Papillon-Lefèvre syndrome
  Haim-Munk syndrome

Secondary immunodeficiencies
  Malnutrition
  Diabetes mellitus
  Crohn disease
  HIV disease

Other acquired causes
  Vitamin C deficiency

Table 7 Causes of Gingival and Oral Mucosal Ulceration in Childhood

Trauma (physical, chemical, radiation, thermal)

Aphthae and associated syndromes
  Recurrent aphthous stomatitis
  Behçet disease
  Others

Infections
  Primary or recurrent herpes simplex virus infection
  Varicella-zoster virus
  Epstein-Barr virus
  Cytomegalovirus
  Coxsackievirus
  Echovirus
  Acute necrotizing ulcerative gingivitis
  Treponema pallidum (may signify sexual abuse)
  Mycobacterium tuberculosis
  Gram-negative infections (rare)
  Atypical mycobacteria
  Chronic mucocutaneous candidiasis

Dermatoses
  Lichen planus
  Mucous membrane pemphigoid
  Pemphigus vulgaris
  Dermatitis herpetiformis
  Erythema multiforme
  Others

Hematologic disorders
  Neutropenia(s)
  Leukemia(s)
  Hematinic deficiencies
  Others

Gastrointestinal disorders
  Crohn disease and related disorders
  Ulcerative colitis

Drugs
  Cytotoxics and others

Malignancy
  Rare (eg, Kaposi sarcoma, non-Hodgkin lymphoma
    [in HIV disease])

Other
  Lipoid proteinosis
  Hypoplasminogenemia

ing of the affected gingivae; later there is gingival bleeding that may arise with tooth cleaning and eventually will occur during eating (Figure 11). Patients with severe acute gingivitis may have oral malodor and complain of dysgeusia (bad taste) and awaking from sleep to find blood on the pillow owing to drooling of bloody saliva. Unlike acute necrotizing ulcerative gingivitis (ANUG), there is no tissue destruction.[35–39]

Chronic. Chronic non-specific gingivitis arises as a sequela to long-standing mild acute gingivitis. The gingivae become variably enlarged and fibrous, and there is often some associated acute gingivitis.

Management of Non-specific Gingivitis. Improvement in oral hygiene is the mainstay of treatment of both acute and chronic non-specific gingivitis. Surgical reduction of any hyperplastic tissue (eg, by gingivectomy) may be required for the treatment of long-standing chronic gingivitis, but this is rarely undertaken in children.

Acute Necrotizing Ulcerative Gingivitis: Acute Ulcerative Gingivitis, Vincent Gingivitis

Acute necrotizing ulcerative gingivitis (ANUG) is a common disorder of adulthood but can arise in children, particularly those who are malnourished

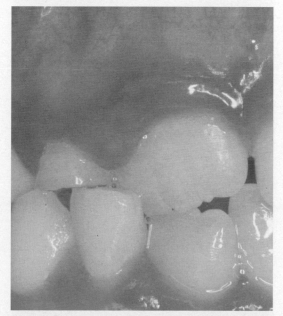

Figure 11 Acute gingitivitis—always due to poor removal of plaque.

or immunocompromised, for example, with human immunodeficiency virus (HIV) disease.[40] ANUG is characterized by notable, painful, necrotic gingival ulceration and edema with bleeding and malodor (Figure 12). The ulceration typically commences interdentally but, in severe disease, may extend to cause ulceration of all marginal areas. The tissue destruction results in irreversible flattening of the interdental papillae. Involvement can be localized or generalized.[39]

Patients may complain of an abnormal, sometimes metallic taste (dysgeusia), and oral malodor. Periodontal destruction is rare, although in severe malnourishment, an ANUG-like disorder (termed noma) can cause ulceration and destruction of the periodontium and adjacent tissues and sometimes perforation of the facial tissues, fistula formation, and eventual orofacial disfigurement.[41] In severe ANUG, there may be cervical lymphadenopathy, pyrexia, and, rarely, malaise.

Poor oral hygiene is the most common cause of ANUG, although viral lymphopenia (particularly upper respiratory virus infections) and, less commonly, immunodeficiency associated with undiagnosed or poorly controlled diabetes mellitus, leukemia, HIV disease, profound malnutrition, and other severe immunocompromised states can be contributing etiologic factors.

There is unlikely to be a specific causative micoorganism, but ANUG is typically associated with *Borrelia vincentii*, fusiform bacteria, *Treponema denticola*, and other gingival spirochetes.[39]

For the management of ANUG, oral hygiene must be improved. Where possible, supragingival deposits and tissue debris should be removed immediately, but subgingival cleaning may be possible until there has been some resolution of the acute disease. Chlorhexidine gel and/or sodium perborate mouthrinses may be helpful, although significant evidence that these topical

agents are effective is lacking. Systemic oral metronidazole or phenoxymethylpenicillin is indicated when the disease is severe and/or there is lymphadenopathy or pyrexia. Appropriate referral (eg, to endocrinology or infectious diseases specialists) may also be warranted.[36–37]

Hereditary Gingival Fibromatosis

Hereditary gingival fibromatosis is usually inherited as an autosomal dominant or recessive disorder (the genetic defects lying on chromosomes 2 and 5), although sporadic disease can occur.[42–43] There is fibrous enlargement affecting many or all gingivae, particularly the free gingiva about the smooth surfaces of the teeth. The disease manifests in early childhood, sometimes causing delayed or partial eruption of teeth, median diastema (spacing of the upper permanent incisors), malocclusion, and prolonged retention of the primary teeth. Syndromic gingival fibromatosis can be a feature of a spectrum of rare syndromes that usually includes deafness, learning disability, and hypertrichosis. Similar gingival enlargement may be seen in a number of rare conditions (see Table 5).

Surgical reduction by gingivectomy or gingivoplasty is usually required to improve esthetics and permit better oral hygiene maintenance. Surgery is more effective postpuberty, when recurrence is unlikely.[39]

Other Congenital Causes of Gingival Enlargement

Sturge-Weber syndrome, can give rise to hemangioma of the gingiva, usually the maxillary gingiva of one side. There is usually an extensive orofacial hemangioma that roughly follows the distribution of one or more of the divisions of the trigeminal nerve and extends into the parietal and occipital lobes of the brain. The maxillary gingivae are often involved, the affected tissue being enlarged, boggy, and purple or blue colored, often covering the crowns of several teeth. The eruption and form of the involved teeth are variably affected. Because epilepsy is a common accompaniment, there may also be phenytoin-induced gingival enlargement. Sturge-Weber syndrome may also include epilepsy, learning disability, hemiplegia, and glaucoma.[44–45]

Tuberous sclerosis may give rise to multiple fibrous enlargements of the gingivae,[46] whereas neurofibromatosis (usually type 1) may give rise to variable numbers of gingival neurofibromas (as well as occasional pigmentation).[43,47] Cowden disease causes multiple gingival fibrous swellings.[48–49]

Other Acquired Causes of Gingival Enlargement

Orofacial Granulomatosis. Orofacial granulomatosis and Crohn disease in childhood may give rise to localized or generalized gingival enlargement. The swelling is diffuse and salmon pink in color, often with a granular surface, and affects the free and attached gingivae. The other oral manifestations of orofacial granulomatosis are discussed later.

Drug-Induced Gingival Enlargement. Gingival enlargement commonly arises with long-term phenytoin, cyclosporin, and calcium channel blockers.[39] The gingival enlargement usually commences interdentally and affects both the labial and the lingual/palatal aspects. The enlargement is most likely in patients who do not maintain good plaque control and in those receiving high-dose regimens. The enlargement associated with phenytoin is fibrous in quality, whereas that associated with cyclosporin and calcium channel blockers is softer and more erythematous. Surgical reduction followed by the maintenance of good plaque control is the mainstay of treatment of drug-induced gingival enlargement.

Periodontal Disease in Childhood

Periodontitis—loss of periodontal attachment—is uncommon in childhood but when present is usually associated with poor plaque control. Periodontitis manifests as increased tooth mobility and migration, and is usually accompanied by features of acute and/or chronic gingivitis. Some loss of alveolar bone may be observed radiographically.

Aggressive periodontitis—periodontal destruction in excess of that expected irrespective of the levels of plaque—is likewise uncommon in childhood (Figure 13) and usually reflects an underlying primary defect of phagocyte number or function, deficiency of cathepsin C (as in Papillon-Lefevre syndrome),[50] a structural defect of cementum (eg, hypophosphatasia) or connective tissue of the periodontium (eg, some types of Ehlers-Danlos syndrome), or HIV disease (see Table 6).[39]

The management of periodontitis of childhood is principally directed toward reducing the infection with *Aggregatibacter actinomycetemcomitans* and other periodontopathic bacteria by thorough subgingival mechanical cleaning, subgingival antimicrobial agents, intermittent use of systemic tetracyclines (typically doxycycline), and, when indicated, periodontal surgery, and perhaps orthodontic movement of malaligned teeth.

ORAL MUCOSAL DISEASE IN CHILDHOOD

Oral mucosal disease in childhood principally encompasses lesions that manifest as ulcers, white or red patches, or pigmentation.[3]

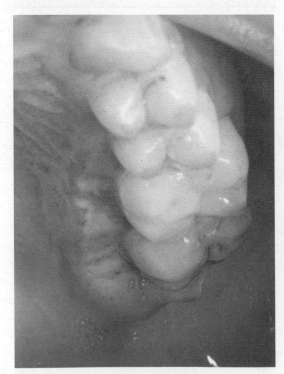

Figure 12 Acute necrotizing ulcerative gingivitis.

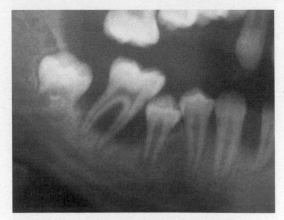

Figure 13 Aggressive periodontitis in childhood.

Oral Mucosal Ulceration in Childhood

The causes of oral and gingival ulceration in childhood are summarized in Table 7.

Traumatic Ulceration

Traumatic ulceration in childhood tends to be due to physical trauma, for example, injury from a toothbrush or orthodontic appliance, or accidents in the home or during play (Figure 14). The ulcers are usually solitary, arise at the site of trauma, and heal within about a week of removal of the cause. Traumatic ulceration of the gingivae, lips, or labial frena may be suggestive of physical abuse, particularly when accompanied by facial bruising, laceration, and bite marks.[3,51–53]

Radiotherapy to the mouth or chemotherapy can give rise to oral mucositis.[54] The mucosa becomes red, painful, necrotic, and ulcerated. The cause of mucositis remains unclear; it may simply reflect damage to the basal cells of the epithelium or infection with Gram-negative bacteria.[54–55] The use of ice pops during radiotherapy or chemotherapy may lessen the severity of the ulceration, as may good plaque control.[54] Combinations of topical antifungal-antibacterial regimens (eg, polymyxin, tobramycin, amphotericin) would seem to be of limited benefit in the treatment of oral mucositis.[56–57] A recent systematic review did not determine an effective therapy of oral mucositis secondary to radiotherapy or chemotherapy, although pain relief with opioids and avoidance of mucosal irritation (eg, by regular, careful tooth cleaning) seem to be cardinal.[58] Recently intravenous keratinocyte growth factor (KGF) has been found to be an effective means of lessening chemotherapy-associated mucositis.[59]

Infectious Causes of Mouth Ulcers in Childhood

Viral infections most commonly cause mouth ulcers in childhood. Details of these and other possible infections giving rise to oral mucosal ulceration are summarized in Table 7.

Recurrent Aphthous Stomatitis

The most common form of non-traumatic ulceration affecting the oral mucosa is recurrent aphthous stomatitis (RAS).[60–62] This condition is characterized by the presence of one or more oral ulcers, which heal within days or sometimes in weeks, only to reappear at regular intervals. The associated constitutional effects may vary from minor discomfort from the ulcers themselves to, more rarely, a severely incapacitating illness caused by persistent oral ulceration. The overall prevalence of the condition is 20 to 30%, and it has been estimated that 30% of affected individuals have their first attack of ulceration by the age of 14, with 10% having ulcers before the age of 10. An associated family history has been demonstrated in 24 to 46% of cases, with a very high incidence in patients whose both parents suffered from the condition.[62] Furthermore, in a study carried out on twins, a 90% concordance between identical twins was found, in contrast to a 57% concordance between nonidentical twins.[63]

RAS may be subdivided into three distinct groups, largely on the basis of the clinical appearance and history of the individual lesions. All three types of RAS may be seen in children and are referred to as minor aphthous ulceration, major aphthous ulceration, and herpetiform ulceration.

Minor aphthous ulcers account for 80% of the total and are most common in patients between 10 and 40 years of age.[62] Ulcers of this type characteristically affect the nonkeratinized oral mucosa of the lips, cheeks, vestibule, and margins of the tongue (Figure 15). The hard palate, gingivae, and dorsum of the tongue are typically unaffected. The appearance of a painful ulcer is frequently preceded by a prodromal phase of 1 to 3 days, during which the patient may complain of a burning or pricking sensation accompanied by a degree of paresthesia at the site of future ulceration. The ulcers, which may occur alone or in crops of three or four during a single episode, usually last between 10 and 14 days but reach a maximum size at 4 to 5 days. Healing is complete, with no residual scarring, but recurrent episodes of ulceration tend to occur regularly at 1- to 4-month intervals. Individual ulcers are shallow, surrounded by an area of reddened mucosa, and vary in shape depending on the site.[64]

In major aphthous ulceration, the ulcers are much larger and more longer lasting than those seen in minor aphthous ulceration. They may appear singly or up to three or four at a time, are very painful, and give rise to extensive tissue destruction. Both keratinized and nonkeratinized oral mucosa may be affected, including the dorsum of the tongue and the oropharynx. Herpetiform ulcers occur with a frequency similar to that of major aphthous ulcers and may also affect the keratinized and non-keratinized oral mucosa, typically floor of the mouth, lateral borders, and ventral surface of the tongue.[62,64] At the outset of an episode of ulceration, numerous discrete ulcers, approximately 1 to 2 mm in diameter, appear. These may later coalesce to form a single, large, painful lesion with a serpiginous outline. The ulcers usually heal within 10 days without mucosal scarring, although recurrent episodes of ulceration may supervene within days. Repeated attacks of this type may give rise to severe dysphagia.

There are no distinguishing histopathologic features. Microscopy reveals an appearance similar to that seen in cases of traumatic ulceration of the oral mucosa.[64] The epithelium shows no diagnostic features, and the underlying connective tissue is infiltrated with inflammatory cells, predominantly lymphocytes and plasma cells.

The precise etiology of RAS is not known. Although there are occasional family patterns of involvement, inheritance does not follow any Mendelian patterns, and no particular human leukocyte antigen (HLA) haplotype is associated with RAS.[62] An infectious etiology also seems unlikely because patients do not have a raised frequency of past or present herpetic infections and associations with *Helicobacter pylori* have not been proven.[65–70] There are tenuous associations between RAS and psychological stress, and no consistent pattern has been demonstrated between episodes of RAS and the menstrual cycle. No significant immunologic defects have been consistently detected in patients with RAS.[62]

Associations between RAS and gastrointestinal disease are tenuous. Certainly, a small number of patients with undiagnosed, or poorly managed, gluten-sensitive enteropathy (GSE) may have oral signs. Usually, up to 66% have superficial oral ulcers similar to those of RAS[71]; however, patients with RAS do not have a significantly increased likelihood of having clinical, serologic, or small bowel features of GSE, and the introduction of a gluten-free diet does not cause resolution of RAS.[72–79] Up to 20% of patients with RAS may have a hematinic deficiency, usually iron.[80] An underlying cause for these deficiencies is rarely found, and replacement therapy infrequently produces any cessation of RAS.[81–82]

A systematic review of the management of RAS is available (Table 8).[83] The investigation of patients with possible RAS should be focused on excluding other causes of acute bouts of ulceration (see Table 7), in particular the exclusion of an underlying hematologic or gastrointestinal disorder.[62]

All patients should be advised to use an oral hygiene procedure that is as atraumatic as

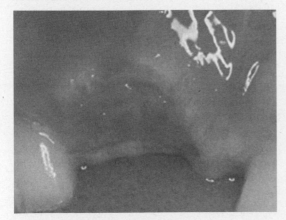

Figure 14 Traumatic ulceration.

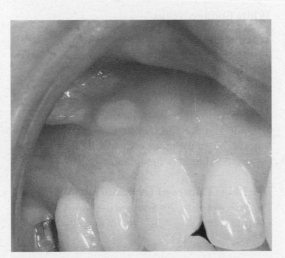

Figure 15 Minor type recurrent aphthous stomatitis.

Table 8   Treatment of Recurrent Aphthous Stomatitis

Antimicrobial
    Chlorhexidine gluconate mouthrinse

Analgesia
    Benzydamine hydrochloride mouthrinse/spray
        (provides symptomatic relief)

Topical corticosteroids
    Triamcinolone acetonide (0.1%) in Orabase
    Betamethasone mouthrinse
    Flucinonide cream/ointment
    Fluticasone cream/spray/inhaler

Systemic therapies
    Systemic corticosteroids
    Corticosteroid-sparing agents

possible, and all dental appliances should fit well and not damage tissue. The correction of any hematinic deficiency is of limited benefit unless the cause is corrected.[82] Topical corticosteroids remain the mainstay of RAS treatment in most countries, although there are few well-controlled studies of their precise efficacy.[83] A wide range of different topical corticosteroids may reduce symptoms.

Benzydamine hydrochloride mouthwash is of no more benefit on ulcer healing than placebo[84]; nevertheless, it (or lidocaine gel) can produce transient relief of pain.

Chlorhexidine used as a 0.2% w/w mouthrinse or 1% gel can reduce the duration of ulcers and increase the number of ulcer-free days.[85–88] Topical tetracyclines (eg, chlortetracycline, tetracycline) may reduce healing times and/or reduce the associated pain of RAS,[89–92] but they may cause dysgeusia, oral candidiasis, and a burning-like sensation of the pharynx and are not suitable for young children, who might ingest them, with resultant tooth staining.

A variety of other topical agents have been suggested to be of some benefit in the management of RAS, but the supportive data are quite sparse. There have been several studies of the efficacy of amlexanox in the management of RAS, including randomized controlled trials, suggesting that the 5% paste may significantly reduce the pain and time of healing of ulceration of RAS.[93–96]

Systemic immunosuppression is rarely warranted in view of the limited efficacy of topical agents and the sometimes profound pain and/or long-standing ulceration. However, although a variety of such agents have been proposed to be clinically useful, there is little supportive evidence.[97]

Thalidomide remains the most effective agent for the management of RAS, producing a remission in almost 50% of treated patients in one randomized controlled trial.[98] Open and double-blind studies of patients with HIV-related oral ulceration and in non–HIV-related RAS and several case studies confirm that thalidomide is of some clinical benefit.[98–106] Thalidomide gives rise to mild adverse side effects (particularly somnolence) in up to 75% of treated patients, and polyneuropathy can arise in about 5%. Clearly, the risk of terato-genicity also limits clinical application of thalidomide in the sexually active adolescents.

Periodic Fever, Aphthous Ulceration, Pharyngitis, and Adenitis (PFAPA).   This is an uncommon disorder of children characterized by fever, pharyngitis, aphthous-like ulceration, and cervical lymphadenopathy. The clinical features last under a week and can be recurrent, the recurrences occurring over variable times of weeks to months. PFAPA seems to arise in early childhood (usually about 2 years of age). The long-term behavior of PFAPA is not known. The etiology is unknown, although interestingly tonsillectomy may cause remission of PFAPA. Cimetidine has been suggested as a possible therapy, although tonsillectomy or systemic corticosteroids seem to cause resolution of episodes of illness.[107–108]

Behcet's Disease

Behcet's disease is clinically characterized by recurrent oral and genital ulceration together with a spectrum of cutaneous, ocular, neurologic, and other systemic manifestations (including gastrointestinal). Although very uncommon in childhood, almost all affected children will have RAS-like oral ulceration.[109–110] The ulcers are clinically and histologically indistinguishable from those seen in RAS, and all three types of RAS may be seen in this closely related condition. The local management of oral ulceration in this condition is similar to that for RAS; however, as with adults, systemic therapies, including thalidomide, may be required.[109]

White Patches of the Oral Mucosa in Childhood

The causes of white patches of the oral mucosa in childhood reflect a wide spectrum of possible pathologies (Table 9).[111] In general, it is possible to consider white patches as being adherent and nonadherent, solitary and multiple. Common causes of oral white patches in children include materia alba (food debris) and acute pseudomembranous candidiasis, although a variety of other disorders can manifest as white lesions of the mouth.

White Sponge Nevus

White sponge nevus (Cannon's disease) is a rare autosomal dominant disorder of genes coding mucosal-specific keratins K4 and K13[112] of otherwise well children and adults. It gives rise to bilateral adherent white or gray thickened patches. Similar lesions may occur on the nasal, anal, or vaginal mucosa. It is generally asymptomatic but may require histopathologic examination to exclude lichen planus.[113]

Infectious Causes of Oral Mucosal White Patches—Acute Pseudomembranous Candidiasis

The most common fungal infections seen in the oral cavity in children are caused by *Candida*

Table 9   Oral Mucosal White Patches in Childhood

Nonadherent
    Pseudomembranous candidosis (thrush)
    Other mycoses
    Food debris
    Furred tongue
    Drug-associated necrotic debris (eg, aspirin, cocaine)

Adherent
    Solitary
        Papillomas (warts—these are rarely of sexual origin)
        White sponge nevus
        Geographic tongue (erythema migrans—red and white lesions
        Oral (idiopathic) leukoplakia
        Frictional keratosis (eg, cheek biting)
        Keratosis owing to smokeless tobacco
        Carcinoma (very rare)
    Multiple
        Traumatic keratosis
        Lichen planus
        Oral hairy leukoplakia
        Chronic mucocutaneous candidiasis
        Others

albicans, which is commensal in the mouths of up to 70% of the general population.[114] Candidiasis may present in a variety of clinical forms but is, in all cases, an opportunistic infection caused by a change in the local or systemic host response. Although *C. albicans* remains the most common fungal commensal of the mouth, there is arising frequency of non-albicans Candida species in the oral cavity, particularly in patients with HIV disease or poorly controlled diabetes mellitus or those receiving iatrogenic immunosuppression. In addition, these patient groups may be liable to carry and transmit azole-resistant fungal infections.[114–116]

Acute pseudomembranous candidiasis (thrush) may occur in the newborn but more typically occurs in children receiving broad-spectrum antibiotics or systemic corticosteroids or in those with some primary or secondary immunodeficiency states (eg, HIV disease). Children receiving corticosteroid inhalers (eg, for asthma) may be particularly liable to thrush. Rarely it may be a feature of undiagnosed or poorly controlled diabetes mellitus.[117] It manifests clinically as asymptomatic soft, creamy-yellow areas raised above the surrounding mucosa, which leave a red-bleeding surface when wiped off. The lesions may be multiple or a confluent mass and may affect all mucosal surfaces, particularly the soft and hard palate, tongue, and vestibule.

Diagnosis is usually based on the clinical picture and history, although, rarely, it can be confirmed by taking a smear of the material; a Gram or periodic acid–Schiff stain of the preparation reveals the typical branching hyphae of Candida. Depending upon the severity and the underlying cause of the candidiasis, topical and/or systemic antifungal agents may be required, although the principal aim of management must be to find the underlying cause.[114]

Chronic Mucocutaneous Candidiasis

Chronic mucocutaneous candidiasis (CMC) is a group of rare immunodeficiencies characterized clinically by recurrent and/or persistent candidal infection of the skin and mucosae. At least four types of CMC have been described: diffuse CMC, sporadic CMC, candidiasis endocrinopathy syndrome, and late-onset CMC. Children with CMC can have widespread and/or recurrent oral pseudomembranous candidiasis, angular cheilitis, and chronic hyperplastic candidiasis. Children with hypoparathyroidism as part of candidiasis endocrinopathy syndrome may have enamel hypoplasia.[118–119]

Antifungal therapy is often difficult in CMC in view of the potential for the azole resistance of Candida to develop. Detailed discussions of CMC can be found elsewhere.[118–119]

Other Types of Candidal Infection—Acute Atrophic Candidiasis

Acute atrophic candidiasis is very occasionally seen in children and is the result of candidal overgrowth in patients being treated with broad-spectrum antibiotics or with immunosuppressive drugs. The mucosa is typically sore, inflamed, and sensitive to hot and spicy foods. Therapy with topical nystatin (eg, pastilles) or amphotericin may be warranted, but signs and symptoms usually resolve on cessation of the causative treatment.[113]

Chronic Atrophic Candidiasis

Chronic atrophic candidiasis, which has also been termed denture-associated candidiasis, is characterized by a red, inflamed mucosa and is precisely limited to the area covered by a well-fitting (usually upper) denture. The condition is often seen in children who are wearing a removable orthodontic appliance, the area of inflammation being confined to the mucosa covered by the acrylic base plate. The acrylic of the appliance has a biofilm that contains *C. albicans* and oral bacteria, the fungal content of which causes the inflammation.[120] Diagnosis is usually easily made from the clinical picture. Microbial culture for fungal infection is not warranted unless the child is immunocompromised, when non-albicans candida species may be present. Treatment usually simply requires improving the hygiene of the appliance together with the application of antifungal gel (eg, miconazole) to the fitting surface of the appliance, as well as the administration of topical nystatin or amphotericin; systemic antifungal agents are rarely warranted.[114]

Angular Cheilitis

Angular cheilitis (stomatitis) presents as reddened folds at the corners of the mouth. Occasionally, there is ulceration. The lesions are usually colonized by *C. albicans* and/or *Staphylococcus aureus*. Although most commonly associated with a reduction in vertical face height in adult denture wearers, angular cheilitis in children may reflect the presence of an iron deficiency, neutropenia, malnutrition, or cell-mediated immunodeficiency, particularly HIV disease. Angular (and median) cheilitis may accompany the labial enlargement of Crohn's disease and orofacial granulomatosis. The diagnosis is usually based on the clinical picture and history; microbiologic studies are usually neither warranted nor helpful. Miconazole gel is usually of some benefit in the treatment of angular cheilitis, although, of course, the underlying cause must be identified and corrected.[114]

Oral Hairy Leukoplakia

Oral hairy leukoplakia manifests as an adherent asymptomatic bilateral white patch on the lateral borders and dorsum of the tongue and sometimes the floor of the mouth. Caused by Epstein-Barr virus, this lesion almost always arises in immunosuppressed patients, typically those with HIV disease and individuals receiving long-term corticosteroids (including inhalers) or other immunosuppressants. Although caused by Epstein-Barr virus, it does not warrant any anti-herpes intervention. The signs often wax and wane and may resolve if the immunosuppression lessens. This lesion is not potentially malignant.[121–122]

Human Papillomavirus Infection

Human papillomavirus manifests as warts or cauliflowerlike white squamous papillomas. The lips, palate, and gums are the most commonly affected sites. The lesions are usually solitary and small, although in immunocompromised children (eg, those with HIV disease and iatrogenic immunosuppression), they can be multiple.[126] Heck's disease (multifocal epithelial hyperplasia) is due to HPV 13 and 32 and presents as multiple white papular lesions, this usually arising in children and adults of Inuit Indian origin.[127] Most human papillomavirus infection of the mouth in children is not sexually associated. The lesions can be removed surgically or with cryotherapy, although topical interferon-α may be an alternative therapy.[128] To date there remain few reports of the efficacy of imiquimod for the treatment of oral HPV infection.

DYSKERATOSIS CONGENITA

Dyskeratosis congenita is an uncommon congenital disorder characterized by the development of adherent white patches of the oral mucosa, cutaneous hyperpigmentation, nail dystrophy, and gradual aplasia of the bone marrow. X-linked recessive, autosomal dominant, and autosomal recessive forms of dyskeratosis congenita occur. In X-linked disease, there is a mutation of *DKC1*, the protein of which (dyskerin) is part of the telomerase complex. There is resultant defective direct translation from internal ribosomal entry site (IRES) elements. The autosomal dominant form of DC is due to mutations of the gene for the RNA component of telomerase (TERC).[123, 124]

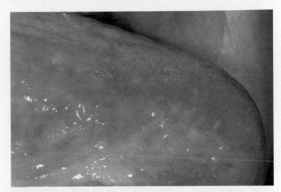

Figure 16 Oral lichen planus.

PACHYONYCHIA CONGENITA

Pachyonychia congenita is an uncommon congenital disorder in a rare genodermatosis keratin clinically characterized by hyperhydrosis, adherent white patches, follicular keratosis, and palmar keratodema. In DC-1 there are mutations in keratins K6a and K16 while in DC-2 there are mutations of K6b and K17. Other oral features of PC include early loss of the primary dentition and rarely the presence of natal teeth.[125]

LICHEN PLANUS

Oral lichen planus is common, affecting 1 to 2% of most populations. It typically arises in middle to late life and has a slight female predominance; nevertheless, disease can occasionally arise in children and young adults. Oral lichen planus gives rise to white patches that typically arise bilaterally on the buccal mucosa, dorsum of the tongue, and/or labial and buccal aspects of the gingival (Figure 16). The white lesions are generally asymptomatic, although patients occasionally report a roughness or dryness of the affected mucosal surfaces. Erosions and/or ulceration can arise within the white patches, giving rise to erosive and ulcerative lichen planus, respectively; these lesions can be notably painful, with symptoms being profound with hot, spicy, or citrus foods.[129–130]

Although lichen planus can be occasionally caused by drug therapy (eg, ß-blockers, sulfonylureas[131]), oral lichen planus in children tends to be idiopathic. Rarely, oral lichen planus will be a complication of chronic graft-versus-host disease.

Unlike most other white patches of the oral mucosa, lichen planus does not give rise to solitary lesions; however, it is often advantageous to confirm the clinical diagnosis by histopathologic examination of lesional tissue.

Oral lichen planus only warrants treatment when lesions are erosive, ulcerative, or bullous, when topical corticosteroids are the mainstays of therapy (see Table 8).[130–132] Based on data of adult patients, topical calcineurin inhibitors such as tacrolimus and pimecrolimus may be of benefit for the treatment of symptomatic oral lichen planus in children recalcitrant to topical corticosteroids.[133–135] Systemic immunosuppressive therapy is rarely warranted for the treatment of oral lichen planus in children or adults. The white lesions of oral lichen planus rarely resolve. It remains unclear if oral lichen planus has a malignant potential; however, in view of the related controversy,[136] careful lifelong clinical follow-up is advisable.

POTENTIALLY MALIGNANT AND MALIGNANT DISEASE OF THE MOUTH IN CHILDHOOD

Oral squamous cell carcinoma is the most common malignant disease of the mouth. Although rare in children, it can still arise and may manifest as a solitary white patch (leukoplakia), speckled area, or ulcer. Any adherent white patch that does not appear to be due to trauma should be examined histopathologically to exclude the, albeit rare, possibility of malignancy.[137]

ORAL MUCOSAL PIGMENTATION

Oral mucosal pigmentation in childhood is usually racial in origin, although a number of local and systemic disorders may give rise to various pigmented areas in the mouth.[3] Children may have localized nevi, which manifest as localized areas of hypermelanotic or blue pigmentation. Malignant melanoma or potentially malignant pigmentatory disorders is rare in the mouths of children[138]; however, when there is any doubt as to the cause of hypermelanotic lesions, histopathologic examination of lesional tissue should always be undertaken.

Amalgam tattoos are more common in adults but may arise in children, presenting as areas of blue macules or, less commonly, papules on the gingivae, floor of the mouth, or buccal mucosa. These lesions are harmless and asymptomatic.[139] Rarely they may warrant removal if unsightly (eg, if on the anterior gingivae).[140]

Kaposi sarcoma is the most common oral malignancy of HIV in childhood. It manifests as

Table 10 Oral Mucosal and Gingival Pigmentation in Childhood

Localized
  Amalgam tattoo
  Nevus
  Freckle (ephelis)
  Melanotic macules
  Kaposi sarcoma (eg, in HIV disease)
  Peutz-Jeghers syndrome
  Malignant melanoma (rare in childhood)
  Laugier-Hunziker syndrome
  Complex of myxomas, spotty pigmentation, and
    endocrine overactivity

Generalized
  Racial
  Addison disease
  Drugs (eg, minocycline)
  Albright syndrome
  Central cyanosis
  Neurofibromatosis
  Hemochromatosis
  Incontinentia pigementi
  Chronic hepatic disease (affects gingivae mainly)

a blue, red, or purple macule, papule, nodule, or ulcer, usually of the hard palate and/or gingivae. These tumors can be locally destructive and often reflect more widespread systemic involvement of the human herpesvirus 8-associated tumor; however, they may regress with effective antiretroviral therapy (ART).[50] Similar, but less extensive, Kaposi sarcoma can occur in the mouths of children receiving long-term iatrogenic immunosuppressive therapy.[141]

Addisonian pigmentation manifests as diffuse hypermelanotic pigmentation of the buccal mucosa.[142–143] More extensive pigmentation can occur but is uncommon. Other causes of oral mucosal pigmentation are indicated in Table 10.

OTHER ORAL MUCOSAL DISORDERS IN CHILDHOOD

Abnormalities of the Lingual or Labial Frenum

Ankyloglossia (Tongue-Tie). Ankylogossia is common, manifesting as an exaggerated lingual frenum that may limit the ability to protrude the tongue. It does not usually cause difficulties with speech development, although it can limit the ability to clean food debris and plaque from the teeth, gums, and vestibules of the mouth. Ankyloglossia requires simple surgical treatment.[8,144–145] Ankyloglossia can be a feature of Opitz syndrome (hypertelorism, hypospodias, and laryngo/tracheal/esophageal abnormalities).[146]

Abnormal Labial Frenum. The frenum of the upper or, less commonly, lower lip can be exaggerated, giving rise to a diastema (space) between the related central incisors and oral notching of the alveolar ridges. This can show a familial pattern of occurrence. Children may have difficulty maintaining good plaque control at this site. Surgical reduction, together with orthodontic care, will correct this common problem.[147]

Defects of the labial frenum are usually isolated, although rarely abnormalities of the labial frenum accompany congenital disease (Table 11).

MAJOR SALIVARY GLAND DISEASE IN CHILDHOOD

Other than mumps, salivary gland disease in childhood is uncommon. Salivary gland disease may manifest as localized swelling (Table 12) and/or xerostomia (Table 13).

Table 11 Syndromes Associated with Abnormalities of the Labial Frenum

Disorder	Abnormality
Ehler-Danlos syndrome	Absence of lower labial frenum (+ possible absence of lingual frenum)
Infantile hypertrophic pyloric stenosis	Hypoplastic or absent lower labial frenum
Holoprosencephaly	Absence of upper labial frenum
Ellis-van Creveld syndrome	Enlarge upper and lower labial frenum. In addition there may be fusion of the upper lip to the upper gingivae
Orofacial digntol syndrome	Enlargement of the labial and buccal frenum
Opitz syndrome	Ankyloglossia
W syndrome	Bifid upper labial frenum
Opitz trigoncephaly syndrome	Multiple enlarged labial and buccal frena

Mumps (Epidemic Parotitis). Mumps is an acute generalized paramyxovirus infection of children and young adults. Mumps typically affects the major salivary glands, although involvement of other structures can occur, including the pancreas, testis, ovaries, brain, breast, liver, joints, and heart.[148]

Mumps is transmitted via the droplet route and has an incubation time of approximately 14 to 18 days. Patients manifest with initial pyrexia, chills, and facial pain. The parotid glands are typically bilaterally enlarged, although this may initially be unilateral. There is often swelling of the submandibular glands together with lymphadenopathy, giving rise to profound facial and neck swelling.

Table 12 Salivary Gland Swelling in Childhood

Mumps
Recurrent parotitis of childhood
Sjögren syndrome and related disorders
Acute suppurative sialadenitis
Duct obstruction (uncommon in children)
Sarcoidosis
Cystic fibrosis
Sialosis (rare—eg, with bulimia nervosa)
HIV disease
Hepatitis C virus disease
Mucoceles

Table 13 Causes of Long-Standing Xerostomia in Childhood

Sjögren syndrome and related disorders
Sarcoidosis
Cystic fibrosis
HIV disease
Hepatitis C virus disease
Drugs
  Anticholinergics
  Antihistamines
  Tricyclic antidepressants
  Serotonin reuptake
  Sympathomimetics
  Phenothiazines
  Occasional cytotoxic drugs
Radiation of the head and neck(when the salivary
  glands lie within the field of radiation)
Chronic graft-versus-host disease
Dehydration (hypercalcemia, diabetes mellitus)
Anxiety
Depression
Salivary gland agenesis

Rarely, sublingual swelling may be so profound as to cause elevation of the tongue, dysphagia, and dysarthria. The salivary swelling tends to diminish after approximately 4 to 5 days and may precede more complicated aspects of illness.

Orchitis may develop approximately 4 to 5 days after the onset of parotitis. Typically, only one testicle is affected, and, occasionally, there can be bilateral involvement. Orchitis tends to arise in postpubertal boys and rarely gives rise to serious, long-standing disease.

Mumps can give rise to a lymphocytic or viral meningitis. This again commences a few days after the development of parotitis, although it can occur in the absence of salivary gland disease. Other neurologic manifestations include retrobulbar neuritis and encephalitis. Deafness is possible but rare. Pancreatic infection may give rise to mild upper abdominal pain, but acute and long-term complications are unusual. Likewise, although cardiac, hepatic, and joint infections can occur, they are rare and do not generally cause notable complications.

The diagnosis of mumps is typically based on the clinical picture; however, it may be confirmed by detection of viral-specific immunoglobulins G and A. Viral culture is possible but generally unnecessary because serologic methods are highly sensitive.

There is no specific treatment for mumps; analgesia and appropriate fluid intake are the mainstays of therapy. It has been suggested that corticosteroids may be effective for profound parotitis, but, generally, these are not required unless the patients have other systemic symptoms, such as orchitis. Mumps can generally be prevented with appropriate vaccination (mumps/measles/rubella).

HIV Salivary Gland Disease. Salivary gland disease can arise in 4 to 8% of adults and children with HIV infection. The salivary gland disease of HIV infection manifests as swelling and/or xerostomia and reflects underlying bacterial sialadenitis, intraparotid lymphadenopathy, primary or metastatic non-Hodgkin lymphoma, or Kaposi sarcoma.[50,150]

The specific disorder of HIV salivary gland disease (HIV-SGD) gives rise to recurrent and/or persistent major salivary gland enlargement and xerostomia. The parotids are most frequently affected; often there is profound bilateral enlargement. Salivary gland disease tends to arise in late HIV infection, although, occasionally, it can be the first manifestation of HIV disease. The cause of HIV-SGD remains unknown, although it may be associated with HLA-DR5 and is part of a more generalized disorder termed diffuse infiltrated lymphocytosis syndrome, which is characterized by CD8+ T-cell infiltration of the lungs, salivary glands, and lacrimal glands.[50,150]

The clinical picture of HIV-SGD mimics that of Sjogren syndrome; however, there are distinct histopathologic and serologic differences between the two disorders. Patients with HIV-SGD generally do not have anti-Ro or anti-La antibodies, but they do have hypergammaglobulinemia.

The diagnosis of HIV-SGD is similar to that of Sjogren syndrome. Fine-needle aspiration biopsy may be particularly useful because it allows rapid exclusion of malignancy.[151]

There is little information regarding the specific management of HIV-SGD. The clinical signs of HIV-SGD are usually nonprogressive; hence, therapy is indicated only if there is notable cosmetic deformity or xerostomia. ART may in some instances cause resolution of the swelling of HIV-SGD. Less practical, suggested therapies are repeated aspiration, tetracycline sclerosis, or surgical removal of an enlarged gland.[152] External radiation may cause transient improvement, although there are no data on the effectiveness for affected children.[153] Xerostomia independent of HIV-SGD may arise in HIV infection as a consequence of some nucleoside analog HIV reverse transcriptase inhibitors or protease inhibitors (see below).[50,154]

Hepatitis C Virus Infection. Although there are no data specific to children, it would be expected that hepatitis C virus (HCV) infection would give rise to HCV-related sialadenitis, which manifests as salivary gland enlargement and xerostomia. The histopathologic features of HCV-associated sialadenitis are similar to those of Sjogren syndrome, although the two disorders are etiologically distinct.[155]

Acute Suppurative Sialadenitis (Suppurative Parotitis). Acute suppurative sialadenitis is an uncommon disorder characterized by painful swelling, usually of parotid glands (suppurative parotitis), purulent discharge from the duct of the affected gland, associated dysgeusia, and cervical lymphadenopathy. When disease is severe, there may be accompanying pyrexia, malaise, and a risk of abscess formation and parapharyngeal space infection, including Ludwig's angina. Rarely, acute suppurative sialadenitis can affect the submandibular glands (independent of sialolithiasis), although can arise in neonates.[156]

Acute suppurative sialadenitis can arise in childhood (prematurity being a possible risk factor),[157] and sialadenitis can occur in newborns.[158] The highest incidence of childhood disease seems to arise in children 3 to 6 years of age.[159] Aseptic sialadenitis has been observed in preterm children receiving long-term orogastric tube feeding. Immunodeficiency and concurrent illness may predispose children to suppurative parotitis.

The causative organism of acute suppurative sialadenitis is often not found. Although facultative anaerobes, particularly *S. aureus* and *Streptococcus viridans*,[160-161] have frequently been reported to be of etiologic significance, a wide range of other bacteria have been implicated[162]— including methycillin-resistant *S. aureus*.[156]

The diagnosis of acute suppurative sialadenitis is based on the history and clinical picture. Microbiologic culture of pus, under both aerobic and anaerobic conditions, may reveal likely causative agents, although specific relevant tests may be useful if a particular infection seems likely.[162]

Additional investigations such as sialography and scintigraphy are rarely warranted, although ultrasonography can be useful, particularly if abscess formation is likely, as can magnetic resonance imaging.

Effective hydration and antibiotics are the mainstays of therapy of uncomplicated acute suppurative sialadenitis.[163] Typically employed antibiotic therapies are anti-staphylococcal penicillins (eg, flucloxacillin, amoxicillin, amoxicillinclavulanate), cephalosporins, or clindamycin, although the precise choice of antibiotic will often depend on any likely causative organism that is identified. Other alternatives may include flurithromycin. Intraductal injection of antibotics is unlikely to be of practical benefit. Surgical drainage should be considered if there is a lack of clinical improvement after 3 to 5 days of antibiotic therapy, any unlikely facial nerve involvement, any involvement of deep fascial spaces, or abscess formation within the parenchyma of the gland.[149] Superficial parotidectomy may be required if disease becomes recurrent or chronic.[163-164] Maintenance of low levels of dental plaque (by good oral hygiene, adequate hydration, and rapid effective treatment of bacterial infection of the oropharynx) may lessen the risk of further episodes of acute suppurative sialadenitis.[162]

Recurrent Parotitis of Childhood. Recurrent parotitis of childhood (juvenile recurrent parotitis and recurrent sialectatic parotitis) gives rise to recurrent parotid inflammation, usually associated with nonobstructive sialectasia of the parotid gland. Recurrent parotitis can arise at any age, but the usual age at onset is 3 to 6 years. While uncommon, it may be the second most common inflammatory disorder of the salivary glands in childhood. The disease is characterized by localized pain and swelling, which may last up to 14 days. Fever and overlying erythema are common, and unlike acute suppurative sialadenitis, pus is rarely expressed from the parotid duct. Recurrent parotitis of childhood tends to be unilateral rather than bilateral. The number of attacks varies from 1 to 5 per year, but some patients may have up to 20 episodes of swelling per year. The frequency of recurrence tends to peak between 5 and 7 years of age, and up to 90% of patients have resolution of disease by puberty.

Sialography and Ultrasonography reveal sialectasia.[165] This feature can also be observed in nonaffected glands of the opposite side. Computed tomography (CT) and magnetic resonance imaging (MRI) may also be of diagnostic benefit.[166]

The precise etiology of recurrent parotitis of childhood is unknown. There is no evidence that viral infection underlies this disorder. Associations with immunodeficiency (hypogammaglobulinaemia, isolated IgG$_3$ deficiency, and selective IgA deficiency) have been observed.[165] It has been proposed that salivary ductile defects (of unknown cause) are susceptible to infection, possibly explaining why abnormal sialographic features can be observed even in nonsymptomatic major salivary glands. A further notion is that salivary stasis (again of unknown cause) predisposes to local infection and resultant ductal damage.[165] Analgesia is the mainstay of therapy. Antibiotics do not shorten attacks. In general, the disease tends to resolve, and there is no need for profound surgical intervention.[167]

Sialolithiasis. Sialolithiasis—calculi within the salivary gland ductal network—is rare in childhood. As in adults, sialolithiasis in children usually affects a submandibular gland giving rise to submandibular pain and swelling on eating. The symptoms usually abate post-prandially. Sialolithiasis of the parotid gland is extremely rare in children.

The diagnosis of sialolithiasis can usually be confirmed by ultrasound scanning or plain radiography of the affected gland, the former being probably more appropriate as it will detect nonradiolucent as well as radiolucent calculi.

Occasionally the calculi will spontaneously pass out of the duct, but the majority of calculi require surgical removal. Calculi in the posterior aspects of the duct may warrant sialoendoscopic retrieval, although there seem to be no reports of the benefits of this for child patients.[168]

Long-Standing Xerostomia (Dry Mouth). Long-standing xerostomia gives rise to a range of disorders of the oral hard and soft tissues (Table 14). Xerostomia can give rise to dysarthria and dysphagia. The oral dryness leads to retention of food on the teeth, mucosa, and gingiva and thus increases the frequency of caries (particularly cervical disease) and acute gingivitis. There is an increased liability to candidal infection, notably acute pseudomembranous candidiasis, and median rhomboid glossitis, chronic atrophic candidiasis (denture-associated stomatitis), and angular cheilitis. Long-standing xerostomia increases the liability to acute suppurative parotitis (see above). The poor salivary output can lead to dysgeusia and loss of taste; many affected persons report that most foodstuffs taste cardboard-like.[169]

Xerostomia is more common in adults than in children; however, children are clearly more likely to manifest the features of salivary gland agenesis than adults and can also be liable to the common causes of acquired salivary gland dysfunction disease.

Salivary Gland Agenesis. Agenesis of one or more of the major salivary glands is extremely uncommon[170] There can be variation in the number of absent salivary glands and hence varying severity of the associated xerostomia. Lack of saliva predisposes the patient to dental caries, gingival inflammation, candidiasis, and acute suppurative sialadenitis, although, in children, rampant dental caries may be the only initial sign of underlying salivary agenesis.[171–173]

The precise incidence of major salivary gland agenesis is difficult to establish owing to the asymptomatic nature of many affected individuals. Familial clustering of salivary gland agenesis has occasionally been reported. Salivary gland aplasia may occur in isolation or be associated with other ectodermal defects, in particular lacrimal apparatus abnormalities. Autosomal dominant aplasia of the lacrimal and salivary glands (ALSG) is due to a defect being loss-of-function mutations in the fibroblast growth factor 10 (FGF10) gene at chromosome 5p13-p12.[174] Associations with hypohidrotic ED[175] and lacrimal-auriclo-dentodigital (LADD; Levy-Hollister syndrome) reflecting defects of *FgF10* gene[176] and ectodactyly-ED syndromes have been reported.[170] There is a recent report of bilateral parotid gland aplasia in a patient with Down's syndrome.[177]

Radiotherapy-Associated Salivary Gland Dysfunction. Brachytherapy of head and neck malignancies can cause profound xerostomia and salivary gland acinar destruction when the radiotherapy is directed through the major salivary glands. The degree of xerostomia clearly reflects the duration and dose of radiotherapy. The xerostomia is irreversible and thus can greatly affect the quality of life of affected children.[148] In adults, orally administered pilocarpine may lessen the severity of radiotherapy-induced xerostomia; however, there are no studies of the effectiveness of this cholinergic agent in children with radiotherapy-associated xerostomia[169] As a consequence, the treatment of long-term oral dryness in children is not specifically directed to enhancing cholinergic stimulation of the salivary glands.[148] Advances in parotid-sparing irradiation techniques (eg, intensity modulated radiotherapy (IMRT) are likely to reduce the frequency and severity of radiotherapy-associated xerostomia and mucositis).[178] Future therapies may include gene therapy (eg, aquaporin).[179]

Sjogren Syndrome. Sjogren syndrome is clinically characterized by xerostomia and xerophthalmia owing to profound lymphocytic infiltrate into the salivary and lacrimal glands.[180]

Sjogren syndrome can be classified as primary disease, of which the principal symptoms and signs affecting the eye and mouth, and secondary Sjogren syndrome, in which there is xerostomia, xerophthalmia, and associated connective tissue disorder, most frequently rheumatoid arthritis or systemic lupus erythematosus.

Although possibly the second most common connective tissue disorder in adults, Sjogren syndrome is an uncommon disorder of childhood.[180–181] The etiology of Sjogren syndrome remains unknown. A viral etiology—human retrovirus 5—was proposed but now seems unlikely; nevertheless, a viral basis cannot be excluded because the salivary features of human T lymphotropic virus 1, HCV, and HIV infection mimic those of Sjogren syndrome. To date there is no evidence of a strong genetic basis for Sjogren syndrome. The pathogenesis of Sjogren syndrome is discussed in detail elsewhere.[180] The investigation of Sjogren syndrome centers on a series of clinical, radiologic, and immunologic tests,[169,180] of which the histopathologic examination of labial gland tissue and the detection of serum anti-Ro and/or anti-La antibodies are cardinal. The management of the oral complications of Sjogren syndrome is similar to that outlined in Table 15.[169] In addition, pilocarpine and other similar agents (eg, cevimeline) may enhance salivary flow. At present, no immunologically based approach (including infliximab, etanercept, or rituximab) has been successful for the treatment of Sjogren syndrome other than perhaps hydroxychloroquine. Interestingly a child with secondary Sjogren's had reduction in symptoms of arthritis (but not oral dryness) with infliximab therapy.[182] All children with confirmed Sjogren syndrome will require lifelong specialist follow-up to ensure the early detection of possible non-Hodgkin lymphoma, particularly mucosa-associated lymphoid tissue lymphoma.

Table 14 Clinical Features of Long-Standing Xerostomia

Symptoms
  Oral dryness
  Dysarthria
  Dysphagia
  Loss of taste (often blunting of taste of all foods)

Signs
  Dryness of the oral mucosa
  Variable lack of saliva
  Depapillation, redness, and crenation of the dorsum of tongue (scrotal tongue)
  Loss of upper denture retention
  Increased liability to gingivitis
  Increased liability to dental decay (eg, cervical caries)
  Increased liability to bacterial sialadenitis (usually of the parotid glands)

Table 15 Management of Long-Standing Xerostomia

Therapy	Comments
Salivary substitutes	
Nonsynthetic agents	Sips of water; convenient but of limited benefit. Soft drinks should be avoided in view of the risk of caries or dental erosion
Synthetic agents	A variety of sprays, mouthrinses, and gels are available; no one agent is better than another; benefit can be transient
Salivary stimulants (salogogues)	
Nonspecific	Nonsucrose confectionary can be of benefit, but there may still be a risk of dental erosion. Sorbitol-containing pastilles may be helpful.
Specific	Pilocarpine (and possibly cevimeline) may be of application, but there are no detailed studies of their application in children with long-standing xerostomia
Oral hygiene care and dietary advice	Minimizes risk of caries and gingivitis
Fluoride supplements	Reduces risk of caries

18. Witkop CJJ. Amelogenesis imperfecta, dentinogenesis imperfect and dentin dysplasia revisited: Problems in classification. Oral Pathol 1989;17:547–53.

19. Shields ED. A proposed classification for heritable human dentine defects with a description of a new entity. Arch Oral Biol 1973;18:543–53.

20. Witkop CJ. Hereditary defects in enamel and dentin. Acta Genet 1957;7:236–9.

21. Kantaputra PN. Dentinogenesis imperfecta-associated syndromes [letter]. Am J Med Genet 2001;104:75–8.

22. Fejerskov O, Kidd E, editors. Dental Caries. The Disease and Its Clinical Management, 1st edition. Oxford: Blackwell Munksgaard; 2003.

23. Ettinger RL. Epidemiology of dental caries. A broad review. Dent Clin North Am 1999;43:679–94.

24. Seow WK. Biological mechanisms of early childhood caries. Community Dent Oral Epidemiol 1998;26:8–27.

25. Moazzez R, Bartlett D, Anggiansah A. Dental erosion, gastro-oesophageal reflux disease and saliva: How are they related? J Dent 2004;32:489–94.

26. Amaechi BT, Higham SM. Dental erosion: Possible approaches to prevention and control. J Dent 2005;33: 243–52.

27. Peres KG, Armenio MF, Peres MA, et al. Dental erosion in 12-year-old schoolchildren: A cross-sectional study in Southern Brazil. Int J Paed Dent 2005;15:249–55.

28. Peak J, Eveson JW, Scully C. Oral manifestations of Rett's syndrome. Br Dent J 1992;172:248–9.

29. Robinson C, Connell S, Kirkham J, et al. The effect of fluoride on the developing tooth. Caries Res 2004;38:268–76.

30. Weerheijm KL. Molar incisor hypomineralization (MIH): Clinical presentation, aetiology and management. Dent Update. 2004;31:9–12.

31. Koch G, Kreiborg S. Eruption and shedding of teeth. In: Koch G, Poulsen S, editors. Pediatric Dentistry. A Clinical Approach. 1st edition. Oxford. Blackwell Munksgaard; 2003. p. 301–19.

32. Oh T-J, Eber R, Wang H-L. Periodontal diseases in the child and adolescent. J Clin Periodontol 2002;29:400–10.

33. Fayle SA, Pollard MA. Congenital erythropoietic porphyria—oral manifestations and dental treatment in childhood: A case report. Quintessence Int 1994;25:551–4.

34. Garcia-Godoy F, Ellacuria J. Effectiveness of Sonicare power to remove chlorhexidine stains. Am J Dent 2002;15:290–2.

35. Clerehugh V, Tugnait A. Periodontal diseases in children and adolescents: I. Aetiology and diagnosis. Dent Update 2001;28:222–30, 232.

36. Coventry J, Griffiths G, Scully C, Tonetti M. ABC of oral health. 3. Periodontal disease. BMJ 2000;321:36–9.

37. Mariotti A. Dental plaque-induced gingival diseases. Ann Periodontol 1999;4:7–19.

38. Kinane DF, Lappin DF. Clinical, pathological and immunological aspects of periodontal disease. Acta Odontol Scand 2001;59:154–60.

39. Porter SR, Scully C. Periodontal Aspects of Systemic Disease—Textbook and Multimedia Package. London: BDJ Publishing (in press).

40. Frezzini C, Leao JC, Porter S. Current trends of HIV disease of the mouth. J Oral Pathol Med 2005;34:513–31.

41. Buchanan JAG, Cedro M, Mirdin A, et al. Necrotizing stomatitis in the developed world. Clin Exper Dermatol 2006;31:372–4.

42. Ye X, Shi L, Cheng Y, et al. A novel locus for autosomal dominant hereditary gingival fibromatosis, GINGF3, maps to chromosome 2p22.3–p23.3. Clinic Genet 2005;68: 239–44.

43. Doufexi A, Mina M, Ioannidou E. Gingival overgrowth in children: Epidemiology, pathogenesis and complications. A literature review. J Periodontol 2005;76:3–10.

44. Cohen MM, Jr. Perspectives on craniofacial asymmetry. VI. The hamartoses. Int J Oral Maxillofac Surg 1995;24:195–200.

45. Mirowski GW, Liu AA, Stone ML, Caldemeyer KS. Sturge-Weber syndrome. J Am Acad Dermatol 1999;41:772–3.

46. Smith D, Porter SR, Scully C. Gingival and other oral manifestations in tuberous sclerosis—a case report. Periodont Clin Investig 1994;15:13–6.

47. Bekisz O, Darimont F, Rompen EH. Diffuse but unilateral gingival enlargement associated with von Recklinghausen neurofibromatosis: A case report. J Clin Periodontol 2000;27:361–5.

48. Porter SR, Cawson RA, Scully C, Eveson JW. Multiple hamartoma syndrome presenting with oral lesions. Oral Surg Oral Med Oral Pathol Oral Radiol Endod 1996;82:295–301.

49. Leao JC, Batista V, Guimaraes PB, et al. Cowden's syndrome affecting the mouth, gastrointestinal and central nervous system: A report and review of the literature. Oral Surg Oral Med Oral Pathol Oral Radiol Endod 2005; 99:569–72.

50. Frezzini C, Leao JC, Porter S. Cathepsin C involvement in the aetiology of Papillon-Lefevre syndrome. Int J Paediatr Dent 2004;14:288–94.

51. Fenton SJ, Bouquot JE, Unkel JH. Orofacial considerations for pediatric, adult and elderly victims of abuse. Emerg Med Clin North Am 2000;18:601–17.

52. Simon PA. Recognizing and reporting the orofacial trauma of child abuse/neglect. Tex Dent J 2000;117:21–32.

53. Lee LY, Ilan J, Mulvey T. Human biting of children and oral manifestations of abuse: A case report and literature review. ASCD J Dent Child 2002;69:92–5.

54. Scully, C, Sonis, S, Diz, PD. Mucosal diseases series: Oral mucositis. Oral Diseases 2006;12:229–41.

55. Singh N, Scully C, Joyston-Bechal S. Oral complications of cancer therapies: Prevention and management. Clin Oncol (R Coll Radiol) 1996;8:15–24.

56. Spijkervet FK, Sonis ST. New frontiers in the management of chemotherapy-induced mucositis. Curr Opin Oncol 1998;10:S23–7.

57. Bez C, Demarosi F, Sardella A, et al. GM-CSF mouthrinses in the treatment of severe oral mucositis: A pilot study. Oral Surg Oral Med Oral Pathol Oral Radiol Endod 1999;88:311–5.

58. Lalla RV, Peterson DE. Treatment of mucositis, including new medications. Cancer J 2006;12:348–54.

59. Radtke ML, Kolesar JM. Palifermin (Kepivance) for the treatment of oral mucositis in patients with haematologic malignancies requiring haematopoietic stell cell support. J Oncol Pharm Pract 2005;11:121–5.

60. Porter SR, Scully C, Pedersen A. Recurrent aphthous stomatitis. Crit Rev Oral Biol Med 1998;9:306–21.

61. Porter SR, Hegarty A, Kaliakatsou F, et al. Recurrent aphthous stomatitis. Clin Dermatol 2000;18:569–78.

62. Jurge S, Kuffer R, Scully C, Porter SR. Mucosal disease series: Recurrent aphthous stomatitis. Oral Dis 2006;12:1–21.

63. Miller MF, Garfunkel AA, Ram C, Ship II. Inheritance patterns in recurrent aphthous ulcers; twin and pedigree data. Oral Surg Oral Med Oral Pathol 1977;43:886–91.

64. Bagan JV, Sauchis JM, Millan MA, et al. Recurrent aphthous stomatitis. A study of the clinical characteristics of lesions of 93 cases. J Oral Pathol Med 1991;20:395–7.

65. Rennie JS, Reade PC, Scully C. Recurrent aphthous stomatitis. Br Dent J 1985;159:361–7.

66. Singh K, Kumar S, Jaiswal MS, et al. Absence of *Helicobacter pylori* in oral mucosal lesions. J Indian Med Assoc 1998;96:177–8.

67. Birek C, Grandhi R, McNeill K, et al. Detection of *Helicobacter pylori* in oral aphthous ulcers. J Oral Pathol Med 1999;28:197–203.

68. Riggio MP, Lennon A, Wray D. Detection of *Helicobacter pylori* DNA in recurrent aphthous stomatitis tissue by PCR. J Oral Pathol Med 2000;29:507–13.

69. Pavelic J, Gall-Troselj K, Jurak I, Mravak-Stipetic M. *Helicobacter pylori* in oral aphthous ulcers. J Oral Pathol Med 2000;29:523–5.

70. Shimoyama T, Horie N, Kato T, et al. *Helicobacter pylori* in oral ulcerations. J Oral Sci 2000;42:225–9.

71. Lahteenoja H, Toivanen A, Viander M, et al. Oral mucosal changes in celiac patients on a gluten-free diet. Eur J Oral Sci 1998;106:899–906.

72. Ferguson R, Basu MJ, Asquith P, Cooke WT. Proceedings: Recurrent aphthous ulceration and its association with coeliac disease. Gut 1975;16:393.

73. Ferguson R, Basu MJ, Asquith P, Cooke WT. Jejunal mucosal abnormalities in patients with recurrent aphthous ulceration. BMJ 1976;1:11–3.

74. Ferguson MM, Wray D, Carmichael HA, et al. Coeliac disease associated with recurrent aphthae. Gut 1980;21:223–6.

75. Hunter IP, Ferguson MM, Scully C, et al. Effects of dietary gluten elimination in patients with recurrent minor aphthous stomatitis and no detectable gluten enteropathy. Oral Surg Oral Med Oral Pathol 1993;75:595–8.

76. Walker DM, Dolby AE, Mead J, et al. Effect of gluten-free diet on recurrent aphthous ulceration. Br J Dermatol 1980;103:111.

77. Veloso FT, Saleiro JV. Small-bowel changes in recurrent ulceration of the mouth. Hepatogastroenterology 1987;34:36–7.

78. O'Farrelly C, O'Mahoney C, Graeme-Cook F, et al. Gliadin antibodies identify gluten-sensitive oral ulceration in the absence of villous atrophy. J Oral Pathol Med 1991;20: 476–8.

79. Sedghizadeh PP, Shuler CF, Allen CM, et al. Celiac disease and recurrent aphthous stomatitis: A report and review of the literature. Oral Surg Oral Med Oral Pathol Oral Radiol Endod 2002;94:474–8.

80. Porter SR, Scully C, Flint S. Hematologic status in recurrent aphthous stomatitis compared with other oral disease. Oral Surg Oral Med Oral Pathol 1988;66:41–4.

81. Wray D, Ferguson MM, Mason DK, et al. Recurrent aphthae treatment with vitamin B12, folic acid and iron. BMJ 1975;2:490–3.

82. Porter SR, Flint S, Scully C, Keith O. Recurrent aphthous stomatitis: The efficacy of replacement therapy in patients with underlying hematinic deficiencies. Ann Dent 1992;51:14–6.

83. Porter SR, Scully C. Aphthous ulcers. Clin Evid 2005;13:1687–94.

84. Matthews RW, Scully CM, Levers BGH, Hislop WS. Clinical evaluation of benzydamine, chlorhexidine and placebo mouthwashes in the management of recurrent aphthous stomatitis. Oral Surg 1987;63:189–91.

85. Addy M, Tapper-Jones L, Seal M. Trial of astringent and antibacterial mouthwashes in the management of recurrent aphthous ulceration. Br Dent J 1974;136:452–5.

86. Addy M, Carpenter R, Roberts WR. Management of recurrent aphthous ulceration—a trial of chlorhexidine gluconate gel. Br Dent J 1976;141:118–20.

87. Addy M. Hibitane in the treatment of recurrent aphthous ulceration. J Clin Periodontol 1977;4:108–16.

88. Hunter L, Addy M. Chlorhexidine gluconate mouthwash in the management of minor aphthous stomatitis. Br Dent J 1987;162:106–10.

89. Guggenheimer J, Brightman VJ, Ship II. Effect of chlortetracycline mouthrinses on the healing of recurrent aphthous ulcers: A double-blind controlled trial. J Oral Therapeut Pharmacol 1968;4:406–8.

90. Graykowski EA, Kingman A. Double-blind trial of tetracycline in recurrent aphthous ulceration. J Oral Pathol 1978;7:376–82.

91. Denman AR, Schiff AA. Recurrent oral ulceration treatment of recurrent aphthous ulceration of the oral cavity. BMJ 1979;1:1248–9.

92. Hayrinen-Immonen R, Sorsa T, Pettila J, et al. Effect of tetracyclines on collagenase activity in patients with recurrent aphthous ulcers. J Oral Pathol Med 1994;23:2 69–72.

93. Greer RO Jr, Lindenmuth JE, Juarez T, Khandwala A. A double-blind study of topically applied 5% amlexanox in the treatment of aphthous ulcers. J Oral Maxillofac Surg 1993;15:243–8.

94. Khandwala A, Van Inwegen RG, Alfano MC. 5% Amlexanox oral paste, a new treatment for recurrent minor aphthous ulcers. Oral Surg Oral Med Oral Pathol 1997;83:222–30.

95. Binnie WH, Curro FA, Khandwala A, Van Inwegen RG. Amlexanox oral paste: A novel treatment that accelerates the healing of aphthous ulcers. Compendium 1997;18:7.

96. Murray, B, McGuinness, N, Biagioni, P, et al. A comparative study of the efficacy of Aphtheal in the management of recurrent minor aphthous ulceration. J Oral Pathol Med 2005;34:413–9.

97. Scully, C. Clinical practice. Aphthous ulceration. N Engl J Med 2006;13:165–72.

98. Revuz J, Guillaume JC, Janier M, et al. Crossover study of thalidomide vs placebo in severe recurrent aphthous stomatitis. Arch Dermatol 1990;126:923–7.

99. Nicolau DP, West TE. Thalidomide: Treatment of severe recurrent aphthous stomatitis in patients with AIDS. DICP 1990;24:1054–6.

100. Paterson DL, Georghiou PR, Allworth AM, Kemp RJ. Thalidomide as treatment of refractory aphthous ulceration related to human immunodeficiency virus infection. Clin Infect Dis 1995;20:250–4.

101. de Wazieres B, Gil H, Magy N, et al. Traiment de l'aphtose recurrente par thalidomide a faible dose. Etude pilote chez 17 patients. Rev Med Interne 1999;20:567–70.

102. Mascaro JM, Lecha M, Torras H. Thalidomide in the treatment of recurrent, necrotic and giant mucocutaneous aphthae and aphthosis. Arch Dermatol 1979;115:636–7.

103. Grinspan D. Significant response of oral aphthosis to thalidomide treatment. J Am Acad Dermatol 1985;12:85–90.

104. Grinspan D, Blanco GF, Aguero S. Treatment of aphthae with thalidomide. J Am Acad Dermatol 1989;20:1060–3.

105. Jacobson JM, Greenspan JS, Spritzler J, et al. Thalidomide for the treatment of oral aphthous ulcers in patients with human immunodeficiency virus infection. National Institute of Allergies and Infectious Diseases AIDS Clinical Trials Group. N Engl J Med 1997;22:1487–93.

106. Jacobson JM, Greenspan JS, Spritzler J, et al. Thalidomide in low intermittent does not prevent recurrence of human immunodeficiency virus-associated aphthous ulcers. J Infect Dis 2001;183:343–6.

107. Atas B, Caksen H, Arslan S, et al. PFAPA syndrome mimicking familial Mediterranean fever: Report of a Turkish child. J Emerg Med 2003; 25:383–5.

108. Tasher D, Somekh E, Dalal I. PFAPA syndrome—new clinical aspects revealed. Arch Dis Child 2006; doi:10.1136/adc.2005.084731.

109. Al-Otaibi LM, Porter SR, Poate TW. Behcet's disease: A review. J Dent Res 2005;84:209–22.

110. Kari JA, Shah V, Dillon MJ. BehCet's disease in UK children: Clinical features and treatment including thalidomide. Rheumatology 2001;40:933–8.

111. Scully C, Porter S. Orofacial disease: Update for the dental clinical team: 3. White lesions. Dent Update 1999;26:123–9.

112. Terrinoni A, Rugg EL, Lane EB, et al. A novel mutation in the keratin 13 gene causing oral white sponge nevus. J Dent Res 2001;80:919–23.

113. deTomas MJ, Bagan JV, Silvestre FJ, et al. White sponge nevus: Presentation of sixteen cases corresponding to six families. Med Oral 1999;4:494–502.

114. Scully C, el-Kabir M, Samaranayake LP. Candida and oral candidosis: A review. Crit Rev Oral Biol Med 1994;5:125–57.

115. Johnson EM, Warnock DW, Luker J, et al. Emergence of azole drug resistance in Candida species from HIV-infected patients receiving prolonged fluconazole therapy for oral candidosis. J Antimicrob Chemother 1995;35:103–14.

116. McCullough MJ, Clemons KV, Stevens DA. Molecular epidemiology of the global and temporal diversity of Candida albicans. Clin Infect Dis 1999;29:1220–5.

117. Manfredi M, McCullough MJ, Polonelli L, et al. In vitro antifungal susceptibility to six antifungal agents of 229 Candida isolates from patients with diabetes mellitus. Oral Microbiol Immunol 2006;21:177–82.

118. Porter SR, Scully C. Chronic mucocutaneous candidosis. In: Samaranayake LM, MacFarlane TW, editors. Oral Candidosis. London: Wright; 1990. p. 200–12.

119. Porter SR, Scully C. Candidiasis endocrinopathy syndrome. Oral Surg Oral Med Oral Pathol 1986;61:573–8.

120. Lamfon H, Al-Karaawi Z, McCullough M, et al. Composition of in vitro denture plaque biofilms and susceptibility to antifungals. FEMS Microbiol Lett 2005;242:345–51.

121. Triantos D, Porter SR, Scully C, Teo CG. Oral hairy leukoplakia: Clinicopathologic features, pathogenesis, diagnosis and clinical significance. Clin Infect Dis 1997;25:1392–6.

122. Teo CG. Viral infections in the mouth. Oral Dis 2002;8:88–90.

123. Walne AJ, Marrone A, Dokal I. Dyskeratosis congenita: A disorder of defective telomere maintenance? Int J Hematol 2005;82:184–9.

124. Yoon A, Peng G, Brandenburg Y, et al. Impaired control of IRES-mediated translation in X-linked dyskeratosis congenita. Science 2006;312:902–6.

125. Leachman SA, Kaspar RL, Fleckman P, et al. Clinical and pathological features of pachyonychia congenita. J Investig Dermatol Symp Proc 2005;10:3–17.

126. Scully C. Oral squamous cell carcinoma; from an hypothesis about a virus, to concern about possible sexual transmission. Oral Oncol 2002;38:227–34.

127. Martins WD, de Lima AA, Vieira S. Focal epithelial hyperplasia (Heck's disease): Report of a case in a girl of Brazilian Indian descent. Int J Paediatr Dent 2006;16:65–8.

128. Kose O, Akar A, Safali M, et al. Focal epithelial hyperplasia treated with interferon alpha-2a. J Dermatol Treat 2001;12:111–3.

129. Lodi G, Scully C, Carrozzo M, et al. Current controversies in oral lichen planus: Report of an international consensus meeting. Part 1. Viral infections and etiopathogenesis. Oral Surg Oral Med Oral Pathol Oral Radiol Endod 2005;100:40–51.

130. Lodi G, Scully C, Carrozzo M, et al. Current controversies in oral lichen planus: Report of an international consensus meeting. Part 2. Clinical management and malignant transformation. Oral Surg Oral Med Oral Pathol Oral Radiol Endod 2005;100:164–78.

131. Porter SR, Scully C. Adverse drug reactions in the mouth. Clin Dermatol 2000;18:525–32.

132. Chan ES, Thornhill M, Zakrzewska J. Interventions for treating oral lichen planus. Cochrane Database Syst Rev 2000;CD001168.

133. Kaliakatsou F, Hodgson TA, Lewsey JD, et al. Management of recalcitrant ulcerative oral lichen planus with topical tacrolimus. J Am Acad Dermatol 2002;46:35–41.

134. Hodgson TA, Sahni N, Kaliakatsou F, et al. Long-term efficacy and safety of topical tacrolimus in the management of ulcerative/erosive oral lichen planus. Eur J Dermatol 2003;13:466–70.

135. Swift JC, Rees TD, Plemons JM, et al. The effectiveness of 1% pimecrolimus cream in the treatment of oral erosive lichen planus. J Periodontol 2005;76:627–35.

136. Mattsson U, Jontell M, Holmstrup P. Oral lichen planus and malignant transformation: Is a recall of patients justified? Crit Rev Oral Biol Med 2002;13:390–6.

137. Porter SR. Clinical manifestations of malignant and potentially malignant oral disease. CPD Dent 2001;2:18–23.

138. Prasad ML, Patel S, Hoshaw-Woodard S, et al. Prognostic factors for malignant melanoma of the squamous mucosa of the head and neck. Am J Surg Pathol 2002;26:883–92.

139. Seward GR. Amalgam tattoo. Br Dent J 1998;184:470–1.

140. Kissel SO, Hanratty JJ. Periodontol treatment of an amalgam tattoo. Compend Contin Educ Dent 2002;23:930–2, 4, 6.

141. Porter SR, Di Alberti L, Kumar N. Human herpes virus 8 (Kaposi's sarcoma herpesvirus). Oral Oncol 1998;34:5–14.

142. Porter SR, Haria S, Scully C, Richards A. Chronic candidiasis, enamel hypoplasia and pigmentary anomalies. Oral Surg Oral Med Oral Pathol 1992;74:312–4.

143. Shah SS, Oh CH, Coffin SE, Yan AC. Addisonian pigmentation of the oral mucosa. Cutis 2005;76:97–9.

144. Ruffoli R, Giambelluca MS, Scavuzzo MC, et al. Ankyloglossia: A morphofunctional investigation in children. Oral Dis 2005;11:170–4.

145. Kupietzky A, Botzer E. Ankyloglossia in the infant and young child: Clinical suggestions for diagnosis and management. Pediatr Dent 2005;27:40–6.

146. Brooks JK, Leonard CO, Coccaro PJ, Jr. Opitz (BBB/G) syndrome: Oral manifestations. Am J Med Genetics 1992;43:595–601.

147. Mintz SM, Siegel MA, Seider PJ. An overview of oral frena and their association with multiple syndromic and nonsyndromic conditions. Oral Surg Oral Med Oral Pathol Oral Radiol Endod 2005;99:321–4.

148. Porter SR. Non-neoplastic salivary gland disease. In: Gleeson M, editor. Scott-Brown's Otorhinolaryngology: Head & Neck Surgery, 7th edition. London: Butterworth-Heinemann (in press).

149. Scully C, Samaranayake L. Clinical virology in oral medicine and dentistry. Cambridge, UK: Cambridge University Press; 1992. p.135–216.

150. Mbopi-Keou FX, Belec T, Teo CG, et al. Synergism between HIV and other viruses in the mouth. Lancet Infect Dis 2002;2:416–24.

151. Chieng DC, Argosino R, McKenna BJ, et al. Utility of fine-needle aspiration in the diagnosis of salivary gland lesions in patients infected with human immunodeficiency virus. Diagn Cytopathol 1999;21:260–4.

152. Lustig LR, Lee KC, Murr A, et al. Doxycycline sclerosis of benign lymphoepithelial cysts in patients infected with HIV. Laryngoscope 1998;198:1199–1205.

153. Bietler JJ, Smith RV, Brook A, et al. Benign parotid hypertrophy on +HIV patients: Limited late failures after external radiation. Int J Radiat Oncol Biol Phys 1999;45:451–5.

154. Porter SR, Scully C. HIV topic update: Protease inhibitor therapy and oral health care. Oral Dis 1998;4:159–63.

155. Leao JC, Teo CG, Porter SR. HCV infection: Aspects of epidemiology and transmission relevant to oral health care workers. Int J Oral Maxillofac Surg 2006;35:295–300.

156. Ryan M, McAdams, Mair EA, Rajnik, M. Neonatal suppurative submandibular sialadenitis: Case report and literature review. Int J Pediat Otorhinolaryngology 2005;69:993–997.

157. Spiegel R, Miron D, Sakran W, Horovitz Y. Acute neonatal suppurative parotitis: Case reports and review. Pediatr Infect Dis 2004;23:76–8.

158. Takahashi R, Chikaoka S, Ito T, et al. Neonatal submandibular suppurative sialadenitis. Eur J Pediatr 2000;159:868.

159. Nusem-Horowitz S, Wolf M, Coret A, Kronenberg J. Acute suppurative parotitis and parotid abscess in children. Int J Pediatr Otorhinolaryngol 1995;32:123–7.

160. Raad II, Sabbagh MF, Caranasos GJ. Acute bacterial sialadenitis: A study of 29 cases and review. Rev Infect Dis 1990;12:591–601.

161. Chiu CH, Lin TY. Clinical and microbiological analysis of six children with acute suppurative parotitis. Acta Paediatr 1996;85:106–8.

162. Brook, I. Acute bacterial suppurative parotitis: Microbiology and management. J Craniofac Surg 2003;14:37–40.

163. Fattahi TT, Lyu PE, Van Sickels JE. Management of acute suppurative parotitis. J Oral Maxillofac Surg 2002;60:446–8.

164. O'Brien CJ, Murrant NJ. Surgical management of chronic parotitis. Head Neck 1993;15:445–9.

165. Leerdam CM, Martin HCO, Isaacs D. Recurrent parotitis of childhood. J Paediatr Child Health 2005;41:631–4.

166. Huisman TA, Holzmann D, Nadal D. MRI of chronic recurrent parotitis in childhood. J Comput Assist Tomogr 2001;25:269–73.

167. Isaacs D. Recurrent parotitis. J Paediatr Child Health 2002;38:92–4.

168. Laskawi F, Schaffranietz C, Arglebe M, Ellies M. Inflammatory diseases of the salivary glands in infants and adolescents. Int J Pediatr Otorhinolaryng 2006;70:129–136.

169. Porter SR, Scully C, Hegarty AM. An update of the etiology and management of xerostomia. Oral Surg Oral Med Oral Pathol Oral Radiol Endod 2004;97:28–46.

170. Hodgson TA, Shah R, Porter SR. The investigation of major salivary gland agenesis: A case report. Pediatr Dent 2001;23:131–4.

171. Fracaro MS, Linnett VM, Hallett KB, Savage NW. Submandibular gland aplasia and progressive dental caries: A case report. Aust Dent J 2002;47:347–50.

172. Antoniades DZ, Markopoulos AK, Deligianni E, Andreadis D. Bilateral aplasia of parotid glands correlated with accessory parotid tissue. J Laryngol Oto 2006;120:327–9

173. Kwon SY, Jung EJ, Kim SH, Kim TK. A case of major salivary gland agenesis. Acta Otolaryngol 2006;126:219–22.

174. Entesarian M, Matsson H, Klar J, et al. Mutations in the gene encoding fibroblast growth factor 10 are associated with aplasia of lacrimal and salivary glands. Nat Genet 2005;37:125–7.

175. Singh P, Warnakulasuriya S. Aplasia of submandibular salivary glands associated with ectodermal dysplasia. J Oral Pathol Med 2004;33:634–6.

176. Milunsky JM, Zhao G, Maher TA, et al. LADD syndrome is caused by FGF10 mutations. Clin Genet 2006;69:349–54.

177. Ferguson MM, Ponnambalam Y. Aplasia of the parotid gland in Down syndrome. Brit J Oral & Maxillofac Surg 2005;43:113–7.

178. Chambers MS, Garden AS, Kies MS, Martin JW. Radiation-induced xerostomia in patients with head and neck cancer: Pathogenesis, impact on quality of life and management. Head Neck 2004;26:796–807.

179. Cotrim AP, Mineshiba F, Sugito T, et al. Salivary gland gene therapy. Dent Clin North Am 2006;50:157–73.

180. Fox RI. Sjogren's syndrome. Lancet 2005;366:321–31.

181. Cimaz R, Casadei A, Rose C, et al. Primary Sjogren syndrome in the paediatric age: A multi-centre survey. Eur J Pediatr 2003;162:661–5.

182. Pessler F, Monash B, Rettig P, et al. Sjogren syndrome in a child: Favorable response of the arthritis to TNFalpha blockade. Clin Rheumatol (in press).

183. Porter SR, Scully C, Kainth B, Ward-Booth P. Multiple salivary mucoceles in a young boy. Int J Paediatr Dent 1998;8:149–51.

184. Roberts MW, Li SH. Oral findings in anorexia nervosa and bulimia nervosa: A study of 47 cases. J Am Dent Assoc 1987;115:407–10.

185. Milosevic A. Eating disorders and the dentist. Br Dent J 1999;186:109–13.

186. Brady WF. The anorexia nervosa syndrome. Oral Surg Oral Med Oral Pathol 1980;50:509–16.

187. Walsh BT, Croft CB, Katz JL. Anorexia nervosa and salivary gland enlargement. Int J Psychiatry Med 1981;11: 255–61.

188. Coleman H, Altini M, Nayler S, Richards A. Sialadenosis: A presenting sign in bulimia. Head Neck 1998;20:758–62.

189. British Nutrition Foundation Task Force. Oral health diet and other factors. Amsterdam: Elsevier; 1999.

190. Oginni FO, Oginni AO, Ugboko VI, Otuyemi OD. A survey of cases of cancrum oris seen in Ile-Ife, Nigeria. Int J Paediatr Dent 1999;9:75–80.

191. Scully C, Monteil R, Sposto MR. Infectious and tropical diseases affecting the human mouth. Periodontology 2000;18:47–70.

192. Enwonwu CO, Edozien JC. Epidemiology of periodontal disease in Western Nigerians in relation to socio-economic status. Arch Oral Biol 1979;15:1231–44.

193. Touyz LZ. Vitamin C, oral scurvy and periodontal disease. S Afr Med J 1984;65:838–42.

194. Ismail AI, Burt BA, Eklund SA. Relation between ascorbic acid intake and periodontal disease in the United States. J Am Dent Assoc 1983;107:927–31.

195. Lamey PJ, Hammond A, Allam BF, McIntosh WB. Vitamin status of patients with burning mouth syndrome and the response to replacement therapy. Br Dent J 1986;160:81–4.

196. Gilman J, Stassey LFA, Lamey P, Fell GS. Geographic tongue: The clinical response to zinc supplementation. J Trace Elements Exp Med 1990;3:205–8.

197. Rugg-Gunn AG. Nutrition and Dental Health. Oxford, UK: Oxford University Press; 1993.

198. Aine L. Dental enamel defects and dental maturity in children and adolescents with coeliac disease. Proc Finn Dent Soc 1986;82:1–71.

199. Aine L, Maki M, Reunala T. Coeliac-type dental enamel defects in patients with dermatitis herpetiformis. Acta Derm Venereol 1992;72:25–7.

200. Martelossi A, Zanatta E, Del Santo E, et al. Dental enamel defects and screening for coeliac disease. Acta Paediatr Suppl 1996;412:47–8.

201. Porter SR, Eveson JW, Scully C. Enamel hypoplasia secondary to candidiasis endocrinopathy syndrome: Case report. Pediatr Dent 1995;17:216–9.

202. Porter SR, Haria S, Scully C, Richards A. Chronic candidiasis, enamel hypoplasia, and pigmentary anomalies. Oral Surg Oral Med Oral Pathol 1992;74:312–4.

203. Field EA, Ellis A, Friedmann PS, et al. Oral tylosis: A re-appraisal. Oral Oncol 1997;33:55–7.

204. Andersson-Wenckert I, Blomquist HK, Fredrikzon B. Oral health in coeliac disease and cow's milk protein intolerance. Swed Dent J 1984;8:9–14.

205. Jokinen J, Peters U, Maki M, et al. Celiac sprue in patients with chronic oral mucosal symptoms. J Clin Gastroenterol 1998;26:23–6.
206. Aine L. Permanent tooth dental enamel defects leading to the diagnosis of coeliac disease. Br Dent J 1994;177:253–4.
207. Aine L. Coeliac-type permanent-tooth enamel defects. Ann Med 1996;28:9–12.
208. Aine L, Reunala T, Maki M. Dental enamel defects in children with dermatitis herpetiformis. J Pediatr 1991;118:572–4.
209. Marsden RA, McKee PH, Bhogal B, et al. A study of benign chronic bullous dermatosis of childhood and comparison with dermatitis herpetiformis and bullous pemphigoid occurring in childhood. Clin Exp Dermatol 1980;5:159–76.
210. Wojnarowska F, Marsden RA, Bhogal B, Black MM. Chronic bullous disease of childhood, childhood cicatricial pemphigoid, and linear IgA disease of adults. A comparative study demonstrating clinical and immunopathologic overlap. J Am Acad Dermatol 1988;19:792–805.
211. Edwards S, Wojnarowska F, Armstrong LM. Chronic bullous disease of childhood with oral mucosal scarring. Clin Exp Dermatol 1991;16:41–3.
212. Primosch RE. Tetracycline discoloration, enamel defects, and dental caries in patients with cystic fibrosis. Oral Surg Oral Med Oral Pathol 1980;50:301–8.
213. Fernald GW, Roberts MW, Boat TF. Cystic fibrosis: A current review. Pediatr Dent 1990;12:72–8.
214. Westbury LW, Najera A. Minocycline-induced intraoral pharmacogenic pigmentation: Case reports and review of the literature. J Periodontol 1997;68:84–91.
215. Cheek CC, Heymann HO. Dental and oral discolorations associated with minocycline and other tetracycline analogs. J Esthet Dent 1999;11:43–8.
216. Barbero GJ, Siblinga MS. Enlargement of the submaxillary glands in cystic fibrosis. Paediatrics 1962;29:788–93.
217. Watman S, Mercadente J, Mandel ID, et al. The occurrence of calculus in normal children, children with cystic fibrosis and children with asthma. J Periodontol 1973;44:278–80.
218. Welsey RK, Delaney JR, Pensler L. Mucocutaneous melanosis and gastrointestinal polyposis (Peutz-Jeghers syndrome): Clinical considerations and report of case. J Dent Child 1977;44:131–4.
219. Dummett CO, Barens G. Oromucosal pigmentation: An updated literary review. J Peridontol 1971;42:726–36.
220. Hasen LS, Silverman S, Jr, Daniels TE. The differential diagnosis of pyostomatitis vegetans and its relation to bowel disease. Oral Surg Oral Med Oral Pathol 1983;55:363–73.
221. Wray D. Pyostomatitis vegetans. Br Dent J 1984;157:316–8.
222. VanHale HM, Rogers RS, III Zone JJ, Greipp PR. Pyostomatitis vegetans. A reactive mucosal marker for inflammatory disease of the gut. Arch Dermatol 1985;121:94–8.
223. Neville BW, Smith SE, Maize JC, et al. Pyostomatitis vegetans. Am J Dermatopathol 1985;7:69–77.
224. Ballo FS, Camisa C, Allen CM. Pyostomatitis vegetans. Report of a case and review of the literature. J Am Acad Dermatol 1989;21:381–7.
225. Chan SW, Scully C, Prime SS, Eveson J. Pyostomatitis vegetans: Oral manifestation of ulcerative colitis. Oral Surg Oral Med Oral Pathol 1991;72:689–92.
226. Thornhill MH, Zakrzewska JM, Gilkes JJ. Pyostomatitis vegetans: Report of three cases and review of the literature. J Oral Pathol Med 1992;21:128–33.
227. Healy CM, Farthing PM, Williams DM, Thornhill MH. Pyostomatitis vegetans and associated systemic disease. A review and two case reports. Oral Surg Oral Med Oral Pathol 1994;78:323–8.
228. Al-Rimawi HS, Hammad MM, Raweily EA, Hammad HM. Pyostomatitis vegetans in childhood. Eur J Pediatr 1998;157:402–5.
229. Chaudhry SI, Philpot NS, Odell EW, et al. Pyostomatitis vegetans associated with asymptomatic ulcerative colitis: A case report. Oral Surg Oral Med Oral Pathol Oral Radiol Endod 1999;87:327–30.
230. Calobrisi SD, Mutasim DF, McDonald JS. Pyostomatitis vegetans associated with ulcerative colitis. Temporary clearance with fluocinonide gel and complete remission after colectomy. Oral Surg Oral Med Oral Pathol Oral Radiol Endod 1995; 79:452–4.
231. Prendiville JS, Israel DM, Wood WS, Dimmick JE. Oral pemphigus vulgaris associated with inflammatory bowel disease and herpetic gingivostomatitis in an 11 year old girl. Pediatr Dermatol 1994;11:145–50.
232. Antoniades K, Eleftheriades I, Karakasis D. The Gardner syndrome. Int J Oral Maxillofac Surg 1987;16:480–3.
233. Kubo K, Miyatani H, Takenoshita Y, et al. Widespread radiopacity of jaw bones in familial adenomatosis coli. J Craniomaxillofac Surg 1989;17:350–3.
234. Katou F, Motegi K, Baba S. Mandibular lesions in patients with adenomatosis coli. J Craniomaxillofac Surg 1989;17:354–8.
235. Jones K, Korzcak P. The diagnostic significance and management of Gardner's syndrome. Br J Oral Maxillofac Surg 1990;28:80–4.
236. Yuasa K, Yonetsu K, Kanda S, et al. Computed tomography of the jaws in familial adenomatosis coli. Oral Surg Oral Med Oral Pathol 1993;76:251–5.
237. Thakker N, Davies R, Horner K, et al. The dental phenotype in familial adenomatous polyposis: Diagnostic application of a clinical manifestations and management. Mouth and esophagus weighted scoring system for changes on dental panoramic radiographs. J Med Genet 1995;32:458–64.
238. Thakker NS, Evans DG, Horner K, et al. Florid oral manifestations in an atypical familial adenomatous polyposis family with late presentation of colorectal polyps. J Oral Pathol Med 1996;25:459–62.
239. Scully C, Porter SR. Oral mucosal disease: A decade of new entities, aetiologies and associations. Int Dent J 1994;44:33–43.
240. Armstrong DK, Burrows D. Orofacial granulomatosis. Int J Dermatol 1995;34:830–3.
241. Eveson JW. Granulomatous disorders of the oral mucosa. Semin Diagn Pathol 1996;13:118–27.
242. Rogers RS, Bekic M. Diseases of the lips. Semin Cutan Med Surg 1997;16:328–36.
243. Leao JC, Hodgson T, Scully C, Porter S. Review article: Orofacial granulomatosis. Aliment Pharmacol Ther 2004; 20:1019–27.
244. Clayden AM, Bleys CM, Jones SF, et al. Orofacial granulomatosis: A diagnostic problem for the unwary and a management dilemma. Aust Dent J 1997;42:228–32.
245. Rees TD. Orofacial granulomatosis and related conditions. Periodontology 2000 1999;21:145–57.
246. Sainsbury CPQ, Dodge JA, Walker DM. Orofacial granulomatosis in childhood. Br Dent J 1987;163:154–7.
247. Scheper JH, Brand HS. Oral aspects of Crohn's disease. Int Dent J 2002;52:163–72.
248. Engel LD, Pasquinelli KL, Leone SA, et al. Abnormal lymphocyte profiles and leukotriene B4 status in a patient with Crohn's disease and severe periodontitis. J Periodontol 1988;59:841–7.
249. Stein SL, Mancini AJ. Melkersson-Rosenthal syndrome in childhood: Successful management with combination steroid and minocycline therapy. J Am Acad Dermatol 1999; 41:746–8.
250. Patton DW, Ferguson MM, Forsyth A, James J. Orofacial granulomatosis: A possible allergic basis. Br J Oral Maxillofac Surg 1985;23:235–42.
251. Sweatman MC, Tasker R, Warner JO, et al. Orofacial granulomatosis. Response to elemental diet and provocation by food additives. Clin Allergy 1986;16:331–8.
252. Lamey PJ, Lewis MAO. Oral medicine in practice: Orofacial allergic reactions. Br Dent J 1990;168:59–63.
253. Hodgson TA, Hegarty AM, Buchanan JAG, Porter SR. Thalidomide for the treatment of recalcitrant oral Crohn disease and orofacial granulomatosis. Oral Surg Oral Med Oral Pathol Oral Radiol Endod 2003;95:576–85.
254. Sanchez AR, Rogers RS, III Sheridan PJ. Oral ulcerations are associated with the loss of response to inflibixmab in Crohn's disease. J Oral Pathol Med 2005;34:447–8.
255. Majewski RF, Hess J, Kabani S, Ramanathan G. Dental findings in a patient with biliary atresia. J Clin Pediatr Dent 1993;1832–7.
256. Zaia AA, Graner E, de Almeida OP, Scully C. Oral changes associated with biliary atresia and liver transplantation. J Clin Pediatr Dent 1993;18:38–42.
257. Seow WK, Shepherd RW, Ong TH. Oral changes associated with end-stage liver disease and liver transplantation: Implications for dental management. ASDC J Dent Child 1991;58:474 80.
258. Morisaki I, Abe K, Tong LS, et al. Dental findings of children with biliary atresia: Report of seven cases. ASDC J Dent Child 1990;57:220–3.
259. Richards A, Rooney J, Prime S, Scully C. Primary biliary cirrhosis. Sole presentation with rampant dental caries. Oral Surg Oral Med Oral Pathol 1994;77:16–8.
260. Porter SR, Scully C. Periodontal aspects of systemic disease. A system of classification. In: Lang N, editor. European Workshop of Periodontology. London: Quintessence; 1999. p. 374–419.

3

Disorders of Deglutition

David N. Tuchman, MD

The pediatric patient with impaired swallowing poses a number of unique problems for the clinician. In contrast to adults, issues such as the growth and development of the swallowing apparatus, the development of normal oromotor reflexes, the maturation of feeding behavior, the importance of oral feeding in the development of parent–child bonding, the acquisition of adequate nutrition for somatic growth, and the effects of nonnutritive sucking on growth must be considered in the approach to this group of patients. In addition, some groups of patients with impaired swallowing lack the cognitive skills necessary to follow specific therapeutic recommendations (eg, those in the infant age group and children with central nervous system disease), a situation that complicates patient management.

NORMAL DEGLUTITION

The swallowing apparatus transports materials from the oral cavity to the stomach without allowing entry of substances into the airway. To accomplish safe swallowing, there must be precise coordination between the oral and pharyngeal phases of swallowing so that the pharyngeal swallow is initiated at the appropriate moment after the onset of bolus movement. The passage of an oral bolus without aspiration is the result of a complex interaction of cranial nerves and muscles of the oral cavity, pharynx, and proximal esophagus.[1,2]

Deglutition is generally divided into three phases based on functional and anatomic characteristics: oral, pharyngeal, and esophageal.[1,2] The oral stage, which is voluntary, involves a preparatory phase. In the unimpaired child, the oral cavity functions as a sensory and motor organ, changing the physical properties of the food bolus to make it safe to swallow. The oral bolus is modified to allow passage through the pharynx without entry into the larynx or the tracheobronchial tree. Physical properties of the food bolus altered by oral activity include size, shape, volume, pH, temperature, and consistency.[3]

The food bolus then moves into the pharynx, where the respiratory and gastrointestinal tracts interface. Passage of food through this region requires an efficient mechanism to safely direct food into the esophagus. During the pharyngeal phase, the swallow is reflexive and involves a complex sequence of coordinated motions. The pharyngeal phase, which lasts for approximately 1 second, generally consists of the elevation of the entire pharyngeal tube,

including the larynx, followed by a descending peristaltic wave. In the adult, this action takes about 100 ms. Food is then injected from the pharynx into the esophagus forcefully, at velocities as high as 100 cm/s.[4,5] Approximately 600 to 900 ms after the onset of the pharyngeal phase, food passes through the upper esophageal sphincter (UES) and enters the esophagus. The cricopharyngeal (CP) muscle, the main component of the UES, relaxes for approximately 500 ms during the swallow to allow passage of the bolus.[6] Normal adults complete the swallow in approximately 1,500 ms[7]; timing data for children are not well described. Following pharyngeal transit, food enters the esophagus and is transported to the stomach via primary peristalsis. Additional discussions of normal and abnormal motility are given in the section on physiology and pathophysiology in Chapter 4, "Esophageal Motility."

UPPER ESOPHAGEAL SPHINCTER: NORMAL FUNCTION

The UES, also known as the pharyngoesophageal segment, is a manometrically defined high-pressure zone located in the region distal to the hypopharynx. Composed of striated muscle, the UES is tonically closed at rest and opens during swallowing, vomiting, or belching.[8] The length of the high-pressure zone in adults is from 2.5 to 4.5 cm, averaging about 3 cm.[8] The length of the CP muscle is about 1 cm; this muscle, therefore, although the main contributor to the UES, is not the only determinant of the high-pressure zone.[8–10] The relative contributions of the inferior pharyngeal constrictor muscle and the muscle fibers of the proximal esophagus to the upper sphincter remain controversial.[11,12]

The structure and function of the UES have been summarized by Lang and Shaker.[13] The cricopharyngeus is structurally and biochemically distinct from the pharyngeal and esophageal musculature. Compared with other striated muscles, the CP muscle is more elastic; it contains large amounts of endomysial connective tissue and sarcolemma, factors that contribute to this elasticity. The length at which the CP muscle reaches its maximal tension is 1.7 times its length; other striated muscles develop maximal tension at resting length. The arrangement of the muscle fibers (parallel and series) and fiber composition may account for the length tension properties. The cricopharyngeus muscle is composed of variably sized fibers that, unlike the fibers of other striated muscle, are not oriented in strict parallel fashion. The structure of the UES allows it to maintain constant basal tone and to rapidly relax during swallowing, belching, and vomiting.[13] The muscle fibers of the UES are not circumferential, but are attached at the anterior end to the lamina of the cricoid cartilage, which functions as the anterior sphincter wall. Because of this connection, the UES moves in conjunction with the laryngeal structures during deglutition.

The pressure profile of the UES is asymmetric, with higher pressures noted in the anterior and posterior directions.[14] Orientation of the recording device must take this into account when pressures are measured in this region. Sleeve manometry has been used to monitor UES pressure in children and to determine the influence of the state of arousal on sphincter pressure values.[15] Table 1 reports normal values for the pharyngoesophageal region of control infants, obtained by using a low-compliance, water-perfused manometry system in which the directional orientation of the catheter is maintained.[16] UES function, including values for UES pressure and relaxation, has also been evaluated in preterm infants greater than 33 weeks gestation.[17]

Neurologic control of the sphincter has been reviewed by Palmer[8] and by Lang and Shaker.[13] The CP muscle is innervated by the vagus nerve via the pharyngoesophageal, superior laryngeal,

Table 1 Pharyngoesophageal Manometric Measurements in Control Infants*		
Resting UES pressure (cm H$_2$O)	28.9 ± 10	(18.0−44.0)
Pharyngeal peristaltic wave		
Amplitude (cm H$_2$O)	74.7 ± 19.9	(37.0−102.0)
Velocity (cm/s)	8.5 ± 3.6	(3.2−15.0)
Duration (s)	0.59 ± 0.18	(0.3−0.86)

Reproduced with permission from reference 16.

UES = upper esophageal sphincter.

*Numbers are mean ± standard deviation; values in parentheses are ranges.

and recurrent laryngeal branches; the glossopharyngeal nerve; and the sympathetic nervous system via the cranial cervical ganglion. Based on functional studies, it is believed that the major motor nerve of the CP muscle is the pharyngoesophageal nerve. Vagal efferents probably reach the muscle by the pharyngeal plexus, using the pharyngeal branch of the vagi.[8] The superior laryngeal nerve may also contribute to motor control of the CP muscle.

Sensory information from the UES is probably provided by the glossopharyngeal nerve and the sympathetic nervous system. Although not completely understood, neurologic connections include visceral afferents that travel to the nucleus solitarius and from there to the nucleus ambiguus. There is probably little or no contribution by the sympathetic nervous system to CP control.[8,18]

The UES responds in a reflexive manner to a variety of stimuli. Balloon distention of the esophagus results in increased UES pressure, which is probably mediated by stimulation of esophageal intramural mechanoreceptors.[19] Motor responses of the UES to esophageal stimuli have been measured following intraesophageal infusion of graded air and liquids (distilled water and apple juice) in healthy preterm infants.[20] A volume-dependent increase in UES pressure was noted for air and liquids. This suggests that UES reflexes are present in the preterm infant to protect the supraesophageal structures. Earlier studies reported that acidification of the esophagus caused an increase in UES tone, suggesting that the UES functions to protect against aspiration following a reflux event. More recent studies have not confirmed this finding. In adult controls and in patients with reflux esophagitis, spontaneous episodes of reflux were not associated with an increase in UES pressure.[21] Similarly, esophageal acidification did not alter UES pressures in either group of individuals. A modified sleeve sensor manometric catheter for measuring UES pressures was used in the latter studies, which might account for differing results.

During deglutition, the function of the pharynx changes from that of an airway to that of a foodway. Simultaneous manometry and videofluorography allow investigators to observe intraluminal bolus movement and measure intraluminal pressures during the act of swallowing.[22,23] During the pharyngeal portion of the swallow, there is velopharyngeal closure, opening of the UES, closure of the laryngeal vestibule, and tongue loading. The bolus is propelled into the esophagus by tongue pulsion and pharyngeal clearance. During swallowing, UES relaxation is associated with upward and anterior motion of the cricoid cartilage, which is pulled in an anterior direction by motion of the hyoid bone and contraction of the thyrohyoid muscle.[24] The response of the UES during swallowing is not stereotypical but may be modified by varying bolus size[24]; as bolus volumes increase, the orad excursion of the UES, the opening of the UES, and the duration of sphincter relaxation all increase. These findings suggest that feedback receptors in the oral

cavity and pharynx provide afferent signals for modulating central nervous system impulses that give rise to the oral and pharyngeal phases of swallowing.[24]

Proposed functions of the UES include prevention of esophageal distention during normal breathing[8] and protection of the airway against aspiration following an episode of acid reflux.[25–27] As previously noted, the latter remains controversial in adults. Studies in infants have demonstrated that UES pressure increases in response to intraesophageal acidification, suggesting that in this group of patients, the UES may function as a dynamic barrier to acid reflux and may protect against aspiration.[16] However, there was no difference in resting UES pressures between control infants and infants with gastroesophageal reflux.[16] In some infants with pulmonary disease, the UES failed to respond following esophageal acidification. Others have documented qualitative abnormalities of UES function in infants with reflux disease.[28]

NEUROLOGY OF DEGLUTITION

Miller provides an excellent review of the neurophysiologic control of swallowing.[29] Swallowing may be evoked by stimulating many different central pathways, including the cortex (the region of the prefrontal gyri), the subcortex, and the brainstem. The swallowing center can be activated by afferent impulses from the cerebral cortex (voluntary swallowing) and from peripheral receptors in the mouth and pharynx (reflex swallowing). The corticobulbar impulses trigger and control the initial phases of swallowing but not the later esophageal stages. The cortex is not essential for the pharyngeal and esophageal phases of swallowing. In the human fetus, swallowing occurs prior to the time when the descending cortical-subcortical pathways have fully innervated the brainstem.[30] Deglutition has been noted to occur in infants, with loss of nervous tissue rostral to the midbrain.[31] Higher pathways, however, are important in allowing the voluntary elicitation of deglutition and in integrating facial and oral movements and other responses to swallowing.[1,29] The neurons important to the pharyngeal and esophageal phases of swallowing are located in different regions of the pons[32,33] and medulla.[1,34,35] Lesions placed in the medulla fractionate the sequence of muscle activity during pharyngeal swallowing, suggesting that interneurons located in this region are important to the pharyngeal and esophageal phases; these core interneurons are termed central pattern generators.[30,36] The deglutition center integrates afferent impulses and coordinates the activity of the motor nuclei of the fifth, seventh, tenth, and twelfth cranial nerves. Other activities, such as respiration, are inhibited during swallowing.[37] Swallowing may be evoked by stimulating the oropharyngeal regions innervated by the pharyngeal branches of the glossopharyngeal nerve (ninth cranial nerve) or by the superior laryngeal and recurrent laryngeal nerves of the vagus (tenth cranial nerve). Sensory fibers from these nerves

synapse in the nucleus tractus solitarius. Multiple receptive sites that elicit swallowing are present in the oral cavity and pharynx.[29] Once activated, the sequence of muscle activity during the pharyngeal phase remains the same in spite of altering the duration of this phase; this is termed a time-locked sequence.[38,39]

All phases of deglutition may be modified by sensory feedback, although each to a different degree. Oral phase activity is modulated by peripheral feedback received from the touch and pressure receptors in the oral cavity and from the mandible and temporomandibular joints.[40] Feedback from sensory receptors modifies the duration of the pharyngeal phase, the intensity of muscle activity, and the threshold necessary to evoke a response.[6,41–45] Sensory feedback may have therapeutic implications in the clinical management of the swallowing-impaired individual. For example, maintaining jaw control during deglutition may facilitate a safe swallow by improving feedback signals from the mandible or temporomandibular joints, whereas modifying the size of an oral bolus may favorably alter the motor response of the pharynx.

PRENATAL DEGLUTITION

Deglutition in utero occurs at approximately 16 to 17 weeks of gestation, although a pharyngeal swallow has been described in a delivered fetus at a gestational age of 12.5 weeks.[46] It is estimated that the normal fetus, at term, swallows approximately 500 to 1,000 mL of amniotic fluid per day. Based on animal studies, the ovine fetus swallows fluid volumes that are greater on a per-kilogram basis than those swallowed by the adult (100 to 300 mL/kg vs 40 to 60 mL/kg).[47] Fetal deglutition plays an important role in amniotic fluid resorption, helping to recirculate urine and lung fluid volumes to the fetus and maintain normal amniotic fluid volume.[48,49] Fetal swallowing may be influenced by a variety of factors, including neurobehavioral changes (such as hypoxia, hypotension, and plasma osmolality), fetal maturation, and volume of amniotic fluid.[47]

POSTNATAL DEVELOPMENT OF DEGLUTITION

Changes in Structure

Most changes in the size and relative location of components of the oral and pharyngeal cavities occur during the postnatal period.[50,51] In general, the central mobile elements of the oropharynx in the infant are large in comparison to their containing chambers. For example, the tongue is large compared to the oral cavity, and the arytenoid mass is nearly mature in size, in contrast to the small-sized vestibule and ventricle of the larynx (Figure 1).[51]

In the infant, the tongue lies entirely within the oral cavity, whereas the larynx is positioned high in the neck, resulting in a small oropharynx.[52]

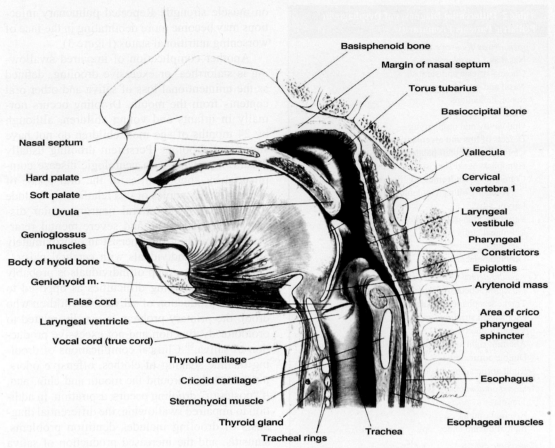

Figure 1 Drawing of postnatal anatomy of the oral and pharyngeal cavities (see text). (Reproduced with permission from reference 51.)

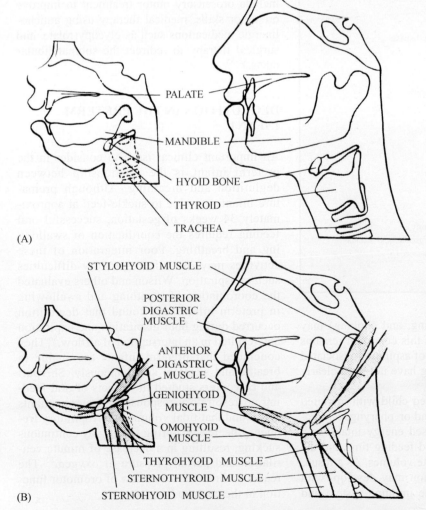

Figure 2 (A) Drawing of infant and adult anatomy shows alteration in shape and orientation of the pharynx that accompanies growth and the descent of the larynx. Laryngeal cartilages and hyoid bone are shown in their relationship to the mandible. The airway is depicted (hatched area). (B) Drawing illustrates change in orientation of muscles (stippled) that suspend the larynx in the infant and the adult. (Reproduced with permission from reference 51.)

Between 2 and 4 years of age, the tongue begins to descend so that by approximately 9 years of age, its posterior third is present in the neck.[52] The larynx also moves in a caudal direction. The larynx descends from the level of the third to the fourth cervical body during the prenatal period, an arrangement that persists during infancy.[53] During childhood, the larynx descends to a level opposite the sixth vertebra and finally to the seventh cervical vertebra level in adulthood. As maturation progresses, the face vertically elongates, and the chambers of the oral cavity and oropharynx enlarge (Figure 2).[51,54]

Developmental Changes in Feeding Behavior

The development of normal feeding behavior in the infant and child has been reviewed in detail.[51,54] Briefly, in the normal infant, the oral phase of swallowing is characterized by a pattern known as suckle-feeding. Developmental changes in the relationship between suck and swallow, such as the suck-to-swallow ratio and differing rhythmic patterns, have been described in the preterm and term infant.[55,56] Feeding behavior in preterm infants has been assessed by using recording devices to measure pharyngeal pressure, oxygen saturation, heart rate, and nasal airflow. Sucking pressure, frequency, and duration were noted to mature with increases in postconceptual age. In younger infants, swallowing occurred during pauses in respiration but, after 35 weeks of age, occurred mainly at the end of inspiration.[57] Suckle-feeding is followed by the development of transitional feeding (ages 6 to 36 months) and eventually mature feeding, characterized by biting and chewing. Maturation of feeding behavior occurs mainly as a result of central nervous system development, with motor activity being directed by higher centers such as the thalamus and cerebral cortex.[54]

Nutritive and Nonnutritive Sucking

The pattern of nutritive sucking is characterized by a series of short bursts and pauses, occurring at approximately one suck per second.[58] Nonnutritive sucking is defined as rhythmic movements on a nonfeeding nipple. The patterns of nonnutritive and nutritive sucking differ. In nonnutritive sucking, short bursts and pauses occur at a faster frequency.[58] Interestingly, nonnutritive sucking may improve weight gain during gavage feeding in preterm infants. Bernbaum and others studied the nutritional effects of nonnutritive sucking in a group of low birth weight infants receiving formula by an enteral tube and found that, compared with control infants, the group engaging in nonnutritive sucking gained relatively more weight.[59] The mechanism accounting for this weight gain is not clear, although it has been hypothesized that non-nutritive sucking results in more efficient nutrient absorption or a decrease in energy requirements secondary to a lessening of infant activity or restlessness.[60,61]

Nonnutritive sucking may have effects on pulmonary function as well. In preterm infants, nonnutritive sucking is associated with increased transcutaneous oxygen tension and respiratory frequency.[62,63] In contrast, lowered oxygen tension may occur during nutritive sucking, although the mechanism for this effect remains unclear and may not be related to the action of sucking per se.[63]

DISORDERS OF DEGLUTITION IN THE PEDIATRIC PATIENT: CLINICAL OVERVIEW

In the pediatric age group, swallowing disorders rarely present as isolated problems but more often occur in infants and children with multiple impairments. Although accurate epidemiologic data are lacking, underlying conditions that predispose to impaired swallowing in childhood include central and peripheral nervous system dysfunction, disease of muscle, and structural anomalies of the oral cavity and pharynx. Structural and motor disorders of the esophagus, which may also present with dysphagia, are discussed elsewhere in the text. Other groups at risk for the development of impaired swallowing and its complications include premature infants with poor coordination of breathing and swallowing, infants with long-term deprivation of oral feeding, and infants with chronic pulmonary disease. The spectrum of pediatric swallowing disorders has been reviewed in detail by others.[51,54,64–69] Table 2 provides a broad list of disorders that result in impaired deglutition in the pediatric age group.[70]

COMPLICATIONS OF IMPAIRED DEGLUTITION

Respiratory complications of impaired swallowing have been reviewed; they include apnea and bradycardia, choking episodes, chronic noisy breathing, reactive airway disease, chronic or recurrent pneumonia, bronchitis, and atelectasis.[71] Aspiration of oral contents may occur directly, that is, in association with a swallow that does not protect the airway. In addition, some patients may be unable to protect the airway from the aspiration of oral secretions. Aspiration may also occur in individuals with impaired swallowing after an episode of gastroesophageal reflux; also, acid reflux may result in bronchospasm, pneumonia, or apnea.[72–74] Aspiration in association with an episode of refluxed gastric contents may occur in individuals with impaired swallowing and occasionally in children without neurologic difficulties.[75]. Isolated swallowing dysfunction has been described in neurologically-intact term infants.[76] This entity is reported to have a good long-term prognosis, although infants may need prolonged nutritional support with enteral feeding provided by gastrostomy tubes.

Unfortunately, in the swallowing-impaired child (and adult), it may be difficult to detect aspiration based on clinical signs and symptoms alone because "silent aspiration" (aspiration

Table 2 Differential Diagnoses of Dysphagia in Pediatric Patients Prematurity

Upper airway-foodway anomalies
  Nasal and nasopharyngeal
  Choanal atresia and stenosis
  Nasal and sinus infections
  Septal deflections
  Tumors
  Oral cavity and oropharynx
  Defects of lips and alveolar processes
  Cleft lip and/or cleft palate
  Hypopharyngeal stenosis and webs
  Craniofacial syndromes (eg, Pierre Robin, Crouzon, Treacher Collins, Goldenhar)
  Laryngeal
  Laryngeal stenosis and webs
  Laryngeal clefts
  Laryngeal paralysis
  Laryngomalacia

Congenital defects of the larynx, trachea, and esophagus
  Laryngotracheoesophageal cleft
  Tracheoesophageal fistula/esophageal atresia
  Esophageal strictures and webs
  Vascular anomalies
  Aberrant right subclavian artery (dysphagia lusorum)
  Double aortic arch
  Right aortic arch with left ligamentum

Acquired anatomic defects
  Trauma
  External trauma
  Intubation and endoscopy

Neurologic defects
  Central nervous system disease
  Head trauma
  Hypoxic brain damage
  Cortical atrophy, microcephaly, anencephaly
  Infections (eg, meningitis, brain abscess)
  Myelomeningocele
  Chiari malformation
  Peripheral nervous system disease
  Traumatic
  Congenital
  Neuromuscular disease
  Myotonic muscular dystrophy
  Myasthenia gravis
  Guillain-Barré syndrome
  Poliomyelitis (bulbar paralysis)
  Miscellaneous
  Achalasia
  Cricopharyngeal achalasia
  Esophageal spasm
  Esophagitis
  Dysautonomia
  Paralysis of esophagus (atony)
  Tracheoesophageal fistula/esophageal atresia– associated nerve defects
  Aberrant cervical thymus
  Conversion dysphagia

without coughing, gagging, and choking) may occur. The prevalence of this condition remains unknown, and predictors of aspiration associated with impaired swallowing have not been clearly defined.

In the severely affected child with impaired swallowing, poor oral and/or pharyngeal function may lead to decreased energy intake as a consequence of prolonged feeding time and the inability to ingest adequate volumes. As a result, protein-energy malnutrition may develop, with deleterious effects on the immune system and

on muscle strength. Repeated pulmonary infections may become more debilitating in the face of worsening nutritional status (Figure 3).

Another complication of impaired swallowing is sialorrhea, or excessive drooling, defined as the unintentional loss of saliva and other oral contents from the mouth. Drooling occurs normally in infants and young children, although by 24 months of age most children do not have significant drooling. Persistent drooling usually occurs in patients with neurologic disease complicated by abnormalities of the oral phase of deglutition. Examples of this relationship include cerebral palsy, peripheral neuromuscular disease, facial paralysis, and severe mental retardation.[77] Drooling may persist in approximately 10 to 38% of individuals with cerebral palsy.[78] Drooling in this group of individuals is probably related to swallowing difficulties as opposed to increased production of saliva.[79] In children who drool, the primary problem is usually related to oromotor dysfunction and not excessive production of saliva.[80] Clinical complications of drooling include soaking of clothes, offensive odors, macerated skin around the mouth and chin, and, if "posterior" drooling occurs, aspiration. In addition to impaired swallowing, the differential diagnosis of drooling includes dentition problems, sinusitis, and the increased production of saliva by the salivary glands. Excellent reviews of this subject include those by Blasco and colleagues[77] and Bailey.[81]

Therapy for the control of drooling may include orosensory motor treatment to improve oromotor skills, medical therapy using anticholinergic medications such as glycopyrrolate, and surgical therapy to redirect the submandibular ducts.[82–85]

DEGLUTITION IN THE PRETERM INFANT

An important clinical issue to consider in the preterm infant is the relationship between deglutition and breathing. Although premature infants are able to suckle-feed at approximately 34 weeks of gestation, successful oral feeding requires the coordination of swallowing and breathing. Poor integration of these activities may result in respiratory difficulties such as aspiration. Wilson and others evaluated the coordination of breathing and swallowing in preterm infants and found that deglutition occurred during both inspiration and expiration and resulted in an interruption of airflow.[86] They concluded that preterm infants are unable to breathe and swallow simultaneously. Shivpuri and coworkers studied the effects of oral feeding on respiratory response in preterm infants and found that tidal volume and respiratory frequency decreased during feeding by continuous sucking, resulting in a decrease of minute ventilation and partial pressure of oxygen.[83] The reader is directed to a review of oromotor function in the neonate.[87]

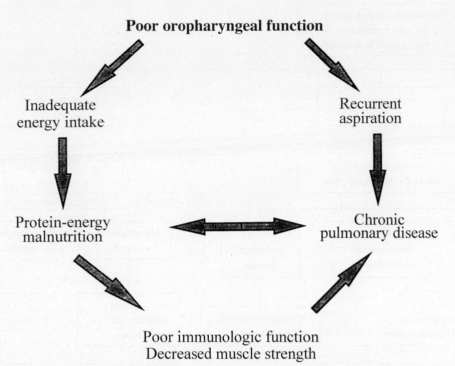

Poor oropharyngeal function

Inadequate
energy intake

Recurrent
aspiration

Protein-energy
malnutrition

Chronic
pulmonary disease

Poor immunologic function
Decreased muscle strength

Figure 3 Clinical sequelae of impaired deglutition. (mouth, thick secretions, urinary retention, flushing) may occur, but these are usually controlled by titrating the dose of medication. Surgical therapy that redirects the flow of saliva posteriorly may increase the flow of liquid to an already compromised swallow and potentially increase the risk of aspiration.

CRITICAL PERIOD OF LEARNING

A critical period of development refers to a segment of time during maturation when a specific stimulus must be applied to produce a particular action. Inadequate oral stimulation during a critical period may result in difficulty in reestablishing successful oral feeding at a later date. The concept of a critical or sensitive period pertaining to feeding behavior has been reviewed by Illingworth and Lister,[85] and cases of infants and children developing resistance to oral feeding after long-term deprivation of oral stimulation have been reported.[86,88] Successful treatment of this problem has been accomplished by a multidisciplinary feeding team using a behavioral approach.[89]

ISOLATED CP DYSFUNCTION AND CP ACHALASIA

CP dysfunction is usually part of a more global disorder of deglutition also involving the oral phase.[10] CP function may be altered by conditions that affect the central nervous system or cranial nerve function or by conditions that locally involve the function of the muscle or movement of the larynx. Achalasia, meaning failure to relax, does not always accurately describe the type of CP dysfunction present. Nonrelaxation of the sphincter resulting from primary CP disease differs from nonopening of the sphincter secondary to weak forces of propulsion in the proximal pharynx.[34]

Isolated CP dysfunction or achalasia is a rare disorder in infants and children.[90–92] Most patients with CP achalasia present at birth with feeding difficulties, although some may present as late as 6 months of age. Drug-induced dysfunction of the UES has also been reported.[93]

The diagnosis of isolated CP dysfunction is difficult when based solely on radiographic studies. A horizontal bar in the proximal esophagus, representing the CP muscle, may be seen in up to 5% of adults undergoing radiographic examinations for all indications and may also be a normal radiologic sign in infants.[94,95] In some patients with a prominent bar seen on radiographic study, manometric studies have demonstrated normal relaxation and decreased UES pressure.[37,92] Alternatively, manometric studies may be normal in patients with clinical or radiologic evidence of CP dysfunction.[37,96,97] Improvement of CP achalasia may occur spontaneously or after dilatation.[97,98] In some cases, CP myotomy may be required after careful assessment of the patient[99]; surgery is usually contraindicated in patients with gastroesophageal reflux or poor pharyngeal peristalsis.

CLINICAL ASSESSMENT

In clinical practice, disorders of swallowing are often considered in the general context of a feeding disorder. Feeding is a complex process that involves a number of phases in addition to the act of swallowing, including the recognition of hunger (appetite), the acquisition of food, and the ability to bring the food to the mouth. The causes of feeding disorders have been extensively reviewed.[96] The classification of feeding disorders includes the broad categories of abnormalities of structure and function, neurologic disorders, and behavioral feeding disorders.[100]

In the spectrum of feeding disorders, food refusal is a common complaint, but a precise definition of food refusal is not well established. Food refusal may be defined as the developmentally inappropriate intake of food (quality or quantity) for more than 8 weeks (R Wachtel, oral communication, March 1998). Associated symptoms may include behavioral problems such as unusual behaviors at meal-time, an abnormal feeding pattern, and mealtimes that are stressful for the family and child. Food refusal may be secondary to a variety of conditions, including impaired swallowing, mucosal disease of the gastrointestinal tract (eg, reflux esophagitis), behavioral difficulties, and chronic disease (eg, renal, cardiac, and endocrine disease).

Successful evaluation and management of the pediatric patient with impaired swallowing and/or a feeding disorder usually require a multidisciplinary approach. Members of a pediatric "dysphagia" or "feeding" team may include a pediatrician, pediatric gastroenterologist, developmental pediatrician, speech-language pathologist, occupational therapist, and pediatric dietitian. The availability of a pediatric radiologist and an otolaryngologist with experience in the field of pediatric swallowing disorders is essential to assist in the diagnostic evaluation.

The American Gastroenterological Association has published a medical position statement on the management of oropharyngeal dysphagia,[101] and an excellent technical review on the management of oropharyngeal dysphagia accompanies this article.[102] Although concerned mainly with the evaluation and management of adults with dysphagia, the clinical objectives of this statement are applicable to children. The main objectives include the following: (1) determine whether oropharyngeal dysphagia is present and, if so, attempt to identify the etiology; (2) identify the structural etiologies of oropharyngeal dysphagia; (3) determine the functional integrity of the swallow; (4) evaluate the risk of aspiration; and (5) determine if the pattern of dysphagia is amenable to therapy. An algorithm for the evaluation and management of the pediatric patient with possible impaired swallowing is shown in Figure 4.

FEEDING HISTORY

The diagnostic approach to the pediatric patient with impaired swallowing begins with the feeding history, but obtaining an accurate feeding history may be difficult for a number of reasons.[103] First, pediatric patients with severe impairment of swallowing frequently include many with limited cognitive abilities, making direct communication with the patient difficult. As a result, the feeding history must be obtained from individuals directly involved in caring for the child, such as a parent or feeding specialist (eg, a speech-language pathologist or an occupational therapist). Second, severely handicapped children with impaired swallowing may aspirate without coughing, a

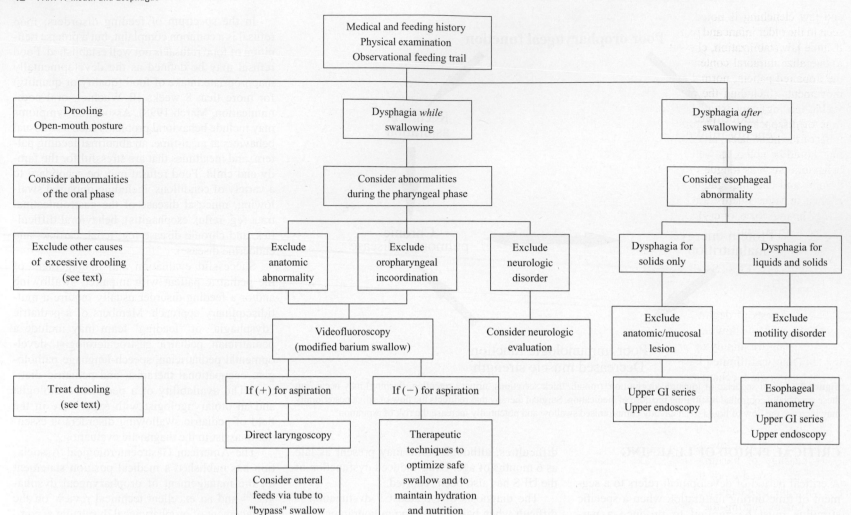

Figure 4 Algorithm for evaluation and management of the pediatric patient with impaired swallowing. GI = gastrointestinal.

phenomenon known as silent aspiration (a similar condition has been described in adults).[104–106] Consequently, it is difficult to accurately predict which food substances are swallowed without aspiration solely on the basis of feeding history or clinical examination.

Areas covered in the feeding history include caretakers involved; location or setting for feeding (the nature of which may differ depending on the location, eg, school versus home); method of feeding (eg, type of feeding utensils used); position of the head, neck, and body during feeding; volume of food offered and volume of food tolerated per swallow; presence or absence of chewing; amount of time required to feed; history of dysphagia or odynophagia; presence or absence of drooling (suggestive of oral phase abnormalities); and history of gagging, choking, or coughing associated with feeding. Determining whether these symptoms occur before, during, or after the swallow helps localize the affected phase.[104] Symptoms that occur prior to the swallow suggest abnormalities of oral control; those that occur during the swallow may indicate pharyngeal phase dysfunction, and gagging and choking just after completion of the swallow probably represent abnormalities of pharyngeal clearance secondary to pharyngeal muscle weakness and/or incoordination or dysfunction of the UES.

In addition to a feeding history, a complete nutritional assessment is essential. Clinical goals should include deter-mining the patient's current nutritional status, estimating energy and protein requirements for establishing optimal growth, and outlining a plan for providing the route and type of feeding. Consultation with a pediatric dietitian will aid in planning a comprehensive nutritional program.

PHYSICAL EXAMINATION

Physical examination should include the structures of the face, oral cavity, and oropharynx. If structural abnormalities are found and/or are suspected in the pharynx, consultation with an otolaryngologist is indicated. Careful attention should be paid to (1) the presence of an intact soft and hard palate, (2) whether the tongue is midline, (3) the size of the tongue relative to the size of the oral cavity (eg, macroglossia), and (4) the size of the mandible (eg, Pierre Robin syndrome). Head control and head and neck position, particularly when feeding, are also important to note during the examination. It is extremely difficult to swallow with a hyperextended neck, a factor that may be important in the patient with neuromuscular disease (eg, cerebral palsy).

The presence or absence of a gag reflex should be noted, including the existence of a "hyperactive" gag reflex. Lack of a gag reflex is a contraindication to oral feeding, whereas a hyperactive gag may result in significant feeding difficulties. "Hypersensitivity" may involve just the face or oral cavity or may be more pervasive. In infants, oral hypersensitivity is suggested by an aversion to nipple-feeding. In older children, irritability with oral activities such as toothbrushing may suggest hypersensitivity. Children with generalized hypersensitivity may become irritable with any type of sensory stimulation (touch, sound, etc). Issues related to hypersensitivity may be seen in children with developmental disabilities such as autism and cerebral palsy.

OBSERVATIONAL FEEDING TRIAL

The diagnostic yield of an observational feeding trial is greatly enhanced if the trial is performed in collaboration with a feeding therapist. During the initial part of the feeding trial, oromotor function is tested by determining the presence or absence of age-appropriate oromotor skills. The acquisition of oral feeding skills and their development have been reviewed in detail by others.[50,107–111] During the feeding trial, the presence of abnormal movements such as jaw thrust, tongue thrust, tonic bite reflex, and jaw clenching is noted. Normal movements seen in the older infant and retained into adulthood include jaw stabilization, chewing, and the ability to lateralize intraoral contents with the tongue. In the impaired patient, normal primitive reflexes or movements (including the phasic bite reflex and suckle-feeding) may extend beyond their expected time of disappearance. During feeding, the positions of the head, neck, and body during swallowing should be noted, as well as abnormal feeding behaviors (such as tongue thrust and averting the mouth) and choking, gagging, or ruminating. A change in voice quality after feeding (such as a "wet," hoarse voice, or cry) suggests soiling of the larynx or aspiration.

DIAGNOSTIC TESTS OF SWALLOWING FUNCTION

Specialized tests of deglutition allow broad categorization of swallowing abnormalities. These examinations are mainly descriptive and provide the clinician with limited data regarding specific pathophysiologic mechanisms.

Videofluoroscopy

Videofluoroscopy, or the modified barium swallow, examines swallowing function by visualizing passage of barium-impregnated liquids, pastes, and pureed foods through the oral cavity, pharynx, and esophagus. This is the procedure of choice for evaluating the patient with impaired swallowing[105,111–113] and provides the best means of determining oral, pharyngeal, and esophageal anatomy and function. This study provides objective evidence of oral and pharyngeal incoordination and detects episodes of aspiration, all of which help identify children in whom oral feeding may be contraindicated. Clinical evaluation by experienced therapists has also been shown to be accurate in detection of fluid aspiration and penetration but, compared to videofluoroscopy, may not be as accurate at detecting aspiration of solids.[114] Videofluoroscopy is usually performed by a feeding therapist, either a speech-language pathologist or an occupational therapist, in conjunction with a pediatric radiologist. During this procedure, a variety of foods, feeding utensils, and different positions of the head and neck are evaluated to help determine optimal and safe swallowing. Using videofluoroscopy, it is possible to determine whether aspiration occurs prior to, during, or following deglutition.[111] Protection of the airway prior to the swallow is dependent on oropharyngeal coordination and laryngeal elevation. Protection during the pharyngeal phase of swallowing is a result of closure of the laryngeal vestibule secondary to laryngeal elevation, closure of the false vocal cords, and anterior tilting of the arytenoids. Following deglutition, pharyngeal clearance mechanisms help prevent aspiration. The clinical significance of small amounts of aspiration noted on videofluoroscopy deglutition remains unknown. Videofluoroscopy is valuable in the management of swallowing-impaired

patients because it aids in determining the bolus characteristics of food that make food safe to swallow (ie, bolus size and consistency).[105] The disadvantages of this procedure include exposure to radiation and lack of quantitative data regarding the function of oral and pharyngeal structures during deglutition. Note that a complete videofluoroscopic examination should include esophagography to evaluate the esophageal phase of swallowing.

Pharyngeal Manometry

Manometry provides quantitative data regarding pharyngeal motor function during deglutition, including the amplitude of peristalsis, the speed of propagation of the pharyngeal wave, the response of the UES following deglutition, and the coordination between pharyngeal peristalsis and UES relaxation.[16,28] Recording the response of the pharyngoesophageal region during deglutition is complicated by a number of factors.[111] First, because motor events in the hypopharynx occur at a more rapid rate than in the esophagus, recording equipment with a rapid response time (usually greater than 300 mm Hg/s) is required.[115] Water-perfused catheters with rapid response times are acceptable, but intraluminal pressure transducers provide the most accurate readings. Second, the asymmetric pressure profile of the UES requires that close attention be given to the spatial orientation of the recording device while recording in the UES. Third, there is significant differential axial movement of the recording catheter and oropharyngeal structures during deglutition, which may result in a significant recording artifact.[116,117] A sleeve sensor has been used to monitor UES pressures over time to minimize the effects of catheter and sphincter movement.[46] Manometry does not provide information regarding intraluminal events, such as the movement of fluid in response to recorded pressure changes. The simultaneous recording of videofluoroscopic images and manometric tracings has allowed investigators to correlate motor events with intraluminal movement of substances.[24,118,119]

Ultrasonography

Ultrasonography represents a relatively new diagnostic modality for the evaluation of the swallowing-impaired individual.[120] The motion of structures in the oral cavity such as the tongue and floor of the mouth may be imaged during feeding and deglutition by placing a transducer in the submental region and aiming the beam toward the tongue. This technique has been used to identify feeding movements of oral structures in healthy breastfed and bottle-fed infants.[121] The disadvantages of ultrasonography include poor visualization of the oropharynx (secondary to an acoustic shadow cast by bony structures in the neck) and the lack of standardized measurements.

Nuclear Scintigraphy

Nuclear scintigraphy involves the patient's swallowing a liquid or solid that is labeled with

a radiopharmaceutical. Technetium-99m, the radionuclide used in swallowing and esophageal scintigraphic studies, is not absorbed after oral administration and does not become attached to gastrointestinal mucosa. Using a gamma counter and computer processing, regions of interest and selection of time intervals are generated that allow the measurement of transit time and the estimation of intraluminal volumes. Exposure to radiation is less than during analogous fluoroscopic procedures. Problems include poor resolution of the image and poor localization. The technique of nuclear scintigraphy has been reviewed by Cowan.[122] Based on a case report, the radionuclide salivagram has also been used to document aspiration of saliva.[123]

Scintigraphy has been used in adults to assess transit of a liquid bolus through the oropharynx.[124–126] Silver and colleagues attempted to use nuclear scintigraphy to detect and quantify aspiration.[127] Unfortunately, this technique proved to have poor sensitivity for detecting aspiration during swallowing in known aspirators. At present, clinical experience with this technique as a test of swallowing function in children is limited.

Other Tests of Swallowing

Using a stethoscope applied to the neck, the technique of cervical auscultation has been used to study the sounds of swallowing in adults and children.[128,129] Sounds denoting pathologic swallowing have been identified. Cervical auscultation is a noninvasive technique, although the limitations include a lack of standardized measurements and reliance on subjective descriptions of sounds. Recently, workers have performed digital signal processing using an accelerometer placed over the neck to graphically display and quantitatively measure sounds.[129]

A new technique, known as fiberoptic endoscopic evaluation of swallowing safety, allows clinicians to directly observe movements of the anatomic structures involved in the pharyngeal phase of swallowing.[130,131] Using this method, laryngeal penetration (material entering the laryngeal vestibule) and aspiration (material falling below the glottis) can be directly visualized. Episodes can be characterized as occurring prior to and/or following the swallow. Using videotape recording, images obtained during endoscopic evaluation of swallowing provide reproducibility and the ability to closely visualize swallowing events.[132]

A related technique, called fiberoptic evaluation of swallowing with sensory testing (FESST), combines endoscopic evaluation of swallowing with a method that determines laryngopharyngeal sensation.[133] This technique has also been used in children for evaluation of pediatric swallowing disorders.[134] Testing laryngeal sensation may also be performed in noncooperative individuals or in those without appropriate cognitive skills.[135]

FESST involves testing the "swallow reflex" which is also known as the laryngeal adductor response. This reflex is initiated by mechanical or chemical stimulation of the laryngeal mucosa, more specifically the supraglottic mucosa in the region of the aryepiglottic fold. The motor response results in closure of the glottis and inhibition of respiration and swallowing. The reflex arc includes sensory information transmitted via the superior laryngeal and glossopharyngeal nerves to the nodose ganglion and subsequently to the nucleus solitarius. The motor response originates at the nucleus ambiguous with impulses traveling via the glossopharyngeal nerve with resultant closure of the glottis and inhibition of respiration with or without swallowing. Testing laryngeal sensation may be important because abnormalities of laryngeal sensation and/or motor response are associated with an alteration of laryngeal protective mechanisms and can lead to complications such as aspiration following an episode of gastroesophageal reflux. The swallow reflex and means of testing for an alteration of laryngeal sensitivity have been reviewed.[136]

It has been suggested that impaired laryngeal sensation may occur as a result of repeated exposure of the laryngeal mucosa to gastric contents secondary to repeated episodes of gastroesophageal reflux. In a retrospective study, Suskind and colleagues evaluated infants with gastroesophageal reflux disease (GERD) and dysphagia and aspiration using flexible endoscopic evaluation of swallowing and sensation testing (FEESST) and/or videofluoroscopy.[137] Following treatment of GERD (either medical or surgical), there was improvement in swallowing function and sensory testing suggesting a causal relationship between laryngopharyngeal reflux (LPR) of gastric contents and decreased laryngeal sensation.

Using the endoscope, air–pulse stimuli are delivered to the pharyngeal mucosa, which is innervated by the superior laryngeal nerves. This allows determination of discrimination thresholds. Laryngopharyngeal sensory capacity is determined by elicitation of the laryngeal adductor reflex, which is a sensorimotor reflex. In adults, FESST is performed at the bedside and has been used as the initial swallowing evaluation for the patient with dysphagia.

TREATMENT

Treatment plans should be developed in the context of a multidisciplinary group. Specific treatment of oral and pharyngeal dysfunction in the neurologically impaired child is not always possible, nor is surgical therapy frequently indicated. Different types of treatment modalities have been discussed in detail by others.[102,134–138] Management techniques involve devising compensatory strategies to minimize swallowing-related complications.[139] Because swallowing abnormalities arise from a diverse group of underlying disorders, management techniques must be individualized. This heterogeneity is also reflected in the fact that patients have differing potentials for recovery. In the patient with

acquired brain injury secondary to head trauma, rehabilitation with possible reacquisition of swallowing skills is a major goal; in contrast, compensatory and adaptive maneuvers form the basis for managing the child with severe cerebral palsy.

The management of dysphagia must be considered in the context of the child's level of development and cognitive abilities. The inability of a child to follow directions limits therapeutic maneuvers to passive procedures (eg, bolus modification). Children with intact cognition have the potential to become actively involved with their therapy and learn specific procedures shown to be effective in promoting a safe swallow (eg, the supraglottic swallow procedure).

In general, therapeutic recommendations are based on the patient's ability to swallow safely (ie, the ability of the patient to transfer food from the oral cavity into the esophagus without entry into the larynx or tracheal airway), the patient's nutritional status, the presence of gastroesophageal reflux, and the enjoyment of feeding for parents and the patient.

For a complete discussion of techniques used to facilitate oromotor function in swallowing-impaired infants and children who are receiving some form of either oral feeding or oral stimulation, the reader is referred to Mueller,[110] Morris,[10,9,140,141] and Ottenbacher and colleagues.[142] Many techniques seek to reduce tactile hypersensitivity, stabilize body position, and optimize the motor response of the oral swallowing mechanism. Modification of the physical characteristics of an oral

bolus remains an important part of therapy. The rheologic properties of food have been measured and described.[3] Table 3 lists some management options used for children with impaired swallowing.[143] It should be noted that because of a paucity of well-controlled clinical trials, the use of many of these therapeutic maneuvers remains empiric.

REFERENCES

1. Miller AJ. Deglutition. Physiol Rev 1982;62:129–84.
2. Morrell RM. The neurology of swallowing. In: Groher ME, editor. Dysphagia and Management. Boston: Butterworths; 1984. p. 3.
3. Coster ST, Schwarz WH. Rheology and the swallow-safe bolus. Dysphagia 1987;1:113–8.
4. Buthpitiva AG, Stroud D, Russell COH. Pharyngeal pump and esophageal transit. Dig Dis Sci 1987;32:1244–8.
5. Fisher MA, Hendrix TR, Hunt JN, Murrills AJ. Relation betweenvolume swallowed and velocity of the bolus ejected from the pharynx into the esophagus. Gastroenterology 1978;74: 1238–40.
6. Shipp T, Deatsch WW, Robertson K. Pharyngo-esophageal muscle activity during swallowing in man. Laryngoscope 1970; 80:1–16.
7. Curtis DJ, Cruess DF, Dachman AH, Maso E. Timing in the normal pharyngeal swallow: Prospective selection and evaluation of 16 normal asymptomatic patients. Invest Radiol 1984;19:523–9.
8. Palmer ED. Disorders of the cricopharyngeus muscle: A review. Gastroenterology 1976;71:510–9.
9. Ellis FH, Jr. Upper esophageal sphincter in health and disease. Surg Clin North Am 1971;51:553–65.
10. Goyal RK. Disorders of the cricopharyngeus muscle. Otolaryngol Clin North Am 1984;17:115–30.
11. Asoh R, Goyal RK. Manometry and electromyography of the upper esophageal sphincter in the opossum. Gastroenterology 1978;74:514–20.
12. Welch RW, et al. Manometry of the normal upper esophageal sphincter and its alteration in laryngectomy. J Clin Invest 1979;63:1036–41.

Table 3 Impaired Swallowing: Management Techniques	
	Desired effect
Postural changes	
Adjust position of head, neck, and, body during deglutition	Optimize muscle function
Provide jaw control and stabilization during deglutition	Position bolus in oral cavity
Chin tuck	Position bolus anteriorly and narrow airway entrance
Tilting head to stronger side	Gravitation forces direct bolus to the stronger side
Head rotation to affected side	Takes advantage of stronger muscles on unaffected side to improve pharyngeal transfer
Alteration of the oral bolus	
Modify volume and physical properties of oral bolus (e.g., viscosity, temperature)	Optimize oral control of bolus
Swallowing maneuver	
Proper intra-oral bolus placement	Position bolus in oral cavity
Tongue resistance/range of motion	Improve tongue control
Sensitization techniques	Decrease oral hypersensitivity/Increase oral hyposensitivity using thermal sensitization/stimulation
Multiple swallows	Residue is cleared with repeated effort
Supra-glottic swallow	Close vocal cords and arytenoids, approximate adducted arytenoids to base of epiglottis. Cough expels any contents which may have penetrated airway
Provide alternate means of enteral nutrition	
Use of valved feeding bottle	Replicates suckle feeding
Naso-gastric tube feeding	Provides hydration and nutrition – short term
Placement of gastrostomy tube (surgical or percutaneous endoscopic)	Provides hydration and nutrition – long term
Surgery	
Cricopharyngeal myotomy	Reduce or abolish resistance to flow of the bolus from the pharynx into the. esophagus

13. Lang IM, Shaker R. Anatomy and physiology of the upper esophageal sphincter. Am J Med 1997;103:50S–5S.
14. Winans CS. The pharyngoesophageal closure mechanism: A manometric study. Gastroenterology 1972;63:768–77.
15. Davidson GP, Dent J, Willing J. Monitoring of upper oesophageal sphincter pressure in children. Gut 1991;32: 607–11.
16. Sondheimer JM. Upper esophageal sphincter and pharyngeal motor function in infants with and without gastroesophageal reflux. Gastroenterology 1983;85:301–5.
17. Omari T, Snel A, Barnett C, et al. Measurement of upper esophageal sphincter tone and relaxation during swallowing in premature infants. Am J Physiol 1999;277: G862–6.
18. Parrish RM. Cricopharyngeus dysfunction and acute dysphagia. Can Med Assoc J 1968;99:1167–71.
19. Gerhardt DC, et al. Human upper esophageal sphincter: response to volume, osmotic, and acid stimuli. Gastroenterology 1978;75:268–74.
20. Jadcherla SR, Duong HQ, Hoffmann RG, Shaker R. Esophageal body and upper esophageal motor responses to esophageal provocation during maturation in preterm newborns. J Pediatr 2003;143:31–8.
21. Vakil NB, Kahrilas PJ, Dodds WJ, Vanagunas A. Absence of an upper esophageal sphincter response to acid reflux. Am J Gastroenterol 1989;84:606–10.
22. Kharilas PJ. Upper esophageal sphincter function during antegrade and retrograde transit. Am J Med 1997;103: 56S–60S.
23. Kahrilas PJ, Logemann JA, Lin S, Ergun GA. Pharyngeal clearance during swallowing: A combined manometric and video-fluoroscopic study. Gastroenterology 1992; 103:128–36.
24. Kahrilas PJ, Dodds WJ, Dent J, et al. Upper esophageal sphincter function during deglutition. Gastroenterology 1988;95:52–62.
25. Hunt PS, Connell AM, Smiley TB. The cricopharyngeal sphincter in gastric reflux. Gut 1970;11:303–6.
26. Gerhardt DC, Shuck TS, Bordeaux RA, Winship DH. Human upper esophageal sphincter: Response to volume, osmotic, and acid stimuli. Gastroenterology 1978;75:268–74.
27. Winship DH. Upper esophageal sphincter: Does it care about reflux? Gastroenterology 1983;85:470–2.
28. Staiano A, Cucchiara S, De Vizia B, et al. Disorders of upper esophageal motility in children. J Pediatr Gastroenterol Nutr 1987;6:892–8.
29. Miller AJ. Neurophysiological basis of swallowing. Dysphagia 1986;1:91 100.
30. Doty RW. Neural organization of deglutition. In: Code CF, editor. Handbook of Physiology, Alimentary Canal. Washington, DC: American Psychological Society; 1968. p. 1861–902.
31. Utter O. Ein fall von anensephalie. Acta Psychiatr Neurol 1928; 3:281–318.
32. Car A, Jean A, Roman C. A pontine primary relay for ascending projections of the superior laryngeal nerve. Exp Brain Res 1975;22:197–210.
33. Sumi T. Reticular ascending activation of frontal cortical neurons in rabbits with special reference to the regulation of deglutition. Brain Res 1972;46:43–54.
34. Car A, Roman C. Deglutitions et contractions oesophaglennes reflexes produit par la stimulation du bulke Rachidien. Exp Brain Res 1970;11:75–92.
35. Miller AJ. Characteristics of the swallowing reflex induced by peripheral nerve and brain stem stimulation. Exp Neurol 1972;34:210–20.
36. Doty RW. Influence of stimulus pattern on reflex deglutition. Am J Physiol 1951;166:142–58.
37. Hellemans J, Pelemans W, Vantrappen G. Pharyngoesophageal swallowing disorders and the pharyngoesophageal sphincter. Med Clin North Am 1981;65:1149–71.
38. Doty RW, Bosma JF. An electromyographic analysis of reflex deglutition. J Neurophysiol 1956;19:44–60.
39. Kawasaki M, Ogura JH, Takenouchi S. Neurophysiologic observations of normal deglutition. I. Its relationship to the respiratory cycle. Laryngoscope 1965;74:1747–65.
40. Dubner RB, Sessle BJ, Storey AT. The Neurological Basis of Oral and Facial Function. New York: Plenum; 1978.
41. Hrychshyn AW, Basmajian JV. Electromyography of the oral stage of swallowing in man. Am J Anat 1972;133:335–40.
42. Mansson I, Sandberg N. Effects of surface anesthesia on deglutition in man. Laryngoscope 1974;84:427–37.
43. Mansson I, Sandberg N. Oro-pharyngeal sensitivity and elicitation of swallowing in man. Acta Otolaryngol (Stockh) 1975; 79:140–5.
44. Mansson I, Sandberg N. Salivary stimulus and swallowing in man. Acta Otolaryngol (Stockh) 1975;79:445–50.
45. Kahrilas PJ, Dent J, Dodds WJ, et al. A method for continuous monitoring of upper esophageal sphincter pressure. Dig Dis Sci 1987;32:121–8.
46. Humphrey T. Reflex activity in the oral and facial arch of the human fetus. In: Bosma JF, editor. Second Symposium on Oral Sensation and Perception. Springfield, IL: Charles C. Thomas; 1967. p. 195.
47. Ross MG, Nijland MJM. Development of ingestive behavior. Am J Physiol 1998;274:R879–93.
48. Pritchard JA. Fetal swallowing and amniotic fluid volume. Obstet Gynecol 1966;28:606–10.
49. Montgomery RK, Mulber AE, Grand RJ. Development of the human gastrointestinal tract: Twenty years of progress. Gastroenterology 1999;116:702–31.
50. Bosma JF. Postnatal ontogeny of performances of the pharynx, larynx, and mouth. Am Rev Respir Dis 1985;131:S10–5.
51. Kramer SS. Special swallowing problems in children. Gastrointest Radiol 1985;10:241–50.
52. Laitman JT, Crelin ES. Postnatal development of the basicranium and vocal tract region in man. In: Bosma JF, editor. Symposium on Development of the Basicranium. Washington, DC: US Government Printing Office; 1976. p. 206.
53. Noback GJ. The developmental topography of the larynx, trachea, and lungs in the fetus, newborn, infant, and child. Am J Dis Child 1923;26:515–33.
54. Bosma JF. Oral-pharyngeal interactions in feeding. Presented at the Symposium on Dysphagia; Feb.1986; Johns Hopkins University.
55. Gewold IH, Vice FL, Schweitzer-Kenny WL, et al. Developmental patterns of rhythmic suck and swallow in preterm infants. Dev Med Child Neurol 2001;43:22–7.
56. Qureshi MA, Vice FL, Taciak VL, et al. Changes in rhythmic suckle feeding patterns in term infants in the first month of life. Dev Med Child Neurol 2002;44:34–9.
57. Mizuno K, Ueda A. The maturation and coordination of sucking, swallowing, and respiration in preterm infants. J Pediatr 2003;142:36–40.
58. Wolff PH. The serial organization of sucking in the young infant. Pediatrics 1968;42:943–56.
59. Bernbaum JC, Periera GR, Watkins JB, Peckham GT. Nonnutritive sucking during gavage feeding enhances growth and maturation in premature infants. Pediatrics 1983;71:41–5.
60. Neely CA. Effects of non-nutritive sucking upon behavior arousal in the newborn. Birth Defects 1979;15:173–200.
61. Field T, Ignatoff E, Stringer S, et al. Non-nutritive sucking during tube feedings: Effects on preterm neonates in an intensive care unit. Pediatrics 1982;70:381–4.
62. Paludetto R, Robertson SS, Hack M, et al. Transcutaneous oxygen tension during non-nutritive sucking in preterm infants. Pediatrics 1984;74:539–42.
63. Paludetto R, Robertson SS, Marting RJ. Interaction between nonnutritive sucking and respiration in preterm infants. Biol Neonate 1986;49:198–203.
64. Illingworth RS. Sucking and swallowing difficulties in infancy: Diagnostic problem of dysphagia. Arch Dis Child 1969;44: 655–65.
65. Fisher SE, Painter M, Milmoe G. Swallowing disorders in infancy. Pediatr Clin North Am 1981;28:845–53.
66. Weiss MH. Dysphagia in infants and children. Otolaryngol Clin North Am 1988;21:727–35.
67. Shapiro J, Healy GB. Dysphagia in infants. Otolaryngol Clin North Am 1988;21:737–41.
68. Arvedson JC, Brodsky L, editors. Pediatric Swallowing and Feeding: Assessment and Management. San Diego: Singular; 1993.
69. Tuchman DN, Walters RS, editors. Pediatric Feeding and Swallowing Disorders: Pathophysiology, Diagnosis, and Treatment. San Diego: Singular; 1994.
70. Cohen SR. Difficulty with swallowing. In: Bluestone CD, Stool SF, editors. Pediatric Otolaryngology. Philadelphia: WB Saunders; 1983.
71. Loughlin GM. Respiratory consequences of dysfunctional swallowing and aspiration. Dysphagia 1989;3:126–30.
72. Mansfield LE, Stein MR. Gastroesophageal reflux and asthma: A possible reflex mechanism. Ann Allergy 1978;41: 224–6.
73. Herbst JJ, Minton SED, Book LS. Gastroesophageal reflux causing respiratory distress and apnea in newborn infants. J Pediatr 1979;95:763–8.
74. Boyle JT, Tuchman DN, Altschuler SM, et al. Mechanisms for the association of gastroesophageal reflux and bronchospasm. Am Rev Respir Dis 1985;131:S16–20.
75. Fung CW, Khong PL, To R, et al. Videofluoroscopic study of swallowing in children with neurodevelopmental disorders. Pediatr Int 2004;46:26–30.
76. Heuschkel RB, Fletcher K, Hill Abuonomo C, et al. Isolated neonatal swallowing dysfunction. Dig Dis Sci 2003 2003;48:30–35.
77. Blasco PA, et al. Consensus statement of the Consortium on Drooling, Kluge Children's Rehabilitation Center, University of Virginia Health Sciences Center, Charlottesville (VA), July 10–11, 1990.
78. Johnson H, Scott A. A Practical Approach to Saliva Control. Tuscon, AZ: Communication Skill Builders, 1993.
79. Senner, Jill E, Logemann J, Zecker S, Gaebler-Spira, D. Drooing saliva production, and swallowing in cererbral palsy. Dev Med Child Neurol 2004;46:801–806.
80. Myer CM. Sialorrhea. Pediatr Clin North Am 1989;36: 1495–500.
81. Bailey CM. Management of the drooling child. Clin Otolaryngol 1988;13:319–22.
82. Bachrach SJ, Walter RS, Trzcinski K. Use of glycopyrrolate and other anticholinergic medication for sialorrhea in children with cerebral palsy. Clin Pediatr 1998;37:485–90.
83. Mankarious LA, Bottrill ID, Huchzermeyer PM, Bailey CM. Long-term follow-up of submandibular duct rerouting for the treatment of sialorrhea in the pediatric population. Otolaryngol Head Neck Surg 1999;120:303–7.
84. Becmeur F, Horta-Geraud P, Brunot B, et al. Diversion of salivary flow to treat drooling in patients with cerebral palsy. J Pediatr Surg 1996;31:1629–33.
85. Crysdale WS, Raveh E, McCann C, et al. Management of drooling in individuals with neurodisability: A surgical experience. Dev Child Neurol 2001;43:379–83.
86. Wilson SL, et al. Coordination of breathing and swallowing in human infants. J Appl Physiol Respir Environ Exer Physiol 1981;50:851–8.
87. Lau C, Schanler RJ. Oral motor function in the neonate. Clin Perinatol 1996;23:161–78.
88. Shivpuri CR, et al. Decreased ventilation in preterm infants during oral feeding. J Pediatr 1983;103:285–9.
89. Blackman JA, Nelson CLA. Reinstituting oral feedings in children fed by gastrostomy tube. Clin Pediatr 1985;24:434–8.
90. Bishop HC. Cricopharyngeal achalasia in childhood. Pediatr Surg 1974;9:775–8.
91. Reichert TJ, Bluestone CD, Stool SE, et al. Congenital cricopharyngeal achalasia. Ann Otol Rhinol Laryngol 1977;86:603–10.
92. Muraji T. Congenital cricopharyngeal achalasia: Diagnosis and surgical management. J Pediatr Surg 2002;37:E12.
93. Wyllie E, et al. The mechanism of nitrazepam-induced drooling and aspiration. N Engl J Med 1986;314:35–8.
94. Seaman WB. Cineroentgenographic observation of the cricopharyngeus. AJR Am J Roentgenol 1966;96:922–31.
95. Gideon A, Nolte K. The non-obstructive pharyngoesophageal cross roll. Ann Radiol 1973;16:129–35.
96. Fisher SE, Painter M, Milmoe G. Swallowing disorders in infancy. Pediatr Clin North Am 1981;28:845–53.
97. Dinari G, et al. Cricopharyngeal dysfunction in childhood: treatment by dilatations. J Pediatr Gastroenterol Nutr 1987;6:212–6.
98. Lernau OZ, et al. Congenital cricopharyngeal achalasia treatment by dilatations. J Pediatr Surg 1984;19:202–3.
99. Berg HM, Jacob JB, Persky MS, Cohen NL. Cricopharyngeal myotomy: A review of surgical results in patients with cricopharyngeal achalasia of neurogenic origin. Laryngoscope 1985;95:1337–40.
100. Burklow KA, Phelps AN, Schultz JR, et al. Classifying complex pediatric feeding disorders. J Pediatr Gastroenterol Nutr 1998;27:143–7.
101. American Gastroenterology Association. American Gastroenterology Association medical position statement on management of oropharyngeal dysphagia. Gastroenterology 1999;116:452–4.
102. Cook IJ, Kahrilas PJ. American Gastroenterology Association technical review on management of the oropharyngeal dysphagia. Gastroenterology 1999;116:455–78.
103. Tuchman DN. Dysfunctional swallowing in the pediatric patient: Clinical considerations. Dysphagia 1988;2:203–8.
104. Logemann JA. Evaluation and treatment of swallowing disorders. San Diego: College-Hill Press; 1983.
105. Linden P, Siebens A. Dysphagia: Predicting laryngeal penetration. Arch Phys Med Rehabil 1983;64:281–4.
106. Splaingard ML, Hutchins B, Sulton LD, Chaudhuri G. Aspiration in rehabilitation patients: Videofluoroscopy vs bedside clinical assessment. Arch Phys Med Rehabil 1988;69:637–40.
107. Bosely E. Development of sucking and swallowing. Cereb Palsy J 1963;24:14–6.
108. Bosma JF. Development of feeding. Clin Nutr 1986;5:210–8.
109. Morris SE. Program Guidelines for Children with Feeding Problems. Madison, WI: Childcraft Education; 1977.
110. Mueller HA. Facilitating feeding and pre-speech. In: Pearson PH, Williams CE, editors. Physical Therapy Services in the Developmental Disabilities. Springfield, IL: Charles C. Thomas; 1972.
111. Curtis DJ, Hudson T. Laryngotracheal aspiration: Analysis of specific neuromuscular factors. Radiology 1983;149: 517–22.
112. Eckberg O, Wahlgren L. Pharyngeal dysfunctions and their interrelationship in patients with dysphagia. Acta Radiol Diagn (Stockh) 1985;26:659–64.

113. Jones B, Kramer SS, Donner MW. Dynamic imaging of the pharynx. Gastrointest Radiol 1985;10:213–24.

114. DeMatteo C, Matovich D, Hjartarson A. Developmental Medicine and Child Neurology 2005;47:149–57.

115. Dodds WJ, et al. Considerations about pharyngeal manometry. Dysphagia 1987;1:209–17.

116. Kahrilas PJ, Lin S, Rademaker AW, Logemann JA. Impaired deglutitive airway protection: A videofluoroscopic analysis of severity and mechanism. Gastroenterology 1997;113:1457–64.

117. Dodds WJ. Instrumentation and methods for intraluminal esophageal manometry. Arch Intern Med 1976;136:515–23.

118. Sokol EM, Heitmann P, Wolf BS, Cohen BR. Simultaneous cineradiographic and manometric study of the pharynx, hypopharynx, and cervical esophagus. Gastroenterology 1966;51:960–74.

119. Hamilton JW, et al. Evaluation of the upper esophageal sphincter using simultaneous pressure measurements with a sleeve device and videofluoroscopy. Gastroenterology 1986;91:1054a.

120. Shawker TH, Sonies BC, Stone M. Sonography of speech and swallowing. In: Sanders RC, Hill M, editors. Ultrasound Annual. New York: Raven Press; 1984. p. 237.

121. Weber F, Woolridge MW, Baum JD. An ultrasonographic study of the organization of sucking and swallowing by newborn infants. Dev Med Child Neurol 1986;28:19–24.

122. Cowan RJ. Radionuclide evaluation of the esophagus in patients with dysphagia. In: Gelfand DW, Richter JE, editors. Dysphagia: Diagnosis and Treatment. New York: Igaku-Shoin; 1989. p. 127–58.

123. Heyman S. Volume dependent pulmonary aspiration of a swallowed radionuclide bolus. J Nucl Med 1997;38:103–4.

124. Hamlet SL, Muz J, Patterson R, Jones L. Pharyngeal transit time: Assessment with videofluoroscopy and scintigraphic techniques. Dysphagia 1989;4:4–7.

125. Holt S, Miron SD, Diaz MC, et al. Scintigraphic measurement of oropharyngeal transit in man. Dig Dis Sci 1990;35:1198–204.

126. Humphreys B, Mathog R, Rosen R, et al. Videofluoroscopic and scintigraphic analysis of dysphagia in the head and neck cancer patient. Laryngoscope 1987;97:25–32.

127. Silver KH, et al. Scintigraphy for the detection and quantification of subglottic aspiration: Preliminary observations. Arch Phys Med Rehabil 1991;72:902–10.

128. Selley WG, Ellis RE, Flack FC, et al. The synchronization of respiration and swallow sounds with videofluoroscopy during swallowing. Dysphagia 1994;9:162–7.

129. Lefton-Greif MA, Loughlin GM. Specialized studies in pediatric dysphagia. Semin Speech Lang Dev 1996;17:311–29.

130. Langmore SE, Schatz K, Olsen N. Fiberoptic endoscopic examination of swallowing safety: A new procedure. Dysphagia 1988;2:216–9.

131. Langmore SE. Endoscopic and videofluoroscopic evaluations of swallowing and aspiration. Ann Otol Rhinol Laryngol 1991;100:678–81.

132. Langmore SE, Hicks DM. Presented at the Symposium on Endoscopy as a Tool for Clinical Evaluation of Swallowing and Voice Disorders, Orlando, FL; March 3–4, 1995.

133. Aviv JE, Kim T, Sacco RL, et al. FEESST: A new bedside endoscopic test of the motor and sensory components of swallowing. Ann Otol Rhinol Laryngol 1998;107:378–87.

134. Willging JP. Endoscopic evaluation swallowing in children. Int J Pediatr Otorhinolaryngol 1995;:S107–8.

135. Aviv JE, Marin JH, Kim T, et al. Ann Otol Rhinol Laryngol 1999;108:725–30.

136. Thompson SM. Am J Med 2003;115:166S–8S.

137. Suskind DL, Thompson DM, Gulati M, et al. Improved infant swallowing after gastroesophageal reflux disease treatment: A function of improved laryngeal sensation? Laryngoscope 2006;116:1397–1403.

138. Griffin KM. Swallowing training for dysphagia patients. Arch Phys Med Rehabil 1974;55:467–70.

139. Helfrich-Miller KR, Rector KL, Straka JA. Dysphagia: Its treatment in the profoundly retarded patient with cerebral palsy. Arch Phys Med Rehabil 1986;67:520–5.

140. Morris SE. Prespeech and Language Programming for the Young Child with Cerebral Palsy. Milwaukee WI: Curative Work-shop; 1975.

141. Morris SE. Developmental implications for the management of feeding problems in neurologically impaired infants. Semin Speech Lang 1985;6:293–314.

142. Ottenbacher K, Bundy A, Short MA. The development of treatment of oral-motor dysfunction: A review of clinical research. Phys Occup Ther Pediatr 1983;3:1–13.

143. Saeian K, Shaker R. Oropharyngeal dysphagia. Curr Treat Options Gastroenterol 2000;3:77–87.

144. Illingworth RS, Lister J. The critical or sensitive period, with special reference to certain feeding problems in infants and children. J Pediatr 1964;65:839–48.

145. Geertsma MA, et al. Feeding resistance after parenteral hyperalimentation. Am J Dis Child 1985;139:255–6.

146. Hurwitz AL, Duranceau A. Upper-esophageal sphincter dysfunction: Pathogenesis and treatment. Dig Dis 1978;23:275–81.

147. Rudolph CD, Link DT. Feeding disorders in infants and children. Pediatr Clin North Am 2002;49:97–112.

148. Isberg A, Nilsson ME, Schiratzki H. Movement of the upper esophageal sphincter and a manometric device during deglutition: A cineradiograhic investigation. Acta Radiol Diagn 1985;26:381–8.

149. Reynolds EW, Vice FL, Bosma JF, Gewolb IH. Cervical accelerometry in preterm infants. Dev Med Child Neurol 2002;44:587–92.

150. Dobie RA. Rehabilitation of swallowing disorders. Am Fam Physician 1978;17:84–95.

151. de Lamma Lazzara G, Lazarus C, Logemann JA. Impact of thermal stimulation on the triggering of the swallowing reflex. Dysphagia 1986;1:73–7.

152. Logemann JA. Treatment for aspiration related to dysphagia. Dysphagia 1986;1:34–8.

153. Groher ME. Bolus management and aspiration pneumonia in patients with pseudobulbar dysphagia. Dysphagia 1987;1:215–6.

Esophageal Motility

4.1. Normal Motility and Development of the Esophageal Neuroenteric System

Salvatore Cucchiara, MD, PhD

Osvaldo Borrelli, MD, PhD

Giovanni Di Nardo, MD

The esophagus acts as a conduit for the aborad transport of food from the mouth to the stomach. It can be identified as a distinct structure from 4 weeks of gestation. At birth, it has approximately a length of 8 cm, which doubles in the first year of extrauterine life. Each of the three germ layers (endoderm, ectoderm, and mesoderm) are responsible for esophageal development; their interactions are crucial for the development of the mucosa, muscular coats, and intrinsic nervous system. During embryogenesis, neuronal precursors derived from the neural crest colonize the lengthening gut and become distributed in concentric plexus within the gut wall to form the enteric nervous system (ENS). Formation of the ENS requires the coordinated migration, proliferation, differentiation, and survival of neuronal precursors. Numerous genes and signaling molecules are involved in these processes.

The esophagus is capable of peristalsis during the first trimester of gestation; however, complex pattern of esophageal motility are clearly detected during the second trimester. At birth, motility of the esophagus functionally consists of three regions, corresponding to the upper esophageal sphincter (UES), body of the esophagus, and lower esophageal sphincter (LES). Each of these regions shows specific motor function, and experimental data in preterm and term infants indicate that with growth they undergo both anatomical and functional development. Knowledge of the embryology and physiology of the esophagus is important in understanding the varied clinical presentation of esophageal diseases.

EMBRYOLOGY

The gastrointestinal tract first appears at 4 weeks of gestation with three major phases of development recognized: (1) an early period of proliferation and morphogenesis; (2) an intermediate period of cell differentiation; and (3) a later period of maturation (transport of luminal contents, digestion, and absorption of nutrients).[1] At the beginning of the fourth week the embryo, a trilaminar germ disk (ectoderm, endoderm,

and mesoderm) undergoes a complex process of embryonic folding that converts it from a flat disk into a three-dimensional structure. This process, induced by differential growth of different embryonic portions, starts in the cephalic and lateral regions on day 22 and in the caudal direction on day 23. As a result, the craniocaudal and lateral edges of the germ disk are brought together along the ventral midline, and each germ layer is fused to the corresponding portion on the opposite side, thereby creating a three-dimensional body form. The process of midline germ layer fusion converts the cranial and the caudal portions of endoderm into two blind-ending tubes, the foregut and the hindgut respectively, separated by the future midgut, opened to the yolk sac.[2] Cranially, the foregut terminates in the oropharyngeal membrane, while caudally the hindgut ends in the cloacal membrane (Figure 1). These membranes then break down to form the

mouth (fourth week) and the orifices of the anus and urogenital system (seventh week).

As the lateral edges of the germ disk layers continue to zipper together along the ventral midline, the midgut is progressively converted into a tube, and the yolk sac, compressed by the folding process of the embryo, is reduced to a slim stalk, called the vitelline duct.[2] At this time, the early digestive tract divides into foregut, midgut, and hindgut.

During embryonic development, the lower respiratory tract, esophagus, and stomach are derived from the same embryonic segment, the foregut.[3] On day 22, the respiratory tree begins to develop as a foregut diverticulum, called the lung bud, first appearing as a ventral outpouching of the foregut endoderm. Subsequently, the lung bud grows ventrocaudally through the splanchnic mesenchyme surrounding the foregut, and between the days 26 and 28 bifurcates into

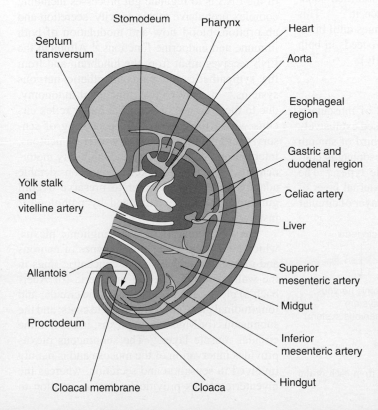

Stomodeum — Pharynx

Septum transversum

Heart

Aorta

Esophageal region

Gastric and duodenal region

Yolk stalk and vitelline artery

Celiac artery

Liver

Allantois

Superior mesenteric artery

Midgut

Proctodeum

Inferior mesenteric artery

Cloacal membrane — Cloaca — Hindgut

Figure 1 Lateral view of a 4-week embryo showing the relationship of primordial gut to yolk sac. The primordial gut is a long tube extending the length of the embryo, and the esophagus corresponds to the small area of endoderm localized between the dilated stomach and the lung bud.

two primary bronchial buds, which are the rudiments of the two lungs.[4] During the fourth week of embryonic development, a mesenchymal "tracheoesophageal septum" evolves and separates the cranial foregut into the laryngotracheal tube and esophagus. Abnormalities in this development result in esophageal atresia and tracheoesophageal fistula.[5–6]

EMBRYONIC ORIGIN OF ESOPHAGEAL STRUCTURES

The esophagus is identified as a distinct structure at 4 weeks of gestation, developing from a small area of endoderm between the dilated stomach and the lung bud. Due to faster cranial growth of the embryonic body, elongation occurs more rapidly than the fetus as a whole.[7] The esophagus reaches its final fetal length between the seventh and eight week of embryonic development, having at birth a length between 8 and 10 cm, which doubles in the first years of extrauterine life.[8]

The esophagus develops from each of the three germ layers (Figure 2): (1) the endoderm which gives rise to the epithelial lining; (2) the ectoderm gives rise to neural components; and (3) the mesoderm that supplies the mesenchymal cell types, such as the muscular layers, connective tissue, and angioblasts.[1]

Esophageal Epithelium

In the early phase of embryonic development, the esophageal epithelium is composed of stratified columnar cells.[9] During the seventh and eighth weeks, the epithelium becomes cuboidal and starts to proliferate, occluding almost completely the foregut lumen; however, complete obliteration of lumen is thought not occur.[10] At 10 weeks, ciliated columnar epithelium appears and, during the fourth month of fetal life, a stratified squamous epithelium begins to replace it.[11–12] This replacement process, which continues until birth, arises in the midesophagus and proceeds in both directions (ie, caudally and cranially).

Esophageal Muscularis Propria

At birth, roughly the upper third of muscularis propria of the esophagus is composed exclusively of skeletal muscle and the distal third of smooth muscle. The middle third of the esophagus consists of a mixture of both muscle types.[13] The musculature coats consist of an external layer of longitudinal fibers and an internal layer of circular

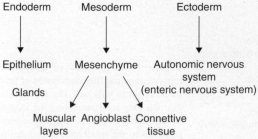

Figure 2 Tissues and cells developing from each of the three germinal layers.

fibers. The circular layer is present from 6 weeks of gestation, whereas the longitudinal layer does not become apparent until 13 weeks of embryonic development.[14] The skeletal muscle of the upper esophagus and the UES, deriving from the branchial arches 4, 5, and 6, are innervated by the vagus nerve (the branchial arch 5 nerve) and by the recurrent laryngeal nerve (a branch of vagus nerve, the branchial arch 6 nerve).[13] Smooth muscle cells and the LES are derived from splanchnic mesenchyme surrounding the foregut; however, the precise genesis of the gastroesophageal junction is still controversial. Gastric rotation, combined with growth of gastric fundus is thought to be involved in the development of the gastroesophageal junction.[13] The middle third of esophagus is a mixture of skeletal and smooth muscle cells, and its origin is not known. Although the two muscle types seem to arise from two different differentiation pathways, it has been suggested that smooth muscle cells undergo a process of transdifferentiation, giving rise to striated muscle cells of the esophagus.[15–16]

Enteric Nervous System

The ENS is defined as the system of neurons and their supporting cells that is present within the wall of the gastrointestinal tract. It extends through the entire gut and is the largest division of the autonomic nervous system, with neuronal density comparable to that of the spinal cord.[17] The ENS is also by far the most complex division in terms of number of different functional types of neurons present (sensory neurons, intrinsic primary afferent neurons, interneurons, excitatory, and inhibitory neurons) and their interactions.[18] The range of neurotransmitters expressed by enteric neurons is also very broad, and most are also found in the central nervous system (CNS).[19–20] The function of the ENS is to regulate gut processes including complex propulsive motor activity, secretion and absorption, blood flow and modulation of both immune and endocrine functions.[21] Although the ENS receives input from the hindbrain and from the sympathetic and parasympathetic nervous systems,[22] it shows great functional autonomy, due to the presence of complete motor reflex circuits within the enteric wall, consisting of sensory neurons, intrinsic primary afferent neurons, interneurons, and excitatory and inhibitory motor-neurons.[21–24] The ENS likely shows considerable adaptive plasticity in order to preserve overall gut function when challenged by pathological insults.[25]

The ENS consists of two ganglionic plexus, which are composed of several types of neurons and glia and arranged as two concentric rings in the wall of the bowel: the myenteric (or Auerbach's) plexus, localized between the circular and longitudinal gastrointestinal muscle coats; and the submucous (or Meissner's) plexus, internal to the circular muscle layer.[26] The submucous plexus provides innervation of the mucosa and is mainly involved in sensation and secretion, whereas the myenteric plexus provides motor innervation to

the muscle coats and submucosal plexus. Myenteric ganglia are present throughout the length of the gastrointestinal tract, but submucosal ganglia are few or absent in some regions, such as the esophagus and stomach.[27]

Due to of a central role in intestinal motility, absorption, and secretion, the ENS is absolutely essential for all stages of postnatal life. Mice lacking enteric neurons throughout the gastrointestinal tract or from particular regions, such as the esophagus or small and large intestines, usually die within 24 hours of birth.[28–30] On the other hand, the ENS is not essential at earlier embryonic stages.[31] Thus, abnormalities of ENS development alone do not contribute to prenatal mortality or morbidity but have great effects on digestive health immediately following birth.

The ENS is derived from the neural crest, which comprises a population of precursor cells, many of that are multipotential.[17] The neural crest arises on the dorsal midline as part of neural tube, later forming the CNS. By controlled migrations, neural crest cells (NCCs) distribute themselves widely and precisely.[32] NCCs differentiate not only into enteric neurons but also into cell types as diverse as pigment cells, connective tissues, and sympathetic neurons.[33] Although this process of NCC migration was suggested over 130 years ago by Wilhelm His, Jr, indirect evidence of the neural crest origin of enteric neurons was achieved 50 years ago, through a series of detailed ablation studies in the dorsal neural primordium of chick embryos.[34] Some 20 years later, Le Douarin and colleagues, by using a chick-quail transplantation technique, established the precise axial origin of the NCC populations which form the ENS.[35]

Many studies have been subsequently performed on migration wave and direction of NCC colonization in the gastrointestinal tract. Yntema and Hammond, performing crest ablation studies in chick embryos at various axial levels, showed that ablations at all levels except one had no effect on the subsequent appearance of enteric neurons.[34,36] However, the ablation of a short region, localized in the hindbrain and extending to the first few cervical segments, resulted in total absence of the ENS over the entire length of the gut. This region, called the vagal neural crest, was at somite levels 1 to 7. As result of these studies, the authors suggested that the source of enteric neurons is the vagal neural crest and that NCCs colonize the gastrointestinal tract in a rostrocaudal direction. Subsequently, an additional source of ENS neurons and glia was identified at the lumbosacral level (lumbosacral neural crest), corresponding in humans to somite 24.[37] Elegant animal experiments have shown that the vagal neural crest is the single source for enteric neurons in the foregut and major part of the midgut, whereas the hindgut and adjacent midgut have an additional lumbosacral source. These findings indicate a complete rostrocaudal wave of colonization of the gut by the NCCs arising from vagal neural crest and an incomplete caudorostral colonization from lumbosacral neural crest.[38,39] NCCs originating from the lumbosacral level do not enter into the hindgut until it has been colonized by vagal crest cells, suggesting some dependency of the former on the presence of the latter.[37] Furthermore, lumbosacral-derived enteric neurons occur principally in the myenteric plexus, with relatively few in the submucosal plexus, and their density is relatively small and declines rostrally.[40]

Recently, Wallace and Burns, studying human embryos, have shown that NCCs from the vagal neural crest enter the foregut at week 4 and colonize the gut in rostrocaudal direction to reach the hindgut by week 7.[14] The latter remains free from NCCs until the migration front of vagal crest-derived cells has colonized the foregut and the midgut. Initially, vagal crest-derived cells are dispersed in the gut mesenchyme, but later they coalesce to form ganglia along a rostrocaudal maturation gradient. The myenteric plexus develops first in the foregut, then in the midgut, and finally in the hindgut. The submucosal plexus appears approximately 2 to 3 weeks after the myenteric plexus, arising from cells that migrate centripetally through the circular muscle layer from the myenteric region.[14] At the present time, the extent of the contribution of lumbosacral NCCs to the ENS in humans has yet to be established.

Although NCCs in each somite are derived from the level of the neural tube closest to that somite, the ENS in each region of the gastrointestinal tract has a mixture of cells from various levels within the neural crest.[41] Nevertheless, a majority of enteric neurons seem to arise from NCCs that migrate through somites 3, 4, and 5, caudal to the branchial arches, with some passing through branchial arch 6.[41] Conversely, using the chick-quail transplantation technique, it has recently been shown that NCCs adjacent to somites 1 to 2 (ie, rostral truncal crest) are the main source of enteric neurons in the esophagus, whereas a smaller number of esophageal neurons originate adjacent to somites 3 to 4, and almost no esophageal neurons are derived from somites 6 and 7.[38,40] Similar data in human embryos are not available.

The gut is colonized in a complex manner involving intricate cell movements along precise pathways, some of which guide cells in opposite directions toward their final destination. During the migration of ENS precursors, signals allow them to proliferate and survive in the gut mesenchyme as well. Furthermore, the cells differentiate into a large variety of neuronal cell types and glial cells, which are organized into ganglionic complexes occupying characteristic positions in the gut wall. Extracellular matrix components provide directional clues for migrating NCCs and, together with neighboring cells, provide signals for crest differentiation.[42] For instance, in humans the appearance of NCCs is preceded by the expression of extracellular matrix molecules, which play a role in both migrational cues and neuronal growth.[43] Undoubtedly, cell–cell signaling mechanisms play a major role in directing vagal NCC migration to and within the gut.

The presence of diffusible chemoattractive molecules, originating in the gut mesenchyme, plays a central role in attracting NCCs. With the advent of molecular biology and gene inactivation studies, numerous genes, cell lineages, and signaling pathways are now implicated in the development of the ENS (Table 1). Among the most important signaling molecules during development of the ENS are GDNF (glial cell line-derived neurotrophic factor) and its functional tyrosine kinase receptor RET. Knockout of either of these genes causes a total loss of enteric neurons and glia within the gut caudal to the esophagus and cardia of the stomach.[31]

In addition to environmental signals, intracellular signaling molecules and transcription factors also control the differentiation of ENS progenitors along the glial and neuronal pathways. Several lines of evidences indicate that members of the transcription factor family, such as Mash1, play a central role in ENS development in the esophagus.[44] Mash1 encodes a transcription factor of the basic helix-loop-helix (bHLH) family, and in mice, is expressed transiently during embryogenesis in the CNS and in NCCs colonizing the gut.[45] Mash1 mutant mice die within 48 hours of birth from difficulties in either feeding or breathing.[29] These mice characteristically lack sympathetic neurons and enteric neurons in the esophagus, as well as neurons mediating LES relaxation. However, extrinsic innervation of the esophagus, arising from the brain stem, is normally present.[46] During the development of Mash1 knockout mice, NCCs migrate to their correct locations, but fail to differentiate into neurons, suggesting that this transcription factor is mandatory for neuronal differentiation.[47] Mash1$^{-/-}$ mice also have a complementary phenotype to Ret$^{-/-}$, GDNF$^{-/-}$ mice; however, Mash1 mutant mice lack enteric neurons in the esophagus only, whereas mice lacking members of the GDNF signaling pathway have neurons in the esophagus but lack neurons in the small bowel and large intestine.[48] Even if the regional divergence between phenotypes is surprising, since Mash1 and Ret belong to the same signaling cascade,

this difference may be related to the different rostrocaudal level of origin of esophageal neurons from enteric neurons localized in more caudal regions of the gut.[49] In lacking nerve fibers in the LES, Mash1$^{-/-}$ mice show features similar to those observed in humans with achalasia of the esophagus, characterized by an absence of LES nitrergic fibers, while extrinsic nerve fibers are not affected.[50] A human homologue of Mash1, which is 95% homologous to rat Mash1, has been isolated and termed HASH1 (human achaete-scute homologue 1).[51] It is expressed by sympathetic neuron precursors early in human embryonic development (weeks 6 to 7), and in fetal pulmonary neuroendocrine cells, as well as in neuroendocrine cells tumors, such as medullary thyroid cancer (MTC), small cell lung cancer, and pheochromocytomas.[52–54] Since Mash1 is expressed only transiently during embryonic development and appears to be required for neuronal differentiation, it is very unlikely that defects in Hash1 cause achalasia of the esophagus in humans.

DEVELOPMENT OF ESOPHAGEAL MOTOR FUNCTION

Motor Activity in the Fetus

Studies in utero document the early development of swallowing, oral, and esophageal motor function. Fetal swallowing of pharyngeal contents, one the first motor response in the pharynx, is detected as early as 11 weeks of gestation, with mounting and sucking movements easily seen at 15 weeks of gestation.[55] Although distinct backward and forward movement of the tongue begin between the 18 and 24 weeks, no significant maturation of sucking occurs in utero between 26 and 29 weeks of gestation.[56] True sucking does not occur effectively until 34 weeks of gestation, when both mouthing movements and disordered sucking burst patterns disappear, and a stable pattern of rhythmic sucking and swallowing is detected.[57] At this time, 30-second bursts of sucking at 2-minute intervals coordinated with swallowing are observed.[58]

Table 1 Genes Involved in the Development of the Enteric Nervous System		
Gene	Location on Human Chromosome	Phenotype of ENS in Mice in Which Gene Is Homozygously Inactivated
RET	10q11.2	Absence of neurons from small and large intestine
GDNF	5p12–13.1	Absence of neurons from small and large intestine
GFRα1	10q25	Absence of neurons from small and large intestine
ET$_B$	13q22	Absence of neurons from distal and large intestine
ET-3	20q13.2–13.3	Absence of neurons from distal large intestine
ECE-1	1p36.1	Absence of neurons from distal large intestine
Phox2b	4p12	Absence of neurons from entire gastrointestinal tract
SOX10	22q13	Absence of neurons from entire gastrointestinal tract
PAX3	2q37	Absence of neurons from small and large intestine
HASH1 (Mash1)	12	Absence of neurons from esophagus
IHH (indian hedgehog)	2q333q35	Absence of neurons from parts of the small and large intestine
SHH (sonic hedgehog)	7q36	Ectopic nerve cell bodies within mucosa
HOX11L1	2p13.1	ENS hyperplasia in colon and hypoplasia in small intestine

The swallowing of amniotic fluid begins slowly at less 10 mL/d around 18 weeks of gestation and increases to as much as 750 mL/d at term.[59] Although it has been suggested that swallowing likely develops in utero only to provide a functional system during the neonatal period, it represents a primary physiological mechanism contributing to fluid homeostasis and development of the fetal gastrointestinal tract.[59]

Investigation of the dynamic aspects of esophageal motor activity in utero has been hampered by lack of persistent patency of the esophageal lumen and by the close proximity of the esophagus to anatomical structures of similar tissue consistency. With the advent of high-frequency ultrasound transducers, a more detailed anatomical description and more detailed motility patterns have been described. Even though the esophagus seems to exhibit some peristalsis during the first trimester, patterns of esophageal motility have only been observed during the second trimester, between 19 and 25 weeks of gestation. During the second trimester, three different esophageal motility patterns have been described.[60] The most common pattern is a simultaneous, synchronized opening of esophageal lumen from the oropharynx to the esophagogastric junction, without propagation of peristaltic waves along the esophageal lumen. The second type is characterized by segmental propulsive peristaltic activity wave, induced by swallowing, which advances from the pharynx, through the mediastinum, into the stomach; in this motility pattern the entire swallowing cycle may be observed, suggesting a well-developed central synaptic control and an appropriate peripheral sensory feedback from receptive fields in the oropharynx and larynx. Finally, the last type

of fetal esophageal motility pattern described is characterized by the abrupt retrograde passage of fluid from the stomach into the pharynx through the esophagogastric junction, indicative of gastroesophageal reflux.[60]

Motor Activity in Newborns, Infants, and Children

At birth, the esophagus has a length of between 8 and 10 cm, which doubles in the first year of extrauterine life.[8] The main purpose of the esophagus is the aboral transport of food from the mouth to the stomach, and functionally consists of three regions: upper esophageal sphincter (UES), esophageal body, and the lower esophageal sphincter (LES).

Upper Esophageal Sphincter. The UES is physiologically defined as a zone of high intraluminal pressure lying in between the pharynx and the cervical esophagus, and comprises functional activity of three adjacent muscles together with cartilage and connective tissue.[61] The main functions of the UES are to provide the most proximal physical barrier of the gastrointestinal tract against pharyngeal and laryngeal reflux during esophageal peristalsis, and to avoid the entry of air into the digestive tract during negative intrathoracic pressure events, such as inspiration. The UES relaxes both transiently during swallowing, in order to allow the entry of a bolus into the esophagus, and during belching and vomiting, in order to allow the egress of gastric contents from the esophageal lumen (Figure 3). Thus, the UES has two basic functions, opening and closing, which imply three muscular responses: tone generation, phasic response activity, and sphincter opening.[62]

At birth, the UES measures ~0.5 to 1 cm in length and increases to ~3 cm (2 to 4 cm) in adults. From an anatomical perspective, the high-pressure zone is approximated, as there are no clear physical landmarks. The UES is a musculocartilaginous structure with its anterior wall formed by the full extent of the posterior surface of the cricoid cartilage and arytenoids and interarytenoid muscles in the upper part.[61] Posteriorly and laterally, the cricopharyngeal muscle is the primary muscular component generating sphincteric tone, even if there is experimental evidence that other muscular components of pharyngoesophageal segment, such as the inferior pharyngeal constrictor and the cervical esophagus, also contribute to some of the UES.[63] Within the pharyngoesophageal segment, the area of highest pressure is located adjacent to the inferior pharyngeal constrictor, while the cricopharyngeal muscle accounts for the distal one-third of the high-pressure zone.[64]

Neural connections of the UES that have been identified are the pharyngeal plexus and recurrent laryngeal nerve.[65] The former is supplied by the pharyngeal branch of the vagus nerve, the superior laryngeal nerve, and the glossopharyngeal nerve. The main motor input is provided by recurrent laryngeal nerve, whereas sensation seems to be mediated by both the superior laryngeal nerve and the glossopharyngeal nerve.[65] The cell bodies of most motor neurons innervating muscles in the UES are located ipsilaterally in the nucleus ambiguus of the medulla.[66] Additional motoneurons of UES muscles are located in various brainstem nuclei outside the nucleus ambiguus (NA), such as the reticular formation.[66] Acetylcholine is the principal neurotransmitter for efferent

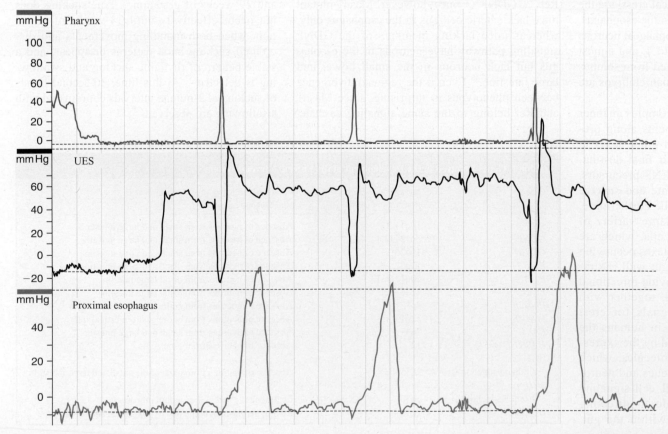

Figure 3 Manometric recording at the level of the oropharyngeal region. The upper channel shows pharyngeal contractions, the middle channel records a profile of the upper esophageal sphincter that exhibits sequential relaxations in coincidence with pharyngeal contractions (oropharyngeal coordination), and the lower channel shows contractions at the level of the proximal esophagus.

innervation of the UES, even if other neuropeptides, such as calcitonin gene-related peptide and substance P, have also been identified in the nerve terminals innervating the UES.[67–68] Pharyngoesophageal afferent fibers, with cell bodies in nodose ganglion, and cervical and thoracic dorsal root ganglia of the spinal cord, terminate in the premotor neurons in the nucleus tractus solitarius (NTS), which, in turn, project onto pharyngeal motoneurons of the NA.[65]

The cricopharyngeal muscle is the primary muscular element that generates tone in the upper sphincter. It arises from the lower part of the dorsolateral aspect of the cricoid cartilage and forms a horizontal loop to attach to the cricoid cartilage on the opposite side.[62] The cricopharyngeal muscle is a striated muscle composed of various-sized small fibers (20 to 25 μm) which are not oriented in strict parallel fashion, as in most other striated muscles.[69] Different from surrounding pharyngeal and laryngeal muscles, the cricopharyngeal muscle is composed by both slow-twitch (type 1, oxidative) and fast-twitch (type 2, glycolytic) muscle fibers; however, the predominant muscle fibers are of slow-twitch type (over 85%).[69] The presence of both types of fibers provides an anatomical basis for UES function, including the maintenance of a constant basal tone and rapid relaxation and contraction during dynamic states, such as swallowing, belching, vomiting, and other reflexes. The cricopharyngeal muscle contains a large amount of connective tissue (40%), resulting in a high degree of elasticity, which serves several functions.[69] For instance, the UES can be opened without the need for active muscular relaxation, by increasing intraluminal pressure, such as exerted by a bolus through the sphincter, or by active distraction, effected by hyoid excursion.[61]

The cellular physiology of other muscles contributing to UES functions has recently been clarified. The cervical esophagus is similar to the cricopharyngeal muscle, containing predominantly slow-twitch-type fibers.[70] As the muscle fibers of the cervical esophagus are about the same size as the adjacent cricopharyngeal muscle, fibers from the cricopharyngeal muscle could directly contribute to the adjacent cervical portion of esophagus. The inferior pharyngeal constrictor contains two muscle layers: an outer layer of predominantly (90%) type II muscle fibers, and an inner layer of predominantly type I fibers (85%). Given structural similarities, all muscular components of the UES closing mechanism likely act in a similar fashion, as a single functional unit.[61–62,69]

Maintenance of basal tone of the UES resting pressure is not entirely the result of myogenic activity, since a component of pressure is the result of passive forces caused by elasticity of the surrounding tissues.[61,62] Furthermore, radial and axial resting pressure asymmetry has been demonstrated: anterior and posterior values are higher than those laterally, with the highest anterior pressure recorded near to the pharynx, while the highest posterior pressure occurs closer to the esophagus.[71] These pressure asymmetries are not observed after laryngectomy, indicating that the rigid laryngeal cartilages forming the anterior wall of the high pressure zone are responsible for the asymmetry.[72]

After resting tone, the next most prominent function of the UES is the relaxation response to swallowing (Figure 3).[73] Opening of UES has two major components: relaxation of high-pressure zone and displacement of the larynx. The former is the result of the cessation of tonic activity at the cricopharyngeal and inferior pharyngeal constrictor muscles, whereas the upward and forward movements of the larynx are the result of active contraction of suprahyoid muscles, such as mylohyoid, thyrohyoid, and geniohyoid muscles.[62] Larynx displacement not only facilitates the opening of the UES, but also enlarges the pharynx to receive the bolus, decreasing the distance the bolus must travel, and protects the larynx against aspiration. Additionally, UES opening is influenced by distending pressure forces of the oncoming food bolus crossing the pharyngoesophageal junction.[74] Bolus viscosity and volume independently also affect the opening mechanism of the UES.[74]

Because of asymmetry and rapid pressure changes as well as brief axial movements, manometric study of the UES has been hampered in the past by recording methods. With modern systems allowing recordings of very rapid pressure changes and with special catheter devices, accurate measurements of the UES pressure at rest and in response to different stimuli have become feasible. In addition to the swallowing reflex, a number of other reflexes have been identified, illustrating the physiological role of this high-pressure zone.[75] During belching, the UES relaxes in the absence of other esophageal motor activity, whereas during retching all muscle components of UES contract prior to full relax if vomiting occurs.[76–79] The slow distension of the esophagus causes an increase in UES tone, whereas the role of intraesophageal acidification, such as acid reflux, is still not defined.[80–81] By contrast, the rapid distension of the esophagus causes UES relaxation, suggesting that this reflex is likely part of belch response.[80] Several other stimuli result in an increase in UES pressure, including gagging, pharyngeal stimulation with water or air, secondary peristalsis beginning in the upper third of the esophagus, and phonation.[61]

As in adults, there is no consensus regarding the "normal values" for UES resting pressure in children. Depending on the measuring method used, a wide range of normal values have been reported in children, varying from 8 mmHg to 70 mmHg.[82–85] The UES is functionally present at birth, although incoordination between the pharynx and esophagus may be observed in the first week of life and in premature infants less than 1,500 g.[86] Using micromanometric assembly with a UES sleeve sensor, a clearly defined UES–high-pressure zone can be detected from 32 weeks of gestational age in premature healthy infant, which promptly relaxes in response to swallowing.[86] In premature infants, UES resting pressure ranges from 2.3 to 26.2 mmHg (mean around 15 mmHg), which is greatly influenced by infant behavior patterns, being lower during periods of apparent comfort and higher during periods of irritability or abdominal straining.[86] Although motor mechanisms involved in UES tone generation as well as the coordination between pharyngeal contraction and UES relaxation appear well developed in preterm infants, it has been clearly shown that there is a maturation of UES motor function during infant growth and development. Recently, Jadcherla and colleagues characterized the motor pattern of the UES at rest and during deglutition in preterm infants, studied longitudinally at 33 and 36 weeks postmenstrual age; preterm data were compared to those in healthy full-term born infants and healthy adult volunteers.[87] With growth, the resting UES pressure rises by over twofold and UES pressure fall after swallowing becomes greater. Additionally, with growth, due to faster UES relaxation and a shorter nadir duration, the time of UES remaining open is markedly reduced.

The development of UES reflexes, protecting against gastroesophageal and esophagopharyngeal reflux, received little interest until recently, because of a lack of suitable micromanometric device to allow fidelity recordings. It is now clear that UES motor responses to abrupt mild midesophageal provocation are present at as early as 33 weeks of postmenstrual age.[88] In response to air and liquid-induced esophageal distension, three types of UES pressure responses are detected: an increase, a decrease, and no change. A contractile response is the most prevalent pattern at both 33 and 36 weeks of postmenstrual age, and its proportion increases significantly with larger volumes of air or liquid during midesophageal provocation. This finding suggests that both afferent and efferent limbs of the reflex arch are functionally present at this stage of development.[88]

Esophageal Body. In children the length of the esophageal body depends on the patient's age, whereas the length in adults is approximately 20 cm (range of 18 to 22 cm).[74] The body of the esophagus begins at the caudal edge of the cricopharyngeal muscle and extends to the rostral limit of the esophagogastric junction.[74] Based on anatomical location, three esophageal segments can be identified: cervical, thoracic, and abdominal. The esophagus is situated in the posterior mediastinum, behind the trachea and left mainstem bronchus, and curves leftward to course behind the heart. The esophagus passes through an opening in the diaphragm, the esophageal hiatus, which is normally straddled by LES, so that the upper part of the sphincter lies in the thoracic cavity, whereas the lower end in the abdomen.[10]

The wall of the esophageal body is composed of the mucosa, submucosa, and muscularis propria.[89] However, no true serosal outer layer is identified. The esophageal mucosa is stratified squamous epithelium, except at gastroesophageal junction where the squamous epithelium joins the columnar epithelium of the gastric cardia. The muscularis propria of the esophageal body is composed of an outer longitudinal muscle layer and an inner circular muscle layer.[90] In adults, the proximal 4 to 5 cm of esophageal muscularis propria (ie, below the cricopharyngeal muscle) is composed of skeletal muscle fibers, which originate from the dorsal surface of cricoid cartilage and are joined by fibers from the cricopharyngeal muscle.[90] A 4 to 8 cm transitional zone (ie, the middle third of the esophagus) consists of both skeletal and smooth muscle cells, with an increasing proportion of smooth muscle cells distally. The caudal half of the esophageal body, the distal 10 to 14 cm, consists entirely of smooth muscle fibers, oriented in a circular or an elliptical fashion.[90]

The skeletal muscle fibers of the esophagus are innervated by myelinated vagal lower motoneurons with cells bodies located in the nucleus retrofacialis and in the nucleus ambiguus that controls swallowing.[91] A small number of cell bodies also arise in the dorsal motor nucleus of the vagus. Some of these nerves accompany the vagus nerve, and other branch out into the pharyngeal nerve at the level of nodose ganglion, ending at the motor end plates of the skeletal muscle fibers.[91-92] Acetylcholine is the primary neurotransmitter involved in the activation of esophageal skeletal muscle.[91]

Smooth muscle cells in the body of the esophagus are innervated by the autonomic nervous system, with contributions from parasympathetic, sympathetic, and enteric divisions. Central control of smooth muscle motor function is provided by preganglionic parasympathetic neurons originating in the dorsal vagal complex located in the dorsomedial hindbrain medulla.[93] It consists of two nuclei, the nucleus tractus solitarius (NTS), which receives the sensory information from the viscera, and the dorsal motor nucleus of the vagus (DMN), which contains preganglionic motor output to the viscera.[91] Axons of preganglionic parasympathetic neurons are carried in the vagus nerve and enter the esophagus at various levels, where they synapse on postganglionic neurons in the enteric esophageal plexus.[94] Cell bodies of the preganglionic sympathetic fibers innervating the esophagus reside in the anterior mediolateral cell columns of the T_1 to T_{10} spinal cord segments.[94] Preganglionic sympathetic fibers reach the celiac ganglion, passing through the great splanchnic nerve network, and synapse with postganglionic neurons at the level of a plexus around the esophagus. Postganglionic axons enter into the esophageal wall, travel few centimeters, and then synapse with the myenteric or submucosal neurons, thereby providing sympathetic innervation to the esophagus.[94]

Sensory afferent neurons of the esophageal body run in the vagal (parasympathetic) and spinal afferent fibers (sympathetic).[95] The cell bodies of parasympathetic afferents are located in the jugular and nodose ganglia, and those of sympathetic afferents in thoracic and dorsal root ganglia, with most of these neurons reaching the NTS.[95] Sensory information carried by the sympathetic neural pathway seems to be relevant to cognitive sensation and the appreciation of symptoms arising from the esophagus.[96] The sequential program of swallowing is organized by a central pattern generator, previously described as the swallowing center,[91-92] which can be subdivided into three functional systems: a sensory afferent system, an efferent motor system, and a brainstem neuronal organizing system that programs the motor pattern. The neurocircuitry of swallowing is initiated by esophageal sensory afferents that project to the premotor neurons of the NTS in the dorsal vagal complex. These project to other clusters of premotor neurons, such as subnucleus centralis, and ultimately reach somatic motor neurons in the nucleus ambiguus and preganglionic motor neurons in the DMV for control of striated and smooth muscle esophageal regions.[91,94,95,97]

Two distinct populations of enteric motor neurons have been described.[98-99] Cholinergic neurons, which are excitatory in nature as they elicit contraction of the smooth muscle cells by releasing acetylcholine and substance P.[100-101] The second set of intrinsic neurons are nitrergic, which mediate nonadrenergic noncholinergic (NANC) inhibition of smooth muscle layers by releasing nitric oxide (NO) and vasoactive intestinal peptide (VIP).[102-103] Cholinergic and nitrergic neurons are innervated by separate sets of preganglionic parasympathetic fibers, giving rise to distinct excitatory and inhibitory pathways. Each pathway consists of preganglionic fibers in the vagus and postganglionic neurons located in the myenteric plexus. The excitatory cholinergic pathway originates in the rostral part of the DMN, whereas the inhibitory nitrergic pathway in the caudal regions of the same nucleus.[89,91] However, postganglionic myenteric motor neurons also receive input from local intramural sensory neurons and, consequently, participate in local mediated reflexes.[89,91]

Although the myenteric plexus is best developed in the smooth muscle region, a ganglionated myenteric network is also found within the skeletal muscle portion of the esophagus, but its role is still largely unknown.[104] The presence of intrinsic neurons at motor endplates in adults may represent a specific holdover from early developmental stages.[105] However, recent data suggest that enteric coinnervation is involved in the smooth-to-striated switch (ie, transdifferentiation process) occurring during development, thereby playing a key role in the ontogeny of skeletal muscle.[106] Additionally, the chemical coding and spatial relationships of enteric coinnervation support an inhibitory modulation of vagally mediated contraction of esophageal skeletal muscle.[107-108] Thus, the central pattern generator controlling esophageal peristalsis may be immature at birth, and the prominent enteric co-innervation in the early postnatal period functionally compensates it by local modulation of skeletal motor activity.[104]

At rest, the musculature of the esophageal body does not exhibit rhythmic or tonic contractions. Intraluminal pressure relative to atmospheric pressure varies from −5 to −15 mm Hg during normal inspiration to −2 to +5 mm Hg during expiration.[109] Primary peristalsis is defined as a reflex esophageal peristaltic contraction wave initiated by swallowing (Figure 4). It results from a sequential contraction of esophageal muscle layers moving down the entire length of the esophagus, appearing shortly after the pharyngeal contraction traverses the UES.[94] Control of esophageal peristalsis in the smooth muscle regions is more complicated than in the adjacent skeletal muscle regions. In the latter, neurons located in the NA (central pattern generator) initiate the peristaltic wave and control the sequencing of the contraction, by a consecutive activation of motor neurons innervating progressively distal segments in the skeletal esophagus (Figure 5).[91] Thus, coordination of skeletal muscle cells is not influenced by intramural enteric plexus and is totally under central control. On the other hand, primary peristalsis in the esophageal smooth muscle segments is under an integrated control, which combines both central and intramural mechanisms (Figure 6).[110] In smooth muscle esophageal segments the CNS is required for activation of the primary peristaltic wave, exerting only some control over the contraction sequencing program, through the modulation of intramural enteric neurons.[111-112] Elegant studies reveal that esophageal peristalsis is largely determined by a neurally mediated intrinsic "latency gradient" of contraction waves along smooth muscle segments.[113] Upon intrinsic neuron stimulation, this coordinated latency gradient relates to the initial release of NANC inhibitory neurotransmitters, causing membrane hyperpolarization.[114] NO is the predominant inhibitory neurotransmitter involved in esophageal peristaltic activity, having a great influence on both the direction and the velocity of propagating waves.[115] The duration of this hyperpolarization is longer aborally, so that the resulting contraction is delayed aborally.[116]

In adults, the contraction amplitude of peristaltic waves is lowest in the midesophagus (between 30 and 40 mm Hg), which corresponds to the transition zone of mixed skeletal and smooth muscle cells, and highest in the lower esophagus (between 50 and 90 mm Hg).[117-118] The efficacy of esophageal emptying is strongly related to the peristaltic amplitude with emptying becoming progressively impaired when the peristaltic amplitude is less than 35 mm Hg.[119] The wave duration increases progressively in the distal parts of the esophagus, whereas wave propagation is faster in the upper esophagus. In adults, peristaltic contractions are lumen-occluding contractions lasting from 2 to 7 seconds and traversing the esophagus at a velocity of about 4 cm/s, taking between 10 and 15 seconds to complete a primary peristaltic activity.[120-121]

Esophageal motor activity is functionally present at birth. Using micromanometric assembly,

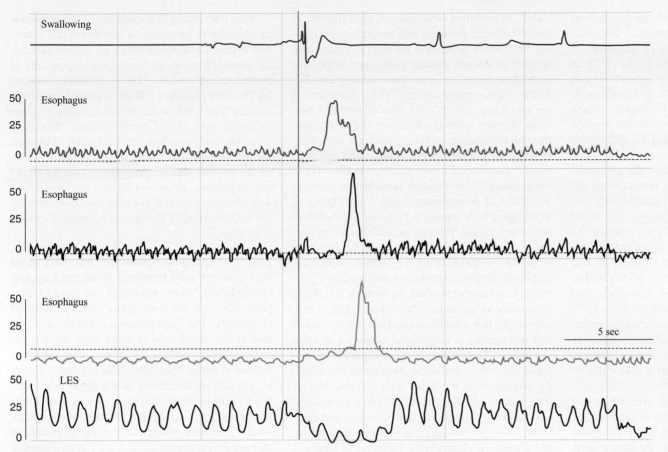

Figure 4 Manometric recording of the esophageal peristalsis (second, third, and fourth channels) and relaxation of the lower esophageal sphincter (fifth channel). The first channel records the swallowing activity.

primary peristalsis that is well-developed at 33 weeks postmenstrual age can be detected as early as 26 weeks of gestation age, indicating full development of the central control of swallow-induced peristalsis.[122–123] In premature infants between 33 and 38 weeks postmenstrual age, two major esophageal motility patterns are identified: a peristaltic sequence and a nonperistaltic sequence.[122] The latter includes synchronous, incomplete, and retrograde pressure wave sequences. Although in premature infants, there is characteristically a high proportion of swallow-unrelated nonperistaltic sequences; the most frequent esophageal motor pattern in response

to swallowing is primary peristalsis. However, during early phases of growth, nonperistaltic sequences may represent motor activity equivalent to the burst of nondeglutitive esophageal

contraction recorded in adults.[124] The motor pattern of esophageal body triggered by deglutition in preterm infants, studying longitudinally at 33 and 36 weeks postmenstrual age, has been

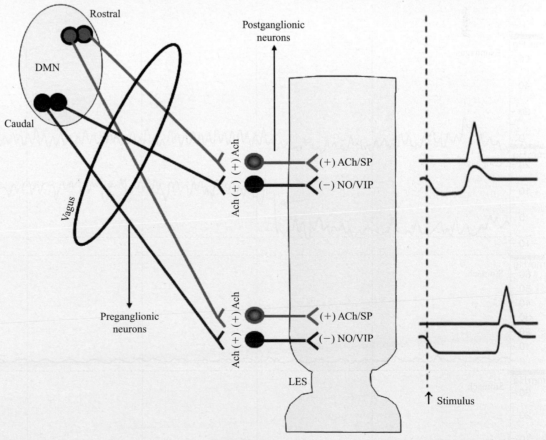

Figure 5 Central control of peristalsis in the striated muscle portion of the esophagus.

Figure 6 Central control, and inhibitory and excitatory innervation of the esophageal smooth muscle. DMN: dorsal motor nucleus of the vagus; Ach: acetylcholine; NO: nitric oxide; SP: substance P; VIP: vasoactive intestinal peptide; LES: lower esophageal sphincter.

compared with findings in both healthy full-term born infants and adult volunteers.[87] Successful coordination and complete propagation of the primary peristaltic sequences occur in 70 to 80% of swallows in neonates (both preterm and full-term infants), whereas 99% of swallows in adults propagate completely. Full-term infants show an esophageal peristaltic velocity twofold greater than preterm babies, but no difference was found in either the amplitude or the duration of peristaltic waves between the two neonatal groups.[87] Compared with neonates, adults exhibit higher amplitude and shorter durations of contraction in the proximal esophagus, and faster peristaltic velocity in the distal esophagus. As in adults, in children the mean amplitude values of peristaltic contractions range between 40 and 89 mm Hg, whereas the duration of peristaltic contractions is between 2.5 and 5 seconds, and the propagation velocity is around 3.0 cm/s.[125,127] These data indicate that the increase in organ growth and muscle mass, enteric neuromuscular coordination, and brain stem maturation, particularly vagal nerve activity, underlie motor development of the esophagus.

Secondary peristalsis can be elicited at any level of the esophagus in response to luminal distension by fluid and air. It does not involve the full swallowing reflex. Usually secondary peristalsis starts at the highest level reached by the refluxed materials into the esophagus and contributes to the esophageal clearance of a bolus not fully cleared by a primary peristaltic wave. The amplitude and velocity of secondary peristalsis are similar to those observed during primary peri-

stalsis. In human skeletal muscle, no difference is found between primary and secondary peristalsis, both being dependent on central vagal pathways.[89] In smooth muscle esophageal segments, secondary peristalsis is an intramural reflex elicited by local sensory nerves.[89] Thus, distension of the esophagus causes activation of intrinsic neurons, eliciting contraction above the distension, through cholinergic excitatory neurons, and relaxation below the distension, through nitrergic neurons.[128] Esophageal motor response to abrupt mild midesophageal provocation is present as early as 33 weeks of postmenstrual age.[88] Two types of esophageal body pressure response are noted in premature infants: primary peristalsis and secondary peristalsis, and the latter is the predominant response compared with the former to both air and liquid distensions. The rate of secondary peristalsis is volume dependent for both air and liquid distension during midesophageal provocation test, suggesting that secondary peristalsis is an important mechanism in esophageal clearance of large volumes.[88] The frequency of completely propagated secondary peristalsis as well as the velocity of peristalsis increases with growth. In preterm infants, the duration of proximal esophageal contractions shortens during neonatal development, whereas propagating velocity during liquid distension significantly increases.[88] Changes in central control mechanisms and enteric neural pathways likely underlie these changes in motility pattern during development. Tertiary contractions occur spontaneously and randomly in the mid and lower esophagus, unrelated to either swallowing or reflux and with no peristaltic function.

One interesting phenomenon of the peristaltic mechanism is "deglutitive inhibition."[129] A second swallow, initiated while an earlier peristaltic contraction, is still progressing, results in complete inhibition of the contraction induced by the first swallow. With repeated swallows at very short intervals, the esophagus remains inhibited and a large "clearing wave" will occur after the last swallow in the series. Although the deglutitive inhibition primarily is a function of the central pattern generator of the swallowing sequences, cessation of neuronal excitatory and inhibitory discharges may also contribute to the interruption of peristalsis in smooth muscle segments.[130]

Lower Esophageal Sphincter. The LES is the high-pressure zone localized at the esophagogastric junction, which regulates the flow of contents between the esophagus and the stomach (Figure 7). The high-pressure zone at the lower end of the esophagus is more than the smooth muscle fibers of the LES, and a poor antireflux barrier is more than low LES pressure. Intrinsic smooth muscle fibers of the distal esophagus (LES) constitute the intrinsic active component of the sphincteric mechanism at the esophagogastric junction, whereas the skeletal muscle of diaphragm represent the extrinsic active component.[131] Since the two components are anatomically superimposed and anchored to each other by the phrenoesophageal ligament that extends from the inferior diaphragmatic surface to the distal esophagus, the LES and crural diaphragm function as a well-coordinated and efficient functional

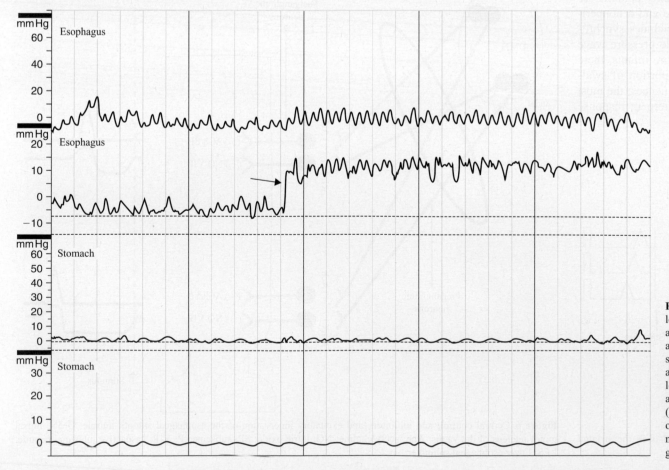

Figure 7 Manometric tracing at the level of the distal esophagus and stomach. From top to bottom: distal esophagus (*first channel*), lower esophageal sphincter (*second channel*), and stomach (*third and fourth channels*). At the level of the second channel, there is a sudden rise in the pressure profile (*arrow*) corresponding to the entrance of the recording side-hole of a manometric catheter into the lower esophageal sphincter.

unit. The muscles of LES are thicker than those of the adjacent esophagus and are not completely arranged in circular fashion; distally, they are split into two segments, one straddles the greater curvature and is parallel to the sling fiber of the stomach, and the other consists of short clasps that straddles the lesser curvature and join the gastric sling fibers, which play a key role in the formation and modulation of the angle of His.[131] The LES is tonically contracted at rest to produce a roughly concentric occlusion. However, the occlusion is not perfectly uniform, showing a radial asymmetry.[109] In adults, the LES is 2 to 4 cm long, whereas in children its length increases with age, ranging from few millimeters in newborns to adult values in adolescents.[8,94] In adults, as in older children, the proximal 1.5 to 2 cm of the sphincter is above the squamocolumnar mucosal junction and completely encircled by the crural diaphragm, whereas the distal 2 cm is below the squamocolumnar mucosal junction.[131] Consequently, the proximal part of the sphincter lies in the esophageal hiatus, the distal 2 cm in the abdominal cavity. Sphincteric exposure to high intra-abdominal pressures likely contribute to the maintenance of EGJ competence. At 8 weeks of gestation, the abdominal portion of sphincter is wide and large; gradually, it shortens so that in newborns the intra-abdominal portion of the sphincter is very short or completely absent, predicting the possibility of developing gastroesophageal reflux.[8] Other mechanisms explaining the greater frequency of gastroesophageal reflux (GER) in infants include the less oblique angle of insertion of the esophagus into the stomach. However, the exact role of these predisposing factors in determining GER in infants is still largely unknown.[132,133]

Afferent sensory information from the LES to the brain runs in both spinal and vagal sensory afferents. Spinal afferents have their cell bodies in the dorsal root ganglia at T1 to L3, whereas vagal afferents have cell bodies in the nodose ganglia.[97,131,134] The afferent stimuli travel to the sensory nucleus, that is, NTS, which is closely connected with the DMN of the vagus nerve.[97,131,134] The latter provides parallel inhibitory and excitatory motor innervation to the LES. The rostral neurons in the DMN preferentially give rise to innervate the excitatory vagal pathway, whereas neurons in the caudal regions give rise to the inhibitory vagal pathway.[134] Excitatory preganglionic neurons are cholinergic in nature and synapse on postganglionic nitrergic inhibitory neurons localized in the myenteric plexus.[134] Inhibitory preganglionic neurons are also cholinergic in nature and synapse on postganglionic cholinergic excitatory neurons localized in the myenteric plexus.[134] Myenteric motor neurons to the LES are also innervated by postganglionic sympathetic neurons. However, the vagus nerve exerts the main regulatory action on the LES, whereas sympathetic neurons exert only a modulatory role.[97,131,134]

One of the main functions of the LES is to create a high-pressure zone for preventing retrograde movement of gastric content into the esophagus. The LES is tonically contracted at rest (Figure 7), exhibiting both radial and axial pressure asymmetry.[135] The LES resting tone is determined by three factors (Figure 8): myogenic properties of sphincteric smooth muscle cells, which are independent of any neural influences and may be produced by ionic movement (ie, calcium) through smooth muscle cell membranes; cholinergic excitatory activity; and nitrergic inhibitory activity.[89,94] Excitatory cholinergic neurons and the tonic myogenic property of LES (the first two factors) stimulate contraction, whereas the inhibitory nitrergic pathway favors relaxation.[89] Thus, the net balance between these factors determines the final resting pressure of the LES.

LES pressure is influenced by several factors (Table 2). It is significantly variable during the interdigestive migrating motor complex (MMC) cycle. There is a pattern of LES contraction closely related to the phase of MMC in the stomach, showing higher LES pressure during MMC phase III than in phase I.[136] Postprandial LES pressure is rather constant at a level comparable with levels measured during phase I of the MMC.[136] LES pressure also shows inspiratory augmentation due to contraction of the crural diaphragm encircling the sphincter.[131] LES pressure is also modified by intra-abdominal pressure, gastric distension, peptides, hormones, various foods, and many drugs.[89,94]

During swallowing and belching, the LES promptly relaxes in order to allow the passage of ingested food or air in appropriate directions (Figure 4). At the time of swallowing, the LES relaxes promptly in response to the initial neural discharge from the swallowing center in order to minimize resistance to flow across the esophagogastric junction.[131] This relaxation starts within 2 seconds after the peristaltic contraction has begun in the proximal esophagus and lasts 5 to 10 seconds until the peristaltic wave reaches the distal esophagus. During relaxation, LES pressure falls to the level of gastric pressure. As the LES relaxes (an active process), it is passively opened by the bolus and propelled by the peristaltic wave. LES relaxation is followed by an aftercontraction of the upper part of the sphincter, which likely represents the end of contraction wave as it reaches the distal esophagus.[94]

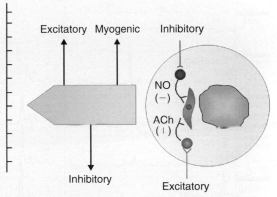

Figure 8 Three mechanisms involved in the regulation of basal LES tone.

Swallow-induced LES relaxation is part of primary peristalsis.[97,131,134] Central control is provided by preganglionic parasympathetic neurons originating in the nuclei of dorsal vagal complex, represented by the NTS, which receives sensory information from the pharynx and by the DMN, which contains preganglionic motor output to the LES.[97,131,134] NO and acetylcholine are the principal neurotransmitters involved in the neural network at the DMN, even though γ-aminobutyric acid (GABA) is involved in the control of preganglionic neurons.[137–138] The axons of preganglionic parasympathetic neurons synapse with intramural inhibitory neurons. Convincing evidence supports the role of NO as the main postganglionic neurotransmitter mediating swallow-induced relaxation of the LES.[138]

Transient relaxation of the LES refers to relaxation that is unrelated to either swallowing or secondary peristalsis (Figure 9). Transient LES relaxations (TLESRs) occur in healthy persons and represent the mechanism by which gas is vented from the stomach during belching.[139] Characteristically, it is associated with inhibition of the crural diaphragm.[140] TLESRs are of longer duration than swallow-induced relaxation of the LES, lasting between 10 and 45 seconds.[141] Manometric criteria for defining TLESR include: (1) the absence of a pharyngeal swallow for 4 seconds before and 2 seconds after the beginning of LES relaxation; (2) LES pressure falls of 1 mm Hg/s; (3) ≤10 seconds to complete the relaxation of the LES; and (4) a nadir pressure during the relaxation

Table 2 Factors Affecting Lower Esophageal Sphincter Pressure (LESP)		
Factor	Increase LESP	Decrease LESP
Hormones	Gastrin, motilin, substance P, bombesin, galanin, pancreatic polypeptide, somatostatin	Secretin, CCK, glucagon, VIP, progesterone, calcitonin gene-related peptide (CGRP)
Neural agents	α-Adrenergic agonist, β-adrenergic antagonist, cholinergic agonist, serotonin	α-Adrenergic antagonist, β-adrenergic agonist, cholinergic antagonist, nitric oxide (NO)
Medications	Metoclopramide, domperidone, cisapride, histamine, prostaglandin F_{2a} erythromycin (motilin receptor agonist)	Nitrates, calcium channel blockers, theophylline, morphine, meperidine, diazepam, sildenafil, prostaglandin E_1, prostaglandin E_2
Food	Protein	Fat, chocolate, ethanol, peppermint

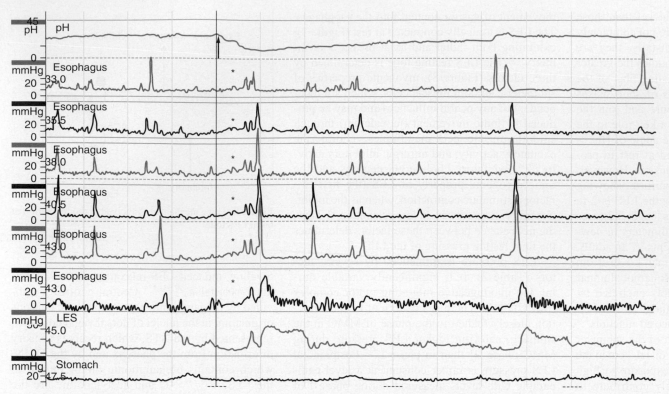

Figure 9 Prolonged recording of the lower esophageal sphincter activity. From top to bottom: pH (*first channel*), esophageal body (*second to seventh channels*), lower esophageal sphincter (*eighth channel*), and stomach (*ninth channel*). A transient lower esophageal sphincter relaxation is evident during the occurrence of a reflux episode (*arrow noted in the pH channel*). During the reflux episode, a common cavity phenomenon (defined as an increase in intraesophageal pressure, indicative of flow into the esophagus) is recorded along the body of the esophagus (*asterisks*).

≤ 2 mm Hg.[141] TLESRs are a neural reflex involving afferent and efferent pathways, and a central pattern generator, corresponding to the nuclei of dorsal vagal complex.[131,134] The afferent pathway is activated by stimulation of tension receptors in the proximal stomach, particularly the subcardial region, as well as by of pharyngeal stimuli. Afferent neurons, through the vagus, travel to the NTS and the DMV via interneurons. The efferent pathway involves the same efferent neural pathways of swallow-induced LES relaxation. However, because of crural diaphragm are also inhibited during TLESRs, the phrenic nerve nucleus located in the spinal cord may also be involved.[131] TLESRs are more frequent in the seated position, with large meals and in response to higher intragastric osmolarity. Although TLESRs are an essential component of belch reflex, they also represent the predominant mechanism underlying gastroesophageal reflux (GER) episodes in both normal and patients with GER disease (GERD). The proportion of reflux episodes attributable to TLESRs ranges between 100% in children with nonerosive reflux disease (NERD) and healthy adults, compared to 60 to 80% in children and adults with erosive esophagitis.[142–145]

In children, LES pressure ranges between 10 and 40 mm Hg.[125,126] LES pressures of 5 mm Hg above intragastric pressure are sufficient to maintain esophagogastric competence.[131,132] Using a perfused side-hole pull-through technique, LES pressure was reported as very low in preterm infants, increasing from ~4 mm Hg in premature infants younger than 29 weeks of age to 18 mm Hg in term infants.[146,147] By employing a micromanometric assembly with a sleeve device, LES pressure can be detected in preterm infants from 26 weeks gestation.[148] In very premature infants, LES pressure ranges between 5 and

20 mm Hg and promptly relaxes with swallowing, indicating full development of the central control of swallow-induced LES relaxation.[123] In addition, LES pressure in premature infants fluctuates substantially over time and significantly decreases after feeding. In both premature infants and term infants, TLESRs are the predominant mechanisms underlying GER episodes, indicating that the neural pathway responsible for transient inhibition of LES tone is already full developed.[148,149] Thus, LES motor patterns in premature infants are almost identical to those recorded in older children and adults.

REFERENCES

1. Larsen WJ. Development of gastrointestinal tract. In: Sherman LS, Potter SS, Scott WJ, editors. Human Embryology, 3rd edition. Philadelphia: Churchill Livingstone; 2001. p. 235–64.
2. Larsen WJ. Embryonic folding. In: Sherman LS, Potter SS, Scott WJ, editors. Human Embryology, 3rd edition. Philadelphia: Churchill Livingstone; 2001. p. 133–4.
3. Mansfield LE. Embryonic origins of the relation of gastroesophageal reflux disease and airway disease. Am J Med. 2001;111:3S–7S.
4. Pringle KC. Human fetal lung development and related animal models. Clin Obstet Gynecol. 1986;29:502–13.
5. Qi BQ, Beasley SW, Williams AK. Evidence of a common pathogenesis for foregut duplications and esophageal atresia with tracheo-esophageal fistula. Anat Rec. 2001;264:93–100.
6. Cardoso WV, Lu J. Regulation of early lung morphogenesis: Questions, facts and controversies. Development. 2006;133:1611–24.
7. Montgomery RK, Mulberg AE, Grand RJ. Development of the human gastrointestinal tract: Twenty years of progress. Gastroenterology 1999;116:702–31.
8. Skandalakis JE, Ellis H. Embryologic and anatomic basis of esophageal surgery. Sur Clin North Am 2000;80:85–155.
9. Menard D, Arsenault P. Maturation of human fetal esophagus maintained in organ culture. Anat Rec. 1987;217:348–54.
10. Long JD, Orlando RC. Anatomy, histology, embryology, and developmental abnormalities of the esophagus. In: Feldman M, Fieldman LS, Sleisenger MH, editors. Gastrointestinal and Liver Disease. Philadelphia: WB Saunders; 2002. p. 551–60.
11. Menard D. Morphological studies of the developing human esophageal epithelium. Microsc Res Tech 1995;31:215–25.
12. Yu WY, Slack JM, Tosh D. Conversion of columnar to stratified squamous epithelium in the developing mouse esophagus. Dev Biol. 2005;284:157–70.
13. Liebermann-Meffert D, Duranceau A. Anatomy and embryology. In: Orringer MB, Zuidema GD, editors. Shackelford's Surgery of the Alimentary Tract, 4th edition. Philadelphia: Saunders. 1996, p. 3–38.
14. Wallace AS, Burns AJ. Development of the enteric nervous system, smooth muscle and interstitial cells of Cajal in the human gastrointestinal tract. Cell Tissue Res 2005; 319:367–82.
15. Patapoutian A, Wold BJ, Wagner RA. Evidence for developmentally programmed transdifferentiation in mouse esophageal muscle. Science 1995;270:1818–21.
16. Stratton CJ, Bayguinov J, Kenton M, et al. Ultrastructural analysis of the transdifferentiation of smooth muscle to skeletal muscle in the murine esophagus. Cell Tissue Res 2000;301:83–298.
17. Gershon MD, Chalazonitis A, Rothman TP. From neural crest to bowel: Development of the enteric nervous system. J Neurobiol 1993;24:199–214.
18. Furness JB. Types of neurons in the enteric nervous system. J Auton Nerv Syst 2000;81:87–96.
19. Galligan JJ, LePard KJ, Schneider DA, et al. Multiple mechanisms of fast excitatory synaptic transmission in the enteric nervous system. J Auton Nerv Syst 2000;81:97–103.
20. Liu MT, Rothstein JD, Gershon MD, et al. Glutamatergic enteric neurons. J Neurosci 1997;17:4764–84.
21. Grundy D, Schemann M. Enteric nervous system. Curr Opin Gastroenterol 2006;22:102–10.
22. Powley TL. Vagal input to the enteric nervous system. Gut 2000;47:30–2.
23. Furness JB, Johnson PJ, Pompolo S, et al. Evidence that enteric motility reflexes can be initiated through entirely intrinsic mechanisms in the guinea-pig small intestine. Neurogastroenterol Motil 1995;7:89–96.
24. Furness JB, Kunze WA, Bertrand PP, et al. Intrinsic primary afferent neurons of the intestine. Prog Neurobiol 1998; 54:1–18.
25. Giaroni C, De Ponti F, Cosentino M, et al. Plasticity in the enteric nervous system. Gastroenterology 1999;117:1438–58.
26. Wood JD, Alpers DH, Andrews PL. Fundamentals of neurogastroenterology. Gut 1999; 45:6–16.
27. Costa M, Brookes SJ, Hennig GW. Anatomy and physiology of the enteric nervous system. Gut 2000;47:15–9.
28. Pattyn A, Morin X, Cremer H, et al. The homeobox gene Phox2b is essential for the development of autonomic neural crest derivatives. Nature 1999;399:366–70.
29. Guillemot F, Lo LC, Johnson JE, et al. Mammalian achaete-scute homolog 1 is required for the early development of olfactory and autonomic neurons. Cell 1993;75:463–76.

30. Schuchardt A, D'Agati V, Larsson-Blomberg L, et al. Defects in the kidney and enteric nervous system of mice lacking the tyrosine kinase receptor Ret. Nature 1994;367:380–3.
31. Newgreen D, Young HM. Enteric nervous system: Development and developmental disturbances—part 1. Pediatr Dev Pathol 2002;5,224–47.
32. Newgreen DF. Establishment of the form of the peripheral nervous system. In: Hendry IA, Hill CE, editors. Development, Regeneration and Plasticity of the Autonomic Nervous System. Switzerland: Harwood Academic Publishers, Chur; 1992. p. 1–94.
33. Smith VV, Milla PJ. Developmental disorders. In: Spiller R, Grundy D, editors. Pathophysiology of the Enteric Nervous System. 1st edition. Oxford: Blackwell Publishing, 2004. p. 47–60.
34. Yntema CL, Hammond WS. The origin of intrinsic ganglia of trunk viscera from vagal neural crest in the chick embryo. J Comp Neurol 1954;101:515–41.
35. Le Douarin NM, Teillet MA. The migration of neural crest cells to the wall of the digestive tract in avian embryo. J Embryol Exp Morphol 1973;30:31–48.
36. Yntema CL, Hammond WS. Experiments on the origin and development of the sacral autonomic nerves in the chick embryo. J Exp Zool 1955;129:375–413.
37. Burns AJ, Le Douarin NM. The sacral neural crest contributes neurons and glia to the post-umbilical gut: Spatiotemporal analysis of the development of the enteric nervous system. Development 1998;125:4335–47.
38. Burns AJ, Champeval D, Le Douarin NM. Sacral neural crest cells colonise aganglionic hindgut in vivo but fail to compensate for lack of enteric ganglia. Dev Biol 2000;219:30–43.
39. Burns AJ, Delalande JM, Le Douarin NM. In ovo transplantation of enteric nervous system precursors from vagal to sacral neural crest results in extensive hindgut colonisation. Development 2002;129:2785–96.
40. Burns AJ. Migration of neural crest-derived enteric nervous system precursor cells to and within the gastrointestinal tract. Int J Dev Biol 2005;49:143–150.
41. Newgreen D, Young HM. Enteric nervous system: Development and developmental disturbances—part 2. Pediatr Dev Pathol 2002;5:329–49.
42. Rauch U, Schafer KH. The extracellular matrix and its role in cell migration and development of the enteric nervous system. Eur J Pediatr Surg 2003;13:158–62.
43. Parikh DH, Tam PK, Van Velzen D, et al. The extracellular matrix components, tenascin and fibronectin, in Hirschsprung's disease: An immunohistochemical study. J Pediatr Surg 1994;29:1302–06.
44. Lo LC, Johnson JE, Wuenschell CW, et al. Mammalian achaete-scute homolog 1 is transiently expressed by spatially restricted subsets of early neuroepithelial and neural crest cells. Genes Dev 1991;5:1524–37.
45. Gershon MD. Genes and lineages and tissue interactions in the formation of the enteric nervous system. Am J Physiol 1998;275:G869–73.
46. Sang Q, Ciampoli D, Greferath U, et al. Innervation of the esophagus in mice that lack MASH1. J Comp Neurol 1999;408:1–10.
47. Sommer L, Shah N, Rao M, et al. The cellular function of MASH1 in autonomic neurogenesis. Neuron 1995;15: 1245–58.
48. Hirsch MR, Tiveron MC, Guillemot F, et al. Control of noradrenergic differentiation and Phox2a expression by MASH1 in the central and peripheral nervous system. Development 1998;125:599–608.
49. Lo LC, Tiveron MC, Anderson DJ. MASH1 activates expression of the paired homeodomain transcription factor Phox2a, and couples pan-neuronal and subtype-specific components of autonomic neuronal identity. Development 1998;125:609–20.
50. Park W, Vaezi MF. Etiology and pathogenesis of achalasia: The current understanding. Am J Gastroenterol 2005;100:1404–14.
51. Ball DW, Azzoli CG, Baylin SB, et al. Identification of a human achaete-scute homolog highly expressed in neuroendocrine tumors. Proc Natl Acad Sci USA 1993;90:5648–52.
52. Gestblom C, Grynfeld A, Ora I, et al. The basic helix-loop-helix transcription factor dHAND, a marker gene for the developing human sympathetic nervous system, is expressed in both high- and low-stage neuroblastomas. Lab Invest 1999;79:67–79.
53. Borges M, Linnoila RI, van de Velde HJ, et al. An achaetescute homologue essential for neuroendocrine differentiation in the lung. Nature 1997;386:852–5.
54. Chen H, Biel MA, Borges MW, et al. Tissue-specific expression of human achaete-scute homologue-1 in neuroendocrine tumors: Transcriptional regulation by dual inhibitory regions. Cell Growth Differ 1997;8:677–86.
55. Bowie JD, Clair MR. Fetal swallowing and regurgitation: Observation of normal and abnormal activity. Radiology 1982;144:877–8.
56. Boyle JT. Motility of upper gastrointestinal tract in the fetus and neonate. In: Polin RA, Fox WW, editors. Fetal and Neonatal Physiology. Philadelphia: WB Saunders; 1998. p. 1028–32.
57. Dumont RC, Rudolph CD. Development of gastrointestinal motility in the infant and child. Gastroenterol Clin North Am 1994;23:655–71.
58. Herbst J. Development of suck and swallow. J Pediatr Gastroentero Nutr 1983;2:131–5.
59. Ross MG, Nijland MJM. Development of ingestive behaviour. Am J Physiol 1998;274:R878–93.
60. Malinger G, Levine A, Rotmensch S. The fetal esophagus: Anatomical and physiological ultrasonographic characterization using a high-resolution linear transducer. Ultrasound Obstet Gynecol 2004;24:500–5.
61. Shaker R. Pharyngeal motor function. In: Leonard R Johnson, editor. Physiology of Gastrointestinal Tract. 4th edition. Burlington, MA: Academic Press; 2006. p. 895–912.
62. Sivarao DV, Gojal RK. Functional anatomy and physiology of the upper esophageal sphincter. Am J Med 2000;108: 27S–37S.
63. Kahrilas PJ, Dodds WJ, Dent J, et al. Upper esophageal sphincter function during deglutition. Gastroenterology 1988;95:52–62.
64. Goyal RK, Martin SB, Shapiro J, et al. The role of cricopharyngeus muscle in pharyngoesophageal disorders. Dysphagia 1993;8:253–8.
65. Mu L, Sanders I. The innervation of the human upper esophageal sphincter. Dysphagia 1996;11:234–8.
66. Yoshida Y, Tanaka Y, Hirano M, et al. Sensory innervation of the pharynx and larynx. Am J Med 2000;108:51S–61S.
67. Malberg L, Ekberg O, Ekstrom J. Effects of drugs and electrical field stimulation on isolated muscle strips from rabbit pharyngoesophageal segment. Dysphagia 1991;6:203–8.
68. Rodrigo J, Polak JM, Fernandez L, et al. Calcitonin gene-related peptide immunoreactive sensory and motor nerves of the rat, cat, and monkey esophagus. Gastroenterology 1985;88:444–51.
69. Mu L, Sanders I. Neuromuscular organization of the human upper esophageal sphincter. Ann Otol Rhinol Laryngol 2001;107:370–7.
70. Mu L, Sanders I. Neuromuscular compartments and fiber-type regionalization in the human inferior pharyngeal constrictor muscle. Anat Rec 2001;264:367–77.
71. Kahrilas PJ, Dent J, Dodds, et al. A method for continuous monitoring of upper esophageal sphincter. Dig Dis Sci 1987;32:121–8.
72. Welch RW, Luckmann K, Ricks PM, et al. Manometry of the normal upper esophageal sphincter and its alterations in laryngectomy. J Clin Ivest 1979;63:1036–41.
73. Kahrilas PJ, Dent J, Dodds, et al. Upper esophageal sphincter function during deglutition. Gastroenterology 1988;95: 52–62.
74. Clouse RE, Diamant NE. Motor function of the esophagus. In: Leonard R Johnson, editor. Physiology of Gastrointestinal Tract, 4th edition. Burlington, MA: Academic Press; 2006. p. 913–26.
75. Lang IM, Sarna, SK, Dodds WJ. The pharyngeal, esophageal, and gastric responses associated with vomiting. Am J Physiol 1993;265:G963–72.
76. Kahrilas PJ, Dodds WJ, Dent J, et al. Upper esophageal function during belching. Gastroenterology 1986;91:133–40.
77. Shaker R, Ren J, Kern M, et al. Mechanisms of airway protection and upper esophageal sphincter opening during belching. Am J Physiol 1992;262:G621–8.
78. Shaker R, Ren J, Xie P, et al. Characterization of the pharyngo-UES contractile reflex in humans. Am J Physiol 1997;273:G854–8.
79. Lang IM, Dana N, Medda BK, et al. Mechanisms of airway protection during retching, vomiting, and swallowing. Am J Physiol 2002;283:G529–36.
80. Lang IM, Medda BK, Shaker R. Mechanisms of reflexes induced by esophageal distension. Am J Physiol 2001;281: G1246–63.
81. Vakil NB, Kahrilas PJ, Dodds WJ, et al. Absence of an upper esophageal sphincter response to acid reflux. Am J Gastroenterol 1989;84:606–10.
82. Sondheimer JM. Upper esophageal sphincter and pharingo-esophageal motor function in infants with or without gastro-esophageal reflux. Gastroenterology 1983;85:301–5.
83. Davidson GP, Dent J, Willing J, et al. Monitoring of upper oesophageal sphincter pressure in children. Gut 1991;32:607–11.
84. Willing J, Davidson GP, Dent J, et al. Effect of gastrooesophageal reflux on upper oesophageal sphincter motility in children. Gut 1993;34:904–10.
85. Willing J, Furukawa Y, Davidson GP, et al. Strain induced augmentation of upper oesophageal sphincter motility in children. Gut 1994;35;159–64.
86. Omari T, Snel A, Barnett C. Measurement of upper esophageal sphincter tone and relaxation during swallowing in premature infants. Am J Physiol 1999; 277:G862–6.
87. Jadcherla SR, Duong HQ, Hoffmann C, et al. Characteristics of upper oesophageal spincter and oesophageal body during maturation in healthy human neonates compared with adults. Neurogastroenterol Motil 2005;17:663–70.
88. Jadcherla SR, Duong HQ, Hoffmann RG, et al. Esophageal body and upper sphincter motor responses to esophageal provocation during maturation in preterm newborns. J Pediatr 2003;143:31–8.
89. Goyal RK, Prasad M, Chang HY. Functional anatomy and physiology of swallowing and esophageal motility. In: Castell DO, Richter JE, editors. The Esophagus, 4th edition. Philadelphia: Lippincott Williams & Wilkins; 2003. p. 1–36.
90. Meyer GW, Austin RM, Brady CE, et al. Muscle anatomy of the human esophagus. J Clin Gastroenterol. 1986;8: 131–4.
91. Jean A. Brain stem control of swallowing: Neuronal network and cellular mechanisms. Physiol Rev 2001;81:829–69.
92. Aziz Q, Rothwell JC, Hamdy S, et al. The topographic representation of esophageal motor function on the human cerebral cortex. Gastroenterology 1996;111:855–62.
93. Broussard DL, Altschuler SM. Brainstem viscerotropic organization of the afferents and efferents involved in the control of swallowing. Am J Med 2000;108:79S–86S.
94. Biancani P, Harnett KM, Behar J. Esophageal motor function. In: Yamada T, editor. Textbook of Gastroenterology, Volume 1, 4th edition. Philadelphia: Lippincott Williams & Wilkins; 1999. p. 166–92.
95. Sengupta JN. An overview of esophageal sensory receptors. Am J Med. 2000;108:87S–9S.
96. Hobson AR, Aziz Q. Brain processing of esophageal sensation in health and disease. Gastroenterol Clin North Am. 2004;33:69–91.
97. Goyal RK, Padmanabhan R, Sang Q. Neural circuits in swallowing and abdominal vagal afferent-mediated lower esophageal sphincter relaxation. Am J Med. 2001;111: 95S–105S.
98. Singaram C, Sengupta A, Sweet MA, et al. Nitrinergic and peptidergic innervation of the human esophagus. Gut 1994;35:1690–96.
99. Singaram C, Sengupta A, Sugarbaker DJ, et al. Peptidergic innervation of the human esophageal smooth muscle. Gastroenterology 1991;101:1256–63.
100. Crist J, Gidda JS, Goyal RK. Intramural mechanisms of esophageal peristalsis: Roles of cholinergic and noncholinergic nerves. Proc Natl Acad Sci USA 1984;81:3595–99.
101. Crist J, Gidda J, Goyal RK. Role of substance P nerves in longitudinal smooth muscle contractions of the esophagus. Am J Physiol 1986;250:G336–43.
102. Yamato S, Spechler SJ, Goyal RK. Role of nitric oxide in esophageal peristalsis in the opossum. Gastroenterology 1992;103:197–204.
103. Murray JA, Ledlow A, Launspach J, et al. The effects of recombinant human hemoglobin on esophageal motor function in humans. Gastroenterology 1995;109:1241–48.
104. Wörl J, Neuhuber WL. Enteric co-innervation of motor endplates in the esophagus: State of the art ten years after. Histochem Cell Biol 2005;123:117–30.
105. Neuhuber WL, Eichhorn U, Worl J. Enteric co-innervation of striated muscle fibers in the esophagus: Just a "hangover"? Anat Rec. 2001;262:41–6.
106. Breuer C, Neuhuber WL, Worl J. Development of neuromuscular junctions in the mouse esophagus: Morphology suggests a role for enteric coinnervation during maturation of vagal myoneural contacts. J Comp Neurol. 2004;475:47–69.
107. Storr M, Geisler F, Neuhuber WL, et al. Characterization of vagal input to the rat esophageal muscle. Auton Neurosci 2001;91:1–9.
108. Izumi N, Matsuyama H, Ko M, et al. Role of intrinsic nitrergic neurones on vagally mediated striated muscle contractions in the hamster esophagus. J Physiol. 2003;551: 287–94.
109. Christensen J. Motor function of the pharynx and esophagus. In: Leonard R Johnson editor. Physiology of the Gastrointestinal Tract, 2nd edition. New York: Raven Press; 1987. p. 595–612.
110. Reynolds RP, El Sharkawy TY, Diamant NE. Lower esophageal sphincter function in the cat: Role of central innervation assessed by transient vagal blockade. Am J Physiol 1984;246:G666–74.
111. Gidda JS, Goyal RK. Influence of successive vagal stimulations on contractions in esophageal smooth muscle of opossum. J Clin Invest 1983;71:1095–103.

112. Gidda JS, Goyal RK. Regional gradient of initial inhibition and refractoriness in esophageal smooth muscle. Gastroenterology 1985;89:843–51.

113. Weisbrodt NW, Christensen J. Gradients of contractions in the opossum esophagus. Gastroenterology 1972;62:1159–66

114. Serio R, Daniel EE. Electrophysiological analysis of responses to intrinsic nerves in circular muscle of opossum esophageal muscle. Am J Physiol 1988;254:G107–16.

115. Anand N, Paterson WG. Role of nitric oxide in esophageal peristalsis. Am J Physiol 1994;266:G123–31.

116. Sifrim D, Janssens J, Vantrappen G. A wave of inhibition precedes primary peristaltic contractions in the human esophagus. Gastroenterology 1992;103:876–82.

117. Richter JE, Wu WC, Johns DN, et al. Esophageal manometry in 95 healthy adult volunteers. Variability of pressures with age and frequency of "abnormal" contractions. Dig Dis Sci. 1987;32:583–92.

118. Hewson EG, Ott DJ, Dalton CB, et al. Manometry and radiology. Complementary studies in the assessment of esophageal motility disorders. Gastroenterology. 1990;98:626–32.

119. Kahrilas PJ, Dodds WJ, Hogan WJ, et al. Peristaltic dysfunction in peptic esophagitis. Gastroenterology 1986;91:897–904.

120. Clouse RE, Hallett JL. Velocity of peristaltic propagation in distal esophageal segments. Dig Dis Sci 1995;40:1311–6.

121. Frobert O, Middelfart HV, Bagger JP, et al. Distal oesophageal motility characteristics in relation to amplitude of contraction in healthy persons. Scand J Gastroenterol 1996;31:966–72.

122. Omari TI, Miki K, Fraser R, et al. Esophageal body and lower esophageal sphincter function in healthy premature infants. Gastroenterology 1995;109:1757–64.

123. Omari TI, Benninga MA, Barnett CP, et al. Characterization of esophageal body and lower esophageal sphincter motor function in the very premature neonate. J Pediatr 1999;135:517–21.

124. Janssen J, Annese V, Vantrappen G. Burst of non-deglutive simultaneous contractions may be a normal oesophagealò motility pattern. Gut 1993;34:1021–24.

125. Hillemeier AC, Grill BB, McCallum R, et al. Esophageal and gastric motor abnormalities in infants with and without gastroesophageal reflux. Gastroenterology 1983;84:741–6.

126. Cucchiara S, Staiano A, Di Lorenzo C, et al. Esophageal motor abnormalities in children with gastroesophageal reflux and peptic esophagitis. J Pediatr 1986;108:907–10.

127. Mahony MJ, Migliavacca M, Spits L, et al. Motor disorders of the esophagus in gastroesophageal reflux. Arch Dis Child 1988;63:1333–38.

128. Bornstein JC, Costa M, Grider JR. Enteric motor and interneuronal circuits controlling motility. Neurogastroenterol Motil 2004;16:34–8.

129. Castell JA, Castell DO. Stationary esophageal manometry. Functional investigation in esophageal disease. In: Modlin IR, Rozen P, and Scarpignato C, editors. Basel: Front Gastrointest Res. Karger; 1994. p. 71–108.

130. Dong H, Loomis CW, Bieger D. Distal and deglutitive inhibition in the rat esophagus: Role of inhibitory neurotransmission in the nucleus tractus solitarii. Gastroenterology 2000;118:328–6.

131. Mittal RK, Balaban DH. The esophagogastric junction. N Engl J Med 1997;336:924–32.

132. Davidson GP, Omari TI. Reflux in children. Baillieres Best Pract Res Clin Gastroenterol 2000;14:839–55.

133. Cresi F, de Sanctis L, Savino F, et al. Relationship between gastroesophageal reflux and gastric activity in newborns assessed by combined intraluminal impedance, pH metry and epigastric impedance. Neurogastroenterol Motil 2006;18:361–8.

134. Hornby PJ, Abrahams TP, Partosoedarso ER. Central mechanisms of lower esophageal sphincter control. Gastroenterol Clin North Am 2002;31:S11–20.

135. Liu J, Parashar VK, Mittal RK. Asymmetry of lower esophageal sphincter pressure: Is it related to the muscle thickness or its shape? Am J Physiol 1997;272:G1509–17.

136. Dent J, Dodds WJ, Sekigushi T, et al. Interdigestive phasic contraction of the human lower esophageal sphincter. Gastroenterology 1983;84:453–60.

137. McDermott CM, Abrahams TP, Partosoedarso E, et al. Site of action of GABA(B) receptor for vagal motor control of the lower esophageal sphincter in ferrets and rats. Gastroenterology 2001;120:1749–62.

138. Yamato S, Saha JK, Goyal RK. Role of nitric oxide in lower esophageal sphincter relaxation to swallowing. Life Sci 1992;50:1263–72.

139. Wyman JB, Dent J, Heddle R, et al. Control of belching by the lower oesophageal sphincter. Gut 1990;31:639–46.

140. Mittal RK, Holloway RH, Penagini R, et al. Transient lower esophageal sphincter relaxation. Gastroenterology 1995;109:601–10.

141. Holloway RH, Penagini R, Ireland AC. Criteria for the objective definition of transient lower esophageal sphincter relaxation. Am J Physiol 1994;268:G128–33.

142. Dodds WJ, Dent J, Hogan WG, et al. Mechanism of gastroesophageal reflux in patients with reflux esophagitis. N Engl J Med 1982;307:1547.

143. Dent J, Dodds WJ, Friedman RH, et al. Mechanism of gastroesophageal reflux in recumbent asymptomatic human subjects. J Clin Invest 1980;65:256–67.

144. Cucchiara S, Bortolotti M, Minella R, et al. Fasting and postprandial mechanisms of gastroesophageal reflux in children with gastroesophageal reflux disease. Dig Dis Sci 1993;38:86–92.

145. Kawahara H, Dent J, Davidson G. Mechanism responsible for gastroesophageal reflux in children. Gastroenterology 1997;113:399–408.

146. Newel SJ, Sarkar PK, Durbin GM, et al. Maturation of the lower esophageal sphincter in the preterm baby. Gut 1988;95:52–62.

147. Boix-Ochoa J, Canals J. Maturation of the lower esophagus. J Pediatr Surg 1976;11:749–56.

148. Omari TI, Barnett C, Snel A, et al. Mechanisms of gastroesophageal reflux in healthy premature infants. J Pediatr 1998;133:650–4.

149. Omari TI, Barnett CP, Benninga MA, et al. Mechanisms of gastroesophageal reflux in preterm and term infants with reflux disease. Gut 2002; 51:475–9.

4.2. Gastroesophageal Reflux

Colin D. Rudolph, MD, PhD
Eric Hassall, MBChB, FRCPC

Gastroesophageal reflux (GER), defined as the passage of gastric contents into the esophagus, is a normal physiologic process that occurs throughout the day in healthy infants, children, and adults[1] In children and adults most episodes of reflux are brief and asymptomatic but occasionally refluxed gastric contents enter the mouth, a phenomenon described as regurgitation. However, in infants episodes of GER are frequently associated with expulsion of gastric contents from the mouth, and this normal, effortless event is known as "spitting, poseting, or spilling." It is almost always benign. GER should be differentiated from vomiting which results from different physiologic mechanisms. However, since both result in passage of gastric contents through the esophagus and out of the mouth, it may be difficult to discriminate normal physiologic GER from vomiting that may be a harbinger of underlying disease. This is particularly true in infants. A list of terminology and definitions is given in Table 1.

Refluxed gastric contents contain acid and digestive enzymes which can be caustic to the mucosal lining of the esophagus, pharynx, and airway. A variety of protective mechanisms prevent damage to the esophagus and airway. Failure of these mechanisms causes a variety of symptoms and signs that comprise gastroesophageal reflux disease (GERD). The diagnostic approach differs depending upon the specific symptom or sign that led to a suspicion of GERD. The optimal treatment approach varies depending upon the specific symptom presentation, possible concurrent diagnosis, and the expected natural history of the disorder that can vary depending upon the age of the patient.

In this chapter the underlying mechanisms of GER and the protective mechanisms that prevent GERD are reviewed. This is followed by a discussion of the epidemiology of both GER and GERD. Finally, diagnostic and treatment strategies are reviewed for each presentation of possible GERD. Details of the differential diagnosis and therapy for esophagitis are discussed in Chapter 5, "Esophagitis."

PHYSIOLOGY OF GER AND NORMAL PROTECTIVE MECHANISMS

Mechanisms of Gastroesophageal Reflux

GER occurs when gastric (intra-abdominal) pressure exceeds esophageal (intrathoracic) pressure. GER is prevented by a combination of a pressure barrier generated by the lower esophageal

---

Table 1 Definitions

Gastroesophageal reflux (GER)
- Passage of gastro/duodenal contents into the esophagus
- Physiologic: common in infants, postprandially in all ages

Gastroesophageal reflux disease (GERD)
- Reflux causing complications, sometimes with *objective* damage (esophagitis, stricture, and Barretts) or systemic, eg, failure to thrive
- Reflux causing *subjective* troublesome symptoms, eg, heartburn or regurgitation or vomiting above some threshold

Regurgitation/"spitting up"/"spilling"
- Reflux into oropharynx or ejected from mouth, usually effortless/nonforceful but may be quite forceful, especially in infants
- Sometimes termed "vomiting"

Vomiting*
- Forceful ejection of gastro/duodenal contents from mouth

*"Vomiting" has an underlying pathophysiology that differs from "regurgitation"/ "spitting up"/ "spilling," but those mechanisms are not evident other than with highly specialized studies. The main difference evident to the observer between vomiting is forcefulness of ejection of contents, which is somewhat subjective. Therefore, the terms often are used synonymously.

---

sphincter (LES), the crus of the diaphragm, and the intra-abdominal esophagus (Figure 1). The LES consists of a segment of specialized muscle, 3 to 4 cm in length in the adult that is contiguous with and just exterior to the smooth muscle of the esophageal body and the stomach. The LES is tonically contracted to form a pressure barrier of about 8 to 30 mm Hg between the stomach and esophagus. The sphincter relaxes during normal swallowing to allow the food bolus to pass antegrade from the esophagus into the stomach. In the term and preterm infant, the length of this smooth muscle segment is about 1 cm, but the magnitude of the pressure barrier is similar to that in the adult.[2]

Skeletal muscle fibers of the crus of the diaphragm sweep around the LES region and contract during inspiration or straining. Thus, these fibers supplement the pressure barrier at the gastroesophageal junction when it is challenged by an increased abdominal-intrathoracic pressure gradient.[3] A further contribution to the pressure barrier consists of an intra-abdominal segment of esophagus, which is squeezed shut as the intra-

abdominal pressure increases. The acuity of the angle at which the tubular esophagus meets the stomach—the angle of His—also is thought to comprise an important component of the mechanical barrier at the GE junction. In patients with hiatal hernia, all of these barriers are disrupted making hiatal hernia an important contributing factor to severe reflux.[4]

Most episodes of GER occur during transient episodes of relaxation of the LES (TLESR) that are not related to swallowing or straining (see Chapter 49, "Gastrointestinal Manometry: Methodology and Indications"). TLESRs are observed in normal individuals and appear to be a mechanism to assure venting from a distended stomach by belching or regurgitating, depending upon whether air or food is located at the gastroesophageal junction. Following stimulation of stretch-sensitive receptors in the cardia of the stomach, a vago-vagal reflex, relaxes the LES. TLESRs occur up to six times per hour in normal adults, being more frequent with gastric distension as seen after eating and rarely occur at night.

Episodes of transient relaxation of the LES (TLESRs) are responsible for more than 90% of episodes of GER in children.[5] This is also the case in both preterm and term infants with more episodes occurring following meals and rarely during sleep.[2] To support their very rapid growth rate, infants consume large volumes of milk relative to their overall size at frequent intervals, leading to more frequent TLESRs. The relatively short esophagus cannot accommodate the refluxate volume, which overflows through the mouth as effortless regurgitation, also referred to as "spitting" or "spilling."[6] This regurgitation is facilitated by the posterior location of the esophagogastric junction in the supine position. It is exacerbated in the "infant seat" or "car seat" position, due to the additional factor of raised intra-abdominal pressure.[7] During episodes of TLESR associated with abdomino-thoracic straining, the frequency of GER also increases.[8]

Esophageal Protective Mechanisms

Following most episodes of GER, a relatively small volume of refluxed gastric contents, enters the esophagus and the upper esophageal sphincter (UES) contracts, preventing passage from the proximal esophagus into the pharynx. Subsequently, a coordinated secondary peristaltic

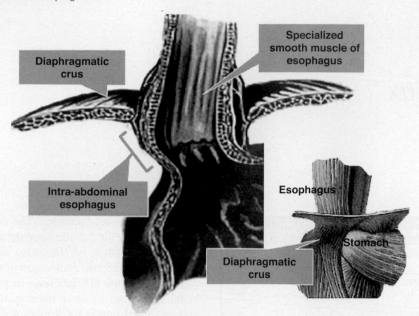

Figure 1 Components of the LES: The lower esophageal sphincter is composed of smooth muscle in the distal portion of the esophagus that maintains a high-resting pressure, the diaphragmatic crus that wraps around the region of the lower esophageal sphincter (see insert) and contracts with inspiration or straining, and the intra-abdominal segment of the esophagus that is compressed with increased intra-abdominal pressure.

Table 2 Protective Mechanisms Against GERD
Protection of the esophagus
Lower esophageal sphincter
Esophageal capacitance and clearance
Mucosal mucus and bicarbonate secretion
Swallowed saliva buffering residual acid
Protection of the airway
Upper esophageal sphincter
Esophageal-glottal closure reflex
Reflex apnea
Pharyngeal clearance
Cough
Ciliary airway clearance

contraction resulting from distension of the esophageal wall propels the refluxed material down the esophagus back into the stomach. Following clearance of most of the refluxed gastric contents, residual acid adherent to the esophageal wall, is neutralized by swallowing of saliva that is secreted in response to esophageal acidification. These mechanisms are likely intact in normal premature infants since clearance time for both acid and nonacid GER are similar to adults.[2] The esophageal mucosa also has a mucus layer and glands that secrete bicarbonate, adding to the barrier that protects the epithelium against refluxed caustic gastric contents. All these mechanisms are present in the normal infant and child. The result is that despite more frequent GER events, damage to the esophageal mucosa is uncommon unless there are concurrent risk factors that compromise these clearance mechanisms. Such factors include esophageal dysmotility, delayed gastric emptying, impaired swallowing and, rarely decreased production of saliva (Table 2).

Airway Protective Mechanisms

Several factors prevent refluxed gastric acid from reaching the proximal esophageal body in most children and normal adults. First, most TLESRs occur after meals, and since meals are usually taken in the upright position, refluxed material does not advance against gravity up the 15 cm or more of esophagus. In contrast, although GER occurs in patterns similar to the adult, the infant usually maintains a horizontal position and the esophagus is shorter (10 cm) with a much smaller capacity than in the adult. Small amounts of reflux into the proximal esophagus promote contraction of the UES, but larger volume episodes (as occur most frequently in the infant) provoke a vagal nerve-mediated relaxation of the upper esophageal

sphincter thereby allowing refluxed material to advance into the pharynx. The same reflex mechanism results in centrally mediated apnea and protective closure of the larynx that prevents aspiration of refluxed material.[9] Thus, brief episodes of apnea may be associated with normal infant physiologic GER.[10] Reflex responses to laryngeal stimulation are age-related, such that a stimulus that provokes apnea in the infant will cause cough in the older child. Infants and children with anatomic defects of the larynx or neurologic disease are more prone to aspiration following GER, most likely, due to failure of these protective mechanisms. When aspiration does occur, the sequelae depend, at least in part, on the volume and nature of the aspirated material. Animal studies[11] show that aspiration of water or saline with a pH that exceeds 2.5 causes bronchospasm, but not an inflammatory response. In contrast, even neutral stomach contents that are aspirated can cause an inflammatory response with pneumonia, particularly if they contain food or milk.[12] Factors that presumably increase the bacterial content of 'aspirates and thereby could increase the risk of pneumonia include dental caries[13] and suppression of gastric acid[14] (Table 2).

EPIDEMIOLOGY AND NATURAL HISTORY

During infancy GER is common and most often manifests as effortless regurgitation. This occurs in 50 to 70% of infants in the first 3 to 6 months of life and then decreases over the first year of life, so that by 12 to 15 months expulsion of gastric contents from the mouth is infrequent[15] The great majority of infants with GER are happy, healthy, and thriving. A symptom survey showed that infants with GER have

no increase in the frequency of ear, sinus, upper respiratory infections, or wheezing compared to a control population although those infants with GER are more likely to have feeding refusal than age-matched controls.[16] Gender, breast-feeding, and environmental tobacco smoke exposure are not significant factors related to infant regurgitation.[15]

It is well-recognized that the GERD is highly prevalent in adults. In contrast, a survey of the parents of 3- to 9-year-old children reported symptoms of heartburn in 2%, epigastric pain in 7%, and regurgitation in 2%.[17] Another study reported regurgitation in 4%, vomiting in 8%, and heartburn in 5% of 9-year-old children.[15] About 5% of adolescents report symptoms of heartburn, epigastric pain, or regurgitation.[17] A large analysis of diagnostic codes from inpatient and outpatient visits to a children's hospital showed that about one-third of patients diagnosed with GERD had an identified risk factor such as cystic fibrosis or morbid obesity.[18] Those children with GERD were also more likely to be diagnosed with sinusitis, laryngitis, asthma, pneumonia, and brochiectasis but were less likely to be diagnosed with otitis media than the control patients. However, this study lacked clear diagnostic criteria for the diagnosis of GERD.

Few longitudinal follow-up studies have been performed to evaluate whether infants with GER are more likely to have persistent symptoms through childhood, or if children with GERD are likely to have persistent symptoms through adulthood. In one study, mothers of infants with GER reported an increased prevalence of feeding problems at 2 years of age compared to nonspitters.[19] Another study[15] reported that infants with frequent spitting up (described as more than 90 days during which they spit up following more than half of their feedings) had increased risk of GERD symptoms at 9 years of age. Pre-pregnancy smoking and smoking in the same room as the child at 9- and 18-months of age is associated with GERD symptoms at 9 years of age. Both of these longitudinal studies could be flawed by recall bias.

A follow-up study of children diagnosed with GERD based on esophageal pH probe studies reported that symptoms persisted at 1 to 8 years following initial diagnosis, such that 6% underwent antireflux surgery, 19% resolved off medication, 62% required continuing medical management, and 12% did not have a change in symptoms.[20] A more recent study examined a cohort of 207 adolescents and adults (median age 19 years and range 10 to 41 years) who had GERD diagnosed at endoscopy at age 5 years or later. Of the 80 respondents to a survey, at least 31% had monthly symptoms and 9% had weekly symptoms. Overall, 30% were currently taking acid-suppressant medications, and about 10% had undergone fundoplication.[21] These findings suggest that children who have demonstrated GERD at 5 years or older have a high prevalence of GERD symptoms in adolescence or young adulthood. However, it is unclear if this represents an increased prevalence of symptoms in those presenting with GERD in childhood, since a similar high prevalence of symptoms is observed in many adult surveys.[22] Another study that contacted adults who had been diagnosed with GERD in infancy or childhood found that those diagnosed with GERD as infants had no increase in GERD symptoms versus controls; however, those diagnosed with GERD in childhood reported somewhat increased GERD symptoms.[23]

AT RISK POPULATIONS FOR GERD

While children who are otherwise quite healthy develop GERD, which on occasion may be severe, the prevalence of severe GERD is much higher among those with certain underlying disorders such as neurologic or neuromotor impairment, previous esophageal surgery (eg, for repaired esophageal atresia or diaphragmatic hernia), chronic lung disease (eg, cystic fibrosis), and chemotherapy,[24] where the normal protective mechanisms that prevent damage from GER are impaired. Hiatal hernia is also an important contributing factor to severe reflux, being found at endoscopy in up to 40% of children with severe esophagitis, whether or not they have an underlying disorder.[24] An additional factor potentially placing children at risk for GERD is obesity. In adults, both obesity and incremental weight gain have been shown to increase the prevalence and severity of GERD, Barrett's esophagus, and esophageal adenocarcinoma.[25]

Familial and genetic factors also play a role in GERD. Clusterings of reflux symptoms, hiatal hernia, erosive esophagitis, Barrett's esophagus, and esophageal adenocarcinoma are observed in families, suggesting heritability of GERD and its complications.[26–29]

Neuromotor Impairment

Neurologically impaired children are at substantially increased risk for GERD, with a prevalence of about 50% in populations with an IQ <50.[30] In a recent series of 166 children with relapsing esophagitis on long-term proton pump inhibitor (PPI) therapy, two-thirds had a underlying neuromotor disorder.[24] In affected individuals, proton pump inhibitor therapy decreases episodes of

vomiting and pneumonia[31–32] and heals the esophagitis.[33] Dosage titration based on symptoms is reported effective,[30] but whether symptom resolution assures healing of esophagitis remains to be established. In patients unable to tolerate oral or gastric feeding due to GERD, enteral feeding can be administered via a gastrojejunal tube,[34] or feeding jejunostomy and esophagitis may be healed then prevented by administration of a PPI. Antireflux surgery is also effective but wrap failure occurs in about 30% of patients within 5 years; mortality is high and the frequency of pneumonia often does not change.[35–36] Alternative surgical approaches such as esophagastric disconnection can be used in highly selected individuals,[37,38] but complications are common with these procedures.[39–40]

Esophageal Anatomic Disorders

At least 50% of children and young adults with repaired esophageal atresia have GERD[41] and recurrent pulmonary disease. This likely is due to abnormal motility of the distal esophagus leading to impaired acid clearance and the frequent presence of a hiatal hernia. Barrett's esophagus or some form of esophageal metaplasia is also quite prevalent in this patient population.[42] In the pre-PPI era, several case series demonstrate a benefit from antireflux surgery but failure rates of fundoplication are high in children with repaired esophageal atresia. Medical therapy with PPIs is highly effective in patients with esophageal atresia and GERD.[24] No studies formally compare outcomes using medical therapy versus surgical antireflux therapy in these children.

There is also an increased risk for esophagitis and Barrett's esophagus following Heller myotomy for achalasia. The benefit of antireflux therapy at the time of myotomy remains controversial.[43] All patients with a history of achalasia or a history of esophageal atresia repair require follow-up for possible complications of GERD since even those who underwent surgical repair are at risk.[44] Endoscopic surveillance may be indicated but no study has yet evaluated the potential benefit of screening of these patient populations.

Pulmonary Disease: Cystic Fibrosis and Postpulmonary Transplant

A higher prevalence of GERD is reported in patients with a variety of chronic respiratory disorders including cystic fibrosis. In cystic fibrosis, there may be an increased risk for Barrett's esophagus,[45] but this has not been shown in other chronic pediatric pulmonary disorders. There is also a high frequency of GERD following lung transplant in children.[46]

Although children with pulmonary disease may benefit from antireflux surgery, wrap failure is more common in this patient population compared to any other group. Combinations of nonpharmacologic and pharmacologic therapies can be considered as alternatives to surgery. Although acid suppression can improve gastrointestinal symptoms and enhance fat absorption

in cystic fibrosis patients, there is no convincing evidence to benefit in overall nutritional status, lung function, or quality of life or long-term survival.[47] Since agents that reduce gastric acid may potentially increase the risk for bacterial pneumonias in some patient groups,[14] PPI treatment could potentially have adverse effects.

Prematurity

Although GERD treatment is frequently administered,[48] the true frequency of peptic esophagitis or pulmonary disease due to GERD is unknown.[49] Most of the physiologic protective mechanisms appear to be intact in the preterm infant.[50] There is no evidence supporting a role for GERD in causing apnea or bradycardias of prematurity. Although GERD may be more common in infants with bronchopulmonary dysplasia, no data suggest that GERD therapy impacts on the clinical course or outcome.[51–52] Infants with GER have slightly longer periods of hospitalization[53] than those without GERD, but except in those infants with severe GERD (reflux index >14) and concomitant disorders such as intraventricular hemorrhage and necrotizing enterocolitis[54] GERD seems to have little impact on overall outcomes.

Acid-reducing therapies including both H_2RA and PPI reduce gastric acid in preterm infants at lower doses than those used in older infants.[55] Also to be considered is the potential that treatment with acid suppressing agents may have adverse consequences in premature infants. For instance, a review of a large database found an association between antecedent H_2RA therapy and higher rates of necrotizing enterocolitis in very low-birth-weight infants.[56] The relative risks and benefits of empiric GERD therapy in premature infants are unclear, but it appears that GERD is frequently diagnosed on inadequate criteria. Reduction of gastric acid is useful for therapy of peptic esophagitis, but behaviors often interpreted as signs of reflux disease in the preterm infant are nonspecific and not predictive of esophagitis.[57] If esophageal pH monitoring shows increased esophageal acid exposure or if esophagoscopy and biopsy shows esophagitis, ranitidine would be a reasonable therapeutic option since good pharmacokinetic data is available for premature infants. Omeprazole (0.7 mg/kg/d) effectively increases gastric and esophageal pH in infants of 34- to 40-week-gestational ages and may provide an alternative therapeutic approach.[55] However, increased acid suppression may increase the likelihood of infection and necrotizing enterocolitis. Use of empiric acid suppression therapies to treat airway symptoms, irritability, or feeding intolerance in premature infants lacks any supporting data.[58–59]

A recent cohort study in Sweden[60] reported a >11-fold increase in the incidence rate for esophageal adenocarcinoma in adults who were born preterm or small for gestational age. By contrast, a subsequent nested case-control study did not confirm a strong association between risk of esophageal cancer and birth weight.[61]

DIAGNOSTIC TESTING FOR GERD

Since GER is a normal physiologic event, the role of diagnostic testing is to determine if GER is causing disease (ie, GERD). Therefore, the value of specific diagnostic tests varies depending on the clinical presentation. An ideal test would determine the likelihood that GER is causing the specific symptom and would predict whether treatment of GERD would alleviate this symptom. Since each test is designed to answer a particular question, it is valuable only when used in the appropriate clinical situation. In general, physiologic GER in infants is easy to recognize and no treatment is necessary other than parental reassurance.

The history and physical alone may be adequate to diagnose GERD and initiate management. However, this depends on the nature of the presenting symptoms and their severity. In infants and children with symptoms or signs potentially due to GERD, the risks and benefits of empiric therapy with acid-suppressant medications versus those of diagnostic testing need to be balanced. History and physical examination are poor predictors of the presence of esophagitis,[62] and more formal symptom questionnaires also do not have adequate sensitivity or specificity for meaningful application in clinical settings.[63-64]

Radiographic upper GI contrast studies are used to detect anatomic abnormalities that can cause respiratory complications, dysphagia, or vomiting. These include aspiration during swallowing, tracheoesophageal fistula, esophageal rings or webs, and gastroduodenal anatomic abnormalities such as antral webs, hiatal hernia, and malrotation. The upper GI series is not useful for the diagnosis of GERD since the observation of gastroesophageal reflux during the study may simply represent normal physiologic GER.

Esophageal pH monitoring determines when the esophageal lumen becomes acidified. This generally results from reflux of acid gastric contents but may also occur when drinking acidic beverages such as fruit juice and carbonated beverages. The protocol utilized for pH probe studies may vary depending on the question being asked. If the study is performed to determine the risk of esophagitis or the potential role of GER in causing asthma, the protocol should be designed to determine the amount of acid exposure during the patient's normal meals and routine activities, including sleep, since this correlates with the risk of GER causing disease. Interpretation of these studies generally involves calculations of the amount of time that the esophageal pH is below 4 and the number and length of episodes. The percentage of time in a 24-hour study that the esophageal pH is <4, also called the reflux index, is considered the most valid measure of reflux because it reflects the cumulative exposure of the esophagus to acid. The mean upper limit of normal reflux index is 12% in infants up to 11 months[65] and 6% in children[66] and adults[67]. However, the intrasubject reproducibility of esophageal pH monitoring studies is suboptimal.[68]

Children with esophagitis are more likely to have an abnormal pH probe, but only about 50% of children with abnormal esophageal pH monitoring studies have esophagitis.[1] Moreover, there is little correlation between the total exposure time and the severity of esophagitis in an individual patient. In patients with persistent, steroid-dependent asthma an abnormal pH probe (especially with nocturnal GER) suggests that a patient may benefit from GERD treatment.[1] Esophageal pH monitoring is also useful to evaluate the efficacy of acid-suppressive treatment in patients unresponsive to standard therapies, or to monitor the adequacy of acid suppression in Barrett's esophagus and in patients with persistent nocturnal symptoms.[69] Esophageal pH monitoring may also be performed to determine if an episodic symptom such as apnea or chest pain is due to GER. In such cases the occurrence of the symptom and esophageal pH should be simultaneously monitored so that a symptom index (% of GER episodes associated with the symptom) can be evaluated.[1]

The predictive value of esophageal pH monitoring to determine if GER causes supraesophageal symptoms such as recurrent pneumonia and laryngeal symptoms is poorly established. New technologies that permit the measurement of pH in the air-filled nasopharynx may provide more meaningful data. Despite the popularity of esophageal pH monitoring, the clinical utility of this test in most clinical scenarios is limited.

Esophageal electrical impedance monitoring is a relatively new test, also known as multichannel intraesophageal impedance, or MII. Electrical impedance changes when a bolus of fluid or air passes between electrical sensors along a catheter. When MII is combined with esophageal pH monitoring, it allows detection of both acid and nonacid episodes of gastroesophageal reflux.[70,71] It enables simultaneous determination of esophageal clearance times and acid exposure. Since a large proportion of GER episodes are nonacid in infants (particularly postprandial GER) and children,[72] it was hoped that this new technology might provide additional useful information that would improve the clinical utility of prolonged esophageal monitoring. Unfortunately, despite the improved detection of GER episodes, this new technology has yet to impact on clinical management approaches in children, especially in those with airway symptoms[73-74] in whom a cause and effect relationship is difficult to establish. Due to the high cost, expertise, and extended time required for interpretation,[75] this test is generally not useful for routine patient management,[76] although it may aid in correlating specific symptoms with GER events.[74] Furthermore, the predictive value of esophageal impedance monitoring for response to GERD therapies is not established.

Upper endoscopy with biopsy evaluates whether GER has caused damage to the esophagus. Endoscopy and biopsy can determine the presence and severity of esophagitis, strictures, and Barrett's esophagus, and can exclude other causes of upper GI symptoms, such as Crohn's disease, webs and eosinophilic or infectious esophagitis, as well as disorders of the stomach and duodenum.[77]

A normal appearance of the esophagus during endoscopy does not reliably exclude histopathological esophagitis. Moreover, there are many causes of esophagitis other than reflux that can present with similar symptoms. Thus, multiple biopsies from different zones of the esophagus, stomach, and duodenum are generally indicated, regardless of the appearance of the mucosa at endoscopy. Recent data in adults suggest that the traditional approach to evaluate esophageal biopsies for GERD, including evaluation of basal cell hyperplasia and papillary elongation, is prone to substantial error.[78] Morphologic features such as dilation of intercellular spaces appear to be more sensitive predictors of GERD in adults with nonerosive GERD.[78] Similar criteria have been studied in children,[79] but the correlation with clinical scenarios and response to treatment have not yet been systematically evaluated.

Laryngoscopy and bronchoscopy is widely used for the assessment of possible supraesophageal symptoms of GERD including hoarseness, chronic cough, and recurrent pneumonia.[80] Laryngoscopic findings of posterior glottic edema, laryngeal erythema, laryngeal hypervascularity, and laryngeal pseudosulcus are proposed to be more frequent with GERD,[81] but variability in the interobserver interpretation of these findings, lack of specificity for GERD, and a lack of correlation with treatment response have led to a reevaluation of the clinical utility of these findings.[82-84]

Bronchoscopy with lavage and evaluation for lipid-laden macrophages may suggest that chronic aspiration during swallowing or with GER is responsible for recurrent pneumonia. However, a lack of specificity and the inability to differentiate between GER and aspiration from above during swallowing limit the value of this study.[85] One promising study showed increased concentrations of pepsin in pulmonary aspirates in children with symptoms of GERD,[86] but this diagnostic approach requires further validation prior to application in the clinical setting.

Nuclear scintigraphy is performed by the oral ingestion or instillation of technetium-labeled formula or food into the stomach. Images are obtained every 20 to 30 seconds for 1 hour, and the number of episodes of postprandial GER or any episodes of aspiration into the lung are observed. Scintigraphy also provides information about gastric emptying, which may be delayed in some children with GERD.[87] However, a lack of standardized techniques, absence of age-specific normative data, and a lack of sensitivity limit the value of this test. In addition, this test, like an upper GI contrast study, offers a nonphysiologic "snapshot" evaluation of reflux. However, scintigraphy can demonstrate pulmonary aspiration in children with refractory respiratory symptoms and normal esophageal pH monitoring, suggesting superior sensitivity to esophageal pH monitoring.[88] However, since some aspiration occurs in normal individuals, the predictive value of this test for treatment responses is not yet established.

Trials of gastric acid antisecretory therapy have been validated in adults as a cost-effective approach for diagnosis of a likely relationship between acid reflux and symptoms of cough,[89] heartburn, and noncardiac chest pain[90] and dyspepsia.[91] Short-term-defined courses of empiric therapy (ie, without diagnostic evaluation) is effective in adult patients.[92] Although there are no data in children, similar short-term, empiric therapy is frequently administered in the pediatric age group. If a trial is initiated, it should be time-limited (eg, 3 to 4 months) to determine if there is a symptomatic response and to evaluate if symptoms relapse off drug. Empiric trials with PPIs should rarely be undertaken in infants, as it is often difficult to ascribe symptoms to GERD; in the first few months of age, placebo responses are substantial and the variability of pharmacokinetics is unknown.

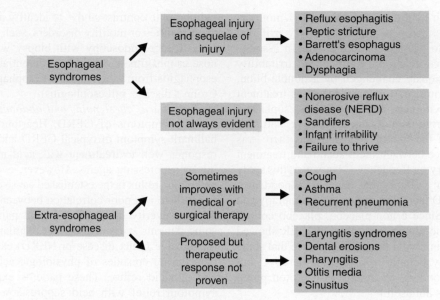

Figure 2 A classification schema for disorders associated with GERD.

SYMPTOMS, SIGNS, AND DISORDERS ASSOCIATED WITH GER

A major challenge in managing GERD is to first determine if it is the cause of a specific presenting symptom or sign. In infants or children with severe neurodevelopmental delays, a decreased ability to describe symptoms further complicates evaluation. A symptom-based approach to GERD diagnosis and management was first proposed by a consensus expert panel and provides a logical construct for approaching individual patients.[1] Symptoms and signs of GERD are listed in Table 3 and a classification schema is shown in Figure 2.

Recurrent vomiting or "spitting" (see Table 1) is difficult to differentiate in infants since physiologic GER is usually associated with expulsion of gastric contents from the mouth in normal infants. In otherwise happy and thriving infants, recurrent spitting is not forceful and it is not accompanied by distress. In contrast, "vomiting" describes emesis that is more forceful and

more often associated with distress, pallor, and retching. In the infant with recurrent vomiting, a thorough history and physical examination with attention to warning signs is usually sufficient to allow a diagnosis of uncomplicated GER. Warning signs of another underlying diagnosis include a history of bilious vomiting, hematemesis, hematochezia, unusually forceful vomiting, or vomiting that is de novo or of increasing severity after age 6 months. Associated failure to thrive, diarrhea, abdominal tenderness, abdominal distension, or constipation should alert the physician to other underlying gastrointestinal disorders. Fever, lethargy, hepatosplenomegaly, a bulging fontanelle, macro- or microcephaly, and seizures indicate a neurologic disorder or systemic illness could be causing vomiting.

In the absence of warning symptoms, no therapy is required. Parental reassurance, education, and anticipatory guidance about the natural history of GER should be adequate. Some infants with milk protein allergy have symptoms that are indistinguishable from GER and, therefore, a 1 to 2 weeks trial of a hypoallergenic formula may be a reasonable consideration.

In infants with physiologic reflux, if the regurgitation is particularly distressing to the parent (since it usually is not bothersome to the infant), then thickening of the formula or administration of a formula designed to thicken upon exposure to gastric acid is acceptable. Supine positioning is recommended since the risk of sudden infant death syndrome (SIDS) is increased with prone positioning.[1] There is no evidence that pharmacological therapy affects the natural history of uncomplicated GER in infants.[93]

If vomiting persists or begins after 24 months of age in an otherwise well child, there is no clear consensus on appropriate diagnostic work-up. Vomiting may result from common conditions such as otitis media, occult urinary tract infections, food sensitivity, postnasal drip, and cough. Although an upper GI contrast study or upper endoscopy and biopsy are often performed, the

likelihood of finding treatable abnormalities is small if the vomiting is not associated with pain or discomfort, is nonbloody, and nonbilious in nature. This type of regurgitation can be a nuisance, or in some instances may disrupt participation in normal childhood activities. Administration of a safe and effective prokinetic agent or cognitive behavioral therapy may be useful for management in this clinical scenario.

Poor weight gain may be associated with GERD, but it is uncommon for calorie loss from GERD alone to limit the ability of an infant or child to gain weight. Usually, there are other associated disorders causing the weight loss or the amount of feedings administered is being limited to prevent benign regurgitation. A careful dietary history to ensure that adequate calories are being offered and ingested is essential prior to considering other etiologies. If an infant is not ingesting adequate calories, potential causes should be explored[1] prior to assuming that GERD is the cause. If an infant with vomiting is not gaining weight despite ingesting adequate calories, then malabsorptive disorders, disorders that increase caloric requirements or genetic disorders associated with impaired growth, must be considered. In those rare cases where calorie loss from vomiting limits weight gain, therapeutic maneuvers include increasing the caloric density of feedings, administration of prokinetic agents, or in severe cases, administration of nighttime nasogastric, nasojejunal feeds or gastrojejunal feeds.[94] A time-limited trial of an elemental formula is reasonable since vomiting can be due to a food protein intolerance.

Infant irritability is frequent and GERD is often considered as a major etiologic factor. Despite this widely held belief, there is little data to support this supposition. One study demonstrated a temporal relationship between reflux, arching, and discomfort in infants, but a causal effect of GERD was not clearly demonstrated.[95] Associations between these behaviors and episodes of GER could not be confirmed in premature infants.[57] Other studies have shown that

Table 3 Symptoms, Signs, and Disorders Associated with GERD in Children	
Well Documented	Poorly Documented
Recurrent regurgitation ("spitting up")	Infant irritability
Poor weight gain	Infant feeding refusal
Heartburn, chest pain, or abdominal pain	Infant sleep apnea
Esophagitis	Hoarseness
Sandifer syndrome	Sinusitis
Vomiting	Otitis media
Hematemesis	Dental erosions
Anemia	
Barretts esophagus	
Asthma or wheezing	
Chronic cough	
Globus sensation	
Acute life-threatening events (especially awake apnea)	
Recurrent pneumonia or interstitial lung disease	

infants with abnormal esophageal pH monitoring or esophagitis are not excessively irritable, compared to age-matched controls. An association between acid reflux and infant irritability is most seriously challenged by a double-blind, placebo-control trial of omeprazole as treatment of infants with persistent irritability. Esophageal pH monitoring demonstrated effective acid suppression in the treatment group, but there was no difference between the placebo and treatment groups in crying frequency.[96] However, this study enrolled only infants that had not responded to other GERD therapies such as H_2RA therapy and cisapride. Since a non-placebo, placebo control trial of famotidine in infants with GER showed reductions in crying time, it is possible that some infants may benefit from H_2RA therapy[97] but in nonresponders, treatment with proton pump inhibitors is not useful.

Normal infants fuss or cry for 2 h/d and some infants cry as much as 6 h/d. Treatment for presumed GERD is often inappropriately instituted in such infants. Nonmedical therapies such as parental education about normal infant behavior, settling techniques, and establishment of routine,[98] or increased infant carrying are alternative effective therapies. Furthermore, a wide range of conditions other than GERD are associated with irritability. Since there are no convincing data to support GERD as a frequent cause of infant irritability, alternative diagnoses and treatment approaches including trial of an elemental formula, parent education, and behavioral management should be considered prior to acid suppressive therapy.

Infant feeding refusal is often ascribed to underlying GERD.[99–100] However, no study has shown improvement with GERD treatment. One study has shown persistence of oromotor deficiencies following treatment of presumed GERD.[101] Another small study suggested an association between dysphagia and GERD due to brain stem abnormalities in children with underlying neurological disorders.[102] A retrospective uncontrolled, multicenter study in infants and toddlers proposed that swallowing and laryngeal sensation improved following various treatments of GERD, but the lack of uniformity in diagnostic criteria and treatment modalities undermine the credibility of these findings.[103] Taken together, the role of GERD as a cause of infant feeding refusal remains unclear. Therefore, empiric therapy for GERD in infants with feeding refusal is generally not recommended. Other possible causes of feeding difficulties should be considered.

Dysphagia is reported to improve in some adults treated for GERD, but only one nonrandomized, uncontrolled trial specifically addresses this issue.[104] A retrospective series evaluated children presenting with dysphagia reported that 75% had GERD and that symptoms resolved with therapy.[105] However, these studies did not discriminate between eosinophilic esophagitis and GERD. In a child or adolescent with dysphagia, the diagnostic evaluation usually begins with a radiographic contrast study[1] to identify anatomic abnormalities or motility disorders, such as achalasia. Upper endoscopy with biopsy will diagnose esophagitis and help to differentiate peptic esophagitis from other causes of esophagitis (eg, Crohn's disease, pill esophagitis).

Heartburn, chest pain, and abdominal pain are all symptoms of GERD. Heartburn is the hallmark symptom of typical GERD and usually responds well to treatment with acid neutralizing or suppressing agents. However, even when pathologic reflux is the established cause of symptoms, there is a poor correlation between the histologic severity of esophagitis and pain. Thus, some patients without esophageal inflammation (nonerosive reflux disease or NERD) experience pain during episodes of physiologic acid reflux and nonacid reflux. These patients experience symptom relief with acid suppression therapy compared with placebo. However, the frequency of response is lower than for patients with erosive esophagitis.[106] NERD may be due to visceral hypersensitivity ("sensitive esophagus") or abnormal motor events.[107] The mechanisms underlying these processes are unclear, but heightened sensory responses due to increased esophageal pain fiber densities, and alterations in tissue resistance due to increased permeability of the epithelial surface, could account for symptoms in the absence of obvious mucosal inflammation.[78] A 5HT-4 receptor antagonist, tegaserod, reduced pain responses to esophageal balloon distension but not esophageal acid exposure in adult NERD,[108] but comparable studies of tegaserod in children with NERD are awaited.

In most cases an empiric treatment trial is the most cost-effective approach for diagnosis of pain due to GERD in adults.[109] Children older than 8 years of age often present with symptoms similar to adults including epigastric or mesogastric abdominal pain, but this is not necessarily the sole presenting symptom.[17,110] If there is no improvement in symptoms following a treatment trial with a proton pump inhibitor, other causes of abdominal or chest pain including cardiac, respiratory, musculoskeletal, pill, or infectious esophagitis should be considered. If symptoms resolve with therapy and then recur following discontinuation of a time-limited course of acid suppression, then an upper endoscopy with biopsy is indicated.[1] As persistent heartburn symptoms can have a substantial negative impact on a patients quality of life, long-term therapy can be continued with either PPI or H_2RA to provide relief from symptoms even in the absence of esophagitis. Episodic meal-induced heartburn in children may be treated with episodic antacid or H_2RA since these have a rapid onset of action. Episodic periods of pain in patients with nonerosive esophagitis may also be managed with on demand PPI therapy.

Sandifer syndrome is a rare complication of GERD in children. Patients present with arching of the back and rigid opisthotonic posturing, mainly involving the neck, back, and upper extremities. The posturing may be misdiagnosed as seizures or a neurologic movement disorder.[111] Esophageal pH monitoring with symptom correlation is a useful test for evaluation, although documentation of esophagitis and treatment initiation is a reasonable alternative approach. Improvement is usually observed with medical therapy although several reports suggest that some patients only improve following surgical intervention.[112]

Hematemesis and/or anemia may result from GERD-induced esophagitis. The diagnostic approach, differential diagnosis, and treatment approaches for esophagitis are discussed in Chapter 5, "Esophagitis."

Barretts esophagus is an acquired metaplastic condition in which the normal squamous mucosa of the esophagus is replaced for part of its length by mucosa that is columnar, villiform, and contains goblet cells that produce acid mucin.[42] The importance of Barretts is that it has a lifetime malignant potential of up to 10%.[113] Barretts esophagus is much less common in children than in adults, but of a highly selected population of 166 children with severe esophagitis requiring long-term PPI therapy, 5% had histologically proven Barretts with goblet cells.[24] Barretts esophagus is usually diagnosed in children over the age of 10 years, with the youngest child reported being 5 years of age.[42] Genetic factors are likely a determinant, which explains why only roughly 10% of individuals with peptic esophagitis develop Barretts esophagus.[114–115]

The process of malignant change usually takes decades, although very rarely esophageal adenocarcinoma has been reported in children and young adults with Barretts esophagus.[116] Therefore, surveillance with multiple stepwise biopsies, beginning at age 10 years, is suggested in those children who have documented Barretts esophagus with specialized mucosa and goblet cells.[24] In patients with established Barretts esophagus, there is some evidence that treatment with PPIs may lower the rate of development of dysplasia (ie, precancerous change),[117] but as yet, there is no definitive evidence that cancer can be prevented by this approach.[118] There is no evidence that PPI treatment or antireflux surgery prevents the development of Barretts esophagus. Therefore, once dysplasia and cancer has been ruled out by multiple biopsies of the metaplastic segment of mucosa, the treatment of Barretts esophagus is the treatment of esophagitis, with either PPIs or antireflux surgery. However, in Barretts esophagus, when the choice has been made to use PPIs rather than surgery, more aggressive PPI *bid* therapy is indicated. This is because in subjects with Barretts esophagus, symptoms are not a reliable guide to the severity of esophagitis[119]; nocturnal acid reflux occurs frequently,[120] and high-dose PPIs may slow the development of dysplasia.[117] In patients with Barretts esophagus, the goal of therapy is to eliminate pathologic reflux, as determined by intraesophageal pH monitoring while receiving high-dose PPI therapy.

Acute life-threatening events (ALTE) in infants are defined as episodes characterized by a combination of apnea, change in color (cyanosis, pallor, rubor, and plethora), change in muscle tone (limpness and stiffness), or choking and gagging that requires intervention by the caretaker.[121] The first event usually occurs between 1 and 2 months, and rarely after 8 months of age. Infants with an ALTE are at risk for subsequent sudden death, so investigation of possible causes of ALTE is generally recommended. These include cardiac,[122] central nervous system,[123] and infectious disorders, or upper airway obstruction or central apnea.[124]

Despite extensive studies a frequent causal relationship between acid or nonacid GER and prolonged apnea or bradycardia in term or preterm infants[59] has yet to be established. However, ALTE episodes due to GER have been documented in awake infants by simultaneous recording of esophageal pH, chest wall movement, and nasal airflow.[125] Most episodes of apnea during sleep are likely due to primary central mechanism, and not GER.

In those infants with GER-associated awake apnea, there is no consensus on appropriate therapy. Most of these infants are able to recover from the apneic episode spontaneously, and the frequency of these episodes decreases as the infant matures. Unfortunately, rare cases of relatively well-documented GER-induced respiratory arrest resulting in death have been reported. Medical therapy is used, but there is no evidence that thickened feedings, acid suppression therapies, or prokinetics agents reduce risk. Prone positioning increases the risk of sudden infant death and is therefore not recommended. Surgical therapy has been reported to be effective in preventing recurrent ALTE.[126] However, treatment decisions must balance the risks of the apneic episodes with those of antireflux surgery. Home monitoring and CPR training for parents provides a comforting option, but the efficacy of these interventions is controversial.[127]

Recurrent pneumonia or interstitial lung disease both may result from GERD. The assumed pathophysiologic mechanism is a failure of the airway protective mechanisms. An association between GER and recurrent bronchopulmonary infection in children has been demonstrated, with improvement following both medical[31] and surgical therapies[128] of GERD. In several interstitial pulmonary disorders, including idiopathic pulmonary fibrosis,[129] cystic fibrosis,[130] or post-lung transplant,[46] GERD may exacerbate disease. Before considering GERD as a potential cause of recurrent pneumonia, other causes such as an anatomic abnormality, aspiration during swallowing, a foreign body, cystic fibrosis, and an underlying immunodeficiency must be ruled out. In a retrospective review of 238 children with recurrent pneumonia (defined as two pneumonia episodes in 1 year or three episodes overall), the underlying cause was aspiration with swallowing in 48%, immunologic disorders in 14%, congenital heart disease in 9%, asthma in 8%, respiratory

tract anatomic abnormalities in 8%, unknown in 8%, and GERD in only 6%.[131]

Determining whether GERD causes recurrent pneumonia in a specific patient is difficult due to the lack of sensitivity and specificity of available diagnostic tests. The ability of any diagnostic test to predict a response to antireflux therapy has not been evaluated prospectively. In certain high-risk populations, such as those with neurological disease and proven peptic esophagitis, therapy with PPI has been shown to decrease the frequency of pneumonia[31] and chronic respiratory symptoms of cough and wheezing.[132] By contrast, in well children, acid-reducing therapies may increase the incidence of community-acquired pneumonia.[14] Therefore, an individual treatment approach must be selected based on a balance between potential benefits versus perceived risks. For example, in patients with severe symptoms or worsening lung function, it may be necessary to proceed with antireflux surgery in an attempt to prevent further pulmonary damage, despite a lack of definitive evidence that GERD is causing the pulmonary disease. Alternatively, if minimal lung disease is present, consideration of medical therapy with careful follow-up of pulmonary function then can be considered. Trials of nasogastric feeding may be used to exclude aspiration during swallowing as a potential cause of recurrent lung disease, whereas trials of nasojejunal therapy may help to demonstrate that surgical therapy of GERD could be beneficial.

Asthma has been reported to be associated with GERD in both affected children and adults. In multiple pediatric reports, the prevalence of symptoms of GERD[133] and abnormal esophageal pH probe monitoring in asthma patients vary widely between 25 and 75%.[1] Proposed pathogenic mechanisms for GER to exacerbate asthma include direct aggravation of airway inflammation or airway hyperresponsiveness triggered by microaspiration of gastric contents and esophago-vagal reflexes that induce airway hyperresponsiveness.[134] Conversely, asthma itself can cause reflux due to an increased intra-abdominal pressure and increased negativity of intrathoracic pressure that occurs in pulmonary disorders. Therefore, for asthma it is often difficult to ascribe a cause and effect with GER. In fact, acid reflux may just be an association in many, or most, patients with reactive airway disease.

Several large well-controlled trials in adults with moderate to severe persistent asthma show no significant improvement following proton pump inhibitor therapy.[134] A double-blind, placebo-control trial of over 700 patients showed no difference in morning FEV1 in those patients treated for 16 weeks with esomeprazole 40 mg twice daily, compared to a placebo group.[135] However, post hoc subgroup analysis showed that in patients with GER symptoms and nocturnal asthma, there was a reduction in FEV1. Another double-blind, placebo-controlled trial in adults with moderate to severe persistent asthma showed no improvement in pulmonary function or albuterol use.[136] Again, a post hoc analysis

revealed a 4% decrease in the number of asthma exacerbations and a 14% decrease in oral corticosteroid use in the treatment group. A small, randomized placebo-controlled trial of 38 children with asthma and abnormal esophageal pH monitoring gave 12 weeks of omeprazole 20 mg once daily or placebo and found no difference between the two groups in asthma symptoms or pulmonary functions.[137] In contrast, a nonrandomized study of 27 children ages 5 to 10 years with persistent asthma and abnormal esophageal pH monitoring described a reduction in asthma medication use in patients receiving either medical or surgical therapy for GERD, whereas those that were not treated had no change in medication requirements.[138] Uncontrolled case series also report that antireflux sugerery is beneficial in children with severe persistent asthma requiring use of either frequent oral corticosteroids or high-dose inhaled steroids.[139]

In summary, both pediatric and adult trials demonstrate that GERD treatment is at best only modestly beneficial for selected patients with moderate to severe asthma. It is likely that those children with corticosteroid-resistant asthma and either a positive esophageal pH monitoring study or symptoms such as heartburn or regurgitation are those who are most likely to benefit from antireflux therapy. However, no test has proven to reliably predict those asthma patients who will respond well to either medical or surgical therapy for GERD.[134,140]

Laryngeal symptoms of hoarseness, chronic cough, and globus sensation have been ascribed to GERD. Typical findings of laryngopharyngeal inflammation include posterior glottic edema, laryngeal erythema, laryngeal hypervascularity, and laryngeal pseudosulcus widely believed to be diagnostic of GERD.[81] However, diagnosis using laryngoscopic criteria has proven unreliable. As an alternative approach, twice daily, PPI as a treatment trial has been recommended for symptomatic adults with potential GERD-related laryngeal symptoms or signs. However, multiple well-designed prospective, placebo-controlled studies in adults[141–144] show minimal, if any, benefit for all laryngeal symptoms[145] except for a small reduction of chronic cough.[146] In addition, those patients that show no improvement in response to medical therapy are unlikely to improve following antireflux surgery.[147]

An increased frequency of GERD or gastropharyngeal reflux (GPR) is reported in infants and children with laryngo-tracheomalacia, subglottic stenosis, and recurrent laryngotracheitis. Increased GERD has also been noted in children with hoarseness, cough, and poor outcomes following surgery for subglottic stensosis.[1] As in adults, no clear cause-and-effect relationship between GERD and any laryngeal symptom has been demonstrated in pediatric patients. No placebo-controlled study has been performed to evaluate the efficacy of GERD medical therapies to reduce laryngeal symptoms in children. Even though one retrospective case series reported resolution of a variety of possible laryngeal symptoms following antireflux surgery, the diagnostic criteria for GERD are poorly described.[148] One case report describes a child with recurrence of subglottic stenosis who underwent fundoplication for laryngeal findings suspected to be due to GER but were later ascribed to a milk protein allergy.[149]

Taken together, there is only weak and circumstantial evidence in support of a relationship between laryngeal disorders and GERD in children. Prior to treating presumed laryngeal symptoms and signs in children with high-dose PPI, other etiologies of laryngeal inflammatory alterations, such as vocal abuse and allergy should be considered and either excluded or appropriately managed.

Sinusitis, otitis media, and otalgia each has been related to GERD in uncontrolled case series.[150,151] High concentrations of pepsin, which is presumed to be of gastric origin, has been found in the middle ear fluid obtained from infants with serous otitis media[152,153] suggesting a role for GERD in the etiology of chronic otitis media. Despite these findings, a prospective study found no evidence of increased sinusitis or otitis media among infants with GERD compared to normal infants without GERD.[19] A retrospective, case-control study found that children over age 2 years with GERD have an increased incidence of sinusitis but not otitis media.[18] Otalgia has been associated with GERD in children and reported to improve following treatment of GERD.[154] Until well-designed, prospective, double-blind, placebo-controlled studies demonstrate the efficacy of treatment of GERD, it cannot yet be concluded that GER contributes to either sinus disease or otitis media.

Dental erosions with enamel loss involving the facial, occlusal, and lingual tooth surfaces are reported to be increased in frequency among children and adolescents with GERD.[155] However, there is no increased incidence of dental erosions in adolescents with abnormal esophageal pH monitoring.[156] There may be an increased risk of dental caries in children with GERD.[157] The prevalence of GERD-related dental disease is not yet known, and the best approach to therapy remains unclear. No studies have evaluated the efficacy of GERD treatment for prevention of acid–relux-related dental disorders.

TREATMENT OF GERD

The approach to treatment of GERD varies depending on the specific symptoms, severity, expected natural history, and presence of concomitant problems (Table 4). The goals of GERD therapy are to relieve symptoms and to prevent and treat complications. It is important to balance the potential risks of GERD with those of the therapy to be employed for each individual patient. For example, reflux of gastric contents into the mouth in an infant may be considered a normal physiologic event, but in an infant with a neurological disorder that compromises airway protective

---

Table 4 Treatment of GERD

Nonpharmacologic
  Position changes (prone sleeping not recommended)
  Formula thickening
  Time-limited trial of hypoallergenic formula
  Higher calorie formulas
  Nasogastric/jejunal feeds if undernourished or
    for airway complications
  Weight loss if overweight

Pharmacologic
  Antacids (usually not recommended in infants)
  Surface agents (eg, sodium alginate, sucralfate)
  Motility agents (eg, domperidone, baclofen)
  Acid-suppressive agents (eg, H_2Ras, PPIs)

Surgical
  Surgical fundoplication (open, laparoscopic)
  Feeding by gastrostomy/jejunostomy
  Esophago-gastric dissociation

---

mechanisms, this same reflux event may lead to aspiration and pneumonia. No treatment is indicated for the normal infant, but aggressive therapeutic approaches such as nasojejunal feeding and/or antireflux surgery may be indicated in the latter case.

Nonpharmacologic Treatments

Nonpharmacologic options for GER therapy in infants include positioning changes, formula changes including thickening, use of hypoallergenic formulas or high calorie formulas, and alterations in mode of feeding. Less episodes of GER occur in the prone position than in the supine or semi-supine position (as in an infant seat). However, prone positioning for infants with GER is associated with a substantial increase in the risk of SIDS and is not recommended.[1]

Thickening of feeds with guar gum or added cereals reduces the number and height of nonacid reflux episodes and regurgitation but does not decrease esophageal acid exposure.[158] Thickening of formulas also increases the work of sucking from a nipple and requires the nipple to be slit. Thickening can also increase coughing or gagging during feeds.[159] Cows milk-based formulas that contain rice starches or locust bean gum that thickens upon acidification in the stomach provide an alternative approach to decrease the number of episodes of regurgitation.[160,161] If these approaches are ineffective, a time-limited trial of hypoallergenic infant formula (such as hydrolyzed protein formula or elemental amino acid formula for 2 weeks) can be used to determine if cows or soy milk protein allergy is the cause of symptoms.[1]

The mode of formula delivery may also provide a therapeutic option for some infants with GERD. Administration of smaller volumes of feeds and thickened feeds decreases the frequency of emesis, but not esophageal acid exposure.[162] The tendency for regurgitation and vomiting is reduced if feedings are administered by continual drip rather than by bolus. This technique has been used as a short-term bridge to promote growth in infants with

---

GERD and growth failure. Furthermore, in infants with pulmonary symptoms from swallowing dysfunction and GERD, continual jejunal tube feeding markedly reduces the risk of aspiration of feedings.[163] However, a nasogastric tube increases the number of episodes of gastroesophageal reflux in preterm infants so that the use of chronic indwelling nasogastric or nasojejunal tubes could actually increase reflux events and worsen problems such as esophagitis.[164] Strategies for intermittent orogastric tube placement with feeds and its removal after feeds or gastrojejunal feeding may minimize reflux events.

For older children and adolescents, nonpharmacologic therapies are similar to those used for adults. Although there is physiologic evidence that exposure to tobacco, alcohol, chocolate, and high-fat meals decreases lower esophageal sphincter pressure, the therapeutic efficacy of dietary measures, smoking, or alcohol cessation has not been demonstrated.[165] In contrast, left-side positioning and elevation of the head of the bed are beneficial in adults and presumably should also be useful in children.[165–166]

Weight loss should be encouraged in overweight children since it improves pH profiles and reduces GERD symptoms in overweight adults.[25] One case series suggests that some children with symptoms suggestive of GERD improve with treatment of constipation,[167] possibly due to slow gastric emptying caused by the constipation.

Pharmacologic Treatments

The primary options for currently available pharmacotherapy all focus on reduction of esophageal acid exposure, either by buffering secreted gastric acid or by reducing secretion of gastric acid. None of the available agents directly improves esophageal peristalsis or acid clearance. Oral antacids buffer gastric acid, while H_2RAs and PPIs suppress the production of gastric acid.

Oral Antacids. Magnesium hydroxide and aluminum hydroxide are as effective as H_2RAs when used at high doses in children with peptic esophagitis.[1] However, the possible adverse effects of increases in plasma aluminum levels in children and infants (eg, osteopenia, microcytic anemia, neurotoxicity) limit their usefulness at the doses required to produce comparable effects to H_2RA. Hypophosphatemic metabolic bone disease (rickets) can occur with chronic use in adults or children, and particular care is required in infants.[168] Thus, in older children with mild or intermittent symptoms, antacids may be useful for on-demand use, but they are not recommended for chronic use due to the associated complications especially in infants.

Surface Agents. Alginate containing antacid formulations form a raft atop the gastric contents with entrapped carbon dioxide that is thought to provide longer-lasting relief than traditional antacids.[169–170] However, studies using impedance technologies to evaluate the efficacy of these agents in infants demonstrated no alterations in the number of reflux events or reflux index. There was a marginal reduction in the height of the refluxed material into the esophagus but no clinically meaningful response was observed.[171] Sucralfate also forms a protective coating on gastroesophageal surfaces and binds to bile acids. It has been shown to be as effective as cimetidine for treatment of childhood esophagitis.[172] However, sucralfate is an aluminum complex and the potential adverse systemic effects of long-term use are of concern, more so in renal disease.[1] In addition, the formulation of sucralfate—a large tablet, or a slurry—makes it poorly accepted by children. The chronic use of these agents in pediatric populations is not recommended.

Agents That Alter Gastrointestinal Motility. The efficacy of a variety of prokinetic agents has been evaluated in pediatric GERD. The dopamine receptor antagonists, metoclopramide and domperidone, have both been used to treat GER in infants and children. Multiple series show that metoclopramide is not useful for treatment of GER and side effects including anxiety, tremors, and dystonia make this agents use even more undesirable.[173] Domperidone has less side effects, but there is not strong evidence of benefit in pediatric GERD,[174] and there are reports of QTc interval prolongation in infants treated with domperidone.[175] Bethanachol had been used for treatment, but efficacy is questionable and the side effects generally outweigh any potential benefit.[176] Cisapride, a serotonin (5HT4) receptor agonist that stimulates postganglionic acetylcholine release in the myenteric plexus appeared to show some efficacy for a reduction of GER symptoms in infants,[1] but it seems likely that this interpretation was at least partially accounted for by publication bias suggesting that it may have no efficacy.[177] Cisapride has been withdrawn from distribution in most of the world due to concerns about cardiac arrhythmia risks. Tegaserod, another newly available serotinergic agent, may reduce esophageal acid exposure, but there are conflicting studies in adults[178–179] and no pediatric studies have been performed. In view of the lack of proven efficacy of any of these agents and the proven risks associated with each agent, none of these agents can be recommended for the treatment of pediatric GERD.

Baclofen, a gamma butyric acid (GABA) receptor agonist, reduces the number of TLESRs and episodes of acid and nonacid GER in adults,[180–182] and a placebo-controlled study in infants also showed a reduction of TLESRs, decreased acid reflux, and acceleration of gastric emptying.[183] Pharmacokinetics appear to be similar in children and adults[184] but infant studies are lacking. Baclofen may be useful as adjunctive therapy for some patients with GERD, but potential side effects limit its use.[185] Baclofen may be particularly well suited for therapy in combination with PPIs for treatment of GERD symptoms in children with concomitant spasticity prior to considering surgical therapy, but no placebo-controlled trials have been conducted.

H2-Receptor Antagonists. H_2RAs act to decrease acid secretion by inhibiting the histamine-2 receptor on the gastric parietal cell. H_2RA agents shown to be effective for treatment of esophagitis in children include cimetidine, ranitidine, nizatidine, and famotidine.[1,97,186] The renal clearance of famotidine is less in infants below 3 months of age compared to older infants.[187] A lower dose of ranitidine is effective in premature infants (0.5 mg/kg/body weight bid) compared to full-term infants (1.5 mg/kg/body weight tid).[188] The side effect profiles of H_2RA agents in children have not been compared, but the best studied agent, famotidine, was shown to possibly cause agitation and signs interpreted as headache in some infants.[97] The quicker onset of action of H_2RA makes their use preferable to PPIs for episodic symptom relief. In many cases tolerance develops to this class of agents in both children and adults on chronic therapy. This tachyphylaxis makes H_2RA less effective than PPI's for long-term therapy of GERD.

Proton Pump Inhibitors. PPIs covalently bind and deactivate the H^+, K^+-ATPase pumps in the stomach, providing more effective gastric suppression compared to H_2RAs.[189] Binding requires protonation in the active secretory canaliculus of the parietal cell. Different PPIs have different rates of activation and plasma half-life leading to variations in their duration of acid inhibition,[189] but these differences have led to only marginal demonstrable differences in clinical efficacy of varied formulations.[190] PPIs are highly efficacious and safe for the treatment of GERD-related symptoms and signs, including the most severe degrees of reflux esophagitis refractory to H_2RA, with rates of symptom relief and cure of esophagitis above 90% for omeprazole,[33,132,191] lanzoprazole,[192–195] pantoprazole,[196–197] and esomeprazole.[198–199] The safety of PPI therapy compares to that in adults, with the longest published experience in pediatrics being with omeprazole.[24]

Children between 1 and 10 years of age generally metabolize PPIs much faster than adults, and therefore have greater requirement for drug on a per kilogram basis.[200] In children below 1 year of age, pharmacokinetics are less predictable and safety is less well validated, so considerable caution is required in prescribing PPI in this age group especially without good evidence of GERD.[201] PPIs should be tapered, not be stopped abruptly, because their discontinuation is followed by acid rebound[202] that may may lead to an exacerbation of symptoms and an incorrect perception that the patient has relapsed and requires another course of PPI. Nocturnal acid breakthrough defined as a recovery of pH to less than 4, for 1 hour or more overnight during PPI therapy is common in both children[203] and adults[204] but despite this, symptoms and healing of esophagitis often continue to improve during therapy. Therefore, suppression of nocturnal acid should not be a therapeutic goal with the possible exception of patients with nocturnal symptoms or with Barretts esophagus.

More so than many drugs, the optimal effectiveness of PPI therapy requires careful attention to details of the timing of administration and formulation. The PPI is best administered as a single dose daily, one-half hour before breakfast so that serum concentration of the drug coincides with activation acid pumps following meal ingestion after an overnight fast. Usually once-daily dosing is adequate to produce symptom relief and healing of esophagitis. If nocturnal symptoms persist on therapy or when Barretts esophagus is present, a twice-daily dosing regimen may be required. In such cases, the second dose should be given half an hour before the evening meal.

In children PPI administration can be particularly challenging due to refusal or inability to ingest medications that are in tablet or capsule form. This is particularly true in children less than about 8 years of age, those with neurodevelopmental problems or swallowing disorders. Since the various PPIs are of equivalent efficacy and safety, the cost and acceptability of a particular PPI preparation may be more important when selecting among them than comparable efficacy. A variety of liquid formulations and orally dissolvable tablets are increasingly available in different marketplaces, making PPI administration simpler in children. Since omeprazole, lanzoprazole, and pantoprazole have undergone studies in children older than age 1 year, these should be used in preference to other agents. Only omeprazole has been studied in premature infants. Intravenous formulations may be used, but are costly, associated with significant resource use, and substantial benefit has not been demonstrated compared to enteral formulations,[205] especially in the case of esophagitis.

Risks of Acid Suppression. Although there is no doubt that acid-suppressive therapies are beneficial in patients with proven GERD, the indiscriminate use of these agents for presumptive treatment of symptoms questionably caused by GER is not advisable since there are now data that show potential adverse consequences of chronic gastric acid suppression. Gastric acid inhibition with PPIs or H_2RA may increase the risk of contracting acute gastroenteritis and community-acquired pneumonia in young children.[14] The risk of candidal infection[206–207] and necrotizing enterocolitis[56] is increased in premature infants treated with acid-suppressive agents. In adults, there is an association between acid suppression and an increased incidence of hospital- and community-acquired *Clostridium difficile* infection,[208–209] vitamin B12 deficiency,[210] and hip fracture.[211] Although long-term acid suppression may cause hyperplasia of enterochromaffin-like (ECL) cells, there is no evidence that it is associated with an increased risk of carcinoid tumors.[212] However, in patients with *Helicobacter pylori* gastritis, long-term acid suppression may accelerate development of atrophic gastritis. Therefore, it is recommended that *H. pylori* testing is performed, and treatment given to eradicate the infection in those who are infected, and are expected to receive long-term acid suppression.[213] The risks and benefits of acid suppressive-therapy can be mitigated by only using them for appropriate indications for a frequency and dose that is adequate to relieve symptoms. Achlorhydria is not the goal of therapy since intermittent gastric acidity should conceivably help to prevent the complications of potent acid suppression.

Antireflux Surgery

Analysis of a national database reported that over 6,000 (10 per 100,000) antireflux procedures were performed per year in children less than 18 years old between 1996 and 2003 in the United States, and of these 45% were in children under 1 year of age.[214] During this period there was a trend toward an increase in the number of fundoplications performed, but there was a reduction in the number of procedures performed in children with neurological impairment (53 to 40%) suggesting that pediatric fundoplication rates increased in children without neurological disease with the advent of laparoscopic surgery.

Complication rates are similar with laparoscopic or open antireflux surgery.[215] Intra- or peri-operative complications with antireflux surgery include splenectomy (0.2%), esophageal laceration (0.2%), and infection.[214] Long-term complications include breakdown of the wrap with recurrent GERD (2.5 to 40%),[216–217] small bowel obstruction, gas bloat syndrome, gastroparesis, and dumping syndrome.[1,218–219] There is a wide variation in reported complication rates that likely reflects differences in patient selection, reliability of follow-up information or differences in surgical experience. The type of fundoplication performed (anterior, posterior, or complete wrap) does not appear to alter complication rates.[217] Furthermore, up to two-thirds of patients that undergo antireflux surgery are reported to have persistent symptoms and continue to receive GERD-related medical therapy at 2 months following the procedure.[220]

The decision to subject a child to the risks of antireflux surgery requires that outcome will be substantially improved compared with medical therapy. Even though recent evidence suggests some risks associated with long-term medical therapy, these risks are small compared to the potential complications of surgery. Current medical therapy almost always provides adequate therapy for esophageal complications of GERD. Therefore, antireflux surgery is most often considered to manage recurrent respiratory problems including severe asthma and recurrent pneumonia. In patients with other potential supraesophageal complications of GER, it is unlikely that antireflux surgery will be beneficial in those that do not respond to medical therapy.[147]

Analysis of a Washington state hospital admissions data set showed that those children that underwent antireflux surgery prior to age 4 showed reduced hospitalizations for GER-related events such as pneumonia following their procedure, whereas those greater than age 4 years had increased hospitalizations for pneumonia.[221] The approach to selecting patients for antireflux surgery could not be determined, so it is unclear if many of these patients may have had similar improvement with more aggressive medical therapy. Studies of children even with severe neurological disease show substantial reductions in pneumonia rates following PPI treatment.[31] Another single center study showed that in severely neurologically impaired children, antireflux surgery decreased vomiting and GI bleeding, but did not change the rates of pneumonia, and recurrence of reflux occurred in 30% of patients, further highlighting the variable efficacy of this procedure for patients with severe neurological disease.[36] Patients with neurodevelopmental disorders who undergo antireflux surgery often can be successfully managed with omeprazole therapy[222] and are more likely to fail a redo fundoplication,[223] findings which further support the contention that medical therapy should be optimized prior to considering antireflux surgery.[219]

Endoscopic approaches to GERD therapy have also been reported in children. One report described endoscopic fundoplication in 17 children 6 to 16 years of age. Early repeat procedures were required in 3, but at 2 years of follow-up most had maintained symptom resolution.[224] However, the risks, benefits, and efficacy of an endoscopic approach to manage GERD remain controversial even in adults.[225] Currently such approaches should be reserved to centers undertaking rigorous clinical trials, evaluating the outcomes of the newer GERD management options.

Esophagogastric dissociation had been used with some success to manage children with severe neurodevelopmental disorders where oral feeding is either unsafe or undesirable[37–38] although others report high complication rates. This procedure has also been used in neurologically normal children when conventional antireflux surgical approaches either fail or are not possible due to the patients anatomy.[226]

REFERENCES

1. Rudolph CD, Mazur LJ, Liptak GS, et al. Guidelines for evaluation and treatment of gastroesophageal reflux in infants and children: Recommendations of the North American Society for Pediatric Gastroenterology and Nutrition. J Pediatr Gastroenterol Nutr 2001;32:S1–31.
2. Omari TI, Barnett C, Snel A, et al. Mechanisms of gastroesophageal reflux in healthy premature infants. J Pediatr 1998;133:650–4.
3. Mittal RK, Holloway RH, Penagini R, et al. Transient lower esophageal sphincter relaxation. Gastroenterology 1995;109:601–10.
4. Carre IJ, Johnston BT, Thomas PS, et al. Familial hiatal hernia in a large five generation family confirming true autosomal dominant inheritance. Gut 1999;45:649–52.
5. Werlin SL, Dodds WJ, Hogan WJ, et al. Mechanisms of gastroesophageal reflux in children. J Pediatr 1980;97:244–9.
6. Davidson GP, Omari TI, Pathophysiological mechanisms of gastroesophageal reflux disease in children. Curr Gastroenterol Rep 2001;3:257–62.
7. Orenstein SR, Whitington PF, and Orenstein DM. The infant seat as treatment for gastroesophageal reflux. N Engl J Med 1983;309:760–3.
8. Omari TI, Barnett CP, Benninga MA, et al. Mechanisms of gastroesophageal reflux in preterm and term infants with reflux disease. Gut 2002;51:475–9.
9. Shaker R. Protective mechanisms against supraesophageal GERD. J Clin Gastroenterol 2000;30:S3–8.
10. Wenzl TG, Schenke S, Peschgens T, et al. Association of apnea and nonacid gastroesophageal reflux in infants: Investigations with the intraluminal impedance technique. Pediatr Pulmonol 2001;31:144–9.
11. Wynne JW, Modell JH. Respiratory aspiration of stomach contents. Ann Intern Med 1977;87:466–74.
12. Schwartz DJ, Wynne JW, Gibbs CP, et al. The pulmonary consequences of aspiration of gastric contents at pH values greater than 2.5. Am Rev Respir Dis 1980;121:119–26.
13. Terpenning M. Geriatric oral health and pneumonia risk. Clin Infect Dis 2005;40:1807–10.
14. Canani RB, Cirillo P, Roggero P, et al. Therapy with gastric acidity inhibitors increases the risk of acute gastroenteritis and community-acquired pneumonia in children. Pediatrics 2006;117:e817–20.
15. Martin AJ, Pratt N, Kennedy JD, et al. Natural history and familial relationships of infant spilling to 9 years of age. Pediatrics 2002;109:1061–7.
16. Nelson SP, Chen EH, Syniar GM, et al. Prevalence of symptoms of gastroesophageal reflux during infancy. A pediatric practice-based survey. Pediatric Practice Research Group. Arch Pediatr Adolesc Med 1997;151:569–72.
17. Nelson SP, Chen EH, Syniar GM, et al. Prevalence of symptoms of gastroesophageal reflux during childhood: A pediatric practice-based survey. Pediatric Practice Research Group. Arch Pediatr Adolesc Med 2000;154:150–4.
18. El-Serag HB, Gilger M, Kuebeler M, et al. Extraesophageal associations of gastroesophageal reflux disease in children without neurologic defects. Gastroenterology 2001;121:1294–9.
19. Nelson SP, Chen EH, Syniar GM, et al. One-year follow-up of symptoms of gastroesophageal reflux during infancy. Pediatric Practice Research Group. Pediatrics 1998;102:E67.
20. Treem WR, Davis PM, Hyams JS. Gastroesophageal reflux in the older child: Presentation, response to treatment long-term follow-up. Clin Pediatr (Phila) 1991;30:435–40.
21. El-Serag HB, Gilger M, Carter J, et al. Childhood GERD is a risk factor for GERD in adolescents and young adults. Am J Gastroenterol 2004;99:806–12.
22. Fujiwara Y, Higuchi K, Watanabe Y, et al. Prevalence of gastroesophageal reflux disease and gastroesophageal reflux disease symptoms in Japan. J Gastroenterol Hepatol 2005;20:26–9.
23. Young RJ, Lyden E, Ward B, et al. A retrospective, case-control pilot study of the natural history of pediatric gastroesophageal reflux. Dig Dis Sci 2007;52:457–62.
24. Hassall E, Kerr W, El-Serag HB Characteristics of children receiving proton pump inhibitors continuously for up to 11 years duration. J Pediatr 2007;150:262–7, 267 e1.
25. Gerson LB. A little weight gain, how much gastroesophageal reflux disease? Gastroenterology 2006;131:1644–6. discussion 1646.
26. Cameron AJ, Lagergren J, Henriksson C, et al. Gastroesophageal reflux disease in monozygotic and dizygotic twins. Gastroenterology 2002;122:55–9.
27. Mohammed I, Cherkas LF, Riley SA, et al. Genetic influences in gastroesophageal reflux disease: A twin study. Gut 2003;52:1085–9.
28. Chak A, Ochs-Balcom H, Falk G, et al. Familiality in Barrett's esophagus, adenocarcinoma of the esophagus, and adenocarcinoma of the gastroesophageal junction. Cancer Epidemiol Biomarkers Prev, 2006;15:1668–73.
29. Casson AG, Zheng Z, Porter GA, et al. Genetic polymorphisms of microsomal epoxide hydroxylase and glutathione S-transferases M1, T1 and P1, interactions with smoking, and risk for esophageal (Barrett) adenocarcinoma. Cancer Detect Prev 2006;30:423–31.
30. Bohmer CJ, Klinkenberg-Knol EC, Niezen-de Boer MC, et al. Gastroesophageal reflux disease in intellectually disabled individuals: How often, how serious, how manageable? Am J Gastroenterol 2000;95:1868–72.
31. Bohmer CJ, Niezen-de Boer RC, Klinkenberg-Knol EC, et al. Omeprazole: Therapy of choice in intellectually disabled children. Arch Pediatr Adolesc Med 1998;152:1113–8.
32. Cheung KM, Tse PW, Ko CH, et al. Clinical efficacy of proton pump inhibitor therapy in neurologically impaired children with gastroesophageal reflux: Prospective study. Hong Kong Med J 2001;7:356–9.
33. Hassall E, Israel D, Shepherd R, et al. Omeprazole for treatment of chronic erosive esophagitis in children: A multicenter study of efficacy, safety, tolerability and dose requirements. International Pediatric Omeprazole Study Group. J Pediatr 2000;137:800–7.

34. Mathus-Vliegen EM, Koning H, Taminiau JA, et al. Percutaneous endoscopic gastrostomy and gastrojejunostomy in psychomotor retarded subjects: A follow-up covering 106 patient years. J Pediatr Gastroenterol Nutr 2001;33:488–94.

35. Martinez DA, Ginn-Pease ME, Caniano DA. Sequelae of antireflux surgery in profoundly disabled children [see comments]. J Pediatr Surg 1992;27:267–71; discussion 271–3.

36. Cheung KM, Tse HW, Tse PW, et al. Nissen fundoplication and gastrostomy in severely neurologically impaired children with gastroesophageal reflux. Hong Kong Med J 2006;12:282–8.

37. Gatti C, di Abriola GF, Villa M, et al. Esophagogastric dissociation versus fundoplication. Which is best for severely neurologically impaired children? J Pediatr Surg 2001;36:677–80.

38. Morabito A, Lall A, Lo Piccolo R, et al. Total esophagogastric dissociation: 10 years' review. J Pediatr Surg 2006;41:919–22.

39. Takamizawa S, Tsugawa C, Nishijima E, et al. Laryngotracheal separation for intractable aspiration pneumonia in neurologically impaired children: Experience with 11 cases. J Pediatr Surg 2003;38:975–7.

40. Islam S, Teitelbaum DH, Buntain WL, et al. Esophagogastric separation for failed fundoplication in neurologically impaired children. J Pediatr Surg 2004;39:287–91; discussion 287–91.

41. Koivusalo A, Pakarinen MP, Rintala RJ. The cumulative incidence of significant gastrooesophageal reflux in patients with oesophageal atresia with a distal fistula–a systematic clinical, pH-metric, and endoscopic follow-up study. J Pediatr Surg 2007;42:370–4.

42. Hassall E. Esophageal metaplasia: Definition and prevalence in childhood. Gastrointest Endosc 2006;64:676–7.

43. Roberts KE, Duffy AJ, Bell RL. Controversies in the treatment of gastroesophageal reflux and achalasia. World J Gastroenterol 2006;12:3155–61.

44. Leeuwenburgh I, Van Dekken H, Scholten P, et al. Oesophagitis is common in patients with achalasia after pneumatic dilatation. Aliment Pharmacol Ther 2006;23:1197–203.

45. Malfroot A, Dab I. New insights on gastroesophageal reflux in cystic fibrosis by longitudinal follow up. Arch Dis Child 1991;66:1339–45.

46. Benden C, Aurora P, Curry J, et al. High prevalence of gastroesophageal reflux in children after lung transplantation. Pediatr Pulmonol 2005;40:68–71.

47. Ng SM, Jones AP. Drug therapies for reducing gastric acidity in people with cystic fibrosis. Cochrane Database Syst Rev 2003; CD003424.

48. Dhillon AS, Ewer AK. Diagnosis and management of gastroesophageal reflux in preterm infants in neonatal intensive care units. Acta Paediatr 2004;93:88–93.

49. Jadcherla SR. Gastroesophageal reflux in the neonate. Clin Perinatol 2002;29:135–58.

50. Jadcherla SR. Manometric evaluation of esophageal-protective reflexes in infants and children. Am J Med 2003;115:157S–160S.

51. Akinola E, Rosenkrantz TS, Pappagallo M, et al. Gastroesophageal reflux in infants < 32 weeks gestational age at birth: Lack of relationship to chronic lung disease. Am J Perinatol 2004;21:57–62.

52. Fuloria M, Hiatt D, Dillard RG, et al. Gastroesophageal reflux in very low birth weight infants: Association with chronic lung disease and outcomes through 1 year of age. J Perinatol 2000;20:235–9.

53. Frakaloss G, Burke G, Sanders MR. Impact of gastroesophageal reflux on growth and hospital stay in premature infants. J Pediatr Gastroenterol Nutr 1998;26:146–50.

54. Khalaf MN, Porat R, Brodsky NL, et al. Clinical correlations in infants in the neonatal intensive care unit with varying severity of gastroesophageal reflux. J Pediatr Gastroenterol Nutr 2001;32:45–9.

55. Omari TI, Haslam RR, Lundborg P, et al. Effect of omeprazole on acid gastroesophageal reflux and gastric acidity in preterm infants with pathological acid reflux. J Pediatr Gastroenterol Nutr 2007;44:41–4.

56. Guillet R, Stoll BJ, Cotten CM, et al. Association of H2-blocker therapy and higher incidence of necrotizing enterocolitis in very low birth weight infants. Pediatrics 2006;117:e137–42.

57. Snel A, Barnett CP, Cresp TL, et al. Behavior and gastroesophageal reflux in the premature neonate. J Pediatr Gastroenterol Nutr 2000;30:18–21.

58. Jadcherla S, Rudolph C. Gastroesophageal reflux in the preterm neonate. Neoreviews 2005;6:e87–98.

59. Poets CF Gastroesophageal reflux: A critical review of its role in preterm infants. Pediatrics 2004;113:e128–32.

60. Kaijser M, Akre O, Cnattingius S, et al. Preterm birth, low birth weight, and risk for esophageal adenocarcinoma. Gastroenterology 2005;128:607–9.

61. Akre O, Forssell L, Kaijser M, et al. Perinatal risk factors for cancer of the esophagus and gastric cardia: A nested case-control study. Cancer Epidemiol Biomarkers Prev 2006;15:867–71.

62. Chadwick LM, Kurinczuk JJ, Hallam LA, et al. Clinical and endoscopic predictors of histological oesophagitis in infants. J Paediatr Child Health 1997;33:388–93.

63. Kleinman L, Revicki DA, Flood E. Validation issues in questionnaires for diagnosis and monitoring of gastroesophageal reflux disease in children. Curr Gastroenterol Rep 2006;8:230–6.

64. Deal L, Gold BD, Gremse DA, et al. Age-specific questionnaires distinguish GERD symptom frequency and severity in infants and young children: Development and initial validation. J Pediatr Gastroenterol Nutr 2005;41:178–85.

65. Vandenplas Y, Goyvaerts H, Helven R, et al. Gastroesophageal reflux, as measured by 24-hour pH monitoring, in 509 healthy infants screened for risk of sudden infant death syndrome. Pediatrics 1991;88:834–40.

66. Boix-Ochoa J, Lafuenta JM, Gil-Vernet JM. Twenty-four hour exophageal pH monitoring in gastroesophageal reflux. J Pediatr Surg 1980;15:74–8.

67. Jamieson JR, Stein HJ, DeMeester TR, et al. Ambulatory 24-h esophageal pH monitoring: Normal values, optimal thresholds, specificity, sensitivity, and reproducibility [see comments]. Am J Gastroenterol 1992;87:1102–11.

68. Mahajan L, Wyllie R, Oliva L, et al. Reproducibility of 24-hour intraesophageal pH monitoring in pediatric patients. Pediatrics 1998;101:260–3.

69. Vakil N, van Zanten SV, Kahrilas P, et al. The Montreal definition and classification of gastroesophageal reflux disease: A global evidence-based consensus. Am J Gastroenterol 2006;101:1900–20.

70. Sifrim D, Castell D, Dent J, et al. Gastroesophageal reflux monitoring: Review and consensus report on detection and definitions of acid, non-acid, and gas reflux. Gut 2004;53:1024–31.

71. Wenzl TG. Evaluation of gastroesophageal reflux events in children using multichannel intraluminal electrical impedance. Am J Med 2003;115:161S–5S.

72. Wenzl TG, Moroder C, Trachterna M, et al. Esophageal pH monitoring and impedance measurement: A comparison of two diagnostic tests for gastroesophageal reflux. J Pediatr Gastroenterol Nutr 2002;34:519–23.

73. Peter CS, Sprodowski N, Bohnhorst B, et al. Gastroesophageal reflux and apnea of prematurity: No temporal relationship. Pediatrics 2002;109:8–11.

74. Condino AA, Sondheimer J, Pan Z, et al. Evaluation of gastroesophageal reflux in pediatric patients with asthma using impedance-pH monitoring. J Pediatr 2006;149:216–9.

75. Peter CS, Sprodowski N, Ahlborn V, et al. Inter- and intraobserver agreement for gastroesophageal reflux detection in infants using multiple intraluminal impedance. Biol Neonate 2004;85:11–4.

76. Vandenplas Y, Salvatore S, Vieira MC, et al. Will esophageal impedance replace pH monitoring? Pediatrics 2007;119:118–22.

77. Gillett P, Hassall E. Pediatric gastrointestinal mucosal biopsy. Special considerations in children. Gastrointest Endosc Clin North Am 2000;10:669–712.

78. Dent J. Microscopic esophageal mucosal injury in nonerosive reflux disease. Clin Gastroenterol Hepatol 2007;5:4–16.

79. Sbarbati A, Deganello A, Bertini M, et al. Reflux esophagitis in children: A scanning and transmission electron microscopy study. J Submicrosc Cytol Pathol 1993;25:603–11.

80. Rudolph CD. Supraesophageal complications of gastroesophageal reflux in children: Challenges in diagnosis and treatment. Am J Med 2003;115:150S–6S.

81. Belafsky PC. Abnormal endoscopic pharyngeal and laryngeal findings attributable to reflux. Am J Med 2003;115:90S–6S.

82. Hicks DM, Ours TM, Abelson TI, et al. The prevalence of hypopharynx findings associated with gastroesophageal reflux in normal volunteers. J Voice 2002;16:564–79.

83. Branski RC, Bhattacharyya N, Shapiro J. The reliability of the assessment of endoscopic laryngeal findings associated with laryngopharyngeal reflux disease. Laryngoscope 2002;112:1019–24.

84. Qadeer MA, Swoger J, Milstein C, et al. Correlation between symptoms and laryngeal signs in laryngopharyngeal reflux. Laryngoscope 2005;115:1947–52.

85. Krishnan U, Mitchell JD, Tobias V, et al. Fat laden macrophages in tracheal aspirates as a marker of reflux aspiration: A negative report. J Pediatr Gastroenterol Nutr 2002;35:309–13.

86. Krishnan U, Mitchell JD, Messina I, et al. Assay of tracheal pepsin as a marker of reflux aspiration. J Pediatr Gastroenterol Nutr 2002;35:303–8.

87. Di Lorenzo C, Piepsz A, Ham H, et al. Gastric emptying with gastroesophageal reflux. Arch Dis Child 1987;62:449–53.

88. Ravelli AM, Panarotto MB, Verdoni L, et al. Pulmonary aspiration shown by scintigraphy in gastroesophageal reflux-related respiratory disease. Chest 2006;130:1520–6.

89. Ours TM, Kavuru MS, Schilz RJ, et al. A prospective evaluation of esophageal testing and a double-blind, randomized study of omeprazole in a diagnostic and therapeutic algorithm for chronic cough. Am J Gastroenterol 1999;94:3131–8.

90. Fass R, Fennerty MB, Ofman JJ, et al. The clinical and economic value of a short course of omeprazole in patients with noncardiac chest pain [see comments]. Gastroenterology 1998;115:42–9.

91. Johnsson F, Weywadt L, Solhaug JH, et al. One-week omeprazole treatment in the diagnosis of gastroesophageal reflux disease. Scand J Gastroenterol 1998;33:15–20.

92. van Pinxteren B, Numans ME, Bonis PA, et al. Short-term treatment with proton pump inhibitors, H2-receptor antagonists and prokinetics for gastroesophageal reflux disease-like symptoms and endoscopy negative reflux disease. Cochrane Database Syst Rev 2000;2:CD001960.

93. Orenstein SR, Shalaby TM, Kelsey SF, et al. Natural history of infant reflux esophagitis: Symptoms and morphometric histology during one year without pharmacotherapy. Am J Gastroenterol 2006;101:628–40.

94. Friedman JN, Ahmed S, Connolly B, et al. Complications associated with image-guided gastrostomy and gastrojejunostomy tubes in children. Pediatrics 2004;114:458–61.

95. Feranchak AP, Orenstein SR, Cohn JF. Behaviors associated with onset of gastroesophageal reflux episodes in infants. Prospective study using split-screen video and pH probe. Clin Pediatr (Phila) 1994;33:654–62.

96. Moore DJ, Tao BS, Lines DR, et al. Double-blind placebo-controlled trial of omeprazole in irritable infants with gastroesophageal reflux. J Pediatr 2003;143:219–23.

97. Orenstein SR, Shalaby TM, Devandry SN, et al. Famotidine for infant gastroesophageal reflux: A multi-centre, randomized, placebo-controlled, withdrawal trial. Aliment Pharmacol Ther 2003;17:1097–107.

98. Armstrong K, Previtera N, McCallum R. Medicalizing normality? Management of irritability in babies. J Paediatr Child Health 2000;36:301–5.

99. Rommel N, De Meyer AM, Feenstra L, et al. The complexity of feeding problems in 700 infants and young children presenting to a tertiary care institution. J Pediatr Gastroenterol Nutr 2003;37:75–84.

100. Shepherd RW, Wren J, Evans S, et al. Gastroesophageal reflux in children. Clinical profile, course and outcome with active therapy in 126 cases. Clin Pediatr (Phila) 1987;26:55–60.

101. Mathisen B, Worrall L, Masel J, et al. Feeding problems in infants with gastroesophageal reflux disease: A controlled study. J Paediatr Child Health 1999;35:163–9.

102. Saito Y, Kawashima Y, Kondo A, et al. Dysphagia-gastroesophageal reflux complex: Complications due to dysfunction of solitary tract nucleus-mediated vago-vagal reflex. Neuropediatrics 2006;37:115–20.

103. Suskind DL, Thompson DM, Gulati M, et al. Improved infant swallowing after gastroesophageal reflux disease treatment: A function of improved laryngeal sensation? Laryngoscope 2006;116:1397–403.

104. Oda K, Iwakiri R, Hara M, et al. Dysphagia associated with gastroesophageal reflux disease is improved by proton pump inhibitor. Dig Dis Sci, 2005;50:1921–6.

105. Catto-Smith AG, Machida H, Butzner JD, et al. The role of gastroesophageal reflux in pediatric dysphagia. J Pediatr Gastroenterol Nutr 1991;12:159–65.

106. Fass R. Erosive esophagitis and nonerosive reflux disease (NERD): Comparison of epidemiologic, physiologic, and therapeutic characteristics. J Clin Gastroenterol 2007;41:131–7.

107. Barlow WJ and Orlando RC. The pathogenesis of heartburn in nonerosive reflux disease: A unifying hypothesis. Gastroenterology 2005;128:771–8.

108. Rodriguez-Stanley S, Zubaidi S, Proskin HM, et al. Effect of tegaserod on esophageal pain threshold, regurgitation, and symptom relief in patients with functional heartburn and mechanical sensitivity. Clin Gastroenterol Hepatol 2006;4:442–50.

109. Fass R, Ofman JJ, Gralnek IM, et al. Clinical and economic assessment of the omeprazole test in patients with symptoms suggestive of gastroesophageal reflux disease. Arch Intern Med 1999;159:2161–8.

110. Gupta SK, Hassall E, Chiu YL, et al. Presenting symptoms of nonerosive and erosive esophagitis in pediatric patients. Dig Dis Sci 2006;51:858–63.

111. Olguner M, Akgur FM, Hakguder G, et al. Gastroesophageal reflux associated with dystonic movements: Sandifer's syndrome. Pediatr Int 1999;41:321–2.

112. Frankel EA, Shalaby TM, Orenstein SR. Sandifer syndrome posturing: Relation to abdominal wall contractions,

gastroesophageal reflux, and fundoplication. Dig Dis Sci 2006;51:635–40.
113. Sharma P, Falk GW, Weston AP, et al. Dysplasia and cancer in a large multicenter cohort of patients with Barrett's esophagus. Clin Gastroenterol Hepatol 2006;4:566–72.
114. Fitzgerald RC. Complex diseases in gastroenterology and hepatology: GERD, Barrett's, and esophageal adenocarcinoma. Clin Gastroenterol Hepatol 2005;3:529–37.
115. Chak A, Lee T, Kinnard MF, et al. Familial aggregation of Barrett's esophagus, oesophageal adenocarcinoma, and oesophagogastric junctional adenocarcinoma in Caucasian adults. Gut 2002;51:323–8.
116. Hassall E, Dimmick JE, Magee JF. Adenocarcinoma in childhood Barrett's esophagus: Case documentation and the need for surveillance in children. Am J Gastroenterol 1993;88:282–8.
117. El-Serag HB, Aguirre TV, Davis S, et al. Proton pump inhibitors are associated with reduced incidence of dysplasia in Barrett's esophagus. Am J Gastroenterol 2004;99:1877–83.
118. McColl KE. Acid inhibitory medication and risk of gastric and oesophageal cancer. Gut 2006;55:1532–3.
119. Sharma P, McQuaid K, Dent J, et al. A critical review of the diagnosis and management of Barrett's esophagus: The AGA Chicago Workshop. Gastroenterology 2004;127:310–30.
120. Katz PO. Review article: Putting immediate-release proton-pump inhibitors into clinical practice–improving nocturnal acid control and avoiding the possible complications of excessive acid exposure. Aliment Pharmacol Ther 2005;22:31–8.
121. Dewolfe CC. Apparent life-threatening event: A review. Pediatr Clin North Am 2005;52:1127–46, ix.
122. Goldhammer EI, Zaid G, Tal V, et al. QT dispersion in infants with apparent life-threatening events syndrome. Pediatr Cardiol 2002;23:605–7.
123. Nunes ML, Appel CC, da Costa JC. Apparent life-threatening episodes as the first manifestation of epilepsy. Clin Pediatr (Phila) 2003;42:19–22.
124. McGovern MC, Smith MB. Causes of apparent life threatening events in infants: A systematic review. Arch Dis Child 2004;89:1043–8.
125. Spitzer AR, Boyle JT, Tuchman DN, et al. Awake apnea associated with gastroesophageal reflux: A specific clinical syndrome. J Pediatr 1984;104:200–5.
126. Jolley SG, Halpern LM, Tunell WP, et al. The risk of sudden infant death from gastroesophageal reflux [see comments]. J Pediatr Surg 1991;26:691–6.
127. Apnea, sudden infant death syndrome, and home monitoring. Pediatrics 2003;111:914–7.
128. Chen PH, Chang MH, Hsu SC. Gastroesophageal reflux in children with chronic recurrent bronchopulmonary infection. J Pediatr Gastroenterol Nutr 1991;13:16–22.
129. Raghu G, Freudenberger TD, Yang S, et al. High prevalence of abnormal acid gastroesophageal reflux in idiopathic pulmonary fibrosis. Eur Respir J 2006;27:136–42.
130. Scott RB, O'Loughlin EV, Gall DG. Gastroesophageal reflux in patients with cystic fibrosis. J Pediatr 1985;106:223–7.
131. Owayed AF, Campbell DM, Wang EE. Underlying causes of recurrent pneumonia in children. Arch Pediatr Adolesc Med 2000;154:190–4.
132. Gunasekaran TS, Hassall EG. Efficacy and safety of omeprazole for severe gastroesophageal reflux in children [see comments]. J Pediatr 1993;123:148–54.
133. Debley JS, Carter ER, Redding GJ. Prevalence and impact of gastroesophageal reflux in adolescents with asthma: A population-based study. Pediatr Pulmonol 2006;41:475–81.
134. Sontag SJ. The spectrum of pulmonary symptoms due to gastroesophageal reflux. Thorac Surg Clin 2005;15:353–68.
135. Kiljander TO, Harding SM, Field SK, et al. Effects of esomeprazole 40 mg twice daily on asthma: A randomized placebo-controlled trial. Am J Respir Crit Care Med 2006;173:1091–7.
136. Littner MR, Leung FW, Ballard ED, II, et al. Effects of 24 weeks of lansoprazole therapy on asthma symptoms, exacerbations, quality of life, and pulmonary function in adult asthmatic patients with acid reflux symptoms. Chest 2005;128:1128–35.
137. Stordal K, Johannesdottir GB, Bentsen BS, et al. Acid suppression does not change respiratory symptoms in children with asthma and gastroesophageal reflux disease. Arch Dis Child 2005;90:956–60.
138. Khoshoo V, Le T, Haydel RM, Jr, et al. Role of gastroesophageal reflux in older children with persistent asthma. Chest 2003;123:1008–13.
139. Mattioli G, Sacco O, Repetto P, et al. Necessity for surgery in children with gastrooesophageal reflux and supraoesophageal symptoms. Eur J Pediatr Surg 2004;14:7–13.
140. Gibson PG, Henry RL, Coughlan JL. Gastroesophageal reflux treatment for asthma in adults and children. Cochrane Database Syst Rev 2003;CD001496.
141. Vaezi MF, Richter JE, Stasney CR, et al. Treatment of chronic posterior laryngitis with esomeprazole. Laryngoscope 2006;116:254–60.
142. Noordzij JP, Khidr A, Evans BA, et al. Evaluation of omeprazole in the treatment of reflux laryngitis: A prospective, placebo-controlled, randomized, double-blind study. Laryngoscope 2001;111:2147–51.
143. Eherer AJ, Habermann W, Hammer HF, et al. Effect of pantoprazole on the course of reflux-associated laryngitis: A placebo-controlled double-blind crossover study. Scand J Gastroenterol 2003;38:462–7.
144. Steward DL, Wilson KM, Kelly DH, et al. Proton pump inhibitor therapy for chronic laryngo-pharyngitis: A randomized placebo-control trial. Otolaryngol Head Neck Surg2004;131:342–50.
145. Qadeer MA, Phillips CO, Lopez AR, et al. Proton pump inhibitor therapy for suspected GERD-related chronic laryngitis: A meta-analysis of randomized controlled trials. Am J Gastroenterol 2006;101:2646–54.
146. Chang AB, Lasserson TJ, Kiljander TO, et al. Systematic review and meta-analysis of randomised controlled trials of gastroesophageal reflux interventions for chronic cough associated with gastroesophageal reflux. BMJ 2006;332:11–7.
147. Swoger J, Ponsky J, Hicks DM, et al. Surgical fundoplication in laryngopharyngeal reflux unresponsive to aggressive acid suppression: A controlled study. Clin Gastroenterol Hepatol 2006;4:433–41.
148. Suskind DL, Zeringue GP, III, Kluka EA, et al. Gastroesophageal reflux and pediatric otolaryngologic disease: The role of antireflux surgery. Arch Otolaryngol Head Neck Surg 2001;127:511–4.
149. Hartnick CJ, Liu JH, Cotton RT, et al. Subglottic stenosis complicated by allergic esophagitis: Case report. Ann Otol Rhinol Laryngol 2002;111:57–60.
150. Phipps CD, Wood WE, Gibson WS, et al. Gastroesophageal reflux contributing to chronic sinus disease in children: A prospective analysis. Arch Otolaryngol Head Neck Surg 2000;126:831–6.
151. Bothwell MR, Parsons DS, Talbot A, et al. Outcome of reflux therapy on pediatric chronic sinusitis. Otolaryngol Head Neck Surg 1999;121:255–62.
152. Lieu JE, Muthappan PG, Uppaluri R. Association of reflux with otitis media in children. Otolaryngol Head Neck Surg 2005;133:357–61.
153. Tasker A, Dettmar PW, Panetti M, et al. Reflux of gastric juice and glue ear in children. Lancet 2002;359:493.
154. Gibson WS, Jr, Cochran W. Otalgia in infants and children—a manifestation of gastroesophageal reflux. Int J Pediatr Otorhinolaryngol 1994;28:213–8.
155. Dahshan A, Patel H, Delaney J, et al. Gastroesophageal reflux disease and dental erosion in children. J Pediatr 2002;140:474–8.
156. O'Sullivan EA, Curzon ME, Roberts GJ, et al. Gastroesophageal reflux in children and its relationship to erosion of primary and permanent teeth. Eur J Oral Sci 1998;106:765–9.
157. Ersin NK, Oncag O, Tumgor G, et al. Oral and dental manifestations of gastroesophageal reflux disease in children: A preliminary study. Pediatr Dent 2006;28:279–84.
158. Wenzl TG, Schneider S, Scheele F, et al. Effects of thickened feeding on gastroesophageal reflux in infants: A placebo-controlled crossover study using intraluminal impedance. Pediatrics 2003;111:e355–9.
159. Orenstein SR, Shalaby TM, Putnam PE. Thickened feedings as a cause of increased coughing when used as therapy for gastroesophageal reflux in infants. J Pediatr 1992;121:913–5.
160. Miyazawa R, Tomomasa T, Kaneko H, et al.. Effect of locust bean gum in anti-regurgitant milk on the regurgitation in uncomplicated gastroesophageal reflux. J Pediatr Gastroenterol Nutr 2004;38:479–83.
161. Vanderhoof JA, Moran JR, Harris CL, et al. Efficacy of a pre-thickened infant formula: A multicenter, double-blind, randomized, placebo-controlled parallel group trial in 104 infants with symptomatic gastroesophageal reflux. Clin Pediatr (Phila) 2003;42:483–95.
162. Khoshoo V, Ross G, Brown S, et al. Smaller volume, thickened formulas in the management of gastroesophageal reflux in thriving infants. J Pediatr Gastroenterol Nutr 2000;31:554–6.
163. Heuschkel RB, Fletcher K, Hill A, et al. Isolated neonatal swallowing dysfunction: A case series and review of the literature. Dig Dis Sci 2003;48:30–5.
164. Peter CS, Wiechers C, Bohnhorst B, et al. Influence of nasogastric tubes on gastroesophageal reflux in preterm infants: A multiple intraluminal impedance study. J Pediatr 2002;141:277–9.
165. Kaltenbach T, Crockett S, Gerson LB. Are lifestyle measures effective in patients with gastroesophageal reflux disease? An evidencebased approach. Arch Intern Med 2006;166:965–71.
166. Castel H, Tiengou LE, Besancon I, et al. What is the risk of nocturnal supine enteral nutrition? Clin Nutr 2005;24:1014–8.
167. Borowitz SM, Sutphen JL. Recurrent vomiting and persistent gastroesophageal reflux caused by unrecognized constipation. Clin Pediatr (Phila) 2004;43:461–6.
168. Robinson RF, Casavant MJ, Nahata MC, et al. Metabolic bone disease after chronic antacid administration in an infant. Ann Pharmacother 2004;38:265–8.
169. Mandel KG, Daggy BP, Brodie DA, et al. Review article: Alginate-raft formulations in the treatment of heartburn and acid reflux. Aliment Pharmacol Ther 2000;14:669–90.
170. Tytgat GN, Simoneau G. Clinical and laboratory studies of the antacid and raft-forming properties of Rennie alginate suspension. Aliment Pharmacol Ther 2006;23:759–65.
171. Del Buono R, Wenzl TG, Ball G, et al. Effect of Gaviscon Infant on gastroesophageal reflux in infants assessed by combined intraluminal impedance/pH. Arch Dis Child 2005;90:460–3.
172. Arguelles-Martin F, Gonzalez-Fernandez F, Gentles MG. Sucralfate versus cimetidine in the treatment of reflux esophagitis in children. Am J Med 1989;86:73–6.
173. Hibbs AM, Lorch SA. Metoclopramide for the treatment of gastroesophageal reflux disease in infants: A systematic review. Pediatrics 2006;118:746–52.
174. Pritchard DS, Baber N, Stephenson T. Should domperidone be used for the treatment of gastroesophageal reflux in children? Systematic review of randomized controlled trials in children aged 1 month to 11 years old. Br J Clin Pharmacol 2005;59:725–9.
175. Rocha CM, Barbosa MM. QT interval prolongation associated with the oral use of domperidone in an infant. Pediatr Cardiol 2005;26:720–3.
176. Orenstein SR, Lofton SW, Orenstein DM. Bethanechol for pediatric gastroesophageal reflux: A prospective, blind, controlled study. J Pediatr Gastroenterol Nutr 1986;5:549–55.
177. Augood C, Gilbert R, Logan S, et al. Cisapride treatment for gastroesophageal reflux in children. Cochrane Database Syst Rev 2002;CD002300.
178. Kahrilas PJ, Quigley EM, Castell DO, et al. The effects of tegaserod (HTF 919) on oesophageal acid exposure in gastroesophageal reflux disease. Aliment Pharmacol Ther 2000;14:1503–9.
179. Tutuian R, Mainie I, Allan R, et al. Effects of a 5-HT(4) receptor agonist on oesophageal function and gastroesophageal reflux: Studies using combined impedance-manometry and combined impedance-pH. Aliment Pharmacol Ther 2006;24:155–62.
180. Kawai M, Kawahara H, Hirayama S, et al. Effect of baclofen on emesis and 24-hour esophageal pH in neurologically impaired children with gastroesophageal reflux disease. J Pediatr Gastroenterol Nutr 2004;38:317–23.
181. Koek GH, Sifrim D, Lerut T, et al. Effect of the GABA(B) agonist baclofen in patients with symptoms and duodeno-gastroesophageal reflux refractory to proton pump inhibitors. Gut 2003;52:1397–402.
182. Vela MF, Tutuian R, Katz PO, et al. Baclofen decreases acid and non-acid post-prandial gastroesophageal reflux measured by combined multichannel intraluminal impedance and pH. Aliment Pharmacol Ther 2003;17:243–51.
183. Omari TI, Benninga MA, Sansom L, et al. Effect of baclofen on esophagogastric motility and gastroesophageal reflux in children with gastroesophageal reflux disease: A randomized controlled trial. J Pediatr 2006;149:468–74.
184. Wiersma HE, van Boxtel CJ, Butter JJ, et al. Pharmacokinetics of a single oral dose of baclofen in pediatric patients with gastroesophageal reflux disease. Ther Drug Monit 2003;25:93–8.
185. Krach LE. Pharmacotherapy of spasticity: Oral medications and intrathecal baclofen. J Child Neurol 2001;16:31–6.
186. Orenstein SR, Gremse DA, Pantaleon CD, et al. Nizatidine for the treatment of pediatric gastroesophageal reflux symptoms: An open-label, multiple-dose, randomized, multicenter clinical trial in 210 children. Clin Ther 2005;27:472–83.
187. Wenning LA, Murphy MG, James LP, et al. Pharmacokinetics of famotidine in infants. Clin Pharmacokinet 2005;44:395–406.
188. Kuusela AL, Ruuska T, Karikoski R, et al. A randomized, controlled study of prophylactic ranitidine in preventing stress-induced gastric mucosal lesions in neonatal intensive care unit patients. Crit Care Med 1997;25:346–51.
189. Sachs G, Shin JM, Howden CW. Review article: The clinical pharmacology of proton pump inhibitors. Aliment Pharmacol Ther 2006;23:2–8.
190. Edwards SJ, Lind T, Lundell L. Systematic review: Proton pump inhibitors (PPIs) for the healing of reflux oesophagitis— a comparison of esomeprazole with other PPIs. Aliment Pharmacol Ther 2006;24:743–50.
191. Andersson T, Hassall E, Lundborg P, et al. Pharmacokinetics of orally administered omeprazole in children. Interna-

tional Pediatric Omeprazole Pharmacokinetic Group. Am J Gastroenterol 2000;95:3101–6.

192. Gremse D, Winter H, Tolia V, et al. Pharmacokinetics and pharmacodynamics of lansoprazole in children with gastroesophageal reflux disease. J Pediatr Gastroenterol Nutr 2002;35:S319–26.

193. Tolia V, Ferry G, Gunasekaran T, et al. Efficacy of lansoprazole in the treatment of gastroesophageal reflux disease in children. J Pediatr Gastroenterol Nutr 2002;35:S308–18.

194. Tolia V, Fitzgerald J, Hassall E, et al. Safety of lansoprazole in the treatment of gastroesophageal reflux disease in children. J Pediatr Gastroenterol Nutr 2002;35:S300–7.

195. Scott LJ. Lansoprazole: In the management of gastroesophageal reflux disease in children. Paediatr Drugs 2003;5:57–61; discussion 62.

196. Tolia V, Bishop PR, Tsou VM, et al. Multicenter, randomized, double-blind study comparing 10, 20 and 40 mg pantoprazole in children (5-11 years) with symptomatic gastroesophageal reflux disease. J Pediatr Gastroenterol Nutr 2006;42:384–91.

197. Tsou VM, Baker R, Book L, et al. Multicenter, randomized, double-blind study comparing 20 and 40 mg of pantoprazole for symptom relief in adolescents (12 to 16 years of age) with gastroesophageal reflux disease (GERD). Clin Pediatr (Phila) 2006;45:741–9.

198. Li J, Zhao J, Hamer-Maansson JE, et al. Pharmacokinetic properties of esomeprazole in adolescent patients aged 12 to 17 years with symptoms of gastroesophageal reflux disease: A randomized, open-label study. Clin Ther 2006;28:419–27.

199. Zhao J, Li J, Hamer-Maansson JE, et al. Pharmacokinetic properties of esomeprazole in children aged 1 to 11 years with symptoms of gastroesophageal reflux disease: A randomized, open-label study. Clin Ther 2006;28:1868–76.

200. Litalien C, Théorê, Faure C. Pharmacokinetics of proton pump inhibitors in children. Clin Pharmacokinet 2005;44:441–6.

201. Hoyo-Vadillo C, Venturelli CR, Gonzalez H, et al. Metabolism of omeprazole after two oral doses in children 1 to 9 months old. Proc West Pharmacol Soc 2005;48:108–9.

202. Fossmark R, Johnsen G, Johanessen E, et al. Rebound acid hypersecretion after long-term inhibition of gastric acid secretion. Aliment Pharmacol Ther 2005;21:149–54.

203. Pfefferkorn MD, Croffie JM, Gupta SK, et al. Nocturnal acid breakthrough in children with reflux esophagitis taking proton pump inhibitors. J Pediatr Gastroenterol Nutr 2006;42:160–5.

204. Ang TL, Fock KM. Nocturnal acid breakthrough: Clinical significance and management. J Gastroenterol Hepatol 2006;21:S125–8.

205. Spiegel BM, Dulai GS, Lim BS, et al. The cost-effectiveness and budget impact of intravenous versus oral proton pump inhibitors in peptic ulcer hemorrhage. Clin Gastroenterol Hepatol 2006;4:988–97.

206. Saiman L, Ludington E, Dawson JD, et al. Risk factors for Candida species colonization of neonatal intensive care unit patients. Pediatr Infect Dis J 2001;20:1119–24.

207. Saiman L, Ludington E, Pfaller M, et al. Risk factors for candidemia in neonatal intensive care unit patients. The National Epidemiology of Mycosis Survey Study Group. Pediatr Infect Dis J 2000;19:319–24.

208. Dial S, Delaney JA, Barkun AN, et al. Use of gastric acid-suppressive agents and the risk of community-acquired *Clostridium difficile*-associated disease. Jama 2005;294:2989–95.

209. Dial S, Delaney JA, Schneider V, et al. Proton pump inhibitor use and risk of community-acquired *Clostridium difficile*-associated disease defined by prescription for oral vancomycin therapy. CMAJ 2006;175:745–8.

210. Valuck RJ,Ruscin JM. A case-control study on adverse effects: H2 blocker or proton pump inhibitor use and risk of vitamin B12 deficiency in older adults. J Clin Epidemiol 2004;57:422–8.

211. Yang YX, Lewis JD, Epstein S, et al. Long-term proton pump inhibitor therapy and risk of hip fracture. JAMA 2006;296:2947–53.

212. Klinkenberg-Knol EC, Nelis F, Dent J, et al. Long-term omeprazole treatment in resistant gastroesophageal reflux disease: Efficacy, safety, and influence on gastric mucosa. Gastroenterology 2000;118:661–9.

213. Bourke B, Ceponis P, Chiba N, et al. Canadian Helicobacter Study Group Consensus Conference: Update on the approach to *Helicobacter pylori* infection in children and adolescents–an evidence-based evaluation. Can J Gastroenterol 2005;19:399–408.

214. Lasser MS, Liao JG, Burd RS. National trends in the use of antireflux procedures for children. Pediatrics 2006;118:1828–35.

215. Lobe TE. The current role of laparoscopic surgery for gastroesophageal reflux disease in infants and children. Surg Endosc 2007;21:167–74.

216. Goessler A, Huber-Zeyringer A, Hoellwarth ME. Recurrent gastroesophageal reflux in neurologically impaired patients after fundoplication. Acta Paediatr 2007;96:87–93.

217. Esposito C, Montupet P, van Der Zee D, et al. Long-term outcome of laparoscopic Nissen, Toupet, and Thal antireflux procedures for neurologically normal children with gastroesophageal reflux disease. Surg Endosc 2006;20:855–8.

218. Bufler P, Ehringhaus C, Koletzko S. Dumping syndrome: A common problem following Nissen fundoplication in young children. Pediatr Surg Int 2001;17:351–5.

219. Hassall E. Outcomes of fundoplication: Causes for concern, newer options. Arch Dis Child 2005;90:1047–52.

220. Gilger MA, Yeh C, Chiang J, et al. Outcomes of surgical fundoplication in children. Clin Gastroenterol Hepatol 2004;2:978–84.

221. Goldin AB, Sawin R, Seidel KD, et al. Do antireflux operations decrease the rate of reflux-related hospitalizations in children? Pediatrics 2006;118:2326–33.

222. Pashankar D, Blair GK, Israel DM. Omeprazole maintenance therapy for gastroesophageal reflux disease after failure of fundoplication. J Pediatr Gastroenterol Nutr 2001;32:145–9.

223. Pacilli M, Eaton S, Maritsi D, et al. Factors predicting failure of redo Nissen fundoplication in children. Pediatr Surg Int 2007.

224. Thomson M, Fritscher-Ravens A, Hall S, et al. Endoluminal gastroplication in children with significant gastroesophageal reflux disease. Gut 2004;53:1745–50.

225. Hogan WJ. Clinical trials evaluating endoscopic GERD treatments: Is it time for a moratorium on the clinical use of these procedures? Am J Gastroenterol 2006;101:437–9.

226. Lall A, Morabito A, Bianchi A. "Total Gastric Dissociation (TGD)" in difficult clinical situations. Eur J Pediatr Surg 2006;16:396–8.

4.3. Other Neuromuscular Disorders

Benjamin D. Gold, MD

Juliana C. Frem, MD

Neuromuscular disorders of the esophagus can be primary or can occur as a result of or associated with (secondary) a variety of conditions (see Tables 1 and 2). Manifestations of these neuromuscular disorders relate to partial or complete failure of normal esophageal function consisting of transporting swallowed food into the stomach and preventing the reflux of gastric contents. Therefore, failure of esophageal function will result in a number of manifestations, in particular, difficulty swallowing or dysphagia in older children or persistent regurgitation of food which can be debilitating and life-threatening, especially in young infants. This chapter considers the primary and secondary causes of esophageal motility disorders, looking at the nature of the dysfunction, associated clinical and diagnostic characteristics and available therapies. The chapter first examines disorders that affect the striated muscle portion of the esophagus (upper esophageal sphincter and upper esophagus) (Table 1), and then describes the disorders that affect the smooth muscle portion of the esophagus (lower esophagus and the lower esophageal sphincter) (see Tables 2 and 3).

Normal deglutition depends on precise coordination between relaxation of the upper esophageal sphincter (UES) and pharyngeal contractions that propel a food bolus through the UES into the esophagus. Subsequently, the esophagus serves to transfer a food bolus from the upper esophagus to the stomach by swallow-induced stimulation of a peristaltic contraction (primary peristalsis) in the esophageal body, which is then associated with lower esophageal sphincter (LES) relaxation. Failure of either UES or LES relaxation leads to an obstruction of bolus passage and dysphagia.[1]

The UES and upper 5% of the esophageal body are made up of striated muscle whereas the distal 50 to 60% of the esophagus and LES are composed of smooth muscle. Between the upper- and midesophagus, there is a transition zone made up of both striated muscle and smooth muscle. Striated muscle is innervated by the central nervous system, whereas the smooth muscle innervation is more complex and involves intermediate neurons in the myenteric plexus of the wall of the esophagus (Figure 1). There are two types of postganglionic nerve fibers originating from the myenteric plexus and innervating the smooth muscle of the distal esophagus and the LES: excitatory fibers that release acetylcholine and inhibitory fibers releasing nitric oxide (NO) and vasoactive intestinal peptide (VIP).[2] Normal esophageal peristalsis and LES relaxation/contraction are the net result of a well coordinated stimulation mediated by the both inhibitory and excitatory postganglionic nerve fibers.[3] Since the neuromuscular anatomy of the proximal and

---

Table 1 Disorders of the Upper Esophageal Sphincter and the Upper Part of the Esophagus

Primary cricopharyngeal dysfunction
  Abnormalities of resting tone
    Hypertension
    Hypotension
  Abnormalities in relaxation
    Incomplete relaxation
    Premature closure
    Delayed relaxation

Secondary cricopharyngeal dysfunction
  Disorders of the striated muscles
    Inflammatory myopathies
    Muscular dystrophies
    Metabolic myopathy
  Neurologic diseases
    Cerebral palsy
    Cerebral vascular events
    Bulbar palsy
    Laryngeal nerve paralysis
    Poliomyelitis
    Botulism
    Multiple sclerosis
    Myasthenia gravis
    Arnold-Chiari malformations
    Cervical spinal cord injury
    Brain tumors
    Pharyngeal-cervical-brachial variant
      Guillain-Barre syndrome
  Syndromes
    CHARGE syndrome
    Fisher syndrome
    Pierre-Robin sequence
    Trisomy 21
    Mitochondrial DNA deletions
  Other
    Post-Norwood procedure
    Postradiation therapy for head and neck cancers
  Medication
    Nitrazepam
    Neuroleptics
    Vincristine
    Calcium-channel blockers
    Anticholinergics

Table 2 Disorders That Affect the LES and the Lower Part of the Esophagus

Primary motility disorders
  See Table 3

Secondary motility disorders
  Congenital malformations
    Esophageal atresia/tracheoesophageal fistula
    Hirschsprung disease
  Gastrointestinal disorders
    Gastroesophageal reflux disease
    Crohin's disease
    Chronic idiopathic intestinal pseudo-obstruction
    Eosinophilic esophagitis
  Collagen vascular disorders
    Scleroderma
    Mixed connective tissue disease
    Systemic lupus erythematosus
  Metabolic disease
    Diabetes mellitus
    Thyroid diseases
  Infectious diseases
    Changas disease
  Malignant tumors
    Esophagogastric
    Extraintestinal: breast and lung cancer
  Benign tumors
    Leiomyoma
  Iatrogenic causes
    Endoscopic band ligation
    Endoscopic sclerotherapy
  Exogenous factors
    Caustic ingestions
    Drugs
    Silicone breast implants
  Esophageal surgery
  Graft vs host disease
  Anorexia nervosa

Table 3 Primary Esophageal Motility Disorders

Inadequate LES relaxation
  Classic achalasia
  Atypical disorders of LES relaxation

Uncoordinated contractions
  Diffuse esophageal spasm

Esophageal hypercontraction
  Nutcracker esophagus
  Isolated hypertensive LES

Esophageal hypocontraction

Ineffective esophageal hypomotility

Nonspecific esophageal motility disorders

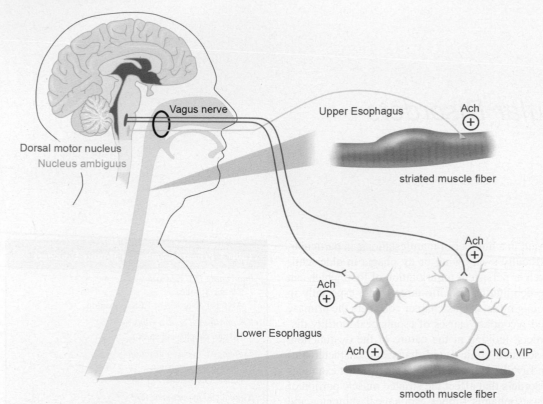

Figure 1 Esophageal motor innervation.

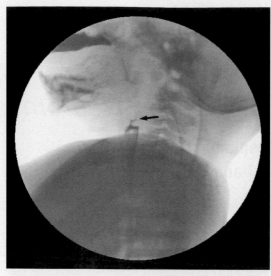

Figure 2 Modified barium swallow study in an infant with cricopharyngeal dysfunction. Note the indentation on the posterior esophageal wall (arrow).

distal portion of the esophagus is different, various diseases can affect either the striated or the smooth muscle portions of the esophagus.

DISORDERS THAT AFFECT THE UPPER ESOPHAGUS

The cricopharyngeal (CP) muscle is a striated muscle that forms the major component of the UES.[4] The CP muscle maintains a constant basal tone and luminal occlusion at rest, enabling rapid relaxations during swallowing. Disorders of the CP muscle are either idiopathic or secondary to inflammatory myopathies, neuromuscular diseases, radiation therapy for head and neck cancers, and medications (Table 1). In idiopathic CP dysfunction, there are two main defects of UES motility: abnormalities in the sphincter resting pressure (UES hypertension or hypotension) and abnormalities in UES relaxation (incomplete relaxation, premature closure, and delayed relaxation).

CRICOPHARYNGEAL DYSFUNCTION

CP dysfunction is characterized by either incomplete or poorly coordinated opening of the UES during the pharyngeal phase of swallowing. CP dysfunction results in hypopharyngeal retention and occasional laryngeal penetration or tracheal aspiration of swallowed food.[4–5] The prevalence, incidence, and epidemiology of CP dysfunction in children are not known since most of the available literature on this subject is limited to case reports.[6–7] For example, Staiano and colleagues

looked at 44 infants with gastroesophageal reflux disease (GERD) and found CP dysfunction in 5 (11%).[7]

Problems with the CP muscle usually present like those of the pharyngeal phase dysfunction. Therefore, it may be difficult to differentiate between the two upper gastrointestinal motility disorders. Symptoms usually appear shortly after birth or during the first 2 months of life. Swallowing difficulties, nasal regurgitation, pharyngeal pooling of saliva, and gagging are common. Repeated aspirations and choking are frequent presenting symptoms and can be life threatening in the affected child. A definitive diagnosis often is missed for several months and patients present with failure to thrive and suffer from the long-term consequences of recurrent episodes of pulmonary aspiration.[8]

Evaluation for CP dysfunction typically includes radiographic studies to assess the oral and upper esophageal anatomy and coordination of the swallow. Videofluoroscopy enables visualization of the CP muscle and laryngeal elevation. CP dysfunction should be suspected in children with pooling of saliva at the back of the pharynx, hold up of barium at the level of the UES, and a posterior indentation in the column of oral contrast at CP level (esophageal bar) (Figure 2). To and fro movements of contrast are frequently seen as the patient attempts to force the contrast distally. Aspiration and nasal reflux may also be noted in a child with CP dysfunction.[8] An esophageal bar is documented in about 5% of contrast studies in normal, asymptomatic individuals.[6] Whether this represents an anatomical variant or if it has any clinical significance is, at present, not clear.

Clinically or radiographically diagnosed "esophageal spasm" does not always correlate with elevated UES pressure measured by manometry. Manometry can be used to evaluate UES dysfunction. Manometry is complementary to videofluoroscopy, and often is less informative than radiography and more challenging to perform, particularly in young children.[9–10] Moreover, the usefulness of UES manometry in the diagnosis of CP dysfunction is not clear. Abnormal manometric findings do not necessarily lead to a change in management.

More recently, fiberendoscopic evaluation of swallowing has provided useful information about the pharyngeal phase of swallowing and compares favorably with videofluoroscopic swallowing studies.[11] Endoscopic swallowing evaluation provides information about oral-pharyngeal handling of foods or liquids before, during, and after the act of swallowing.[11] Pooling of secretions in the hypopharynx can be identified and scored. Penetration of the ingested bolus and aspiration are also assessed as well as the post-swallow residue left in the hypopharynx, which is a potential risk factor for aspiration.[11] The procedure can be performed at the bedside and does not involve radiation.

The optimal approach to the management of CP dysfunction remains to be defined. Spontaneous improvement has been observed in infants, especially with primary CP dysfunction. Thus, conservative treatment of the child with CP dysfunction with nasogastric feeding and speech therapy is an option. Prior to any procedure aimed at relieving UES obstruction, pathological gastroesophageal reflux must be controlled.[12] Reflux of acid can cause spasm of the CP muscle mimicking a primary disorder. Posttherapy, reflux can result in laryngeal complications after weakening of UES tone in response to treatment.[12]

Treatment with balloon catheter dilatation has been used, but experience is limited to case series and case reports in both adults and children.[4,13–14] Results of balloon dilatation are variable with less favorable outcomes in children, with more than half of treated patients experiencing minimal or no benefit.[4,15] In rare circumstances, patients experience long-term relief after just one dilatation. Very few complications of balloon dilatation in patients with CP dysfunction are reported.

In more severe and refractory cases, another option is to undertake myotomy.[13,16] Cricopharyngeal myotomy can relieve pharyngeal obstruction and is successful in 73% of cases reported in the literature. However, the majority of such operations have been performed in adults with CP dysfunction.[12] Prior to myotomy, it is important to assess the adequacy of oral and pharyngeal propulsion and laryngeal function.[12] Traditionally, CP myotomy is performed by an external approach. However, more recently, an endoscopic approach has been reported as a simpler and time-saving approach with reduced morbidity. The original technique described for the treatment of Zenker's diverticulum has been refined by the introduction of an operating microscope, diverticuloscope, (CO_2) laser, and stapler. Lawson and colleagues[5] describe experience with endoscopic CO_2 laser-assisted myotomy in the treatment of adults with CP dysfunction. Pre- and postoperative assessment of 29 adult patients with CP dysfunction included videofluoroscopic and flexible endoscopic evaluations of the swallow as well as patients' subjective ratings for dysphagia and aspiration. All patients improved after the procedure, based on a scoring system for dysphagia, aspiration, flexible fiberoptic endoscopy, and videofluoroscopy. Three patients, at a mean follow-up of 21 months still had intermittent dysphagia and aspiration; however, revision surgery was not necessary.[5] Benefit from CP myotomy was also reported by Yip and colleagues[17] who studied UES opening size pre- and postmyotomy. UES opening size improved from 57% of the size in normal controls to become comparable to controls after the procedure.[17] Complications from CP myotomy appear to be infrequent. Recurrent laryngeal nerve injury and fistulization of the pharynx or esophagus are reported with external CP myotomy.[12] Inadvertent entry into the neck with mediastinitis is the most often reported complication with the endoscopic approach.[12] Failure to relieve the aspiration is also observed after CP myotomy despite improved opening of the UES.[18] Thus, patients should be reevaluated with videofluoroscopy postoperatively, even in the absence of persistent clinical manifestations of CP dysfunction.

More recently, botulinum toxin (BT) has been used for treating CP dysfunction.[19] BT is a neurotoxin produced by the bacterium *Clostridium botulinum*. The BT inhibits the presynaptic release of acetylcholine from cholinergic nerve terminals. Therapeutic effects of BT are usually seen within 3 days of injection but last only weeks to months due to the new development of peripheral neurons.[20] BT has been used for the treatment of CP dysfunction since 1994 with a variety of application techniques including injecting under intraoperative observation, transendoscopic visualization, or percutaneously, with or without electromyography guidance.[20–21] Dosages of injected BT have been quite varied, ranging from 10 to 120 units.[21] Subjective improvement is described in most of the cases. However, objective improvement ranges between 40 and 70% and lasts for 3 to 6 months before recurrence.[19–21] Patients with isolated CP dysfunction are the most responsive to BT.[22] Injection of BT may have a diagnostic value for selection of these patients who will benefit from more definitive treatments, such as myotomy. Clinical and videofluoroscopic responses to BT favor a successful outcome of surgery.[22] However, others found that 8 of the 11 patients who did not benefit from BT still improved after myotomy.[19]

BT injection has proven to be remarkably safe. Diffusion of BT into neighboring structures can occur and may account for reports of mild vocal cord paralysis after BT injection into the UES. Conversely, pharyngeal dysfunction can result after injection for treatment of dysphonia and cervical dystonia. Other local effects due to BT application may be due to the physical trauma associated with the injection rather than the toxin itself. Injection-induced trauma probably is the cause of chest pain after esophageal injections.[22] Other complications of BT application include pharyngeal tears and worsening dysphagia. One case of death secondary to massive aspiration was reported 7 days posttherapy.[19]

In summary, there are no randomized controlled clinical trials comparing one approach to the other for the management of a patient with CP dysfunction. The best approach remains to be determined and is currently based on the preference of the clinician, the disease "phenotype" and the patient. CP myotomy is efficacious and provides long-term relief, especially in secondary causes of CP dysfunction. Balloon catheter dilatation is less invasive, safe, provides long-term relief and may obviate the need for further therapy. BT is also safe but provides only temporary relief.

CRICOPHARYNGEAL ACHALASIA

Cricopharyngeal (CP) achalasia is characterized by incomplete UES relaxation after the majority of swallows or by failure of the UES to open in synchrony with pharyngeal contractions.[10] Failure of the CP muscle to relax will cause accumulation of material in the pyriform sinus. In the patient with CP achalasia, the collected material has great potential to spill over into the airway and be aspirated.

Although rare, CP achalasia is the most commonly described disorder of the UES. Since first described in 4- and 7-week-old patients, almost 40 cases have been reported.[23] CP achalasia can be isolated or associated with other conditions such as prematurity, cerebral palsy, neuromuscular diseases, Arnold-Chiari malformation, congenital suprabulbar palsy and Down syndrome.[10,24–25] The pathogenesis and epidemiology of CP achalasia remain unknown. The condition can resolve spontaneously in neonates, suggesting that immaturity of the swallowing mechanism may be a contributing factor.[10]

Evaluation of CP achalasia is usually undertaken with videofluoroscopic assessment of swallowing. A horizontal indentation on the posterior esophageal wall is noted, with barium passing the muscle slowly and the CP muscle appearing to relax poorly. There is pooling of contrast in the hypopharynx with occasional nasopharyngeal reflux.[13,25–27] At times, there is a complete functional obstruction, and no barium passes into the esophagus.[16] In children, most studies document the abnormal relaxation of the CP muscle by cinefluoroscopy, although manometric abnormalities have also been described.[6,16] When endoscopy is performed, a slight posterior shelf at the level of the UES might be appreciated. In addition, complete obstruction and inability to pass the endoscope are reported.[26–27]

Symptoms of CP achalasia usually begin at birth or shortly thereafter. However, diagnosis of the disorder is often not made until patients are 1 year of age.[27–28] In the literature, only five cases are described of congenital CP achalasia diagnosed during the neonatal period.[25,28] Symptoms are similar to those described in CP dysfunction. It is crucial to evaluate children with recurrent respiratory symptoms for CP achalasia because the diagnosis is often missed, resulting in unnecessary fundoplications.

Experience with the management of CP dysfunction in children is limited. Successful balloon dilatation has been accomplished in cases of CP achalasia and deglutition incoordination.[7,16,26] However, it has failed in other cases.[13] In one series of fifteen patients with CP achalasia, six were managed conservatively with nutrition and positioning, four with myelomeningocele had shunt revision, with subsequent improvement in three patients, four had gastrostomies, and two underwent tracheostomies. Only two children underwent CP myotomy, and only moderate improvement was observed.[25] There are, however, case reports of successful CP myotomy performed in children with CP achalasia.[8,13,25,27] Myotomy has also been employed for children with CP incoordination, with good results reported at short-term follow-up. Experience with BT in children with CP achalasia is limited to a single case report.[27] The possibility of spontaneous improvement of CP achalasia and good responses reported after dilatations in infants and children, suggest a conservative approach. Aggressive nutritional support and dilatations should be reserved for those patients with severe compromise and considering surgery only for the patients who do not respond to conservative management.[7,16,28]

MYOPATHIC DISEASES

Muscular Dystrophies

Dysphagia is rare in most forms of muscular dystrophy, except for three relatively rare types of muscular dystrophies: myotonic muscular dystrophy, merosin-deficient congenital muscular dystrophy, and occulopharyngeal dystrophy. Congenital muscular dystrophy is an autosomal recessive inherited disease, presenting early after birth with hypotonia, muscle weakness, and contractures. Myotonic muscular dystrophy usually has its onset in adulthood but can manifest in infancy or childhood.

Pharyngeal muscle weakness is found in up to 92% of these patients, although symptomatic involvement occurs in less than half.[29–30] Usually, myotonia or other evidence of neuromuscular disease is present for years before the onset of dysphagia. These patients can also have involvement of both striated and smooth muscle of the muscle esophagus.[1] Fourteen patients with merosin-deficient congenital muscular dystrophy reported difficulties at all stages of the feeding process, and all 14 patients had abnormal oral phase of swallowing. Nine of the 14 had abnormal pharyngeal swallowing with laryngeal penetration and tracheal aspiration, as shown by videofluoroscopy and speech therapist evaluation. In the eight children who tolerated pH probe placement, esophageal reflux was demonstrated. All patients had impaired growth and most suffered from frequent respiratory infections.[31]

Pharyngeal weakness of contraction is the predominant finding and reveals itself as barium stasis and hypomotility in the radiograph.[7] The UES may be incompetent and is responsible for the appearance of a continuous column of barium in the pharynx and the upper esophagus.[1] Manometric studies reveal a reduction in basal UES pressure, the duration of contractions in the amplitude, and amplitude progression, as well as dyscoordination of pharyngeal and cricopharyngeal contractions.[1,6,30]

Treatment modalities for patients with muscle disease and swallowing dysfunction include dietary manipulation, enteral feeding, percutaneous endoscopic gastrostomy placement, and surgical intervention by myotomy or upper esophageal dilatation.[31] Studies evaluating these treatments are limited to case series. A recent systematic review of the treatment of swallowing difficulties in adults and children with chronic, noninflammatory muscle diseases concluded that there are no trials that have compared one treatment modality to another.[8] Thus, the benefit of surgical intervention (cricopharyngeal myotomy or upper esophageal dilatation) cannot be precisely determined.[8]

Inflammatory Myopathies

Inflammatory myopathies such as polymyositis, dermatomyositis, and inclusion body myositis affect the striated muscle of the pharynx and esophagus. Juvenile dermatomyositis, although rare, is the most common form of myositis in childhood.[32] Gastrointestinal (GI) involvement is noted in 5% of the patients at presentation of juvenile dermatomyositis and in up to 40% of patients during the course of the disease.[32–33] Dysphagia is the most common GI symptom.[33]

Juvenile dermatomyositis-associated dysphagia is worse while recumbent and if present along with esophageal reflux can lead to aspiration pneumonitis.[32] When present, dysphonia and nasal regurgitation are clues to underlying swallowing dysfunction. Serious GI disease is rare in juvenile dermatomyositis. However, esophageal perforations, a complication of the vasculitis prominent in this disease, can be life threatening.

Gastrointestinal involvement can be due to either underlying vasculopathy or to impairment of muscle function. When dysphagia is present, it is usually secondary to pharyngeal muscle weakness. In adults, manometric studies reveal decreased or normal CP pressure, with normal relaxation of the UES and low amplitude contractions in the pharynx and upper third of the esophagus.[34] Electrophysiological studies, using electromyography, in adult patients with inflammatory myopathies demonstrate either a hyperreflexic or a hyporeflexic CP muscle.

Management is aimed at controlling the underlying disease. Supportive measures, such as nasogastric tube feedings are frequently employed. Experience with CP disruption, particularly in childhood, is minimal. In eight adults who underwent CP dilatation, short- and long-term symptom resolution were 50 and 25%, respectively.[34] Four of the eight patients underwent CP myotomy with further subjective and objective improvement in two.[34]

NEUROLOGIC AND NEUROMUSCULAR OR MUSCULAR DISEASES

Arnold-Chiari Malformation

Arnold-Chiari malformation is a congenital disorder characterized by caudal herniation of the cerebellar tonsils through the foramen magnum. Dysphagia is present in 5 to 30% of affected patients.[24] Dysphagia is the first symptom in up to 30% of the patients with Arnold-Chiari malformation and the only evidence of cranial nerve dysfunction in some. These reports indicate that patients with unexplained CP dysfunction should be evaluated for underlying Chiari malformations. Early recognition of neurogenic dysphagia and expeditious intervention are crucial to ensure a favorable neurologic outcome.[24] Patients demonstrate dysfunction of the swallowing mechanism, with a combination of pharyngoesophageal dysmotility, failure of complete UES relaxation, pharyngo-UES incoordination, nasal regurgitation, tracheal aspiration, and GERD.

Outcomes after surgical decompression of Chiari malformations vary according to the severity of the preoperative symptoms.[24] Arnold-Chiari malformation patients with other signs of brainstem involvement demonstrate poor results postoperatively, whereas those with mild symptoms show an excellent response, with resolution of dysphagia.[1,24]

Myasthenia Gravis

Myasthenia gravis affects the motor end plate of the striated muscle of the body, including the esophagus. In children, the disease presents in three clinical forms: transient neonatal myasthenia gravis, persistent neonatal myasthenia gravis, and juvenile myasthenia gravis.

Dysphagia, choking, and aspiration of food are frequent clinical manifestations of myasthenia gravis and are the presenting symptoms in up to 24% of cases.[35] The description of the swallowing difficulty is unique to this condition: the patient is able to swallow normally at the beginning of the meal, but progressive difficulty appears with each swallow.

During videofluoroscopy, muscle fatigue should be provoked under controlled circumstances. Abnormalities of the oral and pharyngeal phases of swallowing are abnormal in more than half of cases and consist of weak tongue movements, oropharyngeal pooling, delayed pharyngeal phase initiation, abnormal laryngeal elevation, poor UES opening, nasal regurgitation, and aspiration.[36] Manometrically, these patients have contractions of decreased amplitude and prolonged duration, mainly in the upper esophagus.[37] Repetitive simultaneous contractions are noted with low UES pressure. Relaxation and coordination of the UES appear adequate in most patients.[37] The distinguishing feature of the disease is the recovery of the manometric and clinical abnormalities with rest or the administration of anticholinesterases. The intravenous administration of edrophonium chloride (Tensilon), in a dose of 0.2 mg/kg up to a total of 10 mg, produces prompt, but transient, relief of symptoms as well as radiographic and manometric abnormalities. This diagnostic test should be employed in patients who show pharyngeal weakness without any obvious cause, particularly when ptosis is present.

Botulism

Infant botulism results from the absorption of a heat-labile neurotoxin produced in situ by ingested *C. botulinum*. The average annual incidence of infant botulism in the United States is 1.9 of 100,000 live births. Clinical manifestations owe to progressive neuromuscular blockade.[38] Although descending flaccid paralysis of striated muscles is the most striking clinical feature of the syndrome, difficulty in swallowing and delayed evacuation of stools are often initial findings that are frequently overlooked.[39]

The major effect of botulinum toxin on esophageal motility is disruption of UES function and proximal esophageal peristalsis.[39] In a child with botulism, there is a reduction in UES pressure and a marked reduction in the percentage of UES relaxations after swallowing.[39] The hypopharyngeal and proximal esophageal contractions are of low amplitude and poorly coordinated.

Management includes meticulous supportive intensive care that includes mechanical ventilation and administration of botulinum human immune globulin in severe cases.[38]

DISORDERS THAT AFFECT THE LOWER ESOPHAGUS AND THE LES

Primary Esophageal Motility Disorders (Table 3)

Achalasia. Achalasia is a motor disorder of the esophagus that presents as a functional obstruction at the esophagogastric junction. Achalasia is characterized by a lack of esophageal peristalsis, increased lower esophageal sphincter (LES) pressure, and partial or incomplete LES relaxation.[40–42] Overall, achalasia is uncommon, with an estimated incidence of 1 case per 100,000 people.[41] Epidemiologic studies show that the disease varies in frequency around the world and within regions.[43–44] Achalasia is more common in North America, Australia, and Northwestern Europe.[43] In children, the incidence is 0.31 cases per 100,000 children per year in Ireland and 0.11 per 100,000 children per year in England.[44] Fewer than 5% of all patients with achalasia present in the pediatric age group.[44] Achalasia affects males and females equally.[43]

Etiopathogenesis of Achalasia. In idiopathic cases of achalasia, incomplete relaxation of the LES and loss of esophageal peristalsis are believed to be secondary to absent or abnormal inhibitory innervation in the myenteric plexus in the majority of cases.[2] Much less frequently, a central nervous system lesion can cause achalasia.[2] Some of the abnormalities of postganglionic inhibitory nerves include nerves that are absent, reduced in number, functionally impaired, or lacking in central connections.[45] Normal number of ganglion cells is reported in patients with achalasia, especially if the disease is still in its early stages as is the case in children.[2,45] With progression of the disease, progressive ganglion cell degeneration occurs. Other neuropathologic findings that are frequently, although inconsistently, described include chronic inflammatory cell infiltrates in the myenteric plexus and degenerative changes in the smooth muscle and nerve fibers.[2]

These findings are variable in different stages of the disease. In early stages of achalasia, there is myenteric inflammation with ganglionitis without neuronal fibrosis or loss of cells. The disease then progresses to neuronal fibrosis and destruction of inhibitory neurons of the myenteric plexus.[2] Whatever the etiologic trigger of the inflammatory process and the pathological insult causing this destruction of the ganglionic cells in the patient with achalasia, inhibitory neurons appear to be more sensitive to the insult than the cholinergic, excitatory neurons. The end result of the histological changes is a decrease in postganglionic inhibitory cells, which mediate LES relaxation via the release of vasoactive intestinal peptide (VIP) and nitric oxide (NO).[2] Indirect evidence for the lack of inhibitory innervation in patients with achalasia is also provided by hormonal studies. Cholecystokinin-octapeptide (CCK-OP) has opposing effects on the LES, both inhibitory and stimulatory, with a net result of LES relaxation in healthy individuals.[45] Patients with achalasia have a paradoxical increase of LES pressure in response to CCK-OP administration due to the absence of inhibitory neurons, resulting in an unopposed direct excitatory effect of CCK-OP on LES smooth muscle.[45]

Even though the primary pathophysiology of achalasia seems to be neurogenic in origin, minor changes in the smooth muscle of the esophagus have also been noted.[2] Interstitial cells of Cajal are abundant in the LES, and their function is closely integrated with neural activity and muscle function. These cells are fewer in number and more highly modified in patients with achalasia, compared with healthy controls and patients with other esophageal disorders.[46] There is a disruption in contact between nerves and interstitial cells of Cajal, which results in diminished conduction and resultant nerve atrophy.[47] However, it is not certain if these changes are the cause of the disease or simply secondary to the neuronal degeneration. Fibrosis of the intermuscular plane, with normal muscle fibers between the circular and longitudinal musculatures, has been observed in 10 children with achalasia.[46] This fibrosis might impair the mechanical properties of the esophageal wall and thereby contribute to the pathophysiologic features of achalasia.

In some patients, degenerative changes are also found in extraesophageal vagal nerve fibers and in the brainstem vagal motor nuclei.[2,48–49] Thus, patients with achalasia can have functional derangement of other alimentary tract organs, which are under vagal control.[2,48–49] Twenty percent of patients with achalasia have no ganglia in the middle third of the stomach.[50] However, the exact nature of gastric involvement in achalasia is controversial since gastric emptying studies demonstrate variable responses including delayed solid emptying, increased liquid emptying, and normal patterns.[50–51] Abnormal gallbladder emptying and sphincter of Oddi dysfunction are also described.[49,52] Abnormal jejunal motility is reported, including loss of cyclic activity, abnormal migration of phase III migratory motor complex, abnormal fed patterns, and the presence of giant migrating contractions and retrograde contractions.[48] In addition, an increased frequency of constipation, secondary to rectal aganglionosis is reported in patients with achalasia.[53]

An *infectious* etiology of achalasia is suggested by the occurrence of manometric findings of achalasia in patients with Chagas disease.[2] Achalasia is reported to precede infectious diseases such as Guillain-Barre syndrome, poliomyelitis, measles and varicella-zoster virus.[2] However, many patients with achalasia have no evidence of infection and not all patients with measles or varicella zoster virus infections develop achalasia.[2]

An *autoimmune* cause of achalasia is suggested based on the presence of antimyenteric antibodies and CD3 and CD8 positive T-cell lymphocytes in the myenteric plexus.[54] However, antimyenteric antibodies may be a nonspecific reaction to the diseases of the esophagus, and their role in the causation of achalasia is still to be determined.[54] A number of investigators propose an association of achalasia with HLA DQB1*0602, DQA1*0103 and DQB1*0603 alleles.[55–56] Up to 23% of patients with achalasia have the HLA risk alleles DQB1*0502 and DQB1*0601, and 24% have anti-neuronal antibodies.[55] However, there is no correlation among HLA alleles, anti-neuronal antibodies and clinical features of the disease.[55]

The influence of *genetic factors* as a cause of achalasia is suggested by the clustering of achalasia in families and its occurrence in certain syndromes.[57–58] The data are primarily based on case reports where achalasia is reported in monozygotic twins and in children of consanguineous parents.[57–58] On the other hand, there is one study in which there was a lack of concordance of achalasia in monozygotic twins. The role of genetic predisposition to achalasia seemed minimal when large community-based studies failed to identify familial clustering.[41,59]

Conditions Associated with Achalasia. Achalasia is associated with adrenocorticotropic hormone insensitivity and alacrima (Triple A syndrome, AAAS or Allgrove syndrome).[60–61] This is a progressive autosomal recessive disorder resulting from a mutation in the AAAS gene on chromosome 12 q13.[60–61] The gene consists of 16 exons, which encode a 546 amino acid protein, called ALADIN (*a*lacrima-*a*chalasia-a*d*renal *in*sufficiency *n*eurologic disorder).[60] Usually, alacrima is present from birth. Hypoglycemia, frequently associated with Addisonian skin pigmentation, is a common presenting symptom in the first decade of life.[60–61] Glucocorticoid deficiency occurs in the majority of patients. Mineralocorticoid deficiency can also occur but it is less common.[61]

Achalasia can be the presenting symptom or it can present after the cortisol deficiency manifests.[61] Investigation for glucocorticoid deficiency is advised in cases of achalasia when parents are consanguineous or if the age at onset of symptoms is in the first decade of life.[60] Other associated abnormalities include autonomic, peripheral, and central nervous system impairment such as hyperreflexia, muscle weakness, dysarthria and ataxia, optic atrophy, mild mental retardation, and postural hypotension.[61] Short stature, hyperkeratosis, and delayed wound healing are also reported in triple A syndrome.[60]

Achalasia is also associated with an autosomal recessive syndrome consisting of deafness, vitiligo, short stature, and muscle weakness, as well as with familial dysautonomia with hypophosphatemic rickets (Rozychi syndrome).[62] In addition, achalasia may be more frequent in patients with Down syndrome.[58]

Children with Pierre-Robin sequence have abnormal esophageal manometry in 94% of cases, of which 43% have LES hypertonia and 46% a LES that does not relax. These children also have esophageal dyskinesia and UES dysfunction.[63]

Achalasia is also reported in pyloric stenosis, Hodgkin disease, and Hirschsprung disease. However, in a survey of 126 patients with achalasia and their first-degree relatives, there was no increase in these conditions in either patients or their families.[64]

Clinical Presentation of Achalasia. The mean age of presentation of achalasia in children is 8.8 years.[40,65] In 167 children, 57% were older than 6 years, with only 22% between 1 and 5 years, 15% between 30 days and 1 year, and 5.3% less than 30 days of age.[40] The mean duration of symptoms prior to diagnosis is 23 months (range: 1 month to 8 years).[40] Table 4 summarizes the most common symptoms and signs of achalasia in 528 affected children. Younger children with achalasia tend to have symptoms of refusal to eat, although some present as if they have GERD.[66] Respiratory symptoms may predominate in some patients with achalasia, with choking, recurrent pneumonia and nocturnal cough.[65] Older children have symptoms that are more similar to those in adults, with dysphagia, regurgitation, and retrosternal pain being most prominent.[66] Dysphagia caused by achalasia occurs initially with solids and then with liquids, although some studies report dysphagia to both liquids and solids at time of diagnosis.[66] Patients describe the sensation of food getting caught in the middle to lower chest. Affected children commonly are slow eaters and swallow repeatedly to facilitate passage of food into the stomach.[40,42] Vomiting may manifest initially as food remnants on the child's pillow and progresses to severe vomiting and an inability to eat, with consequent weight loss.[65] Regurgitated food usually looks much as it did when it was swallowed and is not mixed with gastric juice.[65] When present, the chest pain associated with achalasia is described as sharp and retrosternal and can be aggravated by the passage of food.

Methods of Diagnosis of Achalasia

Radiography. A barium esophagogram is typically the first imaging study used in the evaluation of dysphagia.[42,65] A scout film may demonstrate a widened mediastinum, a lack of air in the stomach, and an air-fluid level in the esophagus in up to half of cases which may be an initial clue to the underlying diagnosis.[40,66–67] A dilated esophagus with air-fluid levels is more commonly seen in children with achalasia older than 5 years of age.[66] Radiographic features in a barium swallow include variable degrees of esophageal dilatation with tapering at the esophageal junction, referred

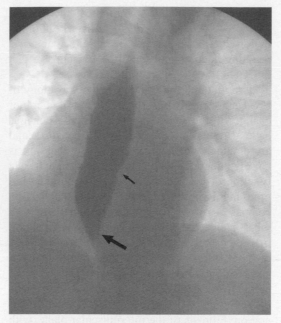

Figure 3 Barium swallow in a child with achalasia. Note the esophageal dilatation and beaking (large arrow) and the tertiary esophageal contractions (small arrow).

to as beaking (Figure 3).[40,66–67] Esophageal dilatation may be severe, with the esophagus occupying the whole mediastinum.[42] In addition, the esophagus may assume an S shape, also called a sigmoid esophagus.[42] There may be delayed clearance of barium, absence of peristalsis, tertiary contractions, and failure of LES relaxation in the barium swallow obtained from the patient with achalasia.[40,65,67] Barium esophagography is normal in less than 10% of cases.[65] Compared to esophageal manometry, the gold standard used for the diagnosis of achalasia, the positive predictive value of a barium swallow for the diagnosis of achalasia is as high as 96%.[68]

Timed-barium esophagograms (TBEs) are also used for the diagnosis of achalasia.[68–69] During TBE, the height of a barium column at 1 and 5 minutes is measured. In most patients with achalasia, there is minimal emptying over this time period.[68] Both barium swallow and TBE correlate poorly with the severity of clinical symptoms of achalasia.[69]

Radionuclide Tests. Nuclear scintigraphy provides information on esophageal transit time and esophageal stasis, particularly important for conditions like achalasia.[70] The most commonly used method involves the ingestion of a liquid or solid meal labeled with technetium 99 m sulfur colloid.[70] Scintigraphy is also useful in the differential diagnosis of achalasia and other conditions, such as progressive systemic sclerosis.[71] The pattern of retention is different between these two conditions: patients with achalasia retaining the tracer even in the upright position, whereas patients with progressive systemic sclerosis do not.[71] The positive predictive value of esophageal transit scintigraphy for the diagnosis of achalasia is 95%, when using manometry as the gold standard.

Endoscopy. The main clinical use of upper endoscopy in patients with suspected achalasia is to exclude other causes of dysphagia (eg, peptic

stricture, eosinophilic esophagitis). Endoscopy can be diagnostic of achalasia in one-third of the cases.[72] In achalasia, esophageal dilatation and food stasis are frequent findings at the time of endoscopy. However, it is not uncommon for the endoscopy to be normal.[40,66–67] During endoscopy, there can be resistance at the gastroesophageal junction that gives away to gentle pressure, as opposed to peptic strictures.[40,42] A role for endoscopic ultrasonography in the diagnosis of achalasia remains to be defined.[73]

Esophageal Manometry. Esophageal manometry remains the study of choice and can lead to the diagnosis in more than 90% of suspected cases (Figure 4).[42,72] Manometry provides quantitative information about the severity of the condition and responses to treatment.[65] The manometry findings proposed for a diagnosis of classic achalasia are as follows:[74]

1. Incomplete or abnormal LES relaxation (<30% of normal) is noted in 85 to 100% of children with achalasia.[40,66–67,75] Much less frequently, there is a complete loss of relaxation.[76]

2. A lack of esophageal peristalsis is the hallmark of the disease.[74] Usually, the abnormal peristalsis involves the entire length of the esophagus, and tertiary waves of low amplitude are described.[40,74,76] If the amplitude of these tertiary contractions is >50 or 60 mm Hg or if three or more pressure waves appear in response to a single swallow, the condition is referred to as "vigorous" achalasia.

Other manometry findings characteristic of achalasia, but are not required for diagnosis include:

3. Increased LES pressure: LES pressure has been described as markedly elevated, usually twice the normal levels, in the majority of patients.[10,40,67,75] Although, as a group, patients with achalasia have higher LES pressure, there is enough overlap with normal values that normal LES pressure alone does not exclude the diagnosis.[66,76]

4. Elevated intraesophageal pressure compared with intragastric pressure: This is the result of the functional obstruction at the level of the LES. In a study of 19 children with achalasia, there was inversion of the normal esophagogastric pressure gradient in 90% of the children.[67]

Manometric abnormalities are found in even the youngest patients.[77] Some patients initially present with nonspecific manometry findings that progress later to achalasia.[78] Manometric findings are also used to identify predictors of success of therapy. A posttherapy LES pressure of less than 10 mm Hg is the best predictor of long-term clinical response.[70] Manometry is also used intraoperatively to identify the high-pressure zone and better assess the length of the myotomy.[70,79] Manometry can be used to reduce the frequency of postoperative dysphagia.[79] Repeat manometry is usually not necessary after therapy,

Table 4 Clinical Symptoms and Signs in 528 Children with Achalasia	
Symptoms	Percent of Children
Vomiting	80
Dysphagia	75
Weight loss	64
Respiratory symptoms	44
Chest pain/odynophagia	45
Failure to thrive	31
Nocturnal regurgitation	21
This table is a compilation of 23 pediatric case series in which symptoms and signs were reported.	

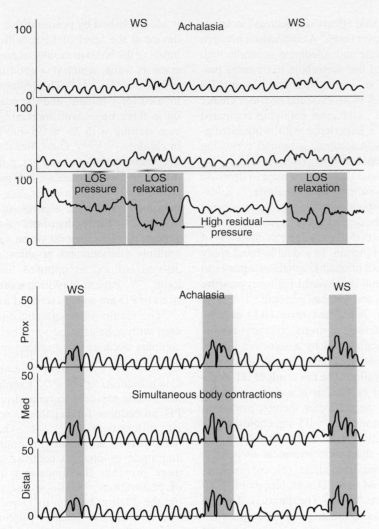

Figure 4 Esophageal manometry tracing from a patient with classic achalasia.

A combined impedancemanometry technique also has been used to assess bolus transit in relation to esophageal motility (Figure 5).[85] This technique evaluates functional aspects of the esophageal contraction by simultaneously measuring bolus transit and esophageal contractions.[86] In patients with achalasia, impedance patterns of bolus transport are variable and include failed swallow-induced bolus transport through the esophagus and evidence of luminal content regurgitation with excessive air trapping.[85] There are differences of baseline esophageal impedance between healthy subjects and achalasia patients thereby allowing a characterization of the esophageal resting state in disease states.[85] The benefit of this combined technique is mainly noted when presumed ineffective low-amplitude esophageal peristaltic contractions of less than 30 mm Hg are shown to be associated with the normal transit of a bolus.[87]

Little information is available on UES function in patients with achalasia. Recent reports have drawn attention to an association between acute airway obstruction and achalasia, prompting speculation that abnormalities of the pharynx and the UES are present.[88–89] Elevated UES residual pressure with incomplete relaxation upon swallowing is noted in achalasia patients, as compared to healthy controls.[89] UES pressure decreases after pneumatic dilatation (PD), suggesting that it might be a secondary phenomenon.[89] In other studies, an abnormal belch reflex was postulated to be the nature of the dysfunction and the cause of respiratory symptoms.[88]

Differential Diagnosis of Achalasia. Achalasia has to be differentiated from other organic causes of esophageal obstruction, particularly malignant tumors in adults. Less common causes of symptoms similar to achalasia are benign tumors and sequelae of surgical procedures at the distal esophagus.[90]

provided that the symptoms have resolved.[75,80–81] In the majority of cases, therapy does not seem to affect esophageal peristalsis or the amplitude of contractions in the esophagus.[82–83] However, there are case reports in which the return of esophageal peristalsis has been described after myotomy.[84]

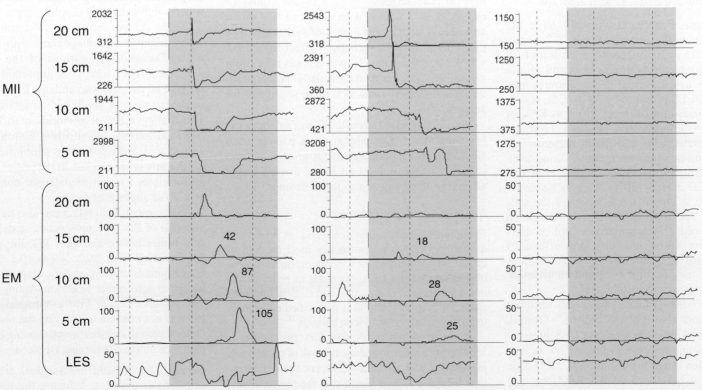

Figure 5 Combined impedance manometry in a patient with achalasia. MII: Multichannel intraluminal impedance; EM: Esophageal manometry

Two children with a clinical diagnosis of achalasia underwent surgical exploration and were found to have leiomyomas of the distal esophagus. In the majority of the cases, only surgical exploration reveals the underlying disease.[90]

Chagas disease is an important consideration in the differential diagnosis in areas where it is endemic, particularly in South America.[91] The disease occurs from neuronal damage caused by the parasite *Trypanosoma cruz*.[92] Esophageal denervation of both excitatory and inhibitory neurons is immune-mediated, with the damage leading to nonspecific contractions in the esophageal body, absent LES relaxation, and dilatation of the esophagus.[91–92] Idiopathic achalasia and Chagas disease have similar clinical presentations.[91] The duration of symptoms prior to diagnosis of Chagas disease seems to be longer and patients tend to have more marked esophageal dilatation.[91] As for manometric findings, patients with Chagas disease are observed to have lower LES basal pressure than achalasia, fewer simultaneous contractions, and shorter contraction duration.[91]

Achalasia can also be mistaken for anorexia nervosa.[93–94] In one study, esophageal motor activity was investigated in 30 consecutive patients meeting the standard criteria for the definition of anorexia nervosa, and 7 patients had achalasia instead of a chronic eating disorder.[94]

Treatment of Achalasia. There is no definitive cure for achalasia. Therefore, therapy is directed toward symptomatic relief by relieving the obstruction at the level of the LES. This is achieved mainly with pneumatic dilation (PD) and esophageal myotomy (EM). Less effective and more temporary measures include pharmacological agents like calcium-channel blockers, nitrates, and botulinum toxin. No therapy is able to restore esophageal peristalsis or the impaired esophageal LES relaxation in the patient with achalasia.

Pharmacologic Treatment. Nitrates have the effect of relaxing the smooth muscle.[95–96] Isosorbide dinitrate (5 to 10 mg) causes significant LES relaxation in patients with achalasia and allows most patients to eat normal meals. Nitrates usually decrease LES pressure by 30 to 65%, resulting in symptom improvement in up to 87% of patients.[96] This improvement has been confirmed both manometrically and with radionuclide esophageal transit measurements.[95] Long-term use of the drug is associated with a high frequency of side effects (50%), such as headache and tolerance.[95] There is one report of the successful short use of an isosorbide dinitrate patch in an 8-year-old.[97] Randomized controlled trials evaluating the short- and long-term effects of nitrates are lacking. Currently, the use of nitrates is limited to temporizing symptoms until more effective therapy can be established.[42]

Calcium channel blockers have been used but their usefulness also remains limited.[98] Overall, calcium channel blockers decrease LES pressure by 13 to 49% and improve symptoms by varying amounts, which range from 0 to 75%.[95–96,98] Side effects such as peripheral edema, headache, and hypotension are reported in up to 30% of patients.[99]

However, these side effects can decrease in severity or disappear over time.[99] A comparison between isosorbide dinitrate and nifedipine in adults with achalasia showed that isosorbide has a more pronounced effect on symptomatic relief, early LES pressure fall (63.5 vs 46.7%), and provides greater improvement of esophageal emptying compared with nifedipine.[95] Experience with using nifedipine in children with achalasia is limited, consisting mainly of case reports.[100]

Recently, *sildenafil* has been used to decrease LES pressure in patients with achalasia.[101] Sildenafil blocks phosphodiesterase type 5, an enzyme responsible for the degradation of cyclic guanosine monophosphate (cGMP), resulting in inhibition of smooth muscle function. In a double-blind study of 14 patients with idiopathic achalasia, ages 21 to 64 years, sildenafil decreased LES tone, pressure wave amplitude, and residual pressure.[101]

In achalasia, *botulinum toxin* (BT) acts by inhibiting excitatory neurons, thereby restoring the imbalance caused by a selective loss of inhibitory innervation in the LES with unopposed excitatory innervation. The net result of BT injection at the distal esophagus is a decrease in the resting tone of the sphincter thereby providing relief of the obstruction.[2,22] BT injection into the LES is an effective, safe, and relatively simple method for the short-term treatment of achalasia.[66,81,102–103] The immediate response rate is comparable to EM and PD with reports of 75 to 100% success rate.[22,104–105] The duration of action of BT lasts weeks to months and depends on the dose as well as the speed of new nerve terminal sprouting.[22,103,106] However, the long-term results (>6 months) are less, with only 35 to 41% of patients remaining symptom-free at 2 years, compared to 87.5% after surgery.[81,105] Effects of BT injection in children with achalasia are published only in case series.[66,103,107–108] In one study, 19 (83%) of 23 children with achalasia had either an improvement or resolution of symptoms. The mean duration of the beneficial effect for the BT was 4.2 ± 4.0 months. However, 16% underwent subsequent balloon dilatation, 16% balloon dilatation and surgery, and 58% were scheduled for surgery.[102]

Serious adverse events to BT therapy have not been reported.[22] Occasional chest pain or transient skin rashes may occur. Of greater concern is that BT injections as an initial therapy might adversely affect future surgical outcomes.[109]

Nonpharmacologic Treatment

Pneumatic Dilatation for Achalasia. A pneumatic dilatation (PD) is a commonly used method of dilatation for achalasia.[40,110] PD produces a controlled tear of the LES, resulting in relief of the distal esophageal obstruction and clinical improvement.[96,111] At present, PD is performed commonly using a graded polyethylene balloon.[112–114]

Careful preparation for this procedure is important in order to reduce the risk of esophageal perforation and aspiration. Preprocedure preparation includes a clear liquid diet for few days and a 12-hour fast prior to the procedure.[40,113,114] PD

is accomplished by positioning a dilating balloon device at the level of LES, with the purpose of inflating the balloon rapidly in an attempt to obliterate its waist, which is a good indicator of procedure success.[111,114] The balloon is maintained inflated for 1 minute, and the procedure repeated up to three times with increasing balloon diameter, starting with 20- to 35-mm Hg size balloon in children.[111–112,114] Outcomes do not depend on the precise technique used but, rather, on the postdilatation LES pressure.[115] A postdilation LES pressure of <10 mm Hg or less than 50% from baseline is a favorable predictor of the success of PD.[116–117] Predictors of poor outcome are male gender, age less than 20 years, patients requiring multiple dilations and, possibly, dilating with a 30-mm balloon as opposed to a 35-mm balloon.[116–117] Patients requiring more than three sessions of PD are usually referred for surgery.[40,66]

The results of pneumatic dilatation in children with achalasia are variable and difficult to compare because of variations in the techniques used.[40,112,113]

Complications after PD. Esophageal perforation risk is reported to range from 0.5 to 6% of PD procedures for achalasia, with a mortality rate of less than 1%.[111,118–119] The presence of a hiatal hernia, esophagitis, malnutrition, or high-amplitude esophageal contractions and one, or more, previous dilatations may increase the risk of perforation.[120] Balloon instability or inflating the dilation balloon to 11 psi or higher may also increase the risk.[120] Symptoms after perforation include severe and persistent chest pain, usually fever and unexplained tachycardia. Dysphagia and subcutaneous emphysema may also be seen.[96] A plain chest radiograph reveals subcutaneous and mediastinal emphysema or a left-sided pleural effusion. A definitive diagnosis of esophageal perforation is made with the use of a water-soluble contrast esophagogram.[96]

Some centers recommend the routine use of a postdilatation esophagogram with gastrograffin.[114] Delayed perforations of the esophagus can occur. Therefore, it is important to closely observe all patients who undergo PD and to obtain or repeat contrast studies if symptoms develop. The management of perforation following PD included parenteral nutrition, neutralization of gastric acid, and intravenous antibiotics.[121] Medical therapy is appropriate in the presence of small perforations without mediastinal contamination and in the absence of sepsis.[121]

Gastroesophageal reflux can also be a late complication of PD. In a prospective study comparing acid reflux before and after PD, the percent pH <4 increased from 2.9 ± 4.9 to 10.2 ± 15.9%.[122] Esophagitis is another complication of PD, caused by either acid reflux from low-resting LES pressure postdilatation or from esophageal stasis if the PD was not efficient at relieving the obstruction.[123] Other reported complications following PD are chest pain, hematomas, fever and, GI bleeding.[116,118–119]

Surgery for Achalasia. Surgical treatment of achalasia is aimed at reducing the pressure gradient across the LES, facilitating gravity-aided esophageal emptying. Treatment options vary, but invariably involve a myotomy, with or without an antireflux procedure.[98,124] The most common esophageal myotomy employed is the Heller myotomy and its variants. A Heller myotomy consists of either a thoracic or an abdominal approach and a vertical incision of the esophagus extending along the serosal surface of the distal esophagus and transecting the circular muscle fibers that make up the LES.[124-125]

In children, successful outcome after EM varies from as low as 10% to as high as 100%.[40,126-128] The youngest patient reported with a successful EM was 6 weeks of age. There are numerous descriptions of successful EM in infants less than 6 months of age.[65,129] In a series of 19 children, 17 had excellent and 2 had good long-term results after a mean follow-up of 9 years.[130] More recent series provide encouraging results with minimally invasive surgery using the laparoscopic approach, with success rates of 70 to 100%.[126-128,131-132]

Simultaneous endoscopy can be performed during EM to provide insufflation and light, which allow the surgeon better visualization of the esophageal wall during EM.[125] The endoscopist can also determine if a complete EM has been accomplished and alert the surgeon if there has been entry into the esophageal or gastric lumen.[125]

When surgery is performed after failed PD or BT, results of EM have also been satisfactory, but previous esophageal surgery for achalasia adversely affects the outcome.[133] Since the overall results after EM in children are very good, the primary treatment for children with achalasia should be surgical.[65] This contention is supported by a review of the literature in adults comparing PD and EM.[134]

There are two main long-term complications after EM: recurrent or persistent dysphagia and GERD.[135] Recurrent or persistent dysphagia results from failure to adequately relieve the LES obstruction and is usually secondary to an inadequate myotomy, postmyotomy stricture or scarring, or excessive fundoplication.[124,135] Inadequate myotomy usually results from failure to carry the myotomy sufficiently far into the stomach (gastric myotomy of 1 cm).[125,135] To avoid this complication, a gastric myotomy of 2 cm adding a partial fundoplication in order to minimize the risk of perforation and reflux has been advised.[125] Postmyotomy stricture forms as a result of failure of separation between the muscle edges of the myotomy.[135] Partial fundoplication can be helpful in preventing this complication.[135] On the other hand, fundoplication can lead to persistent dysphagia. In children, the frequency of postoperative dysphagia varies (roughly 5%), but it is equally distributed between children with and without concomitant fundoplication. Manometry and endoscopy can differentiate between an inadequate myotomy (high-LES pressure) and a complication of surgery (eg, esophagitis and stricture). Management includes BT or PD for moderate dysphagia and either a redo of the EM or a release of the fundoplication for more severe dysphagia.[66,126-127]

GERD can be a serious comorbidity in patients with achalasia both pre- and posttherapy. The aperistaltic esophagus clears the refluxed materials poorly, and patients can develop strictures and Barrett's esophagus.[135] The true prevalence of GERD in achalasia post-EM is unknown but might be related to surgical technique.[42,135-136] In adults, GERD occurs in 10 (47.6%) of 21 patients after EM alone versus just 2 (9.1%) of 22 patients after EM plus fundoplication.[136] There are no randomized studies in children with achalasia comparing EM with or without antireflux surgery. In pediatric case series, there is an overall frequency of GERD of 3.8% with a tendency for a higher frequency in patients who underwent EM alone (4.6%) versus EM with antireflux surgery (2.3%).

Peptic strictures can develop as a complication of GERD in 3 to 6% of achalasia patients.[137] Peptic strictures secondary to disabling GER after EM have also been described in the pediatric literature.[110] Barrett's esophagus has also been reported with incidence rates from as low as 0.5 to 13%.[137-139]

Other Complications. Esophageal perforation occurs intraoperatively due to inadvertent perforation of the mucosa.[135] Such a perforation usually can be closed easily with one or two sutures. Alternatively, a partial fundoplication can cover the repair.[135] Phrenic nerve paralysis, massive GI tract hemorrhage, and necrosis of the stomach or esophagus, owing to herniation, have all been reported.[140]

In summary, the therapy of choice for esophageal achalasia in children often depends on the available expertise at the treating institution.[112]

Long-Term Follow-Up of the Patient with Achalasia Posttherapy. After successful therapy, recurrence of symptomatic achalasia can develop, even after a symptom-free period of many years.[140] Although the reason for recurrent disease is not known, it may be due to slow progression of the underlying degenerative process of the myenteric plexus.[140] Esophageal squamous cell carcinoma is considered as a late complication of achalasia in adults, with a frequency of 0.02 to 5% at a mean age of just 48 years.[138-139] The mean time from diagnosis of the achalasia in adults to the occurrence of the malignancy is 17 years.[141] Currently, there is no information about the incidence of esophageal cancer as a complication of achalasia in children (Table 3).

DIFFUSE ESOPHAGEAL SPASM

Diffuse esophageal spasm (DES) is a primary esophageal motility disorder characterized by high-amplitude, repetitive, nonperistaltic esophageal contractions interrupting normal peristalsis.[142-143] DES is rarely described in children as isolated case reports.[144] In children presenting with noncardiac chest pain, DES was most commonly encountered and accounted for one-third of 83 cases.[145] Altered endogenous nitric oxide synthesis or degradation could explain the beneficial effects of nitrates.[143] Noncardiac chest pain and intermittent dysphagia are the most common presenting symptoms in older children and adults. Chest pain can resemble angina, and is associated with meals but not with exertion and is relieved by nitroglycerine.[142] Dysphagia, to both liquids and solids, is intermittent, nonprogressive and is precipitated by stress and liquids of extreme temperature.[142] In infants, the presentation is usually with apnea and bradycardia.[144] The barium swallow can be normal but when abnormalities are seen, there is a disruption of peristalsis with tertiary contractions producing esophageal segmentation (corkscrew esophagus).[142]

The diagnosis of DES is established manometrically using the following criteria: (1) simultaneous (nonperistaltic) contractions in the distal esophagus associated with at least 20% of wet swallows and (2) mean simultaneous contraction amplitude of more than 30 mm Hg (Figure 6).[142-143] Other common findings include spontaneous contractions, repetitive contractions, multiple peaked contractions, and intermittent normal peristalsis.[142-143]

Treatment can be quite challenging for patients with DES. Large therapeutic studies are lacking, and the literature is limited to small case series.[143] As an initial step, empiric treatment with proton pump inhibitors is advised since GERD can cause esophageal spasm and is a frequent cause of noncardiac chest pain.[142-143] GER was found in 20 to 50% of patients with DES.[142] Smooth mus-

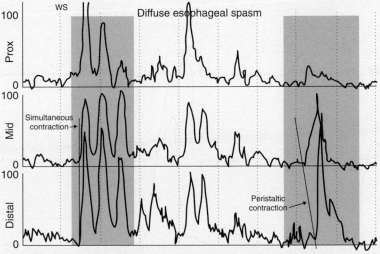

Figure 6 Esophageal manometry tracing from a patient with diffuse esophageal spasm.

cle relaxants such as nitrates, calcium-channel blockers, and botulinum toxin are reported as beneficial.[142–143] These agents decrease high-amplitude contractions but do not consistently relieve chest pain.[143] Antidepressants have also been used with some success by relieving discomfort from chest pain.[142–143] Pneumatic dilatation and longitudinal surgical myotomy are used as a last resort since they do not always provide relief of symptoms.[142–143]

NUTCRACKER ESOPHAGUS

A nutcracker esophagus is a clinical entity characterized by hypercontractility of the esophagus, representing 10% of cases presenting as noncardiac chest pain in children.[145] Patients present with chest pain and, much less commonly, with dysphagia. There is poor temporal correlation between symptoms and manometric findings.[142] The barium swallow and radionuclide emptying scans are usually normal, and the diagnosis is made by manometry (Figure 7). A mean distal esophageal peristaltic wave amplitude >180 mm Hg (measured as the average amplitude of 10 swallows at 2 recording sites positioned 3 and 8 cm above the LES) is the hallmark of this disease.[74] There is usually an increased duration of esophageal waves (>6 seconds) along with normal peristalsis.[142] Resting LES pressure is usually normal but may be elevated in patients categorized as having nutcracker esophagus with a hypertensive LES.[74] Treatment is similar to treatment of DES, and results are just as unpredictable.[142]

INEFFECTIVE ESOPHAGEAL MOTILITY

Ineffective esophageal motility is a term used to describe manometric abnormalities characterized by esophageal hypocontraction. The clinical implication is not certain, but it may place the patient at risk for GERD.[74] Manometric features proposed for the diagnosis of ineffective esophageal motility include: (1) distal esophageal peristaltic wave amplitude <30 mm Hg, (2) simultaneous contractions with amplitudes <30 mm Hg, (3) failed peristalsis in which the peristaltic wave does not traverse the entire length of the distal esophagus, or (4) absent peristalsis.

NONSPECIFIC ESOPHAGEAL MOTILITY DISORDERS

A large number of patients have esophageal motility abnormalities that cannot be classified as one of the above disorders. Pending further understanding of the pathophysiology and clinical implications of such findings, nonspecific esophageal motility abnormalities should be reported descriptively.[74]

SECONDARY ESOPHAGEAL MOTOR DISORDERS

Esophageal Atresia/Tracheoesophageal Fistula

Esophageal atresia/ tracheoesophageal fistula (EA/TEF) is a common congenital anomaly, with an incidence of 1 in 2,400 to 4,500 infants.[146] The cause of esophageal dysmotility in EA is debated. Coordinated peristaltic contractions are documented in response to swallowing between the upper and lower esophageal pouch in EA prior to surgical repair. Thus, dysmotility occurs only after surgical repair and is secondary to vagus nerve damage.[147] On the other hand, the presence of EA/TEF disrupts the normal in utero development of the myenteric plexus in the esophagus, which could lead to abnormal peristalsis and impaired LES function.[146] Structural abnormalities prior to surgical repair are also documented, consisting of disorganized muscle layers and tracheobronchial remnants.[146]

Dysphagia is present in 53 to 92% of adults with a history of EA/TEF accompanied with chocking in 33%. Food impaction may also occur. Patients who require gastric, jejunal, or colonic transposition have a higher risk of dysmotility, dysphagia, GERD, aspiration, and impaired growth, compared to those who do not undergo an interposition procedure.[146] GERD is a frequent complication documented in 35 to 58% of children based on symptoms and in 68% based on pH probe.[146] GERD is secondary to an intrinsic motor dysfunction of the esophagus and a shortened intra-abdominal segment of the esophagus.[146] Esophagitis occurs in 20% of patients and Barrett's esophagus in 6%.[146] Esophageal strictures develop in 6 to 40% of patients, especially those with an esophageal gap longer than 2.5 cm and in those with documented pathologic acid reflux.[146]

Abnormal peristalsis is documented by manometry in 75 to 100% of children with EA/TEF and in all of those with colonic interposition. Findings on manometry include an aperistaltic segment, and both simultaneous and repetitive, low-amplitude esophageal contractions. There is a decrease in LES pressure, baseline esophageal pressure, and peak esophageal pressure, compared to healthy controls.[147] GERD should be treated aggressively with acid suppression or fundoplication. A loose fundoplication is preferred to avoid worsening of dysphagia and the risk of aspiration in the presence of a dyskinetic esophagus.[146]

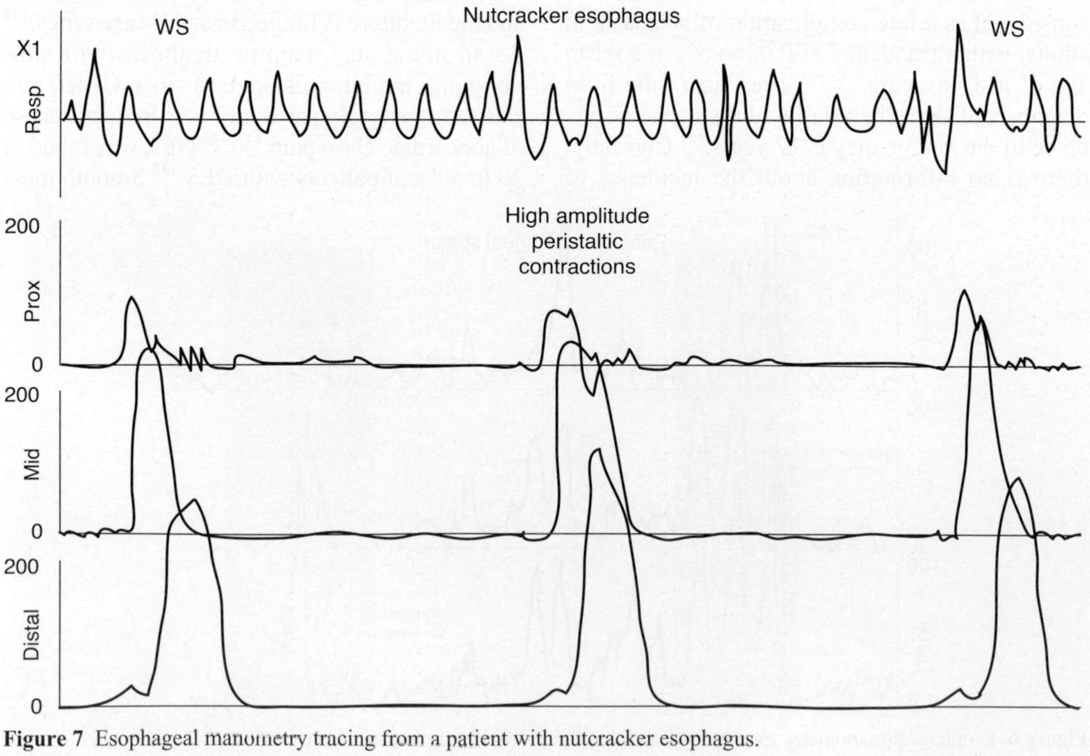

CHRONIC IDIOPATHIC INTESTINAL PSEUDO-OBSTRUCTION (IIP)

IIP syndrome is characterized by intermittent symptoms and signs of intestinal obstruction without evidence of mechanical blockage. Various motility abnormalities throughout the body have been described, with esophageal involvement present in up to 85% of affected patients.[148–149]

Most children exhibit aperistalsis and often decreased or absent LES with failure of the LES to relax with swallowing.[149] Low-amplitude waves occurred in the esophageal body, with lack of propagation and the presence of simultaneous contractions.[148–149] Therefore, esophageal motility can be used as an initial screening test, particularly if small bowel motility studies are not available.

CAUSTIC INGESTION

Ingestion of harmful household compounds is a frequent accident in toddlers and can lead to severe esophagitis and life-threatening acute complications. Damage to the deep muscle esophageal layers with fibrosis seems to be the basis for the motor abnormalities noted in these patients.[150] In the subacute and chronic stages, strictures of the esophagus and dysphagia are common.[151] Abnormal esophageal acid exposure was also found in

Figure 7 Esophageal manometry tracing from a patient with nutcracker esophagus.

68% of patients by 24-hour pH probe.[151] Ingestion of sodium hydroxide is more frequently associated with the development of strictures and, hence, esophageal dysmotility on manometry.[150]

Manometrically, nonperistaltic low-amplitude and long-duration waves are noted as early as 5 days after the insult. There is usually normal UES and LES function.[150–151] Early findings of severe dysmotility are associated with the development of strictures as a late complication.[150] Therefore, esophageal manometry may be used as prognostic indicator.

ENDOSCOPIC VARICEAL SCLEROTHERAPY AND BAND LIGATION

Endoscopic variceal sclerotherapy (EVS) of esophageal varices and endoscopic variceal band ligation (EVBL) both can result in transient esophageal dysmotility and GERD.[152–153]

Following EVS, histological changes in the esophageal wall include thrombosis of the submucosal vessels, esophagitis, and subsequently, fibrosis leading to abnormal peristalsis.[153] GERD results from abnormal esophageal peristalsis, rather than low postsclerotherapy LES pressures. In some studies, these abnormalities have been reversible, suggesting that EVS impairs the motility of the esophagus only transiently.[152]

The majority of patients treated with EVS do not have dysphagia or reflux-related symptoms despite documented esophageal dysmotility and abnormal acid reflux indices. Post-EVS manometry findings include reduced amplitude of contractions, increased duration of peristaltic waves, and propagating simultaneous contractions, but little effect on LES function.[152–153] In a prospective, randomized trial comparing EVS and EVBL, there was no change in reflux indices or manometric findings pre- and post-EVL, whereas there was significantly decreased amplitude of contractions, appearance of simultaneous contractions and GERD in the post-EVS group.[153] A short course of antireflux medication after each therapeutic session is advocated by some.[152–153] Treatment of underlying esophageal dysmotility is less clear.

COLLAGEN VASCULAR DISORDERS

Progressive Systemic Sclerosis (PSS)

Of all of the collagen vascular disorders, PSS shows the most marked esophageal abnormalities. PSS is a systemic disease of unknown etiology characterized by excessive deposition of collagen, and other connective tissue components, in skin and other target organs, most notably the GI tract. Esophageal involvement has been documented in both PSS and cutaneous scleroderma.[154]

PSS is rare in children, with children accounting only for 3% of all cases.[154] Gastrointestinal involvement is present in 90% and is the initial presentation in 10%. The esophagus is the most common organ affected (50 to 90%).[155] Heartburn, dysphagia, and regurgitation are the most common presenting symptoms and are present in 82% of patients with PSS.[155156] Dysphagia is attributed to esophageal dysmotility and acid reflux and is often elicited by both solids and liquids.[156] Acid reflux is present in 54 to 86% of the patients by 24-hour pH monitoring.[154–155] There is poor correlation with symptoms, so it is recommended to evaluate for GERD, even in the absence of clinical symptoms.[154] Endoscopic esophagitis is present in 33 to 63% of patients with PSS and is more frequently observed in those with most severe esophageal manometric findings. Other complications of esophageal disease in PSS are strictures (17 to 29%), perforations, and Candida albicans esophagitis. PSS is not well established as a risk factor for esophageal cancer: Only seven cases are described, four squamous cell carcinomas and three adenocarcinomas of the esophagus. Patients with PSS also have autonomic dysfunction that correlates with the manometric finding of low-esophageal contraction amplitude.[155–156] The presence of autonomic dysfunction (such as inadequate pupillary dilatation, lack of increased heart rate in response to deep inspiration, and a valsalva maneuver) should raise the suspicion of esophageal involvement, even in the absence of relevant symptoms.

Esophageal manometry is the golden standard for diagnosis of esophageal involvement in PSS.[154–155] Findings consist of low-amplitude peristaltic waves in the lower two-thirds of the esophagus that eventually evolves into aperistalsis with reduced LES pressure.[155] These findings are nonspecific, however, and are seen in other connective tissue disorders, severe acid reflux, amyloidosis, and hypothyroidism.[155] On chest radiographs, one can see dilatation and shortening of the esophagus, resulting in a hiatal hernia. Normally, the esophagus collapses and pushes air out but in PSS, air can be seen in the esophagus secondary to esophageal fibrosis. Endoscopy is used to rule out infections and acid reflux-induced esophagitis.[155]

Treatment principles are based on careful monitoring of organ-specific manifestations and early treatment before the occurrence of irreversible fibrotic tissue damage. GERD should be aggressively treated with potent acid suppression and avoiding medications known to cause reflux, such as calcium-channel blockers.

Other Collagen Vascular Diseases

In a study of 150 patients with a variety of rheumatologic disorders who underwent esophageal motility testing, it was common to find involvement of the esophagus.[157] The frequency differs by disease: In PSS, abnormalities were found more frequently in the LES (82%) and in the esophageal body (85%), whereas patients with dermatomyositis and mixed connective tissue disorders overlapped.[157] In systemic lupus erythematosus, there were no abnormalities in the LES, but isolated abnormal peristalsis was noted. The authors conclude that simultaneous involvement of the esophageal body and the LES discriminates between systemic lupus erythematosus and other connective tissue diseases.[157]

Esophageal involvement in mixed connective tissue disease was frequent, with delayed esophageal emptying and esophageal dysmotility noted in 90% of patients tested by scintigraphy. Esophagitis was found in 95% of patients.[158] In a study of four children with mixed connective tissue disease, three had low-LES pressure, two had tertiary waves, and two had weak contractions, but no evidence of aperistalsis.[156]

HIRSCHSPRUNG'S DISEASE

Esophageal dysmotility is described in children with Hirschsprung disease. Manometric findings include higher amplitude of esophageal contractions and the presence of simultaneous contractions or double-peaked waves. No abnormalities of the LES are noted. After the corrective surgery, simultaneous contractions and double-peaked waves persisted but the wave amplitude fell to a level similar to that seen in a control group.[159] The significance of these manometry changes is not well established since patients rarely have esophageal symptoms.[159] There are also isolated case reports of an association between short-segment Hirschsprung disease and achalasia.[160]

EOSINOPHILIC ESOPHAGITIS

Eosinophilic esophagitis is a chronic, relapsing condition characterized by increased eosinophils in the esophageal mucosa (ie, >15 to 20 eosinophils per high power field on biopsies of the mid- and distal esophagus).[161] Clinical presentation with dysphagia and food impaction is common. Esophagograms can be either normal or demonstrate a static, narrowed caliber.[162] Esophageal manometry is abnormal in 41% of 49 cumulative patients reported in the literature. These abnormalities include uncoordinated contractions (30%) with or without LES relaxation, hypercontraction (7%), and ineffective peristalsis (4%). Three patients have been diagnosed with both achalasia and eosinophilic esophagitis.[161] Esophageal dysmotility is attributed to acetylcholine activation by histamine released from mast cells present in the esophageal wall.[161] Management includes dietary modifications (specific allergen elimination vs elemental diet) and corticosteroids (topical and systemic).[161] When these patients undergo esophageal dilatation, usually in undiagnosed cases, they can develop extensive mucosal disruption (linear shearing mucosal tears) of the esophageal body.[161–162]

CROHN'S DISEASE

Crohn's disease is characterized by transmural inflammation which may occur in any part of the digestive tract. Esophageal involvement is rare

(1 to 10%).[163] There are over 100 reports in the English literature of patients suffering from esophageal Crohn's disease. In the few cases where manometry was performed, the findings carried some similarities to those found in achalasia—hypertensive lower esophageal sphincter but with inconsistent findings concerning peristalsis and sphincter relaxation.[163–164] Management is with control of the disease by means of steroids and immunomodulatory agents.

REFERENCES

1. Putnam PE, Orenstein SR, Pang D, et al. Cricopharyngeal dysfunction associated with Chiari malformations. Pediatrics 1992;89:871–6.
2. Park W, Vaezi MF. Etiology and pathogenesis of achalasia: The current understanding. Am J Gastroenterol 2005;100:1404–14.
3. Crist J, Gidda JS, Goyal RK. Intramural mechanism of esophageal peristalsis: Roles of cholinergic and noncholinergic nerves. Proc Natl Acad Sci U S A 1984;81:3595–9.
4. Wang AY, Kadkade R, Kahrilas PJ, Hirano I. Effectiveness of esophageal dilation for symptomatic cricopharyngeal bar. Gastrointest Endosc 2005;61:148–52.
5. Lawson G, Remacle M, Jamart J, Keghian J. Endoscopic CO_2 laser-assisted surgery for cricopharyngeal dysfunction. Eur Arch Otorhinolaryngol 2003;260:475–80.
6. Dinari G, Danziger Y, Mimouni M, et al. Cricopharyngeal dysfunction in childhood: Treatment by dilatations. J Pediatr Gastroenterol Nutr 1987;6:212–6.
7. Staiano A, Cucchiara S, De Vizia B, et al. Disorders of upper esophageal sphincter motility in children. J Pediatr Gastroenterol Nutr 1987;6:892–8.
8. Brooks A, Millar AJ, Rode H. The surgical management of cricopharyngeal achalasia in children. Int J Pediatr Otorhinolaryngol 2000;56:1–7.
9. Cook IJ, Kahrilas PJ. AGA technical review on management of oropharyngeal dysphagia. Gastroenterology 1999;116:455–78.
10. Hussain SZ, Di Lorenzo C. Motility disorders. Diagnosis and treatment for the pediatric patient. Pediatr Clin North Am 2002;49:27–51.
11. Willging JP, Thompson DM. Pediatric FEESST: Fiberoptic endoscopic evaluation of swallowing with sensory testing. Curr Gastroenterol Rep 2005;7:240–3.
12. Kelly JH. Management of upper esophageal sphincter disorders: Indications and complications of myotomy. Am J Med 2000;108:43S–6S.
13. Muraji T, Takamizawa S, Satoh S, et al. Congenital cricopharyngeal achalasia: Diagnosis and surgical management. J Pediatr Surg 2002;37:E12.
14. Zepeda-Gomez S, Montano Loza A, Valdovinos F, et al. Endoscopic balloon catheter dilation for treatment of primary cricopharyngeal dysfunction. Dig Dis Sci 2004;49:1612–4.
15. Solt J, Bajor J, Moizs M, et al. Primary cricopharyngeal dysfunction: Treatment with balloon catheter dilatation. Gastrointest Endosc 2001;54:767–71.
16. De Caluwe D, Nassogne MC, Reding R, et al. Cricopharyngeal achalasia: Case reports and review of the literature. Eur J Pediatr Surg 1999;9:109–12.
17. Yip HT, Leonard R, Kendall KA. Cricopharyngeal myotomy normalizes the opening size of the upper esophageal sphincter in cricopharyngeal dysfunction. Laryngoscope 2006;116:93–6.
18. Munoz AA, Shapiro J, Cuddy LD, et al. Videofluoroscopic findings in dysphagic patients with cricopharyngeal dysfunction: Before and after open cricopharyngeal myotomy. Ann Otol Rhinol Laryngol 2007;116:49–56.
19. Zaninotto G, Marchese Ragona R, Costantini M, et al. The role of botulinum toxin injection and upper esophageal sphincter myotomy in treating oropharyngeal dysphagia. J Gastrointest Surg 2004;8:997–1006.
20. Parameswaran MS, Soliman AM. Endoscopic botulinum toxin injection for cricopharyngeal dysphagia. Ann Otol Rhinol Laryngol 2002;111:871–4.
21. Murry T, Wasserman T, Carrau RL, Castillo. B. Injection of botulinum toxin A for the treatment of dysfunction of the upper esophageal sphincter. Am J Otolaryngol 2005;26:157–62.
22. Zhao X, Pasricha PJ. Botulinum toxin for spastic GI disorders: A systematic review. Gastrointest Endosc 2003;57:219–35.
23. Utian HL, Thomas RG. Cricopharyngeal incoordination in infancy. Pediatrics 1969;43:402–6.
24. Pollack IF, Pang D, Kocoshis S, et al. Neurogenic dysphagia resulting from Chiari malformations. Neurosurgery 1992;30:709–19.
25. Reichert TJ, Bluestone CD, Stool SE, et al. Congenital cricopharyngeal achalasia. Ann Otol Rhinol Laryngol 1977;86:603–10.
26. Davis D, Nowicki M, Giles H. Cricopharyngeal achalasia responsive to balloon dilation in an infant. South Med J 2005;98:472–4.
27. Sewell RK, Bauman NM. Congenital cricopharyngeal achalasia: Management with botulinum toxin before myotomy. Arch Otolaryngol Head Neck Surg 2005;131:451–3.
28. Korakaki E, Hatzidaki E, Manoura A, et al. Feeding difficulties in a neonate with primary cricopharyngeal achalasia treated by cricopharyngeal myotomy. Int J Pediatr Otorhinolaryngol 2004;68:249–53.
29. Eckardt VF, Nix W, Kraus W, et al. Esophageal motor function in patients with muscular dystrophy. Gastroenterology 1986;90:628–35.
30. Lecointe-Besancon I, Leroy F, Devroede G, et al. A comparative study of esophageal and anorectal motility in myotonic dystrophy. Dig Dis Sci 1999;44:1090–9.
31. Philpot J, Bagnall A, King C, et al. Feeding problems in merosin deficient congenital muscular dystrophy. Arch Dis Child 1999;80:542–7.
32. Ramanan AV, Feldman BM. Clinical features and outcomes of juvenile dermatomyositis and other childhood onset myositis syndromes. Rheum Dis Clin North Am 2002;28:833–57.
33. Singh S, Bansal A. Twelve years experience of juvenile dermatomyositis in North India. Rheumatol Int 2006;26:510–5.
34. Williams RB, Grehan MJ, Hersch M, et al. Biomechanics, diagnosis, and treatment outcome in inflammatory myopathy presenting as oropharyngeal dysphagia. Gut 2003;52:471–8.
35. Colton-Hudson A, Koopman WJ, Moosa T, et al. A prospective assessment of the characteristics of dysphagia in myasthenia gravis. Dysphagia 2002;17:147–51.
36. Gates J, Hartnell GG, Gramigna GD. Videofluoroscopy and swallowing studies for neurologic disease: A primer. Radiographics 2006;26:e22.
37. Huang MH, King KL, Chien KY. Esophageal manometric studies in patients with myasthenia gravis. J Thorac Cardiovasc Surg 1988;95:281–5.
38. Brook I. Infant botulism. J Perinatol 2007;27:175–80.
39. Cannon RA. Differential effect of botulinal toxin on esophageal motor function in infants. J Pediatr Gastroenterol Nutr 1985;4:563–7.
40. Berquist WE, Byrne WJ, Ament ME, et al. Achalasia: Diagnosis, management, and clinical course in 16 children. Pediatrics 1983;71:798–805.
41. Podas T, Eaden J, Mayberry M, et al. Achalasia: A critical review of epidemiological studies. Am J Gastroenterol 1998;93:2345–7.
42. Woltman TA, Pellegrini CA, Oelschlager BK. Achalasia. Surg Clin North Am 2005;85:483–93.
43. Mayberry JF. Epidemiology and demographics of achalasia. Gastrointest Endosc Clin N Am 2001;11:235–48.
44. Mayberry JF, Mayell MJ. Epidemiological study of achalasia in children. Gut 1988;29:90–3.
45. Dodds WJ, Dent J, Hogan WJ, et al. Paradoxical lower esophageal sphincter contraction induced by cholecystokinin-octapeptide in patients with achalasia. Gastroenterology 1981;80:327–33.
46. Khelif K, De Laet MH, Chaouachi B, et al. Achalasia of the cardia in Allgrove's (triple A) syndrome: Histopathologic study of 10 cases. Am J Surg Pathol 2003;27:667–72.
47. Watanabe Y, Ando H, Seo T, et al. Attenuated nitrergic inhibitory neurotransmission to interstitial cells of Cajal in the lower esophageal sphincter with esophageal achalasia in children. Pediatr Int 2002;44:145–8.
48. Schmidt T, Pfeiffer A, Hackelsberger N, et al. Dysmotility of the small intestine in achalasia. Neurogastroenterol Motil 1999;11:11–7.
49. Caturelli E, Squillante MM, Fusilli S, et al. Gallbladder emptying in patients with primary achalasia. Digestion 1992;52:152–6.
50. Csendes A, Smok G, Braghetto I, et al. Histological studies of Auerbach's plexuses of the esophagus, stomach, jejunum, and colon in patients with achalasia of the oesophagus: Correlation with gastric acid secretion, presence of parietal cells and gastric emptying of solids. Gut 1992;33:150–4.
51. Benini L, Castellani G, Sembenini C, et al. Gastric emptying of solid meals in achalasic patients after successful pneumatic dilatation of the cardia. Dig Dis Sci 1994;39:733–7.
52. Kobara H, Uchida N, Tsutsui K, et al. Abnormal bile flow in patients with achalasia. J Gastroenterol 2003;38:327–31.
53. Shafik A. Anorectal motility in patients with achalasia of the esophagus: Recognition of an esophago-rectal syndrome. BMC Gastroenterol 2003;3:28.
54. Moses PL, Ellis LM, Anees MR, et al. Antineuronal antibodies in idiopathic achalasia and gastroesophageal reflux disease. Gut 2003;52:629–36.
55. Latiano A, Degiorgio R, Volta U, et al. HLA and enteric antineuronal antibodies in patients with achalasia. Neurogastroenterol Motil 2006;18:520–5.
56. Ruiz-de-Leon A, Mendoza J, Sevilla-Mantilla C, et al. Myenteric antiplexus antibodies and class II HLA in achalasia. Dig Dis Sci 2002;47:15–9.
57. Kaar TK, Waldron R, Ashraf MS, et al. Familial infantile oesophageal achalasia. Arch Dis Child 1991;66:1353–4.
58. Zarate N, Mearin F, Gil-Vernet JM, et al. Achalasia and Down's syndrome: Coincidental association or something else? Am J Gastroenterol 1999;94:1674–7.
59. Mayberry JF, Atkinson M. A study of swallowing difficulties in first degree relatives of patients with achalasia. Thorax 1985;40:391–3.
60. Handschug K, Sperling S, Yoon SJ, et al. Triple A syndrome is caused by mutations in AAAS, a new WD-repeat protein gene. Hum Mol Genet 2001;10:283–90.
61. Prpic I, Huebner A, Persic M, et al. Triple A syndrome: Genotype-phenotype assessment. Clin Genet 2003;63:415–7.
62. Grant DB, Barnes ND, Dumic M, et al. Neurological and adrenal dysfunction in the adrenal insufficiency/alacrima/achalasia (3A) syndrome. Arch Dis Child 1993;68:779–82.
63. Baujat G, Faure C, Zaouche A, et al. Oroesophageal motor disorders in Pierre Robin syndrome. J Pediatr Gastroenterol Nutr 2001;32:297–302.
64. Mayberry JF, Atkinson M. Achalasia and other diseases associated with disorders of gastrointestinal motility. Hepatogastroenterology 1986;33:206–7.
65. Myers NA, Jolley SG, Taylor R. Achalasia of the cardia in children: A worldwide survey. J Pediatr Surg 1994;29:1375–9.
66. Hussain SZ, Thomas R, Tolia V. A review of achalasia in 33 children. Dig Dis Sci 2002;47:2538–43.
67. Viola S, Goutet JM, Audry G, et al. Clinical profile and long-term outcome in children with esophageal achalasia. Arch Pediatr 2005;12:391–6.
68. Kostic SV, Rice TW, Baker ME, et al. Timed barium esophagogram: A simple physiologic assessment for achalasia. J Thorac Cardiovasc Surg 2000;120:935–43.
69. Vaezi MF, Baker ME, Achkar E, et al. Timed barium oesophagram: Better predictor of long term success after pneumatic dilation in achalasia than symptom assessment. Gut 2002;50:765–70.
70. Vaezi MF. Quantitative methods to determine efficacy of treatment in achalasia. Gastrointest Endosc Clin North Am 2001;11:409–24.
71. Russell CO, Hill LD, Holmes ER, et al. Radionuclide transit: A sensitive screening test for esophageal dysfunction. Gastroenterology 1981;80:887–92.
72. Boeckxstaens GE, Jonge WD, van den Wijngaard RM, et al. Achalasia: From new insights in pathophysiology to treatment. J Pediatr Gastroenterol Nutr 2005;41:S36–7.
73. Miller L, Dai Q, Korimilli A, et al. Use of endoluminal ultrasound to evaluate gastrointestinal motility. Dig Dis 2006;24:319–41.
74. Spechler SJ, Castell DO. Classification of oesophageal motility abnormalities. Gut 2001;49:145–51.
75. Tovar JA, Prieto G, Molina M, et al. Esophageal function in achalasia: Preoperative and postoperative manometric studies. J Pediatr Surg 1998;33:834–8.
76. Morera C FV, Jaen D, Pestana E, et al. Are the manometric findings in pediatric achlasia similar to those found in adults? JPGN 2002;35:447–56.
77. Asch MJ, Liebman W, Lachman RS, et al. Esophageal achalasia: Diagnosis and cardiomyotomy in a newborn infant. J Pediatr Surg 1974;9:911–2.
78. Chelimsky G, Hupertz V, Blanchard T. Manometric progression of achalasia. J Pediatr Gastroenterol Nutr 2000;31:303–6.
79. Chapman JR, Joehl RJ, Murayama KM, et al. Achalasia treatment: Improved outcome of laparoscopic myotomy with operative manometry. Arch Surg 2004;139:508–13.
80. Kalicinski P, Dluski E, Drewniak T, et al. Esophageal manometric studies in children with achalasia before and after operative treatment. Pediatr Surg Int 1997;12:571–5.
81. Zaninotto G, Annese V, Costantini M, et al. Randomized controlled trial of botulinum toxin versus laparoscopic heller myotomy for esophageal achalasia. Ann Surg 2004;239:364–70.
82. Gockel I, Junginger T, Eckardt VF. Effects of pneumatic dilation and myotomy on esophageal function and morphology in patients with achalasia. Am Surg 2005;71:128–31.

83. Patti MG, Galvani C, Gorodner MV, et al. Timing of surgical intervention does not influence return of esophageal peristalsis or outcome for patients with achalasia. Surg Endosc 2005;19:1188–92.

84. Cucchiara S, Staiano A, Di Lorenzo C, et al. Return of peristalsis in a child with esophageal achalasia treated by Heller's myotomy. J Pediatr Gastroenterol Nutr 1986;5:150–2.

85. Nguyen HN, Domingues GR, Lammert F. Technological insights: Combined impedance manometry for esophageal motility testing-current results and further implications. World J Gastroenterol 2006;12:6266–73.

86. Cho YK, Choi MG, Park JM, et al. Evaluation of esophageal function in patients with esophageal motor abnormalities using multichannel intraluminal impedance esophageal manometry. World J Gastroenterol 2006;12:6349–54.

87. Tutuian R, Castell DO. Combined multichannel intraluminal impedance and manometry clarifies esophageal function abnormalities: Study in 350 patients. Am J Gastroenterol 2004;99:1011–9.

88. Arcos E, Medina C, Mearin F, et al. Achalasia presenting as acute airway obstruction. Dig Dis Sci 2000;45:2079–83.

89. Yoneyama F, Miyachi M, Nimura Y. Manometric findings of the upper esophageal sphincter in esophageal achalasia. World J Surg 1998;22:1043–6.

90. Gockel I, Eckardt VF, Schmitt T, et al. Pseudoachalasia: A case series and analysis of the literature. Scand J Gastroenterol 2005;40:378–85.

91. Herbella FA, Oliveira DR, Del Grande JC. Are idiopathic and Chagasic achalasia two different diseases? Dig Dis Sci 2004;49:353–60.

92. Meneghelli UG, Peria FM, Darezzo FM, et al. Clinical, radiographic, and manometric evolution of esophageal involvement by Chagas' disease. Dysphagia 2005;20:40–5.

93. Desseilles M, Fuchs S, Ansseau M, et al. Achalasia may mimic anorexia nervosa, compulsive eating disorder, and obesity problems. Psychosomatics 2006;47:270–1.

94. Stacher G, Kiss A, Wiesnagrotzki S, et al. Oesophageal and gastric motility disorders in patients categorised as having primary anorexia nervosa. Gut 1986;27:1120–6.

95. Gelfond M, Rozen P, Gilat T. Isosorbide dinitrate and nifedipine treatment of achalasia: A clinical, manometric and radionuclide evaluation. Gastroenterology 1982;83:963–9.

96. Vaezi MF, Richter JE. Current therapies for achalasia: Comparison and efficacy. J Clin Gastroenterol 1998;27:21–35.

97. Efrati Y, Horne T, Livshitz G, et al. Radionuclide esophageal emptying and long-acting nitrates (Nitroderm) in childhood achalasia. J Pediatr Gastroenterol Nutr 1996;23:312–5.

98. Bruley des Varannes S, Scarpignato C. Current trends in the management of achalasia. Dig Liver Dis 2001;33:266–77.

99. Bassotti G, Annese V. Review article: Pharmacological options in achalasia. Aliment Pharmacol Ther 1999;13:1391–6.

100. Maksimak M, Perlmutter DH, Winter HS. The use of nifedipine for the treatment of achalasia in children. J Pediatr Gastroenterol Nutr 1986;5:883–6.

101. Bortolotti M, Mari C, Lopilato C, et al. Effects of sildenafil on esophageal motility of patients with idiopathic achalasia. Gastroenterology 2000;118:253–7.

102. Hurwitz M, Bahar RJ, Ament ME, et al. Evaluation of the use of botulinum toxin in children with achalasia. J Pediatr Gastroenterol Nutr 2000;30:509–14.

103. Nurko S. Botulinum toxin for achalasia: Are we witnessing the birth of a new era? J Pediatr Gastroenterol Nutr 1997;24:447–9.

104. Bansal R, Nostrant TT, Scheiman JM, et al. Intrasphincteric botulinum toxin versus pneumatic balloon dilation for treatment of primary achalasia. J Clin Gastroenterol 2003;36:209–14.

105. Martinek J, Siroky M, Plottova Z, et al. Treatment of patients with achalasia with botulinum toxin: A multicenter prospective cohort study. Dis Esophagus 2003;16:204–9.

106. Pasricha PJ, Ravich WJ, Hendrix TR, et al. Intrasphincteric botulinum toxin for the treatment of achalasia. N Engl J Med 1995;332:774–8.

107. Ip KS, Cameron DJ, Catto-Smith AG, et al. Botulinum toxin for achalasia in children. J Gastroenterol Hepatol 2000;15:1100–4.

108. Khoshoo V, LaGarde DC, Udall JN, Jr. Intrasphincteric injection of Botulinum toxin for treating achalasia in children. J Pediatr Gastroenterol Nutr 1997;24:439–41.

109. Patti MG, Feo CV, Arcerito M, et al. Effects of previous treatment on results of laparoscopic Heller myotomy for achalasia. Dig Dis Sci 1999;44:2270–6.

110. Nakayama DK, Shorter NA, Boyle JT, et al. Pneumatic dilatation and operative treatment of achalasia in children. J Pediatr Surg 1987;22:619–22.

111. American Society for Gastrointestinal Endoscopy. Esophageal dilation. Gastrointest Endosc 1998;48:702–4.

112. Babu R, Grier D, Cusick E, et al. Pneumatic dilatation for childhood achalasia. Pediatr Surg Int 2001;17:505–7.

113. Khan AA, Shah SW, Alam A, et al. Efficacy of Rigiflex balloon dilatation in 12 children with achalasia: A 6-month prospective study showing weight gain and symptomatic improvement. Dis Esophagus 2002;15:167–70.

114. Vakil N, Kadakia S, Eckardt VF. Pneumatic dilation in achalasia. Endoscopy 2003;35:526–30.

115. Gideon RM, Castell DO, Yarze J. Prospective randomized comparison of pneumatic dilatation technique in patients with idiopathic achalasia. Dig Dis Sci 1999;44:1853–7.

116. Eckardt VF, Gockel I, Bernhard G. Pneumatic dilation for achalasia: Late results of a prospective follow up investigation. Gut 2004;53:629–33.

117. Ghoshal UC, Kumar S, Saraswat VA, et al. Long-term follow-up after pneumatic dilation for achalasia cardia: Factors associated with treatment failure and recurrence. Am J Gastroenterol 2004;99:2304–10.

118. Katsinelos P, Kountouras J, Paroutoglou G, et al. Long-term results of pneumatic dilation for achalasia: A 15 years' experience. World J Gastroenterol 2005;11:5701–5.

119. Khan AA, Shah SW, Alam A, et al. Sixteen years follow up of achalasia: A prospective study of graded dilatation using Rigiflex balloon. Dis Esophagus 2005;18:41–5.

120. Metman EH, Lagasse JP, d'Alteroche L, et al. Risk factors for immediate complications after progressive pneumatic dilation for achalasia. Am J Gastroenterol 1999;94:1179–85.

121. Gershman G, Ament ME, Vargas J. Frequency and medical management of esophageal perforation after pneumatic dilatation in achalasia. J Pediatr Gastroenterol Nutr 1997;25:548–53.

122. Shoenut JP, Duerksen D, Yaffe CS. A prospective assessment of gastroesophageal reflux before and after treatment of achalasia patients: Pneumatic dilation versus transthoracic limited myotomy. Am J Gastroenterol 1997;92:1109–12.

123. Leeuwenburgh I, Van Dekken H, Scholten P, et al. Oesophagitis is common in patients with achalasia after pneumatic dilatation. Aliment Pharmacol Ther 2006;23:1197–203.

124. Abir F, Modlin I, Kidd M, et al. Surgical treatment of achalasia: Current status and controversies. Dig Surg 2004;21:165–76.

125. Bonavina L. Minimally invasive surgery for esophageal achalasia. World J Gastroenterol 2006;12:5921–5.

126. Karnak I, Senocak ME, Tanyel FC, et al. Achalasia in childhood: Surgical treatment and outcome. Eur J Pediatr Surg 2001;11:223–9.

127. Mattioli G, Esposito C, Pini Prato A, et al. Results of the laparoscopic Heller-Dor procedure for pediatric esophageal achalasia. Surg Endosc 2003;17:1650–2.

128. Patti MG, Albanese CT, Holcomb GW, et al. Laparoscopic Heller myotomy and Dor fundoplication for esophageal achalasia in children. J Pediatr Surg 2001;36:1248–51.

129. Elder JB. Achalasia of the cardia in childhood. Digestion 1970;3:90–6.

130. Lelli JL, Jr, Drongowski RA, Coran AG. Efficacy of the transthoracic modified Heller myotomy in children with achalasia–a 21-year experience. J Pediatr Surg 1997;32:338–41.

131. Mehra M, Bahar RJ, Ament ME, et al. Laparoscopic and thoracoscopic esophagomyotomy for children with achalasia. J Pediatr Gastroenterol Nutr 2001;33:466–71.

132. Rothenberg SS, Partrick DA, Bealer JF, et al. Evaluation of minimally invasive approaches to achalasia in children. J Pediatr Surg 2001;36:808–10.

133. Deb S, Deschamps C, Allen MS, et al. Laparoscopic esophageal myotomy for achalasia: Factors affecting functional results. Ann Thorac Surg 2005;80:1191–4.

134. Lopushinsky SR, Urbach DR. Pneumatic dilatation and surgical myotomy for achalasia. JAMA 2006;296:2227–33.

135. Luckey AE, 3rd, DeMeester SR. Complications of achalasia surgery. Thorac Surg Clin 2006;16:95–8.

136. Richards WO, Torquati A, Holzman MD, et al. Heller myotomy versus Heller myotomy with Dor fundoplication for achalasia: A prospective randomized double-blind clinical trial. Ann Surg 2004;240:405–12.

137. Agha FP, Keren DF. Barrett's esophagus complicating achalasia after esophagomyotomy. A clinical, radiologic, and pathologic study of 70 patients with achalasia and related motor disorders. J Clin Gastroenterol 1987;9:232–7.

138. Csendes A, Braghetto I, Burdiles P, et al. Very late results of esophagomyotomy for patients with achalasia: Clinical, endoscopic, histologic, manometric, and acid reflux studies in 67 patients for a mean follow-up of 190 months. Ann Surg 2006;243:196–203.

139. Ruffato A, Mattioli S, Lugaresi ML, et al. Long-term results after Heller-Dor operation for oesophageal achalasia. Eur J Cardiothorac Surg 2006;29:914–9.

140. Vantrappen G, Hellemans J. Treatment of achalasia and related motor disorders. Gastroenterology 1980;79:144–54.

141. Aggestrup S, Holm JC, Sorensen HR. Does achalasia predispose to cancer of the esophagus? Chest 1992;102:1013–6.

142. Richter JE. Oesophageal motility disorders. Lancet 2001;358:823–8.

143. Tutuian R, Castell DO. Review article: Oesophageal spasm—diagnosis and management. Aliment Pharmacol Ther 2006;23:1393–402.

144. Fontan JP, Heldt GP, Heyman MB, et al. Esophageal spasm associated with apnea and bradycardia in an infant. Pediatrics 1984;73:52–5.

145. Glassman MS, Medow MS, Berezin S, et al. Spectrum of esophageal disorders in children with chest pain. Dig Dis Sci 1992;37:663–6.

146. Kovesi T, Rubin S. Long-term complications of congenital esophageal atresia and/or tracheoesophageal fistula. Chest 2004;126:915–25.

147. Dutta HK, Grover VP, Dwivedi SN, et al. Manometric evaluation of postoperative patients of esophageal atresia and tracheo-esophageal fistula. Eur J Pediatr Surg 2001;11:371–6.

148. Boige N, Faure C, Cargill G, et al. Manometrical evaluation in visceral neuropathies in children. J Pediatr Gastroenterol Nutr 1994;19:71–7.

149. Vargas JH, Sachs P, Ament ME. Chronic intestinal pseudo-obstruction syndrome in pediatrics. Results of a national survey by members of the North American Society of Pediatric Gastroenterology and Nutrition. J Pediatr Gastroenterol Nutr 1988;7:323–32.

150. Genc A, Mutaf O. Esophageal motility changes in acute and late periods of caustic esophageal burns and their relation to prognosis in children. J Pediatr Surg 2002;37:1526–8.

151. Bautista A, Varela R, Villanueva A, et al. Motor function of the esophagus after caustic burn. Eur J Pediatr Surg 1996;6:204–7.

152. Fass R, Landau O, Kovacs TO, et al. Esophageal motility abnormalities in cirrhotic patients before and after endoscopic variceal treatment. Am J Gastroenterol 1997;92:941–6.

153. Viazis N, Armonis A, Vlachogiannakos J, et al. Effects of endoscopic variceal treatment on oesophageal function: A prospective, randomized study. Eur J Gastroenterol Hepatol 2002;14:263–9.

154. Murray KJ, Laxer RM. Scleroderma in children and adolescents. Rheum Dis Clin North Am 2002;28:603–24.

155. Ebert EC. Esophageal disease in scleroderma. J Clin Gastroenterol 2006;40:769–75.

156. Flick JA, Boyle JT, Tuchman DN, et al. Esophageal motor abnormalities in children and adolescents with scleroderma and mixed connective tissue disease. Pediatrics 1988;82:107–11.

157. Lapadula G, Muolo P, Semeraro F, et al. Esophageal motility disorders in the rheumatic diseases: A review of 150 patients. Clin Exp Rheumatol 1994;12:515–21.

158. Caleiro MT, Lage LV, Navarro-Rodriguez T, et al. Radionuclide imaging for the assessment of esophageal motility disorders in mixed connective tissue disease patients: Relation to pulmonary impairment. Dis Esophagus 2006;19:394–400.

159. Faure C, Ategbo S, Ferreira GC, et al. Duodenal and esophageal manometry in total colonic aganglionosis. J Pediatr Gastroenterol Nutr 1994;18:193–9.

160. Kohler S, Fitze G, Hosie S, et al. The combination of Hirschsprung's disease and achalasia. J Pediatr Surg 2005;40:E28–30.

161. Sgouros SN, Bergele C, Mantides A. Eosinophilic esophagitis in adults: What is the clinical significance? Endoscopy 2006;38:515–20.

162. Vasilopoulos S, Murphy P, Auerbach A, et al. The small-caliber esophagus: An unappreciated cause of dysphagia for solids in patients with eosinophilic esophagitis. Gastrointest Endosc 2002;55:99–106.

163. Knoblauch C, Netzer P, Scheurer U, et al. Dysphagia in Crohn's disease: A diagnostic challenge. Dig Liver Dis 2002;34:660–4.

164. Treem WR, Ragsdale BD. Crohn's disease of the esophagus: A case report and review of the literature. J Pediatr Gastroenterol Nutr 1988;7:451–5.

5

Esophagitis

Mike Thomson, MB, ChB, DCH, FCRP, FRCPCH, MD

Pathologic processes in the pediatric esophagus have received a disproportionately small amount of attention until recently, when appreciation of their pathophysiology and concordant clinical importance has been highlighted. This increase in interest and exposure is probably a phenomenon secondary to a number of important factors, which include improved diagnostic yield from relatively recent technical advances in areas such as infant and pediatric endoscopy; advances in fields such as mucosal immunology, allowing for the realization that etiopathologic mechanisms for esophagitis are more complex than simple luminal chemical damage; and a shift in clinical opinion recognizing esophageal pathology as a major cause of nonspecific ubiquitous symptoms such as infant colic, feeding disorders, and recurrent abdominal pain among others. A state of knowledge such as this has made pediatric esophagitis, until recently, a relatively underdeveloped area of research and clinical understanding, but this is rapidly changing.[1]

It is now clear, therefore, that esophagitis in infants and children has many responsible etiologic pathways that may have complex interactions and hence requires equally complex diagnostic and therapeutic strategies. Such causative factors are now known to include cow's milk protein (CMP) intolerance or allergy; pH-dependent and -independent gastroesophageal reflux (GER); dysmotility of various causes; and infective, traumatic, and iatrogenic causes, among others. Hence, the term "esophagitis" can be used to describe chemical, infectious, inflammatory, ischemic, immunologic, and degenerative abnormalities.[2] Nevertheless, there remains a minor degree of controversy regarding the definition and significance of esophagitis, as assessed by standard diagnostic techniques, including endoscopy and biopsy.[3,4] This chapter attempts to describe basic etiologies and their interactions, symptomatic presentations, timing and choice of diagnostic measures, current practice of therapeutic interventions, and prognosis of, and for, esophagitis in infancy and childhood.

EPIDEMIOLOGY

This is a relatively gray area in infancy and childhood. Esophagitis occurs throughout the age spectrum of pediatrics and has even been reported as a cause of prenatal gastrointestinal (GI) bleeding.[5] Neonatal esophagitis is well known as a cause of GI bleeding or anemia.[6,7] It is estimated that the prevalence of reflux esophagitis varies between 2 and 5% of the general population[8]; however, few objective data exist to allow determination of esophagitis distribution in childhood. Some limited data are available regarding GER, and in an early study by Carre, 60% of infants were symptom free by 18 months of age, but 10% developed complications.[9] Such studies would now be considered unethical, and, subsequently, other studies assessing outcome with early therapy have indicated that less than 55% would be symptom free by 10 months of age and 81% by 18 months.[10] In a study of 32 older children (3.5 to 16 years) with GER, 50% had esophagitis, and less than 50% underwent complete resolution or marked symptom resolution over the ensuing 1 to 8 years.[11] Forty percent came off medication, and 40% required ongoing medication for control of symptoms. Two children required fundoplication. Unfortunately, no wider studies are available, and other information on the incidence and prevalence of esophagitis comes from adult studies. These indicate that 48 to 79% of those with GER have esophagitis with few having symptoms,[1] which is similar to that quoted for infants.[12]

ETIOLOGY AND PATHOPHYSIOLOGY

The etiologies of esophagitis in infancy and childhood can usefully be divided into the following groups:

1. *Chemical*: (a) owing to refluxed contents from the stomach and duodenum such as gastric acid, pepsin, bile, and trypsin, and (b) owing to swallowed substances, either intended such as medications, or accidental caustic ingestion such as dishwasher liquid
2. *Immunologic*: owing to specific responses to specific antigens such as CMP or multiple food intolerance or allergy
3. *Infective*: associated with organisms as diverse as *Helicobacter pylori* (with associated reflux), *Candida,* cryptosporidiosis, herpes simplex, and cytomegalovirus (CMV)
4. *Traumatic*: secondary to intraluminal trauma (eg, long-term nasogastric tube) or irradiation (eg, as part of bone marrow transplant conditioning)

5. *Systemic disease manifestation*: associated with conditions such as Crohn's disease and chronic granulomatous disease
6. *Miscellaneous*: such as that associated with passive smoking or that occurring in Munchausen syndrome by proxy
7. *Idiopathic*: eosinophilic esophagitis

The etiopathologic role of each of these situations can, therefore, be usefully discussed under each heading, bearing in mind that an individual child or infant may, of course, have more than one factor contributing to the esophageal insult at any one time (eg, GER and cow's milk–associated esophagitis).

Chemical Esophagitis

Gastroesophageal Reflux. This is dealt with in Chapter 4.2, "Gastroesophageal Reflux." Nevertheless, a brief summary of the pathophysiology and etiology of GER is pertinent here.

The natural history of GER is to improve with age. However, one important question arises: Why do infants (and subsequently a hard core of older children) have a greater propensity toward GER? Differences in the function of the lower esophageal sphincter (LES) have been investigated[13,14]; this is an area that is tonically contracted at rest, with relaxation occurring consequently on an esophageal peristaltic wave. Inhibitory neurotransmitter production is integral to LES relaxation, and the nonadrenergic, noncholinergic neurotransmitter nitric oxide (NO) has received attention in animal[15] and human studies.[16,17] Vasoactive intestinal polypeptide is another candidate undergoing investigation, and the importance of the ontogeny of neuropeptides in the human fetus and infant is becoming increasingly apparent.[18] In eosinophilic inflammation of the esophagus, the peptide eosinophil-derived neurotoxin is implicated. Rather than a "weak" LES in infants, it is more likely that a combination of anatomic relationships of the LES precluding effective pressure generation, in combination with inappropriate LES relaxation is responsible for infantile GER, and its subsequent age-related improvement.[19,20] In adults, 90% of the refluxate is cleared in seconds, and the remainder is neutralized by subsequent swallows.[21] Efficiency of esophageal clearance is therefore vitally important in the genesis of esophagitis.

Although work exists suggesting that acid exposure of the distal esophagus induces dysmotility in pediatric patients,[22] allowing the potential for a "vicious cycle" of LES dysfunction to GER to LES dysmotility to further GER to esophagitis and back to LES dysmotility, it is still not clear how an inflamed esophagus further impairs esophageal tone or motility, but emerging work suggests a role for interleukin (IL)-5 and eotaxin (and derived neurotoxin) in allergic neurohumoral modification, and possibly inappropriate gastroesophageal junction (GEJ) relaxation, with an interrelation with mast cell degranulation and histamine release to afferent and then efferent neurons, which control transient lower esophageal sphincter relaxation episodes (TLESRs).[23] Inducible nitric oxide synthetase (iNOS) (which is markedly upregulated in GI inflammatory conditions such as Crohn's disease), is important in relaxation of the LES during TLESRs, which are the single most common mechanism underlying GER, but in one study was not upregulated in the inflamed pediatric esophagus.[24] However, other researchers suggest an increased release of NO in the inflamed esophagus in children.[25] Other factors that affect clearance are posture–gravity interactions; volume, size, and contents of meal, for example, breast milk[26,27]; defective peristalsis of the esophagus; gastric emptying; and increased noxiousness of refluxate.

Acid, particularly when combined with pepsin, which is most active below pH 2 (but importantly still active up to pH 5.5 underlining the recent appreciation of the importance of weak or nonacid reflux), is known to cause severe esophagitis in animals and humans.[28–31] Even a 24-week gestation infant in an intensive care setting has the ability to lower intragastric pH below 2.[32] Pepsin plays a critical role in esophagitis owing to acidic refluxate; animal work has shown that in dogs and rabbits, infusion of hydrochloric acid alone caused no damage, but in combination with low concentrations of pepsin at pH less than 2, severe esophagitis resulted.[33,34] Proteolysis may allow deeper penetration of harmful refluxate, and the simple notion that acid causes epithelial damage must therefore be questioned in favor of a more complex interplay of a number of noxious stimuli in the pathogenesis of reflux esophagitis in infants and children.

Furthermore, the role of duodenogastroesophageal reflux (DGER) remains controversial[35–36] and has not, to date, been adequately studied in pediatrics. What is clear from adult studies is that alkaline reflux does not correlate well with bile reflux, the former being attributable to reasons other than DGER, such as saliva, food, oral infection, or an obstructed esophagus.[35] In fact, in one study, bile acid DGER correlated well with acid reflux, and those with the more severe esophagitis had greater exposure to the simultaneous damaging effects of both acid and bile acids.[33] Perfusion studies of the rabbit esophagus show that conjugated bile acids in an acidic environment produce mucosal injury, whereas unconjugated bile acids and trypsin are more harmful at more neutral pH values (pH 5–8); therefore, the latter are less likely to cause reflux-associated damage because this is usually an acidic phenomenon.[36] It is further suggested by animal work that the hydrochloride-pepsin damage may actually be attenuated by the presence in the esophagus of conjugated bile acids, but if damage is done to the squamous epithelium, the un-ionized forms of conjugated bile acids at a low pH may be allowed access to mucosal cells and cause damage by the dissolution of cell membranes and mucosal tight junctions.[37–40] The histologic appearances typical of luminal chemical-induced esophagitis secondary to GER or GER disease are discussed in the diagnosis section of this chapter.

Chemical Esophagitis Owing to Swallowed Substances. The importance of caustic ingestion into the esophagus is dealt with in Chapter 6, "Traumatic and Toxic Injury of the Esophagus" (Figure 1). Ingested materials are usually household or garden substances and are usually markedly alkaline; the common one is dishwasher fluid, often with a pH of 9 or above. However, fortunately, in most countries, this has been replaced with powder, which is less easy to swallow, and even individually wrapped tablets of powder. Acute perforation, mediastinitis, and subsequent esophageal stricture have frequently been seen. The possibility of nonaccidental injury should not be forgotten in this context. It is notable that the rate of subsequent stricture formation is high, and, more recently, a potentially effective postdilation topical application of an antifibrotic, mitomycin C, has shown promise in preventing restenosis and long-term repeated stricture dilation.[41] Many medications have been associated with esophageal damage and symptoms of esophagitis, and these include tetracyclines (not recommended under the age of 12 years, of course), drugs used in acne therapy, and nonsteroidal anti-inflammatory drugs.[42–45]

Immunologic Esophagitis

Although it is now clear that multiple food antigens may induce esophagitis,[46,47] the most common precipitant is CMP. Standard endoscopic biopsy and histology do not reliably distinguish between primary reflux esophagitis and the emerging clinical entity of cow's milk–associated reflux esophagitis. This variant of cow's milk allergy appears to be a particularly common manifestation in infancy, with symptoms indistinguishable from primary GER but that settle on an exclusion diet.[48] Some differentiation from primary reflux has been suggested on the basis of an esophageal pH testing pattern and a {15β 8}-lactoglobulin antibody response, although the former has not been substantiated by more than one center.[48,49] There is recent evidence that this esophagitis is becoming a more common presentation of infant food allergy within the developed world and, in fact, may be induced by a variety of antigens in addition to cow's milk.[46,47] Many affected infants have sensitized while exclusively breastfed, and a defect in oral tolerance for low doses has been postulated as the underlying cause.[50,51]

Esophageal mucosal eosinophilia has been described in both suspected cow's milk–associated[46] and primary reflux esophagitis (Figure 2),[52] as well as in other conditions, such as idiopathic eosinophilic esophagitis (EE).[53] However, the density of the eosinophilic infiltrate has been used as a differentiator between allergic esophagitis and EE, with the latter defined as more than 20 eosinophils per high-power field (HPF).[54] The clinical significance of eosinophils and their role in the pathogenesis of mucosal injury is poorly understood and the subject of recent debate.[3–4,55] Some have suggested an active role for eosinophils in the inflammatory process of esophagitis and have supported this with the observation of activation of the eosinophils by electron microscopic criteria.[56]

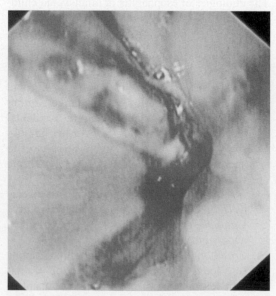

Figure 1 Example of caustic injury to the esophagus.

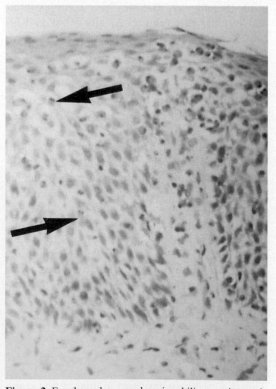

Figure 2 Esophageal mucosal eosinophilia seen in cow's milk–associated and primary reflux esophagitis and primary eosinophilic esophagitis. (Eosinophils marked by arrows.)

In addition to dietary exclusion of cow's milk,[46,48] oral steroids can induce remission of symptoms with decreased mucosal eosinophilia[48,53] suggesting a pathoetiologic role for eosinophils. In addition to eosinophils, intraepithelial T lymphocytes, known as cells with irregular nuclear contours (CINC), have also been implicated as markers of reflux esophagitis.[57,58] In adults, such cells are of memory phenotype and display activation markers,[59] although little is known of their pediatric equivalents.

A variety of immunohistochemical markers have been used to examine the esophageal mucosa, including eotaxin, a recently described eosinophil-specific chemokine (Figure 3),[60] and markers of T-cell lineage and activation. Despite the mild histologic abnormality in CMP-associated esophagitis, an increased expression of eotaxin colocalized with activated T lymphocytes to the basal and papillary epithelium has been shown,[61] distinguishing this from primary reflux esophagitis. The molecular basis of the eotaxin upregulation in cow's milk protein–sensitive enteropathy (CMPSE) is unknown. However, there is evidence from murine models of asthma that antigen-specific upregulation of eotaxin expression can be induced by T cells and blocked by anti-CD3 monoclonal antibodies. This suggests the possibility of a distinct mechanism in CMSE, in which mucosal homing to the esophagus occurs of lymphocytes activated within the small intestine. This may explain the seemingly counterintuitive finding of basal, as opposed to superficial, chemokine expression and the common occurrence of mucosal eosinophilia in this condition. The esophageal motility disturbance of CMSE-associated esophagitis is thus suggested to occur as a neurologic consequence of the inflammatory infiltration induced from lamina propria vessels into the epithelial compartment.[62] This proposed mechanism contrasts with the current concept of luminally induced inflammation found in primary reflux esophagitis and is consistent with the characteristic delayed onset and chronic nature of cow's milk–associated reflux esophagitis. The upregulated expression of epithelial human leukocyte antigen (HLA)-DR suggests that the cytokine secretion profile of these cells includes interferon-{159}, and thus a mixed T helper (Th)1-Th2 pattern is likely (IL-5 secretion is also likely in view of the frequent

mucosal eosinophilia), and it may thus be relevant that small intestinal mucosal lymphocytes in infants with CMSE show both Th2 skewing and low transforming growth factor (TGF)-{158} expression.[63] It seems, therefore, that there is a characteristic esophageal mucosal immuno-histochemical profile in cow's milk–associated reflux esophagitis. Upregulation of basal eotaxin expression and focal distribution of T-cell lineage and activation markers suggest a mechanism of mucosal homing of cow's milk–sensitized cells from the small intestine in the pathogenesis of CMPSE-associated esophageal reflux, in a manner distinct from luminally mediated primary reflux esophagitis. It has also been suggested that increased numbers of mucosal mast cells allow a distinction to be made between allergy-induced and reflux-induced esophagitis.[64] Much work is required in this area and is ongoing.

Infective Esophagitis

The majority of infective esophagitis that occurs is in the immunocompromised child and is due to such agents as herpes simplex, CMV, *Candida,* and others. Mucosal damage owing to physical or chemical causes may predispose the patient to opportunistic infection. Oral herpes or *Candida* may offer some clue to etiology, and the older child will often complain of odynophagia or dysphagia. Diagnosis may be made on endoscopy with biopsy, but brushings may offer a greater diagnostic yield.

Viral esophagitis is usually due to herpes simplex, CMV, and, occasionally, varicella zoster.[65–67] Herpes simplex esophagitis can occur in those with normal immune function[68] but is more often seen in those who are immunocompromised. In one series, 10% of liver or kidney transplant recipients had herpes or CMV esophagitis,[69] and it is also commonly seen in pediatric human immunodeficiency virus (HIV) infection.[70] Use of prophylactic acyclovir/gangcyclovir is conjectural but may be of some benefit.

Diagnosis of herpes esophagitis is often difficult because the characteristic nuclear inclusions and multinucleate giant cells may not be seen in endoscopic biopsies; however, a prominent mononuclear cell infiltrate is described as characteristic (Figure 4).[71] It may be that the

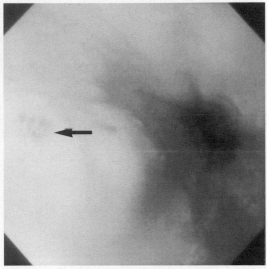

Figure 5 Macroscopic appearances of herpes esophagitis. Roundish distinct disseminated lesions with yellowish borders are seen and have been termed "volcano ulcers" (*arrow*).

esophagus is particularly vulnerable in the GI tract owing to affinity of the herpes virus for stratified epithelium. Typically, roundish distinct disseminated lesions with yellowish borders are seen and have been termed "volcano ulcers" (Figure 5),[72] although early in the presentation, vesicles may be noted. Although the inflammation can resolve spontaneously in the immunocompetent, in those with poor immune function, acyclovir and a high index of suspicion are recommended.[72] Resistance to acyclovir has been described, in which case, foscarnet is the agent of choice.[73] CMV esophagitis is confirmed by basophilic nuclear inclusions on biopsy of the edge of the ulcers, which are similar in appearance to herpetic ones. CMV is predominantly found in immunocompromised individuals, and treatment is with ganciclovir or foscarnet.[67] Hemorrhage, fistulae, and esophageal perforation in adults with viral esophagitis are described.[74,75] Acute HIV infection can also cause esophagitis.[76]

Candida, the most common infectious cause of esophagitis, has the classic appearance of white plaques on the mucosa, which cannot be washed or brushed off, unlike food or milk residue, and which often extend up to the upper third of the esophagus (Figure 6).[77] Oral *Candida* is not predictive of esophageal involvement except in the immunocompromised host, but even in these children, extensive esophageal involvement is seen in the absence of oral candidiasis.[78] Mucositis and a white cell count less than 0.5 {164} 10^6/L predisposes patients with leukemia to candidal esophagitis.[79] Steroid use (even poor technique with inhaled steroids for asthma) or acquired or congenital immunocompromise may be etiologic and may have the appearance of white focal lesions on the esophageal surface (Figure 7). This appearance may be difficult to distinguish from allergic esophagitis. Apart from the macroscopic appearances, diagnosis is confirmed by the presence of hyphae

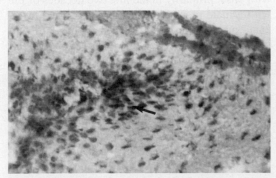

Figure 3 Eotaxin, a recently described eosinophil-specific chemokine. (Darker staining area marked by an arrow.)

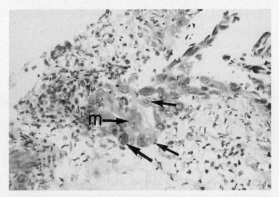

Figure 4 Herpes esophagitis with nuclear inclusions, multinucleate giant cells, and a prominent mononuclear cell infiltrate.

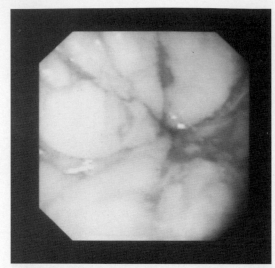

Figure 6 Candidal esophagitis has the classic appearance of white plaques on the mucosa that cannot be washed or brushed off.

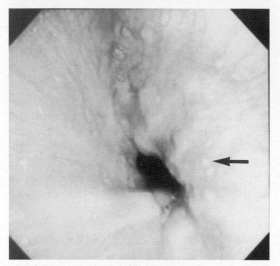

Figure 7 Candidal esophagitis may have the appearance of white focal lesions on the esophagus, which may be difficult to distinguish from allergic esophagitis.

in biopsies (Figure 8). Culture is not helpful because coexistent oral *Candida* can confuse the assessment. Complications include fistulae, perforation, painless stricture formation, esophageal dysmotility, transient achalasia,[80] and systemic candidiasis. A 2- to 6-week course of oral nystatin can be effective in those with normal immune function, but it is more convenient to give fluconazole. Fluconazole or liposomal amphotericin is required, and both are effec-

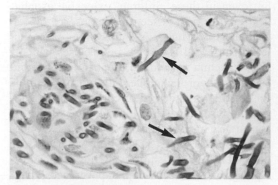

Figure 8 Candidal hyphae (*arrows*).

tive in the immunocompromised child. Esophageal resection and diversion for necrotizing candidal esophagitis have been successful in a 10-year old.[81]

Eradication of *H. pylori* in adults has been associated with increased acid production and hence more noxious gastroesophageal refluxate. However, there does not seem to be any increased incidence of esophagitis in the presence of, or following, the eradication of *H. pylori* in children.[82] Because *H. pylori* affects gastric epithelium, it is not surprising that it has been identified in Barrett's epithelium in a child, in whom symptoms resolved only with addition of amoxicillin to antireflux therapy.[83] Primary bacterial esophagitis is described in immunocompromised patients.[84] Other opportunistic organisms causing esophagitis, such as *Cryptosporidium* and *Acremonium*, have been reported.[85,86]

Traumatic Esophagitis

Trauma causing esophageal pathology could, of course, be accidental, intentional, or iatrogenic. The presence of a nasogastric tube may be associated with abrasive esophagitis, and it has been postulated that the severe esophagitis found in newborn infants in one study, in the absence of other etiologic factors, may have been secondary to enthusiastic upper GI suction at birth.[7] Of particular note was the severity of the esophagitis in the face of relatively minimal symptomatology, such as feeding refusal. Radiation-induced esophageal strictures are described in children receiving mediastinal irradiation (usually greater than 4,000 cGy) and doxorubicin, occurring between 1 and 10 years posttherapy.[87] Radiation-associated esophagitis following bone marrow transplant conditioning is known to occur in the subsequent 1 to 2 weeks but is usually amenable to medical therapy.

Systemic Disease Manifestation

GER occurs more commonly in diverse conditions such as cystic fibrosis, severe combined immunodeficiency, cerebral palsy, raised intracranial pressure, celiac disease, and conditions associated with impaired gastric emptying.[88,89] Certain diseases are, however, associated with esophagitis, which is not via the pathogenetic pathway of reflux. Crohn's disease is a prime example, and Crohn's lesions in the esophagus are usually distinct rounded ulcers, although diffuse disease may also occur (Figure 9). Endoscopic examination with biopsy of the upper GI tract should be part of the diagnostic workup of a child with suspected Crohn's disease.[90] Relapse of the disease may be associated with recurrence of esophageal manifestations.[91] Type 1b glycogen storage disease may present with similar phenotype to Crohn's disease, and severe esophageal involvement has been noted in childhood in this condition.[92] Inflammation and stricturing of the esophagus can occur in chronic granulomatous disease and can involve most of its length, making balloon dilation difficult.[93] Scleroderma and

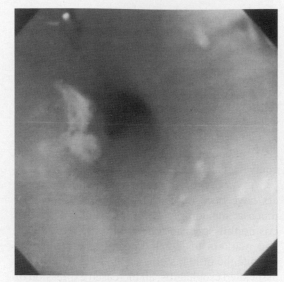

Figure 9 Distinct round ulcers of Crohn's esophagitis.

vasculitic conditions such as polyarteritis nodosa have significant esophageal pathology in adults but are very rare in pediatric populations.

Miscellaneous Causes

Passive smoking has a strong association with esophagitis in childhood. The reasons behind this are not completely understood, but nicotine is known to relax the LES and may decrease mucosal blood flow. The nicotine levels in swallowed saliva may directly injure the esophagus or render it more susceptible to injury from acid exposure. Also, free radicals present in tobacco smoke may reduce antioxidant defenses.[94]

Munchausen syndrome by proxy (dealt with in Chapter 20, "Immune and Inflammatory Disorders") can be at the root of esophagitis in children, but this is usually due to the deliberate introduction into the esophagus by the perpetrator of caustic or irritative substances.[95]

Idiopathic: Eosinophilic Esophagitis

Eosinophilic esophagitis (EE) is characterized by a dense eosinophilic infiltrate in the absence of GER, parasitic infection, or other recognized causes of eosinophilic inflammation.[53,96] The importance of IL-5 and eotaxin, both potent eosinophilic chemokines in the mucosal recruitment of the eosinophilic infiltrate, has recently been recognized.[97] It is an unusual entity and may encompass a wide range of symptoms and histology. EE is a disease with onset primarily in the first two decades of life with a male preponderance, and is defined by its anatomical confinement to the esophagus distinguishing it from eosinophilic enterocolonopathies. Clinical definition is provided by the absence of response of GOR-like symptoms to high-dose proton pump inhibitor use and/or a normal pH study, and the spectrum of clinical symptoms characterizing its presentation, and differentiating it from other esophageal diseases that is in one series 66% of individuals presented with dysphagia compared to only 3% of the control GER group.[98] GER-like symptoms can occur but are often intermittent and refractory to GER management.

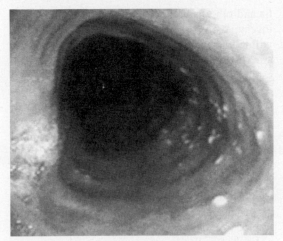

Figure 10 Macroscopic appearances of idiopathic eosinophilic esophagitis: concentric ring indentations and inference of edema and inflammation.

EE is familial in 30 to 40%, and non-GI symptoms may occur such as wheezing, eczema, and allergic rhinitis. It is important to diagnose EE definitively because it may result in narrowing or stricturing of the proximal or mid-esophagus. Macroscopically, it appears as either concentric indentations for most of the length of the esophagus, white plaques, or longitudinal furrows and with the suggestion of background mucosal edema and inferred inflammation, or[99] (Figure 10).[54] Indeed, the suggestion of inflammation has been confirmed by one endosonographic study identifying an increase in the diameter of the submucosa and muscularis layers in children with this increasingly common pathology (Figure 11).[54] In conjunction with this, it is becoming clear that a distinction can be made between EE and simple allergic esophagitis on histology. EE will have more than 20 to 40 eosinophils per HPF, whereas allergic esophagitis will have less than 10 to 15 eosinophils per HPF (Figure 12). It is of particular interest that the prevalence of EE is increasing over the last 5 to 10 years and is clearly not simply acquisition bias. The prevalence is now determined by the order of other chronic GI diseases such as

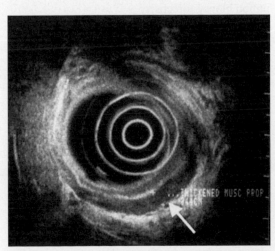

Figure 11 Endosonographic appearances of idiopathic eosinophilic esophagitis: increase in thickness of submucosa and muscularis layers (*arrow*). (Courtesy Dr V. Fox.)

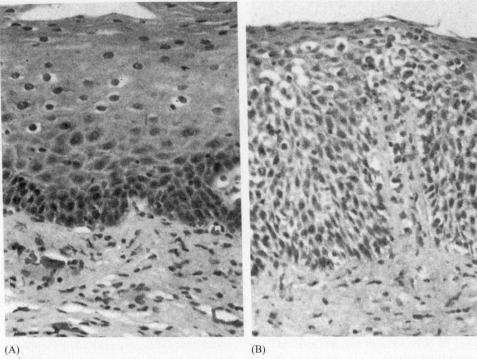

(A)   (B)

Figure 12 Density of eosinophilic infiltrate differs between allergic esophagitis (<10 to 15 eosinophils/high-power field) and idiopathic eosinophilic esophagitis (>20 to 40 eosinophils/high-power field).

Crohn's disease in many developed countries. It is a disease of the developed world, initially recognized in the United States, then also in Australia, Canada, South America, and Europe, and its incidence is now approaching that of Crohn's disease that is 9/100,000 up to 2004 in Australia (when it had been only 0.5/100,000 in 1995), and 10/100,000 up to 2003 in the United States (with a prevalence in this study of 43/100,000), with an apparent rapid upward trend.[98,100] In the latter study only 53 of 381 presented over the age of 15 years, but why this should be is at present unknown. Interestingly, in contradistinction to reflux esophagitis, the distal esophagus may be spared, and proximal esophageal biopsies are always recommended if EE or allergic esophagitis is suspected. Allergy testing does not usually help to identify a responsible allergen because EE, as the name suggests, is idiopathic, but this can sometimes be helpful in allergic esophagitis. Treatment approaches are dealt with in the later section on therapy. In summary, major advances have been made over the past 10 years in the comprehension of this new disease entity, and there seems to be an explosion in incidence of this occurring at present, usually in the first two decades of life with debilitating consequences for the sufferer.

SYMPTOMS

Comparatively little has been validated regarding the appearance, prevalence, or specificity of symptoms of esophagitis. In the infant, parents and the clinician may have differing opinions on what constitutes excessive crying, irritability, and regurgitation, but parents have often learnt to distinguish what is normal and abnormal crying for their infant. It must be remembered, how-

ever, that crying varies with age and often with the time of day, peaking in frequency between 6 weeks and 3 months, with the majority occurring in the evening.[101] Excessive crying or irritability is likely to be associated with pathologic GER or esophagitis over, but not under, 3 months of age,[102] and feed refusal may occur if the infant associates this (consciously or subconsciously) with pain on swallowing.[105] Excessive crying and irritability-causing maternal distress leading to child abuse have been reported in three cases.[106] Visceral hyperalgesia, in which prior painful GER leads to sensory nerve changes, which, in turn, lead to pain with subsequent innocuous stimuli, may be important and may explain in part the lack of a clear correlation of symptoms and esophageal pathology in some cases.[2,104–106] Paroxysmal head posturing, often with torticollis or neck extension, is known as Sandifer-Sutcliffe syndrome (Figure 13).[107] Refractory wheezing as an association of GER rather than esophagitis is well recognized and may be secondary to vagal stimulation at the distal esophagus.[108] GER airway–associated sequelae are noted in

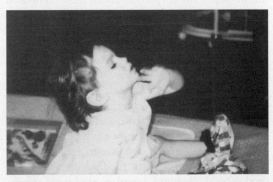

Figure 13 Sandifer-Sutcliffe syndrome, which usually manifests as torticollis, in this case as neck hyperextension that resolved on adequate acid suppression.

Table 1 Common Symptoms/Associations with Esophagitis (Usually Due to Reflux) in Infants

General	Specific
Excessive crying	Hematemesis/melena/fecal occult blood
Irritability	Anemia
"Colic"	Sandifer's syndrome (torticollis)
Feeding refusal	Aspiration
Failure to thrive	Wheezing
Excessive regurgitation	Apnea, stridor
Vomiting	Apparent life-threatening events
	Sudden infant death syndrome

Table 2 Common Symptoms/Associations with Esophagitis in Older Children

Epigastric pain, especially peri-/postprandial and nocturnal
Nausea/regurgitation/vomiting
Anorexia
Food refusal/specific feeding disturbances
Heartburn
"Dyspepsia"/chest pain
Odynophagia
Dysphagia
Early satiety
Hematemesis/melena
Anemia

Table 1 and dealt with more fully in Chapter 4.2, "Gastroesophageal Reflux."

Anemia is uncommonly due to esophagitis in an infant, but hematemesis merits same day endoscopy, if feasible. Fecal occult blood has been noted in only 15% of infants and toddlers with esophagitis, although all patients with pH study evidence of GER had esophagitis when endoscopy was performed for hematemesis.[105] Even prenatal GI bleeding has been reported secondary to esophagitis.[5]

The term "colic" is defined as paroxysms of irritability, fussing, or crying lasting more than 3 hours per day for 3 days per week and has been estimated to occur in up to 25% of infants (see Chapter 13, "Congenital Anomalies Including Hernias"). It probably represents a variant of normal infant development. Pediatricians have a difficult decision to make to determine what is abnormal in this situation, but it would be wise to assume a low threshold of suspicion for reflux esophagitis if the irritability is excessive, according to their judgment or that of the parents,[109] bearing in mind that there is a significant overlap between maternal perceptions of "colic" and what is termed "normal infant distress."[110]

In 34 patients with an endoscopic diagnosis of esophagitis (median age of 6.5 months), Ryan and colleagues recognized the following symptoms: repeated regurgitation (100%), excessive crying and irritability (85%), significant sleep disturbance (79%), failure to thrive (41% below 10th percentile for weight/age), and hematemesis (29%). Maternal distress was a common finding in infants less than 6 months. These were compared with a group of 28 infants with no or minimal esophagitis in whom the respective percentages were 100, 58, 21, 11, and 3%. Hence, regurgitation was not predictive of esophagitis.[106] Tables 1 and 2 outline the common symptom characteristics seen in infancy and in older children.

In the group between 1 and 5 years who are still not able to verbalize and describe their symptoms accurately, there may be a mixture of both constellations of symptoms, but they may remain nonspecific, with feeding disorders and food refusal, sleeping disorders, and more generalized behavioral problems predominating. In the younger age groups, it is important to realize that

there is no clear relationship between symptoms and the severity of the esophagitis. The extent of such symptoms as irritability, crying, failure to thrive, or wheezing does not predict the severity of esophagitis.[1,104,105] It is also important to be aware that GER and associated esophagitis may be secondary phenomena to other pathology outside the GI tract, such as urinary tract infections, raised intracranial pressure, deliberate poisoning, and metabolic conditions.

Older children exhibit symptoms similar to adults and are less of a diagnostic conundrum. Conjecture exists regarding the role of esophagitis in recurrent abdominal pain, and in one series, 38% of such children had esophagitis on endoscopy.[111] However, although this may be true for recurrent epigastric pain, it is not generally thought to account for such a large proportion of classic periumbilical recurrent abdominal pain.

It is reasonable to include endoscopy and esophageal manometry in the diagnostic workup of children with chest pain, as Glassman and colleagues demonstrated esophagitis in 28%, and esophageal spasm and dysmotility in 25% of consecutive children complaining of chest pain.[112] Eleven of 16 children with asthma and chest pain had endoscopic and histologic evidence of esophagitis in a study by Berezin and colleagues, and all 16 had significant GER on pH study.[113] Rarely, hypertrophic osteoarthropathy has been reported with esophagitis in childhood.[114]

DIAGNOSIS

In this context, one is clearly concerned with determining a number of important issues, namely, the presence, severity, extent, etiology, and potential complications of esophagitis. Hence, investigations must be tailored to the question being asked. Indeed, in uncomplicated cases of GER, no investigation may be indicated, and simple therapeutic measures or even a trial of a first-line antireflux medication such as ranitidine may be a first-line diagnostic and therapeutic manouever.[115,116] Ambulant esophageal pH analysis will give an indication of the nature and severity of acid or alkali reflux, whereas endoscopy with biopsy reveals the nature and severity of the esophagi-

tis and other pathology in the upper GI tract, and investigations such as an upper GI barium series will tell us only about anatomic abnormalities and are clearly an inadequate method for looking at esophagitis.

Endoscopy with Biopsy

Endoscopy of the whole upper GI tract (esophagus, stomach, and duodenum) with multiple biopsies is the investigation of choice in evaluation of infants and children with symptoms suggestive of esophagitis.[1,2] This should be performed only by experienced and qualified pediatric endoscopists trained in endoscopy in infants and children. Technology now allows us to perform esophagogastroduodenoscopy in even the smallest infants.[117,118] It is, however, useful only if it will lead to alteration in diagnosis, treatment, or prognosis, and position papers for the North American and European Pediatric Gastroenterology Societies have recently been published.[2,110,113,119,120] Short general anesthetic is preferable to sedation for the procedure for reasons of safety, ease, and success of a complete and comprehensive study.[121]

Macroscopic appearances of the esophagus revealing, for instance, erythema, erosions, or ulceration will guide biopsy acquisition from the areas and lesions most likely to yield highest diagnostic return. A normal endoscopy or an absence of macroscopic lesions does not exclude the presence of histologic esophagitis,[122] and with our increased understanding of the variety of etiologies for esophagitis, biopsies have an enhanced role in altering management; the counterargument to this was previously advanced to defend endoscopy without esophageal biopsy in cases in which no macroscopic lesions existed,[1,3,4] and these authors also suggested that the increase in the cost of endoscopy, when combined with biopsy, may mitigate against the latter in some countries. This is generally held to be an outdated philosophy. No conjecture exists when performing biopsies for detection or surveillance of Barrett's esophagus in which four-quadrant biopsies between 2 and 5 cm from the GEJ can be most helpful—the so-called Seattle protocol, using jumbo biopsy forceps.[123]

Classifications and scoring systems are employed in an attempt to semiquantify the appearances suggestive of esophagitis, which helps to remove interobserver error. The most widely used of these are the modified Savary-Miller criteria (Table 3, Figure 14).[124] The classification of Hetzel and colleagues has also been employed (Table 4); however, a criticism of this is that distinction between grades 0 and 1 is relatively subjective.[120] These classification systems have uses other than introducing objectivity, that is, the pretreatment grade of esophagitis is of value in predicting the pattern and severity of acid reflux and healing rates,[125] and improvement to grade 0 or 1 would be the usual aim, in either classification, of treatment. The specific macroscopic appearances of conditions other than GER esophagitis are noted in the relevant sections on

Table 3 Proposed Endoscopic Classification of Esophagitis	
Grade	Features
0	Normal mucosa
1	Nonconfluent erosions appearing as red patches or striae just above the Z line*
	Erythema or loss of vascular pattern
2	Longitudinal noncircumferent erosions with a hemorrhagic tendency of the mucosa
2a	1 plus bleeding to light touch (friability)
2b	1 plus spontaneous bleeding
3	Circumferent tendency; no strictures
4a	Ulcerations with stricture or metaplasia
4b	Stricture without erosions or ulcerations

Adapted from Savary, Miller.[123]

*Z line defined as junction between columnar gastric fungal mucosa and stratified esophageal mucosa.

pathogenesis above. Hassal suggests that erosions usually found on the tops of esophageal folds are specific for reflux disease, often with a rim of erythema around the white erosions[3]; however, these may mimic, for instance, Crohn's disease (see Figure 9). Gupta and colleagues suggest that vertical lines in the distal esophageal mucosa are a true endoscopic manifestation of reflux esophagitis in children (Figure 15).[126] In severe ulcerated esophagitis, objective proof of recovery following treatment is important, and repeat endoscopy between 3 and 12 weeks later is generally recommended.

Generally, it is held that although the majority of esophagitis is due to reflux, the esophageal appearances themselves do not reliably differentiate between reflux and other causative pathologies. This is perfectly demonstrated in the diagnosis and management of esophagitis in children with cancer, in whom esophagitis is a common occurrence but whose etiology is not predicted accurately by clinical observations (eg, oral candidiasis does not predict for candidal esophagitis) or by macroscopic endoscopic appearances[127]—hence, the requirement for confirmatory biopsy and histology.

Histology

A diagrammatic representation of an esophageal cross section is shown in Figure 16. Nowadays, biopsies are endoscopic, but suction biopsies have been assayed in the past and probably yield a deeper, more satisfactory biopsy.[128] When suction biopsies were added to conventional grasp biopsy technique in a study by Hyams and colleagues, the histologic diagnosis of esophagitis was increased from 60 to 83% of cases, although if one takes more biopsies, one would expect a greater diagnostic yield given the patchy nature of childhood esophagitis; hence, this cannot be used to suggest that suction biopsies are superior in pediatric practice.[105] Friesen and colleagues showed no statistically significant difference in predictive value for esophagitis in infants between the two techniques.[129] Correctly, oriented endoscopic biopsies (eg, immediate orientation on filter paper or nylon mesh in 10% formalin) are, however, perfectly adequate, and so-called "crocodile" biopsy forceps, which allow the operator to biopsy perpendicular to the esophageal lumen, may be preferable. Large-cup ("jumbo") biopsy forceps are increasingly used and are mandatory for the surveillance of Barrett's esophagus using the so-called Seattle protocol (quadrantic biopsies every 1 cm above the GEJ involving the distal 5 cm of the esophagus) because they yield deeper biopsies.[123] The site of biopsy should be above the distal 15% of the esophagus to avoid confusion with normal variance.[105] Biopsies should include epithelium, lamina propria, and muscularis mucosae and be oriented in a perpendicular plane to maximize diagnostic yield, such as evaluating properly the thickness of the basal zone, vascular ingrowth, and the elongation of the stromal papillae. For definitive diagnosis, the presence of two of three of these features is preferable, which will not be possible with poorly oriented tissue.[1,2] In an adult study, failure to use well-defined histologic criteria resulted in only 50% sensitivity for diagnosing esophagitis.[130] The classic histologic findings of GER esophagitis are displayed in Table 5 (Figure 17). Elongation of stromal papillae is a useful indicator of reflux, and basal zone hyperplasia is defined when the papillae are more than 25% of the entire thickness of the epithelium, and if more than 50%, then the papillae are considered to be elongated.[58]

Esophageal mucosal eosinophilia has been described in both suspected cow's milk–associated[46] and primary reflux esophagitis,[52] as well as in other conditions, such as primary eosinophilic esophagitis (see Figures 2 and 12).[53] The clinical significance of eosinophils and their role in the pathogenesis of mucosal injury are poorly understood and are the subject of recent debate.[3,4,55] Some have suggested an active role for eosinophils in the inflammatory process of esophagitis and have supported this with the observation of resolution of symptoms and eosinophils in the esophagus on dietary exclusion of cow's milk[46,48] or with oral steroids,[46,53] both suggesting a pathoetiologic role for eosinophils. The mucosal density of the eosinophils may be important, as noted above, in distinguishing between allergic esophagitis and EE. In addition to eosinophils, intraepithelial T lymphocytes, known as CINC or squiggle cells, have also been implicated as markers of reflux esophagitis (Figure 18).[57,59] However, the degree of intraluminal esophageal acid exposure did not correlate well with the CINC count in one study in children, and the authors use this fact to question the day-to-day reliability of pH-metry in defining the extent of reflux in children.[58] In adults, such cells are of memory phenotype and display activation markers,[59] although little is known of their pediatric equivalents. The finding of mucosal mast cells may also help to differentiate GER from CMP-associated esophagitis, but there is considerable overlap with the presence of eosinophils.[56] Neutrophils also indicate a degree of inflammation,[12] and actual numbers of eosinophils and/or neutrophils per most involved HPF have been used to indicate the severity of esophagitis.[58] Minimal histologic criteria are simultaneous occurrence of elongated papillae and basal zone hyperplasia. Moderate esophagitis is diagnosed if there is ingrowth of vessels in the papillae, and 1 to 19 eosinophils/neutrophils are seen in the most involved HPF. Severe esophagitis is diagnosed if more than 20 eosinophils/neutrophils are seen in the most involved HPF. However, the criteria established by European Society of Pediatric Gastroenterology, Hepatology and Nutrition and displayed in Table 5 are probably the most robust to date.[2]

The important point to realize is that correlation between macroscopic and histologic features is generally poor, partly because the esophagitis may be a patchy lesion but also because histologic esophagitis may exist when the esophagus is macroscopically normal.[122] This is not now merely academic because it does have the potential to direct therapy appropriately, for example, in the case of CMP allergy or intolerance-associated esophagitis when a cow's milk exclusion diet is associated with a better outcome than use of antacid therapy alone, and it is suggested that up to 40% of cases of esophagitis may have CMP intolerance as an etiologic factor.[46,48,61]

Table 4 Endoscopic Classification of Esophagitis	
Grade	Features
0	No mucosal abnormalities
1	Erythema, hyperemia, mucosal friability
2	Longitudinal noncircumferent erosions with a hemorrhagic tendency of the mucosa
3	Superficial erosions or ulceration of 10 to 50% of the mucosal surface of the distal 5 cm of esophageal squamous mucosa
4	Deep peptic ulceration anywhere in the esophagus or confluent erosion of >50% of the mucosal surface of the distal 5 cm of the esophageal squamous mucosa

Adapted from Hetzel et al.[124]

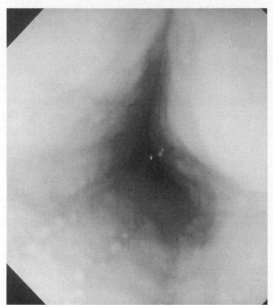

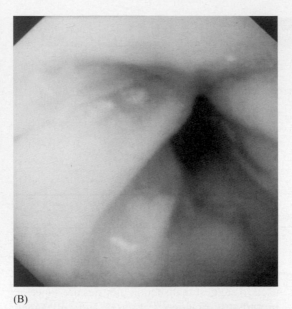

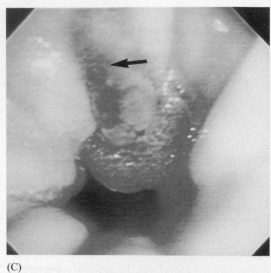

(A)

(B)

(C)

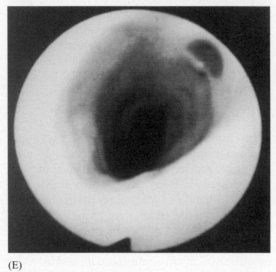

(D)

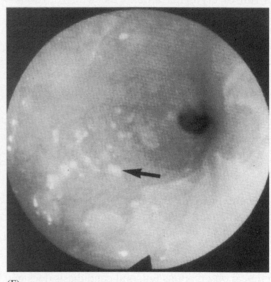

(E)

(F)

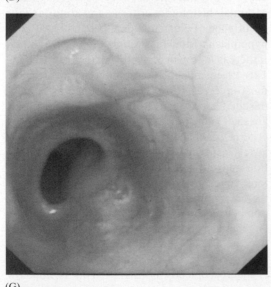

(G)

Figure 14 Savary-Miller–based grading of macroscopic appearances of esophagitis. (A) Grade 1, erythema or loss of vascular pattern. (B) Grade 1, nonconfluent erosions. (C) Grade 2, longitudinal erosions (*arrow*). (D) Grade 3, circumferent erosions. (E) Grade 4a, ulceration. (F) Grade 4a, metaplasia, islands of stratified epithelium within histologically confirmed gastric metaplastic mucosa (*arrow*). (G) Grade 4b, stricture without erosions.

Furthermore, with the advent of more complex diagnostic techniques such as immuno-histochemistry and electron microscopy, the esophagus, which is apparently normal both macroscopically and histologically, may still yield diagnostic information. Standard endoscopic biopsy and histology do not reliably distinguish between, for instance, primary reflux esophagitis and the emerging clinical entity of cow's milk–associated reflux esophagitis. Some differentiation from primary reflux has been suggested on the basis of esophageal pH testing pattern and {158}-lactoglobulin antibody response, although the former has not been substantiated by more than one center.[48,49]

Barrett's esophagus and premalignant or malignant esophageal pathology are dealt with in Chapter 4.2, "Gastroesophageal Reflux." Cytologic esophageal brushings may be helpful in such situations, as they are in candidal esophagitis.[131]

Immunohistochemistry

A variety of immunohistochemical markers have been used to examine the esophageal mucosa. An increase in Ki-67, a proliferation marker, has been shown in the longer papil-

lae seen in GER, suggesting increased cell turnover (Figure 19). Basal focal distribution of CD4 lymphocytes showing expression of the activation markers CD25 and HLA-DR, together with upregulated epithelial HLA-DR expression, has also been reported.[61] Eotaxin

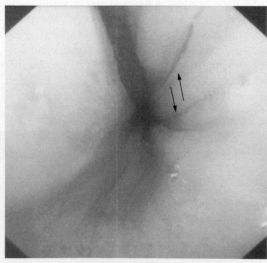

Figure 15 Vertical lines in the distal esophageal mucosa may be an endoscopic manifestation of reflux esophagitis (*arrows*).

Table 5 Grading Criteria for Histologic Appearance of Esophagus

Grade	Histologic Criteria	Clinical Diagnosis
	Normal	Normal
1a	Basal zone hyperplasia	Reflux
1b	Elongated stromal papillae	Reflux
1c	Vascular ingrowth	Reflux
2	Polymorphs in the epithelium ± lamina propria	Esophagitis
3	Polymorphs with epithelial defect	Esophagitis
4	Ulceration	Esophagitis
5	Aberrant columnar epithelium	Esophagitis

guishing this from primary reflux esophagitis (see Figure 3).[61] Inhibitory neurotransmitter production is integral to LES relaxation, and the non-adrenergic, noncholinergic neurotransmitter NO has received recent attention in human studies.[16,17] Increased esophageal expression of iNOS has also been noted,[23,25] although in another study, it was not upregulated in the inflamed pediatric esophagus.[24] Because NO is a powerful smooth muscle relaxant, it is interesting to speculate whether inflammation-induced iNOS may play a role in LES relaxation, leading to more reflux and hence worse inflammation, and so on. An exciting development is that of confocal endomicroscopy in which real time images of the cell ultrastructure can be obtained at endoscopy.

is a recently described eosinophil-specific chemokine,[60] and, despite the mild histologic abnormality in CMP-associated esophagitis, an increased expression of eotaxin colocalized with activated T lymphocytes to the basal and papillary epithelium has been shown, distin-

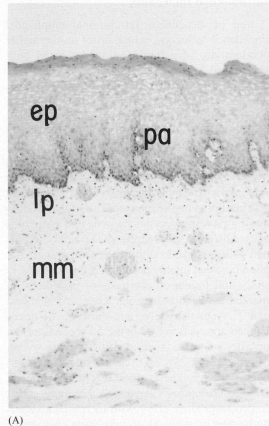

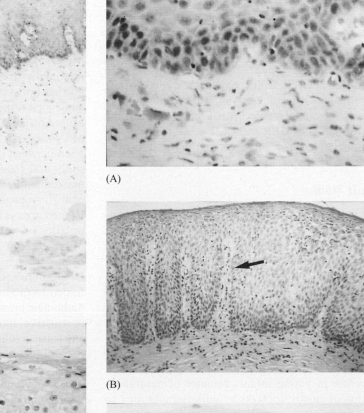

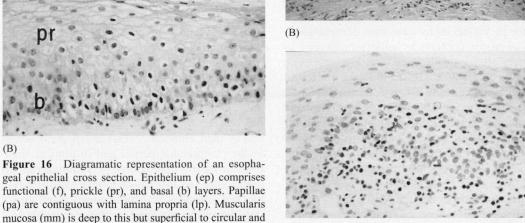

Figure 16 Diagramatic representation of an esophageal epithelial cross section. Epithelium (ep) comprises functional (f), prickle (pr), and basal (b) layers. Papillae (pa) are contiguous with lamina propria (lp). Muscularis mucosa (mm) is deep to this but superficial to circular and longitudinal muscle layers and serosa, not shown.

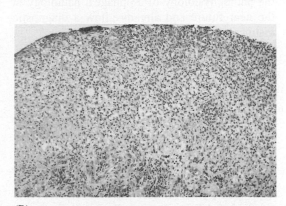

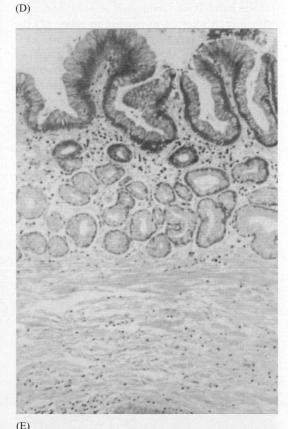

Figure 17 Histologic grading system of esophagitis. (A) Grade 0, normal esophagus. (B) Grade 1a and 1b, basal zone hyperplasia (when the papillae are >25% of the entire thickness of the epithelium) and elongation of papillae (>50%) (*arrow*). (C) Grade 2, polymorphs in the epithelium ± lamina propria. (D) Grade 3, polymorphs with epithelial defect. (E) Grade 4, ulceration, epithelium replaced by granulation tissue.

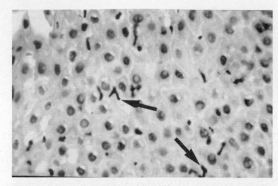

Figure 18 Intraepithelial T lymphocytes, known as cells with irregular nuclear contours or squiggle cells (*arrows*).

Hence, techniques such as immunohisto-chemistry will allow better comprehension of the pathophysiology of esophageal pathology in the near future and already allow a diagnostic distinction to be drawn between etiologies.

Electron Microscopy

Electron microscopy has demonstrated the ultra-structural changes associated with esophagitis, adding to our comprehension of the lesion. Strati-fied squamous nonkeratinizing epithelium line the mucosa, and the surface is composed of large flat cells displaying a regular pattern of parallel microridges 200 nm in thickness. Three layers are visible by transmission electron microscopy: (1) the basal layer, composed of polygonal cells with a high nucleus-to-cytoplasm ratio; (2) the intermediate layer, composed of large prickle cells; and (3) the superficial layer, composed of flattened cells. Three grades of ultrastructural changes in esophagitis in children have been identified: grade I, irregular microridges and reduced intercellular junctions; grade II, of the superficial epithelium only, microvilli instead of microridges that, when present, are distorted, and extruding cells with degeneration and inter-ruptions of the cell membrane; lymphocytes and monocytes occupy the large intercellular spaces in the intermediate layer, and the basal layer is thickened; and grade III, microerosive cytopa-thy, loss of superficial layer microridges with crater-like erosions and abundant cell debris. Degenerating cells are seen in all three layers (Figure 20). Reduced numbers of desmosomes

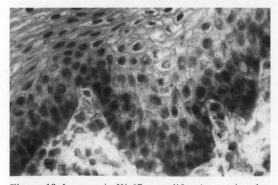

Figure 19 Increase in Ki-67, a proliferation marker, has been shown in the longer papillae seen in gastroesopha-geal reflux, suggesting increased cell turnover.

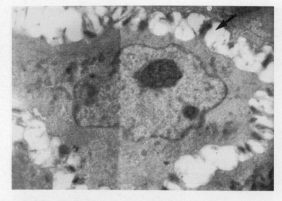

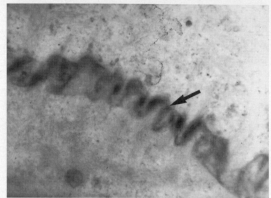

Figure 20 Ultrastructural changes in esophagitis in chil-dren, grade I, irregular desmosomes and reduced intercel-lular junctions.

and large intercellular spaces containing lympho-monocytes are seen. Ultrastructural damage to nuclei, nucleoli, Golgi complex, and endoplasmic reticulum is seen. Activation of eosinophils by electron microscopic criteria has helped in the distinction of GER and CMP-associated esopha-gitis.[56] Hence, a more compelling case can be made for biopsy than previously.

pH Studies

Esophageal pH monitoring has gained gen-eral acceptance as the method for assessment of GER in children and until recently has been regarded as the investigation technique of first choice in infants and children with unusual pre-sentations of GER disease, such as apnea and recurrent respiratory disease.[132–134] However, pH measurements cannot detect GER in the pH range of 4.0 to 7.0 owing to the proximity to the normal esophageal pH.[135,136] Consequently, pH-metry misses many episodes of postprandial reflux in young infants because of neutraliza-tion of gastric contents by milk formula for 1 to 2 hours after a meal. Therefore, the term acid, neutral, or alkaline GER should be preferred over the blanket term GER. A poor correlation exists between morphometry and histology and classic parameters used in pH studies[3,135]; how-ever, this correlation is improved by analysis of esophageal acid exposure using the param-eter area under pH 4.0.[138] Indeed, pH-metry does not detect GER directly but measures the H[+] ion concentration at the sensor site.[139]

Hyams and colleagues found no correlation between any pH parameter (except the acid reflux

in the 2 to 4 hours following a clear liquid feed) and the severity of esophagitis or macroscopic appearances suggesting esophagitis and histo-logic changes, and this has been seen by other groups.[105,122] Ambulant esophageal pH-metry is dealt with in greater detail in Chapter 4.2, "Gastroesophageal Reflux."

Currently, available techniques for the study of reflux that are pH-independent include ultra-sonography,[140] aspiration,[141] scintigraphy,[142] fluoroscopy,[143] bilirubin monitoring,[144] and pH monitoring. However, the disadvantages of these methods include short-term applicability, a high incidence of artifact caused by body move-ment, and the requirement for unphysiologic, nonambulant body positioning. These methods fall far short of the ideal because they measure only a short time window and do not allow for symptom or event temporal correlation.

Intraluminal Impedance

A new pH-dependent, intraluminal esophageal impedance technique, which relies on the higher conductivity of a liquid bolus compared with esophageal muscular wall or air, has been vali-dated in adults. When used in infants with GER who had simultaneous pH measurement for pro-longed periods, intraluminal esophageal imped-ance showed that 73% of all GER occurs during or in the first 2 hours after feeding. Furthermore, this is pH neutral and, therefore, will be missed by pH-metry. Indeed, 75% of GER extends proximally as far as the pharyngeal space, and this has broad implications for the study of GER-associated respiratory phenomena and symptoms caused by gastrolaryngopharyngeal reflux. Wenzl and colleagues re-examined the temporal associ-ation between infant apnea and reflux in a recent study and found, on the basis of impedance, a marked association between these two phenom-ena.[145] Approximately, one-third of all docu-mented apneas occurred in the 30 seconds before or after an impedance-identified reflux event, of which only 23% were acidic reflux events— hence, the hypothesis that GER may stimulate laryngeal receptors. Conversely, they suggest that forced respiratory effort with increased abdomi-nothoracic pressure, as occurs during episodes of obstructive apnea, can overcome LES pressure and cause a reflux episode.

Multichannel intraluminal impedance mea-surements have allowed new insight into the physiology and pathophysiology of gastrointes-tinal function in health and disease.[148] Patterns of antegrade and retrograde bolus movement, length of the swallowed or refluxed bolus, and direction and velocity of bolus movement can be described precisely.[149] Episodes of GER can be characterized by their height in the esophagus and by their duration.[150] This is especially useful in the postprandial period and in clinical situa-tions of gastric hypoacidity.[151] Simultaneous pH monitoring and IMP allow further categorization of GER episodes.[152] Multichannel intraluminal impedance measurement is also a valuable tool for describing the process of GER clearance and swallowing, allowing a distinction to be drawn between the protective events of volume clearance and acid clearance (primarily by swallowing of saliva) in the prevention of GER-associated lower esophageal reflux pathology and associated symptoms. Although normative values for various pediatric age groups remain to be defined, this technique already allows time-related associations to be made for GER and symptoms and allows interventional therapeutic studies to be conducted for the first time on a physiologically appropriate basis. With increasing clinical use of the IMP in children, normative data will soon be available. Until then, IMP can be performed in studies with a crossover design so that individual subjects may act as their own controls. Indeed, this has already occurred with DBPC trials involving such medications as Gaviscon Infant[153] and dietary manipulations as amino acid based milks such as Neocate.[154]

To document symptom association,[151] IMP can be incorporated into other diagnostic systems, for example, manometry[152,155,156] and sleep studies. Technical effort has now developed a portable-recording device for mobile, outpatient impedance studies in all age groups.[157] Semiautomated and soon fully automated software will allow this to emerge from application on a research basis to have clinical day-to-day applicability, and software for IMP has now been developed and improved to aid in detecting characteristic patterns and eliminating artifact, thereby making it more practical for routine clinical use.[158] The importance of independent, long-term assessment of the esophageal and gastric motility is increasingly recognized, especially for pediatric patients. Impedance monitoring is indeed very promising in revolutionizing this aspect of GER investigation. In the next few years, a combination of pH and intraluminal impedance will be adopted as the new gold standard for investigating reflux events in pediatric settings. Future studies will verify and improve the technique and will broaden our understanding of esophageal motility and its disorders and associated supraesophageal phenomena.

Other techniques, such as intraluminal impedance, may offer advantages over pH-metry for assessing nonacid or neutral reflux, which is the predominant type in the postprandial 1 to 2 hours when most GER occurs, and a variety of studies now point clearly to the inadequacy of assessment of simple acid exposure of the esophagus in determining the role of reflux in the genesis of GER.[159] More recently, Tasker and colleagues suggested that reflux of gastric juice could be a major cause of glue ear in children by analyzing middle ear effusion fluid at the time of grommet insertion for the presence of pepsin (which can only have come from the stomach by reflux) and found it to be present in 83% of cases. This elegant study further supports the association of GER with tubotympanal disorders and also suggests that nonacid reflux may be just as important as acid reflux.[160] Furthermore, some recent studies have looked at the predictive value of pepsin

estimation in such situations as postallograft lung rejection.[161]

Manometry

This is useful in limited circumstances in the evaluation of esophagitis per se, although it has a role in the assessment of GER etiology. Berezin and colleagues studied 31 children with mild to moderate esophagitis and concluded that there were no differences compared with 48 normal controls in LES pressure and the amplitude, duration, and velocity of esophageal contractions.[162] Combined pH/impedance/micromanometry catheters are now available and expose the possibility of a more profound comprehension of all of the issues that contribute to the complex process of a reflux event in an infant or child.

Upper GI Barium Series

Barium studies of the upper GI tract are not helpful in assessment of esophagitis except in detecting the presence or absence of anatomic abnormalities, for example, esophageal strictures, gastric outlet obstruction, and small bowel malrotation, for which they are indispensable. Some authors report specific radiologic abnormalities associated with pathologies such as candidal esophagitis, but the technique of choice is obviously endoscopy in such situations.

Blood Tests

Obviously, hemoglobin estimation will allow anemia to be excluded as a complication of esophagitis. Specific etiologies can be elucidated and distinguished by specific blood tests. Examples include a high anti-{158}-lactoglobulin in CMP-associated esophagitis; radioallergosorbent tests for specific allergens; low-quartile immunoglobulin (Ig)A, high IgE, high IgG, and specifically high IgG$_1$ and IgG$_4$ subclasses, all suggestive of CMP-associated GER; herpes or CMV serology; and raised inflammatory markers such as C-reactive protein, erythrocyte sedimentation rate, and platelet count suggestive of more widespread GI inflammation such as occurs in Crohn's disease.

MANAGEMENT AND PROGNOSIS

Management of esophagitis must, of course, be dictated by its etiology, which further underlines the vital nature of obtaining an accurate diagnosis based on upper endoscopy and histologic assessment. Because the vast majority of cases of esophagitis in infants and children will be due to GER, then treatment of GER and treatment of GER-related esophagitis will be very closely linked. Treatment of GER is also dealt with in Chapter 4.2, "Gastroesophageal Reflux," and the emphasis of this section is toward the rationale for treatment of esophagitis but inevitably touches on anti-GER measures also. Other specific treatments for specific pathologies are also dealt with.

It must be borne in mind that spontaneous resolution of reflux esophagitis may occur. The early studies of Carre indicated in infants that if no active therapy is initiated, approximately 60% will be symptom free by 18 months of age, with the greatest improvement by 8 to 10 months, when the child starts to sit upright; 30% will continue to have symptoms during childhood; approximately 5% develop strictures; and 5% will die of pneumonia or malnutrition.[9] In another, more up-to-date study on the outcome of infant GER esophagitis with accurate recognition and treatment (at that stage, only a histamine$_2$ [H$_2$] antagonist), 82% had responded satisfactorily to medical management by 18 months of age, with 51% being able to cease treatment with spontaneous improvement by 8 to 10 months, a proportion similar to Carre's.[10,104] With the advent of effective antireflux therapies, one would expect the figure of 18% who required antireflux surgery in the latter study to be much less. Shepherd and colleagues advocate the early use of endoscopy to detect the degree of esophagitis because the constellation and severity of symptoms do not always reflect the degree of esophagitis.[10] It is important to know the degree of esophagitis (see Tables 3 and 4) because this may allow one to tailor therapy appropriately and, indeed, prognosticate on outcome. One group suggested that more than seven eosinophils per HPF made the success of treatment with ranitidine and cisapride unlikely, although the confounding factor of allergic esophagitis certainly has importance in this situation.[127] Individualized treatment is the goal, but generalizations may be made based on the severity of the esophagitis and, to an extent, the severity of the symptom constellation. In adult studies, the pretreatment severity of esophagitis is of some help in predicting healing rates on antisecretory therapy.[163,164] It also correlates with the duration and pattern of acid reflux in adults,[165] although a poor correlation exists between morphometry/histology/endoscopic appearances and classic parameters used in pH studies in pediatrics,[3,105,122,137] except, perhaps, area under pH 4.0.[138] Hence, the presence of histologic esophagitis alone may not allow prediction of outcome. It is clear also in adult studies that erosive esophagitis is a chronic problem that has an attendant worse prognosis and will tend to relapse off treatment.[166] This is probably the case in pediatrics also, but this question is very difficult to answer because long-term follow-up studies with treated and untreated patients would be required to provide viable answers.[2]

Figure 21 outlines an algorithm for the treatment of GER esophagitis in infants and children. It is generally agreed that for treatment purposes, infants and children with GER esophagitis can be regarded as falling into two main groups: those with normal (grade 0) or mildly erythematous (grade 1) mucosa and only histologic esophagitis and those with esophagitis, which is erosive or worse (grade 2 or more) (see Figure 14). The milder group will generally receive so-called simple measures, which are particularly applicable in

Possetting/mild reflux
↓
1. Simple measures
Position: 30[198] head-elevated left lateral Trendelenburg
Feeds: ↑ frequency, ↓ volume of each feed
Milk-thickening agents (Nestargel, Carobel)/prethick-
ened milks (Enfamil AR, SMA staydown)
Antacids (Infant Gaviscon)
↓
2. Prokinetic agents
Prokinetic agent such as domperidone 0.4 mg/kg/dose,
3 times daily.
H2 antagonist such as ranitidine 1 to– 3 mg/kg/dose,
3 times daily.
↓
3. Investigate
Investigate as individual case dictates (see text),
eg, pH/endoscopy/barium study
↓
4. Consider substituting CMP-based formula with
caseine-hydrolysate milk (eg, Pregestimil,
Nutramagen, Peptijunior)
or elemental milk (eg, Neocate; Neocate Advance)
(ideally, but not necessarily, following small bowel
biopsy evidence of cow's milk–sensitive enteropathy)
↓
If CMPI not considered a contributory factor
↓
5. Consider additional medical therapy
Proton pump inhibitor (eg, omeprazole 0.7 to–
2.7 mg/kg/dose in 1 to– 2 divided daily doses)
(no place yet for metoclopramide or bethanechol)
(use of misoprostol or sucralfate not yet proven)
↓
5. "Maximum medical therapy" for 6 wk to 3 mo
Maximum doses of
Omeprazole
Domperidone
↓
No significant symptom resolution
↓
6. Consideration for surgery
endoscopic gastroplication
or formal open/laparoscopic Nissen or Thal fundoplication
(± gastrostomy if significant feeding disorder)

Figure 21 Gastroesophageal reflux and esophagitis treatment algorithm in infants and young children.

infancy, such as positioning with the head elevated to 30[198] in the left lateral Trendelenburg
position, which may be effective in up to 25%
of infants with simple regurgitation[2]; advice to
increase the frequency and decrease the volume
of each feed; use of milk-thickening agents (eg,
Nestargel, Carobel) or prethickened milks (eg,
Enfamil AR); and the use of antacids (eg, Infant
Gaviscon), which may be effective in mild,
simple GER.[167–168]

For uncomplicated reflux unresponsive to
these measures, a case can be made for the use
of an H₂ antagonist before further investigation.
Unfortunately, cisapride, the noncholinergic prokinetic drug with 5-hydroxytryptamine4 agonist
properties that improves pH-metric variables[169]
and was the drug of first choice in GER, is no longer widely available owing to concerns, rightly
or wrongly, regarding prolongation of the Q–Tc
interval and cardiac dysrhythmias in childhood. It
is metabolized by the cytochrome P-450 3A4 isoenzyme, as are "azole" antifungal agents and the
macrolide antibiotics erythromycin and clarithro-

mycin, and combinations of these drugs with cisapride have produced cardiac dysrhythmias and
prolonged Q–Tc syndrome in some patients. In a
major article purporting to show a prolongation
of the Q–Tc interval, there was no statistical difference between the cisapride group and the control group with regard to Q–Tc interval or J–Tc
interval. However, 16 of the 35 patients reported
have had a prolongation of Q–Tc.[170] There have
been recent reports of prolonged Q–Tc syndrome
in neonates with cisapride alone,[171] but Levine
and colleagues published a report on the use of
cisapride in 30 children, 12 of whom were premature neonates, and no effect on the Q–T interval was seen.[172,173] A useful and rational summary of risk and benefit has been published.[174] Its
active component, termed nor-cisapride, which
is purported to have no effect on the Q–Tc interval, may be available soon. Tegaserod, acting as
a 5HT₄ agonist is available on a named-patient
basis in the UK but is unlicensed in treatment of
GER in children, and its major market focus has
been in adult irritable bowel syndrome.

H₂ blockers can improve esophagitis, but the
effect on GER cannot be assessed by pH because
they neutralize gastric acid. High-dose ranitidine (6
to 7 mg/kg dose 3 times per day) has been shown
to be as effective as omeprazole in refractory reflux
esophagitis in those children with[175] and without[176]
developmental disabilities. A rebound nocturnal
acid secretion has been reported.[177]

For the second group of infants and children who have documented erosive esophagitis
or whose symptoms are refractory to the use of
ranitidine (grade 2 or more), the treatment must
entail a more aggressive approach.[3] Occasionally,
this will pertain to a young child without a prore-
flux condition, but, more usually, this will be in
an older child with a predisposing condition such
as neurologic compromise, cystic fibrosis, and
repaired esophageal atresia. Medical treatment of
the latter has an effect on the duration of reflux
and could decrease the rate of subsequent stricture
formation.[178] Ongoing trials and recent work with
proton pump inhibitors in infants and children
suggest that they are a useful therapeutic strategy
in refractory reflux esophagitis, producing symptom improvement in all and histologic improvement in 40% in a recent study.[179] It has been proposed as the therapy of choice in children with
neurologic compromise.[180] Symptomatic relapse
is an issue on cessation of therapy, however, and
this may be because the underlying lower esophageal dysmotility is unaltered by omeprazole
therapy.[181] Definitive dose-finding studies remain
to be carried out, and a higher dose/kg may be
required than is observed in adults, for example, 0.7 to 2.0 mg/kg/d of omeprazole.[121,182,183]
Esomeoprazole is identified as having possible
advantages of bioavailability over omeprazole.
Lansoprazole has not been widely studied for
GOR/dyspepsia in childhood to date. Domperidone acts similarly to metoclopramide but has
less dystonic reactions or other side effects and
may be helpful for a limited period, but its objective clinical evidence base is limited.[184,185]

The role of surgery is as a last-line therapy
after maximal medical therapy has failed and
significant complications of GER esophagitis
remain. Most fundoplications to date have been
open Nissen procedures, which involve a full
wraparound of the gastric fundus on the distal
esophagus. Thal procedures are performed less
commonly and involve an approximately 80%
circumferential wrap. Fundoplication probably
works because it prevents full LES relaxation
and a reduction in the number of transient LES
relaxations.[186] A large retrospective (20 years)
multicenter study of over 7,000 children showed
that so-called good to excellent results were
achieved in 96 and 85% of normal and neurologically impaired children, respectively. Mortality
was 0.1 and 0.8%, respectively. Recurrent reflux
occurred in 7%, gas bloat in 3.6%, and obstruction in 2.6%. Reoperation was required in 3.6 and
11.8%, respectively.[187] Failed fundoplication is
reported in those with EE.[53] Laparoscopic fundoplication is becoming more widespread. The
results now compare favorably with the open
procedure,[188] and it is associated with a faster
recovery.[189,190]

Of particular interest recently is the advent
of endoscopic antireflux procedures whose efficacy is well documented in the adult literature
but whose use in pediatrics is still in only a few
centers. One such procedure makes use of an
EndoCinch (C.R. Bard Inc. Murray Hill, New
Jersey, United States) sewing machine attached to
the endoscope, which was used to place three pairs
of stitches below the GEJ to create three internal plications of the stomach (Figure 22).[191,192]
Three or four plications are placed circumferentially or longitudinally 0.5 to 1.5 cm below the
gastroesophageal junction (GEJ), which differs
slightly from the reported adult studies in which
various combinations of plications have been
employed (eg, two circumferential, two or three
longitudinal).

The initial results from a pilot study of 17
children suggest that endoluminal gastroplication
is safe and effective in terms of improved quality of life assessed with two validated quality of
life scoring tools, in terms of symptom scores,

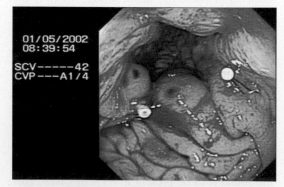

Figure 22 Endoscopic gastroplication (Endocinch) creating three pairs of sutures (plications): either longitudinally
0.5, 1, and 1.5 cm distal to the gastroesophageal junction
(GEJ) and on the lesser curvature; or one each on the
greater and lesser curvatures 1.5 cm distal to the GEJ and
one on the lesser curvature 0.5 cm distal to the GEJ.

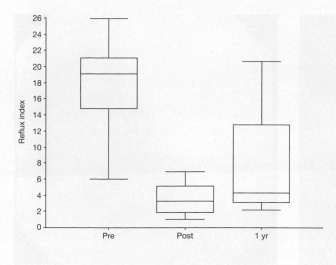

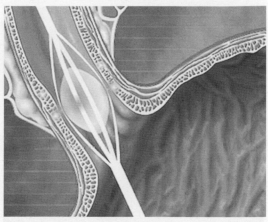

Figure 23 Reflux index of pH pre-, 6 weeks post-, and 36 months postendoscopic gastroplication showing medium-term sustained response. (Wilcoxon rank sum test, and data presented as box and whisker plots with interquartile ranges.)

Figure 25 Delivery of radiofrequency energy to the gastroesophageal junction as an antireflux endoscopic procedure: not performed in children to date.

and objectively with improvement of all analyzed pH parameters in 16 of 16 patients and return to normal values in 9 of 16 patients who underwent pH studies subsequent to endoluminal gastroplication (Figure 23).[193–194]

Questions have been asked regarding the way in which the procedure actually improves the degree of reflux. It may be that the plications help to alter the angle of His, addressing the defective LES, and thereby decrease the amount of refluxate entering the esophagus. Swain and colleagues demonstrated an increase in the length and pressure of the LES.[195] However, other groups have not shown similar findings using esophageal manometry. It may be that the angle of the GEJ is improved or that the number of transient LES relaxations is decreased, and it is known that these are a major contributor to GER disease. Liu and colleagues have shown in porcine and adult human endosonographic studies that tissue remodeling with an increase in the circular smooth muscle layer as a possible "foreign-body" reaction is a putative model of efficacy whereby GEJ compliance is reduced by greater tissue bulk.[196] In addition to this technique is that of the full thickness Plicator whereby a serosa to serosa placation is delivered with a specialized device through which a slim-line 5 mm diameter scope is passed and retroverted in the fundus[197] (Figure 24). These techniques are dealt with in greater detail in the Chapter 46.6, "Interventional Endoscopy: Recent Innovations."

The alternative endoluminal techniques that have been promoted are endoluminal delivery of radiofrequency energy (Figure 25)[198] and endoluminal injection of inert biopolymers (Figure 26)[199]; however, neither of these techniques are reversible and hence not desirable for application in the pediatric patient. As with any new technique, concerns remain about the learning curve of the endoscopist. However, a previous multicenter study in adults does not show a significant difference in the learning curve of endoscopists in different centers.[199]

Removal of CMP from the diet needs to be completed in a case of CMP-associated esophagitis and may occur even in the breastfed infant whose mother is taking dairy produce in her own diet, in which case, these should be excluded from mother's intake, and breastfeeding can continue. CMP-associated symptoms in exclusively breast-fed infants have been reported with a prevalence of 0.37% in a population in which CMP allergy amounts to 1.9%.[200] In those on formula milk, a substitute is required. It is not appropriate to use soy milks because up to 30 to 40% or so of CMP-intolerant infants will also have an intolerance to soy, quite apart from the phytoestrogen effect on young male infants. Classically, an infant will initially improve on the soy formula, and then symptoms similar to those experienced with CMP will ensue some 4 to 6 weeks later. More preferable, and to be recommended as a first-line substitute in this situation, is a casein hydrolysate milk (eg, Pregestimil, Nutramagen, Alimentum) or a whey hydrolysate (eg, Pepti-Junior, Alfa-Ré, Profylac, Hypolac, Nutrilon-Pepti).[201] However, these still contain peptides greater than 15 amino acids in length, which are still capable of precipitating a major histocompatibility complex–mediated immunoreaction. In some instances, it is necessary therefore to go one step further and put the infant exclusively on an elemental milk (eg, Neocate, Neocate Advance, Nutri Junior) containing amino acids, glucose polymer, and long-chain fatty acids. An improvement may be seen within 1 week, but Kelly and colleagues, and other groups, recommend a 6-week trial.[46,202,203] The glucose polymer is used to prevent the osmolality of the milk becoming too high and precipitating osmotic diarrhea. The only drawback of such milks is their unpalatability, but with persistence, infants usually get used to them, especially if introduction occurs early in life. Certain milks may require the addition of calcium to the diet, and involvement of a dietitian is advised. It is normal practice to reintroduce CMP around 12 to 18 months, but some children require dairy exclusion until 3, 4, or more years. Multiple food-associated esophagitis can occur,[47] and in such situations, a few foods diet starting with hypoallergenic components such as rice, potato, green beans, and chicken with stepwise reintroduction may be necessary. A proportion of these infants are also helped by oral sodium cromoglycate, although the evidence base for this is not great.

Infective causes of esophagitis in pediatrics require specific therapies. Viral esophagitis is usually due to herpes simplex, CMV, and,

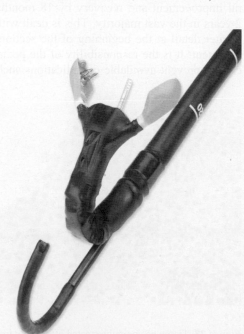

Figure 24 Full thickness plication for GERD.

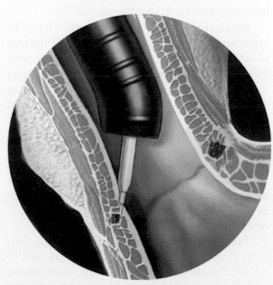

Figure 26 Injection of inert biopolymer into the gastroesophageal junction to act as an antireflux endoscopic procedure: not performed in children to date.

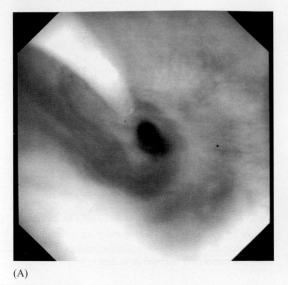

(A)

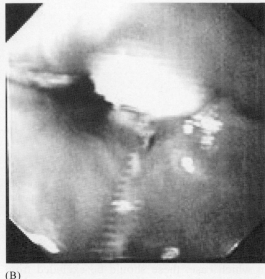

(B)

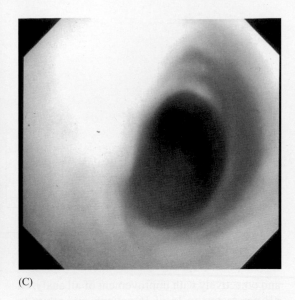

(C)

Figure 27 Application of mitomycin-C antifibrotic agent postdilation in order to prevent restenosis is effective.

occasionally, varicella zoster.[65–67] Although the inflammation can resolve spontaneously in the immunocompetent, in those with poor immune function, acyclovir and a high index of suspicion are recommended.[72] Use of prophylactic acyclovir is conjectural but may be of some benefit posttransplant. Resistance to acyclovir has been described, in which case, foscarnet is the agent of choice.[73] CMV esophagitis is predominantly found in immunocompromised individuals, and treatment is with ganciclovir or foscarnet.[67] Hemorrhage, fistulae, and esophageal perforation in adults with viral esophagitis have been described.[74,75] Acute HIV infection can also cause esophagitis, and antiretroviral regimens are needed.[76]

Candida is the most common infectious cause of esophagitis. A 2- to 6-week course of oral nystatin can be effective in those with normal immune function, but it is more convenient to give fluconazole. Fluconazole and liposomal amphotericin are both effective and are necessary in the immunocompromised child. Esophageal resection and diversion for necrotizing candidal esophagitis have been successful in a 10-year old.[81]

Eradication of *H. pylori* is not likely to improve coexistent esophagitis, and, indeed, in adults, eradication has been associated with increased acid production and hence more noxious gastroesophageal refluxate. However, there does not seem to be any increased incidence of esophagitis in the presence of or following the eradication of *H. pylori* in children.[82] Primary bacterial esophagitis is described in immunocompromised patients and requires appropriate antibiotics dictated by sensitivity testing.[84] Other opportunistic organisms causing esophagitis, such as *Cryptosporidium* and *Acremonium,* have been reported and require appropriate therapy.[85,86]

Treatment of caustic esophagitis is initially conservative, with barium swallow at 4 to 6 weeks postingestion, endoscopic assessment, and, if necessary, stricture dilation. The place of steroids in stricture prevention is controversial and not routine in many centers. Recently, the

use of an antifibrotic, mitomycin C, applied topically to the mucosa poststricture dilation has been used successfully in patients who have required multiple stricture dilations, with prevention of restenosis (Figure 27).[41] Antibiotic therapy for mediastinitis and judicious use of surgery may be employed; these are dealt with in Chapter 4.2, "Gastroesophageal Reflux."

Older children whose esophageal stratified epithelium is exposed to long-term acid may, as with adults, develop gastric metaplasia, eponymously termed Barrett's esophagus.[204–206] This increases the risk for esophageal adenocarcinoma 30 to 40 times. Debate surrounds the relative merits and success rates of antireflux surgery or long-term proton pump inhibitor use, and this is dealt with in greater detail in Chapter 4.2, "Gastroesophageal Reflux."

Prognostication in infant and childhood esophagitis is wholly dependent on etiology; however, fortunately, the most common causes, reflux and allergy, are relatively self-limiting, with a natural improvement and recovery by 18 months to 2 years in the vast majority. This is dealt with in greater detail at the beginning of the section on treatment. It is the responsibility of the pediatrician to prevent avoidable complications such as

peptic strictures occurring during the period of vulnerability until such an age has been reached. A low threshold for diagnosis and intervention is therefore sensible in this population.

Treatment of EE has been varied with variable success. Immunomodulation and anti-inflammatory treatment with MDI-administered (swallowed rather than inhaled) topical steroids such as fluticasone and beclomethasone improve symptoms and eosinophilic infiltration whilst on the therapy, but have esophageal candidiasis as a side effect in some.[53,96,207] Systemic steroids are not recommended as any response is only during treatment and attendant side effects are well documented. Mast cell stabilizers are ineffective, and small studies of leukotriene receptor antagonists have suggested some efficacy.[208] Elemental amino acid based exclusive ingestion for a number of weeks has been shown not only to be therapeutic, but also with the potential to induce a long-term remission of the inflammatory condition.[46] Elimination diets and dietary reintroduction, which are useful in allergic esophagitis, have not until recently been shown to be therapeutic in EE, however a recent study, albeit retrospective, suggests that a six-food elimination diet (cow's milk protein, soya, wheat, egg, fish, and

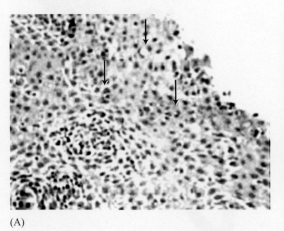

(A)

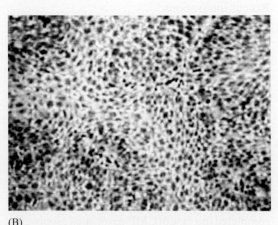

(B)

Figure 28 Tissue eosinophilia treated effectively in the esophagus with anti-IL-5 monoclonal antibody, mepolizumab, in hypereosinophilic syndrome.

peanut) to be as effective as the elemental diet with the obvious advantage of palatability with consequent increased compliance and thereby efficacy.[209] As it is known that excess IL-5 is implicated in the pathoetiology of this condition then it seems reasonable to try anti-IL-5 monoclonal antibody infusions and phase 2 trials in adults and children are beginning with mepolizumab, which has shown efficacy in hypereosinophilic syndromes including one man whose EE as part of this picture was treated effectively at the tissue level (Figure 28).[210]

In summary the pediatric esophagus is no longer regarded as a boring part of the GI tract with little advances or interest accruing clinically or in research terms. The developments in physiologically appropriate tools such as impedance, and the rapid rise in comprehension of issues such as neurohumoral interactions controlling esophageal function, combined with the recent apparent explosion in incidence of new esophageal diseases in children, for example, eosinophilic esophagitis, suggest that the study and clinical care of children with esophageal inflammatory disorders is likely to be of expanding interest to the pediatric gastroenterology community as each year goes by.

REFERENCES

1. Thomson M. The pediatric esophagus comes of age. J Pediatr Gastroenterol Nutr 2002;34:S40–5.
2. Vandenplas Y. Reflux esophagitis in infants and children: A report from the Working Group on Gastro-oesophageal Reflux Disease of the European Society of Paediatric Gastroenterology and Nutrition. J Pediatr Gastroenterol Nutr 1994;18:413–22.
3. Hassal E. Macroscopic versus microscopic diagnosis of reflux esophagitis: Erosions or eosinophils? J Pediatr Gastroenterol Nutr 1996;22:321–5.
4. Vandenplas Y. Reflux esophagitis: Biopsy or not? J Pediatr Gastroenterol Nutr 1996;22:326–7.
5. Bedu A, et al. Prenatal gastrointestinal bleeding caused by esophagitis and gastritis. J Pediatr 1994;125:465–7.
6. Borowitz S. Ulcerative esophagitis. A rare source of upper gastrointestinal bleeding in a neonate. Use of fiberoptic endoscopy for diagnosis. Clin Pediatr 1989;28:89–91.
7. Deneyer M, et al. Esophagitis of likely traumatic origin in newborns. J Pediatr Gastroenterol Nutr 1992;15:81–4.
8. Wienbeck M, Barnert J. Epidemiology of reflux disease and reflux oesophagitis. Scand J Gastroenterol 1989;24:7–13.
9. Carre I. The natural history of the partial thoracic stomach ("hiatal hernia") in children. Arch Dis Child 1959;34:344–53.
10. Shepherd R, Wren J, Evans S, et al. Gastroesophageal reflux in children. Clinical profile, course and outcome with active therapy in 126 cases. Clin Pediatr 1987;26:55–60.
11. Treem W, Davis P, Hyams J. Gastroesophageal reflux in the older child: Presentation, response to treatment, and long-term follow up. Clin Pediatr 1991;30:435–40.
12. Shub M. Esophagitis: A frequent consequence of gastroesophageal reflux in infancy. J Pediatr 1985;107:881–4.
13. Cucchiara S, et al. Pathophysiology of gastroesophageal reflux and distal esophageal motility in children with gastroesophageal reflux disease. J Pediatr Gastroenterol Nutr 1988;7:830–6.
14. Dent J, Holloway R, Toouli J, Dodds W. Mechanisms of lower oesophageal sphincter incompetence in patients with symptomatic gastrooesophageal reflux. Gut 1988;29:1020–8.
15. Murray J, Du C, Ledlow A, et al. Nitric oxide: Mediator of nonadrenergic noncholinergic responses of opossum esophageal muscle. Am J Physiol 1991;261:G401–6.
16. Hitchcock R, Pemble M, Bishop A, et al. Quantitative study of the development and maturation of human oesophageal innervation. J Anatom 1992;180:175–83.
17. Preiksaitis H, Tremblay L, Diamant N. Nitric oxide mediates inhibitory nerve effects in human esophagus and lower esophageal sphincter. Dig Dis Sci 1994;39:770–5.
18. Hitchcock R, Pemble M, Bishop A, et al. The ontogeny and distribution of neuropeptides in the human fetal and infant esophagus. Gastroenterology 1992;102:840–8.
19. Cucchiara S, Bortolotti M, Minella R, Auricchio S. Fasting and post-prandial mechanisms of gastroesophageal reflux in children with gastroesophageal reflux disease. Dig Dis Sci 1993;38:86–92.
20. Hillemeier A, McCallum R, Biancani P. Developmental characteristics of the lower esophageal sphincter in the kitten. Gastroenterology 1985;89:760–6.
21. Helm J, Dodds W, Riedel D. Determinant of esophageal acid clearance in normal subjects. Gastroenterology 1983;85:607–12.
22. Ganatra J, et al. Esophageal dysmotility elicited by acid perfusion in children with esophagitis. Am J Gastroenterol 1995;90:1080–3.
23. Torrente F, Fitzhenry R, Heuschkel R, et al. Cow's milk induces T cell proliferation and mucosal mast cell degranulation with neural tropism in an in vitro organ culture model. J Pediatr Gastroenterol Nutr 2003;36:527.
24. Gupta S, Fitzgerald J, Chong S, et al. Expression of inducible nitric oxide synthase (iNOS) mRNA in inflamed esophageal and colonic mucosa in a pediatric population. Am J Gastroenterol 1998;93:795–8.
25. Zicari A, et al. Increased levels of prostaglandins and nitric oxide in esophageal mucosa of children with reflux esophagitis. J Pediatr Gastroenterol Nutr 1997;26:194–9.
26. Heacock H, Jeffery H, Baker J, Page M. Influence of breast versus formula milk on physiological gastroesophageal reflux in healthy, newborn infants. J Pediatr Gastroenterol Nutr 1992;14:41–6.
27. Ewer A, Durbin G, Morgan M, Booth I. Gastric emptying in preterm infants: A comparison of breast milk and formula. Arch Dis Child 1994;71:F24–7.
28. Ferguson D, et al. Studies on experimental esophagitis. Surgery 1950;28:1022–39.
29. Goldberg H, Dodds W, Gee S, et al. Role of acid and pepsin in acute experimental esophagitis. Gastroenterology 1969;56:223–30.
30. Hirschowitz B. A critical analysis, with appropriate controls, of gastric acid and pepsin secretions in clinical esophagitis. Gastroenterology 1991;101:1149–58.
31. Vaezi M, Singh S, Richter J. Role of acid and duodenogastric reflux in esophageal injury: A review of animal and human studies. Gastroenterology 1995;108:1897–907.
32. Kelly E, Newell S, Brownlee K, et al. Gastric acid production in preterm infants. Early Hum Dev 1993;35:215–20.
33. Redo S, Barnes W, de la Sierra A. Perfusion of the canine esophagus with secretions of the upper gastrointestinal tract. Ann Surg 1959;149:556–64.
34. Lillemoe K, Johnson L, Harmon J. Role of the components of the gastroduodenal contents in experimental acid esophagitis. Surgery 1982;92:276–84.
35. Vaezi M, Richter J. Role of acid and duodenogastroesophageal reflux in gastroesophageal reflux disease. Gastroenterology 1996;111:1192–9.
36. Marshall R, Anggiansah A, Owen W, Owen W. The relationship between acid and bile reflux and symptoms in gastro-oesophageal reflux disease. Gut 1997;40:182–7.
37. Orel R, Markovich S. Bile in the esophagus: A factor in the pathogenesis of reflux esophagitis in children. J Pediatr Gastroenterol Nutr 2003;36:266–73.
38. Singh S, Bradley L, Richter J. Determinants of oesophageal "alkaline" pH environment in controls and patients with gastro-oesophageal reflux disease. Gut 1993;34:309–16.
39. Harman J, Johnson L, Maydonovitch C. Effects of acid and bile salts on the rabbit esophageal mucosa. Dig Dis Sci 1981;26:65–72.
40. Lillemoe K, Johnson L, Harman J. Taurodeoxycholate modulates the effects of pepsin and trypsin in experimental esophagitis. Surgery 1985;97:662–7.
41. Afsal N, Lloyd-Thomas A, Albert D, Thomson M. Treatment of oesophageal strictures in childhood. Lancet 2002;359:1032.
42. Goldberg N, Ott M, Parker-Hartigan L. Medication-induced esophagitis. J Pediatr Health Care 1996;10:35–6.
43. Biller J, Flores A, Buie T, et al. Tetracycline-induced esophagitis in adolescent patients. J Pediatr 1992;120:144–5.
44. Kato S, Komatsu K, Harada Y. Medication-induced esophagitis in children. Gastroenterol Jpn 1990;25:485–8.
45. Holvoet J, Terriere L, Van Hee W, et al. Relation of upper gastrointestinal bleeding to non-steroidal anti-inflammatory drugs and aspirin: A case control study. Gut 1991;32:730–4.
46. Kelly KJ, et al. Eosinophilic esophagitis attributed to gastroesophageal reflux: Improvement with an amino acid-based formula. Gastroenterology 1995;109:1503–12.
47. Hill DJ, Hosking CS. Emerging disease profiles in infants and young children with food allergy. Pediatr Allergy Immunol 1997;8:21–6.
48. Iacono G, et al. Gastroesophageal reflux and cow's milk allergy in infants: A prospective study. J Allergy Clin Immunol 1996;97:822–7.
49. Cavataio F, et al. Clinical and pH-metric characteristics of gastro-oesophageal reflux secondary to cows' milk protein allergy. Arch Dis Child 1996;75:51–6.
50. Murch S. Diabetes and cows' milk. Lancet 1996;348:1656.
51. Walker-Smith JA, Murch SH. Gastrointestinal food allergy. Diseases of the Small Intestine in Childhood, 4th edition. Oxford, UK: Isis Medical Media; 1999. p. 205–34.
52. Winter HS, et al. Intraepithelial eosinophils: A new diagnostic criterion for reflux esophagitis. Gastroenterology 1983;83:818–23.
53. Liacouras CA, et al. Primary eosinophilic esophagitis in children: Successful treatment with oral corticosteroids. J Pediatr Gastroenterol Nutr 1998;26:380–5.
54. Fox VL, Nurko S, Teitelbaum JE, et al. High-resolution EUS in children with eosinophilic "allergic" esophagitis. Gastrointest Endosc 2003;57:30–6.
55. Furuta GT. Eosinophils in the esophagus: Acid is not the only cause. J Pediatr Gastroenterol Nutr 1998;26:468–71.
56. Justinich C, et al. Activated eosinophils in esophagitis in children: A transmission electron microscopic study. J Pediatr Gastroenterol Nutr 1997;25:194–8.
57. Mangano M, et al. Nature and significance of cells with irregular nuclear contours (CINC) in esophageal mucosa. Lab Invest 1991;64:38A.
58. Cucchiara S, et al. Intraepithelial cells with irregular nuclear contours as a marker of esophagitis in children with gastroesophageal reflux disease. Dig Dis Sci 1995;40:2305–11.
59. Wang HH, Mangano MM, Antonioli DA. Evaluation of T-lymphocytes in esophageal mucosal biopsies. Mod Pathol 1994;7:55–8.
60. Garcia-Zepeda EA, et al. Human eotaxin is a specific chemoattractant for eosinophil cells and provides a new mechanism to explain tissue eosinophilia. Nat Med 1996;2:449–56.
61. Butt A, Murch S, Ng C-L, et al. Upregulated eotaxin expression and T-cell infiltration in the basal and papillary epithelium in cow's milk associated reflux oesophagitis. Arch Dis Child 2002;87:124.
62. Collins SM. The immunomodulation of enteric neuromuscular function: Implications for motility and inflammatory disorders. Gastroenterology 1996;111:1683–99.
63. Pérez-Machado MA, Ashwood P, Thomson MA, et al. Reduced transforming growth factor-beta1-producing T cells in the duodenal mucosa of children with food allergy. Eur J Immunol 2003;33:2307–15.
64. Justinich C, et al. Mucosal mast cells distinguish allergic from gastroesophageal reflux-induced esophagitis. J Pediatr Gastroenterol Nutr 1996;23:342–74.
65. Gill R, Gebhard R, Dozeman R, Sumner H. Shingles esophagitis: Endoscopic diagnosis in two patients. Gastrointest Endosc 1984;30:26–7.
66. Agha F, Lee H, Nostrant T. Herpetic esophagitis: A diagnostic challenge in immunocompromised patients. Am J Gastroenterol 1986;81:246–53.
67. Parente F, Bianchi Porro G. Treatment of cytomegalovirus esophagitis in patients with acquired immunodeficiency syndrome: A randomized controlled study of foscarnet versus ganciclovir. The Italian Cytomegalovirus Study Group. Am J Gastroenterol 1998;93:317–22.
68. Springer D, DaCosta L, Beck I. A syndrome of acute self-limiting ulcerative esophagitis in young adults probably due to herpes simplex virus. Dig Dis Sci 1979;24:535–44.
69. Alexander J, et al. Infectious esophagitis following liver and renal transplant. Dig Dis Sci 1988;33:1121–6.
70. Powell K. Guidelines for the care of children and adolescents with HIV infection. Approach to gastrointestinal manifestations in infants and children with HIV infection. J Pediatr 1991;119: S34–40.
71. Greenson J, Beschorner W, Boitnott J, Yardley J. Prominent mononuclear cell infiltrate is characteristic of herpes esophagitis. Hum Pathol 1991;22:541–9.
72. Becker K, Lubke H, Borchard F, Haussinger D. Inflammatory esophageal diseases caused by herpes simplex virus infections—overview and report of 15 personal cases. Z Gastroenterol 1996;34:286–95.
73. Chatis P, Miller C, Schraeger L, Crumpacker C. Successful treatment with foscarnet of an acyclovir-resistant mucocutaneous infection with herpes simplex virus in a patient with acquired immunodeficiency syndrome. N Engl J Med 1989;320:296–300.
74. Rattner H, Cooper D, Zaman M. Severe bleeding from herpes esophagitis. Am J Gastroenterol 1985;80:523–5.
75. Cronstedt J, Bouchama A, Hainau B, et al. Spontaneous esophageal perforation in herpes simplex esophagitis. Am J Gastroenterol 1992;87:124–7.
76. Rabeneck L, Popovic M, Gartner S. Acute HIV infection presenting with painful swallowing and esophageal ulcers. JAMA 1990;263:2318–22.
77. Wigg A, Roberts-Thomson I. *Candida* oesophagitis. J Gastroenterol Hepatol 1998;13:831.

78. Braegger C, Albisetti M, Nadal D. Extensive esophageal candidiasis in the absence of oral lesions in pediatric AIDS. J Pediatr Gastroenterol Nutr 1995;21:104–6.
79. DeGregorio M, Lee W, Ries C. *Candida* infections in patients with acute leukemia: Ineffectiveness of nystatin prophylaxis and relationship between oropharyngeal and systemic candidiasis. Cancer 1982;50:2780–4.
80. Bode C, Schroten H, Koletzko S, et al. Transient achalasia-like esophageal dysmotility disorder after *Candida* esophagitis in a boy with chronic granulomatous disease. J Pediatr Gastroenterol Nutr 1996;23:320–3.
81. Gaissert H, Breuer C, Weissburg A, Mermel L. Surgical management of necrotizing *Candida* esophagitis. Ann Thorac Surg 1999;67:231–3.
82. Rosioru C, Glassman M, Halata M, Schwartz S. Esophagitis and *Helicobacter pylori* in children: Incidence and therapeutic implications. Am J Gastroenterol 1993;88:510–3.
83. De Giacomo C, Fiocca R, Villani L, et al. Barrett's ulcer and *Campylobacter*-like organisms infection in a child. J Pediatr Gastroenterol Nutr 1988;7:766–8.
84. Walsh T, Beltisos N, Hamilton S. Bacterial esophagitis in immunocompromised patients. Arch Intern Med 1986;146:1345–8.
85. Kaslow P, et al. Esophageal cryptosporidiosis in a child with acquired immune deficiency syndrome. Gastroenterology 1986;91:1301–3.
86. Mascarenhas M, McGowan K, Ruchelli E, et al. *Acremonium* infection of the esophagus. J Pediatr Gastroenterol Nutr 1997;24:356–8.
87. Mahboubi S, Silber J. Radiation-induced esophageal strictures in children with cancer. Eur Radiol 1997;7:119–22.
88. Boeck A, Buckley R, Schiff R. Gastroesophageal reflux and severe combined immunodeficiency. J Allergy Clin Immunol 1997;99:420–4.
89. Thomson M, Walker-Smith J. Dyspepsia in infants and children. Baillieres Clin Gastroenterol 1998;12:601–24.
90. Witte A, Veenendaal R, Van Hogezand R, et al. Crohn's disease of the upper gastrointestinal tract: The value of endoscopic examination. Scand J Gastroenterol 1998;225:100–5.
91. D'Haens G, Rutgeerts P, Geboes K, Vantrappen G. The natural history of esophageal Crohn's disease: Three patterns of evolution. Gastrointest Endosc 1994;40: 296–300.
92. Schulman H, Weizman Z, Barki Y, et al. Inflammatory bowel disease in glycogen storage disease type 1B. Pediatr Radiol 1995;25:S160–2.
93. Renner W, Johnson J, Lichtenstein J, Kirks D. Esophageal inflammation and stricture: Complication of chronic granulomatous disease of childhood. Radiology 1991;178: 189–91.
94. Shabib S, Cutz E, Sherman P. Passive smoking is risk factor for esophagitis in children. J Pediatr 1995;127:435–7.
95. Meadow R. Munchausen syndrome by proxy: The hinterland of child abuse. Lancet 1977;ii:343–4.
96. Faubion W, Perrault J, Burgart L, et al. Treatment of eosinophilic esophagitis with inhaled corticosteroids. J Pediatr Gastroenterol Nutr 1998;27:90–3.
97. Mishra A, Hogan S, Brandt E, Rothenberg M. IL-5 promotes eosinophilic trafficking to the eosophagus. J Immunol 2002;168:2464–9.
98. Noel R, Putnam P, Rothenberg M. Eosinophilic esophagitis. N Engl J Med 2004;351:940–1.
99. Ahmed A, Matsui S, Soetiko R. A novel endoscopic appearance of idiopathic eosinophilic esophagitis. Endoscopy 2000;32:S33.
100. Cherian S, Smith NM, Forbes DA. Rapidly increasing prevalence of eosinophilic oesophagitis in Western Australia. Arch Dis Child 2006;91:1000–4.
101. Walker AM, Menahem S. Normal early infant behaviour patterns. J Pediatr Child Health 1994;30:260–2.
102. Heine R, Jaquiery A, Lubitz L, et al. Role of gastro-oesophageal reflux in infant irritability. Arch Dis Child 1995;73:121–5.
103. Dellert S, Hyams J, Treem W, Geertsma M. Feeding resistance: An unappreciated complication of gastroesophageal reflux in infants. J Pediatr Gastroenterol Nutr 1993; 17:66–71.
104. Ryan P, Lander M, Shepherd R. When does reflux oesophagitis occur with gastro-oesophageal reflux in infants? A clinical and endoscopic study, and correlation with outcome. Aust Pediatr J 1983;19:90–3.
105. Hyams J, Ricci A, Leichtner A. Clinical and laboratory correlates of esophagitis in young children. J Pediatr Gastroenterol Nutr 1988;7:52–6.
106. Hyman P. Gastroesophageal reflux: One reason why baby won't eat. J Pediatr 1994;125:S103–9.
107. Sutcliffe J. Torsion spasms and abnormal posture in children with hiatus hernia. Sandifer's syndrome. Prog Pediatr Radiol 1969;2:190–7.
108. Eid N, Shepherd R, Thomson M. Persistent wheezing and gastroesophageal reflux in infants. Pediatr Pulmonol 1994;18:39–44.
109. Berezin S, Glassman M, Bostwick H, Halata M. Esophagitis as a cause of infant colic. Clin Pediatr 1995;34:158–9.
110. St James-Roberts I, Conroy S, Wilsher K. Bases for maternal perceptions of infant crying and colic behaviour. Arch Dis Child 1996;75:375–84.
111. Mavromichalis I, Zaramboukas T, Richman P, Slavin G. Recurrent abdominal pain of gastro-intestinal origin. Eur J Pediatr 1992;151:560–3.
112. Glassman M, Medow M, Berezin S, Newman L. Spectrum of esophageal disorders in children with chest pain. Dig Dis Sci 1992;37:663–6.
113. Berezin S, Medow M, Glassman M, Newman L. Esophageal chest pain in children with asthma. J Pediatr Gastroenterol Nutr 1991;12:52–5.
114. Rosario N, Farias L. Gastroesophageal reflux and esophagitis-associated hypertrophic osteoarthropathy. J Pediatr Gastroenterol Nutr 1998;27:125.
115. Rudolph C, et al. Guidelines for evaluation and treatment of gastroesophageal reflux in infants and children. Recommendations of NASPGAN. J Pediatr Gastroenterol Nutr 2001;32:S1–31.
116. Thomson M. Disorders of the oesophagus and stomach in infants. Baillieres Clin Gastroenterol 1997;11:547–71.
117. Maki M, Ruuska T, Kuusela A, et al. High prevalence of asymptomatic esophageal and gastric lesions in preterm infants in intensive care. Crit Care Med 1993;21:1863–7.
118. deBoissieu D, Dupont C, Barbet J, et al. Distinct features of upper gastrointestinal endoscopy in the newborn. J Pediatr Gastroenterol Nutr 1994;18:334–8.
119. Squires R, Coletti R. Indications for pediatric gastrointestinal endoscopy: A medical position statement of the North American Society for Pediatric Gastroenterology and Nutrition. J Pediatr Gastroenterol Nutr 1996;23:107–10.
120. Hassall E, Israel D, Shepherd R, et al. Omeprazole for treatment of chronic erosive esophagitis in children: A multicenter study of efficacy, safety, tolerability and dose requirements. International Pediatric Omeprazole Study Group. J Pediatr 2000;137:800–7.
121. Biller J, Winter H, Grand R, Allred E. Are endoscopic changes predictive of histologic esophagitis in children? J Pediatr 1983;103:215–8.
122. Sampliner, R, et al. Practice guidelines on the diagnosis, surveillance and therapy of Barrett's esophagus. Am J Gastroenterol 1998;93:1028–32.
123. Savary M, Miller G. L'oesophage: Manuel et Atlas D'endoscopie. Soleure, France: Gasmann AG; 1977.
124. Hetzel D, et al. Healing and relapse of severe peptic esophagitis after treatment with omeprazole. Gastroenterology 1988;95:903–12.
125. Hunt R, et al. Optimizing acid suppression for treatment of acid-related diseases. Dig Dis Sci 1995;40:24S–49S.
126. Gupta S, Fitzgerald J, Chong S, et al. Vertical lines in distal esophageal mucosa (VLEM): A true endoscopic manifestation of esophagitis in children? Gastrointest Endosc 1997;45:485–9.
127. Isaac D, Parham D, Patrick C. The role of esophagoscopy in diagnosis and management of esophagitis in children with cancer. Med Pediatr Oncol 1997;28:299–303.
128. Fink S, Barwick K, Winchenbach C, et al. Reassessment of esophageal histology in normal subjects: A comparison of suction and endoscopic techniques. J Clin Gastroenterol 1983;3:177–83.
129. Friesen C, Zwick D, Streed C, et al. Grasp biopsy, suction biopsy, and clinical history in the evaluation of esophagitis in infants 0-6 months of age. J Pediatr Gastroenterol Nutr 1995;20:300–4.
130. Wienbeck M. Cisapride acts as a motor stimulation in the esophagus. Gastroenterology 1984;86:1298.
131. Geisenger K. Endoscopic biopsies and cytological brushings of the esophagus are diagnostically complementary. Am J Clin Pathol 1995;103:295–9.
132. Vandenplas Y, Belli D, Boige N, et al. A standardised protocol for the methodology or oesophageal pH monitoring and interpretation of the data for the diagnosis of the gastroesophageal reflux. Society statement of a working group of the European Society of Paediatric Gastroenterology and Nutrition. J Pediatr Gastroenterol Nutr 1992;14:467–71.
133. Benhamou PH. Vannerom PY, Kalach N, Dupont C. Diagnostic procedures of GOR in the childhood lung disease. Paediatr Pulmonol 1995;11:116–7.
134. Grill B. Twenty-four hour oesophageal pH monitoring: What's the score? J Paediatr Gastroenterol Nutr 1992;14:249–51.
135. De Ajuriaguerra M, Radvanyi-Bouvet MF, Huon C, Morriette G. Gastroesophageal reflux and apnoea in prematurely born infants during wakefulness and sleep. Am J Dis Child 1991;145:1132–6.
136. Orenstein SR. Controversies in paediatric gastroesophageal reflux. J Paediatr Gastroenterol Nutr 1992;14:338–48.
137. Black D, Haggitt R, Orenstein S, Whitington P. Esophagitis in infants: Morphometric histological diagnosis and correlation with measures of gastroesophageal reflux. Gastroenterology 1990;98:1408–14.
138. Vandenplas Y, Franckx-Goossens A, Pipeleers-Marichal M, et al. Area under pH 4: Advantages of a new parameter in the interpretation of pH monitoring data in infants. J Pediatr Gastroenterol Nutr 1989;9:34–9.
139. Skopnik H, Silny J, Heiber O, et al. Gastroesophageal reflux in infants: Evaluation of a new intraluminal impedance technique. J Pediatr Gastroenterol Nutr 1996;23:591–8.
140. LiVoti G, Tulone V, Bruno R, et al. Ultrasonography and gastric emptying: Evaluation in infants with gastroesophageal reflux. J Paediatr Gastroenterol Nutr 1992;14:397–9.
141. Vaezi MF, Singh S, Richter J. Role of acid and duodenogastric reflux in esophageal mucosal injury: A review of animal and human studies. Gastroenterology 1995;108:1897–907.
142. Velasco N, Pope CE, Gannan RM, et al. Measurement of esophageal reflux by scintigraphy. Dig Dis Soc 1984;29:977–82.
143. Bender G, Makuch R. Double contrast barium examination of the upper gastrointestinal tract with non-endoscopic biopsy: Findings in 100 patients. Radiology 1997;202:1567–70.
144. Just RJ, Leite LP, Castell DO. Changes in overnight fasting intragastric pH show poor correlation with duodenogastric bile reflux in normal subjects. Am J Gastroenterol 1996;91:1567–70.
145. Wenzl T, Schenke S, Peschgens T, et al. Association of apnea and non-acid gastroesophageal reflux in infants: Investigations with the intraluminal impedance technique. Pediatr Pulmonol 2001;31:144–9.
146. Nguyen HN, Silny J, Matern S. Multiple intraluminal electrical impedenancometry for recording of upper gastrointestinal motility: Current results and further implications. Am J Gastroenterol 1999;94:306–17.
147. Frieling T, Hermann S, Kuhlbusch R, et al. Comparison between intraluminal multiple electric impedance measurement and manometry in the human esophagus. Neurogastroenterol Motil 1996;8:45–50.
148. Wenzl TG, Skopnik H. Advances in diagnosing gastroeosophageal reflux in infants—the pH independent intraluminal impedance technique. In: Cadranel S, Scallian M, editors. Disorders of Digestive Motility in Childhood from Theory to Practice. Brussels: Department of Gastroenterology and Hepatology Brussels; 1998.
149. Wenzl TG, Silny J, Schenke S, et al. Gastroesophageal reflux and respiratory phenomena in infants—status of the intraluminal impedance technique. J Pediatr Gastroenterol Nutr 1999;28:423–8.
150. Vandenplas Y, Ashkenazi A, Belli D, et al. A proposition for diagnosis and treatment of gastro-oesophageal reflux disease in children: A report from a working group on gastroesophageal reflux disease. Eur J Pediatr 1993;152:704–11.
151. Corrado G, Cavaliere M, Pacchiaroti C, et al. When is gastroesophageal reflux the cause of symptoms? J Pediatr Gastroenterol Nutr 2000;31:322–3.
152. Fess J, Silny J, Braun J, et al. Measuring esophageal motility with a new intraluminal impedance device. Scand J Gastroenterol 1994;29:693–702.
153. Del Buono R, Wenzl T , Ball G, et al. The Influence of Gaviscon Infant or placebo on gastro-oesophageal reflux in infants: Investigations with the Intraluminal Multiple Electrical Impedance Procedure (IMP). Arch Dis Child 2005;90:460–3.
154. Thomson M, Wenzl TG, Fox AT, Del Buono R. Effect of an amino acid-based milk Neocate on gastro-oesophageal reflux in infants assessed by combined intraluminal impedance/pH. Pediatr Asthma Allergy Immunol 2006; 19:205–213.
155. Cucchiara S, Campanozzi A, Greco L, et al. Predictive value of esophageal manometry and gastroesophageal pH monitoring for the responsiveness of reflux disease to medical therapy in children. Am J Gastroenterol 1996;91:680–5.
156. Gilger MA, Boyle JT, Sonderheimer JM, et al. Indications for pediatric manometry. Statement of the North American Society for Pediatric Gastroenterology and Nutrition (NASPGN). J Pediatr Gastroenterol Nutr 1997;24: 616–8.
157. Sifrim D, Holloway R, Silny J, et al. Acid, nonacid, and gas reflux in patients with gastroesophageal reflux disease during ambulatory 24-hour pH-impedance recordings. Gastroenterology 2001;120:1588–98.
158. Al- Zaben A, Chandra V, Stuebe T. Detection of gastrointestinal tract events from multichannel intraluminal impedance measurements. Biomed Sci Instrum 2001;37:55–61.

159. Skopnik H, Silny J, Heiber O, et al. Gastroesophageal reflux in infants: Evaluation of a new intraluminal impedance technique. J Pediatr Gastroenterol Nutr 1996;23:591–8.

160. Tasker A, Dettmar PW, Pearson JP, et al. Reflux of gastric juice in glue ear. Lancet 2002;359:493.

161. Ward C, Forrest IA, Brownlee IA, et al. Pepsin like activity in bronchoalveolar lavage fluid is suggestive of gastric aspiration in lung allografts. Thorax 2005;60:872–4.

162. Berezin S, Halata M, Newman L, et al. Esophageal manometry in children with esophagitis. Am J Gastroenterol 1993;88:680–2.

163. Ruchelli E, Wenner W, Voytek T, et al. Severity of esophageal eosinophilia predicts response to conventional gastroesophageal reflux therapy. Pediatr Dev Pathol 1999;2:15–8.

164. Tytgat G, Nicolai J, Reman F. Efficacy of different doses of cimetidine in the treatment of reflux esophagitis: A review of three large, double-blind, controlled trials. Gastroenterology 1990;99:629–34.

165. Saraswat V, et al. Correlation of 24 hr esophageal patterns with clinical features and endoscopy in gastroesophageal reflux disease. Dig Dis Sci 1994;39:199–205.

166. Spechler S. Epidemiology and natural history of gastrooesophagitis reflux disease. Digestion 1992;51:24–9.

167. McHardy G. A multicentric randomized clinical trial of Gaviscon in reflux esophagitis. South Med J 1978;71:16–20.

168. Buts J, Barudi C, Otte J. Double-blind controlled study on the efficacy of sodium-alginate in reducing gastroesophageal reflux assessed by 24h continuous pH monitoring in infants and children. Eur J Pediatr 1987;146:156–8.

169. Olafsdottir E. Gastro-oesophageal reflux and chronic respiratory disease in infants and children: Treatment with cisapride. Scand J Gastroenterol 1995;211:32–4.

170. Hill S, et al. Pro-arrhythmia associated with cisapride in children. Paediatrics 1998;101:1053–6.

171. Lupoglazoff J, et al. Allongement de l'espace QT sous cisapride chez le nouveau-ne et le nourrisson. Arch Pediatr 1997;4:509–14.

172. Levine A, et al. QT interval in children and infants receiving cisapride. Paediatrics 1998;101:E9.

173. Ward R, Lemons J, Molteni R. Cisapride: A survey of the frequency of use and adverse events in premature newborns. Pediatrics 1999;103:469–72.

174. Vandenplas Y. Clinical use of cisapride and its risk-benefit in pediatric patients. Eur J Gastroenterol Hepatol 1998;10:871–81.

175. Cucchiara S, et al. Omeprazole and high dose ranitidine in the treatment of refractory reflux oesophagitis. Arch Dis Child 1993;69:655–9.

176. Kaufman S, Loseke C, Young R, Perry D. Ranitidine therapy for esophagitis in children with developmental disabilities. Clin Pediatr 1996;35:451–6.

177. Sutphen J, Dillard V. Effect of ranitidine on twenty-four-hour gastric acidity in infants. J Pediatr 1988;114:472–4.

178. Bergmeijer J, Hazebroek F. Prospective medical and surgical treatment of gastroesophageal reflux in esophageal atresia. J Am Coll Surg 1998;187:153–7.

179. Strauss R, Calenda K, Dayal Y, Mobassaleh M. Histological esophagitis: Clinical and histological response to omeprazole in children. Dig Dis Sci 1999;44:134–9.

180. Bohmer C, Niezen-de Boer R, Klinkenberg-Knol E, Meuwissen S. Omeprazole: Therapy of choice in intellectually disabled children. Arch Pediatr Adolesc Med 1998;152:1113–8.

181. Cucchiara S, et al. Effects of omeprazole on mechanisms of gastroesophageal reflux in childhood. Dig Dis Sci 1997,42.293–9.

182. Gunasekaran T, Hassall E. Efficacy and safety of omeprazole for severe gastroesophageal reflux in children. J Pediatr 1993;123:148–54.

183. Alliët P, Raes M, Gillis P, Zimmermann A. Optimal dose of omeprazole in infants in children. J Pediatr 1994;124:332–3.

184. Grill B, Hillemeyer A, Semeraro L, et al. Effects of domperidone therapy on symptoms and upper gastrointestinal motility in infants with gastroesophageal reflux. J Pediatr 1985;106:311–6.

185. Bines J, Quinlan J, Treves S, et al. Efficacy of domperidone in infants and children with gastroesophageal reflux. J Pediatr Gastroenterol Nutr 1992;14:400–5.

186. Kawahara H, et al. Mechanisms underlying the antireflux effect of Nissen fundoplication in children. J Pediatr Surg 1998;33:1618–22.

187. Fonkalsrud E, et al. Surgical treatment of gastroesophageal reflux in children: A combined hospital study of 7467 patients. Pediatrics 1998;101:419–22.

188. Tovar J, et al. Functional results of laparoscopic fundoplication in children. J Pediatr Gastroenterol Nutr 1998;26:429–31.

189. Georgeson K. Laparoscopic fundoplication. Curr Opin Pediatr 1998;10:318–22.

190. Rothenberg S. Experience with 220 consecutive laparoscopic Nissen fundoplications in infants and children. J Pediatr Surg 1998;33:274–8.

191. Filipi CJ, Lehman GA, Rothstein RI, et al. Transoral, flexible endoscopic suturing for treatment of GERD: A multicenter trial. Gastrointest Endosc 2001;53:416–22.

192. Mahmood Z, McMahon B, Arfin Q, et al. Endocinch therapy for gastro-oesophageal reflux: A one year prospective follow up. Gut 2003;52:34–9.

193. Thomson M, Fritscher-Ravens A, Afsal N, et al. Endoscopic fundoplication for the treatment of paediatric gastro-oesophageal reflux disease. Gut 2004;53:1745–50.

194. Antao B, Thomson M, Fritscher-Ravens A, et al. Long term outcome of endoluminal gastroplication (Endocinch) in children. J Laparoscop Advanced Surg Techniques 2006;16:196.

195. Swain C, Kadairkamanarthann S, Gong F, et al. Endoscopic gastroplasty for gastro-esophageal reflux disease. Gastrointest Endosc 1997;45:AB242.

196. Liu J, Glickman J, Carr-Locke D, et al. Gastroesophageal smooth muscle remodeling after endoluminal gastroplication. Am J Gastroenterol 2004;99:1–7.

197. Pleskow D, Rothstein R, Lo S, et al. Endoscopic full thickness plication for the treatment of GERD: A multicenter trial. Gastrointestin Endosc 2004;59:163–71.

198. Triadafilopoulos G, DiBaise J, Nostrant T, et al. Radiofrequency energy delivery to the gastroesophageal junction for the treatment of GERD. Gastrointest Endosc 2001;53:407–15.

199. Deviere J, Silverman D, Pastorelli A, et al. Endoscopic implantation of a biopolymer in the lower esophageal sphincter for gastroesophageal reflux: A pilot study. Gastrointest Endosc 2002;55:335–41.

200. Jakobsson I, Lindbergh T. A prospective study of cow's milk protein intolerance in Swedish infants. Acta Pediatr 1979;68:853–9.

201. Isolauri E, et al. Efficacy and safety of hydolyzed cow milk and amino acid-derived formulas in infants with cow milk allergy. J Pediatr 1995;127:550–7.

202. Lake A. Beyond hydrolysates: Use of L-amino acid formula in resistant dietary protein-induced intestinal disease in infants. J Pediatr 1997;131:658–60.

203. Vanderhoof J, Murray N, Kaufman S, et al. Intolerance to protein hydrolysate infant formulas: An underrecognized cause of gastrointestinal symptoms in infants. J Pediatr 1997;131:741–4.

204. Hassal E. Barrett's esophagus: New definitions and approaches in childhood. J Pediatr Gastroenterol Nutr 1993;16:345–64.

205. Knuff T, Benjamin S, Worsham F, et al. Histologic evaluation of chronic gastroesophageal reflux an evaluation of biopsy methods and diagnostic criteria. Dig Dis Sci 1984;29:194–201.

206. Leape L. Esophageal biopsy in the diagnosis of reflux esophagitis. J Pediatr Surg 1981;16:379–84.

207. Noel R, Putnam P, Collins M, et al. Clinical and immunopathologic effects of swallowed fluticasone for eosinophilic esophagitis. Clin Gastroenterol Hepatol 2004;2:568–75.

208. Attwood S, Lewis C, Bronder C, et al. Eosinophilic oesophagitis: An novel treatment using Montelukast. Gut 2003;52:181–5.

209. Kagalwalla A, Sentongo T, Ritz S, et al. Effect of six-food elimination diet on clinical and histologic outcomes in eosinophilic esophagitis. Clin Gastroenterol Hepatol 2006;4:1097–102.

210. Garrett J, Jameson S, Thomson B, et al. Anti-interleukin-5 (mepolizumab) therapy for hypereosinophilic syndromes. J Allergy Clin Immunol 2004;113:115–9.

6

Toxic and Traumatic Injury of the Esophagus

Emmanuel Mas, MD, MsC
Jean-Pierre Olives, MD

The management of esophageal diseases has changed dramatically over the last two decades, with the improvement of diagnostic procedures. Nowadays, sophisticated procedures are available in the majority of pediatric hospitals: ultrasonography, computed tomography (CT) (if necessary with three-dimensional reconstruction), nuclear magnetic resonance imaging, and, of course, fiberoptic flexible endoscopy, which allows a thorough examination of the esophagus lumen and also provides the opportunity to perform interventional procedures.[1,2]

Injuries of the esophagus in children are most often due to ingestions and to traumatic lesions secondary to thoracic contusion, crush syndrome, blunt trauma, and iatrogenic perforations occurring during either investigational procedures or surgery.[1,2] Ingestions of foreign bodies, coins, disk batteries, corrosive substances, and drugs are accidental in the majority of cases,[3–6] but child abuse, poisoning, or Munchausen syndrome by proxy should be considered.[2] Retrosternal pain, dysphagia, hypersalivation, and emesis are typical symptoms of esophageal lesions,[3–6] but in the young and nonverbal or developmentally delayed child and sometimes even in older children, esophageal symptoms are not always obvious.[2] For example, large esophageal blunt objects might predominantly cause respiratory symptoms[7–9] and can be misdiagnosed as tracheobronchitis, bronchopneumonia, or asthma.[8] Moreover, small impacted foreign bodies and even intramural perforations or infections can be asymptomatic.[3,10–13]

INGESTED FOREIGN BODIES

Ingestion of foreign bodies is a common pediatric problem, with more than 100,000 cases occurring each year. The vast majority ingestions in children are accidental with an increasing frequency of intentional ingestions in the adolescent age group.[4] The majority of foreign bodies will progress through the gastrointestinal tract without any problem and ultimately will be excreted in the feces. Deaths caused by foreign body ingestion are rarely reported: large series reporting no deaths among 852 adults and just 1 death among 2,206 children.[10,11,14,15] Most studies show either no gender predilection[2] or a slight prevalence of males.[3] Surprisingly, a prospective study from Paul and colleagues reported that 60% of the patients were female.[5]

Infants and young children explore their environment by placing objects in their mouth; around 10% of the children seem to be recidivists.[5] Childhood curiosity and carelessness appear to be the major risk factors for accidental ingestion. Since foreign bodies are often easy for children to reach, caregivers need to place more emphasis on environmental safety. In only 51% of cases reported by Paul and colleagues, was the ingestion witnessed.[5] This suggests that the true frequency of accidental swallowing is, in general, underestimated because the majority of ingested foreign bodies do not cause symptoms. As a consequence, caretakers are not aware of accidental ingestion in number of cases.[11]

Esophageal foreign body impactions should be removed as soon as possible because of an increased risk of perforation and aspiration, especially when lodged in the upper third of the esophagus.[2,6] Foreign objects that arrive into the stomach are likely to be eliminated between 2 and 30 days. Nevertheless, complications are reported with large objects (>5 cm in length and >2.5 cm in diameter), sharp-ended foreign bodies and batteries located either in the stomach or duodenum.[2,3] In considering the outcome of foreign bodies located in the gastrointestinal tract, the composition, size, shape, and number of ingested objects should be taken into account. Also, the existence of a number of specific anatomic barriers should be considered: transit is likely to be retarded or blocked at the cricopharyngeal ring, aortic arch, lower esophageal sphincter, pylorus, duodenal curve, ligament of Treitz, Meckel diverticulum, ileocecal valve, appendix, and rectosigmoid junction.[2,3,14] There exist, as well, associated conditions, such as esophageal stenosis, achalasia, or previous abdominal surgery, that may alter spontaneous passage of an ingested foreign body. The evaluation of children should include a careful clinical history, including age, previous digestive symptoms, the type of ingested object, and the interval from ingestion to consultation.

PHARYNGEAL AND CRICOPHARYNGEAL FOREIGN BODIES

Foreign bodies that lodge in the pharynx or at the level of the cricopharyngeal ring are often coins, tokens, toy parts, and fish bones. Standard fluoroscopy is useful to detect metallic objects; plain films of the neck should be taken in both postero-anterior and lateral views. Flat objects, such as coins or tokens, that lodge in the hypopharynx are seen on edge on the lateral film of the neck, whereas those lodged in the upper airway are seen on edge on the frontal film. The accuracy of a radiologic examination to locate fish bones has been validated for nine species when taped to the neck of a control patient[2] and for 14 fish bones embedded in a tissue phantom.[16] Coins and flat objects are easily removed using a Magill forceps, a Foley catheter,[17,18] a magnet,[3,11] or by suction retrieval.[19] Fish bones usually can be extracted with a curved forceps or with long tweezers.

ESOPHAGEAL FOREIGN BODIES

Children often put inedible objects into their mouths. Sometimes, the object is swallowed and becomes a foreign body when it enters into the gastrointestinal tract. Impaction, obstruction, and perforation most often occur at areas of physiologic narrowing.[14] The esophagus is a natural "filter": the majority of foreign bodies pass spontaneously if they are less than 2 cm in diameter.[2,3,6,20,21] Blunt, long, or sharp-pointed objects are most likely to be retained in the cervical esophagus (Figure 1), at the level of the aortic arch and just above the lower esophageal sphincter. The type of ingested foreign body varies with age: in young children, they are largely coins, toy parts, crayons, jewelry, and ballpoint pen caps, whereas older children and teenagers commonly tend to have problems with meat and bones (Table 1).[2–6,10,11,14,15,20–28]

Small coins (15 to 20 mm) are less likely to get stuck in the esophagus than are larger coins (20 to 35 mm), which lodge at the cricopharyngeal ring in up to 65% of cases (Figure 2), at the level of the aortic arch in 10 to 15% of cases and above the lower esophageal sphincter in 25% of cases. Radiologic investigations show that most coins pass from the esophagus to the stomach between 1 and 20 hours. Another prospective study showed that 62% of the coins were in the stomach 6 hours after ingestion.[2]

Symptoms

In young or noncommunicative (mentally impaired or psychiatrically deranged) children, the sudden onset of dysphagia, wheezing, or

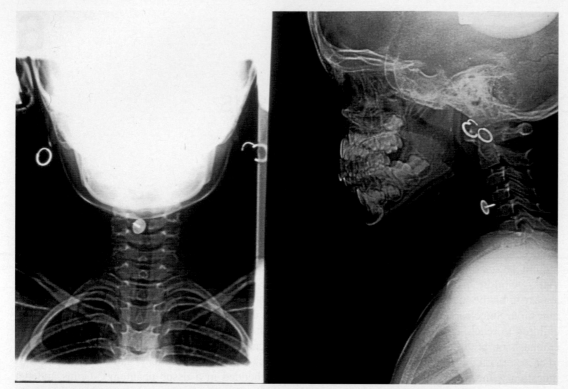

Figure 1 Ingested thumbtack at the level of the cricopharyngeus.

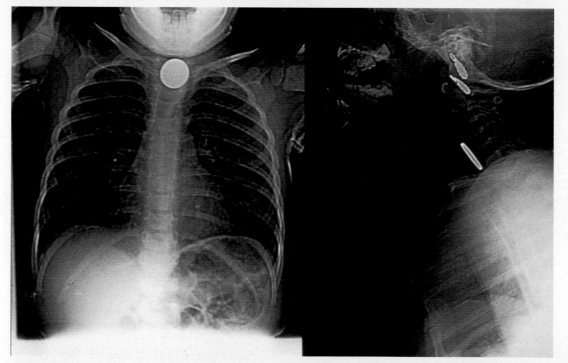

Figure 2 Anteroposterior film showing the flat surface of an ingested coin within the cervical esophagus. Lateral film showing the edge of the coin.

Table 1 Kinds of Foreign Bodies Lodged in the Esophagus
Coins
Buttons, press studs, zips
Bones*
Button battery disks
Crayons
Meat*
Toy parts
Tooth picks*
Fruits
Jewelry
Ballpoint pen caps
Salad vegetable leaves*
Needles
Can pop tops
Nails
Bottle tops
Dental retainers, crowns*
Screws
Marble
Plastic leaves
Safety pins
Stones
Spoons*
Straight pins
Drug vials and bags*
Toothbrushes*
Tacks
Small electric bulbs
Razor blades

*More frequently ingested by teenagers and adults.

respiratory distress can suggest the ingestion of a foreign body. Older children are able to identity the object swallowed and point to the location of discomfort. The most common symptoms of an impacted foreign body are choking, hoarseness, refusal to eat, vomiting, drooling, bloodstained saliva, and respiratory distress. Less common symptoms are pain on swallowing, chest pain, and localization of the level of impaction in the chest, which is usually not reliable. Long-standing esophageal foreign bodies can present as a neck mass, chronic cough or stridor, and dysphagia.

Swelling, erythema, tenderness, and crepitus in the neck region may be present with oropharyngeal and proximal esophageal perforation.[2]

Diagnosis

Radiographs usually identify most true foreign objects, bones, and the majority of complications secondary to perforation, such as pneumomediastinum, pneumothorax, mediastinitis, and pneumoperitoneum.[2,14] Plain films of the neck, chest, and abdomen are generally recommended and should be taken in both posteroanterior and

lateral views.[2,3,20,21] The lateral projection confirms location in the esophagus and may reveal the presence of more than one disk-shaped object (coins, button batteries, and tokens).[10]

Handheld metal detectors are useful to spot the majority of swallowed metallic objects and may be of use as a screening tool in pediatric patients.[23–28] Nevertheless, it depends on the location of the foreign body: in an emergency room study in 14 children the presence or absence of coins was correctly identified by a metal detector in 13.[23] When compared with radiologic studies, the remaining child had a coin lodged in the rectum. Comparable results were published by Saccheti and colleagues; of 20 coins, 1 was missed in the right iliac fossa.[24] More recently, in a large prospective study, radio-opaque metallic foreign bodies were detected by use of a metal detector in 79% of 231 cases, whereas two were not identified by radiologic studies.[26]

If symptoms are not clear or specific, a cautious contrast study may be appropriate to clarify the presence of a foreign body and define its location (Figure 3).[27,28] CT may be necessary in some cases, but can be negative with radiolucent objects; the yield may be improved with the use of three-dimensional reconstruction.[14,29] Drug packings have been studied by radiography, CT, and ultrasonography. Cannabis and cocaine packages are easily detected by plain radiographs and CT scans showing a high-density shadow surrounded by a gas halo. Heroin packages are difficult to localize, but on sonograms they appear as round echogenic structures.[29]

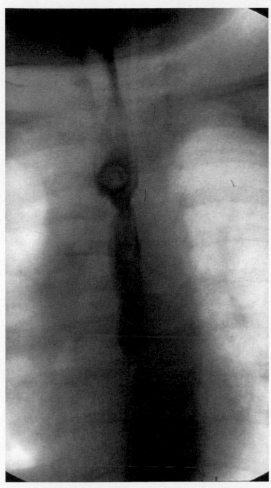

Figure 3 A 9-month-old boy who had an esophageal atresia repair has a plastic pearl impacted at the level of the anastomosis.

Treatment

The management of an esophageal foreign body is influenced by the child's age, body weight, clinical criteria (eg, the size, shape, number, and classification of ingested objects), the anatomic location in which the object is lodged and, finally, the armamentarium, skillfulness, and technical capacities of the endoscopist.

For coin ingestions, in many circumstances, noninterventional protocols are applied. Several studies propose a management based on location and symptoms.[30,31] A radiologic study documented the site of the coin. If present in the upper third of the esophagus (including the cricopharyngeus region), it should be removed urgently. Flexible endoscopy is safe and efficient, but recently safe removal using a Magill forceps has also been reported.[32] If the coin lies in the middle of the lower esophagus, a repeat film should be taken in 12 to 24 hours if the child remains asymptomatic, because most coins will pass into the stomach within 24 hours.[30] If the coin is still in the esophagus after 24 hours, it should be retrieved endoscopically. If the coin is located below the diaphragm or it is not visible, the family can be reassured; the child discharged, and the stools examined and strained to identify the passage of the coin. If, after a week the child has not passed the coin, an abdominal X-ray should be obtained. If the coin remains in the stomach

after a delay of 4 to 6 weeks, it should be removed endoscopically.[2,3,30] In removing a foreign body from the esophagus, the most important point of treatment is the maintenance of an airway at all times.[2,21] For that, anesthesia and endotracheal intubation, prior to endoscopic retrieval, is the safest method. Rat-tooth and alligator-jaws forceps are very efficient to ensure coin retrieval if the child is correctly sedated. If the patient does not have an endotracheal tube, the Trendelenburg position should be used to keep the coin out of the trachea.[21]

A "through-the-scope" balloon can also be used to extract a coin, but this is rarely necessary. Foreign bodies, such as marbles, that cannot be grasped with instruments can be removed easily under direct vision by using through-the-scope esophageal dilating balloons.[21] The Roth retrieval net, which is a polypectomy snare with a net, also can be used to capture round or oval foreign bodies.[2,20,21] If it is difficult to retrieve a foreign body from the esophagus and it is less than 2.0 cm in diameter and 5.0 cm in length, the object can be gently pushed into the stomach, and it should then pass through the rest of the gastrointestinal tract without difficulty.[2,3,14]

An alternative method for removing coins and blunt foreign bodies from the esophagus is the use of a Foley catheter.[33,34] Campbell and colleagues successfully removed blunt foreign bodies from 98 of 100 infants and children using this method.[33] However, the Foley catheter technique provides no control of the foreign body as it is being removed.[2,21] Another disadvantage is that mucosal pathology, if present, cannot be assessed. If the foreign body has been present for longer than 24 hours, or if edema is present, the Foley catheter technique should not be used. Currently, the Foley catheter technique is recommended only if endoscopy expertise is not available. A magnet can be used for the removal of metallic objects, but the disadvantages are identical to those of the Foley catheter. Paulson and Jaffe, however, reported successful removal of metallic foreign bodies in 34 of 36 cases using this technique.[35]

Sharp and pointed foreign bodies, as well as elongated foreign bodies, can be difficult to manage; fortunately, they are not common. When considering sharp and pointed foreign bodies as a separate group, morbidity and mortality figures are higher.[2,4,6,10,15,21] The most common foreign bodies in this group are toothpicks, nails, needles, bones, razor blades, and safety pins. The open safety pin represents a major problem (Figure 4). If a safety pin is in the esophagus with the open end proximal, it is best managed with the flexible endoscope by pushing the pin into the stomach, turning it, and then grasping the hinged end and pulling it out first. An alternative approach is to close the pin using a polypectomy snare. The closed safety pin, once in the stomach, will then pass without difficulty. An overtube or a rigid esophagoscope may be necessary with large, open safety pins.

An ingested razor blade is a challenging experience for both the patient and the endoscopist. This foreign body can be managed with the

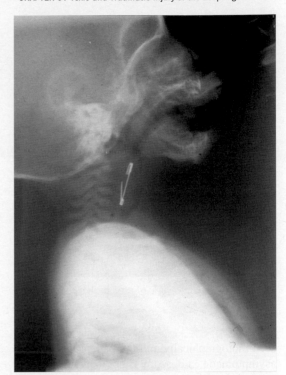

Figure 4 Open safety pin at the level of the cricopharyngeal ring.

rigid esophagoscope by pulling the blade into the instrument. One can also use a rubber hood or a piece of rubber glove on the end of the endoscope to protect the esophagus from sharp or pointed foreign bodies.[2,20,21]

The straight pin ingested by infants and children is an exception. Those longer than 5 cm may fail to pass through the duodenal loops and can perforate with a risk of hepatic hemorrhage or infection.[2,6] The use of an overtube or an endoscopic end protector hood will prevent laceration during removal of the straight pin. Crack tubes or body bags of heroin or cannabis must be retrieved very cautiously using a basket or a net, because grasping with a forceps carries the danger of tearing the bag, with intraluminal release of the narcotic substance.[2]

Recently, several cases of severe intestinal complications following multiple magnet ingestion were reported.[36,37] When more than one magnet is ingested, intestinal injuries can occur, because the magnets are attracted to each other across the bowel wall leading to pressure necrosis, perforation, fistula formation, and intestinal obstruction. Consequently, if more than one magnet is found as a foreign body in the esophagus or in the stomach, they should be removed immediately by endoscopy.

Radiolucent objects such as pieces of glass, bone fragments, aluminum (eg, canned drink pop tabs), plastic, and pieces of wood often are difficult to see in the hypopharynx and cervical esophagus on routine radiographs.[21] It the patient reports swallowing a foreign body and it is not seen on routine radiographs, thin barium is used to try to outline the object.[2] If the foreign body is identified radiographically, endoscopy is performed. If no foreign body is seen radiographically, but the patient remains symptomatic, endoscopy should also be performed (Figure 5). If no foreign body is

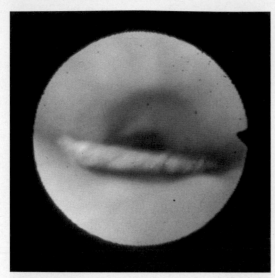

Figure 5 Endoscopic view of a rabbit bone stuck in the esophagus.

seen radiographically and the patient has become asymptomatic, endoscopy is not mandatory.[21]

Complications

Esophageal examination in children with coin ingestions of less than 24 hours in duration shows normal mucosa in the majority, and minimal erythema or abrasions in a minority of cases. Complications increase with the length of time the foreign body remains in the esophagus, with perforations, particularly from sharp bodies, occurring after 24 hours.[2,31] Fewer than 1% of esophageal foreign bodies cannot be retrieved by endoscopy, requiring esophagotomy. Perforation of the esophagus after foreign body and coin ingestions may be either acutely symptomatic or asymptomatic. Aspiration pneumonia, lobar atelectasia, hemoptysis, perforation with neck abscess, mediastinitis with lung abscess, acquired esophageal pouch, pseudodiverticula, tracheoesophageal fistula, esophageal-aortic fistula, perforation of the heart by an open safety pin, and aortic pseudoaneurysm are less common complications, reported to occur months to even years after impaction of the foreign body.[2]

A CT scan is useful in confirming the location of impacted fish bones and radiolucent foreign bodies, as well as identifying inflammatory changes in adjacent structures.[29,38] Indications for thoracotomy to remove a long-retained foreign body are poor endoscopic visualization of the foreign body because of inflammatory tissue and massive bleeding during endoscopy.[2]

Nickel dermatitis and associated gastritis and copper and zinc toxicity have been reported after coin ingestion, usually by retarded or schizophrenic adults.[2,39]

FOOD IMPACTION

Food bolus obstruction can occur in children with an esophageal stricture. If there is no esophageal stenosis identified at endoscopy, underly-

ing motility disorders should be considered (eg, achalasia, primary motor disorders, neuromuscular diseases, scleroderma, infections, and eosinophilic esophagitis). Children who are in severe distress and unable to swallow oral secretions require immediate intervention. If the patient is not uncomfortable, not at risk for aspiration and able to handle secretions, then intervention need not be emergent and can be postponed, because food impactions will often pass spontaneously.[21] However, endoscopic intervention should not be delayed beyond 24 hours from presentation because the risk of complications increases.[6,15,20]

The initial endoscopic examination should verify and locate the site of the impaction. The food bolus can usually be removed either in bloc or in a piecemeal fashion.[14]

An overtube may facilitate multiple passes of the endoscope, protect the esophageal mucosa, and minimize the risk of aspiration. Nevertheless, in small children this technique is difficult to use because of the risk of esophageal injury during insertion of the overtube. Once reduced in size, the bolus often will pass under endoscopic visualization and direction. The high frequency of underlying esophageal pathology in this setting increases the risk associated with the practice of blindly pushing an impacted food bolus with an endoscope or a dilator.[14] The application of a cautery current applied to a bipolar snare to cut into and retrieve an impacted food bolus in the esophagus has been reported.[40,41]

Enzymatic digestion with papain should not be used, because it has been associated with hypernatremia, erosion, and esophageal perforation.[20,21] The administration of glucagon 0.5 to 1.0 mg intravenously, in an attempt to relax the esophagus, is generally safe and may promote spontaneous passage of an impacted food bolus while definitive endoscopic therapy is being coordinated. However, its use should not delay definitive endoscopic removal.[14] The use of a cola beverage has even been suggested to "digest" a food bolus trapped in an esophageal stricture to avoid the need for endoscopy.[42]

FOOD-RELATED ESOPHAGEAL TRAUMA

Food-related trauma of the esophagus in children is rare. In adults, esophageal hematoma or laceration has been reported following impaction of tortilla chips, taco shells, bagels, and bay leaves. Ingestion of hot pepper sauces can cause esophageal burns; inflammation of the mucosa is associated with an increase in esophageal peristalsis.[2]

DISK BATTERY INGESTION

The disk button battery is a single cell usually used to power digital watches, photographic equipment, toys, hearing aids, car electronic keys, handheld calculators, and even musical greeting cards.[2,43] Although these cells are sealed, they

contain corrosive and toxic chemicals. Lodgment in the esophagus can lead to mucosal damage, and exposure to gastric acid is associated with a remote risk of leakage of the cell contents.[44,45]

There are four main types of button cell: mercury, silver, alkaline manganese, and lithium. Lithium cells are mostly used in watches in which replacement is normally by a specialist, thereby limiting access by children. Lithium cells exhibit a potential of 3 V against the 1.5 V of the other systems, but are more resistant to corrosion than other button cells. Used batteries are less toxic than new ones. Discharged cells are less liable to leak and cause tissue injury. In discharged mercury cells, mercuric oxide is largely converted to elemental mercury, which is not absorbed.[43,45] Mechanisms that corrode the cell container also discharge the cell, so the contents of a discharged cell are the most relevant.[43]

With an estimated 510 to 850 ingestions yearly, a National Button Battery Ingestion Study was begun in 1982 in the United States to provide guidelines for therapy. A 1992 update from this registry described 2,382 cases, the authors estimated a minimum of 2,100 battery ingestions per year, based on figures of 2.1 to 8.5 ingestions per million population.[46] The majority of buttons contained silver or mercuric oxide. Less common were magnesium dioxide, zinc or air, or lithium content, with all containing a 20 to 45% solution of potassium or sodium hydroxide. Most frequently ingested were 7.9 mm and 11.6 mm batteries. Ingesters were primarily young, with 71% less than 5 years, and 1 to 2 year olds and males at greatest risk. Nearly half of children find the battery loose or discarded, with a surprising source (44%) from hearing aids. More than one battery was ingested by 8.5% of patients. Older children and adults, while testing the viability of the battery by touching it to the tongue, have inadvertently swallowed it. Lithium batteries, with larger diameters and greater voltage, cause the most severe injuries. Mercuric oxide cells are more likely to fragment.[2,47]

Although 90% of batteries pass spontaneously between 12 hours and 14 days, with 31% requiring more than 48 hours, those lodged in the esophagus (4.2%) require early removal. Most of the batteries lodged in the esophagus are 20 to 23 mm in diameter. Esophageal injury is attributable to electrolyte leakage from the battery, alkali produced from external flow of current causing liquefaction necrosis (it is estimated that when lodged in the esophagus, 26 to 45% will leak sodium or potassium hydroxide), mercury toxicity, pressure necrosis, and direct flow of current causing low-voltage burns.[2] Although most batteries show corrosion, they do not disassemble, but 2% fragment and 11% have either severe crimp dissolution or extensive perforations.[46]

Esophageal damage occurs rapidly, and burns are noted as early as 1 hour after ingestion. Within 4 hours, there may be involvement of all layers of the esophagus. In experimental studies in dogs in whom batteries were placed within the esophagus, by 8 hours there was mucosal abrasion and necrosis under the muscular layer without evidence of battery leakage. In rabbits, esophageal injury was created by placing a 3-V battery in the esophagus for 9 hours that results in more severe damage on the alkaline side when the battery was placed with the cathode directed toward the trachea. More severe damage is produced by a lithium battery than a button alkali battery, with damage occurring within 15 minutes.[2]

Symptoms

Usually, children are asymptomatic after button battery ingestion.[44,46] Nevertheless, immediate symptoms can include coughing, gagging, nausea, vomiting, and chest or abdominal pain.[2]

Diagnosis

The battery must be identified and distinguished from a coin radiologically. In the anterior projection, a battery shows a double-density shadow owing to its bilamellar structure (Figure 6). On lateral films, the edges are round and show a step-off at the junction of anode and cathode.

Treatment

Ipecac is not recommended to induce vomiting, because it may lead to aspiration and impaction of the disk in the respiratory tree or to retrograde movement from the stomach into the esophagus. Ipecac use also carries a risk of perforation of the stomach or esophagus if the battery has caused a mucosal burn.[2] Administration of neutralizing solutions or charcoal has not proven helpful. A treatment protocol recommended by the Button Battery study advocates nothing by mouth and an initial radiologic study to determine the location of the battery.[46] If the battery is lodged within the esophagus, it should be removed immediately.[2,44,46] Endoscopic retrieval rates are 33 to 100% and, in children, endoscopic removal is performed using general anesthesia (to avoid

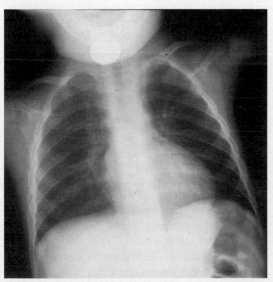

Figure 6 Anteroposterior film of a large disk battery (20 mm) with the halo sign (double-density shadow).

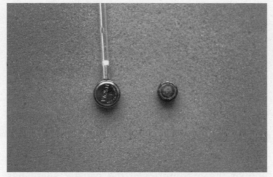

Figure 7 The new battery on the left is attracted with the magnet tube. The battery on the right shows severe corrosion after 6 hours in the upper gastrointestinal tract.

aspiration) and may include the use of a polyp snare, a Roth retrieval net, a basket, or a through-the-endoscope balloon.[2] Endoscopy also permits assessment of the degree of esophageal trauma. If there is evidence of tissue damage, a follow-up barium study should be performed 10 to 14 days later to rule out stricture and fistula formation.[47]

Success for removal of disk batteries lodged in the esophagus has also been reported with the use of a Foley catheter, a balloon, and a magnetized catheter (Figure 7). Button batteries located in the esophagus and stomach are easily extracted with a magnet attached to an orogastric tube: magnetic removal proved successful in 49 of 56 attempts, including all 14 cells lodged in the esophagus.[44] Failure of extraction occurred for 6 batteries located in the duodenum and solely for 1 in the stomach. This type of device is inexpensive (50 dollars) and can be used by pediatricians under fragmentary fluoroscopy.[44]

Management of a battery in the stomach remains controversial; for some authors, the child can be discharged home with normal eating and activity, with the parents instructed to strain the stool for retrieval of the battery and to report pain, fever, and vomiting.[43,45,47] A prokinetic agent or a laxative may hasten battery transit through the stomach and small intestine. If the battery remains within the stomach after 1 week, it should be retrieved by endoscopy. If the battery fails to move through the intestine or if the child develops severe abdominal pain or peritoneal symptoms, it should be removed surgically.[2]

Complications

Reported complications of esophageal lesions are tracheoesophageal fistula, perforation, stricture, and even death.[2,49,50,51] A battery may lodge in a Meckel diverticulum and cause perforation.[2] Mercury toxicity is possible but rare, with only one mild case reported. Elemental mercury is produced by the action of gastric acid and iron from the casing, which, in contrast to mercuric oxide, is readily absorbed. Elevated mercury levels are reported in some patients after battery ingestion, but there are no signs of mercury toxicity.[47] The highest mercury levels found in children in whom the batteries split before or after passage and who have evidence of radiopaque droplets within the

gastrointestinal tract. Rashes owing to presumed nickel hypersensitivity occur in approximately 2% of children. Systemic absorption of lithium following ingestion of a lithium button battery has also been described.[48]

CAUSTIC INGESTIONS

Ingestions of caustic agents occur frequently in young children. The peak incidence is below the age of 5 years. The estimated frequency of admissions for caustic ingestion ranges from 1,000 to 20,000 per year in industrialized countries; the majority of cases are children.[52] Severe caustic injuries have also been reported from developing countries, especially in northern Africa.[53] The male-to-female ratio is usually 1.2 to 1.4:1, although a female preponderance has also been reported, mainly owing to occupational habits. After a rise in frequency in the 1960s, there has been a decreasing incidence owing to legislation and because of an increasing awareness of the hazards of storing caustic products in an inappropriate way, such as within the reach of young children and in food and drink containers.[52] Inappropriate storage occurred in 10 to 15% of the accidental ingestions.[54]

Etiology

In the majority of cases, ingestion of caustic agents in children is accidental.[2,52–54] Only a minority of cases are intentional as an attempt at suicide or, rarely, as an attempt at homicide.[52] Caustic products ingested by children most often are strong alkaline or acidic agents. Liquid forms cause more serious injuries than solid products, which are more irritating and difficult to swallow.[2,55] Strong alkali are used in the household as cleaning agents for the dishwasher (sodium metasilicate, sodium tripolyphosphate), oven, drain, or toilet bowl or as a declogging agent (sodium hydroxide, potassium hydroxide). Sodium hydroxide tablets are used for medical (Clinitest tablets) and sometimes pseudomedical purposes (a homemade mixture to predict gender during pregnancy) and cause caustic as well as thermic injury, leading to devastatingly deep burns.[55] Ammonia causes not only caustic esophageal injury, but also chemical pneumonitis and pulmonary edema. Less frequently, caustic esophagitis is caused by the ingestion of strong acids (eg, hydrochloric, sulfuric, formic, and phosphoric acid used in the household as cleaner for coffee makers, irons, and toilet bowls, but also used as soldering fixes, antirust compounds, battery liquids, and cleaners for swimming pools, milking machines, and slate).

Detergents and bleach are reported to be ingested most commonly by children, but this is not confirmed by many reports. Household bleaches (Na hypochlorite, pH 6.0) are considered an esophageal irritant, but do not cause tissue necrosis because of low concentration (5%) and therefore seldom cause clinically significant esophageal injury.[2,52,54–57] Yarrington studied the effect of sodium hypochlorite bleach on the canine esophagus and concluded that although ingestion of household bleach may induce mucosal burns and edema, extensive necrosis and stricture formation do not occur.[57]

Pathophysiology

The physical form and pH of the corrosive agent play a significant role in the location and type of resultant injuries. Crystalline drain cleaners (lye) or dishwasher powders tend to adhere to the oropharynx or become lodged in the upper esophagus, where they cause the most damage.[55,56] High-density liquid drain cleaners, on the other hand, usually pass rapidly through the oropharynx and upper esophagus to cause more serious in the lower esophagus and stomach. Strong acids also usually pass rapidly through the esophagus and cause damage in the stomach and duodenum.

Since corrosive substance ingestions are rarely fatal and the injured mucosa is seldom removed surgically during the immediate postinjury phase, little histopathologic information is derived from human specimens. Much of what is known is derived from studies in experimental animals where acid burns cause a coagulation necrosis that usually limits acid penetration and results in damage limited to the surface mucosa.[2,56] Both cats and dogs have been used to study the effects of sodium hydroxide on the esophagus. Initially, there is liquefaction necrosis with destruction of the surface epithelium and the submucosal layer. Hemorrhage, thrombosis, and a marked inflammatory response with significant edema are seen within the first 24 hours of injury (as an early acute phase). Depending on the extent of the burn, inflammation may extend through the muscle layer and perforation may occur. After several days, the necrotic tissue is sloughed, edema decreases, and neovascularization begins. This early reparative, or subacute, phase extends from the end of the first week through the second week after injury, and if the insult has been relatively minor, normal esophageal function begins to return. The cicatrization phase begins in the third week when fibroblast proliferation replaces the submucosa and muscularis mucosa and stricture formation begins. During this time, adhesions form and narrowing or obliteration of the esophageal lumen can occur. If there has been a significant penetrating injury, adhesions to surrounding mediastinal tissues may also occur. Reepithelialization begins during the third week and is usually complete by the sixth week after injury.[56]

Symptoms

The clinical presentation of caustic esophageal injury shows a wide spectrum: in many cases, the child will have no complaints, and the physical examination is normal. At the other end of the clinical spectrum, the child can presents in circulatory shock or severe respiratory distress.[58–60] Respiratory distress and stridor following laryngeal injury occur most frequently in children below the age of 2 years, and are not related to the nature of the caustic ingestion. Vomiting, dysphagia, drooling, epigastric pain, abdominal pain, and refusal to drink do not accurately predict either the presence or the severity of esophageal injury.[52] A close inspection of the patient will show irritation or frank burns periorally, on the lips, but also on other parts of the body; for example, on the thorax and or the extremities if the caustic agent has been vomited. Inspection of the mouth and pharynx can show edema, ulceration, or white, fragile, easily bleeding membranes over the buccal mucosa, tongue, uvula, and tonsils. Laryngoscopy can reveal laryngeal edema or more severe lesions. Fever may occur, and in 30% a leukocytosis is present.[52]

Serious esophageal burn and even perforation can occur in the absence of oropharyngeal burns or abdominal complaints. On the other hand, burns in the mouth do not provide evidence of an esophageal burn.[2,52,54,59,60]

Diagnosis

Ingestion of caustic agents by children is often unwitnessed. The first element in diagnosing esophageal burn is a good history taking. Every effort should be made to document the ingested agent, its physical and chemical characteristics and the volume taken to estimate both caustic properties and noncaustic toxicity.[2,52] However, adequate information often is simply not available. The easiest way to obtain such information is to have the product itself.

If there is any suspicion of the ingestion of a caustic agent, the child needs immediate evaluation by a physician. Burns to the mouth or pharynx are inaccurate as indicators of the presence and extent of esophageal injury and, therefore, mandate endoscopy. Conversely, the absence of an oropharyngeal burn should not eliminate the need for endoscopy.[2,52,54,59,60]

Esophagoscopy with a flexible pediatric endoscope, allowing complete examination of both the esophagus and stomach, is the single most accurate method to assess esophageal injury. Upper endoscopy should be performed within 12 to 36 hours after ingestion or suspicion of ingestion.[2,52] Esophagoscopy should be done under general anesthesia. Not all authors, however, agree with the need for systematic endoscopy.[2,52,54,55] Two studies concluded that endoscopy is not mandatory for children living in developed countries who are asymptomatic after nonintentional caustic ingestion.[61,62]

Caustic esophageal lesions are graded endoscopically as grade 0, normal; grade I, erythema and edema; grade II-A, noncircumferential superficial mucosal ulcerations with necrotic tissue and white plaques extending over less than one-third of the esophageal length; grade II-B, the same as grade II, with deep or circumferential ulcerations

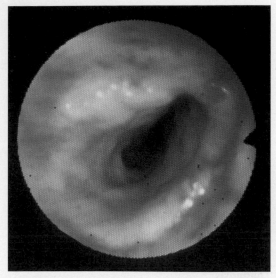

Figure 8 Endoscopic view of a grade III caustic esophagitis.

extending over more than one-third of the esophagus; grade III-A, mucosal ulcerations and area of necrosis in a circumferential pattern extending over less than one-third of the esophagus length; and grade III-B, extensive necrosis over more than one-third of the esophagus.[63] Some authors include a grade IV, that is, with signs of transmural necrosis, shock, coagulopathy, and metabolic acidosis. Others do not take into account the circumferential appearance of the lesions. Distinguishing grade II from grade III then can be difficult endoscopically, however, because there is no clear definition of how the depth of an injury is determined (Figure 8).[52]

Radiology is adequate in the management of caustic esophageal injury.[52,64] Barium swallow, when performed early, is useful in assessing perforation in patients with suggestive symptoms; however, it is rarely sensitive enough to detect early mucosal injury or to allow therapeutic or prognostic decisions. When esophagography is performed 2 to 3 weeks after ingestion, an assessment of stricture formation can be made.[65] Cineesophagography has been recommended as the examination of choice in assessing esophageal damage sufficient to provoke stricture formation: mucosal and submucosal injuries are seen as irregularities along the contact margin. Alterations in esophageal motility, resulting from injury to the myenteric nerve plexuses, are an indication of a severe burn and accurately predict evolution to stricture formation.[65,66]

Outcome

Sequelae of caustic injuries of the esophagus are stricture formation, development of achalasia, brachyesophagus, gastroesophageal reflux and, as a late complication, development of malignancy.[2,52] Esophageal motor function is disordered for days to years after lye ingestion and can present as weak to absent peristaltic contractions, nonpropulsive contractions, gastroesophageal reflux, and dysphagia. Studies with pH monitoring, esophageal manometry, radiology, and esophageal transit scintigraphy with technetium 99m or krypton 81m show that the severity of dysphagia does not correlate with the degree of the residual stenosis, but rather relates to specific patterns of esophageal motility.[66,67] The frequency of esophageal strictures in children ranges from 9 to 18%.[52,59,60,65] Most strictures result from grade III lesions and, to a lesser degree, from grade II-B but, rarely, from grade II-A. Most authors agree that grade I lesions heal without stricture, regardless of treatment, and that grade III lesions progress to stricture, regardless of treatment.[52,54] Acute inflammatory strictures appear at about 21 days (or earlier); complete stricture formation takes roughly 30 to 45 days (Figure 9).[54,56] Pyloric stenosis can occur after gastric lesions, mainly owing to acidic agents.[52,54]

Treatment

Some investigators suggest that patients who are asymptomatic after unintentional ingestions are not at risk for complications and do not necessarily have to undergo endoscopy.[61,62] Many, however, agree that children suspected of caustic ingestion should be admitted to the hospital for observation.[2,52,54,56,60] Intravenous fluids are administered and the child not permitted to drink until the decision for endoscopy is made.[2,52,54,55,65]

If there is a reasonable suspicion of caustic ingestion, regardless of symptomatology, the child should be brought immediately to the emergency department.[52] If medical advice is asked by telephone, the first treatment that should be recommended is not to make the child vomit or to give any acid or alkali to neutralize the agent

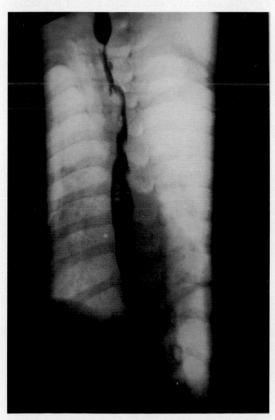

Figure 9 Severe irregular stricture of the upper third of the esophagus.

ingested, as is sometimes recommended on the packaging of caustic agents, since the latter can cause exothermal reactions and additional injury. Water can be used to wash away residual caustic from the buccal mucosa and face.[52,56] There is no role for diluents, emetics, lavage, smectite, aluminum phosphate, or charcoal. The use of a nasogastric tube for gastric lavage is contraindicated, because of the risk of aggravation of esophageal injury and of esophageal perforation. For suspicion of ingestion of bleach or mild household detergents, endoscopy is not mandatory, except when signs or symptoms suggest mucosal injury.[2,52,57,61,62]

After admission to the hospital, when severe symptoms are present in cases of perforation, laryngeal obstruction, and pulmonary edema, immediate treatment consists of resuscitation, airway control, administration of fluids, plasma expanders, and blood. Children with severe lesions should be kept under strict surveillance in an intensive care unit during the first week after the accident. Early surgical treatment in cases of esophageal or gastric perforation or laryngeal edema, or for feeding gastrostomy in cases of very severe injury, is rarely indicated.[65] Emergency esophagectomy is indicated only if massive quantities of a strong caustic agent are ingested with esophageal necrosis, which occurs almost exclusively in the setting of an intentional ingestion. Gastric resection, if indicated, must be sparse and limited to the antrum, if possible.[52]

When no burns or grade I lesions are present on endoscopy, no treatment is indicated, and the patient can be discharged home. Children with grade II-A lesions are usually observed for 1 to 3 days in the hospital. In some centers, they receive no treatment, but elsewhere are given oral broad-spectrum antibiotics and, in some cases, acid suppression medications.

Once evidence of grade II-B or grade III lesions is established, treatment of esophageal lesions is directed toward the prevention of strictures. Optimal nutrition is imperative during the acute healing phase.[2,52,54,56] Liquids are given by mouth as soon as the child is able to swallow. Oral intake, if possible, is started with antacids and dairy products. The diet is progressively increased as tolerated. If the patient is unable to eat, either a feeding gastrostomy or parenteral nutrition is indicated. Total parenteral nutrition is given in grade II and III lesions in some centers for at least 3 weeks and continued if there is still no healing of the lesions.[68]

The specific treatment regimen used for significant caustic esophagitis seems to have less influence on the development of stricture formation than the degree of injury immediately after ingestion. Evidence from animal experiments has shown that systemic or locally injected steroids prevent stricture formation, although there is a high mortality resulting from infections.[52,56,66] Corticosteroid treatment (prednisone) at the dose of 2 mg/kg has since been

widely used in humans, but it is also rejected as a therapy because of lack of proof of efficacy and due to concerns about serious infections.[2,52,54–56] In a review of 10 clinical studies,[69] in which 572 patients were assessed, and in a controlled study,[64] no significant difference were shown in the frequency of esophageal strictures between patients treated with corticosteroids (2 mg/kg/d) and those not treated. Compared with those treated with prednisone 2 mg/kg, patients with severe caustic esophageal lesions treated with dexamethasone 1 g/1.73 m^2/d developed less esophageal strictures.[70] However, patients in the dexamethasone-treated group had less severe lesions than the patients in the other groups. On the other hand, there was a marked reduction in the number of esophageal dilatations used to treat strictures when high-dose dexamethasone was given immediately after the dilatation.[70,71] A multicenter study of the French Speaking Society of Pediatric Hepatology, Gastroenterology, and Nutrition assessed 43 children with severe corrosive esophagitis who were treated with dexamethasone (1 g/1.73 m^2/d), with a 70% success rate in the prevention of stricture formation.[72]

The use of antibiotics also remains controversial.[65] In all cases in which steroids are included as therapy, antibiotics are associated with the prevention of infection.[2,52] In some reports, antibiotics without steroid treatment are used.[52,58,68] However, bacteremia does not occur even in severe reflux esophagitis, and it is rare in caustic lesions, except in those with a perforation. Bacteremia can also occur, although rarely, after esophageal dilatation. If antibiotics are used, generally ampicillin 50 to 100 mg/kg/d is given.[2,52] As caustic injury causes esophageal dysmotility and gastroesophageal reflux,[52,54] acid blockade is also indicated.

The use of an esophageal stent to prevent stricture formation has been tried in cats and in humans,[52] with variable degrees of success in preventing strictures.[2,52,54] The rationale is that stenting inhibits synechial formation in ulcerated zones, inhibits excessive granuloma formation and retraction of fibrous tissue, and facilitates epithelialization. A stent is believed to give a continuous, atraumatic, and early dilatation. It permits early gastric feeding, facilitates later dilatation if necessary and can avoid the need for a gastrostomy. Stenting was performed in the past with a silicone rubber nasogastric tube, but poor tolerance of the stent was reported.[52] More recently, self-expanding plastic or metal stent devices inserted through an endoscope have been tried with success.[73,74] The stent can be kept in situ for 3 to 4 weeks, although durations of up to 3 months have been reported.[73,74] Stenting is also used in combination with corticosteroids. Possible disadvantages of stenting are enhanced gastroesophageal reflux and pro-inflammatory reactions, provoking stenosis delaying healing. Furthermore, there is a risk of perforation when placed in a blinded fashion.[52] Severe ulcerative esophagitis following the placement of a self-expanding metal-stent has been reported in a child.[75]

Gastrostomy, whether or not in combination with a stent, is performed in severe burns to allow feeding and to facilitate dilatations. Additionally, it allows superficial exploration of the stomach.

Endoscopic or radiographic evaluation after 2 to 3 weeks establishes healing of the lesions or the development of a stricture. If no healing of the lesions has occurred, treatment must be continued. If a stricture is developing, dilatation is initiated, but should not be started before 1 to 2 months after ingestion. If performed at high enough frequency, dilatations can prevent major surgery. Dilatations have been performed either in an antegrade way with Eder–Puestow dilators, Savary bougies, and mercury-filled Hurst-Maloney bougies or in a retrograde fashion with Tucker dilators using an endless guidewire via a gastrostomy.[2,52,54,55] Recent studies report no difference between bougienage and balloon dilatation regarding the risk of esophageal perforation, although the balloon technique seems less hazardous and more efficient.[2,52] Dilatation is performed under general anesthesia and is repeated every 2 or 3 weeks, starting at every session with the size that was used when the last session was completed.[52,72] When dilatation progresses, the frequency is reduced and, according to the result, is eventually stopped. The goal of treatment is to dilate the esophageal stricture so that the child is able to take a normal diet by mouth. However, dysphagia, a common symptom in esophageal stricture, does not correlate with esophageal caliber but with the esophageal transit time, as measured by scintigraphy and with the esophageal motor function, as measured by manometry.[66,67] Complications of esophageal dilatations include traumatic perforation and tracheoesophageal fistula. When serious complications occur, the dilatations should be interrupted.[52,72] Dilatation is not indicated in patients showing clear evidence of developing severe extended stenosis, even early after ingestion, or in patients unable to swallow their own saliva. Failure of dilatation is defined as the need for continuous dilatation after completion of a 12- to 18-month dilatation program or when the psychological burden on the child has become too severe.[2] Recent studies report using topical mitomycin C to prevent of restenosis after dilatation in the management of intransigent esophageal strictures.[73,76,77] Alternative ways of stricture treatment include resection of the stenosis, failure to obtain sufficient dilatation is considered an indication for esophageal replacement.[52] However, esophageal replacement should not be performed until at least 6 months of medical treatment.[2,52] Colonic interposition is the most frequent therapeutic procedure, but other techniques, such as gastric interposition and gastric tube formation are also used, but the latter can be performed only if there is no gastric lesion. The transverse colon and the left or right hemicolon are anastomosed in either an isoperistaltic or an antiperistaltic fashion.[2,52] The antiperistaltic anastomosis is preferred by some surgeons because it inhibits gastroesophageal reflux, although, in practice, it appears to make little functional difference. Additionally, a pyloroplasty and fundoplication can be performed to prevent reflux.[52] Perioperative and early postoperative complications include perforation and torsion of the colonic transplant, ischemia of the colon, a tracheal tear, pneumothorax, and cervical hematoma. The most frequent late complications include anastomotic leak or fistula, cervical anastomotic stenosis, anastomotic bleeding, and gastroesophageal reflux. However, pyloric stenosis, transient dumping syndrome, eventration, and mediastinitis are also reported as late complications of surgery. There is some discussion whether esophagectomy should be performed simultaneously with an esophageal replacement.[2,52] As patients with esophageal stricture are at risk for malnutrition, adequate nutritional support during the pre- and postoperative period is crucial.[52]

Risks of Cancer

Carcinoma of the esophagus occurs with a thousandfold increased risk in patients with a history of caustic lesion.[54] The percentage of caustic esophageal lesions in which carcinoma ultimately develops is up to 5%, but figures as high to 30% have been reported.[2,52] In a large series of 846 patients with esophageal squamous cell carcinoma registered between 1941 and 1981, 12 (1.4%) had previously ingested a caustic agent.[78] In another series of 2,414 patients with carcinoma of the esophagus, 63 had previously ingested lye.[79] The time interval between the ingestion and diagnosis of esophageal carcinoma was between 13 and 71 years. The latent time between the corrosive accident and cancer is inversely correlated with age at the time of ingestion.[78,79] Carcinoma can also develop in the isolated strictured esophagus left in situ after replacement therapy.[52] The risk of malignancy has led some authors to strongly advocate early colonic interposition surgery in severe caustic esophageal injury, even in childhood.[2,52] A possible contributory factor in the evolution to malignancy after caustic esophageal injury is repeated stricture dilatations.

THERMIC AND ELECTRIC BURNS

Burns may follow the drinking of hot beverages. In infants, intensive warming up of bottles may induce acute burns in the throat and esophagus. Since microwave ovens rapidly cook through to the center of heated foods, children may suffer esophageal burns, not appreciating that the interior of a heated dish is intensely hot, even though the outer covering is only moderately warm.[80]

Electrical burns of the esophagus in adults occur in situations of esophageal temperature monitoring during general anesthesia. Experimentally, they have been produced during pill electrode transesophageal pacing when current levels above 75 mA are applied over a period of less than 30 minutes. A deliberate electrical burn followed by stricture was reported in a suicide attempt by ingestion of an active electrical wire.[2]

Electrical burns of the esophagus in children are extremely rare. Charged disk-shaped or cylindrical batteries may produce a direct current flow of 1.5 to 3.0 V. Low-voltage burns are described with batteries lodged in the esophagus; endoscopy shows lesions ranging from mucosal edema to necrosis and hemorrhagic deep ulcerations.[2,45] In experimental studies in animals, esophageal damage occurs rapidly, and burns are noted 1 hour after contact with the mucosa; lesions of the submucosa and the muscle layers were observed after 8 hours.[2]

RADIATION-INDUCED INJURY

Because some children need radiation therapy for thoracic tumors, the risk of esophageal damage is a consideration, even though the esophagus has long been considered relatively radioresistant. A deleterious effect is enhanced by the combined effects of chemotherapeutic agents.[81–84]

Pathologic examination of samples of irradiated esophagus shows early degenerative changes: inhibition of mitosis in the germinal cells of the squamous epithelium and dilation of the capillaries with edema and leukocytic infiltration.[81] Epithelial cells may slough, and some glandular cells are distended with secretions, whereas others are atrophic. Endothelial cells proliferate and regeneration begins at the end of therapy and then continues for 3, or more, months. Late effects are dependent on the dose, length of irradiation, and length of the exposed esophagus. Injury results from damage to capillaries and disturbances of microcirculation in the tissues, causing tissue hypoxia, oxidative stress, and loss of parenchymal cells.[2] The most frequent complications are altered motility, mucosal ulceration, pseudodiverticula, and stricture formation owing to fibrosis of the lamina propria and submucosa.[81–83] Secondary changes, such as altered motility and stricture, can occur 10 to 15 years after the exposure to radiation.[83–84] These chronic lesions are secondary to subepithelial and arteriolar-capillary fibrosis, causing epithelial atrophy and ulceration. Esophageal squamous cell carcinoma is a rare late complication and, in one instance, developed 30 years after mediastinal irradiation.[85]

Symptoms

Acute manifestations of radiation-induced damage are mucositis, dysphagia and odynophagia, which generally appear 10 to 12 days after the start of therapy. Some patients experience sharp chest pains that radiate to the back and may be lessened by interruption of radiation treatment for up to 10 days. Radiologic examination of the esophagus at this time shows fine mucosal serrations and an absence of primary peristalsis. Double-contrast radiologic studies performed 13 to 87 days after the initiation of radiation therapy showed multiple, small, discrete ulcers and a granular appearance of the mucosa.[85,86] In 13 asymptomatic patients investigated at the end of this period, 3 (23%) developed significant strictures.[86]

Treatment

Treatment during irradiation with sucralfate has been of limited efficacy in the treatment of esophagitis, particularly if used after the onset of symptoms. The combination of sucralfate with fluconazole initiated during the fourth week of treatment seems to diminish oral discomfort and pain.[2] Treatment for acute esophagitis consists of viscous xylocaine and diphenhydramine for topical anesthesia, and the use of acid suppression or a calcium channel blocker like nifedipine.[2,84] Strictures are treated by stenting, bougienage, and balloon dilatation.

PILL-INDUCED ESOPHAGEAL INJURY

Esophageal injury caused directly by prolonged mucosal contact with tablets or capsules ingested in therapeutic dosages was first reported in adults.[83] Since that time, a variety of drugs have been identified as causing esophagitis (Table 2).[84] Many cases of pill-induced esophageal injury likely are unrecognized and underreported because most patients recover fully. Medication-induced esophageal injury is rare in children, because the presence of an underlying systemic disease or esophageal transit abnormalities is not frequent. Pills and gelatin or cellulose capsules have a great tendency to adhere to the esophageal mucosa. By contrast, aqueous suspensions, syrups and powders are less likely to stick to the mucosa and induce esophageal injury.[89] Nevertheless, some cases of drug-induced esophageal damage are reported in children.[90–92]

In adults, the most common site of esophageal injury is near the level of the aortic arch, an area characterized by external compression from the arch itself, a transition from skeletal to smooth muscle and by a physiologic reduction in the amplitude of esophageal peristaltic waves, all of which can contribute to pill retention.

Table 2 Orally Administered Drugs Causing Esophageal Damage

Doxycycline
Other antibiotics: tetracycline, clindamycin, oxytetracycline minocycline, erythromycin, phenoxymethylpenicillin, lincomycin, tinidazole, rifampin, metronidazole
Ephedrine
Emeprodium bromide
Potassium chloride
Ferrous sulfate or succinate
Bisphosphonates
Alprenolol chloride
Quinidine and chloroquine phosphate
Indomethacin
Aspirin, phenacitin, acetaminophen
Phenylbutazone
Prednisone
Birth control pills
Ascorbic acid

The sharp demarcation of esophageal injury seen in most cases suggests that this injury results from mucosal contact with a potentially caustic agent. This premise is supported by the fact that 25% of patients sense that the swallowed pill had stuck in the chest and, by the occasional observation of pill fragments in a region of injury.[87,88]

About 40% of patients take pills with little or no fluid. A further predisposition to injury is decreased salivation and decreased swallowing if the pill is taken at night and if the patient lies down shortly after its ingestion.[2]

Symptoms

Most commonly, presenting symptoms include continuous retrosternal pain and dysphagia occurring shortly after pill ingestion. Less common symptoms are abdominal pain, weight loss, hematemesis, and dehydration. Lesions of the lower esophagus are less frequent, and their symptoms may be erroneously attributed to gastroesophageal reflux. Doxycycline, ferrous sulfate, and emepronium bromide produce an acid pH (less than 3) even when dissolved in water and may injure the buccal mucosa if held in the mouth for a protracted time. Doxycycline further accumulates in the buccal layer of squamous epithelium. Stricture may be an eventual complication of this type of esophageal burn.[2,87]

Endoscopy shows circumferential lesions, well-delineated ulcers, or a longitudinal exudate with necrotic epithelial shreds covering linear ulcerations. Histologically, changes vary from intense inflammatory reaction to erosions and necrosis.

Conventional barium studies are positive only in cases with deep ulcerations or strictures. Double-contrast studies may show the discrete, clustered, ovoid ulcerations, and more subtle mucosal abnormalities of edema and irregularity.

Treatment

To avoid esophageal injury, pills should be taken when upright rather than supine, with adequate water, and not at bedtime when saliva production and swallowing are decreased.[2,87,88] The offending drug should be either discontinued or given in liquid or parenteral form. In patients with severe symptoms, and in a few truly severe cases, intravenous fluids and nutrition may be required. Strictures that develop require dilation.[2]

TRAUMATIC RUPTURE AND PERFORATION OF THE ESOPHAGUS

Esophageal perforation is a rare occurrence in children that can cause considerable diagnostic difficulty. Two etiologic types of rupture can be defined: traumatic and spontaneous.

Traumatic Rupture

In children, perforation may occur as a complication of operative procedures; for example, during the process of immobilizing the esophagus to effect hiatal hernia repair or vagotomy, impaction of a sharp foreign body when perforation can occur at the time of attempted removal, external penetrating injuries such as gunshot and stab wounds, indirect trauma to the chest and abdomen (eg, automobile injuries), corrosive damage, and compressed air injuries (Figure 10).[93] Cardiac massage, neonatal resuscitation, the Heimlich maneuver, improperly positioned seat belts (even in minor accidents), boxing blows to the stomach, and repeated vomiting have led to rupture of the esophagus.[2]

Traumatic perforation of the esophagus in children is most commonly a complication of instrumentation: endotracheal intubation, nasogastric tubes, biopsy, dilating procedures, variceal sclerosis, and esophagoscopy.[90] Complications arise during a procedure by blind advancement of an endoscope with failure to maintain the tip of the instrument in the midline, particularly when passing it through the cricopharyngeal lumen.[2] The perforation is usually located on the posterior wall of the esophagus. Balloons used for variceal tamponade and for dilating procedures, for stricture or achalasia, are less frequent causes of perforation.[95] Perforation occurs in up to 6% of patients following pneumatic dilation of the esophagus.[93,95] In a review of esophageal damage after pneumatic dilation for achalasia, transmural perforation was reported in 4% and linear mucosal tears in 8% of patients.[95] After dilations for caustic strictures in 195 patients, 75% of perforations occurred during antegrade dilations with a stiff woven dilator, and most occurred in the first three dilatations.[96]

Although uncommon, instances of iatrogenic esophageal perforation in the newborn, particularly preterm babies, have been increasingly reported since the introduction of more intensive resuscitative procedures for low birth weight babies.[97] The injury is usually located in the area of the pharyngoesophageal junction and may be either transmural or intramural (submucosal).

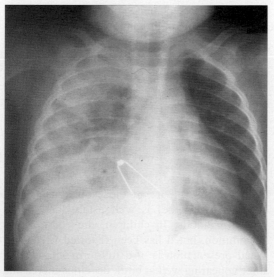

Figure 10 Perforation of the lower esophagus by a large open safety pin ingested 6 weeks ago. Note the enlargement of the mediastinum and the empyema of the right pleura.

Transmural Perforation. A transmural esophageal perforation should be suspected in any newborn developing rapidly increasing respiratory distress. Subcutaneous crepitus of the neck and clinical signs of a pneumothorax may be demonstrable. The esophagus may be torn or perforated by vigorous suctioning of the neonate in which nonregulated wall suction has been implicated as a risk factor.[2,98] Other causes of neonatal perforation include stiff suction catheters, nasogastric tubes, traumatic laryngoscopy, and endotracheal intubation.[98,99] In a review of 12 cases of neonatal pharyngoesophageal perforation, 10 of whom were in premature infants, repeated attempts at postpartum suctioning, airway intubation, and gastric aspiration preceded the perforation.[97] Esophageal atresia was the initial erroneous diagnosis in five cases. Six were treated nonoperatively, five underwent thoracotomy, and one had a gastrostomy. One infant developed an esophageal stricture, and two infants died. A case of esophageal rupture in a 5-month-old following inadvertent placement of a Foley gastrostomy tube into the esophagus at the time of tube change has been reported. Another infant had cervical esophageal rupture as a result of abusive blunt trauma. The esophageal obturator used in cardiopulmonary resuscitation has been the source of perforation owing to distention of the occlusive balloon at the level of the tracheal bifurcation. Similarly, compression of the esophagus by a tracheostomy tube cuff can result in perforation and the creation of a tracheoesophageal fistula.

Intramural (Submucosal) Perforation. In some newborns, esophageal rupture is incomplete and results in a pseudodiverticulum. Following a breach in the mucosa, extensive dissection along the submucosal layer separates the mucosa from the muscle wall.[2] This separation may extend for a considerable distance along the length of the esophagus. Radiologic examination with contrast medium, both the esophageal lumen and the false track may fill, giving the appearance of a double-barreled esophagus.

Clinical presentation simulates that of esophageal atresia, with an outpouring of oral secretions and saliva with immediate choking and cyanosis whenever a feeding is attempted. Aspiration pneumonia is a common complication. It is usually impossible to pass a nasogastric catheter into the stomach. The differential diagnosis from esophageal atresia is important because treatment is nonsurgical.

Spontaneous

Spontaneous rupture of the esophagus (Boerhaave's syndrome) is well established as an entity in adults. In children, the condition is uncommon, but it has been reported.[100–101] The usual presentation is of a full-term infant who, after appearing well at birth, develops increasing respiratory distress and cyanosis within the first 48 hours owing to the development of a tension pneumothorax.[2] There is typically no preceding history of intubation or other resuscitatory interventions. An initial chest radiograph taken with the infant upright reveals a hydropneumothorax or tension pneumothorax; a pneumomediastinum is an unusual finding. Contrast radiography of the esophagus shows extraluminal extravasation of contrast material and enables the site of rupture to be localized, which is almost always located in the lower esophagus just above the hiatus.

Rupture almost always occurs into the right pleural cavity.[2,99] On chest aspiration, serosanguineous fluid is obtained that may be contaminated with either amniotic fluid or orally administered feeding.

Early diagnosis and immediate relief of the tension pneumothorax by intercostal drainage are essential to a successful outcome. These measures need to be followed by prompt surgical closure of the esophageal defect, supplemented by broad-spectrum antibiotics, appropriate intravenous fluids and parenteral nutrition.

In adults, spontaneous rupture usually follows a bout of forceful retching and vomiting. This has led to the theory that the cricopharyngeus fails to relax during the act of vomiting, resulting in a sudden, steep rise in intraluminal pressure sufficient to split the relaxed esophageal wall at its lowest and weakest point; that is, the left posterolateral aspect just above the diaphragm.[2] Infants differ because spontaneous rupture usually occurs into the right pleural cavity, and there is characteristically no preceding history of vomiting.[99] Therefore, in newborn infants, factors other than esophageal overdistention likely are operative. The area of esophagus adjacent to a perforation is avascular and friable and shows changes of a necrotizing esophagitis. Therefore, some form of local devitalizing lesion may be a predisposing factor. It has also been suggested that the cause could be a localized congenital defect in the wall of the esophagus by analogy with cases of spontaneous perforation in the stomach.[99]

Symptoms

Symptoms related to traumatic perforation are immediate, whereas those attributable to iatrogenic causes may not be obvious for an hour, or more. With endoscopic perforation of the esophagus, there is direct extension into the mediastinum, with symptoms and signs of pain and tenderness in the neck, tenderness under the neck, difficulty in swallowing, tachycardia, and fever. Crepitus in the neck usually does not appear for several hours, after fever is evident. Cold water polydypsia is frequent in older patients with cervical perforation in an effort to relieve throat discomfort. Perforations associated with procedures may occur anywhere in the esophagus, and are accompanied by pain, fever, and tachycardia. If the thoracic esophagus is perforated, there is chest pain worsened by inspiration or swallowing and on motion, back pain, fever, dyspnea, and tachycardia.[2]

Diagnosis

The diagnosis is made by plain cervical and chest films, which show mediastinal widening[13] or air in the paracervical region or near the esophagus. An esophagogram using a water-soluble contrast will identify the site of perforation in most patients but in only 62% of those with cervical perforation.[2] A barium study may reveal perforation when studies with water-soluble contrast are unremarkable. CT is helpful in demonstrating extraluminal air, periesophageal fluid, esophageal thickening, extraluminal contrast, and mediastinal fluid and air. Endoscopy is the diagnostic procedure of choice to localize precisely a linear mucosal tear or a bluish submucosal mass bulging in the lumen in case of intramural hematoma.

Treatment

The type of treatment varies with the type and location of the perforation, with the overall condition of the patient and with the time elapsed after injury.[2,97] Pharyngoesophageal perforations can be treated successfully with broad-spectrum, intravenous antibiotic therapy, parenteral nutrition, and no oral feeds. Patients with a penetrating injury of the hypopharynx below the arytenoids or of the cervical esophagus should have neck exploration and drainage.[89] Those with a small esophageal tear and minimal contamination can be treated conservatively. If there is mediastinal air, neck drainage may be necessary. For large perforations and extensive contamination of the mediastinum and pleura, as from gunshot wounds where there is extensive tissue damage, esophageal exclusion through ligation of the distal esophagus, gastrostomy and cervical esophagostomy with parenteral nutrition are the treatment of choice. High gastric fundoplication has also been used effectively to surgically cover a perforation of the lower esophagus. Perforations of the intrathoracic esophagus that are confined to the mediastinum are treated conservatively, and those of the intraabdominal esophagus treated by surgical closure or diversion, even if this requires esophageal resection.[2,93]

Complications

Fulminant mediastinitis is the major threat in esophageal perforation.[12] Although most often attributable to rupture of the thoracic esophagus, mediastinitis can also occur in cervical rupture if drainage is delayed and when infection spreads along the periesophageal planes into the mediastinum. Delayed complications include tracheoesophageal, esophagocutaneous, and carotid-esophageal fistula.

Mortality rates from penetrating perforations of the cervical esophagus range from 9 to 15% for those treated immediately to 25% for those in whom treatment is delayed. Patients with perforation after sclerotherapy for esophageal varices are at particularly high risk owing to their underlying liver disease, where mortality may reach 83%. In children, most cases can be closed primarily and the esophagus salvaged, despite late presentation, with a mortality rate of 4%, which is less than in observed adults (25 to 50%). There is little difference in the mortality between iatrogenic perforation and Boerhaave's syndrome as long as the diagnosis is made early and the treatment is prompt.[2,99]

MALLORY WEISS SYNDROME

Although a laceration of the distal esophagus is reported only in a few children, the frequency is probably mostly underestimated[2,102,103] because the diagnosis can be confirmed only at endoscopy.

Linear fissuring of the esophageal mucosa results from forceful or prolonged vomiting. The laceration is located at the esophagogastric junction and cardia of the stomach. The tear is sometimes double, extending only through the mucosa along the longitudinal axis of the organ. There is little inflammatory reaction or fibrosis, but some granulation tissue is apparent with healing. Bleeding is most intense when both the gastric and the esophageal mucosa are involved.[2]

Symptoms

There is a history of vomiting, either of several episodes or of a duration of several days. Suddenly, the vomitus contains small or large amounts of blood. Dark blood may alternate with bright red blood. In some patients, there is a history of achalasia or hiatus hernia.

Diagnosis

This tear is not detected by radiologic examination. At endoscopy, fresh lesions appear as longitudinal cracks in the mucosa with little inflammatory reaction. The lesion may be so thin as to be missed by the endoscopist, so several passages of the endoscope are often needed to identify them. After 24 hours, the tear appears as a white, raised streak with surrounding erythema and granulation tissue. If a perforation does occur, it involves the distal esophagus.[2]

Treatment

In the majority of children, bleeding stops spontaneously and only rarely does the patient require a blood transfusion, unless there is an underlying coagulopathy. The stomach should be lavaged to prevent gastric distention, and many patients are treated with acid suppression. Endoscopic sclerotherapy, using 1:10,000 adrenaline + 1% polydocanol, is generally successful in achieving hemostasis.[102] If hemostasis does not occur, more aggressive treatment can be undertaken using vasopressin infusion, balloon tamponade, clipping, bicap electrocoagulation, or angiographic embolization of the left gastric artery. In children, management of bleeding is effective with medical treatment; in contrast, up to 25% of adults require surgical control of hemorrhage.[2]

REFERENCES

1. Del Rosario JF, Orenstein SR. Common pediatric esophageal disorders. Gastroenterologist 1998;6:104–21.
2. Olives JP. Injuries of the esophagus. In: Walker WA, Goulet OJ, Kleiman RE, et al., editors. Pediatric Gastrointestinal Disease, 4th edition. Hamilton: BC Decker; 2004. p. 463–80.
3. Olives JP, Breton A, Sokhn M, et al. Ingested foreign bodies in children: Endoscopic management of 395 cases. J Pediatr Gastroenterol Nutr 2000;31:188–9.
4. Kay M, Wyllie R. Pediatric foreign bodies and their management. Curr Gastroenterol Rep 2005;7:212–8.
5. Paul RI, Christoffel KK, Binns HJ, Jaffe DM. Foreign body ingestions in children: Risk of complication varies with site of initial health care contact. Pediatrics 1993;91:121–7.
6. Nandi P, Ong GB. Foreign body in the esophagus: Review of 2394 cases. Br J Surg 1978;63:5–9.
7. Urkin J, Bar-David Y. Respiratory distress secondary to esophageal foreign body: A case report. Scientific World J 2006;6:16–9.
8. Persaud RA, Sudhakaran N, Ong CC, et al. Extraluminal migration of a coin in the esophagus of a child misdiagnosed as asthma. Emerg Med J 2001;18:312–3.
9. Chowdury CR, Bricknell MC, MacIver D. Oesophageal foreign body: An unusual cause of respiratory symptoms in a three-week-old baby. J Laryngol Otol 1992;106:556–7.
10. Cheng W, Tam P. Foreign-body ingestion in children: Experience with 1265 cases. J Pediatr Surg 1999;34:1472–6.
11. Hachimi-Idrissi S, Corne L, Vandenplas Y. Management of ingested foreign bodies in childhood: Our experience and review of the literature. Eur J Emerg Med 1998;5:319–23.
12. Kerschner JE, Beste DJ, Conley SF, et al. Mediastinitis associated with foreign body erosion of the esophagus in children. Int J Pediatr Otorhinolaryngol 2001;59:89–97.
13. Damore DT, Dayan PS. Medical causes of pneumomediastinum in children. Clin Pediatr 2001;40:87–91.
14. American Society for Gastrointestinal Endoscopy. Guideline for the management of ingested foreign bodies. Gastrointest Endosc 2002;55:802–6.
15. Panieri E, Bass DH. The management of ingested foreign bodies in children. A review of 663 cases. Eur J Emerg Med 1995;2:83–7.
16. Elle SR, Sprigg A, Parker A. A multi-observer study examining the radiographic visibility of fishbone foreign bodies. J R Soc Med 1996;89:31–4.
17. Jones NS, Lannigan F, Salama N. Foreign bodies in the throat: A prospective study of 388 cases. J Laryngol Otol 1991;105:104–8.
18. Little DC, Shah SR, St Peter SD, et al. Esophageal foreign bodies in the pediatric population: Our first 500 cases. J Pediatr Surg 2006;41:914–8.
19. Nijhawan S, Shimpi L, Mathur A, et al. Management of ingested foreign bodies in upper gastrointestinal tract: Report on 170 patients. Indian J Gastroenterol. 2003;22:46–8.
20. Grinsberg GG. Management of ingested foreign objects and food bolus impactions. Gastrointest Endosc 1995;41:33–8.
21. Webb WA. Management of foreign bodies of the upper gastrointestinal tract update. Gastrointest Endosc 1995;41:39–51.
22. Kim JK, Kim SS, Kim JI, et al. Management of foreign bodies in the gastrointestinal tract: An analysis of 104 cases in children. Endoscopy 1999;31:302–4.
23. Ros SP, Cetta F. Successful use of a metal detector in locating coins ingested by children. J Pediatr 1992;120:752–3.
24. Saccheti A, Caraccio C, Lichtenstein R. Hand held metal detector identification of foreign objects. Pediatr Emerg Care 1994;10:204–7.
25. Tidey B, Price G GJ, Perez-Avilla CA, Kenney I. The use of a metal detector to locate ingested metallic foreign bodies in children. J Accid Med 1998;13:341–2.
26. Doraiswamy N, Baig H, Hallam L. Metal detector and swallowed metal foreign bodies in children. J Accid Emerg Med 1999;16:123–5.
27. Seikel K, Primm PA, Elizondo B, Remley KL. Handheld metal detector localization of ingested metallic foreign bodies. Arch Pediatr Adolesc Med 1999;153:853–7.
28. Basset KE, Schunk JE, Logan L. Localizing ingested coins with a metal detector. Am J Emerg Med 1999;17:338–41.
29. Takada M, Kashiwagi R, Sagane M, et al. 3 CT diagnosis for ingested foreign bodies. Am J Emerg Med 2000;18: 192–3.
30. Conners GP. Management of asymptomatic coin ingestion. Pediatrics 2005;116:752–3.
31. Waltzman ML, Baskin M, Wypij D, et al. A randomized clinical trial of the management of esophageal coins in children. Pediatrics 2005;3:614–9.
32. Cetinkursun S, Sayan A, Demirbag S, et al. Safe removal of upper esophageal coins by using Magill forceps: Two centers' experience. Clin Pediatr 2006;45:71–3.
33. Campbell JB, Quattromani F, Foley LC. Foley catheter removal of blunt esophageal foreign bodies. Experience with 100 consecutive children. Pediatr Radiol 1983;13:116–9.
34. Little DC, Shah SR, St Peter SD, et al. Esophageal foreign bodies in the pediatric population: Our first 500 cases. J Pediatr Surg 2006;41:914–8.
35. Paulson E, Jaffe RB. Metallic foreign bodies in the stomach: Fibroscopic removal with a magnetic orogastric tube. Radiology 1990;174:191–4.
36. Centers for Disease Control and Prevention (CDC). Gastrointestinal injuries from magnet ingestion in children–United States, 2003 2006. MMWR Morb Mortal Wkly Rep 2006;8;55:1296–300.
37. Wildhaber BE, Le Coultre C, Genin B. Ingestion of magnets: Innocent in solitude, harmful in groups. J Pediatr Surg 2005;40:e33–5.
38. Chee LWW, Sehti DSS. Diagnostic and therapeutic approach to migrating foreign bodies. Ann Otol Rhinol Laryngol 1999;108:177–80.
39. Mahdi G, Israel DM, Hassall E. Nickel dermatitis and associated gastritis after coin ingestion. J Pediatr Gastroenterol Nutr 1996;23:74–6.
40. Nighawan S, Shimpi L, Jain N, Rai RR. Impacted foreign body at the pharyngoesophageal junction: An innovative management. Endoscopy 2002;34:353.
41. Mackenzie T, Antonino S. Bipolar cautery snare capture and removal of esophageal food bolus obstruction. Gastrointest Endosc 1992;38:186–7.
42. Karanjia N, Rees M. The use of Coca-Cola in the management of bolus obstruction in benign esophageal stricture. Ann R Coll Surg Engl 1993;75:94–5.
43. David T, Ferguson AP. Management of children who have swallowed button batteries. Arch Dis Child 1986;61:321–2.
44. Olives JP, Breton A, Sokhn M, et al. Magnetic removal of ingested button batteries in children. J Pediatr Gastroenterol Nutr 2000;31:S187–8.
45. Litovitz T, Butterfield AB, Holloway RR, Marion LI. Button battery ingestion: Assessment of therapeutic modalities and battery discharge state. J Pediatr 1984;105:868–73.
46. Litovitz T, Schmitz BF. Ingestion of cylindrical and button batteries: An analysis of 2382 cases. Pediatrics 1992;89:747–57.
47. Kulig K, Rumack B, Duffy JP. Disc battery ingestion: Elevated urine mercury levels and enema removal of battery fragments. JAMA 1983;249:2502–4.
48. Mallon PT, White JS, Thompson RL. Systemic absorption of lithium following ingestion of a lithium button battery. Hum Exp Toxicol 2004;23:193–5.
49. Blatnick DSS, Toohill R, Jehman R. Fatal complication from an alkaline battery foreign body in the esophagus. Ann Otol Rhinol Laryngal 1977;86:611–5.
50. Imamoglu M, Cay A, Kosucu P, et al. Acquired tracheoesophageal fistulas caused by button battery lodged in the esophagus. Pediatr Surg Int 2004;20:292–4.
51. Alkan M, Buyukyavuz I, Dogru D et al. Tracheoesophageal fistula due to disc-battery ingestion. Eur J Pediatr Surg 2004;14:274–8.
52. Depreterre A R. Caustic esophageal lesions in children. Acta Endosc 1994;24:371–85.
53. Trabelsi M, Loukhil M, Boukthir S, et al. Accidental caustic ingestion in Tunisian children: Review of 125 cases. Pediatrie 1990;45:801–5.
54. Rothstein FC. Caustic injuries to the esophagus in children. Pediatr Clin North Am 1986;33:665–74.
55. Chistesen HBT. Epidemiology and prevention of caustic ingestion in children. Acta Paediatr 1994;83:212–5.
56. Wasserman R, Ginsburg CM. Caustic substance injuries. J Pediatr 1985;107:169–74.
57. Yarrington CT, Jr. The experimental causticity of sodium hypochlorite in the esophagus. Ann Otol 1970;79:895–903.
58. Dogan Y, Erkan T, Cokugras FC, Kutlu T. Caustic gastroesophageal lesions in childhood: An analysis of 473 cases. Clin Pediatr 2006;45:435–8.
59. Crain EF, Gershell JC, Mezey AP. Symptoms as predictors of esophageal injury. Am J Dis Child 1984;138:863–5.
60. Gaudreault P, Parent M, Mickael A, et al. Predictability of esophageal injury from signs and symptoms. Pediatrics 1983;71:767–70.
61. Gupta S SK, Croffie JM, Fitzgerald JF. Is esophagogastro-duodenoscopy necessary in all caustic ingestions? J Pediatr Gastroenterol Nutr 2001;32:50–3.
62. Lamireau T, Rebouissoux XL, Denis D, et al. Accidental caustic ingestion in children: Is endoscopy always mandatory? J Pediatr Gastroenterol Nutr 2001;33:81–4.
63. Zargar SA, Kochbar R, Mehta S, Mehta S SK. The role of fiberoptic endoscopy in the management of corrosive ingestion and modified endoscopic classification of burns. Gastrointest Endosc 1991;37:165–9.

64. Anderson KD, Rouse TM, Randolph JGG. A controlled trial of corticosteroids in children with corrosive injury of the esophagus. N Engl J Med 1990;323:637–40.

65. Ferguson M, Migliore M, Staszak VM, et al. Early evaluation and therapy for caustic esophageal injury. Am J Surg 1989;157:116–20.

66. Bautista A, Varela R, Villamera A, et al. Motor function of the esophagus after caustic burn. Eur J Pediatr Surg 1996;6:204–7.

67. Cadranel S, Di Lorenzo C, Rodesch P, et al. Caustic ingestion and esophageal function. J Pediatr Gastroenterol Nutr 1990;10:164–8.

68. Dabadie A, Roussey M, Oummal M, et al. Accidental caustic ingestion in children. Arch Fr Pediatr 1989;46:217–22.

69. Pelclova D, Navratil T. Do corticosteroids prevent oesophageal stricture after corrosive ingestion? Toxicol Rev 2005;24:125–9.

70. Cadranel S, Scaillon M, Goyens P, Rodesch P. Treatment of esophageal caustic injuries: experience with high-dose dexamethasone. Pediatr Surg Int 1993;8:97–102.

71. Boukthir S, Fetni I, Mrad SM, et al. High doses of steroids in the management of caustic esophageal burns in children. Arch Pediatr 2004;11:13–7.

72. Breton A, Olives JP, Cadranel S, et al. Management of severe caustic oesophageal burns in children with very high doses of steroid. J Pediatr Gastroenterol Nutr 2004;39: S458–9.

73. Broto J, Asensio M, Vernet JM. Results of a new technique in the treatment of severe esophageal stenosis in children: Poliflex stents. J Pediatr Gastroenterol Nutr 2003;37:203–6.

74. Zhang C, Yu JM, Fan GP. The use of a retrievable self-expanding stent in treating childhood benign esophageal strictures. J Pediatr Surg 2005;40:501–4.

75. Mas E, Barange K, Breton A, et al. Ulcerative esophagitis: A complication of a self-expanding metal-stent in a child. J Pediatr Gastroenterol Nutr 2006;42:229–31.

76. Rosseneu S, Afzal N, Yerushalmi B, et al. Topical application of mitomycin-C in oesophageal strictures. J Pediatr Gastroenterol Nutr 2007;44:336–41.

77. Uhlen S, Fayoux P, Vachin F, et al. Mitomycin C: An alternative conservative treatment for refractory esophageal stricture in children? Endoscopy 2006;38:404–7.

78. Hopkins RA, Postlethwait RW. Caustic burns and carcinoma of the esophagus. Ann Surg 1981;194:146–8.

79. Appelqvist P, Salmon S. Lye corrosion carcinoma of the esophagus: Review of 63 cases. Cancer 1980;45:2655–8.

80. Lieberman DA, Keefe EB. Esophageal burn and the microwave oven. Ann Intern Med 1982;97:137.

81. Chwhan NM. Injurious effects of radiation on the esophagus. Ann Thorac Surg 1990;85:115–20.

82. Pavy JJ, Bosset JF. Lake effects of radiations on the esophagus. Cancer Radiother 1997;1:732–4.

83. Yeoh E, Holloway RM, Russo A, et al. Effects of mediastinal irradiation on esophageal function. Gut 1996;38: 166–70.

84. Mahboubi S, Silber JH. Radiation-induced esophageal strictures in children with cancer. Eur Radiol 1997;7:119–22.

85. Abboud B, Bou Jaoude J, Chahine G, et al. Radiation-induced esophageal cancer. Presentation of a case and review of the literature. Gastroenterol Clin Biol 1997;21:987–9.

86. Collazo LA, Levine MS, Rubesin SE, et al. Acute radiation esophagitis: Radiographic findings. Am J Roentgenol 1997;169:1067–70.

87. Kikendall W. Pill esophagitis. J Clin Gastroenterol 1999;28:298–305.

88. Jaspersen D. Drug induced esophageal disorders: Pathogenesis, incidence, prevention and management. Drug Saf 2000;22:237–49.

89. Marvola M, Rajaniemi M, Marhifa E, et al. Effect of dosage form and formulation factors on the adherence of drugs to the esophagus. J Pharm Sci 1983;72:1034–6.

90. Fiedorek SC, Casteel HB. Pediatric medication-induced focal esophagitis. Case report and review. Clin Pediatr 1988;7:762–5.

91. Rives JJ, Olives JP, Ghisolfi J. Acute drug-induced esophagitis. Arch Fr Pediatr 1985;42:33–4.

92. Kato S, Kabagashi M, Sato H, et al. Doxycycline-induced hemorrhagic esophagitis: A pediatric case. J Pediatr Gastroenterol Nutr 1988;7:762–5.

93. Bastos RB, Graeber GM. Esophageal injuries. Chest Surg Clin N Am 1997;7:357–71.

94. Panieri E, Millar A, Rode H, et al. Iatrogenic esophageal perforation in children: Patterns of injury, presentation, management and outcome. J Pediatr Surg 1996;31:890–5.

95. Molina EG, Stollman N, Grauer L, et al. Conservative management of esophageal transmural tears after pneumatic dilation for achalasia. Am. J Gastroenterol 1996;91:15–8.

96. Gershman G, Ament ME, Vargas J. Frequency and medical management of esophageal perforation after pneumatic dilation in achalasia. J Pediatr Gastroenterol Nutr 1997;25: 548–53.

97. Demirbag S, Tiryaki T, Atabek C, et al. Conservative approach to the mediastinitis in childhood secondary to esophageal perforation. Clin Pediatr 2005;44:131–4.

98. Bonnard A, Carricaburu E, Sapin E. Traumatic pharyngo-esophageal perforation in newborn infants. Arch Pediatr 1997;4:737–43.

99. Nagaraj HSS. Iatrogenic perforations of the esophagus in preterm infants. Surgery 1979;86:583–9.

100. Inculet R, Clark C, Girven D. Boerhaave's syndrome and children: A rare and unexpected combination. J Pediatr Surg 1996;31:1300–1.

101. Antonis JH, Poeze M, Van Heurn LW. Boerhaave's syndrome in children: A case report and review of the literature. J Pediatr Surg 2006;41:1620–3.

102. Annunziata GM, Guanasekaran TS, Berman JH, Kraut JR. Cough-induced Mallory-Weiss tear in a child. Clin Pediatr 1996;35:417–9.

103. Bharucha AE, Goustout C, Balm R. Clinical and endoscopic risk factors in the Mallory-Weiss syndrome. Am J Gastroenterol 1997;92:805–8.

Anatomy, Embryology and Congenital Anomalies

Nikhil Thapar, BM(Hon), MRCP, MRCPCH, PhD
Drucilla J. Roberts, MD

7

NORMAL ANATOMY OF THE STOMACH AND DUODENUM

The Stomach

Anatomically, the stomach is divided into four main regions, namely, the *cardia, fundus, body,* and *pylorus* (Figure 1). Given the J shape of the stomach, it consists of a smaller concave medial border called the lesser curvature and a larger convex lateral border called the greater curvature. The *cardia* refers to the area that surrounds the proximal opening of the stomach where it connects to the esophagus. The *fundus* is the domed area anatomically superior to and to the left of the cardia. The gastric *body*, the largest of the regions describes the part of the stomach, interposed between the fundus and pylorus. The *pylorus* leads to the distal opening of the stomach that connects directly to the duodenum. The pylorus can be further divided into the pyloric antrum, which connects it to the gastric body and the pyloric canal, which empties into the duodenum via the pyloric sphincter (PS).

The Duodenum

The duodenum describes the most proximal portion of the small intestine, leading directly from the pylorus of the stomach (Figure 1). It is C shaped and curves around the head of the pancreas. It is divided into four parts all of which are retroperitoneal apart from the most proximal portion of the first part (duodenal cap). The second part (descending) contains the opening of the common bile duct or major papilla. The third part runs horizontally and to the ascending fourth part, which joins the jejunum.

NORMAL EMBRYOLOGIC DEVELOPMENT OF THE STOMACH AND DUODENUM (PATTERN FORMATION AT THE PYLORIC SPHINCTER)

The gastrointestinal tract (or gut) is formed very similarly in all vertebrate species early in embryogenesis. The gut starts out as a simple tube of mesodermal tissue surrounding an endodermal core. Later differentiation results in smooth muscle and epithelial development. Neural tissue in the gut comes from colonization of specialized neural crest cells, which form the enteric nervous system. While these tissues are differentiating, the gut tube develops regional specification in both anatomy (gross and microscopic) and physiology (function). All these events must occur in proper spatial and temporal order to complete a normal (nonanomalous) gut. Although many of these

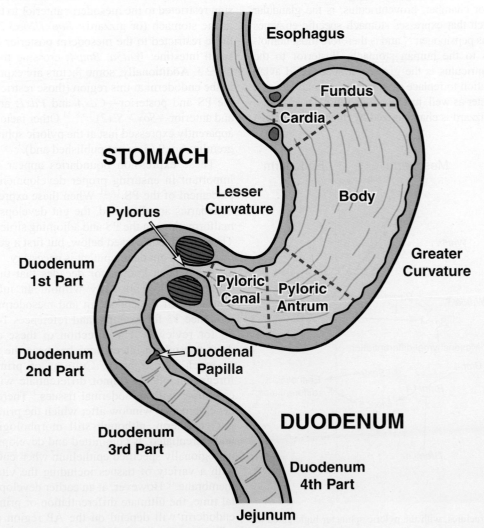

STOMACH

Esophagus

Fundus

Cardia

Lesser Curvature

Body

Pylorus

Pyloric Canal

Pyloric Antrum

Greater Curvature

Duodenum 1st Part

Duodenum 2nd Part

Duodenal Papilla

DUODENUM

Duodenum 3rd Part

Duodenum 4th Part

Jejunum

Figure 1 Gross anatomy of the stomach and duodenum depicting their main regions.

events are understood at the molecular level, much work needs to be done to understand the coordination of these processes to ensure normal development. In this section we will review what is known about the molecular controls of gut development focusing on the development of the stomach and duodenum. Our assumption is that the misregulation of these molecular controls results in anomalous development. Although there is no known specific genetic cause of the congenital anomalies we will discuss, inferences into their etiology can be derived by understanding the normal genetic controls of stomach and duodenal development.

Early gut tube development is choreographed in synchrony with the turning and folding movements of the embryo during and immediately following gastrulation. Critical in early gut formation is the invagination of the definitive endoderm and the subsequent growth and differentiation of the subjacent splanchnic mesenchyme. A sequence of two invaginations, one at the anterior end (anterior intestinal portal, AIP) followed temporally closely by a posterior invagination (caudal intestinal portal, CIP), form the two ends and begin the internalization of the gut. The endoderm of early gut tube stages is remarkably uniform in its morphology along the length of the primitive gut tube. There are no morphologic differences between the portions of tube formed by elongation of the AIP or by the CIP. The primitive gut tube is lined by a single layer of a cuboidal/columnar endoderm/epithelium and encircled by a thin layer of splanchnic mesoderm. As the mesoderm grows and differentiates into smooth muscle, the gut tube alters its gross morphology resulting in clear demarcations that have been categorized as the foregut, midgut, and hindgut. These regions can be defined by embryologic, anatomic, vascular, functional, and molecular criteria. Each of the three major

gut regions is composed of subregions: esophagus and stomach from foregut; small intestines—duodenum, jejunum, and ileum—from midgut; colon from hindgut. Boundaries between these regions typically include valves or sphincters (the PS at the foregut–midgut boundary and the ileocecal valve at the midgut–hindgut boundary). The gross phenotype and the overall "gut plan" along the AP (anterior-posterior) axis is quite well conserved amongst all animal species and remarkably so amongst vertebrates.

Embryologically, the stomach is one of the first structures that differentiates grossly, in nearly all vertebrates, by a left–right axis asymmetry and a hypertrophy/dilatation of the otherwise straight gut tube. The region just caudal to the stomach appears to be clearly demarcated anatomically and molecularly. The small intestines begin distal/posterior to this boundary. The rostral and caudal boundary of the small intestines will be defined in this chapter based on functional and anatomic boundaries which correlate well with molecular expression boundaries,[1] therefore it will be used as the boundaries for this chapter.

As much of the work deciphering the molecular controls of gut development has used the chick embryo as a model system; we will briefly review the chick gut anatomy. The avian species has a specific adaptation in the stomach region. Avian stomachs are composed of two structures, the proventriculus and the gizzard (Figures 2 and 3). The anterior chamber, proventriculus, is the glandular stomach that expresses stomach specific enzymes such as pepsinogen[2–4] and is therefore most homologous to the human stomach. Posterior to the proventriculus is the gizzard, a specialized avian adaptation to replace mastication and may act as a sphincter as well, just due to its muscular anatomy. The gizzard is characterized by thick muscle and a

specialized stratified keratinizing squamous epithelium covered by a thick keratin layer.[5] The gizzard at its posterior most boundary has a specialized region homologous to the human pyloric sphincter (PS). The chick PS can be discerned histologically, anatomically, and molecularly.

The luminal epithelial morphology lags significantly behind the gross gut pattern in its regionally specific differentiation. In some vertebrates the gut epithelium continues to be plastic, often undergoing functional differentiation after birth, before forming the adult phenotype.[6] The gut has the remarkable ability of continued epithelial growth and differentiation throughout the life of the organism along its RADaxis. It is this axis in which the regionalization of the gut is often distinguished as morphologic differences are easily discernable.

The PS lies at the caudal end of the foregut at the foregut–midgut boundary (see above). This structure acts as a valve to control the flow of food from the stomach to the small intestines thereby insuring proper gastric digestion. The anatomic phenotype and physiologic functional importance of this structure varies considerably among species but the development of this boundary appears to be remarkably conserved.[7] The molecular boundary (expression limits) of developmentally important factors shows a "hot spot," of sorts, at the PS (). Many candidate control genes are expressed limited caudally, cranially, or at the PS. Examples include factors with expression restricted to the mesoderm anterior to the PS in the stomach (or gizzard): *Bapx1/Nkx3.2*; and those restricted to the mesoderm posterior in the small intestine: *Wnt5a, Bmp4*; crossing the PS: *Nkx2.5*. Additionally, some factors are expressed in the endoderm at this region (those restricted to the PS and posterior—*CdxA* and *Pdx1*; and PS and anterior—*Sox2, Six2*).[1,5,8–11] Other factors are apparently expressed just at the pyloric sphincter: gremlin, Sox9 (data not published and).[12]

These expression boundaries appear to be important in ensuring proper development and placement of the PS.[1,5,11] When these expression boundaries are disturbed, the gut develops with malformations in the PS and adjoining structures. These will be discussed below, but first a general overview of gut development is necessary.

It has been known for decades that the gut cannot develop normally without an interaction between the endoderm and mesoderm (see reference 13 for example and references 14 and 15 for reviews). The direction of these endoderm–mesoderm interactions has been the focus of much investigation. Cultures of primitive foregut endoderm cannot differentiate without co-culture with mesodermal tissues.[3] There is a developmental window after which the primitive gut endoderm, although still morphologically undifferentiated, is committed and develops into its regionally specified epithelium when cultured with a variety of tissues including the vitelline membrane.[16] However, at an earlier developmental time, the ultimate differentiation of primitive endoderm will depend on the AP region of its adjacent mesoderm. For example, early gizzard

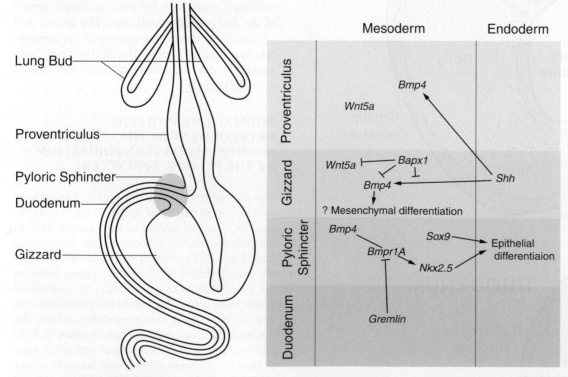

Figure 2 Cartoon of E7 chick foregut-midgut showing the major structures, with the pyloric sphincter highlighted in blue. Mesodermal (*red*) and endodermal (*yellow*) gene expression and proposed model are on the right.

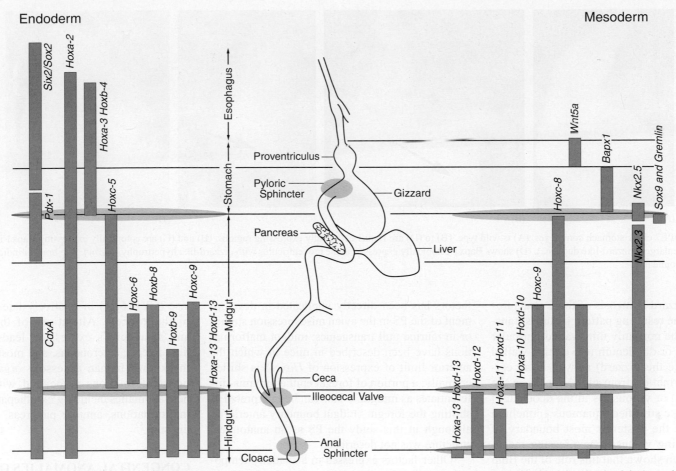

Figure 3 Cartoon outline of an E10 chick gastrointestinal tract showing major structures. Gene expression boundaries are demarcated by black bars on the right (mesodermal expression) and left (endodermal expression). (Adapted from reference 9.)

endoderm can differentiate as proventricular epithelium if cocultured with proventricular mesoderm.[3] Many studies have confirmed that the mesoderm directs the ultimate epithelial pattern in the gut,[14,17–19] but the endoderm also has inductive capacities. Definitive endoderm cocultured with somitic mesoderm stimulates smooth muscle (splanchnic or visceral) rather than skeletal muscle development as assayed by histology and by induction of visceral mesodermal proteins—for example, tenascin[20] and smooth muscle actin.[21,22] Other factors clearly modulate this interaction, including hormonal and basement membrane proteins.[23,24]

The mesodermal influence on endoderm patterning involves primarily specification of morphology that may not include all of the epithelial cytodifferentiation. Most of the endodermal gut regions studied appear plastic to influence from mesoderm in both morphologic and cytologic differentiation, except for the midgut region. Some midgut-specific epithelial cytodifferentiation appears to have cell autonomous/cell specific features. Specific midgut epithelial expression of digestive enzymes is maintained even when influenced by heterologous mesoderm.[2,10,25–27] This difference between the ability of the midgut and foregut endoderm to undergo complete heterologous differentiation may be an endogenous characteristic of the endoderm.

Some of the molecular controls of early endodermal–mesodermal events have been described. *Sonic hedgehog* (*Shh*), a vertebrate homologue

of *Drosophila hedgehog* (*hh*), encodes a signaling molecule implicated in mediating pattern in several regions of the embryo.[28–32] *Shh* is expressed in the endoderm of the gut and its derivatives[10,33–38] and is a candidate for an early endodermally derived inductive signal in gut morphogenesis since its earliest endodermal expression is restricted to the endoderm of the AIP and CIP before invagination occurs.[39] *Shh* is not the signal that initiates the invagination of the AIP or CIP since murine null mutants for *Shh* develop a gut although severe foregut abnormalities are present.[40] These mutants have malformed esophagi with enlarged lumens and disorganized or absent subjacent mesoderm.[35,41] This finding suggests that the endodermally derived signal from *Shh* is involved with mesodermal development, recruitment, or other aspects of mesodermal foregut patterning. Indeed, *Shh* must act as a signal from endoderm to mesoderm since its receptor is present only in the gut mesoderm[10,36,38] and overexpression of *Shh* in the early primitive gut leads to a mesodermal (not endodermal) phenotype.[10]

In each organ in which the endoderm-derived tissue expresses *Shh*, there is closely associated mesenchymal mesoderm that expresses a homolog of *Drosophila's dpp*.[33,39,42] Of the vertebrate homologs of *dpp* expressed in the gut, only *Bmp4* is expressed at the earliest stages of gut development. In the primitive hindgut, at the earliest time *Shh* expression can be detected in the CIP region (even before invagination is apparent), *Bmp4* is expressed in the subjacent mesenchymal

mesoderm.[39] In misexpression studies, *Shh* induces *Bmp4* in the splanchnic mesoderm of the developing gut.[10,38,39] An endodermal role of *Shh* is to induce *Bmp4* expression in the splanchnic mesoderm, which then controls aspects of smooth muscle development in the gut.[10,11,38,39] These aspects of patterning also play a key role in the development of the PS and the foregut–midgut boundary.

At early patterning stages (<E7 in the chick), *Bmp4* is expressed in the mesoderm of all regions of the developing gut mesoderm but is excluded from expression in the primitive gizzard.[1,5,10,42] Several BMP receptors are expressed in the intestinal mesoderm in a position to mediate Bmp signaling in this portion of the gut. The type I receptor, *BMPR1B* is specifically expressed in the gizzard mesoderm from E2.5,[5] despite the fact that no *Bmp* is expressed in the early gizzard mesoderm. With ectopic expression of *Bmp4* early in primitive gizzard development, a thinning of the smooth muscle layer results.[1,10] *Bmp4* may affect the mesoderm by negatively regulating growth and hypertrophy or facilitating differentiation to smooth muscle.[1,11] The factor inhibiting *Bmp4* expression in the gizzard is *Bapx1*, an NK-2 class transcription factor also known as *Nkx3.2*.[1] *Bapx1* has the inverse expression pattern of *Bmp4* in early gut development, expressed only in the gizzard mesoderm from the earliest stages examined.[1] Misexpression of *Bapx1* either anteriorly into the proventriculus or posteriorly into the duodenum

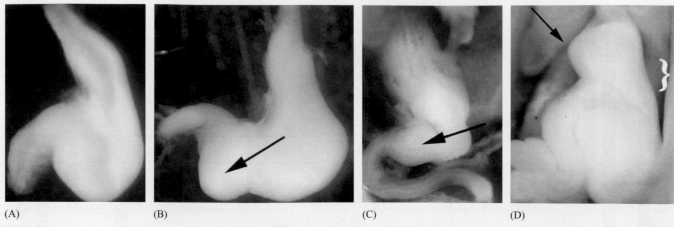

(A) (B) (C) (D)

Figure 4 Panel of E7 chick stomach complexes. (A) is wild type. (B) to (D) are Bapx1 ectopically expressing regions; (B) and (C) are ectopically expressing Bapx1 in the duodenum (*arrows* point to enlarged gizzard-like duodena). (D) shows Bapx1 ectopically expressed in the proventriculus with gizzard-like hypertrophy (*arrow*). The bracket indicates the proventriculus gizzard boundary.

results in a gizzard homeosis of these structures (Figure 4).[1] The resulting pattern includes transformation of the normally thin-walled muscular proventriculus or duodenum into a thick-walled mesoderm (like the gizzard) as well as an epithelial transformation from glandular (as in the proventriculus) or villous (as in the duodenum) into gizzard-like stratified squamous epithelium (Figure 4). At the posterior most boundary of *Bmp4* expressing versus nonexpressing mesoderm it has been shown that this role of the Bmp signaling system is to pattern the foregut midgut boundary, the PS.[5,11] Signaling by Bmp from the avian midgut induces the cells of the adjacent gizzard primordium to form a sphincter,[5] and Bmp signaling is important in the phenotype at this boundary.[1] One of the roles of the Bmp signaling is mediated by induction of a transcription factor necessary for PS formation.

Nkx2.5 is a specific marker for the mesoderm of the PS in the chick embryo (Figure 3). In the early stages, it is expressed adjacent to the *Bmp4* expressing area and overlaps with the posterior expression domain of *BMPR1B*. By misexpressing *Bmp4* into the primitive chick gizzard using a retrovirus containing the *mBMP-4* complementary DNA7 expression of Nkx2.5 was induced and the PS border was anteriorly shifted.[5] If PS mesodermal *Bmp4* expression was inhibited using a *Noggin* (encoding a specific Bmp antagonist) retrovirus, Nkx2.5 was downregulated at the border of the gizzard and the small intestine.[5] As the *Noggin*-infected embryos did not survive long enough to allow morphologic analysis, the presence or absence of the PS could not be determined.[5]

Using the same retroviral misexpression system to extend the expression of *Nkx2.5,* the same alteration of the PS placement resulted if *Nkx2.5* was expanded anteriorly. With posterior infection, no alteration in gut patterning was observed.[11] This suggests that other factors are important in regulating PS patterning or responsiveness to *Nkx2.5*. As there are other known factors expressed differentially at this boundary (Figure 3), one or more of these factors must play a role in PS patterning. Although none of these

factors has been directly implicated in development of the PS in the avian misexpression studies or in murine null transgenics; midgut malformations have been described in mice in which the anterior limit of expression of *Hoxc-8* is shifted cranially: a portion of foregut epithelium mis-differentiates as midgut.[43] This can be interpreted as shifting the foregut–midgut boundary anteriorly, although in this study the PS as an anatomical structure was not described.

Other factors expressed in a spatially temporally mediated manner at or near the PS likely also play a role in the development of this structure. Mutations in any of them may play a role in the development of PS malformations as discussed above.

The gut (and its derivatives) has one of the most prominent left–right asymmetries of all organs in the body. There is a dramatic turning and coiling movement that results in the curvature of the left-sided stomach (and therefore the spleen), right-sided liver, and counterclockwise rotation of the intestines. The factors involved in these events are the same factors involved in setting up the early left–right asymmetry of the body plan and, of course, the heart, and have been well studied and reviewed.[44] Although much more is known about the molecular controls of left–right asymmetry in its earliest manifestations (body turning, heart looping),[45] the gut and heart seem to have coordinated but independent roles in this process.[46] Molecules involved in this process include a hierarchy of genes with asymmetric expression at the primitive streak stage of development (gastrulation) (see Figure 5A and B).[44–51] Although much is known about this signaling, the inciting signal for the cascade has remained elusive.

The foregut turning likely starts the entire process of gut looping and the left–right asymmetry that is so characteristic. Recent advances in the understanding of gut asymmetric control have confirmed the importance of the early foregut induction of the process and have the light on the role of retinoid signaling in this process.[52] This signaling involved genes for retinaldehyde dehydrogenase (RALDH2) and retinoic acid hydroxy-

lase (CYP26A1) in relatively late stage control of this process. Alterations of these agonist's and antagonist's expression leads to malrotation defects, heterotaxias, and most interestingly the known human accessory organ malformations/deformations associated with gut sidedness anomalies including extrahepatic biliary tree malformations, annular pancreas, and pancreas divisum.[52]

CONGENITAL ANOMALIES OF THE STOMACH AND DUODENUM

Congenital anomalies of the stomach are very rare as opposed to those of the duodenum or, indeed, the intestine as a whole. Most gastric or duodenal defects are sporadic, isolated, and of unknown etiology, but some are inherited or form part of recognized syndromes. Notable associations include duodenal atresia and trisomy 21. A careful examination looking for associated defects must therefore be carried out and appropriate management instituted. Clinical presentation is variable and depends on the anomaly. In general, given the proximal position in the gastrointestinal tract, feed-associated symptoms predominate and invariably include vomiting and reflux with or without compromise of the respiratory tract. Presentation may be more subtle and diagnosis delayed even to adult life if anomalies are less conspicuous (eg, gastric diaphragm or diverticulum).

Broadly, congenital anomalies can be divided into the following:

1. *Atresia and stenosis.* Atresia refers to complete obstruction of the gut either by a membrane or fibrous band or complete separation of the adjacent sections. Stenosis refers to incomplete obstruction caused by intrinsic narrowing of the internal lumen of the gut.
2. *Duplications and cysts.* Duplications are cystic or tubular malformations of the gut. They may be multiple and often communicate with and share the blood supply of the adjacent gut. Usually, they are composed of intestinal or ectopic gastric mucosa, submucosa, and

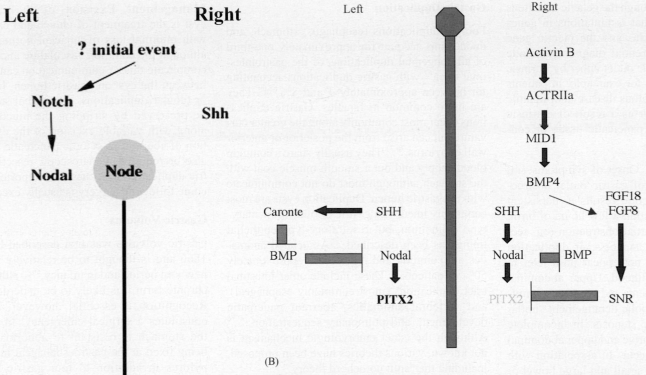

Figure 5 (A) Cartoon of the early events in laterality determination. Dorsal view of a stereotypical embryo with the node and primitive streak. Likely many of these events are epigenetically determined. Lateralization of the HH signaling is directed differently in different vertebrates. In avians, the signal is restricted by H^+/K^+-ATPase activity whereas in the mouse it is likely controlled by the leftward movement of nodal due to nodal flow. The ultimate result of these events is to provide left-sided bias to transfer of the perinodal expression domain of nodal to the lateral plate mesoderm (see reference 45). (B) Genetic cascades of left–right asymmetry in the chick. Cartoon of dorsal aspect of early-stage chick embryo. Sonic hedgehog (SHH) is expressed on both sides of Hensen's node until restricted by bone morphogenetic protein 4 (BMP4). BMP4 is activated by right-sided expression of Activin B and its targets. SHH is thus restricted to the left side and de-inhibits nodal through Caronte's inhibition of BMP4 resulting in expression of PITX2 on the left side. BMP4 is critical in activating right-sided specific genes including FGFs and their target SNR, which inhibits PITX2 on the right side (see reference 45). ACTRIIa = activin receptor IIa; MID1 = midline 1; SNR = snail related.

smooth muscle coats. Presentation may be delayed until enlargement causes compression of adjacent structures or may be revealed following volvulus, intussusception, or investigation of gastrointestinal hemorrhage or perforation. All duplications should be surgically excised to prevent complications.

3. *Abnormal rotation and fixation.* The entire gut assumes its normal postnatal position within the abdominal cavity following a carefully sequenced process of physiologic herniation out of the abdominal cavity in the sixth week of embryonic life. This is followed by elongation, counterclockwise rotation, return into the abdomen in week 10, and fixation of the duodenum and ascending colon to the posterior abdominal wall. Obstruction and volvulus tend to occur when such rotation and fixation are incomplete or abnormal (malrotation) and can lead to ischemia and infarction of the bowel. Total nonrotation results in the duodenojejunal loop on the right and cecocolic loop on the left side of the abdomen. Symptoms and signs at presentation are variable from those of acute obstruction or compromise (eg, volvulus to vague chronic gastrointestinal symptoms).

GENERAL MANAGEMENT

As for most intestinal malformations, surgery is the definitive management. This may be done electively or as an emergency within hours of presentation. Early recognition and diagnosis not only of the defect but also of the clinical state of the child, resuscitation, and stabilization are vital. Valuable time is often lost in stabilizing a child for surgery in whom initial resuscitation has been overlooked or inadequate in the eagerness to diagnose and transfer the child. Intravenous fluid, keeping patients nil by mouth, drainage of gastric or intestinal contents by passage of a nasogastric tube, and careful monitoring are the initial management of almost all children presenting with intestinal malformations. Sepsis must always be considered in an unwell baby or child, appropriate microbiologic cultures taken, and antibiotics commenced. Intestinal perforation or intraoperative spillage of contents may occur, and broad-spectrum antibiotics to cover sepsis from gut organisms are usual during the perioperative period. Postoperative care involves close monitoring and the maintenance of various drains and vascular lines. Recommencement of feeding will depend on the operative procedure undertaken, healing, and clinical signs of recovery of bowel function.

CONGENITAL ANOMALIES OF THE STOMACH

Gastric Atresia or Stenosis

This most commonly affects the pylorus or antrum of the stomach and occurs either as a true atresia of the stomach or secondary to complete or partial occlusion of the lumen by a circumferential mucosal membrane or diaphragm. Hypertrophic pyloric stenosis is not discussed here. Overall, these conditions are extremely rare, with pyloric atresia (PA) accounting for approximately 1% of intestinal atresias, with an incidence of 1 in 100,000 newborns.[53,54] Embryologic events leading to these defects are not clear. Most cases are sporadic, but some may be inherited as autosomal recessive. Although specific genetic causes of these anomalies have yet to be described, one can hypothesize that misregulation of the BMP signaling pathway may play a role because experimental inhibition of signaling results in a hypertrophied muscle in the pylorus.[1,5,11] Defects can be isolated or occur in association with other genetic defects (eg, epidermolysis bullosa (EB), multiple intestinal atresias, Down syndrome, icthyosis, and aplasia cutis congenita).[55–59] Both junctional and simplex forms of EB are most commonly associated with PA although the genetic mutations differ between them that is mutations in genes encoding α6/β4 integrins and the plectin gene respectively.[60,61] Differential diagnoses include obstruction of the gastric outlet either by intrinsic lesions within the wall for examaple, in patients with chronic granulomatous disease and infantile myofibromatosis,[62,63] or as a result of extrinsic pressure from annular pancreatic tissue or congenital peritoneal bands.

Clinical Presentation. Onset of symptoms will depend on the degree of gastric outlet obstruction. Complete obstruction results in persistent nonbilious vomiting within a few hours of birth, whereas in cases of partial obstruction (eg, secondary to membranes, stenosis, or duplication cysts), symptoms may not appear until later in childhood or even adulthood. Upper abdominal distention may be present, and recurrent vomiting may result in metabolic derangement similar to hypertrophic pyloric stenosis. In incomplete obstruction, failure to thrive and upper abdominal discomfort may also occur. In association with multiple atresias of the small and large bowel or with epidermolysis bullosa letalis, the outcome is usually fatal.

Diagnosis. Prenatally, there may be polyhydramnios and both a dilated stomach and narrowed outlet seen on ultrasonography.[57,64] Postnatally, in cases of complete obstruction, plain abdominal radiography reveals a "single bubble" appearance with a large distended stomach and absence of distal intestinal gas. Together with the symptoms this is very suggestive of gastric atresia, and contrast studies are often unnecessary. In partial obstruction additional studies using contrast and/or ultrasonography are valuable. An incomplete prepyloric membrane is seen as a thin, linear filling defect on contrast studies. On a sonogram, this appears as an echogenic band extending centrally from the lesser and greater curvatures in the prepyloric region.[65] Endoscopy may be used to directly visualize the defect, and gastric emptying studies may aid diagnosis.

Management. If the defect is a thin membrane, excision along with pyloroplasty is the treatment of choice. More complex atresias may require resection and formation of a gastroduodenostomy, pyloroplasty, or, less commonly, gastrojejunostomy. More recently, success using gastroduodenal mucosal advancement anastomosis with reconstruction of the PS has been reported.[66] The stomach is kept decompressed post-surgery, and enteral nutrition is commenced in the first week in the absence of complications. If there is little delay of gastric emptying, conservative management consisting of low-residue feeds and gastric-emptying drugs may be successful, although careful long-term follow-up is essential. Gastric webs are traditionally treated by complete excision, although endoscopic transection, balloon dilatation, and laser ablation have emerged as newer therapies. Complications are minimal. Other bowel atresias should be excluded.

Gastric Duplication

Foregut duplications (esophagus, stomach, and duodenum) account for approximately one-third of all congenital duplications of the gastrointestinal tract,[67] with gastric duplications accounting for between approximately 4 and 8%.[68,69] They are more common in females. Gastric duplications occur most commonly along the greater curvature but can arise from the posterior or anterior wall or pylorus.[70,71] They usually share a common blood supply and outer smooth muscle coat with the stomach, although most do not communicate with the gastric lumen. Duplication cysts are most commonly lined with gastric or other alimentary-type epithelium, but respiratory-type epithelial lining has been described.[72] Associated anomalies are common and reported in approximately 50% of patients.[73] These include other intestinal tract duplications (most commonly esophageal), and vertebral anomalies, aberrant pancreatic development, and pulmonary sequestration.[74–76] Although the exact embryologic mechanism is not known, various theories have been proposed, including the "split notochord theory."[73]

Clinical Presentation. Presentation classically occurs in infancy, although presentation at any age is possible. Symptoms depend on the size and location of the cyst and any communication. Common symptoms are vomiting (classically nonbilious), weight loss, failure to thrive, and abdominal pain, and distention. An abdominal mass may be palpable on examination. Pyloric duplication may be mistakenly diagnosed as hypertrophic pyloric stenosis. Enlargement of the cysts can present with obstruction of gastric emptying or compression of adjacent structures. Ulceration, bleeding, or inflammation of the mucosa within the cyst or of the adjacent gut results either in local complications, overt gastrointestinal hemorrhage, or perforation with peritonitis or fistula formation. Pancreatitis can be associated with gastric duplications and most commonly results from their communication with aberrant pancreatic tissue although ectopic intrapancreatic placement has been reported.[77]

Diagnosis. Duplications are often difficult to diagnose preoperatively. Plain abdominal radiography may show a soft tissue mass, and ultrasonography is useful to reveal the cystic nature of the duplication. Contrast studies may reveal the presence of a mass with displacement of adjacent bowel and is useful if a communication exists with the lumen of the gastrointestinal tract. Direct visualization of the mass by endoscopy has also been used.[78] Computed tomography is often used to define the nature and location of duplication cysts, but endoscopic ultrasonography and magnetic resonance imaging are becoming increasingly popular.[79] The presence of an echogenic inner rim and hypoechoeic outer muscle layers is very suggestive of a duplication.[80] Prenatal diagnosis of gastric duplications by ultrasonography or magnetic resonance imaging has been reported.[81–83]

Management. Excision of the duplication cyst is the treatment of choice and can be done with minimal loss of adjacent normal stomach, although the common vasculature and wall often complicate this. A communication can be created between the cyst and gastric lumen. In complete or tubular duplications, the normal stomach can be preserved by stripping the mucosal lining, along with variable excision of the cyst. Resection of aberrant or ectopic pancreatic tissue may also be required. Laparoscopic resection of gastric duplication cysts has been reported.[84,85] Outcome following surgery is usually excellent.

Gastric Volvulus

Gastric volvulus was first described by Berti in 1866 and is thought to be relatively rare in the newborn period and in infancy,[86,87] although in its chronic form it is likely to be underdiagnosed.[88] Recognition is essential, however, because it constitutes a surgical emergency. In normality, the stomach is resistant to abnormal rotation, being fixed at the gastroesophageal junction and pylorus in addition to four gastric ligaments. As a result, congenital gastric volvulus is associated with disruption of one or more of these, although in a proportion no cause is identified.[89] Gastric volvulus is caused by abnormal rotation of one part of the stomach around another, with resulting obstruction at the pylorus or cardia and possible ischemia. This rotation is either organoaxial (around the longitudinal esophagogastropyloric axis), mesentroaxial (around a transverse axis through the greater and lesser curvatures), or combined.[87,90] The majority of congenital gastric volvuli are secondary to gastric malfixation, especially at the gastroesophageal junction, diaphragmatic complications (eg, congenital diaphragmatic hernia), and absence or laxity of gastric ligaments.[87,91–93] Splenic anomalies are commonly associated.[94,95]

Clinical Presentation. Gastric volvulus in childhood tends to present within the first few months of life, with symptoms depending on the degree of rotation and obstruction.[88,96,97] Classic symptoms of Borchardt triad (unproductive retching, localized epigastric distention, inability to pass a nasogastric tube) may be difficult to elicit in younger children, and the diagnosis should be considered in the presence of other chronic symptoms (eg, gastroesophageal reflux, recurrent vomiting, failure to thrive).

Diagnosis. Radiographic features are most reliable for diagnosis, showing abnormalities in the position and contour of the stomach in the abdomen or chest and position of the pylorus in relation to the gastroesophageal junction.[87,98,99] Contrast studies may be most informative.[97]

Management. Acute gastric volvulus, especially intrathoracic, is a surgical emergency to prevent gastric ischemia, necrosis, and perforation and to prevent cardiorespiratory compromise. At surgery, the volvulus is reduced, and the viability of the stomach assessed. If the stomach is viable, it is fixed by gastropexy to the abdominal wall or a gastrostomy is fashioned. The need for a concomitant antireflux procedure is controversial.[97] Repair of any associated defects (eg, diaphragmatic defects) is undertaken. Successful laparoscopic surgery has been reported in acute gastric volvulus.[100] The treatment of chronic cases remains controversial, although surgery is indicated in persistently symptomatic individuals. Gradual improvement over time has been reported in conjunction with conservative treatment (eg, positioning infants in the prone or upright position after meals) in less affected children.[99]

Microgastria

Microgastria results from a failure of gastric enlargement during embryogenesis, resulting in a tubular stomach of reduced capacity. It is extremely rare, with approximately 50 cases described in the literature since its first description in 1842.[101,102] It appears to occur sporadically with a slight female preponderance[101] and is almost always associated with other congenital anomalies. In a review of the literature, Kroes and Festen could identify only 2 of 39 cases in which microgastria appeared to occur as an isolated defect.[103] Associated malformations include intestinal (84%), cardiovascular (43%), pulmonary (33%), skeletal (31%), urogenital (28%), and neuronal (12%) pathologies,[101] many of which share a mesodermal origin. Specific anomalies include intestinal malrotation, asplenia, transverse liver, tracheoesophageal anomalies, atrioventricular septal defects, upper limb and spinal deformities, micrognathia (including Pierre Robin sequence), renal dysplasia or aplasia, corpus callosum agenesis, and anophthalmia.[104–107] Microgastria should be excluded in patients presenting with VACTERL (vertebral, anal, cardiac, tracheal, esophageal, renal, and limb) association and midline defects. The genetic cause of microgastria is unknown, but the BMP signaling pathway may play a role. Overexpression of *Bmp4* results in a microgastria phenotype in the chick.[1,5,11]

Clinical Presentation. Symptoms are mainly related to the markedly reduced capacity of the stomach to retain contents. Thus, postprandial vomiting and gastroesophageal reflux are common, along with aspiration leading to recurrent chest infections and airway damage. Rapid gastric emptying can lead to diarrhea. Nutrition is compromised, and malnutrition, failure to thrive, and growth retardation are very common. Developmental delay is often evident.

Diagnosis. The diagnosis is usually made on the basis of an upper gastrointestinal contrast study, which shows a small, tubular stomach in an abnormal, usually midline, position. A dilated, poorly peristaltic esophagus and gastroesophageal reflux are frequently evident. Attention should be given to excluding associated anomalies with appropriate investigations.

Management. Management is designed to ensure adequate nutrition and prevention of aspiration and, if possible, to create an adequate gastric reservoir. Failure to thrive and gastroesophageal reflux are the greatest problems. Surgery is usually attempted only if a feeding strategy of frequent small-volume, high-calorie feeds fails to achieve adequate growth, or symptoms of reflux are prominent. Nasojejunal or jejunostomy feeding has also been used with variable success.[108] The aim of surgery is to increase the capacity and drainage of the stomach and prevent or resolve dilatation of the esophagus as a compensatory reservoir. This can be achieved by attaching a jejunal pouch to the stomach and forming a distal Roux-en-Y jejunojejunostomy (Hunt-Lawrence pouch).[102,109] Outcome is variable.[103] Associated gastrointestinal anomalies may need correction concurrently.

GASTRIC DIVERTICULUM

Congenital gastric diverticulae are very uncommon. They occur most commonly in the posterior wall, antrum, and pylorus, usually comprising all layers of the stomach wall. They may be associated with hiatus herniae and aberrant pancreatic tissue.[110] Presentation is usually in adult life, although children may present with recurrent abdominal pain and vomiting.[111] Upper gastrointestinal endoscopy or contrast studies revealing the outpouching are usually sufficient to make the diagnosis. It should be differentiated from ulcers and malignancy. Treatment is by surgical excision.

COMPLETE OR PARTIAL ABSENCE OF GASTRIC MUSCLE

This is a rare condition characterized by complete or partial absence of gastric muscle coats. The body of the stomach is most commonly affected. Muscular agenesis likely has many genetic causes, but it is known that in the gut, the hedgehog-bone morphogenetic protein signaling pathway plays a critical role and may be one of the causes of this rare disorder. Gastric perforation is the main complication, often occurring soon after birth. The clinical presentation is of intestinal perforation, often with cardiovascular collapse. Abdominal distention may be marked and may lead to respiratory compromise. Radiography reveals free intraperitoneal air. Fluid resuscitation with or without emergency decompression of intraperitoneal air may be required prior to surgery.

CONGENITAL ANOMALIES OF THE DUODENUM

Congenital duodenal obstruction most commonly results from duodenal atresia. Other causes include extrinsic compression from annular pancreas, Ladd bands or preduodenal portal vein, midgut volvulus, and duodenal webs.

Duodenal Atresia and Stenosis

The duodenum represents one of the most common sites for atresia in the gastrointestinal tract. The reported incidence for duodenal atresia is approximately 1 in 10,000 to 30,000 live births. Most atresias occur at the level of the ampulla of Vater and the obstruction owing to either a complete mucosal membrane or diaphragm without discontinuity of the muscle coats (type 1) or blind-ending proximal and distal segments of duodenum. These segments are either connected by a fibrous band (type 2) or separated by a gap (type 3). Duodenal stenosis is again the most common of gastrointestinal stenoses and occurs when a hole is present through the mucosal diaphragm.

Embryologically, the cause is thought to be a failure of canalization of the duodenum, which normally occurs after the seventh week of gestation. Although gut atresias are thought to be related to ischemic events early in gut development,[112] genetic causes may also play a role.[113–115] Duodenal stenosis has been described in association with congenital rubella and Prader-Willi syndromes.[116,117] Associated anomalies are common and occur in about 50% of cases of atresia. One-third of affected infants have trisomy 21 (Down syndrome). Associated anomalies include esophageal atresia, midgut malrotation, annular pancreas, and biliary tract, anorectal, cardiac, genitourinary, vertebral, and mandibulofacial anomalies.[114,118–120] Prematurity, intrauterine growth retardation, polyhydramnios and umbilical cord ulcers are more common.[119–121] Duodenal obstruction may be secondary to external compression by other congenital anomalies such as an annular pancreas or preduodenal portal vein.[122,123]

Clinical Presentation. Presentation of atresia is within the first few days of life and usually follows the first feed. The major symptom is vomiting, most commonly bile stained, given that most atresias occur distal to the ampulla of Vater. Gastric distention with visible peristalsis may be present but easily decompressed by nasogastric aspiration. Abdominal distention is not usual. There is an increased incidence of jaundice. In duodenal stenosis, presentation may be delayed, and recurrent vomiting and failure to thrive are more common symptoms.

Diagnosis. In atresia, the classic radiographic sign is the "double bubble" sign on abdominal radiography, denoting the higher, larger, left-sided stomach bubble together with the lower, smaller, right-sided bubble of the dilated proximal duodenum. No gas is visible throughout the distal intestine. With such an appearance, there is no need for an upper gastrointestinal series, especially because these contrast studies carry the additional risk of gastrointestinal perforation and aspiration of contrast.[65,120,124] Frequent vomiting may result in an absence of air in the stomach and duodenum, making the diagnosis difficult. To confirm the diagnosis in such cases, a small amount of air can be injected into the stomach via a nasogastric tube prior to radiography.[124] Prenatal diagnosis is possible with the use of ultrasonography to demonstrate the presence of a fluid-filled double bubble in the fetal abdomen in association with polyhydramnios.[125] In such cases, the fetal karyotype and a careful search for other anomalies should be instigated. Direct visualization of defects by endoscopy may be useful in the diagnosis of duodenal stenosis, although contrast studies are most useful. A "windsock" sign on contrast studies may be produced when peristalsis and movement of gut content protrude the membrane distally into the lumen of the third or fourth part of the duodenum or even proximal jejunum. The presence of gastric emphysema or duodenal pneumatosis may suggest a diagnosis of duodenal obstruction.[126,127]

Management. Following resuscitation, surgery is performed at open laparotomy or laparoscopically.[128–130] The entire duodenum is visualized by mobilizing the right colon, allowing identification of the obstruction and exclusion of associated malrotation. In malrotation, peritoneal (Ladd) bands extending from the cecum to the right upper quadrant may obstruct the duodenum. A side-to-side or end-to-side duodenoduodenostomy or duodenojejunostomy is carried out. Traditionally, resection of any obstructing membranes is thought to increase the likelihood of damaging the bile duct or pancreatic duct and therefore usually avoided. More recently duodenal stenosis has been successfully treated by endoscopic membranectomy or balloon dilatation.[131,132] The presence of other small bowel atresias is excluded at operation. The stomach and bowel are kept decompressed postoperatively using nasogastric or nasojejunal tubes, which can also be used for feeding. Survival rates are above 90% in the absence of chromosomal or cardiac defects. Long-term follow-up is needed to monitor development of complications such as ulceration and duodenal stasis.

Duodenal Duplication

Duplications of the duodenum represent the rarest site for intestinal duplications accounting for approximately 5% of such disorders. They tend to occur on the mesenteric border of the first two parts of the duodenum. Gut duplications are fascinating malformations because they are nearly always mesenteric and often have gastric epithelial differentiation.[133] This suggests that the gastric phenotype may be the "default" gut phenotype and occurs when gut development occurs out of the normal spatiotemporal and anatomic controls of development. If this is true, then the molecular controls of stomach development (see Figure 2) may be "ectopically" expressed in duplicated regions of gut. Gastric epithelial differentiation does express embryologic factors when present in adults, as in Barret's esophagus and Meckel diverticulum.[134] Investigation of the expression of these factors in duplications of the gut may help in deciphering their etiology. Duodenal duplication cysts have been described in association with spinal canal abnormalities, possibly as part of the split notochord syndrome.[135]

Clinical Presentation. Presenting symptoms are related to the size and site of the cyst, aberrant communication with the pancreaticobiliary tree and presence of ectopic gastric mucosa.[136–137] The commonest symptoms result from duodenal obstruction but ulceration, hemorrhage within the cyst, pancreatitis, and biliary obstruction may also contribute. Most cases present in the first few years of life, although late presentation is recognized, often with a chronic history of poor feeding and epigastric pain.

Diagnosis. On contrast studies the duodenum may appear to be compressed by a mass in the concavity of the duodenal C loop.[65] Ultrasonography may be useful to further characterize the mass and determine its location, but computed tomography and magnetic resonance imaging provide the best anatomical delineation of the cyst and its relation to the pancreatic and biliary systems. Radioscintigraphic studies using Technetium pertechnate may be useful to detect ectopic gastric mucosa within the lesions, especially in those patients presenting with gastrointestinal hemorrhage.[138] Antenatal diagnosis can be made by ultrasonography.[139,140]

Management. The mainstay of treatment is surgery to excise the duplication in its entirety, but this may be complicated by its close proximity to the pancreatic and biliary tree.[137]

REFERENCES

1. Nielsen C, Murtaugh LC, Chyung JC, et al. Gizzard formation and the role of Bapx1. Dev Biol 2001;231:164–74.
2. Hayashi K, Yasugi S, Mizuno T. Pepsinogen gene transcription induced in heterologous epithelial-mesenchymal recombinations of chicken endoderms and glandular stomach mesenchyme. Development 1988;103:725–31.
3. Koike T, Yasugi S. In vitro analysis of mesenchymal influences on the differentiation of stomach epithelial cells of the chicken embryo. Differentiation 1999;65:13–25.
4. Yasugi S. Regulation of pepsinogen gene expression in epithelial cells of vertebrate stomach during development. Int J Dev Biol 1994;38:273–9.
5. Smith DM, Tabin CJ. BMP signalling specifies the pyloric sphincter. Nature 1999;402:748–9.
6. Rings EHHM, Krasinski SD, Van Beers EH, et al. Restriction of lactase gene expression along the proximal-to-distal axis of rat small intestine occurs during postnatal development. Gastroenterology 1994;106:1223–32.
7. Smith DM, Grasty RC, Theodosiou NA, et al. Evolutionary relationships between the amphibian, avian, and mammalian stomachs. Evol Dev 2000;2:348–59.
8. Grapin-Botton A, Melton DA. Endoderm development: From patterning to organogenesis. Trends Genet 2000;16:124–30.
9. Roberts DJ. Molecular mechanisms of development of the gastrointestinal tract. Dev Dyn 2000;219:109–20.
10. Roberts DJ, Smith DM, Goff DJ, Tabin CJ. Epithelial-mesenchymal signaling during the regionalization of the chick gut. Development 1998;125:2791–801.
11. Smith DM, Nielsen C, Tabin CJ, Roberts DJ. Roles of BMP signaling and Nkx2.5 in patterning at the chick midgut-foregut boundary. Development 2000;127:3671–81.
12. de Santa Barbara P, van den Brink GR, Roberts DJ. Molecular etiology of gut malformations and diseases. Am J Med Genet 2002;115:221–30.
13. Le Douarin N. Etude experimentale de l'organeogenese du tube difestif et du foie chez l'embryon de poulet. Bull Biol France, Belg 1964;98:533–676.
14. Haffen K, Kedinger M, Simon-Assmann P. Mesenchyme-dependent differentiation of epithelial progenitor cells in the gut. J Pediatr Gastroenterol Nutr 1987;6:14–23.
15. Yasugi S. Role of epithelial-mesenchymal interactions in differentiation of epithelium of vertebrate digestive organs. Dev Growth Differ 1993;35:1–9.
16. Sumiya M. Differentiation of the digestive tract epithelium of the chick embryo cultured in vitro enveloped in a fragment of vitelline membrane in the absence of mecenchyme. Roux's Archiv. 1976;197:1–17.
17. Haffen K, Lacroix B, Kedinger M, Simon-Assmann PM. Inductive properties of fibroblastic cell cultures derived from rat intestinal mucosa on epithelial differentiation. Differentiation 1983;23:226–33.
18. Kedinger M, Simon-Asman PM, Lacroix B, et al. Fetal gut mesenchyme induces differentiation of cultured intestinal endodermal and crypt cells. Dev Biol 1986;113:474–83.
19. Kedinger M, Simon-Assman P, Bouziges F, Haffen K. Epithelial-mesenchymal interactions in intestinal epithelial differentiation. Scand J Gastroenterol 1988;23:62–9.
20. Aufderheide E, Ekblom P. Tenascin during gut development: Appearance in the mesenchyme, shift in molecular forms, and dependence on epithelial-mesenchymal interactions. J Cell Biol 1988;107:2341–9.
21. Kedinger M, et al. Smooth muscle actin expression during rat gut development and induction in fetal skin fibroblastic cells associated with intestinal embryonic epithelium. Differentiation 1990;43:87–97.
22. Takahashi Y, Imanaka T, and Takano T. Spatial pattern of smooth muscle differentiation is specified by the epithelium in the stomach of mouse embryo. Dev Dyn 1998; 212:448–60.
23. Kedinger M, Duluc I, Fritsch C, et al. Intestinal epithelial-mesenchymal cell interactions. Ann N Y Acad Sci 1998a; 859:1–17.
24. Kedinger M, Lefebvre O, Duluc I, et al. Cellular and molecular partners involved in gut morphogenesis and differentiation. Philos Trans R Soc Lond B Biol Sci 1998b; 353:847–56.
25. Duluc I, Freund JN, Leberquier C, Kedinger M. Fetal endoderm primarily holds the temporal and positional information required for mammalian intestinal development. J Cell Biol 1994;126:211–21.
26. Yasugi S. Differentiation of avian digestive tract epithelium. Tiss Cult Ress Commun 1995;14:177–184.
27. Yasugi S, Matsushita S, Mizuno T. Gland formation induced in the allantoic and small-intestinal endoderm by the proventricular mesenchyme is not coupled with pepsinogen expression. Differentiation 1985;30:47–52.
28. Goetz JA, Suber LM, Zeng X, Robbins DJ. Sonic Hedgehog as a mediator of long-range signaling. Bioessays 2002;24: 157–65.
29. Matise MP, Joyner AL. Gli genes in development and cancer. Oncogene 1999;18:7852–9.
30. Murone M, Rosenthal A, de Sauvage FJ. Hedgehog signal transduction: From flies to vertebrates. Exp Cell Res 1999;253:25–33.
31. Nybakken K, Perrimon N. Hedgehog signal transduction: Recent findings. Curr Opin Genet Dev 2002;12:503–11.
32. Ruiz i Altaba A. Gli proteins and Hedgehog signaling: Development and cancer. Trends Genet 1999;15:418–25.
33. Bitgood MJ, McMahon AP. Hedgehog and Bmp genes are coexpressed at many diverse sites of cell-cell interaction in the mouse embryo. Dev Biol 1995;172:126–38.
34. Fukuda K, Yasugi S. Versatile roles for sonic hedgehog in gut development. J Gastroenterol 2002;37:239–46.
35. Litingtung Y, Lei L, Westphal H, Chiang C. Sonic hedgehog is essential to foregut development. Nat Genet 1998;20:58–61.
36. Marigo V, Scott MP, Johnson RL, et al. Conservation in hedgehog signaling: Induction of a chicken patched homolog by Sonic hedgehog in the developing limb. Development 1996;122:1225–33.
37. Narita T, Ishii Y, Nohno T, et al. Sonic hedgehog expression in developing chicken digestive organs is regulated by epithelial-mesenchymal interactions. Dev Growth Differ 1998;40:67–74.
38. Sukegawa A, et al. The concentric structure of the developing gut is regulated by Sonic hedgehog derived from endodermal epithelium. Development 2000;127:1971–80.
39. Roberts DJ, et al. Sonic hedgehog is an endodermal signal inducing Bmp-4 and Hox genes during induction and regionalization of the chick hindgut. Development 1995;121:3163–74.
40. Chiang C, et al. Cyclopia and defective axial patterning in mice lacking Sonic hedgehog gene function. Nature 1996;383:407–13.
41. Pepicelli CV, Lewis PM, McMahon AP. Sonic hedgehog regulates branching morphogenesis in the mammalian lung. Curr Biol 1998;8:1083–6.

42. Narita T, et al. BMPs are necessary for stomach gland formation in the chicken embryo: A study using virally induced BMP-2 and Noggin expression. Development 2000;127: 981–8.
43. Pollock RA, Jay G, Bieberich CJ. Altering the boundaries of Hox3.1 expression: Evidence for antipodal gene regulation. Cell 1992;71:911–23.
44. Levin M. Left-right asymmetry in embryonic development: A comprehensive review. Mech Dev 2005;122:3–25.
45. Raya A, Belmonte JC. Left-right asymmetry in the vertebrate embryo: From early information to higher-level integration. Nat Rev Genet 2006;7:283–93.
46. Levin M, et al. Left/right patterning signals and the independent regulation of different aspects of situs in the chick embryo. Dev Biol 1997;189:57–67.
47. Levin M. Left-right asymmetry in vertebrate embryogenesis. Bioessays 1997;19:287–96.
48. Levin M. Left-right asymmetry and the chick embryo. Semin Cell Dev Biol 1998;9:67–76.
49. Levin M. The embryonic origins of left-right asymmetry. Crit Rev Oral Biol Med 2004;15:197–206.
50. Mercola M, Levin M. Left-right asymmetry determination in vertebrates. Annu Rev Cell Dev Biol 2001;17:779–805.
51. Tamura K, Yonei-Tamura S, and Belmonte JC. Molecular basis of left-right asymmetry. Dev Growth Differ 1999; 41:645–56.
52. Lipscomb K, Schmitt C, Sablyak A, et al. Role for retinoid signaling in left-right asymmetric digestive organ morphogenesis. Dev Dyn 2006;235:2266–75.
53. Al-Salem AH. Pyloric atresia associated with duodenal and jejunal atresia and duplication. Pediatr Surg Int 1999;15:512–4.
54. Okoye BO, Parikh DH, Buick RG, Lander AD. Pyloric atresia: Five new cases, a new association, and a review of the literature with guidelines. J Pediatr Surg 2000;35:1242–5.
55. Benjamin B, Jayakumar P, Reddy LA, Abbag F. Gastric outlet obstruction caused by prepyloric web in a case of Down's syndrome. J Pediatr Surg 1996;31:1290–1.
56. Al-Salem A, Nawaz A, Matta H, Jacobsz A. Congenital pyloric atresia: The spectrum. Int Surg 2002;87:147–51.
57. Ilce Z, et al. Pyloric atresia: 15-year review from a single institution. J Pediatr Surg 2003;38:1581–4.
58. Ferguson C, Morabito A, Bianchi A. Duodenal atresia and gastric antral web. A significant lesson to learn. Eur J Pediatr Surg 2004;14:120–2.
59. Darwish AA, et al. Pyloric obstruction, duodenal dilatation, and extrahepatic cholestasis: A neonatal triad suggesting multiple intestinal atresias. J Pediatr Surg 2006;41:1771–3.
60. Nakamura H, et al. Epidermolysis bullosa simplex associated with pyloric atresia is a novel clinical subtype caused by mutations in the plectin gene (PLEC1). J Mol Diagn 2005;7:28–35.
61. Iacovacci S, et al. Novel and recurrent mutations in the integrin beta 4 subunit gene causing lethal junctional epidermolysis bullosa with pyloric atresia. Exp Dermatol 2003;12:716–20.
62. Varma VA, Sessions JT, Kahn LB, Lipper S. Chronic granulomatous disease of childhood presenting as gastric outlet obstruction. Am J Surg Pathol 1982;6:673–6.
63. Rohrer K, Murphy R, Thresher C, et al. Infantile myofibromatosis: A most unusual cause of gastric outlet obstruction. Pediatr Radiol 2005;35:808–11.
64. Hasegawa T, et al. Prenatal diagnosis of congenital pyloric atresia. J Clin Ultrasound 1993;21:278–81.
65. Berrocal T, et al. Congenital anomalies of the upper gastrointestinal tract. Radiographics 1999;19:855–72.
66. Dessanti A, et al. Pyloric atresia: A new operation to reconstruct the pyloric sphincter. J Pediatr Surg 2004;39:297–301.
67. Hocking M, Young DG. Duplications of the alimentary tract. Br J Surg 1981;68:92–6.
68. Pruksapong C, Donovan RJ, Pinit A, Heldrich FJ. Gastric duplication. J Pediatr Surg 1979;14:83–5.
69. Puligandla PS, et al. Gastrointestinal duplications. J Pediatr Surg 2003;38:740–4.
70. Saad DF, Gow KW, Shehata B, Wulkan ML. Pyloric duplication in a term newborn. J Pediatr Surg 2005;40:1209–10.
71. Shah A, More B, Buick R. Pyloric duplication in a neonate: A rare entity. Pediatr Surg Int 2005;21:220–2.
72. Kim DH, Kim JS, Nam ES, Shin HS. Foregut duplication cyst of the stomach. Pathol Int 2000;50:142–5.
73. Wieczorek RL, Seidman I, Ranson JH, Ruoff M. Congenital duplication of the stomach: Case report and review of the English literature. Am J Gastroenterol 1984;79:597–602.
74. Carachi R, Azmy A. Foregut duplications. Pediatr Surg Int 2002;18:371–4.
75. Chen CP, Liu YP, Hsu CY, et al. Prenatal sonography and magnetic resonance imaging of pulmonary sequestration associated with a gastric duplication cyst. Prenat Diagn 2006;26:489–91.
76. Muraoka A, et al. A gastric duplication cyst with an aberrant pancreatic ductal system: Report of a case. Surg Today 2002;32:531–5.
77. Gugig R, Ostroff J, Chen YY, et al. Gastric cystic duplication: A rare cause of recurrent pancreatitis in children. Gastrointest Endosc 2004;59:592–4.
78. Pokorny CS, Cook WJ, Dilley A. Gastric duplication: Endoscopic appearance and clinical features. J Gastroenterol Hepatol 1997;12:719–22.
79. Takahara T, et al. Gastric duplication cyst: Evaluation by endoscopic ultrasonography and magnetic resonance imaging. J Gastroenterol 1996;31:420–4.
80. Segal SR, et al. Ultrasonographic features of gastrointestinal duplications. J Ultrasound Med 1994;13:863–70.
81. Correia-Pinto J, et al. Prenatal diagnosis of abdominal enteric duplications. Prenat Diagn 2000;20:163–7.
82. Granata C, et al. Gastric duplication cyst: Appearance on prenatal US and MRI. Pediatr Radiol 2003;33:148–9.
83. Nakazawa N, Okazaki T, Miyano T. Prenatal detection of isolated gastric duplication cyst. Pediatr Surg Int 2005;21:831–4.
84. Sasaki T, Shimura H, Ryu S, et al. Laparoscopic treatment of a gastric duplication cyst: Report of a case. Int Surg 2003; 88:68–71.
85. Ford WD, Guelfand M, Lopez PJ, Furness ME. Laparoscopic excision of a gastric duplication cyst detected on antenatal ultrasound scan. J Pediatr Surg 2004;39:e8–e10.
86. Idowu J, Aitken DR, Georgeson KE. Gastric volvulus in the newborn. Arch Surg 1980;115:1046–9.
87. al-Salem AH. Intrathoracic gastric volvulus in infancy. Pediatr Radiol 2000;30:842–5.
88. Bautista-Casasnovas A, et al. Chronic gastric volvulus: Is it so rare? Eur J Pediatr Surg 2002;12:111–5.
89. Honna T, Kamii Y, Tsuchida Y. Idiopathic gastric volvulus in infancy and childhood. J Pediatr Surg 1990;25:707–10.
90. Samuel M, Burge DM, Griffiths DM. Gastric volvulus and associated gastroesophageal reflux. Arch Dis Child 1995;73:462–4.
91. Basaran UN, et al. Acute gastric volvulus due to deficiency of the gastrocolic ligament in a newborn. Eur J Pediatr 2002;161:288–90.
92. Kotobi H, et al. Acute mesenteroaxial gastric volvulus and congenital diaphragmatic hernia. Pediatr Surg Int 2005; 21:674–6.
93. Shivanand G, et al. Gastric volvulus: Acute and chronic presentation. Clin Imaging 2003;27:265–8.
94. Aoyama K, Tateishi K. Gastric volvulus in three children with asplenic syndrome. J Pediatr Surg 1986;21:307–10.
95. Okoye BO, Bailey DM, Cusick EL, Spicer RD. Prophylactic gastropexy in the asplenia syndrome. Pediatr Surg Int 1997;12:28–9.
96. Cameron AE, Howard ER. Gastric volvulus in childhood. J Pediatr Surg 1987;22:944–7.
97. Darani A, Mendoza-Sagaon M, Reinberg O. Gastric volvulus in children. J Pediatr Surg 2005;40:855–8.
98. Andiran F, Tanyel FC, Balkanci F, Hicsonmez A. Acute abdomen due to gastric volvulus: Diagnostic value of a single plain radiograph. Pediatr Radiol 1995;25:S240.
99. Elhalaby EA, Mashaly EM. Infants with radiologic diagnosis of gastric volvulus: Are they over-treated? Pediatr Surg Int 2001;17:596–600.
100. Odaka A, et al. Laparoscopic gastropexy for acute gastric volvulus: A case report. J Pediatr Surg 1999;34:477–8.
101. Hernaiz Driever P, et al. Congenital microgastria, growth hormone deficiency and diabetes insipidus. Eur J Pediatr 1997;156:37–40.
102. Menon P, Rao KL, Cutinha HP, et al. Gastric augmentation in isolated congenital microgastria. J Pediatr Surg 2003;38:E4–6.
103. Kroes EJ, Festen C. Congenital microgastria: A case report and review of literature. Pediatr Surg Int 1998;13:416–8.
104. Giurgea I, Raqbi F, Nihoul-Fekete C, et al. Congenital microgastria with Pierre Robin sequence and partial trismus. Clin Dysmorphol 2000;9:307–8.
105. Herman TE, Siegel MJ. Imaging casebook. Asplenia syndrome with congenital microgastria and malrotation. J Perinatol 2004;24:50–2.
106. Sharma SC, Menon P. Congenital microgastria with esophageal stenosis and diaphragmatic hernia. Pediatr Surg Int 2005;21:292–4.
107. Stewart C, Stewart M, Stewart F. Microgastria-limb reduction anomaly with total amelia. Clin Dysmorphol 2002;11: 187–90.
108. Murray KF, Lillehei CW, Duggan C. Congenital microgastria: Treatment with transient jejunal feedings. J Pediatr Gastroenterol Nutr 1999;28:343–5.
109. Neifeld JP, Berman WF, Lawrence W, Jr, et al. Management of congenital microgastria with a jejunal reservoir pouch. J Pediatr Surg 1980;15:882–5.
110. Wolters VM, et al. A gastric diverticulum containing pancreatic tissue and presenting as congenital double pylorus: Case report and review of the literature. J Pediatr Gastroenterol Nutr 2001;33:89–91.
111. Ciftci AO, Tanyel FC, Hicsonmez A. Gastric diverticulum: An uncommon cause of abdominal pain in a 12 year old. J Pediatr Surg 1998;33:529–31.
112. Johnson R. Intestinal atresia and stenosis: A review comparing its etiopathogenesis. Vet Res Commun 1986;10: 95–104.
113. Gahukamble DB, Adnan AR, Al Gadi M. Distal foregut atresias in consecutive siblings and twins in the same family. Pediatr Surg Int 2003;19:288–92.
114. Maegawa GH, et al. Duodenal and biliary atresia associated with facial, thyroid and auditory apparatus abnormalities: A new mandibulofacial dysostosis syndrome? Clin Dysmorphol 2006;15:191–6.
115. Holder-Espinasse M, et al. Familial syndromic duodenal atresia: Feingold syndrome. Eur J Pediatr Surg 2004;14:112–6.
116. Diamanti A, et al. Duodenal stenosis, a new finding on congenital rubella syndrome: Case description and literature review. J Infect 2006;53:e207–10.
117. Vitug-Sales MI, Lemberg DA, Cunningham C, et al. A case of duodenal web occurring in Prader-Willi syndrome. J Paediatr Child Health 2005;41:527–8.
118. Ein SH, Palder SB, Filler RM. Babies with esophageal and duodenal atresia: A 30-year review of a multifaceted problem. J Pediatr Surg 2006;41:530–2.
119. Dalla Vecchia LK, et al. Intestinal atresia and stenosis: A 25-year experience with 277 cases. Arch Surg 133, 490-6; discussion 1998;496–7.
120. Bailey PV, et al. Congenital duodenal obstruction: A 32-year review. J Pediatr Surg 1993;28:92–5.
121. Anami A, et al. Sudden fetal death associated with both duodenal atresia and umbilical cord ulcer: A case report and review. Am J Perinatol 2006;23:183–8.
122. Savino A, Rollo V, Chiarelli F. Congenital duodenal stenosis and annular pancreas: A delayed diagnosis in an adolescent patient with Down syndrome. Eur J Pediatr 2006.
123. Pathak D, Sarin YK. Congenital duodenal obstruction due to a preduodenal portal vein. Indian J Pediatr 2006;73:423–5.
124. Schmidt H, Abolmaali N, Vogl TJ. Double bubble sign. Eur Radiol 2002;12:1849–53.
125. Nelson LH, Clark CE, Fishburne JI, et al. Value of serial sonography in the in utero detection of duodenal atresia. Obstet Gynecol 1982;59:657–60.
126. Alvarez C, Rueda O, Vicente JM, Fraile E. Gastric emphysema in a child with congenital duodenal diaphragm. Pediatr Radiol 1997;27:915–7.
127. Franquet T, Gonzalez A. Gastric and duodenal pneumatosis in a child with annular pancreas. Pediatr Radiol 1987;17:262.
128. Bax NM, Ure BM, van der Zee DC, van Tuijl I. Laparoscopic duodenoduodenostomy for duodenal atresia. Surg Endosc 2001;15:217.
129. Nakajima K, et al. Laparoscopically assisted surgery for congenital gastric or duodenal diaphragm in children. Surg Laparosc Endosc Percutan Tech 2003;13:36–8.
130. Steyaert H, Valla JS, Van Hoorde E. Diaphragmatic duodenal atresia: Laparoscopic repair. Eur J Pediatr Surg 2003; 13:414–6.
131. Torroni F, et al. Endoscopic membranectomy of duodenal diaphragm: Pediatric experience. Gastrointest Endosc 2006; 63:530–1.
132. van Rijn RR, et al. Membranous duodenal stenosis: Initial experience with balloon dilatation in four children. Eur J Radiol 2006;59:29–32.
133. Bajpai M, Mathur M. Duplications of the alimentary tract: Clues to the missing links. J Pediatr Surg 1994;29:1361–5.
134. van den Brink GR, et al. Sonic hedgehog expression correlates with fundic gland differentiation in the adult gastrointestinal tract. Gut 2002;51:628–33.
135. Wakisaka M, Nakada K, Kitagawa H, et al. Giant transdiaphragmatic duodenal duplication with an intraspinal neurenteric cyst as part of the split notochord syndrome: Report of a case. Surg Today 2004;34:459–62.
136. Prasad TR, Tan CE. Duodenal duplication cyst communicating with an aberrant pancreatic duct. Pediatr Surg Int 2005;21:320–2.
137. Merrot T, et al. Duodenal duplications. Clinical characteristics, embryological hypotheses, histological findings, treatment. Eur J Pediatr Surg 2006;16:18–23.
138. Kim W, Willis J, Sohi J, Graham M. Duodenal gastric duplication cyst detection after Roux-en-Y decompression using Tc-99m pertechnetate. Clin Nucl Med 2006;31:164–5.
139. Borgnon J, Durand C, Gourlaouen D, et al. Antenatal detection of a communicating duodenal duplication. Eur J Pediatr Surg 2003;13:130–3.
140. Foley PT, et al. Enteric duplications presenting as antenatally detected abdominal cysts: Is delayed resection appropriate? J Pediatr Surg 2003;38:1810–3.

8

Nausea, Vomiting, and Pyloric Stenosis

B U.K. Li, MD

Nausea and vomiting are among the most common symptoms in children that occur as part of both acute illnesses and chronic disorders originating within and outside the gastrointestinal (GI) tract. For the clinician, these symptoms are important clues to causative underlying disorders, such as common viral enteritis to more serious intestinal obstruction. The presentation of vomiting initiates a broad differential diagnosis, a specific diagnostic approach, treatment approaches aimed at the symptom and/or cause, and prevention of potential complications.

The role of vomiting is to provide for the rapid clearance of ingested toxins. For example, this coordinated GI response occurs promptly in response to ingested *Bacillus cereus* toxin.[1] This patterned response often combines repeated emetic and diarrheal events that act efficiently to clear the entire intestinal tract of toxins in both orad and aboral directions.

Although vomiting during ingestion of toxins is critical to survival, nausea and vomiting can also be the manifestation of a dysfunctional brain-gut response. The Rome III criteria list functional idiopathic nausea, functional vomiting, and cyclic vomiting syndrome, all of which may become highly disabling.[2–4] Although the precise pathogenesis is unknown, the potential role of stress responses has been recently recognized. Based on extensive animal studies, corticotropin-releasing factor is the putative neuroendocrine trigger of vomiting in cyclic vomiting syndrome.[5–6]

The socioeconomic impact of nausea and vomiting, both of specific cause and functional syndromes, has not been formally estimated. In acute enteric infections, the medical cost and economic impact of lost productivity are estimated at $1.25 billion (US) and $21.8 billion (US) in 1980.[7] This figure does not include the cost of care, school absences, and lost parental work days associated with gastroesophageal reflux, postoperative vomiting, and chemotherapy-induced vomiting in children. Although functional syndromes appear less serious, they can also be medically costly, as evidenced by the average annual cost of care for a child with cyclic vomiting syndrome estimated at $17,000 (US).[6]

Despite the development of potent 5-hydroxytryptamine (5-HT$_3$) and neurokinin (NK$_1$) receptor antagonists as antiemetic agents, the treatment efficacy of vomiting associated with both organic and functional conditions remains inadequate. This ineffectiveness highlights the need for further understanding of the pathways and neurotransmitters involved, including the potential role of inhibiting more than one pathway concomitantly and the use of specific agonists.[8] The pathways and neurotransmitters that mediate nausea, other than motion (vection)-induced nausea,[9] remain undelineated and, hence, nausea remains difficult to remedy.[10]

VOMITING

Vomiting (emesis) is a complex behavioral, gastrointestinal, and somatomotor reflex response to a variety of stimuli.[11–12] The emetic reflex has three phases: (1) a prodromal period consisting of the sensation of nausea and signs of autonomic nervous system stimulation, (2) retching, and (3) forceful retrograde expulsion of stomach contents through the oral cavity. Although the overall sequence is patterned, each phase can occur independently of the others. For example, nausea or retching does not always progress to vomiting, and pharyngeal stimulation can induce retching or vomiting without nausea.

Several *GI motor events* coincide with prodromal nausea and autonomic arousal.[11] Gastrointestinal atony and dilation of the proximal stomach occur. Esophageal skeletal muscle shortens longitudinally, pulls the proximal stomach into the thorax, and enables the flow of gastric contents into the esophagus.[13] A single large-amplitude contraction, termed the *retrograde giant contraction* (RGC), is generated in the jejunum and propagated orad at 8 to 10 cm per second.[14] The RGC propels duodenal contents into stomach before retching begins.[13]

These GI motor events are mediated by vagal preganglionic parasympathetic fibers that activate both inhibitory and excitatory pathways in the enteric nervous system.[15] These GI motor events do not appear to be the cause of the sensation of nausea.[16] Moreover, the somatomotor pattern of retching and vomiting persists even when GI motor correlates are obliterated by ablation of vagal efferents.[15]

Although GI motor activity is not necessary for the vomiting act, motor activity may play a functional role in the defense against noxious ingestions.[17] The RGC transfers toxins and alkaline duodenal secretions into the stomach for dilution and buffering (eg, vinegar, hypertonic saline), and gastric accommodation can confine the toxins before being expelled. Buffering of the gastric contents also helps protect the esophagus from acid-induced injury. Finally, proximal positioning of the stomach places it in a beneficial position for compression by the abdominal musculature during emesis.[13]

In *nausea* induced by motion (vection), a different pattern of GI motor activity is observed.[18–19] Just prior to the onset, gastric slow waves increase from 3 to 9 cycles per minute, a phenomenon known as *tachygastria*.[20] Tachygastria is controlled through central cholinergic and α-adrenergic pathways.[9,17] In motion-induced nausea, GI motor activity correlates with the induction of symptoms.[20]

The two major *somatic motor components* of vomiting—retching and expulsion—are produced by a coordinated program of respiratory, abdominal, and pharyngeal muscle contractions that result in rhythmic changes in intrathoracic and intra-abdominal pressures.[21] During each cycle of *retching,* the glottis closes and the diaphragm, external intercostal and abdominal muscles contract,[22] producing large negative intrathoracic and positive intra-abdominal pressures. As the atonic proximal stomach is displaced into the thoracic cavity, normal antireflux mechanisms are overcome, and gastric contents then move in and out of the esophagus with each cycle of retching.[13]

After the onset of retching, *vomiting* is produced by relaxation of the external intercostal muscles and the hiatal diaphragm, and intense contraction of the abdominal muscles and costal diaphragm.[22] These coordinated events produce positive abdominal and thoracic pressures, and, assisted by retrograde contraction of the cervical esophagus, lead to oral expulsion of the gastric contents.[15] Afterwards, antegrade esophageal peristalsis clears the lumen of residual material,[3,23] and the proximal stomach returns to its normal intra-abdominal antireflux configuration.

THE EMETIC REFLEX, PATHWAY, AND MEDIATORS

The emetic reflex consists of an afferent pathway, central integration and control, and an efferent pathway.[10,24–25] A variety of afferent stimuli can trigger vomiting, including visceral pain, inflammation, toxins, motion, pregnancy, radiation exposure, postoperative states, and unpleasant emotions. At least four afferent pathways originate in the *GI tract* (by chemo- and mechanoreceptors), through systemic *blood-borne* exposure, via *vestibular* by real or apparent motion, and from the upper *central nervous system* (eg, stress). Diverse afferent receptors are located within the gut, oropharynx, heart, vestibular system, and central nervous system (eg, area postrema, hypothalamus, cortical regions) to initiate the afferent limb. These afferent pathways appear to be distinct; for example, chemical stimulation of the area postrema by toxins is independent of that induced by either abdominal vagal afferents or motion.

Within the GI tract, both mechanoreceptors and chemoreceptors can initiate the emetic reflex.[26–27] *Mechanoreceptors* located within the muscularis are triggered by changes in bowel wall tension such as are present in bowel obstruction. *Chemoreceptors* within the gastric and small intestinal mucosa respond to a variety of chemical irritants (eg, HCl, copper sulfate, vinegar, hypertonic saline, syrup of ipecac).

Serotonin (hydroxytryptamine, 5-HT) plays a key role in mediating the emetic reflex induced by chemotherapy agents, radiation,[28] and other noxious agents[29–30] in the GI tract. 5-HT released from enterochromaffin cells in response to cisplatin and other noxious substances acts in paracrine fashion on local 5-HT_3 receptors that project via the vagus nerve to the brainstem nucleus tractus solitarus (NTS) and end at the dorsomotor nucleus of the vagus (DMNV) to initiate the reflex.[31–33] This response is blocked by 5-HT_3 receptor antagonists.[32] 5-HT_3 receptors reside on vagal afferent fibers within the GI tract and the presynaptic vagal afferent terminals in the central nervous system, specifically in the NTS and chemotrigger zone in the area postrema.[28,34] Other ligands and receptor subtypes modulate the emetic reflex by either *enhancing* local intestinal 5-HT release—acetylcholine (M_3), noradrenaline (β-adrenoreceptor), histamine and 5-HT, or *diminishing* it—GABA ($GABA_B$), 5-HT (5-HT_4), noradrenaline (α_2-adrenoceptor), VIP, and somatostatin.[8]

Substance P, a neurokinin (tachykinin) peptide, and its NK_1 receptor play an essential role in the emetic response produced by a wide range of stimuli, including intravenous morphine. The site of action is thought to be NK_1 receptors located in NTS and DMNV in the central nervous system.[35] Since pharmacologic blockade of this receptor prevents emesis induced by both peripheral and central acting agents, it has been suggested that NK_1 receptors are crucial to the central integration or effector pathway common to all emesis-inducing stimuli.[36]

Blood-borne toxins and drugs can trigger the emetic reflex through the area postrema which is a permeable region located at the floor of the fourth ventricle that allows cells to detect substances both in the blood and in the cerebrospinal fluid.[37–38] This richly innervated region is also called the *chemotrigger zone* (CTZ) and has multiple receptors types for endogenous neurotransmitters[37] that include dopamine, acetylcholine, enkephalin, peptide YY, and substance P.[39–40] Dopaminergic pathways play a role as demonstrated by the emetic effect of experimental apomorphine mediated by D_2 receptors[41] within the area postrema and the efficacy of D_2

antagonists antiemetic agents metoclopramide, and prochlorperazine. In addition, D_3 receptors may play a role as well.[42]

Bodily motion or apparent motion (vection drum) activates the afferent limb of the vomiting reflex. Motion-induced vomiting results from a sensory mismatch involving the visual, vestibular, and proprioceptive systems[31,43] mediated through histamine (H_1) and cholinergic muscarinic (M_3/M_5) receptors on the afferent limb.[44–45] An intact vestibular system is a necessary component for activation to occur.[46]

Stimuli from upper central nervous system (eg, emotions, trauma, increased intracranial pressure) can also stimulate vomiting. Arousal of higher cortical centers by unpleasant situations (eg, fear) or instances of anticipatory vomiting in chemotherapy also activate the emetic reflex. Although the precise afferent pathways remain unclear, vomiting in these instances can be provoked with minimal nausea. Animal studies convincingly link physical and psychological stress to gastric stasis via central corticotropin-releasing factor (CRF) acting on CRF-R2 at the DMNV.[47] CRF plays an initiating role in stress-induced vomiting as part of the behavioral, neuroendocrine, autonomic, and visceral response to both physical and psychological stressors.[5]

After activation, the afferent systems project centrally principally via vagal 5-HT-mediated pathways.[17] These fibers project mainly to the dorsomedial portion of the NTS and to a lesser extent to the area postrema and the DMNV.[24,27,45,48–49] No single central locus has been identified as a "*vomiting center*."[50] Rather, the integrated motor program of emesis is likely coordinated by several nuclei—NTS, parvicellular reticular formation, and the Bötzinger complex (Lawes, 1990, #321)—with proximate input from the area postrema and effector output through the DMNV.

DIFFERENTIAL DIAGNOSIS

The clinical approach to vomiting begins by distinguishing it from regurgitation and recognizing the temporal (acute, recurrent–chronic, recurrent–cyclic, or episodic) pattern of vomiting. Other variables that help narrow down the diagnostic possibilities include the age of the patient, time of day and proximate events, contents of vomitus, presence or absence of nausea, associated systemic symptoms, and family history. Although one can typically treat empirically, the presence of specific alarm symptoms indicates the need of a more thorough diagnostic evaluation.

VOMITING VERSUS REGURGITATION

In pediatric practice, a preliminary challenge is to differentiate between vomiting and regurgitation. Although both can occur concomitantly (eg, gastroesophageal reflux—see Chapter 4.2 "Gastroesophageal Reflux"), it is important to note that vomiting and regurgitation have distinct mechanics, autonomic signs, and implications (Table 1). Regurgitation represents *effortless* retrograde expulsion of gastric contents unaccompanied by autonomic signs and is usually due to gastroesophageal reflux or rumination (Table 1). In contrast, vomiting is a *forceful* expulsion resulting from a patterned, somatomotor sequence accompanied by autonomic signs (pallor, sweating, and tachycardia) and can be caused by serious disorders with complications and different implications. Vomiting, but not regurgitation, is accompanied by characteristic autonomic signs including pallor, diaphoresis, hypersalivation, listlessness, and tachycardia that can be used as measures of accompanying nausea.[51] Although we are only beginning to appreciate the differences in implications, one example is the presence of vomiting in a child with refractory gastroesophageal reflux predicts persistent postoperative retching dysfunction following fundoplication.[52]

TEMPORAL (INTENSITY VERSUS DURATION) PATTERNS OF VOMITING

There are three temporal patterns of vomiting one *acute* and two recurrent, *chronic* and *cyclic* (or *episodic*) with different diagnostic profiles (Table 2).[53] The *acute* form presents to a pediatric office, urgent care or emergency department with the sudden onset of vomiting in a previously well child. It usually results from enteric infections, extraintestinal infections (eg, urinary tract infections), toxic ingestion (eg, *B. cereus*),[54] and, less commonly, from intestinal obstruction (eg, malrotation with volvulus), or extraintestinal lesions (eg, acute hydronephrosis).[55]

Recurrent vomiting is a common problem encountered in a pediatric gastroenterology practice. In a consecutive series of 106 recurrent vomiting patients, two-thirds could be differentiated into a *chronic*, low frequency, nearly daily vomiting pattern, and one-third into a *cyclic* or *episodic*, an intense, but intermittent one (Table 2).[56] Those with the *chronic* pattern tend to vomit once or twice daily, but never became dehydrated, and were typically discovered to have peptic, bacterial (eg, *Helicobacter pylori*), allergic (eg, eosinophilic

Table 1 Features Differentiating Vomiting from Regurgitation

Feature	Regurgitation	Vomiting
Event	Effortless expulsion	Forceful expulsion of gastric contents
Prodrome	None	Pallor, salivation, tachycardia + retching
Cause(s)	Gastroesophageal reflux, rumination	Many disorders
Complications	Uncommon	Esophagitis, hematemesis
Implications	Few	Post-Nissen retching syndrome

Table 2 Features Distinguishing Acute, Recurrent—Chronic, and Recurrent—Cyclic or Episodic Patterns of Vomiting

Clinical Feature	Acute	Recurren—Chronic	Recurrent—Cyclic or Episodic
Epidemiology	Most common	Two-thirds of recurrent vomiting patients	One-third of recurrent vomiting patients
Vomiting pace	Moderate–severe	Mild ~ 1–2 emeses/h at peak	Severe ~ 6 emeses/h at peak
Stereotype	—	None	98% have similar duration and symptoms, one-half with regular cycles (eg, 4 weeks apart), and one-half irregular episodes
Symptoms	Fever, vomiting, diarrhea	Vomiting, abdominal pain	Pallor, listlessness, nausea, abdominal pain, photophobia
Complications	Dehydration	Uncommon	Dehydration, hematemesis
Family	Sick household contacts	14% positive migraine headaches	72–83% positive migraine headaches
Causes	Viral gastroenteritis	Reflux, gastritis, duodenitis	Cyclic vomiting syndrome (88%)

Adapted in part from Li, Sunku.[169]

esophagitis) or inflammatory (eg, Crohn) esophagitis, gastritis, or duodenitis on upper endoscopy. Those with the *cyclic* pattern tend to have sporadic, intense (> four emeses per h at the peak) attacks of vomiting each of which individually resembles acute vomiting and similarly involves emergent evaluation and intravenous rehydration. Although the cyclic pattern is highly predictive (88%) of cyclic vomiting syndrome, one in eight had treatable organic etiologies such as hydronephrosis, malrotation, Chiari malformation, and brainstem neoplasms, as well as Addison disease and mitochondriopathy, disorders mostly conditions residing outside of the GI tract.[57]

CLINICAL CLUES: AGE, TIME OF DAY, VOMITUS, AND "ALARM" SYMPTOMS

Age

The commonest causes of vomiting vary with the age of the patient (Table 3). In neonates (<1 mo) and infants, vomiting can result from both GI (eg, enteritis) and extra-intestinal infections (eg, pyelonephritis or sepsis). Acid-peptic disease[58] and allergic bowel disorders are also common.[59]

If infectious agents are excluded and time-limited course of empiric therapy is ineffective, anatomic abnormalities of the GI tract, intestinal dysmotility, and inborn metabolic disorders should be considered. Most congenital GI anomalies that cause high-grade obstruction present within the first day of life (eg, duodenal atresia, Hirschsprung) 3 to 6 weeks (pyloric stenosis) or 6 to 12 months (eg, intussusception).[60] However there are other obstructive lesions that can be identified throughout childhood (eg, inguinal hernias, webs, duplications, intermittent volvulus).[61] Metabolic disorders may become unmasked following exposure to expanded diets (eg, organic acidemias, amino acidemias, urea cycle defects,[62] hereditary fructose intolerance) and longer periods of fasting (disorders of fatty acid oxidation,[63–64] mitochondriopathies[65]) with increasing age.

In toddlers, two unusual causes of vomiting include chronic granulomatous disease-induced antral obstruction[66] and cytomegalovirus-associated Ménétrier gastropathy associated with hypoalbuminemia.[67] Recognition of subtentorial brainstem neoplasms (eg, cerebellar medulloblastoma, brainstem glioma) is often delayed.[68]

In school-aged children, ages 5 to 11 years with acute vomiting, infections typical for age continue as leading causes of vomiting. In the emergency setting, acute appendicitis and duodenal hematoma or pancreatitis from abdominal injury should also be considered. In chronic vomiting, mucosal GI injuries including peptic esophagitis, eosinophilic esophagitis, and gastritis from *H. pylori* infection are most common, with celiac disease and Crohn disease infrequently

Table 3 Causes of Vomiting by Temporal Pattern and by Age

Category	Acute	Chronic	Cyclic or Episodic
Infectious	Enteritis* B[†] Otitis media* B Streptococcal pharyngitis* B Acute sinusitis BC Hepatitis BC Urinary tract infection Pyelonephritis Meningitis	Giardiasis BC Chronic sinusitis* BC	Chronic sinusitis* BC
Gastrointestinal	Inguinal hernia Intussusception A Malrotation with volvulus Appendicitis BC Cholecystitis C Pancreatitis BC Surgical adhesions Distal intestinal obstruction syndrome (2° cystic fibrosis)	Anatomic GI obstruction Gastroesophageal reflux disease* Eosinophilic esophagitis* BC *H. pylori* gastritis* BC Peptic duodenitis BC Celiac disease B Achalasia C Cholelithiasis C Gallbladder dyskinesia C Pancreatic pseudocyst BC Superior mesenteric artery syndrome BC	All in the acute category
Genitourinary	Acute hydronephrosis 2° UPJ obstruction	Uremia	Acute hydronephrosis 2† UPJ obstruction
Endocrine, metabolic	Diabetic ketoacidosis BC Organic acidemias A MCAD deficiency AB Aminoacidurias AB Hereditary fructose intolerance A	Adrenal hyperplasia A	All in the acute category Addison disease Partial OTC deficiency AB MELAS syndrome AB Acute intermittent porphyria C
Neurologic	Concussion BC Subdural hematoma BC	Chiari malformation BC Pseudotumor cerebri BC Subtentorial neoplasm B	Cyclic vomiting syndrome* BC Abdominal migraine* BC Migraine headache* BC Subtentorial neoplasm B Hydrocephalus shunt dysfunction
Other	Drug ingestion B Food poisoning	Rumination B Functional vomiting B Bulimia C Pregnancy C	Munchausen-by-proxy (Ipecac) B

Adapted in part from Li, Sunku.[169]

MCAD = medium chain acyl-CoA dehydrogenase deficiency; MELAS = mitochondrial myopathy, encephalopathy, lactic acidosis and stroke-like episodes; OTC = ornithine transcarbamylase deficiency; UPJ = uretero-pelvic junction.
*Most common disorders.
†A = occurs predominantly from 0 to ≤ 1 year of age; B = occurs predominantly from 1 to ≤ 11 years of age;
C = occurs predominantly from 11 to 18 years of age. If no letter appear, the disorder can occur at all ages.

accompanied by vomiting alone. Less common causes include neurological (pseudotumor cerebri and Chiari malformation) and renal disorders. Interestingly, postconcussive vomiting is now considered to be part of an atypical migraine attack.[69–70] Hydronephrosis resulting from acute ureteral–pelvic junction obstruction, so called Dietl crisis, can present with colicky abdominal pain and vomiting.[71] A characteristic cyclic vomiting pattern with recurrent, severe episodes usually indicates cyclic vomiting syndrome (88%) during the elementary school years.[72]

In adolescence, peptic and allergic GI and hepatobiliary disorders come to the fore. Besides acid-peptic disorders, eosinophilic esophagitis and Crohn disease can occasionally present with vomiting and achalasia begins with nonacidic emesis. Hepatobiliary causes include cholelithiasis, cholecystitis, and gallbladder dyskinesia.[73–75] Adolescent pregnancy can present to the both pediatrician and gastroenterologist for diagnosis. Acquired gastroparesis can begin after either long-standing insulin-dependent diabetes mellitus or following an acute viral illness.[76]

Time of Day and Proximate Events

The circadian timing of vomiting and its relationship to proximate oral intake or life events is useful in narrowing the range of diagnoses and identifying aggravating factors. Early morning vomiting, either before or on awakening, is more commonly associated increased intracranial pressure, especially with posterior fossa tumors (eg, cerebellar medulloblastoma), chronic sinusitis, cyclic vomiting syndrome, and pregnancy. Children with acid-peptic disorders, unlike adults, typically experience prandial exacerbation of pain and vomiting. Specific foods may be recurrent triggers: cow or soy milk protein in allergic enteropathy in infants or eosinophilic esophagitis, high protein intake in girls with partial ornithine transcarbamylase deficiency, and sucrose and fructose ingestions in hereditary fructose intolerance. Conversely, repeated occurrences after fasting indicates consideration of mitochondrial dysfunction found in disorders of fatty acid oxidation (eg, medium Co-A dehydrogenase deficiency).[63–64] Stressors, including excitement, are appreciated as common triggers in functional vomiting disorders.

Vomitus

The content of the vomitus provides additional clues as to the underlying cause of vomiting. Undigested, nonacidic emesis indicates the lack of gastric admixture from an esophageal stricture or achalasia. The presence of bile is an alarm sign suggestive of an obstructive lesion distal to the ampulla of Vater (eg, midgut volvulus). However, repeated bouts of nonobstructive vomiting, as occurs in cyclic vomiting syndrome, cause bilious vomiting in over 80% of children.[6]

"Alarm" and Associated Symptoms

Alarm symptoms are those symptoms that suggest a higher likelihood of a specific disease that requires further testing for diagnosis. None have been established for vomiting but those for abdominal pain may be applicable—hematemesis, bilious vomiting (obstruction), weight loss (eg, Crohn, celiac, superior mesenteric artery syndrome),[77] nocturnal vomiting (eg, subtentorial mass), abnormalities on neurological exam (eg, papilledema), and a progressive clinical course.[78]

Accompanying symptoms provide key clinical clues to the underlying etiology. These include fever and other signs of infection or inflammation, abdominal pain or abdominal mass, dysphagia, food- or fasting-induced vomiting, and abnormal neurological findings. Although the absence of nausea is touted as a positive clue for brainstem neoplasms, most affected children have both nausea and vomiting.[79] The absence of other symptoms, physical signs or positive tests may point toward a functional vomiting syndrome, and, rarely, Munchausen-by-proxy from ipecac poisoning.[80]

The presence of prior or systemic disease may provide an underlying diagnosis. For instance, prior surgery can result in paralytic ileus or postoperative adhesions. Small intestinal malrotation is complicated by intermittent volvulus.[81] Hydrocephalus with shunt dysfunction can precipitate acute onset of vomiting. A child with cystic fibrosis may develop distal intestinal obstructive syndrome.[82] Acute or recurrent acute episodes of vomiting can be caused by acute hydronephrosis from ureteral obstruction, cyclic vomiting syndrome, and Addison disease with hyponatremia.[83]

DIAGNOSTIC EVALUATION

Evaluation of the child who presents with *acute vomiting* is usually handled by the primary care pediatrician or emergency room physician. Top priority is to assess the severity (eg, number of emeses), associated symptoms (eg, fever, abdominal pain), hydration status, and potential need for rehydration. If the physical examination reveals signs of an acute abdominal presentation, plain abdominal radiograph or CT and surgical consultation are indicated. When the emesis is frequent, empiric antiemetic ondansetron therapy may reduce the vomiting and need for intravenous fluid therapy.[84–85]

In a child who has *chronic vomiting* once or twice daily without alarm symptoms, the most likely diagnosis is an acid-peptic disorder that can be empirically treated with a course of acid suppression.[56] If a time-limited trial fails to improve symptoms, screening laboratory tests (eg, CBC, ESR, transaminases, amylase, lipase) can be obtained. If these results are unrevealing, definitive tests can be considered including an esophagogastroduodenoscopy (for mucosal injuries), small bowel radiography (for Crohn), and abdominal ultrasound (for cholelithiasis and

hydronephrosis). In one series, sinus evaluation (eg, CT) has a 10% positive yield.[72]

The *cyclic* or *episodic vomiting pattern* often is ultimately diagnosed with cyclic vomiting syndrome. Instead of an exhaustive exclusionary evaluation, based on the NASPGHAN consensus guidelines, a limited evaluation is recommended.[86] Initial screening includes an upper GI radiograph for malrotation and, electrolytes, glucose, blood urea nitrogen, and creatinine during the episode. However, if specific alarm symptoms are present, then further testing is recommended. As test results are generally abnormal only when vomiting, these evaluations should be performed at the beginning of an episode before intravenous fluids are administered.[86]

COMPLICATIONS

The two principal complications of acute vomiting due to a discrete illness (eg, enteritis) or from a recurrence (eg, cyclic vomiting attack) include dehydration with electrolyte abnormalities and hematemesis from the mechanical trauma of vomiting. Combined losses of gastric HCl, pancreatic HCO_3^-, and intestinal NaCl can lead to significant alkalosis, occasionally acidosis, hyponatremia, and hypokalemia. Hyponatremia of less than 130 meq/L can represent Addison disease or inappropriate secretion of antidiuretic hormone. Bleeding more often results from prolapse gastropathy than Mallory-Weiss tear. Usually, no therapy is required.

Although chronic vomiting associated with upper GI disorders injuries usually does not lead to electrolyte disturbance, complications related to the underlying peptic injury include stricture, Barrett esophagus, mucosal ulceration, GI bleeding, perforation, and caloric or protein loss to the point of growth failure. If growth failure is present, nutritional restitution may require continuous nasogastric, transpyloric, or jejunostomy tube feedings. Dental enamel erosions can be severe in the setting of recurrent vomiting.[87]

PHARMACOTHERAPY

Although ideally therapy should be directed toward the specific underlying cause, empiric antiemetic therapy is warranted when the severity of either acute or recurrent vomiting places the child at risk of dehydration and other complications. A comprehensive listing of therapeutic agents by pharmacologic category is presented in Table 4.[88–90] Antihistamines (eg, meclizine) are minimally active antiemetics which have more efficacy in motion sickness because of their effects on vestibular function.[91] Although D_2 receptor antagonists—substituted benzamides (metoclopramide), phenothiazines (promethazine), and butyrophenones (eg, droperidol)—have mild activity in chemotherapy-induced vomiting, their use is limited by the risk of extrapyramidal

Table 4 Antinausea, Antiemetic, and Related Medications

Drug Class and Drug	Mechanism of Action	Indications	Side Effects
Antihistamines	*Minimal antiemetic activity*		
Diphenhydramine	Vestibular suppression, anti-ACh effect, and H_1 antagonist*,†	Motion sickness	Sedation, anti-Ach effects
Hydroxyzine			
Dimenhydrinate			
Meclizine			
Phenothiazines	*Mild–moderate activity*		
Promethazine	D_2 antagonist at CTZ and H_1 antagonist	Chemotherapy-induced vomiting	Anti-ACh effects, extrapyramidal reactions
Prochlorperazine	D_2 receptor antagonist at CTZ		
Chlorpromazine			
Substituted benzamides	*Moderate activity*		
Metoclopramide	D_2 antagonist at CTZ and $5-HT_4$ agonist in gut	GERD, gastroparesis, chemotherapy-induced vomiting	Irritability and extrapyramidal reactions
Trimethobenzamide	D_2 antagonist at CTZ		
Cisapride	$5-HT_4$ agonist, ACh release in gut	GERD, gastroparesis	Diarrhea, abdominal pain, headache, QT prolongation
Benzimidazole derivatives	*Moderate activity*		
Domperidone	D_2 antagonist in gut	Gastroparesis, chemotherapy-induced vomiting	Headaches, not available in United States
$5-HT_3$ receptor antagonists	*High activity*		
Ondansetron	$5-HT_3$ antagonist at CTZ and ↓ vagal afferents from gut	Chemotherapy-, postoperative-induced vomiting, cyclic vomiting	Headache
Granisetron			
Tropisetron			
Tachykinin receptor antagonists	*High activity*		
Aprepitant	NK_1 antagonist on emesis program	Chemotherapy-induced vomiting, effective on delayed phase	Fatigue, dizziness, diarrhea
Anticholinergics	*Minimal-mild activity*		
Scopolamine	Vestibular suppression, anti-Ach	Motion sickness	Sedation, anti-Ach effects
Butyrophenones	*Moderate activity*		
Droperidol	D_2 antagonist at CTZ, anxiolytic action and sedation	Chemotherapy-, postoperative-induced vomiting	Hypotension, sedation, extrapyramidal effects
Benzodiazepines	*Minimal activity*		
Lorazepam	Enhanced central GABA-ergic induction of anxiolysis, sedation and amnesia	Chemotherapy-induced vomiting and cyclic vomiting adjunctive therapy (sedation)	Sedation, respiratory depression
Diazepam			
Antimigraine—abortive triptans			
Sumatriptan	$5-HT_{1B/1D}$ agonist induces cerebral vasoconstriction, relaxes gastric fundus	Abortive approach for migraine, abdominal migraine, cyclic vomiting; SQ, PO, nasal forms	Transient burning sensation in chest and neck
Zolmitriptan		PO, nasal forms	
Frovatriptan		PO, longer half-life	
Other—NSAIDS			
Ketorolac	Cyclooxygenase inhibitor of prostaglandin synthesis	Abortive approach for migraine, cyclic vomiting	GI bleeding
Antimigraine—prophylactic medication			
Cyproheptadine	H_1 antagonist and $5-HT_2$ antagonist	Prevention of migraine, abdominal migraine, cyclic vomiting	Sedation, anti-Ach effects, weight gain 2* appetite stimulation
Pizotyline	$5-HT_2$ antagonist		Not available in United States
Propranolol	β_1, β_2 adrenergic antagonist	Prevention of abdominal migraine, cyclic vomiting	Hypotension, bradycardia, fatigability—monitor pulse
Amitriptyline	$5-HT_2$ antagonist, ↑ synaptic norepinephrine	Prevention of migraine, abdominal migraine, cyclic vomiting	Sedation, anti-ACh effects, QT prolongation
Phenobarbital	$GABA_A$ inhibition results in ↑ Cl^- current	Prevention of cyclic vomiting	Sedation, cognitive learning difficulties
Corticosteroids			
Dexamethasone	Unknown	Chemotherapy-, postoperative-induced vomiting adjunctive therapy	Adrenal suppression
Cannabinoids			
Dronabinol	Acts on CB1R receptors on vagus	Chemotherapy-induced vomiting	Disorientation, vertigo, hallucinations
Nabilone			

ACh = acetylcholine; CBR = cannabinoid receptor; CTZ = chemotrigger zone; D = dopamine; GERD = gastroesophageal reflux disease; H = histamine; 5-HT = 5-hydroxytryptamine; GABA = γ-aminobutyric acid; NK = neurokinin; QT = Q-T interval.

*Anticholinergic effects—blurred vision, dry mouth, hypotension, palpitations, urinary retention.

†Within the same drug class, in the blank space, the same attributes apply from the medication above.

reactions.[92–93] Benzodiazepines (lorazepam) have minimal antiemetic efficacy as a single agent but are useful adjuncts to other antiemetic regimens.[94] Cannabinoids have mild to moderate potency.[95]

The 5-HT$_3$ antagonists have moderate to marked antiemetic efficacy in postoperative and chemotherapy settings.[96–98] Neurokinin$_1$ receptor antagonists also have moderate to marked antiemetic activity, especially in the delayed (>24 h) phase of chemotherapy-induced vomiting.[99] Steroids act both as a single antiemetic agent and to potentiate other treatments.[57] 5-HT$_{1B/1D}$ agonists (eg, triptans) show promise in aborting evolution of cyclic vomiting attacks.[100]

CYCLIC VOMITING SYNDROME

Cyclic vomiting syndrome (CVS) is an especially severe form of functional recurrent vomiting. Based on a 1.9% prevalence in a survey of 5- to 15-year-old children in Aberdeen, Scotland, cyclic vomiting is no longer considered a rare syndrome.[101] Both its original description by Samuel Gee in 1882 and the current consensus diagnostic criteria from 1994 emphasize the hallmark *cyclic pattern* of intermittent, stereotypical episodes of rapid-paced vomiting (q. 5 to 15 min) with return to normal or baseline health between (Table 2).[102] The syndrome refers to those idiopathic cases in whom diagnostic testing is negative and no apparent explanatory cause is found.

Although the pathogenesis remains unknown, CVS is considered to be a brain–gut disorder.[6] There is a strong relationship to migraines based on a positive family history in the majority of cases and common developmental progression from cyclic vomiting to migraine headaches as adolescents.[103] Mitochondrial dysfunction may be a susceptibility factor based upon the matrilineal inheritance pattern and increased rate of heteroplasmic mtDNA.[104] Stress is a known trigger in humans. Based on extensive animal data and Sato subtype (elevated ACTH), Taché has proposed that corticotropin-releasing factor is one neuroendocrine mediator.[5,105] However, an underlying autonomic dysfunction may reflect another predisposing factor.[106–107]

The typical patient is a 5- to 8-year-old girl who has repeated episodes of severe vomiting (median 6 emeses per h and 15 emeses per episode) that begin in the early morning hours, last 1 to 2 days (range: 4 h to 10 d), and occur every 2 to 4 weeks before resuming normal health in the interim.[6,108] The episodes are stereotypic within individuals as related to time of onset, duration, and symptomatology including pallor, listlessness and GI symptoms of unrelenting nausea, retching, and abdominal pain. Typical migraine symptoms of headaches and photophobia affect 30 to 40%. Only half occurs at regular intervals, so called *cyclic,* whereas the other half occurs at varying intervals, *episodic.* More than half require intravenous hydration, and patients miss 3 to 5 weeks of school each year. Because of the acute onset of vomiting and dehydration, most episodes are first diagnosed as acute enteritis. Parents can often identify triggers such as psychological stressors, including birthdays and holidays, intercurrent infections, or foods such as chocolate and cheese. Although this disorder commonly resolves with the onset of adolescence, it is often replaced by migraine headaches.

Cyclic vomiting syndrome remains a diagnosis based upon historical criteria. Although laboratory confirmation of CVS is not possible, a positive response to antimigraine therapy supports the diagnosis.[103]

In the absence of controlled studies, treatment remains empiric and includes lifestyle changes (eg, avoidance of known triggers, regimenting sleep, providing energy snacks), prophylactic therapy, and acute intervention (supportive and abortive approaches). NASPGHAN guidelines recommend prophylactic antimigraine medications agents for frequent and/or prolonged episodes: cyproheptadine in children ≤5 years and amitriptyline in children (>5 years.[86] Other prophylactic agents used include propranolol, phenobarbital, erythromycin, and topirimate. In acute breakthrough episodes, early use of nasal 5-HT$_{1B/1D}$ antimigraine sumatriptan or zolmitriptan may abort the episode in progress.[100] Recommended supportive therapy consists of placing the child in nonstimulating (dark and quiet) environs, replacing fluid with dextrose and electrolytes, antiemetics, sedatives, and nonsteroidal or narcotic analgesics for severe pain. Serotonergic 5-HT$_3$ antagonist antiemetics administered at higher doses (eg, ondansetron 0.3 mg/kg) are more effective than commonly used H$_1$ or D$_2$ antagonist agents.[56,109] With an unpredictable occurrence and course, substantial morbidity and disability, delayed diagnosis and lack of established therapy, parental support and understanding from the medical community is essential to successful management.[86]

FUNCTIONAL VOMITING

The term *psychogenic vomiting* is outdated and has been replaced by more specific Rome III nomenclature for functional gastrointestinal symptoms that, as yet, have no identifiable organic cause. The new diagnostic classification includes CVS in both children and adults and chronic idiopathic nausea and functional vomiting in adults.[110] These diagnostic categories enable clinicians to make a positive diagnosis, rather than one of laboratory exclusion, based on symptom complexes. The new nomenclature acknowledges the interrelationship between brain (eg, central processing, stress response) and gut rather than differentiating disorders into either organic and psychogenic classifications.

Functional symptom patterns range from mild "butterflies" and isolated single emesis ("nervous stomach") under duress to persistent daily ("coalescent") functional vomiting and recurrent CVS with dehydration. Although the underlying mechanisms remain to be elucidated, two pathways appear to be involved: (1) delayed gastric emptying with dysrhythmia that could explain the milder end and (2) vomiting motor program to explain the single or multiple emeses. Stress-induced CRF secretion which, in turn, induces transient gastroparesis in animals via CRF$_2$ receptors[53] potentially causes a range of functional gastroduodenal symptoms.[47,111]

In rare cases, unexplained functional vomiting is perpetrated by parental administration of ipecac that results in bouts of dehydration and hospital admission. Due to its lipid retention, ipecac can be detected on a toxicology screen as long as 2 months after ingestion.[80,95]

There are no published treatment trials of functional vomiting. Treatment should be directed toward restoring the patient to full activity despite persistence of vomiting. A psychologist's key role is to examine various school- and family-related stressors, teach stress-reduction techniques, and develop a graded plan to return the child to school. If the evaluation is unrevealing, a series of medication trials may be warranted (Table 4).

POSTOPERATIVE NAUSEA AND VOMITING

The prevalence of postoperative nausea and vomiting (PONV) in children ranges from 20 to 24%. It is common after elective strabismus repair, tonsillectomy, dental surgery, inguinal herniorrhaphy, and ureter surgery.[112–113] Although the mechanisms have not been elucidated, specific risk factors for the development of PONV include (>2 years of age (ie, less in infants), female gender, certain operations, longer operations, anesthetic use (cyclopropane > halothane > sevoflurorane), nitrous oxide, perioperative opioid use, history of motion sickness, and prior PONV.[114–115] Factors that improve PONV in adults include better perioperative hydration, use of propofol anesthesia, decreased opioid analgesia, shorter operations, laparoscopic surgery, and decompression of the GI tract.

If the susceptible child can be identified from known risk factors, prophylactic therapy is effective. In one study, ondansetron, metoclopramide, and dexamethasone each independently reduced the odds of PONV in children undergoing tonsillectomy.[116] Randomized, blinded, controlled trials established that 5-HT$_3$ antagonists reduce PONV in children undergoing strabismus surgery,[117] tonsillectomy,[118] and other elective operations.[119] Head-to-head comparisons establish the superiority of 5-HT$_3$ antagonists to metoclopramide[120] and droperidol.[121] Although intraoperative doses of either ondansetron[118] or granisetron are

The radiographic test of choice is real-time B-mode ultrasound over barium radiography (Figure 1). Teele and Smith[166] found that the pyloric diameter, wall thickness, and channel length were the most discriminating measures. With a 90% positive predictive value, a diameter of 17 mm, muscle wall of $\geq$4 mm, and a channel of $\geq$17 mm were diagnostic of HPS.[167] In cases where measurements are borderline, a contrast study can demonstrate the classic findings of a narrowed channel and bulge (shoulder) of the pylorus back into the gastric antrum.

Although surgical treatment is the standard approach, preoperative preparation is essential to optimal outcomes. Correcting the dehydration and metabolic alkalosis by replacing fluid and electrolyte deficits can reduce perioperative complications. An initial fluid bolus of normal saline, D5/0.45% NaCl with KCl 40 meq/L infused over 1 to 2 days may be necessary to restore urine output and reduce HCO_3^- below 30 meq/L. Known risk factors for development of alkalosis in HPS include female gender, African-American race, longer duration of illness, and more severe dehydration.

In the preferred Ramsted pyloromyotomy, the pylorus is split longitudinally and the myotomy is carried out by blunt dissection down to the level of the submucosa. Although care is taken to avoid penetrating the duodenal mucosa that complication can occur in 5 to 10% of cases. Surgical outcomes are excellent with few long-term complications and nearly no mortality. In instances where patients continue to have intermittent vomiting, postoperative ultrasonographic or barium studies are not helpful because they are relatively unchanged from the preoperative study. Postoperatively, small amounts of dextrose water can be initiated by 8 hours and advanced to formula.

Success of nonsurgical anticholinergic therapy has been described in Asian children. In a comparison trial, atropine was found to be a less expensive, similarly effective approach with the exception of requiring more time to attain full feedings.[168]

REFERENCES

1. Granum PE, Lund T. Bacillus cereus and its food poisoning toxins. FEMS Microbiol Lett 1997;157:223–8.
2. Rasquin A, Di Lorenzo C, Forbes D, et al. Childhood functional gastrointestinal disorders: Child/adolescent. Gastroenterology 2006;130:1527–37.
3. Drossman DA. The functional gastrointestinal disorders and the Rome III process. Gastroenterology 2006;130:1377–90.
4. Hyman PE, Milla PJ, Benninga MA, et al. Childhood functional gastrointestinal disorders: Neonate/toddler. Gastroenterology 2006;130:1519–26.
5. Taché Y. Cyclic vomiting syndrome: The corticotropin-releasing-factor hypothesis. Dig Dis Sci 1999;44:79S–86S.
6. Li BU, Balint J. Cyclic vomiting syndrome: Evolution in our understanding of a brain-gut disorder. Adv Pediatr 2000;47:117–60.
7. Garthright WE, Archer DL, Kvenberg JE. Estimates of incidence and costs of intestinal infectious diseases in the United States. Public Health Rep 1988;103:107–15.
8. Sanger GJ, Andrews PL. Treatment of nausea and vomiting: Gaps in our knowledge. Auton Neurosci 2006;129:3–16.
9. Hasler WL, Kim MS, Chey WD, et al. Central cholinergic and alpha-adrenergic mediation of gastric slow wave dysrhythmias evoked during motion sickness. Am J Physiol 1995;268:G539–G47.
10. Andrews PLR, Horn CC Signals for nausea and emesis: Implications for models of upper gastrointestinal diseases. Autonomic Neuroscience 2006;125:100–115.
11. Borison HL, Wang SC. Physiology and pharmacology of vomiting. Pharmacol Rev 1953;5:193–230.
12. Lang IM. Digestive tract motor correlates of vomiting and nausea. Can J Physiol Pharmacol 1990;68:242–53.
13. Smith CC, Brizzee KR. Cineradiographic analysis of vomiting in the cat. Gastroenterology 1961;40:654–64.
14. Thompson DG, Malagelada JR. Vomiting and the small intestine. Dig Dis Sci 1982;27:1121–5.
15. Lang IM, Sarna SK, Dodds WJ. Pharyngeal, esophageal, and proximal gastric responses associated with vomiting. Am J Physiol 1993;265:G963–G72.
16. Lang IM, Sarna SK, Condon RE. Gastrointestinal motor correlates of vomiting in the dog: Quantification and characterization as an independent phenomenon. Gastroenterology 1986;90:40–7.
17. Andrews PL. Vomiting: A gastro-intestinal tract defensive reflex. In: Andrews P WJ, editor. The Pathophysiology of Gut and Airways. London: Portland Press Ltd; 1993. p. 97–113.
18. Miller AD. Motion-induced nausea and vomiting. In: Kucharczyk J SD, Miller AD, editors. Nausea and Vomiting: Recent Research and Clinical Advances. Boca Raton, FL: CRC Press; 1991. p. 13.
19. Koch KL. Motion sickness. In: MH S, editor. The Handbook of Nausea and Vomiting. Pawling, NY: Caduceus Medical Publishers Inc.; 1993. p. 43.
20. Stern RM, Koch KL, Stewart WR, Lindblad IM. Spectral analysis of tachygastria recorded during motion sickness. Gastroenterology 1987;92:92–7.
21. Brizzee KR. Mechanics of vomiting: A minireview. Can J Physiol Pharmacol 1990;68:221–9.
22. Abe T, Kieser TM, Tomita T, Easton PA. Respiratory muscle function during emesis in awake canines. J Appl Physiol 1994;76:2552–60.
23. Lumsden K, Holden WS. The act of vomiting in man. Gut 1969;10:173–9.
24. Hornby PJ. Central neurocircuitry associated with emesis. Am J Med 2001;111:106S–12S.
25. Rudd JA, Andrews PL. Mechanisms of Acute Delayed, and Anticipatory Emesis Induced by Anticancer Therapies. Sudbury, MA: Jones and Bartlett; 2005. p. 15–65.
26. Grundy D, Reid K. The physiology of nausea and vomiting. In: LR J, editor. Physiology of the Gastrointestinal Tract. New York, NY: Raven Press; 1994. p. 879–901.
27. Andrews PL, Davis CJ, Bingham S, et al. The abdominal visceral innervation and the emetic reflex: Pathways, pharmacology, and plasticity. Can J Physiol Pharmacol 1990;68:325–45.
28. Naylor RJ, Rudd JA. Mechanisms of chemotherapy/radiotherapy-induced emesis in animal models. Oncology 1996;53:8–17.
29. Fukui H, Yamamoto M, Sasaki S, Sato S. Involvement of 5-HT$_3$ receptors and vagal afferents in copper sulfate- and cisplatin-induced emesis in monkeys. Eur J Pharmacol 1993;249:13–8.
30. Schwartz SM, Goldberg MJ, Gidda JS, Cerimele BJ. Effect of zatosetron on ipecac-induced emesis in dogs and healthy men. J Clin Pharmacol 1994;34:250–4.
31. Launay JM, Callebert J, Bondoux D, et al. Serotonin receptors and therapeutics. Cell Mol Biol 1994;40:327–36.
32. Cubeddu LX. Serotonin mechanisms in chemotherapy-induced emesis in cancer patients. Oncology 1996;53:18–25.
33. Fukui H, Yamamoto M, Ando T, et al. Increase in serotonin levels in the dog ileum and blood by cisplatin as measured by microdialysis. Neuropharmacology 1993;32:959–68.
34. Gale JD. Serotonergic mediation of vomiting. JPGN 1995;21:22–8.
35. Tattersall FD, Rycroft W, Francis B, et al. Tachykinin NK1 receptor antagonists act entrally to inhibit emesis induced by the chemotherapeutic agent cisplatin in ferrets. Neuropharmacology 1996;35:1121–9.
36. Bountra C, Gale JD, Gardner CJ, et al. Towards understanding the aetiology and pathophysiology of the emetic reflex: Novel approaches to antiemetic drugs. Oncology 1996;53:102–9.
37. Miller AD, Leslie RA. The area postrema and vomiting. Front Neuroendocrinol 1994;15:301–20.
38. Borison HL. Area postrema: Chemoreceptor circumventricular organ of the medulla oblongata. Prog Neurobiol 1989;32:351–90.
39. Carpenter DO. Neural mechanisms of emesis. Can J Physiol Pharmacol 1990;68:230–6.
40. Jovanovic-Micic D, Samardzic R, Beleslin DB. The role of adrenergic mechanims within the area postrema in dopamine-induced emesis. Eur J Pharmacol 1995;272:21–30.
41. Stefanini E, Clement-Cormier Y. Detection of dopamine receptors in the area postrema. Eur J Pharmacol 1981;74:257–60.
42. Yoshikawa T, Yoshida N, Hosoki K. Involvement of dopamine D3 receptors in the area postrema in $R(+)$-7-OH-DPAT-induced emesis in the ferret. Eur J Pharmacol 1996;301:143–9.
43. Oman CM. Motion sickness: A synthesis and evaluation of the sensory conflict theory. Can J Physiol Pharmacol 1990;68:294–303.
44. Takeda N, Morita M, Hasegawa S, et al. Neuropharmacology of motion sickness and emesis. A review. Acta Otolaryngol Suppl 1993;501:10–5.
45. Yates BJ, Miller AD, Lucot JB. Physiological basis and pharmacology of motion sickness: An update. Brain Res Bull 1998;47:395–406.
46. Money KE. Motion sickness. Physiol Rev 1970;50:1–39.
47. Taché Y, Martinez V, Million M, Wang L. Stress and the gastrointestinal tract III. Stress related alterations of gut motor function: Role of brain corticotropin-releasing factor receptors. Am J Physiol Gastrointest Liver Physiol 2001;280:G173–G7.
48. Kalia M, Mesulam MM. Brain stem projections of sensory and motor components of the vagus complex in the cat: II. Laryngeal, tracheobronchial, pulmonary, cardiac, and gastrointestinal branches. J Comp Neurol 1980;193:467–508.
49. Gwyn DG, Leslie RA, Hopkins DA. Observations on the afferent and efferent organization of the vagus nerve and the innervation of the stomach in the squirrel monkey. J Comp Neurol 1985;239:163–75.
50. Miller AD, Nonaka S, Jakus J. Brain areas essential or nonessential for emesis. Brain Res 1994;647:255–64.
51. Bellg AJ, Morrow GR, Barry M, et al. Autonomic measures associated with chemotherapy-related nausea: Techniques and issues. Cancer Invest 1995;13:313–23.
52. Richards CA, Milla PJ, Andrews PL, Spitz L. Retching and vomiting in neurologically impaired children after fundoplication: Predictive preoperative factors. J Pediatr Surg 2001;36:1401–4.
53. Li BU. Cyclic vomiting: The pattern and syndrome paradigm. JPGN 1995;21:S6–S10.
54. Ehling-Schulz M, Fricker M, Scherer S. Bacillus cereus, the causative agent of an emetic type of food-borne illness. Mol Nutr Food Res 2004;48:479–87.
55. Tsai JD, Huang FY, Lin CC, et al. Intermittent hydronephrosis secondary to ureteropelvic junction obstruction: Clinical and imaging features. Pediatrics 2006;117:139–46.
56. Pfau BT, Li BU, Murray RD, et al. Differentiating cyclic from chronic vomiting patterns in children: Quantitative criteria and diagnostic implications. Pediatrics 1996;97:364–8.
57. Italian Group for Antiemetic Research. Double-blind, dose-finding study of four intravenous doses of dexamethasone in the prevention of cisplatin-induced acute emesis. J Clin Oncol 1998;16:2937–42.
58. Gupta SK, Hassall E, Chiu YL, et al. Presenting symptoms of nonerosive and erosive esophagitis in pediatric patients. Dig Dis Sci 2006;51:858–63.
59. Liacouras CA, Spergel JM, Ruchelli E, et al. Eosinophilic esophagitis: A 10-year experience in 381 children. Clin Gastroenterol Hepatol 2005;3:1198–206.
60. Reijnen JA, Festen C, Van Roosmalen RP. Intussusception: Factors related to treatment. Arch Dis Child 1990;65:871–3.
61. Brandt ML, Pokorny WJ, McGill CW, Harberg FJ. Late presentations of midgut malrotation in children. Am J Surg 1985;150:767–71.
62. Gordon N. Ornithine transcarbamylase deficiency: A urea cycle defect. Eur J Paediatr Neurol 2003;7:115–21.
63. Rinaldo P, Raymond K, al-Odaib A, Bennett MJ. Clinical and biochemical features of fatty acid oxidation disorders. Curr Opin Pediatr 1998;10:615–21.
64. Rinaldo P, Matern D, Bennett MJ. Fatty acid oxidation disorders. Annu Rev Physiol 2002;64:477–502.
65. Vu TH, Hirano M, DiMauro S. Mitochondrial diseases. Neurol Clin 2002;20:809–39, vii–viii.
66. Dickerman JD, Colletti RB, Tampas JP. Gastric outlet obstruction in chronic granulomatous disease of childhood. Am J Dis Child 1986;140:567–70.
67. Sferra TJ, Pawel BR, Qualman SJ, Li BU. Menetrier disease of childhood: Role of cytomegalovirus and transforming growth factor a. J Pediatr 1996;128:213–9.
68. Dobrovoljac M, Hengartner H, Boltshauser E, Grotzer MA. Delay in the diagnosis of paediatric brain tumours. Eur J Pediatr 2002;161:663–7.
69. Gordon KE, Dooley JM, Wood EP. Is migraine a risk factor for the development of concussion? Br J Sports Med 2006;40:184–5.
70. Jan MM, Camfield PR, Gordon K, Camfield CS. Vomiting after mild head injury is related to migraine. J Pediatr 1997;130:134–7.
71. Swischuk LE. Nausea, vomiting, and diarrhea in an older child. Pediatr Emerg Care 1993;9:307–9.
72. Li BU, Murray RD, Heitlinger LA, et al. Heterogeneity of diagnoses presenting as cyclic vomiting. Pediatrics 1998;102:583–7.

73. Dumont RC, Caniano DA. Hypokinetic gallbladder disease: A cause of chronic abdominal pain in children and adolescents. J Pediatr Surg 1999;34:858–61.
74. Lugo-Vicente HL. Gallbladder dyskinesia in children. J Soc Laparoendosc Surg 1997;1:61–4.
75. Scott Nelson R, Kolts R, Park R, Heikenen J. A comparison of cholecystectomy and observation in children with biliary dyskinesia. J Pediatr Surg 2006;41:1894–8.
76. Sigurdsson L, Flores A, Putnam PE, et al. Postviral gastroparesis: Presentation, treatment, and outcome. J Pediatr 1997;131:751–4.
77. Biank V, Werlin S. Superior mesenteric artery syndrome in children: A 20-year experience. J Pediatr Gastroenterol Nutr 2006;42:522–5.
78. Di Lorenzo C, Colletti RB, Lehmann HP, et al. Chronic Abdominal Pain In Children: A Technical Report of the American Academy of Pediatrics and the North American Society for Pediatric Gastroenterology, Hepatology and Nutrition. J Pediatr Gastroenterol Nutr 2005;40:249–61.
79. Snyder H, Robinson K, Shah D, et al. Signs and symptoms of patients with brain tumors presenting to the emergency department. J Emerg Med 1993;11:253–8.
80. McClung HJ, Murray RD, Braden NJ, et al. Intentional Ipecac poisoning of children. Am J Dis Child 1988; 142:637–9.
81. Kealey WD, McCallion WA, Brown S, Potts SR. Midgut volvulus in children. Br J Surg 1996;83:105–6.
82. Park RW, Grand RJ. Gastrointestinal manifestations of cystic fibrosis: A review. Gastroenterology 1981;81:1143–61.
83. Tobin MV, Aldridge SA, Morris AI, et al. Gastrointestinal manifestations of Addison's disease. Am J Gastroenterol 1989;84:1302–5.
84. Reeves JJ, Shannon MW, Fleisher GR. Ondansetron decreases vomiting associated with acute gastroenteritis: A randomized, controlled trial. Pediatrics 2002;109:e62.
85. Freedman SB, Adler M, Seshadri R, Powell EC. Oral ondansetron for gastroenteritis in a pediatric emergency department. N Engl J Med 2006;354:1698–705.
86. Li BU, Lefevre F, Chelimsky GG, et al. The North American Society for Pediatric Gastroenterology, Hepatology and Nutrition Guideline for the Diagnosis and Management of Cyclic Vomiting Syndrome. J Pediatr Gastroenterol Nutr 2007;45:000–000.
87. Kim SO, Kwak JY, Choi BJ, Lee JH. Oral manifestations of a child with chronic vomiting. J Dent Child (Chic) 2005;72:49–51.
88. Jordan K, Schmoll HJ, Aapro MS. Comparative activity of antiemetic drugs. Crit Rev Oncol Hematol 2007;61:162–75.
89. Quigley EM, Hasler WL, Parkman HP. AGA technical review on nausea and vomiting. Gastroenterology 2001;120:263–86.
90. Hasler WL, Chey WD. Nausea and vomiting. Gastroenterology 2003;125:1860–7.
91. Kris MG, Gralla RJ, Clark RA, et al. Antiemetic control and prevention of side effects of anti-cancer therapy with lorazepam or diphenhydramine when used in combination with metoclopramide plus dexamethasone. A double-blind, randomized trial. Cancer 1987;60:2816–22.
92. Gralla RJ, Itri LM, Pisko SE, et al. Antiemetic efficacy of high-dose metoclopramide: Randomized trials with placebo and prochlorperazine in patients with chemotherapy-induced nausea and vomiting. N Engl J Med 1981;305:905–9.
93. Aapro MS. How do we manage patients with refractory or breakthrough emesis? Support Care Cancer 2002;10:106–9.
94. Aapro MS, Molassiotis A, Olver I. Anticipatory nausea and vomiting. Support Care Cancer 2005;13:117–21.
95. Tramer MR, Carroll D, Campbell FA, et al. Cannabinoids for control of chemotherapy induced nausea and vomiting: Quantitative systematic review. BMJ 2001;323:16–21.
96. Apfel CC, Korttila K, Abdalla M, et al. A factorial trial of six interventions for the prevention of postoperative nausea and vomiting. N Engl J Med 2004;350:2441–51.
97. The Italian Group for Antiemetic Research. Dexamethasone alone or in combination with ondansetron for the prevention of delayed nausea and vomiting induced by chemotherapy. N Engl J Med 2000;342:1554–9.
98. Levitt M, Warr D, Yelle L, et al. Ondansetron compared with dexamethasone and metoclopramide as antiemetics in the chemotherapy of breast cancer with cyclophosphamide, methotrexate, and fluorouracil. N Engl J Med 1993;328: 1081–4.
99. Navari RM, Reinhardt RR, Gralla RJ, et al. Reduction of cisplatin-induced emesis by a selective neurokinin-1-receptor antagonist. L-754,030 Antiemetic Trials Group. N Engl J Med 1999;340:190–5.
100. Benson J, Zorn S, Book L. Sumitriptan [Imitrex] in the treatment of cyclic vomiting. Ann Pharm 1995;29:997–8.
101. Abu-Arafeh IA, Russell G. Cyclical vomiting syndrome in children: A population-based study. JPGN 1995;21:454–8.
102. Li BU. Proceedings of the International Symposium on Cyclic Vomiting Syndrome. J Pediatr Gastroenterol Nutr 1995;21:S1–S62.
103. Li BU, Murray RD, Heitlinger LA, et al. Is cyclic vomiting syndrome related to migraine? J Pediatr 1999;134:567–72.
104. Boles RG, Adams K, Li BU. Maternal inheritance in cyclic vomiting syndrome. Am J Med Genet A 2005;133:71–7.
105. Sato T, Uchigata Y, Uwadana N, Kita K. A syndrome of periodic adrenocorticotropin and vasopressin discharge. J Clin Endocrinol Metab 1982;54:517–22.
106. To J, Issenman RM, Kamath MV. Evaluation of neurocardiac signals in pediatric patients with cyclic vomiting syndrome through power spectral analysis of heart rate variability. J Pediatr 1999;135:363–6.
107. Chelimsky TC, Chelimsky GG. Autonomic abnormalities in cyclic vomiting syndrome. J Pediatr Gastroenterol Nutr 2007;44:326–30.
108. Fleisher D, Matar M. The cyclic vomiting syndrome: A report of 71 cases and literature review. JPGN 1993;17:361–9.
109. Lee WS, Kaur P, Boey CC, Chan KC. Cyclic vomiting syndrome in South-East Asian children. J Paediatr Child Health 1998;34:568–70.
110. Tack J, Talley NJ, Camilleri M, et al. Functional gastroduodenal disorders. Gastroenterology 2006;130:1466–79.
111. Pappas TN, Welton M, Debas HT, et al. Corticotropin-releasing factor inhibits gastric emptying in dogs: studies on its mechanism of action. Peptides 1987;8:1011–4.
112. Kermode J, Walker S, Webb I. Postoperative vomiting in children. Anaesth Intens Care 1995;23:196–9.
113. Sossai R, Johr M, Kistler W, et al. Postoperative vomiting in children. A persisting unsolved problem. Eur J Pediatr Surg 1993;3:206–8.
114. Busoni P, Sarti A, Crescioli M, et al. Motion sickness and postoperative vomiting in children. Paediatr Anaesth 2002;12:65–8.
115. Gan TJ. Risk factors for postoperative nausea and vomiting. Anesth Analg 2006;102:1884–98.
116. Gunter JB, McAuliffe JJ, Beckman EC, et al. A factorial study of ondansetron, metoclopramide, and dexamethasone for emesis prophylaxis after adenotonsillectomy in children. Paediatr Anaesth 2006;16:1153–65.
117. Rose JB, Martin TM, Corddry DH, Zagnoev M. Ondansetron reduces the incidence and severity of poststrabismus repair vomiting in children. Anesth Analg 1994;79:486–9.
118. Rose JB, Brenn BR, Corddry DH, Thomas PC. Preoperative oral ondansetron for pediatric tonsillectomy. Anesth Analg 1996;82:558–62.
119. Rust M, Cohen LA. Single oral dose ondansetron in the prevention of postoperative nausea and emesis. The European and US study groups. Anaesthesia 1994;49:16–23.
120. Furst SR, Rodarte A. Prophylactic antiemetic treatment with ondansetron in children undergoing tonsillectomy. Anesthesiology 1994;81:799–803.
121. Davis PJ, McGowan FXJ, Lansman I, Maloney K. Effect of antiemetic therapy on recovery and hospital discharge time. A double-blind assessment of ondansetron, droperidol, and placebo in pediatric patients undergoing ambulatory surgery. Anesthesiology 1995;83:956–60.
122. Ummenhofer W, Frei FJ, Urwyler A, et al. Effects of ondansetron in the prevention of postoperative nausea and vomiting in children. Anesthesiology 1994;81:804–10.
123. Habib AS, Gan TJ. Combination therapy for postoperative nausea and vomiting—a more effective prophylaxis? Ambul Surg 2001;9:59–71.
124. Splinter WM, Rhine EJ. Low-dose ondansetron with dexamethasone more effectively decreases vomiting after strabismus surgery in children than does high-dose ondansetron. Anesthesiology 1998;88:72–5.
125. Rusy LM, Hoffman GM, Weisman SJ. Electroacupuncture prophylaxis of postoperative nausea and vomiting following pediatric tonsillectomy with or without adenoidectomy. Anesthesiology 2002;96:300–5.
126. Purday JP, Reichert CC, Merrick PM. Comparative effects of three doses of intravenous ketorolac or morphine on emesis and analgesia for restorative dental surgery in children. Can J Anaesth 1996;43:221–5.
127. Grunberg SM, Hesketh PJ. Control of chemotherapy-induced emesis. N Engl J Med 1993;329:1790–6.
128. Matera MG, Di Tullio M, Lucarelli C, et al. Ondansetron, an antagonist of 5-HT_3 receptors, in the treatment of antineoplastic drug-induces nausea and vomiting in children. J Med 1993;24:161–70.
129. Tyc VL, Mulhern RK, Bieberich AA. Anticipatory nausea and vomiting in pediatric cancer patients: An analysis of conditioning and coping variables. J Dev Behav Pediatr 1997;18:27–33.
130. Tyc VL, Mulhern RK, Barclay DR, et al. Variables associated with anticipatory nausea and vomiting in pediatric cancer patients receiving ondansetron antiemetic therapy. J Pediatr Psychol 1997;22:45–58.
131. Figueroa-Moseley C, Jean-Pierre P, Roscoe JA, et al. Behavioral interventions in treating anticipatory nausea and vomiting. J Natl Compr Canc Netw 2007;5:44–50.
132. Cubeddu LX, Hoffmann IS, Fuenmayor NT, Finn AL. Efficacy of ondansetron (GR 38032F) and the role of serotonin in cisplatin-induced nausea and vomiting. N Engl J Med 1990;322:810–6.
133. Dick GS, Meller ST, Pinkerton CR. Randomised comparison of ondansetron and metoclopramide plus dexamethasone for chemotherapy induced emesis. Arch Dis Child 1995;73:243–5.
134. Smith AR, Repka TL, Weigel BJ. Aprepitant for the control of chemotherapy induced nausea and vomiting in adolescents. Pediatr Blood Cancer 2005;45:857–60.
135. Alvarez O, Freeman A, Bedros A, Call SK. Randomized double-blind crossover ondansetron-dexamethasone versus ondansetron-placebo study for the treatment of chemotherapy-induced nausea and vomiting in pediatric patients with malignancies. J Pediatr Hematol Oncol 1995;17:145–50.
136. Roila F, Feyer P, Maranzano E, et al. Antiemetics in children receiving chemotherapy. Support Care Cancer 2005;13:129–31.
137. Antonarakis ES, Evans JL, Heard GF, et al. Prophylaxis of acute chemotherapy-induced nausea and vomiting in children with cancer: What is the evidence? Pediatr Blood Cancer 2004;43:651–8.
138. Pinkerton CR, Williams D, Wootton C, et al. 5-HT_3 antagonist ondansetron—an effective outpatient antiemetic in cancer treatment. Arch Dis Child 1990;65:822–5.
139. Craft AW, Price L, Eden OB, et al. Granisetron as antiemetic therapy in children with cancer. Med Pediatr Oncol 1995;25:28–32.
140. Cappelli C, Ragni G, De Pasquale MD, et al. Tropisetron: Optimal dosage for children in prevention of chemotherapy-induced vomiting. Pediatr Blood Cancer 2005;45:48–53.
141. Brock P, Brichard B, Rechnitzer C, et al. An increased loading dose of ondansetron: A North European, double-blind randomized study in children, comparing 5 mg/m^2 with 10 mg/m^2. Eur J Cancer 1996;32A:1744–8.
142. Miralbell R, Coucke P, Behrouz F, et al. Nausea and vomiting in fractionated radiotherapy: A prospective on-demand trial of tropisetron rescue for non-responders to metocopramide. Eur J Cancer 1995;31A:1461–4.
143. Nathan PC, Tomlinson G, Dupuis LL, et al. A pilot study of ondansetron plus metopimazine vs. ondansetron monotherapy in children receiving highly emetogenic chemotherapy: A Bayesian randomized serial N-of-1 trials design. Support Care Cancer 2006;14:268–76.
144. Lee M, Feldman M. Nausea and vomiting. In: Feldman M SB, Sleisenger M, editors. Gastrointestinal Disease. Philadelphia: WB Saunders; 1998. p. 117–27.
145. Herrington JD, Kwan P, Young RR, et al. Randomized, multicenter comparison of oral granisetron and oral ondansetron for emetogenic chemotherapy. Pharmacotherapy 2000;20:1318–23.
146. Fessele KS. Managing the multiple causes of nausea and vomiting in the patient with cancer. Oncol Nurs Forum 1996;23:1409–15.
147. Koch K. Nausea: An approach to a symptom. Clin Perspect in Gastroenterol 2001:285–97.
148. Challis GB, Stam HJ. A longitudinal study of the development of anticipatory nausea and vomiting in cancer chemotherapy patients: The role of absorption and autonomic perception. Health Psychol 1992;11:181–9.
149. Issenman R, Persad R. What about the queasy teen? Can J CME 2003;August:91–7.
150. Telega G. Biliary dyskinesia in pediatrics. Curr Gastroenterol Rep 2006;8:172–6.
151. Vegunta RK, Raso M, Pollock J, et al. Biliary dyskinesia: The most common indication for cholecystectomy in children. Surgery 2005;138:726–31.
152. Sullivan SD, Hanauer J, Rowe PC, et al. Gastrointestinal symptoms associated with orthostatic intolerance. J Pediatr Gastroenterol Nutr 2005;40:425–8.
153. Lien HC, Sun WM, Chen YH, et al. Effects of ginger on motion sickness and gastric slow-wave dysrhythmias induced by circular vection. Am J Physiol Gastrointest Liver Physiol 2003;284:G481–9.
154. Koch KL, Stern RM, Vasey MW, et al. Neuroendocrine and gastric myoelectrical responses to illusory self-motion in humans. Am J Physiol 1990;258:E304–10.
155. Koch KL, Summy-Long J, Bingaman S, et al. Vasopressin and oxytocin responses to illusory self-motion and nausea in man. J Clin Endocrinol Metab 1990;71:1269–75.

156. Deich RF, Hodges PM. Motion sickness, field dependence, and levels of development. Percept Mot Skills 1973;36:1115–20.

157. Barabas G, Matthews WS, Ferrari M. Childhood migraine and motion sickness. Pediatrics 1983;72:188–90.

158. Lucot JB. Pharmacology of motion sickness. J Vestib Res 1998;8:61–6.

159. Warwick-Evans LA, Masters IJ, Redstone SB. A double-blind placebo controlled evaluation of acupressure in the treatment of motion sickness. Aviat Space Environ Med 1991;62:776–8.

160. Jedd MB, Melton LJ, 3rd, Griffin MR, et al. Trends in infantile hypertrophic pyloric stenosis in Olmsted County, Minnesota, 1950–1984. Paediatr Perinat Epidemiol 1988;2:148–57.

161. Carter CO, Evans KA. Inheritance of congenital pyloric stenosis. J Med Genet 1969;6:233–54.

162. Rollins MD, Shields MD, Quinn RJ, Wooldridge MA. Pyloric stenosis: Congenital or acquired? Arch Dis Child 1989;64:138–9.

163. Vanderwinden JM, Mailleux P, Schiffmann SN, et al. Nitric oxide synthase activity in infantile hypertrophic pyloric stenosis. N Engl J Med 1992;327:511–5.

164. Wattchow DA, Cass DT, Furness JB, et al. Abnormalities of peptide-containing nerve fibers in infantile hypertrophic pyloric stenosis. Gastroenterology 1987;92:443–8.

165. Handelsman JC. The significance of hematemesis in congenital hypertrophic pyloric stenosis. Sinai Hosp J (Balt) 1959;8:143–52.

166. Teele RL, Smith EH. Ultrasound in the diagnosis of idiopathic hypertrophic pyloric stenosis. N Engl J Med 1977;296:1149–50.

167. Lamki N, Athey PA, Round ME, et al. Hypertrophic pyloric stenosis in the neonate–diagnostic criteria revisited. Can Assoc Radiol J 1993;44:21–4.

168. Yamataka A, Tsukada K, Yokoyama-Laws Y, et al. Pyloromyotomy versus atropine sulfate for infantile hypertrophic pyloric stenosis. J Pediatr Surg 2000;35:338–41.

169. Li BU, Sunku BK. Vomiting and nausea. R Wyllie, JS Hyams, M Kay, editors. Pediatric Gastrointestinal and Liver Disease, 3rd edition. New York, NY. Elsevier; 2006. p. 127–49.

Gastritis

9.1. Helicobacter pylori *and Peptic Ulcer Disease*

Marion Rowland, MD, PhD
Billy Bourke, MD, FRCPI
Brendan Drumm, MD, FRCPC, FRCPI

GASTRITIS AND PEPTIC ULCER DISEASE

The surface of the gastric mucosa is lined by a simple mucus-secreting columnar epithelium punctuated by gastric pits within which the gastric glands are situated. From a functional and histologic point of view, the stomach can be divided into three areas: cardia, fundus or oxyntic, and antrum, according to the predominant gland type within each zone (Table 1). In the normal gastric mucosa, the glands are separated by little or no extracellular matrix, and few or no mononuclear cells are present.[1] Gastritis is defined as microscopic evidence of inflammation affecting the gastric mucosa. The intensity of the inflammatory response is variable. Mild mucosal inflammation may be difficult to distinguish from normal mucosa and often requires review by an experienced pathologist.[2,3]

Duodenitis is characterized by the presence of neutrophils in the lamina propria, crypts, or surface epithelium, in addition to an increase in the number of mononuclear cells. There may be associated villous blunting. Duodenitis is graded from mild to severe, depending on the number of neutrophils present. Histologic assessment of the mucosa bordering primary duodenal ulcers usually reveals active duodenitis, and this histologic appearance may also be seen in symptomatic patients without overt ulceration. Therefore,

duodenitis and duodenal ulceration likely represent different manifestations of a disease spectrum sharing a common underlying pathogenesis.

Peptic ulcers, by definition, are deep mucosal lesions that disrupt the muscularis mucosa coat of the gastric or duodenal wall.[4] Peptic erosions, on the other hand, are superficial mucosal lesions that do not penetrate the muscularis mucosae. Most gastric ulcers are located on the lesser curvature of the stomach. More than 90% of duodenal ulcers are found within the duodenal bulb.[5]

Gastritis and peptic ulcer disease can be divided into two major categories, primary and secondary, on the basis of the underlying etiology.[5] This division is relevant because the natural history of primary gastroduodenal inflammation or ulceration is different from that of the secondary type. Most cases of primary or unexplained gastritis are now known to be caused by gastric infection with the organism *Helicobacter pylori*.[6–10] Secondary gastritis and secondary ulceration are clinically and often histologically distinct from primary peptic disease.[5] Secondary ulcers may be gastric or duodenal in location and are discussed in Chapter 9.2, "Acid-Peptic Disease."

Gastritis and peptic ulcer disease were previously considered distinct entities. Over the past 20 years, it has come to be understood that these two conditions are closely related. In 1983,

Warren and Marshall reported an association between the presence of spiral organisms on the gastric mucosa and antral gastritis in adults.[11] Subsequent studies in adults and children have confirmed the etiologic role of *H. pylori* in primary antral gastritis and have demonstrated a strong association between *H. pylori*-associated gastritis and duodenal ulcer disease.[6–10]

Duodenal ulcer disease, unusual prior to the turn of the twentieth century, increased steadily in the 1900s, reaching a peak in the 1950s.[12,13] In the 1950s duodenal ulcer disease was reported as one of the more common chronic diseases in adults, occurring in 5 to 10% of the population. There has been a dramatic decline in the prevalence of peptic ulcer disease in all age groups since the 1950s. The current estimated annual incidence of duodenal ulcer disease is 2 to 3 per 1,000 population,[10] which is in marked contrast to incidence rates of 150 per 1,000 reported in the 1970s.[13,14]

There are no accurate figures on the incidence of peptic ulcer disease in children. Primary duodenal ulcer disease is very rare in children under 10 years of age, but prevalence increases in adolescence.[5] Large medical centers for children typically diagnosed only four to six cases of peptic ulcer disease per year in the 1970s.[5] Anecdotal evidence would suggest that there has been a decline in the prevalence of duodenal ulcer disease children in recent years in developed countries. As the prevalence of *H. pylori* infection decreases, the relative number of non–*H. pylori*-associated duodenal ulcers will increase, but, to date, very few non–*H. pylori*-associated duodenal ulcers have been reported in children.[7,15,16] Primary gastric ulcers rarely, if ever, occur in children.[5]

HISTOLOGIC DIAGNOSIS OF *H. PYLORI* GASTRITIS

In the past, there has been considerable confusion surrounding the histologic terminology used to classify gastritis. This is due to the use of such terms as "acute," "chronic," and "chronic active" to describe gastritis. The Sydney classification of gastritis aims to incorporate topographic,

Table 1 Anatomy and Physiology of the Stomach

Anatomic/Gland Area	Cell Type*	Secretory Products†
Cardiac	Mucous cells	Mucus, pepsinogen
	Endocrine cells	—
Fundus/oxyntic	Parietal cells	Hydrochloric acid
	Chief cells	Pepsinogen
	Enterochromaffin cells	Histamine, serotonin
	G cells	Gastrin
Antral/pyloric	G cells	Gastrin
	D cells	Somatostatin
	Enterochromaffin cells	Histamine, serotonin

Adapted from Soll AH.[4]

*All three anatomic areas contain mucus-secreting cells in addition to endocrine cells.

†Endocrine cells in the stomach produce a variety of different products. For cells such as enterochromaffin cells and D cells, the secretory product has been identified, whereas the function of others is not as well defined.

morphologic, and etiologic information into a clinically relevant scheme.[17,18] This classification and grading, which now incorporates the use of a visual analogue scale,[18] is accepted as the standard research method by which all gastric biopsies from adult patients should be assessed. Classification is based on the location (antrum or corpus) and presence of a number of histologic parameters that are graded semiquantitatively as mild, moderate, or marked. These parameters are inflammation, activity, atrophy, intestinal metaplasia, and *H. pylori* infection.

When the Sydney system is used, it is recommended that two antral biopsies from within 2 to 3 cm of the pylorus, two corpus biopsies, and one biopsy from the incisura be obtained at endoscopy. The usefulness of the updated Sydney classification in a pediatric setting has not been formally assessed, but the underlying principles can be applied.

INFLAMMATION AND ACTIVITY

A precise definition for chronic gastric inflammation is difficult owing to a lack of agreement on the number of mononuclear cells present in the normal gastric mucosa of adults or children.[17] However, chronic inflammation is generally considered to be present if there are more than two to five lymphocytes, plasma cells, and/or macrophages per high-power field.[17] In children with *H. pylori* infection, substantial numbers of plasma cells and lymphocytes are present in mucosal biopsy sections. The inflammatory cell infiltrate is usually superficial in location, with panmucosal inflammation present in a small number of cases.[6,19]

The term "activity" is used to characterize the presence of neutrophils in the gastric biopsy. Neutrophil activity is almost always present in adults in association with *H. pylori* infection, and the density of the intraepithelial neutrophils has been correlated with the extent of mucosal damage.[17] Neutrophils have been identified as early as day 5 in an adult with acute infection,[20] and more recently in a human challenge study acute and chronic changes were demonstrated at the time of first endoscopic assessment 2 weeks after ingestion of the organism in all infected volunteers.[21] In children and animal models, the active or neutrophil component of the histologic response is less than that reported in adults.[6]

ATROPHY

When damage to the gastric glands is such that they lose their ability to regenerate, a repair process consisting of fibroblast recruitment and deposition of extracellular matrix occurs. The space previously occupied by the glands becomes replaced by fibrosis.[1] This loss of glandular tissue is defined as atrophy. However, the presence of an inflammatory infiltrate and lymphoid follicles in the lamina propria may alter the architecture of the gastric mucosa, particularly in the antrum,

where the glands are tortuous. Therefore, it may be difficult to distinguish loss of gastric glands from mere displacement secondary to increased numbers of inflammatory cells. For these reasons, inter- and intraobserver agreement among pathologists for the diagnosis of atrophy is poor.[22] Atrophy of the gastric mucosa is extremely rare in children in Western countries.[19,23] However, research from Japan found that grade 2 to 3 atrophy was present in the antrum of 14 of 131 (10.7%) of infected children, with 2 of these children also having corpus atrophy.[24]

INTESTINAL METAPLASIA AND LYMPHOID FOLLICLES

Intestinal metaplasia is common in adults with chronic gastritis attributable to any cause and increases in prevalence with disease duration.[18] Intestinal metaplasia is an independent process, and although it is often present with atrophy, these conditions may occur independently. Intestinal metaplasia was found in a small number of both infected and noninfected Japanese children.[24]

Lymphoid follicles with germinal centers are very suggestive of *H. pylori* infection in adults and children. If specifically sought, they are found in 100% of adult patients with *H. pylori*,[18] and were reported in 60% of children of Japanese children.[24] However, sampling error may occur unless sufficient biopsy specimens are taken. If lymphoid follicles and inflammation are present in the absence of *H. pylori*, it is likely that the organism has been missed.[18]

H. PYLORI

Colonization of the gastric antrum by *H. pylori* is graded as mild, moderate, or marked. In children, the number of bacteria present on the gastric mucosa is usually less than that in adults. Identification of *H. pylori* is facilitated by the use of special staining techniques (see below).

Successful treatment for *H. pylori* is accompanied by rapid and complete disappearance of bacteria and neutrophils. The presence of even a small number of neutrophils after treatment is very suggestive of treatment failure even if *H. pylori* is not identified.[25] Assessment of biopsy specimens for the presence of small numbers of *H. pylori* is more difficult following treatment.[25] Chronic inflammatory changes may take a year or more to resolve.[25] Lymphoid follicles decrease very slowly and are still present 1 year after treatment. Lymphoid follicles, in the absence of active inflammation in the adjacent mucosa, are strongly suggestive of *H. pylori* eradication.[25]

There has been a suggestion that the Sydney Classification is too cumbersome for use in routine practice and fails to provide clinically relevant information on which to base a treatment strategy for patients with preneoplastic lesions.[26] Rugge and Genta propose to combine the degree of mucosal inflammation and activity in both antral and body biopsies and grade them from

0 (no inflammation) to 4 (very dense infiltration in all biopsies). Similarly, atrophy and intestinal metaplasia would be reported as a composite score for all biopsies from 0 (no atrophy) to 4 (atrophy involving all biopsies).[27] Further validation of a new integrated histology report is currently underway.

DISEASES ASSOCIATED WITH *H. PYLORI* GASTRITIS

H. pylori is a gram-negative spiral flagellated bacterium. It is found within and beneath the mucous layer on the gastric epithelium.[6,7,9] Infection of gastric epithelium has been reported not only in the stomach, but also in areas of gastric metaplasia in the duodenum, esophagus (Barrett esophagus), and ectopic gastric mucosa at various sites in the gastrointestinal tract, including Meckel diverticulum and the rectum.[6] However, *H. pylori* does not colonize tissue of nongastric origin.

There is strong evidence implicating *H. pylori* as a cause of chronic gastritis in children.[6,7] All children colonized with *H. pylori* have chronic gastritis. *H. pylori* is not an opportunistic colonizer of inflamed gastric tissue[28,29] because children with secondary gastritis due to Crohn's disease or eosinophilic gastritis are not consistently colonized with *H. pylori*. Eradication of *H. pylori* from the gastric mucosa results in healing of gastritis in children[6,30] and adults.[8,9] Further evidence implicating *H. pylori* as a gastric pathogen has come from volunteer studies. Adult volunteers who ingested the organism developed gastritis, and gastric colonization was demonstrated.[20,21,31]

Despite the universal presence of chronic gastritis in infected individuals, the majority do not develop any clinical disease and remain asymptomatic throughout their lives. A small proportion of infected individuals will develop peptic ulcer disease with an even smaller proportion developing gastric cancer. In populations with a low prevalence of *H. pylori* infection, the primary goal of clinical investigations should be to determine the cause of the presenting symptoms and not the presence of *H. pylori* infection.[32] The European Pediatric Consensus Statement suggests that if *H. pylori* is identified as an incidental finding at endoscopy the patient should be offered treatment. The question, which needs to be addressed in populations with a low risk of gastric cancer, is should gastric biopsies be taken for the diagnosis of *H. pylori* infection in the absence of gross findings at endoscopy?

DUODENAL ULCER DISEASE

H. pylori is found on the antral mucosa of almost 90% of children with duodenal ulcer disease.[28] Studies on adult patients have similarly indicated that 80% of individuals with duodenal ulcer disease are colonized with *H. pylori*.[8] Eradication of *H. pylori* from the gastric mucosa leads to long-term healing of duodenal ulcer disease in both adults[8–10] and children.[6,7,30] It is not known why a bacterial infection of the antral mucosa is critical in the pathogenesis of duodenal ulcers or why only a minority of those colonized with *H. pylori* develop ulcers. It has been hypothesized that *H. pylori* colonizes areas of ectopic gastric tissue (gastric metaplasia) in the duodenum, with the subsequent development of duodenal inflammation and possibly ulceration. In children, *H. pylori* infection of the antral mucosa and gastric metaplasia in the duodenum were each found to be significant risk factors for duodenal ulceration.[23] The presence of both *H. pylori* in the antrum and gastric metaplasia in the duodenum greatly increases the risk of duodenal disease.[23]

As the prevalence of *H. pylori* is declining with a consequent decline in *H. pylori* associated duodenal ulcer disease, there is a relative increase in the number of non–*H. pylori*-related duodenal ulcers. From a clinical perspective it is important to determine if *H. pylori* is the cause of the duodenal ulcer in an individual patient so that appropriate therapy is instituted and the risk of recurrence of *H. pylori*-associated ulcers eliminated.[10]

GASTRIC ULCER DISEASE

There is also an association between *H. pylori* antral gastritis and gastric ulcer disease in adults.[8–10] The organism is found in approximately 60% of adults with gastric ulceration.[10] This lower correlation may be due to the fact that a significant number of gastric ulcers are secondary, being related to drug and other ingestions. Gastric ulceration is extremely rare in children; when it occurs, it is usually secondary.[6,7] Therefore, there are no studies on any possible association between gastric ulceration and the presence of *H. pylori* on the gastric mucosa in children.

GASTRIC CANCER

Gastric cancer is the fourth most frequent cancer in the world and the second leading cause of death from cancer.[33] Gastric cancer is a multifactorial disease in which bacterial, host, and environmental risk factors play a complex role in the cascade which leads to gastric cancer. Based on data from seroepidemiologic studies which suggested a two- to sixfold increase in risk for gastric cancer among infected individuals,[10,34] *H. pylori* was classified as a group 1 carcinogen in 1994 by the World Health Organization.[35] Early studies may have underestimated the risk of gastric cancer associated with *H. pylori* infection because later studies using immunoblotting or biopsy-based tests to diagnose infection suggest that the risk of gastric carcinoma may be greater.[36] Research in Japan, where the prevalence of gastric cancer is extremely high, suggests that up to 5% of *H. pylori*-infected individuals in Japan will develop gastric cancer in contrast to noninfected controls.[37]

In 1975 Correa first described a multistep process for the precancerous process leading to intestinal-type gastric cancer with the following steps: gastritis, atrophy, intestinal metaplasia (complete type 1 to incomplete type 3), and dysplasia.[38] The histologic diagnosis of atrophy particularly of the antrum is not straightforward and the level of agreement among experienced pathologists is often less than acceptable.[39] The coexistence of loss of glands together with the presence intestinal metaplastic epithelium is now considered to represent true atrophy.[1] While it cannot be disputed that *Helicobacter* is a major trigger of events in this cascade that leads to gastric cancer, *H. pylori* alone is not sufficient to for the development of gastric cancer.[10,40] In adults the pattern and severity of gastritis in a particular individual varies very little over time and those who develop atrophy do so at an early stage in the disease process.[41] In large prospective cohort study from Japan, Watabe et al have shown that patients who had gastric atrophy and were infected with *H. pylori* had a sixfold higher risk of gastric cancer compared to patients who had a normal gastric mucosa. More importantly, however, they showed that patients who had no evidence of gastric atrophy, infection with *H. pylori* did not increase their risk of gastric cancer.[42] Therefore, the development of atrophy is the critical step for the progression to gastric cancer. The key question is which factors in addition to *H. pylori* trigger the development of gastric atrophy.

Research on peptic ulcer disease and gastric cancer has for many years focused on the importance of acid secretion in disease outcome. The risk of gastric cancer is highest in those who have a corpus predominant gastritis with reduced or low gastric acid secretion, while those with an antral predominant gastritis and normal or high acid secretion have a much reduced risk of gastric cancer.[37,42] It is also well established that patients who develop duodenal ulcer disease (normal or high acid producers) do not develop gastric cancer.[37,43] Interleukin 1-beta (IL-1β) is a well-characterized proinflammatory cytokine which is potent inhibitor of gastric acid secretion. It is estimated that IL-1β is a hundred times more potent an inhibitor of gastric acid secretion than proton pump inhibitors (PPIs).[44] el-Omar was the first to examine the role of interlukin-1 gene cluster polymorphisms in the development of hypochlorhydria and gastic cancer.[45] It has now been demonstrated in a number of different populations that *IL-1β*-511T is associated with gastric cancer and that *IL-1RN*2* increases risk of gastric cancer among Caucasians.[10] Interleukin 10 (IL10) and tumor necrosis factor alpha (TNF-α) may also increase risk of gastric cancer.[46–48] Interleukin IL-10 and TNF-α doubled the risk of gastric cancer while multiple proinflammatory polymorphisms of Il-1B, interleukin 1-receptor antagonist (Il-1-RN), and IL10 increased the risk of gastric cancer substantially (OR 27.3, 95% CI 7.4 to 99.8)[10,47]

The prevalence of gastric cancer is much higher in Japan, Korea, China, and Columbia than in Europe and the United States.[33] Familial clustering has been observed in gastric cancer and the risk of gastric cancer is increased threefold in first-degree relatives of gastric cancer patients.[49] Relatives of patients with gastric cancer have a much higher prevalence of gastric atrophy suggesting a genetic predisposition to developing gastric cancer.[49] A study which compared the gastric histology between a group of patients from Japan with an age-matched cohort of patients from the United Kingdom demonstrated that Japanese patients had a more severe gastritis which was present at an earlier age, was corpus predominant with more atrophy and intestinal metaplasia compared to their UK counterparts who had an antral predominant gastritis.[50] These differences were not accounted for by differences in the Cag and Vac pathogenicity of *H. pylori* and may be accounted for in part by differences in the genetic makeup of the two populations.

The role of *H. pylori* in hereditary diffuse gastric cancer has not been defined. The molecular basis for familial gastric cancer was determined by Guilford et al in 1998 when they found germline truncating mutations in the *E-cadherin* gene (*CDH1*) in a Maori kindred with early-onset diffuse gastric cancer.[51] Mutations in the gene have since been reported in hereditary diffuse gastric cancer families from different populations.[52] It has been estimated that mutation in the *E-cadherin* gene is causal in at least 30% of cases of hereditary diffuse gastric cancer with a penetrance of approximately 75 to 80% . Therefore, carriers of the *CDHI* mutation have a 75 to 80% chance of developing gastric cancer.

Much attention is now focused on the possibility that treatment of *H. pylori* infection will prevent the development of gastric cancer. In a Japanese study, Uemura and colleagues suggest that patients who were not infected or who received treatment for *H. pylori* did not develop gastric cancer.[37] However, the duration of follow-up was much shorter in the treatment group of patients compared with the patients who did develop gastric cancer.[37] Whereas a number of studies have suggested that eradication of infection can reverse atrophy and intestinal metaplasia, others suggest that if eradication is to be successful, it must be prior to the development of atrophy because, by definition, atrophy is irreversible.[53–55] Various dietary exposures, including salt, nitrate, and alcohol consumption, have been implicated in the etiology of gastric cancer, but to date there is no clear consensus on the importance of these risk factors. In addition, increased consumption of fruit, vegetables, vitamin, and mineral supplements has not been shown to reduce the risk of gastric cancer.[10,56] Recent research would suggest that smoking increases the risk of stomach cancer in smokers compared to nonsmokers and like other smoking-related diseases the risk is greater in men than women.[56] Randomized trials in adults of *H. pylori* eradication therapy for the prevention of gastric cancer have been limited by difficulties in recruiting sufficient numbers of infected participants. Therefore, strategies aimed at reducing the risk of infection or preventing transmission may now have to be considered in high-risk populations.

MUCOSA-ASSOCIATED LYMPHOID TISSUE LYMPHOMA

H. pylori has been implicated as an etiologic factor in mucosa-associated lymphoid tissue (MALT) lymphomas of the stomach. Normal gastric mucosa is devoid of organized lymphoid tissue. For lymphoma to develop, the gastric wall must first acquire organized lymphoid tissue, which occurs as a reaction to infection with *H. pylori*.[57] Gastric MALT lymphoma is often multifocal, and most tumors are located in the antrum or distal body of the stomach. Eradication of *H. pylori* leads to complete resolution of 75% of gastric MALT lymphomas.[10] Staging of the tumor may help to determine the response to anti–*H. pylori* treatment because only those in the early stages respond to treatment.[10,57] Liu and colleagues demonstrated that MALT lymphomas, regardless of stage of disease, with the translocation t(11;18)(q21;q21) do not respond to *H. pylori* eradication and require conventional chemotherapy.[58] Less commonly, *H. heilmannii* has been implicated as a cause of MALT lymphoma.[57,59] There have been a number of case reports of MALT lymphoma in children.[60–62]

EPIDEMIOLOGY

H. pylori is one of the most common enteric infections worldwide with up to 50% of the world population infected.[9] While up to 80% of children in developing countries are infected, there is a rapid decline in the prevalence of infection in developed countries.[14,63] Recent evidence from Sweden would suggest that the prevalence of infection in children of Swedish parents may be as low as 2%.[64]

H. pylori is acquired in childhood and infection is lifelong unless specifically treated. In the first study specifically designed to examine when children become infected with *H. pylori*, it has been shown that the majority of children become infected before their third birthday.[63] Only one child became infected after the age of 5 years during 416 person-years of follow-up (0.2 per 100 person-years follow-up) compared to 19 under the age of 5 years with 554 person-years of follow-up (3.4 per 100 person-years). It was not possible in this study to determine the earliest age at which infection is acquired because the ^{13}C-UBT is unreliable in children less than 2 years of age. However, it seems likely that children can be infected with *H. pylori* before the age of 2 years. Using stool antigen testing Konno et al, found that four of five children became infected between the age of 12 and 24 months while the fifth child became infected at the age of 4 years.[65] There have been a number of individual case reports of *H. pylori* infection in very young children.[66,67] However, under 1 year of age, children rarely become infected with *H. pylori* even when they are exposed to infected mothers.[66] Many groups have reported a high prevalence of *H. pylori*-specific immunoglobulin (IgG) anti-

bodies in the first few months of life, with subsequent decline by 6 to 12 months.[67,68] Elevated IgG titers in these children reflect maternal transfer of *H. pylori*-specific antibodies to the fetus, but whither maternal antibodies are protective against *H. pylori* infection is unknown.

Adults rarely become infected with *H. pylori*, with seroconversion rates varying between 0.33 and 0.5% per person-year.[69,70] The high prevalence seen in adults is consistent with a birth cohort effect, whereby adults acquired the infection as children because they lived in much poorer socioeconomic circumstances in the last century.[71] As socioeconomic conditions have improved in successive generations in the developed world, the prevalence of *H. pylori* has declined.

Previous studies have shown that low socioeconomic status is a major risk factor for infection and infection is much more common in children from developing countries compared to developed countries.[72,73] In developed countries where the overall prevalence of infection in young children is less than 10%, up to 50% of those children living in poor socioeconomic conditions may be infected.[72] However, some studies from developed countries now suggest that that socioeconomic status and family size are risk factors for infection only when the mother is infected.[63,74] *H. pylori* is clustered in families and having an infected mother[63,74] or an infected older sibling[63,75,76] have been shown to be risk factors for infection. There is conflicting evidence on the role of fathers in the transmission of infection,[63] but in many studies the number of fathers included in the study is often small.

TRANSMISSION

The mode of transmission of *H. pylori* is poorly understood. A clear understanding of the most common route of *H. pylori* transmission would help elucidate the epidemiology of this infection and is essential for the prevention of infection. The only known reservoir for *H. pylori* is the human stomach. Person-to-person spread currently appears to be the most likely mode of transmission. Evidence for person-to-person transmission includes clustering of *H. pylori* in families[29] and in institutions for the mentally handicapped.[77] Whether infection is spread from adult to child or from child to child is unknown. In some studies, strain identification using deoxyribonucleic acid (DNA) digest patterns has shown the same strain infecting different members of the same family, suggesting a common source of infection, whereas others have reported colonization by different strains.[78–80] Indirect evidence from a number of studies has suggested that transmission may be from mother to child,[63,74,81] whereas other studies have suggested that transmission is more likely from father to child. Goodman et al suggested that transmission of infection is from older to younger siblings.[82] However, in this study from Columbia, 61% of firstborn children were also infected, which suggests that

older siblings are not the only source of infection. The first direct evidence of transmission of infection from mother to child has come from a study by Konno et al.[65] They followed a group of five children from birth to 5 years of age and determine when they became infected, and using gastric juice samples, they demonstrated that all five children who became infected were infected with strains having identical DNA fingerprinting patterns to their mothers' strain.[65]

If transmission is from person to person, then the possible routes of transmission are fecal–oral, oral–oral, or gastric–oral. The fastidious growth requirements of *H. pylori* have hindered attempts to establish the relative importance of these potential routes of transmission. Polymerase chain reaction (PCR) is a very sensitive technique for detecting microbial DNA in clinical samples, but the use of PCR on feces, saliva, and dental plaque for the identification of *H. pylori* has limitations. Although a PCR diagnosis confirms the presence of DNA, it does not confirm the presence of viable organisms. Inhibitors present in fecal samples, such as acidic polysaccharides and metabolic products, can interfere with the PCR.[83,84] False-positive reactions can occur because of the presence of unidentified *Helicobacter* species or other urease-producing organisms.

Using a novel approach for stool culture, Thomas and colleagues were the first to report the successful culture of *H. pylori* from feces in 9 of 23 Gambian children under 30 months of age and in 1 adult.[85] Hypochlorhydria occurs in association with acute infection.[20,86,87] It has been speculated that successful culture in these children may have been possible because of gastric hypochlorhydria. In animal studies, Fox and colleagues found that *H. mutelae* could be detected in the feces of infected ferrets when gastric pH was increased using omeprazole but not when acid secretion was normal.[86]

Parsonnet and colleagues failed to culture *H. pylori* from normal stool but cultured *H. pylori* from 7 of 14 infected volunteers following administration of a cathartic.[88] Stools passed late in the catharsis were more likely than early stools to grow *H. pylori*, but the number of organisms present was very low. This further supports the finding of Graham and Osato that *H. pylori* may not survive normal transit through the gastrointestinal tract owing to interference from bile acids.[89]

Oral–oral transmission has also been postulated. *H. pylori* has been cultured on one occasion from saliva,[90] and there are a number of reports of culture from dental plaque.[91,92] The complexity of oral flora is a major draw-back in attempting to isolate *H. pylori* from the oral cavity. Evidence against oral–oral transmission is that there is no increased prevalence in teenagers and that *H. pylori* does not appear to be spread between couples. Furthermore, although gastroenterologists have a higher prevalence of infection than expected,[93] dentists do not,[94,95] suggesting that exposure to oral secretions is not a risk factor for infection.

Gastric oral transmission has been postulated in young children in whom reflux and regurgitation are common occurrences. Leung and colleagues have reported isolation of *H. pylori* from vomitus on one occasion in a 6-year-old child.[96] Culture of *H. pylori* from gastric juice specimens in young children also supports the hypothesis of gastric oral transmission.[65] Parsonnet and colleagues cultured *H. pylori* from all 16 infected adult volunteers with organism growths of greater that 1,000 colony-forming units (CFU)/mL of vomitus.[88] Animal studies in socially housed Rhesus Macaques suggest that gastric oral transmission is much more likely than a fecal–oral route of transmission.[97] Of interest *H. pylori* was never isolated from the saliva of Rhesus Macaques prior to vomiting but was regularly cultured from saliva after emesis.[97]

Waterborne transmission has also been investigated. *H. pylori* has been cultured from waste water in Mexico,[98] and there have been a number of reports of PCR identification of *H. pylori* DNA in water from Peru, Sweden, Mexico, and Japan.[99–101] Water as a source of infection is a possibility where drinking water is untreated. It is unlikely that *H. pylori* can persist in treated drinking water systems under normal disinfectant concentrations.[102] Recent evidence that *H. pylori* can form biofilms on surfaces exposed to water has greatly increased the possibility of water as a source of infection.[103]

REINFECTION

Adults in developed countries rarely become reinfected with *H. pylori* following successful treatment, with reinfection rates being less than 1% per year.[104–106] This low rate of reinfection is not surprising because primary infection in adults is also uncommon. However, a study from Bangladesh suggests that reinfection in adults in developing countries may be as high as 13% per annum.[107] It is important to distinguish true reinfection with a new organism from inadequate treatment of the primary infection. It has been suggested that any evidence of infection in the first year following treatment should be considered recrudescence rather than reinfection.[108–110] Careful consideration must be given to the choice of noninvasive diagnostic test used to determine if treatment for *H. pylori* has been successful. Any borderline ^{13}C-UBT result (2.0 to 5.0 excess delta) should be repeated repeated.[111] In addition, the monoclonal stool antigen test is much more accurate for the diagnosis of infection following treatment than the polyclonal stool antigen test.[112]

There is conflicting evidence in children on the risk of reinfection following treatment for *H. pylori*. Early studies suggested that reinfection in children in developed countries was uncommon,[113–115] but that children under the age of 5 years may be a risk of reinfection.[113] More recent studies from Italy and France suggests that reinfection may be as high as 6 to 13% per year in children following treatment for *H. pylori*

infection.[116,117] However, the number of children included in both studies is small and the duration of follow-up (2 years) was short in the study from Italy. The declining prevalence of *H. pylori* infection in developed countries will make further research from individual centers on the rates of reinfection in children difficult, but this question has important implications for the management of *H. pylori* infection in the pediatric population.

MECHANISMS OF DISEASE

H. pylori lives in the hostile environment of the stomach and displays a very strict host and tissue trophism. Despite a vigorous immune response infection, once established persists for life. In fact much of the damage associated with *H. pylori* infection is a direct consequence of the host's immune response rather than direct bacterial activity.[10] Our understanding of how *H. pylori* causes disease is hampered by the lack of good animal models of infection and there is mounting evidence that in vitro work may not accurately reflect what is happening in vivo. Animal models used in *H. pylori* research have many disadvantages and in many instances do not mimic human disease. For instance, neither the mouse, guinea pig, nor rhesus monkey develops peptic ulcer disease or gastric cancer. While the Mongolian gerbil is possibly the best animal model for *H. pylori* infection, because the gerbil develops both peptic ulcer disease and gastric cancer, the lack of transgenic gerbil is a significant disadvantage to the use of the gerbil for *H. pylori* research. Care must be taken in interpreting research results for the various animal models.[10]

BACTERIAL VIRULENCE FACTORS

There are many potential virulence factors that may contribute to the ability of *H. pylori* to induce gastric inflammation and ulcer disease. These include motility, adherence of the organism to the gastric mucosa, urease activity, toxin production, and subversion of host cell signal transduction.[118] The potent urease activity of *H. pylori* is an important virulence factor for this organism.[119] Urease-negative *H. pylori* mutants are incapable of colonizing the gastric mucosa in animal models.[119] Urease appears to play a vital role in protecting the bacteria against gastric acid.[120] The UreI protein, expressed from a gene of the urease gene cluster, has been identified as a pH-sensitive urea channel.[121] As the external pH falls, UreI increases urea transport to the bacterial cytoplasmic urease complex, providing the organism with a mechanism to maintain a neutral and viable intracellular pH despite the variable and often highly acidic milieu in the stomach.

Flagella are also important for the virulence of *H. pylori*. Flagella confer motility on the organism, allowing it to move through the gastric mucus.[118] Isogenic mutants that do not express flagella are incapable of colonizing gnotobiotic piglets.[118]

The cytotoxin-associated gene *cagA* has been identified as a possible marker for more virulent *H. pylori* strains.[9,49] The CagA protein is a highly immunogenic protein encoded by the *cagA* gene and is present in up to 70% of *H. pylori* strains and is a marker for the Cag pathogenicity island (cag PAI), which encodes up to 34 proteins.[49,122] Patients infected with CagA positive strains usually have a higher inflammatory response and are at increased risk of developing gastric cancer and peptic ulcer disease compared to patients infected with Cag negative strains.[10] Although CagA is an important virulence factor the presence of CagA is not sufficient for the prediction of disease outcome in *H. pylori*.

The Cag pathogenicity island encodes a type IV secretion apparatus that serves to translocate bacterial products, notably CagA, into host gastric epithelial cells.[10,49,122] Subversion of host cell processes is an emerging paradigm among bacterial enteric pathogens. In the case of *H. pylori*, the translocated CagA localizes to the inner surface of the plasma membrane and subsequently undergoes tyrosine phosphorylation which causes cytoskeletal reorganization and arrest of cell growth in the gastric epithelium.[10,123] Structural analysis has shown that the size of the CagA protein varies between different *H. pylori* strains. This size variation is thought to be due to a variation in the number and sequence of tyrosine phosphorylation sites located on the C-terminal region of CagA.[124] Higashi et al have shown that the potential of CagA to disrupt host-cell function, and hence cause disease, depends on the number and sequences of tyrosine phosphorylation sites.[124] Differences exist between CagA proteins in western and East Asian isolates of *H. pylori* in terms of the number of tyrosine phosphorylation motifs present on each molecule, and this may help to explain differences in the incidence of gastric cancer rates between the two regions.[124]

The *vacA* gene of *H. pylori* encodes for VacA, a secreted vacuolating cytotoxin, which induces vacuolation in several cell lines. VacA may facilitate colonization by blocking proliferation of T cells including cell cycle arrest in vivo.[49] The best studied allele is the *s1/m1* which has been associated with an increased risk of developing gastric cancer. As with CagA, gastric cancer may occur in association with VacA-negative strains. While VacA is essential for in vitro growth of *H. pylori*, the physiological relevance of VacA and its role in the development of disease have yet to be clarified in vivo.

Many other outer membrane proteins of *H. pylori* which mediate adhesion to the gastric epithelium have been described including BabA, OipA, SabA, SabB, AlpA, AlpB, Hp-NAP, IceA, and DupA which are reviewed very comprehensively by Kusters et al.[10] Of note DupA (duodenal ulcer promoting gene) is exclusively associated with duodenal ulcer disease and protects against the development of gastric atrophy and gastric cancer.[10,125]

HOST INFLAMMATORY RESPONSE

Following infection with *H. pylori*, the human host mounts a strong local and systemic immune response with the production of various pro- and anti-inflammatory cytokines. Evidence is accumulating for a complex interaction between the organism and host defense mechanisms which allows the organism to persist on the gastric mucosa even in the presence of a vigorous immune response.[10] Many of the animal experimental models suggest that *H. pylori* infection evokes a Th1 immune response which leads to atrophy and intestinal metaplasia.[49] Coinfection of C57BL/6 mice with the parasite *Heligmosomoides polygyrus* and *H. felis* can polarize the immune response toward a Th2 response, thereby decreasing the risk of gastric atrophy.[126] While this may explain the low rates of gastric cancer in Africa, it is not sufficient to explain differences between European and Japanese rates of gastric cancer.

GASTRIC ACID SECRETION

Acute infection with *H. pylori* is associated with a transient hypochlorhydria that may last for several months, as demonstrated by volunteer studies[20] and by reports of accidental infection.[87,127] Hypochlorhydria following acute infection has also been demonstrated in animal models.[128] The mechanism for this hypochlorhydria and its importance in determining colonization of the gastric mucosa are not understood. This acute hypochlorhydria is thought to facilitate transmission of infection.[129]

The gastric antrum plays an important role in the regulation of normal gastric acid secretion (see Table 1). G cells located within the gastric mucosa and duodenum produce gastrin, which, in turn, stimulates parietal cells to produce acid.[130,131] D cells are found within the antral mucosa in close proximity to G cells and also in the fundal mucosa close to parietal cells. D cells secrete somatostatin, a hormone that inhibits gastrin release and, therefore, acid secretion.[130,132] The factors that control acid secretion are regulated through complex pathways. Gastrin release is stimulated by cholinergic innervation, gastrin-releasing peptide, and cytokines. If excessive amounts of acid are produced, then somatostatin is released in response to a low intraluminal pH.

The relationship between chronic *H. pylori* infection and acid secretion is not straightforward.[133] There is a large overlap in the levels of acid production between normal noninfected individuals, individuals with *H. pylori* gastritis alone, and individuals with *H. pylori*-associated peptic ulcer disease.[133] Most researchers now accept the fact that basal acid output does not differ markedly between infected and noninfected healthy controls. However, patients with *H. pylori*-associated duodenal ulcer disease have an increased basal and maximal acid output when compared with infected healthy volunteers, whereas patients who develop

gastric cancer have a reduced gastric acid output.[132,133] Genetic polymorphisms in the *IL-1* gene cluster as discussed above may help to explain the complex interaction between *H. pylori* infection, gastric acid secretion, and disease outcome.

SYMPTOMS

Gastritis

There is no evidence that *H. pylori* gastritis in the absence of duodenal ulcer disease causes symptoms in children. *H. pylori* infection occurs frequently in asymptomatic children both in the developed and the developing world, and its eradication is consistently associated with improved symptoms only in children who have duodenal ulcer disease and not in those with gastritis alone.[134]

Recurrent abdominal pain (RAP) in children is a common condition of childhood, affecting 15% of children between 4 and 16 years of age. Apley and Naish[135] defined RAP as abdominal pain which is present for at least 3 months and interferes the child's normal activities. RAP is a functional disorder and therefore there is no organic cause for the pain. In the search for a possible relationship between RAP and *H. pylori*, it is important that there is a clear definition of RAP, and that both the parent and/or child together with the researcher are unaware of the *H. pylori* status of the child when symptoms are assessed. There is now conclusive evidence from a number of studies that there is no association between *H. pylori* and RAP.[64,136–139] In fact a number of these studies have shown that children who are not infected with *H. pylori* are more likely to complain of abdominal pain.[137,140]

Duodenal Ulcer Disease

Primary duodenal ulcer disease is associated with chronic or recurrent symptoms.[5] Most children present with episodic epigastric pain that is frequently associated with vomiting and nocturnal awakening.[5,30] When only patients with ulcer disease diagnosed at endoscopy are evaluated, up to 90% of children have abdominal pain which is often epigastric in location,[141] and in 55% of these children, abdominal pain is the sole presenting symptom.[5] Nocturnal awakening, which should be differentiated from difficulty in falling asleep, is an important feature in distinguishing abdominal pain associated with peptic ulcer disease from RAP.[134,141,142] Similarly, recurrent vomiting in association with upper abdominal pain should be considered suggestive of ulcer disease.

An acute episode of hematemesis may indicate primary or secondary ulceration. In such patients, a history of recent nonsteroidal anti-inflammatory drug ingestion should be sought. However, hematemesis occurring with a history of chronic abdominal pain is highly suggestive of primary duodenal ulcer disease.

In the past, up to 80% of children with primary peptic ulcer disease had symptoms that persisted into adult life. The discovery of

H. pylori has dramatically altered the prognosis of such patients. Successful treatment of *H. pylori*-infected children who have duodenal ulceration results in long-term healing of the ulcer and complete resolution of symptoms.[30,143]

Nongastrointestinal Manifestations

There have been a number of case reports describing children with refractory sideropenic anemia that responded to treatment only after the eradication of *H. pylori*.[144–146] *H. pylori* eradication therapy has been shown to reverse iron deficiency anemia in both adults and children.[147,148] The mechanisms postulated for iron deficiency anemia in patients infected with *H. pylori* include an increased demand for iron because *H. pylori* requires iron for growth, *H. pylori* may sequester iron, or *H. pylori* infection may result in hypochlorhydria, which would inhibit the reduction of iron to its ferrous state for absorption.[149] Because only 5 to 20% of ingested iron is absorbed, it is unlikely that insufficient iron is available from dietary sources for *H. pylori*. Capurso and colleagues found that 51% of patients with *H. pylori*-associated iron deficiency anemia had a pan-gastritis compared with 20% of *H. pylori*-infected controls.[150] They suggest that this pan-gastritis may be responsible for changes in intragastric pH, which results in suboptimal iron absorption. Although pan-gastritis does occur in adults, there are no reports of pan-gastritis in the pediatric literature. Care must be used in interpreting studies of *H. pylori* and iron deficiency anemia because poor socioeconomic status is an important risk factor for both conditions. Furthermore, many of these studies use different ferritin levels to define anemia, and evidence of a microcytic anemia or reduced hemoglobin levels are often not provided. *H. pylori* may contribute to the severity of iron deficiency anemia but is unlikely to be the principal cause of the anemia.

DIAGNOSIS OF *H. PYLORI* GASTRITIS AND ULCER DISEASE

Upper gastrointestinal endoscopy is the investigation of choice for the diagnosis of peptic ulcer disease.[151] It has been shown to be both safe and effective, even in small infants.[152] The detection of ulcers using radiographic studies is often difficult in children. Single-contrast barium examinations correctly identified only one of seven (14%) endoscopically proven duodenal ulcers in children.[5] Furthermore, the risk of false-positive diagnoses with barium studies is especially high in children. Miller and Doig failed to demonstrate any abnormality at endoscopy in 56 of 89 children with abdominal pain who had peptic ulcers diagnosed by barium meal.[153] Double-contrast barium techniques are more sensitive, but even in adults, this procedure failed to demonstrate 55% of gastric ulcers and 30% of duodenal ulcers.[154] In children, double-contrast barium studies are more difficult to perform, particularly in young children, and such studies involve an unacceptable radiation dose for the child.

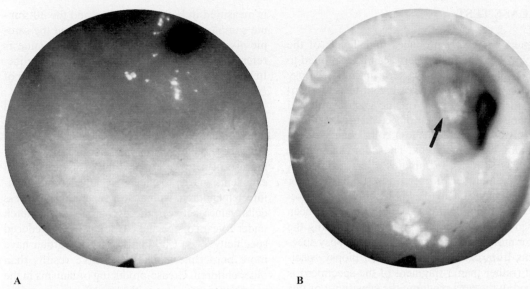

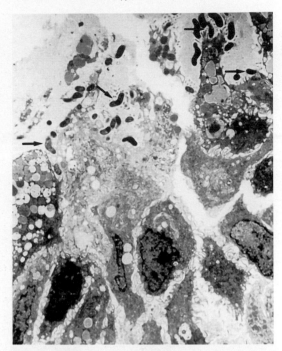

Figure 1 (A) Endoscopic photograph showing normal-appearing antral mucosa: histologic examination of an antral biopsy, however, revealed evidence of acute gastritis and colonization with *Helicobacter pylori*. (B) A duodenal ulcer (*arrow*) is visible through a patent but irregular pyloric channel.

The endoscopic appearance of a peptic ulcer depends on the stage of the disease. Florid, active ulcers are usually round or oval, with a white base composed of debris and fibrin. The ulcer border may be hyperemic and elevated. Duodenal ulcers are often associated with spasm of the pylorus and a deformed pyloric outlet (Figure 1).

The endoscopic appearance of the stomach often correlates poorly with the presence or absence of gastritis.[2,3,5,7] Histologic evidence of mucosal inflammation is essential to establish a diagnosis of gastritis, and it frequently aids in the differential diagnosis of gastritis.

A nodularity of the antral mucosa has been described in association with *H. pylori* gastritis in children.[5,7] These nodules give the antrum a cobblestone appearance (Figure 2). Hassall and Dimmick reported that nodularity of the antrum was present in their study in all 23 children with *H. pylori*-associated duodenal ulcers.[7] Nodularity of the antral mucosa is also seen in the majority of children with *H. pylori*-associated gastritis who do not have duodenal ulceration. The reason

for this appearance of the gastric mucosa in association with *H. pylori* in children is unknown.

HISTOLOGY

The characteristic appearance and unique location of *H. pylori* allow a presumptive diagnosis of *H. pylori* colonization in children to be made by identifying spiral organisms on histologic sections of the gastric mucosa. Historically, the organism has been identified using a Warthin-Starry silver stain (Figure 3).[11,28] Silver stains are usually very sensitive and specific for identifying the presence of *H. pylori* in children, but they are expensive and

Figure 4 Transmission electron photomicrograph of antral mucosa shows spiral-shaped *Helicobacter*-like organisms (*arrow*) adherent to surface epithelial cells and contained in the overlying mucous layer. (Courtesy of Dr Ernest Cutz, Department of Pathology, The Hospital for Sick Children, Toronto, ON.)

difficult to perform. A modified Giemsa stain or a cresyl violet stain is both sensitive and specific for the organism and is much easier to perform than silver staining.[5] The Genta stain allows simultaneous visualization of the bacteria and the histologic features of gastritis.[155] Ultrastructural studies show the spiral morphology of organisms present on gastric epithelium (Figures 4 and 5).

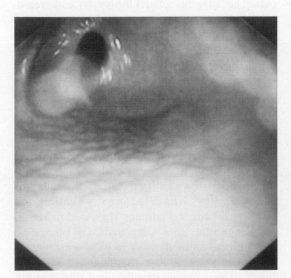

Figure 2 Endoscopic view of nodularity of the gastric antrum, which is seen in association with *Helicobacter pylori* infection.

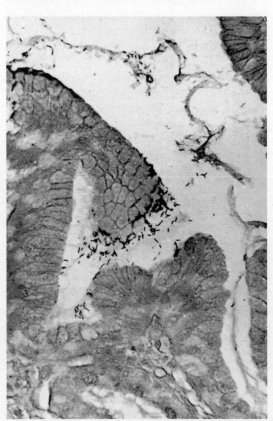

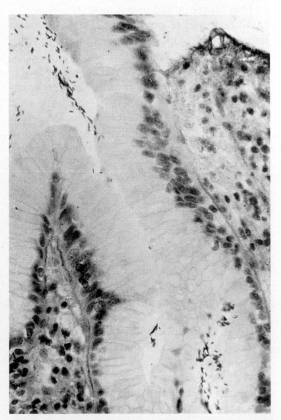

Figure 3 Modified silver impregnation method of antral mucosa (with histologic evidence of active gastritis) demonstrates gastric *Helicobacter*-like organisms. (Reproduced with permission from reference 34.)

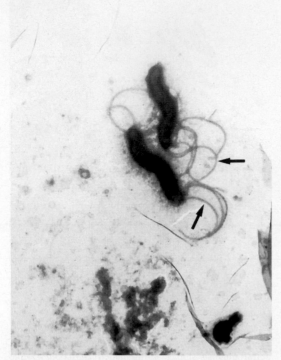

Figure 5 Transmission electron photomicrograph after negative staining of *Helicobacter pylori*. Note the spiral shape of the organism (comparable to intestinal *Campylobacter*) and the presence of flagellae (*arrow*).

CULTURE

Because *H. pylori* is extremely fastidious in its growth requirements, routine culture is difficult in a clinical practice. A more practical "gold standard" for the diagnosis of *H. pylori* is either a positive culture or the identification of *H. pylori* on both histology and urease testing.

Culturing of *H. pylori* is performed by inoculating minced biopsy specimens into blood agar plates that are held under microaerophilic conditions at 37°C. Media that contain nalidixic acid or vancomycin (ie, Skirrow medium) are frequently used to minimize overgrowth of organisms from the oropharyngeal flora. Visible colonies usually require 5 to 7 days of culture. The long incubation period is particularly important in children because the number of organisms present on their gastric mucosa is often very low. The organism is identified as *H. pylori* if it is positive for urease, catalase, and oxidase and produces a negative reaction for hippurate hydrolysis and nitrate reduction.

For optimal recovery rates of *H. pylori* from gastric biopsy specimens, the viability of the organism must be maintained during transportation to the laboratory. It was previously considered necessary for biopsy specimens to be delivered to the microbiology laboratory within 1 hour, but successful culture is possible even after 24 hours when a suitable transport medium is used.[156] It is essential that the biopsy specimens are placed directly into the transport medium and not exposed to room air. When carefully performed, culture of the organism is successful in almost 100% of specimens.[28,29]

UREASE TEST

Because *H. pylori* produces high levels of the enzyme urease, this property can be exploited to detect the presence of bacteria in antral biopsy specimens and also in urea breath tests. To rapidly identify *H. pylori* on the gastric mucosal specimens, a specimen is placed on urea medium; hydrolysis of urea leads to a color change of the medium, from tan to pink. The color change may occur as soon as 30 minutes after inoculation, but if the number of bacteria is small, the color reaction may take up to 24 hours to develop. Urease tests in children occasionally have not been as sensitive as in adults,[28] perhaps reflecting the lower number of bacteria present on biopsy specimens from children. When a full biopsy specimen (rather than a fragment of the specimen) is placed in the urea medium, the sensitivity of this test increases and is close to 100%. Commercial kits based on similar principles are available for use in the endoscopy suite.

UREA BREATH TESTS

The ^{13}C-UBT is a safe and noninvasive method for the diagnosis of *H. pylori* infection in adults and children. Isotopic urea (^{13}C) is ingested by the patient; if *H. pylori* is present in the stomach, breakdown of the labeled urea by *H. pylori* urease results in the production of labeled carbon dioxide, which is measured in the expired air. In contrast to ^{14}C (a radioactive label), ^{13}C urea is labeled with a naturally occurring stable isotope of carbon. Tests using stable isotopes are ideal for use in children, but they are more expensive because they require the use of a mass spectrometer. Numerous test protocols have been examined in both adults and children and the ^{13}C UBT has been shown to be an accurate and highly robust test.[157,158]

The UBT for use in adults usually involves an overnight fast and the administration of a test meal to slow gastric emptying.[159] The use of a prolonged fast and a test meal makes the test difficult to perform in children and limits its usefulness in both research and clinical practice.

We have shown that a simplified test protocol is very successful in children over 2 years of age.[75] After the patient fasts for 2 hours, the UBT is performed by collecting a baseline sample of expired air, followed by ingestion of ^{13}C urea (50 mg for children <50 kg or 75 mg for children >50 kg) with 50 mg of a glucose polymer in 5 to 10 mL of water. It is important that the solution of urea is swallowed quickly and not held in the mouth. This is not a problem in the older child but may present difficulties for younger children. A second breath sample is collected 30 minutes later. In older children, as in adults, samples may be collected by blowing directly with a straw into a glass tube that can be sealed. For younger children, a closed system such as a rebreathing bag with tap (Childerhouse Medical, London) is required, and the expired air is transferred into an evacuated glass tube. The ratio of ^{12}C to ^{13}C

is measured in both the baseline and the 30-minute sample, and the difference between the samples is calculated by subtraction. This value is referred to as excess delta or delta over baseline. In children, an excess delta of 3.5 is indicative of *H. pylori* infection.[75,157]

The UBT was shown to be 100% sensitive and 92% specific for the diagnosis of *H. pylori* infection in older children.[75] The sensitivity and specificity were achieved after a 2-hour fast and without the use of a test meal or drink. This test has an excellent capacity to distinguish infected from noninfected children, with a clear separation of excess delta values between the two groups. In children under 2 years of age, the UBT may have a reduced specificity.[160,161] Children in this age group have more borderline and false-positive results than older children. Urease-producing organisms in the mouth may interfere with the test in very young children.[160,162] When the test was carried out using a nasogastric tube (in situ for clinical indications), there were no false-positive results in children under two years of age.[160]

Samples collected at 15 or 20 minutes often give false-positive results, perhaps because of interference from oral urease-producing organisms.[75] Therefore, the second breath sample should be collected 30 minutes after ingestion of substrate. Because the UBT measures the ratio of ^{12}C to ^{13}C, the volume of expired breath collected is not critical. However, the effect of crying or dead space on the test in young children has not been determined. Breath samples from children are stable for up to at least 7 months; therefore, transport and storage of specimens for analysis at a later time are possible. Following treatment, the UBT is 100% sensitive and specific in assessing *H. pylori* status.[75,157] It has replaced endoscopy as the investigation of choice for assessing treatment success in children. Breath tests should not be carried out for at least 1 month after the completion of treatment and any borderline tests (2.0 to 5.0 delta over baseline) should be repeated.[111] In fact any increase in delta over baseline result following treatment, should be regarded with suspicion because this reflects the presence of urease-producing organism in the gastrointestinal tract. It is important to ensure that the protocol is followed carefully in young children as oral urease-producing organisms can interfere with the test.

STOOL ANTIGEN ENZYME IMMUNOASSAY

The detection of *H. pylori* antigens in stool using monoclonal antibodies provides a noninvasive method for identifying infected adults and children.[32,112,157] The *H. pylori* stool antigen test (HpSA) (Premier Platinum HpSA test, Meridian Diagnostics Inc., Cincinnati, OH) based on a polyclonal antibody is 91 to 98% sensitive and 83 to 100% specific for the diagnosis of infection.[163] The accuracy of polyclonal stool test following treatment for *H. pylori* is reduced, and more recent studies have called into question the overall accuracy of the polyclonal stool antigen test in this situation.[164]

The development of a monoclonal antibody has provided much greater accuracy in stool antigen testing.[157,165] This is particularly so in children in whom the sensitivity, specificity, positive predictive values, and negative predictive values were 98, 99, 98, and 99%, respectively, in a large multicenter European study involving 302 previously untreated children (*H. pylori* CnX, FentoLab, Martinsreid, Germany).[165] Care must be taken to store stool samples at (20(C before testing as the sensitivity of the test declines markedly if stored at room temperature for 2 to 3 days.[32,112] The accuracy of the monoclonal stool antigen test in children following treatment for *H. pylori* or in the diagnosis of infection in children under 2 years of age has not been evaluated adequately to determine if is superior to the ^{13}C-UBT in these situations.[157, 158] However, the cost and convenience of the HpSA makes it a very attractive test for use in clinical practice.

SEROLOGY

Infection with *H. pylori* provokes a specific serum IgG response. The initial antibody response in children is to low-molecular-weight antigens in the 15- to 30-kDa range and may take up to 60 days to develop.[166] The mean antibody levels in young children are significantly lower than in older children and adults.[167,168] Antibody titers in children may not reach their maximum levels until the age of 7 years.[169]

Serologic tests in children must therefore be standardized using children's sera.[169] If the assay is based on adult antibody levels, less than 50% of children will be correctly diagnosed because the cutoff point is higher for adults than for children. Commercially available serologic tests do not have the sensitivity or specificity to accurately diagnose *H. pylori* infection in children under 12 years of age, with second-generation serologic tests failing to diagnose up to 20% of children under the age of 10 years.[170]

Everhart and colleagues have shown that even using adult sera, the reliability of serology on repeat analysis of the same sample is poor and could easily explain the 1 to 2% seroreversion and seroconversion rates reported from adult seroepidemiologic studies.[171] Therefore, in all seroepidemiologic studies, there is a need for caution in interpreting results.

Currently the use of serological tests is not recommended in clinical practice in children and only in certain limited circumstances in adults such as bleeding ulcers or current or recent use of PPIs.[32,157] Furthermore the use of salivary or urinary antibodies to *H. pylori* has no current role in clinical practice.[32] In epidemiological research serological tests are often the only feasible way examining the prevalence of *H. pylori* infection but care must be taken in interpreting the results and only assays which have been validated in children should be used. Measurement of *H. pylori*-specific serum IgA or IgM antibodies in children is not a sensitive indicator of gastric colonization.[32,157]

TREATMENT OF PEPTIC ULCER DISEASE

In adults, both the National Institutes of Health consensus statement[172] and the Maastricht 111 consensus report[32] recommended that *H. pylori* should be eradicated in adults who have *H. pylori*-associated peptic ulcer. The Maastricht 111 consensus report strongly recommends treatment of *H. pylori* infection in patients with MALT lymphoma, atrophic gastritis, after gastric cancer resection, and patients who are first-degree relatives of gastric cancer patients.[32]

Children with peptic ulcer disease who are infected with *H. pylori* should receive treatment to eradicate the infection.[173] However, the majority of children infected with *H. pylori* do not have peptic ulcer disease and are not symptomatic. The diagnosis of *H. pylori* infection is often an incidental finding at endoscopy, and the management of these children is therefore controversial. It is now accepted that there is no evidence demonstrating a link between *H. pylori* gastritis and abdominal pain except in those children in whom an ulcer is present.[173,174] If infection is incidentally diagnosed, it should be treated, but there is currently no indication to screen children for *H. pylori* infection except at endoscopy, when peptic ulcer disease is investigated.

SPECIFIC TREATMENT REGIMENS

Several regimens have been used to treat *H. pylori* in children but a recent meta-analysis of *H. pylori* treatment in children would suggest that the optimal treatment regime for use in children has yet to be determined.[175] Treatment regimens have evolved from using a single antibiotic with a bismuth preparation for 4 to 6 weeks to 1-week treatment regimens using two antibiotics and either bismuth or a PPI. The most frequently used antibiotics in children and adults are amoxicillin, metronidazole, tinidazole, and clarithromycin. Selection of optimal antibiotic combinations should be based on known antibiotic sensitivities in the local population for *H. pylori*. Following treatment, children should have a UBT or stool antigen test carried out to determine if the treatment has been successful.

Adult guidelines recommend a PPI (standard dose bid), clarithromycin (500 mg bid), together with amoxicillin (1,000 mg bid) or metronidazole (400 or 500 mg bid) for 14 days.[32] In children the recommended doses of clarithromycin is 7.5 mg/kg, amoxicillin 25 mg/kg, and omeprazole 0.3 mg/kg. Adult studies suggest that treatment regimens with less than an 75% success rate are unacceptable for use in clinical practice.[176] However, clarithromycin based triple have been shown to be less effective in children with eradication rates of less than 80% in many studies.[175,177,178]

This may be due to the much higher rates of clarithromycin resistance reported in children. Therefore, in children consideration should be given to the use of metronidazole (7.5 mg/kg bid) instead of clarithromycin particularly in areas where there is a high rate of resistance to clarithromycin. Many pediatric studies have used bismuth rather than a PPI and there is some evidence to suggest that bismuth may be more effective than PPI treatment in children.[179] Furthermore Oderda et al have shown that treatment with two antibiotics alone is as effect effective as triple therapy.[180] A sequential treatment regime using omeprazole and amoxicillin for 5 days followed by omeprazole with clarithromycin and tinidazole for 5 days was successful in 97.3% (95% CI 86 to 99.5) of children compared to a 1-week treatment regime of omeprazole, amoxicillin, and metronidazole which eradicated 75% of infections (95% CI 59.8 to 86.7). As in previous pediatric studies the number treated was small (64 children in total) and both arms were not strictly comparable. The combination of clarithromycin and tinidazole was not comparable to metronidazole alone and the longer duration of treatment in the sequential arm could have explained the difference in treatment effect. Treatment for 14 days is now recommended in adult studies because it has been shown to be 12% more effective (95% CI 7 to 17).[32]

TREATMENT FAILURE

Failure of first-line treatment regimes is a major consideration in both adults and children. Numerous factors are responsible for treatment failure, but the most important are poor patient compliance, inadequate drug delivery, and antimicrobial resistance. Ingestion of less than 75% of the prescribed medication results in decreased eradication rates.[181] Walsh and colleagues achieved excellent compliance in children, using special boxes in which the drugs for each dose were compartmentalized.[182] This level of compliance, although desirable, is unlikely in clinical practice.

In treating children, the availability of suitable drug preparations is very important. The strong taste of ammonia from liquid bismuth may reduce compliance in children. In clinical practice, therefore, the treatment regimen with the simplest dosing requirement and fewest side effects is to be preferred, assuming similar eradication rates.

When treatment is unsuccessful, there are a limited number of treatment options available. The Maastricht 111 consensus report recommends a bismuth-based quadruple treatment regime which also includes a PPI, tetracycline, and metronidazole. Alternatively if bismuth is not available, a PPI with amoxicillin and tetracycline is recommended.[32] Claritromycin is not recommended in second-line treatment regimes unless there is genotypic evidence to show that the *H. pylori* strain is susceptible to clarithromycin.[32] Tetracycline is not recommended for use in children under 12 years of age.

A number of other antibiotics including nitrofurantoin, furazolidone, levofloxacin, and rifabutin have been investigated but to date there is little conclusive evidence of their superiority in the management of *H. pylori*. Levofloxacin with amoxicillin and a PPI for 10 days has been suggested as superior to quadruple therapies in adults with less side effects.[183] In children there has been one study which compared two treatment regimes in children where the first-line treatment failed.[184] Nijevitch et al found no difference in eradication rates between a nitrofuran and furazolidone based quadruple treatment. Both groups had achieved a high eradication rate [33 of 37 (89%) vs 34 of 39 (87%)].[184] However, the frequency of severe side effects was greater in the furazolidone with one child having to withdraw because of excessive nausea and vomiting.[184]

Bismuth

Bismuth formulations have been used in the management of peptic ulcer disease for over 100 years. However, the availability of bismuth preparations is declining as manufacturers stop production due to lack of demand. The precise mechanism of action of Bismuth in eradicating *H. pylori* from the gastric mucosa is not known. Bismuth compounds have some antibacterial properties, and bismuth monotherapy clears *H. pylori* from the gastric mucosa in about 50% of cases. The rate of ulcer relapse after bismuth therapy alone is significantly lower than that after treatment with histamine 2 receptor antagonists.

In Europe, colloidal bismuth subcitrate is the bismuth preparation most commonly used to treat *H. pylori* infection, whereas bismuth subsalicylate is used in North America. There has been concern about the use of bismuth salts in children because of potential toxic effects. However, bismuth does not appear to have any toxic effects in children other than those already well described in adults. Encephalopathy and acute renal impairment after chronic use of high dose bismuth are reported, but these side effects, which are reversible, have not been reported in children treated for *H. pylori*-associated gastritis or ulcer disease.[6] Serum bismuth levels remain within the normal range for children when colloidal bismuth subcitrate is prescribed as either 480 mg/1.73 m^2 of body surface area per day or 120 mg twice daily (240 mg twice daily for children over the age of 10 years).

Proton Pump Inhibitors

PPIs inhibit the gastric acid pump (hydrogen–potassium-exchanging adenosine triphosphatase) in a dose-dependent manner.[185,186] PPIs are rapidly absorbed, with peak concentrations occurring 2 to 4 hours after oral administration.[187] The precise mechanism of action of a PPI in inhibiting *H. pylori* is unknown.[187] PPIs have some antibacterial activity in vivo. More important, by inhibiting gastric acid secretion, these drugs may promote the increased effectiveness of acid-sensitive antibiotics, such as clarithromycin, in triple-therapy regimens.

The side effects of omeprazole, which include headache, diarrhea, abdominal pain, and nausea, are self-limiting. Bacterial overgrowth in the stomach and small intestine by oral and colonic flora has been reported.[49] PPIs are metabolized completely by the polymorphic cytochrome P-450 system.[187] Although drug interactions with warfarin, diazepam, and phenytoin theoretically could occur, none have been reported to date.[187]

Concern has been expressed that PPIs may accelerate the progression of gastric atrophy and gastric cancer. Kuipers et al in 1996 were the first to suggest that the progression of atrophic gastritis was greater in patients infected with *H. pylori* who were taking long-term PPIs for reflux esophagitis compared to patients who were taking alternative medication.[188] Similar results have been reported by other investigators.[49,176] It is generally accepted that PPI treatment can change the distribution of *H. pylori* gastritis from antral predominant to corpus predominant gastritis. Furthermore, in a mouse model of *H. pylori* infection mice which overexpress gastrin and were infected with *H. pylori* developed gastric atrophy and gastric cancer.[49] Currently there are no guidelines for the management of children who require long-term PPI therapy. However, the Maastricht 111 Consensus report recommends that adults requiring long-term acid suppression that should be treated prior to commencing therapy.[32]

ANTIBIOTIC RESISTANCE

The development of antibiotic resistance by *H. pylori* is an important variable in the success of treatment regimens. Resistance to antibiotics may be primary, or it may develop during the course of treatment. The development of secondary resistance is usually associated with suboptimal treatment regimens. There is now ample evidence that antibiotic resistance in *H. pylori* is due to chromosomal mutations.[189] The genetic mutations involved are mostly limited to point mutations which allows molecular methods to be used for their detection. However, in routine clinical practice agar dilution and disc diffusion techniques are the methods used routinely for the determination of antibiotic resistance.

Agar dilution is considered the method of choice for resistance testing.[189] Disk diffusion techniques are simple and less expensive but, although less suitable for slow-growing bacteria such as *H. pylori*, are a more realistic option for everyday laboratory use. The E-test is a semiquantitative variant of disk diffusion, and although there is excellent correlation between the different methods when testing for clarithromycin resistance, discrepancies have been reported for metronidazole resistance between E-test and disk diffusion, with rates of metronidazole resistance being higher for E-tests.[190] In determining antibiotic sensitivities, it is recommended that isolates of *H. pylori* should be recovered during the active phase of growth within 3 days and that the inoculum size of 108 CFU/mL (equivalent to McFarland 4) is used.[191] The conditions (anaerobic vs

microaerophilic) under which resistance is determined may also influence the out-come of resistance testing.

Metronidazole resistance greatly reduces the efficacy of metronidazole-based regimens in both adults and children.[189] Primary resistance to metronidazole may be a nonstable phenomenon[189] and may explain why treatment is more successful than anticipated in a number of studies in which metronidazole was used. Rates of metronidazole resistance vary from 10 to 30% in Europe, the United States, and Australia to up to 60% in Singapore.[189] Women are more likely to harbor resistant strains, as are migrants from developing countries. The higher resistance among women and in developing countries may be explained by the use of metronidazole for gynecologic and diarrheal diseases in these groups. In contrast to most other antibiotics the resistance mechanism for metronidazole is not straightforward. The *rdxA* gene and the *frxA* gene are involved but to date a clear set of point mutations for metronidazole resistance have not been identified.[189]

The mechanism of action of clarithromycin is to bind ribosomes and disrupt protein synthesis. The development of resistance is attributed to various point mutations in the two 23S ribosomal ribonucleic acid (rRNA) genes of *H. pylori*. It is thought that clarithromycin needs effective acid control to achieve high eradication rates. Primary clarithromycin resistance is less common in adults than metronidazole resistance and ranges from 10 to 15% of strains. It is now clear that clarithromycin resistance rates are higher in children compared to adults and that clarithromycin resistance has risen from 4 to 6% in the early 1990s[192,193] to 24% in a recent European report.[194] Clarithromycin resistance is thought to be due to the widespread use of clarithromycin in pediatric practice. With this increasing prevalence of resistance to clarithromycin, careful consideration should be given to its inclusion as a first-line treatment in children.

Until recently, it was thought that *H. pylori* did not develop resistance to amoxicillin. Stable amoxicillin resistance has been reported on a number of occasions.[189] To date, amoxicillin resistance in children is extremely rare.[194]

Resistance to tetracycline has also been reported, which may greatly hinder its use as a low-cost first- or second-line treatment. Mutations of the 16S rRNA genes are responsible for resistance, but a number of mutations may be necessary to confer clinically significant resistance.[189]

CONCLUSION

The discovery of *H. pylori* over 30 years ago has revolutionized our knowledge of peptic ulcer disease and gastric cancer. However, it is now clear that the majority of those who become infected with *H. pylori* do not develop any symptoms or disease as a consequence of their infection.

Therefore, evidence of infection should only be sought when there is a clinical suspicion of an *H. pylori*-associated disease. Despite extensive research activity there are still many areas of great uncertainty in relation to the pathogenesis and epidemiology of this infection. *H. pylori* displays marked trophism for gastric tissue, yet we do not understand the mechanism of adherence or the role of the host in adherence of the organism to the gastric mucosa and the development of disease. We know that children become infected at a very young age yet how infection is transmitted is unknown. From a clinical perspective further research on the optimal treatment regimens for children who require treatment is essential.

REFERENCES

1. Genta RM. *Helicobacter pylori*, inflammation, mucosal damage, and apoptosis—pathogenesis and definition of gastric atrophy. Gastroenterology 1997;113:S51– 5.
2. Black DD, Haggitt RC, Whitington PF. Gastroduodenal endoscopic–histologic correlation in pediatric patients. J Pediatr Gastroenterol Nutr 1988;7:353–8.
3. Whitehead R, Truelove SC, Gear MW. The histological diagnosis of chronic gastritis in fibreoptic gastroscope biopsy specimens. J Clin Pathol 1972;25:1–11.
4. Soll A. Gasrointestinal Disease: Pathophysiology, Diagnosis, Management. Philadelphia, PA: WB Saunders; 1993.
5. Drumm B, Rhoads JM, Stringer DA, et al. Peptic ulcer disease in children: Etiology, clinical findings, and clinical course. Pediatrics 1988;82:410–4.
6. Drumm B. *Helicobacter pylori* in the pediatric patient. Gastroenterol Clin North Am 1993;22:169–82.
7. Hassall E, Dimmick JE. Unique features of *Helicobacter pylori* disease in children. Dig Dis Sci 1991;36:417–23.
8. Peterson WL. *Helicobacter pylori* and peptic ulcer disease. N Engl J Med 1991;324:1043–8.
9. Suerbaum S, Michetti P. *Helicobacter pylori* infection. N Engl J Med 2002;347:1175–86.
10. Kusters JG, van Vliet AH, Kuipers EJ. Pathogenesis of *Helicobacter pylori* infection. Clin Microbiol Rev 2006;19:449–90.
11. Warren JR. Unidentified curved bacilli on gastric epithelium in active chronic gastritis. Lancet 1983;i:1273.
12. Susser M, Stein Z. Civilization and peptic ulcer. The Lancet 1962;i:115–9.
13. Coggon D, Lambert P, Langman MJ. 20 years of hospital admissions for peptic ulcer in England and Wales. Lancet 1981;1:1302–4.
14. Sipponen P, Helske T, Jarvinen P, et al. Fall in the prevalence of chronic gastritis over 15 years: Analysis of outpatient series in Finland from 1977, 1985, and 1992. Gut 1994;35:1167–71.
15. Demir H, Gurakan F, Ozen H, et al. Peptic ulcer disease in children without *Helicobacter pylori* infection. Helicobacter 2002;7:111.
16. Elitsur Y, Lawrence Z. Non-*Helicobacter pylori* related duodenal ulcer disease in children. Helicobacter 2001;6:239–43.
17. Price AB. The Sydney System: Histological division. J Gastroenterol Hepatol 1991;6:209–22.
18. Dixon MF, Genta RM, Yardley JH, Correa P. Classification and grading of gastritis. The updated Sydney System. International Workshop on the Histopathology of Gastritis, Houston 1994. Am J Surg Pathol 1996;20:1161–81.
19. Mitchell HM, Bohane TD, Tobias V, et al. *Helicobacter pylori* infection in children: Potential clues to pathogenesis. J Pediatr Gastroenterol Nutr 1993;16:120–5.
20. Morris A, Nicholson G. Ingestion of *Campylobacter pyloridis* causes gastritis and raised fasting gastric pH. Am J Gastroenterol 1987;82:192–9.
21. Graham DY, Opekun AR, Osato MS, et al. Challenge model for *Helicobacter pylori* infection in human volunteers. Gut 2004;53:1235–43.
22. Offerhaus GJ, Price AB, Haot J, et al. Observer agreement on the grading of gastric atrophy. Histopathology 1999;34:320–5.
23. Gormally SM, Kierce BM, Daly LE, et al. Gastric metaplasia and duodenal ulcer disease in children infected by *Helicobacter pylori*. Gut 1996;38:513–7.
24. Kato S, Nakajima S, Nishino Y, et al. Association between gastric atrophy and *Helicobacter pylori* infection in Japanese children: A retrospective multicenter study. Dig Dis Sci 2006;51:99–104.
25. Genta RM, Lew GM, Graham DY. Changes in the gastric mucosa following eradication of *Helicobacter pylori*. Mod Pathol 1993;6:281–9.
26. Rugge M, Genta RM. Staging and grading of chronic gastritis. Hum Pathol 2005;36:228–33.
27. Rugge M, Meggio A, Pennelli G, et al. Gastritis staging in clinical practice: The olga staging system. Gut 2007;56:631–6.
28. Drumm B, Sherman P, Cutz E, Karmali M. Association of *Campylobacter pylori* on the gastric mucosa with antral gastritis in children. N Engl J Med 1987;316:1557–61.
29. Drumm B, Perez-Perez GI, Blaser MJ, Sherman PM. Intrafamilial clustering of *Helicobacter pylori* infection. N Engl J Med 1990;322:359–63.
30. Goggin N, Rowland M, Imrie C, et al. Effect of *Helicobacter pylori* eradication on the natural history of duodenal ulcer disease. Arch Dis Child 1998;79:502–5.
31. Marshall BJ, Armstrong JA, McGechie DB, Glancy RJ. Attempt to fulfill Koch's postulates for pyloric campylobacter. Med J Aust 1985;142:436–9.
32. Malfertheiner P, Megraud F, O'Morain C, et al. Current concepts in the management of *Helicobacter pylori* infection—The Maastricht, III Consensus Report. Gut 2007;56: 772–81.
33. Parkin DM. Global cancer statistics in the year 2000. Lancet Oncol 2001;2:533–43.
34. Imrie C, Rowland M, Bourke B, Drumm B. Is *Helicobacter pylori* infection in childhood a risk factor for gastric cancer? Pediatrics 2001;107:373–80.
35. IARC Working Group on the Evaluation of Carcinogenic Risks to Humans. Schistosomes, liver flukes and *Helicobacter pylori*. IARC Monogr Eval Carcinog Risks Hum 1994;61:1–241.
36. Enroth H, Kraaz W, Rohan T, et al. Does the method of *Helicobacter pylori* detection influence the association with gastric cancer risk? Scand J Gastroenterol 2002;37: 884–90.
37. Uemura N, Okamoto S, Yamamoto S, et al. *Helicobacter pylori* infection and the development of gastric cancer. N Engl J Med 2001;345:784–9.
38. Correa P, Haenszel W, Cuello C, et al. A model for gastric cancer epidemiology. Lancet 1975;2:58–60.
39. El-Zimaity HM, Graham DY, al-Assi MT, et al. Interobserver variation in the histopathological assessment of *Helicobacter pylori* gastritis [see comments]. Hum Pathol 1996;27:35–41.
40. Vauhkonen M, Vauhkonen H, Sipponen P. Pathology and molecular biology of gastric cancer. Best Pract Res Clin Gastroenterol 2006;20:651–74.
41. Kuipers EJ, Uyterlinde AM, Pena AS, et al. Long-term sequelae of *Helicobacter pylori* gastritis. Lancet 1995;345:1525–8.
42. Watabe H, Mitsushima T, Yamaji Y, et al. Predicting the development of gastric cancer from combining *Helicobacter pylori* antibodies and serum pepsinogen status: A prospective endoscopic cohort study. Gut 2005;54:764–8.
43. Hansson LE, Nyren O, Hsing AW, et al. The risk of stomach cancer in patients with gastric or duodenal ulcer disease. N Engl J Med 1996;335:242–9.
44. el-Omar EM, Oien K, El-Nujumi A, et al. *Helicobacter pylori* infection and chronic gastric acid hyposecretion. Gastroenterology 1997;113:15–24.
45. El-Omar EM, Carrington M, Chow WH, et al. Interleukin-1 polymorphisms associated with increased risk of gastric cancer. Nature 2000;404:398–402.
46. El-Omar EM. The importance of interleukin 1beta in *Helicobacter pylori* associated disease. Gut 2001;48:743–7.
47. El-Omar EM, Rabkin CS, Gammon MD, et al. Increased risk of noncardia gastric cancer associated with proinflammatory cytokine gene polymorphisms. Gastroenterology 2003;124:1193–201.
48. Machado JC, Pharoah P, Sousa S, et al. Interleukin 1B and interleukin 1RN polymorphisms are associated with increased risk of gastric carcinoma. Gastroenterology 2001;121:823–9.
49. Fox JG, Wang TC. Inflammation, atrophy, and gastric cancer. J Clin Invest 2007;117:60–9.
50. Naylor GM, Gotoda T, Dixon M, et al. Why does Japan have a high incidence of gastric cancer? Comparison of gastritis between UK and Japanese patients. Gut 2006;55:1545–52.
51. Guilford P, Hopkins J, Harraway J, et al. E-cadherin germline mutations in familial gastric cancer. Nature 1998;392:402–5.
52. Barber M, Fitzgerald RC, Caldas C. Familial gastric cancer—aetiology and pathogenesis. Best Pract Res Clin Gastroenterol 2006;20:721–34.
53. Dixon MF. Prospects for intervention in gastric carcinogenesis: Reversibility of gastric atrophy and intestinal metaplasia. Gut 2001;49:2–4.
54. Yoshida S, Kozu T, Gotoda T, Saito D. Detection and treatment of early cancer in high-risk populations. Best Pract Res Clin Gastroenterol 2006;20:745–65.
55. Kuipers EJ, Sipponen P. *Helicobacter pylori* eradication for the prevention of gastric cancer. Helicobacter 2006;11:52–7.
56. Forman D, Burley VJ. Gastric cancer: Global pattern of the disease and an overview of environmental risk factors. Best Pract Res Clin Gastroenterol 2006;20:633–49.
57. Du MQ, Isaccson PG. Gastric MALT lymphoma: From aetiology to treatment. Lancet Oncol 2002;3:97–104.
58. Liu H, Ye H, Ruskone-Fourmestraux A, et al. T(11;18) is a marker for all stage gastric MALT lymphomas that will not respond to *H. pylori* eradication. Gastroenterology 2002;122:1286–94.
59. Jalava K, On SL, Harrington CS, et al. A cultured strain of "*Helicobacter heilmannii*," a human gastric pathogen, identified as *H. bizzozeronii*: Evidence for zoonotic potential of *Helicobacter*. Emerg Infect Dis 2001;7:1036–8.
60. Ashorn M, Maki M, Ruuska T, et al. Upper gastrointestinal endoscopy in recurrent abdominal pain of childhood. J Pediatr Gastroenterol Nutr 1993;16:273–7.
61. Blecker U, McKeithan TW, Hart J, Kirschner BS. Resolution of *Helicobacter pylori*-associated gastric lymphoproliferative disease in a child. Gastroenterology 1995;109:973–7.
62. Sharon N, Kenet G, Toren A, et al. *Helicobacter pylori*-associated gastric lymphoma in a girl. Pediatr Hematol Oncol 1997;14:177–80.
63. Rowland M, Daly L, Vaughan M, et al. Age-specific incidence of *Helicobacter pylori*. Gastroenterology 2006;130:65–72; quiz 211.
64. Tindberg Y, Nyren O, Blennow M, Granstrom M. *Helicobacter pylori* infection and abdominal symptoms among Swedish school children. J Pediatr Gastroenterol Nutr 2005;41:33–8.
65. Koletzko S, Konstantopoulos N, Bosman D, et al. Evaluation of a novel monoclonal enzyme immunoassay for detection of *Helicobacter pylori* antigen in stool from children. Gut. 2003;52:804–6
66. Ashorn M, Miettinen A, Ruuska T, et al. Seroepidemiological study of *Helicobacter pylori* infection in infancy. Arch Dis Child Fetal Neonatal Ed 1996;74:F141–2.
67. Blecker U, Lanciers S, Lebenthal E, Vandenplas Y. *Helicobacter pylori* infection in infants born from positive mothers. Am J Gastroenterol 1994;89:139–40.
68. Gold BD, Khanna B, Huang LM, et al. *Helicobacter pylori* acquisition in infancy after decline of maternal passive immunity. Pediatr Res 1997;41:641–6.
69. Kuipers EJ, Pena AS, van Kamp G, et al. Seroconversion for *Helicobacter pylori*. Lancet 1993;342:328–31.
70. Cullen DJ, Collins BJ, Christiansen KJ, et al. When is *Helicobacter pylori* infection acquired? Gut 1993;34:1681–2.
71. Banatvala N, Mayo K, Megraud F, et al. The cohort effect and *Helicobacter pylori*. J Infect Dis 1993;168:219–21.
72. Fiedorek SC, Malaty HM, Evans DL, et al. Factors influencing the epidemiology of *Helicobacter pylori* infection in children. Pediatrics 1991;88:578–82.
73. McCallion WA, Murray LJ, Bailie AG, et al. *Helicobacter pylori* infection in children: Relation with current household living conditions. Gut 1996;39:18–21.
74. Tindberg Y, Bengtsson C, Granath F, et al. *Helicobacter pylori* infection in Swedish school children: Lack of evidence of child-to-child transmission outside the family. Gastroenterology 2001;121:310–6.
75. Rowland M, Lambert I, Gormally S, et al. Carbon 13-labeled urea breath test for the diagnosis of *Helicobacter pylori* infection in children. J Pediatr 1997;131:815–20.
76. Goodman KJ, Correa P. *H. pylori* transmission among siblings. Lancet 1999;355:332–3.
77. Berkowicz J, Lee A. Person-to-person transmission of *Campylobacter pylori*. Lancet 1987;2:680–1.
78. Nwokolo CU, Bickley J, Attard AR, et al. Evidence of clonal variants of *Helicobacter pylori* in three generations of a duodenal ulcer disease family. Gut 1992;33:1323–7.
79. Simor AE, Shames B, Drumm B, et al. Typing of *Campylobacter pylori* by bacterial DNA restriction endonuclease analysis and determination of plasmid profile. J Clin Microbiol 1990;28:83–6.
80. Kivi M, Tindberg Y, Sorberg M, et al. Concordance of *Helicobacter pylori* strains within families. J Clin Microbiol 2003;41:5604–8.
81. Rothenbacher D, Winkler M, Gonser T, et al. Role of infected parents in transmission of *Helicobacter pylori* to their children. Pediatr Infect Dis J 2002;21:674–9.
82. Goodman KJ, Correa P, Tengana Aux HJ, et al. *Helicobacter pylori* infection in the Colombian Andes:

A population-based study of transmission pathways. Am J Epidemiol 1996;144:290–9.

83. Monteiro L, Bonnemaison D, Vekris A, et al. Complex polysaccharides as PCR inhibitors in feces: *Helicobacter pylori* model. J Clin Microbiol 1997;35:995–8.

84. van Zwet AA, Thijs JC, Kooistra-Smid AM, Schirm J, Snijder JA. Use of PCR with feces for detection of *Helicobacter pylori* infections in patients. J Clin Microbiol 1994;32:1346–8.

85. Thomas JE, Gibson GR, Darboe MK, et al. Isolation of *Helicobacter pylori* from human faeces. Lancet 1992;340: 1194–5.

86. Fox JG, Blanco MC, Yan L, et al. Role of gastric pH in isolation of *Helicobacter mustelae* from the feces of ferrets. Gastroenterology 1993;104:86–92.

87. Sobala GM, Crabtree JE, Dixon MF, et al. Acute *Helicobacter pylori* infection: Clinical features, local and systemic immune response, gastric mucosal histology, and gastric juice ascorbic acid concentrations. Gut 1991;32:1415–8.

88. Parsonnet J, Shmuely H, Haggerty T. Fecal and oral shedding of *Helicobacter pylori* from healthy infected adults. JAMA 1999;282:2240–5.

89. Graham DY, Osato MS. *H. pylori* in the pathogenesis of duodenal ulcer: Interaction between duodenal acid load, bile, and *H. pylori*. Am J Gastroenterol 2000;95:87–91.

90. Ferguson DA, Jr, Li C, Patel NR, et al. Isolation of *Helicobacter pylori* from saliva. J Clin Microbiol 1993;31:2802–4.

91. Krajden S, Fuksa M, Anderson J, et al. Examination of human stomach biopsies, saliva, and dental plaque for *Campylobacter pylori*. J Clin Microbiol 1989;27:1397–8.

92. Shames B, Krajden S, Fuksa M, et al. Evidence for the occurrence of the same strain of *Campylobacter pylori* in the stomach and dental plaque. J Clin Microbiol 1989;27: 2849–50.

93. Chong J, Marshall BJ, Barkin JS, et al. Occupational exposure to *Helicobacter pylori* for the endoscopy professional: A sera epidemiological study. Am J Gastroenterol 1994;89:1987–92.

94. Malaty HM, Evans DJ, Jr, Abramovitch K, et al. *Helicobacter pylori* infection in dental workers: A seroepidemiology study. Am J Gastroenterol 1992;87:1728–31.

95. Banatvala N, Abdi Y, Clements L, et al. *Helicobacter pylori* infection in dentists—a case-control study. Scand J Infect Dis 1995;27:149–51.

96. Leung WK, Siu KLK, Kwok CKL, et al. Isolation of *H. pylori* from vomitus in children and its implications in gastro–oral transmission. Am J Gastroenterol 1999;94:2881–4.

97. Solnick JV, Fong J, Hansen LM, et al. Acquisition of *Helicobacter pylori* infection in rhesus macaques is most consistent with oral–oral transmission. J Clin Microbiol 2006;44:3799–803.

98. Lu Y, Redlinger TE, Avitia R, et al. Isolation and genotyping of *Helicobacter pylori* from untreated municipal wastewater. Appl Environ Microbiol 2002;68:1436–9.

99. Hulten K, Han SW, Enroth H, et al. *Helicobacter pylori* in the drinking water in Peru. Gastroenterology 1996;110:1031–5.

100. Hulten K, Enroth H, Nystrom T, Engstrand L. Presence of *Helicobacter* species DNA in Swedish water. J Appl Microbiol 1998;85:282–6.

101. Horiuchi T, Ohkusa T, Watanabe M, et al. *Helicobacter pylori* DNA in drinking water in Japan. Microbiol Immunol 2001;45:515–9.

102. Baker KH, Hegarty JP, Redmond B, et al. Effect of oxidizing disinfectants (chlorine, monochloramine, and ozone) on *Helicobacter pylori*. Appl Environ Microbiol 2002;68:981–4.

103. Bunn JE, MacKay WG, Thomas JE, et al. Detection of *Helicobacter pylori* DNA in drinking water biofilms: Implications for transmission in early life. Lett Appl Microbiol 2002;34:450–4.

104. Forbes GM, Glaser ME, Cullen DJ, et al. Duodenal ulcer treated with *Helicobacter pylori* eradication: Seven-year follow-up. Lancet 1994;343:258–60.

105. Borody T, Andrews P, Mancuso N, et al. *Helicobacter pylori* reinfection 4 years post-eradication. Lancet 1992;339:1295.

106. Mitchell HM, Hu P, Chi Y, et al. A low rate of reinfection following effective therapy against *Helicobacter pylori* in a developing nation (China). Gastroenterology 1998;114:256–61.

107. Hildebrand P, Bardhan P, Rossi L, et al. Recrudescence and reinfection with *Helicobacter pylori* after eradication therapy in Bangladeshi adults. Gastroenterology 2001;121:792–8.

108. Bell GD, Powell KU. *Helicobacter pylori* reinfection after apparent eradication—the Ipswich experience. Scand J Gastroenterol Suppl 1996;215:96–104.

109. Okimoto T, Murakami K, Sato R, et al. Is the recurrence of *Helicobacter pylori* infection after eradication therapy resultant from recrudescence or reinfection, in Japan. Helicobacter 2003;8:186–91.

110. Gisbert JP, Luna M, Gomez B, et al. Recurrence of *Helicobacter pylori* infection after several eradication therapies: Long-term follow-up of 1000 patients. Aliment Pharmacol Ther 2006;23:713–9.

111. Gisbert JP, Olivares D, Jimenez I, Pajares JM. Long-term follow-up of ^{13}C-urea breath test results after *Helicobacter pylori* eradication: Frequency and significance of borderline delta^{13}CO$_2$ values. Aliment Pharmacol Ther 2006;23:275–80.

112. Gisbert JP, Pajares JM. Stool antigen test for the diagnosis of *Helicobacter pylori* infection: A systematic review. Helicobacter 2004;9:347–68.

113. Rowland M, Kumar D, Daly L, et al. Low rates of *Helicobacter pylori* reinfection in children. Gastroenterology 1999;117:336–41.

114. Feydt-Schmidt A, Kindermann A, Konstantopoulos N, et al. Reinfection rate in children after successful *Helicobacter pylori* eradication. Eur J Gastroenterol Hepatol 2002;14:1119–23.

115. Kato S, Abukawa D, Furuyama N, Iinuma K. *Helicobacter pylori* reinfection rates in children after eradication therapy. J Pediatr Gastroenterol Nutr 1998;27:543–6.

116. Magista AM, Ierardi E, Castellaneta S, et al. *Helicobacter pylori* status and symptom assessment two years after eradication in pediatric patients from a high prevalence area. J Pediatr Gastroenterol Nutr 2005;40:312–8.

117. Halitim F, Vincent P, Michaud L, et al. High rate of *Helicobacter pylori* reinfection in children and adolescents. Helicobacter 2006;11:168–72.

118. Clyne M, Drumm B. Cell envelope characteristics of *Helicobacter pylori*: Their role in adherence to mucosal surfaces and virulence. FEMS Immunol Med Microbiol 1996;16:141–55.

119. Eaton KA, Brooks CL, Morgan DR, Krakowka S. Essential role of urease in pathogenesis of gastritis induced by *Helicobacter pylori* in gnotobiotic piglets. Infect Immun 1991;59:2470–5.

120. Clyne M, Labigne A, Drumm B. *Helicobacter pylori* requires an acidic environment to survive in the presence of urea. Infect Immun 1995;63:1669–73.

121. Weeks DL, Eskandari S, Scott DR, Sachs G. A H+-gated urea channel: The link between *Helicobacter pylori* urease and gastric colonization. Science 2000;287:482–5.

122. Clyne M, Dolan B, Reeves EP. Bacterial factors that mediate colonization of the stomach and virulence of *Helicobacter pylori*. FEMS Microbiol Lett 2007;268:135–43.

123. Odenbreit S, Puls J, Sedlmaier B, et al. Translocation of *Helicobacter pylori* CagA into gastric epithelial cells by type IV secretion. Science 2000;287:1497–500.

124. Higashi H, Tsutsumi R, Fujita A, et al. Biological activity of the *Helicobacter pylori* virulence factor CagA is determined by variation in the tyrosine phosphorylation sites. Proc Natl Acad Sci U S A 2002;99:14428–33.

125. Lu H, Hsu PI, Graham DY, Yamaoka Y. Duodenal ulcer promoting gene of *Helicobacter pylori*. Gastroenterology 2005;128:833–48.

126. Fox JG, Beck P, Dangler CA, et al. Concurrent enteric helminth infection modulates inflammation and gastric immune responses and reduces *Helicobacter*-induced gastric atrophy. Nat Med 2000;6:536–42.

127. Graham DY, Alpert LC, Smith JL, Yoshimura HH. Iatrogenic *Campylobacter pylori* infection is a cause of epidemic achlorhydria. Am J Gastroenterol 1988;83:974–80.

128. Fox JG, Otto G, Taylor NS, et al. *Helicobacter mustelae*-induced gastritis and elevated gastric pH in the ferret (Mustela putorius furo). Infect Immun 1991;59:1875–80.

129. Fox JG, Paster BJ, Dewhirst FE, et al. *Helicobacter mustelae* isolation from feces of ferrets: Evidence to support fecal–oral transmission of a gastric *Helicobacter*. Infect Immun 1992;60:606–11.

130. Sawada M, Dickinson CJ. The G cell. Annu Rev Physiol 1997;59:273–98.

131. Moss SF, Legon S, Bishop AE, et al. Effect of *Helicobacter pylori* on gastric somatostatin in duodenal ulcer disease. Lancet 1992;340:930–2.

132. McGowan CC, Cover TL, Blaser MJ. *Helicobacter pylori* and gastric acid: Biological and therapeutic implications. Gastroenterology 1996;110:926–38.

133. McColl KE, el-Omar E, Gillen D. *Helicobacter pylori* gastritis and gastric physiology. Gastroenterol Clin North Am 2000;29:687–703, viii.

134. Gormally SM, Prakash N, Durnin MT, et al. Association of symptoms with *Helicobacter pylori* infection in children. J Pediatr 1995;126:753–6.

135. Apley J, Naish N. Recurrent abdominal pains: A field survey of 1,000 school children. Arch Dis Child 1958;33:165–70.

136. Nijevitch AA, Shcherbakov PL. *Helicobacter pylori* and gastrointestinal symptoms in school children in Russia. J Gastroenterol Hepatol 2004;19:490–6.

137. De Giacomo C, Valdambrini V, Lizzoli F, et al. A population-based survey on gastrointestinal tract symptoms and *Helicobacter pylori* infection in children and adolescents. Helicobacter 2002;7:356–63.

138. Kalach N, Mention K, Guimber D, et al. *Helicobacter pylori* infection is not associated with specific symptoms in nonulcer-dyspeptic children. Pediatrics 2005;115:17–21.

139. Macarthur C, Saunders N, Feldman W. *Helicobacter pylori*, gastroduodenal disease, and recurrent abdominal pain in children. JAMA 1995;273:729–34.

140. Bode G, Rothenbacher D, Brenner H, Adler G. *Helicobacter pylori* and abdominal symptoms: A population-based study among preschool children in southern Germany. Pediatrics 1998;101:634–7.

141. Nijevitch AA, Sataev VU, Vakhitov VA, et al. Childhood peptic ulcer in the Ural area of Russia: Clinical status and *Helicobacter pylori*-associated immune response. J Pediatr Gastroenterol Nutr 2001;33:558–64.

142. Drumm B, O'Brien A, Cutz E, Sherman P. *Campylobacter pyloridis*-associated primary gastritis in children. Pediatrics 1987;80:192–5.

143. Huang FC, Chang MH, Hsu HY, et al. Long-term follow-up of duodenal ulcer in children before and after eradication of *Helicobacter pylori*. J Pediatr Gastroenterol Nutr 1999;28:76–80.

144. Dufour C, Brisigotti M, Fabretti G, et al. *Helicobacter pylori* gastric infection and sideropenic refractory anemia. J Pediatr Gastroenterol Nutr 1993;17:225–7.

145. Barabino A, Dufour C, Marino CE, et al. Unexplained refractory iron-deficiency anemia associated with *Helicobacter pylori* gastric infection in children: Further clinical evidence. J Pediatr Gastroenterol Nutr 1999;28:116–9.

146. Marignani M, Angeletti S, Bordi C, et al. Reversal of long standing iron deficiency anaemia after eradication of *Helicobacter pylori*. Scand J Gastroenterol 1997;32:617–22.

147. Annibale B, Marignani M, Monarca B, et al. Reversal of iron deficiency anemia after *Helicobacter pylori* eradication in patients with asymptomatic gastritis. Ann Intern Med 1999;131:668–72.

148. Konno M, Muraoka S, Takahashi M, Imai T. Iron-deficiency anemia associated with *Helicobacter pylori* gastritis. J Pediatr Gastroenterol Nutr 2000;31:52–6.

149. Barabino A. *Helicobacter pylori*-related iron deficiency anemia: A review. Helicobacter 2002;7:71–5.

150. Capurso G, Lahner E, Marcheggiano A, et al. Involvement of the corporal mucosa and related changes in gastric acid secretion characterize patients with iron deficiency anaemia associated with *Helicobacter pylori* infection. Aliment Pharmacol Ther 2001;15:1753–61.

151. Squires RH, Jr, Colletti RB. Indications for pediatric gastrointestinal endoscopy: A medical position statement of the North American Society for Pediatric Gastroenterology and Nutrition. J Pediatr Gastroenterol Nutr 1996;23:107–10.

152. Hargrove CB, Ulshen MH, Shub MD. Upper gastrointestinal endoscopy in infants: Diagnostic usefulness and safety. Pediatrics 1984;74:828–31.

153. Miller V, Doig CM. Upper gastrointestinal tract endoscopy. Arch Dis Child 1984;59:1100–2.

154. Dooley CP, Larson AW, Stace NH, et al. Double-contrast barium meal and upper gastrointestinal endoscopy. A comparative study. Ann Intern Med 1984;101:538–45.

155. Genta RM, Robason GO, Graham DY. Simultaneous visualization of *Helicobacter pylori* and gastric morphology: A new stain. Hum Pathol 1994;25:221–6.

156. Siu LK, Leung WK, Cheng AF, et al. Evaluation of a selective transport medium for gastric biopsy specimens to be cultured for *Helicobacter pylori*. J Clin Microbiol 1998;36:3048–50.

157. Koletzko S. Noninvasive diagnostic tests for *Helicobacter pylori* infection in children. Can J Gastroenterol 2005;19:433–9.

158. Dzierzanowska-Fangrat K, Lehours P, Megraud F, Dzierzanowska D. Diagnosis of *Helicobacter pylori* infection. Helicobacter 2006;11:6–13.

159. Savarino V, Vigneri S, Celle G. The ^{13}C urea breath test in the diagnosis of *Helicobacter pylori* infection. Gut 1999;45: I18–22.

160. Imrie C, Rowland M, Bourke B, Drumm B. Limitations to carbon 13-labeled urea breath testing for *Helicobacter pylori* in infants. J Pediatr 2001;139:734–7.

161. Kindermann A, Demmelmair H, Koletzko B, et al. Influence of age of the ^{13}C-urea breath test results in children. J Pediatr Gastroenterol Nutr 2000;30:85–91.

162. Peng NJ, Lai KH, Liu RS, et al. Clinical significance of oral urease in diagnosis of *Helicobacter pylori* infection by [^{13}C]urea breath test. Dig Dis Sci 2001;46:1772–8.

163. Kabir S. Detection of *Helicobacter pylori* in faeces by culture, PCR and enzyme immunoassay. J Med Microbiol 2001;50:1021–9.

164. Manes G, Balzano A, Iaquinto G, et al. Accuracy of stool antigen test in posteradication assessment of *Helicobacter pylori* infection. Dig Dis Sci 2001;46:2440–4.

165. Koletzko S, Konsstantopoulos N, Bosman DK, et al. Evaluation of a novel monoclonal enzyme immunoassay for detection of *H. pylori* antigen in stool in children. Gut 2003;52:804–6.

166. Mitchell HM, Hazell SL, Kolesnikow T, et al. Antigen recognition during progression from acute to chronic infection with a cagA-positive strain of *Helicobacter pylori.* Infect Immun 1996;64:1166–72.

167. Russell RG, Wassermann SS, O'Donoghue JM, et al. Serologic response to *Helicobacter pylori* among children and teenagers in Northern Chile. Am J Trop Med Hyg 1993;49:189–91.

168. Raymond J, Kalach N, Bergeret M, et al. Evaluation of a serologic test for diagnosis of *Helicobacter pylori* infection in children. Eur J Clin Microbiol Infect Dis 1996;15:415–7.

169. Crabtree JE, Mahony MJ, Taylor JD, et al. Immune responses to *Helicobacter pylori* in children with recurrent abdominal pain. J Clin Pathol 1991;44:768–71.

170. Raymond J, Sauvestre C, Kalach N, et al. Evaluation of a new serologic test for diagnosis of *Helicobacter pylori* infection in children. Eur J Clin Microbiol Infect Dis 1999;18:192–8.

171. Everhart JE, Kruszon-Moran D, Perez-Perez G. Reliability of *Helicobacter pylori* and CagA serological assays. Clin Diagn Lab Immunol 2002;9:412–6.

172. NIH Consensus Development Panel. *Helicobacter pylori* in peptic ulcer disease. NIH Consensus Statement 1994;12:1–19.

173. Drumm B, Koletzko S, Oderda G. *Helicobacter pylori* infection in children: A consensus statement. J Pediatr Gastroenterol Nutr 2000;30:207–13.

174. Bourke B, Ceponis P, Chiba N, et al. Canadian Helicobacter Study Group Consensus Conference: Update on the approach to *Helicobacter pylori* infection in children and adolescents—an evidence-based evaluation. Can J Gastroenterol 2005;19:399–408.

175. Khurana R, Fischbach L, Chiba N, et al. Meta-analysis: *Helicobacter pylori* eradication treatment efficacy in children. Aliment Pharmacol Ther 2007;25:523–36.

176. Malfertheiner P, Megraud F, O'Morain C, et al. Current concepts in the management of *Helicobacter pylori* infection—the Maastricht 2-2000 Consensus Report. Aliment Pharmacol Ther 2002;16:167–80.

177. Gottrand F, Kalach N, Spyckerelle C, et al. Omeprazole combined with amoxicillin and clarithromycin in the eradication of *Helicobacter pylori* in children with gastritis: A prospective randomized double-blind trial. J Pediatr 2001;139:664–8.

178. Tiren U, Sandstedt B, Finkel Y. *Helicobacter pylori* gastritis in children: Efficacy of 2 weeks of treatment with clarithromycin, amoxicillin and omeprazole. Acta Paediatr 1999;88:166–8.

179. Oderda G, Rapa A, Bona G. A systematic review of *Helicobacter pylori* eradication treatment schedules in children. Aliment Pharmacol Ther 2000;14:59–66.

180. Oderda G, Marinello D, Lerro P, et al. Dual vs. triple therapy for childhood *Helicobacter pylori* gastritis: A double-blind randomized multicentre trial. Helicobacter 2004;9:293–301.

181. Graham DY, Lew GM, Malaty HM, et al. Factors influencing the eradication of *Helicobacter pylori* with triple therapy. Gastroenterology 1992;102:493–6.

182. Walsh D, Goggin N, Rowland M, et al. One week treatment for *Helicobacter pylori* infection. Arch Dis Child 1997;76:352–5.

183. Gisbert JP, Morena F. Systematic review and meta-analysis: Levofloxacin-based rescue regimens after *Helicobacter pylori* treatment failure. Aliment Pharmacol Ther 2006;23:35–44.

184. Nijevitch AA, Shcherbakov PL, Sataev VU, et al. *Helicobacter pylori* eradication in childhood after failure of initial treatment: Advantage of quadruple therapy with nifuratel to furazolidone. Aliment Pharmacol Ther 2005;22:881–7.

185. Israel DM, Hassall E. Omerprazole and other proton pump inhibitors: Pharmacology, efficacy, and safety, with special reference to use in children. J Pediatr Gastroenterol Nutr 1998;27:568–79.

186. Walters JK, Zimmermann AE, Souney PF, Katona BG. The use of omeprazole in the pediatric population. Ann Pharmacother 1998;32:478–81.

187. Richardson P, Hawkey CJ, Stack WA. Proton pump inhibitors. Pharmacology and rationale for use in gastrointestinal disorders. Drugs. 1998;56:307–35.

188. Kuipers EJ, Lundell L, Klinkenberg-Knol EC, et al. Atrophic gastritis and *Helicobacter pylori* infection in patients with reflux esophagitis treated with omeprazole or fundoplication. N Engl J Med 1996;334:1018–22.

189. Megraud F. *H. pylori* antibiotic resistance: Prevalence, importance, and advances in testing. Gut 2004;53:1374–84.

190. Glupczynski Y, Megraud F, Lopez-Brea M, Andersen LP. European multicentre survey of in vitro antimicrobial resistance in *Helicobacter pylori*. Eur J Clin Microbiol Infect Dis 2001;20:820–3.

191. McNulty C, Owen R, Tompkins D, et al. *Helicobacter pylori* susceptibility testing by disc diffusion. J Antimicrob Chemother 2002;49:601–9.

192. Raymond J, Kalach N, Bergeret M, et al. Effect of metronidazole resistance on bacterial eradication of *Helicobacter pylori* in infected children. Antimicrob Agents Chemother 1998;42:1334–5.

193. Bontems P, Devaster JM, Corvaglia L, et al. Twelve-year observation of primary and secondary antibiotic-resistant *Helicobacter pylori* strains in children. Pediatr Infect Dis J 2001;20:1033–8.

194. Koletzko S, Richy F, Bontems P, et al. Prospective multicentre study on antibiotic resistance of *Helicobacter pylori* strains obtained from children living in Europe. Gut 2006;55:1711–6.

9.2. Acid-Peptic Disease

Frédéric Gottrand, MD, PhD

The clinical spectrum of acid-peptic disease in children includes reflux esophagitis, gastric and duodenal peptic ulcer disease,[1] gastritis,[2] duodenitis, and rare entities such as Zollinger-Ellison syndrome. Several chapters of this textbook specifically address the pathogenesis, diagnosis, and treatment of some of these diseases (see Chapter 5, "Esophagitis" and Chapter 9.1, "Helicobacter pylori") that will not be considered further here. The purpose of this chapter is also to focus on the pharmacologic aspects of the principal drugs used for acid-peptic diseases, including the mechanism of action, pharmacokinetic and pharmacodynamic data, efficacy, and side effects based mainly on information available from studies on children.

Two major developments have been observed in the management of acid-related disorders during the last 20 years represented by proton pump inhibitors (PPIs) and Helicobacter pylori. PPIs irreversibly bind to the H^+-K^+ adenosine triphosphatase (ATPase) enzyme complex and extensively inhibit acid production, revolutionizing the management of acid-related diseases. H. pylori is the leading cause of primary peptic ulcer and chronic-active (type B) antral gastritis.[3] Eradication of this organism dramatically reduces the recurrence of gastric and duodenal ulcers both in adults and in children. These two factors have profoundly changed the natural history and epidemiology of acid-peptic disorders in adults, mainly gastroesophageal reflux and peptic ulcer diseases, as well as diagnostic tests and therapeutic strategies, demonstrated by a dramatic decrease in surgical indications for this group of diseases in humans.

PATHOPHYSIOLOGY

Gastritis, duodenitis, and peptic ulcer disease in childhood is the result of an imbalance between mucosal defensive and aggressive factors.[4] The degree of inflammation results in varying degrees of gastritis, duodenitis, mucosal erosion, or frank ulceration. These entities are closely related and often associated.

Acid Secretion

By 3 to 4 years of age, gastric acid secretion approximates adult values.[4-5] Stimulation of gastric acid secretion occurs via multiple pathways including neuroendocrine (acetylcholine and vagus nerve), endocrine (gastrin and pepsin), and paracrine (histamine) (Figure 1). Despite the tremendous number of studies published on mucosal ulceration in the stomach and duodenum, the precise role of acid secretion in ulcer and gastritis pathogenesis remains incompletely understood. Gastric ulcer is generally associated with lower acid secretion, while acid production is usually above normal in subjects with duodenal ulceration.[6-7] It has been postulated that gastritis and duodenitis also contribute to the natural history of ulcer development, due to decreased protection of the mucosal barrier lining the stomach and the duodenum, and increased epithelial cell exposure to hydrochloric acid. Data on acid secretion in children are limited and old,[8] and their interpretations complicated by the considerable overlap in acid secretion between children with and without ulcers.[9] In H. pylori infection, several studies demonstrate that levels of serum pepsinogen I (and at a lesser degree pepsinogen II) are elevated, reflecting antral inflammation.[10-11] The expression of gastrin is increased in children with chronic gastritis and duodenal ulcer.[12]

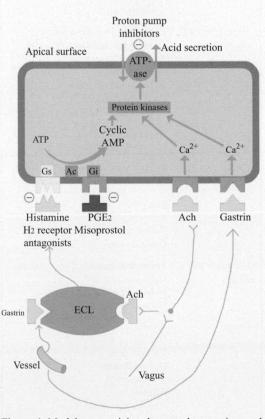

Figure 1 Model summarizing the neural, paracrine, and hormonal regulation of gastric acid secretion. The sites of action of the main antisecretory drugs are shown. Ach: acetylcholine, PGE2: prostaglandin E2, ECL: enterochromaffin-like cells.

Bicarbonate–Mucus Barrier and Mucosal Defense

Disturbances in bicarbonate secretion and the mucus layer overlining gastric and duodenal epithelia are also involved in the pathogenesis of acid-peptic diseases.[4] The mucus layer serves as a barrier to luminal pepsin and hydrochloric acid,[13] preventing access of pepsin to the apical surface of the epithelial cells and neutralizing acid through the presence of bicarbonate secreted into the mucus layer. In the recent years, there have been striking findings regarding trefoil factor peptides, which increase the barrier properties of the preepithelial mucus gel.[14] While prostaglandins stimulate the mucosal production of bicarbonate, nonsteroidal anti-inflammatory drugs (NSAIDs) inhibit bicarbonate secretion. Other host defenses involved in cytoprotection include mucosal blood flow, rapid cell turnover, surface-active hydrophobic phospholipids present in the mucus layer and on the apical membrane of surface epithelial cells, and epidermal growth factor.

Mediators of the Mucosal Inflammation

A number of mediators of mucosal inflammation, which play a role in the development of gastritis and ulcer disease, have been identified. These include platelet-activating factor, cachectin, leukotrienes, free oxygen radicals, lymphokines, and monokines. The relative contribution and role of each of these pro-inflammatory mediators remain to be clarified, specifically in children and could well vary according to the causative agent.

Aggressive Factors

Normal host defenses are continuously confronted by a number of aggressive factors. Many of them are present in the lumen as substances necessary to the normal process of digestion: acid, pepsins, and bile acids. In certain circumstances, they may cause mucosal inflammation. Other factors are exogenous including caustic substances, alcohol, and NSAIDs.

GASTRIC AND DUODENAL ULCER DISEASE

H. pylori infection is now well recognized as a major factor in the development of duodenal ulcers both in adults and in children.[15] In a systematic review of 45 studies published from 1983 to 1994, the prevalence of H. pylori infection in children with duodenal ulcer was high (range, 33 to 100%; median, 92%) compared with children with gastric ulcer (range, 11 to 75%; median, 25%).[15] Epidemiological studies have shown a higher *H. pylori* infection rate in children from developing countries, compared with developed countries;[16] Moreover, with the improved economy in the developed world, the incidence of *H. pylori* infection in children is expected to decrease further. It is postulated, therefore, that the relative number of non-*H. pylori*-related duodenal ulcer diseases will increase. Indeed, recent data suggest that up to 20% of duodenal ulcers in adults have no identified etiology.[17–18] Comparable data in children are limited.[19–20]

Epidemiology

Peptic ulcer disease is a rare feature in childhood and data specifically addressing the issue of its prevalence are scare and mainly arise from small retrospective studies.[19] In spite of a high prevalence of *H. pylori* infection worldwide, the incidence of duodenal ulcer disease in children is low.[20–23] In large medical centers, the incidence of duodenal ulceration in children was estimated at 1 case per 2,500 hospital admissions.[23] Other studies suggest an average of 1 to 6 new cases/hospital/year.[24] In a retrospective review of 112 Taiwanese children undergoing upper GI endoscopy for upper GI bleeding, gastric ulcer was reported in 10%, duodenal ulcer in 15%, and erosive duodenitis in 3%.[25] From 1993 to 2002, 24 Saudi Arabian children of 521 (5%) who presented with upper gastrointestinal tract symptoms were diagnosed by endoscopy to have peptic ulcer disease and 87% were *H. pylori* positive.[26] In another report from Brazil, 15% of symptomatic children had duodenal ulcer; all were *H. pylori* positive.[27] Similar results were reported from Russia where 24% of 129 pediatric outpatients undergoing gastroduodenal endoscopy for evaluation of chronic abdominal pain had a duodenal ulcer (all were *H. pylori* positive).[28] In children, the prevalence of non-*H. pylori*, non-NSAIDs duodenal ulceration is not known. In a retrospective analysis of 622 endoscopic procedures from the United States, mucosal ulceration of the stomach or duodenum was identified in 11 children (1.7%).[19] None of the 11 reported the use of NSAIDs, and only 3 of the children (all with duodenal ulcers) were *H. pylori* positive. Duodenal or gastric ulcer was found in 8/324 (2.5%) of children undergoing upper GI endoscopy in Turkey; 2 of them were *H. pylori* negative.[29] In another retrospective study of 2,550 children undergoing endoscopy in Greece, peptic ulcer was diagnosed in 2% of the patients;[30] 8/10 children with gastric ulcer and 15/42 children with duodenal ulcer were *H. pylori* negative. Taken together, these data suggest that, at least in developed countries, *H. pylori* is no longer the major cause of gastric and duodenal ulcer disease in children, and that other factors likely are responsible for their development.[31]

Causes. Since the discovery of *H. pylori* in 1983, duodenal ulcer disease in humans has been categorized as either *H. pylori* positive or *H. pylori* negative. In children with non-*H. pylori* gastric and duodenal ulcers, the etiology for the development of ulcer disease is not established. Previously, investigators used to categorize peptic ulcer disease into primary and secondary conditions.[32] From a clinical perspective, however, it might be more convenient to classify peptic ulcer disease according to its physiopathology (Table 1). Although the list of possible causes is long, several etiological factors are the most frequent. These include drugs (NSAIDs and corticosteroids), chronic diseases (Crohn's disease), and stress situations.

Primary Ulcer Peptic Disease. While genetic and psychological factors probably play a role,[33] primary peptic ulcer disease remains unexplained.

Table 1 Causes of Acid-Peptic Disease in Children

Mechanism	Etiology
Unknown	Primary peptic ulcer disease
Infectious	Primary gastritis
	– *Helicobacter pylori*
	– *Helicobacter heilmanii*
	– Cytomegalovirus
	– Herpes simplex
	– Influenza A
	– *Treponema pallidum*
	– *Candida albicans*
	– Histoplasmosis
	– Mucormycosis
	– Anisakiasis
Hypersecretory states	Zollinger-Ellison syndrome
	G-cell hyperplasia/hyperfunction
	Systemic mastocytosis
	Cystic fibrosis
	Hyperparathyroidism
	Short bowel syndrome
	Renal failure
Stress	ICU, multiple trauma, neurosurgery
	Hepatic insufficiency/cirrhosis
Granulomatous	Foreign body reaction
	Idiopathic
	Sarcoidosis
	Histiocytosis X
	Tuberculosis
	Crohn disease
Immunologic/allergy	Eosinophilic gastritis/allergic gastritis
	Graft-versus-host disease
	Henoch-Schönlein gastritis
	Celiac disease
Drugs	Aspirin
	NSAIDs
	Valproic acid
	Dexamethasone
	Chemotherapy
	Alcohol
	Potassium chloride
Physical agents	Corrosives
	Bile acid gastropathy
	Exercise induced
	Radiation gastropathy

It is possible that acid hypersecretion may be one factor in some children[8] but is far from a constant feature.

Hypersecretory States. Zollinger-Ellison syndrome and antral G-cell hyperplasia are rare in children.[34–36] These diagnoses should be suspected in severe or recurrent duodenal and gastric ulcers, resistance to PPI treatment, or multiple location of ulcerations (or recurrence in different locations). A family history of ulcers and a history of endocrine diseases are common in these diseases.[37] In Zollinger-Ellison syndrome, a high basal level of gastrinemia (usually >1,000 ng/L) or after pentagastrin stimulation is always found. Other biological markers include high plasma level of chromatogranin A. Calcium, parathyroid hormone, and prolactin are assessed in the plasma to detect other MEN-1 tumors. Radiologic imaging is required to detect the site of primary tumor or metastasis. Computerized tomography, magnetic resonance imaging, radionucleotide octreotide scanning, ultrasound, echoendoscopy, and selective arterial secretin testing are recommended, but over 50% of gastrinomas still are not visualized by preoperative imaging. The location of these gastrinomas is typically in the pancreas, but they may also occur in the stomach and the duodenum. Patients with multiple endocrine neoplasias type 1 (MEN-I) and Zollinger-Ellison syndrome may become symptomatic in childhood. High dosage of PPIs (60 to 80 mg/d or more) is required for acid suppression and symptom relief prior to surgical ablation. A precise preoperative localization of all pancreaticoduodenal lesions, in combination with a surgical exploration and management by experienced surgeons, is curative in patients without distal metastases.[36–37] Antral G-cell hyperplasia is characterized by hyperchlorhydria and an exaggerated postprandial gastrin response, but no response to secretin stimulation.[32,38] It may respond to surgical antrectomy or long-term, high-dosage PPI therapy. Other conditions associated with acid hypersecretion include systemic mastocytosis,[39] short bowel syndrome for the first year after surgical resection,[40] hyperparathyroidism,[41–42] renal failure,[43–44] and cystic fibrosis[45] (Table 1).

Stress-Related Ulcer. The overall prevalence of stress-induced gastritis and ulcers in children is not known.[46] Twenty percent of infants treated in the neonatal intensive care unit have signs of gastrointestinal tract bleeding, with mechanical ventilation being an identified risk factor.[47] In a prospective endoscopic study of mechanically ventilated infants, 53% had remarkable gastric mucosa lesions.[47] A study of stress ulcer prophylaxis showed that nasogastric administration of a PPI suspension had variable efficacy in critically ill children.[48] Half of the study subjects required either dose titrations to achieve adequate gastric acid suppression or did not respond to nasogastric administration of the PPI.[48] Causes of stress-related ulcer in children are similar to those of adults and have been reported in critically ill neonates,[47] after cardiac surgery,[49] organ transplantation,[50] burns, and neurosurgery.

Drug-Induced Ulcers. Numerous pharmacologic agents are noxious to the gastroduodenal mucosa, causing mucosal inflammation and ulceration. The most common, and potentially underdiagnosed, are injuries to the gastroduodenal mucosa caused by NSAIDs. Peptic ulcers are clearly demonstrated in *H. pylori*-negative children receiving NSAIDs for rheumatologic disorders.[51] Acetylsalicylic acid, even at low doses used for antiplatelet therapy in cardiovascular disorders, induces either bleeding ulcers or gastric erosions.[52] Acetylsalicylic acid mediates injury to the gastric and duodenal mucosa via a number of pathophysiological mechanisms including decreasing gastric epithelial cell apical surface pH, modulation of the constituents of the gastric mucus, and decreasing bicarbonate secretion. NSAIDs also increase platelet-activating factor, induce platelet dysfunction, inhibit prostaglandin synthesis, and increase mucosal capillary damage. Due to the decreasing use of acetylsalicylic acid and increasing use of ibuprofen for treatment of fever in children in many countries, the latter probably has become a leading cause of drug-induced gastroduodenal mucosal lesions in children.[53]

Crohn's Disease. (See Chapter 20.5a, "Crohn's Disease"). Gastritis and gastric mucosal ulceration are found in 25 to 40% of children and adults with Crohn's disease. Upper gastrointestinal symptoms are commonly reported in these patients.[54] Upper gastrointestinal endoscopic biopsies can show histological abnormalities in Crohn's disease. In one study, gastritis was demonstrated in 92%, duodenitis in 33%, and a granuloma was present in the proximal GI tract in 40% of children with Crohn's disease.[54] However, presence of gastroduodenal inflammation does not ensure the diagnosis of Crohn's disease since chronic active gastritis and duodenitis can be found in ulcerative colitis.[54]

Diagnosis, Endoscopic Findings

Mucosal ulceration is strictly defined as a mucosal crater that can be deep and involves the mucosa, with an inflamed edge (Figure 2). An erosion is defined as a small (<3 mm), superficial defect in the mucosa that does not penetrate beyond the muscularis mucosa, of a white or yellow color. Peptic ulceration of the stomach or duodenum is almost always accompanied by abnormalities of the gastric mucosa, either a gastritis or a gastropathy.[32] Most gastric ulcers are located on the lesser curvature of the stomach. More than 90% of the duodenal ulcers are found in the duodenal bulb. Upper gastrointestinal contrast studies have very poor accuracy for the diagnosis of ulcer disease and are only indicated in cases of suspected postulcer pyloric stenosis.[55] Fiberoptic endoscopy with biopsies is the first-line procedure when acid-peptic disease is suspected in a child. Endoscopy allows

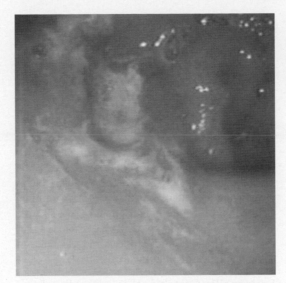

Figure 2 Endoscopic view showing a prepyloric ulcer.

confirmation of the diagnosis, precise definition of the topography and type of lesion, gives prognosis information (eg, the risk of bleeding), information about etiology (nodules of the antrum suggestive of *H. pylori* infection), and elimination of other conditions in the differential diagnosis (eg, Mallory Weiss tear, esophagitis). Endoscopic signs indicating an increased risk of rebleeding were classified in 1974 by Forrest and colleagues (Table 2).[56] Multiple biopsies of the stomach and duodenum should be carefully examined by an experimented pathologist for the possibility of *H. pylori* infection, Crohn disease, or other rare conditions (eg, mastocytosis, *H. helmanii*).

Clinical Presentations

Presenting symptoms and signs include abdominal pain, vomiting, hematemesis, early satiety, anemia, and weight loss. Abdominal pain is the most common presenting symptom of peptic ulcer disease (Table 3). Nevertheless, acid-peptic diseases account for fewer than 5% of children presenting with nonspecific abdominal pain, even in a subspeciality practice.[32] Symptoms of peptic disorders are similar to those seen in adults in children aged more than 8 years, including epigastric pain or discomfort that is meal exacerbated or awakens the child from sleep. Younger children may not be able to localize the pain to the epigastrium and may present with nonspecific anorexia and irritability. Up to

Table 3 Alarm Features Associated with Ulcer Disease and Gastritis in Children

- Epigastric location
- Epigastric tenderness
- Nocturnal pain
- Meal exacerbation
- Early satiety
- Weight loss
- Recurrent vomiting
- Gastrointestinal bleeding,
- Iron deficiency, anemia

25% of children with a duodenal ulcer have a silent presentation with painless upper GI bleeding or iron deficiency anemia.[32]

Complications

Bleeding, perforation, and gastric outlet obstruction are the three main complications of peptic ulcer disease. When severe bleeding occurs and medical treatment (eg, proton pump inhibitors) fails to control bleeding, interventional endoscopy is required. Several techniques (eg, saline or norepinephrine injection, heatprobe, yag laser) have been described.[57] With highly effective acid-suppression medications, operations for peptic disease (eg, vagotomy, antrectomy) have become virtually obsolete.[38,57] Current indications for surgery in peptic disease are perforation of the stomach or duodenum,[38,58–59] active bleeding that cannot be controlled by medical management or endoscopic hemostasis,[60] gastric outlet or duodenal obstruction caused by scarring,[55,61] or the failure of medical treatment in hypersecretory syndromes.[32,36]

GASTRITIS

Gastritis excluding non-peptic acid gastritis and gastropathy that are addressed in the following Chapter 9.3, "Other Causes of Gastritis." There are no accurate figures related to the incidence of gastritis in children. As for ulcer disease, *H. pylori* is probably not the major cause of gastritis. Indeed, in the same systematic review of the 45 studies published from 1983 to 1994 mentioned above, the rate ratio of antral gastritis in children with *H. pylori* infection (compared with uninfected children) ranged from 1.9 to 71.0 (median, 4.6), much lower than for duodenal ulcer and either gastric ulcer.[15] In a recent prospective study of 100 children referred to upper GI endoscopy

Table 2 Risk of Rebleeding According to the Endoscopic Features of Ulcer

Forrest Class	Type of Lesions	Risk of Rebleeding If Untreated (%)
IA	Arterial spurting bleeding	100
IB	Arterial oozing bleeding	55 (17 to 100)
IIA	Visible vessel	43 (8 to 81)
IIB	Sentinel clot	22 (14 to 36)
IIC	Hematin-covered flat spot	10 (0 to 13)
III	No stigmata of hemorrhage	5 (0 to 10)

Adapted from Forest et al[56]

for symptoms of dyspepsia, 79% of them presented with gastritis (none had ulcer disease), of whom only 33% had *H. pylori* infection.[62]

Diagnosis, Endoscopic Findings

Gastritis is defined as microscopic evidence of inflammation affecting the gastric mucosa. Endoscopical aspect of gastritis may vary from normal to erythema, edema, friability, exudate, erosion, atrophy, vascular pattern, and nodularity. However, there is no correlation between endoscopical findings and histological lesions, highlighting the need for multiple and good quality biopsies taken from both the antrum and fundus.[2] The pathological diagnosis of gastritis is often not clear-cut, because there are normally a few chronic inflammatory cells present in the lamina propria. Mild mucosal inflammation may be difficult to distinguish from normal and requires review by an experienced pathologist. Moreover, there are no universally accepted criteria to characterize the presence and severity of gastritis. Gastritis can be divided as active (presence of polymorphonuclear leukocytes), chronic (presence of chronic inflammatory cells without polymorphonuclear leukocytes), chronic-active (increased number of both acute and chronic inflammatory cells), atrophic (loss of gastric glands), and intestinal metaplasia. The updated Sydney system is currently the most widely accepted classification for gastritis even in children.[63] It was, however, established to recognize the importance of *H. pylori* in causing gastritis in adults and includes both endoscopic appearance and histologic findings. The morphology of gastritis is described according to graded variables (mild, moderate, and severe) allowing for standardization among different pathologists and for comparisons between studies.

Causes

See Table 1.

Drug-Induced. In a primary care prospective study, the risk of hospitalization with gastrointestinal bleeding among children receiving short-term treatment with ibuprofen for fever was 17 per 100,000 (95% confidence interval and 3.5 to 49 per 100,000).[64] In another study of 702 patients with juvenile rheumatoid arthritis, mild gastrointestinal disturbances were frequent side effects associated with NSAID therapy, but the number of children ($n = 10$) who experienced clinically significant gastritis was low.[65] In children with juvenile rheumatoid arthritis treated with NSAIDs, epigastric pain strongly correlates with documented gastroduodenal injury. More than 75% of children referred for gastrointestinal symptoms have gastritis, antral erosions, or peptic ulcers. Chemical gastropathy, also known as chemical or reactive gastritis, is characterized by presence of foveolar hyperplasia, vascular congestion, lamina propria edema, and prominent smooth muscle fibers in the absence of inflammatory cells in the gastric antral mucosa. It has been described in children taking NSAIDs.[66]

Stress Gastritis. Many clinical conditions—mainly acutely ill patients with severe stress—are associated with stress gastritis (Table 1). Although abdominal pain is a common presenting feature, up to 75% remain clinically asymptomatic and are revealed by either hematemesis or melena.

Bile Reflux. Duodenogastric reflux of bile has been suggested as a possible cause of gastritis. Except for rare circumstances, such as partial gastrectomy or biliary reconstruction after excision of choledocal cyst, where its etiological role is clearly demonstrated,[67] its occurrence in children is unknown.[68] Pathological changes are specific and include foveolar hyperplasia, edema, vasodilatation in the lamina propria, and a paucity of acute and chronic inflammatory cells.

Eosinophilic Gastritis. It is a rare disorder of unknown etiology that is characterized by an intense eosinophilic infiltration of the gastric mucosa. Often accompanied by a peripheral eosinophilia, it can involve the stomach alone or together with more distal intestinal inflammation (eosinophilic gastroenteritis). Vomiting, abdominal pain, and weight loss are the major presenting features and can be associated with a protein-losing enteropathy responsible for hypoproteinemia and edema.

Ménétrier's Disease. It is a rare condition of unknown etiology characterized by giant hypertrophy of the mucosal folds in the stomach. Vomiting, abdominal pain, anorexia, and edema secondary to the protein loss from the stomach are the most common presenting features. Cytomegalovirus has been implicated in several children.[69–70]

Varioliform Gastritis. Although suggested to have an allergic basis, the underlying cause of varioliform gastritis is unknown. Chronic diffuse varioliform gastritis is an uncommon, subacute, inflammatory gastric mucosal disease characterized by swollen congested rugae, and disseminated mucosal erosions. The entity is exceptionally rare in children.[2]

Lymphocytic Gastritis. It is defined by the recognition of >25 intraepithelial lymphocytes per 100 surface epithelial cells. Approximately 50% of children with untreated celiac disease have lymphocytic gastritis, which mainly involves the gastric antrum and disappears after the introduction of a gluten-free diet.[71] Endoscopic appearance can be either normal or, rarely, suggestive of varioliform gastritis. Dyspeptic symptoms are frequent.

Gastric and Duodenal Anomalies. These are frequently observed in portal hypertension. While gastropathy is mainly related to portal hypertension per se, gastritis is strongly associated with cirrhosis.[72] The prevalence of duodenal ulcer is also increased in children with portal hypertension, independent of the severity of liver disease, *H. pylori* infection, and serum gastrin levels.[73] In addition to esophageal varices, gastric and duodenal pathologies are responsible for episodes of gastrointestinal bleeding.

Atrophic Gastritis

This is a new and controversial area of interest in children.[74] Atrophy is defined as the loss of normal glandular components, including replacement with fibrosis, intestinal metaplasia (IM), and/or pseudopyloric metaplasia of the corpus (identified by the presence of pepsinogen I in mucosa). *H. pylori*-associated gastric cancer arises via a multistage process, with atrophic gastritis being the precursor lesion. Little is known regarding the prevalence of atrophic gastritis in childhood. In a recent study from Korea and Colombia, atrophic gastritis was demonstrated in 16% of 173 children undergoing endoscopy.[75] In this study, all the children with gastric atrophy were *H. pylori* infected. Atrophic gastritis has been occasionally reported in children without *H. pylori* infection[74] (Figure 3). Autoimmune gastritis is a cause of atrophic gastritis, characterized by the presence of systemic autoantibodies directed against either gastric parietal cells or gastrin-producing cells in the antrum of the stomach.[76] The association of autoimmune gastritis with intrinsic factor antibodies, achlorhydria, and pernicious anemia (cobalamin malabsorption) is rare in children.

DUODENITIS

Duodenitis is characterized by the presence of neutrophils in the lamina propria, crypts, or surface epithelium in addition to an increase in the number of mononuclear cells. Duodenitis can be graded from mild to severe depending on the number of neutrophils present. Since histopathological features of duodenitis are the same as those of mucosa bordering a duodenal ulcer, duodenitis and duodenal ulcer are considered to be a different spectrum of the same disease. Gastric metaplasia of the duodenum is an important factor in the pathogenesis of duodenal disease, especially in duodenal ulcer associated with *H. pylori*. At endoscopy, the diagnostic signs include mucosal edema, erythema, erosions, and

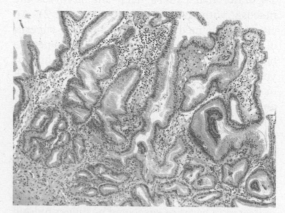

Figure 3 Severe atrophic gastritis associated with foveolar hyperplasia in a child with chronic graft-versus-host reaction (hematoxylin-eosin staining X10). (Courtesy of Pr F Boman.)

friability. The radiological signs of duodenitis at upper GI examination include mucosal-fold thickening, nodularity, and ulceration. Although duodenitis occurs in many diseases (Table 1), Henoch-Schönlein purpura should be considered in acute onset, nonspecific duodenitis in previously healthy children, even in the absence of skin findings.[77]

PROTON PUMP INHIBITORS

PPIs (omeprazole, lansoprazole, pantoprazole, rabeprazole, and esomeprazole) inhibit gastric acid secretion by selectively acting on gastric parietal cell H^+-K^+ ATPase, which is the enzyme involved in the last step of acid secretion by parietal cells (Figure 5).

In contrast to histamine 2 (H_2)-receptor antagonists, inhibition of gastric acid secretion by PPIs is independent of the pathway of stimulation. PPIs are highly selective and effective in their action and have relatively few short- and long-term adverse effects. These pharmacologic features have made the development of PPIs the most significant advancement in the management of acid-peptic–related disorders in the last two decades. Although numerous adult studies have been published, there are still few large studies with significant patients enrolled and no randomized controlled comparative studies in childhood.[78] It should be emphasized that few clinical or pharmacologic data are available in infants under 1 year of age.[79–80] Although several different PPIs are available on the market (Figure 4), omeprazole and lansoprazole are the two that have been the most extensively studied in childhood.

Mode of Action

PPIs form a group of compounds called substituted benzimidazoles, which concentrate within the intracellular canaliculi of parietal cells, irreversibly bind to the H^+-K^+ ATPase enzyme complex, and extensively inhibit acid production. PPIs differ from each other by the molecular structures bound to the pyridine and benzimidazole components of the molecule (Figure 5).[81] This explains differences in pharmacologic properties, but all of the PPIs have the same mechanism of action. Because they are weakly basic compounds (the pKa value of the pyridine nitrogen being close to 4.0), they are maximally protonated in environments of high acidity (which is exclusively found in the intracellular canaliculi of actively secreting parietal cells and within the stomach cavity). PPIs can be considered pro-drugs, because in highly acidic environment, protonation of the molecule results in a series of reactions that ultimately produces the active form of the PPI (Figure 5).[81] The active cyclic sulfenamide then binds permanently to exposed cysteine thiol groups on the luminal surface of the H^+-K^+ ATPase enzyme. Once covalently bound, the H^+-K^+ ATPase enzyme becomes nonfunctional, and activity returns only by parietal cell synthesis of new H^+-K^+ ATPase

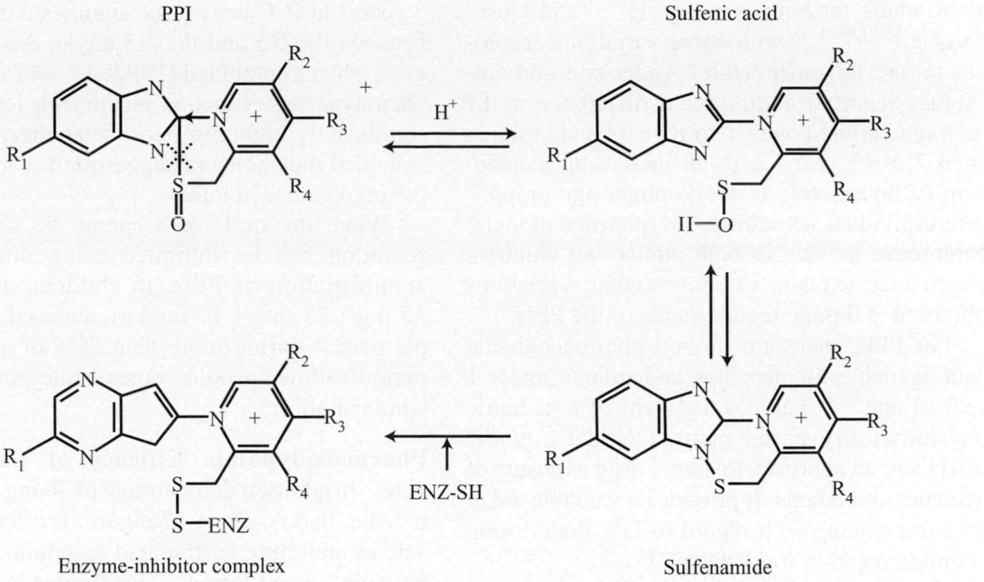

enzyme systems. The turnover of the H^+-K^+ ATPase is constant, with a half-life of about 48 hours in adults. The maturation of turnover is unknown in infants and children. The best access of the drug to the H^+-K^+ ATPase situated on the luminal side of the secretory membrane of the gastric parietal cells is provided by a meal, which is the strongest physiologic event inducing the exteriorization of the H^+-K^+ ATPase.

Given orally, PPIs can be prematurely converted to the active form in the acidic environment of the stomach. Therefore, they are prepared as capsules containing protective enteric-coated granules or as enteric-coated tablets. In these forms, absorption begins only in the higher-pH environment of the duodenum, and they are almost completely absorbed in the small intestine.[81]

Pharmacokinetic Properties

Most of the data on the pharmacokinetics of PPIs were obtained in adult volunteers and adult patients with peptic ulcer disease. However, some studies have provided information regarding the pharmacokinetics for omeprazole and lansoprazole in children.[79–80,82–84] Data are lacking on rabeprazole in children; some data have more recently been published on pantoprazole and esomeprazole.[85-87]

PPIs are metabolized by the hepatocyte cytochrome P-450 isoforms CYP2C19 and CYP3A4 to inactive metabolites (sulfide, sulfone, and hydroxymetabolites) excreted in urine. A comprehensive comparative review on the pharmacokinetics of omeprazole, lansoprazole, pantoprazole, and rabeprazole has been published on adults.[81] Schematically, the drugs are quickly absorbed (T_{max} = 1 to 3 h), with bioavailability varying between them (omeprazole 35 to 65%, lansoprazole 80 to 91%, and pantoprazole 57 to 100%). They are rapidly metabolized (half-time [T1] = 2; 0.6 to 2 h). The antisecretory effect of PPIs is independent of plasma concentration, but correlates with the area under the plasma concentration time curve (AUC).[88]

In older children and adolescents, pharmacokinetic parameters are in roughly the same range

Figure 4 Mechanism of action of antisecretory drugs. ATPase: adenosine triphosphatase, PPI: proton pump inhibitor.

	R_1	R_2	R_3	R_4
Omeprazole/Esomeprazole	CH_3O	CH_3	CH_3O	CH_3
Lansoprazole	H	H	CH_3F_2O	CH_3
Pantoprazole	CF_2HO	H	CH_3O	CH_3O
Rabeprazole	H	H	$CH_3O(CH_2)_3O$	CH_3

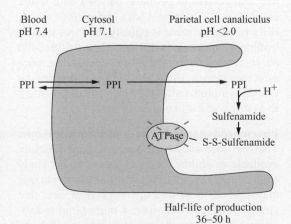

Blood
pH 7.4

Cytosol
pH 7.1

Parietal cell canaliculus
pH <2.0

Sulfenamide

S-S-Sulfenamide

Half-life of production
36–50 h

Figure 5 Chemical formula of proton pump inhibitor (PPIs) and the mechanisms of action of enzyme (H^+-K^+ adenosine triphosphatase inhibitor complex) formation. (Reproduced from Gibbons, Gold.[78])

as in adults for both omeprazole[89,90] and lansoprazole,[83–84,88,91–93] with some variations according to age for omeprazole. Andersson and colleagues reported a significant difference in T1 between children aged 1 to 6 years and children aged 7 to 12 years, with an increasing metabolism of omeprazole in the younger-age group.[90] Interindividual variability of pharmacokinetic parameters is wide in both adults and children, which may explain, to some extent, variations observed in dosage requirements of the PPIs.

For PPIs, there are limited pharmacokinetic data available for neonates and infants under 1 year of age.[79,94] The development of a pediatric physiologically based pharmacokinetic model offers a good approach to assess drug exposure of neonates and infants. It provides a valuable aid to decision making with regard to first-time dosing in children and in study design.[95]

Pharmacokinetic parameters in children may be affected, as in adults, by genetic variability of the enzyme systems.[96] Indeed, CYP2C19 displays a known genetic polymorphism,[97] and differences in pantoprazole, omeprazole, and lansoprazole disposition have been demonstrated with an AUC that is fivefold higher in poor metabolizers than in extensive metabolizers. Clinically, poor metabolizers (a poor metabolizer phenotype occurs in 1% of Blacks, 2 to 6% of Whites, 15% of Chinese, and 23% of Japanese) experience superior acid suppression (with omeprazole and lansoprazole) compared with extensive metabolizers, without an increase in the incidence of adverse effects.[81] Thus far, there is no toxicity issue that warrants a dosage adjustment of PPIs in poor metabolizers.

Other maturation factors may also affect the metabolism of PPIs, such as the rate of renewal of the proton pumps in the parietal cell. In patients with hepatic impairment, AUC values increased to the same extent as observed in poor metabolizers, with no need to adjust the dosage: nevertheless caution should be exercised when giving PPIs to patients with severe hepatic insufficiency.[98] No dosage adjustment of PPIs is required in patients with renal insufficiency or for those on hemodialysis.[99]

Pharmacodynamic Properties

Pharmacodynamic Efficacy of Omepra-zole. Omeprazole is available for oral and in many countries intravenous administration. Oral clearance and apparent volume of distribution in adults are not different than in children (mean age 6 years).[82] In children, most data were obtained after oral administration, and a mean daily dose of 1 mg/kg body weight is required to obtain a sustained efficacy over 24 hours.[82] However, in a multicenter study of children aged 1 to 16 years, using esophageal pH monitoring below a pH of <4 for less than 6% of a 24-hour period, the healing dosage varied from 0.7 to 3.5 mg/kg/d. Overall, in this study, more than 75% of the patients required 1.4 mg/kg as the healing dosage.[90] The pharmacokinetics of omeprazole have been recently studied in children less than

2 years old.[79] There was no significant difference between the 0.5 and the 1.5 mg/kg doses. However, when a combined CYP2C19- and CYP3A4-phenotype was estimated, omeprazole levels were significantly higher in poor metabolizers than in extended metabolizers suggesting the use of the 0.5 mg/kg dose in infants.[79]

When the oral route cannot be used, acid secretion can be inhibited using intravenous administration of PPIs. In children, a dose of 40 mg/1.73 m^2 (1.17 mg/kg) achieved a gastric pH over 4 during more than 90% of a 24-hour period following bolus omeprazole intravenous administration.[89]

Pharmacodynamic Efficacy of Lansopra-zole. In adults, a daily dosage of 30 mg of lansoprazole, that is, about 17 mg/m^2, is effective and safe in inhibiting gastric acid secretion and healing acid-related lesions. This dosage has proven effective in numerous randomized double-blind trials and is recommended for the treatment of duodenal ulcer and reflux esophagitis in adults. In children, as for omeprazole, the efficacy of lansoprazole on gastric acid secretion studied by gastric pH monitoring varies widely among the patients studied: about 40% of children respond to a dose of 0.73 mg/kg (equivalent to the adult dose, ie, 17 mg/m^2), 26% responded to 1.44 mg/kg, but 35% failed to respond to this doubled dose.[88] This variability can be ascribed, in part, to differences in pharmacokinetics: the AUC of lansoprazole shows a significant positive correlation with gastric acid inhibition. Failure to respond to the lower dose may be ascribed to reduced bioavailability and faster metabolism of the drug. Patients with these characteristics likely require a higher dose to achieve the desired antisecretory effect.[88] In a small pharmacokinetic study of children between 13 and 24 months of age with gastroesophageal reflux disease, six of eight children had an improvement in overall GERD symptom severity. The dosage of lansoprazole was increased from 15 mg once daily to 15 mg twice daily in three of the eight children.[84]

Pharmacodynamic Efficacy of Pantopra-zole. Oral pantoprazole (20 mg daily) provides gastric acid control in pediatric patients with reflux esophagitis.[86] Treatment with either 20 or 40 mg daily of pantoprazole is equally effective in controlling symptoms of GERD in 12- to 16-year-old adolescents. The 20 and 40 mg doses were more effective than a 10mg daily dose in improving GERD symptoms after the first week of treatment in 5- to 12-year-old children.[85]

Pharmacodynamic Efficacy of Esomepra-zole. There is just one small pharmacokinetic study available in children 1 to 11 years.[87] This study suggests that the PK properties of esomeprazole may be both dose and age dependent, and that younger children may have a more rapid metabolism of esomeprazole per kilogram of body weight compared with older children. Esomeprazole is well tolerated at doses of 5, 10, and 20 mg in the pediatric patients studied.[87] Another

study performed in adolescents aged 12 to 17 years with symptoms of GERD, showed that PK parameters of esomeprazole were dose- and time-dependent.[100] Both doses of 20 and 40 mg daily were well tolerated.[100]

Clinical Efficacy

The major use of PPIs in pediatrics has been the management of peptic esophagitis and peptic ulcer disease and for the eradication of *H. pylori* infection in triple therapy regimens.[101] Studies which assessed healing of peptic esophagitis have defined the efficacy of omeprazole[102] and lansoprazole.[88, 91,93] More recent studies have focused on control of reflux symptoms rather than healing esophagitis *per se*.[85,87,103] Overall, for both omeprazole and lansoprazole, studies performed in children show that patients with adequate acid suppression (ie, receiving an appropriate dosage) have a healing rate of peptic esophagitis of more than 75% after 4 to 8 weeks of treatment. Relevant clinical symptoms improve over the same time period. PPIs are also used in the treatment of gastric and duodenal peptic ulcers. Low doses (0.3 to 0.7 mg/kg) will achieve ulcer healing. Except for the use of PPI with antibiotics for the eradication of *H. pylori* infection,[104] there is no study on PPI as a sole therapy in the treatment of *H. pylori*-negative gastritis.

Safety

Short-Term Safety. PPIs are well tolerated by most patients. The principal side effects are mild to moderate headaches, abdominal pain, vomiting, and diarrhea.[88] In a double-blind study comparing omeprazole, clarithromycin, and amoxicillin with placebo, clarithromycin, and amoxicillin in *H. pylori*-infected children, adverse events were reported in 24% of patients in both groups but were mild.[104] No adverse effect was reported in children who received a high dose of intravenous omeprazole,[89] but several cases of hepatic toxicity have been reported in adults.[105] Recently, acute interstitial nephritis (AIN) and acute renal failure have been reported in adults receiving various PPIs, suggesting a class effect. Recovery occurs after withdrawal of the drug but is often incomplete. Early diagnosis may be facilitated by clinician awareness of the insidious onset of renal failure, and an elevated erythrocyte sedimentation rate and C-reactive protein.[106–107]

Prolonged periods of achlorrhydria may lead to gastric bacterial overgrowth, as noted in adults and neonates.[108] Studies confirm that proton pump inhibitors do alter bacterial populations in the stomach, but current evidence indicates that this change does not lead to clinical disease.[109] A recent prospective study of children with gastroesophageal reflux disease suggested an increased frequency of both acute enteritis and community-acquired pneumonia during the 4-month follow-up while receiving antisecretory drugs (both ranitidine and omeprazole).[110]

Long-Term Safety. Although PPIs have been available for more than 15 years and are widely used in adults, with an excellent long-term safety profile, few data are available on infants and children regarding long-term use (eg, more than 6 months) of these potent acid-suppressing agents.[111] Long-term acid suppression may promote the production of N-nitrosamine compounds in the stomach secondary to bacterial overgrowth. These compounds are considered carcinogenic. Due to experimental data provided in newborn rats, there are theoretical concerns regarding the consequences and effects on the gastric mucosa of increased gastrin levels (two- to fivefold rise in half of PPI-treated patients). The trophic effects of gastrin lead to stimulation of the enterochromaffin-like cell population and hyperplastic changes in parietal cell mass.[112] Carcinoid tumors have been observed in animals treated lifelong with high-dose omeprazole or an H_2-receptor antagonist. Although enterochromaffin-like hyperplasia has been observed in adults, a carcinoid tumor has been reported only once.[113] Increased endoscopic surveillance and associated sophisticated pathological evaluation of gastric biopsies undoubtedly are responsible for some of the observed increase in the incidence of gastric carcinoid tumors. These data allow no specific role to be assigned to the effects of acid-suppressive medications. Nevertheless, the role of such agents cannot be entirely discounted since the time frame of the increased incidence is comparable to the introduction of these agents as is the known biological effect of gastrin on ECL cell proliferation.[114]

The trophic action of gastrin on gut epithelium has not been implicated in the development of gastric or colonic adenocarcinoma in animal and adult safety studies.[115] However, fundic polyps and nodules have been reported in children who received omeprazole for more than 6 months (Figure 6).[116] The effect of long-term omeprazole therapy (4 to 7 years) on the ratio of G (gastrin secretion) to D cells (somatostatin secretion) was studied in six children.[116] The mean G-cell number and the

ratio of G to D cells showed a significant increase for omeprazole compared with baseline levels. In adults, studies have shown an increased incidence of gastric atrophy associated with long-term use of PPIs, especially in the presence of *H. pylori* infection.[115] However, similar studies are lacking in children.

Suppression of acid secretion may, theoretically, lead to malabsorption of vitamin B12[117–118] and maldigestion of proteins. In children, long-term treatment with PPIs is not considered as a cause of vitamin B12 deficiency.[119] In vitro data have shown that osteoclast activity may be inhibited by omeprazole but without an influence on bone turnover in children during short-term treatment.[78,120] Overall, one should consider that long-term use of PPIs in children is safe but requires ongoing follow-up.[78]

Drug Interactions. Although most PPIs interact with the cytochrome P-450 system, no clinically important interactions have been observed between PPIs and other drugs.[121] However, omeprazole may increase the plasma concentration of diazepam, phenytoin, carbamazepine, and warfarin.[81]

Dosage and Administration

PPIs are available for oral use in capsules containing protective enteric-coated granules or as an enteric-coated tablet. An intravenous formulation is available in many countries for omeprazole, lanzoprazole, and pantoprazole. The granules and tablets should not be crushed, chewed, or dissolved because gastric acid secretion may alter the drug's action. The capsules can be opened and, for those children who are unable to swallow capsules or tablets, the microgranules may be administered *per os* or via a feeding tube, in suspension in an acidic medium such as fruit juice, yogurt, or applesauce. Oral suspensions with different flavors are available increasing taste acceptance and preference.[122] Owing to the activation of the proton pumps by feedings, PPIs should be administered roughly one-half hour before meals. The intravenous formulation should not be administered orally because gastric acid secretion alters the drug.

Omeprazole. The usual recommended starting dosage of omeprazole is 1 mg/kg once daily (eg, 10 mg for children 10 to 20 kg and 20 mg for children weighing more than 20 kg). Although not registered in all countries, intravenous omeprazole is given once daily 40 mg/1.73 m^2 (eg, 1 mg/kg).[89] As the benefit of a loading dose of intravenous omeprazole has been demonstrated in adults, it is suggested to use a loading dose of 40 mg/0.73 m^2 repeated after 12 hours to achieve a rapid antisecretory effect in critical situations in pediatric patients.[89]

Lansoprazole. The usual recommended starting dosage is 1 mg/kg once daily (eg, 15 mg for children <30 kg in weight and 30 mg for those weighing >30 kg[123]). This drug is not yet labeled in all countries for use in children. Intravenous lansoprazole has been administered in children aged 1 to 16 years at a dose of 0.8 to 1.6 mg/kg once a day.

For both omeprazole and lansoprazole, it should be emphasized that the optimal dose may vary among patients. Therefore, in the case of an apparent lack of efficacy, one must be aware that almost 25% of patients may require a double dosage. In the absence of a clinical response to the starting recommended dose, it is suggested to check very carefully with caregivers regarding the mode of administration of the PPIs. If this is correct, doubling the dosage can be suggested as a trial of therapy.

Esomeprazole. Was recently licensed in several European countries and the United States for the adolescents presenting symptoms of GERD at a dose of 20 mg once per day.[100]

Pantoprazole. From data recently obtained in children aged 5 to 11 years with GER, a starting dose of 20 mg (0.6 to 0.9 mg/kg) is recommended, with the possibility of increasing the dose to 40 mg (>1.2 mg/kg) if symptoms do not improve.[85] Data are currently lacking on recommended dosages for intravenous pantoprazole in children.

H_2-RECEPTOR ANTAGONISTS

The first H_2 blocker licensed was cimetidine, in 1976, followed by ranitidine and later famotidine and nizatidine. Experience with other H_2-receptor antagonists, such as roxatidine and ebrotidine, is very limited or nonexistent in children. Although PPIs have now supplanted these drugs for the treatment of acid-peptic diseases because of their greater efficacy and excellent tolerance; the large experience of more than 20 years of use of H_2-receptor antagonists on millions of patients has provided considerable insight regarding efficacy, pharmacology, and long-term tolerance in both adults and children.[124,125] A large number of studies in adults have established that PPIs are more effective in decreasing acid secretion and have better clinical efficacy than H_2-receptor antagonists; however, there are no published articles on children that specifically address this question. Ranitidine, famotidine, and nizatidine are preferred over cimetidine because cimetidine interferes with the cytochrome P-450 enzyme and demonstrates more central nervous system, gastrointestinal, and endocrine side effects than the other H_2 blockers. In parallel with the increase of self-medication of ranitidine in adults, there is also a movement toward the treatment of symptoms in children regardless of the presence or absence of esophagitis. However, the pharmacokinetic and pharmacodynamic effects of over-the-counter H_2-receptor antagonists in the pediatric population remain largely unknown.[125]

Pharmacodynamic Properties

H_2-receptor antagonists are competitive inhibitors of histamine-stimulated acid secretion; however, they have limited effects on acid secretion that is induced by meals or other stimuli. In most pediatric studies, a good correlation is demonstrated between median plasma ranitidine

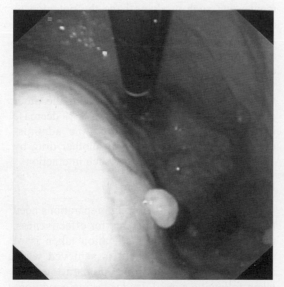

Figure 6 Sessile hyperplastic polyp in the fundus in a neurologically impaired child receiving PPI for 3 years for the treatment of GERD.

concentration and the pharmacodynamic parameter elevation of intragastric pH. The gastric pH typically rises above 4 when the plasma ranitidine concentration approaches 100 ng/mL. In contrast to PPIs, tolerance and rebound effects may occur with the use of H_2-receptor antagonists. Tolerance to the antisecretory effects of H_2-receptor antagonists has been demonstrated in adults and appears to develop quickly. The occurrence of a rebound hypersecretion effect should be taken into account when discontinuing the drugs, which therefore should be progressively withdrawn.

Pharmacokinetic Properties

Studies of pharmacokinetics of H_2-receptor antagonists have been conducted in infants and children.[126] Overall, the parameters are similar to those of adults, with a reasonable absorption after oral dosing. Absorption is not affected by food. Peak blood levels are achieved within 1 to 3 hours after an oral dose. These drugs are well distributed throughout the body and cross the blood-brain barrier. After oral administration, cimetidine, ranitidine, and famotidine undergo "first-pass" hepatic metabolic alteration that reduces their bioavailability by 50%. Protein binding is low (15%). H_2-receptor antagonists are eliminated by a combination of renal excretion and hepatic metabolic degradation. Sixty to 80% of orally administered cimetidine and ranitidine is cleared by the liver. In contrast, after intravenous administration they are eliminated principally through renal excretion. Dose reductions are, therefore, recommended for patients with renal insufficiency.

Clinical Efficacy

Although no controlled trials are available in children, oral ranitidine therapy may be useful in pediatric practice for the treatment of GERD and peptic ulcer diseases. For instance, Cucchiara and colleagues reported that high-dose (20 mg/kg/d) ranitidine is as effective as omeprazole in treating peptic esophagitis.[127]

Tolerability

The majority of pediatric clinical trials with ranitidine reported few side effects and few abnormal laboratory values. As for PPIs, raising the gastric pH may result in the overgrowth of pathogenic bacteria in the digestive tract.[108]

Interactions between H_2 antagonists and other drugs have been extensively reviewed.[128] It is widely held that cimetidine is a more important antagonist of other drugs than the other H_2-receptor antagonists; however, the clinical relevance of many of the interactions with cimetidine is marginal. Cimetidine should be used cautiously in neonates concurrently receiving theophylline, phenytoin, or caffeine because it may prolong the half-life of those drugs.[129]

Dosage and Administration

Ranitidine (5 to 10 mg/kg), given orally daily, divided into two or three doses, produces a symptomatic and endoscopic improvement in erosive esophagitis in children. Pharmacodynamic data on ranitidine suggest that a dosing period of 6 to 9 hours may provide a more effective control of intragastric acidity. In patients with renal impairment, the dosage should be adjusted: if the creatinine clearance is 10 to 50 mL/min, the dosage should be decreased to 75% of normal dosage; if the creatinine clearance is <10 mL/min, the dosage should be decreased to 50% of normal dosage.

The recommended dosages of intravenous cimetidine are 5 to 10 mg/kg/d every 8 to 12 hours in neonates and 10 to 20 mg/kg/d every 6 to 12 hours in infants.[129] Intravenous cimetidine may be infused preferably over 15 to 30 minutes because rapid injection has been associated with cardiac arrhythmias and hypotension. It also may be given by continuous infusion. In premature infants and neonates, ranitidine is usually given intravenously or, rarely, intramuscularly at a dosage of 1 to 2 mg/kg/d divided every 6 hours. The maximal intravenous dosage is 6 mg/kg/d divided every 6 hours. Intravenous continuous infusion is preferred over intermittent dosing at a dosage of 1.44 to 4 mg/kg/d (maximum 6 mg/kg/d).[129] It can be administered in a parenteral nutrition solution. Famotidine can be given intravenously either at a dosage of 0.3 mg/kg every 8 hours (maximum 2.4 mg/kg/d) or by continuous infusion of 1 to 2 mg/kg/d over 24 hours. It can be administered in a parenteral nutrition solution.[129]

ANTACIDS

Antacids include carbonate and bicarbonate salts (eg, $NaHCO_3$ and Ca^- or $MgCO_3$), alkali complexes of aluminum and/or magnesium (eg, aluminum and magnesium hydroxides), aluminum and magnesium phosphates, magnesium trisilicate, and alginate-based raft-forming formulations. They are used for the symptomatic treatment of heartburn and esophagitis. Experience with antacids is limited in infants. Their efficacy in buffering gastric acid is strongly influenced by the time of administration and requires multiple administrations. Simethicone is used in some regions for regurgitation, although there are no reliable studies demonstrating its efficacy in the treatment of gastroesophageal reflux in infants. Although often classified as an antacid, it acts more as a feed thickener, because it contains more than 50% of bean gum and has hardly any acid-neutralizing properties.

Pharmacodynamic Properties

All antacids have a nonsystemic mechanism of action. They chemically neutralize gastric acid. The key therapeutic advantage of antacids is their rapid onset of action. Antacids act within minutes to elevate intragastric pH above 3.5 and, thereby, provide symptomatic relief. Hence, their action is limited by the capacity to maintain an elevated pH in the presence of continued physiologic acid secretion and by normal gastric emptying.

Alginate-based raft-forming preparations have a quite different mode of action. In the presence of gastric acid, alginates precipitate to form a gel. Alginate-based raft-forming formulations usually contain sodium or potassium bicarbonate; in the presence of gastric acid, the bicarbonate is converted to carbon dioxide, which becomes entrapped within the gel precipitate, converting it into a foam that floats on the surface of the gastric surface, providing a relatively pH-neutral barrier.[130]

Clinical Efficacy

Double-blind studies in adults have shown that alginate-based raft-forming preparations are superior to placebo in relieving symptoms of heartburn.[130] However, studies in infants and children remain limited (six studies including a total of 303 patients, only one being double blind) and had various study designs (open-label prospective study, comparison of two different dosages of alginate, comparison of placebo, famotidine, or cisapride). Efficacy as monotherapy or in combination with prokinetics for the management of gastroesophageal reflux disease is not convincing.[131]

Tolerability

Since absorption from aluminum-containing antacids may cause serum aluminum concentrations to approach levels reported to cause osteopenia and neurotoxicity, chronic antacid therapy in children is not recommended. Gaviscon contains a considerable amount of sodium carbonate, so its administration may increase the sodium content of feeds to an undesirable level, especially in preterm infants (1 g of Gaviscon contains 46 mg of sodium, and the suspension contains twice this amount). Occasional formation of large bezoar-like masses of agglutinated intragastric material has been reported in association with Gaviscon use. Side effects include diarrhea with magnesium-rich preparations and excessive absorption of aluminum in infants.[132] The presence of aluminum and magnesium in the majority of antacids means that such products have the potential to chelate drugs in the upper gastrointestinal tract, including quinolones, azithromycin, tetracyclines, and the H_2-recptor antagonists.[128] The effects of antacids on the pharmacokinetics of other drugs vary widely according to the type of antacid and time dosage of the administration of the other drug, ranging from no effect to an 85% decrease in bioavailability.[128] Separating the administration of antacid from that of another drug by 2 hours usually eliminates any such interaction.

Dosage and Administration

As alginate-based raft-forming preparations need to float on the gastric contents for effectiveness, the time at which this medication taken is of importance. Optimal benefit is achieved when alginate-based raft-forming preparations are taken following a meal. Under fasting conditions or when taken just prior to or with a meal, alginate-based raft-forming preparations are reported to empty from the stomach with a T1 of 20 to 30 minutes.[130] When dosed 30 minutes following a meal, alginate-based formulations empty from the stomach with a T1 of 180 minutes.

OTHER DRUGS

Prostaglandin Analogues

Misoprostol is a prostaglandin E1 (PGE1) analogue that is primarily used to prevent NSAID-induced gastropathy in high-risk patients.[133] Although initial animal studies showed considerable promise in the treatment of acid-peptic disease, studies in humans have not confirmed a clear advantage of the PGE1 analogues, and their clinical efficacy is now attributed primarily to their antisecretory activity. Experience in children is limited and mainly focused on children with rheumatologic disease or receiving NSAIDs.[134] Side effects are usually limited to transient diarrhea. Prenatal exposure to misoprostol is associated with an increased risk of Mobius sequence and terminal transverse limb defects.[135]

Coating Agent

The coating agent sucralfate is a basic aluminum salt of sucrose octasulfate. At an acid pH, it polymerizes to form a white paste-like substance that adheres selectively to ulcers or erosions via an electrostatic attraction between negatively charged sucralfate polyanions and positively charged protein moieties exposed by the inflamed mucosa. At these specific sites, sucralfate acts as a protective barrier by slowing back-diffusion of acid, pepsin, and bile salts. It also directly inhibits the binding of pepsin to ulcer proteins and, like cholestyramine, adsorbs free bile salts. Gastric pH does not appear to affect sucralfate binding to the ulcer bed. Other important effects of sucralfate include increased bicarbonate and mucus production, enhanced epithelial cell renewal, and restoration of a normal transmucosal potential difference. Sucralfate also protects the gastric mucosa against damage induced by ethanol, bile acids, and NSAIDs and prevents stress ulceration in critically ill patients. Despite its aluminum hydroxide components, sucralfate does not increase gastric pH or act as an antacid at usual therapeutic doses. The drug has no apparent effects on gastric acid secretion, gastrin release, or upper gastrointestinal tract motility. Thus, hypochlorrhydria and concomitant gastric bacterial overgrowth do not occur. Several studies in adults show that sucralfate (1 g orally before meals and at bedtime) is significantly better than placebo and equivalent to cimetidine and ranitidine in the healing of both duodenal and gastric ulcers. Maintenance therapy with sucralfate decreases the recurrence rate of both gastric and duodenal ulcers. Sucralfate may also protect patients from NSAID-induced gastroduodenal lesions. Sucralafate is effective in the treatment of duodenogastric reflux.[68] Sucralfate can prevent stress ulceration in critically ill patients. Recent data have also shown clinical efficacy of sucralfate topically to treat or prevent mucosal lesions from various origins (ie, stomatitis, mucositis, or pouchitis).[136] Sucralfate is relatively free of side effects, the only major one being constipation, which occurs in about 2 to 3% of patients. Nausea and headaches occur much less frequently. Sucralfate causes bezoars, especially when given to patients in intensive care units (especially in premature and neonates). Aluminum accumulation has been observed in critically ill children with acute renal failure.[137]

Bismuth Compounds

Use of bismuth has progressively declined in the last 30 to 40 years because its mode of action remained unknown and therapeutic benefits unproven. Moreover, reports of encephalopathy associated with ingestion of various bismuth salts in large quantities over long periods in France and Australia in the early 1970s contributed to the dramatic reduction of its use and led to the interdiction of use both in adults and children in several countries by national drug authorities. In the last decade, a renaissance of the use of some bismuth compounds has taken place. Bismuth subsalicylate and colloidal bismuth subcitrate both have been used in the eradication of H. pylori infection in combination with antibiotics and antisecretory drugs.[138] In children, rare cases of acute renal failure after overdose have been reported.[139]

SUMMARY

PPIs have become the first-line treatment of acid-peptic diseases in children, and recent studies have better delineated their pharmacologic characteristics in childhood. Although side effects are mild and uncommon in childhood, long-term safety studies are still required.

REFERENCES

1. Chelimsky G, Czinn S. Peptic ulcer disease in children. Pediatr Rev 2001;22:349–55.
2. Dohil R, Hassall E, Jevon G, Dimmick J. Gastritis and gastropathy of childhood. J Pediatr Gastroenterol Nutr 1999;29:378–94.
3. Sherman P, Czinn S, Drumm B, et al. *Helicobacter pylori* infection in children and adolescents: Working Group Report of the First World Congress of Pediatric Gastroenterology, Hepatology, and Nutrition. J Pediatr Gastroenterol Nutr 2002;35:S128–33.
4. Blecker U, Gold BD. Gastritis and peptic ulcer disease in childhood. Eur J Pediatr 1999;158:541–6.
5. Boyle JT. Acid secretion from birth to adulthood. J Pediatr Gastroenterol Nutr 2003;37:S12–6.
6. Nagita A, Amemoto K, Yoden A, et al. Diurnal variation in intragastric pH in children with and without peptic ulcers. Pediatr Res 1996;40:528–32.
7. Yamashiro Y, Shioya T, Ohtsuka Y, et al. Patterns of 24 h intragastric acidity in duodenal ulcers in children: The importance of monitoring and inhibiting nocturnal acidity. Acta Paediatr Jpn 1995;37:557–61.
8. Hyman PE, Hassall E. Marked basal gastric acid hypersecretion and peptic ulcer disease: Medical management with a combination H₂-histamine receptor antagonist and anticholinergic. J Pediatr Gastroenterol Nutr 1988;7:57–63.
9. Euler AR, Byrne WJ, Campbell MF. Basal and pentagastrin-stimulated gastric acid secretory rates in normal children and in those with peptic ulcer disease. J Pediatr 1983;103:766–8.
10. Lopes AI, Palha A, Lopes T, et al. Relationship among serum pepsinogens, serum gastrin, gastric mucosal histology and *H. pylori* virulence factors in a paediatric population. Scand J Gastroenterol 2006;41:524–31.
11. Fukuda Y, Isomoto H, Ohnita K, et al. Impact of CagA status on serum gastrin and pepsinogen I and II concentrations in Japanese children with *Helicobacter pylori* infection. J Int Med Res 2003;31:247–52.
12. Xie XZ, Zhao ZG, Qi DS, Wang ZM. Assay of gastrin and somatostatin in gastric antrum tissues of children with chronic gastritis and duodenal ulcer. World J Gastroenterol 2006;12:2288–90.
13. Nam SY, Kim N, Lee CS, et al. Gastric mucosal protection via enhancement of MUC5AC and MUC6 by geranylgeranylacetone. Dig Dis Sci 2005;50:2110–20.
14. Bi LC, Kaunitz JD. Gastroduodenal mucosal defense: An integrated protective response. Curr Opin Gastroenterol 2003;19:526–32.
15. Macarthur C, Saunders N, Feldman W. *Helicobacter pylori*, gastroduodenal disease, and recurrent abdominal pain in children. JAMA 1995;273:729–34.
16. Perez-Perez GI, Rothenbacher D, Brenner H. Epidemiology of *Helicobacter pylori* infection. Helicobacter 2004;9:1–6.
17. Laine L, Hopkins RJ, Girardi LS. Has the impact of *Helicobacter pylori* therapy on ulcer recurrence in the United States been overstated? A meta-analysis of rigorously designed trials. Am J Gastroenterol 1998;93:1409–15.
18. Ciociola AA, McSorley DJ, Turner K, et al. *Helicobacter pylori* infection rates in duodenal ulcer patients in the United States may be lower than previously estimated. Am J Gastroenterol 1999;94:1834–40.
19. Elitsur Y, Lawrence Z. Non-*Helicobacter pylori* related duodenal ulcer disease in children. Helicobacter 2001;6:239–43.
20. Koletzko S, Richy F, Bontems P, et al. Prospective multicentre study on antibiotic resistance of *Helicobacter pylori* strains obtained from children living in Europe. Gut 2006;55:1711–1716.
21. Murphy MS, Eastham EJ, Jimenez M, et al. Duodenal ulceration: Review of 110 cases. Arch Dis Child 1987;62:554–8.
22. Oderda G, Vaira D, Holton J, et al. *Helicobacter pylori* in children with peptic ulcer and their families. Dig Dis Sci 1991;36:572–6.
23. Drumm B, Rhoads JM, Stringer DA, et al. Peptic ulcer disease in children: Etiology, clinical findings, and clinical course. Pediatrics 1988;82:410–4.
24. Mezoff AG, Balistreri WF. Peptic ulcer disease in children. Pediatr Rev 1995;16:257–65.
25. Huang IF, Wu TC, Wang KS, et al. Upper gastrointestinal endoscopy in children with upper gastrointestinal bleeding. J Chin Med Assoc 2003;66:271–5.
26. El Mouzan MI, Abdullah AM. Peptic ulcer disease in children and adolescents. J Trop Pediatr 2004;50:328–30.
27. de Oliveira AM, Rocha GA, Queiroz DM, et al. Evaluation of enzyme-linked immunosorbent assay for the diagnosis of *Helicobacter pylori* infection in children from different age groups with and without duodenal ulcer. J Pediatr Gastroenterol Nutr 1999;28:157–61.
28. Nijevitch AA, Sataev VU, Vakhitov VA, et al. Childhood peptic ulcer in the Ural area of Russia: Clinical status and *Helicobacter pylori*-associated immune response. J Pediatr Gastroenterol Nutr 2001;33:558–64.
29. Demir H, Gurakan F, Ozen H, et al. Peptic ulcer disease in children without *Helicobacter pylori* infection. Helicobacter 2002;7:111.
30. Roma E, Kafritsa Y, Panayiotou J, et al. Is peptic ulcer a common cause of upper gastrointestinal symptoms? Eur J Pediatr 2001;160:497–500.
31. Stringer, Veysi VT, Puntis JW, et al. Gastroduodenal ulcers in the *Helicobacter pylori* era. Acta Paediatr 2000;89:1181–5.
32. Dohil R, Hassall E. Peptic ulcer disease in children. Baillieres Best Pract Res Clin Gastroenterol 2000;14:53–73.
33. Levenstein S. Stress and peptic ulcer: Life beyond Helicobacter. BMJ 1998;316:538–41.
34. Wilson SD. Zollinger-Ellison syndrome in children: A 25-year follow-up. Surgery 1991;110:696–702; discussion 702–3.
35. De Giacomo C, Fiocca R, Villani L, et al. Omeprazole treatment of severe peptic disease associated with antral G cell hyperfunction and hyperpepsinogenemia I in an infant. J Pediatr 1990;117:989–93.
36. Quatrini M, Castoldi L, Rossi G, et al. A follow-up study of patients with Zollinger-Ellison syndrome in the period 1966-2002: Effects of surgical and medical treatments on long-term survival. J Clin Gastroenterol 2005;39:376–80.
37. Nikou GC, Toubanakis C, Nikolaou P, et al. Gastrinomas associated with MEN-1 syndrome: New insights for the diagnosis and management in a series of 11 patients. Hepatogastroenterology 2005;52:1668–76.

38. Edwards MJ, Kollenberg SJ, Brandt ML, et al. Surgery for peptic ulcer disease in children in the post-histamine2-blocker era. J Pediatr Surg 2005;40:850–4.
39. Jensen RT. Gastrointestinal abnormalities and involvement in systemic mastocytosis. Hematol Oncol Clin North Am 2000;14:579–623.
40. Tang SJ, Nieto JM, Jensen DM, et al. The novel use of an intravenous proton pump inhibitor in a patient with short bowel syndrome. J Clin Gastroenterol 2002;34:62–3.
41. Bismar HA, El-Bakry AA. Primary hyperparathyroidism. Saudi Med J 2003;24:1214–8.
42. Wise SR, Quigley M, Saxe AW, Zdon MJ. Hyperparathyroidism and cellular mechanisms of gastric acid secretion. Surgery 1990;108:1058–63; discussion 1063–4.
43. Sotoudehmanesh R, Ali Asgari A, Ansari R, Nouraie M. Endoscopic findings in end-stage renal disease. Endoscopy 2003;35:502–5.
44. Marsenic O, Peco-Antic A, Perisic V, et al. Upper gastrointestinal lesions in children on chronic haemodialysis. Nephrol Dial Transplant 2003;18:2687–8.
45. Cox KL, Isenberg JN, Ament ME. Gastric acid hypersecretion in cystic fibrosis. J Pediatr Gastroenterol Nutr 1982;1:559–65.
46. Crill CM, Hak EB. Upper gastrointestinal tract bleeding in critically ill pediatric patients. Pharmacotherapy 1999;19:162–80.
47. Kuusela AL, Maki M, Ruuska T, Laippala P. Stress-induced gastric findings in critically ill newborn infants: Frequency and risk factors. Intensive Care Med 2000;26:1501–6.
48. Haizlip JA, Lugo RA, Cash JJ, Vernon DD. Failure of nasogastric omeprazole suspension in pediatric intensive care patients. Pediatr Crit Care Med 2005;6:182–7.
49. Behrens R, Hofbeck M, Singer H, et al. Frequency of stress lesions of the upper gastrointestinal tract in paediatric patients after cardiac surgery: Effects of prophylaxis. Br Heart J 1994;72:186–9.
50. Kaufman SS, Lyden ER, Brown CR, et al. Omeprazole therapy in pediatric patients after liver and intestinal transplantation. J Pediatr Gastroenterol Nutr 2002;34:194–8.
51. Len C, Hilario MO, Kawakami E, et al. Gastroduodenal lesions in children with juvenile rheumatoid arthritis. Hepatogastroenterology 1999;46:991–6.
52. Guslandi M. Gastric toxicity of antiplatelet therapy with low-dose aspirin. Drugs 1997;53:1–5.
53. Hawkey CJ. Nonsteroidal anti-inflammatory drug gastropathy. Gastroenterology 2000;119:521–35.
54. Tobin JM, Sinha B, Ramani P, et al. Upper gastrointestinal mucosal disease in pediatric Crohn disease and ulcerative colitis: A blinded, controlled study. J Pediatr Gastroenterol Nutr 2001;32:443–8.
55. Feng J, Gu W, Li M, et al. Rare causes of gastric outlet obstruction in children. Pediatr Surg Int 2005;21:635–40.
56. Forrest JA, Finlayson ND, Shearman DJ. Endoscopy in gastrointestinal bleeding. Lancet 1974;2:394–7.
57. Wong BP, Chao NS, Leung MW, et al. Complications of peptic ulcer disease in children and adolescents: Minimally invasive treatments offer feasible surgical options. J Pediatr Surg 2006;41:2073–5.
58. Franciosi CM, Romano F, Caprotti R, Uggeri F. Multiple gastric perforations in an immunodepressed child. Surgery 2002;131:685–6.
59. Morikawa N, Honna T, Kuroda T, et al. Lethal gastric rupture caused by acute gastric ulcer in a 6-year-old girl. Pediatr Surg Int 2005;21:943–6.
60. Agarwal HS, Churchwell KB, Pietsch JB, Little CA. Hemorrhagic stress ulceration in a case of appendicitis. J Pediatr Surg 2006;41:1483–5.
61. Yen JB, Kong MS. Gastric outlet obstruction in pediatric patients. Chang Gung Med J 2006;29:401–5.
62. Kalach N, Mention K, Guimber D, et al. *Helicobacter pylori* infection is not associated with specific symptoms in nonulcer-dyspeptic children. Pediatrics 2005;115:17–21.
63. Dixon MF, Genta RM, Yardley JH, Correa P. Classification and grading of gastritis. The updated Sydney System. International Workshop on the Histopathology of Gastritis, Houston 1994. Am J Surg Pathol 1996;20:1161–81.
64. Lesko SM, Mitchell AA. The safety of acetaminophen and ibuprofen among children younger than two years old. Pediatrics 1999;104:e39.
65. Keenan GF, Giannini EH, Athreya BH. Clinically significant gastropathy associated with nonsteroidal antiinflammatory drug use in children with juvenile rheumatoid arthritis. J Rheumatol 1995;22:1149–51.
66. Pashankar DS, Bishop WP, Mitros FA. Chemical gastropathy: A distinct histopathologic entity in children. J Pediatr Gastroenterol Nutr 2002;35:653–7.
67. Takada K, Hamada Y, Watanabe K, et al. Duodenogastric reflux following biliary reconstruction after excision of choledochal cyst. Pediatr Surg Int 2005;21:1–4.
68. Hermans D, Sokal EM, Collard JM, et al. Primary duodenogastric reflux in children and adolescents. Eur J Pediatr 2003;162:598–602.
69. Black JO, White J, Abramowsky C, Shehata B. Pathologic quiz case. Edema and diarrhea in a 2-year-old boy. Menetrier disease with cytomegalovirus gastritis. Arch Pathol Lab Med 2004;128:e117–9.
70. Tokuhara D, Okano Y, Asou K, et al. Cytomegalovirus and *Helicobacter pylori* co-infection in a child with Menetrier disease. Eur J Pediatr 2007;166:63–5.
71. Drut R, Drut RM. Lymphocytic gastritis in pediatric celiac disease—immunohistochemical study of the intraepithelial lymphocytic component. Med Sci Monit 2004;10: CR38–42.
72. El-Rifai N, Mention K, Guimber L, et al. Gastropathy and gastritis in children with portal hypertension. J Pediatr Gastroenterol Nutr 2007;45:137–40.
73. Hung PY, Ni YH, Hsu HY,Chang MH. Portal hypertension and duodenal ulcer in children. J Pediatr Gastroenterol Nutr 2004;39:158–60.
74. Dimitrov G, Gottrand F. Does gastric atrophy exist in children? World J Gastroenterol 2006;12:6274–9.
75. Ricuarte O, Gutierrez O, Cardona H, et al. Atrophic gastritis in young children and adolescents. J Clin Pathol 2005;58:1189–93.
76. Segni M, Borrelli O, Pucarelli I, et al. Early manifestations of gastric autoimmunity in patients with juvenile autoimmune thyroid diseases. J Clin Endocrinol Metab 2004;89:4944–8.
77. Gunasekaran TS, Berman J, Gonzalez M. Duodenojejunitis: Is it idiopathic or is it Henoch-Schonlein purpura without the purpura? J Pediatr Gastroenterol Nutr 2000;30:22–8.
78. Gibbons TE, Gold BD. The use of proton pump inhibitors in children: A comprehensive review. Paediatr Drugs 2003;5:25–40.
79. Hoyo-Vadillo C, Venturelli CR, Gonzalez H, et al. Metabolism of omeprazole after two oral doses in children 1 to 9 months old. Proc West Pharmacol Soc 2005;48:108–9.
80. Litalien C, Theoret Y, Faure C. Pharmacokinetics of proton pump inhibitors in children. Clin Pharmacokinet 2005;44:441–66.
81. Stedman CA, Barclay ML. Review article: Comparison of the pharmacokinetics, acid suppression and efficacy of proton pump inhibitors. Aliment Pharmacol Ther 2000;14:963–78.
82. Marier JF, Dubuc MC, Drouin E, et al. Pharmacokinetics of omeprazole in healthy adults and in children with gastroesophageal reflux disease. Ther Drug Monit 2004;26:3–8.
83. Gremse D, Winter H, Tolia V, et al. Pharmacokinetics and pharmacodynamics of lansoprazole in children with gastroesophageal reflux disease. J Pediatr Gastroenterol Nutr 2002;35:S319–26.
84. Heyman MB, Zhang W, Huang B, et al. Pharmacokinetics and pharmacodynamics of lansoprazole in children 13 to 24 months old with gastroesophageal reflux disease. J Pediatr Gastroenterol Nutr 2007;44:35–40.
85. Tolia V, Bishop PR, Tsou VM, et al. Multicenter, randomized, double-blind study comparing 10, 20 and 40 mg pantoprazole in children (5–11 years) with symptomatic gastroesophageal reflux disease. J Pediatr Gastroenterol Nutr 2006;42:384–91.
86. Madrazo-de la Garza A, Dibildox M, Vargas A, et al. Efficacy and safety of oral pantoprazole 20 mg given once daily for reflux esophagitis in children. J Pediatr Gastroenterol Nutr 2003;36:261–5.
87. Zhao J, Li J, Hamer-Maansson JE, et al. Pharmacokinetic properties of esomeprazole in children aged 1 to 11 years with symptoms of gastroesophageal reflux disease: A randomized, open-label study. Clin Ther 2006;28:1868–76.
88. Faure C, Michaud L, Shaghaghi EK, et al. Lansoprazole in children: Pharmacokinetics and efficacy in reflux oesophagitis. Aliment Pharmacol Ther 2001;15:1397–402.
89. Faure C, Michaud L, Shaghaghi EK, et al. Intravenous omeprazole in children: Pharmacokinetics and effect on 24-hour intragastric pH. J Pediatr Gastroenterol Nutr 2001;33:144–8.
90. Andersson T, Hassall E, Lundborg P, et al. Pharmacokinetics of orally administered omeprazole in children. International Pediatric Omeprazole Pharmacokinetic Group. Am J Gastroenterol 2000;95:3101–6.
91. Gunasekaran T, Gupta S, Gremse D, et al. Lansoprazole in adolescents with gastroesophageal reflux disease: Pharmacokinetics, pharmacodynamics, symptom relief efficacy, and tolerability. J Pediatr Gastroenterol Nutr 2002;35:S327–35.
92. Tran A, Rey E, Pons G, et al. Pharmacokinetic-pharmacodynamic study of oral lansoprazole in children. Clin Pharmacol Ther 2002;71:359–67.
93. Croom KF, Scott LJ. Lansoprazole: In the treatment of gastro-oesophageal reflux disease in children and adolescents. Drugs 2005;65:2129–35; discussion 2136–7.
94. Omari TI, Haslam RR, Lundborg P,Davidson GP. Effect of omeprazole on acid gastroesophageal reflux and gastric acidity in preterm infants with pathological acid reflux. J Pediatr Gastroenterol Nutr 2007;44:41–4.
95. Johnson TN, Rostami-Hodjegan A, Tucker GT. Prediction of the clearance of eleven drugs and associated variability in neonates, infants and children. Clin Pharmacokinet 2006;45:931–56.
96. Kearns GL, Winter HS. Proton pump inhibitors in pediatrics: Relevant pharmacokinetics and pharmacodynamics. J Pediatr Gastroenterol Nutr 2003;37:S52–9.
97. Furuta T, Ohashi K, Kosuge K, et al. CYP2C19 genotype status and effect of omeprazole on intragastric pH in humans. Clin Pharmacol Ther 1999;65:552–61.
98. Ferron GM, Preston RA, Noveck RJ, et al. Pharmacokinetics of pantoprazole in patients with moderate and severe hepatic dysfunction. Clin Ther 2001;23:1180–92.
99. Keane WF, Swan SK, Grimes I, Humphries TJ. Rabeprazole: Pharmacokinetics and tolerability in patients with stable, end-stage renal failure. J Clin Pharmacol 1999;39:927–33.
100. Li J, Zhao J, Hamer-Maansson JE, et al. Pharmacokinetic properties of esomeprazole in adolescent patients aged 12 to 17 years with symptoms of gastroesophageal reflux disease: A randomized, open-label study. Clin Ther 2006;28: 419–27.
101. Marchetti F, Gerarduzzi T, Ventura A. Proton pump inhibitors in children: A review. Dig Liver Dis 2003;35:738–46.
102. Hassall E, Israel D, Shepherd R, et al. Omeprazole for treatment of chronic erosive esophagitis in children: A multicenter study of efficacy, safety, tolerability and dose requirements. International Pediatric Omeprazole Study Group. J Pediatr 2000;137:800–7.
103. Tsou VM, Baker R, Book L, et al. Multicenter, randomized, double-blind study comparing 20 and 40 mg of pantoprazole for symptom relief in adolescents (12 to 16 years of age) with gastroesophageal reflux disease (GERD). Clin Pediatr (Phila) 2006;45:741–9.
104. Gottrand F, Kalach N, Spyckerelle C, et al. Omeprazole combined with amoxicillin and clarithromycin in the eradication of *Helicobacter pylori* in children with gastritis: A prospective randomized double-blind trial. J Pediatr 2001;139:664–8.
105. Christe C, Stoller R, Vogt N. Omeprazole-induced hepatotoxicity? A case report. Pharmacoepidemiol Drug Saf 1998;7:S41–4.
106. Simpson IJ, Marshall MR, Pilmore H, et al. Proton pump inhibitors and acute interstitial nephritis: Report and analysis of 15 cases. Nephrology (Carlton) 2006;11:381–5.
107. Geevasinga N, Coleman PL, Webster AC, Roger SD. Proton pump inhibitors and acute interstitial nephritis. Clin Gastroenterol Hepatol 2006;4:597–604.
108. Cothran DS, Borowitz SM, Sutphen JL, et al. Alteration of normal gastric flora in neonates receiving ranitidine. J Perinatol 1997;17:383–8.
109. Williams C, McColl KE. Review article: Proton pump inhibitors and bacterial overgrowth. Aliment Pharmacol Ther 2006;23:3–10.
110. Canani RB, Cirillo P, Roggero P, et al. Therapy with gastric acidity inhibitors increases the risk of acute gastroenteritis and community-acquired pneumonia in children. Pediatrics 2006;117:e817–20.
111. Hassall E, Kerr W, El-Serag HB. Characteristics of children receiving proton pump inhibitors continuously for up to 11 years duration. J Pediatr 2007;150:262–7.
112. Jensen RT. Consequences of long-term proton pump blockade: Insights from studies of patients with gastrinomas. Basic Clin Pharmacol Toxicol 2006;98:4–19.
113. Haga Y, Nakatsura T, Shibata Y, et al. Human gastric carcinoid detected during long-term antiulcer therapy of H_2 receptor antagonist and proton pump inhibitor. Dig Dis Sci 1998;43:253–7.
114. Modlin IM, Lye KD, Kidd M. A 50-year analysis of 562 gastric carcinoids: Small tumor or larger problem? Am J Gastroenterol 2004;99:23–32.
115. Klinkenberg-Knol EC, Nelis F, Dent J, et al. Long-term omeprazole treatment in resistant gastroesophageal reflux disease: Efficacy, safety, and influence on gastric mucosa. Gastroenterology 2000;118:661–9.
116. Pashankar DS, Israel DM. Gastric polyps and nodules in children receiving long-term omeprazole therapy. J Pediatr Gastroenterol Nutr 2002;35:658–62.
117. Valuck RJ, Ruscin JM. A case-control study on adverse effects: H_2 blocker or proton pump inhibitor use and risk of vitamin B12 deficiency in older adults. J Clin Epidemiol 2004;57:422–8.
118. Ruscin JM, Page RL, II, Valuck RJ. Vitamin B(12) deficiency associated with histamine(2)-receptor antagonists and a proton-pump inhibitor. Ann Pharmacother 2002;36: 812–6.

119. ter Heide H, Hendriks HJ, Heijmans H, et al. Are children with cystic fibrosis who are treated with a proton-pump inhibitor at risk for vitamin B(12) deficiency? J Pediatr Gastroenterol Nutr 2001;33:342–5.

120. Kocsis I, Arato A, Bodanszky H, et al. Short-term omeprazole treatment does not influence biochemical parameters of bone turnover in children. Calcif Tissue Int 2002;71:129–32.

121. Sachs G, Humphries TJ. Rabeprazole: Pharmacology, pharmacokinetics, and potential for drug interactions. Introduction. Aliment Pharmacol Ther 1999;13:1–2.

122. Tolia V, Johnston G, Stolle J, Lee C. Flavor and taste of lansoprazole strawberry-flavored delayed-release oral suspension preferred over ranitidine peppermint-flavored oral syrup: In children aged between 5-11 years. Paediatr Drugs 2004;6:127–31.

123. Scott LJ. Lansoprazole: In the management of gastroesophageal reflux disease in children. Paediatr Drugs 2003;5:57–61; discussion 62.

124. Ameen VZ, Pobiner BF, Giguere GC, Carter EG Ranitidine (Zantac) syrup versus Ranitidine effervescent tablets (Zantac) EFFERdose) in children: A single-center taste preference study. Paediatr Drugs 2006;8:265–70.

125. Orenstein SR, Blumer JL, Faessel HM, et al. Ranitidine, 75 mg, over-the-counter dose: Pharmacokinetic and pharmacodynamic effects in children with symptoms of gastro-oesophageal reflux. Aliment Pharmacol Ther 2002;16:899–907.

126. Lugo RA, Harrison AM, Cash J, et al. Pharmacokinetics and pharmacodynamics of ranitidine in critically ill children. Crit Care Med 2001;29:759–64.

127. Cucchiara S, Campanozzi A, Greco L, et al. Predictive value of esophageal manometry and gastroesophageal pH monitoring for responsiveness of reflux disease to medical therapy in children. Am J Gastroenterol 1996;91:680–5.

128. Flockhart DA, Desta Z, Mahal SK. Selection of drugs to treat gastro-oesophageal reflux disease: The role of drug interactions. Clin Pharmacokinet 2000;39:295–309.

129. Bell SG. Gastroesophageal reflux and histamine2 antagonists. Neonatal Netw 2003;22:53–7.

130. Mandel KG, Daggy BP, Brodie DA, Jacoby HI. Review article: Alginate-raft formulations in the treatment of heartburn and acid reflux. Aliment Pharmacol Ther 2000;14:669–90.

131. Del Buono R, Wenzl TG, Ball G, et al. Effect of Gaviscon infant on gastro-oesophageal reflux in infants assessed by combined intraluminal impedance/pH. Arch Dis Child 2005;90:460–3.

132. Pattaragarn A, Alon US. Antacid-induced rickets in infancy. Clin Pediatr (Phila) 2001;40:389–93.

133. Hooper L, Brown TJ, Elliott R, et al. The effectiveness of five strategies for the prevention of gastrointestinal toxicity induced by non-steroidal anti-inflammatory drugs: Systematic review. Bmj 2004;329:948.

134. Gazarian M, Berkovitch M, Koren G, et al. Experience with misoprostol therapy for NSAID gastropathy in children. Ann Rheum Dis 1995;54:277–80.

135. da Silva Dal Pizzol T, Knop FP, Mengue SS. Prenatal exposure to misoprostol and congenital anomalies: Systematic review and meta-analysis. Reprod Toxicol 2006;22:666–71.

136. Marini I, Vecchiet F. Sucralfate: A help during oral management in patients with epidermolysis bullosa. J Periodontol 2001;72:691–5.

137. Thorburn K, Samuel M, Smith EA, Baines P. Aluminum accumulation in critically ill children on sucralfate therapy. Pediatr Crit Care Med 2001;2:247–249.

138. Oderda G, Shcherbakov P, Bontems P, et al. Results from the pediatric European register for treatment of Helicobacter pylori (PERTH). Helicobacter 2007;12:150–6.

139. Islek I, Uysal S, Gok F, et al. Reversible nephrotoxicity after overdose of colloidal bismuth subcitrate. Pediatr Nephrol 2001;16:510–4.

9.3. Other Causes of Gastritis

Chee Yee Ooi (Keith), MB, BS, DipPaed
Daniel Avi Lemberg, BSc (Med), MBBS, DipPaed, FRACP
Andrew S. Day, MB, ChB, MD, FRACP

The stomach provides a key role in primary defense against foreign stimuli entering the gastrointestinal tract, and after, delivery of ingested material from the esophagus, is first to encounter pathogens and other ingested antigens. Generic defenses in the stomach include secretion of gastric acid and mucus production. Due to the specific location and specialized roles of the stomach, the stomach can respond in unique ways to stimuli, and this can manifest in various ways.

A manifestation of gastric response to injury is the development of gastritis: inflammatory changes within the stomach evident microscopically. The pattern and intensity of the response vary according to the stimulus and according to the local or systemic nature of the stimulus. Endoscopically visible associations of gastritis include erosions and mucosal ulceration, secondary to inflammatory changes in the mucosa. Erosions are superficial whereas ulcers involve the muscularis mucosa in addition to the superficial layers.

The objective of this chapter is to systematically review the various conditions leading to gastritis and to provide a structured approach to evaluate these disorders.

STRUCTURE AND FUNCTION OF AREAS OF THE STOMACH

The stomach is divided into three main functional areas, the fundus, body, and antrum, which are distinguishable histologically. All areas of the stomach possess mucus-secreting cells as well as more specialized cells. Located in the fundus or body of the stomach are parietal cells, the source of gastric acid. Chief cells (producing pepsinogen) and regulatory enterochromaffin cells are also present in this area. The antrum, situated in the distal portion of the stomach, contains G, D, and enterochomaffin cells. These cells respectively secrete gastrin, somatostatin, and histamine/serotonin. Functionally, this area provides hormonal activity, controlling upper gut digestive activity with important regulatory roles on gastric function; for instance, gastrin and histamine secretion prompt gastric acid secretion, while somatostatin is an important regulator of gastrin release.

CLASSIFICATION OF GASTRITIS

Gastritides and gastropathies can be classified according to the etiologic agent, the endoscopic appearance of the gastric mucosa,[1] and the histopathological pattern of gastric biopsies.[2] The nonspecific and overlapping nature of endoscopic and/or histologic findings of many gastritides and gastropathies make classifications based on only endoscopic and/or histologic findings alone less helpful. Although no single classification or system provides a satisfactory description of all types of gastritis and gastropathy, an etiology-based classification (Table 1) provides a practical approach for directing both further investigations and therapy, and unifies the pediatric endoscopist with the pathologist.

The original and upgraded Sydney systems have been used as standard methods to assess and report gastritis over the last decade.[2–3] Important features of gastric atrophy and cellular infiltrates are included in this system. Subsequent Atrophy Club guidelines include a revised method for the reporting of atrophy and intestinal metaplasia.[4] More recently, Rugge and Genta[5] suggest a modified approach for the staging and grading of gastritis, which includes reporting on the presence and extent of atrophy, along with a semiquantitative assessment of infiltrates of mononuclear and granulocytic cells.

CHANGING PATTERN OF GASTRITIS/PEPTIC ULCERATION

Until recent years, the primary etiology of gastritis and related peptic ulcer disease (PUD) was considered to be infection with *Helicobacter pylori*. Over the last few years, there are increasing reports of non–*H. pylori*-associated gastritis and PUD, reflecting the changing epidemiology of infection with this gastric pathogen in the Western world. Several reports indicate that up to 20% of PUD in adults is not related to *H. pylori* infection or nonsteroidal anti-inflammatory drugs (NSAID).[6] Idiopathic PUD is of low frequency (5%) in studies of European patients,[7] but higher (17%) in Asian subjects.[8]

In North America, Elitsur and Lawrence[9] described 622 pediatric patients who had undergone upper gastrointestinal endoscopy. Eight of 11 children with mucosal ulceration had no evidence of *H. pylori* infection or exposure to nonsteroidal anti-inflammatory drugs, similar to previous reports on non–*H. pylori*/non–NSAID PUD. These authors did not define specific clinical or endoscopic features that permit one to distinguish idiopathic ulcers from others. The etiology of idiopathic PUD and the frequency of this entity are likely to be more clearly elucidated over the coming years.

INFECTIOUS GASTRITIS

Helicobacter pylori

Helicobacter pylori is a gram-negative, microaerophilic bacterium specialized to colonize gastric epithelial cells that is the most common cause of infectious gastritis (as detailed in Chapter 9.1, "Helicobacter Pylori"). The association of *H. pylori* with gastritis was first described some two decades ago in Australia.[10] Infection with *H. pylori* universally leads to a chronic active gastritis, featuring neutrophilic infiltration along with accumulation of lymphocytes and plasma cells. In addition, *H. pylori* infection is associated with disruption of normal gastric functional activity (eg, hypergastrinemia), peptic ulceration, gastric MALT lymphoma, and gastric adenocarcinoma.[11] Despite induction of gastritis, the infection is not cleared and persists throughout the life of the individual, along with ongoing inflammatory changes.

H. pylori is also associated with several distinct patterns of gastritis. These include atrophic, eosinophilic and granulomatous gastritis (GG), and follicular gastritis (ie, an increased number of lymphoid follicles).

Other Bacterial Causes of Gastritis

Several other members of the *Helicobacter* species also colonize the stomach in human hosts. *H. heilmannii,* a large helical-shaped bacterium (Figure 1) that can be transmitted from cats, colonizes the gastric mucosa and leads to chronic active gastritis in children and adults.[12] *H. heilmannii* occurs much less frequently than *H. pylori* and is present in roughly 1% of a large group of children with dyspepsia.[13] Like *H. pylori*, *H. heilmannii* is associated with gastric carcinoma

Table 1 Classification of Gastris/Gastropathy in Children

Infectious
  Viral
  Bacterial
    H. pylori/other *Helicobacters*
    Mycobacterial
    Phlegmonous and emphysematous gastritis
    Other
  Fungal
  Parasitic

Reactive
  Nonsteroidal anti-inflammatory drugs/aspirin
  Other medications
  Bile reflux
  Stress
  Neonatal
  Exercise
  Radiation
  Corrosive
  Traumatic
  Alcohol

Granulomatous
  Noninfectious
    Crohn's disease
    Chronic granulomatous disease
    Sarcoidosis
    Foreign body
    Wegener's granulomatosis
    Langerhans cell histiocytosis (histiocytosis X)
    Vasculitis-associated
    Idiopathic/isolated
  Infectious
    Tuberculosis
    Fungal
    Syphilis
    Histoplasmosis
    Parasitic

Eosinophilic-mediated gastritis
  Allergic gastritis
  Eosinophilic gastritis

Lymphocytic
  Noninfectious
    Celiac disease
    Varioliform gastritis
    Idiopathic
  Infectious
    H. pylori
    Cytomegalovirus

Collagenous
  Collagenous gastritis

Hyperplastic
  Menetrier disease
  Zollinger-Ellison syndrome
  Proton-pump inhibitor gastropathy

Metabolic
  Cysteamine (Cystinosis)

Vascular
  Portal hypertensive gastrompathy

Autoimmune/vasculitic
  Henoch-Schonlein purpura
  Pernicious anemia
  Autoimmune endocrinopathies
  Connective tissue diseases

Miscellaneous
  Graft-Versus-host disease
  Uremic gastropathy

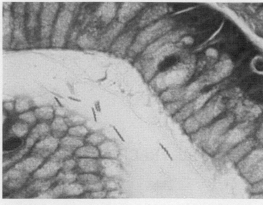

Figure 1 Focally enhanced gastritis. Focal infiltration of neutrophils in the gastric mucosa is a feature of Crohn's disease. Hematoxylin and eosin: original magnification 40×. (Courtesy of Drs Tobias and Sugo, Sydney Children's Hospital, Randwick, Australia.)

and MALT lymphoma, and also responds to anti-*Helicobacter* eradication therapy. Rarely, other *Helicobacter* species have been isolated from the stomach.

Involvement of the stomach is a well described, but uncommon, manifestation of tuberculosis (TB). Due to the pathophysiology of mycobacterial infection, with damage occurring secondary to reactivation of a primary focus, this will less commonly lead to gastritis in children. Five cases of primary gastric TB and two secondary cases were identified among 210 Indian adults with gastric symptoms.[14] Endoscopic features included ulceration and mucosal hypertrophy. In the six patients who completed 6 months of anti-TB therapy, endoscopic and microbiological resolution was noted. Gastritis may occur due to other bacteria; for example, a recent case report described acute necrotizing gastritis due to *Bacillus cereus* infection.[15]

Viral Gastritis

CMV, EBV, TT virus, hepatitis C, human herpes virus 7, measles, varicella, influenza, and herpes virus each are described as being isolated from the stomach. However, gastric manifestations are an uncommon component of the clinical features of these viral infections. Gastric infection with cytomegalovirus (CMV) is described in both immune compromised hosts[16] and otherwise immunocompetent individuals. Moreover, CMV is one of several etiological agents associated with Menetrier's disease.

Hepatitis C may localize to the stomach, where it is associated with a chronic lymphocytic cell infiltrate, and has also been implicated in the development of autoimmune gastritis.[17]

Parasitic and Fungal Gastritis

Various fungal species can infect the stomach, but more commonly in the setting of immunodeficiency. Fungal gastritis can be seen in conjunction with systemic fungal invasion or present solely as local colonization and may lead to significant morbidity and mortality. *Candida albicans* was the most common fungus isolated in a large

Polish series of 293 adult patients undergoing upper endoscopy.[18] Fungal colonization is seen in 54% of those with gastric ulcer and in 10% of patients with chronic gastritis. In this cohort, however, there was poor correlation between the fungal concentrations, the levels of antibodies, and the serum fungal antigen, which was felt to suggest that fungal colonization was secondary.

Cryptosporidiosis is reported rarely in the stomach where it can cause PUD and erosive gastritis.[19] Infection with this organism is almost always associated with immune deficiency. Aspergillus may lead to gastric aspergillosis or emphysematous gastritis. Gastric aspergillus has been reported in one fatal case presenting with upper GI bleeding due to an antral ulcer.[20] Following emergency gastrectomy, pseudomembranous gastritis throughout the stomach was detected.

Gastritis associated with the helmith Anisakis simplex is reported, especially in case reports from Japan.[21] This pathogen, acquired from eating infected fish, is associated with eosinophilic gastritis. The development of gastric mucormycosis is also described in case reports and is associated with emphysematous gastritis.

Although *Giardia lamblia* is found most commonly in the duodenum, these organisms can also inhabit the harsher environment of the stomach. In a series of 567 cases at a single institution, Oberhuber and colleagues[22] located trophozoites on gastric biopsies in 8.7% of cases. *Giardia* infection was associated with various patterns of gastritis, including reactive gastritis, chronic atrophic, gastritis, and chronic active gastritis.

GRANULOMATOUS GASTRITIS

Inflammatory Bowel Disease

Gastritis can be a feature seen in both Crohn's disease (CD) and ulcerative colitis (UC), the main clinical entities comprising the chronic inflammatory bowel diseases (IBD) (see Chapter 20.5, "Chronic Inflammatory Bowel Disease"). Focal gastritis is more characteristic of CD, which is the commonest cause of granulomatous gastritis.

In a series of children and adolescents with CD, reported by Cameron,[23] almost half (46%) had inflammation of the body of the stomach, with less having antral gastritis (36%). Ruuska and colleagues[24] also noted a high prevalence of changes in the upper gastrointestinal tract, including the stomach, both endoscopically (75%) and histologically. Upper gut changes, particularly in the stomach, can help support a diagnosis of CD, compared to UC, thereby altering management strategies. In a recently published cohort of 61 children with CD, 57.4% had endoscopic abnormalities in the stomach and 80.3% had gastritis.[25] More than half the children with otherwise nonspecific pan-colitis had a diagnosis of CD labelled by endoscopic and histologic assessment of the upper gastrointestinal tract. The gastritis seen in CD is characterized as focally enhanced gastritis (FEG) (Figure 2). FEG is present in

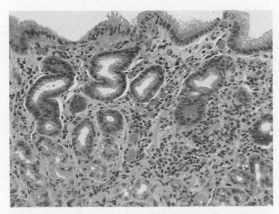

Figure 2 Eosinophilic gastropathy. Infiltration of eosinophils in the lamina propria, muscularis, and superficially in the epithelium of the stomach of a 10-year-old boy diagnosed with eosinophilic gastroenteropathy. Hematoxylin and eosin: original magnification 40×. (Courtesy of Drs Tobias and Sugo, Sydney Children's Hospital, Randwick, Australia.)

76% of adults with CD, compared with 0.8% of healthy controls.[22] Similar data are reported in children, although the differences are not as dramatic as those reported in adults.[26]

More recent reports reveal that between 70 and 93% of children labeled as UC have histological evidence of gastritis.[25,27] Children with UC have evidence of Th2 immune responses in the gastric mucosa, with IL-4 expression and CCR3+ lymphocytes. A similar pattern was seen in the rectal mucosa in these patients, leading the authors to suggest that lymphocytes home from the colon to the gastric mucosa.[27]

Other Causes of Granulomatous Gastritis

Granulomatous gastritis (GG) is a rare feature found in gastric biopsies. In several large series, GG was found in up to 0.35% of patients undergoing upper endoscopy.[28] One retrospective series of granulomatous gastritis cases seen at the Cleveland Clinic over 20 years included 42 patients.[28] Crohn's disease ($n = 23$) and sarcoidosis ($n = 9$) were the largest patient groups in this largely adult cohort.

GG in association with *H. pylori* infection has been described in case reports, predominantly in adult patients, but also in children.[29] One report described a 13-year-old boy presenting with epigastric pain who was found to have GG and *H. pylori* detected histologically.[34] Repeat endoscopy 3 months after *Helicobacter* eradication therapy demonstrated complete resolution of both endoscopic and histologic changes. The mechanisms by which *H. pylori* infection leads to GG have not yet been elucidated.

Chronic granulomatous disease (CGD) is known to present with gastric outlet obstruction (15% in one large series) due to inflammatory thickening in the antral gastric wall leading to obstructive features.[30] CGD may rarely cause a more diffuse gastric involvement.[31]

Other uncommon causes of granulomatous gastritis include vasculitis-associated disease, tuberculosis, syphilis, histoplasmosis, parasitic infection, and foreign body granulomas.[1] Berylliosis, Whipple's disease, and Wegener's granulomatosis are also rarely reported.[28]

In addition, an entity of idiopathic granulomatous gastritis is described, but it is unclear if this is a distinct condition. While the Cleveland Clinic case series of 42 patients did not include any idiopathic GG,[28] isolated case reports have depicted cases of GG with no apparent etiological factors.[32] Histological identification of GG requires consideration of the potential etiological factors, especially exclusion of Crohn's disease and infectious agents. Management relates to the underlying cause.

REACTIVE GASTROPATHY

Reactive gastropathy is a term that describes nonspecific injury to the gastric mucosa with characteristic histopathological features. It has also been referred to as reactive gastritis, chemical gastritis, chemical gastropathy, bile reflux gastritis, or "type C" gastritis.[2] The term "reactive gastropathy" is now preferred because it reflects a reactive change in response to injury from ischemia, chemical agents, or trauma. Endoscopic features are nonspecific and include antral erythema, erosions, and ulceration.[33] Histopathological features include foveolar hyperplasia, mucosal edema and smooth muscle fibers in the lamina propria, vasodilation and congestion of superficial mucosal capillaries, and a paucity of active and chronic inflammatory cells. The involved area varies according to the underlying cause, but the antrum is the most commonly involved site.

NONSTEROIDAL ANTI-INFLAMMATORY DRUG GASTROPATHY

Nonsteroidal anti-inflammatory drugs (NSAIDs) are widely used as analgesic, antipyretic, and anti-inflammatory agents in children, as well as in adults. Unfortunately, there is a relative paucity of literature on NSAID use in children, but NSAID-induced gastroduodenal lesions are well described. In children administered NSAIDs chronically for juvenile idiopathic arthritis, the frequency of clinically significant gastropathy and the risk of developing gastroduodenal injury are comparable to that of adults, with a four- to fivefold increase of gastroduodenal injury following NSAID administration.[34]

NSAIDs cause damage through both pharmacological effects and topical irritant actions. The inhibition of cyclooxygenase (COX) enzymes, of which there are at least two distinct forms (COX-1 and COX-2), is the main underlying mechanism of injury.[35] The role of the recently cloned COX-3 enzyme remains unknown. COX-independent effects in the pathogenesis of NSAID gastropathy have been observed in experimental studies.

NSAIDs inhibit COX enzymes to reduce prostaglandin synthesis. Prostaglandins derived from COX-1 promote gastric mucosal blood flow and production of the mucus-bicarbonate barrier. The main therapeutic effect of NSAIDs is associated with the inhibition of COX-2, which is responsible for the production of prostaglandins at sites of inflammation. The classic understanding that distinguishes COX-1 as a constitutive enzyme and COX-2 as an inducible enzyme at sites of inflammation is no longer considered true, and overlap of features are now known to occur.[35] Studies suggest that COX-2 expressed in inflammatory cells and fibroblasts contribute to tissue healing through induction of growth factors, and COX-2 inhibition increases leukocyte adherence to the vascular endothelium leading to mucosal injury.[35] This concept is supported by the observation that while selective COX-2 inhibitors result in marginally fewer gastroduodenal ulcers and gastrointestinal adverse effects compared to nonselective NSAIDs in adults, these events remain a significant cause of gastrointestinal morbidity in both drug classes.[35]

Symptoms range from asymptomatic to gastric bleeding or perforation. NSAID use should always be asked specifically during the clinical interview, as this information may not be voluntarily given regardless of whether or not a medication history was taken. NSAIDs are easily available over the counter and can be purchased from supermarket shelves in certain countries. Erosions and ulcers may occur acutely with only a single dose of NSAID and with chronic use.[36] Ulceration of the incisura with bleeding is a typical NSAID lesion.[1] The majority of lesions occur in, but are not limited to, the antrum. Histologicin, findings are those of reactive gastropathy or, less frequently, reactive gastritis.[2,33]

There are several approaches to prevention and minimization of NSAID-related gastroduodenal toxicity. These include consideration of alternatives to NSAID therapy, modification of risk factors, use of nitric oxide bound to NSAID, and cotherapy with either gastroprotective or acid suppressive agents. However, a literature regarding this issue is lacking in the pediatric population.

Risk factors for NSAID-related gastroduodenal complications in adults, which may also be considered in children, include a past history of peptic ulceration, high doses of NSAID, concurrent use of aspirin, anticoagulants, or corticosteroids, coagulopathy, and *H. pylori* infection.[35] *H. pylori* infection and NSAID are independent risk factors for ulcer disease, and the risk is additive rather than synergistic.[37] The use of NSAID in the presence of *H. pylori* infection in adults increases the risk of ulcer disease and ulcer bleeding by 3.55- and 6.13-fold, respectively.[37] Therefore, prior to starting long-term NSAID therapy, *H. pylori* infection should be tested for and, if present, eradicated.

Gastroprotection during NSAID or COX-2 therapy using concurrent acid-suppression therapy with proton pump inhibitors (PPIs) or cytoprotection with misoprostol[38] may be helpful in preventing gastrointestinal lesions. Healing rates are similar, but PPI are better tolerated and associated with lower rates of relapse.[38] H2 receptor antagonists do not effectively prevent NSAID-induced gastric ulcers.[39] Experimental therapies based on gastric mucosal protection are currently under evaluation.

OTHER MEDICATIONS, INCLUDING ALCOHOL

Endoscopic changes of erythema, erosions, and subepithelial hemorrhages have been noted with a number of medications, including iron, potassium chloride, cysteamine,[40] corticosteroids, chemotherapeutics, and valproate. Alcohol ingestion is associated with subepithelial hemorrhages seen endoscopically, with a minimal inflammatory component evident histologically.[41] The combination of alcohol with either aspirin or NSAID can lead to significantly greater gastric mucosal damage on endoscopy than with either agent alone.[42]

DUODENOGASTRIC REFLUX

Duodenogastric reflux (DGR) refers to the reflux of duodenal secretions through the pylorus into the stomach. It is also known as bile or alkaline reflux, and as duodenogastroesophageal reflux (DGER) when duodenal and gastric contents together reflux into the esophagus. Reflux of duodenal contents into the stomach is a physiological event, occurring approximately 5% of a 24-hour period in healthy adults.[43]

However, DGR may play a role in the pathogenesis of gastric mucosal inflammation,[44] intestinal metaplasia,[45] and development of gastric carcinoma.[46] The exact mechanisms of gastric mucosal damage from bile reflux are still unclear.

Pathologic DGR is reported in adults after partial gastrectomy, pyloroplasty, and cholecystectomy,[47] but also in adults with an intact stomach.[48] The introduction of 24-hour intragastric bilimetry has increased the recognition of excess bile reflux and a diagnosis of DGR.[49] Similar DGR-related changes have been reported in children both with and without previous abdominal surgery.[50–51]

Clinical features suggestive of DGR include recurrent bilious vomiting, oral bile reflux, and nonspecific acid peptic reflux symptoms, which may be responsive to antacid therapy.[51] Bile is commonly seen during gastroscopy, but this feature is not pathognomonic because the process of inserting an endoscope leads to retropulsive waves and consequent reflux of bile in healthy individuals.[52] Gastric mucosal changes on endoscopy include erythema and erosions. Histological changes are those of a reactive gastropathy.[33] A 24-hour bilimetry study allows monitoring of the duration of bilirubin exposure in the lumen of the stomach,[49] but there are only limited data on its use in children.

PPI therapy decreases DGER, perhaps by decreasing gastric volume and acidity, but their role in the management of DGR is unclear. There is limited evidence to support the use of prokinetic agents, such as cisapride, to improve gastroduodenal coordination,[44,51] or bile acid-binding agents such as sucralfate, cholestyramine, and ursodeoxycholic acid.[51] In patients with severe DGER refractory to medical therapy, surgical Roux-en-Y duodenojejunostomy (duodenal switch) is reported to alleviate clinical symptoms.[53]

STRESS-RELATED MUCOSAL DISEASE

Critically ill children, including preterm infants, who experience severe physiologic stress are at risk of stress-related mucosal disease (SRMD) of the stomach.[54] The term SRMD encompasses a spectrum of mucosal changes from stress erosions to stress ulcers.[55] The frequency of clinically significant upper gastrointestinal bleeding in critically ill patients is relatively low (approximately 1.5 to 2%) and is comparable in children and adults.[54] While the pathogenesis of SRMD is not completely understood, a number of mechanisms have been hypothesized. Under normal physiologic conditions, gastric mucosal integrity is maintained by protective mucosal defense mechanisms. In the setting of physiologic stress with secondary hypoperfusion of the upper gastrointestinal tract, ischemia followed by reperfusion leads to the breakdown of mucosal defenses, predisposing the mucosa to damage by mucosal irritant agents, such as gastric acid.[55] Hypersecretion of gastric acid is not seen in all critically ill patients, suggesting the importance of other factors, such as gastric enzymes and bile salts in the development of mucosal damage.[56]

The main risk factors for clinically significant stress-related gastrointestinal bleeding are respiratory failure, coagulopathy, and a high pediatric risk of mortality score (PRISM; score of 10 or more).[54] The incidence rate of clinically significant upper gastrointestinal bleeding is 0.1% in patients without any or with one risk factor, 2.9% with two risk factors, and 18.8% with three risk factors.[54] Other risk factors associated with bleeding include sepsis, renal failure, hepatic failure, hypotension, multiple trauma, severe burns, head injury, multiorgan failure, and the use of corticosteroids.[57]

SRMD typically occurs in the fundus (ie, acid-secreting areas)[55] but may progress to more diffuse involvement of the stomach. Stress erosions are usually asymptomatic and multiple.[57] Coagulopathy should be suspected when bleeding occurs. Stress ulcers, in contrast, may lead to clinically significant bleeding and perforation.[55,57]

Patients at very high risk for stress-related bleeding should receive potent acid suppression. There is currently limited evidence comparing H_2 receptor antagonist to PPI for the prophylaxis of stress-related bleeding in children. Ranitidine is superior to sucralfate in decreasing the rate of clinically significant bleeding, but neither led to a reduction in mortality.[58]

NEONATAL GASTROPATHY

Various gastropathies have been reported in both sick preterm neonates treated in newborn intensive care units and healthy full-term newborns.[59] A high prevalence of hemorrhagic gastropathy has been reported in critically ill preterm and term infants and may occur in the absence of symptoms.[59–60] Neonatal exposure to indomethacin and dexamethasone are implicated in the development of stress-related bleeding.[61] Gastric perforation has also been reported as a complication of the use of these agents in neonates.[62] Prophylactic short-term therapy with an agent to suppress acid production is associated with a reduction in the rate of gastric mucosal lesions.[60]

Hemorrhagic gastropathy has also been reported in well full-term infants. The etiology is unknown, and several pathogenic hypotheses such as traumatic suctioning of upper gastrointestinal tract, fetal distress, hypergastrinemia associated with maternal stress or antacid use, hyperpepsinogenemia,[63] and cow's milk allergy have been proposed. When present, symptoms are nonspecific and may include feeding difficulties, vomiting, upper gastrointestinal bleeding, and poor weight gain. A variety of endoscopic lesions are described, especially in the fundus. These lesions are usually benign and respond rapidly to acid-suppression therapy, suggesting that endoscopic evaluation should be reserved for patients with significant bleeding or recurrent bleeding despite empiric medical therapy.

Focal foveolar hyperplasia (FFH) has been reported in neonates with duct-dependent congenital heart disease, requiring therapy with high doses of prostaglandin E1.[64–65] Prostaglandins are known to promote elongation and dilatation of gastric foveolae. Cases are often asymptomatic, and spontaneous resolution occurs with discontinuation of prostaglandin therapy.[64] Infants become symptomatic when gastric outlet obstruction develops.[64,65] FFH has also been described with concomitant ectopic pancreas[65] and hypertrophic pyloric stenosis during prostaglandin therapy.[66] Treatment options include cessation of prostaglandin therapy and nasojejunal feeding, or surgical excision with or without pyloroplasty.[64–65,67] Cases of FFH in young infants just beyond the neonatal period have also been reported. Cow's milk protein allergy was implicated in one infant, but no obvious cause was apparent in other reported cases.[67]

EXERCISE-INDUCED GASTROPATHY

Erosive or hemorrhagic gastropathies have been described in athletes.[68] The intensity, type (more prevalent in long-distance running), and duration of exercise appear to be important risk factors.[68–69] The pathophysiology of exercise-related gastropathy likely is similar to stress-related mucosal disease in that splanchnic ischemia plays a key role.[69] Loss of gastric mucosal defense mechanisms due to ischemia predisposes the mucosa to damage by mucosal irritants such as gastric acid, explaining the benefit demonstrated by acid-suppression therapy in preventing gastric mucosal lesions and bleeding.[68] Endoscopic lesions may occur in both fundus and antrum.[68]

RADIATION-INDUCED GASTROPATHY

Radiation-induced gastropathy can occur following intended or unintended gastric exposure during abdominal radiotherapy. A high total dose and large fraction size are associated with a higher rate of gastric complications, but the exact tolerance of the stomach to irradiation is unknown.[70] Gastric erosions and ulceration may progress to bleeding, perforation, fibrosis, and gastric outlet obstruction.[70] Surgical gastric resection has been the preferred treatment in the past, but successful conservative treatment with endoscopic intervention, in particular laser therapy,[71] and hyperbaric oxygen[72] have been reported. There is no current evidence for the use of acid-suppression therapy as a preventative measure.

CORROSIVE GASTROPATHY

Corrosive injuries of the stomach occur with strong acid and alkaline ingestion. Injuries caused by acids are relatively less common than alkalis because of the harsh taste of acids and the greater use of alkali in household products. Acid ingestion primarily causes gastric injury whereas alkalis mainly damage the oropharynx and esophagus. However, isolated cases of esophageal acid and gastric alkaline injuries have been reported.[73–74] The severity of corrosive gastric injury depends on the concentration and amount of ingested agent, the nature of the agent, the length of time in the stomach, and amount of gastric food content at the time of ingestion.[73–74] Acid typically pools in the antrum due to prepyloric spasm thereby leading to gastric burns.[73–74]

Gastroscopy, contraindicated in the presence of perforation, can reveal friability, erythema, ulcers, hemorrhage, and necrosis (black-brown discoloration). Extensive necrosis or perforation is an indication for surgical intervention. Antral and pyloric strictures due to fibrosis may occur with healing resulting in gastric outlet obstruction, with presenting symptoms such as postprandial fullness, nonbilious vomiting, and weight loss as early as 7 days postingestion.[75]

Oral iron, zinc-containing foreign bodies, certain button batteries (lithium or mercuric oxide cells), pine oil cleaner, and oxidizing agents such as hydrogen peroxide and potassium permanganate also cause a corrosive gastropathy.

UREMIC GASTROPATHY

The reported prevalence of upper gastrointestinal diseases in acute and chronic renal failure (ARF, CRF) varies widely.[76–78] Upper gastrointestinal hemorrhage occurs in ARF, with gastric erosions or ulcers found in over half of these patients.[76] The underlying mechanism is thought to be related to physiologic stress, with additional factors that increase the risk of bleeding such as acute uremia, thrombocytopenia, and preexisting liver disease.[76]

Upper gastrointestinal symptoms also are common in patients with CRF. A frequency of 40% was reported in one group of 37 children.[78] Underlying mechanisms and factors contributing to the development of these gastropathies are complex. Gastric hypomotility is demonstrated in CRF patients. Patients with impaired gastric myoelectrical activity and delayed gastric emptying experience more gastrointestinal symptoms.[79] Possible mechanisms for hypomotility include increased levels of hormones involved in gastrointestinal motility, such as cholecystokinin, gastrin, and neurotensin, with reduced renal clearance,[80] and autonomic nervous system dysfunction with uremia.[81] The role of gastric acid secretion in the pathogenesis of uremic gastropathy is not well defined. Hypergastrinemia is commonly seen due to reduced renal clearance but may also be due to a feedback mechanism from gastric acid neutralization with gastric ammonia.[82] This concept is supported by the observation that the frequency and severity of gastropathies increase after CRF treatment.[82–83] Endoscopic abnormalities are more frequent in symptomatic patients but may also be present in asymptomatic individuals with CRF.[78] Hemorrhagic gastropathy is the most common gastric lesion in uremic patients,[83] with gastric lesions predominantly in the antrum.[78,83] An increase in number of bi- and multinucleated parietal cells with vacuolation and fragmentation of the cytoplasm is observed histologically.[84] Peptic ulcers in CRF patients have atypical features: they are more likely to be pain-free, present with bleeding, multiple, located in the postbulbar region, and less likely to have *H. pylori* infection.[77] Gastric angiodysplasia is another recognized cause of gastrointestinal bleeding in CRF patients and may be a cause of recombinant human erythropoietin-resistant anemia.[85]

Peptic ulcer is a significant cause of morbidity and mortality after renal transplantation historically, having accounted for approximately 4% of deaths.[86] However, the use of acid-suppression therapies and corticosteroid-sparing immune-suppressive regimens have reduced the frequency of this complication.[87] The development of hyperplastic gastric polyps postrenal transplant, of which the cause is unknown, has recently been reported.[88]

COLLAGENOUS GASTRITIS

Collagenous gastritis is a rare condition first described in 1989 by Colletti and Trainer.[89] Subsequently, there have only been 6 pediatric and 14 adult cases reported in the literature.[90–91] Collagenous gastritis is characterized by subepithelial collagen fibrosis greater than 10 μm in thickness associated with an inflammatory infiltrate of the lamina propria.[89–91]

The cause and pathogenesis of collagenous gastritis remain unknown but assumed to be similar to collagenous colitis. The more frequently reported (greater than 500 cases) collagenous colitis has been studied in more detail. Several pathogenic mechanisms have been proposed including subepithelial collagen deposition as a consequence of damage caused by intraluminal toxic or infectious agents, previous leakage of plasma proteins and fibrinogen with replacement by collagen in the absence of inflammation, and abnormal pericryptal fibroblast sheath and associated deposition of subepithelial collagen.[90]

The presenting clinical features in children with collagenous gastritis are severe anemia from gastrointestinal bleeding and epigastric pain.[91] Endoscopic features are variable and include erythema, mucosal hemorrhages, erosions, ulcerations, exudate, granularity and nodularity in either the gastric body or, less frequently, in the antrum.[91] Endoscopic appearances resembling varioliform gastritis have also been reported.

Variable symptomatic improvement has been reported with acid-suppression and corticosteroid therapy.[90–91] Follow-up studies have not shown endoscopic or histologic improvement. Symptomatic, endoscopic, and histologic improvements were reported after commencing of a gluten-free diet in a single adult patient with associated celiac disease.[90]

LYMPHOCYTIC GASTRITIS

Lymphocytic gastritis, first described by Haot and colleagues[92] is characterized by an intense lymphocytosis of the foveolar and surface epithelium in association with chronic inflammation in the lamina propria.[92–93] The definition of lymphocytic gastritis varies in the literature in regard to the numbers of intraepithelial lymphocytes (IEL).[92,94–95] Lymphocytic gastritis is reported in association with celiac disease, *H. pylori* gastritis,[93] and chronic varioliform gastritis.[93] Lymphocytic gastritis should be regarded, therefore, as a histopathological finding seen in conjunction with multiple disease entities.

CELIAC GASTRITIS

Celiac disease is an autoimmune gluten sensitive enteropathy with characteristic histological lesions of the small bowel, including villous atrophy, crypt hyperplasia, and elevated numbers of intraepithelial lymphocytes (IEL). Increased numbers of IEL are also observed in the stomach in up to 87% of children with untreated celiac disease.[94–95] Lymphocytic gastritis in children with untreated celiac disease consists of CD8+ intraepithelial T-lymphocytes that differ from T cells found in the duodenojejunal mucosa in untreated adult celiac disease.[96]

It is unclear whether celiac gastritis contributes significantly to the gastrointestinal symptoms of celiac disease. Dyspeptic symptoms may be more prominent in children with celiac disease with lymphocytic gastritis than those without[97] although this was not confirmed in a subsequent study.[95] Celiac-associated lymphocytic gastritis does not have specific endoscopic features. Histopathological changes are those of a lymphocytic gastritis associated with nonspecific chronic gastritis. Lymphocytic gastritis was present in 29 of 33 children with untreated celiac disease.[95] Fifteen of these 29 patients had lymphocytic gastritis in the presence of nonspecific chronic gastritis. Histology normalized after the introduction of a gluten-free diet.[95] A second pediatric study found increased gastric IEL in 16 of 23 children with celiac disease, with significant reductions in the number of gastric IEL following gluten withdrawal.[94]

CHRONIC VARIOLIFORM GASTRITIS

Chronic varioliform (erosive) gastritis is an insidious chronic gastritis that occurs rarely in children. The diagnosis is established by the presence of specific endoscopic features of thickened gastric rugae, nodules, and erosions.[98–99] The nodules, typically, have central erosions. The etiology, clinical significance, and natural history of this condition remain unknown. Increases in IgE containing plasma cells observed in biopsies taken from the edges of varioliform lesions suggest a role for IgE-mediated allergy in disease pathogenesis.[98] However, a more recent study failed to confirm such a relationship.[100] Reported clinical features in children include nonspecific upper gastrointestinal symptoms, gastric bleeding, and protein-losing gastropathy.[99] Superficial hyperplastic gastritis with mixed inflammatory cellular infiltrate is seen on histology.[98] An association with collagenous and lymphocytic gastritis[93] has been described. Successful treatment has been reported with the use of mast cell stabilizers, such as sodium cromoglycate.[98] Adenomatous transformation was reported in an adult patient, suggesting a possible link between varioliform gastritis and gastric neoplasia.[101]

EOSINOPHIL-MEDIATED GASTRITIS

Eosinophil-mediated gastritis is part of the spectrum of allergic gastrointestinal disorders. The pathophysiology remains unclear and likely represents a condition with heterogenous underlying etiologies. Allergic gastritis (AG) and primary eosinophilic gastritis (EG) are conditions that share similar features and are characterized by gastric infiltration with eosinophils.[2,102] Additional causes of gastric eosinophilia include the hypereosinophilic syndrome, infectious gastritis (including *H. pylori*), celiac disease, connective tissue disease (such as scleroderma), IBD, myeloproliferative disorders, vasculitis, drug injury, and drug hypersensitivity reactions.[21]

Allergic Gastritis

Cow's milk protein is considered the food antigen most often implicated in allergic gastritis (AG), but approximately half of these patients are also intolerant to soy-milk protein.[103] Solids such as cereals, vegetables, and poultry have also been implicated.[104] This condition typically presents in young infants.[102] Symptoms include recurrent vomiting, hematemesis, irritability, and poor weight gain.[102] Infants with cow's milk protein allergy may have gastric dysrhythmia and delayed gastric emptying.[105]

A definitive diagnosis of food allergy requires a formal food challenge (double-blind, placebo-controlled, crossover) with or without endoscopic investigation. However, in clinical practice, the diagnosis is often suspected based on allergen elimination with subsequent resolution of symptoms. Depending on the clinical presentation and response to treatment, upper and lower gastrointestinal endoscopy and biopsies may be undertaken. Gastroscopy in infants with cow's milk protein allergy may show erythema, erosion, and friability of the gastric mucosa.[102] Histologically, there is an infiltration of eosinophils into the lamina propria, accompanied by an increase in lymphocytes, plasma cells, and neutrophils.[1,2,102] In contrast to EG, peripheral eosinophilia is not commonly observed in AG.[102] IgE-specific tests such as radioallergosorbent tests (RAST) and skin prick tests often are not helpful and, therefore, are not recommended in infants with suspected cow's milk protein allergy. The atopy patch test may become a potentially valuable complementary test for diagnosing cell-mediated food allergy in infants and children.

Strict dietary elimination of offending allergen(s) is a therapeutic intervention. In infants, this involves the use of a hypoallergenic diet in the form of either an extensively hydrolyzed or amino acid-based formula, and a maternal elimination diet in breastfeeding mothers.[106] Supervision by a dietitian is recommended due to the potential risk of inadequate caloric intake and micronutrient deficiency. The prognosis is excellent with the development of tolerance by 3 years of age.[107]

Eosinophilic Gastritis

Primary eosinophilic gastritis (EG) may present at any age, including preterm infants. Symptoms of EG are nonspecific and vary depending on the severity, anatomic involvement of the gastrointestinal tract, and histological level of eosinophilic infiltration. Mucosal forms present with vomiting, abdominal pain, and blood loss. Muscular involvement produces gastric outlet obstruction[108] and delayed gastric emptying.[109] The serosal form induces eosinophilic ascites.[110] Gastroscopic abnormalities include swollen mucosal folds, nodules, and polyps, particularly in the gastric antrum.[1] Gastric biopsy reveals marked infiltration with eosinophils[2] (Figure 3), but this may not be detected when the eosinophilic involvement is exclusively in the muscle or serosal layers. Peripheral eosinophilia is observed in up to 50% of adult patients.[110] Food sensitization is infrequently identified using skin prick testing and/or radioallergosorbent tests for IgE-mediated

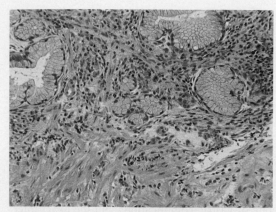

Figure 3 *Helicobacter heilmannii*-associated gastritis. Spiral organisms are seen in the lumen and associated with gastric epithelium of a 7-year-old girl with *H. heilmannii* infection contracted from her cat. At autopsy the cat was shown to have infection with the same organism. Hematoxylin and eosin: original magnification 100×. (Courtesy of Drs Tobias and Sugo, Sydney Children's Hospital, Randwick, Australia.)

types, and atopy patch test for cell-mediated types of eosinophilic gastroenteropathies.

Treatment of eosinophilic gastritis includes hypoallergenic diets, topical or systemic steroids, or antiallergic medications such as leukotriene inhibitors and mast cell stabilizers (eg, sodium cromoglycate and ketotifen). The response to dietary elimination is variable. Immunosuppressive medications, such as azathioprine (or 6-mercaptopurine) or mycophenolate mofetil, and novel therapies such as humanized anti-IL-5 antibody (mepolizumab) have been used in severe, refractory, or steroid-dependent cases.[111] In addition, empiric PPI therapy may provide symptomatic improvement.

The natural course of eosinophilic gastroenteropathies is not well defined. The conditions appear to wax and wane into adulthood, with an element of improvement over time.[110] There is a higher likelihood of remission by late childhood in cases presenting in infancy in association with food sensitization.

PORTAL HYPERTENSIVE GASTROPATHY

Portal hypertensive gastropathy (PHG) is a common complication of portal hypertension both in children and in adults.[112–113] The incidence, severity, response to treatment, and natural history are contentious because of the lack of a uniform diagnostic criteria.[114–115]

PHG occurs in patients with both cirrhotic and non cirrhotic portal hypertension but is more common in cirrhosis.[116] Direct measurements of portal pressure and resolution of PHG after surgical or transjugular intrahepatic portosystemic shunt (TIPS) placement suggest a direct association between portal hypertension and PHG.[117] The progression of PHG is associated with the presence and size of gastroesophageal varices and previous endoscopic variceal therapy.[113] However, the presence or severity of PHG does not have a linear correlation with portal venous

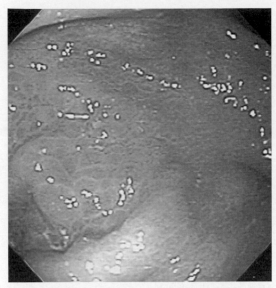

Figure 4 Portal hypertensive gastropathy. Characteristic endoscopic appearance. (Courtesy of Dr S Ling, Hospital for Sick Children, University of Toronto, Canada.)

pressure.[117] Increased gastric blood flow due to chronic increase in portal pressure and splenic circulation is a reasonable underlying explanation, but studies measuring gastric blood flow have provided shown varying results.[118–119] Impaired gastric mucosal defense mechanisms in the presence of portal hypertension (eg, nitric oxide, endothelin-1) have also been suggested in the pathogenesis of PHG in experimental models.[118,120]

PHG presents with symptoms of chronic or massive acute bleeding. A diagnosis of PHG is based on a characteristic endoscopic feature of mosaic-like (or snake-skin) pattern of the gastric mucosa with or without red marks (Figure 4).[112,114] The mosaic-like pattern appears as white reticular network separating areas of raised red or pink mucosa. Red-point lesions and cherry-red spots, collectively called red marks, are often seen in severe PHG. Black-brown spots secondary to intramural bleeding may also be seen.[114] Although mucosal biopsies are rarely indicated, due to the high risk of bleeding, the described histological findings include dilated capillaries and venules in the mucosa and submucosa without erosion, inflammation, or fibrin thrombi.[115] One indication for obtaining mucosal biopsies is to attempt to differentiate PHG from antral vascular ectasia.

Nonselective β-blockers, such as propanolol and nadolol, reduce portal venous pressure and gastric mucosal blood flow and are recommended for prophylaxis of bleeding from PHG.[121] Propanolol may also reduce the development of PHG after endoscopic variceal banding.[122] Somatostatin analogues, such as octreotide and terlipressin, are effective in controlling acute bleeding from PHG.[123–124] Recent studies have demonstrated novel roles in the management of PHG for the angiotensin II receptor antagonist losartan[125] and thalidomide[126] by decreasing portal pressure and by inhibition of tumor necrosis factor-α and angiogenesis, respectively. Endoscopic treatment of PHG bleeding has not been well studied but

is unlikely to play a significant role because the bleeding is usually diffuse in nature. However, an identifiable active focal site of bleeding could be managed by either injection sclerotherapy or heat cauterization. Improvement or resolution of PHG occurs after TIPS placement and shunt surgery. Liver transplantation is also an effective treatment for PHG.

HENOCH-SCHONLEIN GASTRITIS

Henoch-Schonlein purpura (HSP), the commonest vasculitis in children, is a small vessel vasculitis mediated by IgA deposition typically involving the skin, joints, gastrointestinal tract, and kidneys. Mucosal lesions can develop anywhere in the gastrointestinal tract, but the duodenum and small bowel are the most commonly involved sites.[127]

Gastrointestinal symptoms occur in up to 85% of patients and may precede other manifestations in 14% of cases.[128] Although rare, it is increasingly recognized that HSP-related gastrointestinal symptoms can occur in the absence of skin lesions or with a nonpurpuric rash.[129] Gastrointestinal symptoms of HSP include abdominal pain, nausea, vomiting, and bleeding. Complications of involvement of the gastrointestinal tract in HSP include intramural hematomas, intussusception, bowel infarction, bowel perforation, pancreatitis, appendicitis, and cholecystitis.

Esophagogastroduodenoscopy can help to establish a diagnosis of HSP in patients with severe acute or persistent gastrointestinal symptoms when skin lesions are absent,[129] but may also be indicated to define the extent of involvement in classical HSP when gut symptoms predominate. Endoscopic changes include erythema, submucosal hemorrhage, superficial erosions, and ulceration, but there is no specific pattern of gastric involvement.[128,130] Hematoma-like protrusions may be seen in the antrum and duodenum.[127] Histology reveals a leukocytoclastic vasculitis (LCV), similar to that seen in the skin, and inflammatory changes ranging from nonspecific mucosal inflammation to marked lymphoplasmacytic and neutrophilic infiltration of the lamina propria with vascular congestion.[127,129] The frequency of LCV in biopsies correlates with the severity of duodenitis[130] and with ulceration and hematoma-like protrusions.[127] Immunostaining of tissue sections to demonstrate IgA deposits may assist in confirming the diagnosis of HSP, but such deposits are not universally present.[129] Complementary laboratory findings include decreased factor XIII and IgA levels.[129] HSP is generally a benign and self-limiting illness in children, and specific therapy is not usually required.

GRAFT-VERSUS-HOST DISEASE

Acute graft-versus-host disease (GVHD), by definition, occurs within the first 100 days following bone marrow transplantation, during or soon after engraftment (which is defined as

normalization of blood count) and is characterized by damage to the skin, gastrointestinal tract, and liver. Gastrointestinal symptoms, acute gastrointestinal GVHD, are common, but are non-specific, including anorexia, nausea, vomiting, watery diarrhea, abdominal pain, and bleeding. A distinct syndrome of acute upper gastrointestinal tract GVHD is recognized to present with anorexia, nausea, vomiting, dyspepsia, and food intolerance.[131] Conditions such as infections, drug toxicity, radiation toxicity, and preexisting gastrointestinal diseases must also be excluded. When acute GVHD is suspected, endoscopy with biopsy is required to establish the diagnosis.[131–132] It appears that both upper and lower gastrointestinal endoscopy and biopsy should be performed at the same time even in patients without upper gastrointestinal symptoms. Studies report a high diagnostic yield in performing endoscopy with biopsies of the stomach, even when diarrhea is the predominant symptom.[131] Another study found 18% of patients had GVHD limited to the upper gastrointestinal tract. Endoscopy may appear normal or show evidence of mucosal oedema, erythema, erosions, and mucosal sloughing.[132] To increase the diagnostic yield, duodenal and esophageal biopsies should also be performed during esophagogastroduodenoscopy even if the mucosa appears normal. The high frequency of coagulopathy and hence the potential for bleeding from endoscopic biopsies need to be considered.[132] The diagnosis of gastrointestinal GVHD requires the finding of epithelial cell apoptosis (or "crypt cell degeneration") on histology. This may be associated with glandular destruction, granular debris in dilated glands, and a mixed inflammatory infiltrate of lymphocytes, neutrophils, and eosinophils in the lamina propria.[132] However, similar histological changes are noted in viral infections, such as CMV and human immunodeficiency virus, primary immunodeficiency conditions, and within the immediate posttransplant period (<20 days) due to toxicity on the gastrointestinal epithelium by the pretransplant conditioning regimen.[133] Chronic GVHD typically involves the esophagus but generally spares the stomach, small bowel, and colon.

PROTON PUMP INHIBITOR GASTROPATHY

Concerns regarding long-term proton pump inhibitor (PPI) use have generated interest and some controversy over the last decade. Safety data of long-term PPI usage is limited in the pediatric population. Nonetheless, long-term PPI use is associated with gastric polyps and nodules, atrophic gastritis, and gastric bacterial overgrowth.

Graham[134] first proposed a link between gastric polyps and omeprazole. Since then, this association has been reported in both children and adults.[135–136] The underlying mechanism of gastric polyp formation remains unclear. Long-term PPI use leads to hypergastrinemia, gastric mucosal changes such as argyrophil cell hyperplasia,

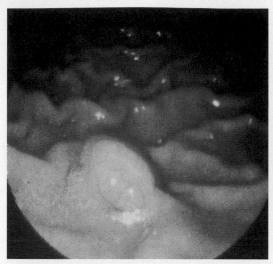

Figure 5 Gastric polyp secondary to proton pump inhibition. Characteristic endoscopic appearance of a pedunculated gastric polyp. (Courtesy of Dr E Hassall, Vancouver, Canada.)

parietal cell hyperplasia, and enterochromaffin-like cell hyperplasia. Such changes could promote the development of mucosal polyps. The natural history and clinical significance of these polyps are unknown, but current evidence indicates a benign nature.[135–136] A retrospective study in children found that 22% (7 out of 31) of children on long-term omeprazole therapy developed polyps and nodules in the gastric body over a mean follow-up period of 28 months.[135] Polyps, either sessile or pedunculated, were noted in isolation or with one or more nodules (Figure 5).

On histological examination, sessile polyps are of the hyperplastic type with findings of glandular dilatation, foveolar hyperplasia, and mild inflammation. Pedunculated polyps are consistent with a fundic gland polyp, with findings of cystic glandular dilatation with cysts lined by chief and parietal cells. All the polyps persisted in this group of children, while the nodules appeared to resolve spontaneously despite ongoing PPI therapy. There are no significant differences between children with and without polyps or nodules of PPI maintenance therapy in regard to age, duration or dose of drug, and serum gastrin levels. Although parietal cell hyperplasia and antral G-cell hyperplasia (with an increase in the ratio of G to D cells) are noted in some children, there are no reports of dysplastic changes in the gastric mucosa, polyps, or nodules.[135] Studies in adults report an incidence of gastric polyps of 7 to 17%, the presence of multiple polyps, and some differences in histological appearance.[136] Cessation of PPI therapy has prompted polyp regression in some adults.[136] Overall, the similarities between the pediatric and adult observations include the persistence of polyps,[136] absence of dysplasia[134,136] and lack of association between polyps and dose of PPI, and elevated serum gastrins.[136]

The loss of the protective acid barrier with hypochlorhydria increases the risk of gastric bacterial overgrowth,[137] but adverse clinical gastrointestinal consequences have not been reported. This may be more of a clinical concern at the extremes of age.

AUTOIMMUNE GASTRITIS

Autoimmune (AI) gastritis, also referred to as atrophic body gastritis, is characterized by hypergastrinemia, achlorhydria, and histological evidence of loss of oxyntic glands.[2] Changes that precede the complete loss of oxyntic glands include lymphoplasmacytic infiltration in the lamina propria with focal gland infiltration, enterochromaffin cell hyperplasia, parietal cell pseudohypertrophy, and epithelial metaplasia.[138] The main immunological marker of AI gastritis is the presence of autoantibodies directed against the parietal cell (anti-parietal cell antibodies: PCA), but antiantral cell antibodies can also be present. Iron deficiency may be seen early, with later development of B12 deficiency (pernicious anemia).

In adults, the primary cause of atrophic gastritis is current or previous *H. pylori* infection.

In children, atrophic gastritis is seen more in the context of other autoimmune conditions, such as diabetes mellitus and autoimmune thyroiditis in the autoimmune polyendocrine syndrome (APS) type 3.[139] AI gastritis is present in up to 30% of patients with autoimmune thyroid disease and in up to 25% of patients with type 1 diabetes mellitus. In a recently reported series of children with autoimmune thyroid disease, 30% of 129 children had positive PCA: roughly half of the children with positive autoantibodies had associated hypergastrinemia.[140] Serum gastrin levels proved to be a more reliable marker of gastric atrophy than clinical symptoms in these children.

MENETRIER'S DISEASE

The primary feature of Menetrier's disease (MD), or transient hypertrophic gastropathy, is of presentation with hypoalbuminemia due to protein loss from hypertrophic gastric folds.[141] MD in children has markedly different features to adults. Whereas adult-type MD is a chronic disease requiring specific therapy, pediatric MD is typically acute in onset, transient, and self-resolving.[141] The precise incidence of MD in children is unknown, but it is thought to be an uncommon event. Several infectious etiologies have been reported including CMV and *H. pylori* and, more rarely, with herpes simplex virus and Mycoplasma.[142–143] Treatment with antiviral agents in MD associated with CMV appears to lead to a more resolution of histological changes.[142] Similarly, anti-*Helicobacter* therapy may lead to resolution of MD in cases where *H. pylori* is detected.[143]

Two additional factors important in the pathogenesis of MD in experimental models are over expression of transforming growth factor (TGF)[144] and signaling via the epidermal growth factor-receptor (EGF-R).[145] A recent report demonstrated rapid improvement in symptoms in an adult with MD following treatment with a monoclonal antibody directed to EGF-R.[145]

MD has also been reported rarely in the neonatal period, as in a recent case report of two infants with onset of disease in the first days of

life.[146] Both infants had characteristic mucosal changes with severe hypoalbuminemia. Interestingly, gastric biopsies taken from both infants showed intense cytoplasmic staining for TGF-β, in a pattern similar to that seen in older patients.

The clinical presentation of MD in children is characteristically one of vomiting, abdominal pain, and hypoalbuminemia appearing over a short-time period. Fever, anorexia, diarrhea, and weight loss have also been reported. Presentation may include peripheral edema, ascites, and pleural effusion related to severe hypoalbuminemia, due to gastric protein losses.

When MD is suspected clinically, other causes of albumin loss should be excluded, and upper gastrointestinal endoscopy is undertaken to define mucosal disease. The endoscopic appearance is of hypertrophic gastric folds, especially in the body. Histologically, the characteristic appearance is of foveolar hyperplasia of the gastric mucosa with hypersecretion of mucus and glandular atrophy. Appropriate investigations to ascertain the presence of infectious agents (as above) are required. MD in childhood is generally a benign and self-limited condition. Accordingly, management is primarily supportive in nature.

MISCELLANEOUS CAUSES

Cytinosis is an autosomal recessive condition characterized by the development of multiorgan damage and, in particular, renal failure due to excessive deposition of intralysosomal cystine. Cysteamine therapy lowers intracellular cystine and reduces the rate of development of end-stage renal failure but is a highly ulcerogenic agent.[40] Cysteamine causes hypergastrinemia and gastric acid hypersecretion.[147] A two- to threefold rise in gastric acid secretion is noted after a single dose of oral cysteamine (11 to 23 mg/kg).[147] Other possible causative factors for ulceration include delayed gastric emptying and diminished duodenal mucosa blood flow with consequent reductions in cytoprotective factors. Endoscopy may reveal a distinctive diffuse fine gastric nodularity. The significance of cystine crystal deposition on histology is unclear but may signify inadequate treatment with cysteamine.[147]

Russell body gastritis is a rarely reported cause of gastritis and has not yet been identified in children. One representative case was an elderly adult with epigastric pain.[148] The fundus was swollen, and histological examination of fundic biopsies showed an infiltration of plasma cells containing so-called Russell bodies. Immunohistochemical staining showed polyclonal expansion of plasma cells. The pathogenesis of this rare gastritis is unclear, as is the management.

Emphysematous gastritis is a rarely described entity featuring intramural gas and thickening of the gastric mucosa.[149] This condition, which has been described in infants and older children, is associated with infection by gas-forming organisms and can progress rapidly to death. Malnutrition and renal failure have been suggested as risk factors.

Phlegmonous gastritis is another rare condition related to rapidly progressive bacterial infection involving the gastric submucosa.[150] α-Hemolytic streptococcus is reported as the most commonly isolated organism, but other etiological agents have included *Escherichia coli*, *Pneumococcus*, *Klebsiella*, and *Staphylococcus*. The majority of reported cases are in adults, but this entity has recently been described in an infant presenting with vomiting, abdominal distension, and fever.[151]

Zollinger-Ellison (ZE) syndrome rarely presents in children: the features of this condition are recurrent and severe peptic ulcer disease with hypersecretion of gastric acid, due to a gastrinoma in the pancreas, stomach, or duodenum.[152] ZE syndrome may be sporadic or in the setting of multiple endocrine neoplasia (MEN) type 1. Histologically, enterochromaffin cell hyperplasia and severe gastritis may be evident. Hypergastrinemia is also seen in a syndrome termed pseudo-Zollinger-Ellison syndrome, where a gastrinoma is not present, and G-cell hyperplasia is evident on biopsies of the body of the stomach.

Various vascular anomalies, such as gastric antral vascular ectasia (watermelon stomach), Dieulafoy lesion, and arteriovenous malformations, may occur in the stomach without causing gastritis.

REFERENCES

1. Dohil R, Hassall E, Jevon G, Dimmick J. Gastritis and gastropathy of childhood. J Pediatr Gastroenterol Nutr 1999; 29:378–94.
2. Dixon MF, Genta RM, Yardley JH, et al. Classification and grading of gastritis: The updated Sydney system. Am J Surg Pathol 1996;20:1161–81.
3. Price AB. The Sydney system: Histological division. J Gastroenterol Hepatol 1991;6:209–22.
4. Rugge M, Correa P, Dixon MF, et al. Gastric mucosal atrophy: Interobserver consistency using new criteria for classification and grading. Aliment Pharmacol Ther 2002; 16:1249–59.
5. Rugge M, Genta RM. Staging and grading of chronic gastritis. Hum Pathol 2005;36:228–33.
6. Ciociola AA, McSorley DJ, Turner K, et al. *Helicobacter pylori* infection rates in duodenal ulcer patients in the United States may be lower than previously estimated. Am J Gastroenterol 1999;94:1834–40.
7. Arents NLA, Thijs JC, van Zwet AA, Kleibeuker JH. Does the declining prevalence of *Helicobacter pylori* unmask patients with idiopathic peptic ulcer disease? Trends over an 8-year period. Eur J Gastroenterol Hepatol 2004;16: 779–83.
8. Xia HHX, Wong BCY, Wong KW, et al. Clinical and endoscopic characteristics of non–*Helicobacter pylori* non-NSAID duodenal ulcers: A long-term prospective study. Aliment Pharmacol Ther 2001;15:1875–82.
9. Elitsur Y, Lawrence Z. Non–*Helicobacter pylori* related duodenal ulcer disease in children. Helicobacter 2001;6: 239–43.
10. Marshall BJ, Warren JR. Unidentified curved bacilli in the stomach of patients with gastritis and peptic ulceration. Lancet 1985;1:1311–5.
11. Jones NL, Day AS, Sherman PM. Determinants of disease outcome following *Helicobacter pylori* infection in children. Can J Gastroenterol 1999;13:613–7.
12. Okiyama Y, Matsuzawa K, Hidaka E, et al. *Helicobacter heilmannii* infection: Clinical, endoscopic and histopathological features in Japanese patients. Pathol Int 2005;55: 398–404.
13. Sykora J, Hejda V, Varvarovska J, et al. *Helicobacter heilmannii* gastroduodenal disease and clinical aspects in children with dyspeptic symptoms. Acta Paediatr 2004;93:707–9.
14. Jain S, Kumar N, Jain SK. Gastric tuberculosis. Endoscopic cytology as a diagnostic tool. Acta Ctol 2000;44:987–92.
15. Le Scanff J, Mohammedi I, Thiebaut A, et al. Necrotising gastritis due to *Bacillus cereus* in an immunocompromised patient. Infection 2006;34:98–9.
16. Peter A, Telkes G, Varga M, et al. Endoscopic diagnosis of cytomegalovirus infection of upper gastrointestinal tract in solid organ transplant recipients: Hungarian single-centre experience. Clin Transplant 2004;18:580–4.
17. Fabbri C, Jaboli MF, Giovanelli S, et al. Gastric autoimmune disorders in patients with chronic hepatitis C before, during and after interferon therapy. World J Gastroenterol 2003;9:1487–90.
18. Zwolinska-Wcislo M, Budak A, Bogdal J, et al. Fungal colonisation of gastric mucosa and its clinical relevance. Med Sci Monit 2001;7:982–8.
19. Clemente CM, Caramori CA, Padula P, Rodrigues MA. Gastric cryptosporidiosis as a clue for the diagnosis of the aquired immunodeficiency syndrome. Arq Gastroenterol 2000;37:180–2.
20. Sanders DL, Pfeiffer RB, Hashimoto LA, et al. Pseudomembraneous gastritis: A complication from aspergillus infection. Am J Surg 2003;69:536–8.
21. Kakizoe S, Kakizoe H, Kakizoe K, et al. Endoscopic findings and clinical manifestation of gastric anisakiasis. Am J Gastroenterol 1995;90:761–3.
22. Oberhuber G, Puspok A, Oesterreicher C, et al. Focally enhanced gastritis: A frequent type of gastritis in patients with Crohn's disease. Gastroenterology 1997;112:698–706.
23. Cameron DJ. Upper and lower gastrointestinal endoscopy in children and adolescents with Crohn's disease: A prospective study. J Gastroenterol Hepatol 1991;6:355–8.
24. Ruuska T, Vaajalahti P, Arajarvi P, Maki M. Prospective evaluation of upper gastrointestinal mucosal lesions in children with ulcerative colitis and Crohn's disease. J Pediatr Gastroenterol Nutr 1994;19:181–6.
25. Lemberg DA, Clarkson C, Bohane T, Day AS. The role of esophagogastroduodenoscopy in the initial assessment of children with IBD. J Gastroenterol Hepatol 2005;20:1696–1700.
26. Sharif F, McDermott M, Dillon M, et al. Focally enhanced gastritis in children with Crohn's disease and ulcerative colitis. Am J Gastroenterol 2002;97:1415–20.
27. Berrebi D, Languepin J, Ferkdadji L, et al. Cytokines, chemokine receptors and homing molecule distribution in the rectum and stomach of pediatric patients with ulcerative colitis. J Pediatr Gastroenterol Nutr 2003;37:300–8.
28. Shapiro JL, Goldblum JR, Petras RE. A clinicopathologic study of 42 patients with granulomatous gastritis. Is there really an "idiopathic" granulomatous gastritis. Am J Surg Pathol 1996;20:462–70.
29. Ozturk Y, Buyukgebiz B, Ozer E, et al. Resolution of *Helicobacter pylori* associated granulomatous gastritis in a child after eradication therapy. J Pediatr Gastroenterol Nutr 2004;39:286–7.
30. Winkelstein JA, Marino MC, Johnston RB, et al. Chronic granulomatous disease. Report on a national registry of 368 patients. Medicine (Baltimore) 2000;79:155–69.
31. Smith FJ, Taves DH. Gastroduodenal involvement in chronic granulomatous disease of childhood. Can Assoc Radiol J 1992;43:215–7.
32. Spinzi G, Meucci G, Radaelli F, et al. Granulomatous gastritis presenting as gastric outlet obstruction: A case report. Ital J Gastroenterol Hepatol 1998;30:410–3.
33. Pashankar DS, Bishop WP, Mitros FA. Chemical gastropathy: A distinct histopathologic entity in children. J Pediatr Gastroenterol Nutr 2002;35:653–7.
34. Hawkey CJ. Nonsteroidal anti-inflammatory drug gastropathy. Gastroenterology 2000;119:521–35.
35. Lazzaroni M, Bianchi Porro G. Gastrointestinal side-effects of traditional non-steroidal anti-inflammatory drugs and new formulations. Aliment Pharmacol Ther 2004;20:S48–58.
36. O'Laughlin JC, Hoftiezer JW, Ivey KJ. Effect of aspirin on the human stomach in normals: Endoscopic comparison of damage produced one hour, 24 hours, and 2 weeks after administration. Scand J Gastroenterol 1981;16:S67:211–4.
37. Sung JJY. Should we eradicate *Helicobacter pylori* in non-steroidal anti-inflammatory drug users? Aliment Pharmacol Ther 2004;20:S65–70.
38. Hawkey CJ, Karrasch JA, Szczepanski L, et al. Omeprazole compared with misoprostol for ulcers associated with nonsteroidal antiinflammatory drugs. N Engl J Med 1998;338:727–34.
39. Taha AS, Hudson N, Hawkey CJ, et al. Famotidine for the prevention of gastric and duodenal ulcers caused by nonsteroidal antiinflammatory drugs. N Engl J Med 1996;334:1435–9.
40. Poulsen SS, Olsen PS, Kirkegaard P. Healing of cysteamine-induced duodenal ulcers in the rat. Dig Dis Sci 1985;30:161–7.
41. Laine L, Weinstein WM. Histology of alcoholic hemorrhagic "gastritis": A prospective evaluation. Gastroenterology 1988; 94:1254–62.
42. Lanza FL, Royer GL, Jr, Nelson RS, et al. Ethanol, aspirin, ibuprofen, and the gastroduodenal mucosa: An endoscopic assessment. Am J Gastroenterol 1985;80:767–9.
43. Bollschweiler E, Wolfgarten E, Putz B, et al. Bile reflux into the stomach and esophagus for volunteers older than 40 years. Digestion 2005;71:65–71.
44. Szarszewski A, Korzon M, Kaminska B, Lass P. Duodenogastric reflux: Clinical and therapeutic aspects. Arch Dis Child 1999;81:16–20.
45. Sobala GM, O'Connor HJ, Dewar EP, et al. Bile reflux and intestinal metaplasia in gastric mucosa. J Clin Pathol 1993;46:235–40.
46. Hashimoto K, Kakegawa T, Takeda J, et al. The effect of bile juice reflux on the development of remnant stomach carcinoma. Kurume Med J 1991;38:5–8.
47. Bonavina L, Incarbone R, Segalin A, et al. Duodeno-gastro-oesophageal reflux after gastric surgery: Surgical therapy and outcome in 42 consecutive patients. Hepato-Gastroenterology 1999;46:92–6.
48. Sobala GM, King RFG, Axon ATR, Dixon MF. Reflux gastritis in the intact stomach. J Clin Pathol 1990;43:303–6.
49. Byrne JP, Romagnoli R, Bechi, et al. Duodenogastric reflux of bile in health: The normal range. Physiol Meas 1999;20:149–58.
50. Takada K, Hamada Y, Watanabe K, et al. Duodenogastric reflux following biliary reconstruction after excision of choledochal cyst. Pediatr Surg Int 2005;21:1–4.
51. Hermans D, Sokal EM, Collard JM, et al. Primary duodenogastric reflux in children and adolescents. Eur J Pediatr 2003;162:598–602.
52. Stein HJ, Smyrk TC, DeMeester TR, et al. Clinical value of endscopy and histology in the diagnosis of duodenogastric reflux disease. Surgery 1992;112:796–803.
53. Klingler PJ, Perdikis G, Wilson P, Hinder RA. Indications, technical modalities and results of the duodenal switch operation for pathologic duodenogastric reflux. Hepatogastroenterology 1999;46:97–102.
54. Chaibou M, Tucci M, Dugas MA, et al. Clinically significant upper gastrointestinal bleeding acquired in a pediatric intensive care unit: A prospective study. Pediatrics 1998; 102:933–8.
55. Spirt MJ. Stress-related mucosal disease: Risk factors and prophylactic therapy. Clin Ther 2004;26:197–213.
56. Navab F, Steingrub J. Stress ulcer: Is routine prophylaxis necessary? Am J Gastroenterol 1995;90:708–12.
57. Beejay U, Wolfe MM. Acute gastrointestinal bleeding in the intensive care unit. The gastroenterologist's perspective. Gastroenterol Clin North Am 2000;29:309–36.
58. Cook DJ, Guyatt GH, Marshall J, et al. A comparison of sucralfate and ranitidine for the prevention of upper gastrointestinal bleeding in patients requiring mechanical ventilation. Canadian Critical Care Trials Group. N Engl J Med 1998;338:791–7.
59. Maki M, Ruuska T, Kuusela AL, et al. High prevalence of asymptomatic esophageal and gastric lesions in preterm infants in intensive care. Crit Care Med 1993;21:1863–7.
60. Kuusela AL, Ruuska T, Karikoski R, et al. A randomized, controlled study of prophylactic ranitidine in preventing stress-induced gastric mucosal lesions in neonatal intensive care unit. Crit Care Med 1997;25:346–51.
61. Ojala R, Ruuska T, Karikoski R, et al. Gastroesophageal endoscopic findings and gastrointestinal symptoms in preterm neonates with and without perinatal indomethacin exposure. J Pediatr Gastroenterol Nutr 2001;32:182–8.
62. Leone RJ, Krasna IH. "Spontaneous" neonatal gastric perforation: Is it really spontaneous? J Pediatr Surg 2000;35: 1066–9.
63. Samloff LM, Stemmermann GN, Heilbrun LK, Nomura A. Elevated serum pepsinogen I and II levels differ as risk factors for duodenal and gastric ulcer. Gastroenterology 1986;90:570–4.
64. Peled N, Dagan O, Babyn P, et al. Gastric-outlet obstruction induced by prostaglandin therapy in neonates. N Engl J Med 1992;327:505–10.
65. Fragoso AC, Correia-Pinto J, Carvalho JL, et al. Ectopic pancreas and foveolar hyperplasia in a newborn: A unifying etiopathogenesis for gastric outlet obstruction. J Pediatr Gastroenterol Nutr 2004;39:92–4.
66. Callahan M, McCauley RGK, Patel H, Hijazi ZM. The development of hypertrophic pyloric stenosis in a patient with prostaglandin-induced foveolar hyperplasia. Pediatr Radiol 1999;29:748–51.
67. Morinville V, Bernard C, Forget S. Foveolar hyperplasia secondary to cow's milk protein hypersensitivity presenting with clinical features of pyloric stenosis. J Pediatr Surg 2004;39:E29–31.
68. Choi SJ, Kim YS, Chae JR, et al. Effects of ranitidine for exercise induced gastric mucosal changes and bleeding. World J Gastroenterol 2006;12:2579–83.

69. Qamar MI, Read AE. Effects of exercise on mesenteric blood flow in man. Gut 1987;28:583–7.
70. Coia LR, Myerson RJ, Tepper JE. Late effects of radiation therapy on the gastrointestinal tract. Int J Radiation Oncology Biol Phys 1995;31:1213–36.
71. Wada S, Tamada K, Tomiyama T, et al. Endoscopic hemostasis for radiation-induced gastritis using argon plasma coagulation. J Gastroenterol Hepatol 2003;18:1215–8.
72. Kernstine KH, Greensmith JE, Johlin FC, et al. Hyperbaric oxygen treatment of hemorrhagic radiation-induced gastritis after esophagectomy. Ann Thorac Surg 2005;80:1115–7.
73. Chong GC, Beahrs OH, Payne SW. Management of corrosive gastritis due to ingested acid. Mayo Clin Proc 1974; 49:861–5.
74. Tekant G, Eroglu E, Erdogan E, et al. Corrosive injury-induced gastric outlet obstruction: A changing spectrum of agents and treatment. J Pediatr Surg 2001;36:1004–7.
75. Ciftci AO, Senocak ME, Buyukpamukcu N, Hicsonmez A. Gastric outlet obstruction due to corrosive ingestion: Incidence and outcome. Pediatr Surg Int 1999;15:88–91.
76. Fiaccadori E, Maggiore U, Clima B, et al. Incidence, risk factors, and prognosis of gastrointestinal hemorrhage complicating acute renal failure. Kidney Int 2001;59:1510–9.
77. Kang JY, Ho KY, Yeoh KG, et al. Peptic ulcer and gastritis in uraemia, with particular reference to the effect of *Helicobacter pylori* infection. J Gastroenterol Hepatol 1999; 14:771–8.
78. Emir S, Bereket G, Boyacroglu S, et al. Gastroduodenal lesions and *Helicobacter pylori* in children with end-stage renal disease. Pediatr Nephrol 2000;14:837–40.
79. Hirako M, Kamiya T, Misu N, et al. Impaired gastric motility and its relationship to gastrointestinal symptoms in patients with chronic renal failure. J Gastroenterol 2005;40: 1116–1122.
80. Sirinek KR, O'Dorisio TM, Gaskill HV, Levine BA. Chronic renal failure: Effect of hemodialysis on gastrointestinal hormones. Am J Surg 1984;148:732–5.
81. Hausberg M, Kosch M, Harmelink P, et al. Sympathetic nerve activity in end-stage renal disease. Circulation 2002; 106:1974–9.
82. Ravelli AM. Gastrointestinal function in chronic renal failure. Pediatr Nephrol 1995;9:756–62.
83. Ala-Kaila K. Upper gastrointestinal findings in chronic renal failure. Scand J Gastroenterol 1987;22:372–6.
84. Misra V, Misra SP, Shukla SK, et al. Endoscopic and histological changes in upper gastrointestinal tract of patients with chronic renal failure. Indian J Pathol Microbiol 2004; 47:170–3.
85. Tomori K, Nakamoto H, Kotaki S, et al. Gastric angiodysplasia in patients undergoing maintenance dialysis. Adv Perit Dial 2003;19:136–42.
86. Kestens PJ, Alexandre GPJ. Gastroduodenal complications after transplantation. Clin Transplant 1988;2:221.
87. Ponticelli C, Passerini P. Gastrointestinal complications in renal transplant recipients. Transpl Int 2005;18:643–50.
88. Amaro R, Neff GW, Karnam US, et al. Acquired hyperplastic gastric polyps in solid organ transplant patients. Am J Gastroenterol 2002;97:2220–4.
89. Colletti RB, Trainer TD. Collagenous gastritis. Gastroenterology 1989;97:1552–5.
90. Stancu M, De Petris G, Palumbo TP, Lev R. Collagenous gastritis associated with lymphocytic gastritis and celiac disease. Arch Pathol Lab Med 2001;125:1579–84.
91. Park S, Kim DH, Choe YH, Suh YL. Collagenous gastritis in a Korean child: A case report. J Korean Med Sci 2005;20:146–9.
92. Haot J, Hamichi L, Wallez L, Mainguet P. Lymphocytic gastritis: A newly described entity: A retrospective endoscopic and histological study. Gut 1988;29:1258–64.
93. Wu TT, Hamilton SR. Lymphocytic gastritis: Association with etiology and topology. Am J Surg Pathol 1999;23:153–8.
94. Alsaigh N, Odze R, Goldman H, et al. Gastric and esophageal intraepithelial lymphocytes in pediatric celiac disease. Am J Surg Pathol 1996;20:865–70.
95. Jevon GP, Dimmick JE, Dohil R, Hassall E. Spectrum of gastritis in celiac disease in childhood. Pediatr Dev Pathol 1999;2:221–6.
96. Drut R, Drut RM. Lymphocytic gastritis in pediatric celiac disease—immunohistochemical study of the intraepithelial lymphocytic component. Med Sci Monit 2004;10: CR38–42.
97. De Giacomo C, Gianatti A, Negrini R, et al. Lymphocytic gastritis: A positive relationship with celiac disease. J Pediatr 1994;124:57–62.
98. Lambert R, Andre C, Moulinier B, Bugnon B. Diffuse varioliform gastritis. Digestion 1978;17:159–67.
99. Vinograd I, Granot E, Ron N, et al. Chronic diffuse varioliform gastritis in a child. Total gastrectomy for acute massive bleeding. J Clin Gastroenterol 1993;16:40–4.
100. Ustundag Y, Oksuzoglu G, Tatar G, et al. Atopy and food allergy in varioliform gastritis. J Clin Gastroenterol 1998; 27:275–6.
101. Cappell MS, Marboe C. Neoplasia in chronic erosive (varioliform) gastritis. Dig Dis Sci 1988;33:1035–9.
102. Machado RS, Kawakami E, Goshima S, et al. Hemorrhagic gastritis due to cow's milk allergy: Report of two cases. J Pediatr (Rio J) 2003;79:363–8.
103. Halpern SR, Sellars WA, Johnson RB, et al. Development of childhood allergy in infants fed breast, soy, or cow milk. J Allergy Clin Immunol 1973;51:139–51.
104. Nowak-Wegrzyn A, Sampson HA, Wood RA, Sicherer SH. Food protein-induced enterocolitis syndrome caused by solid food proteins. Pediatrics 2003;111:829–35.
105. Ravelli AM, Tobanelli P, Sonia V, Ugazio AG. Vomiting and gastric motility in infants with cow's milk allergy. J Pediatr Gastroenterol Nutr 2001;32:59–64.
106. Mofidi S. Nutritional management of pediatric food hypersensitivity. Pediatrics 2003;111:1645–53.
107. Hill DJ, Heine RG, Cameron DJ, et al. The natural history of intolerance to soy and extensively hydolyzed formula in infants with multiple food protein intolerance. J Pediatr 1999;135:118–21.
108. Chaudhary R, Shrivastava RK, Mukhopadhyay HG, et al. Eosinophilic gastritis: An unusual cause of gastric outlet obstruction. Indian J Gastroenterol 2001;20:110.
109. Martin ST, Collins CG, Fitzgibbon J, et al. Gastric motor dysfunction: is eosinophilic mural gastritis a causative factor? Eur J Gastroenterol Hepatol 2005;17:983–6.
110. Talley NJ, Shorter RG, Phillips SF, Zinsmeister AR. Eosinophilic gastroenteritis: A clinicopathological study of patients with disease of the mucosa, muscle layer, and subserosal tissues. Gut 1990;31:54–8.
111. Garrett KJ, Jameson SC, Thomson B, et al. Anti-interleukin-5 (mepolizumab) therapy for hypereosinophilic syndromes. J Allergy Clin Immunol 2004;113:115–9.
112. Hyams JS, Treem WR. Portal hypertensive gastropathy in children. J Pediatr Gastroenterol Nutr 1993;17:13–8.
113. Itha S, Yachha SK. Endoscopic outcome beyond esophageal variceal eradication in children with extrahepatic portal venous obstruction. J Pediatr Gastroenterol Nutr 2006; 42:196–200.
114. Spina GP, Arcidiacono R, Bosch J, et al. Gastric endoscopic features in portal hypertension: Final report of a consensus conference, Milan, Italy, September 19, 1992. J Hepatol 1994;21:461–7.
115. McCormack TT, Sims J, Eyre-Brook I, et al. Gastric lesions in portal hypertension: Inflammatory gastritis or congestive gastropathy? Gut 1985;26:1226–32.
116. Bayraktar Y, Balkanci F, Uzunalimoglu B, et al. Is portal hypertension due to liver cirrhosis a major factor in the development of portal hypertensive gastropathy? Am J Gastroenterol 1996;91:554–8.
117. Iwao T, Toyonaga A, Oho K, et al. Portal-hypertensive gastropathy develops less in patients with cirrhosis and fundal varices. J Hepatol 1997;26:1235–41.
118. Ohta M, Hashizume M, Higashi H, et al. Portal and gastric mucosal hemodynamics in cirrhotic patients with portal hypertensive gastropathy. Hepatology 1994;20:1432–6.
119. Piasecki C, Chin J, Greenslade L, et al. Endoscopic detection of ischemia with a new probe indicates low oxygenation of gastric epithelium in portal hypertensive gastropathy. Gut 1995;36:654–6.
120. Munoz J, Albillos A, Perez-Paramo M, et al. Factors mediating the hemodynamic effects of tumour necrosis factor-alpha in portal hypertensive rats. Am J Physiol 1999;276: 687–93.
121. Merkel C, Marin R, Sacerdoti D, et al. Long-term results of a clinical trial of nadolol with or without isosorbide mononitrate for primary prophylaxis of a variceal bleeding in cirrhosis Hepatology 2000;31:324–9.
122. Lo GH, Lai KH, Cheng JS, et al. The effects of endoscopic variveal ligation and propanolol on portal hypertensive gastropathy: A perspective, controlled trial. Gastrointest Endosc 2001;53:579–84.
123. Kouroumalis EA, Koutroubakis IE, Manousos ON. Somatostatin for acute severe bleeding from portal hypertensive gastropathy. Eur J Gastroenterol Hepatol 1998;10:509–12.
124. Bruha R, Marecek Z, Spicak J, et al. Double-blind randomized, comparative multicenter study of the effect of terlipressin in the treatment of acute esophageal variceal and/or hypertensive gastropathy bleeding. Hepatogastroenterology 2002;49:1161–6.
125. Wagatsuma Y, Naritaka Y, Shimakawa T, et al. Clinical usefulness of the angiotensin II receptor antagonist losartan in patients with portal hypertensive gastropathy. Hepatogastroenterology 2006;53:171–4.
126. Karajeh MA, Hurlstone DP, Stephenson TJ, et al. Refractory bleeding from portal hypertensive gastropathy: A further novel role for thalidomide therapy? Eur J Gastroenterol Hepatol 2006;18:545–8.
127. Esaki M, Matsumoto T, Nakamura, et al. GI involvement in Henoch-Schonlein purpura. Gastrointest Endosc 2002; 56:920–3.
128. Ilona SS. Henoch-Schonlein purpura: When and how to treat. J Rheumatol 1996;23:1661–5.
129. Gunasekaran TS, Berman J, Gonzalez M. Duodenojejunitis: Is it idiopathic or is Henoch-Schonlein purpura without the purpura? J Pediatr Gastroenterol Nutr 2000;30:22–28.
130. Sakagami S, Noda H, Koshino Y, et al. Gastrointestinal tract lesions in a case of Schonlein-Henoch purpura associated with melena and review of 32 cases in Japan. Gastroenterol Endosc 1988;30:1250–4.
131. Appeleton AL, Sviland L, Pearson ADJ, et al. The need for endoscopic biopsy in the diagnosis of upper gastrointestinal graft-versus-host diease. J Pediatr Gastroenterol Nutr 1993 16:183–5.
132. Ponec RJ, Hackman RC, McDonald GB. Endoscopic and histologic diagnosis of intestinal graft-versus-host disease after marrow transplantation. Gastrointest Endosc 1999;49:612–21.
133. Epstein RJ, McDonald GB, Sale GE, et al. The diagnostic accuracy of the rectal biopsy in acute graft-versus-host disease: A prospective study of 13 patients. Gastroenterology 1980;78:764–71.
134. Graham JR. Gastric polyposis: Onset during long-term therapy with omeprazole. Med J Aust 1992;157:287–8.
135. Pashankar DS, Israel DM, Jevon GP, Buchan AMJ. Effect of long-term omeprazole treatment on antral G and D cells in children. J Pediatr Gastroenterol Nutr 2001;33:537–42.
136. Choudhry U, Boyce HW, Jr, Coppola D. Proton pump inhibitor-associated gastric polyps: A retrospective analysis of their frequency, and endoscopic, histologic, and ultrastructural characteristics. Am J Clin Pathol 1998;110:615–21.
137. Theisen J, Nehra D, Citron D, et al. Suppression of gastric acid secretion in patients with gastroesophageal reflux disease results in gastric bacterial overgrowth and deconjugation. J Gastrointest Surg 2000;4:50–4.
138. Torbenson M, Abraham SC, Boitnott J, et al. Autoimmune gastrityis: Distinct histological and immunohistochemical findings before complete loss of oxyntic glands. Mod Pathol 2002;15:102–9.
139. Lam-Tse WK, Batstra MR, Koeleman BP, et al. The association between autoimmune thyroiditis, autoimmune gastritis and type 1 diabetes. Pediatr Endocrinol Rev 2003;1:22–37.
140. Segni M, Borrelli O, Pucarelli I, et al. Early manifestations of gastric autoimmunity in patients with juvenile autoimmune thyroid diseases. J Clin Endocrinol Metab 2004; 89:4944–8.
141. Chouraqui JP, Roy CC, Brochu P, et al. Menetrier's disease in children: Report of a patient and review of sixteen other cases. Gastroenterology 1981;80:1042–7.
142. Hoffer V, Finkelstein Y, Balter J, et al. Ganciclovir treatment in Menetrier's disease. Acta Paediatr 2003;92:982–4.
143. Madisch A, Aust D, Morgner A, et al. Resolution of gastrointestinal protein loss after *Helicobacter pylori* eradication in a patient with hypertrophic lymphocytic gastritis. Helicobacter 2004;9:629–31.
144. Nomura S, Settle SH, Leys CM, et al. Evidence for repatterning of the gastric fundic epithelium associated with Menetrier's disease and TGF alpha overexpression. Gastroenterology 2005;128:1292–305.
145. Settle SH, Washington K, Lind C, et al. Chronic treatment of Menetrier's disease with Erbitux: Clinical efficacy and insight into pathophysiology. Clin Gastroenterol Hepatol 2005;3:654–9.
146. Konstantinidou AE, Morphopoulos G, Korkolopoulou P, et al. Menetrier disease of early infancy: A separate entity? J Pediatr Gastroenterol Nutr 2004;39:177–182.
147. Dohil R, Newbury RO, Sellers ZM, et al. The evaluation and treatment of gastrointestinal disease in children with cytinosis receiving cysteamine. J Pediatr 2003;143: 224–30.
148. Erbersdobler A, Petri S, Lock G. Russell body gastritis: An unusual, tumor-like lesion of the gastric mucosa. Arch Pathol Lab Med 2004;128:915–7.
149. Eisenhut M, Hughes D, Ashworth M. Fatal emphysematous gastritis in a 2-year-old child with chronic renal failure. Pediatr Dev Pathol 2004;7:414–6.
150. Miller AI, Smith B, Rogers AI. Phlegmonous gastritis. Gastroenterology 1975;68:231–8.
151. Feng J, Weng Y, Yuan J, et al. Acute phlegmonous gastritis in an infant. J Pediatr Surg 2005;40:745–7.
152. Quatrini M, Castoldi L, Rossi G, et al. A follow-up study of patients with Zollinger-Ellison syndrome in the period 1966–2002: Effects of surgical and medical treatments on long-term survival. J Clin Gastroenterol 2005;39:376–80.

10

Tumors of the Pediatric Esophagus and Stomach

Fiona Graeme-Cook, MB, FRCP
Gregory Y. Lauwers, MD

The esophagus is a relatively uncommon site for tumors, even in adults. Three tumor types occur with any frequency in the esophagus—small benign mucosal leiomyomas, adenocarcinoma arising in Barrett's esophagus, and squamous cell carcinoma. All these tumor types are reported to occur in children. The latest US cancer surveillance data (SEER) show a measurable but small incidence of esophageal malignancies in the 14- to 18-year-age group. Other tumors, benign or malignant, including papillomas, granular cell tumors, and esophageal sarcoma are unusual in adults, even more so in childhood. A specific pediatric issue related to tumors of the esophagus is the recognition of pathology in childhood that may predispose to adult malignancy. These are summarized in Table 1 and discussed in the specific sections on tumor type. Childhood mediastinal malignancies treated with irradiation may result in various esophageal solid tumors in early adult life. Human papilloma virus infections have been linked both to esophageal papillomas,[1] and less certainly to adult squamous cell carcinoma. Nutritional factors and genetic disorders may manifest as benign pediatric esophageal pathology, predisposing to adult malignancy. Pediatric esophageal tumors may also occur as part of an inherited genetic disorder such as Fanconi's anemia (those relevant to this chapter are listed in Table 2).

ESOPHAGEAL TUMORS

As most benign tumors of the esophagus are small, >50% are asymptomatic and are often discovered incidentally during upper endoscopy performed for unrelated problems. Symptomatic tumors, larger in size (most malignant tumors would be in this category), present with age-specific signs and symptoms—dysphagia occurs in older children, and in infants feeding and respiratory difficulty may be the presenting problem.[2] Bleeding, weight loss, and vomiting are less common and are indicative of a large or aggressive tumor. Mediastinal mass discovered on chest X-ray is a rare presentation.[2-3] Esophageal tumors are investigated using upper gastrointestinal endoscopy, with or without barium esophagram; CT and MR imaging with endoscopic ultrasound help define depth of invasion and degree of spread. Biopsy diagnosis is feasible, and endoscopic procedures may also be curative for small lesions. Surgical resection is the treatment of choice for the remainder. Improved techniques of noninvasive surgery have decreased morbidity for such resections. Data on adjuvant chemo- and radiotherapy for esophageal malignancy in children are not readily available, as malignant tumors are rare.[4]

BENIGN ESOPHAGEAL TUMORS

Epithelial Esophageal Squamous Papilloma

The esophageal squamous papilloma (ESP) is a benign polypoid tumor usually found in the lower esophagus. The reported incidence rates vary, from <0.1 to 0.4%, based on adult autopsy studies.[5] As this polyp is most often asymptomatic and regenerative in nature; these rates may be a large underestimate. ESP is reported in childhood, with similar demographic distribution as in adulthood[6-7] and has also been described in a case of Cowden's syndrome of gastrointestinal hamartomatous polyposis.[8]

For sporadic papillomas, two main groups of etiological factors are reported—physical trauma (including acid reflux, radiation, irritation from chemicals or foreign bodies) and a controversial question of human papilloma virus (HPV) infection. In the lower esophagus, most papillomas are associated with acid reflux and hiatal hernia.[8] In the mid and upper esophagus, and with multiple ESPs, HPV (subtypes 16 > 11) are found in a variable percentage.[8-9]

At endoscopy ESPs are solitary mucosal protrusions without a true stalk. The overlying squamous mucosa is normal or roughened and white due to mucosal keratinization. Most are small (<5 mm), although "giant" ESP (as large as 23 cm in maximum dimension) are reported, rarely in children.

Microscopical examination of ESP reveals a central fibrovascular core covered by benign mature squamous epithelium (Figure 1). Inflammation and reactive epithelial atypia are common. Cytoplasmic clearing and nuclear irregularity (koilocytosis) may indicate the presence of HPV.[8]

The condition known as papillomatosis refers to multiple ESPs distributed throughout the esophagus. This is seen predominantly in the pediatric age group.[10] Human papilloma virus is suspected but only occasionally found.[11] A single case report links these ESP to laryngotracheal papillomatosis.[12] Multiple ESPs are reported with the Goltz syndrome (focal dermal hypoplasia).[13]

Most small ESPs are reactive rather than truly neoplastic and will not recur or progress. The larger and multiple forms of ESP are true benign neoplasms. Multiple recurrence after initial resection is common, with maintainance of benign cytology. Malignant transformation is a concern clinically, particularly with multiple or HPV-related ESP; ESP with HPV subtypes 16 and 18 have been reported to show more aggressive behavior in some instances. This issue is controversial; some reports of ESP with carcinoma may in fact represent papillary squamous carcinoma, and the link between HPV infection and esophageal carcinoma is unclear.[14-15] No cases of malignant ESP are present in the pediatric literature.[5,15]

Table 1 Factors in Pediatric Esophagus Possibly Relating to Adulthood Malignancy

Pathology	Etiology	Tumor
Squamous papilloma	Viral	scc
GERD	BE	aca
Tylosis	Genetic	scc
Achalasia	Inflammatory	scc
TEF	Inflammatory	scc
Radiation	Oxidative stress	Various
Lye	Corrosive	scc
Esophagitis	vit/mineral	sc

scc = squamous cell carcinoma; aca = adenocarcinoma; GERD = gastroesophageal reflux disease; BE = Barrett's esophagus; TEF = tracheoesophageal fistula; vit = vitamins.

Table 2 Esophageal Pathology Associated with Extraesophageal Disease

Esophageal Pathology	Extraesophageal Findings
Cysts	Vertebral anomalies
	Malrotations and TEF
Glycogen acanthosis	Cowden's syndrome
ESP	Cowden's syndrome
Leiomyomatosis	Alport's syndrome
Webs	"Plummer-Vinson" syndrome
SCC	Celiac disease
SCC	Fanconi's anemia
SCC	Cutaneous keratosis
BE	Neurological disease

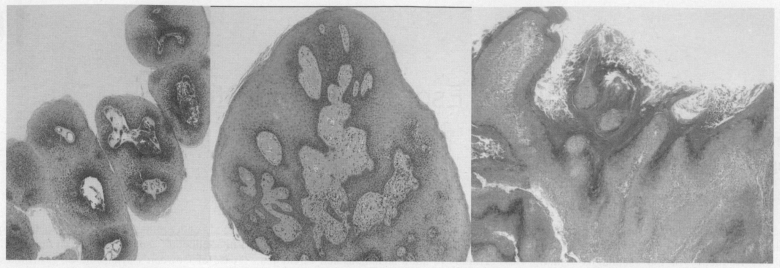

Figure 1 Esophageal squamous papillomas. From left to right: (A) The exophytic form has a branching fibrovascular core, with the "branches" covered by mature, sometimes thin squamous mucosa (H+E × 40). (B) Endophytic papilloma is a sessile polyp with smooth benign squamous epithelium overlying a fibrovascular core into which the deep squamous "rete" extend. It is also occasionally called a "fibroepithelial polyp" (H+E × 100). (C) The "spiked" exophytic ESP, least frequent, is characterized by keratohyaline granules within the superficial keratinocytes and a thick layer of orthokeratin forming hyperkeratotic "spikes" (H+E × 40).

ESOPHAGEAL CYSTS AND REDUPLICATIONS

Gastrointestinal reduplication with resulting cysts and tubules occurs throughout the gastrointestinal tract (GIT). The esophagus is involved in 19% of cases, where spherical/cystic forms are more common. Resulting from a possible abnormality of the notochord, they occur in the lower one-third and toward the right side. The reduplication may extend the entire esophageal length, or communicate with a subdiaphragmatic gastric duplication. Intramural and extramural forms occur, with associated vertebral anomalies (in the form of clefts or fusion) in the extramural form. Most cases present within the first year of life associated with respiratory difficulty; and with increasing age dysphagia or feeding problems become more common.[2,16] The mucosal lining of the cyst may be ciliated columnar (developmental form), gastric, or esophageal squamous, The wall contains smooth muscle, nerves, and blood vessels forming a muscularis propria-like appearance in the wall that may be shared with the adjacent intestinal wall.[17–18] Intramural cysts without muscular components are considered esophageal

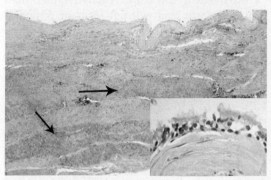

Figure 2 Esophageal reduplication cyst. The partially denuded cyst wall contains muscle layers (arrows) reminiscent of muscularis propria (H+E ×20). Inset: Intact cyst lining has a ciliated columnar appearance (H+E ×200)

cysts if lined by squamous mucosa, and "bronchogenic" if the lining is ciliated columnar and there is cartilage within the cyst wall. The presence of muscularis propria indicates an intestinal reduplication (Figure 2). Communication with a gastric reduplication is relatively common, but only 10% of the cysts communicate with the esophageal lumen.[17]

Treatment is by surgical resection. Extramural forms separate easily from the adjacent esophageal muscularis propria; intramural forms tend to share the muscle wall with the esophagus. Complete excision is recommended, which may be possible by thoracoscopy.[19–20] There is a small risk of malignant transformation in adulthood of the epithelial lining of untreated cysts.[21–22]

PSEUDODIVERTICULOSIS

In this unusual condition, the duct orifices of the esophageal submucosal glands become dilated to form multiple intramural cysts. Achalasia may be present and esophageal dysmotility is the presumptive cause. The pseudodiverticula may involve a segment, usually in the upper esophagus, or be diffuse. Endoscopically, small pit-like openings may be seen on these mural protrusions, but radiological studies may suggest a cystic neoplastic process, particularly in localized disease. Biopsy reveals a squamous lining, commonly with Candidal superinfection.

GLYCOGEN ACANTHOSIS

Glycogen acanthosis (GA) appears as a white patch of esophageal mucosa at upper endoscopy. GA is flat, and although not neoplastic, may be confused with leukoplakia. Biopsy reveals esophageal squamous mucosa with enlarged superficial keratinocytes. The cleared-out appearance of the cytoplasm is due to the accumulation of glycogen

within the cells. GA is usually sporadic, but multiple GA in childhood may indicate the presence of hamartomatous polyposis (Cowden's syndrome and Lhermitte-Duclos syndrome) related to germline mutation in the PTEN gene (coding for a dual phosphatase—protein tyrosine phosphatase and tensin homologue) in 80% of cases, and associated with thyroid and breast malignancy.

BENIGN NON-EPITHELIAL ESOPHAGEAL TUMORS: ESOPHAGEAL LEIOMYOMA

Small mucosal leiomyomas derived from the muscularis mucosa are considered the commonest benign neoplasm of the esophagus. Autopsy studies suggest a steady increase in incidence with longevity.[23] Esophageal leiomyoma (ELM) is an unusual tumor in childhood.[24]

ELM has been reported in children as young as 4 years old, but most are reported in the teenage years. Unlike adults, in childhood they appear more common in females (1.7:1 F:M), and diffuse or multiple forms are more common, with isolated single ELM representing only 9% of cases.[24]

ELMs may occur as part of Alport's syndrome (nephropathy and sensorineural hearing loss).[24] Gastroesophageal reflux disease (GERD) has been reported as an association, possibly reflecting the frequency of GERD, with coincidental ELM. Esophageal diverticulum has been reported with ELM, an association of uncertain significance. Rare cases of congenital stricture with ELM may represent the development of stromal tumors (GIST) in families with inherited mutations of KIT.[25] ELMs have been seen in patients with multiple endocrine neoplasia-1 (MEN-1). The characterisitic gene mutation at 11q13 was demonstrable within these tumors. This mutation does not appear to be responsible for sporadic leiomyomas(LM).[26]

The endoscopic appearance of ELMs is submucosal bumps or sessile polyps. The overlying mucosa is intact. Most ELMs are intramural (97%), with 1% presenting as polyps, and 2% as extramural mediastinal tumors.[28] The commonest site is distal esophagus and gastroesophageal junction (GEJ), with decreasing numbers aborally. ELM form well-circumscribed, non-infiltrative nodules with whorled white-yellow cut surface due to intersecting fascicles of spindle smooth muscle cells without anaplasia. Calcification and cystic degeneration are common in larger forms. Rarely, lesions grow circumferentially round the esophagus forming a stricture.[27–28] In small ELM, origin from the muscularis mucosa is often apparent.[29] Treatment is by enucleation for single tumors and surgical resection for multiple ELMs.[29]

Leiomyomatosis

Multiple ELMs when confluent are sometimes referred to as "diffuse leiomyomatosis." This term has also been used to indicate diffuse hyperplasia of one of the layers of the muscularis propria. These two processes should be clearly delineated, as ELM, though benign, is neoplastic; the etiopathogenesis of the hyperplastic process is unknown.[30] The proliferative form, leiomyomatosis, is seen in familial form in cases of Alport's syndrome. This is relatively frequent in occurrence, representing 22% of ELM in a recent pediatric review.[24]

Alport's Syndrome and Familial Leiomyomatosis

Alport's syndrome, sensorineural hearing loss with nephropathy, is reported in children as young as 2.5 and 5 years old.[24,31] The genetic basis is a mutation in genes responsible for the alpha-5 chain of type 4 collagen (COL4A5). Type 4 collagen is essential for basement membrane synthesis[32] and may play an important role in cell–matrix interaction. Similar mutations have been found in both Alport's syndrome and a familial form of diffuse leiomyomatosis without Alport's syndrome features.[32,33]

GRANULAR CELL TUMOR

The esophageal submucosa is the main site of occurrence of the granular cell tumor (GCT) in the gastrointestinal tract. This unusual mesenchymal tumor is reported in the pediatric population[34] and even in the newborn.[35] Most are small and are found incidentally at upper endoscopy, where a sessile, yellow-white firm nodule is found. The overlying mucosa is intact, and most tumors are 2 cm or less. The lower esophagus is more common a location than the upper, and males and Blacks are more likely to be affected. Occasional reports have linked GCT to neurofibromatosis.

Pathology

The tumor is composed of epithelioid or plump-spindled cells with abundant coarsely granular eosinophilic cytoplasm and small round nuclei without obvious nucleoli. The cytoplasm of the cells is characteristically positive with periodic acid-Schiff (PAS) stain, and both cytoplasm and nucleus are S100 positive by immunohistochemistry, consistent with Schwannian differentiation.[36]. Short fascicles of tumor cells diffusely infiltrate the lamina propria of the esophagus. The overlying squamous mucosa is often markedly hyperplastic with tongues of atypical appearing squamous epithelium extending deeply into the GCT. This "pseudo-epitheliomatous hyperplasia" is a close mimic of invasive squamous cell carcinoma and is a trap for unwary pathologists (Figure 3). Small GCTs have been reported to remain stable in size, but some large GCTs require resection for symptoms.[37] Malignant forms, though exceedingly rare, are reported,[38] although not so far in the pediatric age group.

VASCULAR TUMORS

Hemangioma and lymphangioma have both been reported in the esophagus of children, albeit rarely.[3,39–40] Both are composed of benign vascular channels, and the former may present with bleeding. The lesions are usually apparent at endoscopy.

MALIGNANT ESOPHAGEAL TUMORS

The esophagus and proximal stomach are the site of cancer with the largest and most rapid increase in incidence in the last two decades. Most of these are adenocarcinoma (ACA). In the same time period, the incidence of esophageal squamous cell carcinoma (SCC) has been falling. Squamous cell carcinoma is still more common than adenocarcinoma of the esophagus, but the rise in adenocarcinoma in older White males is alarming, and its cause is not understood. Given the time-course of evolution from preneoplasia to overt carcinoma, many of these tumors may trace their origin to childhood esophageal pathology.

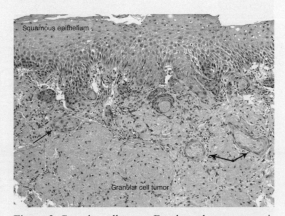

Figure 3 Granular cell tumor. Esophageal squamous epithelium overlies neoplastic cells with abundant amphophilic cytoplasm and small nuclei. Trapped by or infiltrating into the granular cells are tongues of squamous epithelium with dysmaturation (pseudoepitheliomatous hyperplasia) (H+E 200×).

MALIGNANT EPITHELIAL TUMORS: GASTROESOPHAGEAL REFLUX, BARRETT'S ESOPHAGUS, AND ADENOCARCINOMA

ACA arising in Barrett's esophagus (BE) is the most significant topic in neoplasia of the pediatric esophagus (Table 3).

GERD and BE

BE represents glandular mucosa lining the lumen of the esophagus. BE is an acquired defect, the result of chronic mucosal injury, usually from acid reflux, but also possibly from bile, alkali (lye), and other physicochemical causes. Gastroesophageal acid reflux (GER) into the esophagus results in active chronic esophagitis, with injury to esophageal squamous mucosa. Ulceration heals by regrowth from the edges by epithelium from progenitor cells of unknown/disputed derivation. The possibilities include a stem cell from the basal cell region, or residual mucosa, which in dividing rapidly becomes less differentiated. In the stem cell theory, repair after a single episode of damage may be by normal squamous epithelium. Repeated injury and repair in the continuing presence of acid, pepsinogen, or in combination with alkali, may result in differentiation of the covering mucosa to a more resistant type glandular mucosa. The second possibility, regrowth from nearby residual mucosa, requires the repairing mucosa to be glandular in type; origin from the ducts of esophageal mucosal glands has been posited for this pathway. Both of these would explain the cardiac-type nature of "columnar-lined esophagus." BE only occurs in 10% of patients with GERD, implying that other factors, genetic or environmental, play an undetermined role. Familial BE is reported; study of these families should elucidate associated genetic abnormalities.[41–42]

Table 3 Pediatric Issues Relating to Barrett's Esophagus

1 GERD is common in childhood and increasing in incidence
2 GERD is an accepted risk factor for the development of BE in childhood (2.5 to 3% incidence)
3 BE increases the risk of adenocarcinoma of the esophagus 40- to 125-fold
4 Esophageal and proximal gastric adenocarcinoma incidence rates are rising more rapidly over the last two decades than any other carcinoma; both tumors are linked statistically to BE
5 Extrapolation from adult data suggests a 30% incidence of adenocarcinoma in pediatric patients with BE if followed for 50 years
6 Relatively good survival has been reported with early surgical intervention for esophageal ACA
7 Approximately 50% of pediatric BE occurs in the setting of significant other disease, including neurological impairment, where GERD-related symptoms may be absent
8 Some reports suggest endoscopic appearance of BE in childhood may not be classical
9 The reversibility of metaplasia with therapeutic intervention is not well established

Significant comorbidity is common in childhood BE, and a high prevalence of neurological disease or autism is found. This can make the medical management of these cases harder (Table 4).[43]

The development of intestinal metaplasia (IM) is increasingly accepted as a preneoplastic step in a sequence through dysplasia to adenocarcinoma arising in the esophagus. In the adult population, a continuum from GERD to BE through dysplasia to ACA is relatively well documented, but this pathway is less clear in childhood.[44] GERD is a common phenomenon in children, but since adenocarcinoma is rare the issue of risk for dysplasia and screening is unclear.[45–48] Management of acid reflux with medical therapy and/or surgery may not be adequate to reverse the metaplastic process.[49]

Initial reports of pediatric BE have little documentation of the presence of goblet cells in the mucosa. Intestinal metaplasia in GERD/CLE with the appearance of goblet cells within the mucosa increases with age and time, and recent studies suggest that documentable goblet cells in CLE begin to occur at the age of 7 years. Progression from IM through dysplasia to carcinoma has been documented to require approximately 20 years.[50]

The scattered case reports of ACA in reflux-associated BE in children display similar pathological features of malignancy in a setting of dysplastic and metaplastic BE, suggesting that the pathway of GERD–BE–ACA is similar to adults.[51–52]

Endoscopic Appearance

The presentation is similar to adult, with the exception that strictures appear more common in childhood, and malignancy less frequent.[53]

Barrett's esophagus is grossly apparent at endoscopy as velvety-red tongues extending up the esophagus from the proximal gastric fold at the gastroesophageal junction. Within an area of BE, there may be islands of residual white squamous mucosa (Figure 4). Other endoscopic changes include ulceration and nodularity or friability.[50,54] All of these may be related to peptic injury and regeneration but should alert the endoscopist to biopsy generously as these features also occur with dysplasia and adenocarcinoma.[48,55]

Pathology

Historically (pre-endoscopy) BE was recognized as glandular mucosa extending for more than 3 cm from the GEJ. Nomenclature issue related to recognition of anatomical landmarks at endoscopy has been the source of controversy in the adult literature. Many adult pathologists will not diagnose BE now without the presence of goblet cells to indicate intestinal rather than gastric phenotype.[50] The remainder of cases are called columnar-lined esophagus (CLE). This relates to the recognition that the presence of goblet cells (indicating intestinal metaplasia) is generally indicative of progression of the pathological

process, and their presence suggests screening for dysplasia should be instituted. The presence of IM between the proximal gastric fold and 3 cm into the tubular esophagus (in the adult literature termed as short-segment BE [SSBE]) is associated with an increased risk of ACA, although not as high as for standard or long-segment BE (LSBE).[54]

Classical LSBE

The mucosa in BE may show a gastric phenotype with antral or body/fundic type glands and foveolar surface epithelium. Rarely is the mucosa well organized body/fundic type. The presence of hiatal hernia should be suspected if pure body/fundic mucosa is seen. Focal goblet cells are present, resulting in "incomplete intestinal metaplasia." In the absence of goblet cells, the presence of a villiform surface appearance is most suggestive of BE (Figure 5).[56–57] The presence of submucosal glands with mucosal ducts lined by transitional-type mucosa is very good evidence for anatomical localization of the specimen from the tubular esophagus. As goblet cells are often sporadic, and studies have shown that goblet cell "yield" increases with the number of biopsies taken,[44] and also that goblet cells tend to evolve after the first decade in children,[58] it is hard to be dogmatic about the pathological definition of BE. Dysplasia refers to early neoplastic change in the mucosa, and is recognized as changes resembling colonic adenoma formation in the surface epithelium (Figure 5), and is graded as low or high grade. High-grade dysplasia is associated with a high rate of invasive adenocarcinoma within 1 year. Photodynamic therapy is being used to ablate dysplastic mucosa in adult patients; no data is available in children.

Adenocarcinoma

ACA arising in BE usually occurs in the distal esophagus. The reported cases in childhood have shown the presence of surrounding areas of dysplasia and residual BE (Figure 6). Survival is related to stage. Long-term survival is possible with mucosal carcinoma. Submucosal invasion and lymph node metastasis are associated with rapidly diminishing survival.[59]

SQUAMOUS CELL CARCINOMA

Squamous cell carcinoma is a rare tumor in the esophagus in children.[4,60–61] It is more common in Blacks than Whites and in males than females (ratio 3.7:1). The major predisposing factors in the United States are alcohol and tobacco use, but in other regions where the incidence of SCC is very high, such as Linxian in Henan province in China, Northern Iran, South Africa, and areas of India factors such as the ingestion of hot foods, vitamin-deficient diets, mineral deficiencies (zinc), and other dietary problems (foods high in nitrosamines such as pickled vegetables, diet low in fresh food, high intake of benzpyrenes from coal smoke) are key. In these areas, investigation of children in their teens has shown the presence of chronic

Table 4 Benign Tumors of the Pediatric Esophagus

Relatively Frequent	Rare	Not Reported in Children
Leiomyoma	Pseudodiverticulosis	Inflammatory fibroid polyp
Papilloma		Salivary type tumors
Granular cell tumor		
Glycogen acanthosis		
Duplication cysts		

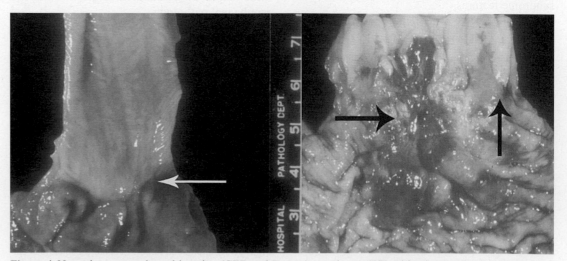

Figure 4 Normal gastroesophageal junction (GEJ) and Barrett's esophagus (BE) with adenocarcinoma. The esophagogastrectomy specimen on the left shows the normal white appearance of squamous esophageal mucosa with a white arrow at the squamocolumnar junction. The specimen on the right shows a GEJ obscured by a carcinoma on the left (black horizontal arrow) with ulceration and raised edges. On the right the normal white mucosa is partially replaced by a tongue of "salmon-pink" BE extending proximally from the GEJ (black vertical arrow).

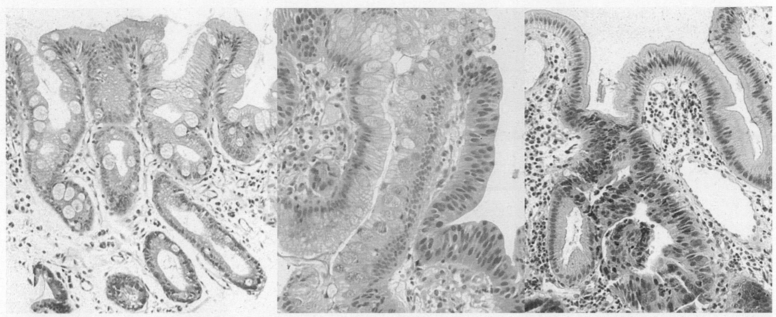

Figure 5 Barrett's mucosa and dysplasia. From left to right: (A) Barrett's esophagus—villiform mucosa with foveolar type cells alternating with goblet cells in "incomplete metaplasia." (B) Low grade dysplasia—metaplastic mucosa is partially replaced by an abrupt focus characterized by cell crowding, pseudostratification, and nuclear hyperchromatism. (C) High-grade dysplasia—the focal area shows increased atypia; nuclei are large with nucleoli. Individual cell necrosis/apoptosis is present. Architectural changes with back-back glands or cribriforming (like a sieve with the gland lumina as the holes) are apparent (H+E ×200).

esophagitis in families with SCC at double the rate of control families.[62] It is unclear as yet the relative importance of genetic over environmental forces in these populations. Some data suggest the regression of the inflammatory changes with vitamin A and zinc supplementation, at least in laboratory animals.[63] Celiac disease is associated with a significant increased risk of esophageal SCC. The pathogenesis is unclear, and the tumor so far has not been reported in childhood.[64]

Fanconi's anemia (FA), associated with high rates of childhood leukemia, is associated with an increase in squamous cell carcinomas at many

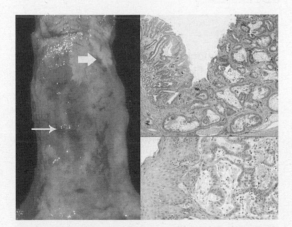

Figure 6 Barrett's esophagus with early adenocarcinoma. The resection specimen shows a long segment of metaplastic mucosa with the squamocolumnar junction now in proximal esophagus (thick arrow). The pink BE mucosa is irregular with areas of reddening and nodularity (thin arrow) corresponding with dysplastic and malignant change. The upper photomicrograph shows benign BE on the left, with intramucosal adenocarcinoma on the right half of the figure. The malignant glands are dilated, and invade into but not through the muscularis mucosa (H+E ×100). The lower photomicrograph shows intact squamous mucosa with infiltrating adenocarcinoma within the lamina propria beneath (H+E ×100).

locations, frequently the esophagus. Patients who survive into young adulthood are at risk of developing SCC of the head, neck, and upper aerodigestive tract. The genetic abnormalities were originally assumed to be due to abnormal DNA repair; subsequent investigtion has shown a complex of abnormalities; one gene associated with FA (FANCD1) was identified as being BRCA2, others have shown DNA helicase and translocase activity. More work is needed to understand the pathophysiology.[65]

Inherited or sporadic genetic disorders, some affecting keratin synthesis, including *palmoplantar keratosis* and *tylosis,* may be associated with very high rates of esophageal SCC. These conditions often manifest in childhood, usually with cutaneous lesions. Mutation in keratin genes or linkage to the tylosis esophageal carcinoma (TEC) gene on 17q25 has been documented.

Accidental caustic ingestion is predominantly a pediatric problem. The resultant chronic inflammatory process is associated with SCC of the esophagus arising later in life. The latency between ingestion and neoplasm is around 40 years, although cases as short as 13 years are reported.[66–67]

The presence of stricture of the esophagus of any cause, by increasing food impaction, irritation, inflammation, ulceration, and repair, increases the risk of esophageal SCC. The presumed pathway is through inflammation, epithelial hyperplasia, accrual of mutations leading to dysplasia, and progression to autonomous neoplasia. Achalasia, dysmotility due to absence or destruction of the distal innervation of the esophagus, whether congenital or acquired, is associated with squamous dysplasia and SCC. SCC has also been reported due to postoperative strictures related to early childhood surgery. Childhood malignancies treated with mediastinal irradiation may also predispose to early SCC.[67]

Endoscopic Appearance

Squamous pre- and early neoplastic lesions form white plaques, nodules, and occasional polyps. Granular surface or ulceration is often associated with higher grades of dysplasia (Figure 7). The mid and lower esophagus are most often affected. Lye-associated neoplasia are usually seen at the site of tracheal bifurcation, where the stricture is located. Although occasionally SCC may be grossly papillary, benign ESPs are not associated with a significant rate of malignant progression in the esophagus.

Pathology

Biopsy of a nodule or plaque may show thickened squamous mucosa with layers of keratin on the surface—benign hyperplasia (Figure 8). Inflammation, both chronic within the lamina propria and acute within the epithelium, is common, and there may be prominent small blood vessels. As dysplasia occurs, maturation to flat squamous phenotype is progressively delayed; when no maturation is seen, carcinoma in situ is present (Figure 8). The next genetic step will result in stromal invasion and early squamous cell carcinoma. The lesion may still have the appearance of a plaque, but as the tumor grows, central ulceration with raised edges or annular stenosing growth may occur. Early invasion into mediastinal soft tissue occurs, with metastasis to regional nodes.

Prognosis and Therapy

Prognosis is grim for advanced tumors, regardless of age. Three-year survival with mucosal carcinoma is >80%. This drops with submucosal invasion to 45% with lymph node metastasis to 17%.[68–69] Death is usually related to local disease. Fistulization into the tracheobronchial tree

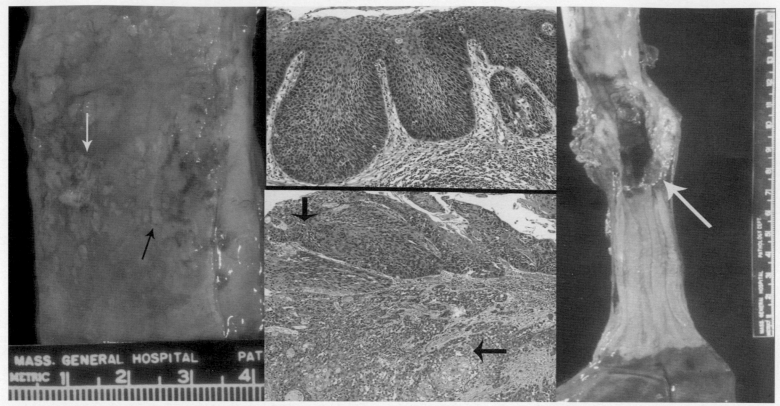

Figure 7 Squamous cell carcinoma of the esophagus. The esophagectomy specimen on the left shows esophageal squamous mucsoa with loss of the normal folds, and with areas of nodularity and redness (vertical arrow) indicating areas of dysplasia and a raised irregular area (horizontal arrow) of early carcinoma. The top photomicrograph shows severe squamous dysplasia with increased cellularity, nuclear enlargement, and loss of maturation until the upper quarter (H+E ×200). The lower photomicrograph shows intraepithelial carcinoma on the right half (vertical arrow), with invasive intramucosal carcinoma on the left (horizontal arrow) (H+E ×100). The resection specimen on the right shows advanced squamous cell carcinoma of the mid esophagus forming a deeply penetrating ulcer extending through the wall of the esophagus (arrow at lower margin of tumor edge).

and hemorrhage occur. Distant spread is a late phenomenon. Surgical resection is often now delayed till after chemoirradiation, though the results are not inconclusive thus far.[60,70]

MALIGNANT MELANOMA

Melanocytes are normally found in small numbers in the esophagus, more numerous distally, and malignant melanoma of the esophagus is reported in young adults.[71] A single case report of malignant melanoma in an 8-year-old boy revealed an aggressive melanin-producing tumor.[72] Whether this case represented a melanoma deriving from

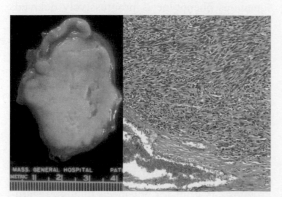

Figure 8 Esophageal sarcoma. Fibrosarcoma postirradiation forms a rubbery well-circumscribed mass deep in the wall of the esophagus, with intact overlying mucosa. The photomicrograph shows a cellular spindle cell proliferation without anaplasia with a pushing rather than infiltrative edge (H+E ×100).

mature melanocytes, or a more primitive precursor, such as a primitive neuroectodermal tumor with melanocytic differentiation is not entirely clear. Melanoma presents with dysphagia and usually forms a sessile polyp in the lower esophagus. The surrounding esophageal squamous mucosa may be heavily pigmented (melanosis). The tumors are often late stage at diagnosis, and curative therapy is rare. Metastasis from cutaneous melanoma to the esophagus needs consideration, although the ileum is the commonest site for secondary melanoma.

NON-EPITHELIAL ESOPHAGEAL MALIGNANT TUMORS

Esophageal sarcomas are very rare; most are the focus of case reports or small series. Rhabdomyosarcoma, malignant Schwannoma, leiomyosarcoma, carcinosarcoma, and malignant gastrointestinal stromal tumor (GIST) are reported. Most present with dysphagia, and large submucosal mass, often with ulceration and necrosis, is found on endoscopy.[73–74]

GIST

This tumor, arising from interstitial cell of Cajal and uniformly expressing KIT (CD117), has not been reported in the pediatric age group. However, germ-line mutations of the KIT gene are associated with a younger age of GIST; in these cases GIST may be seen in the pediatric group.[29]

Leiomyosarcoma

This tumor has not been reported in the pediatric age group. In a recent AFIP review, this was the rarest of the esophageal soft tissue tumors. Uniformly aggressive and bulky, these tumors express smooth muscle markers (SMA), and not CD117.[29,75]

Conclusion

Although tumors of the pediatric esophagus are rare, they are likely to increase in number if the current increase in esophageal adenocarcinoma continues. Guidelines for assessing pediatric patients with GERD for BE may emerge, and agreement, on surveillance for dysplasia. Benign tumors show different patterns of frequency in comparison to tumors in the adult esophagus. Underlying pathophysiological processes are more likely to be apparent in childhood.

GASTRIC NEOPLASMS

Although more frequent than their esophageal counterparts, gastric neoplasms are uncommon in the pediatric population. Reviewing the charts of 4,547 pediatric cancer patients admitted over 44 years, Bethel and colleagues reported only three neoplasms arising in the stomach, making the relative incidence of gastric primaries 0.06%.[76] While malignancies, particularly lymphomas and sarcomas are the most frequent neoplasms, a number of benign tumors can occur, either inflammatory or malformative in nature.[76–79] Since they belong to the differential diagnosis of gastric neoplasms, these tumor-forming lesions will also be reviewed in this chapter. (Carcinoid tumors are reviewed in Chapter 10, with other secretory tumors of the gastrointestinal tract.)

BENIGN TUMORS OF THE STOMACH

Although uncommon, benign gastric neoplasms, either epithelial or stromal in nature, can be observed in children.

Gastric Polyps

Sporadic, or more commonly manifestations of a polyposis syndrome, gastric polyps are less frequent than in the lower gastrointestinal tract. Pathologically, they can be of several types: adenomatous, fundic gland type, juvenile, or hamartomatous.

Familial adenomatous polyposis (FAP) is the most common polyposis syndrome of childhood.[86] The patients frequently develop multiple gastric polyps, fundic gland type more frequently than adenomatous. Fundic gland polyps have been recently shown to be neoplastic in nature with frequent somatic mutations of the APC gene.[80] The development of carcinoma in these lesions remains rare and usually occurs beyond the pediatric age. One case of adenocarcinoma has been diagnosed in a 16-year-old FAP patient.[81–85] Gastric adenomas should be completely excised, and the entire stomach should be examined carefully. Endoscopic follow-up should be initiated since there is a relatively high risk of developing new adenomas. Compared with sporadic cases, fundic gland polyps and adenomas associated with FAP occur at a much younger age. They increase in prevalence with increasing age. Given the risk, regular surveillance is indicated in patients with FAP.

Peutz-Jeghers Syndrome

Forty percent of Peutz-Jeghers patients present with gastric polyps.[86] These hamartomatous polyps are usually silent, although rare presentations may occur such as antral obstruction or in one case auto-amputation. The polyps preferentially affect the antrum. Histologically, the polyps display an arborizing framework of smooth muscle covered by hyperplastic fundic or antral-type mucosa with elongation and cystic change of foveolar epithelium with frequent atrophy of the underlying glands.[87] The risk of malignancy, via the development of dysplasia, is low but not nonexistent with gastric adenocarcinomas reported as early as the second decade.[86,88–89]

Juvenile Polyposis

This type of polyposis sets apart because of its early clinical manifestations with three-fourths of the affected patients presenting during childhood.[86,89] Among the different forms of juvenile polyposis, the stomach is involved in *generalized juvenile polyposis* (with a reported involvement of 13.6% of the cases) and in the usually fatal *juvenile polyposis of infancy* typified by the diffuse involvement of the gastrointestinal tract with patients developing severe diarrhea, hemorrhage, and protein-losing enteropathy.[88–90] Juvenile polyposis of the stomach is limited to that site. Most sessile hamartomatous polyps measure between 5 and 40 mm. They are characterized by large cystic spaces lined by foveolar epithelium and embedded in a lamina propria with mixed inflammatory infiltrate.[87,90] The risk of malignant transformation in the stomach is lower than in the colon.[91] Dysplasia can sometimes be found. Patients with juvenile polyposis should undergo periodic upper endoscopy. In addition to colon and stomach, patients with *Juvenile polyposis* have an increased risk of developing adenocarcinomas in biliary tract and pancreas.

Gastric Teratoma

This rare tumor is composed of mesodermal, endodermal, and ectodermal elements and occurs almost exclusively in the pediatric population. The pathogenesis of gastric teratomas is unknown, but they are thought to arise from a pluripotential cell. Nearly all the patients are male and most are children of less than 2 years of age.[92,93] The patients present with large intra-abdominal masses that may lead to obstruction while younger patients may present with respiratory insufficiency because of the limitation of movements of the diaphragm.[93] Upper GI bleeding, resulting from ulceration of the overlying mucosa, can also be observed. Characteristically, preoperative imaging studies may demonstrate calcifications corresponding to teeth or bone structures developed within the tumor. The histology demonstrates intermixed mature tissue elements such as skin, smooth muscle, bone, cartilage, adipose, and neural tissue. With the exception of a single case reported in an adult, no malignant transformation is reported in the pediatric literature, and excision is curative.[92]

MALIGNANT TUMORS OF THE STOMACH

Adenocarcinoma

Between 2 and 10% of gastric carcinomas are diagnosed in patients younger than 40 years old, and cases seen in the pediatric population are extremely rare. The regional variation in incidence rates seen in gastric adenocarcinoma in adults is not identified, or possibly not identifiable in the pediatric age group.

In a series of 501 gastric cancers in individuals younger than 31 years of age, only 0.4% of cases occurred in children 10 years or younger, 3.4% occurred in children between 11 and 15 years, and 8% occurred in children between 16 and 20 years.[94] A study of 3,079 cases of gastric carcinoma diagnosed in British Columbia over a ten-year period revealed that only 65 cases occurred in younger individuals (under 40 years of age) and that the youngest patient was 24 years of age. No pediatric case was reported. Younger patients exhibited adverse clinical and pathological features compared to older patients.[95] Although no series exist, there are case reports of pediatric gastric adenocarcinoma, one occurring in a child of only 20 months of age.[96–98]

The risk factors for the development of gastric cancers in childhood are not well established. Approximately 10 to 25% of young gastric cancer patients have positive family history suggesting the role of genetic factors.[99] Cases associated with the *familial diffuse gastric carcinoma syndrome* associated with germline mutations in the E-cadherin/*CDH1* gene have been diagnosed in young adults but not in pediatric patients.[100–103] *Helicobacter pylori* infection associated with the development of adult gastric cancer is apparently not reported in pediatric cases. Other precursor lesions such as of intestinal metaplasia, pernicious anemia, and hypertrophic gastropathy, as well as previous gastrectomy are also rare in this population. Several conditions have been linked with gastric cancer. These include IgA deficiency, common variable immunodeficiency syndrome, and ataxia telangiectasia.[104–106] A rare association with Rothmund Thompson syndrome has also been reported.[107] Polyposis syndrome that is familial polyposis coli and Peutz-Jeghers syndrome are associated with the development of adenocarcinomas, although it is usually later in life. Finally, two cases of gastric adenocarcinoma have also been seen as a late complication of individuals previously treated (3.5 and 10 years) for abdominal lymphoma by irradiation and chemotherapy.[108]

In many instances, the presenting symptoms are not different from those of older patients.[98] The most common presenting complaints include pain and vomiting, followed by anorexia and weight loss.[99,109] Abdominal distention is also reported.[98,110] A mass can be palpated in 70% of the patients according to one series.[94] A rare association with tumor thrombotic microangiopathy has been reported.[111]

Although the histologic pattern of gastric cancer in childhood can be similar to the cases reported in adults, some report a predominance of mucinous and signet ring cell carcinoma (Figure 9).

Since there is no large series of children with gastric carcinoma, it is not possible to draw significant conclusion with regard to prognosis. Despite anecdotal reports of cure, the evidence provided suggests that delay in diagnosis usually contribute to limited patient survival.[99] Various protocols, usually based on experience on adult patients, include surgery and various chemotherapy protocols with or without radiotherapy. Lymphatic, vascular, direct extension, and seeding of peritoneal surface/coelomic patterns of metastatic dissemination have been reported.[79,98,99,110–112]

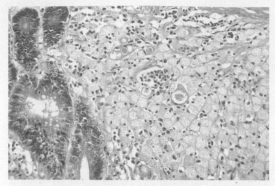

Figure 9 Diffuse type gastric carcinoma in a 17-year-old patient. The tumor is composed of single cells expanding the lamina propria. Rare signet ring cells can be seen. (H+E ×400)

HEMATOPOIETIC NEOPLASMS

Gastric Lymphoma

In the adult population, the stomach is the most common site of gastrointestinal GI lymphomas comprising about 40% of the cases, followed by the small bowel with 27% of the cases. In contrast, in children the small bowel is the predominant site accounting for 40 to 45% of the cases, while gastric lymphoma represents between 2.5 and 17% of the GI non-Hodgkin's lymphomas.[113–116]

Predisposing conditions include primary immunodeficiency such as severe combined immunodeficiency, X-linked agammaglobulinemia, common variable immunodeficiency disease, Wiskott-Aldrich syndrome and ataxia

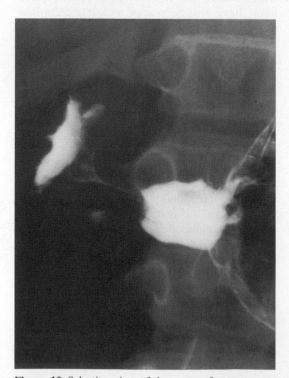

Figure 10 Selective view of the antrum from an upper gastrointestinal series in a 15-year-old boy who presented with hematemesis, weight loss, and right upper quadrant abdominal pain. A mass is seen encircling the antrum and almost completely obstructing it. Endoscopic biopsies revealed a large cell immunoblastic lymphoma. Courtesy of the Teaching Collection, Department of Radiology, The Children's Hospital, Boston.

telangiectasia that are associated with an increased risk of lymphoma.[117, 118]

The mode of clinical presentation may include nonspecific symptoms such as abdominal pain but also the palpation of mass or gastrointestinal bleeding. Gastric outlet obstruction by a lymphoma has been reported (Figure 10).[119] Most gastric lymphomas tumors are cytologically high-grade malignancies either lymphoblastic or large cell anaplastic type.[113–114] Primary treatment includes resection of the tumor, followed by postoperative chemotherapy and/or radiotherapy. Careful medical and surgical management following prompt diagnosis have been shown to offer long survival.[114]

Langerhans cell histiocytosis of the stomach has been reported in a 14-year-old girl. Besides its rarity, the diffuse antral and fundic polyposis and the granulomatous pattern displayed by the histiocytosis are noticeable.[120] To date only a handful of cases with gastric involvement have been reported, all but one in adults. In the case in point the patient remained asymptomatic at 10 months after diagnosis.[120]

MESENCHYMAL NEOPLASMS

Rare reports of benign and malignant mesenchymal lesions can be found in the literature.

Gastrointestinal Stromal Tumor

Gastrointestinal stromal tumors (GISTs) are rare, accounting for less than 1% of all gastrointestinal malignancies. They are uncommon before middle age and extremely rare in children.[121,122] GISTs are defined as spindle and/or epithelioid mesenchymal neoplasms that usually express CD117 and do not have diagnostic features of any other type of mesenchymal tumors.[121,123] Most neoplasms now included in this category would have been previously diagnosed as smooth muscle tumors (leiomyoma, leiomyoblastoma, and leiomyosarcoma), fibromatosis, and schwannomas. The massive amount of information collected on GISTS has been based on the adult experience. Whether it can be translated in the pediatric population is unknown. A recent paper by Bates and colleagues reported that congenital stromal tumors of the gastrointestinal were morphologically similar from the adult but did not express CD117 and carried a favorable prognosis.[124] Pediatric literature from the pre-CD117 era have reported a similar biologic behavior.[107]

Although in most cases they occur sporadically, some GISTs have been described as a component of Carney's triad (gastric epithelioid stromal sarcoma, functioning extra-adrenal paraganglioma, and pulmonary chondroma).[125] Rare myogenic tumors have been reported in AIDS patients. Their pathogenesis is unknown, but the initiating role of the HIV virus but also of EBV has been entertained.[118,126,127]

It has been shown that GISTs share phenotypic similarities with the interstitial cells of

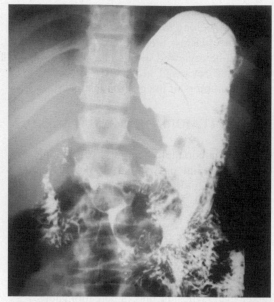

Figure 11 Upper gastrointestinal series in a 10-year-old girl with severe anemia and tarry stools. A large nodular leiomyosarcoma is seen in the gastric antrum. Courtesy of the Teaching Collection, Department of Radiology, The Children's Hospital, Boston.

Cajal, including the expression of C-KIT and CD34.[121,128] These pacemaker cells are now considered to represent the origin of these rare neoplasms. Another important biologic breakthrough has been the demonstration that most GISTs have oncogenic mutations of the *c-kit* gene. This has been translated clinically by the usage of an inhibitor of the tyrosine kinase activity of c-Kit (ST-571), which has shown significant promise in treating patients with metastatic disease.

Most GISTs are diagnosed in the stomach (60 to 70% of the cases). The majority measures between 3 and 15 cm although tumors as small as few millimeters and as large as 30 to 40 cm can be observed. GISTs may present as intraluminal or subserosal masses that may compress regional adjacent organs (Figure 11).[123] Depending on their size, various nonspecific clinical presentations (ie, nausea, vomiting, abdominal pain, bleeding) may be observed. The most common presenting symptoms of GISTs in children are GI bleeding (with frank hematemesis in about 40% of patients and occult bleeding in up to 80%) and symptoms of intestinal obstruction (in about 50% of patients). Abdominal pain, weight loss, fever, and abdominal masses are also reported. GISTs present as firm tan, well-circumscribed masses (Figure 12). Hemorrhage, necrosis, and cystification are seen in large tumors. They are variably cellular and composed of spindle cells and/or epithelioid cells. The spindle cells can be organized in fascicles, storiform and herringbone arrangements, palisading or organoid groupings (Figure 13).[129]

The microscopic characteristics of GISTs are poor indicators of their clinical behavior. A recent workshop sponsored by the National Institute of Health concluded that the benign and malignant behavior of a tumor cannot be predicted on the basis of morphology alone. It is now recommended that all GISTs be considered

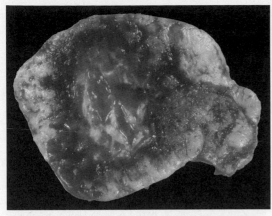

Figure 12 Gastric gastrointestinal stromal tumor. The tumor is well circumscribed but not encapsulated. Note the central necrosis, characteristic of a malignant biologic behavior.

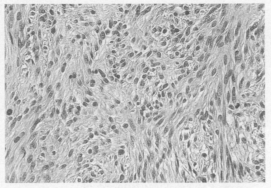

Figure 13 Gastric gastrointestinal stromal tumor. Photomicrograph with typical fascicular arrangement of spindles cells. Scattered mitoses can be seen.

potentially malignant and be classified according to their risk of aggressive behavior based on the size and the number of mitoses in 50 high-power fields.[123]

MISCELLANEOUS

Gastric Hemangioma

Visceral hemangiomas are rare outside of the liver. In the stomach, although hemangiomas can be isolated; they are frequently associated with vascular lesions of the skin and intestine.[130–132] The cases associated with gastrointestinal hemangiomatosis tend to occur at an earlier age with cases discovered in neonatal period.[132] Hematemesis is a frequent initial symptom. Despite their benign nature, these sometimes-large-hemorrhagic masses require surgical therapy ranging from wedge excision to partial and even total gastrectomy.[132]

Gastric Lipoma

Composed of lobules of mature adipose tissue, gastric lipomas are slow-growing tumors. They frequently originate from the submucosa while others are centered on the subserosa. The common antral location of these usually sessile and polypoid lesions accounts for the reports of intussusceptions into the pylorus or the duodenum.[133] Mucosal ulceration with chronic blood loss but also hemorrhage has been reported.[134] On barium swallow, gastric lipomas change of shape with peristalsis and show a preserved mucosal profile, both characteristics of a benign process. MRIs show, on T1 weighted image, a solid hyperintense lesion with a signal corresponding to fat. Finally, on endoscopy, the typical "sinking impression" is felt when the mass is poked with forceps.[133] If small, gastric lipomas can be removed by polypectomy, but larger lesions may necessitate a laparotomy.[134]

Inflammatory Myofibroblastic Tumor

Despite much interest in the pathology literature, the pathogenesis of this unusual process, also known as inflammatory pseudotumor and plasma cell granuloma, remains indeterminate.[135] It preferentially affects children and young adults, and most cases are reported in the lungs while only rare cases have been seen in the stomach. Microscopically, these tumors show a mixed pattern composed of a variable number of spindle-shaped myofibroblasts embedded in a usually collagenized stroma with intermixed chronic inflammatory cells in which plasma cells may be numerous. The spindle cells are CD117 negative and usually positive for SMA.[135] Although usually benign, large size tumor and invasion into surrounding tissues have characterize the aggressive nature of rare cases. Such cases may require several surgical resections.[136]

Gastric Hamartoma

Hamartomas of the gastric wall are benign lesions showing considerable histologic variation. They are composed of abnormal admixture of components of the gastric wall, including hypertrophied bands of muscularis mucosa branching out and dissecting through the mucosa that shows misplaced and cystically distended glands.[137] They should be differentiated from the adenomyomatous variant of ectopic pancreas, which is formed of cystic pancreatobiliary type ducts.[116,138]

Gastric Leiomyosarcoma

Leiomyomas and leiomyosarcomas have been reported in association with Alport's syndrome, acquired immunodeficiency syndrome, pulmonary osteoarthropathy, and Carney's triad (leiomyosarcoma, extra-adrenal paraganglioma, and pulmonary chondroma).

Rare Mesenchymal Lesions of the Stomach

A distinctive malignant gastric mesenchymal tumor sharing some features with *clear cell sarcoma* of soft part has been reported in a 13-year-old boy. This type of tumor, previously observed in the small bowel, displays a distinct nesting pattern formed by medium-sized tumor cells with a clear to acidophilic cytoplasm admixed with osteoclast-like multinucleated cells. Strong positive immunohistochemistry for S-100 protein and t(12;22)(q13;q12) also support the similari-

ties with clear sarcoma of soft part.[139] A case of gastric *rhabdomyosarcoma* with disseminated metastases and death within 2 1/2 months post-diagnosis despite chemotherapy and radiotherapy has also been seen.[79] Uncommon neoplasms of vascular origin, only few cases of *hemangiopericytoma*, have been observed in the stomach. The younger patient was 2 days old when he developed hematemesis and had surgery at day 12. Although these vascular tumors have the potential to behave in a malignant fashion, metastasis of gastric neoplasms seems to be rare, may be because of the usual early diagnosis and treatment.[140] Although less frequent than in adults, *Kaposi sarcoma* has also been reported to affect the stomach of pediatric AIDS patients.[118]

Conclusion

Given their rarity, gastric tumors in childhood are almost always unexpected findings. Nevertheless, the differential diagnosis of upper GI symptoms in childhood must include these rare lesions. It is of obvious clinical importance since in many cases timely treatment is the only hope for good prognosis.

REFERENCES

1. Carr NJ, Bratthauer GL, Lichy JH, et al. Squamous cell papillomas of the esophagus: a study of 23 lesions for human papillomavirus by in situ hybridization and the polymerase chain reaction. Hum Pathol 1994;25:536–40.
2. Sodhi KS, Saxena AK, Narasimha Rao KL, et al. Esophageal duplication cyst:an unusual cause of respiratory distress in infants. Pediatr Emerg Care 2005;21:854–6.
3. Bower RJ, Kiesewetter W.B: Mediastinal masses in infants and children. Arch Surg 1977;112: 1003–9.
4. Eloubeidi MA, Desmond R, Arguedas MR, et al. Prognostic factors for the survival of patients with esophageal carcinoma in the U.S.: the importance of tumor length and lymph node status. Cancer 2002;95:1434–43.
5. Mosca S, Manes G, Monaco R, et al. Squamous papilloma of the esophagus: long-term follow up. J Gastroenterol Hepatol 2001;16:857–61.
6. Arima T, Ikeda K, Satoh T, et al. Squamous cell papilloma of the esophagus in a child. Int Surg 1985;70:177–8.
7. Frootko NJ, Rogers JH. Oesophageal papillomata in the child. J Laryngol Otol 1978;92:823–7.
8. Carr NJ, Monihan JM, Sobin LH. Squamous cell papilloma of the esophagus: a clinicopathologic and follow-up study of 25 cases. Am J Gastroenterol 1994;89:245–8.
9. Odze R, Antonioli D, Shocket D, et al. Esophageal squamous papillomas. A clinicopathologic study of 38 lesions and analysis for human papillomavirus by the polymerase chain reaction. Am J Surg Pathol 1993;17:803–12.
10. Waterfall WE, Somers S, Desa DJ. Benign oesophageal papillomatosis. a case report with a review of the literature. J Clin Pathol 1978;31:111–5.
11. Ravakhah K , Midamba F, West BC. Esophageal papillomatosis from human papilloma virus proven by polymerase chain reaction. Am J Med Sci 1998;316:285–8.
12. Batra PS, Hebert RL II, Haines GK III, Holinger LD. Recurrent respiratory papillomatosis with esophageal involvement. Int J Pediatr Otorhinolaryngol 2001;58: 233–8.
13. Brinson RR, Schuman BM, Mills LR, et al. Multiple squamous papillomas of the esophagus associated with Goltz syndrome. Am J Gastroenterol 1987;82:1177–9.
14. Lagergren J, Wang Z, Bergstrom R, et al. Human papillomavirus infection and esophageal cancer: a nationwide seroepidemiologic case-control study in Sweden. J Natl Cancer Inst 1999;91:156–62.
15. Lavergne D, de Villiers EM. Papillomavirus in esophageal papillomas and carcinomas. Int J Cancer 1999;80:681–4.
16. Moulton MS, Moir C, Matsumoto J, Thompson DM. Esophageal duplication cyst: a rare cause of biphasic stridor and feeding difficulty. Int J Pediatr Otorhinolaryngol 2005;69:1129 – 33.

17. Stringer MD, Spitz L, Abel R, et al. Management of alimentary tract duplication in children. Br J Surg 1995;82:74–8.

18. Perger L, Azzie G, Watch L, Weinsheimer R. Two cases of thoracoscopic resection of esophageal duplication in children. J Laparoendosc Adv Surg tech A 2006;16:418 – 21.

19. Michel JL, Revillon Y, Montupet P, et al. Thoracoscopic treatment of mediastinal cysts in children. J Pediatr Surg 1998;33:1745–8.

20. Cury EK, Schraibman V, De Vasconcelos Macedo AL, Echenique LS. Thoracoscopic esophagectomy in children. J Pediatr Surg 2001;36:E17.

21. McGregor DH, Mills G, Boudet RA. Intramural squamous cell carcinoma of the esophagus. Cancer 1976;37:1556–61.

22. Olsen JB, Clemmensen O, Andersen K. Adenocarcinoma arising in a foregut cyst of the mediastinum. Ann Thorac Surg 1991;51:497–9.

23. Takubo K, Nakagawa H, Tsuchiya S, et al. Seedling leiomyoma of the esophagus and esophagogastric junction zone. Hum Pathol 1981;12:1006–10.

24. Bourque MD, Spigland N, Bensoussan AL, et al. Esophageal leiomyoma in children: Two case reports and review of the literature. J Pediatr Surg 1989;24:1103–7.

25. Cohen SR, Thompson JW, Sherman NJ. Congenital stenosis of the lower esophagus associated with leiomyoma and leiomyosarcoma of the gastrointestinal tract. Ann Otol Rhinol Laryngol 1988;97:454–9.

26. McKeeby JL, Li X, Zhuang Z, et al. Multiple leiomyomas of the esophagus, lung, and uterus in multiple endocrine neoplasia type 1. Am J Pathol 2001;159:1121–7.

27. Al-Bassam A, Al-Rabeeah A, Fouda-Neel K, Mahasin Z. Leiomyoma of the esophagus and bronchus in a child. Pediatr Surg Int 1998;13:45–7.

28. Seremetis MG, Lyons WS, deGuzman VC, Peabody JW Jr. Leiomyomata of the esophagus. An analysis of 838 cases. Cancer 1976;38:2166–77.

29. Miettinen M, Sarlomo-Rikala M, Sobin LH, Lasota J. Esophageal stromal tumors: A clinicopathologic, immunohistochemical, and molecular genetic study of 17 cases and comparison with esophageal leiomyomas and leiomyosarcomas. Am J Surg Pathol 2000;24:211–22.

30. Guest AR, Strouse PJ, Hiew CC, Arca M. Progressive esophageal leiomyomatosis with respiratory compromise. Pediatr Radiol 2000;30:247–50.

31. Federici S, Ceccarelli P, Bernardi F, et al. Esophagealleiomyomatosis in children: A report of a case and review of the literature. Eur J Pediatr Surg 1998;8:358–63.

32. Lee LS, Nance M, Kaiser LR, Kucharczuk JC. Familial massive leiomyoma with esophageal leiomyomatosis; an unusual presentation in a father and his 2 daughters. J pediatr Surg 2005;40:e29–32.

33. Prenzel KL, Schafer E, Stippel D, et al. Multiple giant leiomyomas of the esophagus and stomach. Dis Esophagus 2006;19:504 – 8.

34. Billeret Lebranchu V. Granular cell tumor. Epidemiology of 263 cases. Arch Anat Cytol Pathol 1999;47:26–30.

35. Park SH, Kim TJ, Chi JG. Congenital granular cell tumor with systemic involvement. Immunohistochemical and ultrastructural study. Arch Pathol Lab Med 1991;115:934–8.

36. Lack EE, Worsham GF, Callihan MD, et al. Granular cell tumor: a clinicopathologic study of 110 patients. J Surg Oncol 1980;13:301–16.

37. Goldblum JR, Rice TW, Zuccaro G, Richter JE. Granular cell tumors of the esophagus: A clinical and pathologic study of 13 cases. Ann Thorac Surg 1996;62:860–5.

38. Ohmori T, Arita N, Uraga N, et al. Malignant granular cell tumor of the esophagus. A case report with light and electron microscopic, histochemical, and immunohistochemical study. Acta Pathol Jpn 1987;37:775–83.

39. Farley TJ, Klionsky N. Mixed hemangioma and cystic lymphangioma of the esophagus in a child. J Pediatr Gastroenterol Nutr 1992;15:178–80.

40. Canavese F, Cortese MG, Proietti L, et al. Bulky-pedunculated hemolymphangioma of the esophagus: Rare case in a two-years old girl. Eur J Pediatr Surg 1996;6:170–2.

41. Chak A, Lee T, Kinnard MF, et al. Familial aggregation of Barrett's esophagus, oesophageal adenocarcinoma, and oesophagogastric junctional adenocarcinoma in Caucasian adults. Gut 2002;51:323–8.

42. Jochem VJ, Fuerst PA, Fromkes JJ. Familial Barrett's esophagus associated with adenocarcinoma. Gastroenterology 1992;102:1400–2.

43. Hassall E. Co-morbidities in childhood Barrett's esophagus. J Pediatr Gastroenterol Nutr 1997;25:255–60.

44. Chalasani N, Wo JM, Hunter JG, Waring JP. et al. Significance of intestinal metaplasia in different areas of esophagus including esophagogastric junction. Dig Dis Sci 1997;42:603–7.

45. McDonald ML, Trastek VF, Allen MS, et al. Barretts's esophagus: Does an antireflux procedure reduce the need for endoscopic surveillance? J Thorac Cardiovasc Surg 1996;111:1135-8; discussion 1139–40.

46. Achkar E, Carey W. The cost of surveillance for adenocarcinoma complicating Barrett's esophagus. Am J Gastroenterol 1988. 83:291–4.

47. Siersema PD, Dees J, Tilanus HW, et al. Early detection and treatment of oesophageal and gastric cancer. The Rotterdam Oesophageal Tumour Study Group. Neth J Med 1995;47:76–86.

48. Hassall E. Barrett's esophagus: New definitions and approaches in children. J Pediatr Gastroenterol Nutr 1993;16:345–64.

49. Cheu HW, Grosfeld JL, Heifetz SA, et al. Persistence of Barrett's esophagus in children after antireflux surgery: Influence on follow-up care. J Pediatr Surg 1992;27:260–4; discussion 265–6.

50. Haggitt RC. Barrett's esophagus, dysplasia, and adenocarcinoma. Hum Pathol 1994;25(10):982–93.

51. Hassall E, Dimmick JE, Magee JF. Adenocarcinoma in childhood Barrett's esophagus: case documentation and the need for surveillance in children. Am J Gastroenterol 1993;88:282–8.

52. Adzick NS, Fisher JH, Winter HS, et al. Esophageal adenocarcinoma 20 years after esophageal atresia repair. J Pediatr Surg 1989;24:741–4.

53. Bremner CG. Benign strictures of the esophagus. Curr Probl Surg 1982;19:401–89.

54. Montgomery E, Goldblum JR, Greenson JK, et al. Dysplasia as a predictive marker for invasive carcinoma in Barrett esophagus: A follow-up study based on 138 cases from a diagnostic variability study. Hum Pathol 2001;32:379–88.

55. Hassall E. Columnar-lined esophagus in children. Gastroenterol Clin North Am 1997;26:533–48.

56. Spechler SJ. Barrett's esophagus. Semin Oncol 1994;21:431–7.

57. Spechler SJ, Goyal RK. Barrett's esophagus. N Engl J Med 1986;315:362–71.

58. Qualman SJ, Murray RD, McClung HJ, Lucas J. Intestinal metaplasia is age related in Barrett's esophagus. Arch Pathol Lab Med 1990;114(12): 1236–40.

59. Farrow DC, Vaughan TL. Determinants of survival following the diagnosis of esophageal adenocarcinoma (United States). Cancer Causes Control 1996;7:322–7.

60. Schettini ST, Ganc A, Saba L. Esophageal carcinoma secondary to a chemical injury in a child. Pediatr Surg Int 1998;13:519–20.

61. Shahi UP, Sudarsan, Dattagupta S, et al. Carcinoma esophagus in a 14 year old child: Report of a case and review of literature. Trop Gastroenterol 1989;10:225–8.

62. Lewin KJ. Malignant and premalignant lesions of the esophagus. Keio J Med 1992;41:177–83.

63. Newberne PM, Broitman S, Schrager TF. Esophageal carcinogenesis in the rat: Zinc deficiency, DNA methylation and alkyltransferase activity. Pathobiology 1997;65:253–63.

64. Pricolo VE, Mangi AA, Aswad B, Bland KI. Gastrointestinal malignancies in patients with celiac sprue. Am J Surg 1998;176:344–7.

65. Mathew CG. Fanconi anaemia agenes and susceptibility to cancer. Oncogene 2006;25:5875–84..

66. Appelqvist P, Salmo M. Lye corrosion carcinoma of the esophagus: A review of 63 cases. Cancer 1980;45:2655–8.

67. Ribeiro U, Jr, Posner MC, Safatle-Ribeiro AV, Reynolds JC. Risk factors for squamous cell carcinoma of the esophagus. Br J Surg 1996;83:1174–85.

68. Bremner RM, DeMeester TR. Surgical treatment of esophageal carcinoma. Gastroenterol Clin North Am 1991;20:743–63.

69. Taifu L. Radiotherapy of carcinoma of the esophagus in China—a review. Int J Radiat Oncol Biol Phys 1991;20:875–9.

70. Malhaire JP, Labat JP, Lozac'h P, et al. Preoperative concomitant radiochemotherapy in squamous cell carcinoma of the esophagus: Results of a study of 56 patients. Int J Radiat Oncol Biol Phys 1996;34:429–37.

71. Boulafendis D, Damiani M, Sie E, et al. Primary malignant melanoma of the esophagus in a young adult. Am J Gastroenterol 1985;80:417–20.

72. Basque GJ, Boline JE, Holyoke JB. Malignant melanoma of the esophagus: First reported case in a child. Am J Clin Pathol 1970;53:609–11.

73. Perch SJ, Soffen EM, Whittington R, Brooks JJ. Esophageal sarcomas. J Surg Oncol 1991;48:194–8.

74. McGrath PC, et al. Gastrointestinal sarcomas. Analysis of prognostic factors. Ann Surg 1987;206:706–10.

75. Pramesh CS, et al. Leiomyosarcoma of the esophagus. Dis Esophagus 2003;16:142–4.

76. Bethel CA, Bhattacharyya N, Hutchinson C, et al. Alimentary tract malignancies in children. J Pediatr Surg 1997;1004–8; discussion 1008–9.

77. Skinner MA, Plumley DA, Grosfeld JL, et al. Gastrointestinal tumors in children: An analysis of 39 cases. Ann Surg Oncol 1994;283–9.

78. Ladd AP, Grosfeld JL. Gastrointestinal tumors in children and adolescents. Semin Pediatr Surg 2006;15:37 – 47.

79. Mahour GH, Isaacs H, Jr, Chang L. Primary malignant tumors of the stomach in children. J Pediatr Surg 1980;603–8.

80. Abraham SC, Nobukawa B, Giardiello FM, et al. Fundic gland polyps in familial adenomatous polyposis: Neoplasms with frequent somatic adenomatous polyposis coli gene alterations. Am J Pathol 2000;747–54.

81. Watanabe H, Enjoji M, Yao T, Ohsato K. Gastric lesions in familial adenomatosis coli: Their incidence and histologic analysis. Hum Pathol 1978;269–83.

82. Offerhaus GJ, Entius MM, Giardiello FM. Upper gastrointestinal polyps in familial adenomatous polyposis. Hepatogastroenterology 1999;667–9.

83. Hofgartner WT, Thorp M, Ramus MW, et al. Gastric adenocarcinoma associated with fundic gland polyps in a patient with attenuated familial adenomatous polyposis. Am J Gastroenterol 1999;2275–81.

84. Zwick A, Munir M, Ryan CK, et al. Gastric adenocarcinoma and dysplasia in fundic gland polyps of a patient with attenuated adenomatous polyposis coli. Gastroenterology 1997;659–63.

85. Goedde TA, Rodriguez-Bigas MA, Herrera L, Petrelli NJ. Gastroduodenal polyps in familial adenomatous polyposis. Surg Oncol 1992;357–61.

86. Erdman SH, Barnard JA. Gastrointestinal polyps and polyposis syndromes in children. Curr Opin Pediatr 2002;576–82.

87. Haggitt RC, Reid BJ. Hereditary gastrointestinal polyposis syndromes. Am J Surg Pathol 1986;871–87.

88. Rustgi AK. Hereditary gastrointestinal polyposis and nonpolyposis syndromes. N Engl J Med 1994;1694–702.

89. Coffin M, Pappin AL. Polyps and neoplasms of the gastrointestinal tract in childhood and adolescence. Gastrointest Dis 1997;127–171.

90. Schreibman IR, Baker M, Amos C, McGarrity TJ. The hamartomatous poyposis syndromes: A clinical and molecular review. Am J Gastrenterol. 2005;100:476 – 90.

91. Howe JR, Mitros FA, Summers RW. The risk of gastrointestinal carcinoma in familial juvenile polyposis. Ann Surg Oncol 1998;751–6.

92. Matsukuma S, Wada R, Daibou M, et al. Adenocarcinoma arising from gastric immature teratoma. Report of a case in an adult and a review of the literature. Cancer 1995; 2663–8.

93. Cairo MS, Grosfeld JL, Weetman RM. Gastric teratoma: Unusual cause for bleeding of the upper gastrointestinal tract in the newborn. Pediatrics 1981;721–4.

94. McNeer G. Cancer of the stomach in the young. Am J Roentgenol Rad Therapy Nucl Med 1941;537.

95. Grabiec J, Owen DA. Carcinoma of the stomach in young persons. Cancer 1985;388–96.

96. Koea JB, Karpeh MS, Brennan MF. Gastric cancer in young patients: Demographic, clinicopathological, and prognostic factors in 92 patients. Ann Surg Oncol 2000;346–51.

97. Kokkola A, Sipponen P. Gastric carcinoma in young adults. Hepatogastroenterology 2001;48:1552–5.

98. Siegel SE, Hays DM, Romansky S, Isaacs H. Carcinoma of the stomach in childhood. Cancer 1976;1781–4.

99. Michalek J, Kopecna L, Tuma J, et al. Gastric carcinoma in a 9-year-old boy. Pediatr Hematol Oncol 2000;511–5.

100. Gayther SA, Gorringe KL, Ramus SJ, et al. Identification of germ-line E-cadherin mutations in gastric cancer families of European origin. Cancer Res 1998;4086–9.

101. Keller G, Vogelsang H, Becker I, et al. Diffuse type gastric and lobular breast carcinoma in a familial gastric cancer patient with an E-cadherin germline mutation. Am J Pathol 1999;155:337–42.

102. Guilford PJ, Hopkins JB, Grady WM, et al. E-cadherin germline mutations define an inherited cancer syndrome dominated by diffuse gastric cancer. Hum Mutat 1999;249–55.

103. Caldas C, Carneiro F, Lynch HT, et al. Familial gastric cancer: Overview and guidelines for management. J Med Genet 1999;873–80.

104. Swift M, Morrell D, Massey RB, Chase CL. Incidence of cancer in 161 families affected by ataxia-telangiectasia. N Engl J Med 1991;325:1831–6.

105. Haerer AF, Jackson JF, Evers CG. Ataxia-telangiectasia with gastric adenocarcinoma. Jama 1969;210:1884–7.

106. Fraser KJ, Rankin JG. Selective deficiency of IgA immunoglobulins associated with carcinoma of the stomach. Australas Ann Med 1970;165–7.

107. Black RE. Linitis plastica in a child. J Pediatr Surg 1985;20:86–7.

108. Brumback RA, Gerber JE, Hicks DG, Strauchen JA. Adenocarcinoma of the stomach following irradiation and chemotherapy for lymphoma in young patients. Cancer 1984;54:994–8.

109. McGill TW, Downey EC, Westbrook J, et al. Gastric carcinoma in children. J Pediatr Surg 1993;28:1620–1.

110. Dokucu AI, Ozturk H, Kilinc N, et al. Primary gastric adenocarcinoma in a 2.5-year-old girl. Gastric Cancer 2002;5:237–9.

111. Blaker H, Daum R, Troger J, et al. Adenocarcinoma of the stomach with tumor-thrombotic microangiopathy in an 11-year-old male patient. Eur J Pediatr Surg 2000;10:45–9.

112. Goto S, Ikeda K, Ishii E, et al. Carcinoma of the stomach in a year-old boy—a case report and a review of the literature on children under 10 years of age, Z Kinderchir 1984;137–40.

113. Gurney KA, Cartwright RA, Gilman EA. Descriptive epidemiology of gastrointestinal non-Hodgkin's lymphoma in a population-based registry. Br J Cancer 1999;79:1929–34.

114. Takahashi H, Hansmann ML. Primary gastrointestinal lymphoma in childhood (up to 18 years of age). A morphological, immunohistochemical and clinical study. J Cancer Res Clin Oncol 1990;116:190–6.

115. Jenkin RD, Sonley MJ, Stephens CA, et al. Primary gastrointestinal tract lymphoma in childhood. Radiology 1969;92:763–7.

116. Lewin KJ, Ranchod M, Dorfman RF. Lymphomas of the gastrointestinal tract: A study of 117 cases presenting with gastrointestinal disease. Cancer 1978;42:693–707.

117. Filipovich AH, Mathur A, Kamat D, et al. Lymphoproliferative disorders and other tumors complicating immunodeficiencies. Immunodeficiency 1994;5:91–112.

118. Kahn E. Gastrointestinal manifestations in pediatric AIDS. Pediatr Pathol Lab Med 1997;17:171–208.

119. Ciftci AO, Tanyel FC, Kotiloglu E, Hicsonmez A. Gastric lymphoma causing gastric outlet obstruction. J Pediatr Surg 1996;31:1424–6.

120. Groisman GM, Rosh JR, Harpaz N. Langerhans cell histiocytosis of the stomach. A cause of granulomatous gastritis and gastric polyposis. Arch Pathol Lab Med 1994;118:1232–5.

121. Miettinen M, Monihan JM, Sarlomo-Rikala M, et al. Gastrointestinal stromal tumors/smooth muscle tumors (GISTs) primary in the omentum and mesentery: Clinicopathologic and immunohistochemical study of 26 cases. Am J Surg Pathol 1999;23:1109–18.

122. Kerr JZ, Hicks MJ, Nuchtern JG, et al. Gastrointestinal autonomic nerve tumors in the pediatric population: A report of four cases and a review of the literature. Cancer 1999;85:220–30.

123. Derman J, O'Leary TJ Gastrointestinal stromal tumor workshop. Hum Pathol 2001;32578–82.

124. Bates AW, Feakins RM, Scheimberg I. Congenital gastrointestinal stromal tumour is morphologically indistinguishable from the adult form, but does not express CD117 and carries a favourable prognosis. Histopathology 2000;37:316–22.

125. Carney JA. Gastric stromal sarcoma, pulmonary chondroma, and extra-adrenal paraganglioma (Carney Triad): Natural history, adrenocortical component, and possible familial occurrence. Mayo Clin Proc 1999;543–52.

126. Chadwick EG, Connor EJ, Hanson IC, et al. Tumors of smooth-muscle origin in HIV-infected children. Jama 1990;263:3182–4.

127. Leborgne J, Le Neel JC, Heloury Y, et al. Diffuse esophageal leiomyomatosis. Apropos of 5 cases with 2 familial cases. Chirurgie 1989;115:277–85; discussion 286.

128. Heinrich MC, Blanke CD, Druker BJ, Corless CL. Inhibition of KIT tyrosine kinase activity: A novel molecular approach to the treatment of KIT-positive malignancies. J Clin Oncol 2002;20:1692–703.

129. Miettinen M, Lasota J. Gastrointestinal stromal tumors—definition, clinical, histological, immunohistochemical, and molecular genetic features and differential diagnosis. Virchows Arch 2001;438:1–12.

130. Mellish RW. Multiple hemangiomas of the gastrointestinal tract in children. Am J Surg 1971;121:412–7.

131. Holden KR, Alexander F. Diffuse neonatal hemangiomatosis. Pediatrics 1970;46:411–21.

132. Nagaya M, Kato J, Niimi N, et al. Isolated cavernous hemangioma of the stomach in a neonate. J Pediatr Surg 1998;33:653–4.

133. Alberti D, Grazioli L, Orizio P, et al. Asymptomatic giant gastric lipoma: What to do? Am J Gastroenterol 1999;94:3634–7.

134. Beck NS, Lee SK, Lee HJ, Kim HH. Gastric lipoma in a child with bleeding and intermittent vomiting. J Pediatr Gastroenterol Nutr 1997;24:226–8.

135. Pettinato G, Manivel JC, De Rosa N, Dehner LP. Inflammatory myofibroblastic tumor (plasma cell granuloma). Clinicopathologic study of 20 cases with immunohistochemical and ultrastructural observations. Am J Clin Pathol 1990;94:538–46.

136. Murphy S, Shaw K, Blanchard H. Report of three gastric tumors in children. J Pediatr Surg 1994;29:1202–4.

137. Bogomoletz WV, Cox JN. Hamartoma of the stomach in childhood: Case report and review of the literature. Virchows Arch A Pathol Anat Histol 1975;369:69–79.

138. Appelman HD. The Carney Triad: A lesson in observation, creativity, and perseverance. Mayo Clin Proc 1999;74:638–40.

139. Zambrano E, Reyes-Mugica M, Franchi A, Rosai J. An osteoclast-rich tumor of the gastrointestinal tract with features resembling clear cell sarcoma of soft parts: Reports of 6 cases of a GIST simulator. Int J Surg Pathol 2003;11:75–81.

140. Quinn FM, Brown S, O'Hara D. Hemangiopericytoma of the stomach in a neonate. J Pediatr Surg 1991;26:101–2.

Gastric Motility

11.1. Normal Motility and Development of the Gastric Neuroenteric System

Miguel Saps, MD
Carlo Di Lorenzo, MD

Gastrointestinal motility is responsible for the orderly movement and aboral propulsion of food, chyme, and feces. Coordinated contractions throughout stomach and small bowel facilitate the mixing of food and digestive enzymes and lead to the digestion, and absorption of nutrients and fluids with the elimination of indigestible material. This sophisticated sequence of events requires the coordination of gastrointestinal enteric and autonomic nerves, interstitial cells of Cajal (ICC), and smooth muscle under the modulating effect of hormones and neurotransmitters.

Intrinsic Innervation

Enteric neurons have cell bodies located within the enteric nervous system (ENS). The ENS represents a network composed of neurons, nerve fibers, and supporting cells situated within the walls of the gastrointestinal (GI) tract. These neurons are located in two major ganglionated plexuses throughout the entire length of the bowel: the myenteric plexus and the submucosal plexus. The plexuses form a continuous circumferential network of ganglia and nerve fibers interconnected by nerve bundles. The structure and importance of each plexus vary according to the organ. The myenteric plexus, the predominant plexus in the stomach, is located between the external longitudinal and internal circular muscle layers (Figure 1). The submucosal plexus is actually comprised of two plexuses linked together by nerve fibers and is found between the muscularis mucosa and the circular muscle layer. The ganglia of the plexuses contain tightly packed neurons and glial cells. The absence of a continuous sheath of connective tissue surrounding the ganglia results in the exposure of nerves and glial cells to the extracellular milieu including neurohumoral agents.

The ENS contains all the same classes of neurotransmitters that are present in the central nervous system (CNS), multiple neurons subsets, and more neurons than the spinal cord. It has three functional classes of neurons: sensory, motor, and interneurons. Sensory input is provided by specialized sensory neurons with mechanical, thermal, and chemical receptors. Sensory information is projected along the spinal cord through

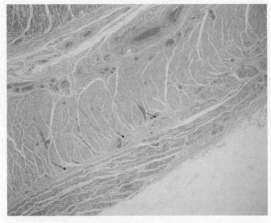

Figure 1 Myenteric plexus shown between the two layer of the muscularis propria (10×, Hematoxylin and Eosin). (Courtesy of Pauline Chou, MD, Children's Memorial Hospital, Chicago, IL.)

afferent neurons to the CNS. The interneurons have synaptic connections with other interneurons, motor, and sensory neurons. The motoneurons that connect with ascending and descending interneurons and the structures that they innervate are in control of initiating, maintaining, and inhibiting mechanical actions.

The ENS has a built-in battery of "programs" corresponding to various motor patterns such as mixing in the postprandial state, aborally migrating interdigestive motility during fasting, and powerful propagated contractions that serve as a defense against infections, food allergens, and enterotoxins. The ENS integrates muscle contractions, secretory function, and intramural blood flow to the muscle, mucosa, and lamina propria to generate appropriate digestive behavior. It controls and coordinates the activity of stomach and intestine by stimulating or inhibiting contractions. In addition, the ENS controls the luminal environment by triggering "cleaning waves," interacts with the immune system to protect the bowel, and modifies the rate of proliferation and growth of mucosal cells. Also known as the "brain of the gut," the ENS acts as a self-reliant engine. Bowel reflexes persist in the absence of CNS input,[1] such as in the case of the transplanted bowel. More than 100 years ago, animal experiments showed

that an increase in pressure in the intestinal lumen results in oral contraction (ascending excitatory reflex) and aboral relaxation (descending inhibitory reflex), followed by a propulsive wave (the "peristaltic reflex") even if all connections to the brain are severed.[2]

The understanding of the multiple factors affecting the function of the ENS has important clinical implications as physiologic and noxious stimuli acting at various levels may affect digestion and the normal propulsion of gut contents. Abnormalities in any of the components or their integration can result in motility disorders manifested by increased or decreased transit or nonpropulsive activity. Motility studies in adult patients with irritable bowel syndrome (IBS) have shown that perturbations of the CNS, such as stress, may alter the modulation of motor activity by the ENS resulting in intestinal motor disturbances that correlate with symptoms.[3] Malfunction of ENS control seems to be a critical factor in several functional gastrointestinal disorders (FGIDs).

CNS

Most of the peripheral input from the gut to the brain does not reach consciousness (a providential occurrence indeed, as a constant update on what is happening within the intestine would be distracting!); however, fullness, satiety, and pain are conscious sensations with important clinical implications. Central projection and integration of visceral information results in a complex neurobehavioral system that is involved in homeostasis, pain perception, and emotional processing. The transfer of nociceptive information from the GI tract to the brain occurs via primary afferents to the spinothalamic tract and postsynaptic dorsal column where it converges with viscerosomatic nociceptive and nonnociceptive afferents and is carried to several thalamic nuclei and cortical structures. As a result, the CNS continuously integrates information from the digestive tract with information from other organs and the environment in order to establish a coordinated and adequate response mediated through the vagus nerve.[4]

Extrinsic Innervation

Neurons with axons or dendrites within the enteric wall that possess cell bodies outside the ENS are classified as extrinsic neurons. The stomach is innervated by both the parasympathetic and sympathetic nervous systems mainly through afferent and efferent fibers of the vagus and splanchnic nerves respectively.

Afferent Transmission. Sensory innervation of the GI tract is achieved by intrinsic sensory neurons located within the wall, intestinofugal fibers that synapse at the prevertebral ganglia, and vagal and spinal afferents that project into the CNS. The information conveyed by the two systems differs. Vagal afferents mainly provide physiological input—including vagovagal reflexes—from the gastrointestinal organs up to the junction of the midgut and hindgut, while spinal afferents encode physiological and noxious events. The cell bodies of vagal and spinal visceral afferents are located at the nodose and dorsal root ganglia and project to the brain stem and spinal cord, respectively. Afferent input converges at multiple levels where it is integrated with information from other regions. At the level of the nucleus tractus solitarium (NTS) in the medulla, vagal information is projected to the cell bodies of the dorsal motor nucleus of the vagus (DMN) located medially and in close proximity. There, it is integrated with information from higher CNS centers including the paraventricular nucleus of the hypothalamus and the limbic structures associated with behavior and emotions. This integration of motility, sensory, and affective input constitutes an important aspect in the understanding of the pathogenesis and treatment of FGIDs.

The sympathetic nerves contain afferent sensory fibers that synapse at the celiac ganglia and plexus. The same receptive fields of neurons involved in visceral response also respond to somatic stimuli. The convergence of both visceral and somatic information at the same level explains the phenomenon of referred pain.[5]

Efferent Transmission. The parasympathetic system is characterized by long preganglionic and short postganglionic efferent fibers. Preganglionic parasympathetic motor fibers arising from the DMN project into the intramural plexuses. From there, fine postganglionic fibers are distributed throughout the smooth muscle layers, endocrine cells, and exocrine glands of the upper and midgut, enabling the regulation of gastric function. Vagal motor pathways are composed of parallel inhibitory and excitatory pathways that are segregated within the DMN. Electrophysiological studies have demonstrated that gastrointestinal projections into the DMN are organized viscerotopically.[6] Functional studies of the lower esophageal sphincter (LES) have shown that stimulation of different areas of the DMN may result in either relaxation or contraction of smooth muscle; with stimulation of the dorsal part of the DMN resulting in relaxation of the sphincter, while stimulation of the rostral area

leads to contraction.[7] Parasympathetic innervations to the stomach that originate in the DMN are carried via the right and left vagus. These nerves form the distal esophageal plexus and give rise to the anterior and posterior vagal trunks that enter the abdomen through the diaphragmatic hiatus carrying preganglionic parasympathetic fibers that synapse with intramural ganglion cells of the plexuses and afferent visceral fibers. Vagal efferents comprise only 10% of vagal nerve fibers and are composed of different fibers. The excitatory pathway consists of cholinergic preganglionic and postganglionic neurons utilizing acetylcholine and substance P as their main neurotransmitters. Excitatory transmission results in increased muscle tone. The inhibitory motor pathway is composed of preganglionic cholinergic neurons and postganglionic nonadrenergic, noncholinergic (NANC) pathways that achieve smooth muscle relaxation via nitric oxide, ATP and vasoactive intestinal polypeptide (VIP) release. The vagus also carries sympathetic fibers. The inhibitory and excitatory vagal motor pathways act independently or in conjunction to produce a complex motor response. The intrinsic myogenic tone is responsible for the persistent basal contraction of the smooth muscle sphincters of the gut. Activation of the inhibitory pathway results in sphincter relaxation whereas activation of the excitatory pathway causes contraction. A sequential activation of both inhibitory and excitatory pathways is responsible for the coordinated sequence of relaxation followed by contraction that allows the bolus to progress. The excitatory contractile response to acetylcholine can be blocked with atropine, a cholinergic muscarinic receptor blocker. Hexamethonium, which blocks nicotinic receptors at the autonomic ganglia, reduces excitatory cholinergic and inhibitory responses. Vagal efferents also innervate and regulate the ICCs. The enteric secretomotor neurons (postganglionic neurons in the vagal pathway) also receive input from enteric neurons, sympathetic nerves, systemic hormones, and local mediators. As the number of postganglionic neurons involved in the vagal pathways is small in relation to the total number of enteric neurons in the gut, each fiber projects extensively within the myenteric plexus of the stomach to establish synapses with excitatory and inhibitory motor neurons innervating the muscle.

In the proximal stomach, vagal efferents modulate the tonic activity of smooth muscles and the vagal inhibitory pathways play an important role in the receptive relaxation reflex after ingestion of a meal. The adaptive relaxation can be generated by a local reflex or vagovagal pathways. This input is conveyed to the NTS and subsequently to the DMN which in turn transmits vagal NANC inhibitory input to the myenteric plexus of the proximal stomach through preganglionic fibers. The vagus modulates the activity of the distal stomach through vagal excitatory pathways. The pyloric sphincter is regulated by vagal excitatory and inhibitory pathways. The vagal excitatory pathway contributes to the closure of the pylorus

during the initial digestive phase when the antrum exhibits strong phasic contractions, while the inhibitory pathway leads to pyloric relaxation to allow the transit of triturated food to the duodenum. Vagal efferent pathways to secretory cells are mostly excitatory and involve acetylcholine and VIP as the postganglionic excitatory neurotransmitters. Direct inhibitory innervation is not present.[8]

The efferent sympathetic system is characterized by short preganglionic fibers proceeding from the CNS and long postganglionic fibers. Major nerve trunks that innervate abdominal organs contain fibers of postganglionic neurons that originate in the celiac ganglion, superior mesenteric ganglion, inferior mesenteric ganglia, hypogastric nerve ganglia and the sympathetic chain ganglia. Sympathetic innervation of the GI tract proceeds predominantly from neurons situated in the prevertebral ganglia (PVG) and, to a lesser degree, from neurons of the paravertebral ganglia. These ganglia constitute centers of integration between the ENS and CNS, with PVG neurons supplying postganglionic sympathetic fibers that travel toward the gut wall to regulate transit, secretion, absorption, and blood flow. The sympathetic innervation of the stomach arises from the intermediolateral column of the thoracic spinal cord (predominantly T6–T8). Most of the preganglionic sympathetic constituents travel in the greater splanchnic nerves. The splanchnic nerves are comprised of preganglionic fibers arising from the T5–T9 ganglia that travel through the crura of the diaphragm into the abdomen and eventually synapse with neurons at the PVG in the celiac ganglia. The splanchnic nerves also contain visceral afferents and postganglionic fibers with cell bodies in the paravertebral ganglia.[9] The postganglionic sympathetic fibers run through the celiac plexus—which also receives some fibers from the vagus—along the vascular supply of the stomach to innervate the intramural nerve plexuses in the stomach. The postganglionic fibers have an inhibitory effect on nonsphincter muscles through β-adrenergic receptors and stimulate contraction of sphincters through α-adrenergic receptors. The sympathetic fibers carry norepinephrine as postganglionic neurotransmitter while acetylcholine is the preganglionic neurotransmitter.

The effects of the extrinsic nerves have been illustrated by studies demonstrating the consequences of nerve ablation and stimulation. Vagotomy results in gastric dysfunction characterized by impaired gastric accommodation,[10] impaired antropyloric coordination and delayed gastric emptying due to abnormal phasic contractility.[11] Electrical vagal stimulation evokes gastric fundic relaxation.[12] Vagotomy in conjunction with the removal of the celiac-superior mesenteric ganglia results in disruption of the interdigestive patterns of upper gastrointestinal myoelectrical activity while interdigestive motility is triggered by vagal stimulation.[13] Patients with long-standing diabetes mellitus may present with autonomic neuropathy characterized by abnormal postprandial proximal

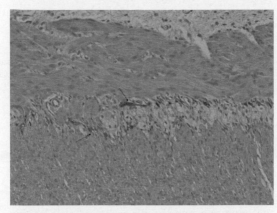

Figure 2 Interstitial cells of Cajal are stained immuno-histochemically with anti-c-Kit (CD117) antibody (×40) and visualized by diaminobenzidine (DAB) as chromogen. ICCs are surrounding the myenteric plexus, which appears as negatively stained areas. (Courtesy of Pauline Chou, MD, Children's Memorial Hospital, Chicago, IL.)

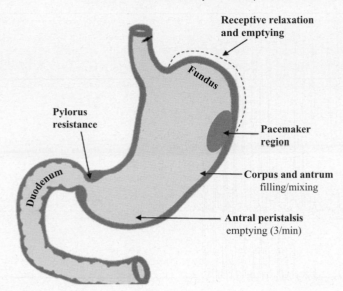

Figure 3 Anatomic and functional areas of the stomach.

gastric accommodation and contractile activity, which result in abnormal retention of solids in the stomach.

Interstitial Cells of Cajal

The ICCs constitute a group of specialized mesenchymal cells distributed throughout the longitudinal and circular muscle layers of the GI tract in close contact with smooth muscle cells and excitatory and inhibitory enteric motor neurons mainly at the level of the myenteric plexus (Figure 2).[14] These cells that are neither neural nor muscle cells are thought to have an essential role in the regulation of gastrointestinal motility and are considered the "gut pacemakers" and/or the mediators of neurotransmission. The ICCs initiate and actively propagate electrical rhythmic activity between nerves and smooth muscles and among muscle cells resulting in gut contractions.[15] ICCs have different morphological functional classes that participate in different aspects of motility. ICCs present in the myenteric plexus of the stomach, small intestine, and colon are pacemaker cells responsible for generating electrical slow waves, while ICCs located along the muscle fibers of the stomach and sphincters seem to be implicated in the modulation of enteric neurotransmission.[16]

Slow waves are spontaneous rhythmic oscillations of the cell membrane potential that control temporal and spatial occurrence of longitudinal and circumferential smooth muscle activity. Slow waves are characterized by an upstroke and a plateau component. A contraction takes place when a spike potential of sufficient magnitude is superimposed on a slow wave. As spike potentials occur only on the crest of the slow wave, the maximum frequency of contractions in the stomach and intestine is determined by the slow waves. Electrical slow wave activity and superimposed action potentials correlate one to one with phasic contractions. In the stomach, slow waves occur at a rate of 3 cycles per minute (cpm); thus there cannot be more than three gastric contractions per minute. Thus, slow waves do not generate

muscular contractions but determine the rate of contractions. The ICC[17,18] control the release of Ca^{2+} in voltage-gated Ca^{2+} channels at the level of the smooth muscle. Cyclic changes in intracellular calcium concentration result in the development of unitary currents[19] leading to the rhythmic electrical slow waves. Summation of unitary currents causes depolarization and propagation of contractions by membrane depolarization via gap junctions between adjacent smooth muscle cells. The duration of each contraction depends upon the period of time that the potential exceeds the electrical threshold for contraction. Contraction amplitude varies based on the effect of neurotransmitters. The ICCs are preferred sites for the release of neurotransmitters[20] from the enteric nerves. Acetylcholine increases the strength of the peristaltic contraction, while sympathetic nerve stimulation, acting through norepinephrine release, decreases the amplitude of contraction.

In the stomach, ICC networks are present mainly in the myenteric plexus where they initiate electrical activity but are also present in lower numbers at the submucosal border.[21] Although the ICCs in the stomach constitute a continuous network from the corpus to the pyloric sphincter, their density varies in relation to the specific motor activities of each area.[22] At the level of the fundus, the ICCs receive innervations from inhibitory neurons, suggesting a role of these cells in fundic relaxation. Animal studies have shown that loss of ICC in the small intestine myenteric plexus correlates with the absence of slow waves.[23] Other studies have shown reduced cholinergic excitatory and nitrergic inhibitory neurotransmission in tissues lacking ICCs.[14] The clinical significance of these cells has been confirmed by reports of severe motor disturbances in pediatric and adult patients lacking ICCs.[21,24]

Gastric Motility

Anatomically defined areas of the stomach (fundus, corpus, antrum, and pylorus) differ from functionally defined areas. The stomach is functionally divided into two regions, the proximal stomach

including the fundus and the proximal one-third of the body, and the distal stomach composed of the distal body and antrum (Figure 3). The proximal stomach is characterized by electrical silence, tonic mechanical activity, and adaptive relaxation, properties that enable accommodation of larger volumes of food without a great increase in luminal pressure. Eventually, as food accumulates, the pressure in the fundus increases, resulting in a sustained contraction that propels the gastric contents toward the antrum. The distal portion is electrically active and able to generate high-pressure contractions that facilitate the trituration of food and passage of chyme to the duodenum. The stomach pacemaker, located in the corpus along the greater curvature near to the proximal one-third of the corpus, generates regular electrical slow waves of depolarization at approximately 3 cpm that spread away, circumferentially and distally, toward the pylorus through the circular muscle layer.[25] The frequency of the slow waves depends on the region of GI tract and varies between 3 in the stomach and 8 to 11 per minute in the small bowel, explaining the difference in rate of contractions among regions. Although an in-depth description of the motility of the rest of the GI tract is beyond the scope of our chapter and will be discussed in other sections of this text, we will discuss some basic motility features in order to emphasize the importance and nature of coordination among different organs.

Interdigestive Period. The gastrointestinal myoelectrical motor activity varies according to the postprandial or fasting state. Motility changes occur in coordination with the motility and secretory functions of other gastrointestinal organs. The migrating motor complex (MMC) is the most recognizable pattern of activity during fasting (Figure 4). Migrating motor complexes can be identified throughout the stomach and small bowel during the interdigestive period. The MMC is a cyclical pattern of electric and mechanical activity initiated almost simultaneously in the stomach and duodenum from where it

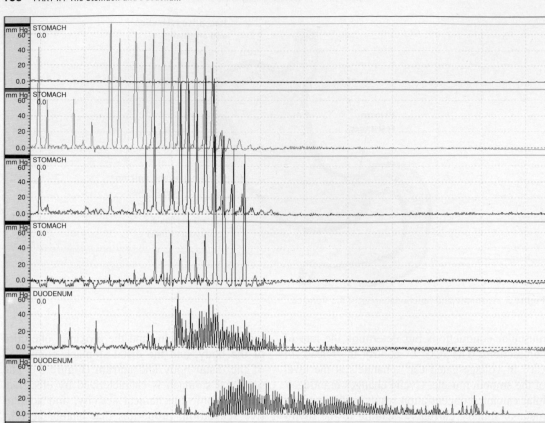

Figure 4 Antroduodenal manometry tracing obtained during fasting showing the phase III of the motor migrating complex, characterized by a propagating cluster of contractions followed by the phase I characterized by motor quiescence. The recording sensors are spaced 3 cm apart and are located within 4 cm in the stomach and 3 cm in the small intestine.

propagates through the small intestine. Unlike the intestine, where cycles of motor activity migrate aborally, gastric cycles do not propagate but start and end simultaneously at all sites. Three phases of mechanical activity that differ mostly by the amplitude and frequency of pressure waves can be identified. Phase I of the MMC is characterized by almost complete motor quiescence lasting approximately 5 to 30 minutes; phase II by a mixture of low- and high-pressure waves lasting 30 to 65 minutes; and phase III by high-amplitude rhythmic contractions with a frequency of 3 cpm in the stomach lasting 3 to 7 minutes. Intestinal phase IIIs ("intestinal housekeepers") are cyclical contraction sequences that propagate aborally, sweep through the small intestine, and terminate in the ileocecal region. These rhythmic contractions last for 10 to 15 minutes with a frequency of approximately 11 cpm in the duodenum and 7 to 8 cpm in the ileum. This sequence of events occurs approximately every 90 minutes.[26]

Postprandial Period. In healthy subjects, ingestion of a meal activates an array of neural responses in the stomach, including a relaxation reflex (accommodation) that expands the volume of the proximal stomach[27] and an excitatory reflex that results in peristaltic contractions in the distal stomach. These reflexes result from inhibitory and excitatory input from intrinsic and central neural pathways. The adaptive relaxation

reflex characterized by relaxation of the proximal stomach in response to gastric antral distension is responsible for creating a pressure gradient that promotes the retropulsion of food ensuring that large food particles are adequately triturated. The duration of the postprandial state pattern is approximately 4 hours after which time the interdigestive motility pattern resumes.

Food ingestion results in release of GI hormones that modulate motor, secretory, and absorptive functions. Feeding results in a postprandial pattern of intestinal motility concomitant with the release of gastrin, cholecystokinin (CCK), and pancreatic polypeptide from the upper gut, glucagon-like peptide-1 and peptide YY from the distal small intestine, and a decline in plasma motilin concentrations.[28] Vagal efferent activity contributes to the maintenance of slow wave rhythmicity and regulates the initiation and maintenance of the postprandial pattern in the upper GI tract and synchronizes the inhibition of the fasting MMC. Vagal activity also results in changes in motilin, gastrin, and pancreatic polypeptide concentrations.[28,29] Vagal blockade results in the replacement of the fed pattern with motor activity similar to MMC activity.[28] The ability to switch from an interdigestive to a digestive pattern is a sign of normal motor function demonstrating the integrity of the enteroenteric reflexes.

Ingestion of a meal results in stimulation of motor activity throughout the gut. When the

fasting MMC is interrupted by a meal, the occurring contractions mimic the phase II pressure waves of the interdigestive period. Gastric function in response to meals varies according to the physical and chemical characteristics and caloric content the meal. Gastric emptying time may vary between 1 and 4 hours depending on the characteristics of the food. While solids are initially retained in the proximal area of the stomach,[30] liquids are distributed throughout the stomach and empty faster,[31,32] with isotonic fluids emptying faster than hypertonic fluids.[33,34] The caloric content of a liquid also determines the emptying rate,[35] with carbohydrates leaving the stomach first, followed by proteins[36] and then fats, which have the slowest emptying.[37,38] High acidity of the chyme,[39] L-tryptophan,[40,41] and rectal and colonic distention[42] also delay gastric emptying (the "colo-gastric inhibitory reflex"). Gastric emptying of liquids is characterized by an exponential curve that is transformed into linear if the caloric content is increased, a phenomenon explained by a longer period of gastric to and fro movements that result in slower emptying with high-caloric meals.[43] The pylorus regulates the gastric emptying of the stomach by contracting and slowing stomach output when nutrients enter the duodenum.[44] Feeding of a solid meal generates neural and humoral feedback that results in an early phase of receptive relaxation of the stomach body, suppression of antral contractions, and increased tonic and phasic pyloric motor activity followed by coordinated phasic contractions in the body, antrum, and pylorus. Gastric proximal accommodation is regulated by mechanosensitive nonneural stretch reflexes involving ICCs participation[45] and vagally mediated neural reflexes.[46] Neural related receptive relaxation involves inhibition by fundic intrinsic neurons through nitric oxide (NO) production that, once released, diffuses to the smooth muscle cells. Fundic relaxation is followed by a fundic tonic contraction that propels the food to the antrum and by the onset of regular phasic contractions of the antrum that mix food with acid and pepsin to form a suspension (chyme) and triturate the solid bolus into smaller particles less than 2 to 3 mm in diameter. The antropyloric region has the ability to discriminate the size of particles allowing only the emptying of particles smaller than 1 to 2 mm.

Gastric emptying of solids occurs in two phases, a lag phase that starts with the ingestion of the meal and correlates with grinding during which solids remain in the stomach and a linear phase when small particulate solids are released into the duodenum (Figure 5).[47] The trituration of the bolus and enhanced fat emulsification is the result of the coordinated action of high amplitude antral contractions acting on a closed pylorus. Pyloric phasic contractions disappear gradually while synchronized contractions remain in the body and antrum.[48] Once the appropriate particle size is achieved, a late phase of pumping of chyme into the duodenum begins. This late phase is characterized by opening of the pylorus in coordination with high amplitude contractions

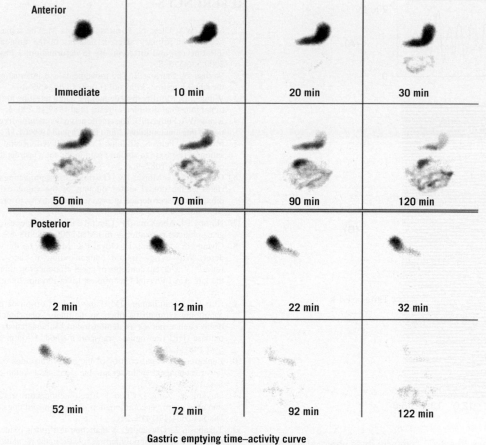

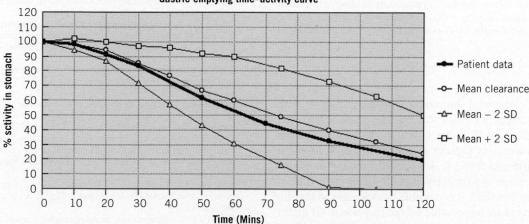

Figure 5 Gastric emptying of a solid meal consisting of 2 large scrambled eggs, 1 piece of toast, and 1 tablespoonful of butter. Images taken at time 0, 10, 20, 30, 40, 50, 60, 75, 90, 105, and 120 min. Normal value plotted as percentage activity in stomach over 120 min is represented by mean ±2 standard deviations (SD). Normal solid emptying is characterized by an initial lag phase followed by a linear emptying time course. (Reproduced with permission from reference 47.)

an intense mechanical activity characterized by increased tone in the proximal areas and superimposed spike electrical waves that result in gastric contractions. A combination of increased basal tone and superimposed phasic contractions of the lower esophageal sphincter prevent the occurrence of gastroesophageal reflux at times of intense contractions and increased pressure within the stomach. The colon and rectum also respond to eating by increasing colonic and rectal tone, the gastrocolonic and gastrorectal response. The gastrocolonic response consists of two phases, a gastric phase generated by mechanoreceptors responding to gastric distention through cholinergic pathways and a nutrient-specific intestinal phase that independently of CCK responds to the stimulation of chemoreceptors mainly by fat.[55]

Gastric Motility in Premature and Term Infants

Amniotic fluid swallowing has been demonstrated as early as 11 to 12 weeks of gestation. Nonnutritive sucking is present at approximately 18 to 24 weeks of gestation while nutritive sucking develops by 34 to 35 weeks. The initiation of nutritive sucking is associated with increase in gastric growth and maturation of gastric and small bowel motility. Prospective studies of neonates of different ages demonstrated that gastric electrical activity and emptying mature gradually with gestational age.[56] As a result, gastrointestinal motor patterns differ in preterm infants from those seen in older children and adults. Fetal gastric emptying has been noted between 24 and 25 weeks.[57,58] The presence of normal electrical rhythm at 3 cpm has been detected by 32 weeks of gestational age.[59] However, this activity only becomes dominant at around 35 weeks of gestational age (Figure 6). The occurrence of the phase III of the MMC, the amplitude of antral contractions,[60,61] and the proportion of antral waves associated with duodenal contractions increase with postnatal age.[62,63] The duodenal motor response to feeding differs between preterm and term infants.[64] Motor quiescence during fasting is rare in the first week of life but increases with postnatal age.[65] Motor migrating complexes are poorly formed in preterm infants.[66] However, another study showed similar interdigestive antral contractile activity in preterm and term infants,[63] and studies of gastric myoelectrical activity revealed a similar prevalence of bradygastria and tachygastria in premature and full-term neonates.[67] Studies of postprandial antropyloric motility in premature infants have demonstrated adequate coordination of antropyloric motility, gastric emptying,[61] and appropriate intestinal motor response to feeding at 30 weeks of postconceptional age, even in infants with immature fasting patterns.[66] The information provided by the latter studies may explain the ability of premature infants to tolerate enteral feedings despite an immature motility pattern.

Neonatal GI hormonal secretions are influenced by the type and route of feeding. Enteral feeding triggers mechanisms of adaptation in

throughout the body and antrum that result in linear emptying, similar to that which occurs with liquids in gastric emptying studies.

Fat ingestion stimulates CCK release resulting in gallbladder contraction and delayed gastric emptying while stimulating pancreatic secretions.[49] In addition, fat ingestion and increased caloric intake also affects motility by direct contact with small bowel mucosa resulting in negative feedback inhibition possibly via increased plasma levels of peptide YY and enteroglucagon.[50] The duodenum acts as an additional brake to gastric contents by increasing tonic resistance.[51] The small bowel has five types of receptors that regulate gastric emptying by small intestinal feedback inhibition: fat receptors, amino acid receptors, glucose receptors, and pH

and osmoreceptors that stimulate vagal afferent fibers to produce a negative feedback control by regulating myenteric and submucosal neurons,[52] although other neural pathways may also be involved. Infusion of fat into the small intestine results in relaxation of the proximal stomach,[53] decreased antral contractility, increased pyloric pressure, and delayed gastric emptying and small bowel motility with longer small bowel transit time (the "ileal brake"). CCK or NO antagonists, vagotomy and sympathectomy can block the intestinal feedback that leads to delayed gastric emptying.[54] Once the digestive phase is finalized, any indigestible solid remaining in the stomach is emptied at the time of return of fasting MMC activity during phase III. As a phase III occurs in the proximal duodenum, the stomach develops

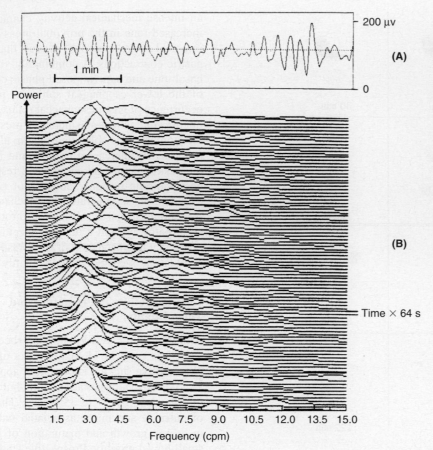

Figure 6 Example of a running spectral analysis from a full-term infant. Regular 3 cpm activity is observed for most of the recording time. The *x* axis indicates the frequency of the signal cpm; the *y* axis indicates time where the running spectral analysis represents consecutive segments of the electrogastrography. A short extract of the cutaneous tracing is reported. (Reproduced with permission from reference 58.)

the gut and changes in metabolism that can be partially explained by alterations in gastrointestinal hormonal secretions. An increase in plasma concentrations of gut hormones including enteroglucagon, gastrin, motilin, neurotensin, gastrointestinal peptide, and pancreatic polypeptide have been demonstrated after minimal amounts of enteral feeding in preterm and term infants.[68] The physiological adaptation to extrauterine nutrition may also be influenced by genetic factors, composition of enteral nutrients, secretions, bacteria, and exogenous hormones present in breast milk.[69] Human milk contains high concentrations of motilin and gastrin that may be an important factor in the development and maturation of gastrointestinal function and motility especially in immature babies. During early postnatal life, gastric emptying is a function of age and composition of formula. Gastric emptying and intestinal transit are rapid during the first week of life in preterm and term infants probably due to the effect of gut hormones. The amount of milk emptied from the stomach varies according to the composition, volume, and energy content. A study of gastric emptying of infants at 33-week gestational age, showed 50% emptying by 25 minutes in those fed with human milk compared to 51 min in those fed an artificial formula.[70] In term infants, half-emptying times average 48 minutes when fed expressed breast milk and 78 minutes with infant formula.[71]

Postnatal hormonal surges correlate with changes in GI function. Gastrin, a gastric hormone with growth factor effect on the gastrointestinal mucosa, is present in higher concentrations at birth and first 3 to 4 weeks of life than in adults. A surge in gastrin levels is also seen at the time of the first feed. It is possible that changes in motilin levels are responsible for the increase in GI motor activity occurring in neonates. Motilin cord blood concentrations are low at birth with basal concentrations increasing at 2 weeks of gestational age.[68] Developmental changes may explain differences in response to erythromycin (a motilin agonist) at various ages, with infants younger than 31 weeks gestation reacting to the drug with uncoordinated antral contractions and failing to produce the phase III of the MMC.[72,73] Although some studies have demonstrated the presence of functioning motilin receptors in infants younger than 32 weeks,[74] others have shown that hormonal modulation of MMC in the neonates by motilin and pancreatic polypeptide is not present at this age.[62] Neurotensin, an ileal peptide with inhibitory effects on gastric secretion and motility, is present in higher concentration in term infants than preterm and adults.[75] Neurotensin may have a unique effect on early life adaptation to enteral nutrition by regulating gastric emptying and the rate of passage of the acidic chyme to the duodenum enhancing absorption.

REFERENCES

1. Kunze WA, Clerc N, Furness JB, Gola M. The soma and neurites of primary afferent neurons in the guinea-pig intestine respond differentially to deformation. J Physiol 2000;526:375–85.
2. Bayliss W, Starling E. The movements and innervation of the small intestine. J Physiol (Lond) 1899;24:99–143.
3. Wingate D. Motility disorders of the small intestine in functional intestinal disorders. Presse Med 1989;18:290–3.
4. Kunze WA, Furness JB. The enteric nervous system and regulation of intestinal motility. Annu Rev Physiol 1999;61:117–42.
5. Miranda A, Peles S, Rudolph C, et al. Altered visceral sensation in response to somatic pain in the rat. Gastroenterology 2004;126:1082–9.
6. Grabauskas G, Moises HC. Gastrointestinal-projecting neurones in the dorsal motor nucleus of the vagus exhibit direct and viscerotopically organized sensitivity to orexin. J Physiol 2003;549:37–56.
7. Hornby PJ, Abrahams TP. Central control of lower esophageal sphincter relaxation. Am J Med 2000;108:90S–8S.
8. Chang HY, Mashimo H, Goyal RK. Musings on the wanderer: What's new in our understanding of vago-vagal reflex? IV. Current concepts of vagal efferent projections to the gut. Am J Physiol Gastrointest Liver Physiol 2003;284: G357–66.
9. Kuo DC, Krauthamer GM. Paravertebral origin of postganglionic sympathetic fibers in the major splanchnic and distal coeliac nerves as demonstrated by horseradish peroxidase (HRP) retrograde transport method. J Auton Nerv Syst 1981;4:25–32.
10. Lundgren O. Vagal control of the motor functions of the lower esophageal sphincter and the stomach. J Auton Nerv Syst 1983;9:185–97.
11. Ouyang H, Xing J, Chen J. Electroacupuncture restores impaired gastric accommodation in vagotomized dogs. Dig Dis Sci 2004;49:1418–24.
12. Takahashi T, Owyang C. Vagal control of nitric oxide and vasoactive intestinal polypeptide release in the regulation of gastric relaxation in rat. J Physiol 1995;484:481–92.
13. Tanaka T, Kendrick ML, Zyromski NJ, et al. Vagal innervation modulates motor pattern but not initiation of canine gastric migrating motor complex. Am J Physiol Gastrointest Liver Physiol 2001;281:G283–92.
14. Ward SM, Sanders KM. Interstitial cells of Cajal: Primary targets of enteric motor innervation. Anat Rec 2001;262: 125–35.
15. Der-Silaphet T, Malysz J, Hagel S, et al. Interstitial cells of cajal direct normal propulsive contractile activity in the mouse small intestine. Gastroenterology 1998;114:724–36.
16. Ward SM, McLaren GJ, Sanders KM. Interstitial cells of Cajal in the deep muscular plexus mediate enteric motor neurotransmission in the mouse small intestine. J Physiol 2006;573:147–59.
17. Thomson AB, Drozdowski L, Iordache C, et al. Small bowel review: Normal physiology, part 2. Dig Dis Sci 2003; 48:1565–81.
18. Daniel EE. Communication between interstitial cells of Cajal and gastrointestinal muscle. Neurogastroenterol Motil 2004;16:118–22.
19. Sanders KM, Koh SD, Ward SM. Interstitial cells of cajal as pacemakers in the gastrointestinal tract. Annu Rev Physiol 2006;68:307–43.
20. Shuttleworth CW, Xue C, Ward SM, et al. Immunohistochemical localization of 3',5'-cyclic guanosine monophosphate in the canine proximal colon: Responses to nitric oxide and electrical stimulation of enteric inhibitory neurons. Neuroscience 1993;56:513–22.
21. Lyford GL, He CL, Soffer E, et al. Pan-colonic decrease in interstitial cells of Cajal in patients with slow transit constipation. Gut 2002;51:496–501.
22. Ibba Manneschi L, Pacini S, Corsani L, et al. Interstitial cells of Cajal in the human stomach: Distribution and relationship with enteric innervation. Histol Histopathol 2004;19:1153–64.
23. Hara Y, Kubota M, Szurszewski JH. Electrophysiology of smooth muscle of the small intestine of some mammals. J Physiol 1986;372:501–20.
24. Sabri M, Barksdale E, Di Lorenzo C. Constipation and lack of colonic interstitial cells of Cajal. Dig Dis Sci 2003; 48:849–53.
25. Collard JM, Romagnoli R. Human stomach has a recordable mechanical activity at a rate of about three cycles/minute. Eur J Surg 2001;167:188–94.
26. Di Lorenzo C, Hillemeier C, Hyman P, et al. Manometry studies in children: Minimum standards for procedures. Neurogastroenterol Motil 2002;14:411–20.

27. Hennig GW, Brookes SJ, Costa M. Excitatory and inhibitory motor reflexes in the isolated guinea-pig stomach. J Physiol 1997;501:197–212.

28. Hall KE, Diamant NE, El-Sharkawy TY, Greenberg GR. Effect of pancreatic polypeptide on canine migrating motor complex and plasma motilin. Am J Physiol 1983;245:G178–85.

29. Hall KE, el-Sharkawy TY, Diamant NE. Vagal control of canine postprandial upper gastrointestinal motility. Am J Physiol 1986;250:G501–10.

30. Collins PJ, Houghton LA, Read NW, et al. Role of the proximal and distal stomach in mixed solid and liquid meal emptying. Gut 1991;32:615–9.

31. Siegel JA, Urbain JL, Adler LP, et al. Biphasic nature of gastric emptying. Gut 1988;29:85–9.

32. Camilleri M, Malagelada JR, Brown ML, et al. Relation between antral motility and gastric emptying of solids and liquids in humans. Am J Physiol 1985;249:G580–5.

33. Paraskevopoulos JA, Houghton LA, Eyre-Brooke I, et al. Effect of composition of gastric contents on resistance to emptying of liquids from stomach in humans. Dig Dis Sci 1988;33:914–8.

34. Vist GE, Maughan RJ. The effect of osmolality and carbohydrate content on the rate of gastric emptying of liquids in man. J Physiol 1995;486:523–31.

35. Hunt JN, Smith JL, Jiang CL. Effect of meal volume and energy density on the gastric emptying of carbohydrates. Gastroenterology 1985;89:1326–30.

36. Burn-Murdoch RA, Fisher MA, Hunt JN. The slowing of gastric emptying by proteins in test meals. J Physiol 1978;274:477–85.

37. Houghton LA, Mangnall YF, Read NW. Effect of incorporating fat into a liquid test meal on the relation between intragastric distribution and gastric emptying in human volunteers. Gut 1990;31:1226–9.

38. Heddle R, Dent J, Read NW, et al. Antropyloroduodenal motor responses to intraduodenal lipid infusion in healthy volunteers. Am J Physiol 1988;254:G671–9.

39. Chaw CS, Yazaki E, Evans DF. The effect of pH change on the gastric emptying of liquids measured by electrical impedance tomography and pH-sensitive radiotelemetry capsule. Int J Pharm 2001;227:167–75.

40. Stephens JR, Woolson RF, Cooke AR. Osmolyte and tryptophan receptors controlling gastric emptying in the dog. Am J Physiol 1976;231:848–53.

41. Mangel AW, Koegel A. Effects of peptides on gastric emptying. Am J Physiol 1984;246:G342–5.

42. Martinez V, Wang L, Tache Y. Proximal colon distension induces Fos expression in the brain and inhibits gastric emptying through capsaicin-sensitive pathways in conscious rats. Brain Res 2006;1086:168–80.

43. Boulby P, Moore R, Gowland P, Spiller RC. Fat delays emptying but increases forward and backward antral flow as assessed by flow-sensitive magnetic resonance imaging. Neurogastroenterol Motil 1999;11:27–36.

44. Treacy PJ, Jamieson GG, Dent J. The importance of the pylorus as a regulator of solid and liquid emptying from the stomach. J Gastroenterol Hepatol 1995;10:639–45.

45. Won KJ, Sanders KM, Ward SM. Interstitial cells of Cajal mediate mechanosensitive responses in the stomach. Proc Natl Acad Sci U S A 2005;102:14913–8.

46. Azpiroz F, Malagelada JR. Vagally mediated gastric relaxation induced by intestinal nutrients in the dog. Am J Physiol 1986;251:G727–35.

47. Lin HC, Prather C, Fisher RS, et al. Measurement of GI transit. Dig Dis Sci 2005;50:989–1004.

48. Ueno T, Uemura K, Harris MB, et al. Role of vagus nerve in postprandial antropyloric coordination in conscious dogs. Am J Physiol Gastrointest Liver Physiol 2005;288:G487–95.

49. Fried M, Erlacher U, Schwizer W, et al. Role of cholecystokinin in the regulation of gastric emptying and pancreatic enzyme secretion in humans. Studies with the cholecystokinin-receptor antagonist loxiglumide. Gastroenterology 1991;101:503–11.

50. Ohtani N, Sasaki I, Naito H, et al. Mediators for fat-induced ileal brake are different between stomach and proximal small intestine in conscious dogs. J Gastrointest Surg 2001;5:377–82.

51. Rao SS, Lu C, Schulze-Delrieu K. Duodenum as a immediate brake to gastric outflow: A videofluoroscopic and manometric assessment. Gastroenterology 1996;110:740–7.

52. Schwartz GJ, Moran TH. Duodenal nutrient exposure elicits nutrient-specific gut motility and vagal afferent signals in rat. Am J Physiol 1998;274:R1236–42.

53. Heddle R, Collins PJ, Dent J, et al. Motor mechanisms associated with slowing of the gastric emptying of a solid meal by an intraduodenal lipid infusion. J Gastroenterol Hepatol 1989;4:437–47.

54. Orihata M, Sarna SK. Inhibition of nitric oxide synthase delays gastric emptying of solid meals. J Pharmacol Exp Ther 1994;271:660–70.

55. Wiley J, Tatum D, Keinath R, Chung OY. Participation of gastric mechanoreceptors and intestinal chemoreceptors in the gastrocolonic response. Gastroenterology 1988;94:1144–9.

56. Riezzo G, Indrio F, Montagna O, et al. Gastric electrical activity and gastric emptying in term and preterm newborns. Neurogastroenterol Motil 2000;12:223–9.

57. Sase M, Miwa I, Sumie M, et al. Gastric emptying cycles in the human fetus. Am J Obstet Gynecol 2005;193:1000–4.

58. Sase M, Nakata M, Tasima R, Kato H. Development of gastric emptying in the human fetus. Ultrasound Obstet Gynecol 2000;16:56–9.

59. Cucchiara S, Salvia G, Scarcella A, et al. Gestational maturation of electrical activity of the stomach. Dig Dis Sci 1999;44:2008–13.

60. Tomomasa T, Itoh Z, Koizumi T, et al. Nonmigrating rhythmic activity in the stomach and duodenum of neonates. Biol Neonate 1985;48:1–9.

61. Hassan BB, Butler R, Davidson GP, et al. Patterns of antropyloric motility in fed healthy preterm infants. Arch Dis Child Fetal Neonatal Ed 2002;87:F95–9.

62. Jadcherla SR, Berseth CL. Effect of erythromycin on gastroduodenal contractile activity in developing neonates. J Pediatr Gastroenterol Nutr 2002;34:16–22.

63. Ittmann PI, Amarnath R, Berseth CL. Maturation of antroduodenal motor activity in preterm and term infants. Dig Dis Sci 1992;37:14–9.

64. Al Tawil Y, Berseth CL. Gestational and postnatal maturation of duodenal motor responses to intragastric feeding. J Pediatr 1996;129:374–81.

65. Baker J, Berseth CL. Postnatal change in inhibitory regulation of intestinal motor activity in human and canine neonates. Pediatr Res 1995;38:133–9.

66. Berseth CL. Neonatal small intestinal motility: Motor responses to feeding in term and preterm infants. J Pediatr 1990;117:777–82.

67. Precioso AR, Pereira GR, Vaz FA. Gastric myoelectrical activity in neonates of different gestational ages by means of electrogastrography. Rev Hosp Clin Fac Med Sao Paulo 2003;58:81–90.

68. Lucas A, Bloom SR, Aynsley-Green A. Postnatal surges in plasma gut hormones in term and preterm infants. Biol Neonate 1982;41:63–7.

69. Lucas A, Bloom SR, Green AA. Gastrointestinal peptides and the adaptation to extrauterine nutrition. Can J Physiol Pharmacol 1985;63:527–37.

70. Cavell B. Gastric emptying in preterm infants. Acta Paediatr Scand 1979;68:725–30.

71. Cavell B. Reservoir and emptying function of the stomach of the premature infant. Acta Paediatr Scand Suppl 1982;296:60–1.

72. Steffen RM. Effect of erythromycin on gastroduodenal contractile activity in developing neonates. Clin Pediatr (Phila) 2002;41:448–9.

73. Tomomasa T, Kuroume T, Arai H, et al. Erythromycin induces migrating motor complex in human gastrointestinal tract. Dig Dis Sci 1986;31:157–61.

74. Tomomasa T, Miyazaki M, Koizumi T, Koroung T. Erythromycin increases gastric antral motility in human premature infants. Biol Neonate 1993;63:349–52.

75. Lucas A, Aynsley-Green A, Blackburn AM, et al. Plasma neurotensin in term and preterm neonates. Acta Paediatr Scand 1981;70:201–6.

11.2. Motility Disorders

Miguel Saps, MD
Carlo Di Lorenzo, MD

EVALUATION OF GASTRIC MOTOR FUNCTION

The number of diagnostic tests available to evaluate gastric function is steadily increasing. Until a few years ago information about gastric motility could be obtained only by evaluating the emptying into the duodenum of barium or radioactive material. It is now possible to measure tonic and phasic pressure changes in different areas of the stomach, detect its electrical activity and assess its sensory function. In view of the inconsistent correlation between symptoms and specific motor abnormalities, a combination of several testing modalities is often required in the evaluation of the child with suspected gastric dysfunction. The clinician must integrate testing results with basic physiological and pathological notions of visceral motility and sensation in order to optimize patient care.

Radiology

The study of a patient with suspected dysmotility usually begins with a radiologic study. Radiologic contrast studies provide essential information on anatomical abnormalities, such as the presence of malrotation or a superior mesenteric artery that compresses the lumen of the small intestine. Radiologic evidence of megaduodenum, megajejunum, intestinal diverticula, or dilated, aperistaltic, and fluid filled bowel in the absence of a lumen-occluding lesion may signal the presence of severe small intestine dysmotility. However, barium studies are generally unsuitable to diagnose a specific gastrointestinal motor abnormality or identify the etiology for disordered motility and are unreliable to assess transit time. There is poor correlation between transit measured by scintigraphic and radiologic methods.[1] A possible explanation for this phenomenon is that barium adheres to the gastric mucosa, leaving the stomach at a different rate than food.

Scintigraphy

Scintigraphy is considered the reference standard for measuring gastric emptying. Nuclear scintigraphy is minimally invasive, requires relatively low levels of exposure to radiation, and is available at most institutions. In this test, a liquid or solid food is labeled with a radionuclide that binds to the test meal. The labeled meal is then tracked as it passes through the stomach using a gamma camera. Ideally, patients should be studied with a dual-labeled meal able to differentiate solid and liquid emptying as different symptoms may relate to abnormal emptying of each phase. Dysfunction of the fundus of the stomach affects preferentially gastric emptying of fluids, while abnormal antral motility leads to delayed emptying of solids. Repeated scintigraphic images are obtained in order to assess the rate of gastric emptying. Although the test can be performed over different periods of time and with single or multiple isotopes, a technique using two isotopes and prolonged evaluation over 4 to 8 hours has been recently proposed in order to sequentially quantify gastric emptying, small bowel transit, and colonic transit.[2] Meal composition, timing of imaging, and report method vary by center. As variations in isotopes, methods of scanning and analysis, and the patient's position may modify results, each nuclear medicine facility should establish a standardized protocol and assess its own control population in order to establish normal reference values. Ideally, the meal should be palatable and representative in volume and composition of an ordinary meal for the age and size of the children studied. Commonly employed isotopes and meals are ^{99m}Technetium sulfur colloid labeled scrambled eggs to mimic a solid meal and ^{111}In-ΔPTA to label the liquid meal. Other centers use ^{99m}Technetium to label formula or milk. The test should identify halftime emptying times, lag time, and postlag emptying slope. Scintigraphic techniques are a sensitive and specific mean to identify and monitor gastric motility disorders.[3] However, interpretation of results in adult patients is limited by a poor correlation between the diagnosis of gastroparesis and symptoms or quality of life[4] and the inability to predict therapeutic effects of prokinetic medications based on the results of the study. A solid phase meal can provide the most useful clinical information as emptying of liquids is characterized by a lesser sensitivity.

Antroduodenal Manometry

Conventional manometric testing is performed through pneumo-hydraulic perfusion of degassed water into a system of capillary tubing that provides high resistance to flow. Multilumen catheters, usually consisting of 6 to 8 radially oriented orifices, spaced 1, 3, or 5 cm apart, are placed in the gastric antrum and duodenum. The spacing between recording sites varies based on the child's size and the area of the gastrointestinal tract under investigation. The evaluation of antrum and pylorus requires closely located sensors ($1 \propto 3$ cm apart), while the small bowel can be better studied with sensors spaced further. Water is infused through the catheters at a low, constant rate. Manometric readings are obtained by measuring the resistance to the water flow.

The recorded signals are a representation of the pressure present within the viscus. A computerized system transforms the pressure recordings into a graphic tracing in which peaks represent contractions and deflections below baseline correspond to relaxations. Newer computerized systems have been designed that utilize solid-state sensors without the need for water infusion, which also allow their use in an "ambulatory" setting. However, the use of solid-state ambulatory systems in pediatrics is not yet widespread and most of the published data in children are derived from water-perfused systems. Because resistance to the flow of water is required to achieve accurate measurements, the accurate determination of luminal occlusion is more difficult in the fundus which has a larger diameter and slow tonic changes in pressure. Thus, fundic recordings are of limited value and usually not obtained when using manometry. Manometry catheters are placed through the nose or a gastrostomy by fluoroscopic or endoscopic technique. The test begins after the child recovers from sedation. Measurements are obtained during fasting, after ingestion of a meal and following the administration of test drugs such as erythromycin or octreotide. In young patients, at least one motor migrating complex (MMC) is usually identified during 4 hours of fasting recording. Postprandial recording lasts at least 1 hour. A trained technician is present throughout the study for safety, to provide information on symptoms and their correlation with the manometric findings, and to observe the family dynamics and assess parental response to the child's symptoms.

Antroduodenal manometry provides direct information on the amplitude, duration, frequency, and direction of propagation of gastrointestinal

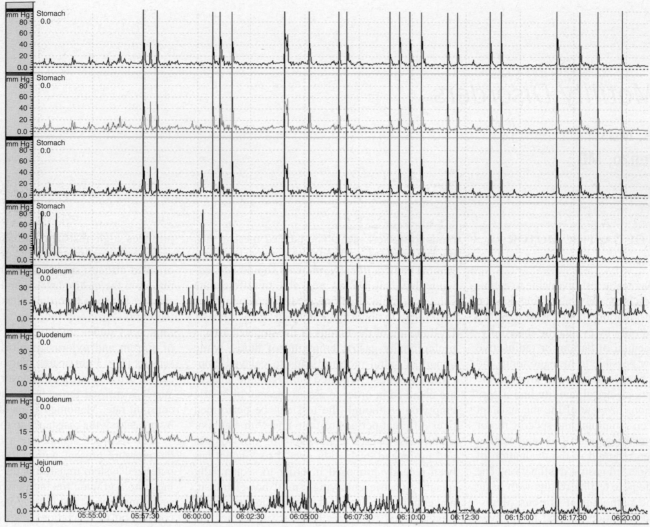

Figure 1 Antroduodenal motility tracing from an adolescent girl with rumination syndrome. There are four recording sites in the stomach and four in the small bowel. The vertical lines represent regurgitation episodes which are associated with simultaneous pressure increases across all the recoding sites.

contractions, by assessing the temporal and spatial distribution of intraluminal pressure changes. There is evidence that manometric studies in children provide information that facilitates clinical management and predicts outcome by aiding in diagnosis and assessing potential therapeutic benefit of medications.[5–8] Manometry should be used in combination with other tests to investigate unexplained symptoms such as nausea, vomiting, abdominal pain, and abdominal distention.[9] In patients with suspected enteric neuromuscular disorders, antroduodenal manometry is an essential aid in determining the presence of a motility disorder.[10]

Gastrointestinal manometry can identify distinct patterns that suggest an underlying neuropathy, myopathy, a mixed disorder, or presence of a mechanical obstruction.[11] While neuropathic processes are characterized by normal amplitude contractions with abnormal propagation or uncoordinated phasic pressure waves, myopathic processes portray a pattern of widespread low-amplitude but well-coordinated contractions. Delayed gastric emptying may result from either impaired antral peristalsis leading to poor propulsive effort or intestinal dysmotility leading to increased resistance to flow into the small bowel. Both myopathic and neuropathic conditions may

result in similarly delayed gastric emptying and prolonged small bowel transit time.[12] Postprandial antral hypomotility often follows a viral infection and is associated with prolonged gastric emptying of solids.[13] Small intestine obstruction is characterized by a sustained pattern of simultaneous, prolonged contractions separated by periods of motor quiescence.[14] Children with mitochondrial disorders may present with gastrointestinal symptoms long before the involvement of the central nervous system becomes apparent. In these children, manometry has shown neuropathic abnormalities including nonpropagated antral bursts, absent MMC, postprandial antral hypomotility, and retrograde and tonic contractions.[15] Scleroderma has been associated with gut hypomotility and a myopathic or mixed pattern in manometric studies.[16] Chronic intestinal pseudo-obstruction can present with various manometric patterns. Patients with myopathic variety may have absent or low-amplitude contractions.[17] Patients with neuropathic variety may have nonpropagated bursts of phasic pressure activity of various duration in the fasting and/or postprandial periods or absence of the phase III of the MMC.[18,19] In patients with rumination syndrome, antroduodenal manometry testing can confirm the diagnosis by demonstrating "r" waves, a

postprandial pattern of increase in pressure that simultaneously occurs in all recording sites as a result of abdominal and diaphragmatic muscle contraction (Figure 1).[20] This pattern is characteristic of this condition and differs from the manometric findings of other causes of vomiting which are usually associated with retrograde antral contractions (Figure 2).

Manometric features that have been shown to be associated with pediatric gastrointestinal motility disorders also include abnormal migration of phase III of the MMC, short intervals between phase III episodes, sustained tonic-phasic contractions and persistent low-amplitude contractions.[21] Patients with manometric evidence of antral hypomotility are likely to benefit from enteral feedings, while in patients with an enteric myopathy, prokinetic medications, and drip feedings have a more unpredictable outcome. Presence of MMC during fasting has been associated with a favorable response to cisapride use and the ability to be weaned from parenteral nutrition.[22]

Breath Tests

Breath testing using ^{13}C-octanoate breath test, a stable isotope, is a sensitive and specific method to measure gastric emptying.[23] Although not readily available in most institutions, this test has

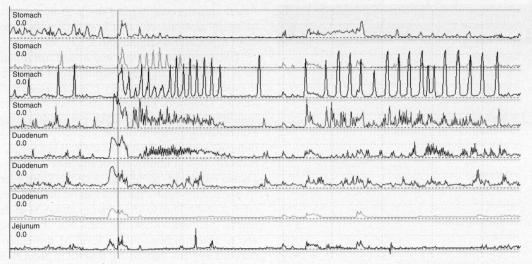

Figure 2 Antroduodenal motility tracing from a boy with chronic vomiting. There are three recording sites in the stomach and five in the small bowel. The vertical line represents an episode of vomiting associated with a retrograde pressure wave migrating from the small bowel to the stomach.

the advantage of being noninvasive, simple, inexpensive, and devoid of ionizing radiation exposure. The test is performed by ingesting a meal labeled with ^{13}C-octanoate acid. Exhaled air samples are obtained before and periodically after the test meal to measure labeled carbon dioxide by mass spectrometry. Breath testing is based on the principle that a single event in the process of absorption and metabolism of the tracer constitutes the limiting step. Gastric emptying constitutes the rate-limiting step in the absorption of ^{13}C-octanoate from the small intestine. The results have a good correlation with those obtained by scintigraphy.

External Electrogastrography (EGG)

EGG is a noninvasive technique that assesses the gastric myoelectrical activity via external electrodes applied to the skin. This technique has the benefit of being noninvasive and therefore can be used repeatedly under different circumstances in children of various ages, including premature neonates. The EGG device is portable and can be utilized at the bedside.[24] Limitations of this technique relate to its fair reproducibility,[25] low correlation of the electrical signal with gastric contractile activity and symptoms, and difficulty in separating artifacts from true abnormal electric rhythm.[26] The signal measured represents a combination of the gastric signal and "noise elements" composed of respiratory and motion artifacts and electrical activity of the small bowel, colon, and heart. Studies conducted in children have demonstrated that EGG correlates poorly with scintigraphic gastric emptying studies.[27] Currently, its use is mostly limited to the research setting.

Barostat

The electronic barostat is now considered the most suitable instrument to investigate fundic tone. The barostat test involves the insertion of a polyethylene balloon connected to a computerized pump through the mouth into the proximal stomach. The intraballoon change in volume

at a fixed pressure reflects variations in fundic tone. Meal-induced fundic relaxation is defined as the difference in volume between the average preprandial and postprandial volumes. Barostat technology is invasive, stressful, and difficult to perform especially in young children, limiting its clinical use. The fundic balloon may also interfere with normal physiology as it provides a positive pressure to the gastric wall that may result in gastric distention. In order to compensate for these shortcomings, alternative techniques have been developed.

Single-Photon Emission Computed Tomography (SPECT)

SPECT is a technology that utilizes the intravenous injection of radiolabeled ^{99m}Tcertechnetate in order to measure gastric emptying and assess gastric accommodation. A dual-isotope SPECT that combines injection of ^{99m}Tc pertechnetate and ingestion of a labeled meal allows the periodic assessment of both gastric dimensions and gastric emptying.[28] The technique has the benefit of being well tolerated and able to identify single or combined pathophysiologic disturbances. The test is based in the principle that the ^{99m}Tc radionuclide accumulates in the gastric mucosa allowing a three-dimensional visualization of the stomach by a gamma camera. The obtained images permit the calculation of total and regional stomach volumes. Changes in volume in relation to a meal are a reflection of gastric accommodation. SPECT-assessed evaluation of gastric emptying can be obtained following ingestion of ^{111}In-ΔPTA In-diethylenetriaminepentaacetic acid in a liquid nutrient drink or an ^{111}In-ΔPTA In-oxine-labeled egg sandwich. Acquiring images at 20-minute intervals allows for a calculation of percent nucleotide retention in the stomach as a function of time. SPECT has been shown to detect changes in postprandial volume similar to those obtained with the gastric barostat.[29] However, another study comparing SPECT scanning to barostat technology demonstrated that SPECT measured

lower volumes, possibly due to the absence of the distending pressure on the stomach by the balloon used in barostat studies.[30] The gastric volumes measured by SPECT reflect intragastric content composed by swallowed air, intragastric secretions, and ingested foods or liquids. A study in adolescents has shown impaired gastric accommodation abnormalities, delayed gastric emptying and increased postprandial symptoms by using this methodology.[31]

Water Load Test

The water load test is a diagnostic technique that provides indirect evaluation of gastric perception and function. The test measures satiation by asking the patient to ingest the largest possible volume of liquids by drinking at a constant speed for a certain period of time. Different fluids and caloric content drinks have been used but the ingestion of water has the advantage of restricting satiety variables to gastric distension, gastric sensitivity, and psychological determinants of fullness.[32] The results of this physiologic test show a good correlation with the gastric barostat study in measuring sensation and accommodation with the advantage of being simple, low cost, noninvasive, and allowing assessment of distensibility of the whole stomach and not only the fundus.[33,34] The drink test enables determination of impaired fundic relaxation in response to meals and visceral hypersensitivity, two elements that seem to play an important role in the pathogenesis of functional dyspepsia.[34] However, the correlation of test results with physiological variables remains controversial as the test is characterized by substantial intra- and intersubject variability with both sensory and psychological factors affecting the results.[32] Despite its shortcomings, the water load test is being increasingly adopted as pediatric studies demonstrate its ability to reproduce symptoms in children with functional gastrointestinal disorders.[35] Normal reference values for children of different size and age have been published.[33]

Ambulatory Diagnostic Test Pill

The *SmartPill* (SmartPill Corporation, Buffalo, NY) has been recently approved by the Food and Drug Administration (FDA). It is a radio telemetry capsule that is able to assess and record pH, pressure, and temperature of the entire gastrointestinal tract in ambulatory subjects for more than 3 days. In addition to the 26 mm × 13 mm ingestible capsule equipped with an internal power supply and capability to transmit radio frequency, the system includes a receiver, a docking station, and specialized software. A change of pH from acid to alkaline indicates the passage from the stomach to the duodenum allowing the assessment of gastric emptying. A study designed to assess the accuracy of the test has shown a sensitivity of 71% and a specificity of 86% in determining gastric emptying.[36] A limitation of the *SmartPill* is its inability to provide an accurate assessment of gastric emptying under physiological conditions, as the indigestible solids empty differently than a standardized meal.

Others

Gastric emptying can also be measured by ultrasonography and magnetic resonance imaging (MRI). Each of these techniques has advantages and shortcomings. While ultrasonography is widely available, it requires a liquid test meal and an experienced operator. In appropriate settings, it may provide an adequate alternative to scintigraphy.[37] The use of MRI is limited by expense and availability. By labeling the meal with gadolinium, MRI allows studying gastric accommodation through tridimensional reconstruction of gastric volumes and comparison of fasting to postprandial images.[38] Upper gastrointestinal endoscopy is usually normal in patients with disordered gastric function but important nevertheless in order to exclude outlet obstruction and peptic disease. In the most severe cases of gastroparesis, endoscopy may reveal the presence of bezoars.

DYSMOTILITY

Although symptoms related to gastric dysfunction are relatively common, primary motility disorders of the foregut defined by an isolated myoneural pathology are rare. Disorders of gastrointestinal motility may result in delayed or accelerated transit. Delayed transit disorders may involve only the stomach (gastroparesis) or be part of a more generalized gastrointestinal disorder (postoperative ileus, intestinal pseudo-obstruction). Cystic fibrosis[39] and surgical interventions such as fundoplication[40] or gastric drainage procedures may result in acceleration of gastric emptying,

GASTROPARESIS

Abnormalities in gastric myoelectrical activity may result in gastric dysmotility and delayed gastric emptying. Gastroparesis is characterized by delayed gastric emptying in the absence of a mechanical obstruction. Patients with gastroparesis may present with a combination of symptoms including nausea, early satiety, vomiting, postprandial abdominal distention and pain, and weight loss. Vomiting is characterized by being postprandial and delayed 30 minutes to several hours after meal ingestion and containing undigested food from previous meals. These vomiting episodes differ from those associated with central nervous disorders in which the emesis is projectile, often abrupt, precipitated by movement, associated with headaches, and usually does not contain undigested food. As patients with gastroparesis frequently modify the diet to ingest only small amounts of food, vomiting may become less prevalent with time. The weak correlation between symptoms, type and severity of disordered gastric motor function suggests that symptoms often have a multifactorial etiology.

Table 1 Most Frequent Causes of Gastroparesis in Children
Prematurity
Drug-induced
Opioids
Anticholinergics
Metabolic/electrolyte disorders
Acidosis
Hypokalemia
Hypothyroidism
Postsurgical
Vagotomy (ie, post-fundoplication)
Postviral
Neuronal dysfunction
Acidosis
Diabetes mellitus
Intestinal pseudo-obstruction
Cerebral palsy
Familial dysautonomia
Spinal cord injury
Eosinophilic gastroenteropathy
Connective tissue disorders
Scleroderma
Muscular dystrophy

The prevalence and causes of gastroparesis differ in children from adults. Common pediatric etiologies of gastroparesis include postsurgical conditions (eg, vagotomy at the time of a fundoplication), prolonged recovery from infections and drugs (eg, narcotics, anticholinergic agents), with many instances having no identifiable etiology (Table 1). Gastroparesis may also result from degenerative processes that affect gastric enteric neurons, smooth muscle, and/or interstitial cells of Cajal (ICC). Loss of ICCs may lead to clinical disorders characterized by altered gastric function. A case report of ICC loss, possibly by an autoimmune mechanism, has been reported in an adult patient with gastroparesis and delayed small intestinal transit.[41] A case series described 11 children with persistent gastroparesis and postprandial antral hypomotility following an acute viral illness. Most of the children had confirmed rotavirus infection. All of them recovered within 6 to 24 months.[13] Adult series of patients with postviral gastroparesis have also showed an excellent prognosis. The pathogenesis of this condition is unknown, although a prolonged infection of the myenteric plexus or an autoimmune response triggered by an infection have been postulated.

Gastrointestinal motor dysfunction leading to vomiting, abdominal distention, constipation, and dysphagia may result from disorders at every anatomic levels of the extrinsic innervation.[42] Neuropathic disorders, including autonomic dysfunction and diabetes, and myopathic conditions, such as connective tissue diseases (eg, scleroderma), although less common than in adults can be found in children as well. Patients with scleroderma may also complain of dysphagia due to esophageal involvement, and intestinal symptoms due to gut hypomotility, characterized by a myopathic or mixed pattern on manometry.

Acute spinal cord injuries result in a generally transient gastroparesis that improves with metoclopramide and erythromycin.[43]

Gastroparesis can be found in preterm infants with immaturity of the gastrointestinal tract and in cases of allergy to dietary proteins. In allergic infants, cow milk provokes gastrointestinal dysmotility that results in delayed gastric emptying, exacerbating gastroesophageal reflux (GER), and inducing vomiting.[44] Use of a hydrolyzed formula leads to clinical improvement and acceleration of gastric emptying.[45] Children with CNS disorders frequently develop abnormal gastric motility and GER possibly due to abnormal modulation of the enteric nervous system by the CNS or secondary to abnormalities at the level of the enteric nervous system caused by a similar process to the one affecting the CNS.[46] Physical stress has been shown to decrease the amplitude of gastric contractions, decrease the number of propagated antral and duodenal pressure waves, increase the number of isolated pyloric pressure waves, trigger retrograde movement of a solid meal from the distal to the proximal stomach, and delay gastric emptying in healthy subjects.[47] Emotional stress has also been associated with a delay in gastric emptying,[48] a phenomenon which seems to be mediated by corticotropin releasing factor through the vagus nerve.[49]

The motor mechanisms associated with gastroparesis are not yet completely understood. In patients with gastroparesis, a reduction of fundic accommodation can be found in combination with retention of liquids and solids in the antrum. Patients with symptoms suggestive of gastroparesis can be studied with various techniques to confirm delayed emptying of the stomach and to identify other conditions that can present with similar symptoms such as GER, peptic ulcer disease, rumination syndrome, mechanical obstruction, and bulimia.

The main goals of treatment for gastroparesis are to alleviate symptoms, maintain adequate fluids and nutrition, and to resume sufficient oral intake of liquids and solids. Therapies for gastroparesis include dietary modifications, behavioral changes, prokinetic drugs and, in the most severe cases, gastric electrical stimulation and surgery. Dietary changes may not be required if symptoms are mild. However, if symptoms are severe, only liquids may be tolerated. Slow ingestion of small-volume, fat-free, low-fiber, liquid meals is ideal. Diet should be tailored to each individual and modified according to the progression of symptoms. In the most severe cases, jejunal feedings or parenteral nutrition may be required.

Prokinetic agents, such as metoclopramide, erythromycin, domperidone, cisapride, and tegaserod, represent the core of pharmacological therapy due to their effects on gastric motility, and will be discussed in detail later in the chapter. In severe cases, a combination of drugs with different mechanism of action is needed. Potential problems such as delivery of medication to the absorption site, tachyphylaxis, and adverse effects should be considered before their use. Serotonin (5-HT) receptors are prevalent in the central nervous system and gut and are involved in the induction of emesis. Although 5-HT3 antagonists are safe and potent antiemetic agents, they are less efficacious in treating delayed vomiting. Nausea may be a debilitating symptom in gastroparesis. Scopolamine, an older drug that has proven to be effective in randomized controlled trials in preventing motion sickness,[50] may be helpful in severe cases of nausea. The use of transdermal scopolamine patches enables adequate absorption of the drug despite vomiting. One should be aware of a reported pediatric case of central anticholinergic syndrome resulting in hallucinations and incontinence that resolved with the removal of the patch.[51]

Gastric electrical stimulation (gastric pacing) constitutes a novel alternative therapy in patients with gastroparesis unresponsive to dietary and medical treatment.[52] Electrical stimulation is provided through a neurostimulator that delivers electrical impulses through leads implanted in the stomach wall. The pacemaker can be placed via laparotomy or laparoscopy (Figure 3). Gastric electrical stimulation has proven to be effective in entraining gastric electrical activity and improving contractility.[53,54] Forward pacing and retrograde pacing can be achieved by pacing in the midcorpus near the region of the natural gastric pacemaker or near the pylorus respectively,[55] although other pacing sites have been proposed. A wide range of frequencies has been employed to stimulate the stomach by different investigators. While some investigators have used frequencies similar to the physiologic rate (3 cycles per minute or c/pm), others have used very high frequencies that are several times the basal rate. In addition, the pulse width of stimulation varies among researchers ranging from 300 μs to 300 ms. By inducing gastric electrical pacing at a rate slightly higher than the physiological pacing, it is possible to entrain and pace the gastric slow waves, accelerating gastric emptying and improving dyspeptic symptoms. Electrical pacing with high-frequency, low-energy, and short-pulse-duration stimulation has shown to ameliorate symptoms with little effect on gastric emptying, possibly acting on afferent nerves. Although there is agreement that higher frequencies can entrain the gastric slow wave, there seems to be a maximum limit in the ability of the electrical stimulation to trigger slow waves. High-frequency gastric electric stimulation at 12 cpm has been considered medically necessary and effective by the FDA which in 1999 approved the use of a device using such frequency as a "humanitarian exemption" in the treatment of chronic intractable nausea and vomiting secondary to diabetic or idiopathic gastroparesis.[56] The gastric pacemaker can be placed surgically in a subcutaneous pouch below the rib cage or endoscopically on the luminal side when planned to be used transiently.[57,58] Gastric pacing seems to affect gastric motility at least partially through an increase in plasma motilin levels.[59] Electrical stimulation has shown beneficial effects by restoring gastric motility, improving symptoms, decreasing the need for prokinetic drugs, and improving quality of life and nutritional status in adult patients.[60] Pacing seems to improve symptoms of nausea and vomiting more than it does gastric emptying. A double-blind randomized study with the pacer turned on and off for 1 month in adults with chronic symptomatic gastroparesis unresponsive to standard medical therapy showed a reduction in symptoms severity, vomiting, and quality of life.[61] A long-term follow-up study of adult patients receiving gastric electrical stimulation for refractory gastroparesis has also shown a significant decrease in hospitalization days and use of medications in per protocol and intention to treat analysis after 3 years.[62] Six out of 55 patients had the devices removed. Although the technique is generally believed to be safe, its effectiveness has not been proved in children and adolescents with different etiologies of gastroparesis and a case series study reported two postoperative complications out of 16 patients.[60] While infection remains the most common complication,[61] a case of stomach wall perforation has also been reported.[63]

Botulinum toxin A injected into the pyloric sphincter constitutes an effective but transient therapy for gastroparesis.[64] Botulinum toxin is a potent neurotoxin produced by the bacteria *Clostridium botulinum*. Two different mechanisms seem to be responsible for the effect of botulinum toxin in pyloric sphincter contractility. At low concentration, botulinum toxin seems to decreases electrically induced contractile stimulation by binding to presynaptic acetylcholine terminals preventing cholinergic transmission, while at higher concentrations it appears to provoke direct inhibition of the contractility of the smooth muscle.[64] As a consequence, there is muscle relaxation and reduction of fasting and postprandial phasic and tonic pyloric contractions.[64] A study of 63 adult patients with gastroparesis showed improvement or resolution of symptoms after endoscopic injection of botulinum toxin into the pylorus. In 43% of cases the effect lasted an average of 5 months.[65] Adult studies have shown improvement of symptoms with circumferential injection at the pylorus at doses of 100 to 200 units.[66,67] Isolated case reports have been published in children demonstrating improvement in gastric emptying after intrapyloric injection.[68]

The "Relief Band" is a device that acts on the P6 Neiguan acupuncture point on the wrist and it may constitute a useful adjunct in the treatment of nausea. Although no pediatric studies have been published, there are reports of improvement of

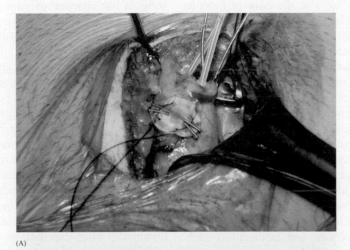

(A)

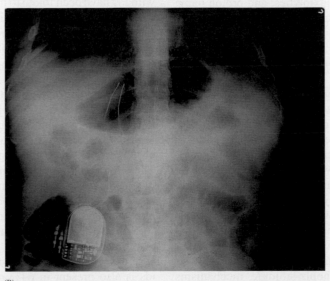

(B)

Figure 3 (A) Intraoperative picture of the gastric pacemaker being inserted with the leads on the serosal side of the stomach. (B) Abdominal radiograph of a patient with an implanted gastric pacemaker. (Courtesy of R.E. Schmieg, Jr, MD, and Thomas L. Abell, MD, University of Mississippi Medical Center, Jackson, MS.)

symptoms, increase serum levels of pancreatic polypeptide and increasing percentage of normal EGG in diabetic patients treated with acupuncture.[69]

In selective cases of refractory gastroparesis, surgery may be considered as a therapeutic option. Surgical interventions include procedures designed to administer nutrients downstream from the stomach such as jejunostomies, or aimed at improving gastric drainage, such as pyloromyotomy or pyloroplasty and partial or total gastrectomy. Surgery is only performed in extreme cases as, with the exception of few case series,[70] the results of surgical interventions in patients with poor motility generally have been disappointing. Although a complete gastrectomy seems to be effective in providing symptoms relief in postsurgical gastroparesis, it should be used with caution as it may result in significant complications.[71] It is our opinion that surgery should be reserved only for children who have required parenteral nutrition for several months and who have failed trials of gastrostomy and jejunostomy feedings.

RUMINATION

Rumination syndrome constitutes a functional gastrointestinal disorder (FGID) characterized by effortless repetitive regurgitation of undigested food from the stomach into the oropharynx. The food is then partially or completely rechewed, reswallowed, or ejected.[72]

The Rome III criteria define two different presentations of rumination syndrome. Infant rumination syndrome is defined as "repetitive contractions of the abdominal muscles, diaphragm and tongue that result in regurgitation of gastric contents into the mouth from where it is either rechewed and reswallowed or expectorated, with an onset between 3 and 8 months, not associated with signs of nausea or distress, not occurring during sleep or when the infant is engaged in social interaction and unresponsive to the usual management of GER, anticholinergics, formula changes, hand restraints, gastrostomy feeding or gavage."[73] Rumination syndrome in infants, unlike in healthy adults and adolescents, constitutes a form of self-stimulation with potential life-threatening psychiatric implications and has been linked to social deprivation.[74] Bonding problems with the mother are frequently described. The Rome III criteria define adolescent rumination as "repeated painless episodes of regurgitation and rechewing or expulsion of food occurring soon after a meal, in the absence of retching, exclusively while awake, unresponsive to usual therapy of gastroesophageal reflux disease, with no organic basis and occurring at least once a week for a minimum of 2 months."[75] Regurgitation is immediately preceded by a sensation of belching. The hallmark of this condition is the regurgitation of material without retching or nausea.

In patients with rumination as opposed to gastroparesis, regurgitation usually occurs during or within minutes from meal ingestion and differently from cases of gastroesophageal reflux disease (GERD) is generally not associated with heartburn, discomfort, or esophagitis. In addition, most patients with rumination do not have postprandial antral hypomotility and delayed gastric emptying, features that are common in patients with gastroparesis. Rumination is relatively common in developmentally delayed infants and toddlers but is increasingly recognized also in otherwise healthy children and adolescents.[76] This problem is frequently unrecognized by parents and often misdiagnosed by physicians due to lack of awareness. Patients with rumination are commonly misdiagnosed as having a motility disorder, GERD, bulimia, or cyclic vomiting syndrome. Rumination syndrome should always be considered in the differential diagnosis of patients with long-standing postprandial vomiting without nausea. In the largest published pediatric series it was reported that the mean age at diagnosis was 15 years. Symptom duration before diagnosis was longer than 2 years, 73% missed school/work, and 46% had been hospitalized because of symptoms. Before diagnosis, 11% underwent surgery for evaluation or management of symptoms and 16% had psychiatric disorders.[77] Thus, there seems to be a very high morbidity associated with this condition.

Rumination is considered a behavioral problem (similar to a "tic") in the case of healthy older children.[78] The affected patients seem to develop the behavior of rumination in response to discomfort associated with food ingestion. As a group, patients with rumination syndrome display higher gastric sensitivity and more frequent lower esophageal sphincter relaxations during gastric distension. A subgroup also has absent postprandial accommodation.[79] Therapy of rumination should be individualized according to the needs of each patient, identifying situations and emotions that may trigger the episodes and excluding possible affective disorders. Therapy includes a combination of aversive behavior modification in infants[80] and cognitive therapy with biofeedback or relaxation techniques, and medications such as antidepressants, anxiolytics, and proton pump inhibitors in older children.[76]

DYSPEPSIA

Functional dyspepsia (FD) has been defined as an FGID characterized by persistent or recurrent pain or discomfort centered in the upper abdomen, that is, not relieved by defecation or associated with changes in stool characteristics occurring at least once a week for at least 2 months in the absence of organic diseases.[75] As currently defined, FD probably represents a heterogeneous group of gastrointestinal disorders, with patients who experience chronic nausea, postprandial bloating, and epigastric pain all fitting in the same group, even though it is likely that they have different pathophysiologic mechanisms and require different diagnostic evaluations and treatment interventions. A new proposal for different subgroups of dyspeptic patients has been suggested as part of the Rome III adult classifications[81] and has been endorsed by the pediatric committee.[75]

Proposed pathophysiological mechanisms underlying FD include gastric dysmotility,[82] impaired fundic function,[83] lower threshold to perceive distention,[84,85] impaired duodenal acid clearance and duodenal motor response to acid infusion,[86] nervous system dysregulation,[87] inflammation,[88] and psychological distress.[89] Delayed gastric emptying is found in 30 to 40% of FD patients.[82] Other pediatric and adult studies have shown accelerated emptying in a subgroup of patients.[2,90] Although symptoms associated with dyspepsia cannot be explained exclusively by alterations in motility, several abnormalities in antroduodenal function and impaired accommodation have been described in children with FD.[2,91] EGG studies conducted in dyspeptic patients have demonstrated irregularities in gastric electrical activity including tachygastria, bradygastria, and mixed arrhythmias during fasting and postprandial states.[92,93] In the most severe cases of FD, the manometric findings resemble those of chronic intestinal pseudo-obstruction.[93] Adult studies in patients with FD have found an association between delayed emptying of solids with postprandial fullness, nausea, and vomiting in the absence of pain as a predominant symptom.[94] Patients with dyspepsia have more symptoms after reaching satiation. The inability to tolerate low volumes of fundic distention in a subset of dyspeptic patients and the current understanding of the role of cholinergic transmission in receptive relaxation, point toward a possible therapeutic role of drugs targeting accommodation in this condition.[95] Although these findings suggest that dyspepsia is more a problem of impaired accommodation rather than visceral hypersensitivity, the pathogenesis of this condition is still not completely understood. Real-time ultrasonography in children with FD has shown increased distension of the antral area 60 and 90 minutes after ingestion of a meal.[96] Patients with FD have been found to have higher scores for anxiety, depression, neuroticism, and tendency to pessimism when compared with community controls.[97] In dyspeptic adults, a correlation was found between the severity of stressful life events and interpersonal sensitivity with disturbance of gastric myoelectrical activity.[89] An adult study using EGG, drink test, solid phase gastric emptying, and symptom and psychological questionnaires revealed significant associations between psychiatric distress and digestive symptoms.[98] Thus, FD seems to be a complex disorder where there is a possible interaction among dysfunction at the level of different regions of the gastrointestinal tract and central mechanisms.

The pathophysiologic abnormalities previously mentioned are hardly specific for patients with dyspepsia. Delayed gastric emptying of solids is also present in 64% of patients with irritable bowel syndrome.[99] A community study has shown that 63% of subjects with symptoms of reflux also had symptoms of dyspepsia.[100]

The possible role of *Helicobacter pylori* (*H. pylori*) in functional dyspepsia remains controversial. A study has shown that out of 405 adult patients diagnosed with dyspepsia 211 tested positive for *H. pylori*.[101] A 7-year follow-up of the subgroup of patients in which *H. pylori* had been eradicated, showed that although the symptoms were slightly improved after eradication, a large percentage of patients that originally improved experienced recurrence of dyspeptic symptoms.[101] Similarly, eradication of *H. Pylori* in children has only a small therapeutic benefit. A pediatric study showed that most children with dyspepsia do not have *H. pylori* infection and most subjects with functional dyspepsia have improvement of symptoms independent of the cause of dyspepsia.[102] A long-term cohort follow-up study of asymptomatic preschool and school-age children showed that children acquiring *H. pylori* infection do not complain more often of abdominal pain or other dyspeptic symptoms.[103] However, another small prospective study concluded that eradication of *H. pylori* may lead to a significant long-term improvement in dyspepsia in children.[104]

In view of heterogeneity of symptoms and pathophysiologic mechanisms, it is not surprising that treatment of dyspepsia remains challenging. Currently there is no FDA-approved drug for treatment of FD. There is a lack of evidence regarding the efficacy of psychological interventions or the combination of pharmacological and psychological therapies in treating FD.[97] The Rome criteria and the technical report endorsed by the American Academy of Pediatrics and the North American Society for Pediatric Gastroenterology, Hepatology, and Nutrition on childhood abdominal pain found insufficient evidence to recommend the use of commonly employed drugs in the management of dyspepsia.[75,105] In patients with dyspepsia, avoidance of nonsteroidal anti-inflammatory agents, spicy and fatty foods, and caffeinated or carbonated beverages is generally recommended. A double-blind, placebo-controlled trial designed to determine the efficacy of famotidine in children with abdominal pain and dyspepsia found that the drug was beneficial only in the subjective symptom of global improvement with no significant effect in objective quantitative assessment.[106] The study also showed that there was significant improvement in symptoms during the first treatment period regardless of the use of medication or placebo.

A study of 127 children referred to pediatric gastroenterology clinics for dyspeptic symptoms reported that 62% did not have an organic disorder.[102] The low prevalence of organic disease found supports the use of reassurance and empiric therapy as initial treatment. In 56 patients that were evaluated by esophagogastroduodenoscopy and biopsy, the most common cause of organic disorder was mucosal inflammation (38%) with *H. pylori* being positive only in 5 patients. The Rome committee recommends that an upper gastrointestinal endoscopy should be performed in the presence of dysphagia, persistence of symptoms despite the use of acid reducing medications, or in patients with recurrent symptoms after discontinuing such medications.[75] There is lack of evidence that performing a gastric emptying study is cost effective in managing dyspepsia.[107]

Despite the scant evidence, antisecretory agents are frequently recommended in the treatment of patients with a predominant complaint of pain, while prokinetic agents are frequently used for bloating and early satiety. Cisapride has been shown to increase accommodation[108] with tegaserod having a similar effect.[109] Drugs that relax the gastric fundus by binding to 5-HT1 receptors, such as buspirone or sumatriptan, have been proposed as potentially beneficial agents in patients with altered accommodation.[110] Although not FDA approved for the use in children, tegaserod may have potentially a role in treating dyspepsia due to its effects of increasing gastric antral motility, gastric fundic accommodation, and acceleration of gastric emptying.[111]

CHRONIC INTESTINAL PSEUDO-OBSTRUCTION

A detailed description of chronic intestinal pseudo-obstruction (CIPO) is beyond the scope of this chapter, but we will briefly discuss it here due to the frequent gastric involvement in this condition and the importance of evaluating gastric function when children with CIPO present for possible small bowel transplantation. Pseudo-obstruction is characterized by impaired gastrointestinal propulsion resulting in signs and symptoms of bowel obstruction in the absence of a mechanical blockage. In contrast to adult cases, where CIPO is generally secondary to systemic diseases, most of the cases presenting in children are considered primary, idiopathic, and nonfamilial.[112] Since any segment of the digestive tract may be involved, the clinical presentation of CIPO varies depending on the areas affected at the time of diagnosis. Nausea, vomiting, and weight loss are predominant symptoms when CIPO affects the upper gastrointestinal tract while diffuse abdominal pain and distension, and constipation are suggestive of distal gut involvement. Ineffective gut motility may result in bacterial overgrowth and diarrhea. CIPO may also involve the urinary system with megacystis, megaurethra, dysuria, and recurrent urinary tract infections. Pseudo-obstruction can result from abnormalities at the level of the visceral smooth muscle, the enteric nerves, or the visceral autonomic nervous system.

The diagnosis of CIPO is based on clinical suspicion and confirmed by radiological or endoscopic exclusion of mechanical causes. Antroduodenal manometry may substantiate the clinical findings and can be helpful in differentiating between myopathic and neuropathic diseases. A review of 85 children with CIPO studied by manometry suggested the presence of an underlying neuropathy in 56% of children, myopathy in 38%, and undefined disease in 6%.[112] Radiologic examination may reveal dilatation of the esophagus, stomach, duodenum, and bowel, and air–fluid levels within the small intestine. Postprandial motility may be difficult to assess in patients with CIPO due to vomiting and inability to tolerate ingestion of a test meal. In children, the presence of the phase III complex of the MMC is associated with a better prognosis and successful use of enteral nutrition.[113] Affected patients rarely have normal gastric motility and scintigraphy generally confirms delayed gastric emptying. Gastric dysrhythmias, including tachygastria, bradygastria, irregular activity, or mixed abnormalities are found in almost all patients with CIPO.[114]

Treatment is best carried out within the context of a multidisciplinary team, which includes pediatric gastroenterologists, pain management specialists, and psychologists.[113] Patients with CIPO benefit from dietary modifications including low-lactose and low-fiber feedings, use of hydrolyzed proteins and supplementation with vitamins, minerals and oligoelements. The lack of effective motility often results in intestinal failure leading most patients with CIPO to require either partial or total parenteral nutrition to satisfy their nutrition and fluid needs. Placement of a gastrostomy may constitute the most helpful therapeutic intervention. The gastrostomy can be used to provide supplemental nutrition or decompress the distended stomach, resulting in reduction of emesis and abdominal pain. Prokinetics, antibiotics to treat bacterial overgrowth or sepsis, tricyclic antidepressants in cases of severe pain, and steroids in specific cases of inflammatory ganglionitis or myositis may be beneficial.[115] Fundoplication is of little benefit for symptom reduction in cases of poor foregut motility and it may just change vomiting to chronic and debilitating retching.

DUMPING SYNDROME

Dumping syndrome constitutes a clinically defined entity characterized by a constellation of gastrointestinal and systemic symptoms that follow the ingestion of food. Dumping syndrome has been described as a complication of various gastric surgical procedures, such as vagotomy, pyloroplasty, gastric resections, gastrojejunostomy, and Nissen fundoplication. Dumping may present as an early and a late form, with early dumping occurring within 30 to 60 minutes of eating and late dumping occurring 2 to 4 hours after a carbohydrate-rich meal.

Early dumping, which is more common, may present with both gastrointestinal and vasomotor symptoms, while late dumping typically presents exclusively with vasomotor symptoms. Gastrointestinal symptoms associated with dumping syndrome include postprandial fullness, colicky abdominal pain, nausea, vomiting, and explosive diarrhea, while vasomotor symptoms include weakness, dizziness, diaphoresis, pallor, flushing, palpitations, and tachycardia. Dumping syndrome results from postsurgical disturbances in the reservoir and transportation function of the stomach. Symptoms of early dumping are a consequence of accelerated emptying of chyme leading to rapid delivery of hyperosmolar liquids and solids into the small intestine, a phenomenon which causes abnormal fluid absorption, gut distention, and diarrhea. Gastrointestinal hormones may play a role in the pathogenesis of symptoms of early dumping. An excessive release of insulin explains the hypoglycemia that characterizes the syndrome. Increases of various vasoactive peptides including enteroglucagon, peptide YY, pancreatic polypeptide, VIP, and neurotensin have been described. The rapid delivery of glucose to the proximal small bowel seems to be involved in the mechanisms leading to peripheral and splanchnic vasodilatation and blood pooling and may also play a role in the vasomotor symptoms of early dumping.

Symptoms of late dumping are generally attributed to reactive hypoglycemia, although low glucose levels cannot always be documented, and symptoms often improve with glucose administration.

Although dumping syndrome is commonly described in adults following Nissen fundoplication and bariatric surgery,[116,117] it is a rare complication in children undergoing antireflux surgery.[118] Diagnosis is confirmed through the oral glucose tolerance test and gastric emptying study by scintigraphy.[119] High levels of HbA1C may be also found. The provocation tests that are commonly used to confirm the diagnosis of dumping syndrome and assess vagal integrity are considered safe and sensitive. In adults, a heart rate rise greater of 10 beats in the first hour following the ingestion of 50 g of oral glucose corroborates the diagnosis. The onset of delayed vasomotor symptoms confirms late phase dumping. Assessment of vagal integrity and nerve function can be obtained by noninvasive means by testing the pancreatic polypeptide (PP) response to a sham feeding.[120] An increase greater than 50% in the PP level within 30 minutes of sham feeding is a sensitive and specific indication of vagal integrity.[121]

The management of dumping syndrome relies on dietary measurements, medications, and surgical revision in refractory cases. Meals should be small, high in protein and fat content and low in carbohydrates. Liquid intake with the meals should be limited. The addition of uncooked starch has been proven to be beneficial in the management of dumping syndrome in children.[122] Viscosity of the meal can be increased by adding fiber. Treatment with octreotide is a promising alternative although side effects may limit chronic use.[123]

MEDICATIONS

The prokinetic agents most widely used to improve gastric motility include dopamine-2 receptor (D2) antagonists such as metoclopramide and domperidone, motilin agonists such as erythromycin, 5-HT4 receptor agonists such as tegaserod, and the mixed 5-HT4 receptor agonist and 5-HT3 receptor antagonist cisapride.

Metoclopramide

Metoclopramide is one of the most widely used antiemetic and prokinetic drugs. Large amounts of dopamine are present in the gastrointestinal wall. Dopamine binding to dopamine-1 (D1) and D2 receptors results in inhibition of motility, although there is also evidence of an interaction of dopamine with adrenoceptors.[124] Dopamine inhibits the release of acetylcholine from myenteric plexus motoneurons by binding to D2 receptors, leading to decreased lower esophageal sphincter and gastric tone, inhibition of antroduodenal coordination, decreased gastric emptying and intestinal peristalsis.[125]

Metoclopramide acts as a central and peripheral D2 receptor antagonist blocking the inhibitory effect of dopaminergic transmission. Metoclopramide increases the tone and amplitude of antral and intestinal contractions, relaxes the pyloric sphincter and duodenal bulb and reduces fundic relaxation. As a result, there is stimulation of gastrointestinal motility with acceleration of gastric emptying and small intestinal transit. Although its main effect is derived from its direct antidopaminergic properties, metoclopramide has the additional cholinergic effect of augmenting acetylcholine release from the myenteric plexus by affecting 5-HT synthesis or by acting on 5-HT4 receptors.[126] Its effect on serotonin elicits an additional effect on smooth muscle contractions.[127]

The effect of metoclopramide on central D2 receptors located in the area postrema is responsible for its antiemetic effect and may result in undesired extrapyramidal dystonic reactions. Metoclopramide inhibits dopamine transmission in the basal ganglia and has been linked with alarming extrapyramidal side effects including tardive dyskinesia as well as dystonic reactions that respond rapidly to the discontinuation of the drug.[128] Metoclopramide[129,130] and domperidone[131] are associated with QTc prolongation, life-threatening ventricular tachyarrhythmias such as torsade de pointes, and cardiac arrest. Subcutaneous administration of metoclopramide allows guaranteed absorption in patients with frequent vomiting.[132]

Domperidone

Domperidone is a peripheral D2 receptor antagonist with antiemetic and prokinetic properties with an effect on gastric and small intestinal smooth muscle motility. Animal studies have shown that intracerebroventricular injection of dopamine results in emesis, which can be abolished after ablation of the area postrema.[133] The main mechanism of domperidone is the blockade of D2 receptors in the chemoreceptor trigger zone at the area postrema located outside the blood brain barrier on the dorsal surface of the medulla oblongata.[134] A meta-analysis designed to determine the efficacy of domperidone in functional dyspepsia showed that it was effective in improving global assessment of symptoms, a less than optimal outcome measure.[135] A review of controlled clinical trials concluded that domperidone was superior to placebo in providing relief of

symptoms (anorexia, nausea, vomiting, abdominal pain, early satiety, bloating, distension) in patients with diabetic gastropathy.[136] A study of children with insulin-dependent diabetes demonstrated a significant benefit of domperidone when compared to cisapride in reducing gastric emptying time, normalizing gastric electrical activity and improving gastric dysrhythmia.[137] Domperidone does not easily cross the blood–brain barrier and therefore has a different side effect profile than metoclopramide. While all antidopaminergic prokinetic agents may result in hyperprolactinemia via their effect on the pituitary gland, located outside the blood–brain barrier, extrapyramidal dystonic reactions do not occur with drugs such as domperidone that are not able to cross the barrier. Both metoclopramide and domperidone have been used as galactogogues to aid in the initiation and maintenance of milk production.[138] Domperidone is not approved by the FDA for regular use in the United States but is available in most other countries.

Erythromycin

Motilin is a peptide hormone released by enteroendocrine cells of the gastrointestinal tract that amplifies and may induce antral phase III of the MMC resulting in peristalsis and facilitation of gastric emptying.[139] Erythromycin is a macrolide antibiotic that affects antral contractility by two mechanisms. It exerts an inotropic effect on specific smooth muscle motilin receptors[140] and a cholinergic chronotropic effect through neuronal motilin receptors.[141] The effects of erythromycin are variable and complex and include modification of the timing, duration, amplitude, and distribution of gastric MMC. Erythromycin administration improves gastric emptying and accelerates small bowel and colonic transit.[142] The gastrokinetic effect of erythromycin is characterized by the initiation and strengthening of gastric contractions in combination with pyloric relaxation.[143] A randomized, double-blinded, placebo-controlled trial has shown that oral erythromycin is safe and efficacious in preterm infants <35 weeks' gestation with feeding intolerance. The study demonstrated that erythromycin provided a significant benefit in decreasing time to full feeding,[144] the primary study outcome, without increasing episodes of sepsis, necrotizing enterocolitis, and cholestasis. However, the number of patients in the treatment group may have been too small to evaluate for less frequent complications. A study on the safety and efficacy of prolonged administration of intravenous erythromycin in an ambulatory setting conducted on adults with severe gastroparesis, refractory to oral prokinetics, showed that the regimen was feasible, well tolerated, and effective.[145] A study of 100 consecutive patients undergoing antroduodenal manometry reported a beneficial effect of infusing erythromycin 3 mg/kg intravenously over 1 hour, in order to facilitate the passage of a catheter through the pylorus into the duodenum.[146] A manometric study conducted in infants found that while the administration of low-dose erythromycin enhances gastric motor activity, higher doses induce continuous high amplitude contractions or motor quiescence 20 to 40 minutes after oral or intravenous administration.[147]

Two uncontrolled studies using erythromycin for prolonged postoperative ileus have been published. A case series study of 7 preterm infants with severe intestinal dysmotility established full enteral feeding within 2 weeks of commencing treatment with erythromycin.[148] A second study showed transition to full feeds within 3 weeks in 4 infants receiving prolonged parenteral nutrition for severe intestinal dysmotility following gastrointestinal surgery.[149] However, a multicenter, randomized, double-blind, placebo-controlled trial evaluating the progress after repair of gastroschisis in 32 infants receiving enteral erythromycin (3 mg/kg/dose 4 times daily) and 30 controls did not show a significant difference in duration of parenteral nutrition, incidence of catheter-related sepsis and time to discharge between the groups.[150] An uncontrolled trial of 24 children with cyclical vomiting has suggested that erythromycin may be beneficial in the treatment of this group of patients.[151]

Erythromycin also enhances fasting and postprandial proximal gastric tone by a mechanism unrelated to motilin.[152] Its effect on fundic tone, a pathophysiologic mechanism linked to dyspeptic symptoms, in combination with the occurrence of tachyphylaxis limits the efficacy of the drug for long-term use. Although the effect and safety of erythromycin has been established for both oral and intravenous administration, its prokinetic effect is more reliable when administered intravenously.[142] When used as a prokinetic agent, a lower dose seems to be necessary than when an antibiotic effect is pursued.

A causal role of erythromycin in the pathogenesis of infantile hypertrophic pyloric stenosis has been suggested.[153] Neonates receiving erythromycin seem to have a higher risk of developing pyloric stenosis than expected. Two clusters of cases of pyloric hypertrophy linked to erythromycin use have been reported in neonates. Five cases were reported in a naval hospital after erythromycin exposure of infants[154] and seven cases were reported in a community hospital among neonates who had received prophylactic erythromycin for possible exposure to whooping cough.[153] It was hypothesized that at large doses a marked increase in motility may result in hypertrophy of the pyloric muscle. There is debate regarding the possible association between prenatal maternal erythromycin exposures and increased risk of pyloric stenosis in infants.[155] A study of the Danish Birth Registry and the County's hospital discharge registry showed an association between breastfeeding mothers receiving macrolides and pyloric stenosis in infants based on an increased odds ratio (OR = 10.3) among female infants of mothers who used antibiotics in comparison with controls.[156] Erythromycin, has also been linked to the onset of torsade de pointes and other ventricular arrhythmias.[157] Some authors have cautioned against the use of antibiotics as prokinetic agents due to increasing problems with antibiotic-resistant bacteria in hospitals.[158]

Cisapride

Cisapride is a mixed 5-HT3 receptor antagonist and 5-HT4 receptor agonist compound with prokinetic effects throughout the entire gastrointestinal tract. Cisapride administration results in improvement of symptoms with a sustained long-term effect in patients with functional dyspepsia and gastroparesis.[159] A study assessing the possible benefits of using cisapride and domperidone in patients with dyspepsia determined that although both medications were effective in global assessment, cisapride was more efficacious than domperidone in relation to most of the symptoms evaluated.[135] A study of gastric emptying using MRI in patients with diabetic gastroparesis showed that cisapride accelerates liquid gastric emptying.[160] The role of cisapride on gastric sensitivity and accommodation is controversial.[161] A study evaluating gastric relaxation and volume with barostat technology showed that cisapride augments the perception of gastric distension and increases gastric relaxation in response to meal ingestion, prompting the authors to propose a propose role for cisapride in the treatment of patients with abnormal postprandial fundic relaxation.[108] Although, it is chemically related to metoclopramide, cisapride does not have central depressant or antidopaminergic effects.[159] Adverse effects related to the drug are generally transient, mild, and mostly related to its gastrointestinal effect, with abdominal cramping, borborygmi, and diarrhea being the most frequently reported symptoms.[159] Cisapride is not available for routine use in the United States because of rare toxicity from QTC prolongation, torsade de pointes, other ventricular arrhythmias, and sudden death.[162]

Octreotide

Octreotide is a long-acting somatostatin analogue that has proven to be an effective modulator of gastrointestinal function in children with dysmotility.[163] The effects of octreotide are complex due to its differential effects when administered after meals or during fasting and because changes in motility do not necessarily predict changes in transit. Subcutaneous injection of octreotide during fasting results in decreased antral motility and gallbladder contractility,[164] induction of intestinal phase III of the MMC and inhibition of phase II activity,[165] the latter explaining the delay in small bowel transit.[166] Overall, octreotide delays gastric emptying of liquids and has less predictable effects on total gut transit in both healthy volunteers and patients with dysmotility. Octreotide has shown to be beneficial in reducing bacterial overgrowth and abdominal symptoms in patients with scleroderma.[167] It may also be beneficial in patients with neuropathic CIPO, presenting with secretory diarrhea.[168] Because of its inhibitory effect on gastric motility, octreotide may be best used in children receiving jejunal feedings or in combination with erythromycin which may overcome the inhibition of gastric motility.[142] There is recent evidence that octreotide has hypoalgesic effects in patients with IBS.[169] Patients undergoing Nissen fundoplication may develop dumping syndrome partially characterized by hypoglycemia secondary to hypersecretion of insulin. An effect of somatostatin is to decrease the release of insulin and vasomotor hormones responsible of some of the systemic effects seen in dumping syndrome. Because it also delays gastric emptying, octreotide is an efficacious agent in individuals experiencing dumping syndrome. Potential side effects related to its use are hypoglycemia, diarrhea, steatorrhea, and gallstones.

Serotonergic Agents

Agonists and antagonists of 5-HT receptors are currently being used in the treatment of various FGID mostly due to their effects on the gut. Tegaserod is a peripherally acting partial 5-HT4 receptor agonist and potent 5-HT2B receptor antagonist[170] that differs chemically and in safety profile from other nonselective serotonergic agents, such as cisapride.[171] Tegaserod is indicated for the treatment of chronic constipation and constipation predominant IBS in adults. It elicits its prokinetic effect by activation of 5-HT4 receptors at similar[172] concentration that elicits its 5-HT2B effect.[170] Tegaserod increases gastric emptying and intestinal peristalsis and accelerates colonic transit.[173] Two randomized, placebo-controlled, double-blinded, studies reported that tegaserod significantly improved gastric emptying rate, small bowel and colonic transit after oral and intravenous administration, with the greatest effects being observed in the upper gastrointestinal tract.[174,175] Tegaserod's properties as a partial rather than a full agonist may potentially be protective against receptor desensitization and result in the maintenance of its pharmacological effect during prolonged treatment.[176] It is known that 5-HT may play a role in mediating sensations such as discomfort and pain.[177] However, the beneficial effect of tegaserod on visceral sensitivity is not completely understood, as it persists even after blocking 5-HT4 and 5-HT2B receptors.[178] In the gastric fundus, tegaserod inhibits the contractile response by its 5-HT2B receptor antagonist effects.[179] A barostat study using tegaserod showed that the compound enhanced fasting gastric compliance and allowed for larger intraballoon volumes both before and after a meal.[109] The combination of its prokinetic and gastric accommodation effects makes tegaserod a potentially beneficial drug in the treatment of dyspepsia. Tegaserod can be used safely in patients with mild to moderate hepatic or renal impairment,[180] has no electrocardiographic effects[181] and has no clinically relevant drug–drug interactions.[182] Thus, tegaserod constitutes a promising drug due its effects on both the upper and lower gastrointestinal tract and its reassuring safety record. The most commonly reported side effects are diarrhea and headaches. Tegaserod has not yet been approved by the FDA for use in children and is contraindicated in patients with hepatic and renal failure, biliary disease, or abdominal adhesions.

Much like tegaserod, 5-HT1 agonists such as the antianxiety agent buspirone[183] and sumatriptan,[184] used for treatment of migraine headache, also have an effect on fundic relaxation making them potentially useful drugs in the treatment of dyspepsia.

Others

Selective Serotonin Reuptake Inhibitors (SSRIs). Serotonin stimulates smooth muscle contractions by a direct effect on the muscle cells and indirectly by stimulating excitatory neurons of the enteric nervous system. Fluoxetine, an SSRI, affects gastric motility by increasing gastric contractions predominantly at the level of the fundus with less pronounced effect in the antrum and pylorus.[185] A controlled study of 16 healthy volunteers undergoing a gastric barostat study before and after pretreatment with paroxetine (another SSRI) or placebo showed that paroxetine significantly enhanced the amplitude of meal-induced fundic relaxation.[186] These findings suggest that the release of serotonin is involved in the accommodation reflex in humans and that SSRIs may be beneficial for improving symptoms in patients with impaired fundic relaxation. A retrospective review of patients receiving fluoxetine or paroxetine for depression revealed that patients did not develop significant gastrointestinal side effects, with the exception of loss of appetite in patients receiving paroxetine.[187] Insomnia and nausea are common side effects of SSRIs in children. Somnolence, a common side effect in adults, has been rarely reported in pediatrics.[188]

Tricyclic Antidepressants. Tricyclic antidepressants seem to be effective in improving abdominal pain and global symptoms in adults with FGIDs associated with pain (eg, IBS and functional dyspepsia). Although the mechanism of this benefit is unknown, a CNS action is suspected.[189] Tricyclic antidepressants have a mixed mechanism of action involving serotonin, norepinephrine, and dopamine pathways and elicit an anticholinergic effect. Amitriptyline inhibits antral contractility in response to electrical stimulation and acetylcholine release probably by an inhibitory effect on the smooth muscle.[190] Amitriptyline also reduces gastric acid secretion.[191]

Clonidine affects gastric fundus contractility probably by acting on alpha-2 receptors on cholinergic nerves resulting in reduction of acetylcholine release.[190] It has been shown to relax the stomach and reduce gastric sensation without inhibiting accommodation or emptying.[192] Clonidine also increases absorption and decreases intestinal motility providing an antidiarrheal effect,[193] but its use is limited by its antihypertensive action.

Botulinum neurotoxin binds irreversibly to presynaptic cholinergic nerve endings where it blocks acetylcholine release leading to paralysis of the muscle through functional denervation. Therapy with botulinum toxin is currently used in smooth muscles and sphincters, such as the lower esophageal sphincter to treat esophageal achalasia, the pylorus in patients with gastroparesis,[64] or the internal anal sphincter to treat anal achalasia[194] and anal fissures. However, its effects are transient, lasting only for a few months as the neuromuscular blockade of botulinum toxin is reversed by developing terminal axons that form new synapses. In order to achieve long-term effects, botulinum toxin must be injected at regular intervals.

REFERENCES

1. Griffith GH, Owen GM, Kirkman S, et al. Measurement of rate of gastric emptying using chromium-51. Lancet 1966;1:1244–5.
2. Chitkara DK, Delgado-Aros S, Bredenoord AJ, et al. Functional dyspepsia, upper gastrointestinal symptoms, and transit in children. J Pediatr 2003;143:609–13.
3. Camilleri M, Zinsmeister AR, Greydanus MP, et al. Towards a less costly but accurate test of gastric emptying and small bowel transit. Dig Dis Sci 1991;36:609–15.
4. Talley NJ, Locke GR 3rd, Lahr BD, et al. Functional dyspepsia, delayed gastric emptying, and impaired quality of life. Gut 2006;55:933–9.
5. Hyman PE, Napolitano JA, Diego A, et al. Antroduodenal manometry in the evaluation of chronic functional gastrointestinal symptoms. Pediatrics 1990;86:39–44.
6. Di Lorenzo C, Flores AF, Reddy SN, et al. Use of colonic manometry to differentiate causes of intractable constipation in children. J Pediatr 1992;120:690–5.
7. Pensabene L, Youssef NN, Griffiths JM, et al. Colonic manometry in children with defecatory disorders. Role in diagnosis and management. Am J Gastroenterol 2003;98:1052–7.
8. Milla P, Cucchiara S, DiLorenzo C, et al. Motility disorders in childhood: Working Group Report of the First World Congress of Pediatric Gastroenterology, Hepatology, and Nutrition. J Pediatr Gastroenterol Nutr 2002;35:S187–95.
9. Di Lorenzo C, Hillemeier C, Hyman P, et al. Manometry studies in children: Minimum standards for procedures. Neurogastroenterol Motil 2002;14:411–20.
10. Cucchiara S, Borrelli O, Salvia G, et al. A normal gastrointestinal motility excludes chronic intestinal pseudoobstruction in children. Dig Dis Sci 2000;45:258–64.
11. Camilleri M, Hasler WL, Parkman HP, et al. Measurement of gastrointestinal motility in the GI laboratory. Gastroenterology 1998;115:747–62.
12. Greydanus MP, Camilleri M, Colemont LJ, et al. Ileocolonic transfer of solid chyme in small intestinal neuropathies and myopathies. Gastroenterology 1990;99:158–64.
13. Sigurdsson L, Flores A, Putnam PE, et al. Postviral gastroparesis: Presentation, treatment, and outcome. J Pediatr 1997;131:751–4.
14. Jadcherla SR, Sty JR, Rudolph CD. Mechanical small bowel obstruction in premature infants diagnosed by intestinal manometry. J Pediatr Gastroenterol Nutr 2005;41:247–50.
15. Chitkara DK, Nurko S, Shoffner JM, et al. Abnormalities in gastrointestinal motility are associated with diseases of oxidative phosphorylation in children. Am J Gastroenterol 2003;98:871–7.
16. Weston S, Thumshirn M, Wiste J, et al. Clinical and upper gastrointestinal motility features in systemic sclerosis and related disorders. Am J Gastroenterol 1998;93:1085–9.
17. Goulet O, Jobert-Giraud A, Michel JL, et al. Chronic intestinal pseudo-obstruction syndrome in pediatric patients. Eur J Pediatr Surg 1999;9:83–9.
18. Hyman PE, McDiarmid SV, Napolitano J, et al. Antroduodenal motility in children with chronic intestinal pseudo-obstruction. J Pediatr 1988;112:899–905.
19. Connor FL, Di Lorenzo C. Chronic intestinal pseudo-obstruction: Assessment and management. Gastroenterology 2006;130:S29–36.
20. Amarnath RP, Abell TL, Malagelada JR. The rumination syndrome in adults. A characteristic manometric pattern. Ann Intern Med 1986;105:513–8.
21. Tomomasa T, DiLorenzo C, Morikawa A, et al. Analysis of fasting antroduodenal manometry in children. Dig Dis Sci 1996;41:2195–203.
22. Hyman PE, Di Lorenzo C, McAdams L, et al. Predicting the clinical response to cisapride in children with chronic intestinal pseudo-obstruction. Am J Gastroenterol 1993;88:832–6.
23. Bromer MQ, Kantor SB, Wagner DA, et al. Simultaneous measurement of gastric emptying with a simple muffin meal using [13C]octanoate breath test and scintigraphy in normal subjects and patients with dyspeptic symptoms. Dig Dis Sci 2002;47:1657–63.
24. Precioso AR, Pereira GR, Vaz FA. Gastric myoelectrical activity in neonates of different gestational ages by means of electrogastrography. Rev Hosp Clin Fac Med Sao Paulo 2003;58:81–90.
25. Jonderko K, Kasicka-Jonderko A, Krusiec-Swidergol B, et al. How reproducible is cutaneous electrogastrography? An in-depth evidence-based study. Neurogastroenterol Motil 2005;17:800–9.
26. Di Lorenzo C. EGG like EKG: Are we there yet? J Pediatr Gastroenterol Nutr 2000;30:134–6.
27. Barbar M, Steffen R, Wyllie R, et al. Electrogastrography versus gastric emptying scintigraphy in children with symptoms suggestive of gastric motility disorders. J Pediatr Gastroenterol Nutr 2000;30:193–7.
28. Simonian HP, Maurer AH, Knight LC, et al. Simultaneous assessment of gastric accommodation and emptying: Studies with liquid and solid meals. J Nucl Med 2004;45:1155–60.
29. Bouras EP, Delgado-Aros S, Camilleri M, et al. SPECT imaging of the stomach: Comparison with barostat, and effects of sex, age, body mass index, and fundoplication. Single photon emission computed tomography. Gut 2002;51:781–6.
30. van den Elzen BD, Bennink RJ, Wieringa RE, et al. Fundic accommodation assessed by SPECT scanning: Comparison with the gastric barostat. Gut 2003;52:1548–54.
31. Chitkara DK, Camilleri M, Zinsmeister AR, et al. Gastric sensory and motor dysfunction in adolescents with functional dyspepsia. J Pediatr 2005;146:500–5.
32. Jones MP, Hoffman S, Shah D, et al. The water load test: Observations from healthy controls and patients with functional dyspepsia. Am J Physiol Gastrointest Liver Physiol 2003;284:G896–904.
33. Sood MR, Schwankovsky LM, Rowhani A, et al. Water load test in children. J Pediatr Gastroenterol Nutr 2002;35:199–201.
34. Boeckxstaens G, Hirsch D, Berkhout B, et al. Is a drink test a valuable tool to study proximal function? Gastroenterology 1999;116:A960.
35. Walker LS, Williams SE, Smith CA, et al. Validation of a symptom provocation test for laboratory studies of abdominal pain and discomfort in children and adolescents. J Pediatr Psychol 2006;31:70–71.
36. Kuo B, McCallum R, Kock K, et al. Smarpill, a novel ambulatory diagnostic test for measuring gastric emptying in health and disease. Gastroenterology 2006;130:A434.
37. Gomes H, Hornoy P, Liehn JC. Ultrasonography and gastric emptying in children: Validation of a sonographic method and determination of physiological and pathological patterns. Pediatr Radiol 2003;33:522–9.
38. Schwizer W, Fraser R, Borovicka J, et al. Measurement of gastric emptying and gastric motility by magnetic resonance imaging (MRI). Dig Dis Sci 1994;39:101S–3S.
39. Collins CE, Francis JL, Thomas P, et al. Gastric emptying time is faster in cystic fibrosis. J Pediatr Gastroenterol Nutr 1997;25:492–8.
40. Jamieson GG, Maddern GJ, Myers JC. Gastric emptying after fundoplication with and without proximal gastric vagotomy. Arch Surg 1991;126:1414–7.
41. Pardi DS, Miller SM, Miller DL, et al. Paraneoplastic dysmotility: Loss of interstitial cells of Cajal. Am J Gastroenterol 2002;97:1828–33.
42. Camilleri M, Bharucha AE. Gastrointestinal dysfunction in neurologic disease. Semin Neurol 1996;16:203–16.
43. Clanton LJ, Jr, Bender J. Refractory spinal cord injury induced gastroparesis: Resolution with erythromycin lactobionate, a case report. J Spinal Cord Med 1999;22:236–8.
44. Ravelli AM, Tobanelli P, Volpi S, et al. Vomiting and gastric motility in infants with cow's milk allergy. J Pediatr Gastroenterol Nutr 2001;32:59–64.
45. Garzi A, Messina M, Frati F, et al. An extensively hydrolysed cow's milk formula improves clinical symptoms of gastroesophageal reflux and reduces the gastric emptying time in infants. Allergol Immunopathol (Madr) 2002;30:36–41.
46. Ravelli AM, Milla PJ. Vomiting and gastroesophageal motor activity in children with disorders of the central nervous system. J Pediatr Gastroenterol Nutr 1998;26:56–63.
47. Fone DR, Horowitz M, Maddox A, et al. Gastroduodenal motility during the delayed gastric emptying induced by cold stress. Gastroenterology 1990;98:1155–61.
48. Mistiaen W, Blockx P, Van Hee R, et al. The effect of stress on gastric emptying rate measured with a radionuclide tracer. Hepatogastroenterology 2002;49:1457–60.

49. Lee C, Sarna SK. Central regulation of gastric emptying of solid nutrient meals by corticotropin releasing factor. Neurogastroenterol Motil 1997;9:221–9.

50. Spinks AB, Wasiak J, Villanueva EV, et al. Scopolamine for preventing and treating motion sickness. Cochrane Database Syst Rev 2004:CD002851.

51. Holland MS. Central anticholinergic syndrome in a pediatric patient following transdermal scopolamine patch placement. Nurse Anesth 1992;3:121–4.

52. Mason RJ, Lipham J, Eckerling G, et al. Gastric electrical stimulation: An alternative surgical therapy for patients with gastroparesis. Arch Surg 2005;140:841–6.

53. Chen J, Lin Z, Edmunds M, et al. Optimization of electrical stimulation and its effects on gastric myoelectrical activitie in humans. Gastroenterology 1995;108:A582.

54. Bellahsene BE, Lind CD, Schirmer BD, et al. Acceleration of gastric emptying with electrical stimulation in a canine model of gastroparesis. Am J Physiol 1992;262:G826–34.

55. Sarna SK, Bowes KL, Daniel EE. Gastric pacemakers. Gastroenterology 1976;70:226–31.

56. Abell TL, Minocha A. Gastroparesis and the gastric pacemaker: A revolutionary treatment for an old disease. J Miss State Med Assoc 2002;43:369–75.

57. Liu J, Hou X, Song G, et al. Gastric electrical stimulation using endoscopically placed mucosal electrodes reduces food intake in humans. Am J Gastroenterol 2006;101:798–803.

58. Ayinala S, Batista O, Goyal A, et al. Temporary gastric electrical stimulation with orally or PEG-placed electrodes in patients with drug refractory gastroparesis. Gastrointest Endosc 2005;61:455–61.

59. Yang M, Fang DC, Li QW, et al. Effects of gastric pacing on gastric emptying and plasma motilin. World J Gastroenterol 2004;10:419–23.

60. de Csepel J, Goldfarb B, Shapsis A, et al. Electrical stimulation for gastroparesis. Gastric motility restored. Surg Endosc 2006;20:302–6.

61. Abell T, McCallum R, Hocking M, et al. Gastric electrical stimulation for medically refractory gastroparesis. Gastroenterology 2003;125:421–8.

62. Lin Z, Sarosiek I, Forster J, et al. Symptom responses, long-term outcomes and adverse events beyond 3 years of high-frequency gastric electrical stimulation for gastroparesis. Neurogastroenterol Motil 2006;18:18–27.

63. Becker JC, Dietl KH, Konturek JW, et al. Gastric wall perforation: A rare complication of gastric electrical stimulation. Gastrointest Endosc 2004;59:584–6.

64. James AN, Ryan JP, Parkman HP. Inhibitory effects of botulinum toxin on pyloric and antral smooth muscle. Am J Physiol Gastrointest Liver Physiol 2003;285:G291–7.

65. Bromer MQ, Friedenberg F, Miller LS, et al. Endoscopic pyloric injection of botulinum toxin A for the treatment of refractory gastroparesis. Gastrointest Endosc 2005;61:833–9.

66. Miller LS, Szych GA, Kantor SB, et al. Treatment of idiopathic gastroparesis with injection of botulinum toxin into the pyloric sphincter muscle. Am J Gastroenterol 2002;97:1653–60.

67. Lacy BE, Zayat EN, Crowell MD, et al. Botulinum toxin for the treatment of gastroparesis: A preliminary report. Am J Gastroenterol 2002;97:1548–52.

68. Woodward MN, Spicer RD. Intrapyloric botulinum toxin injection improves gastric emptying. J Pediatr Gastroenterol Nutr 2003;37:201–2.

69. Chang CS, Ko CW, Wu CY, et al. Effect of electrical stimulation on acupuncture points in diabetic patients with gastric dysrhythmia: A pilot study. Digestion 2001;64:184–90.

70. Watkins PJ, Buxton-Thomas MS, Howard ER. Long-term outcome after gastrectomy for intractable diabetic gastroparesis. Diabet Med 2003;20:58–63.

71. Jones MP, Maganti K. A systematic review of surgical therapy for gastroparesis. Am J Gastroenterol 2003;98:2122–9.

72. O'Brien MD, Bruce BK, Camilleri M. The rumination syndrome: Clinical features rather than manometric diagnosis. Gastroenterology 1995;108:1024–9.

73. Hyman PE, Milla PJ, Benninga MA, et al. Childhood functional gastrointestinal disorders: Neonate/toddler. Gastroenterology 2006;130:1519–26.

74. Whitehead WE, Drescher VM, Morrill-Corbin E, et al. Rumination syndrome in children treated by increased holding. J Pediatr Gastroenterol Nutr 1985;4:550–6.

75. Rasquin A, Di Lorenzo C, Forbes D, et al. Childhood functional gastrointestinal disorders: Child/adolescent. Gastroenterology 2006;130:1527–37.

76. Khan S, Hyman PE, Cocjin J, et al. Rumination syndrome in adolescents. J Pediatr 2000;136:528–31.

77. Chial HJ, Camilleri M, Williams DE, et al. Rumination syndrome in children and adolescents: Diagnosis, treatment, and prognosis. Pediatrics 2003;111:158–62.

78. Olden KW. Rumination. Curr Treat Options Gastroenterol 2001;4:351–8.

79. Thumshirn M, Camilleri M, Hanson RB, et al. Gastric mechanosensory and lower esophageal sphincter function in rumination syndrome. Am J Physiol 1998;275:G314–21.

80. Mestre JR, Resnick RJ, Berman WF. Behavior modification in the treatment of rumination. Clin Pediatr (Phila) 1983;22:488–91.

81. Tack J, Talley NJ, Camilleri M, et al. Functional gastroduodenal disorders. Gastroenterology 2006;130:1466–79.

82. Quartero AO, de Wit NJ, Lodder AC, et al. Disturbed solid-phase gastric emptying in functional dyspepsia: A meta-analysis. Dig Dis Sci 1998;43:2028–33.

83. Tack J, Piessevaux H, Coulie B, et al. Role of impaired gastric accommodation to a meal in functional dyspepsia. Gastroenterology 1998;115:1346–52.

84. Mertz H, Fullerton S, Naliboff B, et al. Symptoms and visceral perception in severe functional and organic dyspepsia. Gut 1998;42:814–22.

85. Hausken T, Gilja OH, Undeland KA, et al. Timing of postprandial dyspeptic symptoms and transpyloric passage of gastric contents. Scand J Gastroenterol 1998;33:822–7.

86. Samsom M, Verhagen MA, vanBerge Henegouwen GP, et al. Abnormal clearance of exogenous acid and increased acid sensitivity of the proximal duodenum in dyspeptic patients. Gastroenterology 1999;116:515–20.

87. Lorena SL, Figueiredo MJ, Almeida JR, et al. Autonomic function in patients with functional dyspepsia assessed by 24-hour heart rate variability. Dig Dis Sci 2002;47:27–31.

88. Sykora J, Malan A, Zahlava J, et al. Gastric emptying of solids in children with H. pylori-positive and H. pylori-negative non-ulcer dyspepsia. J Pediatr Gastroenterol Nutr 2004;39:246–52.

89. Chen TS, Lee YC, Chang FY, et al. Psychosocial distress is associated with abnormal gastric myoelectrical activity in patients with functional dyspepsia. Scand J Gastroenterol 2006;41:791–6.

90. Delgado-Aros S, Camilleri M, Cremonini F, et al. Contributions of gastric volumes and gastric emptying to meal size and postmeal symptoms in functional dyspepsia. Gastroenterology 2004;127:1685–94.

91. Riezzo G, Chiloiro M, Guerra V, et al. Comparison of gastric electrical activity and gastric emptying in healthy and dyspeptic children. Dig Dis Sci 2000;45:517–24.

92. Cucchiara S, Riezzo G, Minella R, et al. Electrogastrography in non-ulcer dyspepsia. Arch Dis Child 1992;67:613–7.

93. Di Lorenzo C, Hyman PE, Flores AF, et al. Antroduodenal manometry in children and adults with severe non-ulcer dyspepsia. Scand J Gastroenterol 1994;29:799–806.

94. Stanghellini V, Tosetti C, Paternicó A, et al. Risk indicators of delayed gastric emptying of solids in patients with functional dyspepsia. Gastroenterology 1996;110:1036–42.

95. Bouin M, Lupien F, Riberdy-Poitras M, et al. Tolerance to gastric distension in patients with functional dyspepsia: Modulation by a cholinergic and nitrergic method. Eur J Gastroenterol Hepatol 2006;18:63–8.

96. Cucchiara S, Minella R, Iorio R, et al. Real-time ultrasound reveals gastric motor abnormalities in children investigated for dyspeptic symptoms. J Pediatr Gastroenterol Nutr 1995;21:446–53.

97. Soo S, Moayyedi P, Deeks J, et al. Psychological interventions for non-ulcer dyspepsia. Cochrane Database Syst Rev 2005:CD002301.

98. Jones MP, Maganti K. Symptoms, gastric function, and psychosocial factors in functional dyspepsia. J Clin Gastroenterol 2004;38:866–72.

99. Caballero-Plasencia AM, Valenzuela-Barranco M, Herrerias-Gutierrez JM, et al. Altered gastric emptying in patients with irritable bowel syndrome. Eur J Nucl Med 1999;26:404–9.

100. Haque M, Wyeth JW, Stace NH, et al. Prevalence, severity and associated features of gastroesophageal reflux and dyspepsia: A population-based study. N Z Med J 2000;113:178–81.

101. di Mario F, Stefani N, Bo ND, et al. Natural course of functional dyspepsia after Helicobacter pylori eradication: A seven-year survey. Dig Dis Sci 2005;50:2286–95.

102. Hyams JS, Davis P, Sylvester FA, et al. Dyspepsia in children and adolescents: A prospective study. J Pediatr Gastroenterol Nutr 2000;30:413–8.

103. Ozen A, Ertem D, Pehlivanoglu E. Natural history and symptomatology of Helicobacter pylori in childhood and factors determining the epidemiology of infection. J Pediatr Gastroenterol Nutr 2006;42:398–404.

104. Farrell S, Milliken I, Murphy JL, et al. Nonulcer dyspepsia and Helicobacter pylori eradication in children. J Pediatr Surg 2005;40:1547–50.

105. Di Lorenzo C, Colletti RB, Lehmann HP, et al. Chronic abdominal pain in children: A technical report of the American Academy of Pediatrics and the North American Society for Pediatric Gastroenterology, Hepatology and Nutrition. J Pediatr Gastroenterol Nutr 2005;40:249–61.

106. See MC, Birnbaum AH, Schechter CB, et al. Double-blind, placebo-controlled trial of famotidine in children with abdominal pain and dyspepsia: Global and quantitative assessment. Dig Dis Sci 2001;46:985–92.

107. Talley NJ, Vakil N. Guidelines for the management of dyspepsia. Am J Gastroenterol 2005;100:2324–37.

108. Tack J, Broeckaert D, Coulie B, et al. The influence of cisapride on gastric tone and the perception of gastric distension. Aliment Pharmacol Ther 1998;12:761–6.

109. Tack J, Vos R, Janssens J, et al. Influence of tegaserod on proximal gastric tone and on the perception of gastric distension. Aliment Pharmacol Ther 2003;18:1031–7.

110. Malatesta MG, Fascetti E, Ciccaglione AF, et al. 5-HT1-receptor agonist sumatriptan modifies gastric size after 500 ml of water in dyspeptic patients and normal subjects. Dig Dis Sci 2002;47:2591–5.

111. Saad R, Chey W. Review article: Current and emerging therapies for funcational dyspepsia. Aliment Pharmacol Ther 2006;24:475–92.

112. Mousa H, Hyman PE, Cocjin J, et al. Long-term outcome of congenital intestinal pseudoobstruction. Dig Dis Sci 2002;47:2298–305.

113. Hyman PE. Chronic intestinal pseudo-obstruction in childhood: Progress in diagnosis and treatment. Scand J Gastroenterol Suppl 1995;213:39–46.

114. Debinski HS, Ahmed S, Milla PJ, et al. Electrogastrography in chronic intestinal pseudoobstruction. Dig Dis Sci 1996;41:1292–7.

115. Ginies JL, Francois H, Joseph MG, et al. A curable cause of chronic idiopathic intestinal pseudo-obstruction in children: Idiopathic myositis of the small intestine. J Pediatr Gastroenterol Nutr 1996;23:426–9.

116. Ukleja A. Dumping syndrome: Pathophysiology and treatment. Nutr Clin Pract 2005;20:517–25.

117. Abell TL, Minocha A. Gastrointestinal complications of bariatric surgery: Diagnosis and therapy. Am J Med Sci 2006;331:214–8.

118. Gilger MA, Yeh C, Chiang J, et al. Outcomes of surgical fundoplication in children. Clin Gastroenterol Hepatol 2004;2:978–84.

119. Samuk I, Afriat R, Horne T, et al. Dumping syndrome following Nissen fundoplication, diagnosis, and treatment. J Pediatr Gastroenterol Nutr 1996;23:235–40.

120. Taylor IL, Feldman M, Richardson CT, et al. Gastric and cephalic stimulation of human pancreatic polypeptide release. Gastroenterology 1978;75:432–7.

121. Balaji NS, Crookes PF, Banki F, et al. A safe and non-invasive test for vagal integrity revisited. Arch Surg 2002;137:954–8. discussion 8–9.

122. Borovoy J, Furuta L, Nurko S. Benefit of uncooked cornstarch in the management of children with dumping syndrome fed exclusively by gastrostomy. Am J Gastroenterol 1998;93:814–8.

123. Vecht J, Lamers CB, Masclee AA. Long-term results of octreotide-therapy in severe dumping syndrome. Clin Endocrinol (Oxf) 1999;51:619–24.

124. Tonini M, Cipollina L, Poluzzi E, et al. Review article: Clinical implications of enteric and central D2 receptor blockade by antidopaminergic gastrointestinal prokinetics. Aliment Pharmacol Ther 2004;19:379–90.

125. Pasricha P. Treatment of disorders of bowel motility and water flux; antiemetics; agents used in biliary and pancreatic disease. In: Goodman L, Gilman A, Burunton L, et al, editors. Goodman & Gilman's The Pharmacological Basis of Therapeutics, 11th edition. New York: McGraw-Hill, 2006; pp. 983–1008.

126. Clayton NM, Gale JD. 5-HT4 receptors are not involved in the control of small intestinal transit in the fasted conscious rat. Neurogastroenterol Motil 1996;8:1–8.

127. Kilbinger H, Pfeuffer-Friederich I. Two types of receptors for 5-hydroxytryptamine on the cholinergic nerves of the guinea-pig myenteric plexus. Br J Pharmacol 1985;85:529–39.

128. Pinder RM, Brogden RN, Sawyer PR, et al. Metoclopramide: A review of its pharmacological properties and clinical use. Drugs 1976;12:81–131.

129. Bentsen G, Stubhaug A. Cardiac arrest after intravenous metoclopramide—a case of five repeated injections of metoclopramide causing five episodes of cardiac arrest. Acta Anaesthesiol Scand 2002;46:908–10.

130. Ellidokuz E, Kaya D. The effect of metoclopramide on QT dynamicity: Double-blind, placebo-controlled, cross-over study in healthy male volunteers. Aliment Pharmacol Ther 2003;18:151–5.

131. Drolet B, Rousseau G, Daleau P, et al. Domperidone should not be considered a no-risk alternative to cisapride in the treatment of gastrointestinal motility disorders. Circulation 2000;102:1883–5.

132. Bruera E, Seifert L, Watanabe S, et al. Chronic nausea in advanced cancer patients: A retrospective assessment of a

metoclopramide-based antiemetic regimen. J Pain Symptom Manage 1996;11:147–53.

133. Yoshikawa T, Yoshida N, Hosoki K. Involvement of dopamine D3 receptors in the area postrema in R(+)-7-OH-DPAT-induced emesis in the ferret. Eur J Pharmacol 1996;301:143–9.

134. Brogden RN, Carmine AA, Heel RC, et al. Domperidone. A review of its pharmacological activity, pharmacokinetics and therapeutic efficacy in the symptomatic treatment of chronic dyspepsia and as an antiemetic. Drugs 1982;24:360–400.

135. Veldhuyzen van Zanten SJ, Jones MJ, Verlinden M, et al. Efficacy of cisapride and domperidone in functional (non-ulcer) dyspepsia: A meta-analysis. Am J Gastroenterol 2001;96:689–96.

136. Silvers D, Kipnes M, Broadstone V, et al. Domperidone in the management of symptoms of diabetic gastroparesis: Efficacy, tolerability, and quality-of-life outcomes in a multicenter controlled trial. DOM-USA-5 Study Group. Clin Ther 1998;20:438–53.

137. Franzese A, Borrelli O, Corrado G, et al. Domperidone is more effective than cisapride in children with diabetic gastroparesis. Aliment Pharmacol Ther 2002;16:951–7.

138. Gabay MP. Galactogogues: Medications that induce lactation. J Hum Lact 2002;18:274–9.

139. Luiking YC, Akkermans LM, Peeters TL, et al. Effects of motilin on human interdigestive gastrointestinal and gallbladder motility, and involvement of 5HT3 receptors. Neurogastroenterol Motil 2002;14:151–9.

140. Peeters T, Matthijs G, Depoortere I, et al. Erythromycin is a motilin receptor agonist. Am J Physiol 1989;257:G470–4.

141. Parkman HP, Pagano AP, Vozzelli MA, et al. Gastrokinetic effects of erythromycin: Myogenic and neurogenic mechanisms of action in rabbit stomach. Am J Physiol 1995;269: G418–26.

142. Di Lorenzo C, Lucanto C, Flores AF, et al. Effect of sequential erythromycin and octreotide on antroduodenal manometry. J Pediatr Gastroenterol Nutr 1999;29:293–6.

143. Nakabayashi T, Mochiki E, Kamiyama Y, et al. Erythromycin induces pyloric relaxation accompanied by a contraction of the gastric body after pylorus-preserving gastrectomy. Surgery 2003;133:647–55.

144. Nuntnarumit P, Kiatchoosakun P, Tantiprapa W, et al. Efficacy of oral erythromycin for treatment of feeding intolerance in preterm infants. J Pediatr 2006;148:600–5.

145. DiBaise JK, Quigley EM. Efficacy of prolonged administration of intravenous erythromycin in an ambulatory setting as treatment of severe gastroparesis: One center's experience. J Clin Gastroenterol 1999;28:131–4.

146. Di Lorenzo C, Lachman R, Hyman PE. Intravenous erythromycin for postpyloric intubation. J Pediatr Gastroenterol Nutr 1990;11:45–7.

147. Jadcherla SR, Klee G, Berseth CL. Regulation of migrating motor complexes by motilin and pancreatic polypeptide in human infants. Pediatr Res 1997;42:365–9.

148. Ng PC, Fok TF, Lee CH, et al. Erythromycin treatment for gastrointestinal dysmotility in preterm infants. J Paediatr Child Health 1997;33:148–50.

149. Simkiss DE, Adams IP, Myrdal U, et al. Erythromycin in neonatal postoperative intestinal dysmotility. Arch Dis Child 1994;71:F128–9.

150. Curry JI, Lander AD, Stringer MD. A multicenter, randomized, double-blind, placebo-controlled trial of the prokinetic agent erythromycin in the postoperative recovery of infants with gastroschisis. J Pediatr Surg 2004;39:565–9.

151. Vanderhoof JA, Young R, Kaufman SS, et al. Treatment of cyclic vomiting in childhood with erythromycin. J Pediatr Gastroenterol Nutr 1995;21:S60–2.

152. Bruley des Varannes S, Parys V, Ropert A, et al. Erythromycin enhances fasting and postprandial proximal gastric tone in humans. Gastroenterology 1995;109:32–9.

153. Honein MA, Paulozzi LJ, Himelright IM, et al. Infantile hypertrophic pyloric stenosis after pertussis prophylaxis with erythromycin: A case review and cohort study. Lancet 1999;354:2101–5.

154. SanFilippo A. Infantile hypertrophic pyloric stenosis related to ingestion of erythromycine estolate: A report of five cases. J Pediatr Surg 1976;11:177–80.

155. MacMahon B. The continuing enigma of pyloric stenosis of infancy: A review. Epidemiology 2006;17:195–201.

156. Sorensen HT, Skriver MV, Pedersen L, et al. Risk of infantile hypertrophic pyloric stenosis after maternal postnatal use of macrolides. Scand J Infect Dis 2003;35:104–6.

157. Kdesh A, McPherson CA, Yaylali Y, et al. Effect of erythromycin on myocardial repolarization in patients with community-acquired pneumonia. South Med J 1999;92:1178–82.

158. Dall'antonia M, Wilks M, Coen PG, et al. Erythromycin for prokinesis: Imprudent prescribing? Crit Care 2005;10:112.

159. Wiseman LR, Faulds D. Cisapride. An updated review of its pharmacology and therapeutic efficacy as a prokinetic agent in gastrointestinal motility disorders. Drugs 1994;47:116–52.

160. Borovicka J, Lehmann R, Kunz P, et al. Evaluation of gastric emptying and motility in diabetic gastroparesis with magnetic resonance imaging: Effects of cisapride. Am J Gastroenterol 1999;94:2866–73.

161. Manes G, Dominguez-Munoz JE, Leodolter A, et al. Effect of cisapride on gastric sensitivity to distension, gastric compliance and duodeno-gastric reflexes in healthy humans. Dig Liver Dis 2001;33:407–13.

162. Benatar A, Feenstra A, Decraene T, et al. Cisapride plasma levels and corrected QT interval in infants undergoing routine polysomnography. J Pediatr Gastroenterol Nutr 2001;33:41–6.

163. Di Lorenzo C, Lucanto C, Flores AF, et al. Effect of octreotide on gastrointestinal motility in children with functional gastrointestinal symptoms. J Pediatr Gastroenterol Nutr 1998;27:508–12.

164. Londong W, Angerer M, Kutz K, et al. Diminishing efficacy of octreotide (SMS 201–995) on gastric functions of healthy subjects during one-week administration. Gastroenterology 1989;96:713–22.

165. Peeters TL, Romanski KW, Janssens J, et al. Effect of the long-acting somatostatin analogue SMS 201–995 on small-intestinal interdigestive motility in the dog. Scand J Gastroenterol 1988;23:769–74.

166. von der Ohe MR, Camilleri M, Thomforde GM, et al. Differential regional effects of octreotide on human gastrointestinal motor function. Gut 1995;36:743–8.

167. Soudah HC, Hasler WL, Owyang C. Effect of octreotide on intestinal motility and bacterial overgrowth in scleroderma. N Engl J Med 1991;325:1461–7.

168. Panganamamula KV, Parkman HP. Chronic intestinal pseudo-obstruction. Curr Treat Options Gastroenterol 2005;8:3–11.

169. Bradette M, Delvaux M, Staumont G, et al. Octreotide increases thresholds of colonic visceral perception in IBS patients without modifying muscle tone. Dig Dis Sci 1994;39:1171–8.

170. Beattie DT, Smith JA, Marquess D, et al. The 5-HT4 receptor agonist, tegaserod, is a potent 5-HT2B receptor antagonist in vitro and in vivo. Br J Pharmacol 2004;143:549–60.

171. Roberts DJ, Banh HL, Hall RI. Use of novel prokinetic agents to facilitate return of gastrointestinal motility in adult critically ill patients. Curr Opin Crit Care 2006;12: 295–302.

172. Crowell M, Mathis C, Schettler V, et al. The effects of tegaserod, a 5-HT receptor agonist, on gastric emptying in a murine model of diabetes mellitus. Neurogastroenterol Motil 2005;17:138–743.

173. Hansen MB. Neurohumoral control of gastrointestinal motility. Physiol Res 2003;52:1–30.

174. Degen L, Matzinger D, Merz M, et al. Tegaserod, a 5-HT4 receptor partial agonist, accelerates gastric emptying and gastrointestinal transit in healthy male subjects. Aliment Pharmacol Ther 2001;15:1745–51.

175. Degen L, Petrig C, Studer D, et al. Effect of tegaserod on gut transit in male and female subjects. Neurogastroenterol Motil 2005;17:821–6.

176. Galligan JJ, Vanner S. Basic and clinical pharmacology of new motility promoting agents. Neurogastroenterol Motil 2005;17:643–53.

177. Kirkup AJ, Brunsden AM, Grundy D. Receptors and transmission in the brain-gut axis: Potential for novel therapies. I. Receptors on visceral afferents. Am J Physiol Gastrointest Liver Physiol 2001;280:G787–94.

178. Grundy D. 5-HT receptors and visceral hypersensitivity—2B or not 2B, that is the question? Neurogastroenterol Motil 2006;18:339–42.

179. McCullough JL, Armstrong SR, Hegde SS, et al. The 5-HT2B antagonist and 5-HT4 agonist activities of tegaserod in the anaesthetized rat. Pharmacol Res 2006;53:353–8.

180. Swan SK, Zhou H, Horowitz A, et al. Tegaserod pharmacokinetics are similar in patients with severe renal insufficiency and in healthy subjects. J Clin Pharmacol 2003; 43:359–64.

181. Morganroth J, Ruegg PC, Dunger-Baldauf C, et al. Tegaserod, a 5-hydroxytryptamine type 4 receptor partial agonist, is devoid of electrocardiographic effects. Am J Gastroenterol 2002;97:2321–7.

182. Appel-Dingemanse S. Clinical pharmacokinetics of tegaserod, a serotonin 5-HT(4) receptor partial agonist with promotile activity. Clin Pharmacokinet 2002;41:1021–42.

183. Tack J. Functional dyspepsia: Impaired fundic accommodation. Curr Treat Options Gastroenterol 2000;3:287–94.

184. Sarnelli G, Janssens J, Tack J. Effect of intranasal sumatriptan on gastric tone and sensitivity to distension. Dig Dis Sci 2001;46:1591–5.

185. James AN, Ryan JP, Parkman HP. Effects of the selective serotonin reuptake inhibitor, fluoxetine, on regional gastric contractility. Neurogastroenterol Motil 2005;17:76–82.

186. Tack J, Broekaert D, Coulie B, et al. Influence of the selective serotonin re-uptake inhibitor, paroxetine, on gastric sensorimotor function in humans. Aliment Pharmacol Ther 2003;17:603–8.

187. Linden RD, Wilcox CS, Heiser JF, et al. Are selective serotonin reuptake inhibitors well tolerated in somatizing depressives? Psychopharmacol Bull 1994;30:151–6.

188. Safer DJ, Zito JM. Treatment-emergent adverse events from selective serotonin reuptake inhibitors by age group: Children versus adolescents. J Child Adolesc Psychopharmacol 2006;16:159–69.

189. Morgan V, Pickens D, Gautam S, et al. Amitriptyline reduces rectal pain related activation of the anterior cingulate cortex in patients with irritable bowel syndrome. Gut 2005;54:601–7.

190. James AN, Ryan JP, Parkman HP. Effects of clonidine and tricyclic antidepressants on gastric smooth muscle contractility. Neurogastroenterol Motil 2004;16:143–53.

191. Sen T, Abdulsalam CA, Pal S, et al. Effect of amitriptyline on gastric ulceration. Fundam Clin Pharmacol 2002;16:311–5.

192. Thumshirn M, Camilleri M, Choi MG, et al. Modulation of gastric sensory and motor functions by nitrergic and alpha2-adrenergic agents in humans. Gastroenterology 1999;116:573–85.

193. Schiller LR, Santa Ana CA, Morawski SG, et al. Studies of the antidiarrheal action of clonidine. Effects on motility and intestinal absorption. Gastroenterology 1985;89:982–8.

194. Ciamarra P, Nurko S, Barksdale E, et al. Internal anal sphincter achalasia in children: Clinical characteristics and treatment with *Clostridium botulinum* toxin. J Pediatr Gastroenterol Nutr 2003;37:315–9.

12

Anatomy and Embryology

Pascal de Santa Barbara, PhD

ANATOMY

The intestines are a vital and specialized organ characterized by its exceptional length and its morphological and functional rostro–caudal regionalization. The intestines are located into the body wall and can be separated in two regions: the small intestine and the colon. The main functions ensured by the intestines are the absorption of nutriment and water, the immune defense, the transit of the feces, and their elimination. Histologically, the intestines present the same tissue layer organization and their differences are mainly observed in the mucosa (Figure 1).

Organization of the Intestine

The intestines can be divided into four different functional layers from innermost to outermost layers: the mucosa, the submucosa, the muscularis propria, and the adventitia.[2] Closest to the lumen, the mucosa is made up with the epithelium, a supporting lamina propria and a thin smooth muscle layer, the muscularis mucosae. The main differences between the small intestine and the colon are present in this layer. In the small intestine, the mucosal surface forms the villi that project into the lumen and the crypts (also called crypts of Lieberkühn) at the base of the villi. In the colon, the mucosa is arranged in

closely straight tubular crypts (Figure 1). The submucosa layer is a connective tissue that supports the mucosa. It contains large blood vessels, lymphatic, and submucosal enteric nervous plexuses (also referred as Meissner's plexus). The muscularis propria consists of smooth muscle, which is organized as an inner circular layer and an outer longitudinal layer. Large clusters of enteric nervous cells are found between these two smooth muscle layers, and are named myenteric plexus (also referred as Auerbach's plexus). The two muscular layers in association with myenteric plexus allow the transit of the feces through the gut via a process of propulsion termed peristalsis. The visceral smooth muscle is the most abundant

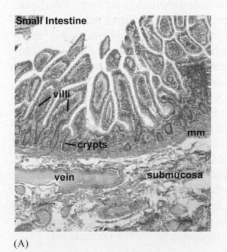

(A)

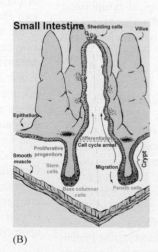

(B)

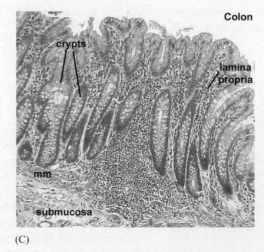

(C)

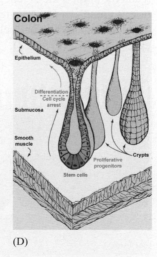

(D)

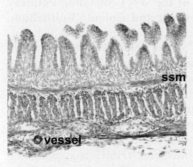

(E)

Figure 1 Structures of human adult small intestine and colon. The mucosa is the innermost layer, closest to the lumen, made up with the epithelium, a supporting lamina propria and a thin smooth muscle layer, the muscularis mucosae. In the small intestine (A, B), the mucosal surface forms the villi that project into the lumen and the crypts (also called crypts of Lieberkühn) at the base of the villi. Stem cells reside above the Paneth cells. Progenitors stop proliferating at the crypt–villus junction and differentiate in enteroendocrine, absorptive and muco-secretin cells that migrate upward, whereas Paneth cells migrate downward. In the colon (C, D), the mucosa is arranged in closely straight tubular crypts. The submucosa is a connective tissue that supports the mucosa. It contains large blood vessels, lymphatic and submucosal enteric plexus. Stem cell resides at the crypt bottom. Progenitors are amplified by constant division and will give rise to enterocyte and goblet cell. mm = muscularis mucosae. ((A, C) From Granier G. and de Santa Barbara P., unpublished. (B, D) Adapted with permission from Sancho, Battle.[1])

contributor of the smooth muscles in the human body and represents 70% of the total (between 1,000 and 1,600 g).[3] The outer layer of the intestine, the adventitia or serosa is a supportive tissue that conducts major vessels and nerves.

Small Intestine

The small intestine is about 5 to 6 m long and is divided into *duodenum*, *jejunum*, and *ileum*. The function of small intestine is digestion and absorption of nutrients. Therefore, the epithelial cells are highly specialized and metabolically active (Figure 1). These cells undergo a relatively rapid generation and death continuously throughout the life of the organism. The cells are derived from a stem cell located in the middle of the crypt.[4] Asymmetric division is essential to insure maintenance of stem cell number and final homeostasis of the intestinal epithelium. The stem cells have a high proliferative rate with embryonic cell-like features. They can be morphologically identified by a large nucleus compartment with diffuse chromatin and a cytoplasm with few small organelles. The number of stem cells in the small intestine is estimated at around 4 to 6 per crypt. This cell produces progenitors, which appear undifferentiated in the crypt but eventually produce four cell types: enterocytes, enteroendocrine cells, Paneth cells, and goblet cells. Cellular position along the crypt–villous unit is different following the differentiation state of its cells (bottom for undifferentiated cells, and top for more differentiated cells), with exception of Paneth cells that always are located at the bottom of the crypts. Morphological changes are achieved during migration from the stem cell to the crypt–villous junction. When these cells reach the crypt–villous junction, their differentiation is complete. Enterocytes are the most abundant intestinal epithelial cells (up to 80% of all epithelial cells) (Figure 2).

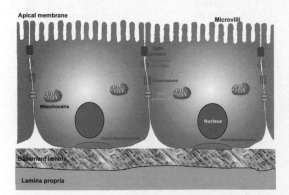

Figure 2 Ultrastructure of enterocyte cells. The absorptive cell (enterocyte) is the most numerous cell types covering the small intestinal villus. These epithelial cells have three surface domains: the apical, lateral, and basal domains. The apical domains toward lumen have microvilli that increase contact surface. The lateral domains have special attachments that allow communication and junction between enterocyte cells. Different complexes are presents: the anchoring junctions (tight junctions, desmosomes) and the communication junctions (gap junctions). The basal domains anchor the epithelium to the mucosa. Hemi-desmosomes attach the enterocyte cells to the basement lamina.

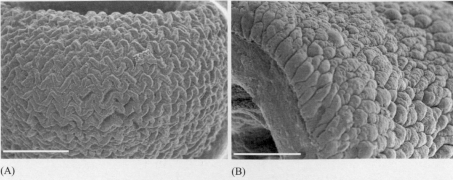

Figure 3 Scanning electron microscopy photos showing small intestine (A) and colon (B) from chicks 17-day-old embryos. (A) The mucosa of the small intestine presents thin, long, and regular villi arranged in Z. (B) The mucosa of the colon presents thick and flat villi. (Scale bars represent 225 μm). (From de Santa Barbara P., unpublished.)

Enterocytes are columnar cells with apical microvilli that greatly increase the absorptive surface, and lateral junctions with neighbor cells. The enterocytes have hydrolytic and absorptive functions and are responsible for degradation of nutrients. The turnover of enterocytes is estimated in mouse at around 3 days. The enterocytes are characteristic of the small intestine and are the main absorptive cell of the intestine. Goblet cells are scattered from the middle of the crypt to the tip of the villus. They represent 5% of the small intestine epithelial cells. They are characterized by specific mucous granules found in the cytoplasm. The mucus constitutes a barrier against the intestinal contents. Goblet cell turnover is quick, around 3 days. Enteroendocrine cells represent a small percentage of the small intestine epithelial cells. They produce numerous hormones that assist in regulating gastrointestinal motility. Paneth cells, in contrast of the three other intestinal epithelial cell types, have a longer turnover period of about 20 days. Mature Paneth cells are columnar epithelial cells with apical cytoplasmic granules. Around 10 Paneth cells are present per crypt. Paneth function is mostly associated with the antimicrobial defense of the intestine.

The pattern of the different cell types in the small intestine is such that the midcrypt position of the stem cell produces progenitor cells, rapidly dividing, committed but undifferentiated, that "move" lumenally to the villous (Figure 1). At the crypt–villous junction, these cells differentiate. Their luminal migration is both passive due to being "pushed" by newly "born" progenitors from the crypts, apoptotic loss of cells from the villous tip, and from newly described epithelial cell–cell and epithelial–mesenchymal interaction signals (described below). In the small intestine, the Paneth cell is the only cell type that apparently disregards this rule, as it is uniquely located at the base of the crypts, apparently migrating "downward."

The Colon

The colon, also called the large intestine, is the part of the intestine from the cecum to the rectum. It can be divided in six parts: the cecum, the ascending colon, the transverse colon, the descending colon, the sigmoid colon, and the rectum. The colon measures approximately 1.5 m in length. The principal function of the adult colon is to extract water from feces. Transient formation of colonic villi is present in embryonic proximal intestine (Figure 3), but in human these villi are flattened by birth. The mature colon epithelium has mainly two differentiated cell types: the enterocyte and goblet cell.[5] The goblet cells are mainly found in the midcrypt, whereas the absorptive enterocytes (or colonocytes) are found at the surface (or top of the crypt), the surface between the crypt is called the "intercrypt table" and consists mainly of enterocytes. The colon also has endocrine cells. Endocrine cells are found in highest numbers at the base of the crypt.[6] The stem cell and proliferating compartment in the colonic epithelium reside at the base of the crypt. All cellular "movements" are toward the lumen.

Molecular Pathways in the Intestine

The genetic control of intestinal and colonic epithelial patterns has been intensively studied over the last decades (Figure 4). The fundamental pattern in adult gut epithelium is the crypt–villus axis, with the progenitor/proliferative cells being deep to the differentiated/functional/and finally apoptotic cells being luminal.[7] The formation of this pattern occurs embryologically, but it is maintained in the adult organ and involves cellular reciprocal interactions between mesenchymal–epithelial layers and between epithelial cells. Disruption of this pattern results in dysfunctional bowel and can lead to malignant growth. Many of the same factors shown to be important in embryologic pattern formation of the gut continue in their importance in pattern formation of the adult organ. The different pathways and factors involved in the control of cell fate decisions, cellular differentiation, and apoptosis, respectively, will be commented.

Interventions of the WNT Signaling Pathway in Adult Intestinal and Colonic Epithelium.

WNT genes encode secreted proteins, which control numerous developmental processes. *WNT* genes are included on the same family, but can be distinguished in two different functional groups: the WNT/β-catenin signaling pathway and the WNT/Ca^{2+} signaling pathway.[8] In the first group, WNT expression leads to the nuclear translocation of β-catenin and its association with T-cell factor (TCF) family members (HMG box-containing DNA-binding proteins). These β-catenin/TCFs

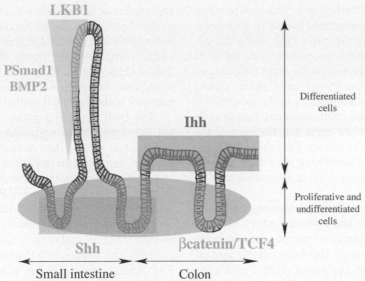

Small intestine   Colon

Figure 4 Pathways involved in cell differentiation, homeostasis and apoptosis in the adult intestinal epithelium. β-catenin and TCF4 are expressed in the proliferative compartment, where are located the intestinal epithelial stem cells. The β-catenin/TCF4 complex mediates WNT signaling pathway by transcriptional activation of target genes (*C-MYC*, *BMP4*, *EphB2*, *EphB3*; other genes are reviewed in http://www.stanford.edu/~rnusse/wntwindow.html). β-Catenin/TCF4 pathway is important in maintaining the proliferative compartment of the adult intestinal epithelium. Two members of the hedgehog family are expressed in the adult intestinal epithelium. *Shh* is expressed in the base of the small intestinal crypt and could positively regulate precursor cell proliferation. *Ihh* is expressed in the differentiated colonic cells and could regulate the maturation of the enterocytes. LKB1, a Ser/Thr kinase, regulates specific p53-dependent apoptosis pathways in the intestinal epithelium. Its gradient expression pattern along the villus axis highly suggests a function of LKB1 in the natural apoptosis of the intestinal epithelial cells. The activation of the BMP signaling pathway (via this morphogene BMP2 and the activated phosphorylated Smad1, 2, and 8 (termed PSmad1) proteins) presents a gradient expression pattern along the villus axis highly similar of LKB1 expression pattern.

complexes mediate WNT signaling pathway by transcriptional activation of WNT target genes. This pathway is important in gut epithelial development. New data have implicated the Wnt/β-catenin/TCF4 pathway as critically important in maintaining the proliferative compartment of the adult gut epithelium (Figure 4, Table 1).

Expression of *Wnt* genes during mouse and chick gut development suggested possible roles in gut patterning.[9–11] These publications have shown *Wnt* expression in the developing gut mesoderm and suggest a role in controlling AP boundaries. Recently, Gregorieff and colleagues have shown specific WNT factor expression in the adult gut, significant evidence documents that its pathway is important at the crypt.[12] WNT proteins signal via complexes formed with β-catenin. After expression of WNT morphogens, WNT binds to its membranous receptor Frizzled and activates it. These stimulation leads to the inhibition of GSK-3 β activity and to cytoplasmic and nuclear β-catenin accumulations. The consensual model states that nuclear β-catenin interacts and binds to TCF factors to activate Wnt target genes.[13] In the digestive epithelium, β-catenin is present in all membranes along the crypt–villus unit, but nuclear accumulation of β-catenin is specifically found in the epithelial cells located from the bottom third of the small intestine crypt to the bottom and at the bottom of the colonic crypt.[14,15] The effector of the WNT/β-catenin signaling pathway, *Tcf4* is found expressed in the gut epithelium throughout life.[16,17] Tcf4 is expressed in a gradient highest in the cells at the base of the crypt.[18,19] *Tcf4* knockout mice appear to lose

the intestinal epithelial progenitor and stem cell population and die before crypt formation is evident.[17] These data suggest that TCF4 functions in intestinal epithelial stem cell maintenance. The experiments identified new signaling pathways

involved in the intestinal epithelium and demonstrate a central role of β-catenin/TCF4 in the maintenance of the crypt progenitor cells.[14,15,20,21] A direct target of the β-catenin/TCF4 is the *Cdx1* gene, one of the mouse *Drosophila caudal* homologues.[22] *Cdx1* is expressed in the developing intestine endoderm[23] and its product finally localizes in the proliferative crypt compartment during differentiation.[24] After WNT stimulation, it was demonstrated that Cdx1 expression is stimulated and let us hypothesize that its homeobox gene is one of the WNT signaling pathway effector involved in the maintenance of the proliferative intestinal compartment.

Genetic Control of Cellular Patterning in the Intestinal and Colonic Epithelium. The Rho GTPase family members play a central role in all eukaryotic cells by controlling the organization of the actin cytoskeleton.[25] These proteins integrate information from different signaling pathways and act as effectors to mediate effects on migration, proliferation, and differentiation.[26] Rac1 is a member of the Rho family of GTP-binding proteins that can activate the Jun N-terminal kinase (JNK) and p38 mitogen-activated-protein (MAP) kinase pathways.[27] Expressions of either constitutively active and/or dominant-negative Rac1 forms in mice result in perturbation of cell differentiation in the intestinal epithelium.[28] Sustained Rac1 activation leads to an early differentiation of Paneth and enterocyte cells within the small intestine intervillus epithelium in late fetal mice, but no impact was observed on Goblet and enteroendocrine cells. These data strongly suggest that Paneth and enterocyte cell fate choice involve

Table 1 Factors Expressed in the Intestinal Epithelium

Gene	Cell Type/Compartment	Gene Function
TCF4	Stem cells	HMG containing domain-transcription factor
c-Myc	Proliferative, mainly bottom two third of crypts	Proto-oncogene
CD44	Proliferative cells	Cell surface receptor
Musashi-1	Stem cells and base columnars cells	RNA-binding protein
EphB3	Stem cells and base columnars cells	Ephrin receptor
EphB2	Decreasing gradient from bottom tp top of crypt	Ephrin receptor
Math1	Goblet, enteroendocrine, Paneth precursors	Basic helix-loop-helix transcription factor
Hes1	Proliferative cells	Basic helix-loop-helix transcription factor
Ngn3	Enteroendocrine precursors	Basic helix-loop-helix transcription factor
P21waf/Cip1	Cell cycle arrested cells	Cyclin-dependent kinase inhibitor
Ephrin-B1	Gradient from surface	Ephrin ligand
IHH	Top third and surface epithelium in colon	Hedgehog morphogen
Phospho-Smad1/5/8	Differentiated cells in villus	Intracellular trasnducer of BMP ligands
Villin	Microvilli-increasing gradient from crypt to villus	Calcium-regulated, actin-binding protein
Fabpi	Enterocytes	Fatty acid-binding protein
Sucrase isomaltase	Enterocytes-brush border	Enzyme
Muc2	Goblet cells	
NeuroD/beta	Enteroendocrine cells	Basic helix-loop-helix transcription factor
Synaptophysin	Enteroendocrine cells	Integral membrane protein
Secretin	Enteroendocrine cells	Hormone
Serotonin	Enteroendocrine cells	Neurotransmitter
Lysozyme	Paneth cells	Anti-bacterial enzyme
Cryptdins	Paneth cells	Anti-microbial peptide

Adapted with permission from Sancho, Battle.[1]

the Rho GTPase pathway. In adult, forced Rac1 activation increases cell proliferation in intestinal crypts and leads to unusually wide villi.[29] Activated Rac1 specifically increases phosphorylation of JNK in both intervillus and villus epithelial cells and alters the actin cytoskeleton.[29] The cytoskeleton is also involved in cell migration. The position of cells along the crypt–villous axis is one of the important factors thought to play a role in cellular differentiation.[30]

A fundamental pathway utilized by many systems to direct cellular differentiation is the Notch–Delta receptor-ligand signaling system.[31] Adult gut epithelial cells use this system to affect cell fate in the proliferative zone of the crypt–villous unit. The Notch pathway affects cell fate decisions by using lateral inhibition in cell–cell interactions with its cell membrane based receptor Delta.[32] Feedback amplification of relative differences in Notch and Delta results in subsets of cells with high levels of Notch and others with high Delta levels. Elevated cellular Notch levels induce expression of transcription factors, such as *Hes1*.[33] *Hes1* is a transcriptional repressor, and *Hes1* positive cells have been shown to remain in the precursor population.[34] Downstream targets of *Hes1* have been recently described to include *Math1*, a basic helix-loop-helix transcription factor.[35] *Math1* expression is present in both developing and mature mouse intestinal epithelium and colocalizes with proliferating markers in the progenitor region of the crypt in small intestinal epithelium. *Math1* null mice have increased reporter expression in crypt cells, lack intestinal goblet, Paneth, and enteroendocrine cells, and show no increased apoptosis. These findings suggest that *Math1* is involved in early epithelial cell fate decisions. *Math1* expression is needed for cells to make their first lineage specifying choice. *Math1* nonexpressing cells remain in the progenitor pool and can only become enterocytes. These results are informative not only in that *Math1* is an early cell fate determining factor, but also that there are apparently two progenitor cell types—a *Math1* dependent progenitor for goblet, Paneth, and enteroendocrine cells and a *Math1* independent progenitor for enterocytes.

During embryonic development, Eph receptors, and their ephrin ligands (Eph/ephrin) have been shown to be essential for migration of many cell types[36] and pattern boundaries.[37] Eph receptors constitute a large family of transmembrane tyrosine kinase receptors.[38] Binding and activation of Eph receptors to ephrin ligands require cell–cell interaction.[39] Eph–ephrin signaling converges to regulate the cytoskeleton.[40] Members of the Eph–ephrin signaling pathway were found expressed in the small intestine epithelium.[15] EphB2 and EphB3 receptors are expressed in the proliferative compartment, whereas their ligand ephrin-B1 is expressed in adjacent differentiated cells. This suggests that the Eph–ephrin system may regulate epithelial cell migration, therefore position in the crypt–villous axis, which is critical in determining cell fate. The neonatal intestinal epithelium of *EphB2/EphB3* double-mutant mice presents perturbation in the proliferative/differentiated compartment boundary with presence of ectopic proliferative cells along the villus. In adults, EphB3 receptor is restricted in its gut epithelial expression to the crypt base columnar cells, where the Paneth cells reside. *EphB3* null mice show abnormalities in the localization of the Paneth cells, with scattered Paneth cells throughout the entire crypt and the base of the villus. These results support the role of the Eph–ephrin system in maintaining the integrity of the epithelial cell pattern in the crypt–villous axis.

Functions of the Hedgehog Signaling Pathways in Adult Intestinal and Colonic Epithelium.

The hedgehog (Hh) family of morphogens includes three members in most vertebrates, Sonic Hedgehog (Shh), Indian Hedgehog (Ihh), and Desert Hedgehog. All hedgehogs can bind two common homologous receptors: Patched (Ptc)-1 and -2. In the unbound state, these receptors negatively regulate the activity of a seven-pass transmembrane receptor Smoothened (Smo) by a so far unresolved mechanism.[41] Upon binding of Ptc by Hh, the suppression of Smo is relieved and pathway activation through the Gli family of transcription factors ensues. Both Shh and Ihh are important endodermal signals in gut tube differentiation and are involved in patterning events along all four axes of its development. Shh expression is downregulated in the developing small intestine in two phases. Initially, Shh expression is lost in the prospective pancreatic endoderm and this loss is critical for normal pancreas formation[42]; in a second phase Shh expression is downregulated along the length of the small intestine. Experiments in *Xenopus* suggest that this phase may be critical to normal small intestinal epithelial differentiation.[43] The *Shh* null mouse shows overgrowth of villi that are abnormally innervated, whereas growth of villi in the *Ihh* mouse is strongly diminished and often lacks innervation.[44] In the adult small intestine, *Shh* mRNA is detected at the base of the crypts around the presumed location of the small intestinal stem cell.[45] Inhibition of the Hedgehog pathway suggests that Shh positively regulates precursor cell proliferation.[46] In the adult colon, *Shh* mRNA is observed in a few cells at the base of the colonic crypts.[45] In the adult, Ihh is expressed by the differentiated colonic enterocytes and seems to be involved in their maturation.[47]

Genetic Control of Apoptosis in Adult Intestinal Epithelium.

Homeostasis of the intestinal epithelium requires tight control and balance of the different processes of proliferation, differentiation, migration, and apoptosis. This coordination requires intervention of numerous and well-timed pathways. Perturbations of the balance between proliferation and apoptosis could be the base of cancer predisposition and development.[48] Recently, new data showed involvement of the *LKB1* gene, a serine/threonine kinase mutated in Peutz-Jegher syndrome,[49,50] in the natural apoptosis of the gut epithelium.[51] The cytoplasmic expression of LBK1 shows a gradient pattern along the villus. LKB1 expression is higher in older epithelial cells (located near the top of the villus) compare to the newly differentiated epithelial cells (Figure 4). LKB1 has been shown to regulate the specific p53-dependent cell death pathway in the intestinal epithelium.

The BMP signaling pathway is involved in gut development (as reviewed below). In addition, human genetic data have demonstrated that this pathway plays an important role in intestinal epithelial homeostasis. Recently, mutations in different members of the BMP signaling pathway were found associated with the human precancerous Juvenile Polyposis Syndrome (JPS). A specific *SMAD4* mutation is found in some JPS patients and results in a truncated protein.[52,53] The Smad4 protein is the common shuttle of both Transforming Growth Factor-beta (TGF-β and BMP(s) signaling pathways. *SMAD4* mutations associated with JPS leads to the hypothesis that other members of TGF-β or BMP signaling pathways may be involved in the JPS patients without the specific SMAD4 mutation. In fact, in some germline nonsense mutations were found in the bone morphogenetic protein receptor 1A (*BMPR1A*) gene.[54] These mutations resulted in protein truncation due to a deletion of the intracellular serine–threonine kinase domain necessary for Smad protein phosphorylation and signal transduction. These genetic studies show that perturbation of the BMP signaling pathway is associated with intestinal hamartomous polyps. This suggests that BMP signaling is involved in normal epithelial differentiation and homeostasis in the gut. In vertebrate, expressions of phosphorylated and activated forms of Smad1/5/8 proteins are found in the intestinal epithelial cells and in the lamina propria stromal cells of the neonate and adult small intestine and colon (Figure 4).[55,56] In addition, ectopic expression of the BMP antagonist Noggin inhibits apoptosis and decreases β-catenin expression in vivo suggesting that BMP signaling pathway activation is able to promote apoptosis in mature colonic epithelial cells.[57]

EMBRYOLOGY

Development of the Primitive Intestine

The intestinal tract is a remarkably complex, specialized, and vital organ system derived from a primitive and undifferentiated structure. In all vertebrates, the intestinal tube is composed of the three germ layers—endoderm (which will give rise to the epithelial lining of the lumen), mesoderm (which will develop into the smooth muscle layers and the myofibroblat cells), and ectoderm (which will contribute to the most posterior luminal digestive structure and to the enteric nervous system (ENS)). The human primitive gut is formed at 4 weeks and is divided into three embryological structures along the cranio–caudal axis: the foregut, the midgut, and the hindgut. The midgut forms the small intestine and the

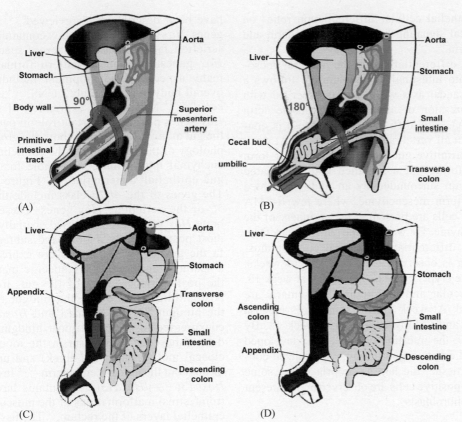

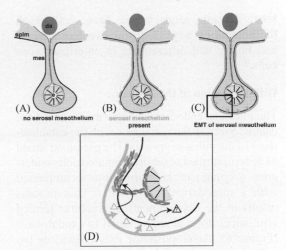

Figure 7 Origin of the gut vasculature during mouse development. The serosal mesothelium gives rise to mural cells of gut vasculature. (A) At E9.5, the primitive gut is not covered by a mesothelium, but a vascular plexus (*red*) runs between endoderm and mesoderm, and within the mesentery. Endoderm (e); dorsal aorta (da); splanchnic mesoderm (splm). (B) At E10.5, the serosal mesothelium (*green*) starts to cover the mesentery and, subsequently, by E11.5, coats the entire gut. (C) Serosal mesothelial cells undergo EMT into the subserosal space (*open green triangles*). (D) Progeny of the serosal mesothelial cells differentiate into smooth muscle cells surrounding the blood vessels (*red*) that form in the subserosal space. A subset of these progeny differentiates into, as yet unidentified, nonvessel cells (*triangle with question mark*). (Adapted with permission from Wilm et al.[58])

Figure 5 Development of the intestinal loop in human embryos. (A) By sixth week the rapid elongation of intestines cause their herniation out the umbilical cord. In addition, the intestines rotate 90° around the superior mesenteric artery in a counterclockwise direction. (B) By eighth to tenth week during the retraction of the intestinal loop into the abdominal cavity, the small intestine undergoes another 180° rotation counterclockwise around the mesenteric artery. (C) By eleventh week the cecum is present in the right upper position of the abdomen. The cecum is then moved downwards, attracting in the same direction the proximal part of the posterior intestine. (D) The position of the intestines is maintained during the entire life.

hindgut will form the colon and the rectum. The primitive gut is localized in the coelomic cavity into the body wall and is connected to the dorsal mesentere. At week 6, the length of the ileum rapidly increases and brings out a part of the intestine (Figure 5). By eighth to tenth week, the intestinal loop rotates around the mesenteric artery and moves back to the body wall. Finally, by eleventh week, the cecum moves downward, attracting the proximal part of the posterior intestine and the intestines reach their adult final position (Figure 5).

During this period, the intestinal endoderm remains uniform in its morphology (undifferentiated appearing stratified cuboidal cells) throughout all axes of the gut until midgestation in most vertebrates when epithelial–mesenchymal interactions direct endodermal differentiation (Figure 6). Finally, the endoderm differentiates from signals provided by the mesoderm directed by its rostro–caudal location and the endodermal pattern becomes phenotypically specific in rostro–caudal axis. The mature gut epithelia conserve their morphologic and functional patterns during all the adult life (Figure 1).

Lateral splanchnic mesoderm will contribute to the visceral mesoderm and will enroll the endoderm to form the primitive tube. At this stage, the visceral mesoderm is a poorly organized mesenchyme and the ENS is not present in the primitive gut. The origin of vascular cells of the digestive tube was unknown until recent new findings. By combination of genetic and embryologic approaches, Wilm and colleagues demonstrated that the serosal mesothelium is the major source of vasculogenic cells in the developing gut.[58] Serosal mesothelial cells first colonize the entire primitive gut and one subset of these cells undergoes epithelial–mesenchymal transition to differentiate into smooth muscle cells surrounding the blood vessels (Figure 7).[58] The ENS arises from the neural crest cells that delaminate from the dorsal region of the neural tube and colonize the whole gut to establish its innervation.[59,60] At week 4, the neural crest derived cells migrate into the gut mesoderm layer and colonize the gut

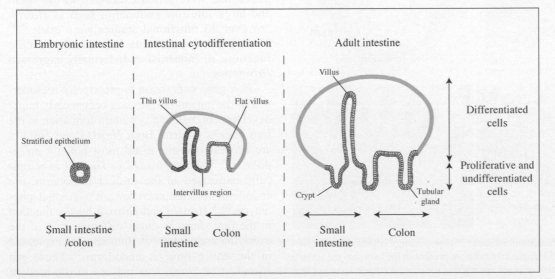

Figure 6 From development to differentiation of the intestinal epithelium. During early embryonic development, the visceral endoderm appears uniform and presents stratified cell layer. Intestinal epithelial cytodifferentiation occurs during foetal development and is marked by mesodermal growing into the lumen and villi formations. These villi are separated by proliferative intervillus epithelium. AP axis differences appear and are characterized by long and thin villi in the small intestine and by transitory wide and flat villi in the colon. The intervillus epithelium of the small intestine is reshaped downward forming crypts. In human, final architecture of the small intestine is reached before birth and is characterized by the crypt–villus unit. The colonic villi disappeared at the time of birth and the mature colonic epithelium present tubular glands (crypts).

along a cranio–caudal wage. These cells reach the hindgut by week 7, forms two cluster rings and finally will differentiate in enteric nervous cells.[61]

Differentiation of the Intestine

The intestinal endoderm layer forms the intestinal characterized in the radial axis with the establishment of the villus–crypt axis. The pseudostratified endoderm formed of undifferentiated cells undergoes a columnar transformation accompanied with a mesodermal outgrowth.[5] This process results in the development of structures termed villi, which form along a cranial to caudal wave (Figure 6). Anteroposterior axis influences the radial axis in morphologic and epithelial cellular differentiation. In late fetal life, small intestine epithelium is characterized by long and thin villi, whereas colon epithelium shows wide and flat villi (Figure 1). These villi are separated by a proliferating intervillus epithelium (Figure 6). As the gut develops the intervillus epithelium is reshaped downward forming crypts. The crypt villous unit allows for a great increase in surface area for absorption. Small intestines conserve their villus–crypt unit throughout life (Figures 1 and 6). In many species (including human but not in chick), the embryonic villi will be lost in adult colonic epithelium. Transient formation of colonic villi is present in embryonic proximal intestine, but in human these villi are flattened by birth. Human colon has a relatively flat epithelium separated regularly by crypts (Figures 1 and 6). The formation of these crypt–villous structures

and epithelial cellular differentiation relies on reciprocal signaling between the endoderm and mesoderm.[62]

The differentiation of the visceral mesoderm into intestinal smooth muscle follows a rostro–caudal axis wave, and is observed with the expression of alpha-smooth muscle actin (α-SMA). This differentiation process is conserved in all vertebrates (Figure 8).[61,63] At week 7, the primitive gut has a simple tubular form and is formed of a stratified undifferentiated epithelium surrounded by an undifferentiated and uniform mesenchyme, where few α-SMA positive cells are present at the periphery of the mesenchyme. By week 9, the villi start to form and the differentiating external circular muscle layer is observed. Around 12 to 14 weeks, primitive crypts begin to appear and at week 13, both circular and longitudinal muscularis are observed. At week 16, the muscularis mucosa appears and is fully organized at week 18. By week 20, the intestine displays well-developed villi and crypts supported by a specialized connective tissue, the lamina propria where some α-SMA positive cells are observed and represent the myofibroblasts.

Molecular Pathwas in the Developing Intestine

Transcription Factors Involved During Intestinal Development.
Genetic controls of intestinal development have been less well studied compare to the other organs.[64] Some factors involved in the specification of this structure

have been described and reviewed[65-67] as *Hox* genes. *Hox* genes are homeobox containing transcription factors conserved across species.[68,69] *Hox* genes function in pattern formation of many aspects of development including the overall body plan,[70,71] limb,[72] CNS,[73,74] and viscera.[10,75-77] Mesodermal expression of specific *Hox* genes play an important role in patterning the gut along the AP axis in both the gross morphology of the gut and later the epithelial–mesenchymal interactions responsible for normal gut epithelial differentiation (Figure 9).[10,78] The genes of the *AbdB* class include the most 5_ of the vertebrate *Hox* genes. These vertebrate *Hox* genes are expressed spatially in the most posterior body regions and subregions.[75] In the gut, these *Hox* genes are expressed in a spatially and temporally specific manner in the posterior mesoderm of the gut, from the postumbilical portion of the midgut through the hindgut.[10,75,76,78] *Hoxa13* and *Hoxd13* are coexpressed in the distal most hindgut mesoderm (anorectal mesoderm in the mouse and cloacal mesoderm in the chick) and uniquely throughout the hindgut endoderm.[10,78] In mouse, *Hoxa13*(+/−)/*Hoxd13*(−/−) mutants have gastrointestinal malformations of the muscular and epithelial layers of the rectum.[77] The tissue specific roles of these genes were not dissected. The role of *Hoxa13* in the posterior endoderm was investigated using the avian system. A *Hoxa13* mutant protein, which behaves as a dominant-negative, was specifically expressed in the early developing chick posterior endoderm.[78] This resulted in decreased wild-type protein and the chicks developed with a dramatic malformation in the gut and genitourinary system with atresia of the hindgut anterior to the cloaca, cystic mesonephric maldevelopment, and atresia of the distal Müllerian ducts. This was the first time that a specific endodermal function of a *Hox* gene was described. Different *Hox* genes also were found expressed in the small and large intestine endoderm, such as *Hoxa8*, however no functional studies were made.[79,80] Their expressions let us hypothesize specific functions of intestinal endodermally expressed *Hox* genes.

Hox gene expression is principally mesodermal in the gut, and expression occurs early in gut development, before any pattern formation in the four axes is evident. Both *Hoxd13* and *Hoxa13* are expressed in the distal most hindgut mesoderm.[75,76,81] When *Hoxd13* or *Hoxa13* is ectopically expressed in the midgut mesoderm, the endoderm differentiated toward a hindgut phenotype.[10,78] *Hoxd13* and *Hoxa13* have a function in the mesoderm to direct differentiation of the overlying endoderm.[10,78] Both are also expressed in the entire hindgut endoderm.[78] These put *Hoxd13* and *Hoxa13* as players in the hindgut mesoderm to endoderm signaling that has been shown to direct the final epithelial phenotype. Recently, the mesodermal–endodermal *HOX* crosstalk pathway was also observed in mouse[82] and shows a strong conserved function of *Hox* genes in GI tract differentiation.

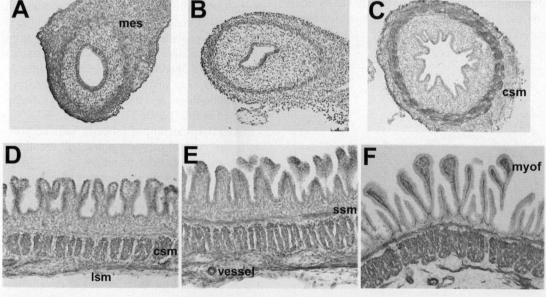

Figure 8 Visceral smooth muscle cell differentiation in the chick small intestine. Development of αSMA-immunopositive layers at 6-, 9-, 13-, 15-, 16-, and 18-day-old stages. (A) SMA positive cells are present in the unorganized smooth muscle cells in chick 6-day-old small intestine. (B) SMA positive cells are observed in the smooth muscle layer in chick 9-day-old small intestine. (C) SMA positive cells are observed in the circular smooth muscle layer in chick 13-day-old small intestine. (D) SMA positive cells are present in the longitudinal and circular smooth muscle layers in chick 15-day-old small intestine. Note the presence of some unorganized smooth muscle cells. (E) SMA positive cells are present in the longitudinal, circular, and submucosal smooth muscle layers in chick 16-day-old small intestine. (F) In addition, SMA positive cells are present in the lamina propria and represent myofibroblast cells in chick 18-day-old small intestine. csm = circular smooth muscle; lsm = longitudinal smooth muscle; mes = mesenchyme; myof = myofibroblast; SMA = smooth muscle actin. (From de Santa Barbara P., unpublished.)

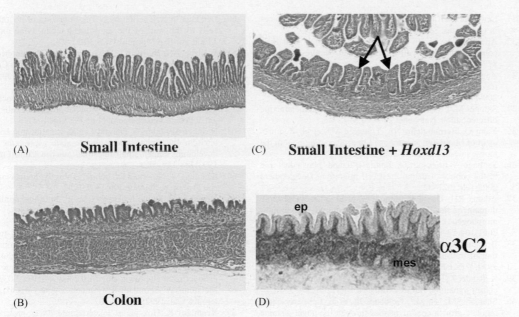

(A) **Small Intestine**   (C) **Small Intestine + *Hoxd13***

(B) **Colon**   (D)

Figure 9 Epithelial–mesenchymal interactions control the regionalization of the intestinal epithelium. Hematoxylin and Eosin stained sections of chick 18-day-old control (A, B) or retroviral Hoxd13 infected (C) guts. (A) Normal small intestine presents thin and long villi. (B) Normal colon has flat and short villi. (C) *Hoxd13* mesodermally infected small intestine shows colonic-like epithelial transformation (as shown by *arrows*). (D) Small intestine retroviral infection shows presence of virus in only the mesodermal layer (detected by a specific avian retrovirus antibody, α3C2). ep = epithelium; mes = mesenchyme. (Adapted from reference 78.)

Signaling Pathways Involved During Intestinal Development. The Hedgehog pathway in *Drosophila* and vertebrates is conserved and known to play an important role in gut development.[83–85] *Shh* is an important factor implicated in the first phase of endoderm–mesoderm signaling in the gut.[75,86] *Shh* is expressed early in the posterior and anterior endoderms.[75,87,88] As the gut tube forms and undergoes morphogenesis, *Shh* expression expands and is maintained in the gut endoderm with the exception of the GI tract derivates.[88–90] One other member of the Hedgehog family, *Ihh*, is expressed later in the gut endoderm in a partially overlapping pattern.[44] The function of Hedgehog signaling in the early gut endoderm layer is not well defined, but its action in the adjacent mesoderm was demonstrated. Endodermally secreted *Shh* acts via its mesodemal expressed receptor *Patched* (*Ptc*) to induce mesodermal expression of *Bmp4*.[10,75] Early endodermal *Shh* expression was suggested to act as a signal in epithelial–mesenchymal interaction in the earliest stage of hindgut formation.[75] In addition, inactivation of the complete Hedgehog signaling pathway impairs visceral smooth muscle development.[44] In agreement with old findings, these data suggest that Hedgehog pathway regulates gut smooth muscle pathway through epithelial–mesenchymal interaction process.[44,91] Both *Ihh* and *Shh* are expressed in the colon during development and may have partially overlapping functions (Figure 4). The *Ihh* null mouse has a colonic phenotype that is reminiscent of Hirschprung's disease with dilatation of parts of the colon and a thin wall with a reduced small muscle layer that lacks innervation at the sites of dilatation.[44] The *Shh* null mutant and several mutants of the Gli family of transcription factors show a spectrum of anorectal malformations.[91]

BMPs are members of the TGF-β superfamily of signaling molecules that play important roles during embryogenesis and organogenesis. BMP ligands were initially identified as regulators of bone formation,[92] but subsequent analyses have suggested that these ligands regulate a spectrum of developmental processes throughout embryogenesis and organogenesis.[93] BMPs are tightly regulated growth and differentiation morphogens, therefore to truly understand what their function any one system may be, it is extremely useful to localize the tissue/cells in which their actions are occurring.[94] BMP ligands act via specific receptors in a complex, which ultimately, by phosphorylation, activates a target molecule, SMAD1/5 and 8, that in turn moves to the nucleus to activate transcription of target genes.[95] Due to the high degree of complexity of the BMP signaling pathway (numerous ligands, receptors, and processing regulations), the detection of the phosphorylated forms of Smad1/5/8 was used to give an endogenous cartography of the BMP activation in *Xenopus*[95] and chick,[96] that could not be predicted from ligand and antagonist expression patterns. Smad1/5/8 phosphorylations are activated in the ventral part of the foregut endoderm.[96] These data suggest an unexpected and early role of BMP signaling in the development and patterning of the endodermal AIP structure formation. Recent investigations have highlighted the roles of BMP in patterning the gut during development. Anti-phospho-Smad1/5/8 antibodies were used to study the endogenous BMP pathway activation in the developing gastrointestinal tract in chick.[55] Endogenous activation of this pathway is specifically found in the

gut mesenchyme layer, but also in the developing endoderm. The localization of activated Smad1 in the mesoderm of the midgut is consistent with the expression of *Bmp-4* at this stage,[10] but the additional activation of Smad1 observed in the endoderm suggests that either diffusion of *Bmp*-4 from the mesoderm induces Smad1/5/8 phosphorylations in the endoderm, or that additional BMPs are expressed in the endoderm.[97] Regional differences in BMP pathway activation also are present in the AP axis. Smad1/5/8 phosphorylations are present in the midgut endoderm, but not in the hindgut endoderm. Activated BMP signaling is present in the all undifferentiated gut mesoderm with the exception of the gizzard mesoderm during the early gut development period.[55] BMP signaling is also activated during the differentiation of the gut mesoderm into visceral smooth muscle. Once the smooth muscle cell differentiation is completed, a pronounced downregulation of BMP pathway activity occurs. In the colon, the maintain of BMP activity perturbed the differentiation of this tissue, leaving undifferentiated mesenchyme in place of visceral smooth muscle.[55] These experiments demonstrate that downregulation of BMP signaling activity may be required for the differentiation of visceral mesoderm into smooth muscle. The ontology of the gastrointestinal musculature is less known compared to the formation of the skeletal, cardiac, and vascular musculatures. In most studies devoted to the development of the digestive tract, the pattern of visceral smooth muscle formation has poorly studied. Only few pathways have been reported to regulate the differentiation of the intestinal smooth muscle cells.[98,99] Since decades, the differentiation status of the visceral mesoderm into visceral smooth muscle cells is characterized by the expression profile of these markers: SMA and Tenascin-C.[63] In addition, RhoA and Cadherin 6B expressions are induced in chick visceral smooth muscle cells at a time point that corresponds with muscle differentiation.[100,101] As reported, tightly regulated BMP activity is need to ensure visceral smooth muscle cell differentiation and place the BMP signaling pathway as a key pathway for these processes.[55]

ACKNOWLEDGMENTS

The author thanks Drucilla Jane Roberts for fruitful discussions and helpful comments on gut development over the last years and Sandrine Faure for constant support. P.d.S.B. is member of the French National Institute of Health (INSERM) and is supported by the "Association Française contre les Myopathies" (AFM) and the "Association pour la Recherche sur le Cancer" (ARC) grants.

REFERENCES

1. Sancho E, Batlle E, Clevers H. Signaling pathways in intestinal development and cancer. Annu Rev Cell Dev Biol 2004;20:695–723.

2. Roberts DJ. Molecular mechanisms of development of the gastrointestinal tract. Dev Dyn 2000;219:109–20.
3. Gabella G. Development of visceral smooth muscle. Results Probl Cell Differ 2002;38:1–37.
4. Radtke F, Clevers H. Self-renewal and cancer of the gut: Two sides of a coin. Science 2005;307:1904–9.
5. de Santa Barbara P, van den Brink GR, Roberts DJ. Development and differentiation of the intestinal epithelium. Cell Mol Life Sci 2003;60:1322–32.
6. Chang WW, Leblond CP. Renewal of the epithelium in the descending colon of the mouse. I. Presence of three cell populations: Vacuolated-columnar, mucous and argentaffin. Am J Anat 1971;131:73–99.
7. Potten CS. Epithelial cell growth and differentiation. II. Intestinal apoptosis. Am J Physiol 1997;273:253–7.
8. Wodarz A, Nusse R. Mechanisms of Wnt signaling in development. Annu Rev Cell Dev Biol 1998;14:59–88.
9. Wells JM, Melton DA. Vertebrate endoderm development. Annu Rev Cell Dev Biol 1999;15:393–410.
10. Roberts DJ, Smith DM, Goff DJ, et al. Epithelial–mesenchymal signaling during the regionalization of the chick gut. Development 1998;125:2791–801.
11. Lickert H, Kispert A, Kutsch S, et al. Expression patterns of Wnt genes in mouse gut development. Mech Dev 2001;105:181–4.
12. Gregorieff A, Pinto D, Begthel H, et al. Expression pattern of Wnt signaling components in the adult intestine. Gastroenterology 2005;129:626–38.
13. van Noort M, Clevers H. TCF transcription factors, mediators of Wnt-signaling in development and cancer. Dev Biol 2002;244:1–8.
14. van de Wetering M, Sancho E, Verweij C, et al. The β-catenin/TCF4 complex controls the proliferation/differentiation switch in colon epithelium through c-MYC-mediated repression of p21CIP1/WAF1. Cell 2002;111:241–50.
15. Batlle E, Henderson JT, Beghtel H, et al. β-Catenin and TCF mediate cell positioning in the intestinal epithelium by controlling the expression of the EPHB/EphrinB system. Cell 2002;111:241–63.
16. Korinek V, Barker N, Morin PJ, et al. Constitutive transcriptional activation by a beta-catenin-Tcf complex in APC–/– colon carcinoma. Science 1997;275:1784–7.
17. Korinek V, Barker N, Moerer P, et al. Depletion of epithelial stem-cell compartments in the small intestine of mice lacking Tcf-4. Nat Genet 1998;19:379–83.
18. Barker N, Huls G, Korinek V, et al. Restricted high level expression of Tcf-4 p rotein in intestinal and mammary gland epithelium. Am J Pathol 1999;154:29–35.
19. Lee YJ, Swencki B, Shoichet S, et al. A possible role for the high mobility group box transcription factor Tcf-4 in vertebrate gut epithelial cell differentiation. J Biol Chem 199;274:1566–72.
20. Willert J, Epping M, Pollack JR, et al. A transcriptional response to Wnt protein in human embryonic carcinoma cells. BMC Dev Biol 2002;2:8.
21. Kim JS, Crooks H, Dracheva T, et al. Oncogenic beta-catenin is required for bone morphogenetic protein 4 expression in human cancer cells. Cancer Res 2002;62:2744–8.
22. Lickert H, Domon C, Huls G, et al. Wnt/(beta)-catenin signaling regulates the expression of the homeobox gene Cdx1 in embryonic intestine. Development 2000;127:3805–13.
23. Duprey P, Chowdhury K, Dressler GR, et al. A mouse gene homologous to the Drosophila gene caudal is expressed in epithelial cells from the embryonic intestine. Genes Dev 1998;2:1647–54.
24. Subramanian V, Meyer B, Evans GS. The murine Cdx1 gene product localises to the proliferative compartment in the developing and regenerating intestinal epithelium. Differentiation 1998;64:11–8.
25. Machesky LM, Hall A. Role of actin polymerization and adhesion to extracellular matrix in Rac- and Rho-induced cytoskeletal reorganization. J Cell Biol 1997;138:913–26.
26. Mackay DJ, Hall A. Rho GTPases. J Biol Chem 1998;273: 20685–8.
27. Van Aelst L, D'Souza-Schorey C. Rho GTPases and signaling networks. Genes Dev 1997;11:2295–322.
28. Stappenbeck TS, Gordon JI. Rac1 mutations produce aberrant epithelial differentiation in the developing and adult mouse small intestine. Development 2000;127:2629–42.
29. Stappenbeck TS, Gordon JI. Extranuclear sequestration of phospho-Jun N-terminal kinase and distorted villi produced by activated Rac1 in the intestinal epithelium of chimeric mice. Development 2001;128:2603–14.
30. Hermiston ML, Wong MH, Gordon JI. Forced expression of E-cadherin in the mouse intestinal epithelium slows cell migration and provides evidence for nonautonomous regulation of cell fate in a self-renewing system. Genes Dev 1996;10:985–96.
31. Lewis J. Notch signalling and the control of cell fate choices in vertebrates. Semin Cell Dev Biol 1998;9:583–9.
32. Apelqvist A, Li H, Sommer L, et al. Notch signalling controls pancreatic cell differentiation. Nature 1999;400: 877–81.
33. Kageyama R, Ohtsuka T, Tomita K. The bHLH gene Hes1 regulates differentiation of multiple cell types. Mol Cells 2000;10:1–7.
34. Skipper M, Lewis J. Getting to the guts of enteroendocrine differentiation. Nat Genet 2000;24:3–4.
35. Yang Q, Bermingham NA, Finegold MJ, et al. Requirement of Math1 for secretory cell lineage commitment in the mouse intestine. Science 2001;294:2155–8.
36. Santiago A, Erickson CA. Ephrin-B ligands play a dual role in the control of neural crest cell migration. Development 2002;129:3621–32.
37. Adams RH, Diella F, Hennig S, et al. The cytoplasmic domain of the ligand ephrinB2 is required for vascular morphogenesis but not cranial neural crest migration. Cell 2001;104:57–69.
38. Bruckner K, Pasquale EB, Klein R. Tyrosine phosphorylation of transmembrane ligands for Eph receptors. Science 1997;275:1640–3.
39. Kullander K, Klein R. Mechanisms and functions of Eph and ephrin signalling. Nat Rev Mol Cell Biol 2002;3:475–86.
40. Shamah SM, Lin MZ, Goldberg JL, et al. EphA receptors regulate growth cone dynamics through the novel guanine nucleotide exchange factor ephexin. Cell 2001;105:233–44.
41. Taipale J, Cooper MK, Maiti T, et al. Patched acts catalytically to suppress the activity of Smoothened. Nature 2002;418:892–7.
42. Hebrok M, Kim SK, Melton DA. Notochord repression of endodermal Sonic hedgehog permits pancreas development. Genes Dev 1998;12:1705–13.
43. Zhang J, Rosenthal A, de Sauvage FJ, et al. Downregulation of Hedgehog signaling is required for organogenesis of the small intestine in Xenopus. Dev Biol 2001;229:188–202.
44. Ramalho-Santos M, Melton DA, McMahon AP. Hedgehog signals regulate multiple aspects of gastrointestinal development. Development 2000;127:2763–72.
45. van Den Brink GR, Hardwick JC, Nielsen C, et al. Sonic hedgehog expression correlates with fundic gland differentiation in the adult gastrointestinal tract. Gut 2002;51: 628–33.
46. van den Brink GR, Hardwick JC, Tytgat GN, et al. Sonic hedgehog regulates gastric gland morphogenesis in man and mouse. Gastroenterology 2001;121:317–28.
47. van den Brink GR, Bleuming SA, Hardwick JC, et al. Indian Hedgehog is an antagonist of Wnt signaling in colonic epithelial cell differentiation. Nat Genet 2004;36:277–82.
48. Hanahan D, Weinberg RA. The hallmarks of cancer. Cell 2000;100:57–70.
49. Hemminki A, Markie D, Tomlinson I, et al. A serine/threonine kinase gene defective in Peutz-Jeghers syndrome. Nature 1998;391:184–7.
50. Jenne DE, Reimann H, Nezu J, et al. Peutz-Jeghers syndrome is caused by mutations in a novel serine threonine kinase. Nat Genet 1998;18:38–43.
51. Karuman P, Gozani O, Odze RD, et al. The Peutz-Jegher gene product LKB1 is a mediator of p53-dependent cell death. Mol Cell 2001;7:1307–19.
52. Houlston R, Bevan S, Williams A, et al. Mutations in DPC4 (SMAD4) cause juvenile polyposis syndrome, but only account for a minority of cases. Hum Mol Genet 1998;7: 1907–12.
53. Howe JR, Roth S, Ringold JC, et al. Mutations in the SMAD4/DPC4 gene in juvenile polyposis. Science 1998;280: 1086–8.
54. Howe JR, Bair JL, Sayed MG, et al. Germline mutations of the gene encoding bone morphogenetic protein receptor 1A in juvenile polyposis. Nat Genet 2001;28:184–7.
55. de Santa Barbara P, Williams J, Goldstein AM, et al. Bone morphogenetic protein signaling pathway plays multiple roles during gastrointestinal tract development. Dev Dyn 2005;234:312–22.
56. Hardwick JC, Van Den Brink GR, Bleuming SA, et al. Bone morphogenetic protein 2 is expressed by, and acts upon, mature epithelial cells in the colon. Gastroenterology 2004;126:111–21.
57. Haramis AP, Begthel H, van den Born M, et al. De novo crypt formation and juvenile polyposis on BMP inhibition in mouse intestine. Science 2004;303:1684–6.
58. Wilm B, Ipenberg A, Hastie ND, et al. The serosal mesothelium is a major source of smooth muscle cells of the gut vasculature. Development 2005;132:5317–28.
59. Yntema C, Hammond WS. The origin of intrinsec ganglia of trunk viscera from vagal neural crest in the chick embryo. J Comp Neurol 1954;101:515–41.
60. Le Douarin N, Theillet MA. The migration of neural crest cells to the wall of the digestive tract in avian embryo. J Embryol Exp Morphol 1973;30:31–48.
61. Wallace AS, Burns AJ. Development of the enteric nervous system, smooth muscle and interstitial cells of Cajal in the human gastrointestinal tract. Cell Tissue Res 2005;319: 367–82.
62. Haffen K, Kedinger M, Simon-Assmann P. Mesenchyme-dependent differentiation of epithelial progenitor cells in the gut. J Pediatr Gastroenterol Nutr 1987;6:14–23.
63. Beaulieu JF, Jutras S, Durand J, et al. Relationship between tenascin and alpha-smooth muscle actin expression in the developing human small intestinal mucosa. Anat Embryol 1993;188:149–58.
64. Stainier DY. No organ left behind: Tales of gut development and evolution. Science 2005;307:1902–4.
65. Kedinger M, Duluc I, Fritsch C, et al. Intestinal epithelial–mesenchymal cell interactions. Ann N Y Acad Sci 1998; 859:1–17.
66. Kedinger M, Lefebvre O, Duluc I, et al. Cellular and molecular partners involved in gut morphogenesis and differentiation. Philos Trans R Soc Lond B Biol Sci 1998;353:847–56.
67. Shivdasani RA. Molecular regulation of vertebrate early endoderm development. Dev Biol 2002;249:191–203.
68. McGinnis W, Krumlauf R. Homeobox genes and axial patterning. Cell 1992;68:283–302.
69. Krumlauf R. Hox genes in vertebrate development. Cell 1994;78:191–201.
70. Prince V. The Hox Paradox: More complex(es) than imagined. Dev Biol 2002;249:1–15.
71. Dressler GR, Gruss P. Anterior boundaries of Hox gene expression in mesoderm-derived structures correlate with the linear gene order along the chromosome. Differentiation 1989;41:193–201.
72. Morgan BA, Izpisua-Belmonte JC, Duboule D, et al. Targeted misexpression of Hox-4.6 in the avian limb bud causes apparent homeotic transformations. Nature 1992;358: 236–9.
73. Carpenter EM. Hox genes and spinal cord development. Dev Neurosci 2002;24:24–34.
74. Awgulewitsch A, Utset MF, Hart CP, et al. Spatial restriction in expression of a mouse homoeo box locus within the central nervous system. Nature 1986;320:328–35.
75. Roberts DJ, Johnson RL, Burke AC, et al. Sonic hedgehog is an endodermal signal inducing Bmp-4 and Hox genes during induction and regionalization of the chick hindgut. Development 1995;121:3163–74.
76. Yokouchi Y, Sakiyama J, Kuroiwa A. Coordinated expression of Abd-B subfamily genes of the HoxA cluster in the developing digestive tract of chick embryo. Dev Biol 1995;169:76–89.
77. Warot X, Fromental-Ramain C, Fraulob V, et al. Gene dosage-dependent effects of the Hoxa-13 and Hoxd-13 mutations on morphogenesis of the terminal parts of the digestive and urogenital tracts. Development 1997;124:4781–91.
78. de Santa Barbara P, Roberts DJ. Tail gut endoderm and gut/genitourinary/tail development: A new tissue-specific role for Hoxa13. Development 2002;129:551–61.
79. Beck F, Tata F, Chawengsaksophak K. Homeobox genes and gut development. Bioessays 2000;22:431–41.
80. Sekimoto T, Yoshinobu K, Yoshida M, et al. Region-specific expression of murine Hox genes implies the Hox code-mediated patterning of the digestive tract. Genes Cells 1998;3:51–64.
81. Kondo T, Dolle P, Zakany J, et al. Function of posterior HoxD genes in the morphogenesis of the anal sphincter. Development 1996;122:2651–9.
82. Aubin J, Dery U, Lemieux M, et al. Stomach regional specification requires Hoxa5-driven mesenchymal–epithelial signaling. Development 2002;129:4075–87.
83. Bitgood MJ, McMahon AP. Hedgehog and Bmp genes are coexpressed at many diverse sites of cell–cell interaction in the mouse embryo. Dev Biol 1995;172:126–38.
84. Bilder D, Scott MP. Hedgehog and wingless induce metameric pattern in the Drosophila visceral mesoderm. Dev Biol 1998;201:43–56.
85. Murone M, Rosenthal A, de Sauvage FJ. Hedgehog signal transduction: From flies to vertebrates. Exp Cell Res 1999;253:25–33.
86. Litingtung Y, Lei L, Westphal H, et al. Sonic hedgehog is essential to foregut development. Nat Genet 1998;20: 58–61.
87. Levin M, Johnson RL, Stern CD, et al. A molecular pathway determining left–right asymmetry in chick embryogenesis. Cell 1995;82:803–14.
88. Grapin-Botton A, Melton DA. Endoderm development: From patterning to organogenesis. Trends Genet 2000;16: 124–30.

89. Sukegawa A, Narita T, Kameda T, et al. The concentric structure of the developing gut is regulated by Sonic hedgehog derived from endodermal epithelium. Development 2000;127:1971–80.

90. Apelqvist A, Ahlgren U, Edlund H. Sonic hedgehog directs specialised mesoderm differentiation in the intestine and pancreas. Curr Biol 1997;7:801–4.

91. Mo R, Kim JH, Zhang J, et al. Anorectal malformations caused by defects in sonic hedgehog signaling. Am J Pathol 2001;159:765–74.

92. Urist MR, Mikulski A, Lietze A. Solubilized and insolubilized bone morphogenetic protein. Proc Natl Acad Sci U S A 1979;76:1828–32.

93. Hogan BL. Bone morphogenetic proteins in development. Curr Opin Genet Dev 1996;6:432–8.

94. Whitman M. Smads and early developmental signaling by the TGFbeta superfamily. Genes Dev 1998;12:2445–62.

95. Faure S, Lee MA, Keller T, et al. Endogenous patterns of TGFbeta superfamily signaling during early Xenopus development. Development 2000;127:2917–31.

96. Faure S, de Santa Barbara P, Roberts DJ, et al. Endogenous patterns of BMP signaling during early chick development. Dev Biol 2002;244:44–65.

97. Moniot B, Biau S, Faure S, et al. SOX9 specifies the pyloric sphincter epithelium through mesenchymal–epithelial signals. Development 2004;131:3795–804.

98. Fukuda K, Tanigawa Y, Fujii G, et al. cFKBP/SMAP; a novel molecule involved in the regulation of smooth muscle differentiation. Development 1998;125:3535–42.

99. de Santa Barbara P, van den Brink GR, Roberts DJ. The molecular etiology of gut malformations and diseases. Am J Med Genet 2002;115:221–30.

100. Carson JA, Culberson DE, Thompson RW, et al. Smooth muscle gamma-actin promoter regulation by RhoA and serum response factor signaling. Biochim Biophys Acta 2003;1628:133–9.

101. Chimori Y, Hayashi K, Kimura K, et al. Phenotype-dependent expression of cadherin 6B in vascular and visceral smooth muscle cells. FEBS Lett 2000;469:67–71.

13

Congenital Anomalies Including Hernias

David Allden Lloyd, MChir, FRCS, FCS(SA), FRCSC (Ped Surg), FACS
Simon Edward Kenny, BSc (Hons), MB ChB (Hons), MD, FRCS (Paed Surg), FAAP

INTRODUCTION

Most congenital anomalies of the intestine that require surgical management present in the newborn period and their preoperative care is provided by neonatologists, pediatricians, and pediatric surgeons. The pediatric gastroenterologist has a role in the diagnosis of congenital conditions not recognized during the neonatal period, for example, duodenal stenosis or Hirschsprung disease, and in the long-term management of the consequences of congenital anomalies and their management. Examples of the latter include intestinal failure following extensive loss of intestine (due for example to necrotizing enterocolitis, gastroschisis, intestinal atresia, or midgut volvulus); liver failure related to long-term parenteral nutrition; and chronic constipation associated with developmental abnormalities of the colon, rectum, and anal sphincter.

EMBRYOLOGY OF THE GUT

An understanding of the embryological development of the gastrointestinal tract is essential to grasp the origins and anatomical basis of congenital anomalies of the bowel. The gut develops during the fourth week of gestation by division of the primitive yolk sac into primitive gut and yolk sac proper. These two structures remain in continuity through the vitelline (omphalomesenteric) duct until the duct obliterates during the seventh week. Most of the epithelial attachments to the gut, including the liver and the pancreas, arise from the endoderm of the primitive gut. Connective tissue elements of the gut, such as smooth muscle, are of splanchnic mesenchymal origin. Cells of the enteric nervous system are not generated from the gut. Instead, they arise from the migration of somatic neural crest cells from the vagal region of the hindbrain into the developing esophagus and subsequently migrate caudally to populate the gut to the anal canal. This process is complete by 12 weeks gestation. The gut also becomes populated by intramural extensions of branches of the vagus, pelvic, and mesenteric nerves.

The primitive gut is divided into three parts: foregut, midgut, and hindgut.

The foregut gives rise to the pharynx, lower respiratory system, esophagus, stomach, proximal duodenum down to the level of the bile duct, liver, pancreas, and biliary system. The blood supply is derived from the foregut artery, which later becomes the celiac artery.

The midgut gives rise to the small intestine beyond the opening of the bile duct, the cecum, appendix, and ascending and proximal transverse colon. The midgut blood supply is from the midgut artery, which subsequently becomes the superior mesenteric artery. Between the sixth and twelfth weeks of gestation, the developing midgut herniates into the umbilical cord and then, by a complex series of stereotyped rotational movements, probably reflecting differential growth, returns into the peritoneal cavity and assumes the postnatal position (see section "Midgut Malrotation")

The hindgut derivatives are the distal third of the transverse colon, descending colon, sigmoid colon, rectum, and rostral portion of the anal canal. The distal end of the hindgut ends in the cloaca. This is separated from the ectoderm of the anal canal by the cloacal membrane. As the hindgut differentiates, a sheet of mesenchyme, the urogenital septum, divides the distal hindgut into dorsal and ventral parts. When separation is complete, the ventral component forms the urogenital sinus and the dorsal component forms the anorectal canal. The epithelium of the anal canal therefore is derived from the endoderm of the hindgut rostrally and ectoderm caudally, as demarcated by the pectinate line. Organs derived from the hindgut are supplied by the inferior mesenteric artery.

Functionally, bile enters the duodenum after the thirteenth week of gestation, giving meconium its characteristic dark-green color. Although all components of the gut wall are present by the middle of the second trimester, cyclical regular electrical activity and propulsive activity are relatively late phenomena. Fetal ultrasound studies suggest the onset of regular stomach contractions at around the twenty-fourth week; mature patterns of gut motility in the premature infant occur at 34 weeks, the same time as the development of an effective suck reflex. The late onset of effective contractile activity probably explains why most congenital obstructive intestinal anomalies are not detected antenatally.

ANTENATAL DIAGNOSIS OF CONGENITAL ABNORMALITIES

Prenatal ultrasonography will identify the major abdominal wall defects, exomphalos and gastroschisis (Figure 1), and occasionally gastric

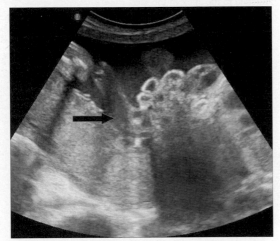

Figure 1 Antenatal ultrasound scan showing the umbilical cord (arrow), to the right of which prolapsed loops of intestine lie outside the abdominal cavity, characteristic of gastroschisis.

or small bowel distention suggestive of intestinal obstruction. The distinctive "double bubble" characteristic of duodenal atresia may be seen, and associated anomalies may be present, notably cardiac. Polyhydramnios raises the possibility of esophageal atresia and upper gastrointestinal obstruction. Abdominal wall defects may be associated with elevated maternal serum α-fetoprotein levels. Fetal karyotyping may be considered in abnormalities with a high risk of chromosomal disorders, such as exomphalos. Prenatal diagnosis provides the opportunity for parental counseling and allows arrangements to be made for prompt postnatal surgical care.[1] However, prenatal diagnosis is not uniformly accurate, and precise diagnosis will be performed after birth.

ABDOMINAL WALL DEFECTS AND HERNIAE

Exomphalos

Exomphalos is a midline developmental defect of the anterior abdominal wall, as a result of which some of the abdominal organs lie outside the abdominal cavity. The incidence is approximately 1 in 3,000.[2-4] The eviscerated abdominal organs are contained within a membranous sac derived from the amniotic membrane. Depending on the size of the lesion, the sac may contain stomach, intestine, liver, and spleen. Somewhat arbitrarily, exomphalos is subcategorized according to the size of the

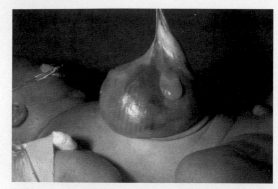

Figure 2 Exomphalos major: the sac is intact and contains intestine and liver; typically, the umbilical cord is attached to the apex of the sac.

abdominal wall defect; those greater than 4 cm are termed major and may contain liver (Figure 2) while those less than 4 cm in diameter are termed minor. Herniation of intestine confined to the base of the umbilical cord, often referred to as a hernia of the cord, may have a different etiology (see section "Gastroschisis") (Figure 3). More complex developmental abnormalities include upper abdominal midline defects, in which exomphalos coexists with defects of the diaphragm, sternum, pericardium, and heart (pentalogy of Cantrell), and lower abdominal midline defects associated with bladder exstrophy. Cloacal exstrophy is a very rare complex lower midline abnormality comprising exomphalos, bladder exstrophy (in which the bladder is in two halves separated by an open colonic plate with ileal prolapse proximally and absence of the anus distally), and abnormalities of the genitalia and sacrum. Up to 75% of infants with exomphalos major have significant associated structural

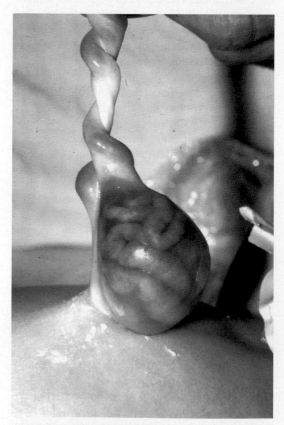

Figure 3 Hernia of the cord: the sac is on the right side of the umbilical cord. Rupture of the sac in utero may produce the typical gastroschisis anomaly.

abnormalities, of which congenital cardiac defects are the most common, or chromosomal anomalies, notably trisomy 13, 18, or 21, which may determine the outcome.[5] It is particularly important to promptly diagnose infants with Beckwith-Wiedemann syndrome, characterized by exomphalos, macroglossia, and hypoglycemia associated with pancreatic islet cell hyperplasia, in order to avoid the serious and avoidable complications of profound, persistent hypoglycemia.[6]

Accurate diagnosis of exomphalos is possible with antenatal ultrasonography and is essential to ensure optimal management.[5] When exomphalos is confirmed, amniocentesis and karyotyping may be appropriate because of the high risk of associated anomalies, and termination of pregnancy may be a consideration.[5]

Surgical management aims to close the abdominal wall defect. There is no urgency to operate if the sac is intact and not infected. For a ruptured exomphalos, urgent operation is required to cover the eviscerated organs to minimize fluid and heat losses and protect against infection. Primary closure of the defect may be possible depending on the volume of the herniated viscera relative to the capacity of the abdominal cavity; closure under tension will impair movement of the diaphragm, compromising ventilation, and may also impair blood flow in the abdominal cavity. After primary closure infants usually will require postoperative positive pressure ventilation. When primary closure is not appropriate, the eviscerated organs are placed in an artificial bag (silo) fashioned from a sheet of reinforced silastic that is sutured to the abdominal wall. Giant exomphalos, where there is a large defect and displacement of most of the abdominal viscera, is a particular problem because the capacity of the abdominal cavity is inadequate and the liver has an abnormal globular shape that does not allow it to fit comfortably into the abdominal cavity. Several operations may be required, including skin grafting, before abdominal closure is achieved. Infection is a major cause of morbidity, and antiseptic care and prophylactic antibiotics are important. Establishment of gastrointestinal function may be slow, and intravenous feeding usually is required.

The outcome is largely dependent on the presence or absence of associated abnormalities; in the absence of these, most infants survive to lead a normal life.[7]

Gastroschisis

In the United Kingdom the incidence of gastroschisis is 4.4 per 10,000 births.[8–9] Several recent studies have reported an increasing incidence over the past decades[8,10–12]; risk factors include young maternal age and ethnic origin.[13]

With gastroschisis, the abdominal muscles appear to be normal and the stomach and intestine are eviscerated through a defect on the right side of the base of the umbilical cord (Figure 4). There is no enveloping sac, and evisceration of other organs is rare. Abnormalities of the intestine, notably atresia, occur in up to 10% of infants but chromosomal and extra-abdominal anomalies are rare,

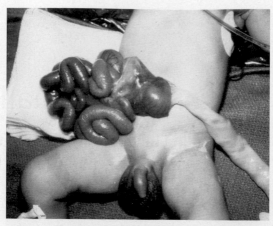

Figure 4 Gastroschisis. The abdominal wall defect is to the right of the umbilical cord, and there is no sac covering the viscera. The stomach and small intestine have prolapsed but not the solid organs.

suggesting a fundamentally different pathogenesis from exomphalos.[14] This is reflected in differences in epidemiology; unlike exomphalos, gastroschisis is associated with young maternal age, lower socioeconomic status, smoking, and cocaine use.[15] The likely mechanism for the development of gastroschisis, supported by evidence from serial antenatal sonograms, is prenatal rupture of a small hernia at the base of the umbilical cord (hernia of the cord)[16] (Figure 3). This defect at the base of the cord may result from obliteration of the right omphalomesenteric artery or from failure of the fetal umbilical hernia to reduce fully during the early development of the abdominal cavity.[16–17]

In utero the eviscerated intestine is exposed to the chemical effects of the amniotic fluid and typically a serositis develops to varying degrees. In extreme cases the loops of intestine become matted together and covered by a fibrinous "peel"; attempts to dissect this carries a risk of damage to the intestine. There is a high risk of short bowel syndrome in neonates with gastroschisis as the result of resection for ischemia or bowel injury.[10,12–13]

As with exomphalos, accurate diagnosis of gastroschisis with antenatal ultrasonography is essential for optimal management.[5] Fetal cardiac instability may develop prompting early delivery, and careful monitoring of the fetus during the third trimester with serial cardiotocography may reduce the high incidence of intrauterine death (10 to 15%).[18] Delivery should take place in a specialist unit. There are differing views on the optimal method of delivery.[19–20] In general, cesarean section is recommended for infants with cardiac instability, but stable infants with gastroschisis may be delivered safely *per vaginam*.

Following birth, urgent operation is required to cover the eviscerated organs to minimize fluid and heat losses and protect against infection. Hypovolemia due loss of protein-rich fluids from the eviscerated bowel is common and preoperative correction of hypovolemia with boluses of saline or albumin is essential (see the section "Intravenous Fluids"). Primary closure of the defect may be possible; because of the increase in intra-abdominal pressure, postoperative positive pressure ventilation will be required. When primary closure is not

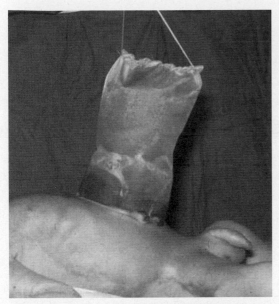

Figure 5 Silo used to cover the viscera temporarily until they can be reduced into the abdominal cavity.

appropriate, the eviscerated organs are placed in a silo of reinforced silastic that is sutured to the abdominal wall (Figure 5). This is progressively reduced in size each day, allowing secondary closure of the abdomen after 7 to 10 days. A commercial spring-loaded silo that can be introduced into the defect has been developed.[21] Infection is a major cause of morbidity, and antiseptic care and prophylactic antibiotics are important. Establishment of gastrointestinal function is often slow and prolonged intravenous feeding is often required. Postoperative problems include adhesive obstruction and short bowel gut syndrome. The overall survival for gastroschisis is greater than 90%.

Omphalomesenteric Duct Remnants

Failure of the omphalomesenteric duct to regress[22] results in an intestinal fistula that presents with a persistent umbilical discharge, commonly with a patch of ectopic intestinal mucosal at the umbilicus. The differential diagnosis includes the far more common umbilical granuloma and rare patent urachus (persistent allantois). The diagnosis is confirmed by passing a fine catheter through the fistula and aspirating small bowel content or injecting radiopaque contrast which enters the ileum (Figure 6). The entire fistula is resected

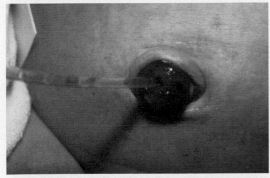

Figure 6 Ectopic intestinal mucosa at the umbilicus with patent omphalomesenteric duct. The bile-colored fluid in the catheter indicates that it has entered the ileum via a patent omphalomesenteric duct.

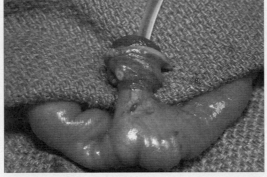

Figure 7 Patent omphalomesenteric duct and Meckel's diverticulum arising from distal ileum. At the top of the specimen, the ectopic mucosa at the umbilicus has been excised. The Meckel's diverticulum will be resected from the small intestine.

through a subumbilical incision (Figure 7). More commonly, the omphalomesenteric duct obliterates but persists as a "Meckel's band" between the umbilicus and small intestine, around which the small intestine may become wrapped, leading to obstruction and ischemia of the volvulus.

The most common remnant of the omphalomesenteric duct is persistence of the enteral end as a Meckel's diverticulum (Figure 8). This is lined by ileal mucosa, but may also contain islands of ectopic gastric mucosa that may lead to ulceration of the adjacent ileal mucosa with bleeding or perforation.[23] Meckel's diverticulum occurs in 2 to 4% of people and is three to five times more prevalent in males than females. Ectopic gastric tissue may be identified by [99m]technetium scanning (Figure 9), which has an 85% sensitivity and a 95% speci-

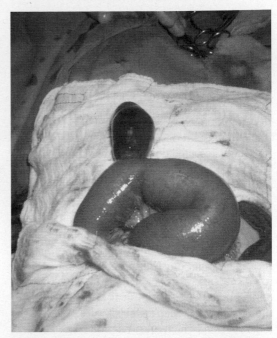

Figure 8 Meckel's diverticulum showing features of inflammation.

ficity.[23] Other complications include diverticulitis, which clinically is indistinguishable from acute appendicitis (Figure 8). Intestinal obstruction may result from intussusception of the diverticulum or from small bowel volvulus around a "Meckel's band." In all these situations, the Meckel's diverticulum is resected with the adjacent segment of ileum. There is no sound evidence to support routine resection of an asymptomatic diverticulum encountered incidentally at operation.

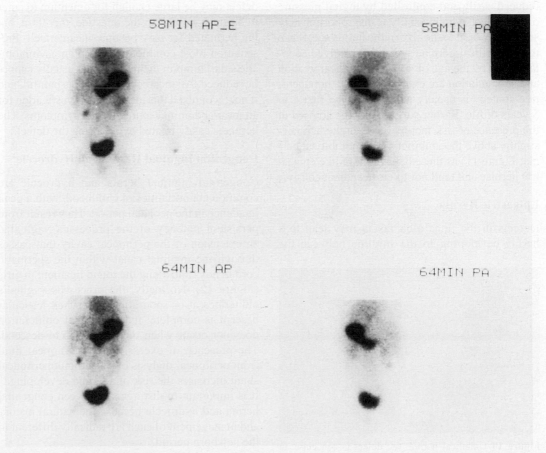

Figure 9 Technetium scan showing uptake by ectopic gastric mucosa in a Meckel's diverticulum in the right lower abdomen. Anteroposterior images on the left, posteroanterior images on the right, at 58 min (*above*) and 64 min (*below*).

At the umbilicus, an isolated remnant of ectopic ileal mucosa will present as a nodule of glossy pink tissue. It must be distinguished from the more common umbilical granuloma and is suspected when the "granuloma" fails to respond to topical treatment. Treatment is excision of the ectopic mucosa. A limited exploration beneath the umbilicus is recommended to exclude an omphalomesenteric (Meckel's) band which, if present, is resected down to the ileum.

Umbilical Granuloma

An umbilical granuloma is a nodule of pink granulation tissue at the umbilicus caused by low-grade infection of the stump of the umbilical cord. It must be distinguished from an omphalomesenteric duct mucosal remnant. Topical treatment suffices, with local antiseptic cleansing and applications of either topical steroids or silver nitrate. The latter carries a risk of damage to the adjacent skin, which must be protected.

Umbilical Hernia

Following separation of the umbilical cord after birth, the umbilical defect forms a scar that contracts to obliterate the opening through the abdominal wall fascia. An umbilical hernia arises when closure of the defect is incomplete or weak; the risk is increased with connective tissue disorders such Ehlers-Danlos syndrome[24] and with peritoneal dialysis.[25] The peritoneal hernia sac is covered by subcutaneous tissue and skin and is more prominent during crying or coughing (Figure 10). On examination the hernia can be reduced easily and controlled by digital pressure on the defect, which usually is disproportionately small compared to the size of the hernia sac. Since most umbilical herniae will have resolved spontaneously by the age of 4 years, and incarceration and strangulation are extremely rare, a nonoperative strategy is usually adopted for the first 4 to 5 years of life. Earlier surgery may be advised in the presence of risk factors or when the hernia is slightly above the umbilicus (supraumbilical hernia; Figure 11) as these behave more like epigastric herniae and tend not to close spontaneously.

Epigastric Hernia

Defects in the linea alba fascia may lead to a hernia developing in the midline between the

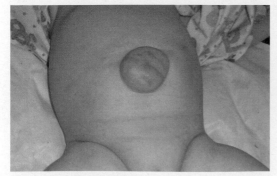

Figure 10 Umbilical hernia: the defect is concentric in the center of the umbilicus and is very likely to close spontaneously.

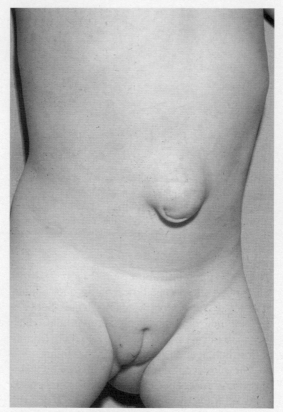

Figure 11 Supraumbilical hernia: the defect is at the upper margin of the umbilicus and is less likely to close spontaneously.

xiphisternum and the umbilicus. Such a hernia contains experitoneal fatty tissue connected to the falciform ligament; there is no communication with the peritoneal cavity although rarely the defect may be large enough for omentum to enter it. There is no risk to the intestine, therefore, but the herniated fat may become incarcerated. Presentation most commonly is with an asymptomatic small lump in the midline that usually cannot be reduced. An incarcerated hernia is painful, and if not recognized this may lead to investigation for an intra-abdominal source for the symptoms. The hernia is easily treated by repairing the defect.

Congenital Inguinal Hernia and Hydrocele

Congenital inguinal hernia and hydrocele are common abnormalities of childhood, with a peak incidence in the neonatal period. They result from persistent patency of the processus vaginalis, an extension of the peritoneal cavity that passes through the inguinal canal within the spermatic cord in boys and along the round ligament in girls (Figure 12). Normally, the processus vaginalis obliterates at or soon after birth when testicular descent is complete; it follows that obliteration does not occur when the testis fails to descend. The presence of excessive intraperitoneal fluid from peritoneal dialysis or a ventriculoperitoneal shunt increases the risk of a hernia developing.[26] It is important to distinguish between congenital hernia and hydrocele because the natural history and management of each are radically different in the newborn period.

Congenital inguinal hernia (indirect inguinal hernia) is the presence of an abdominal viscus,

usually the small intestine, in the patent processus vaginalis (hernia sac). Presentation is with a lump in the groin that may disappear when the infant is quiet and relaxed (Figure 13). A complete or inguinoscrotal hernia is one that extends down to the scrotum (Figure 14). The diagnosis is confirmed clinically by reducing the hernia. The scrotum must be examined to confirm the presence of a testis, since the lump in the groin may be an undescended testis with or without an associated hernia, and will not reduce. Should the hernia not be visible at the time of examination, it is usually possible get the infant to push it out by increasing the intra-abdominal pressure by tickling the infant or by holding its arms above the head, which it will resist. Spontaneous resolution of a hernia does not occur, and there is a risk of it becoming incarcerated (nonreducible) and strangulated. This risk is highest during the first 6 months of life, therefore when a hernia is diagnosed in a newborn infant prompt operation is advised. In a girl the ovary may herniate and present as a firm mobile mass in the groin, often confused with a lymph node. The ovary is difficult to reduce, and excessive attempts to do so may damage it. The herniated ovary may undergo torsion at any time leading to ischemia, and early repair is advisable to avoid this.

An infant with an incarcerated hernia requires urgent admission to hospital. An incarcerated hernia may be painful and infants often become distressed during attempts to reduce the hernia. The infant therefore is sedated, and once it has relaxed, an attempt is made to reduce the hernia by taxis, using very gentle pressure. If reduction is achieved, repair of the hernia is undertaken after an interval of 2 days to allow the tissue swelling in the groin to resolve; this facilitates handling the friable inguinal tissues. If the hernia cannot easily be reduced by taxis, the attempt at reduction is abandoned and immediate operation is undertaken to reduce and repair the hernia. When strangulation of the hernia has occurred, the infant is irritable and feverish and shows features of intestinal obstruction. The hernia itself is acutely tender and the overlying skin may be inflamed. Urgent resuscitation with intravenous fluids, gastric decompression, and antibiotics is followed by emergency repair of the hernia, potentially an extremely difficult operation because of the friability of the tissues. In addition to causing ischemia of the incarcerated intestine, a strangulated hernia may compress the spermatic cord resulting in ischemia and subsequent atrophy of the testis[27] (Figure 15).

Operative treatment of inguinal hernia aims to close the patent processus vaginalis after reducing the hernia. This is done under general anesthesia through a small incision in the groin. There is a risk of impaired fertility arising from injury to the structures in the spermatic cord, namely the testicular artery and vein and the vas deferens. The processus vaginalis must be separated these structures by delicate dissection. The reported risk of vascular injury is 1%, but the true incidences of vascular and vasal injuries are not known. The

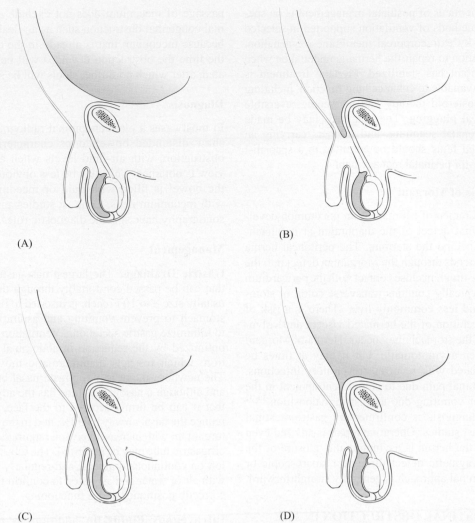

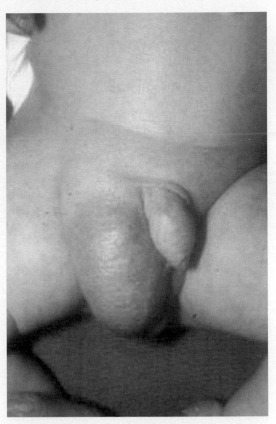

Figure 12 Inguinal hernia and hydrocele. (A) Normal situation after obliteration of the processus: there is no communication between the peritoneal cavity and the tunica vaginalis in the scrotum. (B) Incomplete inguinal hernia: the proximal processus vaginalis remains patent in the groin. (C) Complete inguinal hernia: the whole processus vaginalis remains widely patent leaving an open passage to the scrotum for the intestine to occupy. (D) The processus vaginalis remains patent but is narrow, so that fluid only can enter to form a hydrocele.

Figure 14 Inguinoscrotal hernia: a complete hernia extending to the scrotum.

operation is more difficult, and the risk of complications, including life-threatening perioperative sepsis, is increased when the hernia is strangulated. In an infant with a unilateral inguinal hernia, there are differing views as to whether the contralateral side should be explored (either by open operation or laparoscopically) at the time of hernia repair in order to ligate a patent processus vaginalis if present. There is increasing recognition that an asymptomatic patent processus vaginalis does not necessarily lead to a hernia developing, and

prophylactic ligation does carry a risk to the cord structures. In our view, contralateral exploration is justified only in the presence of risk factors for a hernia developing, or when there are other factors such as prematurity with a high anesthetic risk or difficulty in returning promptly to hospital should a contralateral hernia develop.

Congenital hydrocele occurs when there is a narrow patent processus vaginalis that fills with peritoneal fluid forming a painless swelling in the scrotum that cannot be reduced by taxis. Typically a hydrocele transilluminates brilliantly and examination reveals a normal spermatic cord in the groin above the scrotal swelling, thus differentiating it from a hernia. It may be difficult to exclude a hernia in an infant with a tense swelling that extends from the groin to the scrotum, and ultrasound scanning may be helpful in these circumstances. In most infants the processus vaginalis will obliterate spontaneously during the first 6 months of life and the hydrocele will resolve. Because there is no risk of incarceration, treatment is expectant. A hydrocele that is still present after 2 years of age is not likely to close spontaneously, and operative closure of the processus vaginalis is recommended.

Direct Inguinal Hernia

A direct inguinal hernia is due to a weakness of the posterior wall of the inguinal canal. This allows a knuckle of peritoneum containing intestine to bulge into the inguinal canal. It is rare in infancy. The direct inguinal hernia presents with a lump in the groin that is very difficult to distinguish from the indirect congenital inguinal hernia described above. Usually, the direct type of hernia is first recognized at operation for a presumed indirect hernia or when the patient returns with a "recurrence" after operation for an indirect hernia.[28] Treatment is to repair the fascial weakness through a groin approach.

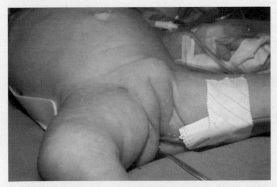

Figure 13 Inguinal hernia: an incomplete hernia extending only to the groin.

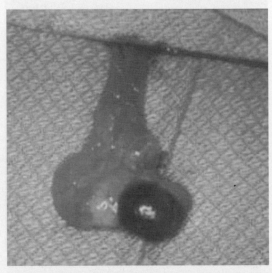

Figure 15 Testicular ischemia due to compression of the testicular blood supply by a strangulated inguinal hernia.

Femoral Hernia

A femoral hernia arises when a knuckle of peritoneum finds its way through the femoral ring, the space beneath the medial end of the inguinal ligament through which the femoral vessels and nerve pass. The hernia lies medial to the femoral vein and may contain omentum and/or small intestine. Presentation is with a lump in the groin below the inguinal ligament and medial to the femoral pulse. Femoral hernia is rare in childhood and must be distinguished from the more common pathological inguinal node. Diagnosis is difficult in an infant and as with a direct hernia, frequently is not made until operation for a suspected inguinal hernia or a "recurrent" hernia.[29]

Congenital Diaphragmatic Hernia

Congenital diaphragmatic hernia is a developmental defect in which intra-abdominal organs herniate into the chest through a posterolateral diaphragmatic defect (Figure 16). Abnormalities of the herniated viscera are rare; there may be associated abnormal rotation of the intestine but most surgeons do not attempt to correct this. Part of the liver may be adherent to the mediastinum but this is not of functional significance. The defect in the diaphragm typically can be repaired directly with sutures, but for large defects a synthetic patch may be required.

The importance of a congenital diaphragmatic hernia lies with the associated abnormalities that account for the high mortality rate of over 60%. These are pulmonary hypoplasia, as a result of which respiration may be seriously compromised, and abnormalities of the pulmonary vasculature resulting in pulmonary hypertension and cardiopulmonary shunting. The net effects of these are varying degrees of respiratory failure that may be irreversible. Immediate operation to repair the hernia is now recognized to be potentially harmful,

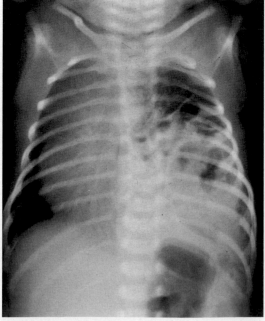

Figure 16 Chest X-ray showing loops of intestine in the left hemithorax, typical of a congenital posterolateral diaphragmatic hernia.

and the focus of postnatal management is on specific methods of ventilation supported in selected cases by extracorporeal membrane oxygenation. Operation to repair the hernia is undertaken when the infant has stabilized. Prenatal treatment is now available to enhance lung function, including corticosteroid therapy and fetoscopic reversible tracheal plugging. The diagnosis may be made on prenatal scanning, and mothers carrying an affected fetus should be admitted to a specialist center for perinatal management.

Hernia of Morgani

The foramen of Morgani is an uncommon developmental defect of the diaphragm at its attachment behind the sternum. The peritoneal hernia sac extends through the Morganian defect into the mediastinum in close contact with the pericardium and typically contains transverse colon or stomach and less commonly liver. There is a risk of incarceration of the herniated viscera and volvulus of the stomach may occur. Hernia of Morgani is often asymptomatic, but it may at times be associated with recurrent respiratory infections, abdominal pain due to colonic entrapment in the sac, or vomiting due to gastric malposition.[30–31] The diagnosis is confirmed by gastrointestinal contrast studies. Operative repair is advised even when the hernia is asymptomatic; closure of the diaphragmatic defect through a laparoscopic or abdominal approach is generally straightforward.

INTESTINAL OBSTRUCTION IN THE NEWBORN INFANT

Congenital intestinal abnormalities present most commonly with intestinal obstruction. From the clinical presentation, notably the presence or absence of vomiting, abdominal distension, and the passage of stool, it may be possible to differentiate proximal from distal obstruction. The following general observations are fundamental to the diagnosis and management of these infants.

Clinical Features

Vomiting. Bile-stained (green) vomiting is a characteristic of intestinal obstruction distal to the ampulla of Vater, and, if present, a mechanical obstruction must be excluded. Non–bile-stained vomiting may be due to obstruction at the pylorus or in the proximal duodenum and must be distinguished from gastroesophageal reflux.

Abdominal Distention. This will depend on the level of obstruction. It is most marked with distal intestinal obstruction where the large and small intestine may be distended, and least apparent with duodenal atresia, where the distention is confined to the epigastrium. Visible peristalsis may be apparent. Abdominal colic is not a characteristic of congenital intestinal obstruction.

Failure to Pass Stools. The normal infant should pass meconium within 36 hours of birth. Failure to pass stool in association with abdominal distention suggests colonic, rectal, or anal obstruction. The

passage of meconium does not exclude a proximal congenital obstruction such as an ileal atresia because meconium that is already in the colon at the time the obstruction develops will be evacuated, after which no further stools will be seen.

Diagnosis

In most cases a plain abdominal radiograph will show distended bowel loops characteristic of obstruction, with air-fluid levels when an erect view is obtained. This may be less obvious when the bowel is filled with fluid or meconium, as with meconium ileus. Contrast studies and ultrasonography have specific diagnostic roles.

Management

Gastric Drainage. The largest nasogastric tube that can be passed comfortably through the nose, usually size 8 to 10 French, is inserted to drain the stomach to prevent vomiting and aspiration and to minimize gastric secretions. Ventilation will be optimized by the reduction in abdominal distention, which restricts diaphragmatic movement. The newborn infant is an obligate nasal breather, and although a nasogastric tube has the advantage that it can be firmly secured to the face, it does reduce the nasal airway by 50%, and in the premature infant with increased oxygen requirements, an orogastric tube may be preferred. The tube must be left on continuous drainage, and regularly flushed with air or water and aspirated to confirm that it is correctly positioned and is functioning.

Intravenous Fluids. In addition to maintenance requirements, there are fluid and electrolyte losses into the stomach and intestine to be replaced. Gastric aspirates are measured and replaced volume for volume with normal saline. Losses into the obstructed intestine will increase sodium, potassium, and chloride requirements, which cannot be measured and are not adequately compensated for by standard "maintenance" solutions containing 0.18% sodium chloride. In anticipation of these additional requirements, we use 0.45% sodium chloride (half normal saline) with potassium chloride 10 to 20 mmol/L as the basic maintenance fluid. The fluid volume is increased for the same reason, with a starting rate of 4 to 5 mL/kg/h for full-term infants and 5 to 6 mL/kg/h for premature infants, depending on the degree of dehydration of the infant. With severe hypovolemia, as occurs with gastroschisis, 10 mL/kg boluses of crystalloid or albumin may be required in addition. Hydration is monitored by clinical assessment of the peripheral circulation, skin turgor, and anterior fontanelle tension and by accurately monitoring the urine volume (normal in a neonate is 2 mL/kg/h) and concentration (ideal specific gravity is 1,008–1,012 although this can be affected by the presence of solutes, notably glucose, aminoacids, blood and bilirubin). Serum electrolytes and acid-base balance are monitored, and urine sodium estimations are useful for interpreting renal function. Based on these findings, the volume of intravenous fluid is adjusted every 4 to 8 hours, the actual frequency of assessment depending on the individual clinical situation. The use of 10% dextrose solutions reduces the risk of hypoglycemia, but regular monitoring of the blood sugar level is important.

Intravenous Antibiotics. Consideration should be given to administration of broad spectrum antibiotics that incorporate anaerobic and aerobic cover for gastrointestinal pathogens, particularly in situations such as midgut volvulus or Hirschsprung enterocolitis (see below), where the physical integrity of the bowel wall is likely to be compromised and bacterial translocation into the peritoneal cavity may occur.

VOMITING IN THE NEWBORN INFANT

Some surgical causes of congenital intestinal obstruction are shown in Table 1. Nonsurgical causes of vomiting must be excluded, including feeding difficulties (under- or overfeeding), systemic infection, urinary tract infection, raised intracranial pressure, food allergy, and adrenogenital syndrome.

Duodenal Atresia

The site of obstruction is typically at the level of the ampulla of Vater and may take the form of an atresia or an intact membrane across the lumen causing a complete obstruction, or a stenosis or fenestrated membrane causing a partial obstruction. At the level of the atresia, there is a marked decrease in the caliber of the distal duodenum; occasionally the obstructing membrane will bulge distally forming the windsock anomaly, as a result of which the change in caliber will suggest that the site of obstruction is further distal than it actually is. The common bile duct usually opens on the membrane and is vulnerable if an attempt is made to excise the membrane.

The incidence of duodenal atresia is about 1 in 5,000 live births.[32] Prematurity is common, and associated anomalies include trisomy 21 (Down syndrome), congenital cardiac disease, esophageal atresia, anorectal abnormalities, and malrotation. The cause of the anomaly is not understood; its occurrence at a complex site of development of the duodenum, pancreas, and biliary and pancreatic ducts and the association with trisomy 21 suggest a genetic origin.[33]

Table 1 Causes of Congenital Intestinal Obstruction
Vomiting in the newborn infant
Duodenal atresia
Malrotation
Jejunoileal atresia
Meconium ileus
Duplication cyst
Incarcerated inguinal hernia
Failure to pass stool in the newborn infant
Anorectal malformation
Hirschsprung disease
Meconium plug syndrome
Intestinal pseudo-obstruction syndrome
Colonic atresia

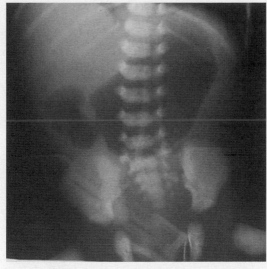

Figure 17 Duodenal atresia: abdominal radiograph showing the characteristic "double bubble" sign owing to gas in the distended stomach and duodenum proximal to the atresia.

The diagnosis may be suspected prenatally when the fetal sonogram shows hydramnios and a distended stomach and duodenum (Figure 1). Because of the association with trisomy 21, these findings may prompt fetal karyotyping, particularly if termination of pregnancy is a consideration.[34] Following birth, the typical presentation is with bilious vomiting and epigastric distention, but vomiting may be nonbilious if the ampulla of Vater opens distal to the atresia. A plain abdominal radiograph shows the characteristic double bubble representing the distended stomach and proximal duodenum (Figure 17). An upper gastrointestinal contrast radiograph or ultrasonography may be required to distinguish this from malrotation. The pediatric gastroenterologist may encounter older patients with partial duodenal obstruction due to a fenestrated membrane who are able to tolerate feeds to such an extent that the diagnosis is not be recognized for months or years until persistent postprandial vomiting prompts a contrast radiograph or endoscopy.

Preoperative management includes gastric decompression and correction of fluid and electrolyte abnormalities. The duodenum is approached through a supraumbilical right transverse incision. The nasogastric tube is pushed distally into the duodenum to define the site of obstruction and exclude a "windsock" abnormality. An annular pancreas may encircle the duodenum at the point of atresia but often is not the primary cause of the obstruction.

Because of the risk of injury to the ampulla of Vater, the preferred procedure for duodenal atresia is a duodenoduodenal anastomosis, bypassing the obstruction. The "diamond" incision described by Kimura and colleagues uses a transverse incision in the dilated upper pouch and a longitudinal incision in the narrow distal duodenum to optimize patency of the anastomosis.[35] Postoperative ileus may be prolonged, and intravenous feeding is often needed; if this is not available, a transanastomotic nasoduodenal feeding tube is passed at operation under direct vision to enable early postoperative enteral feeding.[36]

For duodenal stenosis or a fenestrated diaphragm, the duodenum is entered proximal to the point of obstruction through a longitudinal incision that is extended across the stenosis, taking care to avoid the ampulla of Vater by placing the incision anterolaterally. The incision is closed transversally. Survival rates for duodenal atresia and stenosis are over 90% and depend largely on the influence of associated anomalies.[37] Long-term outcomes are usually good although late obstructive symptoms have been described and attributed to a persistent atonic-dilated proximal duodenum requiring plication or resection.[38]

Midgut Malrotation

Malrotation describes a situation in which the intestine lies in an abnormal position in the peritoneal cavity, putting it at risk of undergoing torsion around the superior mesenteric artery axis. Volvulus of the midgut (small intestine, cecum, and proximal colon) occurs most commonly in the neonatal period, and the resultant intestinal ischemia may be fatal if not recognized and treated immediately. It therefore behooves those caring for newborn infants to be aware of the condition.

The process whereby the gut acquires its position in the abdominal cavity is described in three stages[39] (Figure 18). During normal embryonic development, rapid growth of the gut in the fifth and sixth weeks of gestation forces the gut to herniate through the umbilical ring into the base of the umbilical cord (stage 1). Between the eighth and eleventh weeks (stage 2), the midgut returns to the abdominal cavity in an orderly way, beginning with the proximal small bowel. As it does so, the stomach and duodenum rotate in an anticlockwise direction around the midgut (superior mesenteric) artery, with the result that the duodenum initially lies toward the right and then curves to the left where it is fixed by a peritoneal fold, the ligament of Trietz, to the left of the vertebral column. In the third stage, the distal part of the midgut returns to the abdomen, also rotating in an anticlockwise direction bringing the cecum to its final position in the right lower abdomen where it is fixed by peritoneum to the posterior abdominal wall (Figure 19A). This process may reflect differential growth, but the true mechanism is not understood.[40]

Traditionally, malrotation is attributed to failure of the intestine to "rotate" to its normal position when it moves from the umbilical cord hernia back into the peritoneal cavity during the first trimester. Several configurations of abnormal gut rotation have been described.[39] The common form is the position of "nonrotation," in which the duodenum lies to the right of the vertebral column instead of curving across to the left, with the result that the ligament of Trietz lies to the right of the midline, and the cecum lies in the upper abdomen to the left of duodenum (Figure 19B). A band of peritoneum (Ladd's band) passes from the cecum across the duodenum to be attached to posterior abdominal wall to the right of the duodenum; this may cause

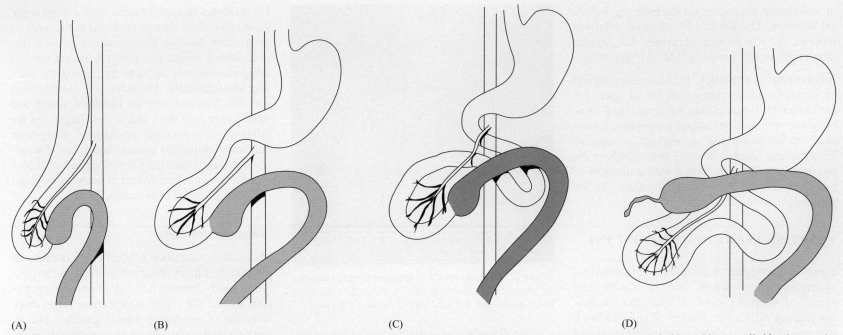

Figure 18 Process of normal rotation of the gastrointestinal tract. (A) Lateral view: gestational week 5, showing the developing stomach, the primitive midgut supplied by the superior mesenteric artery and the colon (*stippled*). (B) Anterior view: by week 6 the stomach and duodenum have rotated 90° clockwise. (C) Anterior view: week 8, duodenum and jejunum have returned to the abdomen and rotated anticlockwise to take up position behind the artery. (D) Anterior view: week 11, colon has completed 270° rotation anterior to the artery and will continue to its final position in the right lower quadrant.

an extrinsic obstruction of the duodenum. The midgut, which normally has a long attachment through its mesentery obliquely to the posterior abdominal wall, is instead suspended from a narrow attachment confined to the base of the superior mesenteric artery (Figure 19B). A volvulus occurs when the midgut twists around this narrow pedicle, usually in a clockwise direction; this may happen at any time but is most common in the neonatal period (Figure 20). Volvulus will lead to potentially fatal midgut ischemia if not promptly corrected (Figure 21). Other forms of malrotation are uncommon and may lead to internal hernia formation with a risk of incarceration and obstruction. Failure of the cecum to be fixed to the posterior abdomen (nonfixation) will allow it to flip from side to side in the abdomen and become intermittently obstructed; in this situation the duodenum may have rotated normally.

The true incidence of malrotation in the general population is not known because the anomaly may remain asymptomatic throughout life.

The clinical presentation of malrotation will depend on whether the abnormality is an acute midgut volvulus or a less severe intermittent obstruction of the gut. Acute midgut volvulus, most frequently encountered in the newborn infant, presents with bilious vomiting, abdominal pain, and progressive abdominal distention and tenderness. Stools may be passed in the early stages; the passage of blood suggests intestinal ischemia. With progressive midgut ischemia, the infant's condition rapidly deteriorates with hypovolemia and persistent metabolic acidosis despite fluid resuscitation. A plain abdominal radiograph may show features of duodenal obstruction; beyond this, the bowel may contain more fluid than air, with resultant opacification

of the abdominal cavity. When the diagnosis is suspected, a pediatric surgeon must be consulted immediately. If the situation allows, an upper gastrointestinal contrast radiograph will show the abnormal configuration of the duodenum (Figure 22) and an ultrasound scan may reveal the abnormal anatomical relationship of the superior mesenteric artery and vein. Time is of the essence and should not be wasted on diagnostic

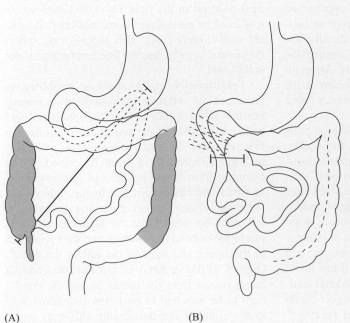

Figure 19 (A) Normal rotation of the intestine. The small bowel mesentery is attached to the posterior abdominal wall obliquely from the ligament of Trietz to the ileocecal junction, so preventing the small bowel from twisting. The ascending and descending colon are fixed by a covering of peritoneum. (B) Nonrotation of the intestine. The duodenum lies to the right of the vertebral column and the cecum lies to the left of the duodenum. Ladd's bands cross from the cecum in front of the duodenum. The mesenteric attachment is very narrow and confined to the origin of the superior mesenteric artery, around which the midgut may twist.

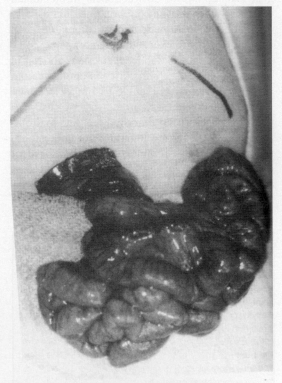

Figure 20 Midgut malrotation with volvulus. The midgut (small bowel, cecum, and right half of the colon) has twisted in a clockwise direction around the pedicle of the superior mesenteric vessels. In this example the midgut is still viable.

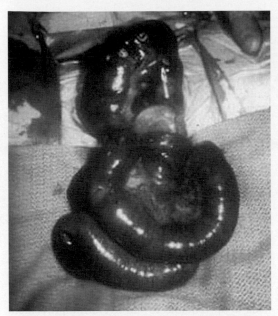

Figure 21 Midgut malrotation with volvulus: there is irreversible ischemic necrosis of the midgut.

procedures when it is clear that immediate laparotomy is required. After rapid attention to fluid and electrolyte abnormalities, a generous supraumbilical transverse incision is used to allow delivery and inspection of the whole of the small and large bowel. If a volvulus is confirmed, it is derotated, usually in an anticlockwise direction, to allow restoration of the mesenteric circulation. This will reveal the typical nonrotation configuration of the gut with the duodenum on the right and the cecum adjacent to it. If the intestine is viable, the Ladd's bands extending from the cecum across the duodenum are divided; this enables the cecum to be mobilized toward the left to widen the mesenteric pedicle in order to reduce

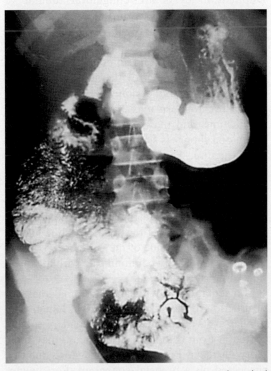

Figure 22 Midgut malrotation: an upper gastrointestinal contrast study showing the duodenum and small intestine lying to the right of the vertebral column.

the risk of the volvulus recurring (Ladd's procedure). The intestine is returned to the abdominal cavity in the position of nonrotation with the cecum on the left side and the small intestine on the right side; the appendix may be removed to avoid diagnostic confusion in the event of appendicitis in the future. When the volvulus clearly is not viable (Figure 21) the prognosis is extremely poor and there is a case for not undertaking any further procedure; should the necrotic midgut be resected, this will result in severe short-gut syndrome and the inevitable consequences of long-term intravenous feeding, notably cholestatic liver disease.[41] When the viability of the bowel is uncertain, any bowel that is obviously not viable is resected, stomas are made to defunction the remaining intestine and the abdomen is closed. A second laparotomy is done after an interval of 24 to 36 hours to re-examine the bowel; the amount of viable bowel remaining will determine further management.

The gastroenterologist is more likely to encounter malrotation in patients at any age presenting with subacute symptoms of intermittent abdominal pain with or without bile-stained vomiting; there may be associated failure to thrive and malabsorption. A contrast upper gastrointestinal contrast radiograph with follow-through must be obtained. If the characteristic features of malrotation are demonstrated (Figure 22), recurrent midgut volvulus must be presumed and operation (Ladd's procedure) is essential to prevent further episodes of volvulus. Because of the risk of volvulus, Ladd's procedure is recommended for all patients found to have nonrotation even if not symptomatic. Should the radiograph not reveal malrotation of the duodenum or signs of an internal hernia, a contrast enema is required. If the cecum is not in its normal position, nonfixation with intermittent torsion is a possibility and may require surgery to fix or resect the right colon. A potential pitfall arises when the contrast enema is normal; this does not exclude nonfixation of the cecum which may have returned to its normal position when the radiograph was taken. In the face of recurring symptoms, it is essential that the radiographs be repeated, preferably while the child is symptomatic.

Jejunoileal Atresia

Congenital obstruction of the jejunum or ileum due to atresia or stenosis develops as a result of ischemia of a segment of fetal intestine. This was first demonstrated experimentally in a fetal dog model by Louw and Barnard in 1955, who created classic small bowel atresia in pups following in utero ligation of branches of the small bowel mesentery.[42] The incidence is approximately 3 per 10,000 live births, and it is associated with low birth weight for gestational age and multiparity.[43]

Patterns of small bowel atresia are shown in Figure 23.[44] These are atresia in continuity (type I) (Figure 24), atresia with connecting band and mesenteric defect (type II), atresia with no continuity and with adjacent mesenteric defect

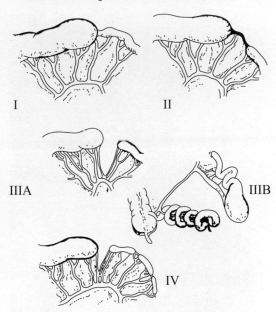

Figure 23 Classification of jejunoileal atresia. (See text for explanation.)

(type IIIA) or extensive mesenteric defect and "apple peel" bowel configuration (type IIIB; Figure 25), and multiple atresias (type IV). Presentation is with bilious vomiting and abdominal distention. Meconium stool that is already in the colon before the atresia develops may be passed, confirming that the obstruction develops after the secretion of bile into the embryonic gastrointestinal tract. The diagnosis is confirmed by plain abdominal radiography, which shows multiple dilated loops of intestine with air fluid levels. Distal ileal atresia must be distinguished from meconium ileus and long-segment Hirschsprung disease; a contrast enema may be required for this.

Preoperative preparation is as described above. At operation, the site of obstruction is easily identified by the abrupt change in caliber from the dilated proximal intestine to the narrow distal small bowel. In type IIIA atresia, there is a defect in the adjacent mesentery. The grossly dilated termination of the proximal bowel is resected, and continuity is restored by end-to-end or end-to-back anastomosis. In the case of multiple atresias (type IV), as many segments as possible should be salvaged to avoid short-gut syndrome. Postoperative recovery may be prolonged, and parenteral nutrition may be required. Survival rates over the past two decades have ranged from 78 to 100%.[44]

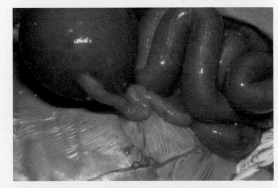

Figure 24 jejunoileal atresia type I showing the typical dilated proximal bowel and narrow distal bowel.

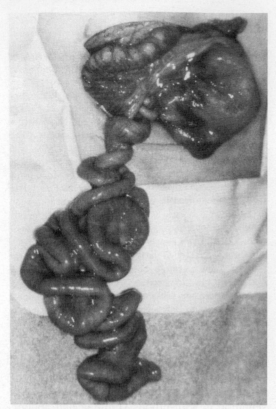

Figure 25 Jejunoileal atresia type IIIB. There is an extensive mesenteric defect and an "apple peel" bowel coiled around the long marginal artery. There is a risk of the bowel twisting and obstructing the tenuous blood supply.

Postoperative complications include anastomotic leak or stenosis and functional intestinal obstruction at the anastomosis. Extensive loss of small bowel attributable to multiple atresias (type IV) or a precarious blood supply (type IIIB) may result in short bowel syndrome.

Where there are concerns about the safety of the anastomosis, either because of impaired vascularity or possible distal obstruction, stomas may be created but at the expense of high fluid and electrolyte losses from the proximal stoma. This may be ameliorated by refeeding the effluent into the distal stoma and has the additional advantage of promoting growth of the distal intestine.[45] With proximal jejunal atresia, resection of the dilated bowel is not possible, and tapering of the proximal jejunum by antimesenteric excision or inversion facilitates construction of the anastomosis and may enhance postoperative transit.

Meconium Ileus

This is a misnomer because the obstruction is not functional, as the name implies, but mechanical. As a result of pancreatic enzyme deficiency, the distal ileum becomes plugged by viscid meconium with a high albumin content. This deficiency of pancreatic enzymes is, with rare exceptions, associated with cystic fibrosis. Up to 20% of newborn infants with cystic fibrosis present with meconium ileus. The diagnosis is suspected when there is a family history of cystic fibrosis and is confirmed by chromosomal analysis, which in 85% of patients will demonstrate the DF508 mutation, a three-base pair deletion from

chromosome 7.[46] Mutations result in defective chloride transport in the apical membrane of epithelial cells and an abnormally high excretion of chloride from the skin.[47] This can be measured by iontophoresis (the sweat test) that remains as the gold standard diagnostic test in mature infants.

The characteristic intestinal features in meconium ileus are a dilated distal ileum containing meconium that is abnormally tenacious and adherent to the intestinal mucosa, with an abrupt transition to a narrow terminal ileum containing multiple pellets of meconium, often nonpigmented. The colon is empty and contracted (microcolon). Presentation is with distal ileal obstruction, which must be distinguished from ileal atresia and long-segment Hirschsprung disease. Abdominal radiographs show air fluid levels in the proximal small bowel but not in the dilated meconium-filled terminal ileum which appears opaque and typically contains multiple translucencies owing to entrapped fat globules, the "soap bubble" appearance. Meconium ileus may be complicated by volvulus of a dilated meconium-filled loop of distal ileum, which may in turn result in intestinal atresia or may perforate, leading to meconium peritonitis. The latter is seen on abdominal radiography as multiple extraintestinal calcifications in the peritoneal cavity.

Following nasogastric decompression and correction of fluid and electrolyte abnormalities, the diagnosis is confirmed by isotonic water-soluble contrast enema, which will show the microcolon, the meconium pellets in the distal ileum, and the dilated proximal ileum (Figure 26). By

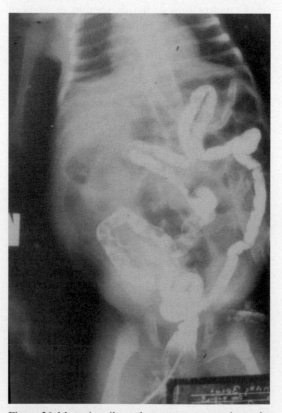

Figure 26 Meconium ileus: the contrast enema shows the typical microcolon, the cecum displaced toward the midline, and the filling defects in the terminal ileum representing meconium pellets.

switching to a Gastrografin enema, it is possible in over 50% of cases for the radiologist to clear the obstructing meconium.[48] Gastrografin has an osmolality of approximately 1,800 mOsm/L, and great care must be taken to anticipate and replace extracellular fluid losses into the intestine during radiography. At operation for uncomplicated meconium ileus, the dilated ileum is opened and the meconium is removed using saline irrigation, not an easy procedure owing to the adherence of the meconium of the intestinal mucosa. Simple enterostomy and resection of the dilated or compromised intestine with primary anastomosis are safe options when the bowel wall is healthy and the distal obstruction has been cleared with certainty. Alternatively, proximal and distal stomas should be created.

The survival rate for meconium ileus has improved from 30% in the 1960s to over 90%.[49] This is attributable to the overall improvement in perioperative respiratory care, increasingly successful nonoperative management, and avoidance of stomas. The gastroenterologist is likely to be involved with older children in whom episodic obstruction due to inspissated meconium may occur (meconium ileus equivalent, distal intestinal obstruction syndrome). This may be associated with underhydration and altered enzyme replacement needs. Presentation is with colicky abdominal pain, and there may be tenderness in the right iliac fossa, where the obstructed bowel may be palpated. This mass must be distinguished from an appendix mass, ovarian tumor, and inflammatory bowel disease. In most children, oral Gastrografin will relieve the obstruction.[50]

Duplication Cysts

Duplication cysts are congenital tubular or spherical cysts attached to the alimentary canal anywhere between the mouth and the anus, most commonly in the ileocecal region. The cysts have a muscle layer and an epithelial lining that usually resembles that of the adjacent gastrointestinal tract. In the abdomen, nodules of ectopic gastric mucosa may be present within the duplications and may lead to peptic ulceration. The blood supply is shared with the adjacent normal structure. Thoracic duplications may communicate through the diaphragm with the intra-abdominal gastrointestinal tract, from which the blood supply is derived (a potential pitfall for the unwary surgeon). Intestinal duplications lie on the mesenteric side of the small intestine and on the antimesenteric side of the large bowel. Tubular duplications may communicate with the intestinal lumen.[51]

Presentation is with an abdominal mass or obstruction of the adjacent intestinal lumen. In a tubular cyst, peptic ulceration secondary to acid secretion from ectopic gastric mucosa may present with rectal bleeding. The diagnosis may be suspected on a prenatal sonogram. For diagnosis, ultrasonography and plain or contrast radiography may be helpful, depending on the site

Table 2 Classification of Congenital Anorectal Anomalies

Males	Females
Cutaneous fistula, bucket-handle malformation, anal stenosis, anal membrane	Cutaneous (perineal) fistula
Rectourethral bulbar fistula	Vestibular fistula
Rectourethral prostatic fistula	
Rectovesical (bladder neck) fistula	Persistent cloaca
Imperforate anus without fistula	Imperforate anus without fistula
Rectal atresia/stenosis	Rectal atresia/stenosis

of the lesion. Computed tomography or magnetic resonance imaging will help to distinguish the duplication from an ovarian or mesenteric cyst. Complete excision of the cyst with preservation of the viscus from which it is arising is the treatment of choice. Where this is not possible, partial excision of the cyst and removal of the mucosal lining from the remaining cyst wall, or resection of the duplication with the adjacent intestine, are options, avoiding if possible an extensive resection that may result in short-gut syndrome.

FAILURE TO PASS STOOL IN THE NEWBORN INFANT

Causes of failure to pass stool are shown in Table 1.

Anorectal Anomalies

These occur in approximately 1 in 2,500 live births.[32,43,52] The embryologic events surrounding hindgut development remain poorly understood. The cloaca forms at approximately 21 days gestation and is a cavity into which hindgut, tailgut, allantois, and mesonephric ducts open. By 6 weeks, a combination of programed cell death and differential growth results in the formation of an anterior urogenital cavity and a posterior anorectal cavity. When this process is disrupted, an anorectal malformation may result. The anatomic findings in children with anorectal malformations vary considerably, and a number of complex classification systems have been proposed. The pragmatic classification of Pena and Hong (Table 2) conveniently summarizes most commonly encountered variants.[53] The cutaneous fistula is a "low" lesion where the rectum has passed through the anal sphincter and the anomaly is distal to this. The cutaneous fistula discharges meconium and can occur anywhere in the perineal midline anterior to the presumptive site of the anus, including the scrotum and penis (Figure 27). Occasionally, it is recognizable as a chain of whitish pearl-like nodules. The remaining lesions are considered to be "intermediate" or "high," where the rectum has not passed completely through the anal sphincter. Examples are the rectourethral fistula in a boy (Figure 28) and the rectovaginal fistula in a girl (Figure 29). The cause of anorectal anomalies is unknown. Although prenatal dosing of rats with the antimitotic agent doxorubicin can result in anorectal malformations,[54] there is little evidence for

environmental factors playing a major causative role in humans.

Anorectal anomalies are most often detected during routine postnatal examination, although with some anomalies, the perineum may appear relatively normal to casual inspection. Anatomically, the lesion is usually associated with a fistulous communication between the rectum and either the genitourinary tract or perineum; the spectrum of abnormalities ranges from simple anterior malposition of the anus to complex anal agenesis. In the latter, typically the anus is absent or represented by a shallow pit, the infant's buttocks are flattened, and the sacrum and anorectal innervation are deficient. The degree of abdominal distention is variable, and intestinal perforation is rare. About 60% of infants will have malformations affecting other organ systems, most commonly cardiac, gastrointestinal, genitourinary, or vertebral in origin.[43,52] These may coexist as the VACTERL (vertebral, anorectal, cardiac, tracheoesophageal, renal, limb) sequence of anomalies.[52]

A structured approach to the assessment of these infants needs to be adopted. Thorough physical examination is essential. Echocardiography, renal tract and spinal ultrasonography, plain spinal radiography, and karyotyping all need to be performed. Neonates with multiple anomalies may require assessment by a range of specialists, including clinical geneticists, neonatologists, orthopedic surgeons, otolaryngologists, neurologists, and neurosurgeons. The infant should be maintained on urinary tract antibiotic prophylaxis until micturating cystourethrography, often performed following definitive reconstructive surgery, has excluded vesicoureteric reflux.

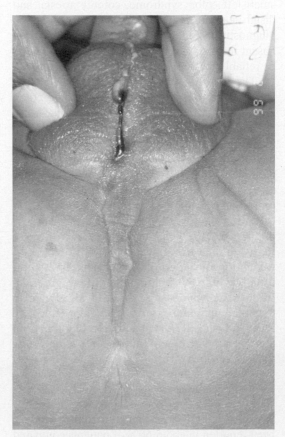

Figure 27 Anorectal malformation: cutaneous fistula. The anus is covered by a skin cap from which meconium is tracking along the fistula anteriorly in the midline onto the scrotum.

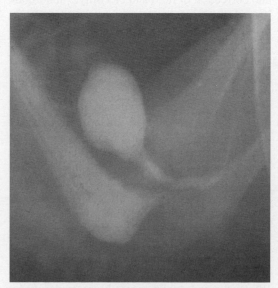

Figure 28 Anorectal malformation: rectourethral fistula. Contrast study via a distal colostomy showing the rectum terminating as a fistula entering the posterior urethra.

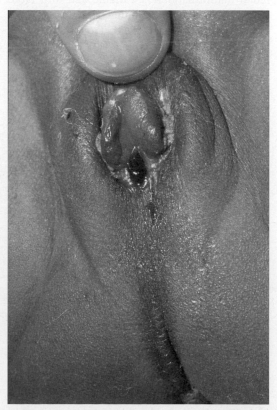

Figure 29 Anorectal malformation: discharge of meconium from the vagina in an infant girl with a rectovaginal fistula.

The principles underlying the initial management of infants with imperforate anus are relief of the distal bowel obstruction and protection of the anal sphincter mechanism from inappropriate surgery. Initial resuscitation should include passage of a nasogastric tube (this will also exclude esophageal atresia) and establishment of intravenous access. Surgical options are to form a colostomy or to perform definitive reconstruction. Only infants presenting with a low lesion such as a cutaneous fistula, in which the anomaly clearly is distal to the anal sphincter, are amenable to relatively straightforward perineal reconstructive procedures without a diverting colostomy. In all other cases, or when there is doubt, it is advisable to perform a temporary diverting colostomy followed by a staged reconstructive procedure after the infant has been fully assessed. A sigmoid colostomy is suitable for most cases of imperforate anus, but for a cloacal anomaly, a transverse colostomy is recommended.

Most anorectal anomalies are amenable to reconstruction via a posterior sagittal approach[55] although a laparotomy is often required in boys with rectovesical fistula and girls with a cloacal anomaly. The two main steps in the reconstruction are, first, mobilization and ligation of the fistula and, second, creation of the neoanus. In girls with a cloacal anomaly, genitourinary reconstruction is also required. Meticulous surgical technique is essential to optimize the long-term outcome. More recently, laparoscopic anorectal reconstruction has been advocated, and long-term outcome data are awaited.[56–57] Following reconstruction, the parents are taught to dilate the infant's anus to avoid stenosis.

The long-term outcome for children with anorectal malformations is variable and to a large extent dependent on the initial anatomy and subsequent clinical management. Troublesome constipation can occur in children with "low" lesions. Careful follow-up and parental support are necessary to ensure that constipation and development of a dilated megarectum are avoided. Children with "high" malformations tend to have a poorer outcome, with higher rates of fecal incontinence.[58] The psychological effects of incontinence and constipation in this group of children and their families as they grow up are considerable.[59] In the last decade, the antegrade continence enema procedure (ACE) has been found to be useful in establishing independent continence.[60] In later life, females will need specialist obstetric assessment and advice in choosing the most appropriate form of delivery.

Hirschsprung Disease and Related Disorders

Hirschsprung disease affects 1 in 5,000 newborns and is defined as an absence of ganglion cells (aganglionosis) in a variable length of distal bowel (see Chapter 24.2b, "Hirschsprung Disease").[61–62] In 80% of infants, the aganglionosis is confined to the sigmoid colon and rectum including the internal sphincter (short-segment disease), but it may extend to encompass the entire colon (total colonic) or rarely affect the entire intestine. Although macroscopically normal, the affected gut is unable to relax, causing a functional bowel obstruction with dilatation of the proximal intestine. The male/female ratio is 4:1 in short-segment disease and approximately 1:1 in long-segment disease.[63–65]

In the embryo, ganglion cells of the enteric nervous system are derived from the vagal neural crest from where they migrate, during the first trimester, into the esophagus and then colonize the developing gut in a craniocaudal direction. Aganglionosis can result from a failure of migration, differentiation, or survival of these cells. Mutations in several genes can cause aganglionosis. The receptor tyrosine kinase gene RET is the most common gene in which a mutation may be found.[66–67] The main mutation predisposing to Hirschsprung disease lies within a noncoding enhancer region of the gene that has different effects according to sex.[68] Significantly, mutations in RET have been found in multiple endocrine neoplasia syndrome types IIA and IIB and familial medullary thyroid carcinoma; a careful family history should, therefore, be taken, and genetic counseling offered to families at risk.[69] Hirschsprung disease is also more common in children with trisomy 21 (Down syndrome).[65]

Hirschsprung disease should be suspected in all infants who have not passed meconium within 48 hours of birth and all infants presenting with features of bowel obstruction for which there is no obvious cause. Constipation and abdominal distention are the most common presenting signs, but affected children may also present with bile-stained vomiting, failure to thrive, or cardiovascular collapse owing to Hirschsprung enterocolitis. A minority of children will present later in life with intractable chronic constipation. Plain abdominal radiographs will show distended loops of bowel, although in neonates it is often impossible to distinguish large from small bowel obstruction. Initial management should be directed at establishment of intravenous access and correction of fluid and electrolyte abnormalities, and passage of a nasogastric tube. When the abdomen is very distended, gentle anal dilatation and rectal washouts with 0.9% saline solution can often result in dramatic decompression and improvement in the physical condition of the child.

The diagnosis is made by suction rectal biopsy of the submucosal plexus, a procedure that can be performed on the ward with minimum discomfort and distress to the infant using custommade biopsy forceps. Multiple biopsies should be obtained at 2 and 4 cm above the anal verge. Histopathology examination will reveal an absence of ganglion cells and the presence of thickened nerve trunks that often extend into the lamina propria. Increased acetylcholinesterase staining is also present and can aid diagnosis. Availability of an experienced pediatric pathologist is essential. Where there is doubt, repeat biopsies should be obtained and the need for a full-thickness biopsy that includes the myenteric plexus considered. A

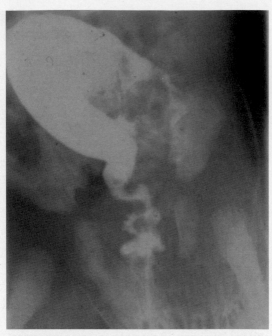

Figure 30 Hirschsprung disease: contrast enema showing the transitional zone from dilated to contracted colon at the level of the sigmoid colon.

contrast enema may be useful in determining the extent of aganglionosis if a clear transitional zone from dilated ganglionic to contracted aganglionic colon is seen (Figure 30); however, false-positives can occur, and Hirschsprung disease should not be diagnosed on the basis of a contrast enema alone. Radiologically, Hirschsprung disease must be distinguished from meconium plug syndrome, small left colon syndrome, colonic atresia, and distal ileal atresia. Anorectal manometry can be diagnostic in older children on the basis of an absent rectoanal inhibitory reflex, but this cannot be reliably performed in neonates.

The principles of definitive surgical reconstruction are excision of the aganglionic colon and "pull-through" of ganglionic colon with a coloanal anastomosis, leaving the anal sphincter mechanism intact. Several methods for this have been described. The traditional operative approach is to perform a colostomy in the neonatal period at the distal limit of ganglionic bowel (confirmed histologically by staged biopsies at operation) followed by staged surgical procedures over 3 to 9 months (Figure 31). Increasingly, infants are managed initially by rectal washouts until definitive surgical treatment, usually within the first month of life (Figure 32). Initial data would suggest little difference in eventual outcome from either approach.[70] A recent advance has been adoption of a transanal approach, with or without laparoscopic assistance.[71] Frozen section biopsies are used to determine the presence of ganglion cells at the level of resection.

Following definitive operation for Hirschsprung disease, fecal incontinence has been reported in about 60% of patients compared with age-matched controls,[72] and the incidence was higher when evaluation was carried out by a psychologist.[73] Most patients have constipation

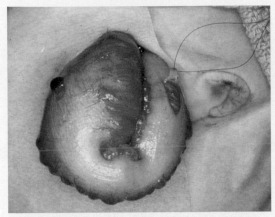

Figure 31 Hirschsprung disease: the transitional zone seen at operation showing the dilated proximal ganglionic colon and contracted distal aganglionic colon from which a seromuscular biopsy is being taken.

with soiling that appears to improve with age, but 9 to 40% are severely incontinent.[72–74] The reasons for these poor results are multifactorial. Incomplete excision of the aganglionic segment, internal sphincter dysfunction, external sphincter damage, and dysmotility of the apparently normal ganglionic bowel may all play a role, and children need careful follow-up into adulthood. The internal sphincter is aganglionic, and the need to preserve this undoubtedly has an important impact on the outcome of surgical treatment, highlighting the need for therapy directed at anorectal innervations. This has led to the search for alternatives to conventional surgery. The recent isolation of multipotent enteric nervous system

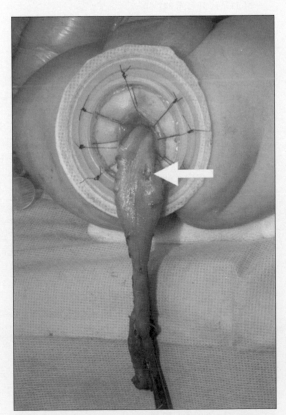

Figure 32 Transanal coloanal pull-through for Hirschsprung disease. The arrow indicates the site of the laparoscopic biopsy; below this the transitional zone can be clearly seen.

progenitor cells that have the capacity to form an enteric nervous system raises the prospect of autologous stem cell therapy as a novel treatment for Hirschsprung disease.[75–77]

Hirschsprung enterocolitis, characterized by malaise, pyrexia, abdominal distention, constipation, or diarrhea, is a potentially life-threatening complication that can occur before or following corrective operation. The pathologic basis of Hirschsprung enterocolitis is poorly understood and may represent alterations of bacterial flora, relative gut stasis, and impaired mucosal or neuronal immunity. Current treatment is empiric, consisting of rectal washouts, antibiotics (vancomycin or metronidazole), probiotics,[78] and sodium cromoglycate.[79] Chemical relaxation of the internal anal sphincter using botulinum toxin[80] or topical glyceryl trinitrate,[81] or surgical internal sphincterotomy, may be of benefit in reducing the risk of relapses. Occasionally, in an acutely ill patient it is necessary to perform an urgent colostomy. The occurrence of necrotizing enterocolitis in a full-term baby without risk factors should suggest the possibility of Hirschsprung disease.

There is a further small group of children who present with symptoms of Hirschsprung disease but who have ganglion cells on rectal biopsy. Often their symptoms are transient. Some investigators have found histopathologic features such as altered numbers of ganglion cells and increased acetylcholinesterase activity and labeled this intestinal neuronal dysplasia.[82–83] Others feel that such findings are part of the spectrum of normality in infants and neonates, and in one blinded study diagnostic concordance between pathologists was found to be low.[84] Other children continue to have pseudo-obstructive symptoms throughout life. It is difficult to define whether histopathologic abnormalities are responsible for their obstructive symptoms or secondary to them. However, it should be noted that a number of gene knockout animals exist with features of hypo- or hyperganglionosis, although no analogous mutations have been seen in humans.[85–87]

In 80% of infants, the aganglionosis is confined to the rectum and sigmoid, but it may extend to encompass the entire colon (total colonic aganglionosis) or very rarely (less than 1% of Hirschsprung disease) affect the entire intestine. When the normal ganglionic small bowel measures less than 50 cm, the likelihood of permanent parenteral nutrition dependency is high. Surgical procedures such as reverse loops, the Kimura procedure or longitudinal myomectomy are not effective options for improving intestinal absorption.[74,88–90] Total colonic aganglionosis with jejunoileal involvement therefore is equivalent to short bowel syndrome without colon, and small bowel transplantation is the ultimate therapeutic option.[89–93]

Meconium Plug Syndrome

Occasionally, when a rectal examination or contrast enema is performed in neonates with

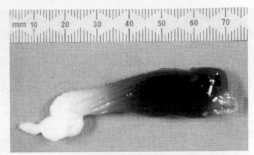

Figure 33 A typical meconium plug consisting of thick meconium proximally and pale epithelial cells distally evacuated from the rectum during contrast enema. Presentation was with distal colonic obstruction, which was relieved by the contrast enema.

symptoms suggestive of Hirschsprung disease, a whitish "plug" of epithelial cells is expressed followed by brisk passage of meconium and flatus, with relief of symptoms (Figure 33). This condition is called meconium plug syndrome and is common in premature infants, possibly owing to relative immaturity of their ganglion cell development. Cystic fibrosis and Hirschsprung disease should be positively excluded in children with meconium plug syndrome. Neonatal small left colon syndrome, often associated with the offspring of diabetic mothers, can be diagnosed after excluding Hirschsprung disease and treated with contrast enemas[94]; occasionally a temporary diverting colostomy is required.

Colonic Atresia

This rare cause of distal intestinal obstruction presents with abdominal distention, failure to pass stool, and vomiting. A contrast enema will distinguish it from distal ileal atresia, with which it may coexist, and Hirschsprung disease. Management is local excision of the atretic segment.

Intestinal Pseudo-obstruction Syndrome

Chronic intestinal pseudo-obstruction syndrome (CIPOS) refers to a group of potentially lethal disorders characterized by intestinal obstruction for which there is no clear pathological explanation.[95] Presentation may be acute in the newborn period or the disease may be chronic and present at an older age. Formation of enterostomies and resection of obviously dilated intestinal segments generally are not beneficial (Chapter 24.2c, "Other Dysmotilities Including Chronic Intestinal Pseudo-Obstruction Syndrome"). Associated megacystis may be seen antenatally and is helpful in suspecting the diagnosis of CIPOS.

TRANSPORTING THE SURGICAL NEWBORN INFANT

Ideally, infants known from prenatal screening to have a major surgical anomaly should be delivered in a specialist center. Postnatal transfer is safe provided that attention is paid to the key points in Table 3.[96]

Table 3 Essential Requirements for Neonatal Transfer

- Trained nursing staff (and if necessary medical staff) must accompany the patient
- Resuscitation equipment must be available for use en route
- Temperature control using a transport incubator to prevent hypothermia
- Intubation and ventilation must be established before transfer of infants with respiratory distress
- Intravenous infusions appropriate for the needs of the infant must be established and secured prior to transfer
- Nasogastric drainage is essential for infants with abdominal disorders, with the tube on open drainage and regular aspiration during transport
- Send with patient:

  Maternal blood sample for cross-matching

  Documentation of medications given, notably vitamin K and antibiotics

  Results of investigations and copies of radiographs

  Consent signed by the mother for operation (where appropriate)

REFERENCES

1. Kemp J, Davenport M, Pernet A. Antenatally diagnosed surgical anomalies: The 87 psychological effect of parental antenatal counseling. J Pediatr Surg 1998;33:1376–9.
2. Salihu H, Pierre-Louis B, Druschel C, Kirby R. Omphalocele and gastroschisis in the State of New York 1992–1999. Birth Defects Res A Clin Mol Teratol 2003;67:630–6.
3. Goldkrand J, Causey T, Hull E. The changing face of gastroschisis and omphalocele in southeast Georgia. J Matern Fetal Neonatal Med 2004;15:331–5.
4. McDonnell R, Delany V, Dack P, Johnson H. Changing trend in congenital abdominal wall defects in eastern region of Ireland. Ir Med J 2002;95:236–8.
5. Langer JC. Abdominal wall defects. World J Surg 2003; 27:117–24.
6. Elliott M, Maher ER. Beckwith-Wiedemann syndrome. J Med Genet 1994;31:560–4.
7. Langer JC. Gastroschisis and omphalocele. Semin Pediatr Surg 1996;5:124–8.
8. Rankin J, Pattenden S, Abramsky L, et al. Prevalence of congenital anomalies in five British regions. Arch Dis Child 2005;5:F374–9.
9. Donaldson L. Gastroschisis: A Growing Concern. London: Department of Health; 2004.
10. Garne E, Loane M, Dolk H, et al. Prenatal diagnosis of severe structural congenital malformations in Europe. Ultrasound Obstet Gynecol 2005;25:6–11.
11. Williams L, Kucik J, Alverson C, et al. Epidemiology of gastroschisis in metropolitan Atlanta, 1968 through 2000. Birth Defects Res Part A Clin Mol Teratol 2005;73:177–83.
12. Arnold M. Is the incidence of gastroschisis rising in South Africa in accordance with international trends? A retrospective analysis at Pretoria Academic and Kalafong Hospitals 1981–2001. S Afr J Surg 2004;42:86–8.
13. Salihu H, Aliyu Z, Pierre-Louis B, et al. Omphalocele and gastroschisis: Black-white disparity in infant survival. Birth Defects Res Part A Clin Mol Teratol 2004;70:586–91.
14. Driver CP, Bruce J, Bianchi A, et al. The contemporary outcome of gastroschisis. J Pediatr Surg 2000;35:1719–23.
15. Torfs CP, Velie EM, Oechsli FW, et al. A population-based study of gastroschisis: Demographic, pregnancy, and lifestyle risk factors. Teratology 1994;50:44–53.
16. Glick PL, Harrison MR, Adzick NS, et al. The missing link in the pathogenesis of gastroschisis. J Pediatr Surg 1985;20:406–9.
17. Hoyme HE, Jones MC, Jones KL. Gastroschisis: Abdominal wall disruption secondary to early gestational interruption of the omphalomesenteric artery. Semin Perinatol 1983;7: 294–8.
18. Brantberg A, Blaas HG, Salvesen KA, et al. Surveillance and outcome of fetuses with gastroschisis. Ultrasound Obstet Gynecol 2004;23:4–13.
19. Salomon L, Mahieu-Caputo D, Jouvet P, et al. Fetal home monitoring for the prenatal mnanagement of gastroschisis. Acta Obstet Gynecol Scand 2004;83:1061–4.
20. Salihu H, Emusu D, Aliyu Z, et al. Mode of delivery and neonatal survival of infants with isolated gastroschisis. Obstet Gynecol 2004;104:768–83.
21. Minkes RK, Langer JC, Mazziotti MV, et al. Routine insertion of a silastic spring-loaded silo for infants with gastroschisis. J Pediatr Surg 2000;35:843–6.
22. Vermeij-Keers C, Hartwig NG, van der Werff JF. Embryonic development of the ventral body wall and its congenital malformations. Semin Pediatr Surg 1996;5:82–9.
23. Moore TC. Omphalomesenteric duct malformations. Semin Pediatr Surg 1996;5:116–23.
24. Colige A, Sieron AL, Li SW, et al. Human Ehlers-Danlos syndrome type VII C and bovine dermatosparaxis are caused by mutations in the procollagen I N-proteinase gene. Am J Hum Genet 1999;65:308–17.
25. Stone MM, Fonkalsrud EW, Salusky IB, et al. Surgical management of peritoneal dialysis catheters in children: Five-year experience with 1,800 patient-month follow-up. J Pediatr Surg 1986;21:1177–81.
26. Grosfeld JL, Cooney DR, Smith J, Campbell RL. Intra-abdominal complications following ventriculoperitoneal shunt procedures. Pediatrics 1974;54:791–6.
27. Phelps S, Agrawal M. Morbidity after neonatal inguinal herniotomy. J Pediatr Surg 1997;32:445–7.
28. Wright J. Direct hernia in childhood. Pediatr Surg Int 1994;9:161–3.
29. Wright J. Femoral hernia in childhood. Pediatr Surg Int 1994;9:167–9.
30. Al-Salem AH, Nawaz A, Matta H, Jacobsz A. Herniation through the foramen of Morgagni: Early diagnosis and treatment. Pediatr Surg Int 2002;18:93–7.
31. Berman L, Stringer D, Ein SH, Shandling B. The late-presenting pediatric Morgagni hernia: A benign condition. J Pediatr Surg 1989;24:970–2.
32. Kyyronen P, Hemminki K. Gastro-intestinal atresias in Finland in 1970-79, indicating time-place clustering. J Epidemiol Community Health 1988;42:257–65.
33. Torfs CP, Christianson RE. Anomalies in Down syndrome individuals in a large population-based registry. Am J Med Genet 1998;77:431–8.
34. Lawrence MJ, Ford WD, Furness ME, et al. Congenital duodenal obstruction: Early antenatal ultrasound diagnosis. Pediatr Surg Int 2000;16:342–5.
35. Kimura K, Mukohara N, Nishijima E, et al. Diamond-shaped anastomosis for duodenal atresia: An experience with 44 patients over 15 years. J Pediatr Surg 1990;25:977–9.
36. Suri S, Eradi B, Chowdhary SK, et al. Early postoperative feeding and outcome in neonates. Nutrition 2002;18: 380–2.
37. Murshed R, Nicholls G, Spitz L. Intrinsic duodenal obstruction: Trends in management and outcome over 45 years (1951-1995) with relevance to prenatal counselling. Br J Obstet Gynaecol 1999;106:1197–9.
38. Escobar MA, Ladd AP, Grosfeld JL, et al. Duodenal atresia and stenosis: Long-term follow-up over 30 years. J Pediatr Surg 2004;39:867–71; discussion 867–71.
39. Filston HC, Kirks DR. Malrotation—the ubiquitous anomaly. J Pediatr Surg 1981;16:614–20.
40. Kluth D, Kaestner M, Tibboel D, Lambrecht W. Rotation of the gut: Fact or fantasy? J Pediatr Surg 1995;30:448–53.
41. Kelly DA. Intestinal failure-associated liver disease: What do we know today? Gastroenterology 2006;130:S70–7.
42. Louw D, Barnard C. Congenital intestinal atresia: Observations on its origin. Lancet 1955;2:1065–7.
43. Forrester M, Merz R. Population-based study of small intestinal atresia and stenosis, Hawaii, 1986-2000. Public Health 2004;118:434–8.
44. Grosfeld J. Jejunoileal atresia and stenosis. In: O'Neill JA RM, Grosfeld JL, Fonkalsrud EW, Coran AG, editors. Pediatric Surgery, vol 2. St Louis: Mosby; 1998. p. 1145–58.
45. Al-Harbi K, Walton JM, Gardner V, et al. Mucous fistula refeeding in neonates with short bowel syndrome. J Pediatr Surg 1999;34:1100–3.
46. Kerem B, Buchanan J, Markiewicz D, et al. DNA marker haplotype association with pancreatic insufficiency in cystic fibrosis. Am J Hum Genet 1989;44:827–34.
47. Schwiebert E, Egan M, Hwang T, et al. CFTR regulates outwardly rectifying chloride channels through an autocrine mechanism involving ATP. Cell 1995;81:1063–73.
48. Kao S, Franken E. Nonoperative treatment of simple meconium ileus: A survey of the Society for Pediatric Radiology. Pediatr Radiol 1995;25:97–100.
49. Mushtaq I, Wright VM, Drake DP, et al. Meconium ileus secondary to cystic fibrosis. The East London experience. Pediatr Surg Int 1998;13:365–9.
50. O'Halloran SM, Gilbert J, McKendrick OM, et al. Gastrografin in acute meconium ileus equivalent. Arch Dis Child 1986;61:1128–30.
51. Wardell S, Vidican DE. Ileal duplication cyst causing massive bleeding in a child. J Clin Gastroenterol 1990;12:681–4.
52. Cuschieri A. Descriptive epidemiology of isolated anal anomalies: A survey of 4.6 million births in Europe. Am J Med Genet 2001;103:207–15.
53. Pena A, Hong A. Advances in the management of anorectal malformations. Am J Surg 2000;180:370–6.
54. Merei JM. Embryogenesis of adriamycin-induced hindgut atresia in rats. Pediatr Surg Int 2002;18:36–9.
55. Pena A. Anorectal malformations. Semin Pediatr Surg 1995;4:35–47.
56. Georgeson KE, Inge TH, Albanese CT. Laparoscopically assisted anorectal pull-through for high imperforate anus—a new technique. J Pediatr Surg 2000;35:927–30; discussion 930–21.
57. Kudou S, Iwanaka T, Kawashima H, et al. Midterm follow-up study of high-type imperforate anus after laparoscopically assisted anorectoplasty. J Pediatr Surg 2005;40: 1923–6.
58. Goyal A, Williams JM, Kenny SE, et al. Functional outcome and quality of life in anorectal malformations. J Pediatr Surg 2006;41:318–22.
59. Ludman L, Spitz L. Psychosocial adjustment of children treated for anorectal anomalies. J Pediatr Surg 1995;30: 495–9.
60. Malone PS, Curry JI, Osborne A. The antegrade continence enema procedure why, when and how? World J Urol 1998;16:274–8.
61. Godberg E. An epidemiological study of Hirschsprung's disease. Int J Epidemiol 1985;13:479–85.
62. Orr J, Scobie W. Presentation and incidence of Hirschsprung's disease. Br Med J 1983;287:1671.
63. Russell MB, Russell CA, Niebuhr E. An epidemiological study of Hirschsprung's disease and additional anomalies. Acta Paediatr 1994;83:68–71.
64. Russell MB, Russell CA, Fenger K, Niebuhr E. Familial occurrence of Hirschsprung's disease. Clin Genet 1994; 45:231–5.
65. Torfs CP, Christianson RE. Maternal risk factors and major associated defects in infants with Down syndrome. Epidemiology 1999;10:264–70.
66. Angrist M, Bolk S, Thiel B, et al. Mutation analysis of the RET receptor tyrosine kinase in Hirschsprung disease. Hum Mol Genet 1995;4: 821–30.
67. Plaza-Menacho I, Burzynski GM, de Groot JW, et al. Current concepts in RET-related genetics, signaling and therapeutics. Trends Genet 2006;22:627–36.
68. Emison ES, McCallion AS, Kashuk CS, et al. A common sex-dependent mutation in a RET enhancer underlies Hirschsprung disease risk. Nature 2005;434:857–63.
69. Decker RA, Peacock ML. Occurrence of MEN 2a in familial Hirschsprung's disease: A new indication for genetic testing of the RET proto-oncogene. J Pediatr Surg 1998;33:207–14.
70. Teitelbaum DH, Cilley RE, Sherman NJ, et al. A decade of experience with the primary pull-through for Hirschsprung disease in the newborn period: A multicenter analysis of outcomes. Ann Surg 2000;232:372–80.
71. Georgeson KE, Cohen RD, Hebra A, et al. Primary laparoscopic-assisted endorectal colon pull-through for Hirschsprung's disease: A new gold standard. Ann Surg 1999;229:678–82; discussion 682–73.
72. Baillie C, Kenny S, Williams J, et al. Long term functional outcome and colonic motility following the Duhamel procedure for Hirschsprung's disease. J Pediatr Surg 1999;34:325–30.
73. Ludman L, Spitz L, Tsuji H, Pierro A. Hirschsprung's disease: Functional and psychological follow up comparing total colonic and rectosigmoid aganglionosis. Arch Dis Child 2002;86:348–51.
74. Marty TL, Seo T, Matlak ME, et al. Gastrointestinal function after surgical correction of Hirschsprung's disease: Long-term follow-up in 135 patients. J Pediatr Surg 1995;30:655–8.
75. Bondurand N, Natarajan D, Thapar N, et al. Neuron and glia generating progenitors of the mammalian enteric nervous system isolated from foetal and postnatal gut cultures. Development 2003;130:6387–400.
76. Almond S, Lindley RM, Kenny SE, et al. Characterisation and transplantation of enteric nervous system progenitor cells. Gut 2007;56:489–96.
77. Belkin-Gerson J, Graeme-Cook F, Winter H. Enteric nervous system disease and recovery, plasticity and regeneration. J Pediatr Gastroenterol Nutr 2006;42:343–50.

78. Herek O. Saccharomyces boulardii: A possible addition to the standard treatment and prophylaxis of enterocolitis in Hirschsprung's disease ? Pediatr Surg Int 2002;18:567.

79. Rintala RJ, Lindahl H. Sodium cromoglycate in the management of chronic or recurrent enterocolitis in patients with Hirschsprung's disease. J Pediatr Surg 2001;36:1032–5.

80. Minkes RK, Langer JC. A prospective study of botulinum toxin for internal anal sphincter hypertonicity in children with Hirschsprung's disease. J Pediatr Surg 2000;35:1733–6.

81. Millar AJ, Steinberg RM, Raad J, Rode H. Anal achalasia after pull-through operations for Hirschsprung's disease—preliminary experience with topical nitric oxide. Eur J Pediatr Surg 2002;12:207–11.

82. Scharli AF, Meier-Ruge W. Localized and disseminated forms of neuronal intestinal dysplasia mimicking Hirschsprung's disease. J Pediatr Surg 1981;16:164–70.

83. Holschneider A, Puri P. Intestinal neuronal dysplasia. In: Holschneider A, Puri P, editors. Hirschsprung's Disease and Allied Disorders. Amsterdam: Harwood Academic Publishers; 2000. p. 147–52.

84. Koletzko S, Jesch I, Faus-Kebetaler T, et al. Rectal biopsy for diagnosis of intestinal neuronal dysplasia in children: A prospective multicentre study on interobserver variation and clinical outcome. Gut 1999;44:853–61.

85. Bates M, Dunagan D, Welch L, et al. The Hlx homeobox transcription factor is required earli in enteric nervous system development. BMC Dev Biol 2006;6:33.

86. Anderson R, Turner K, Nikonenko A, et al. The cell adhesion molecule l1 is reuired for chain migration of neural crest stem cells in the developing mouse gut. Gastroenterology 2006;130:1221–32.

87. Taketomi T, Yoshiga D, Taniguchi K, et al. Loss of mammalian Sprouty2 leads to enteric neuronal hyperplasia and esophageal achalasia. Nat Neurosci 2005;8:855–7.

88. Fortuna RS, Weber TR, Tracy TF, Jr, et al. Critical analysis of the operative treatment of Hirschsprung's disease. Arch Surg 1996;131:520–4; discussion 524–5.

89. Ziegler MM, Royal RE, Brandt J, et al. Extended myectomy-myotomy. A therapeutic alternative for total intestinal aganglionosis. Ann Surg 1993;218:504–9; discussion 509–11.

90. Saxton ML, Ein SH, Hoehner J, Kim PC. Near-total intestinal aganglionosis: Long-term follow-up of a morbid condition. J Pediatr Surg 2000;35:669–72.

91. Fouquet V, De Lagausie P, Faure C, et al. Do prognostic factors exist for total colonic aganglionosis with ileal involvement? J Pediatr Surg 2002;37:71–5.

92. Sharif K, Beath SV, Kelly DA, et al. New perspective for the management of near-total or total intestinal aganglionosis in infants. J Pediatr Surg 2003;38:25–8; discussion 25–8.

93. Revillon Y, Aigrain Y, Jan D, et al. Improved quality of life by combined transplantation in Hirschsprung's disease with a very long aganglionic segment. J Pediatr Surg 2003; 38:422–4.

94. Rangecroft L. Neonatal small left colon syndrome. Arch Dis Child 1979;54:635–7.

95. Goulet O, Jobert-Giraud A, Michel JL, et al. Chronic intestinal pseudo-obstruction syndrome in pediatric patients. Eur J Pediatr Surg 1999;9:83–9.

96. Lloyd DA. Transport of the surgical newborn infant. Semin Neonatol 1996;1:241–8.

14

Lymphatic Disorders

Pierre-Yves von der Weid, PhD

This chapter describes the lymphatic system in the specific context of gastrointestinal (GI) function and elaborates on known and potential roles of this system in GI pathologies in children. The first part of this chapter provides a comprehensive description of current knowledge of the characteristics and functions of the lymphatic system. Explicit reference to the GI tract is provided wherever available.

LYMPHATIC SYSTEM

Historical Perspective

The lymphatic system is an indispensable element of integrated human and animal physiology. It has frequently been ignored or thought of as unimportant, even though the existence of lymph itself has been recognized since the historical beginnings of medicine. Hippocrates (460 to 377 BC) identified "white blood," or "chyle," and referred to the "lymphatic temperament" as a personality type based on balance of bodily fluids (reviewed by Chikly[1]). It was the Greek philosopher, Aristotle, who first referred to the vessels containing the colorless bodily fluid, which was later given the name "lymph," Latin for "milk."

Lymphatic vessels were not differentiated from veins until 1622 when Asellius observed the mesenteric lacteals in a well-fed dog. It was not until 1653 that Olof Rudbeck and Thomas Bartholin independently discovered that lymphatics made up a vast vascular network that was an integrated system of the entire body (reviewed by Chikly[1]). Despite the widespread recognition of the existence of lymph and components of the lymphatic system, few made the effort to conduct further investigations.

Lymphatic clearance of interstitial fluid was historically thought of as a process involving passive absorption of fluid and proteins filtered across the blood capillary wall by hydrostatic and oncotic pressures.[2] As more sophisticated research techniques became available, making access to lymphatic structures easier, knowledge of the lymphatic system and concepts of lymphatic physiology are slowly becoming more complete. This increase in knowledge is especially exemplified by a surge in the scientific interest of lymphatic biology that has occurred since the mid-1990s, which has led to scientific advances, particularly in lymphangiogenesis and function of the lymphatic endothelium. Importantly, it has also become recognized that lymphatic function is tightly regulated, which has become the subject of intense scientific investigation.

Lymphatic Structure and Anatomy

The lymphatic system is composed of numerous vessels connecting interstitial tissue space to blood circulation and to lymphoid organs such as lymph nodes, the spleen, and other lymphoid structures, such as Peyer's patches in the small intestine. The lymphatic vessels, or lymphatics, are widely distributed throughout the body and are particularly abundant in the gut. They are organized into a network that is more extensive than blood capillaries. The vessels lie in close proximity to the blood capillaries, picking up fluid and proteins that leave the cardiovascular system in order to maintain tissue fluid balance. Unlike the cardiovascular system, which is a close circuit relying on a central pump to move blood, lymphatic vessels form a one-way system that collects lymph from the extremities, propels it via the pumping action of individual lymphatic chambers and empties its contents into the venous circulation.

Initial Lymphatics. Lymphatic vessels serve as a drainage system for the pool of fluid that accumulates in the interstitium. This interstitial fluid, along with various cellular components and proteins, enters the vessels through the blind-ended structures known as *initial lymphatics*. The initial lymphatic vessels—also called *terminal* or *peripheral lymphatics*, or *lymphatic capillaries*—have walls composed of a single layer of flattened, nonfenestrated endothelial cells.[3,4] They are usually significantly larger than blood capillaries, being tens to hundreds of micrometers in diameter, are found in the intestinal mucosa and commonly are asymmetrical in shape.[5–7] In humans and other mammals, initial lymphatics are devoid of muscle cells or pericytes and have an incomplete basement membrane. Adhesion between endothelial cells is poorly developed, and cells may be separated by open intercellular junctions; this provides gaps by which macromolecules can pass into the vessel lumen. Collagenous fibrils, called anchoring filaments, attach to the surface of the endothelial cells to prevent the thin-walled vessels from collapsing under high interstitial pressure.[8,9] The overlapping endothelial junctions between adjacent cells in the initial lymphatics to serve as a primary valve system that improves the interstitial-to-lymph fluid flow by minimizing leakage back into the interstitial space.[5,10]

Along the alimentary tract, the best-described lymphatics are those in the small intestine, where initials occupying the central portion of the intestinal villi are identified as *central lacteals* (Figures 1 and 2). They are surrounded by the mucosal capillaries, with their end sitting just below the basement membrane of enterocytes[11]

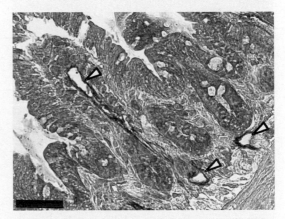

(A)

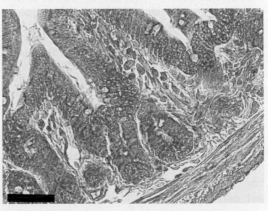

(B)

Figure 1 Lacteals and submucosal lymphatics in the mouse ileum. LYVE-1 immunostaining of initial lymphatics (arrowheads) in the villi (lacteals) and the submucosa (A), and negative control (no primary antibody) (B). Scale bars = 20 μm.

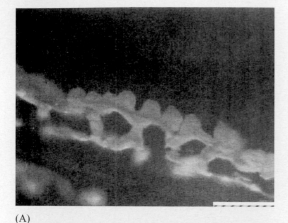

(A)

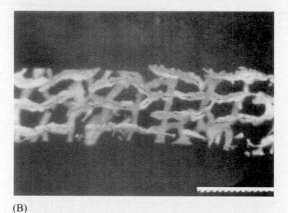

(B)

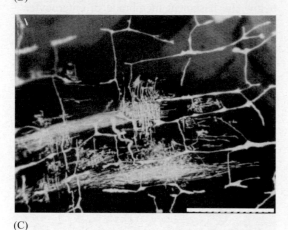

(C)

Figure 2 Scanning electron micrographs of intestinal lymphatic vessels from rat. (A) Villus lacteals, (B) intervillus lacteal connections, and (C) muscle layer lymphatics. Cast were made by single point injection of Microfil into villus lacteal, submucosal lymphatic, or muscle layer lymphatic, respectively. Lacteals of each villus are fused to form a larger lymphatic at base of villi. Structures projecting downward from fused base connect villus lacteals with submucosal lymphatics. Large lymphatic at villus base interconnects lacteals of adjacent villi as seen in (A and B). In (C), lymphatics are oriented parallel to both layers of muscle fibers. Although numerous connections exist between muscle layer lymphatics, valve-like structures are not observed. Scale bars = 500 µm. (Adapted from reference 13, used with permission.)

and thereby strategically positioned to drain fluid not only leaking from the capillaries, but also absorbed through the mucosa. As illustrated in Figure 2, these vessels interconnect, form sinuses, and fuse into larger vessels in the submucosa and muscular layers to emerge in the mesentery as collecting lymphatics, which have smooth muscle in their walls (see description below).[6,12,13] In

the colon, lymphatics have been identified only in the deeper mucosal layers and lacteals are absent, suggesting a lesser role in drainage of absorbed large intestinal fluid.[14,15]

Gastric initials are found in all layers of the stomach. They surround the base of the gastric glands in the mucosa and communicate with the dense networks of vessels of the submucosa and the muscular layers.[16] In the pancreas and salivary glands, initial vessels are found in close apposition to the basement membrane of the actinal epithelium. However, little information is currently available. Initial lymphatics do not appear to be present in liver lobules; however, it is assumed that fluid coming from these areas contributes substantially to liver lymph. Lymphatic vessels are found in portal tracts and in central veins. The reader will find more detailed descriptions of these GI lymphatics in several recent reviews.[2,8,17]

Collecting Lymphatics. Initial lymphatics empty their contents into collecting lymphatics, which have, as their most important difference with the initials, layers of smooth muscle in their wall that are responsible for spontaneous contractions (see Figure 3).[18] Thus, the collecting vessels contain three different layers: an intimal monolayer of endothelial cells surrounded by a basement membrane, a media comprised of one to three layers of smooth muscle cells intermixed with collagen and elastic fibers, and an adventitia made of fibroblasts and connective tissue elements containing axons that innervate the vessel.[17] Tissue and species differences exist and, in smaller vessels, the three layers may not be easy

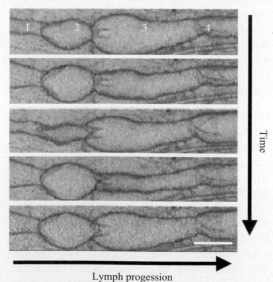

Figure 3 Illustration of rhythmical contractions in a collecting lymphatic vessel. Chronological sequences of video images showing four successive chambers or lymphangions (1 to 4) of a mesenteric lymphatic vessel from guinea pig undergoing sequential contractions. In the third sequence, eg, chamber 2, filled by chamber 1, is contracting and filling chamber 3. The unidirectional valve (particularly visible between chambers 2 and 3) is open. Chamber 3 then contracts, moving its lymph content forward. The valve is now closed to prevent backfilling. Scale bar = 100 µm. (Adapted from reference 20, used with permission from Elsevier.)

to distinguish. However, as vessels progress centrally, the amount of smooth muscle increases, with fibers lying in a more circular way.[19] In the small intestine, all lymphatic vessels embedded in the mucosal and muscular coat are initials; they become collectors (ie, acquiring a muscle layer) once reaching the mesenteric border.[13] Collecting lymphatic vessels coalesce to form larger and larger vessels (ducts and trunks) and drain into lymph nodes along their path. The filtered fluid leaves the lymph nodes via an efferent lymphatic and is returned to the venous circulation when draining into the right and left subclavian veins at the root of the neck via the thoracic and the right lymphatic ducts.

Collecting lymphatics are separated into functional units, termed lymphatic chamber or *lymphangions*,[21] by unidirectional valves, which promote centripetal flow of lymph, macromolecules, antigenic substances, and lipids into the adjacent chambers in a pulsatile manner (Figure 3). Thanks to the intrinsic contractile activity of the lymphatic muscle, each chamber is transiently and independently compressed and thereby propels lymph into the next chamber. The ability of the lymphatic vessels to exhibit spontaneous phasic constrictions is the mechanism by which the system performs its essential functions. Lymphatic contractile mechanisms are discussed in section on Lymph Transport.

Lymph Nodes and Lymphoid Structures. Lymph nodes are the structures in which adaptive immune responses to antigens are initiated in most body parts. Many lymph nodes are spread along the lymphatic vessel network. They are also numerous within the GI tract. Two to six pancreaticoduodenal lymph nodes are located in the angle between the pylorus of the stomach and the duodenum through which lymph from the pancreas, duodenum, and some efferent vessels of the liver is drained. The left, middle, and right colic nodes located along the descending, transverse, and ascending colon connect to lymphatics from their respective location of the colon. An aggregate of nodes, the ileocolic nodes, is located at the junction of the ileum and cecum, the afferent vessels of which drain these structures. As well, there is a group of cecal lymph nodes lying within the mesentery between the ileum and cecum that collect lymph from these areas. Jejunal and cranial mesenteric groups of lymph nodes lie near the root of the mesentery of the small intestine, close to one another and often fusing together. Afferent vessels of the cranial mesenteric lymph nodes drain all lymph from the intestine, except the descending colon.[22]

Lymph nodes are subdivided into three compartments: the lymphatic system, the blood circulation, and the parenchyma, which is further subdivided into B-cell follicles and the T-cell area that together form the cortex and the medulla. Cellular and molecular traffic between these compartments is an essential aspect of lymph node physiology.

In areas in direct contact with the outside world, like the GI mucosa, additional lymphoid structures help to organize the host immune response and often are the first to be stimulated. In the gut wall, secondary lymphoid structures are part of the gut-associated lymphoid tissue (GALT), which can be divided into aggregated lymph nodules (Peyer's patches) and solitary lymph nodules (also referred to as lymphoid follicles). GALT is a local protection system responsible for inducing adaptive immune responses and lymphocyte proliferation and differentiation following stimulation by microbes and other enteric antigens. The immune response is initiated in these structures by specialized M cells, which sample luminal antigens and pass them to underlying dendritic cells (DCs), macrophages, and T cells. It is commonly believed that T cells generate IgA and are carried to the bloodstream though the lymph.[23,24] In the human child, Peyer's patches are abundant in the small intestine, where their dome-like shape protrudes between the villi in the gut lumen.[25] Solitary lymphoid follicles are predominant in the colon. Lymphoid follicles are wrapped by a network of submucosal lymphatic vessels, considered to have a high absorption capacity[26] and which are connected to the muscular network and the mesenteric prenodal collectors. A very detailed morphological and functional description of these structures is provided in a recent review.[25]

Lymphatic Embryology

The embryogenesis of the lymphatic system remained unclear until the beginning of the twentieth century, when two hypotheses were proposed. *The centrifugal* theory of Florence Sabin proposed—based on detailed ink-injection experiments in pigs—that initial lymph sacs are derived by budding from embryonic veins and that these primitive lymphatics then further spread throughout the body to form the lymphatic networks in most organs.[27,28] The *centripetal* model proposed by Huntington and McClure[29] hypothesized that the first lymphatics arise from differentiation of mesenchymal precursors independent from the vein endothelium. A third theory, integrating elements of the two others, has been proposed by van der Jagt,[30] where the main lymphatic trunks sprout out of the grand veins, whereas all the other lymphatics arise independently from the venous system through canalization of connective tissues clefts.

With the recent discovery of reliable molecular markers to specifically detect lymphatic vessels, such as Prox1, LYVE-1, and podoplanin, progress in understanding of the origin and development of lymphatic vessels could be made and these theories tested. Studies of mice deficient in the homeodomain protein Prox1[31,32] revealed that Prox1 is critical for the development of the lymphatic vascular system, since the lymphatic development was halted at day 11.5 and the mice were not viable. Thus Prox1 is required for a subset of venous endothelial cells in the embryonic cardinal veins to migrate out and to form the initial lymphatic vessels during early embryogenesis. Recent studies of avian development indicate that independent lymphangioblasts might contribute to the formation of the lymphatic vascular system in the early wing buds, limb buds, and the chorioallantoic membrane of birds.[33–36] Whether lymphangioblasts also contribute to lymphangiogenesis in mammals remains to be demonstrated.

Vascular endothelial growth factor A (VEGF-A) is known as the primary angiogenic growth factor.[37] However, factors essential for lymphangiogenesis are less well characterized. vascular endothelial growth factor C (VEGF-C) and vascular endothelial growth factor D (VEGF-D) are important via interaction with vascular endothelial growth factor receptor 3 (VEGFR3). It was recently demonstrated that VEGF-C is required for sprouting of the first lymphatic vessels from embryonic veins.[38] In VEGF-C null mice, endothelial cells committed to the lymphatic lineage but did not further develop to form lymph vessels. As a result, the entire lymphatic system does not develop and embryos are not viable. Vessel development, via sprouting, returned upon addition of VEGF-C and was suggested to be a paracrine factor essential for lymphangiogenesis. Yet, VEGF-C also promotes early angiogenesis, which indicates overlapping function.[39]

The expression of the homeobox gene Prox-1 in endothelium provides essential signals for lymphatic endothelial differentiation.[31] In addition, angiopoietin-2 (Ang-2) and podoplanin are required for lymphatic development, whereas VEGF-A, VEGF-C, VEGF-D, fibroblast growth factor, and Ang-1 are implicated in postnatal lymphangiogenesis.[40,41] Further, it has been demonstrated that the adaptor protein SLP-76 and the tyrosine kinase Syk, both mainly expressed in hematopoietic cells, contribute to anatomical separation of lymphatic from blood vasculature during embryogenesis and postnatal development.[42] Without either of these factors, mice have disorganized blood and lymphatic vessels, and as a result, arteriovenous-lymphatic shunts that lead to enlargement of the heart and mixing of blood and lymph.

Endothelium-derived signals mediate the recruitment of lymphatic muscle cells to the nascent vessel to form collecting vessels and promote the maturation of the functional lymphatic system. The embryologic origin of lymphatic muscle cells and their recruitment and investiture into the developing lymphatic vessels is an area about which very little is currently known. If lymphatic muscle development follows the course of vascular smooth muscle, the cells generally will have a mesodermal origin with local variations.[43] For example, vascular smooth muscle of the great arteries and cardinal veins differentiate from cells of the cardiac neural crest.[44] One of the few studies documenting lymphatic muscle development provides evidence in the postnatal rat diaphragm that lymphatic muscle cells arise from mesenchymal progenitors in this fashion.[45] Another possible route of lymphatic muscle development in cardiac lymphatics may follow that of the vascular smooth muscle cells of the coronary circulation, where muscle cells differentiate from proepicardial cells.[43,46] This route of development fits with similarities seen in the molecular characteristics of cardiac and lymphatic muscle, as well as the role of lymphatic muscle in the phasic contractile lymph pump. This potential route of lymphatic development may also be related to the primitive lymphatic hearts that are seen in lower vertebrate species that contain both smooth and striated muscle.[47]

Lymphangiogenesis

Lymphangiogenesis is the growth and formation of new lymphatic vessels. It occurs in normally developing tissues and in pathological processes like inflammation, wound healing, lymphedema, and cancer. Understanding the formation of the lymphatic system as a biological regulation system transporting tissue fluid, immune cells, and fatty nutrients in the GI tract, as well as in diseases involving lymphangiogenesis is important. Yet, the molecular mechanisms of lymphangiogenesis are still not clear. The emergence of new molecular markers (5′-nucleotidase, VEGFR-3, podoplanin, Prox1, and LYVE-1), relatively specific to the lymphatic endothelium, has helped improving knowledge about these processes. The understanding of the molecular mechanism of lymphangiogenesis and an elucidation of the development of normal and pathological tissues will lead to the development of novel therapies for problematic diseases, such as malignant tumors and lymphedema.

Analysis of lymphatic organization and lymphangiogenesis during individual development and tissue repair in the GI lymphatic system has also been facilitated by identification of the specific lymphatic endothelial markers described above. The dense lymphatic network in the intestinal muscle coat develops by vascular sprouting consisting of thin lymphatic endothelial projections and splitting of vessels. Lymphatic regeneration during tissue repair is attributable to sprouting from preexisting lymphatics, and it progresses with vascular maturation. During regrowth, lymphatic endothelial cells exhibit structural changes indicating a high migratory potential and a close association with regenerating stromal cells.[48] Upregulation of the specific lymphangiogenic molecule VEGF-C in a subpopulation of stromal cells probably contributes to lymphatic regeneration by activating its receptor, VEGFR-3, on regrowing lymphatic endothelial cells.

FUNCTIONS OF THE LYMPHATIC SYSTEM WITH SPECIAL EMPHASIS ON THE GASTROINTESTINAL SYSTEM

The lymphatic system serves three main functions: maintaining tissue fluid balance to prevent tissue edema, combating foreign body invasion and infection and in the GI tract, serving as a conduit for lipid absorption and distribution throughout the body.

Tissue Fluid Balance

In spite of daily variations in water and salt content, extracellular fluid volume is maintained remarkably constant. This consistency relies heavily on the control of transport of salts and fluid across the capillary wall, and the return of fluid to the plasma. Most fluid that leaks out of the cardiovascular system (about 90%) is reabsorbed into the venous system, with the remaining 10% entering initial lymphatics to form lymph. This amounts to about 5 to 6 L of fluid that is circulated through the human body everyday via lymphatic vessels.[49] The importance of the lymphatic system in fluid balance is obvious in a case of lymphatic failure. One of the most common clinical consequences of inadequate lymphatic functioning is lymphedema. This affliction, which is described in section on Lymphedema, is a swelling of the tissues caused by an accumulation of fluid and proteins.[50] Lymphedema occurs when the amount of fluid leaking from the capillary wall exceeds the volume that lymphatics are capable of removing. When the lymphatic system is unable to compensate for excess fluid in the tissues, clinical manifestations of lymphatic failure occur. In addition, lymphatics are responsible for the daily clearance of about 60% of vascular proteins, most of this performed by lymphatics of the alimentary tract. Thus, in addition to removing fluid leaking from blood capillaries, intestinal lymphatics have the responsibility of transporting macromolecules synthesized in the digestive system, as well as fluid and nutrients absorbed through the mucosa, particularly lipids in the form of chylomicrons.[8] More than 50% of total lymph is formed in the abdominal viscera, particularly in the intestine, which is propelled through the mesenteric lymphatic vessels before reaching the thoracic duct and the venous circulation.[51,52] The mesentery then not only provides protection and structural support for the digestive organs, and a route for nerves and blood vessels to reach the digestive viscera, but it also contain a dense network of collecting lymphatics, which are necessary for draining the abdominal viscera.

The largest determinants of fluid flux are the Starling forces across the capillary wall, namely, *hydrostatic* and *colloid osmotic pressures*. Plasma and interstitial colloid osmotic pressure is determined by the concentration of solute molecules in these fluids. A higher plasma colloid osmotic pressure will favor osmotic absorption of fluid into the capillary, because water will tend to move into an area of higher solute concentration. A high interstitial colloid osmotic pressure, on the other hand, will favor an outward fluid flux in order to balance colloid concentrations across the wall. Hydrostatic pressure is determined by the pressure that is applied to the wall of the capillary by surrounding fluid. Net pressure on the wall (ie, the difference between pressure applied to the inside wall of the capillary and pressure applied to the wall from the interstitial fluid) in one direction promotes filtration of fluid in the same direction (favoring fluid movement from the blood to the interstitium if the intestinal pressure is lower and capillary absorption in the opposite is true). In most tissues, net colloid osmotic pressure drives fluid into the capillary, and the overall hydrostatic pressure forces fluid out into the tissue. The resulting net balance of forces tends to direct fluid out of capillaries and into the interstitium. Since lymphatic loading is directly proportional to interstitial fluid volume, the amount of lymph that is propelled in the vessels is also determined by the plasma volume filtrated into the interstitium. The greater this volume, the larger the amount of fluid that is transported via the lymphatics back into the bloodstream.

Protein transport out of capillaries must also be balanced with the same amount of proteins leaving the interstitium via the lymphatics. An inability to transport filtered proteins out of the interstitium results in edema. Proteins move across the capillary membrane by means of both diffusion and convection. There are several determinants of transvascular protein transfer, some that relate to characteristics of the capillary membrane itself, and others related to the relative concentrations of protein across the membrane. The flux of proteins across the capillary wall is regulated by a complex set of physiological mechanisms. This is important because fluid flux depends largely on osmotic pressure, and protein concentration can have a large impact on fluid volumes. As in fluid loading in lymphatics, the amount of protein loaded into the initial lymphatics is determined by interstitial protein concentrations. Lymph formation must match the net transcapillary flux of fluid and solutes in order to prevent excessive tissue swelling and edema.[49]

Lymph Transport

Due to the large intercellular spaces in the wall of initial lymphatics, the composition of lymph is quite similar to that of the surrounding interstitial fluid. Fluid, electrolytes, proteins, and cellular elements, such as immune cells, freely enter the vessels. However, fluid does not just passively drift into the lumen; there is a driving force that influences filling, although the exact mechanisms are still not clear. Some proposed mechanisms of vessel filling include vesicular transport, hydraulic pressure gradients and osmotic pressure gradients. Interstitial fluid pressure seems to be the main driving force behind vessel filling.[49] As fluid accumulates and tissue swells, the tension on the fibers attached to lymphatic capillaries cause the walls of the initial lymphatics to be pulled apart, allowing fluid to enter the lymphatic vessels (see section on Initial Lymphatics). Fluid movement through the tissue toward the lymphatic vessel lumen is vital to maintain vessel filling, and can only be preserved if the downstream lymphatic vessels continue to drain fluid away. The centripetal drainage is maintained by the one-way valves that separate each chamber and via both active and passive compression of the vessels. Lymph propulsion is secondarily provided by extrinsic forces, such as skeletal muscle or inspiration movements, blood vessel vasomotion, and suction effect due to blood flow in the subclavian veins.[53] Although these forces contribute to the movement of lymph, the primary mechanism of lymph propulsion is the rhythmical contractions of the lymphatic chambers. Such activity, generated within the muscles of the vessel wall, has been reported in most mammalian species, including humans.[54] Contractile movements, as observed in the mesentery where no surrounding structures are present to compress the vessels, are likely intrinsic to the vessels themselves (see Figure 3). Moreover, persistence of contractions in the presence of tetrodotoxin and in the absence of endothelium confirm their origin in muscle.[55,56] This muscular contractile activity is essential for the normal propulsion of intestinal lymph.[57] Spontaneous and rhythmical origin of lymphatic vasomotion requires the occurrence of a pacemaker event transiently depolarizing the muscle membrane potential to a level where action potentials are evoked, leading to calcium entry and phasic contractions.[58,59] In guinea pig and sheep lymphatics, the putative pacemaker depends on spontaneous transient depolarization, electrical events reflecting the release of calcium from intracellular stores, which activate ion channels permeable to chloride.[58-60] Intrinsic, lymphatic pumping and the underlying pacemaker are highly regulated (see section on Modulation of Lymphatic Pumping). Physical forces including stretch/distension, flow/shear stress and temperature are predominant modulators. Thus, an increase in fluid load, as that occurs during edema, is a major determinant of lymph flow. Chemical modulation is also critical with multiple vasoactive substances and inflammatory mediators able to regulate contractility.[20,58,61,62]

Digestive Functions

It first became clear that lymphatics play a key role in digestion when Asselli observed and described an extensive network of interconnecting white vessels in the mesentery following digestion (*venae albae et lacteae*), indicating that the system played a role in absorption (reviewed by Chikly[1]). It is now well recognized that intestinal lymphatics are crucial to the absorption of dietary lipids. The process of lipid digestion is only briefly described here and the reader is referred to more complete reviews of this topic.[63-66] Fat absorption involves emulsification of bile salts, hydrolysis of long-chain triglyceride species by lipase, passive and or transporter-mediated diffusion into enterocytes, resynthesis in these cells, and, finally, repackaging into chylomicrons, large triacylglycerol-rich lipoproteins, for transport into intestinal lymphatics. Chylomicrons enter the lymphatic system through lacteals in the villi of the small intestine. These initials empty into submucosal lymphatics and then into mesenteric collecting lymphatics.

The concentration of lipids in intestinal lymph is approximately 1 to 2%[63,67] and is highly dependent on feeding patterns. Intestinal lymph flow is greatly enhanced following fat feeding.[68,69] This action can be interpreted as a way to accommodate the increased lipid load and to help propel it through the lymphatic vessels for distribution throughout the body. However, the precise mechanisms by which this occurs and the impact of lipid metabolism on lymphatic function is poorly understood. Lipid absorption has also been linked to the special roles of intestinal lymphatics in terms of immune cell trafficking.[70-72]

Lymphatic System and Intestinal Immunity

The lymphatic system is strongly implicated in the adaptive immune response. It is responsible for transporting and sequestering antigens in lymphoid tissues to bring about immune responses during disease and in response to infection. Immune cells, fluid, and other macromolecules enter lymph nodes from tissues via afferent lymphatic vessels or from the cardiovascular network via high endothelial venules. Antigens present in fluid entering the lymph node can effectively elicit an immune response by activation of resident naive T and B cells. Immune cells exit the lymphatic system and eventually return to the bloodstream, where lymphocytes are transported to tissues throughout the body and act as patrols on the lookout for foreign antigens.

The lymphatic vasculature provides an exclusive environment where immune cells can respond to foreign antigens, and also has the role of proliferating and circulating lymphocytes and returning them to the bloodstream. The lymphatic system also functions as a one-way communication system for molecular messages, such as chemokines, which can be transmitted to cellular constituents in lymph nodes. These messengers are certainly also potential candidates for control of lymph flow, but no investigations formally addressing this possibility have been performed.

Afferent lymph transports antigen and antigen-presenting DCs from peripheral tissues to draining lymph nodes. During cell trafficking, DC and their precursors enter lymph nodes through afferent lymphatics, although access through the high endothelial venule portion of lymph nodes may also occur. Due to their ability to capture and present antigens, DC are intimately involved in the initiation of both tolerogenic and immunogenic intestinal immune responses. The anatomical location and local environment in which DC acquire antigen is likely crucial in determining the nature of the subsequent response. DC process and present antigen from peripheral tissues and are essential for antigen-specific priming of naive T cells in lymph nodes.

DC must first traffic to secondary lymphoid organs, a path that has been assumed to occur through lymphatics. This idea is supported by observations of high numbers of immune cell subpopulations, such as monocytes, macrophages, and DC, found in prenodal lymph, but not to any significant degree in postnodal lymph.[73] This observation certainly indicates a role for lymphatics in transporting these antigen-presenting cells to the lymph node where they confer their antigen-specific information to lymphocytes. It has also been noted that prenodal lymph contains a much lower proportion of B cells than postnodal lymph. Additional evidence supporting this concept is the strong expression of SLC/CCL21 by the lymphatic endothelium.[74-77] SLC/CCL21 attracts and binds mature DC that express CCR7.[75] Presumably, DC migrate to the lymphatic vessel and enter the flow stream of lymph to be carried to the next lymph node. This underscores the importance of lymph flow in the microlymphatic to DC nodal homing and, thus, overall immune function. However, the precise mechanisms and adhesion molecules by which the DC bind to the lymphatic vessel and cross the wall of the lymphatic remain to be determined. The possibility that immune cells modulate lymphatic contractility and lymph flow is essentially unstudied.

Once inside the lymphatic, DC travel along with lymph flow until entering the lymph node. Inside the lymph node, chemokines expressed by the mature antigen-presenting DC, MIP-3b, and CCL18, recruit naive T lymphocytes while monocyte chemoattractant protein, MIP-1α, CCL17, and CCL22 attract activated and memory T lymphocytes, as well as B lymphocytes. This process allows the interaction of lymphocytes with the antigen-presenting DC. The precise involvement of the lymphatic sinuses, lymph flow, and the impact of these chemokines on lymphatic cells is likely to be important, but is as yet unknown. Naive and central memory lymphocytes continuously enter lymph nodes through high endothelial venules, enter the paracortex of lymph nodes, migrate rapidly in random directions, and contact numerous DC in search of a stimulating antigen. Activated T lymphocytes then undergo clonal expansion and acquire tissue-specific homing patterns. Lymphocytes then exit lymph nodes, presumably through the efferent lymphatics, and travel with lymph flow back to the bloodstream where they engage in their immune functions. The interested reader will find supplemental information on DC trafficking in recent comprehensive reviews.[78,79] It is nonetheless important to consider DC and their preferred lymphatic route in the decision-making process distinguishing between immune responses to combat pathogenic organisms and oral tolerance mechanisms to avoid harmless substances or cells.[80,81]

The role of the lymphatic network is especially important during bacterial translocation, a phenomenon characterized by the passage of viable bacteria from the intestinal lumen, through the mucosa and muscle coat to extraintestinal sites, such as the mesenteric lymph nodes, liver, spleen, and the bloodstream. Bacterial translocation is promoted by intestinal bacterial overgrowth, deficiencies in host immune defenses, and increased permeability of the intestinal mucosal barrier.[80] The strategic location and abundance of lymphatic vessels in the intestine, in particular, make them critical in this process, as translocating bacteria travel via the lymph to the mesenteric lymph nodes. Yet, little is known about the elements involved in bacterial entry into lymphatics or the possible alteration of lymph flow by bacteria, or bacterial products. A report recently demonstrated the expression of Toll-like receptors (TLRs 2 and 4), which are part of the innate immune system sensing pathogen-associated molecular patterns (PAMPs) on lymphatic vessels in the human small intestine; specifically, on lymphatic capillaries expressing the chemokine SLC/CCL21 in the lamina propria mucosae.[82] This observation suggests that the lymphatic endothelium has recognition mechanisms for PAMPs by TLRs and that the expression of SLC/CCL21 and TLRs 2 and 4 is induced in the peripheral lymphatic endothelium of the small bowel microcirculation. The lymphatic endothelium may also allow DCs to home into secondary lymphoid tissues through the expression of TLRs, the ligand engagements of which result in the induction of chemokines, such as SLC/CCL21.[82]

Several findings are also of particular interest to the involvement of lymphatics in intestinal and immune functions. Lipid absorption has been shown to increase lymphocyte transport in rat mesenteric lymphatics[71] and functions of intestinal DCs are differentially modulated by long- and medium-chain fatty acids. In particular, the chemotactic ability of mature DC toward SLC/CCL21 is abrogated by long-chain fatty acids.[83] Presumably, this modulation occurs in the lymphatic vessel lumen, where lipids and DC coexist in the lymph. The silent chemoattractant receptor D6, which acts as a decoy and scavenger for inflammatory CC chemokines[84] may also be an important player in the lymphatic immune function, since it is almost exclusively expressed by lymphatic endothelium of afferent lymphatic vessels in skin gut and lung,[85,86] D6 is then strategically located to dampen inflammation in tissues and draining lymph nodes.

MODULATION OF LYMPHATIC PUMPING

Lymphatic vessels have the ability to contract spontaneously. This property, intrinsic to the smooth muscle, is subject to regulation by various physiological factors. These include both mechanical and chemical (humoral, neural, and endothelial) factors.

Mechanical Regulation

The lymph pump is controlled by various mechanical stimuli, including both extrinsic and intrinsic factors. Forces due to the motion of skeletal muscles and surrounding tissues, the suction effects of inspiration, and even the beating of nearby blood vessels and gut movements are factors that can influence the function of lymphatic vessels. For example, skeletal muscle contractions aid lymph flow by squeezing lymphatics, while sustained muscle activity decreases flow.[87]

One important mechanism for maintaining the fluid-balancing function of the lymphatic system is the ability of the lymph pump to autoregulate their force and frequency of contraction in response to fluid load. Under normal conditions, an increase in interstitial and intraluminal lymphatic pressures cause a corresponding rise in contraction frequency to a maximum value, beyond which flow will drop due to a decrease in stroke volume.[88–90] Such typical bell-shaped curves for the pressure/pumping relationship are observed in different regions and for different animal species. More peripheral and smaller lymphatics have higher values of transmural pressure at which maximum lymphatic pumping occurs,[91] suggesting that more peripheral lymphatics can develop much higher pressures to prevail over the greater outflow resistance. Newer evidence demonstrates that all lymphatics have an optimal pumping condition at relatively low transmural pressures[56] and that these pressures tend to be higher in more peripheral lymphatic vessels. For instance, mesenteric lymphatics have the highest fractional pumping (6 to 8 volumes/min at optimal pressure levels).

Lymph flow also affects the contraction frequency of lymphatic vessels. Benoit and colleagues.[56] increased lymph flow in situ in rat mesenteric lymphatics by elevating lymph formation and, accordingly, lymph flow rates as a result of plasma dilution. The authors found increased parameters of active lymph contractility in mesenteric lymphatics during periods of increased lymph flow. They also noted that the pressure in the lymphatic network became less pulsatile at high lymph flow states. Although such experiments give important information on lymphatic contractile behavior, it is difficult to clearly separate the effects of increased flow from the well-known effects of increased transmural pressure. A study on rat iliac microlymphatics showed that increases in perfusate flow correspond to an increase in contraction frequency, and a decrease in the amplitude of contractions.[92] Inhibition of both amplitude and frequency of contraction are observed during increases in imposed flow in rat lymphatics.[93,94] However, it is difficult to conclude that such imposed flow-dependent inhibition of the active lymph pump decreases total lymph flow in vivo. At high levels of lymph formation, passive lymph flow could become a greater driving force to move lymph than the active lymph pump. Flow-dependent inhibition of the active lymph pump in such situations could be a reasonable physiological mechanism to save metabolic energy by temporarily decreasing, or stopping, contractions during the time when the lymphatic does not need it. Inhibition of the lymph pump under these circumstances could also reduce lymph outflow resistance, as a result of a net increase in average lymphatic diameter when contractions are inhibited. This reduction in outflow resistance could ease the removal of fluid from the affected compartment that is producing high lymph flows and thereby facilitate the resolution of edema.[93]

Chemical Regulation

A wealth of experimental evidence has accumulated regarding both circulating and interstitial modulators of lymphatic pumping. Factors affecting vessel contractility are present in the lymph or in fluid surrounding the vessel, after being released from nerves or cells present in the interstitium, the vessel itself or from blood. These factors include inflammatory mediators such as histamine, serotonin and prostaglandins, endothelium-derived factors such as nitric oxide (NO), neurotransmitters such as norepinephrine, calcitonin gene-related peptide (CGRP) and vasoactive intestinal peptide (VIP), as well as many of the circulating hormones. This aspect has been dealt with in detail in several reviews to which the reader is referred.[20,95,96] The sections below describe the effects of those mediators that are related to inflammation and digestive functions.

Inflammatory Mediators. It is difficult to determine whether a lymphatic response is due to either direct stimulation by inflammatory mediators, or to secondary consequences of the inflammatory response, such as edema and vessel filling. Inflammatory mediators stimulate vascular leakage, causing net flow of fluid into the interstitial space, which in itself enhances lymphatic contractility. Whatever the primary cause, multiple inflammatory mediators modulate lymphatic contractility.

Prostanoids. Arachidonic acid metabolites are among the most important regulators of lymphatic vessel function, and because they are also important mediators of inflammation, they likely also play an important role in lymphatic dysfunction in the setting of inflammation. Numerous metabolites are produced from arachidonic acid, and depending on which one, it will lead to variable lymphatic responses. In addition to arachidonic acid, processing in inflammatory cells and surrounding tissues, lymphatic vessels themselves are capable of producing arachidonate metabolites.

Early studies using cyclooxygenase (COX) inhibitors and inhibitors of other arachidonate metabolism pathways showed that spontaneous lymphatic pumping is abolished when these metabolic mediators are repressed.[97] The same study also showed that application of leukotrienes, as well as a PGH_2/thromboxane A_2 (TXA_2) mimetic, induces rhythmic constriction in noncontracting lymphatic vessels. In a study of rat iliac lymphatics, arachidonic acid caused a significant decrease in vessel diameter. These effects were blocked by indomethacin, and significantly reduced by removal of the endothelial layer, suggesting that these metabolites were produced through COX, at least in part, in the endothelium.[98] Constrictions caused by arachidonic acid are converted to dilations when PGH_2/TXA_2 receptors are blocked by antagonists, and dilation is mimicked by exogenous PGE_2.[98] A role for prostaglandins is also illustrated in studies looking at the effect of substance P and ATP, where both enhanced the rate of constriction in guinea pig mesenteric lymphatics, with the effect attenuated by indomethacin.[99,100] These findings indicate that prostanoid PGH_2/TXA_2 release from the endothelium is activated by both substance P and ATP. More recently, Chan and colleagues[101] showed that the decrease in lymphatic pumping induced by the proteinase-activated receptor 2, another potent inflammatory mediator,[102] also involves prostaglandins as the effects are blocked by indomethacin and mimicked by PGE_2 and prostacyclin.

Histamine. Histamine release during the inflammatory response causes an increase in microvascular permeability, leading to an accumulation of fluid in the surrounding interstitial space. Lymph formation and vessel filling must increase, therefore, as a consequence in order to maintain tissue fluid homeostasis. Systemic administration of histamine increases lymph flow,[103–107] an effect partly due to increased microvascular permeability.[104,107] As histamine is also present in the interstitium during inflammation, and is detected in lymph draining injured tissues it could well directly stimulate lymphatic vessels.[108] Indeed, histamine has a direct effect on lymphatic contractile activity and, depending on species and vessel location, it increases the frequency and decreases the amplitude of lymphatic pumping via activation of H_1 receptors located on smooth muscle cells,[109–111] decreases contraction frequency via H_2 receptor stimulation,[109,111] or via an indirect effect mediated by the endothelium.[110] Histamine is also predominant in mast cell granules and is the main mediator of increased lymphatic pumping caused by mast cell activation, as demonstrated in a milk-sensitized animal model, a model of food allergy.[112]

Serotonin. Serotonin, or 5-hydroxytryptamine (5-HT) is also a significant player in both normal and pathophysiological lymph circulation. The mediator is involved in changes in blood flow, vascular permeability, and microcirculatory adjustments.[113] As with other modulators of vascular function, 5-HT also has an impact on lymphatic physiology (see reference 96). In most quiescent lymphatic vessels, 5-HT produced an increase in tone[114–118] and induces an increase in spontaneous contractions in bovine mesenteric vessels.[119] However, when vessels are preconstricted, 5-HT causes a relaxation[119] or an inhibition of spontaneous contractions in both guinea pig and sheep mesenteric vessels.[120,121] Pharmacological characterization of the receptors indicates that increase in tone and contraction frequency are mediated by 5-HT_2 receptors present in the lymphatic vessel wall,[113,119] whereas relaxation and decreases in contraction frequency are due to the activation of 5-HT_4 and 5-HT_7 receptors.[119–121]

Nitric oxide. Previously identified as endothelium-derived relaxing factor, the gaseous molecule NO is involved in many different physiological processes. Vasoactive substances, such as NO, are continuously released from blood vessel walls to affect the tone of cardiovascular smooth muscle. More recently, it has been shown that NO also affects lymphatic muscle tone. Studies conducted using several different animal species have shown that NO abolishes spontaneous constrictions and dilations that are seen in resting conditions.[98] In addition, nitric oxide synthase inhibitors increase the rhythm and amplitude of vessel contraction.[122] Taken together, these findings indicate that smooth muscle tone of lymphatics is continuously modulated by endothelium-derived NO. In inflammatory situations, other cells, such as macrophages, able to synthesize NO can alter lymphatic contractility.[123] NO inhibits vasomotion through arresting pacemaker calcium release associated with spontaneous transient depolarizations. Intracellular microelectrode recordings in guinea pig mesenteric lymphatic vessels showed that endothelium-derived or exogenously applied NO decreased frequency and amplitude of STDs, but not in the presence of ODQ, a guanylate cyclase (GC) blocker. This finding suggests that inhibition of pumping by NO involves activation of GC, and cGMP- and cAMP-dependent protein kinases.[124]

Neural Regulation. Neural regulation of the lymphatic system was described as early as the eighteenth century, when Wrisberg reported that thoracic ganglion and left splanchnic nerve innervated the thoracic duct.[125] More advanced techniques of investigation have been applied to show finer complexities of nervous innervation. Guinea pig mesenteric lymphatics are sparsely innervated, with evidence of both cholinergic and adrenergic nerves. Nerve fibers run lengthwise, with a number of nerve fiber varicosities.[126] Even with sparse innervation in comparison to neighboring blood vessels, neural regulation plays a role in the maintenance of lymphatic contractility.[125,127] Neurotransmitters and neuromodulators have been shown to modify lymphatic contractility, and modify the rate of lymph formation.

Adrenergic Innervation. Localized adrenergic and cholinergic nerve fibers are identified histochemically around initial and collecting guinea pig mesenteric lymphatic vessels.[126,127] Electrical stimulation of sympathetic nerves increases contraction frequency, an effect that is blocked by tetrodotoxin.[125] This effect is due to the release of norepinephrine, which stimulates both excitatory α-adrenoreceptor and inhibitory β-adrenoreceptor depending on the class of adrenergic receptors expressed in the tissue.[125] Further advancement in receptor classification has occurred, and lymphatic investigations indicate the presence of both α receptor subtypes (α_1 and α_2) and β-receptor subtypes (β_1 and β_2).[128–130]

Cholinergic Innervation. Acetylcholine (ACh) causes a dose-dependent relaxation, which was abolished with removal of the endothelium.[131] In vivo, ACh is released from nerve endings and stimulates the endothelium to produce NO, which causes an attenuation of vessel contraction.[124]

Peptidergic Innervation. Wang and colleagues[132,133] identified at least four different axon terminals forming synaptic connections with the submucosal plexus of guinea pig intestinal lymphatic vessels. Immunoreactivity to substance P,

CGRP, VIP, and somatostatin indicates that some lymphatic vessels possess not only autonomic, but also peptidergic innervation. The terminals of these peptidergic nerves are closely adherent to the outer walls of lymphatic vessels, with some appearing to protrude into the lumen. Ultrastructurally, only a thin layer of basal lamina and collagen fibrils is present between the endothelia of lymphatic vessels and these neurons. The endothelium likely is the target of action of these peptides, in line with findings that substance P and CGRP act through the endothelium to exert their effect on lymphatic vessel contractility via production of prostanoids.[99,100] The preferred location of these neurons in the ileum and jejunum suggests a possible link with the regulatory roles of specific activities in these two regions, for instance lymphatic transport of absorbed material.[132,133]

Gastrointestinal Hormones. Whether digestive hormones have inhibitory or excitatory effects on lymphatic contractility is an area of lymphatic regulation that is not as well studied and certainly deserves more attention. Indeed, the presence of chemical mediators in the vicinity of the vessels is expected. Moreover, enteric peptides, such as gastrin, neurotensin, VIP, and substance P are found in the intestinal lymph of conscious dogs and their concentrations increase after feeding.[134] The potential endothelial sensitivity to neuropeptides (and other peptides such as VIP, somatostatin, and cholecystokinin) is suggested by the close physical proximity between nerve terminals and lymphatic endothelium.[132,133] In guinea pig mesenteric lymphatic vessels, strong pumping inhibition is caused by VIP (von der Weid PY, unpublished data); however, no effect is observed when the same vessels are stimulated by octreotide (a metabolically stable analog of somatostatin).[135] Recent findings also demonstrate that GLP-1 reduces intestinal lymph flow, triglyceride absorption, and apolipoprotein production in rats.[136] Future research will likely reveal a more extensive, and complicated, mechanism of regulation of lymphatic contractility and lymph flow via GI hormones.

ROLE OF THE LYMPHATIC SYSTEM IN SELECTED GASTROINTESTINAL PATHOLOGIES

The implication of the lymphatic system is poorly evaluated in GI diseases, particularly mention in children. The following sections highlight instances where diseases have been correlated with lymphatic dysfunction.

Lymphedema

Interstitial edema is largely attributed to an increased leakage of fluid and proteins from the capillaries and venules into the interstitium. However, the critical role of lymphatic clearance of interstitial fluid and proteins is generally minimized or ignored. Clearly, lymphatic function cannot be overlooked when regarding the balance

of tissue fluids. Indeed, the lymphatic system has been described as one of the principal safety factors preventing edema.[137] As demonstrated in the rat, lymph flow increases in response to edemagenic stress created by plasma dilution, attributed, at least in part, to augmented interstitial fluid characterized by both an increase in contraction frequency and stroke volume.[57]

When lymphatics fail to clear interstitial fluid, tissue swelling occurs due to an accumulation of protein-rich interstitial fluid. Persistency of this state leads to situation known as lymphedema. Lymphedema is categorized as *primary* (congenital) if the abnormality preventing lymph flow exists in the lymph vessels or lymph nodes or as *secondary* (acquired) if the disease obstructing or obliterating the lymph conducting pathways began elsewhere.[138] Lymphedema mainly involves abnormalities in the regional lymphatic drainage of the extremities (either upper or lower or both), although visceral lymphatic abnormalities can also occur.[139] In contrast to venous edema in which enhanced capillary pressure indirectly stimulates lymph production, lymphedema is caused by a reduction in lymphatic transport. This can be the result of anatomic problems, including lymphatic hypoplasia and functional insufficiency or absence of lymphatic valves.[140] Some patients have impaired intrinsic contractility of the lymphangions.[140] Indeed, if lymphatic endothelial dysfunctions are present, lymphatic smooth muscle dysfunction is likely to follow. Impaired lymphatic drainage fosters the accumulation of protein and cellular metabolites, followed by an increase in tissue colloid osmotic pressure, which leads to water accumulation and increased interstitial hydraulic pressure. Once a chronic state is reached, an increase in the number of fibroblasts, adipocytes, and keratinocytes in the edematous tissues is observed. Macrophages often denote the chronic inflammatory response.[141] Increased collagen deposition, with adipose and connective tissue overgrowth in and around the edematous tissue (usually skin) also occurs, leading to progressive fibrosis.[139]

Primary Lymphedema. Recent advance in the genetic investigation of hereditary lymphedemas has permitted the identification of forkhead transcription factor FOXC2 as a candidate gene for lymphedema-distachiasis.[142] FOXC2 is involved in abnormal interactions between lymphatic endothelial cells and pericytes as well as valve defects, which are characteristic of the pathology of lymphedema-distachiasis.[143] Hereditary primary lymphedema (also referred to as Milroy's disease) is attributed to a mutation that inactivates VEGFR-3 tyrosine kinase signaling important mainly in lymphatic vessels.[144,145]

Secondary Lymphedema. Secondary lymphedema is much more common than the primary form. It develops after disruption or obstruction of lymphatic pathways by surgical, traumatic, inflammatory, and neoplastic disease processes. Edema of the arm after excision of axillary lymph node, a classical treatment during breast cancer surgery, is probably the most common cause of lymphedema in the United States,[146] although its global incidence is overshadowed by lymphatic filariasis. A mouse model of acute, acquired lymphedema closely simulates the volume response, histopathology, and lymphoscintigraphic characteristics of human acquired lymphedema, and the response is accompanied by an increase in the number and size of microlymphatic structures in the lymphedematous cutaneous tissues.[147]

Lymphatic Filariasis. Lymphatic filariasis is the most common cause of secondary lymphedema in the world and is a major public health problem throughout many regions of the tropics. The disease is caused by several species of filarial nematode the most common of which, *Wuchereria bancrofti*, affects an estimated 120 million people worldwide.[148] Parasites are transmitted by mosquitoes and infective larvae develop into adult worms in afferent lymphatic vessels, causing severe distortion of the lymphatic system. Adult *Wuchereria* can release millions of larvae into the blood over their lifespan of several years and often lodged in the lymphatics of the spermatic cord, causing scrotal damage and swelling. Elephantiasis—a painful, disfiguring swelling of the limbs—is a classic sign of late-stage disease. In addition to these chronic pathologies, infected people experience several episodes of acute inflammatory disease each year, associated with the death of adult worms and infection with opportunistic organisms invading damaged and dysfunctional lymphatics and surrounding tissues. Until recently, understanding of filarial disease was considered to be due to complex interactions between the parasite, host immune responses and opportunistic infections. Studies aiming at characterizing the molecular nature of the inflammatory stimuli derived from filarial nematodes has revealed the critical role played by the worms' symbiont *Wolbachia*.[149,150] Indeed, LPS-like molecules from these intracellular bacteria are responsible for potent pro-inflammatory responses by macrophages in animal models of filarial disease.[151] *Wolbachia* has also been associated with severe inflammatory reactions to filarial chemotherapy, being released into the blood following death of the parasite. Recent studies in animal models even implicate *Wolbachia* in the onset of lymphedema. Taken together, these studies imply a major role for *Wolbachia* in the pathogenesis of filarial disease. It may be possible, through the use of antibiotic therapy, to clear worms of their symbiotic bacteria, with the intent that this approach will prevent the development of filarial pathology.

While the precise pathological mechanisms that produce lymphedema during filariasis are not completely understood, symptoms including lymphangitis, dilated lymphatics, and decreased lymphatic contractile function both in situ and ex vivo point to an inhibition of lymphatic muscle function leading to a loss of lymphatic contractile activity and ultimately, the development of lymphedema.[152]

Inflammatory Bowel Diseases

Despite the cardinal function of adapting contractile activity to changes in fluid load, lymphatic vessels are still not often considered as active players in inflammatory pathologies where edema is a hallmark. In these inflammatory situations, mediators of inflammation, released in the vicinity of lymphatic vessels, directly affect lymphatic smooth muscle and alter lymphatic pumping. Keeping in mind that similar situations may occur in other inflammatory pathologies, such as heart and renal failures and pulmonary edema, dysfunction of lymphatic pumping and impairment of lymph flow could well be involved in chronic inflammatory bowel diseases (IBD).

Although the etiologic aspects of tissue reactions in IBD remain uncertain, some of the most consistent pathological features observed in patients suffering from Crohn's disease (CD) and ulcerative colitis (UC) are mucosal exudation and interstitial (submucosal) edema leading to extensive dilation of lacteals (see Figure 4).[153–155] Lymphatic obstruction is reported in IBD patients undergoing surgery.[156] Lymphatic vessel dilatation and edema suggest poor lymph drainage consequent to either lymphatic obstruction or impaired contractile function.[154,156] This concept is supported by earlier experimental studies where injection of sclerotic agents into canine and porcine mesenteric lymphatic vessels or lymph nodes to obstruct them led to lesions similar to those seen in human IBD.[157,158]

Due to increases in vascular permeability and resultant interstitial fluid, lymph flow increases during inflammatory reactions. Indeed, mesenteric lymphatic pumping is increased during edemagenic stress caused by dilution of plasma in rats in vivo.[57] This is due to an increase in distension of the lymphatic wall, which may be the situation when lymphatics are overloaded in cases of edema. Thus, the lymphatic system must play a crucial role in edema resolution during IBD.

Although the involvement of lymphatic vessels was demonstrated in earlier investigations, the study of lymphatics in human IBD was not pursued until recently. A proportion of granulomas seen in CD patients is associated with initial lymphatic vessels (Figure 5), leading to the suggestion that "granulomatous lymphangitis is a primary lesion of CD, and the consequence of the localization of granulomatous inflammation is the submucosal edema and fibrosis that gives rise to many of the ... histological features of the disease."[160] Antigens that cause CD may be taken up by macrophages, which then enter the lymphatic system. Proliferation of initial lymphatics has been demonstrated in the colonic mucosa of patients with UC, but not in healthy controls.[161,162] In the colon, lymphatics, which are normally distributed beneath the muscularis mucosa, proliferate into the lamina propria and submucosa in patients with UC in proportion to the severity of the disease.[161] In addition, the integrity of the lamina propria, with regards to lymphatic distribution, is restored with disease

resolution. Like in UC, proliferation of lymphatic initials is also observed in CD, where it can occur in each layer of the inflamed small and large bowel (Figure 4).[159] Lymphatic capillaries are prominent lymphoid aggregates (Figure 5) and also observed in fibrotic areas. These findings suggested that lymphangiogenesis in IBD may be triggered by chronic inflammation and is maintained in fibrotic end-stage disease.[159] Demonstration of lymphangiogenesis has also been made in other inflammatory situations.[163–166] A study examining the role of collecting lymphatics in IBD suggested that CD is caused by a congenital lack of mesenteric lymphatic collectors

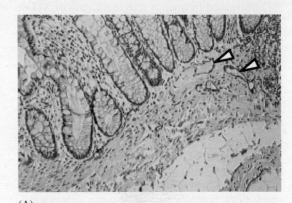

(A)

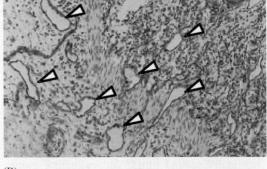

(B)

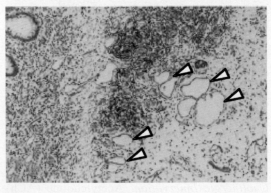

(C)

Figure 4 Distribution of lymphatics (arrowheads) in the small intestinal mucosa and submucosa in normal sections and in those from patients with IBD. Immunostaining with anti-human podoplanin reveals far less lymphatic capillaries in the control sample (A), compared to many tortuous, dilated vessels in sections from patients with CD (B) and UC (C). In addition, numerous lymphatic capillaries are located in areas of the submucosa rich in mononuclear cells (B and C). (Adapted from reference 159 used with kind permission of Springer Science and Business Media.)

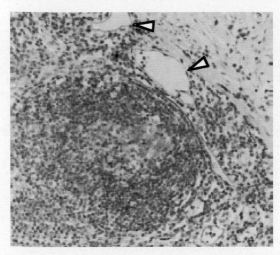

(A)

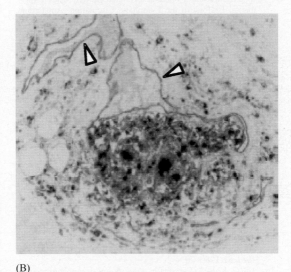

(B)

Figure 5 Prominent lymphoid aggregates/granulomas in the submucosa of small intestine of CD patient. They contain numerous thin and often dilated podoplanin-positive lymphatic capillaries (arrowheads) (A), which can also be colocalized in epithelioid cell granulomas that contain CD68-positive giant cells (B). (Adapted from reference 159 used with kind permission of Springer Science and Business Media.)

leading to the inability to take up toxic bacterial substances, and consequently causing lymph stasis, lymphangitis, and GI inflammation.[167] Although provocative, this study lends support to the hypothesis that the lymphatic system plays a role in the development of IBD.

Recent findings reveal that the contractile function of mesenteric collecting lymphatics in an animal model of intestinal ileitis is impaired both in vivo and in vitro, with a strong correlation to the degree of mucosal inflammation.[168] Dysfunction was partially, but significantly, reduced in the presence of COX inhibitors, suggesting the involvement of arachidonic acid metabolites.

Taken together, these studies provide evidence that the lymphatic system is intimately involved in and highly altered during inflammatory diseases in the gut. Release of inflammatory mediators, in addition to increasing vascular permeability during inflammation, is thought to play a pivotal role in modulating lymphatic vessel

function. Although the exact role of lymphatics is not yet known and failure in the lymphatic system is probably not the direct cause of the ailment, inflammation has a significant effect in impairing normal vessel function. Intervention at the level of the lymphatic system could well serve to ease some of the symptoms of IBD.

Cancer-Induced Lymphangiogenesis and Tumor Spreading

The role of the lymphatic system in the development of tumors has evolved from being rather passive, as perceived 10 years ago, to an active interaction. An improved understanding of the molecular biology of lymphatic endothelial cells and the regulation of lymphangiogenesis has enlightened the active interaction between tumors and lymphatics in inducing lymphangiogenesis. New vessels invading or surrounding a tumor can favor the entry of tumor cells into the lymphatic vasculature, their subsequent transport to regional lymph nodes and promote the formation of metastases. Such findings revealing tumor-induced lymphangiogenesis is an important new target in the fight against metastatic cancers.[169]

Recent studies in animal models provide direct experimental evidence that increased levels of VEGF-C and VEGF-D promote active tumor lymphangiogenesis and lymphatic tumor spread to regional lymph nodes. Moreover, these effects can be suppressed by blocking VEGFR-3 signaling.[170–173] VEGF-A also acts as a potent tumor lymphangiogenesis factor and tumor-derived VEGF-A promotes expansion of the lymphatic network within draining sentinel lymph nodes, even before the tumors metastasize.[174] These findings indicate that lymph node lymphangiogenesis contributes to further metastatic tumor spread beyond a sentinel lymph node. A large number of clinicopathological studies have shown a direct correlation between expression of VEGF-C or VEGF-D by tumor cells and metastatic tumor spread in many human cancers, indicating an important role of lymphangiogenesis in tumor progression.[175] A detailed discussion focusing on current evidence for the role of VEGF-C and VEGF-D and their signaling receptors for the common sites of malignancy of the GI tract is found in a recent review.[176]

Protein-Losing Enteropathy, Lymphangiectasia, and Hypoplasia

Protein-losing enteropathy (PLE) is characterized by enteric losses of plasma proteins in abnormal amounts. PLE can be caused by a large group of diseases. One of them, primary intestinal lymphangiectasia is the most widely known cause of intestinal protein loss in children.[177] Intestinal lymphangiectasia is characterized by asymmetrical peripheral edema, ascites, immunologic deficiencies, lymphocytopenia, hypoalbuminemia, impaired lymphocyte transformation, GI symptoms, and impaired growth. It is the result of abnormal, distorted and obstructed lymphatic

vessels. The back-flow of lymph then causes rupture of intestinal lacteals and leakage of nutrient-laden lymph into the lumen of the bowel. The presence of these abnormally dilated lymphatics is a feature of the disease and correlates with lymphatic dysfunction.

Another, less-recognized cause of neonatal PLE is intestinal lymphatic hypoplasia, which shares many clinical features with primary intestinal lymphangiectasia but is typically associated with a normal lymphocyte count.[178,179] Lymphatic hypoplasia is characterized by the absence or marked lack of lymphatics. However, diagnosis is difficult because identification of lymphatic vessels in the mucosa requires antibodies specific to lymphatic antigens. The recent availability of antibodies against lymphatic markers has improved the diagnosis of lymphatic hypoplasia. In a study performed at the Royal Children's Hospital in Melbourne, Australia, over a 15-year period, immunostaining with D2-40, a mouse monoclonal antibody demonstrated to react with a sialoglycoprotein found on human lymphatic endothelium[180] was analyzed in mucosal and muscular biopsies from the alimentary tract of children in normal and disease conditions (including both lymphangiectasia and intestinal lymphatic hypoplasia patients).[181] The study showed that lymphatic vessels are preserved, and sometimes increased, in many common alimentary tract diseases of children, confirming what has been reported in adult IBD.[161,162] In young patients with lymphatic hypoplasia, D2-40 immunostaining confirmed the absence, or marked paucity, of lymphatic vessels in the small intestine. Lymphatic vessels were not detected in the duodenal mucosal biopsy of a patient whose sibling had confirmed lymphatic hypoplasia and in another patient with similar clinical and laboratory findings in whom lymphatic vessels could not be identified by electron microscopy. Among these patients, the degree and extent of lymphatic hypoplasia were variable, but suggested to be related to the severity of the disease.[181] In intestinal lymphangiectasia, extensive dilatation of lymphatic vessels containing foamy macrophages allows a confident diagnosis to be made. However, this feature is inconsistent and the observation of occasional mildly dilated lymphatic is only suggestive and could also be related to other diseases where prominent dilatation of lymphatic vessels occurs, such as celiac disease[182] or incomplete fasting prior to securing the intestinal biopsy.

Food Allergy

Food allergy is a prominent disease of children.[183] Most allergies (over 90%) are caused by foods including cow milk, hens egg, soy, peanuts, tree nuts, wheat, fish, and shellfish. Although clinical manifestations are often observed at the skin level (urticaria and angioedema), intestinal symptoms, such as vomiting and diarrhea, are also frequent. The involvement of the lymphatic system in food allergy has been neglected. A recent study investigating lymphatic contractile function in a model of food allergy reveals that contractility of mesenteric lymphatic vessels is increased in animals sensitized to the cow milk protein *b*-lactoglobulin. This effect is mediated by histamine and dependent on the activation of mast cells.[112] Increased lymphatic contractility and, presumably, lymph flow during allergic reaction could well have an impact on the way host immune responses are initiated.

Gut Lymphatic System and Multiple Organ Failure

Studies by Deitch and colleagues[184–190] reveal that the mesenteric lymphatic system is critical in setting of major trauma, shock and burn injury that can lead to acute systemic inflammation as well as to multiple organ failure. Although the gut has been experimentally and clinically implicated in the development of these syndromes, its exact role remains controversial. Based on recent experimental evidence, it appears that unique gut-derived factors carried in the intestinal lymph (but not the portal vein) lead to acute injury- and shock-induced systemic inflammation and multiple organ failure.[188] These observations have led to the gut-lymph hypothesis, where gut-derived factors present in intestinal (mesenteric) lymph serve as the triggers to initiate the systemic inflammatory and tissue injurious responses observed after major trauma or episodes of shock.[185,187] A similar role has been attributed to the intestinal/mesenteric lymphatic system in the development of gut and lung injuries following experimental intestinal ischemia/reperfusion.[191,192] These studies suggest TNF-α, produced in the gut during ischemia/reperfusion, as a likely mediator of the injuries.

Neonatal Necrotizing Enterocolitis

Necrotizing enterocolitis (NEC) is one of the most common intestinal emergencies in newborn infants. The disease mainly affects premature infants and leads to high morbidity and mortality rates.[193] The pathophysiology of NEC remains poorly understood. Possible causes include developmental immaturity of key functions such as intestinal motility, digestive ability, circulatory regulation, intestinal barrier function, and immune defences.[194] Hypoxic-ischemic injury, feeding with formula milk, and colonization by pathological bacteria are other potential contributing factors. The involvement of the lymphatic system in NEC has not been carefully addressed. In a study of small neonatal piglets in which intestinal ischemia is produced by ligation of mesenteric vessels (arteries, veins, and lymphatics), Sibbons and colleagues[195] observed that arterial plus lymphatic occlusion produces a unique combination of histopathological features (mucosal stripping, hemorrhage, submucosal disruption, full-thickness necrosis, inflammatory infiltration, and pneumatosis) resembling the pathology of NEC in humans. Lymphatic occlusion alone causes complete NEC in very small neonatal

piglets. Intriguingly, pneumatosis intestinalis, the single most important hallmark in the radiological diagnosis of NEC,[194] appears to originate in lymphatic vessels of the submucosa in this experimental model of NEC, as lymphatics appear distended and follow the shape and distribution of typical pneumatosis.[195] The authors postulated that anaerobic bacteria could gain access to distended lymphatics, which contain ideal substrates for proliferation of bacteria and the production of hydrogen gas that results in pneumatosis in neonatal NEC. Shut down of the mesenteric lymph node by bacterial translocation would further exacerbate lymphatic obstruction and cause progression of the disease process. It is assumed that at a certain stage in the development of NEC, hypoxia and decreased perfusion of the bowel wall leads to circumstances resembling the ischemia/reperfusion cascade and production of toxic superoxide free radicals.[195] These superoxides causing injury to enterocytes and breakage of intercellular connections would favor translocation of enteric bacteria from the gut lumen into the capillaries, lymphatic vessels, and lymph node.[196,197]

Chylous Disorders

Chylous disorders, including chylous ascites and chylothorax, are uncommon but problematic conditions in children. They are consequent to accumulation of intestinal lymph in the abdominal cavity (or the thoracic cavity in case of chylothorax).[198] Chylous disorders can be divided into primary and secondary disorders. Primary disorders are spontaneous leaks due to congenitally weak lymphatic vessels presenting in the early newborn period or related to congenital lymphangectasia. Secondary chylous disorders are seen as a result of operative damage and trauma to lymphatic vessels, such as after abdominal surgery. It can also occur with advanced malignant or obstructive diseases, presumably as a result of obstruction of the lymphatic system with proximal disruption of vessels and leakage of fluid. Lymphatic vessels become dilated, with incompetent valves allowing lymph to reflux into cavities, the lower limbs, or genitalia. Reflux causes delayed lymph transport and chronic lymphedema then frequently develops. Rupture of mesenteric lymphatics results in chylous ascites and rupture of intestinal lacteals into the bowel lumen can cause PLE. Leaks from thoracic vessels lead to chylothorax. Diagnosis is mainly assessed by lymphoscintigraphy and lymphangiography. Technically demanding surgical intervention is required in more than half of cases with primary disorder.[198]

ACKNOWLEDGMENTS

The author would like to thank Theresa Wu and Kelly Plaku for their assistance in compiling the literature related to this chapter and Jenny Cai for her help in carrying out the immunohistochemistry experiments.

REFERENCES

1. Chikly B. Who discovered the lymphatic system. Lymphology 1997;30:186–93.
2. Barrowman JA. Physiology of the Gastro-Intestinal Lymphatic System. London: Cambridge University Press; 1978.
3. Azzali G, Arcari ML. Ultrastructural and three dimensional aspects of the lymphatic vessels of the absorbing peripheral lymphatic apparatus in Peyer's patches of the rabbit. Anat Rec 2000;258:71–9.
4. Casley-Smith JR. The role of the endothelial intercellular junctions in the functioning of the initial lymphatics. Angiologica 1972;9:106–31.
5. Leak LV. The structure of lymphatic capillaries in lymph formation. Fed Proc 1976;35:1863–71.
6. Ushiki T. The three-dimensional organization and ultrastructure of lymphatics in the rat intestinal mucosa as revealed by scanning electron microscopy after KOH-collagenase treatment. Arch Histol Cytol 1990;53:127–36.
7. Lee JS. Lymph capillary pressure of rat intestinal villi during fluid absorption. Am J Physiol 1979;237:E301–7.
8. Barrowman JA, Tso P, Kvietys PR, Granger DN. Gastrointestinal Lymph and lymphatics. In: Johnston MG, editor. Experimental Biology of the Lymphatic Circulation. Amsterdam, New York: Elsevier Science Publishers; 1985. p. 327–54.
9. Casley-Smith JR. Electron microscopical observations on the dilated lymphatics in oedematous regions and their collapse following hyaluronidase administration. Br J Exp Pathol 1967;48:680–6.
10. Trzewik J, Mallipattu SK, Artmann GM, et al. Evidence for a second valve system in lymphatics: Endothelial microvalves. FASEB J 2001;15:1711–7.
11. Granger DN. Intestinal microcirculation and transmucosal fluid transport. Am J Physiol 1981;240:G343–9.
12. Ohtani O. Three-dimensional organization of lymphatics and its relationship to blood vessels in rat small intestine. Cell Tissue Res 1987;248:365–74.
13. Unthank JL, Bohlen HG. Lymphatic pathways and role of valves in lymph propulsion from small intestine. Am J Physiol 1988;254: G389–98.
14. Hirashima T, Kuwahara D, Nishi M. Morphology of lymphatics in the canine large intestine. Lymphology 1984;17: 69–72.
15. Kvietys PR, Wilborn WH, Granger DN. Effects of net transmucosal volume flux on lymph flow in the canine colon. Structural-functional relationship. Gastroenterology 1981;81:1080–90.
16. Ji RC, Kato S. Lymphatic network and lymphangiogenesis in the gastric wall. J Histochem Cytochem 2003;51:331–8.
17. Yoffey JM, Courtice FC. Lymphatics, Lymph and the Lymphomyeloid Complex. London: Academic Press; 1970.
18. Ryan TJ. Structure and function of lymphatics. J Invest Dermatol 1989;93:18S–24S.
19. Horstmann E. Uber die funktionelle Struktur der mesenterialen Lymphgefasse. Morphol Jahrb 1952;91:483–510.
20. von der Weid P-Y, Zawieja DC. Lymphatic smooth muscle: The motor unit of lymph drainage. Int J Biochem Cell Biol 2004;36:1147–53.
21. Florey HW. Observations on the contractility of lacteals. Part I. J Physiol 1927;62:267–72.
21. Cooper G, Schiller AL. Anatomy of the Guinea Pig. Cambridge, MA: Harvard University Press; 1975.
23. Azzali G. Transendothelial transport and migration in vessels of the apparatus lymphaticus periphericus absorbens (ALPA). Int Rev Cytol 2003;230:41–87.
24. Jeurissen SH, Sminia T, Kraal G. Selective emigration of suppressor T cells from Peyer's patches. Cell Immunol 1984;85:264–9.
25. Azzali G. Structure, lymphatic vascularization and lymphocyte migration in mucosa-associated lymphoid tissue. Immunol Rev 2003;195:178–89.
26. Ottaviani G, Azzali G. Ultrastructure of lymphatic vessels in some functional conditions. Acta Anat Suppl (Basel) 1969;56:325–36.
27. Sabin FR. On the development of the superficial lymphatics in the skin of the pig. Am J Anat 1904;3:183–95.
28. Sabin FR. On the origin of the lymphatic system from the veins and the development of the lymph hearts and thoracic duct in the pig. Am J Anat 1902;1:367–91.
29. Huntington GS, McClure CFW. The anatomy and development of the jugular lymph sac in the domestic cat (*Felis domestica*). Am J Anat 1910;10:177–311.
30. van der Jagt ER. The origin and development of the anterior lymph sacs in the sea turtle (*Thalassochelys caretta*). Q J Microbiol Sci 1932;75:151–65.
31. Wigle JT, Oliver G. Prox1 function is required for the development of the murine lymphatic system. Cell 1999;98:769–78.
32. Wigle JT, Harvey N, Detmar M, et al. An essential role for Prox1 in the induction of the lymphatic endothelial cell phenotype. EMBO J 2002;21:1505–13.

33. He L, Papoutsi M, Huang R, et al. Three different fates of cells migrating from somites into the limb bud. Anat Embryol (Berl) 2003;207:29–34.

34. Papoutsi M, Tomarev SI, Eichmann A, et al. Endogenous origin of the lymphatics in the avian chorioallantoic membrane. Dev Dyn 2001;222:238–51.

35. Schneider M, Othman-Hassan K, Christ B, Wilting J. Lymphangioblasts in the avian wing bud. Dev Dyn 1999; 216:311–9.

36. Wilting J, Papoutsi M, Othman-Hassan K, et al. Development of the avian lymphatic system. Microsc Res Tech 2001;55:81–91.

37. Rafii S, Skobe M. Splitting vessels: Keeping lymph apart from blood. Nat Med 2003;9:166–8.

38. Karkkainen MJ, Haiko P, Sainio K, et al. Vascular endothelial growth factor C is required for sprouting of the first lymphatic vessels from embryonic veins. Nat Immunol 2004; 5:74–80.

39. Shibuya M, Claesson-Welsh L. Signal transduction by VEGF receptors in regulation of angiogenesis and lymphangiogenesis. Exp Cell Res 2006;312:549–60.

40. Saharinen P, Tammela T, Karkkainen MJ, Alitalo K. Lymphatic vasculature: Development, molecular regulation and role in tumor metastasis and inflammation. Trends Immunol 2004;25:387–95.

41. Tammela T, Petrova TV, Alitalo K. Molecular lymphangiogenesis: New players. Trends Cell Biol 2005;15:434–41.

42. Abtahian F, Guerriero A, Sebzda E, et al. Regulation of blood and lymphatic vascular separation by signaling proteins SLP-76 and Syk. Science 2003;299:247–51.

43. Hungerford JE, Little CD. Developmental biology of the vascular smooth muscle cell: Building a multilayered vessel wall. J Vasc Res 1999;36:2–27.

44. Bergwerff M, Verberne ME, DeRuiter MC, et al. Neural crest cell contribution to the developing circulatory system: Implications for vascular morphology? Circ Res 1998; 82:221–31.

45. Ohtani Y, Ohtani O. Postnatal development of lymphatic vessels and their smooth muscle cells in the rat diaphragm: A confocal microscopic study. Arch Histol Cytol 2001;64:513–22.

46. Mikawa T, Gourdie RG. Pericardial mesoderm generates a population of coronary smooth muscle cells migrating into the heart along with ingrowth of the epicardial organ. Dev Biol 1996;174:221–32.

47. Wilting J, Neeff H, Christ B. Embryonic lymphangiogenesis. Cell Tissue Res 1999;297:1–11.

48. Shimoda H, Kato S. A model for lymphatic regeneration in tissue repair of the intestinal muscle coat. Int Rev Cytol 2006;250:73–108.

49. Aukland K, Reed RK. Interstitial-lymphatic mechanisms in the control of extracellular fluid volume. Physiol Rev 1993;73:1–78.

50. Harwood CA, Mortimer PS. Causes and clinical manifestations of lymphatic failure. Clin Dermatol 1995;13:459–71.

51. Zawieja DC, Barber BJ. Lymph protein concentration in initial and collecting lymphatics of the rat. Am J Physiol 1987;252:G602–6.

52. Morris B. The hepatic and intestinal contributions to the thoracic duct lymph. Q J Exp Physiol Cogn Med Sci 1956; 41:318–25.

53. Ganong WF. Review of Medical Physiology, 15th edition. Norwalk: Appleton & Lange; 1991.

54. Gashev AA, Zawieja DC. Physiology of human lymphatic contractility: A historical perspective. Lymphology 2001; 34:124–34.

55. McHale NG, Roddie IC, Thornbury KD. Nervous modulation of spontaneous contractions in bovine mesenteric lymphatics. J Physiol (Lond) 1980;309:461–72.

56. Hanley CA, Elias RM, Johnston MG. Is endothelium necessary for transmural pressure-induced contractions of bovine truncal lymphatics? Microvasc Res 1992;43:134–46.

57. Benoit JN, Zawieja DC, Goodman AH, Granger HJ. Characterization of intact mesenteric lymphatic pump and its responsiveness to acute edemagenic stress. Am J Physiol 1989;257:H2059–69.

58. van Helden DF, Zhao J. Lymphatic vasomotion. Clin Exp Pharmacol Physiol 2000;27:1014–8.

59. van Helden DF, von der Weid P-Y, Crowe MJ. Intracellular Ca^{2+} release: A basis for electrical pacemaking in lymphatic smooth muscle. In: Tomita T and Bolton TB, editors. Smooth Muscle Excitation. London: Academic Press; 1996. p. 355–73.

60. van Helden DF. Pacemaker potentials in lymphatic smooth muscle of the guinea-pig mesentery. J Physiol 1993;471: 465–79.

61. Johnston MG, Elias R. The regulation of lymphatic pumping. Lymphology 1987;20:215–8.

62. Johnston MG. Interaction of inflammatory mediators with the lymphatic vessel. Pathol Immunopathol Res 1987;6:177–89.

63. Tso P, Balint JA. Formation and transport of chylomicrons by enterocytes to the lymphatics. Am J Physiol 1986;250: G715–26.

64. Phan CT, Tso P. Intestinal lipid absorption and transport. Front Biosci 2001;6:D299–319.

65. Nordskog BK, Phan CT, Nutting DF, Tso P. An examination of the factors affecting intestinal lymphatic transport of dietary lipids. Adv Drug Deliv Rev 2001;50:21–44.

66. Tso P, Nauli A, Lo CM. Enterocyte fatty acid uptake and intestinal fatty acid-binding protein. Biochem Soc Trans 2004;32:75–8.

67. Tso P, Pitts V, Granger DN. Role of lymph flow in intestinal chylomicron transport. Am J Physiol 1985;249:G21–8.

68. Borgstrom B, Laurell CB. Studies of lymph and lymph-proteins during absorption of fat and saline by rats. Acta Physiol Scand 1953;29:264–80.

69. Simmonds WJ. The effect of fluid, electrolyte and food intake on thoracic duct lymph flow in unanaesthetized rats. Aust J Exp Biol Med Sci 1954;32:285–99.

70. Rothkotter HJ, Hriesik C, Pabst R. Many newly formed T lymphocytes leave the small intestinal mucosa via lymphatics. Adv Exp Med Biol 1994;355:261–3.

71. Miura S, Sekizuka E, Nagata H, et al. Increased lymphocyte transport by lipid absorption in rat mesenteric lymphatics. Am J Physiol 1987;253:G596–600.

72. Husband AJ, Dunkley ML. Lack of site of origin effects on distribution of IgA antibody-containing cells. Immunology 1985;54:215–21.

73. Hay JB, Andrade WN. Lymphocyte recirculation, exercise, and immune responses. Can J Physiol Pharmacol 1998;76:490–6.

74. Gunn MD, Kyuwa S, Tam C, et al. Mice lacking expression of secondary lymphoid organ chemokine have defects in lymphocyte homing and dendritic cell localization. J Exp Med 1999;189:451–60.

75. Kriehuber E, Breiteneder-Geleff S, Groeger M, et al. Isolation and characterization of dermal lymphatic and blood endothelial cells reveal stable and functionally specialized cell lineages. J Exp Med 2001;194:797–808.

76. Mancardi S, Vecile E, Dusetti N, et al. Evidence of CXC, CC and C chemokine production by lymphatic endothelial cells. Immunology 2003;108:523–30.

77. Saeki H, Moore AM, Brown MJ, Hwang ST. Cutting edge: Secondary lymphoid-tissue chemokine (SLC) and CC chemokine receptor 7 (CCR7) participate in the emigration pathway of mature dendritic cells from the skin to regional lymph nodes. J Immunol 1999;162:2472–5.

78. Randolph GJ, Sanchez-Schmitz G, Angeli V. Factors and signals that govern the migration of dendritic cells via lymphatics: Recent advances. Springer Semin Immunopathol 2005;26:273–87.

79. Randolph GJ, Angeli V, Swartz MA. Dendritic-cell trafficking to lymph nodes through lymphatic vessels. Nat Rev Immunol 2005;5:617–28.

80. Berg RD. Bacterial translocation from the gastrointestinal tract. Adv Exp Med Biol 1999;473:11–30.

81. Strobel S, Mowat AM. Oral tolerance and allergic responses to food proteins. Curr Opin Allergy Clin Immunol 2006; 6:207–13.

82. Kuroshima S, Sawa Y, Kawamoto T, et al. Expression of Toll-like receptors 2 and 4 on human intestinal lymphatic vessels. Microvasc Res 2004;67:90–5.

83. Tsuzuki Y, Miyazaki J, Matsuzaki K, et al. Differential modulation in the functions of intestinal dendritic cells by long- and medium-chain fatty acids. J Gastroenterol 2006; 41:209–16.

84. Locati M, Torre YM, Galliera E, et al. Silent chemoattractant receptors: D6 as a decoy and scavenger receptor for inflammatory CC chemokines. Cytokine Growth Factor Rev 2005;16:679–86.

85. Nibbs RJ, Wylie SM, Pragnell IB, Graham GJ. Cloning and characterization of a novel murine beta chemokine receptor, D6. Comparison to three other related macrophage inflammatory protein-1alpha receptors, CCR-1, CCR-3, and CCR-5. J Biol Chem 1997;272:12495–504.

86. Nibbs RJ, Kriehuber E, Ponath PD, et al. The beta-chemokine receptor D6 is expressed by lymphatic endothelium and a subset of vascular tumors. Am J Pathol 2001;158:867–77.

87. Olszewski WL, Engeset A. Intrinsic contractility of prenodal lymph vessels and lymph flow in human leg. Am J Physiol 1980;239:H775–83.

88. McHale NG, Roddie IC. The effect of transmural pressure on pumping activity in isolated bovine lymphatic vessels. J Physiol (Lond) 1976;261:255–69.

89. McHale NG. The lymphatic circulation. Ir J Med Sci 1992;161:483–6.

90. Ohhashi T, Azuma T, Sakaguchi M. Active and passive mechanical characteristics of bovine mesenteric lymphatics. Am J Physiol 1980;239:H88–95.

91. Eisenhoffer J, Lee S, Johnston MG. Pressure-flow relationships in isolated sheep prenodal lymphatic vessels. Am J Physiol 1994;267:H938–43.

92. Koller A, Mizuno R, Kaley G. Flow reduces the amplitude and increases the frequency of lymphatic vasomotion: Role of endothelial prostanoids. Am J Physiol 1999;277: R1683–9.

93. Gashev AA, Davis MJ, Zawieja DC. Inhibition of the active lymph pump by flow in rat mesenteric lymphatics and thoracic duct. J Physiol 2002;540:1023–37.

94. Gashev AA, Davis MJ, Delp MD, Zawieja DC. Regional variations of contractile activity in isolated rat lymphatics. Microcirculation 2004;11:477–92.

95. Johnston MG. Involvement of lymphatic collecting ducts in the physiology and pathophysiology of lymph flow. In: Johnston MG, editor. Experimental Biology of the Lymphatic Circulation. Amsterdam, New York: Elsevier Science Publishers; 1985. p. 81–120.

96. von der Weid P-Y. Lymphatic vessel pumping and inflammation—the role of spontaneous constrictions and underlying electrical pacemaker potentials. Aliment Pharmacol Ther 2001;15:1115–29.

97. Johnston MG, Gordon JL. Regulation of lymphatic contractility by arachidonate metabolites. Nature 1981;293:294–7.

98. Mizuno R, Koller A, Kaley G. Regulation of the vasomotor activity of lymph microvessels by nitric oxide and prostaglandins. Am J Physiol 1998;274:R790–6.

99. Gao J, Zhao J, Rayner SE, van Helden DF. Evidence that the ATP-induced increase in vasomotion of guinea-pig mesenteric lymphatics involves an endothelium-dependent release of thromboxane A2. Br J Pharmacol 1999;127:1597–602.

100. Zhao J, van Helden DF. ATP-induced endothelium-independent enhancement of lymphatic vasomotion in guinea-pig mesentery involves P(2X) and P(2Y) receptors. Br J Pharmacol 2002;137:477–87.

101. Chan AK, Vergnolle N, Hollenberg MD, von der Weid P-Y. Proteinase-activated receptor 2 modulates guinea-pig mesenteric lymphatic vessel pacemaker potential and contractile activity. J Physiol 2004;560:563–76.

102. Vergnolle N, Wallace JL, Bunnett NW, Hollenberg MD. Protease-activated receptors in inflammation, neuronal signaling and pain. Trends Pharmacol Sci 2001;22:146–52.

103. Lewis GP, Winsey NJ. The action of pharmacologically active substances on the flow and composition of cat hind limb lymph. Br J Pharmacol 1970;40:446–60.

104. Haddy FJ, Scott JB, Grega GJ. Effects of histamine on lymph protein concentration and flow in the dog forelimb. Am J Physiol 1972;223:1172–7.

105. Amelang E, Prasad CM, Raymond RM, Grega GJ. Interactions among inflammatory mediators on edema formation in the canine forelimb. Circ Res 1981;49:298–306.

106. McNamee JE. Histamine decreases selectivity of sheep lung blood-lymph barrier. J Appl Physiol 1983;54:914–8.

107. Svensjo E, Adamski SW, Su K, Grega GJ. Quantitative physiological and morphological aspects of microvascular permeability changes induced by histamine and inhibited by terbutaline. Acta Physiol Scand 1982;116:265–73.

108. Edery H, Lewis GP. Kinin-forming activity and histamine in lymph after tissue injury. J Physiol 1963;169:568–83.

109. Fox JL, von der Weid P-Y. Effects of histamine on the contractile and electrical activity in isolated lymphatic vessels of the guinea-pig mesentery. Br J Pharmacol 2002;136: 1210–8.

110. Reeder LB, DeFilippi VJ, Ferguson MK. Characterization of the effects of histamine in porcine tracheobronchial lymph vessels. Am J Physiol 1996;271:H2501–7.

111. Watanabe N, Kawai Y, Ohhashi T. Dual effects of histamine on spontaneous activity in isolated bovine mesenteric lymphatics. Microvasc Res 1988;36:239–49.

112. Plaku KJ, von der Weid PY. Mast cell degranulation alters lymphatic contractile activity through action of histamine. Microcirculation 2006;13:219–27.

113. Dobbins DE. Receptor mechanisms of serotonin-induced prenodal lymphatic constriction in the canine forelimb. Am J Physiol 1998;274:H650–4.

114. Takahashi N, Kawai Y, Ohhashi T. Effects of vasoconstrictive and vasodilative agents on lymphatic smooth muscles in isolated canine thoracic ducts. J Pharmacol Exp Ther 1990;254:165–70.

115. Ohhashi T, Kawai Y, Azuma T. The response of lymphatic smooth muscles to vasoactive substances. Pflugers Arch 1978;375:183–8.

116. Ferguson MK, Williams UE, Leff AR, Mitchell RW. Heterogeneity of tracheobronchial lymphatic smooth muscle responses to histamine and 5-hydroxytryptamine. Lymphology 1993;26:113–9.

117. Hashimoto S, Kawai Y, Ohhashi T. Effects of vasoactive substances on the pig isolated hepatic lymph vessels. J Pharmacol Exp Ther 1994;269:482–8.

118. Williamson IM. Some responses of bovine mesenteric arteries, veins and lymphatics. J Physiol (Lond) 1969;202: 112P+.
119. Miyahara H, Kawai Y, Ohhashi T. 5-Hydroxytryptamine-2 and -4 receptors located on bovine isolated mesenteric lymphatics. J Pharmacol Exp Ther 1994;271:379–85.
120. McHale NG, Thornbury KD, Hollywood MA. 5-HT inhibits spontaneous contractility of isolated sheep mesenteric lymphatics via activation of 5-HT(4) receptors. Microvasc Res 2000;60(3):261–8.
121. Chan AK, von der Weid P-Y. 5-HT decreases contractile and electrical activities in lymphatic vessels of the guinea-pig mesentery: Role of 5-HT 7-receptors. Br J Pharmacol 2003;139:243–54.
122. von der Weid P-Y, Crowe MJ, van Helden DF. Endothelium-dependent modulation of pacemaking in lymphatic vessels of the guinea-pig mesentery. J Physiol 1996;493:563–75.
123. Wang H. Activated macrophage-mediated endogenous prosteglandin and nitric oxide-dependent relaxation of lymphatic smooh muscles. Jap J Physiol 1997;47:93–100.
124. von der Weid P-Y, Zhao J, van Helden DF. Nitric oxide decreases pacemaker activity in lymphatic vessels of guinea pig mesentery. Am J Physiol 2001;280:H2707–16.
125. McHale NG. Lymphatic innervation. Blood Vessels 1990;27:127–36.
126. Alessandrini C, Gerli R, Sacchi G, et al. Cholinergic and adrenergic innervation of mesenterial lymph vessels in guinea pig. Lymphology 1981;14:1–6.
127. Russell JA, Zimmerman K, Middendorf WF. Evidence for alpha-adrenergic innervation of the isolated canine thoracic duct. J Appl Physiol 1980;49:1010–5.
128. Allen JM, McCarron JG, McHale NG, Thornbury KD. Release of [3H]-noradrenaline from the sympathetic nerves to bovine mesenteric lymphatic vessels and its modification by alpha-agonists and antagonists. Br J Pharmacol 1988;94:823–33.
129. Dobbins DE. Catecholamine-mediated lymphatic constriction: Involvement of both alpha 1- and alpha 2-adrenoreceptors. Am J Physiol 1992;263:H473–8.
130. Ikomi F, Kawai Y, Ohhashi T. Beta-1 and beta-2 adrenoceptors mediate smooth muscle relaxation in bovine isolated mesenteric lymphatics. J Pharmacol Exp Ther 1991; 259:365–70.
131. Ohhashi T, Takahashi N. Acetylcholine-induced release of endothelium-derived relaxing factor from lymphatic endothelial cells. Am J Physiol 1991;260:H1172–8.
132. Wang XY, Wong WC, Ling EA. Studies of the lymphatic vessel-associated neurons in the intestine of the guinea pig. J Anat 1994;185:65–74.
133. Wang XY, Wong WC, Ling EA. Ultrastructural localisation of substance P, vasoactive intestinal peptide and somatostatin immunoreactivities in the submucous plexus of guinea pig ileum. J Anat 1995;186:187–96.
134. Chen YK, Richter HM, Kelly KA, et al. Postprandial gastrin, neurotensin, vasoactive intestinal pepetide, substance P and bombesin output in canine thoracic duct lymph. Gastroenterology 1984;86:1046.
135. Makhija S, von der Weid PY, Meddings J, et al. Octreotide in intestinal lymphangiectasia: Lack of a clinical response and failure to alter lymphatic function in a guinea pig model. Can J Gastroenterol 2004;18:681–5.
136. Qin X, Shen H, Liu M, et al. GLP-1 reduces intestinal lymph flow, triglyceride absorption, and apolipoprotein production in rats. Am J Physiol Gastrointest Liver Physiol 2005;288: G943–9.
137. Taylor AE. The lymphatic edema safety factor: The role of edema dependent lymphatic factors (EDLF). Lymphology 1990;23:111–23.
138. Szuba A, Rockson SG. Lymphedema: Classification, diagnosis and therapy. Vasc Med 1998;3:145–56.
139. Rockson SG. Lymphedema. Am J Med 2001;110:288–95.
140. Browse NL, Stewart G. Lymphoedema: pathophysiology and classification. J Cardiovasc Surg (Torino) 1985;26: 91–106.
141. Piller NB. Lymphoedema, macrophages and benzopyrones. Lymphology 1980;13:109–19.
142. Kriederman BM, Myloyde TL, Witte MH, et al. FOXC2 haploinsufficient mice are a model for human autosomal dominant lymphedema-distichiasis syndrome. Hum Mol Genet 2003;12:1179–85.
143. Petrova TV, Karpanen T, Norrmen C, et al. Defective valves and abnormal mural cell recruitment underlie lymphatic vascular failure in lymphedema distichiasis. Nat Med 2004; 10:974–81.
144. Ferrell RE, Levinson KL, Esman JH, et al. Hereditary lymphedema: Evidence for linkage and genetic heterogeneity. Hum Mol Genet 1998;7:2073–8.
145. Irrthum A, Karkkainen MJ, Devriendt K, et al. Congenital hereditary lymphedema caused by a mutation that inactivates VEGFR3 tyrosine kinase. Am J Hum Genet 2000;67:295–301.
146. Segerstrom K, Bjerle P, Graffman S, Nystrom A. Factors that influence the incidence of brachial oedema after treatment of breast cancer. Scand J Plast Reconstr Surg Hand Surg 1992;26:223–7.
147. Tabibiazar R, Cheung L, Han J, et al. Inflammatory manifestations of experimental lymphatic insufficiency. PLoS Med 2006;3:e254.
148. Taylor MJ. A new insight into the pathogenesis of filarial disease. Curr Mol Med 2002;2:299–302.
149. Taylor MJ, Hoerauf A. Wolbachia bacteria of filarial nematodes. Parasitol Today 1999;15:437–42.
150. Taylor MJ, Hoerauf A. A new approach to the treatment of filariasis. Curr Opin Infect Dis 2001;14(6):727–31.
151. Taylor MJ, Cross HF, Bilo K. Inflammatory responses induced by the filarial nematode *Brugia malayi* are mediated by lipopolysaccharide-like activity from endosymbiotic Wolbachia bacteria. J Exp Med 2000;191:1429–36.
152. Kaiser L, Mupanomunda M, Williams JF. Brugia pahangi-induced contractility of bovine mesenteric lymphatics studied in vitro: A role for filarial factors in the development of lymphedema? Am J Trop Med Hyg 1996;54:386–90.
153. Kirsner JB. Observations on the etiology and pathogenesis of inflammatory bowel disease. In: Bockus H, editor. Gastroenterology. Philadelphia: Saunders; 1976. p. 521–39.
154. Kovi J, Duong HD, Hoang CT. Ultrastructure of intestinal lymphatics in Crohn's disease. Am J Clin Pathol 1981;76:385–94.
155. Robb-Smith AH. A bird's-eye view of Crohn's disease. Proc R Soc Med 1971;64:157–61.
156. Heatley RV, Bolton PM, Hughes LE, Owen EW. Mesenteric lymphatic obstruction in Crohn's disease. Digestion 1980;20:307–13.
157. Kalima TV, Saloniemi H, Rahko T. Experimental regional enteritis in pigs. Scand J Gastroenterol 1976;11:353–62.
158. Reichert FL, Mathes ME. Experimental lymphedema of the intestinal tract and its relation to regional cicatrizing enteritis. Annals Surg 1936;104:610–6.
159. Geleff S, Schoppmann SF, Oberhuber G. Increase in podoplanin-expressing intestinal lymphatic vessels in inflammatory bowel disease. Virchows Arch 2003;442:231–7.
160. Mooney EE, Walker J, Hourihane DO. Relation of granulomas to lymphatic vessels in Crohn's disease. J Clin Pathol 1995;48:335–8.
161. Fogt F, Pascha TL, Zhang PJ, et al. Proliferation of D2-40-expressing intestinal lymphatic vessels in the lamina propria in inflammatory bowel disease. Int J Mol Med 2004;13:211–4.
162. Kaiserling E, Krober S, Geleff S. Lymphatic vessels in the colonic mucosa in ulcerative colitis. Lymphology 2003;36:52–61.
163. Cursiefen C, Chen L, Borges LP, et al. VEGF-A stimulates lymphangiogenesis and hemangiogenesis in inflammatory neovascularization via macrophage recruitment. J Clin Invest 2004;113:1040–50.
164. Baluk P, Tammela T, Ator E, et al. Pathogenesis of persistent lymphatic vessel hyperplasia in chronic airway inflammation. J Clin Invest 2005;115:247–57.
165. Mouta C, Heroult M. Inflammatory triggers of lymphangiogenesis. Lymphat Res Biol 2003;1:201–18.
166. Maruyama K, Ii M, Cursiefen C, et al. Inflammation-induced lymphangiogenesis in the cornea arises from CD11b-positive macrophages. J Clin Invest 2005;115:2363–72.
167. Tonelli P. New developments in Crohn's disease: Solution of doctrinal mysteries and reinstatement as a surgically treatable disease. 1. The process is not a form of enteritis but lymphedema contaminated by intestinal contents. Chir Ital 2000;52:109–21.
168. Wu TF, Carati CJ, Macnaughton WK, von der Weid PY. Contractile activity of lymphatic vessels is altered in the TNBS model of guinea pig ileitis. Am J Physiol Gastrointest Liver Physiol 2006;291:G566–74.
169. Sleeman JP. The relationship between tumors and the lymphatics: What more is there to know? Lymphology 2006;39:62–8.
170. Stacker SA, Caesar C, Baldwin ME, et al. VEGF-D promotes the metastatic spread of tumor cells via the lymphatics. Nat Med 2001;7:186–91.
171. Skobe M, Hawighorst T, Jackson DG, et al. Induction of tumor lymphangiogenesis by VEGF-C promotes breast cancer metastasis. Nat Med 2001;7:192–8.
172. Mandriota SJ, Jussila L, Jeltsch M, et al. Vascular endothelial growth factor-C-mediated lymphangiogenesis promotes tumour metastasis. EMBO J 2001;20:672–82.
173. He Y, Kozaki K, Karpanen T, et al. Suppression of tumor lymphangiogenesis and lymph node metastasis by blocking vascular endothelial growth factor receptor 3 signaling. J Natl Cancer Inst 2002;94:819–25.
174. Hirakawa S, Kodama S, Kunstfeld R, et al. VEGF-A induces tumor and sentinel lymph node lymphangiogenesis and promotes lymphatic metastasis. J Exp Med 2005;201: 1089–99.
175. Stacker SA, Baldwin ME, Achen MG. The role of tumor lymphangiogenesis in metastatic spread. FASEB J 2002;16:922–34.
176. Duff SE, Li C, Jeziorska M, et al. Vascular endothelial growth factors C and D and lymphangiogenesis in gastrointestinal tract malignancy. Br J Cancer 2003;89: 426–30.
177. Walker-Smith JA, Murch S. Disease of the small intestine in childhood, 4th edition. Oxford: ISIS; 1999.
178. Hardikar W, Smith AL, Chow CW. Neonatal protein-losing enteropathy caused by intestinal lymphatic hypoplasia in siblings. J Pediatr Gastroenterol Nutr 1997;25: 217–21.
179. Stormon MO, Mitchell JD, Smoleniec JS, et al. Congenital intestinal lymphatic hypoplasia presenting as non-immune hydrops in utero, and subsequent neonatal protein-losing enteropathy. J Pediatr Gastroenterol Nutr 2002;35: 691–4.
180. Kahn HJ, Marks A. A new monoclonal antibody, D2-40, for detection of lymphatic invasion in primary tumors. Lab Invest 2002;82:1255–7.
181. Zeng Y, Wang F, Williams ED, Chow CW. Lymphatics in the alimentary tract of children in health and disease: Study on mucosal biopsies using the monoclonal antibody d2-40. Pediatr Dev Pathol 2005;8:541–9.
182. Tomei E, Diacinti D, Marini M, et al. Abdominal CT findings may suggest coeliac disease. Dig Liver Dis 2005;37:402–6.
183. Sampson HA. 9. Food allergy. J Allergy Clin Immunol 2003;111:S540–7.
184. Adams CA, Jr, Hauser CJ, Adams JM, et al. Trauma-hemorrhage-induced neutrophil priming is prevented by mesenteric lymph duct ligation. Shock 2002;18:513–7.
185. Deitch EA. Role of the gut lymphatic system in multiple organ failure. Curr Opin Crit Care 2001;7:92–8.
186. Deitch EA. Bacterial translocation or lymphatic drainage of toxic products from the gut: What is important in human beings? Surgery 2002;131:241–4.
187. Deitch EA, Xu D, Kaise VL. Role of the gut in the development of injury- and shock induced SIRS and MODS: The gut-lymph hypothesis, a review. Front Biosci 2006;11: 520–8.
188. Magnotti LJ, Upperman JS, Xu DZ, et al. Gut-derived mesenteric lymph but not portal blood increases endothelial cell permeability and promotes lung injury after hemorrhagic shock. Ann Surg 1998;228:518–27.
189. Magnotti LJ, Xu DZ, Lu Q, Deitch EA. Gut-derived mesenteric lymph: A link between burn and lung injury. Arch Surg 1999;134:1333–40; discussion 1340–1.
190. Sambol JT, Xu DZ, Adams CA, et al. Mesenteric lymph duct ligation provides long term protection against hemorrhagic shock-induced lung injury. Shock 2000;14:416–9; discussion 419–20.
191. Cavriani G, Domingos HV, Soares AL, et al. Lymphatic system as a path underlying the spread of lung and gut injury after intestinal ischemia/reperfusion in rats. Shock 2005;23:330–6.
192. Cavriani G, Domingos HV, Oliveira-Filho RM, et al. Lymphatic thoracic duct ligation modulates the serum levels of IL-1beta and IL-10 after intestinal ischemia/reperfusion in rats with the involvement of tumor necrosis factor alpha and nitric oxide. Shock 2007;27:209–13.
193. Anand RJ, Leaphart CL, Mollen KP, Hackam DJ. The role of the intestinal barrier in the pathogenesis of necrotizing enterocolitis. Shock 2007;27:124–33.
194. Lin PW, Stoll BJ. Necrotising enterocolitis. Lancet 2006; 368:1271–83.
195. Sibbons P, Spitz L, van Velzen D. The role of lymphatics in the pathogenesis of pneumatosis in experimental bowel ischemia. J Pediatr Surg 1992;27:339–42; discussion 342–3.
196. Deitch EA. Role of bacterial translocation in necrotizing enterocolitis. Acta Paediatr Suppl 1994;396:33–6.
197. Sonntag J, Wagner MH, Waldschmidt J, et al. Multisystem organ failure and capillary leak syndrome in severe necrotizing enterocolitis of very low birth weight infants. J Pediatr Surg 1998;33:481–4.
198. Noel AA, Gloviczki P, Bender CE, et al. Treatment of symptomatic primary chylous disorders. J Vasc Surg 2001;34:785–91.

Absorption and Digestion

15.1. Normal Physiology of Intestinal Digestion and Absorption

Jean Pierre Cézard, MD, PhD

The knowledge of mechanisms of intestinal digestion and absorption had been developed mainly during the second period of the last century, due to the widespread use of intestinal biopsy, the emergence of basic concepts, such as lipolysis at an interface, miscellar solubilization, Na$^+$-coupled solute transport, and brush border as a digestive–absorptive organelle permitting the breakdown of digestion and absorption into the many different steps in hydrolysis or transport of mineral and nutrients. This allowed also to characterize malabsorption and maldigestion syndromes into specific different pathologic situations, such as those characterized by exocrine pancreatic insufficiency (eg, cystic fibrosis), intestinal villous atrophy (eg, celiac disease), specific hydrolysis (eg, congenital lipase or sucrase deficiencies), or transport (eg, glucose–galactose malabsorption) defects. In order to understand how the clinician should interpret chronic diarrhea, the main symptom of these disease states, and how to orient the approach to the precise defect involved, it is necessary to recall the physiology of digestion and absorption.

CARBOHYDRATES

Physiology of Digestion and Absorption

Carbohydrates in food comprise mainly starch (50 to 60% of total energy supplied by carbohydrates), sucrose (30 to 40%), and lactose (from 0 to 20% in adults, 40 to 50% in infants). Only starch molecules (amylose and amylopectin), which are glucose polymers of high molecular weight (MW), require preliminary intraluminal digestion by salivary and (predominantly) pancreatic amylases. These structurally related endoamylases only split alpha$_{1-4}$ bonds at some distance from the ends of the glycosidic chains and from the branching (alpha$_{1-6}$) positions. They release mainly maltose, maltotriose, and residues of higher degree of polymerization (branched-alpha-limit dextrins, if the substrate is amylopectin) but no glucose.[1] Intraluminal alpha-amylase activity is 10 times that required for digesting the amount of starch ingested daily.[2]

The final hydrolysis of di- and oligosaccharides occurs at the brush border of enterocytes where act three main glycoproteins of high MW (greater than 200 kDa), the disaccharidases (Table 1): two a-glycosidases—(1) sucrase–isomaltase (S–I), which accounts for 75 to 80% of the hydrolysis of maltose in the intestinal mucosa, the total hydrolysis of sucrose, and the nearly total hydrolysis of isomaltose (alpha$_{1-6}$); (2) glucoamylase, an exoamylase that is responsible for 20 to 25% of total mucosal maltase activity and releases glucose from glucose polymers of four or more residues; one β-galactosidase lactase-phlorizin hydrolase, which accounts for over 95% of lactase activity in the intestinal mucosa and for the hydrolysis of glycosyl ceramides, complex glycolipids that are important constituents of milk globule membranes.[3] Sucrase–isomaltase and lactase activities are highest in the proximal intestine whereas glucoamylase activity is highest in the ileum.[4] The ingested disaccharides, which physiologically are not absorbed as such, are thus ultimately broken down into their constituent monosaccharides: glucose, galactose, and fructose.

Entry into the enterocytes through the brush border membrane occurs via carrier molecules. Entry of glucose and of galactose, occurring through the same carrier (SGTL$_1$), is linked to the entry of Na$^+$ along its electrochemical gradient; the latter blocks glucose exit from the cell and eventually provides the energy necessary for its accumulation in the cell against a concentration gradient.[1] The electrochemical Na$^+$ gradient is maintained by Na$^+$, K$^+$-adenosinetriphosphatase (ATPase) located in the basolateral membrane of the enterocyte. Thus, glucose and galactose absorptions are indirectly active. Mutations of the gene coding for SGTL$_1$ are the cause of congenital glucose–galactose malabsorption.[5] Entry of fructose occurs through another specific carrier (GLUT5). It is not Na$^+$ dependent.[6] Fructose is more metabolized in the enterocyte than glucose; exit from the cell of both monosaccharides occurs via a facilitated transport system (a carrier) similar to the one present in red blood cell membranes (GLUT2).[1]

Final hydrolysis and absorption of carbohydrates are closely integrated in the brush border so that when sucrose is perfused into the jejunum, no or low amounts of glucose diffuse back into the intestinal lumen. Perfusion studies in adults as in children have shown that the limiting factor in the overall process of disaccharide absorption is absorption of glucose and fructose in the case of sucrose and of maltose, but lactase activity in the case of lactose. This relationship is not modified in cases of mucosal atrophy.[7]

Pathophysiology

Pancreatic amylase insufficiency occurs normally in newborns, whose amylase activity remains extremely low during the first weeks of life. However, early development of salivary amylase and brush border glucoamylase allowed substantial amounts of starch (greater than 40 g/m^2/d) to be

Table 1 Human Brush Border Proteins with Carbohydrate Activity

Protein	Size of Protein Chain (kDa)	Size of B–B Protein Chains (kDa)	Site of Protein Cleavage	Specificity — Substrates	Specificity — Products
Sucrase isomaltase	240	$S = 130$	Extra cellular (trypsin)	Sucrose	Glucose
				Maltose	Fructose
		$I = 145$		Limit—dextrine	
Lactase-phlorizin hydrolase	230	$L = 160$	Intra and extracellular	Lactose	Glu+Gal
		pH = 160		Glucoside ceramide	
Glucoamylase	335	335	None	α(1-4)-Dextrine	Glu
				Amidon	
Trehalase	65	75	None	Trehalose	Glu

given to 1-month-old infants before fermentation, the sign of carbohydrate malabsorption, occurs.[8] Similarly, in cases of exocrine pancreatic insufficiency (cystic fibrosis or Shwachman syndrome), symptoms related to amylase insufficiency are modest and occurs when activity level are reduced to below 10% of normal. Defects of intestinal digestion and absorption of oligosaccharides are mainly acquired. They lead to a major digestive symptom: fermentative diarrhea, characterized by watery stools with an acidic smell, resembling that of rotten apples or of vinegar. They have an acidic pH (5.5 to 4.0) and usually contain unabsorbed reducing sugars or undigested disaccharides.

The main causes of acquired oligosaccharides maldigestion or absorption are acute severe infectious diarrhea (transient lactose deficiency) and immuno allergic diseases (cow milk allergy and celiac disease) because of villous atrophy. Congenital enzyme deficiencies (S.I and glucose galactose) are exceptional.[9,10]

Excluding the malabsorbed carbohydrate(s) from the diet stops diarrhea in a few hours; it is again triggered in a similar short period of time if the malabsorbed oligosaccharide is reintroduced in the diet.

PROTEINS

Physiology

Dietary aminoacids are ingested predominantly as proteins. Their digestion starts in the lumen of the stomach, where gastric acid denatures them and activates pepsinogens I and II into the corresponding pepsins. The latter are inactive at pH of more than 5 and have a broad specificity, splitting peptide bonds mostly involving phenylalanine, tyrosine, and leucine.[11,12] In view of the buffering capacity of food, it is unlikely that gastric secretion plays a major role in protein digestion. This is illustrated by the fact that partial or total gastrectomy have no impairment on protein digestion and absorption.

In contrast, the efficiency of pancreatic proteolysis is demonstrated by the fact that as soon as 15 minutes after a test meal, about half of amino acids in the lumen are free or in the form of small peptides.[11] After activation by enterokinase, a glycoprotein of high molecular weight synthesized by and anchored in the brush border membrane of enterocytes in the proximal small intestine,[13] trypsinogen is converted into trypsin, which, in its turn, activates the other zymogens into active proteases. The endopeptidases—trypsin, chymotrypsin, and elastase—are serine proteases of similar MW (25 to 28 kDa) but with different and strictly defined specificities. Trypsin splits only bonds involving at the amino end basic amino acids (lysine and arginine); chymotrypsin splits those involving aromatic amino acids (phenylalanine, tyrosine, and tryptophan); and elastase splits those involving uncharged small amino acids (such as alanine, glycine, and serine), which amino acids are left at the carboxy end of the newly formed peptide. They are released

by exopeptidases: carboxypeptidase A, which releases from a peptide its last amino acid when it is aromatic, neutral, or acid, and by carboxypeptidase B, when the last amino acid is basic. The action of the pancreatic enzymes on protein produces a mixture of oligopeptides (60–70%) anf free aminoacids (Figure 1).[11,14]

In contrast to carbohydrates, peptides enter enterocytes either after preliminary digestion by brush border peptidases into amino acids, or as such, in the case of di- or tripeptides which are then split inside the cell by cytoplasmic peptidases.[15–22] In humans, the following brush border peptidases are now well defined: several aminopeptidases (oligoaminopeptidase or neutral aminopeptidase, the main brush border peptidase, acid aminopeptidase, dipeptidyl-peptidase IV, an ileal NAALDASE L (N-acyetylated a-linked acidic dipeptidase) with DPP IV activity[15]), two carboxy-peptidases (carboxypeptidase P and angiotensin-converting enzyme (ACE)), two endopeptidases (including para-aminobenzoic acid (PABA) peptidase), and gamma-glutamyl transpeptidase.

These enzymes are glycoproteins of MW somewhat lower than that of disaccharidases and altogether are able to hydrolyze all peptide bonds

except those involving a proline at the carboxyl side.[11] Their highest activities are in the ileum.[4,16] The released amino acids are absorbed through the following systems: neutral amino acids enter the enterocytes mainly through the B, Na$^+$-dependent system, whose defect is responsible for Hartnup disease[22]; they can also use at least two other systems shared with basic amino acids: B$^{+,0}$ Na$^+$ -independent and b$^{+,0}$ Na$^+$-dependent, defective in type I cystinuria.[18] Proline and hydroxyproline mainly use the Na$^+$, Cl$^-$-dependent IMINO carrier and also, in a lesser proportion (~30%), the B^0 carrier to enter the enterocyte. Bicarboxylic acids enter through a specific Na$^+$-dependent, electroneutral X$^-_{AG}$ system whose defect is responsible for dicarboxylic aminoaciduria.[18]

Small peptides are the form in which amino acids are, in general, the more readily absorbed. Even when a di- or tripeptide is susceptible to rapid hydrolysis by brush border peptidases, an important proportion of it (30 to 50% depending on its concentration) is directly absorbed as such. Thus, peptides represent the main physiologic route of entry of amino acids in the enterocytes.

Di- and tripeptides cross the brush border membrane as such via a (main) peptide transport system (PEPTS) that has been shown to have a

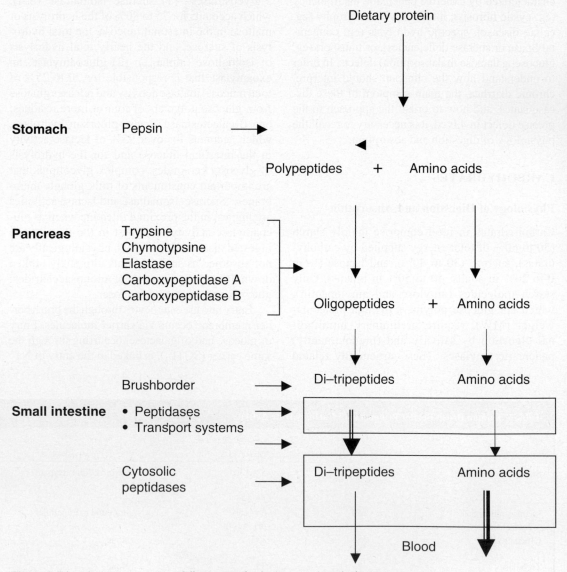

Figure 1 Digestion and absorption of dietary proteins in the gastrointestinal tract.

broad specificity.[23] This carrier protein is able to transport dibasic as well as diacid peptides and di- as well as tripeptides (but no tetrapeptides).[20,21] Transport of peptide is coupled to a proton (H^+) gradient. The human transporter has been cloned and has on chromosome molecular weight of 79kDa.[11,19,20,21]

Once in the absorbing cell, di- and tripeptides are split into amino acids by soluble peptidases of which are known gly-leu dipeptidase, a prolidase hydrolyzing X-Pro bonds, and a tripeptidase[11]

At the basolateral membrane, neutral amino acids leave the enteroyte using the Na^+-dependent L system; basic amino acids use Na^+-dependent y^+ and y^{+L} systems which also accept neutral amino acids.[11] Mutations in the gene coding for a subunit of y^{+L}, y^{+LAT} are the cause of lysinuric protein intolerance.[24] Ubiquitous Na^+-dependent A and ASC systems, of high specificity and low capacity, are probably more involved in the metabolism of the enterocytes than in protein absorption. Recently, a peptide transporter has been characterized in basolateral membranes of Caco-2 cells.[23]

Pathophysiology

In adults, nitrogen absorption is not affected by gastrectomy, which indicates that gastric acid and pepsins do not play a critical role in protein digestion.

In contrast, in children with selective absence of pancreatic protease activities (eg, congenital enterokinase[25] deficiency) or global pancreatic exocrine insufficiency such as in cystic fibrosis, severe malnutrition, failure to thrive, and chronic diarrhea with fecal losses of nitrogen occur.

In patients with global pancreatic exocrine insufficiency, significant losses of energy in the stools are due to the defect in starch digestion and, mostly, in fat digestion with massive steatorrhea.

No specific congenital defect of peptide digestion or absorption by the intestinal mucosa is known. This is not surprising considering that amino acids and peptides enter enterocytes by two routes of roughly similar physiologic importance: when one is blocked, the other one still can be used. Specific absorption defects involving neutral (Hartnup disease), basic (cystinuria), or imino (prolinuria) acids are well known. They have been recognized not because of digestive symptoms, which do not exist in these conditions, but because of associated specific aminoaciduria, reflecting defective tubular reabsorption of the homologous amino acids by the kidney.[20] Indeed, the only known disease affecting amino acid absorption in which diarrhea is a real problem, often associated with severe malnutrition, is protein intolerance with lysinuria (or lysinuric protein intolerance). In this condition, the congenital defect affects the exit of arginine, lysine, and ornithine—out of the cell through the basolateral membrane.[26] Diarrhea is usually liquid, being probably mainly osmotic in its mechanism.

Nonspecific inflammatory alterations of the intestinal mucosa, such as those seen in celiac disease, is associated with symptoms of protein or peptide maldigestion and absorption mostly edema with hypoalmuninemia.

FAT

Physiology

Unlike carbohydrates and proteins, fats are insoluble in water; while they diffuse through the lipid phases of the brush border and basolateral membranes of enterocytes, they have to be "wrapped" in outwardly hydrophilic, inwardly lipophilic particles: bile salt micelles in the gut lumen, and chylomicrons in the absorbing cell and circulation to reach their site of metabolic use (Figure 2).[27]

Digestion of fat starts in the stomach, acted on by a lipase that has been shown recently to originate exclusively from the gastric fundus in humans,[28] whereas it is produced by the serous glands of Ebner at the base of the tongue in the rat (hence the often-used term lingual lipase). In humans, this lipase has an acidic optimum pH (4.5 to 5.5); at the pH of the stomach, it hydrolyzes medium-chain triglycerides (MCT) at the same rate as long-chain triglycerides (LCT), it preferentially splits the outer ester bonds of triglycerides (TG), and it is not dependent on bile salts. It is inhibited by them and is resistant to pepsine. It acts as a "starter" of pancreatic lipolysis by favoring emulsification of lipid droplets by the free fatty acids it releases. It plays a particularly important role in neonates whose pancreatic lipase activity is low.[29]

In the duodenum, pancreatic lipase acts only at the oil/water interface, adsorbed to the lipid droplets. Bile salts both increase the interface by emulsifying the ingested lipid droplets, thus favoring lipase activity, and, on the contrary, by forming a film between oil and lipase, inhibit its action. Colipase restores lipase activity by anchoring lipase to the interface and by keeping its active site open, giving it access to its substrate.[30] In the presence of bile salts, pancreatic lipase has an optimum pH of 8. It has an absolute specificity for the outer ester bonds (positions 1 and 3) of the triglyceride molecule and releases free fatty acids (FFA) and 2-monoglycerides (2 MGs).[30] Other lipolytic enzymes are secreted by the pancreas: (1) carboxylesterhydrolase, whose structure resembles that of human milk, is a bile-salt–dependent lipase, and acts on soluble substrates. In the presence of bile salts, it becomes active toward cholesterol esters and esters of vitamins A and E, whose absorption is thus dependent on normal bile salt secretion[31]; (2) phospholipase A_2 releases lysophosphoglycerides and fatty acids from phosphoglycerides, major membrane constituents.

From the onset of lipolysis, FFAs and 2 MGs are solubilized in bile salt micelles, forming bigger "mixed micelles," which, in their turn, can solubilize more hydrophobic lipids, such as diglycerides, unionized FFA, cholesterol esters, and lipid-soluble vitamins whose absorption is therefore improved when ingested with other fats.

Primary bile acids (cholic and chenodeoxycholic acids) are synthesized in the liver from cholesterol; they are glyco- and tauroconjugated, excreted, and later transformed by colonic bacteria into secondary acids (deoxycholic and lithocholic acids). Because of their lower pKa, conjugated bile acids allow a much better micellar solubilization of the products of lipolysis[22] Bile acids, whose pool amounts to 1 to 2.5 g, are efficiently reabsorbed in the distal ileum by a Na^+-dependent, carrier-mediated process that is responsible for the reabsorption (and recirculation) of 95% of the bile salts secreted in bile.[32]

Micelles diffuse from the gut lumen through the unstirred water layers lining the luminal surface of brush borders, where the products of lipolysis are liberated. They diffuse across the apical cell membrane. At low concentrations, there is evidence that FFAs can enter enterocytes by a fatty acid binding membrane protein with high affinity for saturated or unsaturated LCFA[33,34]; entry of cholesterol is also mediated by brush border membrane lipid exchange proteins.[35] In enterocytes FFAs of 12 carbon atoms or more bind to small carrier proteins, the fatty acid-binding proteins (I [ileal, majority] and L [liver] FABP).[36] In the smooth endoplasmic reticulum, long-chain FA are activated in acyl–CoA before entering the monoglyceride pathway responsible for at least 70% of postprandial TG resynthesis (while the role of glycerophosphate pathway in TG resynthesis increases between meals and during fast).[27] Microsomal TG transfer protein (MTP) transfers resynthesized TG in the rough endoplasmic reticulum where, together with phospholipids and cholesterol, TG is joined by newly synthesized apolipoproteins AI, AIV, and B48. The absence of one of the MTP subunits, but not of B48,[37] has been shown to be responsible for abetalipoproteinemia.[38] Chylomicron formation is then completed in the Golgi apparatus. Chylomicron-containing Golgi vesicles are released from the Golgi apparatus. After fusion of these vesicles with the basolateral membrane, chylomicrons are excreted by exocytosis into the intercellular spaces, from which they reach the lymphatics and, by the thoracic duct, the systemic circulation.[39]

Pathophysiology

Because of their hydrophobicity, digestion and absorption of dietary fats are dependent on many auxiliary molecules other than enzymes and carriers: bile salts, colipase, FABPs, and apolipoproteins. It is thus remarkable that, given this complexity, more than 95% of ingested fat are ultimately absorbed in children over the age of 1 year.

However, these auxiliary mechanisms are also sites for potential disturbances; indeed, causes of fat malabsorption and steatorrhea are much more numerous than those of carbohydrate and protein malabsorption. Fat malabsorption may result from lipase and/or colipase deficiency(ies) isolated[40,41] or global exocrine pancreatic insufficiency, abnormal bile salt synthesis,[42] excretion, deconjugation, and reabsorption[43]; impaired TG

Tissue origin	Enzyme	Substrates	Products
Stomach	Gastric lipase pH 4–5.5	LCT MCT	FFA LCT DG MCT
Pancreas	Pancreatic lipase MW 49 kDa pH 6–6.5 With colipase	LCT MCT DG	FFA MG
	Colipase MW 10 kDa Binding to LCT and lipase (cofactor of lipase)	LCT MCT DG	
	Phospholipase A2 MW 13.6 kDa	Phospholipid	Lysophopholipid FA
	Cholesterol esterase MW 40 kDa	TG sterol Vitamin ester	Cholesterol Esta zetinol
Liver	Bile salts: cholic and chenodeoxycholic acid Essential to pancreatic Enzyme fat digestion	Micellar formation	FFA MG cholesterol ester Lisolecithine liposoluble vitamins
Enterocyte	Brush border	Passive absorption of micelle, MCT cholesterol, vitamins, and bile acids (active in ileum)	
	Cytosol (FABPs)	Binding of FFA	
	Endosplasmic Reticulum + golgi		
	• Glycoerol-3-phosphate and monoglyceral phosphate pathway	Triglycerides synthesis phospholipid	
	• Apolipoprotein synthesis MTP	Chylomicron (LCT, A1, A2, A4, B48 cholesterol)	MCT + liposoluble vitamins
Portal and lymphatic circulation		Lymphactic (chylomicron)	Portal vein (MCT, liposoluble vitamins)

LCT = Long-chain triglycéride FA = Fatty acid	MCT = Medium-chain triglyceride MG = Monoglyceride	DG = Diglyceride MPT = Microsomal transfer	FFA = Free fatty acid TG = Protein

Figure 2 Schematic digestion absorption and secretion of dietary fat.

resynthesis; chylomicron formation and/or excretion (abetalipoproteinemia, Anderson disease[37,38]) or abnormal or obstruction of intestinal lymphatics (lymphangiectasia).[44]

In most cases, fat malabsorption with steatorrhea is part of a more general pathologic condition. Absorption of fat-soluble vitamins is also impaired which could occasionally, determine rickets. Bile salts may also be deconjugated

(bacterial overgrowth) or not be absorbed because of a congenital defect[43] or ileal disease (Crohn's disease) or because of ileal resection with two consequences: on the one hand, abnormally high amounts of nonabsorbed bile salts reach the colon where they inhibit Na$^+$ and water absorption; on the other hand, depletion of the bile salt pool progressively leads to poor micellar solubilization and steatorrhea. In this situation, however,

the direct effect of bile salts on colonic mucosa is probably more responsible for the abnormal loose or watery stools than is the increased fecal loss of fat.

Intestinal mucosal abnormalities never affect only fat absorption. Most frequently fat malabsorption is secondary to intestinal mucosal atrophy, as observed in celiac disease or cow's milk protein intolerance and exceptionnaly autoimmune enteropathies.[45–47] In these conditions, malabsorption of fat, as of other nutrients, results both from decreased absorptive surface and from disturbed enterocyte metabolism. It is not clear whether lipids in the stools originate directly from ingested fat or indirectly from desquamated enterocytes. In any case, fat lost in the stools is mainly FFA partly hydroxylated by the colonic flora, which accounts for at least 1 g daily of obligatory loss of fat in the stools. Steatorrhea is usually far less severe in intestinal mucosal disorders than in exocrine pancreatic insufficiency. The moderate steatorrhea observed in conditions with subtotal villous atrophy is usually not sufficient to make the stools grossly greasy; in fact, stool features in these situations result more from the degree of associated carbohydrate fermentation and bile salt malabsorption than from the degree of steatorrhea.[45]

Similarly, in intestinal lymphangiectasia, reflux of absorbed fat into the intestinal lumen because of blocked lymph flow is never isolated, and steatorrhoea, usually moderate, is associated with signs of enteric loss of the other constituents of intestinal lymph: albumin, immunoglobulins, and T lymphocytes.[44]

PRACTICAL APPROACH TO MALDIGESTION AND MALABSORPTION

The main clinical expression of malabsorption is diarrhea. It is the direct consequence of malabsorption, which, in its turn, when chronic, may result in malnutrition and failure to thrive, the usual other features of malabsorption syndromes. This part of the chapter focuses on chronic diarrhea, or more properly on abnormal stools, as the main clue to the diagnosis and etiology of malabsorption.

RECOGNIZING CHRONIC DIARRHEA

Chronic diarrhea is usually defined as diarrhea lasting for more than 14 days. In toddlers who already control their stools, abnormal stools are not missed by the family. On the contrary, when diarrhea starts from birth or soon after, the abnormal features of the stools are less easily recognized, especially if the infant is breast-fed and is the first child in the family.

For many years balance studies with recording of ingested foods and collection of the stools during at least 3 days have been useful in ascertaining malabsorption and showing that chronic diarrhea had different biochemical features, explaining its macroscopic characteristics (consistence, volume, smell, pH, etc), according to its pathophysiologic mechanism: impaired intraluminal digestion, intestinal malabsorption, or fermentation.

A careful clinical history remains the most important step in getting to the diagnosis of malabsorption. The fluidity, number, size, color, and smell of the stools should first be ascertained. Stools may be as liquid as water and mistaken for urine in infants[48–51] passed noisily with flatus, be loose and bulky; or pasty and yellowish. The number of stools may vary from 2 (bulky) to 10 or more (small and liquid). Stools may be homogeneous or, on the contrary, may contain undigested pieces of vegetables and mucus. Whether the stools are greasy or not is often difficult to ascertain; the less liquid the stools are, the easier it is. Liquid stools may be odorless, or they may have an acidic smell due to fermentation. Finally, the course of diarrhea should be recorded: stools may be abnormal every day or periodically.[52,53]

RECOGNIZING THE CAUSE OF CHRONIC DIARRHEA

The necessary time, then, should be spent in trying to correlate the occurrence of diarrhea with modifications in the diet introduction or elimination of cow's milk proteins, wheat flour, lactose, sucrose, and vegetables, for example. Associated symptoms should be systematically looked for: anorexia (intestinal malabsorption), increased appetite (exocrine pancreatic insufficiency), thirst (when diarrhea is fluid and severe as in sugar intolerance), abdominal pain, cramps, discomfort, bloating (indicative of fermentation), vomiting (protein intolerance), and asthenia, weakness (celiac disease, Crohn's disease).

Equally important is to establish whether the growth of the child is normal or not by recording carefully his growth charts from birth, for height and weight. Clinical examination will appreciate the activity and psychomotor development of the child. One should look for abdominal distention, best observed in the standing position in profile, taking into account the physiologic distention in toddlers. It is important to evaluate the state of nutrition by recording skinfold thickness, muscle tone and volume, paleness of the skin and conjunctiva, color and quality of hair, and dryness of the skin.

At the end of this clinical evaluation, the most frequent cause of chronic diarrhea in childhood "irritable bowel syndrome" or "toddler's diarrhea" (characterized by periods of frequent, heterogeneous (with vegetable matter) often mucus-containing, foul smelling stools, often alternating with periods of normal stools or even constipation, and a normal state of nutrition) has been eliminated.[54] Frequently, the clinical history, the growth chart, and the physical examination of the child allow to evoke one of the three main mechanisms of malabsorption.

To confirm the diagnosis (see Chapter 6, "Traumatic and Toxic Injury of the Esophagus") balance studies are nowadays rarely used except simple tests on stools, such as research of infectious agents, electrolytes concentration, pH and reducing agent for fermentation steatorrhea, or more precise for pancreatic insufficiency elastase in stools. Noninvasive breath test are mainly used for carbohydrate malabsorption or bacterial overgrowth. The most useful and used complementary exam is now endoscopy with biopsies completed eventually by imaging and genetic studies if necessary.

DIARRHEA DUE TO IMPAIRED INTRALUMINAL DIGESTION (IID)

Diarrhea due to exocrine pancreatic insufficiency (EPI), the predominant cause of IID, is remarkable by the macroscopic appearance of the stools: they are more frequently loose and pasty than liquid, homogeneous, and often obviously greasy. The volume of the stools is rather constant from one day to another. Fecal elastase 1 rather than steatorrhea is the simplest as well as the most sensitive and specific test for assessing exocrine pancreatic function.[55]

Apart from acquired surgical conditions (short-bowel syndrome, hypomotile and distended intestinal loop, and intestinal pseudo-obstruction), such a massive fecal loss of the three classes of nutrients can only be explained by EPI, whose most frequent cause in children is, by far, cystic fibrosis. The sweat test and genetic studies confirm the diagnosis. If chloride concentration in sweat is normal, EPI is due to hypoplasia of the pancreas often associated with congenital lipomatous infiltration. Such is the case when EPI is part of several syndromes, the most frequent of which is Shwachman syndrome genetically defined.[56,57] Rarer is Johanson-Blizzard syndrome, in which EPI is associated with phenotypic abnormalities.[58,59] In both cases, MRI may be useful in showing the typical fatty infiltration of the pancreas. In Pearson syndrome, pancreatic hypoplasia is linked to fibrosis and EPI is associated with refractory sideroblastic anemia and vacuolization of marrow precursors. This syndrome was shown to be due to mitochondrial DNA deletions.[60] Finally, in children, EPI due to long-lasting chronic pancreatitis or pancreatectomy is rare (Table 2).

Impaired intraluminal digestion rarely involves only one class of nutrient, such as exceptional isolated congenital lipase or colipase deficiency.[40,41,61] Normal lipase activity would orient the diagnosis toward defective micellar solubilization due to congenital absence of bile acid synthesis,[42,62] abnormal biliary excretion (congenital biliary atresia),[63] interrupted bile acid enterohepatic circulation because of bacterial overgrowth, ileal resection, Crohn's disease, or congenital bile acid malabsorption.[43] Bile acid assay, in blood or the duodenal juice, may lead to one of these diagnostic possibilities. Congenital trypsinogen deficiency or congenital enterokinase deficiency has been also described[25] (see Table 2).

DIARRHEA DUE TO INTESTINAL MALABSORPTION

In patients with diarrhea from intestinal malabsorption stools are loose or liquid, often with an acidic smell, typical of fermentation but rarely greasy.

Table 2 Diarrhea Due to Impaired Intraluminal Digestion

	Diagnosis	
Pathophysiology	Suspected	Evidence for Probable or Certain Diagnosis
Impaired digestion affecting all nutrients	Cystic fibrosis	Sweat test positive
	Pancreatic hypoplasia with lipomatosis (Schwachman syndrome)	Neutropenia
	Metaphyseal chondrodysplasia	Squelettal abnormalities
	Johanson-Blizzard syndrome	Facial dysmorphy
	Fibrosis, (Pearson syndrome)	Sideroblastic anemia, mitochondrial cytopathy
	Cystinosis	Tubular acidosis
Impaired digestion affecting fat proteins	Isolated lipase or colipase deficiency	Direct assay in duodenal juice
Fat	Abnormal micellar solubilization	Bile acid assay in blood, genetic cholestasis
	Impaired bile acid synthesis	Clinical history
	Bile duct atresia	Clinical history
	Interrupted enterohepatic circulation	Bile acid assay in blood, duodenal juice, stools
	Ileal resection	Clinical history, H_2 breath test
	Crohn's disease	
	Congenital malabsorption of bile acids	
	Blind loop syndrome	
Proteins	Congenital trypsinogen deficiency	Direct assay in duodenal juice
	Congenital enterokinase deficiency	Assay in duodenal mucosa

Such a diarrhea in a child with abdominal distension and suboptimal growth should evoke celiac disease, the most common cause of intestinal malabsorption. Whereas tests of malabsorption (xylose test) or blood markers of malnutrition have long been used to assess the jejunal absorption function before the necessary small intestinal biopsy, serological markers of celiac disease (see Chapter 16.1, "Celiac Disease") are now by far more reliable tests to perform before prescribing a biopsy of the jejunal mucosa (nearly 100% sensitivity and specificity) of celiac disease. The intestinal biopsy mandatory in such clinical situation discloses a flat mucosa (total villous atrophy) ascertaining the diagnosis.[64,65]

When the serological tests specific for celiac disease are negative, the intestinal biopsy may be anyway necessary to assess for other causes of intestinal malabsorption. Nonspecific inflammatory alterations leading to partial villous atrophy in an infant of less than 6 months of age is most often secondary to sensitization to food proteins, most often to cow's milk proteins, more rarely to soya, rice, or wheat proteins. Given the lack of a reliable laboratory test to confirm such a sensitization, proof of it relies mainly on the curative effect of an exclusion diet and eventually on relapse of symptoms after challenge with the suspected protein.[66] Partial villous atrophy may also occur in the postgastroenteritis syndrome, or in Giardia lamblia infestation. Finally, partial villous atrophy and chronic diarrhea may reveal a state of immune activation[67] or immune deficiency (eg, hypogammaglobulinemia or combined immunodeficiency syndromes) of which some may be linked to the absence of expression of human leukocyte antigens (HLA) (see Chap-

ter 15.2b, "Persistent Diarrhea"). A combination of several factors, food sensitization, depressed immune status, bacterial overgrowth,[68] probably explains the partial villous atrophy often observed in children with protracted diarrhea (Table 3).

In other, much rarer cases, the intestinal biopsy reveals specific lesions. The mucosal architecture is normal, but enterocytes appear full of lipid droplets that reflect abnormal chylomicron assembly or excretion. Such a disorder may reveal a-betalipoproteinemia,[69] or Anderson's disease (chylomicron retention disease).[70,71] In other cases lymphangiectasia may be observed as distorting the core of villi. Protein losing enteropathy is responsible for hypoalbuminemia sometimes associated with edema, and is confirmed by measurement of alpha$_1$-antitrypsine clearance.[44] Lymphopenia and hypogammaglobulinemia are usually associated and characteristic of lymphatic

Table 3 Diarrhea Due to Intestinal Malabsorption

	Diagnosis	
Pathophysiology	Suspected	Evidence for Probable or Certain Diagnosis
Intestinal biopsy: nonspecific		
Inflammatory lesions		
Total villous atrophy (flat mucosa)	Celiac disease	Antigliadin antibodies, relaspse at gluten challenge
Partial villous atrophy*	Sensitization to food proteins: CMP, rice, soya, wheat	Relapse at challenge
	Dermatitis herpetiformis	Derma igA deposit
	Giardia lamblia infestation	*Giardia* on biopsy specimen
	Immunodeficiency status, among these, absence of HLA expression	HLA typing
	Bacterial overgrowth	Bacterial counts in duodenal juice, H_2 test
	"Protracted diarrhea" syndrome (may be postgastroenteritis)	Clinical history
Intestinal biopsy: specific lesions		
Fat-filled enterocytes	Abetalipoproteinemia	Absence of plasma LDL, apo B, acanthocytosis
	Andersen's disease	Decreased levels of plasma LDL, apo B
Villi distorted by ecstatic Lymphatic	Lymphangectasia	Lymphopenia, hypoalbuminemia Increased alpha, PI clearance
Dense monomorphic lymphoplasmocytic infiltrate	Alpha-chain disease	Monoclonal abnormal IgA in plasma
Normal intestinal biopsy	Lysinuric protein intolerance	Dibasic aminoaciduria Severe ostoeporosis

CMP = cow's milk protein.

*In severe cases, villous atrophy may be total.

Table 4 Diarrhea Due to Fermentation

	Diagnosis	
Pathophysiology	Suspected	Evidence for Probable or Certain Diagnosis
Intestinal biopsy: normal of subnormal intestinal mucosa	CSID Congenital lactase deficiency Late-onset lactase deficiency Congenital trehalase deficiency Congenital glucose-galactose malabsorption	Assay of saccharidases in mucosal homogenate: one activity affected, breath test Absence of glucose-induced short-circuit current in Ussing chamber, genetic

Intestinal biopsy: nonspecific inflammatory lesions	All causes of villous atrophy (cf Table 3), mainly:
	  Celiac disease
	  CMPI
	  Postgastroenteritis syndrome
		All saccharidase activities affected
		  Cf Table 3
		  Cf Table 3
		  Cf Table 3

CMPI = cow's milk protein intolerance; CSID = congenital sucrose-isomaltase deficency.

disorders in a context of protein losing enteropathy while steatorrhea is moderate.

When the lamina propria of the intestinal mucosa is infiltrated by a monomorphic lymphoplasmocytic population, composed of packed plasma cells or later of lymphoblasts, which disrupts crypts and widens and flattens villi whose epithelium is barely altered, autoimmune or alpha-chain disease should be suspected (see Table 3).[67,72]

DIARRHEA DUE TO FERMENTATION

Diarrhea due to fermentation is liquid often passed with flatus, acid (pH less than 5.5).

Overexcretion of H_2 in breath after an oral load of a suspected sugar may orient the diagnosis, confirmed by an intestinal biopsy. The intestinal mucosa appears normal on histologic sections in cases of congenital (or primary) sugar intolerance. The assay of disaccharidase activities in a homogenate of the mucosa detects sucrase–isomaltase deficiency,[73,74] the most frequent of these intolerances, more often than glucoamylase deficiency[75] or congenital lactase deficiency.[76] In children or adolescents of non-Caucasian origin, late-onset lactase deficiency[77] is, on the contrary, frequently the cause of a mild lactose intolerance. Normal enzyme activities, as well as clinical trials with differ-

ent sugars, lead to the possibility of congenital glucose–galactose malabsorption, which can be confirmed by studies in an Ussing chamber (glucose does not trigger any short-circuit current as it should) with brush border vesicles (glucose is not taken up even in the presence of Na^+),[78] eventually using molecular genetics[5] (Table 4).

However, much more frequently, the intestinal mucosa looks abnormal with more or less severe villous atrophy. Disaccharidase activities are, like peptidase activities, nonspecifically decreased as a consequence of mucosal damage. Sugar intolerance and fermentation are, then, secondary to villous atrophy, as in celiac disease or severe acute infectious diarrhea.[79]

CHRONIC DIARRHEA OF NEONATAL ONSET

Diarrhea starting during the early neonatal period is usually extremely severe, leading rapidly to life-threatening malnutrition. The features of a malabsorption syndrome are thus gathered, although in some of the conditions characterized by such a diarrhea, malabsorption may involve only one ion or brush border digestion enzyme or nutrient transporter (Table 5).[48,49,73–75] Congenital chloride diarrhea (CLD) or congenital sodium diarrhea (CSD) are usually associated with hydramnios

as well as blood and stool electrolytes disorders (9 to 11).[48,49] CLD is a rare, autosomal recessive disorder of intestinal Cl/HCO_3 exchange caused by mutations in the *SLC26A3* gene and characterized by persistent Cl-rich diarrhea from birth. Patients with CLD present with lifetime watery diarrhea with a high Cl^- content and low pH, causing dehydration and hypochloremic metabolic alkalosis. Chloride is low in urine and very high in stools ($Cl > 150$ mmol/L > sodium). CSD is caused by defective sodium/proton exchange with only few sporadic cases reported.[49] The genetics of the disease have not been established. Patients with CSD have acidosis and hyponatremia and stools with high concentrations of HCO_3^- and sodium (150 mmol/L). Glucose–galactose malabsorption is an autosomal recessive disease that presents in newborn infants as a life-threatening diarrhea (12). The diarrhea ceases within 1 h of removing oral intake of lactose, glucose, and galactose, but promptly returns with the introduction of one or more of the offending sugars into the diet.

In rare cases "intractable diarrhea" (persisting despite nothing by mouth) is present. Most of them are due to congenital enterocyte defects: microvillous atrophy, tufting enteropathy, syndromatic diarrhea) (see Chapter 45, "Congenital Enteropathy Involving Mucosa Development). Long-term parenteral nutrition is necessary for

Table 5 Chronic Diarrhea of Neonatal Onset

Conditions (in Order of Decreasing Severity)			
Congenital microvillous atrophy	Intractable† watery diarrhea	Intestinal biopsy (PAS stain)	Total Parenteral nutrition
Tufting enteropathy	Intractable watery diarrhea	Intestinal biopsy	Total Parenteral nutrition
Intractable diarrhea with phenotypic abnormalities	Intractable watery diarrhea LBW	Immune system investigations	Total Parenteral nutrition
Congenital glucose–galactose malabsorption	Acid diarrhea with reducing sugars	Intestinal biopsy (Ussing chamber, brush border vesicles)	Replacement of glucose and galactose by fructose in the diet
Congenital lactase deficiency	Acid diarrhea with reducing sugars	Intestinal biopsy (assay of activity)	Lactose-free diet
Congenital chloride diarrhea	Hydramnios, neonatal intractable watery diarrhea	Assay of electrolytes in stools	IV then oral Cl supplementation
Congenital defective jejunal Na^+/H^+ exchange	Hydramnios, neonatal intractable watery diarrhea	Assay of electrolytes in stools	IV then oral Na1 supplementation
Congenital bile acid malabsorption	Steatorrhea	Bile acid assay in plasma, genetic	MCT, cholestyramine
Congenital enterokinase deficiency	Failure to thrive, edema	Intestinal biopsy (assay of kinase activity)	Protein hydrolysate

PAS = periodic acid–Schiff; MCT = medium-chain triglyceride; LBW = low birth weight.

*Neonatal = within the first week of life.

†Intractable = persisting despite nothing by mouth.

survival and most of these patients become candidate for intestinal transplantation.[50,51,80–85]

REFERENCES

1. Traber PG. Carbohydrate assimilation. In: Yamada T, Alpers DH, Laine L, Owyang C, Powel DW, editors, Textbook of Gastroenterology, Vol. 1, 3rd edition. New York: Lippincott, Williams & Wilkins; 1999. p. 404–56.
2. Fogel MR, Gray GM. Starch hydrolysis in man: An intraluminal process not requiring membrane digestion. J Appl Physiol 1973;35:263–7.
3. Semenza G. Anchoring and biosynthesis of stalked brush border membrane proteins: Glycosidases and peptidases of enterocytes and renal tubuli. Annu Rev Cell Biol 1986;2:255–313.
4. Triadou N, Bataille J, Schmitz J. Longitudinal study of the human intestinal brush border membrane proteins. Distribution of the main disaccharidases and peptidases. Gastroenterology 1983;85:1326–32.
5. Wright EM. Genetic disorders of membrane transport. Glucose Galactose malabsorption, Am J Physiol 1998;275:G879–82.
6. Corpe CP, Burant CF, Hoekstra JH. Intestinal fructose absorption: Clinical and molecular aspects. J Pediatr Gastroenterol Nutr 1999;28:364–74.
7. Gray GM, Santiago NA. Disaccharide absorption in normal and diseased human intestine. Gastroenterology 1966;51:489–98.
8. De Vizia B, Ciccimara, De'Cicco, Auricchio S. Digestibility of starches in infants and children. J Pediatr 1975;86:50–5.
9. Arola H, Tamm A. Metabolism of lactose in the human body. Scand J Gastroenterol 1994;29:21–5.
10. Naim NY, Roth J, Sterrhi, et al. Sucrase isomaltase deficiency in human. J Clin Invest 1988;82:667.
11. Ganopathy V, Leibach FH. Protein digestion and assimilation. In: Yamada T, Alpers DH, Laine L, et al, editors. Textbook of Gastroenterology, Vol. 1, 3rd edition. New York: Lippincott, Williams & Wilkins; 1999. p. 456–67.
12. Defize J, Meuwissen SGM. Pepsinogens: An update of biochemical, physiological, and clinical aspects. J Pediatr Gastroenterol Nutr 1987;6:493–508.
13. Kitamoto Y, Veile RA, Donis-Keller, Sadler JE. cDNA sequence and chromosomal localization of human enterokinase, the proteolytic activator of trypsinogen. Biochemistry 1995;34:4562–8.
14. Lowe ME. The structure and function of pancreatic enzymes. In Johnson LR, editor. Physiology of the Gastrointestinal Tract, 3rd edition. New York: Raven Press, 1994; p. 1531–1542.
15. Pangalos MN, et al. Isolation and expression of novel human glutamate carboxypeptidases with *N*-acetylated a-linked acidic dipeptidase and dipeptidyl peptidase IV activity. J Biol Chem 1999;274:8470–83.
16. Darmoul D, et al. Regional expression of epithelial dipeptidyl peptidase IV in the human intestines. Biochem Biophys Res Com 1994;230:1224–9.
17. Kekuda R, et al. Cloning of the sodium-dependent, broad-scope, neutral amino acid transporter B^0 from a human placental choriocarcinoma cell line. J Biol Chem 1996;271:18657–61.
18. Palacin M, et al. Molecular biology of mammalian plasma membrane amino acid transporters. Physiol Rev 1998;78:969–1054.
19. Adibi SA. The oligopeptide transporter (Pept-1) in human intestine: Biology and function. Gastroenterology 1997;113:332–40.
20. Leibach FH, Ganapathy V. Peptide transporters in the intestine and the kidney. Annu Rev Nutr 1996;16:99–119.
21. Liang R, et al. Human intestinal H^+/peptide cotransporter. J Biol Chem 1995;270:6456–63.
22. Steinhardt HJ, Adibi SA. Kinetics and characteristics of absorption from an equimolar mixture of 12 glycyl-dipeptides in human jejunum. Gastroenterology 1986;90:577–82.
23. Terada T, et al. Functional characteristics of basolateral peptide transporter in the human intestinal cell line Caco-2. Am J Physiol 1999;276:G1435–41.
24. Torrents D, et al. Identification of SLC7A7, encoding y^+LAT-1, as the lysinuric protein intolerance gene. Nature Genetics 1999;21:293–6.
25. Green JR, et al. Primary intestinal enteropeptidase deficiency. J Pediatr Gastroenterol Nutr 1984;3:630–3.
26. Desjeux JF, et al. Lysine fluxes across the jejunal epithelium in lysinuric protein intolerance. J Clin Invest 1990;65:1382–7.
27. Davidson NO. Intestinal lipid absorption. In: Yamada T, Alpers DH, Laine L, et al, editors, Textbook of Gastroenterology, Vol. 1, 3rd edition. New York: Lippincott, Williams & Wilkins; 1999. p. 428–56.
28. Moreau H, et al. Human preduodenal lipase is entirely of gastric fundic origin. Gastroenterology 1988;95:1221–6.
29. Bernbäck S, Bläckberg L, Hernell O. The complete digestion of human milk triacylglycerol in vitro requires gastric lipase, pancreatic colipase-dependent lipase, and bile salt-stimulated lipase. J Clin Invest 1990;85:1221–6.
30. Lowe ME. Pancreatic triglyceride lipase and colipase: Insights into dietary fat digestion. Gastroenterology 1994;107:1524–36.
31. Lombardo D, Guy O. Studies on the substrate specificity of a carboxyl ester hydrolase from human pancreatic juice. II. Action on cholesterol esters and lipid-soluble vitamin esters. Biochim Biophys Acta 1980;611:147–55.
32. Craddock AL, et al. Expression and transport properties of the human ileal and renal sodium-dependent bile acid transporter. Am J Physiol 1998;274:G157–69.
33. Stremmel W. Uptake of fatty acids by jejunal mucosal cells is mediated by a fatty acid binding membrane protein. J Clin Invest 1988;82:2001–10.
34. Abumrad N, Harmon C, Ibrahimi A. Membrane transport of long-chain fatty acids: Evidence for a facilitated process. J Lipid Res 1998;39:2309–18.
35. Lipka G, et al. Characterization of lipid exchange proteins isolated from small intestinal brush border membrane. J Biol Chem 1995;270:5917–25.
36. Hsu KT, Storch J. Fatty acid transfer from liver and intestinal fatty acid-binding proteins to membrane occurs by different mechanisms. J Biol Chem 1996;271:13317–23.
37. Wetterau JR, Lin MCM, Jamil H. Microsomal triglyceride transfer protein. Biochim Biophys Acta 1997;1345:136–50.
38. Wetterau JR, et al. Absence of microsomal triglyceride transfer protein in individuals with abetalipoproteinemia. Science 1992;258:999–1001.
39. Hussain MM, et al. Chylomicron assembly and catabolism: Role of apolipoproteins and receptors. Biochim Biophys Acta 1996;1300:151–70.
40. Figarella C, et al. Congenital pancreatic lipase deficiency. J Pediatr 1980;96:412–6.
41. Hildebrand H, et al. Isolated co-lipase deficiency in two brothers. Gut 1982;23:243–6.
42. Jacquemin E, et al. 3 b-hydroxysteroid-dehydrogenase/isomerase deficiency in children: A new cause of progressive familial intrahepatic cholestasis. J Pediatr 1994;125:379–84.
43. Oelkers P, et al. Primary bile acid malabsorption caused by mutations in the ileal sodium-dependent bile acid transporter gene (SLC10A2). J Clin Invest 1997;99:1880–7.
44. Schmitz J. Protein-losing enteropathies. In: Milla PJ, Muller DPR, editors. Harries' Paediatric Gastroenterology. London: Churchill Livingstone; 1988, p. 260.
45. Hamilton JR, Lynch MJ, Reilly BJ. Active coeliac disease in childhood: Clinical and laboratory findings of forty-two cases, Q J Med 1969;38:135–58.
46. Shek LP, Bardina L, Castro R, et al. Humoral and cellular responses to cow milk proteins in patients with milk-induced IgE-mediated and non–IgE-mediated disorders. Allergy 2005;60:912–9.
47. Goulet O, Brousse N, Canioni D, et al. Syndrome of intractable diarrhoea with persistent villous atrophy in early childhood: A clinicopathological survey of 47 cases. J Pediatr Gastroenterol Nutr 1998;26:151–61.
48. Hihnala S, Hoglund P, Lammi L, et al. Long-term clinical outcome in patients with congenital chloride diarrhea. J Pediatr Gastroenterol Nutr 2006;42:369–75.
49. Muller T, Wijmenga C, Phillips AD, et al. Congenital sodium diarrhea is an autosomal recessive disorder of sodium/proton exchange but unrelated to known candidate genes. Gastroenterology 2000;119:1506–13.
50. Goulet O, et al. Intractable diarrhea of infancy with epithelial and basement membrane abnormalities. J Pediatr 1995;127:212–9.
51. Phillips AD, Schmitz J. Familial microvillous atrophy: A clinicopathological survey of 23 cases. J Pediatr Gastroenterol Nutr 1992;14:380–96.
52. Anderson CM. The child with persistently abnormal stools. In: Gracey M Burke V, editors. Paediatric Gastroenterology and Hepatology. London: Blackwell Scientific; 1993, p. 373.
53. Shmerling DH, Forrer JCW, Prader A. Fecal fat and nitrogen in healthy children and in children with malabsorption or maldigestion. Pediatrics 1970;46:690–5.
54. Hyman PE, Milla PJ, Benninga MA, et al. Childhood functional gastrointestinal disorders: Neonate/toddler. Gastroenterology 2006;130:1519–26.
55. Soldan W, Henker J, Sprössig C. Sensitivity and specificity of quantitative determination of pancratic elastase 1 in feces of children. J Pediatr Gastroenterol Nutr 1997;24:53–5.
56. Ginzberg H, et al. Schwachman syndrome: Phenotypic manifestations of sibling sets and isolated cases in a large patient cohort are similar. J Pediatr 1999;135:81–8.
57. Boock Gr, Morrison JA, Popovic M, et al. Mutations in SBDS are associated with Shwachman-Diamond syndrome. Nat Genet 2003;33:97–101.
58. Johanson A, Blizzard R. A syndrome of congenital aplasia of the alae nasi, deafness, hypothyroidism, dwarfism, absent permanent teeth, and malabsorption. J Pediatr 1971;79: 982–7.
59. Guzman C, Carranza A. Two siblings with exocrine pancreatic hypoplasia and orofacial malformations (Donlan syndrome and Johanson-Blizzard syndrome). J Pediatr Gastroenterol Nutr 1997;25:350–3.
60. Rötig A, et al. Pearson's marrow-pancreas syndrome. A multisystem mitochondrial disorder in infancy. J Clin Invest 1990;86:1601–8.
61. Ligumsky M, et al. Isolated lipase and colipase deficiency in two brother. Gut 1990;31:1416–8.
62. Vanderpas JB, et al. Malabsorption of liposoluble vitamins in a child with bile acid deficiency. J Pediatr Gastroenterol Nutr 1987;6:33–41.
63. Kobayashi A, Ohbe Y, Yonekubo A. Fat absorption in patients with surgically repaired biliary atresia. Helv Pediatr Acta 1983;38:307–14.
64. Fasano A. Tissue transglutaminase: The holy grail for the diagnosis of celiac disease, at last? J Pediatr 1999;134:134–5.
65. Report of Working Group of European Society of Paediatric Gastroenterology and Nutrition: Revised criteria for diagnosis of coeliac disease. Arch Dis Child 1990;65:909–1011.
66. The European Society for Paediatric Gastroenterology and Nutrition Working Group for the Diagnostic Criteria for Food Allergy. J Pediatr Gastroenterol Nutr 1992;14:108–12.
67. Cuenod B, et al. Classification of intractable diarrhea in infancy using clinical and immunohistological criteria. Gastroenterology 1990;99:1037–43.
68. Davidson GP, Robby TA, Kirubakaran CP. Bacterial contamination of the small intestine as an important cause of chronic diarrhea and abdominal pain: Diagnosis by breath hydrogen test. Pediatrics 1984;74:229–35.
69. Narcisi T, et al. Mutations of the microsomal triglyceride-transfer-protein gene in abetalipoproteinemia. Am J Hum Genet 1995;57:1298–310.
70. Bouma ME, et al. Hypobetalipoproteinemia with accumulation of an apoprotein B-like protein in intestinal cells: Immunoenzymatic and biochemical characterization of seven cases of Anderson's disease. J Clin Invest 1986;78:398–410.
71. Roy CC, et al. Malabsorption, hypocholesterolemia, and fat-filled enterocytes with increased intestinal apoprotein B: Chylomicron retention disease. Gastroenterology 1987;92:390–9.
72. Rambaud JC. Small intestinal lymphomas and alpha-chain disease. Clin Gastroenterol 1983;12:743–66.
73. Naim HY, et al. Sucrase–isomaltase deficiency in humans: Different mutations disrupt intracellular transport, processing, and function of an intestinal brush border enzyme. J Clin Invest 1988;82:667–79.
74. Ouwendijk J, et al. Congenital sucrase–isomaltase deficiency. Identification of a glutamine to proline substitution that leads to a transport block of sucrase–isomaltase in a pre-Golgi compartment. J Clin Invest 1996;97:633–41.
75. Wright EM, Turk E, Martin MG. Molecular basis for glucose–galactose malabsorption. Cell Biochem Biophys. 2002;36:115–21.
76. Savilahti E, Launiala K, Kuitunen P. Congenital lactase deficiency: A clinical study on 16 patients. Arch Dis Child 1983;58:246–52.
77. Maiuri L, et al. Mosaic pattern of lactase expression by villous enterocytes in human adult-type hypolactasia. Gastroenterology 1991;100:359–69.
78. Booth IW, et al. Glucose–galactose malabsorption: Demonstration of specific jejunal brush border membrane defect. Gut 1988;29:1661–5.
79. Berg NO, et al. Correlation between morphological alterations and enzyme activities in the mucosa of the small intestine. Scand J Gastroenterol 1973;8:703–12.
80. Giraut D, et al. Intractable dirrhoea syndrome associated with phenotypic abnormalities and immune deficiency. J Pediatr 1994;125:36–42.
81. Goulet O, Ruemmele F, Lacaille F, Colomb V. Irreversible intestinal failure. J Pediatr Gastroenterol Nutr 2004;38:250–69.
82. Martinez-Vinson C, Goulet O, Berrebi D, et al. Syndromatic diarrhea in children. Report of 8 cases. J Pediatr Gastroenterol Nutr 2005;40:651.
83. Lachaux A, bouvier R, Loras-Duclaux J, et al. Isolated deficient alpha6beta4 integrin expression in the gut associated with intractable diarrhea. J Pediatr Gastroenterol Nutr 1999;29:395–401.
84. Phililips AD, Brown A, Hichks S, et al. Acetylated sialic acid residues and blood group anti-gens localise within the epithelium in microvillous atrophty indicating internal accumulatin of the glycocalyx. Gut 2004;53:1764–71.
85. Ruemmele FM, Jan D, Lacaille F, et al. New perspectives for children with microvillous inclusion disease: Early small bowel transplantation. Transplantation 2004;77:1024–8.

15.2a. Acute Diarrhea

Stefano Guandalini, MD

Stacy A. Kahn, MD

DEFINITION AND EPIDEMIOLOGY

Acute diarrhea can be defined as the sudden onset of increased fluid content of the stool above normal. In infants and toddlers, "normal" is approximately 10 mL/kg/d, while in the older child and adolescent normal is up to 200 g/d. From a practical standpoint, one can define diarrhea as a decrease in consistency (to loose or liquid) and an increase in frequency of bowel movements to ≥3 per day. The familiar term "gastroenteritis" is inappropriate, because (1) not every instance of acute diarrhea is due to an inflammation of the GI tract as the term implies; and (2) even when an infection causes the symptom, the involvement of the stomach, as the term would imply, is far from constant. The augmented water content of the stools is the result of an imbalance in the function of the small and large intestinal processes involved in the absorption and secretion of electrolytes, organic substrates, and thus water.

Diarrheal episodes of acute onset are most often the result of infections of the gastrointestinal tract, and they continue to be a major problem for worldwide child health. Although in developed countries its prevalence and severity have declined, acute diarrhea remains an extremely common and often severe problem. In developing countries, an average of three episodes per child per year in children below 5 years of age is reported, but there are areas with six to eight episodes per year per child. In these settings, not only malnutrition is an important additional risk factor for diarrhea, but also recurrent episodes of diarrhea lead to growth faltering.[1] Childhood mortality associated with diarrhea has constantly but slowly declined during the past two decades, mostly because of the widespread use of oral rehydration solutions (ORSs),[2,3] but still remains high, with the most recent estimates having diarrhea as the second cause of childhood mortality with 18% of the 10.6 million yearly deaths in children younger than 5 years.[4] However, despite this progressive reduction in global diarrheal disease mortality, diarrhea morbidity in published reports from 1990 through 2000 has slightly increased worldwide compared with previous reports.[5] Furthermore, we should not ignore that in countries where the toll of diarrhea is highest, poverty also adds an enormous additional burden, and long-term consequences of the vicious cycle of enteric infections, diarrhea, and malnutrition are devastating.[3,6]

Diarrheal episodes are classically distinguished into acute and chronic (or persistent) based on their duration: acute diarrhea is thus defined as an episode that has an acute onset and lasts no longer than 14 days; while chronic or persistent diarrhea is defined as an episode that lasts longer than 14 days. The distinction, supported by the World Health Organization (WHO)[7,8] has implications not only for classification and epidemiological studies, but also from a practical standpoint, as protracted diarrhea has often a different set of causes, poses different problems of management, and has a different prognosis (see Chapter 15.2b, "Persistent Diarrhea").

In the United States, a recent estimate assumes a cumulative incidence of 1 hospitalization for diarrhea per 23 to 27 children by age 5,[9] with more than 50,000 hospitalizations in 2000. By these estimates, rotavirus is associated with 4 to 5% of all childhood hospitalizations, and 1 in 67 to 1 in 85 children will be hospitalized with rotavirus by 5 years of age.[9] Furthermore, acute diarrhea causes 20% of physician referrals for children below the age of 2 years and 10% for those below the age of 3 years.[10]

Even though gastrointestinal infections are by far the most common cause of acute diarrhea, the sudden onset of increased stool fluid output can indeed be caused by many different disorders. Table 1 lists these potential causes in their approximate order of frequency. Many different pathogens can be responsible for infectious diarrhea. Table 2 lists the main agents known to infect the intestine and cause acute diarrhea in children. In a multicenter investigation conducted over a period of 1 year in several European countries, we identified a pathogen in 65.6% of 287 children, most commonly Rotavirus (35.1%).[11] The prevalence of individual pathogens varies widely between different geographic areas and different age groups. For instance, bacteria are generally more common in the first few months of life and then again in school-age children. Rotavirus, the single most pervasive cause of infectious diarrhea worldwide, peaks between the ages of 6 and 24 months. A recent report indicates that, surprisingly, diarrheagenic *Escherichia coli* occur frequently as sporadic causes of diarrhea in the United States, and they may well be currently the most common bacterial cause of acute diarrhea in all ages.[12] In developed countries, intestinal infections are usually sporadic, but outbreaks of foodborne or waterborne infections are well described and

continue to occur. Recently, a growing epidemiologic role for Norwalk-like virus has been reported. Norwalk-like virus is now considered to cause an impressive 10% of sporadic cases in developed countries.[13] In patients with immune disorders, and especially with acquired immune deficiency syndrome (AIDS), a much wider array of pathogens is seen. Etiologic diagnosis, not considered necessary in the vast majority of sporadic cases occurring in immunocompetent children, in subjects with human immunodeficiency virus (HIV) infection is very important for treatment, and it is currently thought that endoscopy is necessary.[14] See Chapter 19.2, "Infections," for a detailed presentation of individual enteric infections.

Also extra-intestinal infections (eg, middle ear, lung, and urinary tract infections) can result

---

Table 1 Causes of Acute Diarrhea

Infections
  Enteric infections (including food poisoning)
  Extraintestinal infections

Drug induced
  Antibiotic associated
  Laxatives
  Antacids that contain magnesium
  Opiate withdrawal
  Other drugs

Food allergies or intolerances
  Cow's milk protein allergy
  Soy protein allergy
  Multiple food allergies
  Olestra
  Methylxantines (caffeine, theobromine, theophylline)

Disorders of digestive/absorptive processes
  Sucrase-isomaltase deficiency
  Late-onset (or "adult type") hypolactasia resulting in lactose intolerance

Chemotherapy or radiation-induced enteritis
  "Surgical" conditions
    Acute appendicitis
    Intussusception

Vitamin deficiencies
  Niacin deficiency
  Folate deficiency

Vitamin toxicity
  Vitamin C
  Niacin, vitamin B3

Ingestion of heavy metals or toxins
  Copper, tin, zinc
  Plants such as hyacinths, daffodils, azalea, mistletoe, Amanita species mushrooms

Table 2 Main Causes of Acute Infectious Diarrhea in Developed Countries

Pathogen	Approximate Frequencies in Cases of Sporadic Diarrhea (%)
Viruses	
Rotavirus	25–40
Calicivirus	1–20
Norwalk-like virus	10
Astrovirus	4–9
Enteric-type adenovirus	2–4
Bacteria	
Campylobacter jejuni	6–8
Salmonella	3–7
Escherichia coli	3–5
Enterotoxigenic	
Enteropathogenic	
Enteroaggregative	
Enteroinvasive	
Enterohemorragic	
Diffusely adherent	
Shigella	0–3
Yersinia enterocolitica	1–2
Clostridium difficile	0–2
Vibrio parahaemolyticus	0–1
Vibrio cholerae 01	Unknown
Vibrio cholerae non-01	Unknown
Aeromonas hydrophila	
Aeromonas caviae	
Aeromonas veronii	0–2
biotype sobria	
Parasites	
Cryptosporidium	1–3
Giardia lamblia	1–3

in acute diarrhea, which is usually mild and self-limited, but the mechanisms for such a relationship are not understood.

Many drugs can induce acute diarrhea as a side effect. Among them, antibiotics have a special place because their administration is frequently followed by diarrhea. Although *Clostridium difficile*[15] is a pathogen often responsible for antibiotic-associated diarrhea in adults and in the setting of nosocomial diarrhea, it should be noticed that in children, the majority of episodes of diarrhea secondary to antibiotic use are not related to *C. difficile*.

The incidence of food allergies has risen during the past decade. Presently, it is assumed that about 3% of all infants are affected by food allergies, of which by far the most common is cow's milk protein allergy (CMPA). A vast array of signs and symptoms are linked to CMPA, but acute diarrhea (often accompanied by vomiting) is a very common modality of onset. Thus, CMPA should be taken into consideration in the differential diagnosis of acute-onset diarrhea, particularly when the diarrhea fails to resolve within 10 to 14 days.

Although disorders of digestive and absorptive processes are more commonly considered causes of chronic diarrhea or malabsorption syndromes (see Chapter 15.3, "Congenital Disorders" and Chapter 16, "Immune Enteropathies"), it is worth mentioning that sucrase-isomaltase deficiency may be mistaken for an acute diarrheal illness

if the relationship with the intake of sucrose is not detected by accurate history taking. Likewise, lactose intolerance of the older child may not be distinguishable from other forms of diarrhea with an acute onset. More in general, the child presenting with acute or persistent diarrhea may be showing the early symptoms of a chronic malabsorption syndrome. Fructose "intolerance" is often quoted as a cause of diarrhea, but the term is definitely inappropriate: fructose absorption is physiologically a relatively inefficient process in infants and toddlers, and a high intake of this monosaccharide can therefore result in osmotic diarrhea (see later in this chapter for an explanation of osmotic diarrhea), without any underlying abnormality.

In patients treated for cancer by chemotherapy or radiation therapy, acute diarrhea may also ensue as a result of the damage to the intestinal absorptive area.

Several "surgical" conditions (eg, appendicitis[16]) can also present with acute diarrhea as the most obvious clinical sign. This should always be kept in mind when approaching a child with acute-onset diarrhea.

Much rarer disorders resulting in acute diarrhea are niacin deficiency and ingestion of heavy metals.

Finally, it should be noted that despite an aggressive search for the cause of acute diarrhea in children, only in 60 to 70% of cases is it possible to make a diagnosis (usually an intestinal infection). Whatever the cause, typically acute diarrhea in developed countries runs a mild course and resolves, by definition, in less than 14 days. In the previously mentioned study, we found that acute-onset diarrhea lasted a mean of 5.0 ± 2.2 days.[12] Overall, only about 10% of all children had a course more prolonged than 7 days.

PATHOGENESIS

All the various causes briefly summarized in the above section lead to a common endpoint: diarrhea resulting from an imbalance in the intestinal handling of water and electrolytes. We shall therefore outline how this derangement is brought about, and what constitutes a physiological status of fluid absorption.

Under normal circumstances, the small intestine absorbs large quantities of sodium, chloride, and bicarbonate. It also secretes H^+ ions and, to a lesser extent, bicarbonate and chloride. Water then passively follows the net transport of solutes. The overall absorption of water, sodium, and chloride can therefore be viewed as the result of two opposing unidirectional fluxes of ions, one absorptive and the other secretory. These two processes are in part anatomically separated, with absorption taking place mostly in the mature epithelial cells lining the villi, whereas secretion is predominantly a crypt process. However, both absorption and secretion do occur in villi and crypts.[17] Because the absorptive capacity of the enterocytes quantitatively far exceeds secretory

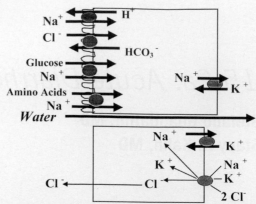

Figure 1 Main intestinal absorptive/secretory processes for electrolytes. In the villous cell (top panel), Na, K adenosine triphosphatase (ATPase) actively extrudes Na in exchange for K, thus maintaining the low intracellular Na concentration, which allows the "downhill" entry of the ionic pair Na–Cl and of the Na-coupled nutrients such as glucose and amino acids. It can also be seen that the entry of the ionic pair Na–Cl is in reality, across most of the intestinal tract, the result of a double antiport, Na being exchanged with H and Cl with HCO₃. In the crypt cell (bottom panel), the low Na cell concentration maintained by Na, K ATPase builds a Na gradient between the extracellular compartment and the cell. Energized by this gradient, a carrier in the basolateral membrane (lower part of the figure) couples the flow of one Na, two Cl, and one K from the serosal compartment into the crypt cell. As a result, Cl accumulates above its electrochemical equilibrium and under physiologic circumstances leaks into the lumen across a semipermeable apical membrane. Because absorptive activity in the villous cell quantitatively far exceeds the minor secretion from the crypts (as suggested in the figure by the *arrows* sizes), the net result is absorption of electrolytes and nutrients. Water absorption then passively follows, mainly through the intercellular tight junctions.

activity, the net result in health is absorption of water and electrolytes.

The basic cellular mechanisms that determine electrolyte absorption and secretion and therefore, when altered, the presence of diarrhea are schematically illustrated in Figure 1. The most important ion in drawing net water and nutrient absorption in the gut is sodium. Three different processes of sodium absorption have been described, all driven by Na, K adenosine triphosphatase (ATPase), a basolateral membrane enzyme with a key role in intestinal absorption of ions and nutrients. In fact, Na, K ATPase generates and maintains a Na electrochemical gradient between the gut lumen and the interior of the intestinal epithelial cell, which allows Na to enter the cell downhill along one of the following three paths.

SODIUM ABSORPTION COUPLED TO NUTRIENTS

The entry of glucose and of several groups of amino acids is coupled with high affinity to that of Na throughout the small intestine. A specific carrier called sodium-glucose transporter 1 (SGLT-1)[18] is involved in coupling the entry of glucose (and galactose) across the brush border to that of Na. Furthermore, several, but not all, carriers for different categories of amino acids also couple their entry into the enterocyte with the downhill transport of Na.[19,20] Dipeptide absorption, on the other hand, is not directly coupled to Na absorption but is nevertheless an electrogenic, active process, due to a carrier—denominated PEPT1—that has affinity for a large number of di- and tri-peptides[21] and is inhibited by chronic intestinal inflammation.[22] Di- and tri-peptide transport across the brush border is coupled to the entry of a proton ion (H^+) across the brush border. The existence of the Na-coupled glucose absorption, and its substantial integrity during most acute diarrheal disorders, is considered the pathophysiological basis for the use of orally administered hydration solutions in children with diarrhea.

ELECTROGENIC, AMYLORIDE-SENSITIVE Na ABSORPTION

This process allows sodium to enter the cell down its electrochemical gradient, through selective channels, uncoupled to other substrates in the ileum and throughout the colon, where it is preponderant. In the large intestine, electrogenic Na^+ absorption via the epithelial Na^+ channel takes place in the surface epithelium and upper crypts of the distal colon.

It should also be noted that Cl is absorbed throughout the gastrointestinal tract whenever a potential difference is created (serosal side positive) as a result of electrogenic Na absorption through either of the two pathways described above.

NEUTRAL NaCl ABSORPTION

By far the most important process involved in vectorial absorption of Na (and Cl) is the Na–Cl cotransport. This transport process operates throughout the gastrointestinal tract, but it predominates in the small intestine. Transport of the ionic pair NaCl is actually mediated by two coupled antiports; one exchanges Na^+/H^+ (cation exchanger), and the other exchanges Cl^-/HCO_3^- (anion exchanger). Two Cl^-/HCO_3^- anion exchangers have been identified and are named SLC26A6; and SLC26A3 or DRA ("down-regulated in adenoma").[23] The Na^+/H^+ antiport operates via specific carriers that have been identified in the past several years and are named the Na-hydrogen exchangers (NHEs). There are nine isoforms of NHE (1 to 9)[24,25]: in the gastrointestinal tract of multiple species, there are resident plasma membrane isoforms including NHE1 (basolateral) and NHE2 (apical), recycling isoforms (NHE3), as well as intracellular isoforms (NHE6, 7, 9). NHE3 recycles between the intracellular compartment and the apical plasma membrane and functions in both locations. NHE2 and especially NHE3 are thought to be the main isoforms involved in the small intestinal and colonic transepithelial absorption

of Na. The isoform NHE1 is mostly involved in maintaining intracellular pH.[26]

ANION SECRETION

Chloride and HCO_3[27] are the major anions being actively secreted into the gut lumen. Such secretion takes place mainly in the crypts and is electrogenic. The cystic fibrosis transmembrane conductance regulator (CFTR) is responsible for chloride secretion and is expressed throughout the intestinal epithelium, predominantly in the crypts.

As a result of this anion secretion, passive diffusion of a cation (mostly Na) and water follow, from the serosal compartment into the lumen. As mentioned, this secretory activity is overall of modest entity, so that the end result of the absorptive and secretory processes described is in the direction of net absorption.

A number of regulatory mechanisms, involving the enteric nervous system, cells in the lamina propria, and the epithelial cells, continuously finely tune the intestinal transport of water and electrolytes through a complex interplay. The regulatory agents released and ultimately responsible for the maintenance of this homeostasis include hormone peptides, active amines, arachidonic acid metabolites, and nitric oxide.[28] When an inflammatory state occurs, more players intervene in regulating ion transport: cytokines, tachykinins, reactive oxygen metabolites, as well as substances released from neutrophils, macrophages, mast cells, and platelets (Table 3).

Under normal circumstances, such complex interactions eventually act on the intestinal epithelial cells, affecting the described ion transport processes and ultimately resulting in net water and electrolyte absorption. The bulk of absorbed water crosses the intestinal epithelium between the cells (across the tight junctions), following the osmotic gradient generated by the transport of nutrients and electrolytes.

Diarrhea, therefore, is the reversal of this normal net absorptive status to secretion. Such a derangement can be the result of either an osmotic force that acts in the lumen to drive water into the gut or the result of an active secretory state induced in the enterocytes. In the former case, diarrhea is osmolar in nature, as observed after the ingestion of nonabsorbable sugars such as lactulose or of lactose in lactose malabsorbers. In the typical active secretory state, there is an enhanced anion secretion mostly by the crypt cell compartment, best exemplified by enterotoxin-induced diarrhea.

OSMOTIC DIARRHEA

These two basic pathogenetic mechanisms are summarized in Figure 2. In osmotic diarrhea, the intestinal mucosa cannot digest and/or absorb one or more nutrients. This can be either the result of an abnormality of the digestive/absorptive processes, or of a load of a solute in excess of the normal digestive/absorptive capacity. As a consequence, these solutes exert an osmotic force, proportional to their concentration, which drives water, mainly across the permeable tight junctions, into the lumen. Furthermore, if the unabsorbed nutrient is a carbohydrate, when it reaches the colon it undergoes further digestion by the resident microflora, generating smaller particles and, hence, further contributing to the osmotic drive of fluid into the lumen. The main features of osmotic diarrhea are described in Figure 2. Stool output is proportional to the intake of the unabsorbable substrate and is usually not massive; diarrheal stools promptly regress with discontinuation of the offending nutrient, and the stool ion gap is high, exceeding 100 mOsm/kg. In fact, the fecal osmolality in this circumstance is accounted for not only by the electrolytes but also by the unabsorbed nutrient(s) and their degradation products. The ion gap is obtained by

Table 3 Endogenous Regulators of Intestinal Fluid and Electrolyte Transport		
Source	Stimulate Absorption	Stimulate Secretion
Mucosal epithelial cells	Somatostatin	Serotonin
		Gastrin
		Cholecystokinin
		Neurotensin
	Nitric oxide	Guanylin
		Nitric oxide
Lamina propria cells	?	Arachidonic acid metabolites
		Nitric oxide
		Several cytokines
		Bradykinin
Enteric neurons	Norepinephrine	Acetylcholine
	Neuropeptide Y	Serotonin
		Vasoactive intestinal polypeptide
		Nitric oxide
		Substance P
		Purinergic agonists
Blood	Epinephrine	Vasoactive intestinal polypeptide
	Corticosteroids	Calcitonin
	Mineralocorticosteroids	Prostaglandins
		Atrial natriuretic peptide

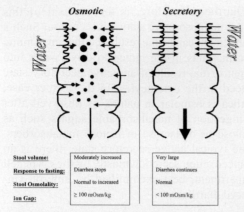

Figure 2 Scheme of osmotic and secretory diarrhea. The left panel shows the situation in osmotically induced diarrhea. Undigested or unabsorbed substrates remain in the gut lumen and exert an osmotic force proportional to their concentration that drives fluid into the lumen. In the case of unabsorbed carbohydrates, colonic flora enzymes may partially digest them, thus further contributing to the osmotic load and water flow into the lumen. Stool vole secretory diarrhea (right panel) is characterized by a state of active secretion of anions by the enterocytes. In vivo, equivalent amounts of cations also passively follow, and the result is net secretion of water and electrolytes. The role of the colon varies ion gap: according to the cause of the secretion.

subtracting the concentration of the electrolytes from total osmolality, according to the formula:
$$\text{ion gap} = \text{osmolality} - [(\text{Na} + \text{K}) \times 2].$$

SECRETORY DIARRHEA

In secretory diarrhea, the epithelial cells' ion transport processes are turned into a state of active secretion. This situation can occur as a result of many processes. When dealing with acute secretory diarrhea, the most common cause is a bacterial infection of the gut. Several mechanisms may be at work.[29] After colonization, enteric pathogens may adhere to or invade the epithelium; they may produce enterotoxins (exotoxins that elicit secretion by increasing an intracellular second messenger) or cytotoxins. They also may trigger release of cytokines attracting inflammatory cells, which, in turn, contribute to the activated secretion by inducing the release of agents such as prostaglandins or platelet-activating factor. Features of secretory diarrhea, reported in Figure 2, are a high purging rate, a lack of response to fasting, and a normal stool ion gap (≤ 100 mOsm/kg), indicating that nutrient absorption is intact.

The role of the colon in secretory diarrhea varies with the causes.[30] Generally speaking, the colonic mucosa's absorptive capacity is maximized; thus, the large intestine partially compensates for the increased small intestinal water loss. However, there are instances in which the colon is either directly involved in the stimulated secretion (ie, when the secretion is the result of a bacterial infection involving the colon) or, even if not challenged topically by a pathogen, may be put in a secretory state via the enteric nervous system as a result of enterotoxin-stimulated secretion going on in the small intestine.[29,31]

Three intracellular second messengers (cyclic adenosine monophosphate [cAMP], cyclic guanosine monophosphate [cGMP], and Ca^{2+}/protein kinase C) have long been recognized as key mediators of secretion (see Table 3). The secretagogues that activate them are both endogenous, physiological as well as exogenous, pathological, the latter notably bacterial enterotoxins. Increases in any of these second messengers result in a series of biochemical events that activate protein kinases, which act directly on ion channels, inhibiting on one side the NaCl-coupled influx and increasing on the other side the Cl efflux (Figure 3). The final common secretory pathway, the chloride channel, is represented by the CFTR: its phosphorylation opens the channel and Cl flows down its electrochemical gradient, as the interior of the cell is electronegative (-40 to -60 mV) relative to the extracellular environment. Enterotoxins elaborated by bacterial pathogens selectively and specifically increase either cAMP (eg, cholera toxin and *E. coli* heat-labile toxin) or cGMP (eg, enterotoxigenic *E. coli* [ETEC], enteroaggregative *E. coli* [EAEC], or Klebsiella heat-stable enterotoxin—STa). In the mature villous cells, cAMP and cGMP appear to be equally powerful inhibitors of NaCl entry, whereas cAMP is more potent than cGMP in stimulating anion secretion. In the crypts, several components are involved in the cyclic nucleotide and Ca-dependent electrogenic anion secretion. Na, K ATPase in the basolateral membrane maintains a low intracellular Na concentration, thereby allowing a gradient favorable to Na entry from the extracellular environment. Because of this gradient, one Na, two Cl, and one K flow via a carrier in the basolateral membrane from the serosal fluid into the cell (see Figure 3). Whereas Na and K may recycle out of the cell, Cl accumulates in the cell above its electrochemical equilibrium. Protein kinases, activated by these cyclic nucleotides and by Ca, then open Cl channels, allowing anions to leave the cell down a favorable electrochemical gradient. As mentioned, the major Cl channel, sensitive to all of the described second messengers, is the CFTR protein.[32]

There appears to be additionally another mechanism for intestinal fluid secretion, not related to the known intracellular mediators of secretions, that has become apparent from studies of the zonula occludens toxin from *Vibrio cholerae*.[33] This toxin in fact loosens tight junctions between small intestinal enterocytes,[34] and this in turn leads to fluid secretion into the lumen.

Although examples of purely osmolar and purely secretory diarrheas do occur, in most acute-onset diarrhea, both mechanisms coexist. For example, in rotaviral enteritis, a serious disruption of absorptive functions occurs as a result of the selective invasion of the mature enterocytes by the invading organisms, resulting in osmolar diarrhea. In vitro studies have shown that rotavirus acts on epithelial cells by altering protein trafficking and distribution, disrupting cell–cell interactions, and by damaging tight junctions thereby increasing paracellular permeability.[35,36] The reduction

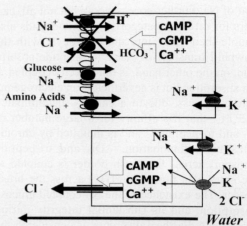

Figure 3 Secretory changes induced by second messengers. Cyclic adenosine monophosphate (cAMP), cyclic guanosine monophosphate (cGMP), and Ca^{2+}/protein kinase C have similar effects. In the mature villous cell (top panel), they inhibit the electrically neutral, coupled influx of Na and Cl (which results from the double antiport of Na/H and Cl/HCO_3). In the undifferentiated crypt cell, cAMP, cGMP, and Ca^{2+}/protein kinase C act by opening Cl channels (mainly the cystic fibrosis transmembrane conductance regulator) in the luminal membrane. As a consequence, Cl leaves the cell moving down its electrochemical gradient. Because the epithelium cannot secrete only anions, cations (Na) flow across the paracellular pathway, driven by the electrical gradient created by the secretory transport of Cl. Thus, antiabsorptive (mostly but not exclusively in the villous cell) and prosecretory (mostly but not exclusively in the crypt cell) forces combine to shift ions, and with them water, from absorption to secretion.

of absorptive cells in the gut lining also unmasks the secretion in the crypts, and a secretory component is superimposed. Furthermore, the secretory nature of rotavirus diarrhea is also augmented by an enterotoxin, the nonstructural protein NSP4, which acts as a viral enterotoxin to induce diarrhea, causing Ca^{2+}-dependent transepithelial Cl secretion.[37] Of interest, recently a second example of an enterotoxin-like action by a viral protein has been found, the HIV-1 Tat protein, which acts on ion secretion and on cell proliferation in human intestinal epithelial cells.[38]

Table 4 summarizes the main pathogenic mechanisms displayed by the most common agents of infectious diarrhea, along with their predominant site of action within the gut. Chapter 19.2, "Infections," contains additional information on the pathogenesis of viral, bacterial, parasitic, and fungal infections.

CLINICAL FEATURES

Acute diarrhea in developed countries is almost invariably a benign, self-limited condition, subsiding within a few days. The clinical presentation and course of illness are dependent on the etiology of the diarrhea and on the host. For example, a recent study examining the impact of acute rotavirus gastroenteritis in the United States found that rotavirus was responsible for 40% of the cases and was more commonly associated with vomiting, fever, and greater number of work days lost than non-rotavirus gastroenteritis.[39] A recent

Table 4 Pathogenic Mechanisms and Localization of the Main Intestinal Pathogens

Predominant Pathogenesis*	Site of Infection	Agent	Clinical Features
Direct cytopathic effect	Proximal small intestine	Rotavirus Enteric-type adenovirus Calicivirus Norovirus EPEC	Copious watery diarrhea, vomiting, mild to severe dehydration; frequent lactose malabsorption, no hematochezia Course may be severe
Enterotoxigenicity	Small intestine	Giardia Vibrio cholerae ETEC EAggEC Klebsiella pneumoniae Citrobacter freundii Cryptosporidium	Watery diarrhea (can be copious in cholera or ETEC), but usually mild course; no hematochezia
Invasiveness	Distal ileum and colon	Salmonella Shigella Yersinia Campylobacter EIEC Amoeba	Dysentery: very frequent stools, cramps, pain, fever, and often hematochezia with white blood cells in stools. Variable dehydration Course may be protracted
Cytotoxicity	Colon	Clostridium difficile EHEC Shigella	Dysentery, abdominal cramps, fever, hematochezia EHEC or Shigella may be followed by hemolytic uremic syndrome

EAggEC = enteroaggregative *Escherichia coli*; EIEC = enteroinvasive *Escherichia coli*; EHEC = enterohemorragic *Escherichia coli*; EPEC = enteropathogenic *Escherichia coli*; ETEC = enterotoxigenic *Escherichia coli*.

*Elaboration of various types of enterotoxins affecting ion transport has been demonstrated as an additional virulence factor for almost all of the bacterial pathogens.

prospective study conducted in the United States in 604 children 3 to 36 months of age in community settings[40] found that the highest incidence of diarrhea of acute onset was in January and August with an overall incidence of 2.21 episodes per person-year. Close to 90% were acute, ie, lasting <14 days, with a median duration of 2 days and a median of six stools per day. Table 5 summarizes the characteristics of the 611 diarrheal episodes that were evaluated.

Age and nutritional status appear to be the most important host factors in determining the severity and the duration of diarrhea. In fact, the younger the child, the higher is the risk for severe, life-threatening dehydration as a result of the high body water turnover and limited renal compensatory capacity of very young children. Whether younger age also means a risk of running a prolonged course is an unsettled issue. In developing countries, it has been reported that persistent postenteritis diarrhea (PPD) shows a strong inverse correlation with age.[41,42] Nutrition plays an essential role in determining the severity of the diarrheal episode, an effect mediated by several factors, including an altered small intestinal mucosal permeability.[43]

As for the infecting organism, the different pathogenic mechanisms deployed by different infectious agents result in a variable pattern of clinical features (see Table 4). Table 6 reports clinical features at admission in the previously quoted series of 287 patients.[11] It can be seen that this group of well-nourished children with acute diarrhea from 10 European centers presented mainly with watery or loose stools, often with vomiting and fever. They were mostly in good or fair condition and with either mild or no dehydration in almost 80%. By looking at the clinical features of children grouped according to the pathogen identified, it is evident that these features do vary according to etiology, as one would expect based on the varying pathophysiology. Table 7 reports data pooled from our recent series[11] and from a previous series of 154 children,[44] 3 months to 5 years of age. Only patients in whom a single pathogen was identified are reported. When compared with children with either invasive etiology or enterotoxigenic bacteria, it is obvious that patients with rotaviral diarrhea tend to have severe dehydration, vomiting, and watery stools. Fever, crampy abdominal pain, and blood mixed with stools are more common in patients with invasive pathogens such as *Salmonella, Shigella, Yersinia, Campylobacter,* and *Entamoeba histolytica.* The smaller group of children affected by STa-producing ETEC had milder illness, with fecal

Table 5 Characteristics of 611 Diarrhea Episodes in 604 Children 3 to 36 Months Old in Community Settings in the United States

Feature	
Feature	
Median duration (d)	2 [1.0–5.0]*
Median number of stools/episode	6 [3.0–18.0]
Associated signs and symptoms	
Loss of appetite	320 (52.4)†
Cold symptoms	283 (46.3)
Fever	173 (28.3)
Abdominal pain	114 (18.7)
Vomiting	102 (16.7)
Mucous in stool	98 (16.3)
Blood in stool	5 (0.8)
Received antibiotics within 10 d of onset	75 (12.3)
Sick contact in home with diarrhea <2 wk before onset	135 (22.1)
Medications given	
Electrolyte solution	63 (10.3)
Bismuth subsalicylate	15 (2.5)
Antibiotics	7 (1.1)
Loperamide	4 (0.7)
Probiotics	2 (0.3)
Herbal products	0 (0)
Medical care received	
Physician/ER visit	59 (9.7)
Hospitalized	2 (0.3)
Child missed day care/preschool	62 (25.2)

Adapted from Guandalini et al.[11]

*Numbers in square brackets, 25th and 75th percentiles.

†Numbers in parentheses, percent.

Table 6 Clinical Features at Presentation of Acute Diarrhea in 287 Children 3 Months to 5-Year-Old in Europe

Feature	Mean ± SD OR%
Feature	
Age (months)	12.3 ± 4.1
Sex (% females)	39
Weight (kg)	8.8 ± 1.6
Height (cm)	73.7 ± 8.4
Weight/height (percentile)	32 ± 18
Partially breast-fed (%)	22.5
Stool characteristics (%)	
Watery	71
Loose	20.8
Mucousy	28.5
Bloody	8.3
Vomiting	60
Fever	59.3
Condition (%)	
Good	50.2
Fair	7.7
Poor	41.3
Dehydration (%)	
Absent	29
Mild	48.5
Moderate	21.8
Severe	0.7

Adapted from Guandalini et al.[11]

Table 7 Comparison of Clinical Features Associated with Specific Pathogens in 306 European Children 3 Months to 5-Year-Old with Acute Infectious Diarrhea

Symptom/Sign	Rotavirus ($N = 180$) (%)	Invasive Pathogens* ($N = 104$) (%)	Enterotoxigenic *Escherichia coli* ($N = 22$)
Shock	2	—	—
Dehydration (moderate to severe)	62	29	18
Vomiting	71	35	14
Fever	26	68	23
Abdominal crampy pain	25	51	32
Watery stools	81	47	64
Hematochezia	5	47	4

*Invasive pathogens combine *Salmonella* ($n = 41$), *Shigella* ($n = 6$), *Campylobacter* ($n = 38$), *Yersinia enterocolitica* ($n = 8$), *Entamoeba* ($n = 11$).

electrolyte content consistent with a secretory pathogenesis.[45]

In 2003 the Center for Disease Control (CDC) put forth new recommendations for the management of acute pediatric diarrhea in both the outpatient and inpatient settings including indication for referral.[46] Table 8 outlines the indications for medical evaluation of children with acute diarrhea. The report also includes information on assessment of dehydration and what steps should be taken to treat adequately (see Table 9).

In developed countries, diarrhea is basically a self-limited condition. If the proper replenishment of water and electrolytes lost with the stools is provided on an ongoing basis, hydration will be maintained, and the condition will fade within a few days. Sometimes diarrhea fails to subside and undergoes a prolonged course. See Chapter 15.2b, "Persistent Diarrhea," for a detailed presentation of this entity.

PRINCIPLES OF MANAGEMENT
REHYDRATION

The obvious major risk in acute diarrhea is the loss of water and electrolytes with consequent dehydration and possibly even loss of Na homeostasis. Rehydration or maintenance of hydration is therefore the cornerstone of treatment. Until the mid-1960s, this was accomplished almost exclusively via the intravenous route. Subsequently, the expanded understanding of the pathophysiologic events in intestinal transport processes allowed a dramatic change of approach. In fact, it became apparent that enterotoxigenic bacteria such as *V. cholerae* or ETEC leave intact small intestinal mucosal morphology and absorptive functions. In particular, the glucose-coupled Na influx was found to be fully functional in cholera toxin and other cAMP-induced secretory diarrheas, studied in vitro and in vivo.[47–49] This was later confirmed for the other cyclic nucleotide, cGMP, and its related heat-stable enterotoxins.[50] Thus, the ongoing absorption of Na and glucose during secretion promotes fluid absorption and allows rehydration to take place in spite of the ongoing fluid loss seen in enterotoxigenic diarrheas. It must be noted that ORSs have been found to be effective even in situations such as rotavirus enteritis, despite a diffuse damage to the epithelium, which in vitro results in the inhibition of nutrient transport. Numerous studies, analyzed in a recent meta-analysis published in the Cochrane Library,[51] had shown convincingly that ORT could safely be used to rehydrate children both in developed and developing countries, with fewer than 5% of children failing ORT and requiring intravenous fluids, regardless of the etiology of acute diarrhea.[51,52]

These concepts provided the pathophysiologic basis for the WHO–UNICEF-supported and highly successful global program for oral rehydration therapy (ORT). ORSs have proved both safe and effective worldwide in hospital settings and also in the home to prevent dehydration. For about three decades, the WHO has recommended a standard formulation of glucose-based ORS with 90 mmol/L of sodium and 111 mmol/L of glucose, with a total osmolarity of 311 mmol/ L. However, many in vitro and in vivo studies during the late 1980s and 1990s had consistently shown that lower concentrations of sodium and glucose enhance solute-induced water absorption and might therefore be superior to the solution with a higher osmolarity.[53]

Reduced-osmolarity solutions have concentrations of glucose and Na inferior to those in the traditional WHO solution: glucose ranges between 75 and 100 and Na between 60 and 75 mmol/L, so osmolarity is maintained at 225 to 260 mOsm/L, and the ratio between glucose and Na close to 1:1. The use of such ORSs in children of developed countries was originally proposed in 1992 by an ad hoc committee of the European Society of Pediatric Gastroenterology, Hepatology and Nutrition (ESPGHAN).[54] Hypo-osmolar ORSs appear to have the additional advantage of allowing a reduced stool output while being just as effective in obtaining and maintaining rehydration and can be safely given throughout the duration of diarrhea, as shown in both developed and in developing countries. Indeed, in 2002 a large meta-analysis of all published controlled trials comparing low-osmolarity solutions with standard WHO formulas appearing in the Cochrane Library concluded that in children hospitalized for diarrhea, reduced osmolarity ORS compared to WHO standard ORS is associated with fewer

Table 8 Indications for Medical Evaluation of Children with Acute Diarrhea

Age <3 mo
Weight <8 kg
History of premature birth, chronic medical conditions, or concurrent illness
Fever ≥38°C for infants <3 mo or ≥39°C for children 3 to 36 mo
Visible blood in the stool
High output diarrhea
Persistent emesis
Signs of dehydration as reported by caregiver-sunken eyes, decreased tears, dry mucous membranes, decreased urine output
Mental status changes
Inadequate response to or Caregiver unable to administer ORT

Adapted from King et al.[46]

Table 9 Treatment of Dehydration due to Diarrhea

Degree of Dehydration	Rehydration Therapy	Replacement of Losses
Minimal or no dehydration	Not applicable	<10 kg body weight: 60–120 mL ORS for each diarrhea stool or vomiting episode >10 kg body weight: 120–140 mL ORS for each diarrheal stool or vomiting episode
Mild to moderate dehydration	ORS, 50–100 mL/kg Same body weight over 3–4 h	
Severe dehydration	Lactated Ringer's solution or normal saline in 20 mL/kg body weight intravenous amounts until perfusion and mental status improve Then administer 100 mL/kg body weight ORS over 4 h or 5% dextrose 1/2 normal saline intravenously at twice maintenance fluid rates	Same, if unable to drink administer through nasogastric tube or administer 5% dextrose 1/4 normal saline with 20 meq/L potassium chloride intravenously

Adapted from King et al.[46]

Table 10 Composition of Oral Rehydration Solutions			
Ingredient	ESPGHAN-ORS (mmol/L)	WHO-ORS 1975 (mmol/L)	WHO-ORS 2002 (mmol/L)
Glucose	74–111	111	75
Na	60	90	75
K	20	20	20
Base	10 (citrate)	30	30
Cl	60	80	65
Osmolality	225–260	331	245

unscheduled intravenous fluid infusions, lower stool volume, and less vomiting, without additional risks of hyponatremia.[55] More recently, evidence has been provided that hypo-osmolar ORS can be used safely and effectively even in newborns and young infants.[56]

Accepting all the evidence accumulated until then, in 2002 the WHO announced the adoption of a new ORS formulation consistent with these recommendations, with 75 meq/L sodium, 75 mmol/L glucose, and a total osmolarity of 245 mOsm/L.[57] This hypotonic WHO-ORS is also recommended for use in adults and children with cholera, a condition characterized as we have seen by a marked stool loss of Na, but further studies are under way to confirm the safety of this indication. A large meta-analysis published in the Cochrane Library[58] confirmed the safety, efficacy, and clinical superiority of low-osmolality ORS. Table 10 reports the composition of these various ORS.

In constant search of a "super-ORS" that would not only be efficacious for rehydration but also could result in a substantial improvement in reducing the stool volume, in recent years the possibility has been advanced that adding to ORS starches resistant to small intestinal hydrolysis by amylase, could be beneficial by allowing an added stimulus to colonic water absorption due to release of fatty acids by the fermenting microflora. This concept was originally tested in adolescents and adults with cholera, where the solution was found able to reduce fecal fluid loss and to shorten the duration of diarrhea.[59] Subsequently, ORSs with amylase-resistant starches have been tried in children, with conflicting results: while a multicenter study of a starch-added ORS in Europe had not provided support for their use,[60] a subsequent study in 178 children aged 3 months to 6 years found the solution to result in a shorter duration of diarrhea.[61] Of interest, initial evidence from the laboratory animal seems to suggest that such solutions may prove even more beneficial if associated with a low-osmolarity ORS.[62]

In summary, ORT with a glucose-based ORS must be viewed as by far the safest, most physiologic, and most effective way to provide rehydration and maintain hydration in children with acute diarrhea worldwide, as recommended by the WHO, by the ad hoc committee of ESPGHAN,[54,63] and by the American Academy of Pediatrics.[64] In spite of this however, the global use of ORT is still insufficient. Particularly developed countries, and among them especially the United States, seem to be lagging behind, in the face of studies showing beyond doubts the efficacy of ORT in the emergency care settings,[65] where intravenous rehydration continues, unduly, to be widely privileged.

We should also mention briefly that the composition of almost all other beverages (carbonated or not) commercially available and frequently used in children with diarrhea is completely inadequate for rehydration or for maintaining hydration, in consideration of a Na content that is invariably extremely low, and of an osmolarity that is often dangerously elevated. For instance, Coca-Cola, Pepsi-Cola, and apple juice have an osmolarity, respectively, of 493, 576, and 694 to 773 mOsm/kg.

REFEEDING

It has been clear for many years that, when affected by gastroenteritis, breastfed infants should be continued on breast milk without any need for interruption. In fact, breastfeeding not only has a well-known protective effect against the development of enteritis,[66,67] it also promotes faster recovery and provides improved nutrition.[68,69] This is even more important in developing countries, where withdrawal of breastfeeding during diarrhea has been shown to have a deleterious effect on the development of dehydration in infants with acute watery diarrhea.[70]

What is the right approach in artificially fed infants who experience acute-onset diarrhea? In the past and for a long time, the popular remedy for acute diarrhea had been that of fasting, on the intuitive basis that "gut rest" would be beneficial. This long-held view has been challenged during the past several years to the point that today the evidence in favor of rapid refeeding is overwhelming. In fact, many well-conducted studies have provided evidence that in weaned children not severely dehydrated or acidotic, a rapid return to full feeding after having completed oral rehydration in the first 4 to 6 hours is well tolerated.[71,72] Indeed, ORT itself has a beneficial effect on nutrition by stimulating the child's appetite as a result of the improved water and potassium balance. Furthermore, rapid refeeding after adequate ORT has been shown to allow a faster recovery from the abnormally increased intestinal permeability owing to induced enteritis.[73]

Furthermore, evidence has been provided that even in the United States, delaying reintroduction of normal feeds in diarrheic children may have devastating nutritional effects.[74] The Working Group on Acute Diarrhea of ESPGHAN evaluated in a multicenter study the effect of early versus delayed resumption of full feedings in European children with acute diarrhea.[72] The children were first orally rehydrated with a reduced-osmolality solution, formulated according to the previous recommendations,[54] and were then assigned to either the "gradual" or the "early" refeeding group. Two hundred thirty patients (mean age 14 months) were examined; their profile on entry into study showed no statistically significant difference between the two groups. After 4 hours of ORT, the patients who were "early" fed resumed their normal diet, including lactose-containing formulas, whereas the "late feeders" continued to receive only ORS for 24 hours before returning to normal foods. Weight gain proved significantly greater in patients refed early, not only during the first 1 or 2 days after rehydration but also throughout hospitalization, and persisted as late as at day 14 postenrolment. Most important, the two groups did not differ in the incidence of emesis and watery stools. Of note, by day 5, no patient in either group had lactose intolerance.

Should formulas with reduced lactose content be used? Lactose intolerance was once thought to be a major problem in children with diarrhea and a reason to delay refeeding milk-based formulas. In reality, and in spite of the common occurrence of reducing substances in the stools of infants with diarrhea, it is believed that lactose intolerance is not a clinical concern for the vast majority of patients in developed countries. In the ESPGHAN study, only 3% of the children at admission had signs of lactose malabsorption and none at day 5 postenrolment after receiving a normal, lactose-containing formula.[72] The occurrence of clinically significant lactose intolerance however must not be completely disregarded: rarely, and more so in malnourished children, diarrhea may worsen on reintroduction of milk or "normal" formulas. If fecal pH decreases and 1% or more reducing substances are found in the stools, lactose intolerance should at that point be diagnosed and a lactose-free formula employed at least temporarily to prevent persistent diarrhea PPD.[68,75–78]

Fermented milks (yogurts) feedings have traditionally been considered very appropriate for infants and young children with acute diarrhea. The concept of having their lactose being digested in vivo by lactic acid bacteria offers an attractive alternative to the use of normal formulas. Few clinical trials are available to compare adequately yogurts versus normal milks; it would appear however that in the subset of infants with carbohydrate malabsorption during diarrhea, yogurt feeding is associated with a clinically relevant decrease in stool frequency and duration of diarrhea.[79]

In the United States, a specific diet introduced in 1926 (the BRAT [bananas, rice, applesauce, and toast] diet) has been widely recommended for decades, and still enjoys some popularity. Although green bananas and pectin have been shown to be useful in infants with persistent diarrhea,[80] the BRAT diet should not be recommended: it has not been proven useful, it is unnecessarily restrictive and can result in poor nutrition.

Thus, to sum up the evidence in terms of the nutritional handling of infants and children with acute-onset diarrhea, we can conclude that rapid refeeding for most infants beyond the first 3 months of age is safe and effective in acute diarrhea. Based on this evidence, including the large meta-analysis by Brown and colleagues of the published trials comparing different refeeding regimens,[78] it can be recommended that the optimal management of mild-to-moderately dehydrated children consist of oral rehydration with ORS over about 4 hours, followed by the rapid reintroduction of normal feeding thereafter." [46,76,77,81]

OTHER TREATMENTS: ANTIBIOTICS, ZINC, IMMUNOGLOBULINS, DRUGS, AND PROBIOTICS

Despite a long search for a single curative treatment, supportive care and prevention remain the cornerstone of therapy. Appropriate management of dehydration, electrolyte status, and nutrition are the critical components of therapy.

Antibiotics

In suspected or proven bacterial enteritis, the decision to treat a child with antibiotics is not easy, as antibiotic treatment may be associated with prolongation of illness, increased carrier state, and increased morbidity. For instance, antibiotic treatment of EHEC has long been debated as there is evidence that it may favor the onset of hemolytic-uremic syndrome (HUS). This complication has been reported in as many as 50% of children who received antibiotic treatment for *E. coli* O157:H7 and it was estimated that antibiotic use was associated with a relative risk of 13.4 to 17.7 of developing HUS.[82] Limited data concerning the efficacy and safety of antibiotics to treat acute childhood diarrhea exist. There is a small but increasing body of literature to support the safe use of fluoroquinolones in pediatrics. Leibovitz et al found that empiric oral ciprofloxacin was as safe and effective as intramuscular ceftriaxone in treating acute invasive diarrhea in the pediatric outpatient population.[83]

In terms of recommended antimicrobial treatment in the immuno-competent host, enteric bacterial and protozoan pathogens can be grouped as follows:

1. Agents for whom antimicrobial therapy is always indicated. The consensus includes in this category only *V. cholerae, Shigella,* and *Giardia lamblia;*

2. Agents for whom antimicrobial therapy is indicated only in selected circumstances:

a. Infections by enteropathogenic *E. coli,* when running a prolonged course;

b. Enteroinvasive *E. coli* (EIEC), based on the serologic, genetic, and pathogenic similarities with *Shigella;*

c. *Yersinia* infections in subjects with sickle cell disease; and

d. *Salmonella* infections in the very young infants, if febrile, or with positive blood culture.[84]

Zinc

Micronutrient deficiencies found in malnourished children with diarrhea include zinc deficiency. In the past few years, a great deal of interest has been generated by the possible role of zinc supplementation in either the prevention or the treatment of acute diarrhea in developing countries, particularly in India and Bangladesh. In a double-blind, controlled study in Bangladesh, Roy and colleagues showed that the supplementation of 20 mg/d of elemental zinc to malnourished children with acute diarrhea resulted in shorter duration of diarrhea, lesser stool output, better weight gain, and improved zinc serum status.[85] All of these changes were again more evident in initially zinc-deficient subjects. Further evidence was subsequently provided in support of the role of zinc supplementation to prevent and treat acute diarrheal diseases in children of developing countries.[86–90]

Considering all the evidence available therefore, in 2004 the WHO and UNICEF issued a joint statement,[91] supporting the use of zinc supplementation for acute diarrhea. In addition to preventing dehydration, continuing or increasing feeding and breastfeeding and providing ORS, WHO/UNICEF in fact recommended providing infants less than 6 months old with 10 mg/d and children with 20 mg/d of zinc supplementation, in the form of either syrup or dispersible tablets (that appear to be acceptable by children in field trials[92]) for 10 to 14 days. It appears that the higher dose can be associated with an increased risk of vomiting and regurgitation, but this is a transient phenomenon not impinging on the efficacy of the overall treatment.[93] In spite of a predominant evidence of effectiveness, still some doubts persist in infants less than 6 months old: a study by Fischer Walker et al looking at infants 28 days to 5 months old, found in fact that infants receiving zinc supplements had no benefit and had a trend to increased duration of diarrhea that was not significant.[94]

Immunoglobulins

Several articles have documented, either in case series or in small uncontrolled trials, the efficacy of oral or enteral immunoglobulin in the treatment of rotavirus diarrhea.[95–98] Although these data are interesting and may apply to certain patients with severe, protracted rotavirus diarrhea (immunocompromised or immunocompetent), it does not appear that the cost-benefit ratio would justify this approach on a wider basis. Interestingly, a recent meta-analysis appearing in the Cochrane Library addressed the issue of possible use of oral immunoglobulin to prevent rotavirus infections in low-birth infants at risk.[99] In fact, epidemics with the

newer P(6)G9 strains have been reported in neonatal units worldwide, and it is known that these strains can cause severe symptoms in infected infants. Although only one article fulfilling the inclusion criteria was found,[100] showing only borderline evidence that immunoglobulin administration was associated with delayed excretion of rotavirus and with milder symptoms of infection, the authors of the meta-analysis concluded that "researchers should be encouraged to conduct well-designed trials in neonates at risk for rotavirus infections using the newer preparations of antirotaviral immunoglobulins. Such trials should also include cost effectiveness evaluations."[99]

Drugs

The search for the ideal drug to treat acute diarrhea is certainly not new. Considering the burden of morbidity of this condition, it is obvious that having a safe and effective drug would be beneficial. This quest has, however, been largely unsuccessful, and all current guidelines warn against the use of drugs that may be more harmful than useful. Even the impressive search that has taken place in the past two decades as a result of the increased knowledge on the pathophysiology of intestinal secretion has been disappointing because most of the antisecretory agents (such as chlorpromazine, loperamide, and octreotide, reviewed in reference 28) have a limited effect and/or are not devoid of potentially hazardous side effects, making them not an option for acute diarrhea. Among these antisecretory agents, the somatostatin analog octreotide seems however to have a role in the treatment of patients with persistent high-volume diarrhea postchemotherapy or in AIDS.[101] Recently, however, a new investigational drug has appeared that does show some promise: the enkephalinase inhibitor acetorphan, later renamed racecadotril.[102] In fact, it is thought that enkephalins are endogenous pro-absorptive agents that directly inhibit the activity of adenylate cyclase on the enterocyte basolateral membrane. Enkephalins are rapidly degraded by a membrane-bound metalloproteinase, enkephalinase, an enzyme abundant in the gastrointestinal tract. Racecadotril is a synthetic, potent inhibitor of enkephalinase, devoid of any effect on intestinal motility, thus without the potential to induce the bloating that can be associated with enteropooling.

The drug has been tested in vitro and in vivo,[103,104] where it has been found effective in reducing jejunal secretion stimulated by cholera toxin.[105] Subsequently, a number of randomized controlled trials have been completed in adults and children, including comparisons with standard antidiarrheal therapy such as loperamide. In a large multinational comparison of racecadotril with loperamide in about 1,000 adult patients, while the duration of diarrhea was similar, symptoms such as abdominal pain, distension and constipation were less frequent with racecadotril.[106] Similar results were found in a similar more recent adult trial.[107]

As for children, a few double-blinded, placebo-controlled clinical trials have now been performed with racecadotril,[108–110] in patients with acute diarrhea most often due to rotavirus. From them, it would appear that the drug reduced the duration of diarrhea and also significantly reduced stool output.

In summary, with the exception of racecadotril that appears to be a relatively safe (an adverse event has recently been reported[111]) and effective drug requiring however larger clinical trials, in general it can be concluded that no antidiarrheal drug can and should be presently recommended in children with acute-onset diarrhea.

Probiotics

One of the most rapidly expanding areas in the treatment and prevention of diarrheal disease has been the use of "probiotics," live microflora supposed to have a beneficial effect on the host.[112] See Chapters 19.1a, "Probiotics," and 19.1b "Prebiotics, Symbiotics, and Fermented Productions," for a full analysis of these products and their role in pediatric gastroenterology. The use of several strains of lactic acid bacteria to treat human diseases is not new; indeed, lactobacilli are among the most commonly employed bacterial species used to promote health and counteract intestinal infections. Table 11 lists the most thoroughly investigated probiotics as well as newer probiotic strains currently being investigated. Among them, *Lactobacillus rhamnosus* strain GG (ATCC 53103) is by far the most widely investigated. The capacity of this strain to transiently colonize the human gut, unlike the strains employed for the production of commonly marketed yogurts and dairy products, is well established.[113]

Lactobacillus GG has a number of diverse, potentially beneficial, biologic effects, and in multiple well-conducted clinical trials, it proved effective in the treatment of acute diarrheal disease in children[11,114] and in adults. Indeed, a growing number of rigorous meta-analyses have appeared on the efficacy of probiotics, especially *Lactobacillus* GG, in the treatment and prevention of acute infectious diarrhea in children. Their conclusions at present can be summarized as follows[114]:

- Probiotics administered to children with acute diarrhea in developed countries are safe and result in a shorter duration of diarrhea of approximately 1 day. Robust evidence of efficacy in developing countries is currently lacking.
- The effect is seen particularly in young children, and when the probiotics are administered early in the course of the illness and at doses of at least 1 billion CFU/d.
- The single probiotic most consistently effective is Lactobacillus GG.
- The efficacy of probiotics is evident in viral diarrheas (and especially in infections by rotavirus) of mild to moderate degree; whereas efficacy is less or absent in invasive, bacterial diarrheas.

Additionally, a meta-analysis conducted in 2002[115] found a statistically significant inverse

Table 11 Probiotic Microorganisms
Lactic acid bacteria
Lactobacilli
Lactobacillus acidophilus
Lactobacillus brevis
Lactobacillus cellobiosus
Lactobacillus fermentum
Lactobacillus crispatus
Lactobacillus curvatus
Lactobacillus rhamnosus aka *Lactobacillus* GG
Lactobacillus salivarus
Lactobacillus gasseri
Lactobacillus casei
Lactobacillus reuteri
Lactobacillus plantarum
Lactobacillus bulgaricus
Lactobacillus johnsoni
Lactobacillus lactis
Bifidobacteria
Bifidiobacterium animalis
Bifidobacterium thermophilum
Bifidobacterium lactis
Bifidobacterium bifidum
Bifidobacterium longum
Bifidobacterium breve
Bifidobacterium infantis
Bifidobacterium adolescentis
Others
Bacteria
Escherichia coli
Enterococcus fecalis
Enterococcus faecium
Lactococcus lactis
Streptococcus thermophilus
Yeasts
Saccharomyces boulardii

correlation between the dose of lactobacilli administered and the duration of diarrhea, thus indicating the possibility that there could well be a dose-effect pattern that still is largely to be understood. These data are of importance as they point to our need to learn more about the pharmacokinetics of these agents in order to employ them effectively.

If the effect of some probiotics in shortening the duration of acute-onset diarrhea in children can now be considered ascertained, what can be said about their ability to prevent its onset? This issue has been investigated in the areas of community-acquired, nosocomial and antibiotic-associated diarrhea.

In the first instance, three randomized clinical trials are available that suggest a modest protective effect. One study[116] assessed the prevalence of acute diarrhea in over 900 infants in a child care setting fed for a prolonged period a formula enriched by *Bifidobacterium breve* and *Streptococcus thermophilus 065*. Although the results showed that incidence, duration of diarrhea episodes, and number of hospital admissions did not differ significantly between the study group and placebo fed a standard formula, the episodes were significantly less severe in the probiotic-supplemented group, with fewer cases of dehydration medical consultations and prescriptions or oral rehydration.

A multicenter clinical trial[117] evaluated the efficacy of a formula supplemented with *B. lactis*

strain Bb 12 (BbF) in the prevention of acute diarrhea in young infants living in residential nurseries or foster-care centers. Again, the formula supplemented with *B. lactis* did not reduce the prevalence of diarrhea when compared with administration of a placebo, with the only significant difference being the number of days with diarrhea (0.84 vs 2.3).

Finally, a study in an indigent community was performed in undernourished Peruvian infants, in an area with a high burden of diarrheal diseases.[118] In this investigation, the children who randomly received *Lactobacillus* GG for 15 months had significantly fewer episodes of diarrhea, especially the non-breast fed ones, and those in the 18- to 29-month age group. Thus, although it is obviously impossible to draw any general conclusions on the effects of probiotics on community-acquired diarrhea in children, the data so far available are not particularly encouraging.

Probiotics efficacy in preventing the spreading of nosocomial infectious diarrhea (defined as any diarrhea that a patient contracts while in a health-care institution) is controversial.

Rotavirus is by far the most common cause of such condition in children, although other enteric pathogens, especially *C. difficile*, can be responsible. The incidence of nosocomial diarrhea ranges from 4.54 to 22.65 episodes per 100 admissions. Three clinical trials evaluated the use of probiotics to prevent diarrhea in infants and young children admitted to hospitals for reasons other than diarrhea. Two of them used L-GG to prevent diarrhea in young children hospitalized for relatively short stays, producing conflicting results. In fact, a double-blind study involving children aged 1 to 36 months[119] showed that L-GG significantly reduced the risk of nosocomial diarrhea, that in this study was predominantly due to Rotavirus.

The second trial however comparing L-GG with placebo in 220 breast-fed infants 1 to 18 months, failed to show any significant effect.[120]

The third area where probiotics have been studied as preventative of diarrhea of acute onset is that of antibiotic-associated diarrhea. In fact, probiotics, primarily *Saccharomyces boulardii* and *Lactobacillus* GG, have repeatedly been shown to be effective in the prevention of antibiotic-associated diarrhea and *C. difficile*-associated diarrhea.[121–128] A recent meta-analysis of six placebo-controlled trials including 766 children found that probiotics reduced the risk of antibiotic-associated diarrhea from 28.5 to 11.9% compared to placebo; for every seven patients that would develop diarrhea while being treated with antibiotics, only fewer will develop it if also receiving probiotics.[129] When pooling, also data regarding adults, a recent meta-analysis assessing 25 published clinical trials concluded that three types of probiotics (*Saccharomyces boulardii*, *Lactobacillus* GG, and probiotic mixtures) significantly reduced the development of antibiotic-associated diarrhea, but only *S. boulardii* was effective for *C. difficile* diarrhea.[130] As more and more candidate probiotics are proposed, it is evident that each one must be studied individually and extensively to prove its efficacy and safety before use in acute diarrhea is recommended.

Several rigorous meta-analyses have confirmed that probiotics are effective and safe in immunocompetent patients. The safety of probiotics in immunocompromised patients however is less clear. Recently, case reports of immunocompromised patients receiving probiotic therapy have emerged documenting bacteremia, fungemia, and sepsis with the same probiotic strain administered.[131–133]

Table 12 summarizes the approach suggested to evaluate and manage a child with acute-onset diarrhea.

Table 12 Summary of the Suggested Approach to the Child with Acute Diarrhea

Assess general status and hydration

Admit if:
- >10% dehydration
- Signs of shock
- Lethargy or unconsciousness
- Presence of ileus
- Inability to deliver or failure to respond to ORS

Manage dehydration

Estimate severity of dehydration and rehydrate accordingly (see Table 9) over 3–4 h

Nutritional management
- Continue breast feeding at all times, even while rehydration is being accomplished
- Rapidly reintroduce an age appropriate normal diet (including solids), soon after completing rehydration with low-osmolarity ORS.
- Routine use of a diluted or special formula is unjustified

Tests

Stool cultures should be performed only in:
- Inpatients;
- When suspecting the presence of treatable pathogens such as *Vibrio cholerae*, *Shigella*, *Entamoeba histolytica*, *Giardia lamblia*; or *Salmonella* in young infants;
- Patients with hemoglobinopathies, neoplasms, chronic diseases of the gastrointestinal tract or immunocompromised.

Tests such as Clinitest or pH are not necessary unless refeeding with a lactose-containing formula is followed by worsening of diarrheal output.

Pharmacological therapy

Antiemetics and antidiarrheal drugs should not be routinely given to infants and children for the indication of acute diarrhea.

Antimicrobial therapy is generally recommended for:
- Shigellosis
- Cholera
- *Yersinia* infections in patients with hemoglobinopathies;
- Symptomatic infection with *Entamoeba histolytica*
- Laboratory-proven symptomatic infection with *Giardia lamblia*
- Infections with enteroinvasive bacteria in patients with an increased risk of invasive disease (see previous heading)

Probiotics

In immunocompetent infants and children, consider the use of probiotics such as *Lactobacillus* GG, in the amount of at least 10^{10} CFU/d, early in the course of an episode of acute diarrhea, whenever abbreviating its course is deemed important. In immunocompetent patients about to undergo a course of antibiotics consider the use of either *Lactobacillus* GG or *Saccharomyces boulardii*.

PREVENTION

With the toll of mortality and morbidity from acute-onset diarrhea still being so high (see introduction), it is understandable that global efforts to reduce diarrheal disease have been led by the WHO and the CDC. Several areas have been targeted for prevention: education, sanitation, hygiene, breastfeeding, food safety, appropriate use of oral rehydration therapy, probiotics, and development of vaccinations.

Simple hand-washing with plain soap has been shown to decrease the incidence of diarrhea by more than 50% in children less than 15 years old.[134] Other education campaigns focused on food safety have also been effective, by decreasing the incidence of diarrhea by more than 50%.[135] In addition, global efforts to educate families about the importance and value of breast feeding have proven successful in decreasing the burden of diarrheal disease in infancy. A healthcare program in Pakistan that promoted breastfeeding, appropriate use of ORS, and continued feeding during diarrheal illnesses, found a significant decrease in infantile diarrhea disease as well as an improvement in linear growth.[136]

Perhaps the most exciting recent addition to standard prevention measures is the reintroduction of the rotavirus vaccine. The original tetravalent rhesus-human reassortant rotavirus vaccine, RotaShield (Wyeth Laboratories) was introduced in 1998 but withdrawn in the fall of 1999 due to concerns of increased risk of intussusceptions. In January 2006, two landmark studies were published establishing the safety and efficacy of two new rotavirus vaccines, Rotarix (GlaxoSmithKline Biologicals) and RotaTeq (Merck and Company).[137,138] Rotarix is a live-attenuated G1[P8] human rotavirus vaccine highly protective against rotavirus serotypes G1, G3, and G9 with partial protection against serotype G2. In a phase 3 trial 31,673 infants in Latin American and Finland received two oral doses of Rotarix at 2 and 4 months of age. The efficacy was evaluated in 20,169 infants, approximately half receiving the vaccine and half receiving placebo. Rotarix was associated with a 85% efficacy against severe rotavirus diarrhea and a 85% reduction in hospitalizations due to rotavirus. RotaTeq is a live pentavalent G1, G2, G3, G4, P[8] bovine-human oral vaccine. In the phase 3 trial, three oral doses of RotaTeq were administered to 70,301 infants aged 6 to 12 weeks in the United States, Latin America, Europe, and Asia. RotaTeq was found to be highly efficacious, preventing 98% of severe rotavirus gastroenteritis and 96% of rotavirus hospitalizations. Both vaccines were safe and were not associated with increased risk of intussusception. In February 2006, RotaTeq was licensed in the United States and abroad. Rotarix is currently licensed in Mexico, Latin America, and Europe.[137,139]

REFERENCES

1. Assis AM, et al. Growth faltering in childhood related to diarrhea: A longitudinal community based study. Eur J Clin Nutr 2005;59:1317–23.
2. Victora CG, et al. Reducing deaths from diarrhoea through oral rehydration therapy. Bull World Health Organ 2000;78:1246–55.
3. Guerrant RL, Carneiro-Filho BA, Dillingham RA. Cholera, diarrhea, and oral rehydration therapy: Triumph and indictment. Clin Infect Dis 2003;37:398–405.
4. Bryce J, et al. WHO estimates of the causes of death in children. Lancet 2005;365:1147–52.
5. Bern C, et al. The magnitude of the global problem of diarrhoeal disease: A ten-year update. Bull World Health Organ 1992;70:705–14.
6. Guerrant RL, et al. Magnitude and impact of diarrheal diseases. Arch Med Res 2002;33:351–5.
7. WHO, DDC. Persistent Diarrhea in Children. Geneva: WHO; 1985.
8. WHO. The Treatment of Diarrhea. A Manual for Physicians and Other Senior Health Workers. Geneva: WHO; 2005. p. WHO/CDD/SER/80.2.
9. Malek MA, et al. Diarrhea- and rotavirus-associated hospitalizations among children less than 5 years of age: United States, 1997 and 2000. Pediatrics 2006;117:1887–92.
10. Avendano P, et al. Costs associated with office visits for diarrhea in infants and toddlers. Pediatr Infect Dis J 1993; 12:897–902.
11. Guandalini S, et al. *Lactobacillus* GG administered in oral rehydration solution to children with acute diarrhea: A multicenter European trial. J Pediatr Gastroenterol Nutr 2000;30:54–60.
12. Nataro JP, et al. Diarrheagenic *Escherichia coli* infection in Baltimore, Maryland, and New Haven, Connecticut. Clin Infect Dis 2006;43:402–7.
13. Bresee J, et al. Foodborne viral gastroenteritis: Challenges and opportunities. Clin Infect Dis 2002;35:748–53.
14. Cohen J, West A, Bini E. Infectious diarrhea in human immunodeficiency virus. Gastroenterol Clin North Am 2001;30:637–64.
15. McFarland L, Brandmarker S, Guandalini S. Pediatric *Clostridium difficile*: A phantom menace or clinical reality? J Pediatr Gastroenterol Nutr 2000;31:220–31.
16. Enav B, et al. Acute appendicitis presenting as secretory diarrhea. J Pediatr Surg 2002;37:928–9.
17. Kockerling A, Fromm M. Origin of cAMP-dependent Cl_2 secretion from both crypts and surface epithelia of rat intestine. Am J Physiol Cell Physiol 1993;264:C1294–301.
18. Wright E. et al. Regulation of Na^+/glucose cotransporters. J Exp Biol 1997;200:287–93.
19. Mailliard M, Stevens B, Mann G, Amino acid transport by small intestinal, hepatic, and pancreatic epithelia. Gastroenterology 1995;108:888–910.
20. Munck L, Munck B. Amino acid transport in the small intestine. Physiol Res 1994;43:335–46.
21. Terada T, et al. Expression profiles of various transporters for oligopeptides, amino acids and organic ions along the human digestive tract. Biochem Pharmacol 2005;70: 1756–63.
22. Sundaram U, Wisel S, Coon S. Mechanism of inhibition of proton: Dipeptide co-transport during chronic enteritis in the mammalian small intestine. Biochim Biophys Acta 2005;1714:134–40.
23. Seidler U, et al. Molecular mechanisms of disturbed electrolyte transport in intestinal inflammation. Ann N Y Acad Sci 2006;1072:262–75.
24. Burckhardt G, Di Sole F, Helmle-Kolb C. The Na^+/H^+ exchanger gene family. J Nephrol 2002;15 :S3–21.
25. Zachos NC, Tse M, Donowitz M. Molecular physiology of intestinal Na^+/H^+ exchange. Annu Rev Physiol 2005;67:411–43.
26. Putney L, Denker S, Barber D. Na^+/H^+ exchanger, NHE1: Structure, regulation, and cellular actions. Annu Rev Pharmacol Toxicol 2002;42:527–52.
27. Binder HJ, et al. Bicarbonate secretion: A neglected aspect of colonic ion transport. J Clin Gastroenterol 2005;39: S53–8.
28. Farthing MJ. Antisecretory drugs for diarrheal disease. Dig Dis 2006;24:47–58.
29. Guerrant R, et al. How intestinal bacteria cause disease. J Infect Dis 1999;179 :S331–7.
30. Kunzelmann K, Mal LM. Electrolyte transport in the mammalian colon: Mechanisms and implications for disease. Physiol Rev 2002;82:245–89.
31. Nocerino A, Iafusco M, Guandalini S. Cholera toxin-induced small intestinal secretion has a secretory effect on the colon of the rat. Gastroenterology 1995;108:34–9.
32. Kunzelmann K. The cystic fibrosis transmembrane conductance regulator and its function in epithelial transport. Rev Physiol Biochem Pharmacol 1999;137:1–70.
33. Fasano A, Baudry B, Pumplin D. Vibrio cholerae produces a second enterotoxin, which affects intestinal tight junctions. Proc Natl Acad Sci U S A 1991;88:5242–6.

34. Fasano A, et al. The enterotoxic effect of zonula occludens toxin on rabbit small intestine involves the paracellular pathway. Gastroenterology 1997;112:839–46.
35. Estes MK, et al. Pathogenesis of rotavirus gastroenteritis. Novartis Found Symp 2001;238:82–96; discussion 96–100.
36. Obert G, Peiffer I, Servin AL. Rotavirus-induced structural and functional alterations in tight junctions of polarized intestinal Caco-2 cell monolayers. J Virol 2000;74:4645–51.
37. Dong Y, et al. The rotavirus enterotoxin NSP4 mobilizes intracellular calcium in human intestinal cells by stimulating phospholipase C-mediated inositol 1,4,5-trisphosphate production. Proc Natl Acad Sci U S A 1997;94:3960–5.
38. Canani RB, et al. Effects of HIV-1 Tat protein on ion secretion and on cell proliferation in human intestinal epithelial cells. Gastroenterology 2003;124:368–76.
39. Coffin SE, et al. Impact of acute rotavirus gastroenteritis on pediatric outpatient practices in the United States. Pediatr Infect Dis J 2006;25:584–9.
40. Vernacchio L, et al. Diarrhea in American infants and young children in the community setting: Incidence, clinical presentation and microbiology. Pediatr Infect Dis J 2006;25:2–7.
41. Fauveau V, et al. Effect on mortality of community-based maternity-care programme in rural Bangladesh. Lancet 1991;338:1183–6.
42. Victora CG, et al. Deaths due to dysentery, acute and persistent diarrhoea among Brazilian infants. Acta Paediatr 1992;381:7–11.
43. Kukuruzovic RH, Brewster DR. Small bowel intestinal permeability in Australian aboriginal children. J Pediatr Gastroenterol Nutr 2002;35:206–12.
44. Guandalini S, Mazzarella G, Fontana M. Childhood acute diarrhoea in Italy [abstract]. Pediatr Res 1988;24:A414.
45. Guarino A, et al. Heat stable enterotoxin produced by *Escherichia coli* in acute diarrhoea. Arch Dis Child 1989;64:808–13.
46. King CK, et al. Managing acute gastroenteritis among children: Oral rehydration, maintenance, and nutritional therapy. MMWR Recomm Rep 2003;52:1–16.
47. Cash RA, et al. Rapid correction of acidosis and dehydration of cholera with oral electrolyte and glucose solution. Lancet 1970;2:549–50.
48. Field M, et al. Effect of cholera enterotoxin on ion transport across isolated ileal mucosa. J Clin Invest 1972;51:796–804.
49. Hirschhorn N, et al. Decrease in net stool output in cholera during intestinal perfusion with glucose-containing solutions. N Engl J Med 1968;279:176–81.
50. Guandalini S, et al. Cyclic guanosine monophosphate effects on nutrient and electrolyte transport in rabbit ileum. Gastroenterology 1982;83:15–21.
51. Hartling L, et al. Oral versus intravenous rehydration for treating dehydration due to gastroenteritis in children. Cochrane Database Syst Rev 2006;3:CD004390.
52. Bellemare, S, et al. Oral rehydration versus intravenous therapy for treating dehydration due to gastroenteritis in children: A meta-analysis of randomised controlled trials. BMC Med 2004;2:11.
53. Thillainayagam AV, Hunt JB, Farthing MJ. Enhancing clinical efficacy of oral rehydration therapy: Is low osmolality the key? Gastroenterology 1998;114:197–210.
54. Booth I, et al. Recommendations for composition of oral rehydration solutions for the children of Europe. J Pediatr Gastroenterol Nutr 1992;14:113–5.
55. Hahn S, Kim S, Garner P. Reduced osmolarity oral rehydration solution for treating dehydration caused by acute diarrhoea in children. Cochrane Database Syst Rev 2002: CD002847.
56. Khan AM, et al. Low osmolar oral rehydration salts solution in the treatment of acute watery diarrhoea in neonates and young infants: A randomized, controlled clinical trial. J Health Popul Nutr 2005;23:52–7.
57. World Health Organization. Oral Rehydration Salts (ORS): A New Reduced Osmolarity Formulation. Geneva: WHO; 2002.
58. Murphy C, Hahn S, Volmink J. Reduced osmolarity oral rehydration solution for treating cholera. Cochrane Database Syst Rev 2004:CD003754.
59. Ramakrishna BS, et al. Amylase-resistant starch plus oral rehydration solution for cholera. N Engl J Med 2000;342: 308–13.
60. Hoekstra JH, et al. Oral rehydration solution containing a mixture of non-digestible carbohydrates in the treatment of acute diarrhea: A multicenter randomized placebo controlled study on behalf of the ESPGHAN working group on intestinal infections. J Pediatr Gastroenterol Nutr 2004;39:239–45.
61. Raghupathy P, et al. Amylase-resistant starch as adjunct to oral rehydration therapy in children with diarrhea. J Pediatr Gastroenterol Nutr 2006;42:362–8.
62. Subramanya S, et al. Evaluation of oral rehydration solution by whole-gut perfusion in rats: Effect of osmolarity, sodium concentration and resistant starch. J Pediatr Gastroenterol Nutr 2006;43:568–75.
63. Szajewska H, Hoekstra JH, Sandhu B. Management of acute gastroenteritis in Europe and the impact of the new recommendations: A multicenter study. The Working Group on acute Diarrhoea of the European Society for Paediatric Gastroenterology, Hepatology, and Nutrition. J Pediatr Gastroenterol Nutr 2000;30:522–7.
64. Provisional Committee on Quality Improvement Subcommittee on Acute Gastroenteritis. Practice parameter: The management of acute gastroenteritis in young children. Pediatrics 1996;97:423–36.
65. Spandorfer PR, et al. Oral versus intravenous rehydration of moderately dehydrated children: A randomized, controlled trial. Pediatrics 2005;115:295–301.
66. Morrow AL, Rangel JM. Human milk protection against infectious diarrhea: Implications for prevention and clinical care. Semin Pediatr Infect Dis 2004;15:221–8.
67. Morrow AL, et al. Human milk oligosaccharides are associated with protection against diarrhea in breast-fed infants. J Pediatr 2004;145:297–303.
68. Brown KH. Dietary management of acute diarrheal disease: Contemporary scientific issues. J Nutr 1994;124: 1455S–60S.
69. Bhandari N, et al. Effect of community-based promotion of exclusive breastfeeding on diarrhoeal illness and growth: A cluster randomised controlled trial. Lancet 2003;361:1418–23.
70. Bhattacharya SK, et al. Risk factors for development of dehydration in young children with acute watery diarrhoea: A case-control study. Acta Paediatr 1995;84:160–4.
71. Isolauri E, et al. Milk versus no milk in rapid refeeding after acute gastroenteritis. J Pediatr Gastroenterol Nutr 1986;5:254–61.
72. Sandhu BK, et al. A multicentre study on behalf of the European Society of Paediatric Gastroenterology and Nutrition Working Group on Acute Diarrhoea. Early feeding in childhood gastroenteritis. J Pediatr Gastroenterol Nutr 1997;24:522–7.
73. Isolauri E, et al. Intestinal permeability changes in acute gastroenteritis: Effects of clinical factors and nutritional management. J Pediatr Gastroenterol Nutr 1989;8:466–73.
74. Baker SS, Davis AM. Hypocaloric oral therapy during an episode of diarrhea and vomiting can lead to severe malnutrition. J Pediatr Gastroenterol Nutr 1998;27:1–5.
75. Penny ME, Brown KH. Lactose feeding during persistent diarrhoea. Acta Paediatr;381:133–8.
76. Walker-Smith JA, et al. Guidelines prepared by the ESPGAN Working Group on Acute Diarrhoea. Recommendations for feeding in childhood gastroenteritis. European Society of Pediatric Gastroenterology and Nutrition. J Pediatr Gastroenterol Nutr 1997;24:619–20.
77. Sandhu BK. Rationale for early feeding in childhood gastroenteritis. J Pediatr Gastroenterol Nutr 2001;33 :S13–6.
78. Brown KH, Peerson JM, Fontaine O. Use of nonhuman milks in the dietary management of young children with acute diarrhea: A meta-analysis of clinical trials. Pediatrics 1994;93:17–27.
79. Boudraa G, et al. Effect of feeding yogurt versus milk in children with acute diarrhea and carbohydrate malabsorption. J Pediatr Gastroenterol Nutr 2001;33:307–13.
80. Rabbani GH, et al. Clinical studies in persistent diarrhea: Dietary management with green banana or pectin in Bangladeshi children. Gastroenterology 2001;121:554–60.
81. Sandhu B, et al. Practical guidelines for the management of gastroenteritis in children. J Pediatr Gastroenterol Nutr 2001;33:S36–9.
82. Wong CS, et al. The risk of the hemolytic-uremic syndrome after antibiotic treatment of Escherichia coli O157:H7 infections. N Engl J Med 2000;342:1930–6.
83. Leibovitz E, et al. Oral ciprofloxacin vs. intramuscular ceftriaxone as empiric treatment of acute invasive diarrhea in children. Pediatr Infect Dis J 2000;19:1060–7.
84. Geme JW, III, et al. Consensus: Management of Salmonella infection in the first year of life. Pediatr Infect Dis J 1988;7:615–21.
85. Roy SK, et al. Randomised controlled trial of zinc supplementation in malnourished Bangladeshi children with acute diarrhoea. Arch Dis Child 1997;77:196–200.
86. Bahl R, et al. Efficacy of zinc-fortified oral rehydration solution in 6- to 35-month-old children with acute diarrhea. J Pediatr 2002;141:677–82.
87. Baqui AH, et al. Effect of zinc supplementation started during diarrhoea on morbidity and mortality in Bangladeshi children: Community randomised trial. BMJ 2002;325: 1059.
88. Bhandari N, et al. Substantial reduction in severe diarrheal morbidity by daily zinc supplementation in young north Indian children. Pediatrics 2002;109:e86.
89. Robberstad B, et al. Cost-effectiveness of zinc as adjunct therapy for acute childhood diarrhoea in developing countries. Bull World Health Organ 2004;82:523–31.
90. Strand TA, et al. Effectiveness and efficacy of zinc for the treatment of acute diarrhea in young children. Pediatrics 2002;109:898–903.
91. Joint Statement World Health Organization and UNICEF. Clinical management of acute diarrhoea. WHO Bulletin 2004.
92. Nasrin D, et al. Acceptability of and adherence to dispersible zinc tablet in the treatment of acute childhood diarrhoea. J Health Popul Nutr 2005;23:215–21.
93. Larson CP, et al. Initiation of zinc treatment for acute childhood diarrhoea and risk for vomiting or regurgitation: A randomized, double-blind, placebo-controlled trial. J Health Popul Nutr 2005;23:311–9.
94. Fischer Walker CL, et al. Zinc supplementation for the treatment of diarrhea in infants in Pakistan, India and Ethiopia. J Pediatr Gastroenterol Nutr 2006;43:357–63.
95. Guarino A, et al. Oral immunoglobulins for treatment of acute rotaviral gastroenteritis. Pediatrics 1994;93:12–6.
96. Guarino A, et al. Enteral immunoglobulins for treatment of protracted rotaviral diarrhea. Pediatr Infect Dis J 1991;10:612–4.
97. Kanfer EJ, et al. Severe rotavirus-associated diarrhoea following bone marrow transplantation: Treatment with oral immunoglobulin. Bone Marrow Transplant 1994;14:651–2.
98. Sarker SA, et al. Successful treatment of rotavirus diarrhea in children with immunoglobulin from immunized bovine colostrum. Pediatr Infect Dis J 1998;17:1149–54.
99. Mohan P, Haque K. Oral immunoglobulin for the prevention of rotavirus infection in low birth weight infants. Cochrane Database Syst Rev 2003:CD003740.
100. Barnes GL, et al. A randomised trial of oral gammaglobulin in low-birth-weight infants infected with rotavirus. Lancet 1982;1:1371–3.
101. Szilagyi A, Shrier I. Systematic review: The use of somatostatin or octreotide in refractory diarrhoea. Aliment Pharmacol Ther 2001;15:189–197.
102. Matheson A, Noble S. Racecadotril. Drugs 2000;59:829–35.
103. Primi M, et al. Racecadotril demonstrates intestinal antisecretory activity in vivo. Aliment Pharmacol Ther 1999;13:3–7.
104. Turvill J, Farthing M. Enkephalins and enkephalinase inhibitors in intestinal fluid and electrolyte transport. Eur J Gastro Hepatol 1997;9:877–880.
105. Hinterleitner T, Petritsch W, Dimsity G. Acetorphan prevents cholera-toxin-induced water and electrolyte secretion in the human jejunum. Eur J Gastroenterol Hepatol 1997;9:887–91.
106. Prado D. A multinational comparison of racecadotril and loperamide in the treatment of watery diarrhoea in adults. Scand J Gastroenterol 2002;37:656–661.
107. Wang HH, Shieh MJ, Liao KF. A blind, randomized comparison of racecadotril and loperamide for stopping acute diarrhea in adults. World J Gastroenterol 2005;11:1540–3.
108. Cezard J, Duhamel J, Meyer M. Efficacy and tolerability of racecadotril in acute diarrhea in children. Gastroenterology 2001;120:799–805.
109. Salazar-Lindo E, et al. Racecadotril in the treatment of acute watery diarrhea in children. N Engl J Med 2000;343:463–7.
110. Turck D, et al. Comparison of racecadotril and loperamide in children with acute diarrhoea. Aliment Pharmacol Ther 1999;13: 27–32.
111. Nucera E, et al. Hypersensitivity to racecadotril: A case report. Eur J Pediatr 2006:1–2.
112. Bengmark S. Ecological control of the gastrointestinal tract. The role of probiotic flora. Gut 1998;42:2–7.
113. Goldin B, Gorbach S, Saxelin M. Survival of Lactobacillus species (strain GG) in human gastrointestinal tract. Dig Dis Sci 1992;37:121–8.
114. Guandalini S. Probiotics for children: Use in diarrhea. J Clin Gastroenterol 2006;40:244–8.
115. Van Niel CW, et al. Lactobacillus therapy for acute infectious diarrhea in children: A meta-analysis. Pediatrics 2002;109:678–84.
116. Thibault H, Aubert-Jacquin C, Goulet O. Effects of long-term consumption of a fermented infant formula (with *Bifidobacterium breve* c50 and *Streptococcus thermophilus* 065) on acute diarrhea in healthy infants. J Pediatr Gastroenterol Nutr 2004;39:147–52.
117. Chouraqui JP, Van Egroo LD, Fichot MC. Acidified milk formula supplemented with bifidobacterium lactis: Impact on infant diarrhea in residential care settings. J Pediatr Gastroenterol Nutr 2004;38:288–92.
118. Oberhelman RA, et al. A placebo-controlled trial of *Lactobacillus* GG to prevent diarrhea in undernourished Peruvian children. J Pediatr 1999;134:15–20.
119. Szajewska H, et al. Efficacy of *Lactobacillus* GG in prevention of nosocomial diarrhea in infants. J Pediatr 2001;138:361–5.

120. Mastretta E, et al. Effect of *Lactobacillus* GG and breast-feeding in the prevention of rotavirus nosocomial infection. J Pediatr Gastroenterol Nutr 2002;35:527–31.

121. Can M, et al. Prophylactic *Saccharomyces boulardii* in the prevention of antibiotic-associated diarrhea: A prospective study. Med Sci Monit 2006;12:PI19–22.

122. Correa NB, et al. A randomized formula controlled trial of *Bifidobacterium lactis* and *Streptococcus thermophilus* for prevention of antibiotic-associated diarrhea in infants. J Clin Gastroenterol 2005;39:385–9.

123. Dendukuri N, et al. Probiotic therapy for the prevention and treatment of *Clostridium difficile*-associated diarrhea: A systematic review. CMAJ 2005;173:167–70.

124. Duman DG, et al. Efficacy and safety of *Saccharomyces boulardii* in prevention of antibiotic-associated diarrhoea due to *Helicobacterpylori eradication*. Eur J Gastroenterol Hepatol 2005;17:1357–61.

125. Erdeve O, Tiras U, Dallar Y. The probiotic effect of *Saccharomyces boulardii* in a pediatric age group. J Trop Pediatr 2004;50:234–6.

126. Kotowska M, Albrecht P, Szajewska H. *Saccharomyces boulardii* in the prevention of antibiotic-associated diarrhoea in children: A randomized double-blind placebo-controlled trial. Aliment Pharmacol Ther 2005;21:583–90.

127. Vanderhoof JA, et al. *Lactobacillus* GG in the prevention of antibiotic-associated diarrhea in children. J Pediatr 1999;135:564–8.

128. Arvola T, et al. Prophylactic *Lactobacillus* GG reduces antibiotic-associated diarrhea in children with respiratory infections: A randomized study. Pediatrics 1999;104:e64.

129. Szajewska H, Ruszczynski M, Radzikowski A. Probiotics in the prevention of antibiotic-associated diarrhea in children: A meta-analysis of randomized controlled trials. J Pediatr 2006;149:367–72.

130. McFarland LV. Meta-analysis of probiotics for the prevention of antibiotic associated diarrhea and the treatment of *Clostridium difficile* disease. Am J Gastroenterol 2006;101:812–22.

131. Land MH, et al. *Lactobacillus sepsis* associated with probiotic therapy. Pediatrics 2005;115:178–81.

132. Riquelme AJ, et al. *Saccharomyces cerevisiae* fungemia after *Saccharomyces boulardii* treatment in immunocompromised patients. J Clin Gastroenterol 2003;36:41–3.

133. Kunz AN, Noel JM, Fairchok MP. Two cases of *Lactobacillus bacteremia* during probiotic treatment of short gut syndrome. J Pediatr Gastroenterol Nutr 2004;38:457–8.

134. Luby SP, et al. Effect of handwashing on child health: A randomised controlled trial. Lancet 2005;366:225–33.

135. Sheth M, Obrah M. Diarrhea prevention through food safety education. Indian J Pediatr 2004;71:879–82.

136. Saleemi MA, et al. Feeding patterns, diarrhoeal illness and linear growth in 0-24-month-old children. J Trop Pediatr 2004;50:164–9.

137. O'Ryan M, Matson DO. New rotavirus vaccines: Renewed optimism. J Pediatr 2006;149:448–51.

138. Vesikari T, et al. Safety and efficacy of a pentavalent human-bovine (WC3) reassortant rotavirus vaccine. N Engl J Med 2006;354:23–33.

139. Dennehy PH. Rotavirus vaccines: An update. Pediatr Infect Dis J 2006;25:839–40.

15.2b. Persistent Diarrhea

Alfredo Guarino, MD
Giulio De Marco, MD

Diarrheal disorders are a major health problem in children worldwide.[1] Studies published in the last ten years, indicate that the global incidence remains unchanged at about 3.2 episodes per child year, despite reduction in mortality.[1,2] Most diarrheal diseases resolve in 1 week but a small, although consistent number of cases, persist beyond this time. Especially in developing countries, these cases are associated with a relatively high risk of mortality, accounting for most of diarrheal-associated fatalities.[2]

Persistent diarrhea is defined as a diarrheal episode that lasts for 14 days or more.[3,4] However the concept of persistent diarrhea is evolving and different definitions have been applied to different clinical conditions. The classical definition of persistent diarrhea was intended to exclude specific causes of chronic diarrhea such as celiac disease or inflammatory bowel diseases. The difficulties in differentiating diarrhea at its onset and predicting its duration, and the possibility that a chronic diarrhea may begin acutely, support the concept that persistent diarrhea is mainly defined by its eventual duration. In this respect, persistent diarrhea is not different from chronic diarrhea whose conventional duration is at least 14 days. However, the term persistent diarrhea is more related to an acute onset diarrhea that continues behind the expected duration of an infectious diarrhea. Narrowing the spectrum, persistent diarrhea may be defined as a protracted diarrhea, ie, diarrhea that persists for more than 2 weeks and is associated with weight loss, ultimately leading to severe nutritional impairment, which may require clinical nutrition and, in selected cases, intestinal transplantation. The definition of persistent diarrhea thus encompasses a wide spectrum of conditions ranging from long-lasting infectious diarrhea to intractable diarrhea, which implies, in its classical definition, a high risk of death.

As persistent diarrhea is a clinical condition resulting from many different causes, many etiologies are only briefly cited in the present chapter and are reported with more detail in other chapters of the textbook.

EPIDEMIOLOGY

The incidence and prevalence of persistent diarrhea show a distinct pattern in developing and developed countries. Studies from Asia, Latin America, and Africa, support an average incidence of persistent diarrhea as high as 10% of all cases of diarrhea, ranging from 5 to 25% in different settings.[5-7] In the light of the burden of infectious diarrhea, persistent diarrhea has a major impact in developing countries. In developed countries, the incidence of persistent diarrhea is inadequately documented. A report from the United Kingdom indicates an incidence of 3 to 5%[8] but a recent study in a cohort of US children reports that more than 8% of diarrheal episodes last more than 14 days.[9] More importantly, mortality rates associated to persistent diarrhea are dramatically high in developing countries (23 to 62%) and are responsible for most of diarrhea-associated deaths. Limited data on the general incidence of persistent diarrhea-related fatal outcomes are available in western countries. However recent observations suggest a generally benign illness,[9] with the exception of the so-called intractable diarrhea syndrome.[10] These epidemiological differences clearly indicate that persistent diarrhea is a distinct disease in developing and developed countries. The concept of two substantially different clinical conditions is supported by studies on primary causes, and on risk factors responsible for persistent diarrhea in the two socioeconomical and environmental settings.

PATHOPHYSIOLOGY

The pathophysiologic mechanisms of persistent diarrhea are generally divided into secretory and osmotic but, in several cases, diarrhea is the result of both mechanisms. Secretory diarrhea is usually associated with large volumes of watery stools, and persists even when oral food is withdrawn. In contrast, osmotic diarrhea is dependent on oral feeding, and stool volumes are usually not as massive as in secretory diarrhea.

Secretory Diarrhea

It is characterized by increased electrolyte and water fluxes toward the intestinal lumen, resulting from either the inhibition of neutral NaCl absorption by villous enterocytes and the increase in electrogenic chloride secretion by secretory crypt cells. The classic example of secretory diarrhea is that induced by *Vibrio cholerae* and enterotoxigenic *E. coli* (ETEC). Cholera toxin produced by *V. cholerae* binds to specific enterocyte membrane receptors activating the adenyl cyclase, through the stimulation of an enterocyte G protein. The resulting increase in intracellular cAMP, in turn, activates specific signaling proteins, inducing the opening of chloride channels. Intestinal fluid secretion predominantly results from electrogenic chloride secretion through the activation of the cystic fibrosis transmembrane regulator (CFTR) chloride channel, located on the apical membrane of the enterocyte. The other components of the enterocyte ion secretory machinery are (Figure 1): (1) the Na:K:2Cl cotransporter for the electroneutral chloride entrance into the enterocyte; (2) the Na:K pump, which decreases the intracellular Na^+ concentration, determining the driving gradient for further Na^+ inlet; (3) the K^+ selective channel, that enables intracellular K^+, once entered because of coupled Na^+ movement, to return to the extracellular fluid.

Chloride secretion, in response to cholera or cholera-like toxins, is mediated by the upregulation of intracellular concentration of cAMP. Other enterotoxins induce intestinal secretion through the activation of cGMP or a rise in intracellular calcium concentration. Recently, another intracellular mediator, nitric oxide, was proposed as a key factor controlling chloride secretion.[11] The classic concept that only bacteria induce secretory diarrhea has now been challenged by the evidence of similar ion secretion pathways induced by viruses and protozoan agents. Rotavirus, the most frequent agent of infectious diarrhea produces a nonstructural protein (NSP4) that stimulates calcium-mediated chloride secretion.[12] Also HIV induces secretory diarrhea: a protein expressed by HIV, the trans-activating transfer factor Tat, acts as an enterotoxin upregulating intracellular calcium concentration.[13] Eukaryotic microorganisms may also produce enterotoxins. The protozoan *Cryptosporidium parvum*, a major agent of severe and protracted diarrhea in immunocompromised children,[14] induces secretory diarrhea through an enterotoxic activity that has been detected in stools, and is able to induce chloride secretion, through a calcium-mediated pathway.[15] Secretory diarrhea may also be of noninfectious nature. Several hormones and neurotransmitters have been implicated in intestinal secretion, as part of a complex neuroendocrine network which integrates the intestinal response to external stimuli.[16] Electrolyte secretion can be activated by microbial enterotoxins or by other secretagogues of endocrine or nonendocrine origin (Table 1). Also inflammatory cytokines, such

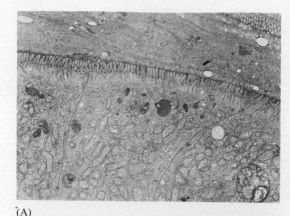

(A)

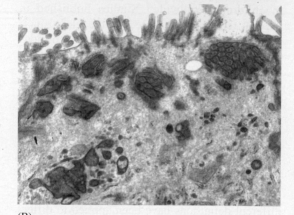

(B)

Figure 1 Components of the secretory machinery in the intestinal epithelial cell. The intestinal crypt cells maintain a secretory tone by a balanced movement of anions and cations through the epithelial monolayer. The Na:K:2Cl cotransporter is responsible for the elecroneutral chloride entrance, from the basolateral membrane, into the enterocyte. The Na:K pump decreases the intracellular Na^+ concentration, indirectly determining a driving gradient for chloride entrance, and the K^+ selective channel enables intracellular K^+ to return to the extracellular fluid. The upregulation of cAMP, cGMP, or Ca^{2+} induces active chloride secretion of the enterocyte, through chloride channels, such as the cystic fibrosis transmembrane regulator (CFTR), located onto the apical membrane of the enterocyte.

as IL1, may exert a direct secretory effect on the enterocyte[17] (Table 1). In microvillous inclusion disease, a genetic developmental disorder involving the brush border, functioning absorptive surface is reduced, and a severe secretory diarrhea is present (Figure 2).

A different mechanism of secretory diarrhea is the inhibition of the electroneutral NaCl-coupled pathway that involves the Na^+–H^+ and the Cl^-–HCO_3^- antiporters. Defects in the genes of the Na^+–H^+ and the Cl^-–HCO_3^- exchangers are responsible for congenital Na^+ and Cl^- diarrhea, respectively.[18]

Osmotic Diarrhea

Osmotic diarrhea is caused by the presence of nonabsorbed nutrients in the gastrointestinal tract, and is generally associated with an intestinal damage. The osmotic force driving water into the lumen is provided by nonabsorbed solutes either deriving from food or from injured mucosa. A classic example of osmotic diarrhea is lactose intolerance associated to congenital or acquired lactose intolerance. Lactose, being not absorbed in the

small intestine, reaches the colon in its intact form. The colonic microflora ferment the sugar to short-chain organic acids, generating an osmotic load which drives water into the lumen. The ingestion of sugar-containing carbonated fluids exceeding the transport capacity, as well as the ingestion of magnesium salts and sorbitol, both not absorbed, also results in an osmotic load.

In general, osmotic diarrhea occurs whenever digestion and/or absorption are impaired. Reduction or absence of pancreatic enzymes, and bile acid disorders are responsible for impaired digestion. Intestinal villi are blunted in overt celiac disease because of antigen-driven immune response. In short bowel syndrome, surgical removal of a large portion of the intestine leaves just not enough of absorbing intestine. Intestinal absorption depends on intact epithelium but also on adequate time for digestion and contact between the nutrients and the absorptive surface. Thus, alterations in intestinal transit times, particularly reductions in small intestinal and whole gut transit times, may result in impaired nutrient, electrolyte, and water intestinal absorption. Finally, increased gut permeability,

Figure 2 Ultrastructural evaluation of enterocytes. (A) Enterocytes show signs of mild, nonspecific damage; microvilli look shorter than normal; cytoplasm is normal with the exception of an increased vacuolization. (Courtesy of M. Morroni, Ancona, Italy.) (B) Microvillous inclusion disease is characterized by loss and disorganization of microvilli of the brush border. In the cytoplasm secretory granules and inclusion bodies with microvilli are evident. (Courtesy of A. Phillips, London, UK.)

secondary to inflammation or cytotoxic agents, is responsible for excessive protein loss as in protein-losing enteropathies. Infectious agents induce diarrhea with an osmotic mechanism when they are responsible of a direct epithelial or mucosal damage as in case of enteroadherent (EAEC) or enteropathogenic *E. coli* (EPEC) (Figure 3).

However various pathways generally contribute to persistent diarrhea, intersecting each other and often producing a synergic vicious circle. A paradigm of the complex pathophysiology of persistent diarrhea is provided by HIV infection. Chronic diarrhea is considered as an AIDS-defining condition in the classification scheme for pediatric HIV infection.[19] Malnutrition can be an early manifestation of HIV infection and is associated with a rapid decrease in CD4+ cell number and an increased rate of opportunistic infections.[20] A long list of combined dysfunctions of the digestive–absorptive processes is observed in 60 to 80% of children with HIV infection naïve to antiretroviral therapy, and may involve the intestine, the liver, and the pancreas.[21] Clinical manifestations of the so-called HIV enteropathy may be limited but iron and lactose malabsorption are very common features.[22] Overall nutrient malabsorption certainly contributes to malnutrition, and eventually to wasting, the terminal feature of HIV

Table 1 Main Factors Determining Electrolyte and Water Secretion

Cyclic adenosine monophosphate (cAMP)-dependent
   Bacterial enterotoxins: *Vibrio cholerae*, *E. coli* (heat-labile), *Shigella*, *Salmonella*, *Campylobacter*, *Pseudomonas*
   Hormones: vasoactive intestinal peptide (VIP), gastrin, secretin
   Anion surfactants: bile acids, ricinoleic acid

Cyclic guanosine monophosphate (cGMP)-dependent
   Bacterial enterotoxins: *E. coli* (heat-stable) enterotoxin, *Klebsiella pneumoniae*, *Citrobacter freundii*, *Yersinia enterocolitica* enterotoxin
   Hormones: guanylin

Calcium-dependent
   Bacterial enterotoxin: *Clostridium*
   Protozoal enterotoxin: *Cryptosporidium*
   Viral enterotoxins: Rotavirus NSP4, HIV Tat
   Endogenous factors: hystamin, IL1β, IL8, bradykinin, cholecystokinin
   Neurohormones: acetylcholine, serotonin, galanin

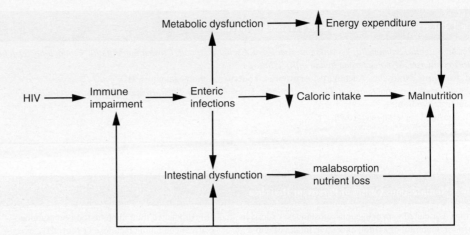

Figure 4 Pathways of malnutrition in HIV-infected children. A complex interplay exists among several conditions, leading to malnutrition in HIV-infected children. Enteric infections and intestinal dysfunction are major determinants of wasting, an AIDS defining condition.

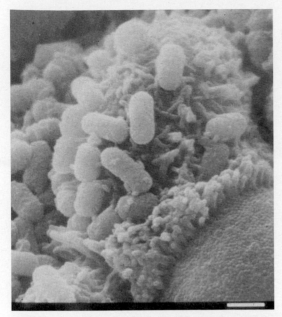

Figure 3 Enteropathogenic *E. coli* adhesion to intestinal epithelial cells. Adherence is the first stage of Enteropathogenic *E. coli* (EPEC)-induced diarrhea. Following that, a number of bacterial proteins are translocated by a type III secretion system, driving the enterocyte effacement, pedestal formation, and intimate bacterial attachment to the host cell. (Courtesy of A. Phillips, London, UK.)

infection. The pathophysiology of intestinal dysfunction is complex and involves multiple factors. There is little evidence of a role of specific enteric pathogens in HIV-associated intestinal dysfunction, even though Cryptosporidium is specifically responsible for intestinal inflammation and secondary digestive abnormalities in these children.[23] A role by HIV itself has been hypothesized, and recent data showed that Tat protein released by the virus, functions both as a viral cytotoxin and as an enterotoxin, directly interacting with the enterocyte to impair cell growth and proliferation, as well as ion transport and glucose absorption.[13,24] The role of HIV in intestinal dysfunction is supported by the finding that children shifted to highly active antiretroviral therapy showed a rapid normalization of intestinal function tests, in parallel with a decrease in viral load and an increase in CD4+ cell number.[25] Interestingly, it was also shown that nutritional rehabilitation is effective in the improvement of the immune status, thus supporting the cause–effect relationship between malnutrition, intestinal dysfunction and immune derangement.[26] Thus HIV-associated intestinal dysfunction, malnutrition, and immune impairment produce a vicious circle, and represent the paradigm of the high risk for persistent diarrhea and its high mortality in poor countries, following intestinal infections (Figure 4).

RISK FACTORS FOR PERSISTENT DIARRHEA

Most studies on risk factors for persistent diarrhea have been performed in developing countries. Protein energy malnutrition appears to be the most relevant risk factor for an intestinal

infection to evolve into persistent diarrhea. The coexistence of malnutrition in children with infectious diarrhea consistently increases the probability of a protracted duration, with an inverse correlation between nutritional status and severity of diarrhea.[27,28] Also specific micronutrient deficiencies are related to persistent diarrhea. Vitamin A and zinc deficiencies are significantly associated with persistent diarrhea, and clinical trials assessing the efficacy of their supplementation support these observations.[29–34] Infants who are not breast fed are at increased risk of persistent diarrhea, whereas prolonged breast feeding is a protective factor.[28–35] As malnutrition is also associated with extraintestinal infections, persistent diarrhea is significantly associated with a broad range of health problems such as pneumonia, urinary tract infections, and anemia.[36] Prior illnesses have also been implicated in triggering protracted diarrhea and, among them, measles carries an increased risk for diarrhea, which may persist as long as 6 months, because of its immunosuppressive effect.[37] The major etiology of acquired immune suppression, the HIV infection, is the leading underlying condition of persistent diarrhea in developing countries, where access to effective antiretroviral therapies is limited or not available.[38] Classic enteropathogenic agents, including Shigella and Enterotoxigenic *E. coli*, have been implicated as agents of persistent diarrhea in developing countries.[39,40] In contrast, in the United States, rotavirus and norovirus were associated with long-lasting diarrhea.[9]

A diarrhea presenting with increased severity at its onset may be associated with an increased risk of long duration, especially when malnutrition is present.[41] Persistent diarrhea is generally more frequent in males with a male/female ratio between 1.2/1 and 2.6/1, and in the age range of 6 to 24 months.[6,28,39] Mother's age may also be a determinant of persistent diarrhea, with an increased risk found in children born to younger mothers.[42,43] The use of antibiotics for acute gastroenteritis is not generally recommended and has been reported as a specific risk for persistent diarrhea.[28] Recently, a deficiency of mannose-binding lectin, a component of the

innate immune system, was associated with *Cryptosporidium*-associated persistent diarrhea.[44]

On the other side, risk factors for persistent diarrhea also exists in developed countries and depend on the specific etiology of persistent diarrhea. As already mentioned, selected viruses have been associated with persistent diarrhea.[9] For selected genetic diseases such as congenital Na+ or Cl− diarrhea, a history of intractable diarrhea in the family may be reported. A family history of fatal diarrhea was identified as a risk factor for the intractable diarrhea syndrome in a population of 32 consecutive children admitted to receive parenteral nutrition.[45] In the same population, the lack of breast feeding, parental atopy, and early (less than 3 months) onset of symptoms had an increased incidence compared to controls.[45]

ETIOLOGY AND SPECIFIC CLINICAL FEATURES

The overall prevalent etiologic pattern of persistent or chronic diarrhea is substantially different in the two distinct socioenvironmental settings considered. Persistent diarrhea in developing countries has its own epidemiology, risk factors and, more importantly, a peculiar etiologic pattern, different from that seen in children living in industrialized countries. These differences can be mainly ascribed to the overwhelming rate of intestinal infections observed in developing and transitional countries, where other causes of persistent diarrhea are almost negligible. In addition, diagnostic facilities are not easily accessible in developing countries, raising problems in diagnosing the rare diseases that are responsible for persistent diarrhea in industrialized countries. A list of the main causes of persistent diarrhea is reported in Tables 2 and 3. Etiologies of persistent diarrhea encompass infectious (Table 2) and noninfectious agents (Table 3), including foods and drugs that may induce diarrhea and a long list of primary intestinal disorders and neoplastic diseases.

Enteric infections are by far the most frequent cause of persistent diarrhea, both in developing and industrialized countries. In the former extensive efforts have been made to identify specific

Table 2 Infectious-Related Etiologies of Persistent Diarrhea

Bacterial: *Shigella, Salmonella, Yersinia enterocolitica, Escherichia coli, Clostridium difficile, Campylobacter jejuni, Vibrio cholerae, Mycobacterium avium intracellulare*
Viral: Rotavirus, Norovirus, Adenovirus, Astrovirus, Torovirus, Cytomegalovirus, HIV
Parasitic: *Cryptosporidium parvum, Guardia lamblia, Entamoeba hystolitica, Isospora belli, Strongyloides*
Postenteritis syndrome
Small intestinal bacterial overgrowth
Tropical sprue

Table 3 Noninfectious Causes of Persistent Diarrhea

Diarrhea associated with exogenous substances: excessive intake of carbonated fluid, dietetic foods containing sorbitol, mannitol or xylitol; excessive intake of antiacids or laxatives containing lactulose or $Mg(OH)_2$; excessive intake of methylxanthines-containing drinks (cola, tea, and coffee)
Abnormal digestive processes: Cystic fibrosis, Schwachman-Diamond syndrome, isolated pancreatic enzyme pancreatitis, chronic pancreatitis, Pearson's syndrome, trypsin/chymotrypsin, enterokinase deficiency
Disorders of bile acids: chronic cholestasis, use of bile acids sequestrants, primary bile acid malabsorption, terminal ileum resection
Carbohydrate malabsorption: congenital or acquired sucrase–isomaltase deficiency; congenital or acquired lactase deficiency; glucose–galactose malabsorption; fructose malabsorption
Immune-based disorders: food allergy, celiac disease, eosinophilic gastroenteritis, inflammatory bowel disease, IPEX syndrome and autoimmune enteropathy, primary immunodeficiencies
Structural defects: microvillus inclusion disease, tufting enteropathy, phenotypic diarrhea, heparan-sulfate deficiency, $\alpha_2\beta_1$ and $\alpha_6\beta_4$ integrin deficiency, lymphangectasia
Defects in electrolyte and metabolite transport: congenital chloride diarrhea, congenital sodium diarrhea, acrodermatitis enteropathica, selective folate deficiency, abetalipoproteinemia
Motility disorders: Hirschsprung's disease, intestinal pseudoobstruction (neurogenic and myophatic), thyreotoxicosis, neurogenin-3 disease
Surgical causes: congenital or acquired short bowel (secondary to stenosis, segmental atresia, malrotation)
Neoplastic diseases: neuroendocrine hormone-producing tumors, VIPoma, apudomas, mastocytosis

pathogens responsible for persistent diarrhea.[46] The results are scattered through different geographic regions. Consecutive cultures during episodes of persistent diarrhea have shown that the same organism is not always found during prolonged illness, suggesting that sequential infections with the same or a different pathogen may be responsible for prolonged symptoms.[47] Enteroadherent *E. coli* (EAEC) have been specifically implicated in persistent diarrhea[48–50] (Figure 3). Less compelling evidence suggest a role for *Shigella*, Enterotoxigenic *E. coli*, and *Campylobacter jejunii*.[39,40] *Cryptosporidium* was often found in persistent episodes in Bangladesh but not in Peru.[47,51] Intractable diarrhea-induced by *Cryptosporidium* was associated with a specific deficiency in γ-interferon production.[52]

Giardia lamblia shows similar incidence rates in acute and persistent diarrhea. In developed countries, the vast majority of cases of persistent diarrhea have a benign course and, in contrast with the etiology in developing countries, are induced by enteric viruses, mainly Rotavirus and Norovirus (Table 4).[9,41,53–55] Rotavirus has been associated with severe and protracted diarrhea,[47,56] and implicated in life-threatening intractable diarrhea syndrome also in developed countries.[57] Cytomegalovirus is a possible cause of intractable diarrhea, also in the immunocompetent child.[58] Also, torovirus and astrovirus have been associated with persistent diarrhea in children.[59–61]

Opportunistic agents are a major cause of persistent diarrhea in children with AIDS. Opportunistic agents are defined as microorganisms that

induce diarrhea exclusively, or in unusually severe forms, in target populations, such as immunocompromised children. Enteric cryptosporidiosis is the most frequent cause of severe and protracted diarrhea in HIV-infected children.[14] Infections with *Blastocystis hominis*, *Coccidia*, *Mycobacterium avium*, *Isospora belli*, and *Candida albicans* should be specifically considered in children with AIDS and persistent diarrhea.[62,63] Finally, HIV may be directly responsible for diarrhea and the so-called HIV enteropathy.[13,24]

Postenteritis syndrome is a clinical–pathological condition in which small intestinal mucosal damage persists following acute gastroenteritis. Sensitization to food antigens and secondary disaccharidase deficiency were classically considered as responsible for postenteritis syndrome. More recent studies have demonstrated that the incidence of disaccharidase deficiency is very low following acute diarrhea.[63–65] Similarly, sensitization to food antigens has a lower incidence than previously thought, and international guidelines discourage the use of hypoallergenic or diluted milk formulas during acute gastroenteritis.[66,67] A third mechanism of postenteritis syndrome is believed to be an infection or reinfection with an enteric pathogen. However, the pathophysiology of postenteritis diarrhea remain to be fully clarified.

Small bowel bacterial overgrowth induces persistent diarrhea through multiple mechanisms. In normal conditions, bacterial load in the proximal jejunal fluid does not exceed 10^4 colony forming units (CFU)/mL of aerobic bacteria. An increase over 10^5 CFU/mL in duodenal fluid, or the presence of anaerobic bacterial species, which are normally detected only in more distal intestinal segments, is believed to be responsible for severe impairment of digestive and absorptive processes. Diarrhea may be the result of either a direct interaction between a microorganism and the enterocyte or the consequence of deconjugation and dehydroxylation of bile salts, and hydroxylation of fatty acids operated by enteric bacteria.

Persistent diarrhea may be the result of maldigestion due to *pancreatic disorders*. In most patients with cystic fibrosis, pancreatic insufficiency results in fat and protein malabsorption. In the Schwachman syndrome, exocrine pancreatic hypoplasia can be associated with neutropenia, bone changes, and intestinal protein loss. Specific isolated pancreatic enzyme defects result in fat or protein malabsorption. Familial pancreatitis, associated with a mutation in the trypsinogen gene, may be associated with pancreatic insufficiency and persistent diarrhea.

Liver disorders, such as cholestasis, may lead to a reduction in the bile acid pool with fat malabsorption. Bile acid loss may be associated with terminal ileum diseases, such as Crohn's disease or with terminal ileum resection. A rare disease is primary bile acid malabsorption due to mutations of the ileal bile acid transporter,[68] and neonates and young infants present with fat malabsorption and chronic diarrhea. Long-term use of bile acid binders such as cholestiramine may be responsible

Table 4 Prevalence of Microorganisms in Baseline and Persistent Diarrheal Stool Specimens in Children from the United States

	Baseline Specimens (% Positive, $n = 484$)	Persistent Diarrhea Specimens (% Positive, $n = 40$)	Relative Risk
Bacteria			
C. difficile	3.5	2.6	0.7
E Agg *E. Coli*	3.7	5.0	1.3
Atypical *E. Coli*	12.2	17.5	1.4
Viruses			
Astrovirus	1.4	2.6	1.8
Norovirus	0.8	10.3	12.4
Rotavirus	1.5	10	6.9
Sapovirus	0.8	5.1	6.2

Adapted from Vernacchio et al.[9]

of continued bile acid loss in the stools and secondary decreased bile acid pool size.

Increased intraluminal osmolarity and subsequent diarrhea, are the endpoints of *excessive sugar-containing carbonated fluid* or fruit juice intake, which exceeds the transport capacities of the small intestine in younger infants. Excessive intake of sorbitol, magnesium hydroxide and lactulose are also responsible for persistent diarrhea. Persistent diarrhea may also be the manifestation of *carbohydrate malabsorption*, because of specific molecular defects. These include lactose intolerance, sucrase–isomaltase deficiency, and congenital glucose–galactose malabsorption. Lactose intolerance may be associated with congenital lactase deficiency but it is more frequently a consequence of lactase deficiency due to mucosal damage. A progressive loss of lactase activity, which affects about 80% of the non-Caucasian population, may be responsible for persistent diarrhea in older children receiving cow's milk.[69]

The extreme severity spectrum of persistent diarrhea includes a number of heterogeneous conditions leading to the so-called *intractable diarrhea syndrome*. This was originally described by Avery et al as a diarrhea lasting more than 2 weeks, with no detectable infectious etiology, starting in the first 3 months of age, and loaded with high mortality rate.[10] More recent definitions reflect the concept that the syndrome, in its typical setting, is the result of a permanent defect in the structure or function of intestine, leading to progressive intestinal failure with the need of parenteral nutrition for survival.[70] The intractable diarrhea syndrome has an evolving etiologic spectrum in which enteric infections and food intolerances have been replaced by more rare congenital conditions.[45,61,62] The main groups of diseases causing severe and protracted diarrhea include: structural enterocyte defects, motility disorders, immune-based disorders, short gut, and multiple food intolerance.[62,70] This classification is based on the main disorder responsible for diarrhea and has implications on the outcome of the disease.[62,70] However the etiology of persistent diarrhea includes a larger number of specific diseases that are herein briefly described.

An increasing number of molecular defects are responsible for a wide variety of *electrolyte transport defects* (see Chapter 15.3c, "Congenital Intestinal Transport Defects"). In congenital chloride diarrhea, a mutation in the solute carrier family 26 member 3 gene (SLC26A3) leads to severe intestinal Cl^- malabsorption due to the defect or absence of the Cl^-/HCO_3^- exchanger.[71,72] The consequent defect in HCO_3^- secretion leads to metabolic alkalosis and acidification of the intestinal content, with further inhibition of Na^+/H^+ exchanger-dependent Na^+ absorption. Patients with congenital sodium diarrhea show similar clinical features, because of a defective Na^+/H^+ exchanger in all segments of the small and large intestine, the presence of extremely high Na^+ fecal concentration, and severe acidosis.[73]

Structural enterocyte defects, based on specific, yet largely unknown molecular defects, are responsible for early onset, severe diarrhea[74] (see Chapter 15.3b, "Congenital Enteropathies"). In *microvillus inclusion disease* there is a net reduction of the absorptive surface area, associated with massive secretion of electrolytes in the stools. The ultrastructural hallmark of the disease is the lack of microvilli on the apical enterocyte surface and the presence of secretory granules and membrane bound inclusions lined by microvilli[75] (Figure 2). Evidence has been obtained that inclusion bodies originate from autophagocytosis of the apical membrane of enterocytes, with engulfing of microvilli.[76] *Intestinal epithelial dysplasia* (or *tufting enteropathy*) is characterized by various degrees of morphological abnormalities mainly localized in the epithelial layer, including disorganization of surface enterocytes with focal crowding and formation of tufts[77] (Figure 5). Abnormal laminin, and heparan sulfate proteoglycan deposition on the basement membrane have been detected in intestinal epithelia from infants with tufting enteropathy.[78] A defect in the distribution of integrins has also been reported.[78] These ubiquitous proteins are involved in cell–cell and cell–matrix interactions, and play a crucial role in cell differentiation and tissue development. An abnormal intestinal distribution of $\alpha_2\beta_1$ and $\alpha_6\beta_4$ integrins has been implicated in tufting enteropathy.[79] Congenital heparan sulfate deficiency is an extremely rare disorder with severe enteric albumin loss presenting within the first weeks of life.[80] Heparan sulfate is a glycosaminoglycan (GAG) component of the basement membrane with multiple roles in the intestine, including restriction of charged macromolecules within the vascular lumen.

Phenotypic diarrhea is characterized by immunodeficiency and facial abnormalities, woolly hair, and intractable diarrhea with a typical familiar pattern[81] (see Chapter 15.3b, "Congenital Enteropathies").

Persistent diarrhea may have an *immune/allergic pathogenesis*. Cow's milk protein allergy, as well as other food allergies, may determine abnormalities of the small intestinal mucosa. *Multiple food intolerance* is included in most series of intractable diarrhea syndrome. However, this is usually an exclusion diagnosis based on a relationship between any ingested food and diarrhea. In most cases, multiple food intolerance is not eventually confirmed by oral challenge (see Chapter 16.2, "Food Allergic Enteropathy").

The intestine may be the target of specific autoimmune processes that are responsible for persistent diarrhea and, in more severe cases, for intestinal failure. *Autoimmune enteropathy* is characterized by the production of antienterocyte antibodies, primarily IgG, directed against components of enterocyte brush border or cytoplasm. In association, a cell-mediated autoimmune response is detected with a mucosal T-cell activation[82,83] (see Chapter 16.3, "Autoimmune Enteropathy and IPEX Syndrome"). Recently, a syndrome with X-linked immune dysregulation, polyendocrinopaty, and enteropathy (*IPEX syndrome*) was characterized and shown to be associated with variable phenotypes of persistent diarrhea.[84–86]

Abnormal immune function, as seen in patients with agammaglobulinemia, isolated immunoglobulin A deficiency, and combined immunodeficiency disorders can result in persistent diarrhea induced by a wide spectrum of microorganisms, as in AIDS.

Disorders of intestinal motility is an emerging group of intestinal diseases associated with persistent diarrhea. Motility disorders include alterations of the enteric nervous system development and function, such as in Hirschsprung's disease, aganglionosis, and chronic intestinal pseudoobstruction (which encompasses either the neurogenic and the myogenic form).[87,88] Alterations of the connective-tissue plexus layer which roots circular and longitudinal intestinal muscles, have been identified in children with chronic intestinal pseudoobstruction.[89] Other motility disorders may be secondary to extraintestinal disorders, such as in hyperthyroidism. Motility disorders are associated with either or both constipation and diarrhea, with the former usually dominating the clinical picture (see Chapter 24.2c, "Other Dysmotilites Including Chronic Intestinal Pseudo-Obstruction Syndrome").

Alterations in the development of enteroendocrine cells may be responsible for severe forms of persistent diarrhea. *Enteroendocrine tumors* may be characterized by the overproduction of intestinal neurotransmitters with secretory effects which in turn lead to diarrhea.[90] A newly discovered disorder is secondary to *mutations of the*

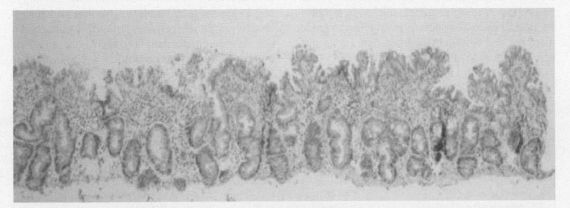

Figure 5 Small intestinal mucosal histology of a child with tufting enteropathy. The epithelial layer appears partially detached by the basal membrane. On tips of villi, enterocytes are focally crowded with formation of typical tufts. (Courtesy of A. Barabino and C. Marino, G. Gaslini Hospital, Genoa, Italy.)

neurogenin-3 transcription factor.[91] The lack of activity of this factor is responsible for a deficiency in the development of intestinal enteroendocrine cells, which is associated with malabsorption and diarrhea.[91]

Short gut syndrome is associated with persistent diarrhea. All intestinal abnormalities such as stenosis, segmental atresia, and malrotation may require surgical resection. In these conditions, the residual intestine may be insufficient to carry on its normal digestive–absorptive functions. Alternatively, small bowel bacterial overgrowth may be the main mechanism involved in diarrhea, such as in blind loop syndrome.

In rare cases of severe persistent diarrhea, the gastrointestinal symptoms may be the initial manifestation of a *mithocondrial disease*.[92] Finally, in cases in which a cause of diarrhea is not detected and the clinical course is inconsistent, *Munchausen by proxy* should be considered.

The natural history of intractable diarrhea is related to the primary intestinal disease.[54,83] Food intolerances generally resolve in few weeks or months, as does autoimmune enteropathy, when appropriate immune suppression is started. Children with motility disorders show more severe, long-lasting symptoms but a less severe course, whereas those with structural enterocyte defects never recover, undergo a more severe course, generally needing parenteral nutrition, and often becoming candidates for intestinal transplantation.[54,83,93,94]

APPROACH TO THE CHILD WITH PERSISTENT DIARRHEA

Because of the wide etiologic spectrum of persistent diarrhea in children, medical decisions should be based on diagnostic algorithms that begin with the age of the child, then consider clinical and epidemiological factors, and always take into account the results of microbiological investigations.

Specific clues in the family and personal history may provide useful indications. History of chronic/intractable diarrhea in a relative, suggests a genetic disease, particularly if presentation occurred in the first months of life. A family history positive for autoimmune or atopic diseases points toward allergy or autoimmunity.

The presence of polyhidramnios is consistent with congenital chloride or sodium diarrhea. A previous episode of acute gastroenteritis is suggestive of postenteritis syndrome, whereas the association of diarrhea with ingestion of specific foods should always be looked for possible intolerance to one or more food antigens.

Initial clinical examination should include the evaluation of general and nutritional status. It is not rare to face critical clinical condition with dehydration / marasmus or kwashiorkor, requiring prompt supportive interventions to stabilize the patient. The presence of eczema or asthma is associated with an allergic disorder, and specific extraintestinal manifestations (arthritis, diabetes,

thrombocytopenia, etc) may suggest an autoimmune disease. Specific skin lesions may be suggestive of enteropathic acrodermatitis. Typical facial abnormalities, and wholly hair are associated with phenotipic diarrhea.

If the child with persistent diarrhea lives in a developing country or comes from a poor social setting where the typical risk factors for persistent diarrhea, including malnutrition, are common, an intestinal infection should be suspected. However, in all cases of persistent diarrhea, irrespective of risk factors, the diagnostic approach should include stool cultures, search for parasites and for Rotavirus and other enteric viruses.

The evaluation of nutritional status is crucial to establish the need for rapid intervention. It should start with the evaluation of the weight and height curves, and of the weight for height index, to determine the impact of diarrhea on growth. Malnutrition may precede the onset of diarrhea, thus contributing to its long duration, or it could be the consequence of the disease, suggesting the presence of intestinal malabsorption. Weight gain is generally impaired before height growth but—with time—also linear growth is affected, and both parameters may be equally abnormal in the long term. Assessment of nutritional status includes dietary history, biochemical and nutritional investigations. Caloric intake should be quantitatively determined. Biochemical markers include albumin (half-life 20 days), prealbumin (half-life 2 days), retinol binding protein (half-life 12 hours), transferrin (half-life 8 days), serum iron, iron binding capacity, and micronutrient concentrations. The half-life of serum proteins may help distinguishing short- and long-term malnutrition. Assessment of body composition may be performed by measuring midarm circumference and triceps skinfold thickness or, more accurately, by bioelectrical impedance analysis or dual emission X-ray absorptiometry (DEXA) scans.

The relationship between weight modifications and energy intake should be carefully considered. In infants and children who are apparently thriving or overweight while suffering from chronic diarrhea, a 1-week dietary record may be used to explore the hypothesis that the youngster is being overfed or is drinking excessive amounts of juices or beverages with high sucrose content. Conversely a child with persistent diarrhea and suspected malabsorption, may be receiving diluted hypocaloric formula or even clear liquids in an effort to reduce diarrhea, and persistent diarrhea may be an indirect consequence of ongoing malnutrition.

Search for etiology may be based on the pathophysiology of diarrhea. Electrolyte concentrations

in fecal samples discriminate between secretory and osmotic diarrhea and may provide important information for guiding the subsequent diagnostic approach (Table 5). In selected cases, a fruitful approach would include a complete bowel rest, leaving the child on total parenteral nutrition, in order to better define the nature of diarrhea. In parallel, a noninvasive assessment both for intestinal function and the presence of inflammation may be performed and has a key intestinal role in the diagnostic approach (Table 6). Overall, a stepwise diagnostic algorithm is proposed in Table 7.

Microbiological investigation of stool samples should include a thorough list of agents, and may provide valuable information. Search for proximal intestinal bacterial overgrowth is part of microbiological investigation. The breath hydrogen test, after glucose oral load, may identify an abnormal bacterial proliferation in the small bowel. Breath test can also be used for detecting carbohydrate malabsorption.

Diagnostic work-up of persistent diarrhea is largely based on the specific diagnostic tools available, however endoscopy and histology provide essential information. Small intestinal biopsy was effective in detecting a primary intestinal etiology in more than 90% of cases of chronic diarrhea.[95] Colonoscopy should be performed in all cases of chronic diarrhea in which gross or occult blood is detected in the stools, or when an increased frequency of mucoid stools and abdominal pain suggest colonic involvement. Biopsies should be performed at multiple sites, even in a normal appearing intestine, because at least 5% of apparently normal colons will yield specimens positive for colitis, when a disease characterized by patchy lesions is responsible for the observed symptoms. Histology is important to establish the degree of mucosal involvement, through grading of intestinal damage and the presence of associated abnormalities, such as inflammatory infiltration of the lamina propria. Morphometry provides additional quantitative information of epithelial changes. In selected cases, light microscopy may help identifying specific intracellular agents, such as cytomegalovirus, from the presence of large inclusion bodies in infected cells[58] or intracellular parasites. Electron microscopy is indicated in all cases of intractable diarrhea of unknown etiology, and is essential to detect microvillous inclusion disease or other cellular structural abnormalities. Immunohistochemistry allows the study of mucosal immune activation as well as of other cell types (smooth muscle cell and enterocyte) as well as components of the basal membrane.

Table 5 Stool Features Supporting the Differential Diagnosis Between Secretory and Osmotic Diarrhea

	Secretory	Osmotic
Osmotic gap	<50 mOsm/kg	>135 mOsm/kg
Cl⁻ concentration	>40 meq/L	<35 meq/L
pH	>6.0	<5.5
Na⁺ concentration	>70 meq/L	<70 meq/L

Table 6 Noninvasive Tests for the Assessment of Intestinal Function and Inflammation

Test	Normal Values	Implication	Reference
α_1–Antitripsin concentration	<0.9 mg/g	Increased intestinal permeability/protein loss	Catassi C et al. J Pediatr 1986;109:500–2
Steatocrit	<2.5% (older than 2 yr) Fold increase over age-related values (below 2 yr)	Fat malabsorption	Guarino A et al. J Pediatr Gastroenterol Nutr 1992;14:268–74
Fecal reducing substances	Absent	Carbohydrate malabsorption	Lindquist BL et al. Arch Dis Child 1976;51:319–21
Elastase concentration	>200 µg/g	Pancreas function	Carroccio A et al. Gut 1998;43:558–63
Chymotripsin concentration	>7.5 U/g >375 U/24 h	Pancreas function	Carroccio A et al. Gastroenterology 1997;112:1839–44
Fecal occult blood	Absent	Fecal blood loss	Fine KD. N Engl J Med 1996;334:1163–7
Calprotectin concentration	<50 µg/g (older than 4 years)	Intestinal inflammation	Fagerberg UL et al. J Pediatr Gastroenterol Nutr 2003;37:468–72
Fecal leukocytes	<5/microscopic field	Colonic inflammation	Harris JC et al. 1972;76:697–703
Nitric oxide in rectal dyalisate	<5 µM of NO_2^-/NO_3^-	Rectal inflammation	Berni Canani R et al. Am J Gastroenterol 2002;97:1574–6

Table 7 Stepwise Diagnostic Work-Up for Children with Persistent Diarrhea

Step 1	Intestinal microbiology	– Stool cultures
		– Microscopy for parasites
		– Viruses
	Noninvasive tests for:	– Fecal osmotic gap, Cl^- and Na^+ concentrations
	• intestinal function	– Dual sugar permeability
		– (α_1–Antitripsin concentration
		– Steatocrit
		– Fecal reducing substances
		– Fecal occult blood
	• pancreatic function	– tripsin
		– Elastase concentration
		– Chymotripsin concentration
	• intestinal inflammation	– Calprotectin concentration
		– Fecal leukocytes
		– Nitric oxide in rectal dyalisate
Step 2	Intestinal morphology	– Standard jejunal histology
		– PAS staining
		– Electron microscopy
Step 3	Special investigations	– Intestinal immunohistochemistry
		– Serum chromogranin and catecholamines
		– Autoantibodies
		– [75]SeHCAT measurement
		– Brush border enzymatic activities
		– Motility and electrophysiological studies

Adapted from De Marco et al.[70]

An immunohistological classification of intractable diarrhea, having prognostic implications, was originally proposed by Cuenod et al.[96] The authors recognized a group of children with severe immune activation and epithelial damage, and another group with no mucosal damage and likely affected by inborn defects of enterocyte differentiation.

Imaging has a major role in the diagnostic approach to persistent diarrhea. A preliminary plain abdominal X-ray is useful for detection of gaseous distension, suggestive of a gastrointestinal obstruction. Intramural or biliary gas may be seen in necrotizing enterocolitis or intestinal invagination. Structural abnormalities such as diverticula, malrotation, stenosis, blind loop, as well as motility disorders, may be appreciated after a barium meal and an entire bowel follow-through examination.

Specific investigations should be carried on when specific diagnostic suspect is posed. A valuable tool in the diagnosis of bile acid malabsorption is the measure of retention, in the enterohepatic circulation, of the bile acid analog [75]Sehomocholic acid-taurine ([75]SeHCAT) as an index of ileal bile acid absorption.[97] A scintigraphic examination, with radio-labeled octreotide, is indicated in case of suspected APUD cell neoplastic proliferation.[98] In other diseases, specific imaging techniques such as computed tomography or magnetic resonance imaging (MRI), may have an important diagnostic value.

Once infections have been excluded, a stepwise approach to the child with persistent diarrhea may be applied (Table 7). The main etiologies of persistent diarrhea should be investigated, based on the features of diarrhea, and their predominant or selective intestinal dysfunction (Figure 6). A step by step diagnostic approach is important to minimize the invasiveness to the child, and the overall costs, while optimizing the yield of the diagnostic work-up.

THERAPY

Persistent diarrhea associated with impaired nutritional status should always be considered a serious disease, and therapy should be promptly started. Treatment of persistent diarrhea can be schematically divided in general supportive measures, nutritional rehabilitation, and drug treatment. The latter includes therapies for specific etiologies as well as treatment aimed at counteracting fluid secretion and/or promoting restoration of disrupted intestinal epithelium.

Because death in most instances is caused by dehydration, replacement of fluid, and electrolyte losses, is the major early intervention. Rehydration is best performed with oral rehydration solution (ORS), and recent meta-analyses demonstrate the efficacy and safety of the oral versus the intravenous route.[99,100] Studies provide data on the efficacy of hypotonic ORS rather than isotonic solutions.[101,102] The addition of aminoacids to glucose-based ORS, or the substitution of rice gruel or cereal for glucose, has been proposed to create a "super ORS," which may provide advantages over the pure glucose and electrolyte conventional WHO ORS.[103,104] Amylase-resistant starch (pectin), added to ORS, is not digested and absorbed in the upper bowel but reaches the colon where bacteria brake it down to short-chain fatty acids, having fluid absorptive effects.[105,106] Starch may be added to ORS to specifically counteract secretory diarrheas, even tough a European multicenter trial failed to show the efficacy of this approach, especially for the scarce palatability of these ORS.[107]

In malnourished children, nutritional rehabilitation is essential, also when an enteric infection is documented. A sufficient number of calories should always be provided. Caloric intake may be progressively increased to 50% or more above the RDA for age and sex. In children who do not tolerate high feeding volumes, caloric density may be increased by adding fat or carbohydrate. However, the intestinal absorbing capacity should be monitored by digestive function tests. In children with steatorrhea, medium-chain tryglicerides may be the main source of lipids, as they are easily absorbed. Even though a disaccharidase deficiency is no longer recognized as major cause of persistent diarrhea, hypolactasia is often secondary to intestinal damage and malnutrition, irrespective to its primary etiology.

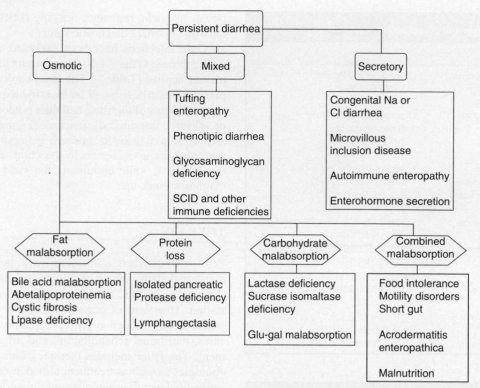

Figure 6 Scheme of specific etiologies of persistent diarrhea according to its pathophysiology. Assessment of the secretory, osmotic, or mixed mechanism of diarrhea, and of predominant nutrient malabsorption may help identifying the primary etiology thereby directing the diagnostic work-up through specific investigations.

Lactose-free diet should be started in all children with persistent diarrhea, and is included in a treatment algorithm designed by WHO.[108] Lactose is generally replaced by maltodextrins or a combination of other carbohydrates. Sucrose-free formula is indicated in sucrase–isomaltase deficiency. Exclusion diets are usually administered with the double purpose of overcoming food intolerance, which may be the primary cause of persistent diarrhea, or its complication. The sequence of elimination should be graded from less to more restricted diets, ie, cow's milk protein hydrolysate to aminoacid-based formula or vice versa, depending on child conditions. If the latter are severely compromised, it may be convenient to start with aminoacids-based feeding.

In several cases, clinical nutrition should be considered: this includes enteral or parenteral nutrition. Enteral nutrition may be performed via nasogastric or gastrostomy tube, and is indicated in a child who is not able to be fed through the oral route, either because of primary intestinal diseases or because of extreme weakness. Continuous enteral nutrition is effective in children with a reduced absorptive function. The rationale of continuous enteral nutrition is based on the increase of time/absorptive surface ratio. A reduced surface functioning for extended time increases daily nutrient absorption. In children with extreme wasting, enteral nutrition may not be sufficient. In such cases, parenteral nutrition may be a life saving procedure. Parenteral nutrition should be undertaken at an early phase, as soon as other less invasive nutritional approaches have been unsuccessfully attempted.

Nutritional rehabilitation has a general beneficial effect on general condition, intestinal function, and immune response. Continuous enteral nutrition was used in children with HIV and intestinal malabsorption and was effective in increasing their body weight while restoring intestinal absorptive function, and inducing a rise in CD4 cell number.[26]

Micronutrient and vitamin supplementation is part of nutritional rehabilitation and prevents further problems, especially in malnourished children from developing countries.[31,32] The fundamental role of zinc in cellular metabolism and immune response has recently emerged at the clinical level.[109,110] Zinc supplementation is an important issue in both prevention and therapy of persistent diarrhea, given its ideal features to counteract diarrhea and malnutrition.[31-34,111] Pooled analysis demonstrated a significant effect of zinc in the treatment as well as in the reduction of fatal events in children with persistent diarrhea.[111]

Specific therapy includes antiinfective drugs, immune suppression, and drugs that may inhibit fluid loss and promote cell growth. When a specific infectious agent is detected, specific treatment should be undertaken. In case of bacterial intestinal infection, antibiotic therapy can be administered.

In Rotavirus-induced diarrhea, oral administration of human immunoglobulins was effective both in immunocompetent and immunocompromised children and should be considered for treatment in severe or protracted diarrhea.[112,113] Human serum immunoglobulins, available in preparations for intravenous use, may be administered through the oral route at the dose of 300 mg/kg of body weight, in a single oral dose. The rationale of passive immunotherapy is based on the demonstration of neutralizing antibodies against all viruses of medical importance in the preparations for intravenous use.[112]

Diarrheal diseases are consistently associated with modifications of intestinal microflora. Thus attempts at modifying intestinal microflora may be worth considering, even when an infectious cause is suspected, but not proved. Two distinct strategies are available: the administration of probiotic bacteria, and the administration of antibiotics. Large and reliable meta-analyses demonstrated an efficacy of probiotic administration both in the prevention and treatment of acute, and protracted diarrhea.[114-116] Alternatively, empiric antibiotic therapy may be undertaken in children with either small bowel bacterial overgrowth or with suspected bacterial diarrhea. A specific efficacy against persistent diarrhea has been shown for trimethoprim-sulfamethoxazole.[117] Metronidazole and Albendazole are a reasonable alternative for the broad pattern of target agents, including parasites.[118] The so-called bowel cocktail (metronidazole, colestiramine, and high dose gentamycin given orally) has been proposed for severe protracted diarrhea of suspected infectious etiology, although conclusive proof of efficacy is lacking.[119] Nitazoxanide, a broad-spectrum antiparasitic drug, was shown to be effective also in rotavirus diarrhea, and could thus be considered as a valuable option for the empiric therapy of persistent diarrhea.[120]

Specific therapy with immune suppressive drugs should be considered in selected conditions such as autoimmune enteropathy. Azathioprine, cyclosporine, and tacrolimus have been used in severe protracted diarrhea of immune origin. Autoimmune enteropathy may be successfully controlled by immune suppression, allowing withdrawal of parenteral nutrition.[54,121]

Treatment may also be directed at modifying specific pathophysiologic processes. Most secretory diarrheas are infectious but intestinal ion secretion is also the most common mechanism of the intractable diarrhea syndrome of infancy. In these cases, the use of drugs active on ion transport may be considered.[122] Among proabsorptive agents, the enkephalinase inhibitor racecadotril inhibits the breakdown of natural endogenous opiates (enkephalins) by intestinal tissue, and has been effective in controlled clinical trials in acute diarrhea.[123] In severe secretory diarrheas, such as in neuroendocrine tumors, microvillus inclusion disease, and enterotoxin-induced severe diarrhea, a trial with somatostatin and its analog octreotide may be considered.[124] Octreotide has been used in diarrhea secondary to neoplastic diseases as well as in intestinal infections. Subcutaneous administration of octreotide was effective in reducing fecal output in HIV-infected children with severe cryptosporidiosis, and a specific antagonist effect against the enterotoxic activity associated with *Cryptosporidium* has been shown in vitro.[125] Loperamide and chlorpromazine have also been used in children with severe and protracted diarrhea, but they are loaded with several major side effects, particularly in children. Growth hormone has been used as a trophic factor in the short gut syndrome and may have an additional beneficial effect in secretory diarrhea, since it inhibits chloride secretion and promotes sodium absorption through a direct effect on the enterocyte.[126–128] Growth hormone may be an ideal drug in case of severe and protracted diarrhea when both epithelial atrophy and ion secretion are associated.

However, when other attempts have failed, the only option may be parenteral nutrition or surgery, including intestinal transplantation.[129]

CONCLUSIONS

Persistent diarrhea still is a major problem worldwide, but with two distinct presentations. In developing and transitional countries, persistent diarrhea is a relatively frequent outcome of intestinal infections and is loaded with high case/fatality ratio, mainly because of the combined effect of enteric infections, intestinal dysfunction, malnutrition, and immune suppression. In industrialized countries persistent diarrhea usually has a benign course with viral infections playing a major role. However, the etiologic spectrum may be broader with an increase of early-onset severe cases, generally evolving toward irreversible intestinal diseases. In these cases, optimal diagnostic approach and general management require advanced knowledge and technology, and should be carried on in tertiary care centers or through a close interaction among experts in gastroenterology, nutrition, infectious diseases, and pediatric surgery.

REFERENCES

1. Lopez AD, Mathers CD, Ezzati M, et al. Global and regional burden of disease and risk factors, 2001: Systematic analysis of population health data. Lancet 2006;367:1747–57.
2. Kosek M, Bern C, Guerrant RL. The global burden of diarrheal disease as estimated from studies published between 1990 and 2000. Bull WHO 2003;81:197–204.
3. Bhutta ZA, Ghishan F, Lindly K, et al. Persistent and chronic diarrhea and malabsorption: Working group report of the Second World Congress of pediatric gastroenterology, Hepatology and Nutrition. J Pediatr Gastroenterol Nutr 2004;39:S711–6.
4. World Health Organization. Diarrhoeal Disease Control. Persistent diarrhoea in children. CCD/DDM/85.1. Geneva: World Health Organization.
5. Huttly SR, Hoque BA, Aziz KM, et al. Persistent diarrhoea in a rural area of Bangladesh: A community-based longitudinal study. Int J Epidemiol 1898;18:964–9.
6. Mbori-Ngacha DA, Otieno JA, Njeru EK, et al. Prevalence of persistent diarrhoea in children aged 3–36 months at the Kenyatta National Hospital, Nairobbi, Kenia. East Afr Med J 1995;72:711–4.
7. Ketama L, Lulseged S. Persistent diarrhoea: Socio-demographic and clinical profile of 264 children seen at a referral hospital in Addis Ababa. Ethiop Med J 1997;35:161–8.
8. Trounce JQ, Walker-Smith JA. Sugar intolerance complicating acute gastroenteritis. Arch Dis Child 1985; 60:986–90.
9. Vernacchio L, Vezina RM, Mitchell AA, et al. Characteristics of persistent diarrhea in a community-based cohort of young US children. J Pediatr Gastroenterol Nutr 2006; 43:52–8.
10. Avery GB, Villavicencio O, Lilly JR, et al. Intractable diarrhea in early infancy. Pediatrics 1968;41:712–22.
11. Berni Canani R, Cirillo P, Buccigrossi V, et al. Nitric oxide produced by the enterocyte is involved in the cellular regulation of ion transport. Pediatr Res 2003;54:1–5.
12. Ball JM, Tian P, Zeng CQ, et al. Age-dependent diarrhea induced by a rotaviral nonstructural glycoprotein. Science 1996; 272:101–4.
13. Berni Canani R, Cirillo P, Mallardo G, et al. Effects of HIV-1 Tat protein on ion secretion and on cell proliferation in human intestinal epithelial cells. Gastroenterology 2003;124:368–76.
14. Guarino A, Castaldo A, Russo S, et al. Enteric cryptosporidiosis in pediatric HIV infection. J Pediatr Gastroenterol Nutr 1997;25:182–7.
15. Guarino A, Berni Canani R, Pozio E, et al. Enterotoxic effect of stool supernatant of Cryptosporidium infected calves on human jejunum. Gastroenterology 1994;106:28–34.
16. Farthing MJ. Novel targets for the control of secretory diarrhoea. Gut 2002;50:III,15–8.
17. Bode H, Schmitz H, Fromm M, et al. IL-1beta and TNF-alpha, but not IFN-alpha, IFN-gamma, IL-6 or IL-8, are secretory mediators in human distal colon. Cytokine 1998;10:457–65.
18. Kere J, Hoglund P. Inherited disorders of ion transport in the intestine. Curr Opin Genet Dev 2000;10:306–9.
19. Centers for Disease Control and Prevention. 1994 Revised Classification system for human immunodeficiency virus infection in children less than 13 years of age. Morb Mortal Wkly Rep 1994;43:1–10.
20. Tovo PA, de Martino M, Gabiano C, et al. Prognostic factors and survival in children with perinatal HIV-1 infection. Lancet 1992;339:1249–53.
21. Guarino A, Bruzzese E, De Marco G, Buccigrossi V. Management of gastrointestinal disorders in children with HIV infection Pediatric Drugs 2004;6:347–62.
22. Castaldo A, Tarallo L, Palomba E. Iron deficiency and intestinal malabsorption in HIV disease. J Pediatr Gastroenterol Nutr 1996;22:359–63.
23. Chen XM, Keithly JS, Paya CV, LaRusso NF. Cryptosporidiosis. N Engl J Med 2002;346:1723–31.
24. Berni Canani R, De Marco G, Passariello A, et al. Inhibitory effect of HIV-1 Tat protein on the sodium-D-glucose symporter of human intestinal epithelial cells. AIDS 2006; 20:5–10.
25. Berni Canani R, Spagnuolo MI, Cirillo P, et al. Ritonavir combination therapy restores intestinal function in children with advanced HIV disease. J AIDS 1999;21:307–12.
26. Guarino A, Spagnuolo MI, Giacomet V, et al. Effects of nutritional rehabilitation on intestinal function and on CD4 cell number in children with HIV. J Pediatr Gastroenterol Nutr 2002;34:366–71.
27. Bahandari N, Bhan NK, Sazawal S, et al. Association of antecedent malnutrition with persistent diarrhoea: A case-control study. BMJ 1989;298:1284–87.
28. Karim AS, Akhter S, Rahman MA, et al. Risk factors of persistent diarrhea in children below five years of age. Indian J Gastroenterol 2001;20:59–61.
29. Usha N, Sankaranarayanan A, Walia BN, et al. Assessment of preclinical vitamin A deficiency in children with persistent diarrhea. J Pediatr Gastroenterol Nutr 1991;13:168–75.
30. Black RE. Zinc deficiency, infectious disease and mortality in the developing world. J Nutr 2003;133:1485S–9S.
31. Bahan MK, Bhandari N. The role of zinc and vitamin A in persistent diarrhea in infants and young children. J Pediatr Gastroenterol Nutr 1998;26:446–53.
32. Rahman MM, Vermund SH, Wahed MA, et al. Simultaneous zinc and vitamin A supplementation in Bangladeshi children: Randomised double blind controlled trial. Br Med J 2001;323:314–8.
33. Kathun UH, Malek MA, Black RE, et al. A randomized controlled clinical trial of zinc, vitamin A or both in undernourished children with persistent diarrhea in Bangladesh. Acta Paediatr 201;90:376–80.
34. Penny ME, Peerson JM, Marin RM, et al. Randomized, community-based trial of the effect of zinc supplementation, with and without other micronutrients, on the duration of persistent childhood diarrhea in Lima, Peru. J Pediatr 1999;135:208–17.
35. Sazawal S, Bhan MK, Bhandari N. Type of milk feeding during acute diarrhoea and the risk of persistent diarrhoea: A case-control study. Acta Paediatr Suppl 1992;381:93–7.
36. Patwari AK, Anand VK, Aneja S, et al. Persistent diarrhea: Management in a diarrhea treatment unit. Indian Pediatr 1995;32:277–84.
37. Feachem RG, Koblinsky MA. Intervention for the control of diarrhoeal disease among young children: Measles immunization. Bull World Health Organ 1983;61:641–52.
38. Amadi B, Kelly P, Mwiya M, et al. Intestinal and systemic infection, HIV, and mortality in Zambian children with persistent diarrhea and malnutrition. J Pediatr Gastroenterol Nutr 2001;32:550–4.
39. Ngan PK, Khan NG, Tuong CV, et al. Persistent diarrhea in Vietnamese children: A preliminary report. Acta Paediatr 1992;81:124–6.
40. Ahmed F, Ansaruzzaman M, Haqua E, et al. Epidemiology of postshigellosis persistent diarrhea in young children. Pediatr Infect Dis J 2001;20:525–30.
41. Bhutta ZA, Nizami SQ, Thobani S, et al. Factors determining recovery during nutritional therapy of persistent diarrhoea: The impact of diarrhoea severity and intercurrent infections. Acta Paediatr 1997;86:796–802.
42. Araya M, Baiocchi N, Espinoza J, et al. Persistent diarrhoea in the community. Characteristics and risk factors. Acta Paediatr Scand 1991;80:181–9.
43. Fraser D, Dgan R, Porat N, et al. Persistent diarrhea in a cohort of Israeli Bedouin infants: Role of enteric pathogens and family and environmental factors. J Infect Dis 1998;178:1081–8.
44. Kirkpatrick BD, Huston CD, Wagner D, et al. Serum mannose-binding lectin deficiency is associated with cryptosporidiosis in young Haitian children, Clin Infect Dis 2006;43:295–6.
45. Catassi C, Fabiani E, Spagnuolo MI, et al. Severe and protracted diarrhea: Results of the 3-year SIGEP multicenter survey. J Pediatr Gastroenterol Nutr 1999;29:63–8.
46. Nataro JP, Sears JL. Infectious causes of persistent diarrhea. Pediatr Infect Dis J 2001;20:195–6.
47. Baqui AH, Sacj RB, Black RE, et al. Enteropathogens associated with acute and persistent diarrea in Bangladeshi children less than 5 years of age. J Infect Dis 1992;166:792–6.
48. Cravioto A, Tello A, Navarro A, et al. Association of Escherichia coli Hep-2 adherence pattern with type and duration of diarrhea. Lancet 1991;337:262–4.
49. Chan KN, Phillips AD, Knutton S, et al. Enteroaggregative *Escherichia coli*: Another cause of acute and chronic diarrhoea in England? J Pediatr Gastroenterol Nutr 1994;18:87–91.
50. Okeke IN, Nataro JP. Enteroaggregative Escherichia coli. Lancet Infect Dis 2001;1:304–13.
51. Lanata CF, Black RE, Maurtua D, et al. Etiologic agents in acute vs persistent diarrhea in children under three years of age in peri-urban Lima, Peru. Acta Paediatr Scand 1992;381:32–8.
52. Gomez-Morales MA, Ausiello CM, Guarino A, et al. Severe, protracted intestinal cryptosporidiosis associated with interferon-gamma deficiency: A pediatric case. Clin Infect Dis 1996;22:848–50.
53. Guarino A, Spagnuolo MI, Russo S, et al. Etiology and risk factors of severe and protracted diarrhea. J Pediatr Gastroenterol Nutr 1995;20:173–8.
54. Guarino A, De Marco G for the Italian National Network for Pediatric Intestinal Failure. Natural history of intestinal failure, investigated through a network-based approach. J Pediatr Gastroenterol Nutr 2003;37:136–41.
55. Vernacchio L, Vezina RM, Mitchell AA, et al. Diarrhea in American infants and young children in the community setting. Incidence, clinical presentation and microbiology. Pediatr Infect Dis J 2006;25:2–7.
56. Khoshoo V, Bhan MK, Jayashree S, et al. Rotavirus infection and persistent diarrhoea in young children. Lancet 1990;336:1314–5.
57. Guarino A, Guandalini S, Albano F, et al. Enteral immunoglobulin for treatment of protracted Rotaviral diarrhea. Pediatr Infect Dis J 1991;10:612–4.
58. Fox LM, Gerber MA, Penix L, et al. Intractable diarrhea from cytomegalovirus enterocolitis in an immunocompetent infant. Pediatrics 1999;103:1–3.
59. Koopmans MP, Goosen ES, Lima AA, et al. Association of torovirus with acute and persistent diarrhea in children. Pediatr Infect Dis J 1997;16:504–7.
60. Unicomb LE, Banu NN, Azim T, et al. Astrovirus infection in association with acute, persistent and nosocomial diarrhea in Bangladesh. Pediatr Infect Dis J 1998;17:611–4.
61. Caballero S, Guix S, El-Senousy WM, et al. Persistent gastroenteritis in children infected with astrovirus: Association with serotype-3 strains. J Med Virol 2003;71:245–50.
62. Keusch GT, Thea DM, Kamenga M, et al. Persistent diarrhea associated with AIDS. Acta Paediatr Scand 1992;381:45–8.
63. Germani Y, Minssart P, Vohito M, et al. Etiologies of acute, persistent, and dysenteric diarrheas in adults in Bangui, Central African Republic, in relation to human immunodeficiency virus serostatus. Am J Trop Med Hyg 1998;59:1008–14.
64. Anonymous. What has happened to carbohydrate intolerance following gastroenteritis? Lancet 1987;1:23–4.
65. Walker-Smith JA, Sandhu BK, Isolauri E, et al. Guidelines prepared by the ESPGAN Working Group on Acute Diarrhoea. Recommendations for feeding in childhood gastroenteritis. European Society of Pediatric Gastroenterology and Nutrition. J Pediatr Gastroenterol Nutr 1997;24:619–20.
66. Guarino A, Albano F. Guidelines for the approach to outpatient children with acute diarrhoea. Acta Paediatr 2001;90:1087–95.
67. American Academy of Pediatrics. Practice parameter: The management of acute gastroenteritis in young children. Provisional committee on quality improvement, Subcommitte on acute gastroenteritis. Pediatrics 1996;97:424–33.
68. Oelkers P, Kirby LC, Heubi JE, et al. Primary bile acid malabsorption caused by mutations in the sodium-dependent

bile acid transporter gene (SLC10A2). J Clin Invest 1997;99:1880–7.

69. Rings EH, Grand RJ, Buller HA. Lactose intolerance and lactase deficiency in children. Curr Opin Pediatr 1994;6:562–7.

70. De Marco G, Barabino A, Gambarara M, et al. The Network approach to the child with primary intestinal failure. J Pediatr Gastroenterol Nutr 2006;43:S61–7.

71. Makela S, Kere J, Holmberg C, et al. SLC26A3 mutations in congenital chloride diarrhea. Hum Mutat 2002;20:425–38.

72. Hihnala S, Hoglund P, Lammi L, et al. Long-term clinical outcome in patients with congenital chloride diarrhea. J Pediatr Gastroenterol Nutr 2006;42:369–75.

73. Muller T, Wijmenga C, Phillips AD, et al. Congenital sodium diarrhea is an autosomal recessive disorder of sodium/proton exchange but unrelated to known candidate genes. Gastroenterology 2000;119:1506–13.

74. Murch SH. The molecular basis of intractable diarrhea of infancy. Bailliere's Clinical Gastroenterology 1998;11:413–40.

75. Goulet OJ, Brousse N, Canioni D, et al. Syndrome of intractable diarrhoea with persistent villous atrophy in early childhood: A clinic-pathological survey of 47 cases. J Pediatr Gastroenterol Nutr 1998;26:151–61.

76. Reinshagen K, Naim HY, Zimmer KP. Autophagocytosis of the apical membrane in microvillus inclusion disease. Gut 2002;51:514–21.

77. Reifen RM, Cutz E, Groffiths AM, et al. Tufting enteropathy: A newly recognized clinicopathological entity associated with refractory diarrhea in infants. J Pediatr Gastroenterol Nutr 1994;18:379–85.

78. Patey N, Scoazec JY, Cuenod-Jabri B, et al. Distribution of cell adhesion molecules in infants with intestinal epithelial displasia (tufting enteropathy). Gastroenterology 1997;113:833–43.

79. Goulet O, Salomon J, Ruemmele F, et al. Intestinal epithelial dysplasia (tufting enteropathy). Orphanet J Rare Dis 2007;2:20.

80. Murch SH, Winyard PJ, Koletzko S, et al. Congenital enterocyte heparan sulphate deficiency with massive albumin loss, secretory diarrhea, and malnutrition. Lancet 1996;347:1299–301.

81. Girault D, Goulet O, Le Deist F, et al. Intractable infant diarrhea associated with phenotypic abnormalities and immunodeficiency. J Pediatr 1994;125:36–42.

82. Walker-Smith JA, Unsworth DJ, Hurchins P, et al. Autoantibodies against gut epithelium in child with small intestinal enteropathy. Lancet 1982;319:566–7.

83. Sherman PM, Mitchell DJ, Cutz E. Neonatal enteropathies: Defining the causes of protracted diarrhea of infancy. J Pediatr Gastroenterol Nutr 2004;38:16–26.

84. Bennett CL, Christie J, Ramsdell F, et al. The immune dysregulation, polyendocrinopathy, enteropathy, X-linked syndrome (IPEX) is caused by mutations of FOXP3. Nat Genet 2001;27:20–1.

85. De Benedetti F, Insalaco A, Diamanti A, et al. Mechanistic associations of a mild phenotype of immunodysregulation, polyendocrinopaty, enteropaty, x-linked syndrome. Clin Gastroenterol Hepatol 2006;4:653–9.

86. Torgerson TR, Linane A, Moes N, et al. Severe food allergy as a variant of IPEX syndrome caused by a deletion in a noncoding region of the FOXP3 gene. Gastroenterology 2007;132:1705–17.

87. Kapur RP. Developmental disorders of the enteric nervous system. Gut 2000;47:81–3.

88. Swenson O. Hirschsprung's disease: A review. Pediatrics 2002;109:914–8.

89. Meier-Ruge WA, Holschneider AM, Scharli AF. New pathogenic aspects of gut dysmotility in aplastic and hypoplastic desmosis of early childhood. Pediatr Surg Int 2001;17:140–3.

90. Warner RR. Enteroendocrine tumors other than carcinoid: A review of clinical significant advances. Gastroenterology 2005;128:1668–84.

91. Wang J, Cortina G, Wu SV, et al. Mutant neurogenin-3 in congenital malabsorptive diarrhea. N Engl J Med. 2006;355:270–80.

92. Chinnery PF, Jones S, Sviland L, et al. Mithocondrial enteropathy: The primary pathology may not be within the gastrointestinal tract. Gut 2001;48:121–4.

93. Pironi L, Hebuterne X, Van Gossum A, et al. Candidates for intestinal transplantation: A multicenter survey in Europe. Am J Gastroenterol 2006;101:1633–43.

94. Sauvat F, Dupic L, Caldari D, et al. Factors influencing outcome after intestinal transplantation in children. Transplant Proc 2006;38:1689–91.

95. Thomas AG, Phillips AD, Walker-Smith JA. The value of proximal small intestinal biopsy in the differential diagnosis of chronic diarrhoea. Arch Dis Child 1992;67:741–3.

96. Cuenod B, Brousse N, Goulet O, et al. Classification of intractable diarrhea in infancy using clinical and immunohistological criteria. Gastroenterology 1990;99:1037–43.

97. Galatola G, Jazrawi RP, Bridges C, et al. Direct measurement of first-pass ileal clearance of a bile acid in humans. Gastroenterology 1991;100;1100–5.

98. Borsato N, Chierichetti F, Zanco P, et al. The role of 111In-octreotide scintigraphy in the detection of APUD tumours: Our experience in eighteen patients. Q J Nucl Med 1995;39:113–5.

99. Bellemare S, Hartling L, Wiebe N, et al. Oral rehydration versus intravenous therapy for treating dehydration due to gastroenteritis in children: A meta-analysis of randomised controlled trials. BMC Med 2004;15:2–11.

100. Hartling L, Bellemare S, Wiebe N, et al. Oral versus intravenous rehydration for treating dehydration due to gastroenteritis in children. Cochrane Database Syst Rev 2006;3: CD004390.

101. Choice Study Group. Multicenter, randomized, double-blind clinical trial to evaluate the efficacy and safety of a reduced osmolarity oral rehydration salts solution in children with acute watery diarrhea. Pediatrics 2001;107:613.

102. Sarker SA, Mahalanabis D, Alam NH, et al. Reduced osmolarity oral rehydration solution for persistent diarrhea in infants: A randomized controlled clinical trial. J Pediatr 2001;138:532.

103. Guarino A. Oral rehydration for infantile diarrhoea: Toward a modified solution for the children of the world. Acta Paediatr 2000;89:764–7.

104. Fontaine O, Gore SM, Pierce NF. Rice-based oral rehydration solution for treating diarrhoea. Cochrane Library 2001;CD001264.

105. Ramakrishna BS, Venkataraman S, Srinivasan P, et al. Amylase-resistent starch plus oral rehydration solution for cholera. N Engl J Med 2000;342:308.

106. Rabbani GH, Teka T, Zaman B, et al. Clinical studies in persistent diarrhea: Dietary management with green banana or pectin in Bangladeshi children. Gastroenterology 2001;121:554–60.

107. Hoekstra JH, Szajewska H, Zikri MA, et al. Oral rehydration solution containing a misture of non-digestible carbohydrates in the treatment of acute diarrhea: A multicenter randomized placebo controlled study on behalf of the ESPGHAN working group on intestinal infections. J Pediatr Gastroenterol Nutr 2004;39:239–45.

108. World Health Organization. Evaluation of an algorithm for the treatment of persistent diarrhoea: A multicenter study. International Working Group on persistent diarrhoea. World Health Organ Bull 1996;74:479–89.

109. Bhatnagar S, Natchu UC. Zinc in child health and disease. Indian J Pediatr 2004;71:991–5.

110. Penny ME, Marin RM, Duran A, et al. Randomized controlled trial or the effect of daily supplementation with zinc or multiple micronutrients on the morbidity, growth, and micronutrient status in young Peruvian children. Am J Clin Nutr 2004;79:457–65.

111. Bhutta ZA, Bird SM, Black RE, et al. Therapeutic effects of oral zinc in acute and persistent diarrhea in children in developing countries: Pooled analysis of randomized controlled trials. Am J Clin Nutr 2000;72:1516–22.

112. Guarino A, Berni Canani R, Russo S, et al. Oral immunoglobulins for treatment of acute rotaviral gastroenteritis. Pediatrics 1994;93:12–6.

113. Guarino A, Albano F, Berni Canani R, et al. HIV, fatal rotavirus infection, and treatment option. Lancet 2002;359:74.

114. Berni Canani R, Cirillo P, Terrin G, et al. Probiotics for the treatment of acute gastroenteritis: A randomized clinical trial with five different preparations. BMJ 2007;335:60.

115. Gaon D, Garcia H, Winter L, et al. Effect of Lactobacillus strains and Saccharomyces boulardii on persistent diarrhea in children. Medicina (B Aires) 2003;63:293–8.

116. Szajewska H, Setty M, Mrukowicz J, Guandalini S. Probiotics in gastrointestinal diseases in children: Hard and not-so-hard evidence of efficacy, J Pediatr Gastroenterol Nutr 2006;42:454–75.

117. Alam NH, Bardhan PK, Haider R, et al. Trimethoprimsulphamethoxazole in the treatment of persistent diarrhoea: A double blind placebo controlled clinical trial. Arch Dis Child 1995;72:483–6.

118. Garg P. Evaluation of an algorithm for persistent/chronic diarrhea in children at a community hospital adjoining slums in Agra, North India. Southeast Asian J Trop Med Public Health 2006;37:508–14.

119. Tedeschi A, Scorza A, Sferlazzas C, et al. Bowel cocktail and severe persistent diarrhea. J Pediatr Gastroenterol Nutr 1990;10:270–1.

120. Rossignol JF, Abu-Zekry M, Hussein A, Santoro MG. Effect of nitazoxanide for treatment of severe rotavirus diarrhoea: Randomised double-blind placebo-controlled trial. Lancet 2006;368:124–9.

121. Bousvaros A, Leichtner AM, Book L, et al. Treatment of pediatric autoimmune enteropathy with tacrolimus (FK506). Gastroenterology 1996;111:237–43.

122. Farthing MJ. Antisecretory drugs for diarrheal disease. Dig Dis 2006;26:67.

123. Cezard JP, Duhamel JF, Meyer M, et al. Efficacy and tolerability of racecadotril in acute diarrhea in children. Gastroenterology 2001;120:799–805.

124. Bisset WM, Jenkins H, Booth I, et al. The effect of somatostatin on small intestinal transport in intractable diarrhoea of infancy. J Pediatr Gastroenterol Nutr 1993;17:169–75.

125. Guarino A, Berni Canani R, Spagnuolo MI, et al. In vivo and in vitro efficacy of octreotide for treatment of enteric cryptosporidiosis. Dig Dis Sci 1998;43:436–41.

126. Scolapio JS, Camilleri M, Fleming CR, et al. Effect of growth hormone, glutamine, and diet on adaptation in short-bowel syndrome: A randomized, controlled study. Gastroenterology 1997;113:1074–81.

127. Szkudlarek J, Jeppesen PB, Mortensen PB. Effect of high dose growth hormone with glutamine and no change in diet on intestinal absorption in short bowel patients: A randomised, double blind, crossover, placebo controlled study. Gut. 2000;47:199–205.

128. Guarino A, Berni Canani R, Iafusco M, et al. In vivo and in vitro effect of growth hormone on rat intestinal ion transport. Pediatr Res 1995;37:1–5.

129. Goulet O, Ruemmele F. Causes and management of intestinal failure in children. Gastroenterology 2006;130:S3–4.

15.3 Congenital Disorders

15.3a. Genetically Determined Disaccharidase Deficiency

Hassan Y. Naim, PhD

Klaus-Peter Zimmer, MD

The hydrolysis of carbohydrates, essential constituents of mammalian diet, in the intestinal lumen is achieved by a family of microvillar enzymes, the disaccharidases. Prominent members of this family are the enzymes sucrase–isomaltase (SI), maltase–glucoamylase (MGA), and lactase–phlorizin hydrolase (LPH).[1–5] Starch, glycogen, sucrose, and maltose are examples of well-known diet carbohydrates that comprise monosaccharides associated with each other through α-glycosidic linkages and are hydrolyzed by SI and MGA to monosaccharides, which are eventually transported across the brush border membrane of epithelial cells into the cell interior. Only a few examples of β-glycosidically linked monosaccharides are known, such as that present in one of the major and most essential carbohydrates in mammalian milk, lactose, which constitutes the primary diet source for the newborn.[6]

The digestive enzymes are membrane-bound glycoproteins that are efficiently expressed at the apical or microvillus membrane of the enterocytes.[2–4] The absence of these enzymes in the intestinal lumen is associated with carbohydrate malabsorption. Malabsorption following maldigestion causes diarrhea with soft to watery, often acid, but rarely fatty, stools. Osmotic diarrhea arises when the intestine cannot digest and/or absorb one or more nutrients. Molecules (especially those of smaller size) cause an osmotic force, which drives water into the gut lumen. Stool volumes are smaller than in secretory diarrhea and depend on the amount (and size) of undigested and unabsorbed molecules (mainly carbohydrates) concentrated in the bowel. Osmotic diarrhea regresses with discontinuation of oral feeding. Ion gap and osmolarity are increased in the stool while the pH is below 6.0.

Bacterial flora of the colon salvage carbohydrates, which were not digested and absorbed in the small intestine, by fermentation to gases (hydrogen, methane, and carbon dioxide) and to lactic acid as well as to volatile short-chain fatty acids (acetic, propionic, butyric, isobutyric, valeric, and isovaleric), the last being absorbed by the colonic mucosa.[7] Indeed, fermentative diarrhea develops when the salvaging capacity of the colonic flora to an undigested carbohydrate is exhausted.

Diarrhea attributable to carbohydrate malabsorption is usually more severe in children (especially infants) than in adults because the intestinal passage of nutrients is more rapid in children. Further impact of unabsorbed carbohydrates on intestinal motility consists of inhibition of gastric emptying and acceleration of small intestinal transit.[8] These effects are more tremendous when malabsorption is associated with conditions such as irritable bowel syndrome[9,10] that are known to accelerate bowel transit.

Diagnosing a disaccharidase deficiency starts with a precise nutritional history, which often points the way to the diagnostic and therapeutic approach. The onset of clinical features often coincides with the introduction of specific disaccharides, such as sucrose and lactose. The parents may already have started a dietary restriction based on empiric observations. In contrast, the causal needs of some patients are suitable to overestimate some unspecific complaints. The assessment of symptoms associated with disaccharidase deficiencies, such as vomiting, abdominal pain, meteorism, and diarrhea, can be difficult because the clinical features show a broad heterogeneity and change with age. Therefore, it is important to evaluate noninvasive tests such as stool examinations (pH and reducing substances), oral tolerance, and, preferentially, hydrogen breath test in the context of specific loads with suspected disaccharides. Breath testing uses the bacterial carbohydrate metabolism in the colon with the production of hydrogen, which is absorbed by the mucosa of the colon and excreted in breath. The (invasive) determination of enzyme activities from homogenates of proximal small intestinal biopsies is required independent of the clinical (therapeutic) relevance. Finally, the therapeutic (long-term) effect of disaccharide restriction must be considered in the conclusive consultation of the patient. Taken together, the diagnosis of a disaccharide deficiency should not be founded only on the result of one of the mentioned diagnostic approaches but in the context of the patients' complaints and sensitive and specific laboratory evaluations.

SUCRASE–ISOMALTASE

Structure, Biosynthesis, and Polarized Sorting of SI

The SI enzyme complex (EC 3.2.1.48-10), the most abundant glycoprotein in the intestinal brush border membrane, is an integral membrane protein that is composed of two subunits, sucrase and isomaltase (isomaltase ~145 kDa and sucrase ~130 kDa).[11] Sucrase and isomaltase are enzymatically active toward α-glycosidically linked carbohydrates, the most abundant sugars in mammalian diet. Sucrase digests primarily 1,2-α- and 1,4-α-glucopyranosidic bonds and is responsible for the terminal digestion of dietary sucrose and starch. Isomaltase hydrolyzes mainly α-1,6 linkages. By virtue of these hydrolytic properties, the SI enzyme complex belongs to a superfamily of α-glucosidases in higher organisms, including, for example, brush border MGA (see later), mammalian lysosomal α-glucosidase, invertase and glucoamylase of *Saccharomyces cerevisiae*, and glucoamylase of *Schwanniomyces occidentalis*.[12]

SI is a type II membrane glycoprotein in which the N-terminal end exhibits a cytosolic orientation and the C-terminal extrudes into the lumen, that is, SI has an N_{in}/C_{out} orientation. The transmembrane domain in this type of membrane proteins also comprises the signal sequence required for translocation of the newly synthesized protein into the endoplasmic reticulum (ER). Figure 1 depicts a schematic presentation of the structure and biosynthesis of SI).[13] An interesting structural feature of SI is a heavily *O*-glycosylated serine/threonine-rich stalk domain in the immediate vicinity of the membrane.[3,13] The extensive *O*-glycosylation of this short domain imposes rigidity and inflexibility, resembling that of a stalk. These structural features may play a role in protecting SI from being digested by pancreatic secretions at the membrane interface (thus decreasing the turnover rate), thus prolonging the life cycle of this molecule in the intestinal lumen. Another important region is the cytoplasmic tail, which contains 12-amino acid residues and has been proposed to undergo phosphorylation in vivo at the conserved Ser_6, raising the possibility that this posttranslational event may be implicated in essential regulatory processes of the protein.[14] Cloning of full-length complementary deoxyribonucleic acids (cDNAs) encoding the rabbit and human species of SI have shown that 38% of the amino acid sequences of sucrase and isomaltase are identical, and an additional 34% show conservative changes.[13] The striking similarity between the two subunits has led to the concept that SI has emerged from one cycle of duplication of a single gene. Furthermore, sequence comparison of SI

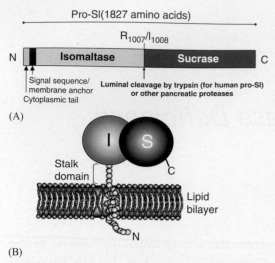

Pro-SI(1827 amino acids)

Figure 1 Structure and biosynthesis of pro-sucrase–isomaltase (pro-SI) in human small intestinal cells. (A) Pro-SI is a type II integral membrane glycoprotein that is synthesized with an uncleavable signal sequence for translocation into the endoplasmic reticulum and consists of 1,827 amino acids. Pro-SI therefore has an N_{in}/C_{out} orientation. The N-terminal starts with a cytoplasmic tail (Met_1-Ser_{12}) followed by a membrane anchor that also contains the signal sequence Leu_{13}-Ala_{32}. A serine/threonine-rich stalk region encompasses the sequences Thr_{33}-Ser_{61} and is the site of extensive O-glycosylation of pro-SI. Isomaltase ends with amino acid residue Arg_{1007}, and sucrase starts immediately thereafter with Ile_{1008}. The Arg/Ile peptide sequence between isomaltase and sucrase is a trypsin site where the mature large precursor pro-SI is cleaved in the intestinal lumen by pancreatic secretions. The human enzyme is cleaved by pancreatic secretions (trypsin in the case of the human enzyme and elastase for the rat enzyme). Sucrase and isomaltase remain strongly associated with each other through ionic interactions. The membrane orientation of pro-SI is depicted in (B) with the cytosolic N-terminal, a luminal C-terminal, and the stalk domain next to the membrane. I = isomaltase; S = sucrase.

with the human lysosomal α-glucosidase and the glucoamylase from the yeast *S. occidentalis* suggests that these proteins have evolved from the same ancestral gene.[12] Although no three-dimensional structure of this large protein is so far available, the striking sequence similarities between sucrase and isomaltase and algorithmic predictions suggest the existence of subdomains within the two species that reveal similar folding patterns, and the native folded state of the SI enzyme complex can be referred to as a pseudodimer.[13] This is further favored by the behavior of sucrase and isomaltase toward proteases. With the exception of the major extracellular cleavage step of the mature precursor form, pro-SI, by luminal trypsin (see later), both species are resistant toward pancreatic proteases and do not reveal altered proteolytic maps, as would be expected for differently folded proteins.[3] It is likely that both subunits can function as autonomous and independent units within the same polypeptide precursor. Nevertheless, individual expression of the subunits in heterologous transfection systems revealed the necessity of isomaltase for the presence of sucrase, which functions as a C-terminally located intramolecular chaperone in the folding of isomaltase.[15] In contrast, it is indepen-

dent of the presence of isomaltase and acquires correct folding, enzymatic activity, and competent intracellular transport. The enzyme complex is expressed and synthesized exclusively by differentiated intestinal epithelial cells initially as a mannose-rich polypeptide precursor of an apparent molecular mass of 210 kDa. The transport of this form from the ER to the Golgi cisternae occurs at a relatively slow rate (half-time of ~105 to 110 minutes) (for comparison, the intestinal proteins dipeptidyl peptidase IV and aminopeptidase N are transported at a half-time of ~15 and 20 minutes, respectively).[3,4] Major posttranslational processing of pro-SI occurs in the Golgi apparatus, leading to the generation of a complex N- and O-glycosylated mature pro-SI.[3] In particular, O-glycosylation is an essential modification that has implications on the further transport of pro-SI to the brush border membrane. Initial evaluation of the role of O-glycans on the sorting of pro-SI employed the inhibitor of O-glycosylation, benzyl-N-acetyl-β-D-galactoseaminide (benzyl-N-acetylgalactosamine), in the intestinal cell line Caco-2 cells.[16] This reagent leads to a drastic reduction in the size of pro-SI owing to impaired O-glycosylation. Concomitantly, the sorting behavior is dramatically altered from an efficient exclusive apical targeting to a random delivery of the modified pro-SI glycoform to both membranes, the apical and basolateral.[16] Deletion analyses have enabled the identification of the apical sorting signal within the stalk region of pro-SI.[17] The mechanism by which the sorting of pro-SI occurs is through association of SI with detergent-insoluble membrane microdomains enriched in glycosphingolipids and cholesterol, known as lipid rafts. In fact, inhibition of sphingolipid synthesis by fumonisin results in a random delivery of pro-SI to the apical and the basolateral membranes. A direct involvement of O-linked glycans in the association of pro-SI with lipid rafts is likely to be the driving mechanism for apical sorting of pro-SI.[16,17] The final step in the trafficking of pro-SI is its budding from the TGN in a special type of carriers that is enriched in cholesterol and sphingolipids and are associated with annexin II, myosin Ia, and alpha-kinase 1.[18,19] These carriers are transported to the cell surface via the actin cytoskeleton.[20] Inhibition of actin polymerization by latrunculin or cytochalasin D results in an intracellular accumulation of pro-SI in the *trans*-Golgi network.

The isomaltase and the sucrase subunits are O-glycosylated. Moreover, O-glycosylation of the sucrase subunit is heterogeneous, as revealed by the presence of at least four glycoforms of differently O-glycosylated sucrase species, whereas the O-glycosylation pattern of the isomaltase subunit is more unique, suggesting a more efficient and consistent glycosylation of isomaltase compared with that of sucrase.[3] The variations in the O-glycosylation pattern of the subunits are presumably the consequence of spatial constraints, whereby isomaltase is readily O-glycosylated because it contains a serine/threonine-rich stalk region that is located in immediate proximity

of the membrane, whereas the sucrase is more distal.[13] O-Glycosylation of pro-SI is not only required for correct targeting of pro-SI to the apical membrane, but also modulates the activity of isomaltase, which increases concomitantly with O-glycosylation.[3]

The final step along the biosynthetic pathway of pro-SI is the proteolytic cleavage in the intestinal lumen of the fully glycosylated precursor (pro-SIc; c stands for complex glycosylated, 245 kDa) by trypsin[11] or other pancreatic proteases into its two mature, enzymatically active subunits, sucrase (Sc, 130 kDa) and isomaltase (Ic, 145 kDa). These two subunits remain associated with each other through noncovalent strong ionic interactions.

The expression of pro-SI depends exclusively on the differentiated state of the intestine. In many tissues, cell differentiation is associated with altered gene expression owing to activation or repression of gene transcription. Gene activation and subsequent expression by tissue-specific transcription factors generate novel cellular phenotypic markers that are associated with significant morphologic and functional alterations of the differentiated cell. Differentiation of intestinal crypt cells to columnar epithelial cells, for example, results in the generation of two structurally and functionally different domains, the apical and basolateral domains,[21] and is characterized by the expression of genes encoding cell surface proteins that are implicated in the final steps of digestion of micromolecular nutrients, transports, and receptors. Among these genes are those encoding the disaccharidases SI, LPH, and MGA.[22] Functional, immunohistochemical, and in situ hybridization studies have demonstrated that the pattern of expression of these disaccharidases, which are barely detectable in the crypts, reaches maximum levels between the lower and midvillus and decreases at the villus tip.[4,23]

Meanwhile, the structure and sequence of the SI gene are known.[24] Much of the information about the structure of the SI gene has described 5'-flanking regions and their role in transcription and regulation.[25] In addition to this, the sequences of the full-length cDNAs of the chicken, rabbit, rat, and human species are known.[25–28] One of the intriguing features of the gene structure of SI, which is perhaps unique for this enzyme, is that its first exon is untranslated, and the second exon starts with the initiation ATG codon.

Molecular Basis of Congenital Sucrase–Isomaltase Deficiency

The expression of SI and its activity increase during weaning and persist at high levels in adulthood.[29] The regulation of the SI activity is a transcriptional event that implicates SI- and intestine-specific nuclear factors. Meanwhile, several studies have identified several of these factors, as well as the structure of the SI gene. The SI gene consists of 48 exons, many of which reveal a predicted β-sheet or β/α-barrel secondary structures. A very similar exon/intron organization reveals the gene of MGA, suggesting a close evolutionary structural and functional relation between the two genes.[24] A critical factor in regulating the SI promoter is *Cdx2*, an intestine-specific caudal-related homeobox gene that may also have a broader role in intestinal development and morphogenesis.[22]

Expression studies of promoter regions of the SI gene have assigned the intestine-specific promoter elements to a region between −183 and +54. On the other hand, several stretches within the sequence −3424 to +54 have an inhibitory effect on the level of transcription of SI. Assessment of the interaction of nuclear proteins with the promoter by footprint analyses has identified three specific footprints for SI (denoted SIF1, SIF2, and SIF3 for SI footprints 1, 2, and 3, respectively).[30,31] Only SIF1 was found to be intestine specific because it was not identified in the nonintestinal cell line HepG2, in contrast to SIF2 and SIF3. Nevertheless, all three elements are implicated in positive regulation of SI gene transcription.[30]

Negative regulation of SI expression is potentially possible. Modulatory effects of certain additives, such as glucose, on the expression levels of SI in the intestinal cell line Caco-2 cells proposed negative regulatory mechanisms that operate at the messenger ribonucleic acid (mRNA) level of SI.[25] Fructose has also been reported to suppress posttranslationally the expression of brush border enzymes.[32]

Posttranslational regulation is the most common mechanism that significantly affects the physiology and cellular expression of SI. These effects are elicited by altered structural features: impaired, defective, or abnormal posttranslational processing of an otherwise normally expressed SI protein and aberrant distribution of SI on the apical and basolateral domains of the enterocytes. These abnormalities in the cell biology and protein chemistry of SI constitute the basis for the congenital sucrase–isomaltase deficiency (CSID) in humans.[30,32–35] In addition to its clinical relevance, CSID has been used as a promising approach to characterize various steps in the biosynthesis, transport, and sorting of SI as a general model for cell surface membrane proteins and highly polarized proteins in epithelial cells.

Substantial progress has been made to elucidate the molecular basis of CSID. Different molecular defects or mutations in the SI gene have been proposed to be responsible for CSID. A number of studies with duodenal biopsy specimens from patients with this disorder at the subcellular and molecular levels have led to the identification of several phenotypes of SI in CSID that could be discriminated on the basis of subcellular localization, type, and nature of the mutation or residual enzymatic activities (Table 1 and Figure 2).[33–35] The emerging concept from all these studies is that these phenotypes are generated by point mutations in the coding region of the SI protein. Our group was the first to successfully clone and characterize a cDNA encoding SI from a biopsy sample of a patient with CSID and to identify a single point mutation that is responsible for the impaired transport behavior of SI in phenotype II.[37] In the meantime, mutations correlating with other CSID phenotypes have been identified, and in what follows, a survey of the features of the individual phenotypes is presented (see also Table 1 and Figures 2 and 3).

Phenotype I Is Blocked in the ER. Phenotype I is characterized by a misfolded immature form of SI that is not capable of passing through the quality control machinery and is blocked in the ER as a mannose-rich glycosylated protein that is ultimately degraded.[33] Immunoprecipitation with several epitope-specific monoclonal anti-SI antibodies followed by enzymatic measurements demonstrated that the activity of this phenotype is below the detection limit. This phenotype is the predominant one among the CSID phenotypes. Most of the mutations that affect the trafficking of SI generate a misfolded form that is blocked in the ER. Recently, a CSID case with properties similar to those of phenotype I has been analyzed at the molecular and cellular levels (Ritz and colleagues, unpublished data). Whereas biosynthetic labelings of an intestinal biopsy specimen and

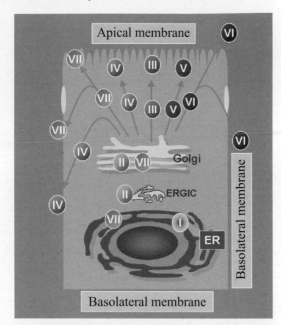

Figure 2 Schematic representation of the phenotypes of congenital sucrase-isomaltase deficiency. Phenotype I is blocked in the endoplasmic reticulum (ER) and phenotype II in the ER/*cis*-Golgi intermediate compartment and *cis*-Golgi.[35,37,41] Phenotype III is transported normally to the cell surface, but the sucrase subunit is enzymatically inactive.[35] Phenotype IV is randomly distributed on the apical and basolateral membranes.[33,38] In phenotype V, only the isomaltase subunit is transported to the apical membrane, whereas sucrase undergoes intracellular degradation.[33] Phenotype VI is characterized by an intracellular cleavage of pro-SI in the ER, generating a pro-sucrase–isomaltase that lacks its membrane-anchoring domain and stalk region and is secreted from both sides of the membranes of the enterocytes as an active protein.[39]

immunoelectron microscopy reveal predominant localization of SI in the ER and hence are similar to phenotype I, a partial conversion of the SI protein to a complex glycosylated mature form suggests a classification of this case as a subtype of phenotype I. The SI cDNA in this phenotype revealed a point mutation that results in an exchange of a leucine by a proline at position 620 (L620P) of the isomaltase subunit.[36] The expression of this mutation in a heterologous cell line generates a protein with similar characteristics

Phenotype	Cellular Localization of SI	Enzymatic Activity	Molecular Forms	Mutation	Reference
I	ER	Completely inactive	Mannose-rich 210 kDa pro-SI	L620P	33–35, 36
II	ER, ER-Golgi intermediate compartment (ERGIC) and *cis*-Golgi	Completely inactive	Predominant mannose-rich 210 kDa pro-SI and partial complex 245 kDa pro-SI	Q1098P	33, 35, 37
III	Brush border membrane	Completely inactive	Mannose-rich 210 kDa pro-SI and complex 245 kDa pro-SI	Not identified	35
IV	Random on apical as well as basolateral membranes	Active sucrase and isomaltase	Mannose-rich 210 kDa pro-SI and complex 245 kDa pro-SI	Q117R	33, 38
V	Intracellular cleavage, degradation of sucrase, isomaltase is correctly located at the apical membrane	Active isomaltase and absent sucrase activity	Mannose-rich 210 kDa pro-SI, complex 245 kDa pro-SI and 150 kDa isomaltase	Not identified	33
VI	Intracellular cleavage, enzyme secreted	Active sucrase and isomaltase	Mannose-rich 210 kDa pro-SI and mannose-rich 207 kDa cleaved pro-SI and complex glycosylated 240 kDa cleaved pro-SI	L340P	39
VII	ER, random cell surface distribution at the apical as well as basolateral membranes	Decreased sucrase activity and absent isomaltase	Predominant mannose-rich 210 kDa pro-SI and partial complex 245 kDa pro-SI	C635R	40

Table 1 Naturally Occurring Phenotypes of Congenital Sucrase Isomaltase Deficiency (CSID)

Control

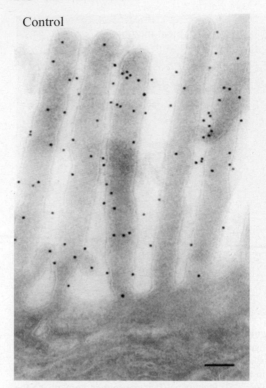

CSID

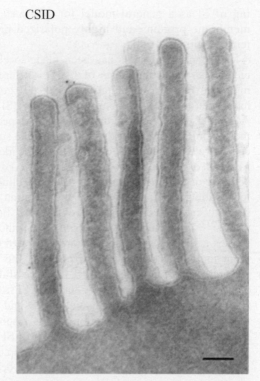

Figure 3 Immunogold labeling of sucrase–isomaltase (SI) within a thin frozen section of a duodenal biopsy of a control and a patient with congenital sucrase–isomaltase deficiency (CSID). Strong immunogold labeling corresponding to SI could be detected at the microvillar membrane of enterocytes from normal controls. In one case of CSID, the microvillar membrane was devoid of immunogold labeling owing to a defective intracellular transport behavior of SI. The absence of SI at the apical membrane could be observed in CSID phenotypes I, II, and VI.[35,37,41,39] Phenotype III is characterized by normal levels of SI in the brush border membrane,[35] whereas phenotype IV reveals marked reduction in the appearance of SI in the apical membrane, with the concomitant labeling of the basolateral membrane.[33,38] In phenotype V, only isomaltase could be detected in the brush border membrane.[33]

and intracellular localization to the intestinal phenotype. Thus, it was partially complex glycosylated and localized predominantly in the ER and, to a lesser extent, at the cell surface. In addition, examination of the folding pattern in a proteolytic sensitivity assay results in an entire degradation of this mutant with the protease trypsin owing to additionally exposed cleavage sites in the malfolded protein.

Phenotype II Is Blocked in the *cis*-Golgi and ER Golgi Intermediate Compartments. The second most common phenotype of CSID is phenotype II. One of the most significant cellular features of phenotype II is an intracellular accumulation in the Golgi apparatus.[33] Some cases of CSID reveal the SI protein in the *cis*-Golgi in addition to the ER and the ER/*cis*-Golgi intermediate compartment (ERGIC), and in other cases, an accumulation in the medial and *trans*-Golgi has been observed.[34] In all of these cases, an enzymatically inactive mannose-rich polypeptide could be immunoisolated. Naim and colleagues have identified a mutation in this phenotype that results in a substitution of a glutamine by a proline in the sucrase subunit of SI at amino acid 1098 (Q1098P).[37] One of the consequences of this mutation is the synthesis of a temperature-sensitive form of SI that accumulates in the *cis*-Golgi and ERGIC.[42] This observation and type of localization are surprising for membrane proteins because the consensus has emerged that proteins fulfilling the requirements of the quality control machinery in the ER and exiting this

organelle acquire transport competence up to their final destination. For SI, this destination should be the cell surface; in phenotype II, however, the SI protein is blocked in the *cis*-Golgi. As such, this observation has important implications for current concepts of membrane and protein transport because this suggests that the Q1098P mutation generates a recognition site for a protein involved in a hypothetical quality control mechanism that operates beyond the ER, and such an event has not yet been described. The Q1098P substitution has therefore been investigated in more detail, and we could demonstrate that it is not only functional in intestinal epithelial cells, but also produces a similar phenotype when expressed in nonpolarized COS-1 cells.[41] It is apparent therefore that (1) the Q1098P mutation is responsible for the generation of the SI phenotype II and (2) the onset of this CSID phenotype does not involve cellular factors specifically expressed in the small intestine. One important observation is that the folding state of the mutant SI protein is not as stable as its wild-type counterpart and is degraded within a relatively short period of time. The interesting aspect of these folding experiments is that the sucrase and the isomaltase subunits in the mutant phenotype II are degraded. Although malfolding of the sucrase subunit as a result of the mutation Q1098P is plausible, the altered structure of the isomaltase in the context of SI suggests that the association between sucrase and isomaltase takes place very early in the ER, whereby the sucrase subunit plays a decisive role in the folding of iso-

maltase and could be designated an intramolecular chaperone. In fact, more recent evidence has proven this hypothesis and provided further data in which an alternating association between the ER chaperones BiP and calnexin, together with sucrase, occurs during the folding process of isomaltase.[15] Therefore, it is clear that sucrase is an important and crucial player in the acquisition of isomaltase to its physiologic function and transport competence within the cell on its way to the cell surface.

One of the interesting features of the Q1098P mutation is its presence in a region that shares striking homologies among human, rat, and rabbit sucrase and isomaltase variants, as well as human lysosomal α-glucosidase and *S. occidentalis* glucoamylase.[12] The fact that all these proteins, which have been suggested to have evolved from a common ancestral gene, are transported along the secretory pathway to their final destinations proposes a key role for the region containing the Q1098P mutation in the sorting of these proteins from the ER and proposes a common function of this or structurally similar regions in other proteins along the secretory pathway. Indeed, we could show that the Q1098P mutation of sucrase elicits a similar effect when introduced at the corresponding amino acid position 244 in lysosomal α-glucosidase.[41] The mutated lysosomal α-glucosidase precursor does not undergo maturation in the Golgi, is not cleaved into mature enzyme, and is not transported through the Golgi cisternae. It is therefore conceivable that the Q1098P mutation has introduced a retention signal for the *cis*-Golgi or the mutation has led to a structural alteration in lysosomal α-glucosidase that functions as a recognition site for a quality control machinery operating in the intermediate compartment or *cis*-Golgi. The components of this hypothetical machinery must be unraveled.

Phenotype II Is a Temperature-Sensitive Mutant. One striking feature of phenotype II, in addition to the unusual block of SI in the *cis*-Golgi and ERGIC, is that the mutation Q1098P generates a temperature-sensitive mutant SI protein. In fact, biochemical and confocal microscopy analyses could unequivocally demonstrate that correct folding, intracellular transport, and full enzymatic activity can be restored by expression of the mutant SI (indicated $SI_{Q/P}$) at the permissive temperature of 20°C instead of 37°C.[42] Moreover, the acquisition of normal protein trafficking and function appears to use several cycles of anterograde and retrograde steps between the ER and the Golgi, implicating the molecular chaperones calnexin and BiP. A similar temperature-sensitive feature has also been proposed to be generated by the main genetic alteration in cystic fibrosis, the DF508 deletion in the cystic fibrosis transmembrane regulator.[43] However, the Q1098P mutation in phenotype II of SI is the first of its kind to generate a temperature-sensitive mutant implicated in an intestinal enzyme deficiency or an intestinal disorder.

Normal Intracellular Protein Transport and Absent Enzymatic Activity in phenotype III.

In sharp contrast to the phenotypes I and II is phenotype III. Here SI is transported to the cell surface with kinetics similar to that of the wild-type protein. It is correctly folded because it reacted efficiently with different epitope-specific monoclonal antibodies and is correctly sorted to the apical membrane.[35] These criteria are adequate to propose that gross structural alterations did not occur in this specific phenotype of SI. Although further information about the location of the putative mutation in this phenotype is lacking, it is reasonable to assume that the mutation has immediately affected the catalytic site of sucrase, Asp,[1349] or is located in immediate vicinity of the catalytic domain of sucrase, which is the DGL-WIDMNE stretch.[13] The isomaltase subunit, on the other hand, expresses normal activity and is therefore not affected in this phenotype.

Random Delivery of SI to the Apical and the Basolateral Membranes Is the Characteristic of Phenotype IV.

SI is almost exclusively (95%) located at the apical membrane of intestinal epithelial cells. This striking polarity and high sorting fidelity are required for an efficient function of the protein in the intestinal lumen. Deviation from this polarity pattern and an impaired sorting profile are associated with reduced function of SI and subsequent malabsorption. Analysis of two cases of CSID using immunoelectron microscopy demonstrated an altered distribution of SI from an exclusive apical to a random localization at the apical membrane and basolateral membranes.[33,38] Molecular characterization of this novel phenotype revealed a point mutation in the coding region of the SI gene that results in an amino acid substitution of a glutamine by arginine at residue 117 (Q117R) of the isomaltase subunit.[38] This amino acid exchange is located in a domain revealing features of a trefoil motif or a P domain in the immediate vicinity of the heavily O-glycosylated stalk domain. In wild-type SI, the stalk domain itself is directly involved in the targeting of the SI molecule to the apical membrane through an interaction of its O-glycosylated carbohydrate content with a putative lectin receptor that recruits SI to lipid rafts.[16] Although the location of the mutation in the P domain of SI did not affect O-glycosylation of the mutant SI protein per se, random targeting of SI to the apical and basolateral membranes occurred. Unlike wild-type SI, the mutant protein is completely extractable with Triton X-100, despite the presence of O-glycans, which are required for the association of SI with detergent-insoluble lipid microdomains. This finding indicated that the O-glycan units were not adequately recognized in the context of the mutant SI by a putative lectin-like sorting receptor owing to a sterical hindrance or altered folding of the P domain generated by the mutation Q117R. Importantly, this naturally occurring mutant phenotype was the first of its kind of an apically sorted protein; moreover, it provided strong support to the notion of an active apical sorting mediated by sorting signals and a corresponding receptor.

Intracellular Proteolytic Cleavage at Two Different Sites in Phenotypes V and VI.

Human SI is transported to the brush border membrane as a single-chain polypeptide, pro-SI, which is cleaved in the intestinal lumen by pancreatic trypsin to isomaltase and sucrase.[3] In phenotypes V and VI, the pro-SI precursor is intracellularly cleaved.[33,39] The cleavage sites are, however, different. In phenotype V, the cleavage occurs relatively late in the biosynthesis, in the trans-Golgi or trans-Golgi network.[33] In fact, biosynthetic labeling of an intestinal biopsy specimen and immunoisolation of SI revealed normal levels of the ER-located, mannose-rich polypeptide at an early labeling time point of 30 minutes. Within 4 hours of labeling, the complex glycosylated mature SI appears to be concomitant with the detection of a polypeptide of an apparent molecular weight similar to that of isomaltase.[33] The sucrase subunit was not detected by immunoprecipitation with monoclonal antisucrase antibodies. This observation was supported by immunolabeling of intestinal biopsy specimens. Here only the isomaltase subunit was detected at the apical membrane with an antiisomaltase antibody. Obviously, the sucrase subunit in this phenotype undergoes an intracellular degradation immediately after being proteolytically processed from the precursor protein, whereas the isomaltase is transported correctly to the apical membrane. This phenotype provided the first indication that the isomaltase contains all of the necessary information required for apical transport of SI. Later, this hypothesis was experimentally verified, and the signals for apical sorting were identified in the O-glycosylated stalk region, and the membrane-anchoring domain and both domains were located in the isomaltase subunit.[16,17] The putative mutation in this phenotype has not yet been identified. Another mode of cleavage characterizes phenotype VI.[39] Biosynthesis of SI in intestinal explants revealed, in addition to the mannose-rich pro-SI polypeptide precursor, another band of smaller apparent molecular weight. The glycosylation pattern of this species was also of the mannose-rich type, suggesting that this band is a truncated form of the mannose-rich polypeptide and that the cleavage occurs within the ER. This view was supported by cDNA cloning of the SI from this phenotype and identification of the point mutation, as well as expression of the mutant cDNA in COS cells. The molecular basis of this phenotype is a point mutation isomaltase subunit that converts a leucine to proline at residue 340 of isomaltase. Expression of the mutant in COS cells and biosynthetic pulse-chase experiments revealed that pro-SI is cleaved early in the biosynthesis, in the ER, and the cleaved protein is transported efficiently along the secretory pathway, processed in the Golgi apparatus, and ultimately secreted into the exterior milieu as an active enzyme. This is a novel pathogenetic mechanism of a disorder that is elicited by the conversion of an integral membrane glycoprotein into a secreted species that is lost from the cell surface.

Altered Folding, Sorting, and Increased Turnover Are the Characteristics of Phenotype VII.

Recently, we could identify a novel case of CSID in which a cysteine was substituted by an arginine at amino acid residue 635 of the isomaltase subunit.[40] This mutation affects disulphide bond formation and leads subsequently to alterations in the folding pattern of pro-SI and subsequent reduction in the stability of the protein as assessed by its increased turnover rates to about 36 hours which renders a half life of about 50% of the wild-type protein. Another major consequence of altered folding is the partial transport of the mutant protein to the basolateral membrane (Figure 4). Furthermore, the enzymatic activity of the mutant towards the substrate sucrose is substantially decreased and the activity of isomaltase is below detection limit. These measurements are indicative of an altered folding at least around the activity centers of the isomaltase and sucrase subunits.

Heterozygosity in Novel Cases of CSID.

While all CSID cases so far analyzed conformed exclusively to the "homozygous single mutation concept," several novel CSID cases from Eastern Europe and therefore different ethnic origin have revealed a new type of pathogenetic mechanism that is based on heterozygous mutations that act together to elicit CSID.[44]

However, further biochemical and cell biological analysis is required to evaluate the role of these mutations in the pathogenesis of the disease.

EPIDEMIOLOGY OF CSID

The prevalence of CSID is 0.2% in individuals of European descent[45] and appears to be much higher in Greenland, Alaskan, and Canadian native people. It has been estimated to be 5% in indigenous Greenlanders.[46] Heterozygotes, which are defined as sucrase activity level below the lower limit for the normal population and with normal small bowel morphology, represent about 2 to 9% of European Americans.[47,48] CSID is transmitted by autosomal recessive inheritance. Recently compound heterozygous mutations have been demonstrated in CSID.[44] It was first described by Weijers and colleagues.[49]

Pathophysiology of CSID

Several factors, some of them less favorably present in infants, contribute to the development and extent of symptoms in CSID patients.

Residual Enzyme Activity.

Amount of fed carbohydrate (in association with other foods)

- Gastric emptying
- Small bowel transit
- Degree of fermentation of unabsorbed carbohydrates by colonic bacteria
- Absorption of the colon

Sucrase hydrolyzes α-1,2- and α-1,4-glucosidic bonds, whereas isomaltase cleaves

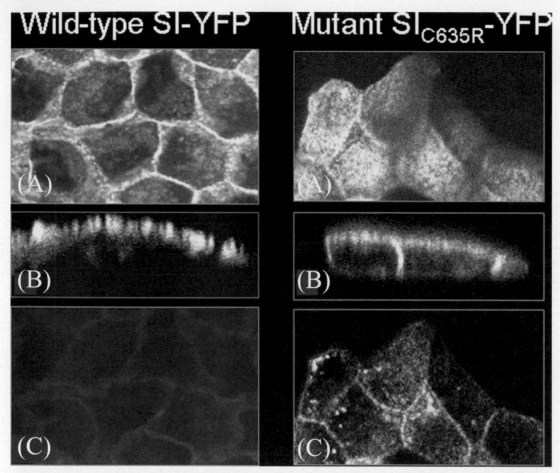

Figure 4 Polarized targeting of SI and SI_{C635R}.[40] Shown is an analysis by confocal laser microscopy of YFP-tagged versions of wild-type SI (SI-YFP) and mutant SI_{C635R} (SI_{C635R}-YFP) that were stably expressed in polarized MDCK II cells. The images show an exclusive localization of wild-type SI at the apical membrane, while a marked distribution of the SI_{C635R}-YFP mutant at the basolateral membrane is observed.

α-1,6-linkages. SI overlaps with MGA, which digests the end and intermediary products of α-amylolysis of starch, such as maltose, maltotriose, and low- and high-molecular-weight branched dextrins, by hydrolyzing α-1,4-glucosidic linkages. However, only 20% of maltase activity is covered by MGA and 80% by SI.[5] Several factors led to the observation that patients with CSID tolerate starch better than sucrose:

1. MGA activity is preserved.

2. Starch fed by infants and toddlers has a low amount of α-1,6-glucosidic bonds, which may by sufficiently hydrolyzed by the residual isomaltase activity.

3. Colonic bacteria ferment starch in infants by 6 months of age.

Clinical Features of CSID

SI-deficient infants receiving human milk and lactose-containing formulas do not develop symptoms. Some parents introduced empirically a low-sucrose diet. Populations such as the Greenland Eskimos use traditionally low-carbohydrate diets with a high amount of protein and fat. Later, introduction of sucrose and its reduction in quantity led to a delay in the onset of diarrhea.[50] Characteristic symptoms of patients with CSID are crying spells, vomiting, meteorism, watery diarrhea, mild steatorrhea, and chronic diarrhea.[51] Occasionally, dehydration, malnutrition, failure to thrive and to grow, developmental retardation, and muscular hypotonia were observed, indicating broad clinical heterogeneity.[45,52]

Presenting symptoms depend more on age and the amount of ingested sucrose than on the intestinal levels of SI activity. Symptoms and especially starch tolerance spontaneously improve with age. Chronic watery diarrhea and failure to thrive are common in infants and toddlers, chronic diarrhea with normal growth is usually found in preschool children, and irritable bowel syndrome and recurrent abdominal pain are typical symptoms of schoolchildren.[45] Adult patients present with refractory diarrhea or unspecific complaints.[53–55] Symptoms may present at the time of puberty, possibly unmasked by gastroenteritis. Onset of symptoms in adulthood with diagnosis up to the age of 59 years has been reported.[56]

Clinical heterogeneity includes (adult) patients with CSID who do not develop diarrhea following ingestion of large amounts of sucrose. In a few cases, CSID was associated with nephrocalcinosis, renal calculi,[53,55] metabolic acidosis, and hypercalcemia.[55–57]

The diagnosis of CSID is often missed or delayed because diseases such as food allergy, cystic fibrosis, and celiac disease or other causes of recurrent diarrhea are suggested.

Transient hypoglycemia, acidosis, and lethargy may even lead one to consider inborn errors of metabolism.

Diagnostic Evaluation of CSID

A major step in diagnosing CSID is to recognize the complaints and clinical features of patients in relation to age-dependent alterations and composition of nutrition; sometimes, the parents started an empiric low sucrose diet.

Stool and urine examinations serve as screening methods with limited sensitivity and specificity. A stool pH between 5.0 and 6.0 is an indicative but, finally, unreliable screening test for the diagnosis of sugar malabsorption.[58] The detection of reducing substances estimated with Clinitest tablets (normal <0.5%) in stool, whose sucrose is hydrolyzed by boiling with 0.1 N HCl, has been proposed as a screening test for the diagnosis of CSID.[59] However, this method is not specific for sucrose.[58] Stool pH and reducing substances are falsely negative as soon as nonabsorbed carbohydrates are totally fermented in the colon. In contrast, reducing substances tend to be falsely positive in neonates and patients who have undergone a colectomy. The differential urinary excretion of sucrose in relation to lactulose can be used to diagnose SI deficiency[60]; however, this noninvasive sugar absorption test has not been approved in a larger series of patients.

A rise of blood glucose of less than 20 mg/dL after a 2.0 g/kg sucrose load indicates sucrose intolerance. Capillary blood samples show higher peak rises up to 25 mg/dL in blood glucose compared with venous samples.[61] Oral tolerance tests produce false-positive results between 24 and 33% owing to delayed gastric emptying.[62] False-positive results are also due to increased intestinal transit time. Monitoring of symptoms and determination of reducing substances in the stools within 6 hours improve the diagnostic values of this method.

Patients with CSID show a rise of breath hydrogen of more than 20 ppm over baseline between 90 and 180 (240) minutes after an oral load of 2.0 g/kg sucrose.[63,64] False-negative results are obtained by a delay in gastric emptying, the acid milieu of the colon (unrestricted diet prior to the test),[65] and nonhydrogen producers (following antibiotic therapy).[66,67] Up to 18% of patients who are referred for the evaluation of lactose intolerance are hydrogen nonexcretors.[68] Fast intestinal transit produces false-positive results on the breath test. The sucrose tolerance test, the hydrogen breath test, and sucrase activity did not strictly correlate in children who suffered from chronic diarrhea.[69]

The diagnosis of CSID requires the determination of SI activity with normal histology of the mucosa and the level of other disaccharidases (lactase, MGA, and alkaline phosphatase) in the normal range (DD: secondary deficiency owing to general mucosa damage). Enterocytes of patients with CSID lack the sucrase activity of the enzyme SI, whereas the isomaltase activity can vary from absent to practically normal. Disaccharidase activities show a 40% reduction in the duodenum compared with the proximal jejunum.[70,71] In some SI-deficient patients, MGA activity is reduced in addition to isomaltase activity.[72] Combined deficiency of sucrase, lactase, and MGA, which seems to be caused by pleiotropic regulatory factors, has recently been described.[73] The differential diagnosis of CSID is broad, including the various causes of chronic diarrhea in childhood.

Therapy of CSID

Lifelong sucrose restriction is an effective therapeutic option for patients with CSID; it works well and is cheaper (as supplementation with sucrase). Because patients with CSID tolerate smaller or larger amounts of sucrose, the degree of restriction finally depends on the individual complaints of a patient. Foods with nutrients with high sucrose concentrations are beetroot (6.0), pea (4.5), honey (3.0), soybean flour (4.5), and onion (2.9 g/100 g edible parts). Care has to be taken with sucrose included in glucose polymer formulas[74] and medications. Because isomaltase function is also affected, the diet also excludes starch and glucose polymers, that is, foods with high amylopectin content such as wheat (cereals, bread, and pasta) and potatoes, especially in the first years of life. Tolerance to starch improves during the first 3 to 4 years. Rice starch and maize starch are the best digested. Arguing with compliance problems of a sucrose-restricted diet, it has to be considered that no short- or long-term complications of noncompliance are known, with the exception of severe (missed) cases.[55]

Lyophilized baker's yeast (*S. cerevisiae*), which is not very palatable, possesses sucrase activity, low isomaltase and maltase activity, and virtually no lactase activity. It has been shown that viable yeast cells reduce hydrogen excretion by 70%, with loss or reduction of clinical symptoms.[75]

Recently, sacrosidase (invertase), a liquid preparation produced from *S. cerevisiae* (Sucraid) that has already been used to hydrolyze unrefined sucrose solutions, has been successfully used in the treatment of patients with CSID.[76] It is a β-fructofuranosidase that is tasteless and resistant to pH changes down to 1.5, but it has no activity with oligosaccharides containing α-1,6-glucosyl bonds.

LACTASE–PHLORIZIN HYDROLASE

Structure, Biosynthesis, and Polarized Sorting of LPH

LPH (EC 3.2.1.23/62) is a type I integral membrane glycoprotein of the intestinal brush border membrane that comprises two major hydrolytic activities[77]: lactase activity, which is responsible for the hydrolysis of milk sugar lactose, the main carbohydrate in mammalian milk, and phlorizin hydrolase, which digests β-glycosylceramides, which are part of the diet of most vertebrates. A physiologic role of phlorhizin hydrolase activity is still unknown.[77]

The LPH gene is located on chromosome 2 and consists of 17 coding domains, or exons.[78–80] The amino acid sequence deduced from the cDNA encoding LPH consists of 1,927 amino acids (Figure 5 summarizes the structural and biosynthetic features of LPH). The LPH molecule is highly *N*- and *O*-glycosylated. The primary sequence of the human enzyme predicted 15 potential *N*-glycosylation sites (the rabbit and rat enzymes possess 14 and 15, respectively). *N*- and *O*-Glycosylation are crucial in the folding, maturation, and enzymatic activity of LPH.[81,82] A study of the effect of glycosylation on the intracellular transport of human LPH in biopsy samples in the presence or absence of glycosidase inhibitors demonstrated that carbohydrate modification affects the transport rates from the ER to the *cis*-Golgi, but is not important in the transport of LPH from the *cis*-Golgi to the cell surface.[2,82] Moreover, processing of N-linked carbohydrates has direct effects on the *O*-glycosylation of LPH, which is essential for the acquisition of LPH to an efficient enzymatic function. In fact, a mature *N*- and *O*-glycosylated LPH protein is almost fourfold more active than a LPH glycoform that is only *N*-glycosylated.[82]

All cloned LPH species have shown that the molecule consists of four highly conserved structural and functional regions.[80] These domains, denoted I to IV, reveal 38 to 55% identity to one another. The catalytic activity of lactase is localized to Gln_{1273} in the homologous region III and of phlorizin hydrolase is localized to Gln_{1749} in the homologous region IV.[83] Because of the four homologous regions, LPH may have arisen from two subsequent duplications of one ancestral gene.[80] An evolutionary and developmental example supporting this notion is given by the sequence similarities of LPH and each of its homologous regions with β-glycosidases from archebacteria, eubacteria, and fungi. It is possible that LPH belongs to a superfamily of β-glucosidases and β-galactosidases. The prokaryotic β-glycosidases are, on average, about 50 kDa in size, which corresponds to approximately one-fourth of the size of full-length LPH or roughly to the size of one homologous region (I to IV).

The biosynthesis and processing of LPH in several mammalian intestinal epithelial cells follow essentially similar pathways.[2,84,85] In what follows, the posttranslational processing of the human enzyme most relevant to this book is described in Figure 5. LPH is synthesized as a single-chain 215 kDa pro-LPH precursor that is *N*-glycosylated while translocating into the ER. *N*-Glycosylation is a critical covalent modification that is directly implicated in the attainment of pro-LPH to a correct protein folding, which, in turn, is a prerequisite for homodimerization, another modification step that takes place in the ER and is absolutely required for pro-LPH to exit the ER.[88,89] Dimerization is not only important for efficient transport from the ER, it is also crucial for the acquisition of enzymatic activity.[89] A correctly folded monomeric pro-LPH is not sufficient per se for a functional protein. The transmembrane domain of pro-LPH is a crucial structure in the dimerization event of pro-LPH, and its elimination results in a monomeric, inactive pro-LPH. Complex *N*- and *O*-glycosylation of pro-LPH in the Golgi apparatus precedes a proteolytic cleavage step that takes place in a late Golgi compartment, most likely the *trans*-Golgi network, and eliminates the large profragment LPHα at Arg_{734}/Leu_{735}, leaving the membrane-bound $LPHβ_{initial}$, which extends from Leu_{735} to Tyr_{1927}.[86,87] $LPHβ_{initial}$ is sorted with high fidelity to the apical membrane, where it is cleaved by pancreatic trypsin at Arg_{868}/Ala_{869} to $LPHβ_{final}$ (Ala_{869}–Tyr_{1927}), which comprises the functional domains of the enzyme and is also known as mature brush border LPH of 160 kDa.[2,84,85] The proteolytic cleavage of pro-LPH neither activates LPH nor is required for the correct transport of LPH to the brush border membrane.[90–92] The profragment LPHα undergoes intracellular degradation immediately after intracellular cleavage, as has been shown in pulse-chase experiments of intestinal biopsy samples.[93] The LPHα polypeptide is neither *N*-glycosylated, despite the presence of five potential *N*-glycosylation sites, nor *O*-glycosylated. This, together with its high content of hydrophobic amino acids and its tendency to form a compact, rigid, and trypsin-resistant structure immediately after translation, endows LPHα with the characteristics of an intramolecular chaperone that is directly involved in the folding of the $LPHβ_{initial}$ domain. Individual expression of a cDNA encoding $LPHβ_{initial}$ generated a protein that was not as transport competent as pro-LPH. Only when $LPHβ_{initial}$ was coexpressed with LPHα were correct folding and enzymatic activity of $LPHβ_{initial}$ restored.[94] It is clear, therefore, that LPHα is required in the context of correct folding of pro-LPH. Finally, LPHα does not express enzymatic activities toward lactose, despite the strong structural homologies between regions LPHα and LPHβ.[92]

To achieve its physiologic function, pro-LPH or its membrane-bound form must be transported to the luminal surface of epithelial cells, that is, to the brush border membrane. The sorting to the apical membrane of proteins such as LPH is signal mediated. Until present, several types of signals have been described; some of them are associated with membrane detergent-insoluble glycophosphatidylinositol (DIG)/cholesterol membrane microdomains,[90] whereas some do not associate with DIGs. LPH is not associated with microdomains, and its sorting is not mediated through *O*-glycans as SI.[16,95,96] Recent observations have strongly suggested that putative sorting signals of pro-LPH are exclusively located in the domain corresponding to the brush border-associated $LPHβ_{final}$, precisely in the homologous region IV that also harbors the catalytic domain of LPH.[91,97]

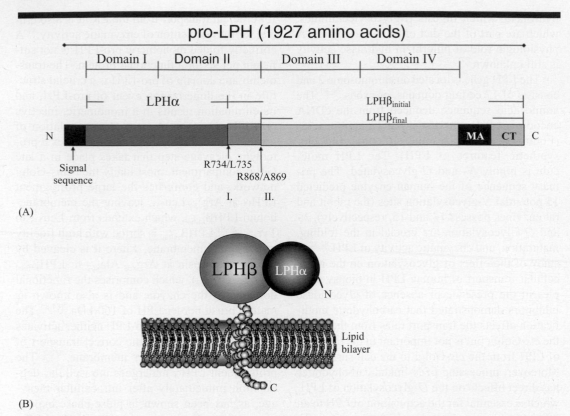

Figure 5 Schematic representation of the structure of pro-lactase–phlorhizin hydrolase (LPH) in human small intestinal cells and the two constructs LPHβ and LPHα. (A) Some important structural features of pro-LPH in human small intestinal cells. Shown is the cleavable sequence Met^1-Gly^{19} at the N-terminal. The ectodomain encompasses amino acid residues Ser^{20} to Thr^{1882}. Four internal homology domains within the pro-LPH amino acid sequence are indicated. The intracellular proteolytic cleavage takes place between Arg^{734} and Leu^{735} to generate LPH $β_{initial}$. The luminal extracellular cleavage occurs at Arg^{868} to generate the brush border mature enzyme, LPH $β_{final}$ (Arg^{868}-Phe^{1927}).[86,87] (B) Schematic drawing of the membrane orientation of pro-LPH. The C-terminal on the cytosolic side of the membrane, the luminal N-terminal, and the subunits LPHα and LPHβ are depicted. CT = cytoplasmic tail; MA = membrane anchoring.

Epidemiology of Adult-Type Hypolactasia

Primary adult-type hypolactasia affects the majority of the world's human population. More than 75% of the human adult population shows a decline to about 5 to 10% of the level at birth during childhood and adolescence ("post-weaning decline"). The incidence of adult-type hypolactasia varies between different populations because the expression of lactase is genetically determined. Up to 80% of Blacks Arabs, and Latinos, as well as up to 100% of American Indians and Asians, reveal adult-type hypolactasia; the lowest prevalences (<5%) are detected in populations in northwestern Europe.[98] The persistence of lactase activity is most likely a consequence of a dominant gene defect with failure to repress the synthesis of lactase after weaning in regions with an abundant milk supply, which implies the "culture historical hypothesis."[99]

Molecular Basis of Adult-Type Hypolactasia

Genetic analysis of homozygotes and heterozygotes of lactase-persistent and lactase-nonpersistent families supported the initial idea that lactase activity is inherited as a single autosomal dominant gene.[100] There are currently several ideas that attempt to explain the late onset of lactase activity. Initial concepts suggested that lactase regulation may be a posttranslational event, as

is the case in CSID (see above). Alterations in the structural features of LPH itself may generate an inactive protein or lead to a defective post-translational processing and possibly intracellular degradation of the protein. This hypothesis was later discussed when the mRNA levels of lactase in the intestine of adult rats were found to be almost similar to the mRNA levels in fetal rats.[101] Another study used biopsy material to demonstrate that appreciable levels of lactase mRNA were detected in the intestines of hypolactasic individuals in southern Italy.[102] These observations were compatible with posttranslational regulatory mechanisms of adult-type hypolactasia.

A study of a race- and sex-balanced cohort in which levels of jejunal lactase protein, activity, and mRNA were measured showed that black heritage predicts low lactose-digesting capacity (LDC) and white heritage predicts high LDC.[103] A decisive criterion in these studies was the assessment of the lactase-to-sucrase ratio (L:S) in jejunal biopsy specimens. All subjects with a high LDC had an L:S ratio >0.5, immunodetectable LPH protein, and measurably higher LPH mRNA levels than subjects with low LDC. Further, LPH mRNA levels correlated highly with lactase-specific activity ($r = .80$) and L:S ratio ($r = .88$). The direct correlation between LPH mRNA levels and lactase expression argues that the gene responsible for the human lactase polymorphism regulates the level of LPH mRNA.

Similarly, studies in the rat small intestine have essentially described a similar coordinate pattern of interrelationship between mRNA and protein levels of LPH.[101] The regional distribution of lactase activity, although clearly dependent on the presence of the LPH mRNA pattern, did not absolutely correlate with the mRNA and protein levels along the proximal–distal axis. This suggests that additional secondary mechanisms, perhaps posttranslational, influence the lactase activity. One potential modification is O-glycosylation that commences in the cis-Golgi and increases the activity of LPH fourfold.[82] It is known that variations in the extent of O-glycans are associated with the differentiation state of intestinal cells to polarized enterocytes. These events are associated with dramatic alterations in the gene expression of intestinal proteins and increased enzymatic activities of typical intestinal markers such as SI and LPH. Along this, a regulatory mechanism of the enzymatic function of LPH (and also SI) that depends on the carbohydrate moiety and therefore the differentiation state of the intestinal cell cannot be excluded. Despite this, the major mechanism of regulation of LPH is transcriptional because the majority of the accumulated data have clearly demonstrated that adequate levels of LPH mRNA must be present to detect LPH activities.[100,103,104] Meanwhile, the structure of the LPH gene has been published, as well as data on the interaction of specific regulatory elements with 5′-flanking regions of the gene. The gene for LPH is approximately 55 kb and is made out of 17 exons, which all encode LPH.[78] Transcription factors such as CTF/NF-1 and AP2 bind to regions in the LPH gene located within 1 kb of the 5′-flanking region of rat and human genes.[105] The lactase activity has been demonstrated to be enhanced in rats by glucocorticoids during the first weeks in life. Glucocorticoids also have regulatory effects on human lactase.[106] Responsive elements to glucocorticoids have not been, however, in the 5′-flanking region of LPH. Analysis of 5′-flanking sequences employed, fused to human growth hormone as a reporter gene in transfected Caco-2 cells or the nonintestinal cell line HepG2, has demonstrated the exclusive and specific function of these sequences in cells of intestinal lineage.[107] Footprint analysis of the promoter region has led to the identification of a nuclear protein (NF-LPH1) that binds to a 15 bp region just upstream from the transcription site (between −54 and −40), which is functional in the adenocarcinoma cell line Caco-2 and is probably involved in regulation of lactase activity.[105,108]

A specific region in the LPH promoter, CE-LPH1, has been identified that interacts with NF-LPH1 and is strongly associated with the regulation of gene transcription of LPH.[108,109] Nevertheless, differences in the promoter region of LPH between individuals with low LDC and those with high LDC have not been detected. Likewise, there is no evidence that describes variations in the levels of particular transcription factors associated with low or high LDC. Also, sequence analyses of the coding and promoter regions of the gene encoding LPH did not reveal DNA variations associated with low LDC. More recently, however, Enattah and colleagues identified a variant associated with adult-type hypolactasia.[110] Linkage dysequilibrium and haplotype analyses of nine extended Finnish families, the locus to a 47 kb interval on chromosome 2q21, were restricted. Sequence analysis revealed a DNA variant, C/T-13910, about 14 kb upstream from the gene locus of LPH that associates with low LDC in Finnish families and 236 individuals from four different populations. Another variant, G/A-22018, 8 kb telomeric to C/T-13910, is also associated with adult-type hypolactasia in 229 of 236 cases. Significant effects of these variants on the levels of LPH mRNA and the L:S ratio were demonstrated. Here the expression of LPH mRNA in the intestinal mucosa in individuals with T(-13910), A(-22018) alleles was found to be manyfold higher than that found in individuals with C(-13910), G(-22018) alleles.[111] Likewise, a significant elevation of the L:S ratio in the T(-13910), A(-22018) allele could be observed.

Clinical Features of Adult-Type Hypolactasia

Symptoms of adult-type hypolactasia increase with age, with many patients developing signs of lactose intolerance in adolescence and adulthood. They start briefly after consumption of milk, causing abdominal discomfort (colicky pain), flatulence, loose stools, diarrhea, and flatus. Symptoms are related to the amount of lactose administered, showing a broad heterogeneity in response among patients.

A major issue is the clinical relevance of lactose intolerance. The milk rejection rate has been 31% among the lactose malabsorbers and 12% among the lactose-tolerant individuals. However, 70% of the lactose-intolerant patients drink some milk.[112] Fifty-nine to 75% of lactose malabsorbers develop symptoms within 3 or 4 hours after ingesting 12 g of lactose (equivalent to 240 mL of milk) or less, 2 of 20 subjects had symptoms with 3 g of lactose, and 5 of 20 subjects had symptoms with 24 to 96 g of lactose.[112,113] Individuals with low lactase levels have revealed persistently low polyethylene glycol concentrations, representing fluid accumulation in the jejunum of 6 g of fed lactose and in the ileum of 12 and 24 g of fed lactose.[113] This study found no consistent correlation between jejunal lactase levels and the threshold for lactose-inducted symptoms. Symptoms in most lactose malabsorbers do not appear to be caused by small amounts (0.5 to 7.0 g) of lactose.[114] Other studies have identified lactose malabsorbers who tolerate one (240 mL) or even two cups of milk per day.[115,116]

The question has been raised as to whether symptomatic lactose malabsorbers have an additional gastrointestinal affection, such as irritable bowel syndrome.[115,117] Because about 70% of patients with milk intolerance and patients with irritable bowel syndrome revealed a positive lactose hydrogen breath test[118] and bowel transit is increased in irritable bowel syndrome,[9,10] it is hypothesized that fast intestinal transit contributes to the complaints of lactose malabsorbers.

Diagnostic Evaluation of Adult-Type Hypolactasia

Symptoms and nutritional history lead to the diagnosis of adult-type hypolactasia. Laboratory assessment of this diagnosis includes, preferentially, a lactose hydrogen breath test and, exceptionally, confirmation by lactase activity of a duodenal biopsy. The diagnostic values of other procedures, such as reducing substances, which are positive in the feces of patients with lactose malabsorption, implying no specificity for lactose malabsorption, are limited and depend more on the context of the patients' complaints and the results of additional laboratory evaluations. The lactose tolerance test is considered to be less sensitive than the lactose breath test. The latter does not reliably predict tolerance toward lactose in infants recovering from diarrhea.[69,118] Another study has found the relationship between the lactose breath hydrogen test and lactase activities not to be uniform.[119] A bad correlation among the lactose tolerance test, lactase activity, and hydrogen breath test has been found in children who suffered from chronic diarrhea.[69]

Lactose tolerance and hydrogen breath tests using an oral load of 2.0 g/kg lactose (<50 g) must be performed after a 6-hour (overnight) fast. The monitoring of symptoms (abdominal discomfort, flatulence, and diarrhea) is crucial during and after testing. Conditions that cause false-positive results are a low gastric emptying rate[62,120] and fast intestinal transit time.[121] False-negative results of the breath test are obtained by hydrogen nonexcretors or are due to prior treatment with antibiotics. Hydrogen breath tests are falsely negative in nonexcretors because hydrogen is metabolized by bacteria to methane. The daytime breath hydrogen profile, which includes breath sampling at home at half-hour intervals during 1 day from awakening until bedtime, was abnormal in children with abdominal pain and diarrhea,[122] suggesting that the prevalence of lactose malabsorption underlying these conditions is high.

Diagnosis of adult-type hypolactasia on the enzyme level requires lactase activity in jejunal (duodenal) biopsies of less than 8 U/g protein or 0.7 U/g wet weight.[119] Disaccharidase activities are reduced in the duodenum compared with the proximal jejunum.[70,71] Other disaccharidase activities, as well as the morphology of the mucosa, must be in the normal range to exclude a secondary lactase deficiency. Therefore, the ratios of maltase to lactase and sucrase to lactase have been proposed as additional parameters.[123] Disaccharidase (lactase, sucrase, and maltase) activity in aspirated fluid correlates with that measured in the mucosal microvillus membrane,[124] but this method has not been widely adopted.

The value of the C/T-13910 genotype,[110,125,126] which is associated with adult-type hypolactasia, for the decision to initiate a lactose-free diet, is questionable. Sub-Saharan pastoralists tolerate milk instead of being C/C-13910 positive. In-vitro experiments showed that C-13910 actually enhances (but less than T-13910) lactase promotor activity.[127,128] Furthermore, the T/T-13910 genotype does not allow the exclusion of a secondary lactose intolerance.

Concerning the clinical relevance of lactose intolerance, it is a crucial diagnostic step to determine the response of the patient to a lactose-reduced diet. It allows one to estimate which symptoms are solely caused by lactose intolerance and not to additional affections, such as irritable bowel syndrome. The differential diagnosis of adult-type hypolactasia includes other causes of chronic diarrhea in childhood, especially infectious, immunologic (cow's milk allergy), and inflammatory disorders of the intestinal mucosa, many of them causing secondary lactase deficiency owing to mucosal damage. A reduction of duodenal lactase ($p = .024$) and pathologic lactose breath testing ($p = .005$) has been reported in patients with active Crohn's disease in contrast to Crohn's disease patients in remission.[129] Another study has not found lactase activity levels to be different in a cohort of patients with inflammatory bowel disease (37%) in comparison with control patients with chronic abdominal pain.[129,130]

Therapeutic Aspects of Hypolactasia

An increased frequency of osteoporosis have been reported in lactose malabsorbers that is due to the dietary calcium restriction as a consequence of milk avoidance.[131,132] Total calcium consumption is lower among non–milk-drinkers by about 18%.[133] Calcium is essential for adequate mineralization of bone matrix. Because lactose malabsorbers cannot use the main source of calcium, that is, dairy products, they need calcium supplementation to prevent osteoporosis.[134] Two hundred forty milliliters of milk contains 300 mg of calcium, with linkage to casein and optimal bioavailability. The National Academy of Science recommends a dietary calcium intake of 210 mg/d for age 0 to 6 months, 270 mg/d for age 6 months to 1 year, 500 mg/d for age 1 to 3 years, 800 mg/d for age 4 to 8 years, and 1,300 mg/d for age 9 to 18 years.[135] Recently the Committee on Nutrition of the American Academy of Pediatrics released guidances to improve the daily intake of calcium in children and adolescents to reduce the risk of osteoporosis.[136,137] Many lactose malabsorbers tolerate small amounts of milk without complaints so that they can improve calcium intake by solid cheeses and yogurt. In contrast to food allergy or celiac disease lactose intolerance allows to titrate the amount of lactose tolerated by the malabsorber. Yogurt is a fermented milk product containing live active culture of *Lactobacillus bulgaricus* and *Streptococcus thermophilus*, which reveal lactase activity. The lactase of yogurt, cultured buttermilk, and curds ferments lactose to lactic acid; however, pasteurization of these products reduces digestion of lactose. *Lactobacillus acidophilus* also possesses lactase activity and is available as "sweet acidophilus milk," with a taste similar to that of milk.[138] Alternatives to dairy products represent calcium-fortified fruit (orange) juice, vegetables, or lactose-free milks.

Lactase (β-galactosidase) is produced from yeast (*Kluyveromyces lactis*) or fungi (*Aspergillus oryzae*). Preincubation of milk with lactase was associated with a significant lower breath hydrogen and crying time in infants with colic compared with placebo.[139] Formulation of stable lactase microparticles with enteric release seems to preserve the activity of acid-labile lactase for enteric release.[140] However, warming of breast milk and formulas treated with lactase for 15 minutes significantly increases osmolality by 87 to 122 mOsm/kg owing to hydrolysis of lactose.[141]

Addition of lactase to a preterm formula may enhance weight gain.[142] Preterm infants have relative lactose malabsorption because lactase activity is only 30% of its full-term level by 26 to 34 weeks gestation.[143] Lactase activity is depressed in rabbit fetuses with intrauterine growth retardation.[144] Hypoxia in newborn rats causes delayed maturation of lactase.[145] Enteral feeding of preterm infants is suggested to increase lactase activity,[146] which has been confirmed in preterm pigs.[147] Sphingomyelin, the major phospholipid of human milk, reduces lactase in the intestine of 2-week-old rats, promoting enzymatic and morphologic maturation of the neonatal gut.[148]

Gene technological strategies to lower the lactose content in milk are developed[149] because more than 75% of the adult human population is affected by hypolactasia, and long-term complications of lactose malabsorption, such as osteoporosis, represent an endemic disease. There are inconsistent studies regarding the hypothesis that lactase deficiency protects against parasite infections such as malaria.[150,151] The strategy to reduce the lactose content in milk includes benefits even for individuals without lactase deficiency, taking into account that the potentially harmful effects of lactose consumption, such as arteriosclerosis and ovarian cancer, can be overcome. A high incidence of galactose-induced senile (cortical) cataracts has been found in lactose absorbers.[152,153] Ischemic heart disease and ovarian cancer have also been attributed to the consumption of high amounts of lactose (galactose).[154–156] In contrast, there is some evidence that lactose may be beneficial against lower intestinal diseases such as Crohn's disease because of its prebiotic potential.[157] Prebiotics are essential for the establishment of intestinal colonization of newborns. On the other hand, *Bifidobacterium bifidum*, as well as conventional colonization of the germ-free intestine, induces biochemical maturation of enterocytes in gnotobiotic mice, promoting the postnatal decline of lactase activity.[158]

Congenital Lactase Deficiency (Alactasia)

Congenital lactase deficiency is a rare disorder inherited by an autosomal recessive mode. Since the first report in 1959,[159] few cases of this disease

have been described.[160,161] To date, the molecular basis of this deficiency is still obscure. However, posttranslational mechanisms are likely to be implicated in the lactase activity in these cases, as has been described for CSID (see above). In 32 Finish patients, a homozygous nonsense mutation (Y1390X), called "Fin(major)," was detected in 84% of the cases; the other mutations were early trunctions (S166fsX1722, S218fsX224) and point mutations (Q268H and G1363S), which were compound heterozygous for Y1390X.[162]

The typical symptoms of congenital lactase deficiency start from a few days after birth with the onset of breastfeeding (or lactose-containing formula feeding). They consist of liquid and acid diarrhea, meteorism, and severe malnutrition. The patients are hungry; vomiting is rarely noted. Some patients present with hypercalcemia and nephrocalcinosis, which may be provoked by the metabolic acidosis and/or the calcium absorption-increasing effect of lactose.[163]

When congenital lactase deficiency is suspected, a lactose-free diet should be started. In the case of a positive effect, this diagnosis is further confirmed. Finally, the diagnosis needs to be based on a deficient lactase activity in a duodenal or jejunal biopsy. Other disaccharidases, as well as the morphology of the intestinal mucosa, should be in the normal range. Molecular genetics offers an additional diagnostic approach.[162]

Because of the severe symptoms, congenital lactase deficiency requires a strong restriction to a lactose-free diet (see above). In the further course of the disease, some patients may cope well with lactase supplementation.

MALTASE–GLUCOAMYLASE

Structure and Biosynthesis of MGA

Another brush border enzyme with digestive properties similar to those of isomaltase, MGA (EC 3.2.1. 20 and 3.2.1.3) contributes to the overall digestion of α-glycosidic linkages of carbohydrates. MGA compensates the lack of SI in a number of cases of CSID. MGA activity has been proposed to serve as an alternate pathway for starch digestion when luminal α-amylase activity is reduced because of immaturity or malnutrition, whereby MGA plays a unique role in the digestion of malted dietary oligosaccharides.[24] Similar to SI, MGA is a type II integral membrane glycoprotein of the intestinal. Immunoprecipitation with specific monoclonal antibodies and electrophoretic analysis of the precipitates under denaturing conditions reveal a 335 kDa single polypeptide in the presence or absence of reducing agents.[1] Examination of the quaternary structure of MGA by cross-linking analyses demonstrated a monomeric form of MGA in the brush border membrane. Biosynthetic studies in intestinal biopsy samples revealed two forms of MGA: the ER 285 kDa mannose-rich polypeptide and the mature, complex, glycosylated 335 kDa brush border protein. Unlike SI, mature MGA does not undergo extracellular cleavage in the brush bor-

der membrane by pancreatic secretions because the 335 kDa polypeptide was the dominant form in the presence or absence of pancreatic secretions. In a fashion similar to SI, MGA is heavily *N*- and *O*-glycosylated, and it is likely that its trafficking to the brush border membrane is mediated by *O*-glycan units located in the stalk region—again, a structural similarity with SI.

The cDNA of human small intestinal MGA cDNA has recently been isolated from mRNA using reverse-transcriptase polymerase chain reaction.[164] The deduced amino acid sequence of 1,857 amino acids corresponds to an unglycosylated protein of an apparent molecular mass of 210 kDa. The substantial difference between this size and the biosynthetic forms of MGA in biopsy samples is probably due to glycosylation and the electrophoretic behavior of the glycoforms on SDS-polyacrylamide gel electrophoresis. It is also possible that splice variants of MGA exist. MGA and SI are strikingly homologous (59% homology) and, correspondingly, share several common structural features, such as the presence of an *O*-glycosylated stalk region immediately following the membrane-anchoring domain, a trefoil or P domain, and two identical catalytic sites.[164]

The recent cloning and sequencing of the human MGA gene could demonstrate its close evolutionary relationship to SI. The gene is located at chromosome 7q34 and consists of 58 exons.[24] Expression of the gene product results in a protein that hydrolyzes maltose and starch, but not sucrose, and is thus distinct from SI. Another similarity of both genes is their identical exon structures. These similarities strongly support the notion that MGA and SI have evolved by duplication of an ancestral gene, which itself had already undergone a gene duplication.

Molecular Basis of MGA Deficiency

The hypothesis that villus atrophy accounts for the reduced maltase enzyme was examined in mucosal biopsy specimens.[165] It was observed that the drastic reduction in the maltase activity and the MGA mRNA levels of about 45% paralleled the reduction in the villin mRNA used as a marker for villus integrity. Likewise, the levels of the SI mRNA were also decreased in proportion to villus atrophy of malnourished infants. Congenital cases of MGA deficiency are rare, and one case has recently been characterized at the molecular level.[73] In this case, however, sucrase deficiency and lactase deficiency have also been detected. Isolation and sequencing of the MGA cDNA revealed homozygosity for a nucleotide change in the patient that resulted in a substitution of serine by leucine at amino acid residue 542 (S542L), very close to the catalytic site aspartic acid. Analysis of the function of this mutation by its introduction into the wild-type MGA cDNA did not reveal any alteration in the biosynthesis, processing, and enzymatic activity of mutant MGA. The promoter region of MGA in this patient was also analyzed, and no nucleotide changes could be observed. This case led to the conclusion that the reduced activities of MGA, SI, and LPH are caused by shared, pleiotropic regulatory factors.

Clinical Implications of MGA Deficiency

In 1994, glucoamylase deficiency was reported in a large group of children suffering from chronic diarrhea; the morphology of their mucosa was normal.[166] The incidence was estimated to be 1.8% among children with chronic diarrhea. Although these patients have revealed normal pancreatic amylase activities, other disaccharidases, most notably isomaltase, have shown marked reduced activities in addition to glucoamylase. This could be due to the known overlap of isomaltase and glucoamylase activities toward maltose as a substrate.

Primary MGA deficiency should be suspected in the differential diagnosis of chronic diarrhea of infants and toddlers. Besides diarrhea, patients present with abdominal distention and bloating. Symptoms start with the introduction of starch and formula containing short polymers of starch at 4 to 6 months of age or later until the fifth year of life.

Some of these MGA-deficient patients show a positive response to challenge with 2 to 4 g/kg starch and to reelimination of starch. The starch digestive capacity can be evaluated by the $^{13}CO_2$ breath test using ^{13}C-starch oligomers as a loading substrate.[73,167] Reducing substances are inconsistently found to be positive. The diagnosis is established by low activity of glucoamylase of a duodenal biopsy and evidence of a normal pancreatic amylase. A high percentage of glucoamylase-deficient subjects have been found in a group of dyspeptic children with normal duodenal histology, some of them presenting additionally with low activity of sucrase and lactase.[168]

An elimination diet excluding starches and short polymers of glucose within lactose-free infant formulas should be given for 3 to 4 weeks, documenting any relief of symptoms. When symptoms regress following the introduction of the diet, patients should stick to this diet to an extent, which keeps them free of symptoms.

TREHALASE

Structure and Function of Trehalase

Trehalase is another member of α-glucosidases of the small intestine.[169] It is also present in the human serum.[170] Because plasma trehalase activity is increased in diabetes[171] and reduced in rheumatoid arthritis,[172] it is not used to diagnose trehalase deficiency. Its substrate, trehalose, is a disaccharide composed of two glucose molecules. It is contained in mushrooms, lower plants (algae), insects, *Ascaris lumbricoides*, and *Artemia salina*. Because trehalose improves the quality of dried food, it became a food additive.

A complete cDNA clone encoding human trehalase has been isolated from a human kidney library.[173] The protein is composed of 583 amino acids with a calculated molecular weight of 66,595 kDa. The enzyme is a type I membrane glycoprotein that is synthesized with a typical cleavable signal peptide at amino terminus and contains five potential glycosylation sites. Trehalase is associated with the membrane via a glycosylphosphatidylinositol type of membrane anchor. The sequence similarity of the human enzyme with those of the rabbit, silkworm, *Tenebrio molitor*, *Escherichia coli*, and yeast suggested a common old ancestral gene. The small intestine trehalase is also expressed in the liver and the kidney.

Trehalase Deficiency

The first case of trehalase deficiency, which is inherited as an autosomal recessive disorder, was reported in 1971.[174] Two years later, it was described in a family.[175] An autosomal recessive inheritance has been suggested as a genetic background owing to trehalase deficiency. Other brush border enzymes are not affected. Trehalase deficiency is found in 8% of Greenlanders.[176,177] It is rare in white Americans.[48] Only a few cases have been described in other populations. The implications and significance of this observation on molecular pathophysiology of the intestine are unclear, however.

The major source of trehalose for humans is young mushrooms.[178] Symptoms resembling those of lactose intolerance consist mainly of vomiting, abdominal pain, meteorism, and diarrhea. Two trehalase-deficient patients developed no symptoms after trehalose load and proclaimed themselves mushroom tolerant.[178]

Because the increases in breath hydrogen and blood glucose did not differ between trehalose-intolerant and -tolerant subjects, oral tolerance and breath tests seem to be unsuitable for diagnostic investigation.[178] Trehalase deficiency requires the performance of a duodenal biopsy with determination of trehalase activity. The normal range (mean ± 2 SD) of trehalase activity is 4.79 to 37.12 U/g protein.[177] Trehalase deficiency is diagnosed when the activity of duodenal trehalase is less than 8 U/g protein.[176] The activities of other brush border enzymes, as well as the duodenal histology, are normal, ruling out the presence of a general mucosa damage as an underlying cause of trehalase deficiency. The few studies performed indicate that there is a poor correlation among patient complaints, results of oral tolerance and breath testing, and trehalase activities.

The only available therapy is trehalose restriction, which includes reducing the consumption of mushrooms and trehalose-containing food additives. At present, several applications of trehalose in human nutrition are considered by the food industry.[179]

REFERENCES

1. Naim HY, Sterchi EE, Lentze MJ. Structure, biosynthesis, and glycosylation of human small intestinal maltase-glucoamylase. J Biol Chem 1988;263:19709–17.
2. Naim HY, Sterchi EE, Lentze MJ. Biosynthesis and maturation of lactase–phlorizin hydrolase in the human small intestinal epithelial cells. Biochem J 1987;241:427–34.
3. Naim HY, Sterchi EE, Lentze MJ. Biosynthesis of the human sucrase–isomaltase complex. Differential *O*-glycosylation of the sucrase subunit correlates with its position within the enzyme complex. J Biol Chem 1988;263:7242–53.
4. Hauri HP, Sterchi EE, Bienz D, et al. Expression and intracellular transport of microvillus membrane hydrolases in human intestinal epithelial cells. J Cell Biol 1985;101:838–51.
5. Kelly JJ, Alpers DH. Properties of human intestinal glucoamylase. Biochim Biophys Acta 1973;315:113–22.
6. Debongnie JC, Newcomer AD, McGill DB, Phillips SF. Absorption of nutrients in lactase deficiency. Dig Dis Sci 1979;24:225–31.
7. Cummings JH, Englyst HN. Fermentation in the human large intestine and the available substrates. Am J Clin Nutr 1987;45:1243–55.
8. Launiala K. The effect of unabsorbed sucrose and mannitol on the small intestinal flow rate and mean transit time. Scand J Gastroenterol 1968;3:665–71.
9. Houghton LA, Atkinson W, Whitaker RP, et al. Increased platelet depleted plasma 5-hydroxytryptamic concentration following meal ingestion in symptomatic female subjects with diarrhoea predominant irritable bowel syndrome. Gut 2003;52:663–70.
10. Wackerbauer R, Schmidt T. Symbolic dynamics of jejunal motility in the irritable bowel. Chaos 1999;9:805–11.
11. Hauri HP, Quaroni A, Isselbacher KJ. Biogenesis of intestinal plasma membrane: Posttranslational route and cleavage of sucrase–isomaltase. Proc Natl Acad Sci U S A 1979;76:5183–6.
12. Naim HY, Niermann T, Kleinhans U, et al. Striking structural and functional similarities suggest that intestinal sucrase–isomaltase, human lysosomal alpha-glucosidase and Schwanniomyces occidentalis glucoamylase are derived from a common ancestral gene. FEBS Lett 1991;294:109–12.
13. Hunziker W, Spiess M, Semenza G, Lodish HF. The sucrase–isomaltase complex: Primary structure, membrane-orientation, and evolution of a stalked, intrinsic brush border protein. Cell 1986;46:227–34.
14. Keller P, Semenza G, Shaltiel S. Phosphorylation of the N-terminal intracellular tail of sucrase–isomaltase by cAMP-dependent protein kinase. Eur J Biochem 1995;233:963–8.
15. Jacob R, Purschel B, Naim HY. Sucrase is an intramolecular chaperone located at the C-terminal end of the sucrase–isomaltase enzyme complex. J Biol Chem 2002;277:32141–8.
16. Alfalah M, Jacob R, Preuss U, et al. O-linked glycans mediate apical sorting of human intestinal sucrase–isomaltase through association with lipid rafts. Curr Biol 1999;9:593–6.
17. Jacob R, Alfalah M, Grunberg J, et al. Structural determinants required for apical sorting of an intestinal brush-border membrane protein. J Biol Chem 2000;275:6566–72.
18. Heine M, Cramm-Behrens CI, Ansari A, et al. Alpha-kinase 1, a new component in apical protein transport. J Biol Chem 2005;280:25637–43.
19. Jacob R, Heine M, Eikemeyer J, et al. Annexin II is required for apical transport in polarized epithelial cells. J Biol Chem 2004;279:3680-4.
20. Jacob R, Heine M, Alfalah M, Naim HY. Distinct cytoskeletal tracks direct individual vesicle populations to the apical membrane of epithelial cells. Curr Biol 2003;13:607–12.
21. Traber PG, Silberg DG. Intestine-specific gene transcription. Annu Rev Physiol 1996;58:275–97.
22. Olsen WA, Lloyd M, Korsmo H, He YZ. Regulation of sucrase and lactase in Caco-2 cells: Relationship to nuclear factors SIF-1 and NF-LPH-1. Am J Physiol 1996;271:G707–13.
23. Rings EH, de Boer PA, Moorman AF, et al. Lactase gene expression during early development of rat small intestine. Gastroenterology 1992;103:1154–61.
24. Nichols BL, Avery S, Sen P, et al. The maltase–glucoamylase gene: Common ancestry to sucrase–isomaltase with complementary starch digestion activities. Proc Natl Acad Sci U S A 2003;100:1432–7.
25. Chantret I, Lacasa M, Chevalier G, et al. Sequence of the complete cDNA and the 5_ structure of the human sucrase–isomaltase gene. Possible homology with a yeast glucoamylase. Biochem J 1992;285:915–23.
26. Uni Z. Research notes: Identification and isolation of chicken sucrase–isomaltase cDNA sequence. Poult Sci 1998;77:140–4.
27. Pothoulakis C, Gilbert RJ, Cladaras C, et al. Rabbit sucrase-isomaltase contains a functional intestinal receptor for Clostridium difficile toxin A. J Clin Invest 1996;98:641–9.
28. Chandrasena G, Osterholm DE, Sunitha I, Henning SJ. Cloning and sequencing of a full-length rat sucrase-isomaltase-encoding cDNA. Gene 1994;150:355–60.
29. van Beers EH, Rings EH, Taminiau JA, et al. Regulation of lactase and sucrase–isomaltase gene expression in the duodenum during childhood. J Pediatr Gastroenterol Nutr 1998;27:37–46.

30. Wu GD, Chen L, Forslund K, Traber PG. Hepatocyte nuclear factor-1 alpha (HNF-1 alpha) and HNF-1 beta regulate transcription via two elements in an intestine-specific promoter. J Biol Chem 1994;269:17080–5.

31. Traber PG, Wu GD, Wang W. Novel DNA-binding proteins regulate intestine-specific transcription of the sucrase–isomaltase gene. Mol Cell Biol 1992;12:3614–27.

32. Danielsen EM. Post-translational suppression of expression of intestinal brush border enzymes by fructose. J Biol Chem 1989;264:13726–9.

33. Fransen JA, Hauri HP, Ginsel LA, Naim HY. Naturally occurring mutations in intestinal sucrase–isomaltase provide evidence for the existence of an intracellular sorting signal in the isomaltase subunit. J Cell Biol 1991;115:45–57.

34. Hauri HP, Roth J, Sterchi EE, Lentze MJ. Transport to cell surface of intestinal sucrase–isomaltase is blocked in the Golgi apparatus in a patient with congenital sucrase–isomaltase deficiency. Proc Natl Acad Sci U S A 1985; 82:4423–7.

35. Naim HY, Roth J, Sterchi EE, et al. Sucrase–isomaltase deficiency in humans. Different mutations disrupt intracellular transport, processing, and function of an intestinal brush border enzyme. J Clin Invest 1988;82:667–79.

36. Ritz V, Alfalah M, Zimmer KP, et al. Congenital sucrase–isomaltase deficiency because of an accumulation of the mutant enzyme in the endoplasmic reticulum. Gastroenterology 2003;125:1678–85.

37. Ouwendijk J, Moolenaar CE, Peters WJ, et al. Congenital sucrase–isomaltase deficiency. Identification of a glutamine to proline substitution that leads to a transport block of sucrase–isomaltase in a pre-Golgi compartment. J Clin Invest 1996;97:633–41.

38. Spodsberg N, Jacob R, Alfalah M, et al. Molecular basis of aberrant apical protein transport in an intestinal enzyme disorder. J Biol Chem 2001;276:23506–10.

39. Jacob R, Zimmer KP, Schmitz J, Naim HY. Congenital sucrase–isomaltase deficiency arising from cleavage and secretion of a mutant form of the enzyme. J Clin Invest 2000;106:281–7.

40. Keiser M, Alfalah M, Propsting MJ, et al. Altered folding, turnover, and polarized sorting act in concert to define a novel pathomechanism of congenital sucrase–isomaltase deficiency. J Biol Chem 2006;281:14393–9.

41. Moolenaar CE, Ouwendijk J, Wittpoth M, et al. A mutation in a highly conserved region in brush-border sucrase–isomaltase and lysosomal alpha-glucosidase results in Golgi retention. J Cell Sci 1997;110:557–67.

42. Propsting MJ, Jacob R, Naim HY. A glutamine to proline exchange at amino acid residue 1098 in sucrase causes a temperature-sensitive arrest of sucrase–isomaltase in the endoplasmic reticulum and cis-Golgi. J Biol Chem 2003;278:16310–4.

43. Cheng SH, Gregory RJ, Marshall J, et al. Defective intracellular transport and processing of CFTR is the molecular basis of most cystic fibrosis. Cell 1990;63:827–34.

44. Sander P, Alfalah M, Keiser M, et al. Novel mutations in the human sucrase–isomaltase gene (SI) that cause congenital carbohydrate malabsorption. Hum Mutat 2006;27:119.

45. Treem WR. Congenital sucrase–isomaltase deficiency. J Pediatr Gastroenterol Nutr 1995;21:1–14.

46. Gudmand-Hoyer E, Fenger HJ, Kern-Hansen P, Madsen PR. Sucrase deficiency in Greenland. Incidence and genetic aspects. Scand J Gastroenterol 1987;22:24–8.

47. Peterson ML, Herber R. Intestinal sucrase deficiency. Trans Assoc Am Physicians 1967;80:275–83.

48. Welsh JD, Poley JR, Bhatia M, Stevenson DE. Intestinal disaccharidase activities in relation to age, race, and mucosal damage. Gastroenterology 1978;75:847–55.

49. Weijers HA, va de Kamer JH, Mossel DA, Dicke WK. Diarrhoea caused by deficiency of sugar-splitting enzymes. Lancet 1960;2:296–7.

50. Baudon JJ, Veinberg F, Thioulouse E, et al. Sucrase–isomaltase deficiency: Changing pattern over two decades. J Pediatr Gastroenterol Nutr 1996;22:284–8.

51. Gudmand-Hoyer E, Krasilnikoff PA. The effect of sucrose malabsorption on the growth pattern in children. Scand J Gastroenterol 1977;12:103–7.

52. Antonowicz I, Lloyd-Still JD, Khaw KT, Shwachman H. Congenital sucrase–isomaltase deficiency. Observations over a period of 6 years. Pediatrics 1972;49:847–53.

53. Cooper BT, Scott J, Hopkins J, Peters TJ. Adult onset sucrase–isomaltase deficiency with secondary disaccharidase deficiency resulting from severe dietary carbohydrate restriction. Dig Dis Sci 1983;28:473–7.

54. Neale G, Clark M, Levin B. Intestinal sucrase deficiency presenting as sucrose intolerance in adult life. Br Med J 1965;2:1223–5.

55. Starnes CW, Welsh JD. Intestinal sucrase–isomaltase deficiency and renal calculi. N Engl J Med 1970;282:1023–4.

56. Muldoon C, Maguire P, Gleeson F. Onset of sucrase–isomaltase deficiency in late adulthood. Am J Gastroenterol 1999;94:2298–9.

57. Belmont JW, Reid B, Taylor W, et al. Congenital sucrase–isomaltase deficiency presenting with failure to thrive, hypercalcemia, and nephrocalcinosis. BMC Pediatr 2002;2:4.

58. Soeparto P, Stobo EA, Walker-Smith JA. Role of chemical examination of the stool in diagnosis of sugar malabsorption in children. Arch Dis Child 1972;47:56–61.

59. Kerry KR, Anderson CM. A ward test for sugar in faeces. Lancet 1964;41:981.

60. Maxton DG, Catt SD, Menzies IS. Combined assessment of intestinal disaccharidases in congenital asucrasia by differential urinary disaccharide excretion. J Clin Pathol 1990;43:406–9.

61. McGill DB, Newcomer AD. Comparison of venous and capillary blood samples in lactose tolerance testing. Gastroenterology 1967;53:371–4.

62. Krasilnikoff PA, Gudman-Hoyer E, Moltke HH. Diagnostic value of disaccharide tolerance tests in children. Acta Paediatr Scand 1975;64:693–8.

63. Ford RP, Barnes GL. Breath hydrogen test and sucrase isomaltase deficiency. Arch Dis Child 1983;58:595–7.

64. Perman JA, Barr RG, Watkins JB. Sucrose malabsorption in children: Noninvasive diagnosis by interval breath hydrogen determination. J Pediatr 1978;93:17–22.

65. Perman JA, Modler S, Olson AC. Role of pH in production of hydrogen from carbohydrates by colonic bacterial flora. Studies in vivo and in vitro. J Clin Invest 1981;67:643–50.

66. Gardiner AJ, Tarlow MJ, Symonds J, et al. Failure of the hydrogen breath test to detect pulmonary sugar malabsorption. Arch Dis Child 1981;56:368–72.

67. Joseph F, Jr Rosenberg AJ. Breath hydrogen testing: Diseased versus normal patients. J Pediatr Gastroenterol Nutr 1988;7:787–8.

68. Hammer HF, Petritsch W, Pristautz H, Krejs GJ. Assessment of the influence of hydrogen nonexcretion on the usefulness of the hydrogen breath test and lactose tolerance test. Wien Klin Wochenschr 1996;108:137–41.

69. Davidson GP, Robb TA. Value of breath hydrogen analysis in management of diarrheal illness in childhood: Comparison with duodenal biopsy. J Pediatr Gastroenterol Nutr 1985;4:381–7.

70. Rana SV, Bhasin DK, Katyal R, Singh K. Comparison of duodenal and jejunal disaccharidase levels in patients with non ulcer dyspepsia. Trop Gastroenterol 2001;22:135–6.

71. Smith JA, Mayberry JF, Ansell ID, Long RG. Small bowel biopsy for disaccharidase levels: Evidence that endoscopic forceps biopsy can replace the Crosby capsule. Clin Chim Acta 1989;183:317–21.

72. Skovbjerg H, Krasilnikoff PA. Maltase–glucoamylase and residual isomaltase in sucrose intolerant patients. J Pediatr Gastroenterol Nutr 1986;5:365–71.

73. Nichols BL, Avery SE, Karnsakul W, et al. Congenital maltase–glucoamylase deficiency associated with lactase and sucrase deficiencies. J Pediatr Gastroenterol Nutr 2002;35:573–9.

74. Newton T, Murphy MS, Booth IW. Glucose polymer as a cause of protracted diarrhea in infants with unsuspected congenital sucrase–isomaltase deficiency. J Pediatr 1996;128:753–6.

75. Harms HK, Bertele-Harms RM, Bruer-Kleis D. Enzyme-substitution therapy with the yeast Saccharomyces cerevisiae in congenital sucrase–isomaltase deficiency. N Engl J Med 1987;316:1306–1309.

76. Treem WR, McAdams L, Stanford L, et al. Sacrosidase therapy for congenital sucrase–isomaltase deficiency. J Pediatr Gastroenterol Nutr 1999;28:137–42.

77. Colombo V, Lorenz-Meyer H, Semenza G. Small intestinal phlorizin hydrolase: The "beta-glycosidase complex." Biochim Biophys Acta 1973;327:412–24.

78. Boll W, Wagner P, Mantei N. Structure of the chromosomal gene and cDNAs coding for lactase–phlorizin hydrolase in humans with adult-type hypolactasia or persistence of lactase. Am J Hum Genet 1991;48:889–902.

79. Kruse TA, Bolund L, Grzeschik KH, et al. The human lactase–phlorizin hydrolase gene is located on chromosome 2. FEBS Lett 1988;240:123–6.

80. Mantei N, Villa M, Enzler T, et al. Complete primary structure of human and rabbit lactase–phlorizin hydrolase: Implications for biosynthesis, membrane anchoring and evolution of the enzyme. EMBO J 1988;7:2705–13.

81. Jacob R, Weiner JR, Stadge S, Naim HY. Additional N-glycosylation and its impact on the folding of intestinal lactase–phlorizin hydrolase. J Biol Chem 2000;275:10630–7.

82. Naim HY, Lentze MJ. Impact of O-glycosylation on the function of human intestinal lactase–phlorizin hydrolase. Characterization of glycoforms varying in enzyme activity and localization of O-glycoside addition. J Biol Chem 1992;267:25494–504.

83. Wacker H, Keller P, Falchetto R, et al. Location of the two catalytic sites in intestinal lactase–phlorizin hydrolase. Comparison with sucrase–isomaltase and with other glycosidases, the membrane anchor of lactase–phlorizin hydrolase. J Biol Chem 1992;267:18744–52.

84. Buller HA, Montgomery RK, Sasak WV, Grand RJ. Biosynthesis, glycosylation, and intracellular transport of intestinal lactase–phlorizin hydrolase in rat. J Biol Chem 1987;262:17206–11.

85. Danielsen EM, Skovbjerg H, Noren O, Sjostrom H. Biosynthesis of intestinal microvillar proteins. Intracellular processing of lactase–phlorizin hydrolase. Biochem Biophys Res Commun 1984;122:82–90.

86. Jacob R, Radebach I, Wuthrich M, et al. Maturation of human intestinal lactase–phlorizin hydrolase: Generation of the brush border form of the enzyme involves at least two proteolytic cleavage steps. Eur J Biochem 1996;236:789–95.

87. Wuthrich M, Grunberg J, Hahn D, et al. Proteolytic processing of human lactase–phlorizin hydrolase is a two-step event: Identification of the cleavage sites. Arch Biochem Biophys 1996;336:27–34.

88. Danielsen EM. Biosynthesis of intestinal microvillar proteins. Dimerization of aminopeptidase N and lactase–phlorizin hydrolase. Biochemistry 1990;29:305–8.

89. Naim HY, Naim H. Dimerization of lactase–phlorizin hydrolase occurs in the endoplasmic reticulum, involves the putative membrane spanning domain and is required for an efficient transport of the enzyme to the cell surface. Eur J Cell Biol 1996;70:198–208.

90. Jacob R, Brewer C, Fransen JA, Naim HY. Transport, function, and sorting of lactase–phlorizin hydrolase in Madin–Darby canine kidney cells. J Biol Chem 1994;269:2712–21.

91. Jacob R, Zimmer KP, Naim H, Naim HY. The apical sorting of lactase–phlorizin hydrolase implicates sorting sequences found in the mature domain. Eur J Cell Biol 1997;72:54–60.

92. Naim HY. The pro-region of human intestinal lactase–phlorizin hydrolase is enzymatically inactive towards lactose. Biol Chem Hoppe Seyler 1995;376:255–8.

93. Naim HY, Jacob R, Naim H, et al. The pro region of human intestinal lactase–phlorizin hydrolase. J Biol Chem 1994;269:26933–43.

94. Jacob R, Peters K, Naim HY. The prosequence of human lactase–phlorizin hydrolase modulates the folding of the mature enzyme. J Biol Chem 2002;277:8217–25.

95. Jacob R, Preuss U, Panzer P, et al. Hierarchy of sorting signals in chimeras of intestinal lactase–phlorizin hydrolase and the influenza virus hemagglutinin. J Biol Chem 1999;274:8061–7.

96. Naim HY. Processing and transport of human small intestinal lactase–phlorizin hydrolase (LPH). Role of N-linked oligosaccharide modification. FEBS Lett 1994;342:302–7.

97. Panzer P, Preuss U, Joberty G, Naim HY. Protein domains implicated in intracellular transport and sorting of lactase–phlorizin hydrolase. J Biol Chem 1998;273:13861–9.

98. Sahi T. Genetics and epidemiology of adult-type hypolactasia. Scand J Gastroenterol Suppl 1994;202:7–20.

99. Simoons FJ. Primary adult lactose intolerance and the milking habit: A problem in biologic and cultural interrelations. II. A culture historical hypothesis. Am J Dig Dis 1970;15:695–710.

100. Harvey CB, Wang Y, Hughes LA, et al. Studies on the expression of intestinal lactase in different individuals. Gut 1995;36:28–33.

101. Buller HA, Kothe MJ, Goldman DA, et al. Coordinate expression of lactase–phlorizin hydrolase mRNA and enzyme levels in rat intestine during development. J Biol Chem 1990;265:6978–83.

102. Rossi M, Maiuri L, Fusco MI, et al. Lactase persistence versus decline in human adults: Multifactorial events are involved in down-regulation after weaning. Gastroenterology 1997;112:1506–14.

103. Fajardo O, Naim HY, Lacey SW. The polymorphic expression of lactase in adults is regulated at the messenger RNA level. Gastroenterology 1994;106:1233–41.

104. Krasinski SD, Estrada G, Yeh KY, et al. Transcriptional regulation of intestinal hydrolase biosynthesis during postnatal development in rats. Am J Physiol 1994;267:G584–94.

105. Troelsen JT, Olsen J, Mitchelmore C, et al. Two intestinal specific nuclear factors binding to the lactase–phlorizin hydrolase and sucrase–isomaltase promoters are functionally related oligomeric molecules. FEBS Lett 1994;342:297–301.

106. Yeh KY, Yeh M, Holt PR. Intestinal lactase expression and epithelial cell transit in hormone-treated suckling rats. Am J Physiol 1991;260:G379–84.

107. Markowitz AJ, Wu GD, Bader A, et al. Regulation of lineage-specific transcription of the sucrase–isomaltase gene in transgenic mice and cell lines. Am J Physiol 1995;269: G925–39.

108. Troelsen JT, Olsen J, Noren O, Sjostrom H. A novel intestinal trans-factor (NF-LPH1) interacts with the lactase–phlorizin hydrolase promoter and co-varies with the enzymatic activity. J Biol Chem 1992;267:20407–11.

109. Troelsen JT, Mitchelmore C, Spodsberg N, et al. Regulation of lactase–phlorizin hydrolase gene expression by the caudal-related homoeodomain protein Cdx-2. Biochem J 1997;322:833–8.

110. Enattah NS, Sahi T, Savilahti E, et al. Identification of a variant associated with adult-type hypolactasia. Nat Genet 2002;30:233–237.

111. Kuokkanen M, Enattah NS, Oksanen A, Savilahti E, Orpana A, Jarvela I. Transcriptional regulation of the lactase–phlorizin hydrolase gene by polymorphisms associated with adult-type hypolactasia. Gut 2003;52:647–52.

112. Bayless TM, Rothfeld B, Massa C, et al. Lactose and milk intolerance: Clinical implications. N Engl J Med 1975;292:1156–9.

113. Bedine MS, Bayless TM. Intolerance of small amounts of lactose by individuals with low lactase levels. Gastroenterology 1973;65:735–43.

114. Vesa TH, Korpela RA, Sahi T. Tolerance to small amounts of lactose in lactose maldigesters. Am J Clin Nutr 1996;64:197–201.

115. Suarez FL, Savaiano DA, Levitt MD. A comparison of symptoms after the consumption of milk or lactose-hydrolyzed milk by people with self-reported severe lactose intolerance. N Engl J Med 1995;333:1–4.

116. Suarez FL, Savaiano D, Arbisi P, Levitt MD. Tolerance to the daily ingestion of two cups of milk by individuals claiming lactose intolerance. Am J Clin Nutr 1997;65:1502–6.

117. Malagelada JR. Lactose intolerance. N Engl J Med 1995;333:53–4.

118. Lifschitz CH, Bautista A, Gopalakrishna GS, et al. Absorption and tolerance of lactose in infants recovering from severe diarrhea. J Pediatr Gastroenterol Nutr 1985;4:942–8.

119. Forget P, Lombet J, Grandfils C, et al. Lactase insufficiency revisited. J Pediatr Gastroenterol Nutr 1985;4:868–72.

120. Newcomer AD, McGill DB. Lactose tolerance tests in adults with normal lactase activity. Gastroenterology 1966;50:340–6.

121. Vonk RJ, Priebe MG, Koetse HA, et al. Lactose intolerance: Analysis of underlying factors. Eur J Clin Invest 2003;33:70–5.

122. Kneepkens CM, Bijleveld CM, Vonk RJ, Fernandes J. The daytime breath hydrogen profile in children with abdominal symptoms and diarrhoea. Acta Paediatr Scand 1986;75:632–8.

123. Newcomer AD, McGill DB. Distribution of disaccharidase activity in the small bowel of normal and lactase-deficient subjects. Gastroenterology 1966;51:481–8.

124. Aramayo LA, De Silva DG, Hughes CA, et al. Disaccharidase activities in jejunal fluid. Arch Dis Child 1983;58:686–91.

125. Rasinpera H, Savilahti E, Enattah NS, et al. A genetic test which can be used to diagnose adult-type hypolactasia in children. Gut 2004;53:1571–6.

126. Poulter M, Hollox E, Harvey CB, et al. The causal element for the lactase persistence/non-persistence polymorphism is located in a 1 Mb region of linkage disequilibrium in Europeans. Ann Hum Genet 2003;67:298–311.

127. Troelsen JT, Olsen J, Moller J, Sjostrom H. An upstream polymorphism associated with lactase persistence has increased enhancer activity. Gastroenterology 2003; 125:1686–94.

128. Olds LC, Sibley E. Lactase persistence DNA variant enhances lactase promoter activity in vitro: Functional role as a cis regulatory element. Hum Mol Genet 2003; 12:2333–40.

129. von Tirpitz C, Kohn C, Steinkamp M, et al. Lactose intolerance in active Crohn's disease: Clinical value of duodenal lactase analysis. J Clin Gastroenterol 2002;34:49–53.

130. Pfefferkorn MD, Fitzgerald JF, Croffie JM, et al. Lactase deficiency: Not more common in pediatric patients with inflammatory bowel disease than in patients with chronic abdominal pain. J Pediatr Gastroenterol Nutr 2002;35:339–43.

131. Birge SJ, Jr Keutmann HT, Cuatrecasas P, Whedon GD. Osteoporosis, intestinal lactase deficiency and low dietary calcium intake. N Engl J Med 1967;276:445–8.

132. Newcomer AD, Hodgson SF, McGill DB, Thomas PJ. Lactase deficiency: Prevalence in osteoporosis. Ann Intern Med 1978;89:218–20.

133. Gugatschka M, Dobnig H, Fahrleitner-Pammer A, et al. Molecularly-defined lactose malabsorption, milk consumption and anthropometric differences in adult males. QJM 2005;98:857–63.

134. Jarvis JK, Miller GD. Overcoming the barrier of lactose intolerance to reduce health disparities. J Natl Med Assoc 2002;94:55–66.

135. Baker SS, Cochran WJ, Flores CA, et al. American Academy of Pediatrics. Committee on Nutrition. Calcium requirements of infants, children, and adolescents. Pediatrics 1999;104:1152–7.

136. Greer FR, Krebs NF. Optimizing bone health and calcium intakes of infants, children, and adolescents. Pediatrics 2006;117:578–85.

137. Heyman MB. Lactose intolerance in infants, children, and adolescents. Pediatrics 2006;118:1279–86.

138. Montes RG, Bayless TM, Saavedra JM, Perman JA. Effect of milks inoculated with Lactobacillus acidophilus or a yogurt starter culture in lactose-maldigesting children. J Dairy Sci 1995;78:1657–64.

139. Kanabar D, Randhawa M, Clayton P. Improvement of symptoms in infant colic following reduction of lactose load with lactase. J Hum Nutr Diet 2001;14:359–63.

140. Alavi AK, Squillante E, III, Mehta KA. Formulation of enterosoluble microparticles for an acid labile protein. J Pharm Pharm Sci 2002;5:234–44.

141. Fenton TR, Belik J. Routine handling of milk fed to preterm infants can significantly increase osmolality. J Pediatr Gastroenterol Nutr 2002;35:298–302.

142. Erasmus HD, Ludwig-Auser HM, Paterson PG, et al. Enhanced weight gain in preterm infants receiving lactase-treated feeds: A randomized, double-blind, controlled trial. J Pediatr 2002;141:532–7.

143. Antonowicz I, Lebenthal E. Developmental pattern of small intestinal enterokinase and disaccharidase activities in the human fetus. Gastroenterology 1977;72:1299–303.

144. Buchmiller-Crair TL, Gregg JP, Rivera FA, Jr et al. Delayed disaccharidase development in a rabbit model of intrauterine growth retardation. Pediatr Res 2001;50:520–4.

145. Lee PC, Struve M, Raff H. Effects of hypoxia on the development of intestinal enzymes in neonatal and juvenile rats. Exp Biol Med (Maywood) 2003;228:717–23.

146. McClure RJ, Newell SJ. Randomized controlled study of digestive enzyme activity following trophic feeding. Acta Paediatr 2002;91:292–6.

147. Sangild PT, Petersen YM, Schmidt M, et al. Preterm birth affects the intestinal response to parenteral and enteral nutrition in newborn pigs. J Nutr 2002;132:3786–94.

148. Motouri M, Matsuyama H, Yamamura J, et al. Milk sphingomyelin accelerates enzymatic and morphological maturation of the intestine in artificially reared rats. J Pediatr Gastroenterol Nutr 2003;36:241–7.

149. Vilotte JL. Lowering the milk lactose content in vivo: Potential interests, strategies and physiological consequences. Reprod Nutr Dev 2002;42:127–32.

150. Anderson B, Vullo C. Did malaria select for primary adult lactase deficiency? Gut 1994;35:1487–9.

151. Meloni T, Colombo C, Ogana A, et al. Lactose absorption in patients with glucose 6-phosphate dehydrogenase deficiency with and without favism. Gut 1996;39:210–3.

152. Rinaldi E, Albini L, Costagliola C, et al. High frequency of lactose absorbers among adults with idiopathic senile and presenile cataract in a population with a high prevalence of primary adult lactose malabsorption. Lancet 1984;1:355–7.

153. Simoons FJ. A geographic approach to senile cataracts: Possible links with milk consumption, lactase activity, and galactose metabolism. Dig Dis Sci 1982;27:257–64.

154. Cramer DW. Lactase persistence and milk consumption as determinants of ovarian cancer risk. Am J Epidemiol 1989;130:904–10.

155. Meloni GF, Colombo C, La Vecchia C, et al. Lactose absorption in patients with ovarian cancer. Am J Epidemiol 1999;150:183–6.

156. Segall JJ. Dietary lactose as a possible risk factor for ischaemic heart disease: Review of epidemiology. Int J Cardiol 1994;46:197–207.

157. Szilagyi A. Review article: Lactose—a potential prebiotic. Aliment Pharmacol Ther 2002;16:1591–602.

158. Kozakova H, Rehakova Z, Kolinska J. Bifidobacterium bifidum monoassociation of gnotobiotic mice: Effect on enterocyte brush-border enzymes. Folia Microbiol (Praha) 2001;46:573–6.

159. Holzel A, Schwarz V, Sutcliffe KW. Defective lactose absorption causing malnutrition in infancy. Lancet 1959;1:1126–8.

160. Lifshitz F. Congenital lactase deficiency. J Pediatr 1966;69:229–37.

161. Savilahti E, Launiala K, Kuitunen P. Congenital lactase deficiency. A clinical study on 16 patients. Arch Dis Child 1983;58:246–52.

162. Kuokkanen M, Kokkonen J, Enattah NS, et al. Mutations in the Translated Region of the Lactase Gene (LCT) Underlie Congenital Lactase Deficiency. Am J Hum Genet 2006;78:339–44.

163. Saarela T, Simila S, Koivisto M. Hypercalcemia and nephrocalcinosis in patients with congenital lactase deficiency. J Pediatr 1995;127:920–3.

164. Nichols BL, Eldering J, Avery S, et al. Human small intestinal maltase–glucoamylase cDNA cloning. Homology to sucrase–isomaltase. J Biol Chem 1998;273:3076–81.

165. Nichols BL, Nichols VN, Putman M, et al. Contribution of villous atrophy to reduced intestinal maltase in infants with malnutrition. J Pediatr Gastroenterol Nutr 2000;30:494–502.

166. Lebenthal E, Khin MU, Zheng BY, et al. Small intestinal glucoamylase deficiency and starch malabsorption: A newly recognized alpha-glucosidase deficiency in children. J Pediatr 1994;124:541–6.

167. Lifshitz CH, Boutton TW, Carrazza F, et al. A carbon-13 breath test to characterize glucose absorption and utilization in children. J Pediatr Gastroenterol Nutr 1988;7: 842–7.

168. Karnsakul W, Luginbuehl U, Hahn D, et al. Disaccharidase activities in dyspeptic children: Biochemical and molecular investigations of maltase–glucoamylase activity. J Pediatr Gastroenterol Nutr 2002;35:551–6.

169. Galand G. Brush border membrane sucrase–isomaltase, maltase–glucoamylase and trehalase in mammals. Comparative development, effects of glucocorticoids, molecular mechanisms, and phylogenetic implications. Comp Biochem Physiol B 1989;94:1–11.

170. Sacktor B, Berger SJ. Formation of trehalose from glucose in the renal cortex. Biochem Biophys Res Commun 1969;35:796–800.

171. Eze LC. Plasma trehalase activity and diabetes mellitus. Biochem Genet 1989;27:487–95.

172. Yoshida K, Mizukawa H, Haruki E. Serum trehalase activity in patients with rheumatoid arthritis. Clin Chim Acta 1993;215:123–4.

173. Ishihara R, Taketani S, Sasai-Takedatsu M, et al. Molecular cloning, sequencing and expression of cDNA encoding human trehalase. Gene 1997;202:69–74.

174. Bergoz R. Trehalose malabsorption causing intolerance to mushrooms. Report of a probable case. Gastroenterology 1971;60:909–12.

175. Madzarovova-Nohejlova J. Trehalase deficiency in a family. Gastroenterology 1973;65:130–3.

176. Gudmand-Hoyer E, Fenger HJ, Skovbjerg H, et al. Trehalase deficiency in Greenland. Scand J Gastroenterol 1988;23:775–8.

177. Murray IA, Coupland K, Smith JA, et al. Intestinal trehalase activity in a UK population: Establishing a normal range and the effect of disease. Br J Nutr 2000;83:241–5.

178. Arola H, Koivula T, Karvonen AL, et al. Low trehalase activity is associated with abdominal symptoms caused by edible mushrooms. Scand J Gastroenterol 1999;34: 898–903.

179. Schiraldi C, Di L, I, De Rosa M. Trehalose production: Exploiting novel approaches. Trends Biotechnol 2002;20:420–5.

15.3b. Congenital Intestinal Transport Defects

Martín G. Martín, MD, MPP

Ernest M. Wright, PhD, DSc, FRS

Disorders of intestinal nutrient and ion assimilation can lead to clinical symptoms that range from severe life-threatening diarrhea in a neonate to multisystem deficits in adulthood. With the exception of lactose intolerance, most disorders of nutrient assimilation are both exceptionally rare and inherited in an autosomal recessive manner. However, milder forms of each disorder may be rather subtle clinical signs and not diagnosed until well into adulthood. Disorders of nutrient assimilation should be entertained particularly when there is a history of consanguinity, even in the absence of other similarly afflicted family members.

Chronic diarrhea is the most common clinical symptom of disorders that are secondary to abnormalities of nutrient assimilation.[1] Categorizing the type of diarrhea into either malabsorptive or secretory is a useful initial step in the evaluation of any patient with chronic diarrhea. Classifying the type of diarrhea may be done with either a trial of fasting, or by analysis of stool electrolytes while on a complete diet. To compute the stool osmotic gap, either cations such as Na^+ and K^+ or anions such as Cl^- and HCO_3^- may be measured in liquid fecal samples.[2,3] If the sum of twice the value of cations (or anions) is lower <50 mOsm) than the obligatory fecal osmolarity of ~290 mOsm, an osmotic gap provided by the ingested osmotically active nutrient or nonmeasured ion (ie, Mg^{2+}) likely accounts for the gap (Figure 1). Short-chain fatty acids (SCFA) are osmotic anions that are products of fermented carbohydrates formed by the intestinal microflora may contribute to the final osmotic load if insufficiently absorbed by colonocytes. In contrast, a low osmotic gap (<50 mOsm) is seen in secretory diarrheas, which are generally large volume (2 to 3 L) and fail to subside with fasting.

Nutrient-specific malabsorption is an important characteristic of all inherited transport disorders and is generally not a feature of some of the more common chronic diarrheal disorders (Figure 2 and Table 1). However, defects of pancreatic and brush border enzyme function share many of the clinical characteristics seen in transport defects and will also result in the maldigestion of specific complex nutrients. In contrast, generalized malabsorption (ie, not nutrient specific) occurs in the clinical setting where the overall intestinal absorptive capacity is insufficient to appropriately process a dietary load that is required to maintain appropriate growth and development.[4] Nonspecific abnormalities of intestinal nutrient assimilation most often occur when either small bowel surface area is inadequate (ie, short bowel syndrome) or when intestinal transit time is too short to allow for adequate nutrient assimilation (Figure 2 and Table 1). For instance, enteropathies such as celiac disease, microvillus inclusion disease (Mendelian inheritance in man [MIM] #251850), and immunodysregulation, polyendocrinopathy, enteropathy X-linked (IPEX) (MIM #304790), generally present with features of nutrient nonspecific malassimilation.[5,6] In fact, the majority of patients with abnormal intestinal histology have a mixed form of diarrhea that has both osmotic and secretory components. Therefore, a thorough evaluation of small bowel histology is an indispensable part of the evaluation of all patients with presumed defects of nutrient assimilation.

Secretory diarrhea is due to an imbalance between absorption and secretion of noningested electrolytes, with consequential luminal ions driving the influx of water in order to reach the obligatory isomolar requirements of stool (Figure 2 and Table 1). During early infancy, chronic diarrhea that is purely secretory in character is due almost exclusively to a small number of transport disorders and, as such, is not secondary to defects of enzymatic function, as is frequently seen in maldigestive diarrhea. Several hormone-secreting tumors may present with severe secretory diarrhea and need to be distinguished from two disorders of intestinal transport, namely, congenital chloride diarrhea (MIM #214700) and congenital sodium diarrhea (CSD) (MIM #270420).[7,8]

DISORDERS OF CARBOHYDRATE ABSORPTION

Complex sugars are digested by salivary and pancreatic α-amylases and further by brush border enzymes into monosaccharides that are absorbed in the small intestine (Figure 3). Enterocytes, which are renewed every week, express the enzymes and transporters needed for carbohydrate digestion and absorption. The enterocytes apical brush border membrane contains various saccharidases including glucoamylase, sucrase-isomaltase and lactase-phlorhizin hydrolase (LPH), the Na^+-dependent glucose-galactose cotransporter (SGLT1), and the fructose uniporter (GLUT5). The basolateral membrane contains the glucose-galactose-fructose uniporter (GLUT2) and the Na^+, K^+-adenosine triphosphatase

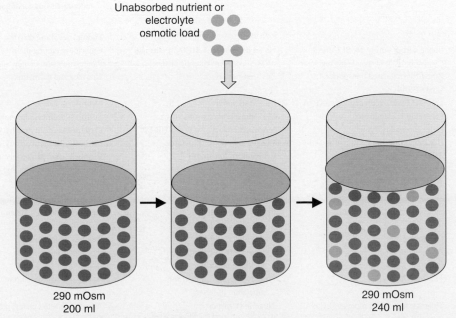

Figure 1 Stool osmolarity is always isosmolar (290 mOsm). The addition of an increased osmotic load (ie, nutrient or electrolyte) will result in an increase stool volume such that isosmolarity is maintained.

Unabsorbed nutrient or electrolyte osmotic load

290 mOsm
200 ml

290 mOsm
240 ml

Table 1 Molecular Basis of Disorders of Nutrient Assimilation and Ion/Metal Transport.

Clinical Disorder	MIM No.	IP	CHR	Gene/Protein (HUGO No.)	Function	Symptoms
Carbohydrate digestion						
Congenital lactase deficiency	223000	AR	2q21	Lactase-phlorhizin hydrolase	Hydrolyzes lactose	Lactose-induced diarrhea
Hypolactasia	223100	AR	2q21	Lactase-phlorhizin hydrolase	Hydrolyzes lactose	Lactose-induced diarrhea
Congenital sucrase-isomaltase deficiency	222900	AR	3q25	Sucrase-isomaltase	Hydrolyzes lactose	Sucrose-induced diarrhea
Carbohydrate absorption						
Glucose galactose malabsorption	182380	AR	22q13	Na^+–glucose-galactose cotransport (SGLT1); SLC5A1	Apical glucose-galactose transporter	Glucose-induced diarrhea
Fructose malabsorption	~	AR	1p36	Facilitative fructose transport (GLUT5); SLC2A5	Apical fructose transporter	Fructose-induced diarrhea
Fanconi-Bickel syndrome	227810	AR	3q26	Facilitative glucose transport (GLUT2); SLC2A2	Basolateral glucose transporter	Diarrhea and nephropathy
Protein digestion						
Enterokinase deficiency	226200	AR	21q21	Serine protease 7	Proenterokinase—hydrolyzes trypsinogen	Protein-induced diarrhea; edema
Trypsinogen deficiency	276000	AR	7q35	Trypsinogen	Hydrolyzes endo- and exopeptidases	Protein-induced diarrhea; edema
Amino acid absorption						
Cystinuria type I	220100	AR	2p16	rBAT; SLC3A1	Heavy-chain cysteine, dibasic and neutral AA apical transport	Nephrolithiasis
Cystinuria type II/III	600918	AR	19q13.1	$b^{0,+}AT$; SLC7A9	Light-chain cysteine, dibasic and neutral apical AA transport	Nephrolithiasis
Lysinuric protein intolerance	222700	AR	14q11	y^+ L-type AA transporter 1; SLC7A7	y^+L-type AA basolateral transport	Vomiting, diarrhea, neurologic delay
Hartnup disorder neurologic delay	234500	AR	5p21	BOAT1	Na^+-neutral AA transport	Dermatitis
Iminoglycinuria	242600	AR	~	?	Imino AA transport	Neurologic delay
Fat digestion						
Pancreatic lipase deficiency	246600	AR	10q26	Pancreatic lipase	Hydrolyzes dietary triglycerides to fatty acids	Steatorrhea
Fat assimilation						
Abetalipoproteinemia	200100	AR	4q22	Microsomal triglyceride transfer protein	Transfers lipids to apolipoprotein B	Steatorrhea
Hypobetalipoproteinemia	107730	AD/AR	2p24	Apolipoprotein B	Apolipoprotein that forms chylomicrons	Steatorrhea
Chylomicron retention disease	246700	AR	5q31	Sar1-ADP-ribosylation factor family GTPases vesicles	Targets intracellular protein-coated	Steatorrhea
Primary bile acid malabsorption	601295	AR	13q33	Sodium–bile acid transporter; SLC10A2	Ileal Na^+-bile acid transporter	Steatorrhea/bile acid diarrhea
Tangier disease	205400	AR	9q	ATP–binding cassette transporter 1	Controls intracellular cholesterol	Liver, spleen, lymph transport node enlargement
Sitosterolemia	21250	AR	2q21	ATP binding cassette, subfamily G, member 8; ABCG8	Dietary sterol absorption	Atherosclerosis
Generalized malabsorption						
Enteric anendocrinosis	610370	AR	10q21.3	Neurogenin-3	Endocrine cell fate determination	Generalized malabsorption Diabetes (MODY)
Enteric dysendocrinosis	~	AR	?	?	?	Generalized malabsorption No diabetes
Proprotein convertase 1 deficiency	600955	AR	5q15-q21	Prohormone convertase-1	Impaired Processing of Prohormone	Generalized malabsorption Hypocortisolemia, obesity
Polyglandular syndrome, type 1	240300	AR	21q22.3	Autoimmune regulator gene (AIRE)	Central immune tolerance	Generalized malabsorption mucocutaneous candidiasis
Ion and metal absorption						
Congenital sodium diarrhea	270420	AR		~	? ?	Sodium-secreting diarrhea
Congenital chloride diarrhea	214700	AR	7q22	Solute carrier family 26; SLC26A3	Na^+-independent Cl^-/HCO_3^- exchanger	Chloride-secreting diarrhea
Cystic fibrosis	219700	AR	7q31.2	Cystic fibrosis transmembrane regulator	cAMP-dependent chloride channel	Pancreatic insufficiency; ileus
Acrodermatitis enteropathica	201100	AR	8q24.3	Zinc-/iron-regulated transporter 4; SLC39A4	Zn^+ transporter	Diarrhea and dermatitis
Menkes disease	309400	XR	Xq12	Cu^{2+} ATPase, α-polypeptide; ATP7A	Cu^{2+} transporter	Neurologic delay
Primary hypomagnesemia	248250	AR/X	3q27	Paracellin 1; claudin 16	Mg^+ transporter/sensor	Seizures, deafness, and polyuria
Classic hemochromatosis	235200	AR	6p21.3	Hemochromatosis gene	Modulates endocytosis of the $TfR-Fe^{2+}$	Cirrhosis, cardiomyopathy, diabetes
Juvenile hemochromatosis	602390	AR	19q13	Hepcidin	Hepatic antimicrobial peptide	Cirrhosis, cardiomyopathy, diabetes
Hemochromatosis type III	604250	AR	7q22	TfR2	Receptor for transferrin	Cirrhosis, cardiomyopathy, diabetes
Hemochromatosis type IV	606069	AD	2q32	Ferroportin; SLC11A3	Basolateral Fe^{2+} transporter	Cirrhosis, cardiomyopathy, diabetes
Vitamin absorption						
Folate malabsorption	229050	AR	~	~		Anemia; diarrhea; neurologic delay
Congenital pernicious anemia	261000	AR	11q13	Intrinsic factor	Required for binding of cobalamin to cubilin	Anemia; neurologic delay
Imerslund-Graesbeck syndrome (Finland)	261100	AR	10p12.1	Cubilin	IF-cobalamin receptor	Anemia; proteinuria
Imerslund-Graesbeck syndrome (Norway)	261100	AR	14q32	Amnionless	Targets the IF-cobalamin and cubilin to endosomes	Anemia; proteinuria
Congenital deficit of transcobalamin II	275350	AR	22q11.2	Transcobalamin II	Primary transport protein for cobalamin in serum	Anemia; diarrhea; neurologic delay
Thiamine-responsive megaloblastic anemia	249270	AR	1q23.3	Thiamine transporter protein; SLC19A2	Thiamine transporter	Anemia; diabetes; cranial nerve defects
Familial retinol-binding protein deficiency	180250	AR	10q24	Retinol-binding protein 4	Binding protein for retinol transfer	Ophthalmologic problems
Selective vitamin E deficiency	277460	AR	8q13.1	α-Tocopherol transfer protein	Binding protein that adds vitamin E to VLDL	Vitamin E malabsorption

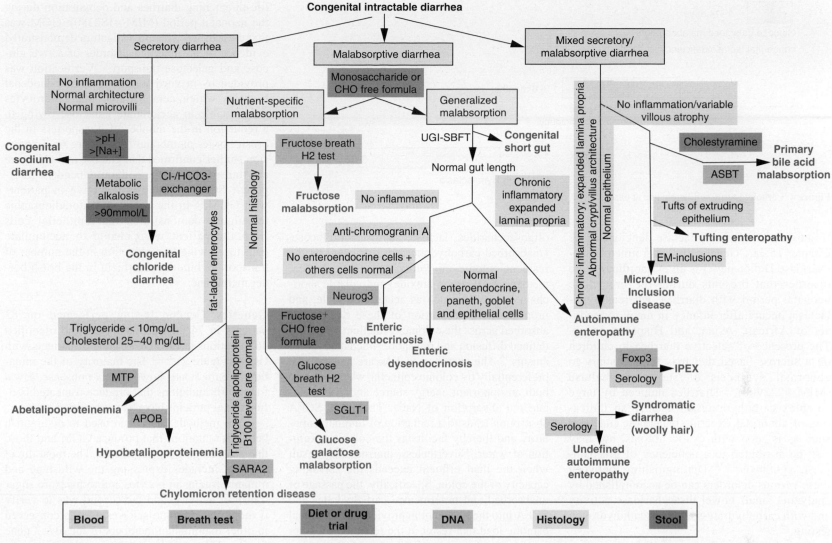

Figure 2 Diagnostic algorithm for the evaluation of an infant with congenital intractable diarrhea.

(Na,K-ATPase) pump which maintains the low intracellular Na$^+$ concentration by extruding Na$^+$ into the blood in exchange for K$^+$.[9] This Na,K-ATPase pump provides the potential energy required for the movement of sugars and amino acids up their steep concentration gradients across the enterocytes apical membrane. For instance, the low intracellular concentration of Na$^+$ provided by the pump, allows for the influx of Na$^+$ to be coupled to the movement of glucose up its own osmotic gradient via the active transporter SGLT1. In contrast, fructose is passively transported, moving down its own osmotic gradient, across the intestine by the brush border uniporter (GLUT5) and by the basolateral GLUT2 uniporter.

Disturbances of carbohydrate assimilation may be secondary to defective enzymatic processing of complex sugars and disaccharides or failure to transport monosaccharides across the apical membrane (Figure 3 and Table 1). Abnormalities of carbohydrate assimilation may be categorized into three general forms: ontogenic forms that result from the normal immaturity of the digestive functions during the early stages of life, genetic forms that are congenital conditions, and an acquired form that is preceded by

a period of normal function. The age at onset of clinical symptoms is an important characteristic to consider when evaluating the basis of carbohydrate-induced diarrhea (Figure 4). Defective

synthesis of lactase-phlorhizin hydrolase (LPH) may lead to chronic diarrhea, resulting from either primary lactase deficiency (MIM #223000) or hypolactasia (MIM #223100)

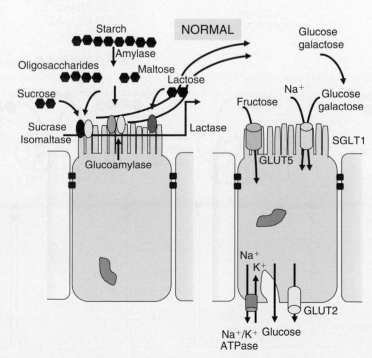

Figure 3 Normal assimilation of carbohydrates in the intestine.

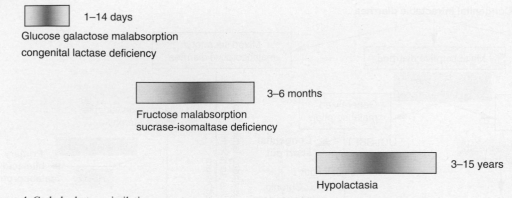

Figure 4 Carbohydrate assimilation: age at onset.

(Figure 5).[10–11] Primary lactase deficiency (see Chapter 15.3a, "Genetically Determined Disaccharidase Deficiency") is an extraordinary rare disorder that presents during the immediate neonatal period with diarrhea, whereas hypolactasia occurs after infancy in many individuals of African, Asian, and Hispanic origin. The presence of selective diarrhea in children on a sucrose-based diet may be secondary to abnormal synthesis of sucrase-isomaltase (MIM #222900).[12] Diarrhea induced by large complex carbohydrates is usually an indication of abnormal exocrine pancreatic function, such as is seen with cystic fibrosis, but may also be attributed to a deficiency of glucoamylase synthesis.[13,14] Distinguishing between these various disorders can be accomplished by analyzing small bowel disaccharidase activity and with carbohydrate-specific breath hydrogen testing.[15]

Carbohydrate intolerance of all forms is characterized by diarrhea that subsides shortly after carbohydrates are reduced or eliminated from the diet. Therefore, abnormal carbohydrate assimilation results in the presence of major osmotic forces in colonic luminal fluid derived from oligosaccharides, lactose, sucrose, or glucose. Unabsorbed carbohydrates are fermented by the resident colonic microflora to gas (hydrogen, methane, and carbon dioxide) and volatile short-chain fatty acids such as acetate, butyrate, and propionate. A proportion of these SCFAs are absorbed across the colonic epithelium by poorly defined diffusion and transporter-mediated mechanisms.[16] The absorbed SCFAs are metabolized preferentially by colonic epithelia, where they are both an important energy source and also facilitate the absorption of NaCl. Therefore, SCFA absorption leads to a reduction of luminal osmolarity and thereby facilitates the colonic absorption of water. Nevertheless, diarrhea may result when the ileal effluent exceeds the salvaging capacity of the colon. Specifically, the passage of unabsorbed and unfermented carbohydrates and SCFA into the distal colon provides an additional osmotic load that result in the retention of water in the gut and subsequent diarrhea.

Glucose Galactose Malabsorption

Glucose galactose malabsorption (GGM) is a rare autosomal recessive disorder that causes severe life-threatening diarrhea and dehydration during the neonatal period (MIM #182380). GGM was first established when investigators demonstrated evidence of an inherited disorder of active glucose and galactose transport.[17] Verification was provided by in vitro studies on GGM duodenal biopsies which demonstrated that enterocytes were unable to accumulate galactose owing to a reduction in the number of transporters in the brush border membrane[18–20] (Figure 6). Expression studies confirmed that glucose and galactose are transported by the sodium-dependent transporter, SGLT1, which is defective in patients with GGM.[21] In these studies, autoradiographic techniques demonstrated that epithelial cells from the patient were unable to accumulate galactose owing to a reduction in the number of transporters binding phlorhizin in the brush border membrane.

Genetics. Genetic testing performed on 82 patients in 74 unrelated families and identified 46 mutations in the *SGLT1* gene of patients with GGM (Figure 7).[22–25] The majority of the mutations are missense; however, six nonsense, seven frameshift mutations that produce truncated nonfunctional proteins have been identified.

Two methods have been used to distinguish between mutations that produce GGM and those that are benign polymorphisms. The most direct analysis includes expressing the wild-type and mutant proteins in oocytes and to measure sugar transport activity, and the second was to verify if the mutated amino acid reside was conserved in other mammalian members of the *SGLT* gene family (Figure 7).[22–25] All missense mutations that caused a defect in sugar transport were in amino acids that were conserved within the 18 closely related genes, including eight *SGLT1*s from different species. However, the two missense mutations that do not impair sugar

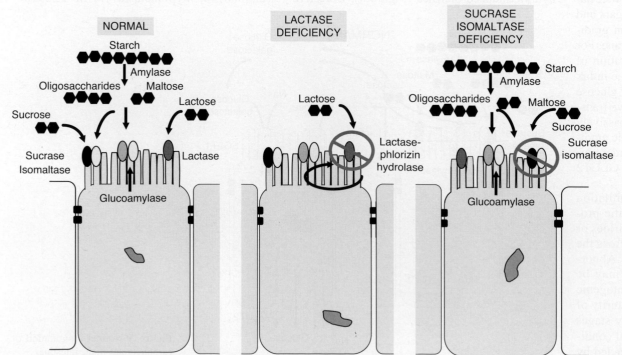

Figure 5 Disorders of disaccharidase deficiency.

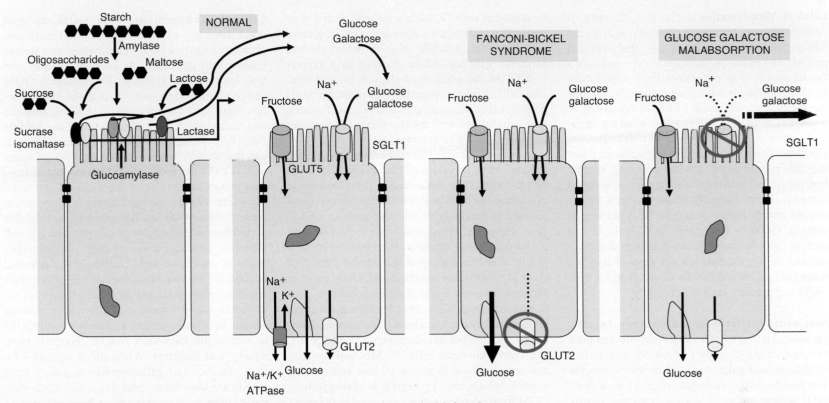

Figure 6 Carbohydrate absorption in normal, glucose galactose malabsorption, and Fanconi-Bickel syndrome.

transport, Phe405Ser and His615Gln, are not conserved and rarely occur in the general population. In contrast, the Asn51Ser variant occurs in the general population at a frequency of 4% in over 552 alleles analyzed. On this basis, we also suggest that Ala12Val is a benign polymorphism, whereas the other eight untested mutants are mutations that may be responsible for the impaired sugar transport in these GGM patients.

Molecular Pathophysiology. The primary carbohydrate present in breast milk is lactose (50 to 90 g/L) that is hydrolyzed by lactase on the external surface of the intestinal brush border.

The liberated glucose and galactose are then transported across the brush border membrane by SGLT1 and accumulated within the enterocyte. Complex carbohydrates provide the major source of glucose in older children and adults. Until recently, the facilitated carrier GLUT2 was believed to be responsible for transport of glucose and galactose across the basolateral membrane; however, this is now doubtful in light of studies on humans and mice with mutations of GLUT2 and no evidence of osmotic diarrhea.[26,27]

SGLT1 is responsible for the tight coupling of two Na^+ ions and one sugar molecule across the membrane during one catalytic turnover.

The basolateral Na,K-ATPase pump maintains the low intracellular sodium concentration by pumping sodium out of the cell, and this results in the net absorption of sodium (chloride and bicarbonate), sugar, and water across the epithelium.[28] Because the osmolarity of stool in both secretory and malabsorptive diarrhea is always identical to serum (~290 mOsm), the addition of undigested solutes (glucose and galactose) and SCFA that reach the colon of patients with GGM will result in an excessive amount of water loss in order to maintain the obligatory fecal osmolarity.

Glucose stimulates salt and water absorption, and this is possible by the coupling of Na^+ and glucose transport across the brush border, and the subsequent pumping of Na^+ out of the enterocyte across the basolateral membrane by the Na,K-ATPase pump. It was generally believed that water follows solute absorption by local osmosis; or local osmotic gradients that formed in the spaces between epithelial cells which drive water transport across the epithelial layer. However, it has been postulated that there is a more direct link between sodium, sugar, and water transport across the brush border membrane, water cotransport, but this is not broadly accepted.[29] These studies provide evidence that the SGLT1 functions as low conductance water channel that is coupled with sugar transport. In vitro estimates of water transport suggest that one-third of the transport occurred via Na^+-glucose cotransport, while the remaining occurred by local osmosis. This link between salt, sugar, and water absorption provides the rationale for the use of oral rehydration therapy in patients with various forms of acute diarrhea including those of infectious origin.[30]

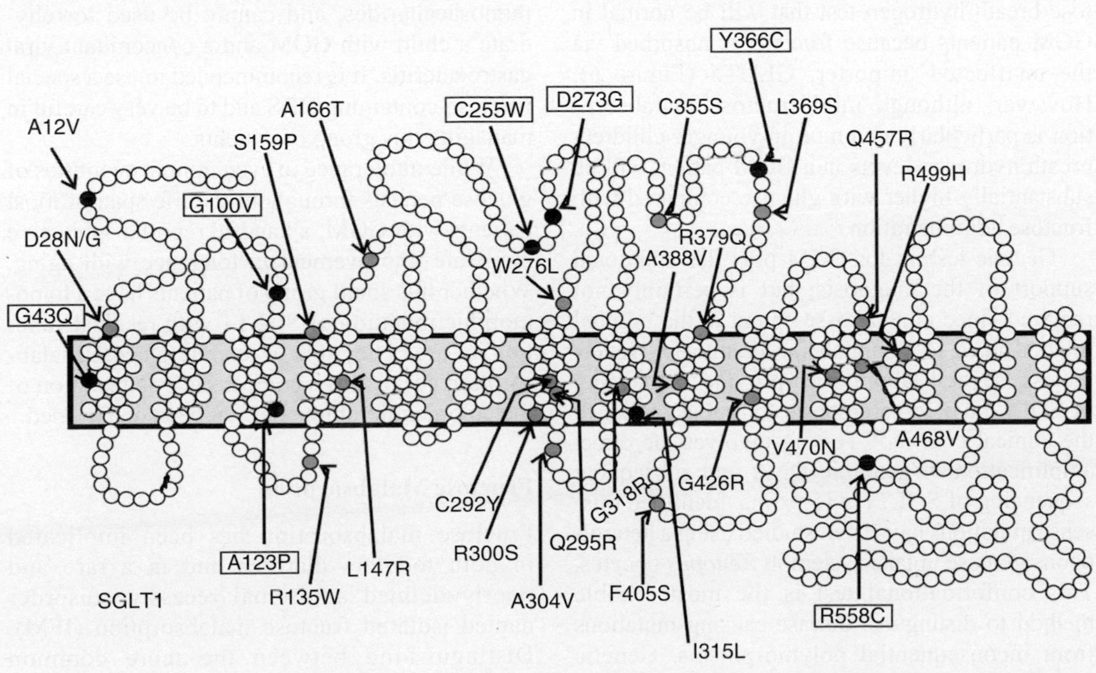

Figure 7 Location of missense mutations in sodium-coupled glucose transporter (SGLT1) in patients with glucose galactose malabsorption.

Clinical Manifestations. The vast majority of patients with GGM present clinically with severe life-threatening diarrhea during the neonatal period; however, on extremely rare occasions the diagnosis was not established until adulthood.[31] Diarrhea is most frequently detected during the first several week of life in breast-fed or bottle-fed child, and will result in a severe metabolic acidosis and hyperosmolar dehydration. Diarrhea ceases at bowel rest and resumes when the child receives again the same feeding, protein hydrolysate or elemental diet (amino acid–based formula). If not properly diagnosed in a timely manner and if dietary management is not implemented, GGM is frequently fatal. Isolated and profuse carbohydrate malabsorption is distinctly unusual during the first several days of life, but when present, should initiate the workup for both GGM and primary lactase deficiency.

Diagnostic Criteria or Laboratory Investigations. Two crucial evaluations are required to establish the diagnosis of GGM: elimination of glucose and galactose (and lactose) from the diet results in the complete resolution of diarrheal symptoms and a normal intestinal biopsy (Figure 2). Abnormal glucose breath hydrogen test and SGLT1 DNA sequencing are useful, but not required to establish the formal diagnosis of GGM. When considering the diagnosis, several stool tests should be performed including measurement of pH, occult blood, leukocyte analysis, and reducing and nonreducing sugars (Clinitest). Carbohydrate malabsorption and subsequent colonic bacterial fermentation result in the synthesis of high concentrations of SCFAs and lactic acid, which leads to the acidification of stool (pH <5.3).[2]

Establishing the diagnosis of GGM will inevitably require a systematic trial of various modular diets with careful assessment of stool volume (Figure 2). Placement of a Foley catheter into the urinary system provides definitive separation of stool and urine and facilitates the measurement of fecal content. One useful approach would be to challenge the infant with ad lib access to glucose-based oral rehydration solution (ie, Pedialyte), and carefully assess stool volume, pH, and reducing substances. Such a challenge in a patient with GGM will produce severe diarrhea (generally 100 to 70 mL/kg/d) and may result in significant hypokalemia and a metabolic acidosis, and therefore intravenous fluid and electrolyte administration is generally recommended during these trials. Ad lib bolus feeds should be encouraged as this approach is most likely to provide indisputable results particularly when a catheter is used to distinguish stool from urine (unpublished observations).

If diarrhea ensues from such a trial, clinicians may consider challenging with one of several carbohydrate-free formulas, including Ross Carbohydrate Free Formula (Ross Products, Columbus, OH) or Galactomin 19 (Nutricia, Holland). Ad lib bolus feeds with such a formula and no added carbohydrate will be well tolerated by a patient with GGM, but not one with a generalized malabsorptive disorder such as enteric anendocrinosis.[32] While these carbohydrate-free formulas will not induce diarrhea in a subject with GGM, the addition of glucose, but not fructose will. Direct comparison of stool volumes unmistakably demonstrates dramatic differences when challenged with the two forms of monosaccharides (glucose or fructose).

Since the clinical assessment is the optimal method used to establish the diagnosis, small bowel biopsies are not essential if the diagnostic evaluation has been well done and the results demonstrate an indisputable selective glucose intolerance. However, when small bowel biopsies are performed in the evaluation of an infant with congenital diarrhea, they provide several important clues in establishing the diagnosis. GGM patients should have normal-appearing microvilli on electron microscopy, with normal villus architecture on light microscopy, including the normal distribution and number of enterocytes, Paneth, goblet, and enteroendocrine cells.[32,33] Mucosal biopsies can also be used to assess lactase and sucrase activity, which may be helpful in distinguishing GGM from primary lactase or sucrase deficiency.

Breath hydrogen testing is an easily performed test that may assist in the diagnosis of GGM (Figure 2). The test relies on the colonic fermentation of unabsorbed carbohydrate by bacteria that produce methane, hydrogen, and carbon dioxide gas. This gas chromatographic analysis quantifies the level of hydrogen gas in exhaled air following the administration of either glucose (or galactose) at 1 g/kg body weight or a maximum of 25 g. Although an elevation of more than 20 ppm above the fasting baseline is consistent with the diagnosis of glucose malabsorption, most patients with GGM have levels that are frequently higher than 100 ppm (unpublished observations).[34] The specificity of an abnormal glucose breath hydrogen test may be confirmed by performing a fructose breath hydrogen test that will be normal in GGM patients because fructose is absorbed via the unaffected uniporter, GLUT5 (Figure 6). However, although mild fructose malabsorption is particularly common in younger children, breath hydrogen levels in a GGM patient will be substantially higher with glucose compared with fructose administration.[35]

Genetic testing for GGM provides additional support of the diagnosis, but is certainly not required since clinical assessment is the optimal method used to establish the diagnosis. Nevertheless, several laboratories provide sequencing of SGLT on a research basis for subjects that fit the clinical criteria.[22] Testing involves the direct amplification of genomic DNA and subsequent sequencing of SGLT1's 15 exons. Identified missense mutations have been studied using a heterologous glucose uptake system in *Xenopus* oocytes. This conformational test is the most reliable method to distinguish disease-causing mutations from inconsequential polymorphisms. Genetic testing has been used successfully to perform prenatal diagnosis on a family at risk for GGM.[36]

Clinical Management. With GGM, as with other disorders of carbohydrate malabsorption, symptoms resolve on an elimination diet free of glucose and galactose. As outlined earlier, several formulas are available for managing GGM patients during early infancy, including Ross Carbohydrate Free Formula (RCF) in North America and Galactomin 19 in Europe and the Middle East. RCF is supplied as a liquid, in a 390 mL can that should be diluted with 360 mL of water and 54 g (4 tablespoons and 2 teaspoons) of fructose mixed to develop a 0.6 Kcal/mL formula. Such formulas are required during infancy, and in some children their use has extended beyond this period because of a lack of suitable alternatives. However, prolonged use of these specialty formulas is expensive and is certainly not required beyond the first several years of life. Since milk and other dairy products are a rich-dietary source of calcium and vitamin D, alternative sources should be recommended to patients with GGM to reduce the long-term risk of abnormal bone density and fractures. While the obligatory life-long glucose- and galactose-free diet may have significant long-term renal, bone and cardiovascular consequences; none have been reported in adult patients.

The dietary management of GGM becomes particularly challenging as children enter into late infancy and begin to exert more independence. Guidance from a well-trained dietitian is frequently invaluable, and all parents would benefit from dietary manuals that list the sugar content of selected foods. Furthermore, instructing caretakers how to read food labels and avoid items with anymore than the lowest amount of carbohydrates is recommended. Most liquid medicines share a similar solvent that is high in sugar and frequently leads to worsening diarrhea in a child with GGM. The use of sugar-free medicines should be encouraged in this group of patients. Finally, most ORS solutions contain the either glucose polymers or monosaccharides, and cannot be used to rehydrate a child with GGM and a concomitant viral gastroenteritis. It is recommended to use a special fructose-containing ORS and to be very careful in managing this group of patients.

While intolerance to even minute quantities of glucose persists throughout the life span of most patients with GGM, a handful report a subjective moderate improvement in tolerance with aging. Whether this small group of patients have a hypomorphic mutation of SGLT1 with residual function, or are better able to tolerate glucose malabsorption because of a compensatory adaptation of the colonic microbiota has not been determined.

Fructose Malabsorption

Fructose malabsorption has been implicated in both toddlers diarrhea and in a rare and poorly defined autosomal recessive disorder named isolated fructose malabsorption (IFM). Distinguishing between the more common toddler's diarrhea and IFM is particularly difficult, and it is unclear if they represent distinct disorders. The clinical and genetic features of IFM are not as well defined as its other counterpart carbohydrate transport disorder, GGM. Although the ability of GLUT5 to transport fructose has been demonstrated, there remains insufficient information confirming that GLUT5 represents the main fructose facilitative carrier in the intestine (Figure 6).[37] Recent studies have identified GLUT7 as a high affinity glucose and fructose carrier on the brush border membrane of enterocytes located in the distal intestine.[38] New studies are also emerging in rats implying that brush border GLUT2 plays a major role in the absorption of fructose.[39]

Genetics and Molecular Pathophysiology. Eight patients with clinical evidence suggestive of IFM were previously evaluated for mutations in the *GLUT5* gene.[40] Analysis of both the coding region and intron and exon boundaries of the *GLUT5* gene failed to identify a deleterious mutation that could account for defective transport.

Current data suggest that fructose absorption in the small intestine occurs via GLUT5, since it has a much higher K_m (and thereby higher capacity) for fructose than GLUT7.[41–42] Fructose absorption is independent of glucose absorption and remains intact in patients with GGM. Studies performed primarily in rodents have confirmed that GLUT5 expression is regulated in a tissue- and development-specific manner and is induced by dietary fructose.[43] Specifically, GLUT5 messenger ribonucleic acid and protein levels are found at very low levels prior to weaning and increase dramatically in the proximal small intestine in weaned animals. An analysis of the age dependence of GLUT5 levels in human intestine has not been performed; however, fructose malabsorption as determined by the breath hydrogen test is certainly more common during early infancy when compared to adults.[35] Likewise, whether or not the fructose malabsorption that is so common in toddler's diarrhea is secondary to insufficient GLUT5 expression has yet to be formally established.

Clinical Manifestations. Fructose is the primary monosaccharide found in fruits and fruit juices. Fruit juices that contain a high proportion of fructose to glucose or an excessive amount of the nonabsorbable carbohydrate sorbitol have been associated with infant diarrhea and abdominal pain.[44,45] Malabsorption of fruit juices is dose-dependent, with diarrheal symptoms associated with the daily consumption of juice that exceeds 15 mL/kg. Whether children with toddler's diarrhea have a reduced capacity to absorb fructose than other similarly aged children has yet to be defined. Intolerance to dietary fructose has also been identified in infants with colic and adults with irritable bowel syndrome.[46,47] It should be noted that IFM is a disorder that is distinct from hereditary fructose intolerance (MIM #229600), which results from a deficiency of aldolase B and the subsequent accumulation of fructose-1-phosphate in the cytoplasm.

Diagnostic Criteria or Laboratory Investigations. Fructose malabsorption can be assessed by either placing the patient on a fructose elimination diet or performing a fructose breath hydrogen test. Fructose given at 1 g/kg body weight or a maximum of 25 g can be used to perform these studies[15] (Figure 2). Concomitant administration of glucose can attenuate the malabsorption of fructose as assessed by breath testing presumably by improving solvent drag.[48] To determine whether the malabsorption is fructose-specific, intestinal biopsies should reveal normal intestinal histology, and malabsorption should be limited to fructose and not other monosaccharides.

Clinical Management. Patients experiencing significant fructose-induced diarrhea should either reduce or eliminate their dietary fructose load to resolve symptoms. It has been established in rodent models that GLUT5 levels are dependent on the chronic load of dietary fructose; therefore, it is conceivable that fructose malabsorption may resolve by initiating a feeding regimen of incrementally increasing amounts of fructose. Because fructose malabsorption is generally limited to early infancy, attempts to reintroduce fructose should be considered as patients enter into the school-age years.

Fanconi-Bickel Syndrome

Fanconi-Bickel syndrome (FBS; MIM #227810) is a very rare autosomal recessive disorder that is characterized by carbohydrate malabsorption, tubular nephropathy, hepatomegaly and abnormal glycogen accumulation, failure to thrive, and fasting hypoglycemia.[49–50]

Genetics and Molecular Pathophysiology. Homozygote mutations in the facilitative glucose transporter, *GLUT2*, has been identified in over 60 patients with FBS (Figure 6).[27] Although most of the mutations are nonsense and result in a truncated transporter, several missense mutations were also identified. In vitro functional studies have not been performed to confirm that these mutations adversely alter the transport capabilities of the GLUT2 protein.

The mechanism by which mutation in the facilitative carrier, GLUT2, alters the fasting- and feeding-induced changes in serum glucose is not well understood; however, impaired hepatocyte transport and glucose-sensing mechanism by pancreatic β cells are possible explanations.[50] In the small intestine, GLUT2 is restricted to the basolateral membrane and was previously believed to be the primary method of monosaccharide exit from the enterocyte (Figure 6). However, severe osmotic diarrhea is generally not associated with FBS, and mice containing a targeted deletion of *Glut2* also retain monosaccharide transport across the basolateral membrane, suggesting that a GLUT2-independent pathway for glucose transport exists in enterocytes.[51]

Clinical Manifestations. The diagnosis of FBS should be considered in patients with hepatomegaly and evidence of a renal tubulopathy. Although

carbohydrate malabsorption has been reported in some but not all cases of FBS, it is certainly not a dominant feature of the disorder, however, failure to thrive, rickets, and osteoporosis are clinical characteristics that are found in most patients with FBS.[50]

Diagnostic Criteria or Laboratory Investigations and Treatment. Urine analysis generally shows evidence of glycosuria, a generalized aminoaciduria, and excessive urinary losses of phosphate and calcium. Histologic analysis of the small bowel, liver, and kidney generally reveals excessive glycogen stores. Abdominal ultrasonography is useful to confirm the relative enlargement of the liver and kidney. Management is primarily focused on supplementing urinary electrolyte losses. Uncooked cornstarch has been used to prevent hypoglycemia and to minimize postprandial hyperglycemia, and since abnormalities in fructose absorption and metabolism has not been described, it is a reasonable alternative in the therapy of FBS.[52]

DISORDERS OF AMINO ACID AND PEPTIDE ASSIMILATION

The complex process of dietary protein assimilation begins with proteolytic hydrolysis to small peptides and amino acids by multiple gastric, pancreatic, and brush border proteases. Small peptides (di- and tripeptides) and amino acids are transported into enterocytes across the brush border membrane through a series of transporters with overlapping specificities based on the characteristics of substrate size and charge (Figure 8). Di- and tripeptides are hydrolyzed by intracellular peptidases to single amino acids, which efflux across the basolateral membrane through a second series of transporters. The 21 common amino acids add to the variety of dietary proteins whose digestion requires a host of endopeptidases and exopeptidases with precise yet overlapping specificities. Passive and ion-mediated transepithelial absorption is mediated by a diverse group of transporters with broad amino acid specificities.[53–55] The redundant role of these enzyme and transport systems minimizes the physiologic consequences of a single deficiency in almost any component of this process (Table 1).

Protein digestion is initiated in the stomach by a family of pepsin proteases that are secreted by chief cells in the inactive form as pepsinogen (Figure 8). Pepsinogen becomes activated by the acidic content of the stomach, where it produces nonabsorbable peptides. Under most conditions, however, gastric hydrolysis is not necessary for protein digestion. Dietary proteins that get to the intestine are further hydrolyzed into smaller peptides by a family of endopeptidases (trypsin, chymotrypsin, and elastase) and exopeptidases (carboxypeptidase A and B) that are secreted in their dormant form by the exocrine pancreas.

Enterokinase, a serine protease situated on the brush border membrane of enterocytes in the duodenum, converts the proenzyme trypsinogen to

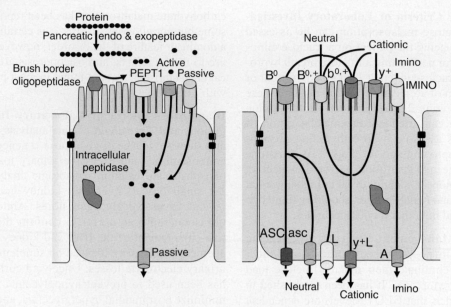

Figure 8 Protein and amino acid assimilation in the small intestine.

trypsin. Trypsin consequently cleaves the precursor form of other endo- and exopeptidases to their active counterpart. The oligopeptides undergo further hydrolysis by another large family of oligopeptidases (aminopeptidase and carboxypeptidase) located on the brush border membrane. These proteolytic enzymes have distinct substrate specificity and hydrolyze the dietary protein into either dipeptides or single amino acids that are consequently transported by a group of uniporters.

Disorders of protein digestion are unusual but should be considered when evaluating a patient for a potential defect of amino acid transport (Table 1). The best characterized disorder of specific protein malabsorption is a deficiency of enterokinase synthesis (MIM #226200).[56] Individuals with enterokinase deficiency present with diarrhea, failure to thrive, and hypoproteinemic edema while on a diet of intact dietary proteins; while symptoms resolve on an amino acid–based diet. Primary trypsinogen deficiency has also been reported and results in clinical symptoms that resemble enterokinase deficiency.[57] Nearly 90% of patients with cystic fibrosis (MIM #219700) have clinical evidence of exocrine pancreatic dysfunction that results in the impaired digestion of complex dietary protein, fat, and carbohydrates.[13,14] A similar type of generalized malabsorptive condition also occurs in the late stages of other disorders that result in chronic pancreatitis, including hereditary pancreatitis (MIM #167800).[58]

A large group of amino acid transporters have been isolated and characterized, and these are expressed either on the apical or basolateral membrane of the enterocyte (Figure 8).[53,54] The brush border membrane contains the B^0, B0AT1, and $B^{0,+}$ Na^+-dependent systems that transport neutral amino acids.[59] Anionic and cationic amino acids are selectively transported via system xc^- and y^+, respectively. Proline and hydroxyproline are selectively transported by the proline IMINO transporter system Sodium/Imino-acid Transporter 1 (SIT1).[60] In contrast, cationic and neutral

(cysteine) amino acids are transported by the Na-independent system $b^{0,+}$, which is defective in cystinuria (MIM #220100), an autosomal recessive aminoaciduria that is not associated with a major gastrointestinal phenotype.[61] Although the $b^{0,+}$ system is expressed in the kidney and intestine, in patients with cystinuria dietary cysteine may still be absorbed as a component of oligopeptides via the H^+-oligopeptide cotransporter (PEPT1).[62] Proton-coupled amino acid transporters, PAT1 and PAT2, have been identified and PAT1 is found expressed in the brush border small intestine.[63,64] The relative contributions of SIT1 and PAT1 to imino acid absorption and iminoaciduria have yet to be resolved.

Intracellular neutral amino acids efflux across the basolateral membrane in a size-dependent manner; with system L carrying the larger and system ASC the smaller amino acids (Figure 9). Small neutral amino acids also cross the basolateral membrane via a Na^+-dependent ASC system, whereas the A system is selective for both neutral and imino acids. In contrast, cationic amino acids are transported by the Na^+-dependent system y^+L, which is defective in lysinuric protein intolerance (LPI). Although the redundancy in the transport specificity of these various systems essentially minimizes gastrointestinal and nutritional consequences that are observed when an individual transport system is disrupted, LPI patients do experience significant gastrointestinal symptoms.

Lysinuric Protein Intolerance

Lysinuric protein intolerance (LPI) (MIM #222700) is an autosomal recessive disorder that results from mutations in the *SLC7A7* gene, which encodes for the cationic amino acid transporter y^+LAT-1 (Figure 9).[65,66] The y^+LAT-1 transporter is situated on the basolateral membrane of the enterocyte and renal tubules and transports cytoplasmic dibasic amino acids such as lysine, arginine, and ornithine in exchange for Na^+ and neutral amino acids.[67] Several gastrointestinal symptoms, including failure to thrive, diarrhea, vomiting and pancreatitis, are the main clinical symptoms associated with LPI.

Genetics and Molecular Pathophysiology. Approximately 30 mutations have been identified in the *LPI* gene in more than 100 patients with LPI.[65,66,68,69] Founder mutations have been identified in Finnish, Japanese, and Italian kindreds in whom the incidence of LPI is particularly common. Ornithine and arginine are important urea cycle intermediates that fail to exit the intestinal and renal epithelium of patients with LPI. Their relative deficiency, particularly during a high-protein diet meal, results in urea cycle dysfunction that leads to hyperammonemia and subsequent alterations in mental status.[70]

Clinical Manifestations. Undiagnosed patients with LPI generally present with failure to thrive and a self-imposed restriction of dietary protein. Although diarrhea, emesis, and abdominal pain are frequent symptoms, the distinguishing feature of LPI is that high-protein diets result in

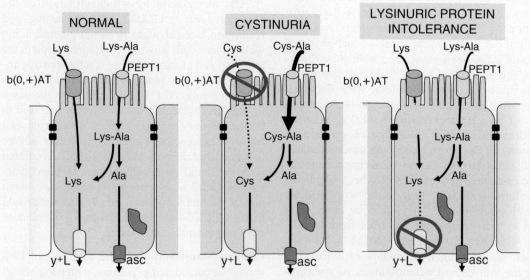

Figure 9 Amino acid transport in the small intestine of normal, LPI, and cystinuria patients.

hyperammonemia and dramatic changes in mental status, and chronic exposure to dietary protein is usually associated with various degrees of mental retardation. Marked hepatosplenomegaly and frequent bone fractures are also characteristic of LPI, and life spans are generally limited by complications associated with alveolar proteinosis and osteoporosis.[71–72]

Diagnostic Criteria, Laboratory Investigations, and Management. Quantitative plasma amino acids and urinary organic acids provide useful clues in the detection of LPI as plasma levels of diamino acids are low, whereas urinary levels of lysine and orotic acid are elevated.[67] The diagnosis can commonly be recognized by testing with an enteral bolus of dietary protein. Such a challenge would result in the rapid impairment of motor function and alteration of mental status that result from hyperammonemia. Citrulline supplements (200 mg/kg/d) and dietary protein restriction <1.5 g/kg/d) are used to manage patients with LPI.[70] Mealtime supplements of citrulline are readily absorbed and lessen postprandial hyperammonemia following a protein meal. Oral carnitine supplementation has been shown to be significant in a subset of patients described with LPI and hypocarnitinemia.[73]

Hartnup's Disease

Hartnup's disease (MIM #234500) and iminoglycinuria (MIM #242600) are two other autosomal recessive disorders that have been well characterized clinically.[74,75] Hartnup's disease is characterized by a malabsorption and renal excretion of neutral amino acids (neutral aminoaciduria) and a heterogeneous set of symptoms ranging from a pellagra-like rash to neurologic disorders (Figure 9).[59] Through linkage analysis a candidate gene, *B0AT1* (SLC6A19), was identified and sequencing of affected individuals found variants that included splice site, deletions and nonsense mutations that produce a truncated protein and missense mutations. Testing of the missense mutant proteins expressed in *Xenopus laevis* oocytes eliminated amino acid transport.[76–77] B0AT1 is a sodium-dependent and chloride-independent neutral amino acid transporter that is expressed in the intestine and kidney.

Other Defects of Amino Acid Transport

A second disturbance of amino acid transport has been characterized to date: system b$^{0,+}$, which is defective in cystinuria (MIM #220100) and is selective for cationic and neutral amino acid transport across the brush border membrane (Figure 9).[61] The diagnosis of these disorders can be established with analysis of urine amino acid profiles, and both disorders present with either neurologic or renal symptoms and a lack of noteworthy gastrointestinal complications. There is only one report of impaired proline absorption that may be due to mutations in the imino transporter SIT1.[75,78]

DISORDERS OF FAT ASSIMILATION

Assimilation of dietary fats requires hydrolysis and subsequent repackaging of lipids by an intricate group of intraluminal and intracellular events.[79] The clinical consequences of disorders of fat assimilation include failure to thrive, steatorrhea, and neurologic deficits that result from the malabsorption of fat-soluble vitamins (Figure 2 and Table 1). Lipolysis is initiated by gastric lipase in the stomach and concludes in the intestine through the action of pancreatic lipase. Because pancreatic exocrine function is particularly not fully formed during early infancy, fat absorption in this age group primarily depends on the action of gastric lipase.[80] A congenital deficiency of pancreatic lipase (MIM #246600) is an exceedingly rare autosomal recessive disorder that leads to fat malabsorption.[81]

Fatty acid and diglyceride are the products of triglyceride hydrolysis, and their solubilization to the aqueous phase of luminal content requires adequate levels of conjugated bile salts, and therefore various disorders of intrahepatic and extrahepatic cholestasis will impede the delivery of luminal bile salts and result in fat malabsorption. Bile salts are particularly important in the emulsification of long-chain fatty acids because of their lower aqueous solubility when compared with their medium-chain (12 to 6 carbons) counterpart.

A fatty acid transport protein (FATP4) that has been localized to the brush border membrane appears to play an essential role in the absorption of long-chain fatty acids.[82–83] Analysis of *Fatp4* null mice demonstrates a 40% reduction in fatty acid uptake and a neonatal lethal restrictive dermopathy.[84–86] In contrast, the apical cholesterol transporter named Niemann-Pick C1-like protein (NPC1L1) was identified using a genomic-bioinformatics approach,[87] and *NPC1L1* null mice absorbed only 30% of luminal cholesterol.[88] Ezetimibe is a potent selective inhibitor of NPC1L1, and may have a significant role in restricting the absorption of dietary cholesterol in patients with hypercholesterolemia.[89,90] The cholesterol export across the epithelial layer was recently established to occur via an adenosine triphosphate (ATP)-binding cassette transporter, ABCA1. The role of ABCA1 in cholesterol and phospholipid transport was confirmed when linkage analysis established it as the gene defective in Tangier disease (MIM #205400).[91,92] Tangier disease patients have a deficiency of high-density lipoproteins, which predisposes to the development of premature coronary heart disease despite hypocholesterolemia, in addition to the accumulation of cholesterol in tissue such as the liver, spleen, lymph node, and small intestine. Patients with sitosterolemia (MIM #210250) have the peculiar ability to absorb an excessive amount of the main plant sterol, sitosterol. Mutations in the ABC transporter, ABCG5 and ABCG8, have been associated with sitosterolemia.[93] These proteins form a heterodimer, which serves as the primary sterol efflux mechanism in the intestine. In spite of defective processing of cholesterol and

sterol, patients with Tangier disease and sitosterolemia have no noteworthy gastrointestinal phenotype apart from hepatosplenomegaly. In contrast, disorders that result in defective packaging of reesterified lipids into apolipoprotein-rich chylomicrons and very-low-density lipoprotein (VLDL) particles normally lead to fat malabsorption and failure to thrive.

Abetalipoproteinemia

Abetalipoproteinemia (ABL) (MIM #200100) is the classic and most well-characterized disorder of fat absorption and results from failure to reassemble dietary fat in the form of β-lipoproteins. Triglyceride and cholesterol esters are principally transported in the plasma via β-lipoproteins; therefore, ABL patients have a severe shortage of both of these neutral lipids. Patients generally present shortly after birth with failure to thrive and steatorrhea and if untreated will develop irreversible neurologic problems in late infancy. However, milder variants have been identified in asymptomatic adult patients who were recognized by routine cholesterol screening.

Genetics and Molecular Pathophysiology. Homozygote mutations in the *MTP* gene have been identified in patients with ABL, and the MTP protein is a 97 kDa subunit that forms a heterodimer with a 55 kDa protein named disulfide isomerase (PDI).[94–95] Only a handful of missense mutations have been identified in ABL patients, and the majority result from a truncated or nonfunctional MTP, and no mutations have been reported in the gene encoding the PDI protein.[96] Serum lipoproteins in patients with ABL are deficient in triglycerides and cholesterol-rich apolipoproteins B-100 and B-48, which form VLDL and chylomicrons. Apolipoprotein B-100 is synthesized by hepatocytes that produce VLDL, whereas the truncated protein (apolipoprotein B-48) is formed by enterocytes and is necessary for chylomicron formation.

The role of MTP in chylomicron formation has been definitively established by investigating the consequences of ABL-causing mutations.[95,97–99] These studies reveal that apolipoprotein B single-handedly is incapable of initiating lipoprotein formation and that MTP is specifically required to complete proper assembly. The protein component of apolipoproteins B-100 and B-48 is synthesized in the endoplasmic reticulum and must fold properly to form a complex with lipids. Consequently, MTP has two discrete roles in lipoprotein assembly: first, to move lipids such as cholesterol and triglycerides into the lumen of the smooth endoplasmic reticulum and, second, to transfer small quantities of these lipids to the newly formed and unstable apolipoprotein B protein in a process that has been termed "lipidation."[98] In the absence of lipoprotein assembly, lipid droplets accumulate in the endoplasmic reticulum and are not transported to the *trans*-Golgi apparatus in the enterocyte and hepatocytes.[100]

Clinical Manifestations. The typical clinical presentation is often failure to thrive, emesis, and low-volume diarrhea. Poor growth despite adequate caloric intake is an early clinical characteristic that should hasten the assessment of a possible defect of fat malabsorption. In the long-term, patients may develop an aversion to fatty meals as a way to diminish their diarrheal symptoms. The first evidence of neuromuscular abnormalities is frequently the loss of deep tendon reflexes which results from prolonged vitamin E deficiency; additional neuromuscular manifestations, including retinitis pigmentosa, ataxia, and spinocerebellar degeneration, may be mistaken for various forms of Friedreich ataxia.

Diagnostic Criteria, Laboratory Investigations, and Medical Management. Serum samples should be analyzed for evidence of β-lipoprotein (VLDL and chylomicron) deficiencies. Specifically, plasma triglyceride levels are generally low <10 mg/dL), whereas cholesterol levels range from 25 to 40 mg/dL (Figure 2). Acanthocytosis is usually seen in peripheral blood smears and results from abnormal lipoproteins in the plasma membrane of erythrocytes. Endoscopic evaluation of the small bowel can show yellow discoloration, and biopsies have characteristic fat-laden enterocytes located in the upper portion of the villus (Figure 10). Fat droplets within the cytoplasmic compartment of the enterocyte may be established by electron microscopy.

To minimize diarrheal symptoms, ABL patients may be managed on a low-fat diet (~15 g/d), and serum levels of fat-soluble vitamins should be monitored periodically. Sufficient serum levels of vitamins A and K can be achieved with supplementation of moderate oral doses; though, absorption of tocopherol is severely impaired and may require massive doses (2,000 mg in infants, and 10,000 mg in older children and adults) of tocopherol to diminish the neuromuscular manifestations of vitamin E insufficiency.

Hypobetalipoproteinemia

Hypobetalipoproteinemia (HBL; MIM #107730) is another very well-characterized disorder of fat absorption that results from the formation of abnormally truncated forms of apolipoprotein B.[101,102] The heterozygote state has been estimated to occur in approximately 1 in every 3,000 Americans.[102]

Genetics and Molecular Pathophysiology. The chief difference between ABL and HBL is that the obligate ABL heterozygotes have normal cholesterol and triglycerides levels, whereas HBL heterozygotes have low lipoprotein levels.[103] Therefore, HBL is inherited in an autosomal dominant manner; however, patients with only a single defective allele generally have no gastrointestinal and only minimal, if any, neuromuscular abnormalities. In contrast, individuals with two defective alleles are indistinguishable from ABL patients based on both physical and laboratory assessment.

Many mutations have been described in the *APOB* gene in patients with HBL.[104] The mutations all result in proteins that are

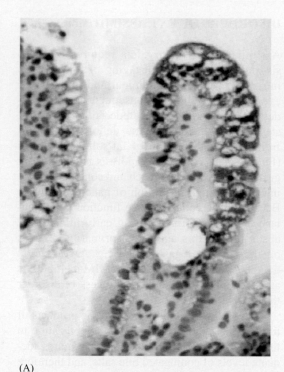
(A)

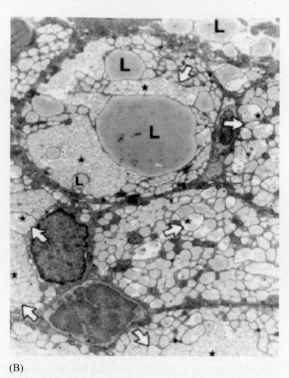
(B)

Figure 10 Classic lipid enterocytes seen in patients with abetalipoproteinemia, hypobetalipoproteinemia, and chylomicron retention disease. (A) Intestinal biopsies from patients show vacuolization and marked staining with Oil Red O when examined by light microscopy. (B) Electron microscopy of biopsies from patients shows the accumulation of large lipid droplets, free in the cytoplasm (L), and smaller chylomicrons and very low density lipoprotein sized particles (*stars*) in membrane-bound vesicles (*arrows*). (Courtesy of Dr Marie-Elisabeh Samson-Bouma, Faculté de Médecine X. Bichat, 100.)

truncated either because of a nonsense or frameshift mutation that leads to a premature downstream stop codon. Several kindreds have been described that are clinically indistinguishable from HBL and ABL; however, mutations in either the apolipoprotein B or MTP alleles have not been identified. Various models have shown that truncation of the carboxy terminal of the apolipoprotein B protein influences the process of lipidation, as described earlier. Therefore, the inadequate addition of neutral lipids to the shortened apolipoprotein B protein leads to instability of the protein and its eventual degradation.

Clinical Manifestations. The clinical manifestations of patients with homozygote mutations of the *APOB* gene are identical to what was described in the ABL section of this chapter. In contrast, defects in a single allele (heterozygotes) may have subtle neurologic findings indicative of mild vitamin E deficiency.

Diagnostic Criteria or Laboratory Investigations and Treatment. In heterozygote patients, cholesterol, triglyceride, and low-density lipoprotein levels are lower than in other unaffected members of the same kindred. In contrast, patients with homozygote mutations in the *APOB* allele have cholesterol, triglyceride, chylomicron, and VLDL levels that are similar to what was previously described in ABL patients (Figure 2). Moreover, characteristic findings such as acanthocytosis and fat-laden enterocytes are also seen (Figure 10). Homozygote HBL patients should be managed as described in the ABL section,

including the restriction of dietary fat and the supplementation of vitamin E. In contrast, the heterozygote patient should be given modest doses of vitamin E.

Chylomicron Retention Disease

Chylomicron retention disease (CMRD; MIM #246700), or Andersen disease, is the least common of the classic disorders of lipid packaging in the intestine.[105,106] CMRD is an autosomal recessive disorder in which apolipoprotein B and MTP are produced; however, there is failure to secrete chylomicrons across the enterocyte's basolateral membrane.

Genetics and Molecular Pathophysiology. CMRD was recently found to be secondary to a defect in the a gene named *SARA2* which encodes for the Sar1b protein and a member of the Sar1–adenosine diphosphate–ribosylation factor family of small guanosine triphosphatases.[107] This family of proteins have an important role in the process of intracellular trafficking, and suggest that when defective, chylomicron trafficking to the *trans*-Golgi apparatus may be disrupted.[108] While some nonsense mutations were identified, all the missense mutations alter a highly conserved residue in the guanine nucleotide-binding motif, which would presumably interfere with guanosine triphosphate binding. This domain of the Sar1b protein interacts with a series of Sec proteins (including Sec12 and Sec23) that eventually leads to membrane deformation, budding, and the eventual transport of chylomicron through the secretory pathway.[109]

Clinical Manifestations and Diagnostic Criteria or Laboratory Investigations and Treatment.

Patients have been reported to present as neonates with severe diarrhea but may also first come to medical attention in early adolescence with neuromuscular manifestations of vitamin E deficiency. However, the retinitis pigmentosa and neuromuscular manifestations are less severe when compared with either HBL or ABL (Figure 2). Unlike patients with HBL and ABL, triglyceride apolipoprotein B100 levels are normal in this condition. Enterocytes are also laden with fat, as is seen in HBL and ABL (Figure 10). Treatment consists of restricting dietary fats and supplementation of vitamin E.

Primary Bile Acid Malabsorption

Proficient digestion and absorption of dietary lipids and lipid-soluble vitamins require their emulsification by bile salts (taurocholate) within the intestinal lumen.[110] The majority of dietary fats are absorbed in the jejunum, and residual bile salts are reabsorbed primarily by ileal enterocytes that express a Na^+-dependent bile salt transporter, ASBT (*SLC10A2*), on its apical membrane. Primary bile acid malabsorption (PBAM; MIM #601295) is a rare autosomal recessive disorder that results from an impairment of bile acid reabsorption secondary to a defect in the function of the ASBT transporter.[111,112] Taurocholate malabsorption more frequently results from the loss of an adequate amount of ileum, which may occur either because of surgical resection or because of extensive inflammation secondary to disorders such as Crohn's disease.[113,114] The diarrhea that accompanies both primary and secondary forms of bile acid malabsorption may be attributed to both fat malabsorption and bile acid stimulation of colonocyte secretion of ions and fluid. Idiopathic adult-onset bile acid malabsorption has also been described in patients with presumably normal ileal function.[115]

Genetics and Molecular Pathophysiology.

Dawson identified three missense (Ala171Ser, Leu243Pro, Thr262Met) and a splice site mutation the *SLC10A2* gene in patients with PBAM.[111] In vitro analysis of these missense mutations failed to alter the proper targeting of ASBT to the cell membrane, however; the Leu243Pro and Thr262Met mutations impaired taurocholate transport.[116] The Ala171Ser mutation was found in 28% of asymptomatic individuals and appears to represent a benign polymorphism because bile acid absorption was not impaired by in vitro analysis. A missense mutation (Pro290Ser) was identified on a single ASBT allele (heterozygote), a patient with Crohns disease.[117] The Pro290Ser mutation abolishes taurocholate transport and in heterozygote carriers may influence cholesterol homeostasis and bile acid metabolism; however, the frequency and role of this and other polymorphisms in the general population await further investigations. No significant genomic mutations were identified in a large cohort of adult patients with idiopathic bile acid malabsorption.[115]

The Na^+-dependent bile salt transporter ASBT is expressed on cholangiocytes and ileocytes and therefore plays an essential role in the enteric and hepatic phases of the enterohepatic circulation. Taurocholate is excreted in the biliary tree, where it is initially stored in the gallbladder and eventually enters the duodenum after cholecystokinin-induced gallbladder contraction in response to a meal. A small fraction of taurocholate is passively absorbed in the jejunum and colon. Along the horizontal axis of the intestine, ASBT expression is limited to the ileum, where it transports taurocholate via an electrogenic, Na^+-dependent mechanism. The reabsorption of taurocholate is about 95% efficient, and the 5% loss is replaced by hepatocyte conversion of cholesterol to bile salts.

Differential expression of orphan solute transporters in *SLC10A2* null mice was recently used to identify the putative basolateral taurocholate transporter.[118] The heteromeric organic solute transporter α-β, Ostα-Ostβ, is expressed in the kidney and intestine and localized by immunohistochemistry at the basolateral surface. Both proteins are required to get correct targeting of the complex to the basolateral membrane in order to facilitate to taurocholate efflux in the ileum. Eventually, taurocholate enters the portal circulation and are transported across the hepatocytes sinusoidal membrane by a Na^+-dependent taurocholate cotransport polypeptide, NTCP (*SLC10A1*). Transport of recycled and newly formed taurocholate out of the hepatocyte occurs across the canalicular membrane via an ATP-dependent bile salt export pump, BSEP.

Clinical Manifestations.

Patients with PBAM present during infancy with diarrhea, steatorrhea, failure to thrive, and low plasma levels of low-density lipoprotein cholesterol.[111,112] The diarrhea is generally secretory (persists while fasting) in character and is exacerbated by the addition of dietary fats.

Diagnostic Criteria or Laboratory Investigations and Treatment.

The small intestine of patients with PBAM should be normal in length and architecture, and the extent of the diarrhea should improve with a trial of cholestyramine and a low-fat diet (Figure 2). Bile acid absorption by the ileum may be measured using the bile acid analogue ^{75}Se-homocholic acid–taurine test.

DISORDERS OF GENERALIZED MALABSORPTION

Nonspecific diminution in intestinal absorption capacity most often occurs when small bowel surface area declines either from a reduction in gut length, villus, or microvillus, or when pancreatic exocrine function is impaired (Figure 2). For instance, congenital or surgical-induced short bowel syndrome, or enteropathies such as hypersensitivity to proteins, and even more unusual disorders, such as autoimmune enteropathy (IPEX) and microvillus inclusion disease

have features of generalized (or nonspecific) malabsorption.[5,6] Cystic fibrosis results in impairment of pancreatic exocrine function and generalized malabsorptive symptoms, as pancreatic enzymes hydrolyze dietary fats and complex carbohydrates.[119] However, disorders of pancreatic insufficiency are not associated with malabsorption of either monosaccharide (glucose, galactose, or fructose) or amino acids.

Diarrhea induced by the malabsorption of specific nutrients, an important characteristic of all inherited disorders of nutrient assimilation, and is not a feature of disorders associated with a decline in intestinal surface area. Defects of enzymatic function, both from the exocrine pancreas or intestinal brush border, share many of the clinical characteristics seen in mucosal transport defects and result in the malabsorption of specific nutrients. In contrast, generalized malabsorption (ie, not nutrient specific) occurs in the clinical setting where the intestinal absorptive capacity is insufficient to appropriately handle a normal dietary load.[4,120,121] A large proportion of children with congenital diarrhea have a generalized malabsorptive form that has not been well characterized clinically, and its molecular basis had not been elucidated until recently.

Enteric Anendocrinosis

Enteric anendocrinosis is an exceeding rare autosomal recessive disorder that presents with a generalized malabsorptive disorder during the initial month of life, and results from mutation of Neurogenin-3 (*NEUROG3*) and an absence of intestinal endocrine cells (MIM #610370).[32,33] Neurogenin-3 is a basic-helix-loop-helix (bHLH) transcriptional factor. Murine studies have demonstrated that Neurog3 drives endocrine cell fate determination both in the pancreas and the intestine, and that Neurogenin-1 and -2 drives neuronal cell fate determination.

Until the description of this novel disorder, only defects in the structure and function of enterocytes and inflammatory cells of the gut have been associated with diarrhea and alteration of ion and nutrient absorption and secretion. The crypt-villus axis of the small bowel is populated by four well-differentiated cell populations including absorptive epithelial cells, and a secretory population comprised of mucus-secreting goblet cells, antimicrobial Paneth cells, and hormone-secreting enteroendocrine cells (Figure 11).[122–124] Stems cells located at the base of the crypt-villus axis provide uncommitted progeny situated in the proliferative zone that eventually differentiates into absorptive or secretory cells.[125] Recent studies have begun to elucidate the molecular basis of small bowel stem cell differentiation to these four functional cell types.

Cell fate determination within the uncommitted progeny of stem cells occurs by NOTCH-mediated lateral inhibition, a process that has been well described in neuronal development

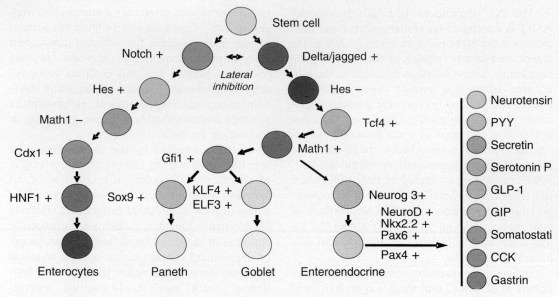

Figure 11 The transcription factors that drive cell fate determination in the gut.

(Figure 11).[126–127] In the small bowel, several isotypes of the NOTCH receptor and its ligands, Jagged and Delta, are differentially expressed in undifferentiated stem cell progeny and triggers a signaling cascade dominated by sequential expression of numerous basic helix-loop-helix (bHLH) transcriptional factors.[128,129] Cells expressing the NOTCH receptor are stimulated by adjacent cells containing the membrane-bound Delta or Jagged ligands, resulting in cleavage of the intracellular NOTCH domain which interacts with RBP-Jk to activate transcriptional expression of several isoforms of hairy and enhancer of split (Hes).[126,129] Hes1 is a potent inhibitor of this cascade of bHLH transcription factors in the intestine and results in the exclusive development of epithelial cells, as the intestine of *Hes1* null mice is overpopulated by enteroendocrine and goblet cells, while depleted of the absorptive lineage.[129] Mouse atonal homolog 1 (Math1) is the immediate downstream target of Hes1, and in Jagged/Delta but not NOTCH expressing stem progeny, Math1 initiates a transcriptional factor cascade that leads to the secretory cell fate determination.[130] *Neurog3* null mice are devoid of all islet cells, including insulin-producing β cells of the pancreas, and enteroendocrine cells in the small and large bowel, and presumably succumb eventually to diabetes during the first several days of life.[131–135] Neurogenin-3 is a bHLH activator of NeuroD1, another bHLH transcription factor that directly stimulates insulin synthesis, and is essential for differentiation of a subset of enteroendocrine cells (Figure 11).[136] Despite extensive studies evaluating the signals responsible for intestinal cell fate determination, the physiologic consequences of disturbing the balance of the four differentiated cell populations of the small bowel in either mouse or man had not been evaluated until recently.

The gastrointestinal tract is populated by 10 or more different types of enteroendocrine cells that can be characterized by the types of hormones and paracrine factors that they secrete, and their distribution along the rostrocaudal axis (Figure 11).[137] For instance, endocrine cells expressing ghrelin and gastrin are primarily confined to the stomach, while CCK and secretin-secreting endocrine cells are located in the proximal small bowel. GLP-1 and 2 and peptide YY cells are primarily limited to the distal small bowel and colon, while endocrine cells that secrete other hormones (substance P, serotonin, and somatostatin) are located throughout the gastrointestinal tract.[138]

Small bowel biopsies of patients with enteric anendocrinosis reveal normal villus structure, crypt–villus axis without pathological inflammatory cell infiltration.[32,33] Extensive evaluation of the small bowel mucosa demonstrates profound enteroendocrine cell dysgenesis; while the remaining mucosa is otherwise normal and showed no abnormality of Paneth and goblet cells appearance as assessed by PAS and lysozyme immunohistochemistry. Chromogranin A staining of the index case revealed only one aberrant enteroendocrine cell in over 350 small bowel crypts examined, and none in the colon; compared to 5 to 6 enteroendocrine cells per crypt in normal mucosa. Staining with various antibodies that are toward multiple gut hormones confirmed the generalized absence enteroendocrine cells. Electron microscopic evaluation has a normal brush border and microvilli, normal appearing intracellular mitochondria and tight junctions, and an occasional lipid-laden enterocytes that was limited to the one-third of the villus.

Genetics and Molecular Pathophysiology. Sequencing of the *neurogenin-3* gene of the index case revealed the presence of a homozygote missense mutation that changed residue 107 located in the first helix, from an arginine to a serine (Arg107Ser).[32] The remaining cases also had a homozygote missense mutation that altered amino acid 93 from an arginine to leucine (Arg93Leu). This amino acid is located just upstream of the first helix in the basic DNA binding domain. The two changed amino acids are strictly conserved in the entire neurogenin (ie, NEUROG1 to 3) family of proteins from humans to *Caenorhabditis elegans*. These missense mutations result in loss-of-function of NEUROGENIN-3 given both their location and the extent to which these residues are conserved among a wide range of species, and additional in vitro and in vivo data support this claim. What remains unclear is the role that enteroendocrine cells have in facilitating the absorption of simple nutrients.

Clinical Manifestations, Diagnostic Criteria, Laboratory Investigations, and Medical Management. The severity of the diarrhea in patients with enteric anendocrinosis is in the range of 80 to 120 cc kg^{-1} d^{-1} (normal: <20 cc kg^{-1} d^{-1}) and it ceased while fasting.[32] While water was well tolerated, glucose-based oral rehydration solution led to diarrhea. However, unlike patients with GGM, these children continued to experience diarrhea while on a carbohydrate-free cow's milk-based formula (Figure 2). The addition of either fructose or glucose to this formula exacerbated the severity of the diarrhea. Several amino acid–based formulas, including one without carbohydrates, were attempted without resolution of diarrheal symptoms. These infants may be optimally managed with limited quantities of low osmotic formula's and lifelong parenteral nutrition. Several studies have shown that Neurogenin-3 is critical in the development of pancreatic islet cells, and patients with enteric anendocrinosis develop clinical evidence of diabetes (without anti-islet antibodies) between 4 and 10 years of age[131–135] (unpublished observations).

Other Disorders of Generalized Malabsorption

We have recently identified a larger subset of children with nonspecific malabsorption that have many of the features of enteric anendocrinosis, save the presence of normal appearing enteroendocrine cells and an absence of *Neurogenin-3* mutations (unpublished observations). The generalized malabsorption necessitates the use of chronic parenteral nutrition to sustain normal growth, and in the majority of patients was continued life-long. We believe that the pathophysiology in this group of patients is that the enteroendocrine cells are dysfunctional, and that the elucidation of the molecular basis of this disorder will provide insight into how the enteroendocrine cell products augment nutrient absorption. We have tentatively named this disorder enteric dysendocrinosis, and unlike enteric anendocrinosis, it is not associated with insulin-dependent diabetes (Table 1) (unpublished observations).

A homozygote loss-of-function mutation of prohormone convertase 1 (PC1) has been reported to result in a generalized malabsorption, obesity, hypoadrenalism, hypogonadotropic hypogonadism, primary amenorrhea, and elevated levels of prohormones with a related depletion of mature hormones[139] (MIM #600955). The PC family of enzymes are located in enteroendocrine and other endocrine cells, and convert inactive peptide hormone precursors into their mature functional forms.[140] Like enteric anendocrinosis, these patients present during the early neonatal periods with generalized malabsorption and are generally TPN dependent; however, they develop a set of general endocrine abnormalities that are unique to this disorder, and are not seen in patients with either enteric anendocrinosis or dysendocrinosis.[32-33]

A transient depletion of enteroendocrine cells was reported in an adult patient with temporary malabsorption and autoimmune polyglandular syndrome type I (APS-1), and clinical symptoms resolved following the spontaneous recovery of enteroendocrine cells[141] (MIM #240300). We have also identified a small group of children who had no evidence of diarrhea or failure to thrive until their sudden onset during the childhood period. These children also experienced a transient depletion of enteroendocrine cells that corresponded to the period of time when they had severe malabsorptive diarrhea. Mutations in the gene named AIRE (autoimmune regulator) that is responsible for APS-1 was seen in only a single patient, suggesting that the other children have a disorder other than APS-1 (unpublished observations).

DISORDERS OF MINERAL AND ELECTROLYTE ABSORPTION AND SECRETION

Congenital Chloride Diarrhea

The most common cause of severe congenital secretory diarrhea in the presence of normal intestinal mucosa is the autosomal recessive disorder congenital chloride diarrhea (CCD; MIM #214700) (Figure 12).[142] Nearly half the reported cases have been confined to Finland, where it has been estimated to occur in 1 in 20,000 of the population, whereas it has been estimated

to occur in 1 in 32,000 live births in the Persian Gulf.[143] The gene defective in CCD is *SLC26A3* which encodes a Na^+-independent Cl^-/HCO_3^- exchanger that is expressed primarily in the apical brush border membrane of ileal enterocytes and colonic epithelium (Figure 12).[144]

Genetics and Molecular Pathophysiology. The founder mutations in the *SLC26A3* gene in patients of Finnish descent with CCD is the Val317del nonsense mutation.[142,144-145] Over 30 disease-related mutations have been identified in over 100 patients studied with CCD.[142] Two other prominent founder mutations have been identified that account for the majority of cases of CCD in Poland (Ile675-676ins), Saudi Arabia, and Kuwait (Gly187X).[143] A small number of patients have been identified that fit the clinical characteristics of CCD but do not have detectable mutations in the *SLC26A3* gene, suggesting the possibility of a second allele.

SLC26A3's main role as a Cl^-/HCO_3^- exchanger is to reabsorb chloride in exchange for bicarbonate along the length of the distal small bowel and colon (Figure 12).[146] In the distal intestine and colon, salt (NaCl) absorption is secondary to SLC26A3 transport of chloride and Na^+-H^+ exchange (NHE-3) transport of sodium. In normal physiologic settings, the expression of NHE-3 in the proximal small intestine is low, and the Cl^-/HCO_3^- exchanger secretes bicarbonate into the lumen while absorbing chloride produced by gastric acid.[147,148] Consequently, the exchanger neutralizes the acidity of gastric secretion once it reaches the proximal small bowel. CFTR is a chloride channel whose primary role in the small intestine is to secrete chloride, which is then absorbed in the distal intestine and colon by the Cl^-/HCO_3^- exchanger.[149] Thus, impaired Cl^-/HCO_3^- exchanger function in CCD patients would disrupt the neutralization of gastric acid in the proximal small bowel and impair luminal chloride reabsorption in the distal small intestine and colon.

Clinical Manifestations. The earliest clinical symptoms may occur in utero with severe

polyhydramnios and dilated loops of small bowel detectible by ultrasonography that may resemble a distal intestinal obstruction.[150] The severity of the polyhydramnios frequently leads to preterm labor or planned premature delivery by cesarean section. Patients with CCD generally present during the first weeks of life with severe life-threatening secretory diarrhea. The serum electrolytes prior to treatment are unique among the various congenital diarrheal disorders and include metabolic alkalosis, hypochloremia, hypokalemia, and hyponatremia.

Diagnostic Criteria, Laboratory Investigations, and Medical Management. The diagnosis of CCD would be suggestive if fecal chloride concentration is high (>90 mmol/L) and exceeds the concentration of cations (Na^+ and K^+)[151] (Figure 2). This classic characteristic of CCD suggests that fecal HCO_3^- levels are particularly low and that another cation, presumably accounted for by H^+, contributes to the excessive electroneutral transfer of HCl. The mainstay of therapy is life-long enteral administration of KCl and NaCl supplements, in the range of 2.8 mmol/kg/d for infants, and 3 to 4 mmol/kg/d for adults.[151] However, occasional assessment of serum and urine electrolyte and pH balance is recommended to optimize the Cl^- replacement doses.

Once the diagnosis is established and maintenance electrolyte initiated, subsequent hospitalizations for bouts of dehydration become significantly less frequent despite life-long large-volume diarrhea. A unique classic characteristic of CCD is the severe exacerbation of diarrheal symptoms that is associated with most febrile illnesses, including upper respiratory infections. Such episodes are generally accompanied by emesis, and are a common cause of severe dehydration and electrolyte abnormalities that frequently necessitate hospitalizations. Recurrent episodes are believed to contribute to the renal insufficiency and systemic hypertension that are common in this group of patients.[151]

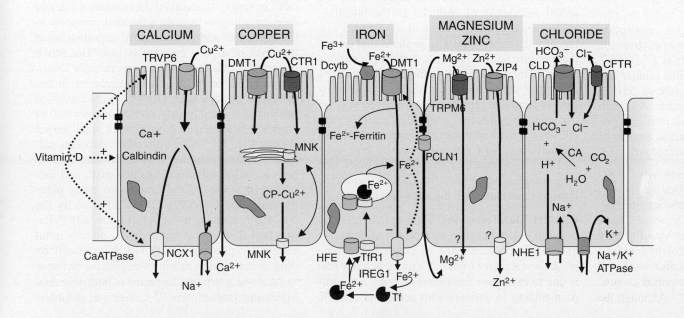

Figure 12 Ion and metal transport in the small intestine. ATPase = adenosine triphosphatase; CFTR = cystic fibrosis transmembrane regulator; CLD = congenital chloride diarrhea; CTR = copper transporter; Dcytb = duodenal cytochrome b; DMT = divalent metal transporter; FPN = ferroportin; HFE = hemochromatosis; IF = intrinsic factor; MNK = Menkes syndrome transport protein; NCX = Na^+-Ca^{2+} exchanger; NHE = Na^+-H^+ exchange; PCLN = paracellin; TfR = transferrin receptor; TRPV = transient receptor potential voltage; ZIP = zinc- and iron-regulated protein.

The administration of proton pump inhibitors slightly diminishes the severity of diarrhea, presumably by inhibiting meal-induced gastric acid secretion.[152] Cholestyramine administrated with oral electrolytes has been reported to transiently diminish stool volume. More recently, orally administered butyrate has been shown to dramatically improve stool volume and electrolyte depletion in a single patient with CCD in a dose-dependent manner.[153] Luminal butyrate can increase NaCl absorption by activation of the Cl^-/butyrate exchanger and by reducing both basal and cAMP-mediated chloride secretion.

Congenital Sodium Diarrhea

Congenital sodium diarrhea (CSD, MIM #270420) is an exceedingly rare autosomal recessive disorder that presents with secretory diarrhea and many of the same clinical characteristics seen in patients with CCD.[154,155] Currently, only six cases of CSD have been described in the literature, and the molecular basis of this condition has not been fully established.[156] Nevertheless, the available information suggests that the disorder results from impaired function of the intestinal Na^+-H^+ exchanger (Figure 12). The gastrointestinal tract expresses primarily three Na^+-H^+ exchangers: NHE-2, -3, and -4.[157] NHE-4 is expressed largely by gastric mucosa, whereas both NHE-2 and -3 are present in the small intestine.

Genetics and Molecular Pathophysiology. A kindred with five CSD-affected children from a remote rural community in Austria was enabled to investigate the potential involvement of known candidate genes encoding for sodium/proton exchangers.[156] These children belonged to two families linked by inbreeding, strongly suggesting that CSD is transmitted as an autosomal recessive disease. Using homozygosity mapping and multipoint linkage analysis, they excluded the known sodium/proton exchangers as being causative for CSD in this large pedigree.

Vesicle transport studies performed on brush border membrane samples confirmed that CSD is the result of a faulty Na^+-H^+ exchanger.[154] The NHE-3 exchanger is considered to be the primary transporter responsible for Na^+ absorption because deletion of the *Nhe-3* gene in mice results in sodium secretory that resembles CSD.[158,159] These mice also had a mild proximal tubular acidosis that was secondary to the role of NHE-3 in renal Na^+ and HCO_3^- reabsorption. Although mild diarrhea was reported in these mice, the primary finding in the gut was an excess amount of luminal fluids and an expanded surface area.

Clinical Manifestations. Patients with CSD have high-volume secretory diarrhea that is very alkaline and contains high concentrations of Na^+ (Figure 2). Therefore, patients generally have hyponatremia, low or normal excretion of urinary Na^+, and metabolic acidosis. Polyhydramnios resulting from in utero diarrhea is also associated with CSD, and a recent report described choanal atresia in two patients with CSD.[156] Although the

intestinal biopsies of patients with selective impairment of transport function are generally considered to be normal, biopsies from three recently described cases that fit the clinical characteristics of CSD showed partial villous atrophy and a decreased villus-to-crypt ratio, suggesting the possibility of a distinct disorder.[156] Electromicroscopy demonstrated unexpected membranous whorls located in lysosomal bodies, vacuoles, and mitochondria.

Diagnostic Criteria, Laboratory Investigations, and Treatment. The diagnosis of CSD should be considered in patients who present as newborns with high-output secretory diarrhea and can be established by confirming the presence of elevated levels of fecal Na^+ and HCO_3^-. Unlike patients with CCD who have metabolic alkalosis, metabolic acidosis is typically found in CSD and in all other forms of congenital diarrhea. The medical management of CSD patients is to maintain their fluid and electrolyte balance with the use of oral fluids and salts. These patients will experience life-long large-volume diarrhea; therapeutic options to minimize the severity of the diarrhea have not been proposed.

Acrodermatitis Enteropathica

Primary acrodermatitis enteropathica (AE; MIM #201100) is a rare autosomal recessive disorder of impaired intestinal absorption of zinc (Figure 12).[160,161] Even though secondary deficiencies in trace elements such as zinc and selenium are a frequent complication of chronic diarrhea, patients with AE present in early infancy with profound depletion of total body zinc.

Genetics and Molecular Pathophysiology. Genome-wide screening for the AE allele was performed on two large consanguineous families, which led to the identification of a candidate gene that encodes for a member of the zinc- and iron-regulated transporter family of proteins (ZIP4; Figure 12).[162,163] Sequencing of the *ZIP4* gene identified five missense mutations that altered highly conserved and critical amino acid residues in the family of zinc transporters in patients with AE. ZIP4 is expressed on the apical membrane of epithelia in the intestine, colon, stomach, and kidney, and is a member of a recently described family of proteins that directs the transport of zinc into the cytoplasm of various cells.[164] During periods of zinc deficiency, ZIP4 content of the brush border increases as expression is increased, and the protein is recruited to the apical membrane.[165] Although patients with AE have a markedly reduced capacity to absorb luminal zinc, their responsiveness to high-dose oral zinc supplements raises the possibility that they retain a redundant, but less efficient zinc transport mechanism in the intestine (Figure 12).

Clinical Manifestations. Zinc deficiency may develop either because of a principal defect in absorption or secondary to either inadequate intake or excessive losses.[160] Zinc deficiency that is due to excessive fecal losses is a common finding in patients with acute and chronic

diarrhea, and short-term oral supplement of zinc has been shown to reduce the duration and severity of diarrhea.[166] Severe zinc deficiency can present with anorexia, diarrhea, and severe failure to thrive.[160] The dermatitis located on the hands, feet, and perirectal and oral regions has a vesicobullous character, and the alopecia of the scalp and face is also a striking feature that occurs in patients with prolonged zinc deficiency. Humoral and cell-mediated immunodeficiencies have been reported in association with AE and may contribute to both poor wound healing and recurrent infections. Poorly characterized neurologic features such as mental lethargy and neurosensory abnormalities may also be present.

Diagnostic Criteria, Laboratory Investigations, and Medical Management. Zinc deficiency results in low levels of serum alkaline phosphatase, a zinc-dependent metalloenzyme. Alkaline phosphatase levels decline with age, and lower than expected levels should raise the possibility of zinc deficiency. Both serum and urinary zinc concentrations are significantly reduced in untreated patients with AE. Radiolabeled zinc has been used to assess the absorptive capacity of the intestine using both mucosal biopsy samples and in vivo uptake studies.[160] Histology of the small intestine has shown several abnormalities that may represent the consequence of inadequate zinc concentrations in patients with AE. Paneth cells and enterocytes of the small bowel have been shown to have inclusion bodies and abnormal intracellular organelles; villus atrophy has also been reported.[160] Patients with AE can be managed with large oral doses, ~1 mg elemental zinc/kg/d, of zinc supplements. Chronic supplementations with adequate doses of zinc will resolve the clinical and laboratory features of this disorder.

Calcium Absorption

Calcium absorption in the small intestine occurs by both active and passive transport mechanisms.[167] Passive absorption of dietary calcium takes place paracellularly along the entire length of the small bowel, and this pathway is predominant when the calcium supply is abundant. In contrast, the active calcium transport system is located primarily in the duodenum and is particularly important when the level of dietary calcium is low. The active transcellular transport system was recently identified as a member of the transient receptor potential cation channel 6, or TRPV6, and is expressed primarily on the brush border membrane of enterocytes located in the proximal small bowel (Figure 12).[168,169] Once within the cytoplasm, calcium forms a complex with a calcium-binding protein called calbindinD9k, or CaBP, and calcium efflux out of the enterocyte takes place by either the CaATPase (PMCA1b) or by the Na^+-Ca^{2+} exchanger NCX1 (Figure 12). Vitamin D (1,25-dihydroxyvitamin D3) directly influences the expression of both TRPV6 and CaBP by directly activating vitamin D-responsive elements in the immediate promoter region of both genes and increasing transcription.[168] Congenital disorders that impair calcium absorption include pseudo-vitamin D deficiency rickets (MIM #264700), which is secondary to a defective synthesis of 25-hydroxyvitamin D3 1α-hydroxylase.[170] Specific inherited defects in the transporters that control dietary calcium absorption have yet to be described.[171]

Disorders of Magnesium Transport

Magnesium absorption in the gut occurs primarily in the small intestine by two different pathways: a nonsaturable paracellular passive and saturable active transcellular transport processes. Primary hypomagnesemia with hypercalciuria and nephrocalcinosis (FHHNC, MIM #248250) is a rare autosomal recessive disorder that presents clinically with neonatal seizures and tetany, and is associated with impaired absorption of dietary magnesium and a renal tubular defect of magnesium transport (Figure 12).[172]

Hypocalcemia secondary to low parathyroid hormone and 1,25-dihydroxyvitamin D_3 levels is common and may result in tetany. The molecular basis of primary hypomagnesemia was elucidated several years ago when linkage analysis led to the identification of a tight junction protein named paracellin 1 (PCLN1).[173] Mutations in the gene encoding the PCLN protein (also called claudin 16) were identified in 10 kindreds, and the protein was located in the tight junction region of the thick ascending limb of Henle. Whether paracellin is expressed by small intestinal epithelium has not been reported, yet it accounts for the nonsaturable paracellular magnesium transport system that is particularly active at high intraluminal concentrations. Although paracellin may serve as a selective paracellular transporter of magnesium, it may also represent a sensor of magnesium concentration.

Active transcellular transport of magnesium occurs via a transient receptor potential (TRP) family of cation channels named TRPM6. Various missense and nonsense mutations of the *TRPM6* gene have been identified in patients with hypomagnesemia with secondary hypocalcemia (HSH, MIM #602014).[174,175] TRPM6 is located along the entire gut and in the distal tubule cells of the kidney, where immunofluorescence studies have localized it to the apical membrane.[176] The life-long oral administration of high-dose magnesium supplementation can be used to sustain near normal serum magnesium and calcium levels in this group of patients.

Disorders of Copper Transport

Copper is an important cofactor required for the synthesis and function of many proteins whose roles vary from antioxidants to enzymes required for mitochondrial function. The diet is a significant source of copper, and our understanding of the complex process of copper absorption, intracellular processing, and efflux has improved by investigating the basis of two disorders of copper transport, Menkes syndrome and Wilson disease.[177,178] Menkes syndrome (MIM #309400) is a rare (1 in 100,000) X-linked recessive disorder of copper deficiency resulting from defective synthesis of the Menkes syndrome transport protein (MNK) (Figure 12).[179] In contrast, Wilson disease (WD; MIM #277900) is a more common autosomal recessive disorder that is the consequence of copper accumulation secondary to malfunctioning of the WD transporter.[180] Both transporters have been localized to the membranes of the *trans*-Golgi network (TGN), where they modulate copper transport into the network. When intracellular copper levels increase, both transporters redistribute to small vesicles and the plasma membrane, where they presumably control the efflux of copper out of the cell. MNK is expressed primarily by enterocytes and cells of the placenta and central nervous system, whereas expression of the WD transporter is limited mainly to hepatocytes. Given their tissue-specific pattern of expression, defects in the function of MNK result in inadequate efflux of copper from the gut, whereas an alteration of WD results in failure to excrete copper to bile, which subsequently accumulates in the liver.[177]

The mechanism of dietary copper absorption has not been definitively established; however, two active transporters located on the apical membrane of the enterocyte have been implicated (Figure 12). The H^+-divalent metal transporter (DMT1) has a broad range of substrates, including copper, iron, manganese, and cobalt.[181] A more specific family of high-affinity copper transporters, Ctr1 and -2, has been isolated and is expressed in a broad variety of tissue, including the intestine.[182] Within the intracellular compartment of the enterocyte, copper may be either incorporated into copper-containing proteins or traffic into the TGN by way of the MNK transporter.[177,178] Copper binds ceruloplasmin within the TGN and subsequently enters the systemic circulation bound primarily to ceruloplasmin. Although copper levels do not influence the production of ceruloplasmin, it has a shorter half-life during copper-deficient states, resulting in low ceruloplasmin levels. Because defects of both MNK and WD lead to impaired trafficking of copper across the TGN membrane, Menkes syndrome and WD are both associated with hypoceruloplasminemia.

Genotype–phenotype relationships have been established in Menkes syndrome, and the clinical consequences of mutations in MNK are primarily the result of a copper-deficient state that leads to improper synthesis of copper-containing proteins. Patients generally present during early infancy with failure to thrive, various neurologic symptoms, hyperpigmentation, and morphologic changes of the hair. Most children with Menkes syndrome die during early infancy, and while copper supplementation has not been shown to be efficacious, anecdotal reports suggest that copper-histidine may delay the onset of various symptoms.[183] In contrast, WD generally presents during early adolescence with either neurologic or hepatic consequences of copper overload.

Chelation therapy with D-penicillamine or ammonium tetrathiomolybdate augments renal excretion of copper while improving its positive balance in the liver and brain.[184] Oral administration of zinc has been shown to inhibit dietary intake of copper, presumably by competing for transport into the enterocyte via the DMT (Figure 12).[181,184]

Disorders of Iron Transport

Our understanding of mechanism of iron absorption has improved significantly over the last decade with the discovery of the molecular basis of hereditary hemochromatosis (HH; MIM #235200).[185–186] HH is an autosomal recessive disorder characterized by excessive intestinal iron absorption and secondary multiorgan failure related to excessive tissue iron content. Hemochromatosis is the most common genetic disorder among individuals of European ancestry, with an estimated carrier frequency of about one in eight.[185,187] The most common form of HH is secondary to mutations in the gene that encodes a major histocompatibility class I–like protein, *HFE*. Several mutations, including Cys282Tyr, His63Asn, and Ser65Cys, account for the majority of abnormal alleles in the *HFE* gene.[185,186]

The role of HFE in iron absorption was elucidated when HFE was found to interact with the transferrin receptor (TfR) with an affinity that was comparable to the diferric transferrins' interaction with the receptor (Figure 12). Immunohistochemical analysis also confirmed that HFE and TfR were localized to both the basolateral membrane and the intracellular compartment of crypt cells of the intestine. It is believed that HFE facilitates the interaction of diferric transferrin and TfR, resulting in endocytosis in clathrin-coated vesicles and the eventual release of iron into the cell cytoplasm.

The primary apical iron transporter, DMT1, was isolated by expression cloning and also transports copper, another divalent cation (Figure 12).[181] Since the absorption of dietary iron is limited to the reduced ferric (Fe^{2+}) form, the reduction of the oxidized form (Fe^{3+}) by the brush border enzyme duodenal cytochrome b (CYBRD1) prepares it for transport. Within the enterocyte, iron can be stored in ferritin or effluxed across the basolateral membrane by the transporter, Ferroportin 1 (IREG1).[188] At the basolateral membrane, hephaestin facilitates the export of iron with its ferroxidase activity. Both apical and basolateral iron transporters are expressed primarily in duodenal enterocytes located along the upper portion of the villus, and their expression is dramatically upregulated in iron-deficient states.

The common HFE mutations appear to inhibit its interaction with its heterodimeric partner, $β_2$-microglobulin, and diminish the level of HFE on the basolateral membrane. Because the endocytosis of the transferrin-TfR-Fe^{2+} complex requires adequate levels of HFE, mutations of the HFE protein would reduce cytoplasmic iron levels while augmenting the expression of DMT1 and FPN1 and increasing iron intake.[189,190] In contrast, in iron-abundant states associated with wild-type HFE, the endocytosis of the Fe^{2+}-containing complex would increase the cellular stores of iron and thereby reduce the synthesis of DMT1 and FPN1.

Deficiencies of proteins other than HFE have recently been implicated in the pathogenesis of other forms of hemochromatosis. Mutations in the gene encoding Ferroportin 1 have been identified in an autosomal dominant form of hemochromatosis (MIM #606069).[191] Hepcidin, Tfr2, and Hemojuvelin are three proteins expressed by hepatocytes that regulate the intestinal absorption of iron.[192] Defects in TfR2 have also been identified in several kindreds (MIM #604250), whereas a juvenile form of hemochromatosis (MIM #602390) has been associated with mutations of either hepcidin, an antimicrobial peptide synthesized by hepatocytes that appears to negatively modulate intestinal absorption of iron, or Hemojuvelin.[193–196] Hepcidin responds to iron body stores and inflammation and regulates iron efflux by binding to the iron exporter, Ferroportin.[197] Moreover, hepcidin production is increased by IL-6 and appears to explain the anemia of chronic inflammation.[198]

Recent studies have elucidated the mechanism by which heme-containing iron is transported in the intestine. Heme carrier protein 1 (HCP1) is located on the apical membrane of enterocytes of the duodenum and transports the heme iron complex intact.[199] Once within the enterocyte the complex dissociates, probably by heme oxygenase, releasing iron which is transferred to the circulation by the basolateral transporter Ferroportin. While the abundance of HCP1 was not altered by the iron status of the host, its expression was dramatically upregulated by hypoxia. Interestingly, in iron-depleted states, HCP1 occupies the apical brush border membrane, while in iron-plentiful conditions move to internal cellular compartments and thereby interrupts luminal absorption.[199]

DISORDERS OF VITAMIN ABSORPTION

Folate Malabsorption

Dietary folate is found primarily in green leafy vegetables, organ meats, and grains as polyglutamylated folates. Glutamate carboxypeptidase II (GCP-II), expressed on the brush border membrane of small bowel enterocytes, hydrolyzes folylpolyglutamates to a form (monoglutamyl folates) that can be transported by the reduced folate transporter 1 (RFC-1) (Figure 13). Once within the enterocyte, folylmonoglutamate is converted to 5-methyltetrahydrofolate (5-MTHF), which exits the basolateral membrane via the RFC-1 transporter. The folate-binding protein mediates the transport of 5-MTHF in hepatocytes, where it is stored in the form of polyglutamylated folates, an essential cofactor for nucleic and amino acid synthesis.

Folate deficiency generally results in hyperhomocysteinemia because 5-MTHF is required to synthesize methionine from homocysteine. A sufficient level of methionine is required for the synthesis of S-adenosylmethionine, an enzyme critical for DNA methylation. Congenital folate malabsorption (MIM #229050) is a rare autosomal recessive disorder associated with the clinical symptoms of diarrhea, glossitis, and seizures in the face of pancytopenia.[200] The underlying mechanism of the congenital form of folate deficiency has not been identified. Folic acid deficiency has been definitively associated with neural tube defects in neonates and an increased risk of cardiovascular disease in adults with elevated levels of homocysteine.[201] Serum folate and homocysteine levels are readily available assays that may be used to assess adequate folate stores.

Vitamin B12 Malabsorption

The absorption of vitamin B_{12} (cobalamin) is a complex process that is initiated by gastric acidity which removes cobalamin from dietary proteins and transfers it to a binding protein called haptocorrin.[7] Intrinsic factor (IF), produced by parietal cells, binds cobalamin after pancreatic proteases hydrolyze the cobalamin-haptocorrin complex in the duodenum. The enterocytes of the ileum express cubilin, which forms a heterodimer with amnionless, forming a receptor for the cobalamin-IF complex (Figure 13).[202] Amnionless role is to direct the receptor–vitamin complex to the endosomes, where it encounters a second receptor, megalin.[203] The cobalamin-IF complex is cleaved within the endosome, resulting in the formation of a cobalamin-transcobalamin-2 complex, which transverses the enterocyte and enters the systemic circulation.

The clinical consequences of vitamin B12 and folate deficiency overlap because cobalamin is a cofactor for methionine synthase, which uses a methyl group from 5-MTHF to convert homocysteine to methionine.[204] Hyperhomocysteinemia is thus the consequence of both vitamin B12 and folate deficiency. Defects of cobalamin absorption are, however, uniquely associated with methylmalonicacidemia because adenosylcobalamin is required for appropriate mitochondrial fatty acid metabolism.[205]

Because of the complexity of vitamin B12 assimilation, deficiency may be secondary to numerous problems, ranging from inadequate intake to disruption of any of the various steps required for absorption.[204] Primary or secondary achlorhydria is commonly associated with cobalamin deficiency because gastric acidity is required for the formation of the cobalamin-haptocorrin complex. Bacterial overgrowth in the small intestine may also disrupt the cobalamin-IF complex and lead to a decline in cobalamin levels. Because cobalamin is absorbed exclusively in the ileum, disorders resulting in an inadequate ileal absorptive capacity will also result in vitamin B12 deficiency.

There are three rare yet well-described autosomal recessive disorders linked with congenital forms of cobalamin deficiency. Congenital pernicious anemia (MIM #261000) is associated with an absence of IF, which facilitates the binding of cobalamin to the cubilin-amnionless receptor.[206] Imerslund-Grasbeck syndrome (MIM #261100) was originally described in both Finland and Norway, and linkage analysis of the Finnish patients identified mutations in the cubilin receptor[207]; whereas the Norwegian cases were recently identified to be secondary to mutations in the amnionless gene.[202,208] Finally, congenital defects of transcobalamin 2 (MIM #275350) have also been shown to result in inadequate levels of vitamin B12 and in both bone marrow failure and a range of neurologic deficits.[209] Measurement of serum vitamin B12 levels and evidence of homocysteine and methylmalonic acid may be used to assess vitamin B12 stores. The Schilling test is particularly useful in assessing the various origins of cobalamin deficiency.[205]

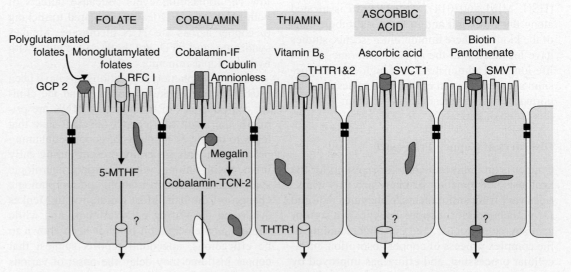

Figure 13 Water-soluble vitamin absorption in the small intestine. GCP = glutamate carboxypeptidase; MTHF = methyltetrahydrofolate; RFC = reduced folate transporter; SMVT = sodium multivitamin transporter; SVCT = sodium vitamin cotransporter; TCN = transcobalamin; THTR = thiamine transporter protein.

Absorption of Various Water-Soluble Vitamins

The molecular basis of several water-soluble vitamins has recently been elucidated. Vitamin C, or L-ascorbic acid, has been found to be transported across the intestinal epithelial layer by the Na^+-dependent vitamin C transporter, SVCT1 (Figure 13).[210,211] Ascorbic acid transport via SVCT1 appears to be critical during the perinatal period because null SVCT1 null mice succumb immediately after birth.[212] While dietary deficiency of ascorbic acid is common, inherited forms of a congenital deficiency have not been reported. Although the pyridoxine (vitamin B6) transporter has not been identified, recent reports have begun to determine various characteristics of this pH-dependent carrier-mediated system.[213]

The Na^+-dependent multivitamin transporter (SMVT) was also identified to transport pantothenate (vitamin B5) and lipoate at high affinity (Figure 13).[214] An abnormality of biotin transport was recently described in an encephalopathic child; however, the molecular mechanism has not been described.[215] Thiamin (vitamin B1) absorption across the intestinal brush border membrane is facilitated by two thiamin transporter proteins-1 and -2 (THTR-1 and THTR-2). Both transporters are abundantly expressed in enterocytes, and while THTR-1 has been localized to both the apical and basolateral membrane, THTR-2 is limited to the apical surface. The thiamin transporters resemble the structure of the folate transporter RFC-1, and mutations of THTR-1 have been associated with a thiamin-responsive megaloblastic anemia syndrome (MIM #249270).[216,217] This is a rare autosomal recessive disorder that is associated with megaloblastic anemia, diabetes mellitus, and deafness.

Absorption of Various Fat-Soluble Vitamins

The most common cause of a generalized deficiency of fat-soluble vitamins includes specific dietary restrictions and a wide assortment of gastrointestinal disorders that impair fat absorption. All fat-soluble vitamins are absorbed by enterocytes primarily by passive diffusion, a process that is facilitated by the emulsification of fats by bile salts. Selective deficiencies are certainly more unusual and may suggest a defect in the interaction of the vitamin with a specific transfer protein. For instance, vitamin A (retinol) is packaged in chylomicrons in the enterocyte and is eventually taken up by hepatocytes, where it is either stored or remains bound to retinol-binding protein for transfer to other cells. A rare inherited disorder of retinol-binding protein deficiency (MIM #180250) has been described and leads to an assortment of ophthalmologic findings and a low serum level of vitamin A.[218] A selective vitamin E deficiency (MIM #277460) has also been identified that is secondary to mutations in the α-tocopherol transfer protein and results in a form of spinocerebellar ataxia and undetectable serum vitamin E levels.[219]

REFERENCES

1. Fine KD, Schiller LR. AGA technical review on the evaluation and management of chronic diarrhea. Gastroenterology 1999;116:1464–86.
2. Eherer AJ, Fordtran JS. Fecal osmotic gap and pH in experimental diarrhea of various causes. Gastroenterology 1992;103:545–51.
3. Duncan A, Robertson C, Russell RI. The fecal osmotic gap: Technical aspects regarding its calculation. J Lab Clin Med 1992;119:359–63.
4. Lam MM, O'Connor TP, Diamond J. Loads, capacities and safety factors of maltase and the glucose transporter SGLT1 in mouse intestinal brush border. J Physiol 2002;542:493–500.
5. Bennett CL, Ochs HD. IPEX is a unique X-linked syndrome characterized by immune dysfunction, polyendocrinopathy, enteropathy, and a variety of autoimmune phenomena. Curr Opin Pediatr 2001;13:533–8.
6. Cutz E, Rhoads JM, Drumm B, et al. Microvillus inclusion disease: An inherited defect of brush-border assembly and differentiation. N Engl J Med 1989;320:646–51.
7. Udall JN, Jr Secretory diarrhea in children—Newly recognized toxins and hormone-secreting tumors. Pediatr Clin North Am 1996;43:333–53.
8. Modlin IM, Kidd M, Latich I, et al. Current status of gastrointestinal carcinoids. Gastroenterology 2005;128:1717–51.
9. Freel RW, Goldner AM. Sodium-coupled nonelectrolyte transport across epithelia: Emerging concepts and directions. Am J Physiol 1981;241:G451–60.
10. Savilahti E, Launiala K, Kuitunen P. Congenital lactase deficiency. A clinical study on 16 patients. Arch Dis Child 1983;58:246–52.
11. Enattah NS, Sahi T, Savilahti E, et al. Identification of a variant associated with adult-type hypolactasia. Nat Genet 2002;30:233–7.
12. Ouwendijk J, Moolenaar CE, Peters WJ, et al. Congenital sucrase-isomaltase deficiency. Identification of a glutamine to proline substitution that leads to a transport block of sucrase-isomaltase in a pre-Golgi compartment. J Clin Invest 1996;97:633–41.
13. Lebenthal E, Khin-Maung-U, Zheng B-Y, et al. Small intestinal glucoamylase deficiency and starch malabsorption: A newly recognized alpha-glucosidase deficiency in children. J Pediatr 1994;124:541–6.
14. Etemad B, Whitcomb DC. Chronic pancreatitis: Diagnosis, classification, and new genetic developments. Gastroenterology 2001;120:682–707.
15. Romagnuolo J, Schiller D, Bailey RJ. Using breath tests wisely in a gastroenterology practice: An evidence-based review of indications and pitfalls in interpretation. Am J Gastroenterol 2002;97:1113–26.
16. Kunzelmann K, Mall M. Electrolyte transport in the mammalian colon: Mechanisms and implications for disease. Physiol Rev 2002;82:245–89.
17. Lindquist B, Meeuwisse GW. Chronic diarrhoea caused by monosaccharide malabsorption. Acta Paediatr 1962;51:674–85.
18. Schneider AJ, Kinter WB, Stirling CE. Glucose-galactose malabsorption. Report of a case with autoradiographic studies of a mucosal biopsy. N Engl J Med 1966;274:305–12.
19. Meeuwisse GW, Dahlqvist A. Glucose-galactose malabsorption. A study with biopsy of the small intestinal mucosa. Acta Paediatr Scand 1968;57:273–80.
20. Stirling CE, Schneider AJ, Wong M-D, Kinter WB. Quantitative radioautography of sugar transport in intestinal biopsies from normal humans and a patient with glucose-galactose malabsorption. J Clin Invest 1972;51:438–51.
21. Hediger MA, Coady MJ, Ikeda TS, Wright EM. Expression cloning and cDNA sequencing of the Na+/glucose cotransporter. Nature 1987;330:379–81.
22. Martin MG, Turk E, Lostao MP, et al. Defects in Na+ glucose cotransporter (SGLT1) trafficking and function cause glucose-galactose malabsorption. Nature Genet 1996;12:216–20.
23. Martin MG, Lostao MP, Turk E, et al. Compound missense mutations in the sodium/D-glucose cotransporter result in trafficking defects. Gastroenterology 1997;112:1206–12.
24. Lam JT, Martin MG, Turk E, et al. Missense mutations in SGLT1 cause glucose-galactose malabsorption by trafficking defects. Biochim Biophy Acta—Molecular Basis of Disease 1999;1453:297–303.
25. Turk E, Zabel B, Mundlos S, et al. Glucose/galactose malabsorption caused by a defect in the Na+/glucose cotransporter. Nature 1991;350:354–6.
26. Stumpel F, Burcelin R, Jungermann K, Thorens B. Normal kinetics of intestinal glucose absorption in the absence of GLUT2: Evidence for a transport pathway requiring glucose phosphorylation and transfer into the endoplasmic reticulum. Proc Natl Acad Sci U S A 2001;98:11330–5.
27. Santer R, Groth S, Kinner M, et al. The mutation spectrum of the facilitative glucose transporter gene SLC2A2 (GLUT2) in patients with Fanconi-Bickel syndrome. Hum Genet 2002;110:21–9.
28. Loo DDF, Zeuthen T, Chandy G, Wright EM. Cotransport of water by the Na+/glucose cotransporter. PNAS 1996;93:13367–70.
29. Loo DD, Wright EM, Zeuthen T. Water pumps. J Physiol 2002;542:53–60.
30. Wright EM, Hirayama BA, Loo DF. Active sugar transport in health and disease. J Intern Med 2007;261:32–43.
31. Hughes WS, Senior JR. The glucose-galactose malabsorption syndrome in a 23-year-old woman. Gastroenterology 1975;68:142–5.
32. Wang J, Cortina G, Wu SV, et al. Mutant neurogenin-3 in congenital malabsorptive diarrhea. N Engl J Med 2006;355:270–80.
33. Cortina G, Smart CN, Farmer DG, et al. Enteroendocrine cell dysgenesis and malabsorption, a histopathologic and immunohistochemical characterization. Hum Pathol 2007;38:570–80.
34. Montes RG, Gottal RF, Bayless TM, et al. Breath hydrogen testing as a physiology laboratory exercise for medical students. Am J Physiol 1992;262:S25–8.
35. Barnes G, McKellar W, Lawrance S. Detection of fructose malabsorption by breath hydrogen test in a child with diarrhea. J Pediatr 1983;103:575–7.
36. Martin MG, Turk E, Kerner C, et al. Prenatal identification of a heterozygous status in two fetuses at risk for glucose-galactose malabsorption. Prenat Diagn 1996;16:458–62.
37. Rand EB, Depaoli AM, Davidson NO, et al. Sequence, tissue distribution, and functional characterization of the rat fructose transporter GLUT5. Am J Physiol Gastrointest Liver Physiol 1993;264:G1169–76.
38. Li Q, Manolescu A, Ritzel M, et al. Cloning and functional characterization of the human GLUT7 isoform SLC2A7 from the small intestine. Am J Physiol Gastrointest Liver Physiol 2004;287:G236–42.
39. Kellett GL, Brot-Laroche E. Apical GLUT2: A major pathway of intestinal sugar absorption. Diabetes 2005;54:3056–62.
40. Wasserman D, Hoekstra JH, Tolia V, et al. Molecular analysis of the fructose transporter gene (GLUT5) in isolated fructose malabsorption. J Clin Invest 1996;98:2398–402.
41. Beaudet AL, Tsui L-C. A suggested nomenclature for designating mutations. Hum Mutat 1993; 2:245–8.
42. Ferraris RP. Dietary and developmental regulation of intestinal sugar transport. Biochem J 2001;360:265–76.
43. Cui XL, Soteropoulos P, Tolias P, Ferraris RP. Fructose-responsive genes in the small intestine of neonatal rats. Physiol Genomics 2004;18:206–17.
44. Nobigrot T, Chasalow FI, Lifshitz F. Carbohydrate absorption from one serving of fruit juice in young children: Age and carbohydrate composition effects. J Am Coll Nutr 1997;16:152–8.
45. Hoekstra JH. Fructose breath hydrogen tests in infants with chronic non-specific diarrhoea. Eur J Pediatr 1995;154:362–4.
46. Fernandez-Banares F, Esteve-Pardo M, De Leon R, et al. Sugar malabsorption in functional bowel disease: Clinical implications. Am J Gastroenterol 1993;88:2044–50.
47. Duro D, Rising R, Cedillo M, Lifshitz F. Association between infantile colic and carbohydrate malabsorption from fruit juices in infancy. Pediatrics 2002;109:797–805.
48. Kellett GL. The facilitated component of intestinal glucose absorption. J Physiol 2001;531:585–95.
49. Santer R, Steinmann B, Schaub J. Fanconi-Bickel syndrome—a congenital defect of facilitative glucose transport. Curr Mol Med 2002;2:213–27.
50. Santer R, Schneppenheim R, Suter D, et al. Fanconi-Bickel syndrome—the original patient and his natural history, historical steps leading to the primary defect, and a review of the literature. Eur J Pediatr 1998;157:783–97.
51. Santer R, Hillebrand G, Steinmann B, Schaub J. Intestinal glucose transport: Evidence for a membrane traffic-based pathway in humans. Gastroenterology 2003;124:34–9.
52. Lee PJ, Van't Hoff WG, Leonard JV. Catch-up growth in Fanconi-Bickel syndrome with uncooked cornstarch. J Inherit Metab Dis 1995;18:153–6.
53. Chillaron J, Roca R, Valencia A, et al. Heteromeric amino acid transporters: Biochemistry, genetics, and physiology. Am J Physiol Renal Physiol 2001;281:F995–1018.
54. Palacin M, Estevez R, Bertran J, Zorzano A. Molecular biology of mammalian plasma membrane amino acid transporters. Physiol Rev 1998;78:969–1054.
55. Stevens BR, Ross HJ, Wright EM. Multiple transport pathways for neutral amino acids in rabbit jejunal brush border vesicles. J Membr Biol 1982;66:213–25.
56. Holzinger A, Maier EM, Buck C, et al. Mutations in the proenteropeptidase gene are the molecular cause of congenital enteropeptidase deficiency. Am J Hum Genet 2002;70:20–5.

57. Townes PL. Trypsinogen deficiency disease. J Pediatr 1965;66:275–85.
58. Whitcomb DC, Gorry MC, Preston RA, et al. Hereditary pancreatitis is caused by a mutation in the cationic trypsinogen gene. Nature Genet 1996;14:141–5.
59. Broer A, Klingel K, Kowalczuk S, et al. Molecular cloning of mouse amino acid transport system B0, a neutral amino acid transporter related to Hartnup disorder. J Biol Chem 2004;279:24467–76.
60. Takanaga H, Mackenzie B, Suzuki Y, Hediger MA. Identification of mammalian proline transporter SIT1 (SLC6A20) with characteristics of classical system imino. J Biol Chem 2005;280:8974–84.
61. Calonge MJ, Gasparini P, Chillarón J, et al. Cystinuria caused by mutations in *rBAT*, a gene involved in the transport of cystine. Nature Genet 1994;6:420–5.
62. Fei Y-J, Kanai Y, Nussberger S, et al. Expression cloning of a mammalian proton-coupled oligopeptide transporter. Nature 1994;368:563–6.
63. Anderson CM, Grenade DS, Boll M, et al. H+/amino acid transporter 1 (PAT1) is the imino acid carrier: An intestinal nutrient/drug transporter in human and rat. Gastroenterology 2004;127:1410–22.
64. Boll M, Daniel H, Gasnier B. The SLC36 family: Proton-coupled transporters for the absorption of selected amino acids from extracellular and intracellular proteolysis. Pflugers Arch 2004;447:776–9.
65. Borsani G, Bassi MT, Sperandeo MP, et al. *SLC7A7*, encoding a putative permease-related protein, is mutated in patients with lysinuric protein intolerance. Nature Genet 1999;21:297–301.
66. Torrents D, Mykkänen J, Pineda M, et al. Identification of *SLC7A7*, encoding y^+LAT-1, as the lysinuric protein intolerance gene. Nature Genet 1999;21:293–6.
67. Rajantie J, Simell O, Perheentupa J. Lysinuric protein intolerance. Basolateral transport defect in renal tubuli. J Clin Invest 1981;67:1078–82.
68. Sperandeo MP, Bassi MT, Riboni M, et al. Structure of the SLC7A7 gene and mutational analysis of patients affected by lysinuric protein intolerance. Am J Hum Genet 2000;66:92–9.
69. Palacin M, Borsani G, Sebastio G. The molecular bases of cystinuria and lysinuric protein intolerance. Curr Opin Genet Dev 2001;11:328–35.
70. Rajantie J, Simell O, Perheentupa J. Oral administration of urea cycle intermediates in lysinuric protein intolerance: Effect on plasma and urinary arginine and ornithine. Metabolism 1983;32:49–51.
71. Parto K, Penttinen R, Paronen I, et al. Osteoporosis in lysinuric protein intolerance. J Inherit Metab Dis 1993;16:441–50.
72. Kerem E, Elpelg ON, Shalev RS, et al. Lysinuric protein intolerance with chronic interstitial lung disease and pulmonary cholesterol granulomas at onset. J Pediatr 1993;123:275–8.
73. Korman SH, Raas-Rothschild A, Elpeleg O, Gutman A. Hypocarnitinemia in lysinuric protein intolerance. Mol Genet Metab 2002;76:81–3.
74. Scriver CR, Mahon B, Levy HL, et al. Hyperdibasicaminoaciduria: An inherited disorder of amino acid transport. Pediatr Res 1968;2:525–34.
75. Goodman SI, McIntyre CA, Jr, O'Brien D. Impaired intestinal transport of proline in a patient with familial iminoaciduria. J Pediatr 1967;71:246–9.
76. Seow HF, Broer S, Broer A, et al. Hartnup disorder is caused by mutations in the gene encoding the neutral amino acid transporter SLC6A19. Nat Genet 2004;36:1003–7.
77. Kleta R, Romeo E, Ristic Z, et al. Mutations in SLC6A19, encoding B0AT1, cause Hartnup disorder. Nat Genet 2004;36:999–1002.
78. Takanaga H, Mackenzie B, Suzuki Y, Hediger MA. Identification of mammalian proline transporter SIT1 (SLC6A20) with characteristics of classical system imino. J Biol Chem 2005;280:8974–84.
79. Lammert F, Wang DQ. New insights into the genetic regulation of intestinal cholesterol absorption. Gastroenterology 2005;129:718–34.
80. McClean P, Weaver LT. Ontogeny of human pancreatic exocrine function. Arch Dis Child 1993;68:62–5.
81. Figarella C, De Caro A, Leupold D, Poley JR. Congenital pancreatic lipase deficiency. J Pediatr 1980;96:412–6.
82. Stahl A, Hirsch DJ, Gimeno RE, et al. Identification of the major intestinal fatty acid transport protein. Mol Cell 1999;4:299–308.
83. Hirsch D, Stahl A, Lodish HF. A family of fatty acid transporters conserved from mycobacterium to man. Proc Natl Acad Sci U S A 1998;95:8625–9.
84. Gimeno RE, Hirsch DJ, Punreddy S, et al. Targeted deletion of fatty acid transport protein-4 results in early embryonic lethality. J Biol Chem 2003;278:49512–6.
85. Herrmann T, van der HF, Grone HJ, et al. Mice with targeted disruption of the fatty acid transport protein 4 (Fatp 4, Slc27a4) gene show features of lethal restrictive dermopathy. J Cell Biol 2003;161:1105–15.
86. Moulson CL, Martin DR, Lugus JJ, et al. Cloning of wrinkle-free, a previously uncharacterized mouse mutation, reveals crucial roles for fatty acid transport protein 4 in skin and hair development. Proc Natl Acad Sci U S A 2003; 100:5274–9.
87. Altmann SW, Davis HR, Jr, Zhu LJ, et al. Niemann-Pick C1 Like 1 protein is critical for intestinal cholesterol absorption. Science 2004;303:1201–4.
88. Davies JP, Scott C, Oishi K, et al. Inactivation of NPC1L1 causes multiple lipid transport defects and protects against diet-induced hypercholesterolemia. J Biol Chem 2005;280:12710–20.
89. Garcia-Calvo M, Lisnock J, Bull HG, et al. The target of ezetimibe is Niemann-Pick C1-Like 1 (NPC1L1). Proc Natl Acad Sci U A 2005;102:8132–7.
90. Davis HR, Jr, Zhu LJ, Hoos LM, et al. Niemann-Pick C1 Like 1 (NPC1L1) is the intestinal phytosterol and cholesterol transporter and a key modulator of whole-body cholesterol homeostasis. J Biol Chem 2004;279:33586–92.
91. Bodzioch M, Orsó E, Klucken T, et al. The gene encoding ATP-binding cassette transporter 1 is mutated in Tangier disease. Nature Genet 1999;22:347–51.
92. Brooks-Wilson A, Marcil M, Clee SM, et al. Mutations in *ABC1* in Tangier disease and familial high-density lipoprotein deficiency. Nature Genet 1999;22:336–45.
93. Berge KE, Tian H, Graf GA, et al. Accumulation of dietary cholesterol in sitosterolemia caused by mutations in adjacent ABC transporters. Science 2000;290:1771–5.
94. Wetterau JR, Aggerbeck LP, Bouma ME, et al. Absence of microsomal triglyceride transfer protein in individuals with abetalipoproteinemia. Science 1992;258:999–1001.
95. Gordon DA, Jamil H. Progress towards understanding the role of microsomal triglyceride transfer protein in apolipoprotein-B lipoprotein assembly. Biochim Biophys Acta 2000;1486:72–83.
96. Ohashi K, Ishibashi S, Osuga J, et al. Novel mutations in the microsomal triglyceride transfer protein gene causing abetalipoproteinemia. J Lipid Res 2000;41:1199–204.
97. Raabe M, Flynn LM, Zlot CH, et al. Knockout of the abetalipoproteinemia gene in mice: Reduced lipoprotein secretion in heterozygotes and embryonic lethality in homozygotes. Proc Natl Acad Sci U S A 1998;95:8686–91.
98. Raabe M, Véniant MM, Sullivan MA, et al. Analysis of the role of microsomal triglyceride transfer protein in the liver of tissue-specific knockout mice. J ClinInvest 1999;103:1287–98.
99. Read J, Anderson TA, Ritchie PJ, et al. A mechanism of membrane neutral lipid acquisition by the microsomal triglyceride transfer protein. J Biol Chem 2000;275: 30372–7.
100. Berriot-Varoqueaux N, Dannoura AH, Moreau A, et al. Apolipoprotein B48 glycosylation in abetalipoproteinemia and Anderson's disease. Gastroenterology 2001;121:1101–8.
101. Steinberg D, Grundy SM, Mok HY, et al. Metabolic studies in an unusual case of asymptomatic familial hypobetalipoproteinemia with hypolphalipoproteinemia and fasting chylomicronemia. J Clin Invest 1979;64:292–301.
102. Schonfeld G. Familial hypobetalipoproteinemia: A review. J Lipid Res 2003;44:878–83.
103. Wolff JA, Bauman WA. Stidies concerning acanthocytosis: A new genetic syndrome with absent beta lipoprotein. Am J Dis Child 1961;102:478–9.
104. Linton MF, Farese RV, Jr, Young SG. Familial hypobetalipoproteinemia. J Lipid Res 1993;34:521–41.
105. Roy CC, Levy E, Green PHR, et al. Malabsorption, hypocholesterolemia, and fat-filled enterocytes with increased intestinal apoprotein B. Chylomicron retention disease. Gastroenterology 1987;92:390–9.
106. Shoulders CC, Stephens DJ, Jones B. The intracellular transport of chylomicrons requires the small GTPase, Sar1b. Curr Opin Lipidol 2004;15:191–7.
107. Jones B, Jones EL, Bonney SA, et al. Mutations in a Sar1 GTPase of COPII vesicles are associated with lipid absorption disorders. Nat Genet 2003;34:29–31.
108. Schekman R, Orci L. Coat proteins and vesicle budding. Science 1996;271:1526–33.
109. Bi X, Corpina RA, Goldberg J. Structure of the Sec23/24-Sar1 pre-budding complex of the COPII vesicle coat. Nature 2002;419:271–7.
110. Hofmann AF, Schteingart CD, Lillienau J. Biological and medical aspects of active ileal transport of bile acids. Ann Med 1991;23:169–75.
111. Oelkers P, Kirby LC, Heubi JE, Dawson PA. Primary bile acid malabsorption caused by mutations in the ileal sodium-dependent bile acid transporter gene (*SLC10A2*). J Clin Invest 1997;99:1880–7.
112. Heubi JE, Balistreri WF, Fondacaro JD, et al. Primary bile acid malabsorption: Defective in vitro ileal active bile acid transport. Gastroenterology 1982;83:804–11.
113. Marcus SN, Schteingart CD, Marquez ML, et al. Active absorption of conjugated bile acids in vivo. Kinetic parameters and molecular specificity of the ileal transport system in the rat. Gastroenterology 1991;100:212–21.
114. Hofmann AF, Poley JR. Role of bile acid malabsorption in pathogenesis of diarrhea and steatorrhea in patients with ileal resection. I. Response to cholestyramine or replacement of dietary long chain triglyceride by medium chain triglyceride. Gastroenterology 1972;62:918–34.
115. Montagnani M, Love MW, Rossel P, et al. Absence of dysfunctional ileal sodium-bile acid cotransporter gene mutations in patients with adult-onset idiopathic bile acid malabsorption. Scand J Gastroenterol 2001;36:1077–80.
116. Wong MH, Oelkers P, Craddock AL, Dawson PA. Expression cloning and characterization of the hamster ileal sodium-dependent bile acid transporter. J Biol Chem 1994;269:1340–7.
117. Wong MH, Oelkers P, Dawson PA. Identification of a mutation in the ileal sodium-dependent bile acid transporter gene that abolishes transport activity. J Bioll Chem 1995;270:27228–34.
118. Dawson PA, Hubbert M, Haywood J, et al. The heteromeric organic solute transporter alpha-beta, Ostalpha-Ostbeta, is an ileal basolateral bile acid transporter. J Biol Chem 2005;280:6960–8.
119. Quinton PM. Cystic fibrosis: A disease in electrolyte transport. FASEB J 1990;4:2709–17.
120. O'Connor TP, Lam MM, Diamond J. Magnitude of functional adaptation after intestinal resection. Am J Physiol Regul Integr Comp Physiol 1999;276:R1265–75.
121. O'Connor TP, Diamond J. Ontogeny of intestinal safety factors: Lactase capacities and lactose loads. Am J Physiol Regul Integr Comp Physiol 1999;276:R753–65.
122. Bjerknes M, Cheng H. Clonal analysis of mouse intestinal epithelial progenitors. Gastroenterology 1999;116:7–14.
123. Bjerknes M, Cheng H. Gastrointestinal stem cells. II. Intestinal stem cells. Am J Physiol Gastrointest Liver Physiol 2005;289:G381–7.
124. Bjerknes M, Cheng H. The stem-cell zone of the small intestinal epithelium. V. Evidence for controls over orientation of boundaries between the stem-cell zone, proliferative zone, and the maturation zone. Am J Anat 1981;160:105–12.
125. Leedham SJ, Brittan M, McDonald SA, Wright NA. Intestinal stem cells. J Cell Mol Med 2005;9:11–24.
126. Lai EC. Notch signaling: Control of cell communication and cell fate. Development 2004;131:965–73.
127. Sternberg PW. Lateral inhibition during vulval induction in *Caenorhabditis elegans*. Nature 1988;335:551–4.
128. Schroder N, Gossler A. Expression of Notch pathway components in fetal and adult mouse small intestine. Gene Expr Patterns 2002;2:247–50.
129. Jensen J, Pedersen EE, Galante P, et al. Control of endodermal endocrine development by Hes-1. Nat Genet 2000;24:36–44.
130. Yang Q, Bermingham NA, Finegold MJ, Zoghbi HY. Requirement of Math1 for secretory cell lineage commitment in the mouse intestine. Science 2001;294:2155–8.
131. Gradwohl G, Dierich A, LeMeur M, Guillemot F. Neurogenin3 is required for the development of the four endocrine cell lineages of the pancreas. Proc Natl Acad Sci U S A 2000;97:1607–11.
132. Lee CS, Perreault N, Brestelli JE, Kaestner KH. Neurogenin 3 is essential for the proper specification of gastric enteroendocrine cells and the maintenance of gastric epithelial cell identity. Genes Dev 2002;16:1488–97.
133. Mellitzer G, Martin M, Sidhoum-Jenny M, et al. Pancreatic islet progenitor cells in neurogenin 3-yellow fluorescent protein knock-add-on mice. Mol Endocrinol 2004; 18:2765–76.
134. Schonhoff SE, Giel-Moloney M, Leiter AB. Neurogenin 3-expressing progenitor cells in the gastrointestinal tract differentiate into both endocrine and non-endocrine cell types. Dev Biol 2004;270:443–54.
135. Watada H. Neurogenin 3 is a key transcription factor for differentiation of the endocrine pancreas. Endocr J 2004;51:255–64.
136. Peyton M, Stellrecht CM, Naya FJ, et al. BETA3, a novel helix-loop-helix protein, can act as a negative regulator of BETA2 and MyoD-responsive genes. Mol Cell Biol 1996;16:626–33.
137. Schonhoff SE, Giel-Moloney M, Leiter AB. Minireview: Development and differentiation of gut endocrine cells. Endocrinology 2004;145:2639–44.
138. Rindi G, Leiter AB, Kopin AS, et al. The "normal" endocrine cell of the gut: Changing concepts and new evidences. Ann N Y Acad Sci 2004;1014:1–12.

139. Jackson RS, Creemers JW, Farooqi IS, et al. Small-intestinal dysfunction accompanies the complex endocrinopathy of human proprotein convertase 1 deficiency. J Clin Invest 2003;112:1550–60.
140. Jackson RS, Creemers JW, Ohagi S, et al. Obesity and impaired prohormone processing associated with mutations in the human prohormone convertase 1 gene. Nat Genet 1997;16:303–6.
141. Hogenauer C, Meyer RL, Netto GJ, et al. Malabsorption due to cholecystokinin deficiency in a patient with autoimmune polyglandular syndrome type I. N Engl J Med 2001;344:270–4.
142. Makela S, Kere J, Holmberg C, Hoglund P. SLC26A3 mutations in congenital chloride diarrhea. Hum Mutat 2002;20:425–38.
143. Hoglund P, Auranen M, Socha J, et al. Genetic background of congenital chloride diarrhea in high-incidence populations: Finland, Poland, and Saudi Arabia and Kuwait. Am J Hum Genet 1998;63:760–8.
144. Hoglund P, Haila S, Socha J, et al. Mutations of the Down-regulated in adenoma (DRA) gene cause congenital chloride diarrhoea. Nat Genet 1996;14:316–9.
145. Moseley RH, Hoglund P, Wu GD, et al. Downregulated in adenoma gene encodes a chloride transporter defective in congenital chloride diarrhea. Am J Physiol 1999;276:G185–92.
146. Kere J, Sistonen P, Holmberg C, de la CA. The gene for congenital chloride diarrhea maps close to but is distinct from the gene for cystic fibrosis transmembrane conductance regulator. Proc Natl Acad Sci U S A 1993;90:10686–9.
147. Bieberdorf FA, Gorden P, Fordtran JS. Pathogenesis of congenital alkalosis with diarrhea. Implications for the physiology of normal ileal electrolyte absorption and secretion. J Clin Invest 1972;51:1958–68.
148. Turnberg LA, Bieberdorf FA, Fordtran JS. Electrolyte transport in the human ileum. Gut 1969;10:1044.
149. Schweinfest CW, Spyropoulos DD, Henderson KW, et al. slc26a3 (dra)-deficient mice display chloride-losing diarrhea, enhanced colonic proliferation, and distinct up-regulation of ion transporters in the colon. J Biol Chem 2006;281:37962–71.
150. Hartikainen-Sorri AL, Tuimala R, Koivisto M. Congenital chloride diarrhea: Possibility for prenatal diagnosis. Acta Paediatr Scand 1980;69:807–8.
151. Hihnala S, Hoglund P, Lammi L, et al. Long-term clinical outcome in patients with congenital chloride diarrhea. J Pediatr Gastroenterol Nutr 2006;42:369–75.
152. Aichbichler BW, Zerr CH, Santa Ana CA, et al. Proton-pump inhibition of gastric chloride secretion in congenital chloridorrhea. N Engl J Med 1997;336:106–9.
153. Canani RB, Terrin G, Cirillo P, et al. Butyrate as an effective treatment of congenital chloride diarrhea. Gastroenterology 2004;127:630–4.
154. Booth IW, Stange G, Murer H, et al. Defective jejunal brush-border Na+/H+ exchange: A cause of congenital secretory diarrhoea. Lancet 1985;1:1066–9.
155. Holmberg C, Perheentupa J. Congenital Na+ diarrhea: A new type of secretory diarrhea. J Pediatr 1985;106:56–61.
156. Muller T, Wijmenga C, Phillips AD, et al. Congenital sodium diarrhea is an autosomal recessive disorder of sodium/proton exchange but unrelated to known candidate genes. Gastroenterology 2000;119:1506–13.
157. Orlowski J, Grinstein S. Diversity of the mammalian sodium/proton exchanger SLC9 gene family. Pflugers Arch 2004;447:549–65.
158. Gawenis LR, Stien X, Shull GE, et al. Intestinal NaCl transport in NHE2 and NHE3 knockout mice. Am J Physiol Gastrointest Liver Physiol 2002;282:G776–84.
159. Woo AL, Gildea LA, Tack LM, et al. In vivo evidence for interferon-gamma-mediated homeostatic mechanisms in small intestine of the NHE3 Na+/H+ exchanger knockout model of congenital diarrhea. J Biol Chem 2002;277:49036–46.
160. van Wouwe JP. Clinical and laboratory diagnosis of acrodermatitis enteropathica. Eur J Pediatr 1989;149:2–8.
161. Aggett PJ. Acrodermatitis enteropathica. J Inherit Metab Dis 1983;6:39–43.
162. Kury S, Kharfi M, Kamoun R, et al. Mutation spectrum of human SLC39A4 in a panel of patients with acrodermatitis enteropathica. Hum Mutat 2003;22:337–8.
163. Kury S, Dreno B, Bezieau S, et al. Identification of SLC39A4, a gene involved in acrodermatitis enteropathica. Nat Genet 2002;31:239–40.
164. Dufner-Beattie J, Wang F, Kuo YM, et al. The acrodermatitis enteropathica gene ZIP4 encodes a tissue-specific, zinc-regulated zinc transporter in mice. J Biol Chem 2003;278:33474–81.
165. Dufner-Beattie J, Wang F, Kuo YM, et al. The acrodermatitis enteropathica gene ZIP4 encodes a tissue-specific, zinc-regulated zinc transporter in mice. J Biol Chem 2003;278:33474–81.
166. Sazawal S, Black RE, Bhan MK, et al. Zinc supplementation in young children with acute diarrhea in India. N Engl J Med 1995;333:839–44.
167. Bronner F. Mechanisms of intestinal calcium absorption. J Cell Biochem 2003;88:387–93.
168. den Dekker E, Hoenderop JG, Nilius B, Bindels RJ. The epithelial calcium channels, TRPV5 & TRPV6: From identification towards regulation. Cell Calcium 2003;33:497–507.
169. Hoenderop JG, Nilius B, Bindels RJ. Calcium absorption across epithelia. Physiol Rev 2005;85:373–422.
170. Kitanaka S, Takeyama K, Murayama A, et al. Inactivating mutations in the 25-hydroxyvitamin D3 1alpha-hydroxylase gene in patients with pseudovitamin D-deficiency rickets. N Engl J Med 1998;338:653–61.
171. Nijenhuis T, Hoenderop JG, Nilius B, Bindels RJ. (Patho)physiological implications of the novel epithelial Ca2+ channels TRPV5 and TRPV6. Pflugers Arch 2003;446:401–9.
172. Stromme JH, Steen-Johnsen J, Harnaes K, et al. Familial hypomagnesemia—a follow-up examination of three patients after 9 to 12 years of treatment. Pediatr Res 1981;15:1134–9.
173. Simon DB, Lu Y, Choate KA, et al. Paracellin-1, a renal tight junction protein required for paracellular Mg2+ resorption. Science 1999;285:103–6.
174. Schlingmann KP, Weber S, Peters M, et al. Hypomagnesemia with secondary hypocalcemia is caused by mutations in TRPM6, a new member of the TRPM gene family. Nat Genet 2002;31:166–70.
175. Schlingmann KP, Konrad M, Seyberth HW. Genetics of hereditary disorders of magnesium homeostasis. Pediatr Nephrol 2004;19:13–25.
176. Voets T, Nilius B, Hoefs S, et al. TRPM6 forms the Mg2+ influx channel involved in intestinal and renal Mg2+ absorption. J Biol Chem 2004;279:19–25.
177. Shim H, Harris ZL. Genetic defects in copper metabolism. J Nutr 2003;133:1527S–31S.
178. Mercer JF, Llanos RM. Molecular and cellular aspects of copper transport in developing mammals. J Nutr 2003;133:1481S–4S.
179. Chelly J, Tümer Z, Tønnesen T, et al. Isolation of a candidate gene for Menkes disease that encodes a potential heavy metal binding protein [see comments]. Nat Genet 1993;3:14–9.
180. Bull PC, Thomas GR, Rommens JM, et al. The Wilson disease gene is a putative copper transporting P-type ATPase similar to the Menkes gene. Nature Genet 1993;5:327–37.
181. Gunshin H, Mackenzie B, Berger UV, et al. Cloning and characterization of a mammaliian proton-coupled metal-ion transporter. Nature 1997;388:482–8.
182. Zhou B, Gitschier J. hCTR1: A human gene for copper uptake identified by complementation in yeast. Proc Natl Acad Sci U S A 1997;94:7481–6.
183. Tumer Z, Horn N, Tonnesen T, et al. Early Copper-histidine treatment for Menkes Disease. Nature Genet 1996;12:11–3.
184. Brewer GJ, Hedera P, Kluin KJ, et al. Treatment of Wilson disease with ammonium tetrathiomolybdate: III. Initial therapy in a total of 55 neurologically affected patients and follow-up with zinc therapy. Arch Neurol 2003;60:379–85.
185. Feder JN, Gnirke A, Thomas W, et al. A novel MHC class I-like gene is mutated in patients with hereditary haemochromatosis. Nature Genet 1996;13:399–408.
186. Jazwinska EC, Cullen LM, Busfield F, et al. Haemochromatosis and HLA-H. Nat Genet 1996;14:249–51.
187. Harrison SA, Bacon BR. Hereditary hemochromatosis: Update for 2003. J Hepatol 2003;38:S14–23.
188. Donovan A, Brownlie A, Zhou Y, et al. Positional cloning of zebrafish ferroportin1 identifies a conserved vertebrate iron exporter. Nature 2000;403:776–81.
189. Ramalingam TS, West AP, Jr, Lebron JA, et al. Binding to the transferrin receptor is required for endocytosis of HFE and regulation of iron homeostasis. Nat Cell Biol 2000;2:953–7.
190. Waheed A, Grubb JH, Zhou XY, et al. Regulation of transferrin-mediated iron uptake by HFE, the protein defective in hereditary hemochromatosis. Proc Natl Acad Sci U S A 2002;99:3117–22.
191. Njajou OT, Vaessen N, Joosse M, et al. A mutation in *SLC11A3* is associated with autosomal dominant hemochromatosis. Nature Genet 2001;28:213–4.
192. Fleming RE, Bacon BR. Orchestration of iron homeostasis. N Engl J Med 2005;352:1741–4.
193. Camaschella C, Roetto A, Cali A, et al. The gene TFR2 is mutated in a new type of haemochromatosis mapping to 7q22. Nat Genet 2000;25:14–5.
194. Roetto A, Papanikolaou G, Politou M, et al. Mutant antimicrobial peptide hepcidin is associated with severe juvenile hemochromatosis. Nat Genet 2003;33:21–2.
195. Frazer DM, Inglis HR, Wilkins SJ, et al. Delayed hepcidin response explains the lag period in iron absorption following a stimulus to increase erythropoiesis. Gut 2004;53:1509–15.
196. Papanikolaou G, Samuels ME, Ludwig EH, et al. Mutations in HFE2 cause iron overload in chromosome 1q-linked juvenile hemochromatosis. Nat Genet 2004;36:77–82.
197. Nemeth E, Tuttle MS, Powelson J, et al. Hepcidin regulates cellular iron efflux by binding to ferroportin and inducing its internalization. Science 2004;306:2090–3.
198. Ganz T. Hepcidin—a peptide hormone at the interface of innate immunity and iron metabolism. Curr Top Microbiol Immunol 2006;306:183–98.
199. Shayeghi M, Latunde-Dada GO, Oakhill JS, et al. Identification of an intestinal heme transporter. Cell 2005;122:789–801.
200. Corbeel L, Van den BG, Jaeken J, et al. Congenital folate malabsorption. Eur J Pediatr 1985;143:284–90.
201. Bjorke Monsen AL, Ueland PM. Homocysteine and methylmalonic acid in diagnosis and risk assessment from infancy to adolescence. Am J Clin Nutr 2003;78:7–21.
202. Fyfe JC, Madsen M, Hojrup P, et al. The functional cobalamin (vitamin B12)-intrinsic factor receptor is a novel complex of cubilin and amnionless. Blood 2004;103:1573–9.
203. Christensen EI, Birn H. Megalin and cubilin: Multifunctional endocytic receptors. Nat Rev Mol Cell Biol 2002;3:256–66.
204. Rasmussen SA, Fernhoff PM, Scanlon KS. Vitamin B12 deficiency in children and adolescents. J Pediatr 2001;138:10–7.
205. Ward PC. Modern approaches to the investigation of vitamin B12 deficiency. Clin Lab Med 2002;22:435–45.
206. Katz M, Lee SK, Cooper BA. Vitamin B 12 malabsorption due to a biologically inert intrinsic factor. N Engl J Med 1972;287:425–9.
207. Aminoff M, Carter JE, Chadwick RB, et al. Mutations in *CUBN*, encoding the intrinsic factor-vitamin B12 receptor, cubilin, cause hereditary megaloblastic anaemia 1. Nature Genet 1999;21:309–13.
208. Tanner SM, Aminoff M, Wright FA, et al. Amnionless, essential for mouse gastrulation, is mutated in recessive hereditary megaloblastic anemia. Nat Genet 2003;33:426–9.
209. Li N, Rosenblatt DS, Kamen BA, et al. Identification of two mutant alleles of transcobalamin II in an affected family. Hum Mol Genet 1994;3:1835–40.
210. Tsukaguchi H, Tokui T, Mackenzie B, et al. A family of mammalian Na+-dependent L-ascorbic acid transporters. Nature 1999;399:70–5.
211. Said HM. Recent advances in carrier-mediated intestinal absorption of water-soluble vitamins. Annu Rev Physiol 2004;66:419–46.
212. Sotiriou S, Gispert S, Cheng J, et al. Ascorbic-acid transporter Slc23a1 is essential for vitamin C transport into the brain and for perinatal survival. Nat Med 2002;8:514–7.
213. Said HM, Ortiz A, Ma TY. A carrier-mediated mechanism for pyridoxine uptake by human intestinal epithelial Caco-2 cells: Regulation by a PKA-mediated pathway. Am J Physiol Cell Physiol 2003;285:C1219–25.
214. Prasad PD, Wang H, Kekuda R, et al. Cloning and functional expression of a cDNA encoding a mammalian sodium-dependent vitamin transporter mediating the uptake of pantothenate, biotin, and lipoate. J Biol Chem 1998;273:7501–6.
215. Mardach R, Zempleni J, Wolf B, et al. Biotin dependency due to a defect in biotin transport. J Clin Invest 2002;109:1617–23.
216. Labay V, Raz T, Baron D, et al. Mutations in SLC19A2 cause thiamine-responsive megaloblastic anaemia associated with diabetes mellitus and deafness. Nat Genet 1999;22:300–4.
217. Fleming JC, Tartaglini E, Steinkamp MP, et al. The gene mutated in thiamine-responsive anaemia with diabetes and deafness (TRMA) encodes a functional thiamine transporter. Nat Genet 1999;22:305–8.
218. Seeliger MW, Biesalski HK, Wissinger B, et al. Phenotype in retinol deficiency due to a hereditary defect in retinol binding protein synthesis. Invest Ophthalmol Vis Sci 1999;40:3–11.
219. Ouahchi K, Arita M, Kayden H, et al. Ataxia with isolated vitamin E deficiency is caused by mutations in the α-tocopherol transfer protein. Nature Genet 1995;9:141–5.

15.3c. Congenital Enteropathies

Olivier J. Goulet, MD, PhD

Alan David Phillips, BA, PhD, FRCPCH

The syndrome of intractable diarrhea of infancy was first described by Avery and colleagues in 1968 with the following features: diarrhea of more than 2 weeks' duration, age less than 3 months, and three or more negative stool cultures for bacterial pathogens.[1] All cases were managed with intravenous fluids and despite hospital management, diarrhea was persistent and intractable with a high mortality rate from infection or malnutrition.[1–2] Most of the time no specific diagnosis was made. The definition, presentation, and outcome of intractable diarrhea have changed considerably during the last three decades because of major improvements in nutritional management and better understanding of the pathology of the small bowel mucosa. The term "intractable diarrhea in infancy" (IDI), as previously used, embraced a heterogeneous syndrome of diverse etiology. Guarino and colleagues[3] and Catassi and colleagues[4] proposed the term "severe diarrhea requiring parenteral nutrition." Within this group of diarrhea, it seems possible to differentiate "protracted diarrhea of infancy" (PDI) which resolves despite its initial severity and "intractable diarrhea of infancy" (IDI), which continues despite treatment. The so-called "protracted diarrhea of infancy" is due to either a specific immune deficiency or a sensitization to a common food protein (eg, cow's milk and gluten), to severe infection of the digestive tract, or to the lack of a diagnosis where a specific treatment is available, for example, celiac disease in a developing country. Three studies have shown that IDI is clearly different from protracted diarrhea or severe colitis of infancy even if the onset may be sometimes similar.[3–5] Intractable diarrhea of infancy with persistent villous atrophy alludes to children whose diarrhea starts within the first 2 years of life is abundant (=100 mL/kg/d) and persists despite bowel rest. Rapidly, it becomes life threatening, and long-term total parenteral nutrition (TPN) is required. It is associated with a persistent histological intestinal lesion and continues for years despite various therapeutic trials. These characteristics clearly differentiate intractable diarrhea of infancy from protracted diarrhea of infancy which responds to bowel rest and/or enteral feeding and always recovers even after several weeks or months of parenteral and/or enteral nutrition.

ATTEMPT AT CLASSIFICATION OF INTRACTABLE DIARRHEA OF INFANCY

Conditions within the heterogeneous group of patients with IDI such as autoimmune enteropathy[7] and microvillous atrophy (microvillous inclusion disease)[8] were recognized at an early stage. The difference in the enteropathy in these conditions prompted an attempt to classify intractable diarrhea according to immunohistological criteria which emphasized the involvement or not of activated T cells in the intestinal mucosa.[9] Finally, a work performed within ESPGHAN collected cases of IDI and villous atrophy and applied precisely defined light microscopic characteristics that allowed several types of IDI to be characterized.[6] The aim of the survey was to analyze the clinical, histological, biological, and immunological features, and the outcome of the syndrome of IDI, microvillous inclusion disease being excluded as it had been considered previously.[10] The main diagnostic criteria to identify IDI were severe life-threatening diarrhea occurring within the first 24 months of life and requiring TPN, persistent villous atrophy demonstrated in consecutive biopsies, and resistance to several therapeutic trials.

Histological analysis included the degree of villous atrophy (mild, moderate, severe); crypt size and appearance (hyperplastic or normoplastic), necrotic or branched, and the presence of crypt abscesses; epithelial cell height and appearance (an epithelial cell tuft was defined as a focal crowding and disorganization of surface enterocytes); the mononuclear cellularity of the lamina propria; the density of intraepithelial lymphocytes; an increased number of neutrophils and eosinophils either in the epithelium or in the lamina propria; and the uniform or patchy nature of the enteropathy.

According to clinical and histological analysis, several groups were delineated: the first one presented with extradigestive symptoms suggestive of autoimmune enteropathy, including arthritis, diabetes, nephrotic syndrome, dermatitis, anemia, thrombocytopenia, and tended to have a later onset of diarrhea which was of larger volume compared to a group of patients who had only gastrointestinal symptoms and gut autoantibodies. Two other groups included patients who did not present with mononuclear cell infiltration of the lamina propria. Some patients were small for gestational

age and presented with phenotypic abnormalities corresponding to the previously described "syndromatic diarrhea."[11] Some other infants presented with mucosal changes including mild to moderate villous atrophy, epithelial cell tufts, branching, and/or pseudocystic glands.[12] Family history was noted in 40% of these patients. The last group included infants with villous atrophy in which histological analysis did not result in specific features being recognized.

Histological analysis seems to be the most important point for the diagnosis of IDI. Patients present histologically in two clearly different forms: the first one is characterized by a mononuclear cells infiltration of the lamina propria and is considered to be associated with activated T cells. A well-recognized and distinct entity of severe enteropathy is in form of "autoimmune enteropathy (AIE)"[13] (see Chapter 16.3, "Autoimmune Enteropathy and IPEX Syndrome" by F. Ruemmele, Nicole Brousse, and O. Goulet). The second pattern includes early onset of severe intractable diarrhea with villous atrophy without mononuclear cell infiltration of the lamina propria, but with specific histological abnormalities involving the epithelium. This chapter aims to review such entities that are considered as congenital enteropathies affecting the development of the intestinal mucosa. Early onset of severe watery diarrhea is immediately suggestive of intestinal disease involving the intestinal epithelium. To date, several types of primary epithelial abnormalities inducing IDI have been described. The first described was microvillus atrophy (MVA) or microvillus inclusion disease (MIVD), and more recently tufting enteropathy or epithelial dysplasia.

MICROVILLOUS ATROPHY/ MICROVILLOUS INCLUSION DISEASE

Microvillous atrophy, first described in 1978,[14] was the first clinical entity identified on a morphological basis as being responsible for the so-called protracted or intractable diarrhea syndrome.[15] Microvillous inclusion disease (MVID) or microvillous atrophy (MVA) is a congenital and constitutive disorder of intestinal epithelial cells.[10,15–17] It is characterized by the neonatal onset of abundant watery diarrhea persisting despite total bowel rest. Onset most often occurs within the first days of life. The diagnosis is based on typical morphological abnormalities detected through a combination of light and electron microscopic (EM) analysis of proximal small bowel biopsies.[10,15–18] Standard histology reveals a variable degree of villous atrophy without marked crypt hyperplasia, although epithelial cell mitotic activity and apoptosis is increased,[10,20] in addition to an abnormal accumulation of periodic acid schiff (PAS) positive material in the apical cytoplasm of upper crypt and mature enterocytes and an absent neutral PAS staining of the enterocyte brush border membrane; the acidic alcian blue-positive staining on the surface of the brush border remains in place.[21] These findings are completed by EM with the detection of atrophic or completely absent microvilli on mature enterocytes (see below) along with so-called microvillous inclusions (vacuoles lined by microvilli) and the finding of electron dense "secretory granules" in the same distribution as the abnormal PAS positive accumulation.

Epidemiology

MVID is an extremely rare congenital disorder. To date, no prevalence data are available; however, it can be estimated that there are no more than a few hundred children with MVID in Europe. The prevalence is higher in countries with a high degree of consanguinity, suggesting an autosomal recessive transmission.

Clinical Presentation

Pregnancy and delivery are uneventful; in general, there is no notion of polyhydramnios except in rare isolated cases. Severe watery diarrhea starts within the first days of life.[10] This diarrhea becomes so abundant that within 24 hours the children can loose up to 30% of their body weight, resulting in profound metabolic acidosis and severe dehydration. MVID is most often severe and life threatening. and many children die within the first year of life. Accurate quantification of the stool volumes reveals 150 to over 300 mL/kg/d, with a high sodium content (100 to 130 mmol/L). Stools usually contain noticeable quantities of mucus. Complete and prolonged bowel rest reduces stool volume moderately, but volumes nearly always remain above 150 mL/kg/d. Inappropriate parenteral nutrition with steadily increasing intravenous fluids may significantly aggravate stool output. Secondary to the marked diarrhea, children with MVID rapidly develop metabolic acidosis and signs of hypotonic dehydration. No other biological signs are associated with this disorder; however, most children are at risk of developing cholestasis and liver failure. Stool examination reveals fecal sodium concentrations between 100 and 130 mmol/L, normal α-1 antitrypsin clearance, and no fecal inflammatory parameters.

No additional clinical signs are associated with MVID; in particular, there are no malformations or involvement of other organs such as liver, kidney, etc. However, a small number of children have a massive pruritus secondary to marked

elevations in the concentrations of biliary acids in the blood. Initially, no specific findings can be detected except enormous abdominal distension with fluid-filled intestinal and colonic loops. All children with congenital MVID urgently require total parental nutrition (TPN), which often causes rapidly evolving cholestasis and liver disease.

A detailed multicenter analysis of 23 patients with MVID[10] allowed two different forms and presentations of MVID to be distinguished on a clinical and morphological basis: congenital early-onset MVID (starting within the first days of life) and late-onset MVID (with first symptoms appearing after 2 or 3 months of life).

Histopathological Presentation

The gold standard in the diagnosis of MVID is a combined light/electron microscopic histological analysis of small bowel biopsies obtained during diagnostic gastrointestinal endoscopy. Macroscopic endoscopic analysis of the entire gastrointestinal tract remains completely normal, besides nonspecific minimal alterations, such as mild mucosal erythema or, in rare cases, indirect signs of villous atrophy. In contrast, histological analysis reveals major alterations of the entire small bowel and, to a lesser degree, also of the colon. Standard histology shows a variable degree of villous atrophy without marked crypt hyperplasia, appearing as "thin mucosa."[10,20] The accumulation of PAS positive granules within the apical cytoplasm of immature enterocytes in the

upper crypt is highly characteristic of MVID.[22–23] In parallel, on PAS staining (light microscopy), the brush border membrane looks pathological, with an enlarged intracytoplasmic band along the apical pole of enterocytes (largely corresponding to secretory granules plus autophagocytic vacuoles and microvillous inclusion bodies revealed by EM) and an atrophic band instead of the normally well-defined small line representing the brush border (Figure 1).

Immunostaining techniques directed against CD10, a neutral membrane-associated peptidase, can further help the diagnosis of MVID,[18–14] since the small linear band of the brush border appears markedly enlarged and as a double band in MVID patients (Figure 1). This abnormal staining pattern (PAS or CD10) on the apical pole of enterocytes appears first in upper crypt epithelial cells in congenital MVID with early onset, whereas late-onset MVID has abnormal enterocyte structures within the lower villous part. Based on the morphological presentation of abnormal PAS stain in low crypt cells, an atypical form of MVID was also described.[10] On EM, upper crypt epithelial cells show a reduced to completely absent microvillus profile on the apical membrane, increased numbers of autophagic vacuoles and vastly increased quantities of secretory granules; in contrast, the diagnostic and characteristic microvillus inclusions are very infrequent.[10] In a noticeable contrast to the clearly abnormal crypt cells, surface lumi-

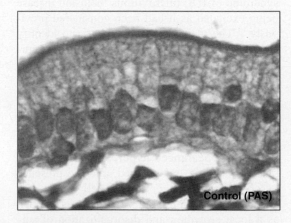
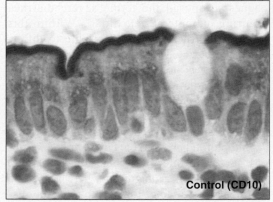
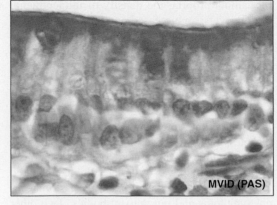
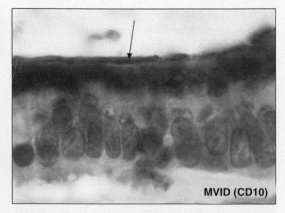

Figure 1 High power magnification of a duodenal section of a patient with typical MVA after periodic schiff acid (PAS) staining or anti-CD10 immunohistochemistry. Compared to normal controls, in MVA an enlarged intracytoplasmic band (arrow) along the apical pole of enterocytes is observed along with an atrophic band instead of the normally well-defined small line representing the brush border.

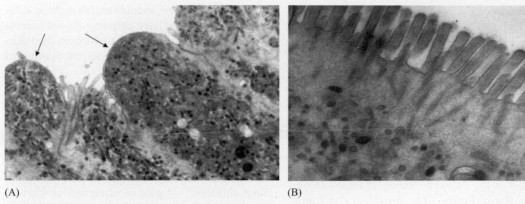

Figure 2 (A) Upper crypt epithelium showing absence of microvilli (arrow) and greatly increased presence of secretory granules in the apical cytoplasm. (B) Villous epithelium showing presence of microvilli and a decreased presence of secretory granules. (From reference 10.)

nal exposed mature enterocytes may possess microvilli and appear more normal on EM, apart from an increased number of secretory granules, indicating that the microvillous abnormality is temporary and can be reversed later on in the epithelial life cycle (Figure 2A and B).[10] Thus, the diagnosis of MVID is difficult and should be performed, or at the very least confirmed, by particularly skilled pathologists who most often can make this diagnosis on light microscopy after PAS or CD10 staining (characteristic alterations in the apical pole of immature and mature enterocytes). However, the diagnosis is formally confirmed by the finding of microvillous inclusion bodies within the cytoplasm along with atrophic microvilli on EM. Since microvilli on immature crypt cells are most often normal, isolated EM analysis of these cells should not be performed as it could lead to a false-negative diagnosis. In addition, the isolated finding of rudimentary or absent microvilli on enterocytes is a nonspecific finding and is found in many enteropathies.

Etiopathogenesis

The precise etiology of MVID is still unknown. A major defect in membrane trafficking in enterocytes has been proposed as a pathogenetic mechanism of MVID, probably secondary to an altered structure of the cytoskeleton.[19] However, the observation of morphologically normal microvilli on immature crypt cells in children with MVID indicate that the microvillous changes seen in differentiating and mature cells are of a secondary nature or are a consequence of yet unidentified events within the cell. These events could include membrane recycling or mechanisms controlling endo- or exocytosis.[25–26] However, analysis of the membrane targeting of disaccharidases, such as sucrase-isomaltase, revealed no abnormalities of the direct or indirect constitutive pathway (Figure 3). Recent observations indicate a selective defect in exocytosis of the glycocalyx or epithelial glycoproteins in patients with MVID.[21] These findings need further confirmation. Another hypothesis suggesting a defect in the autophagocytosis pathway was proposed to explain the morphological and functional abnormalities in MVID.[27]

Management and Outcome

As a result of the severe diarrhea, acute episodes of dehydration and metabolic decompensation are common complications of MVID. Hypovolemia often causes temporary ischemia; therefore, neurological and psychological symptoms such as developmental retardation can occur.[10] Impaired renal function is also a frequent complication, together with nephrocalcinosis. TPN is extremely difficult to adapt and requires vast experience, especially for the initial stabilization of small babies with MVID. Major complications of TPN such as cholestasis or liver failure are normally avoidable, but still very frequent. Infectious complications of the central catheter resulting in sepsis are the most frequent cause of death, followed by liver failure.

MVID is a constitutive intestinal epithelial cell disease that causes an irreversible diarrheal disorder leading to permanent and definitive intestinal failure.[10,17] Children with MVID are dependent on exclusive parenteral nutrition throughout their lives. Oral alimentation and appropriate oral caloric intake are impossible. There is no hope for improvement with age for the vast majority of cases, and only one child has been described in which the disease appeared to resolve with time.[28] A large number of patients do not survive

the first 3 years of life as a result of infectious complications or rapid evolution of liver failure. Those children with MVID who survive often have mental retardation and renal complications. In contrast to children with early-onset MVID, the diarrhea is often less severe in children with the late-onset form of the disease. With age, children with late-onset MVID can acquire partial intestinal autonomy, resulting in a reduction of the number of perfusions of parental nutrition to one or two a week.

To date, no causal treatment exists for MVID. Trials with anti-inflammatory drugs including steroids and antisecretory medications (such as sandostatin or loperamide) did not significantly change stool volumes over a prolonged period.[10] Therefore, all patients are dependent on supportive measures such as parenteral nutrition, which is the only way of stabilizing them. However, this treatment is often difficult to administer successfully as the diarrhea is very abundant and the patients can rapidly succumb to metabolic decompensation. Therefore, it is important that children with MVID are transferred to highly specialized pediatric gastroenterology centers. As discussed, the long-term outcome is rather poor for children treated with parenteral nutrition. New treatment strategies for the management of MVID are needed.[29] Intestinal transplantation is a clear alternative to parenteral nutrition for children with MVID.[30–33] It can be performed as isolated small bowel or combined liver–small bowel transplantation if significant liver disease exists. A recent study in a national referral center for IDI revealed that the outcome for children who had undergone small bowel transplantation for MVID was much better than that for children undergoing small bowel transplantation for other indications.[33] Based on this observation and the fact that prolonged parenteral nutrition has a rather poor outcome, it is now appropriate to consider early small bowel transplantation as a first choice treatment of early-onset MVID, allowing the patients to obtain full intestinal autonomy. However, it is hoped that a curative treatment will be available in the future.

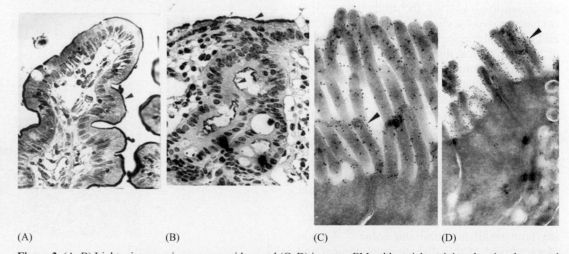

Figure 3 (A, B) Light microsopy immunoperoxidase and (C, D) immuno-EM gold particle staining showing the normal localization of S-IM in the apical membrane in both normal (A, C) and microvillous atrophy (B, D) (arrow heads). (From reference 21.

Genetic Counseling

The observations that the incidence of MVID is higher in families with a preexisting case of MVID[15,34] and that there is a high rate of consanguinity in parents of children with MVID,[35] clearly indicate a genetic basis for this disorder, which is probably inherited on an autosomal recessive basis. It is particularly striking to note the large number of children of Turkish origin with MVID and a high degree of consanguinity in this population. As a genetic defect has not been identified, no genetic counseling or prenatal diagnosis is possible.

Recent work has described a mouse knockout model that resembles aspects of MVA[36] and brings the hope that identification of a genetic basis of the disease is getting closer. In this model, the deletion of the gene *rab8* demonstrated that it is involved in locating apical membrane proteins in intestinal epithelium. On transmission EM the mice showed shortened microvilli, increased autophagic vacuoles, and microvillous inclusions in enterocytes that is some of the hallmarks of microvillous atrophy. The microvillous inclusions appeared to develop from endocytosis of the apical membrane. Diarrhea developed from 3 weeks of age and the mice died at 5 weeks. Brush border enzymes (eg, sucrase isomaltase, alkaline phosphatase) were reduced and accumulated in the cytoplasm. No changes were apparent in the liver. Despite the morphological similarities to microvillous atrophy, no mutations in the exons of *rab8* were identified in patients of either early-onset (two cases) or late-onset (one case) form, although one of the patients with MVA showed a marked decrease in the level of rab8 protein in the small intestine by immunohistochemistry.[36]

INTESTINAL EPITHELIAL DYSPLASIA

Intestinal epithelial dysplasia (IED), also known as tufting enteropathy, is a newly described clinicopathologic entity with early-onset severe intractable diarrhea and persistent villous atrophy with low or normal mononuclear cell infiltration of the lamina propria but specific histological abnormalities involving the epithelium.[6,9] IED is characterized by clinical and histological heterogeneity and association with malformations or other epithelial diseases. It is thought to be related to abnormal enterocytes development and/or differentiation.

Three cases of neonatal severe diarrhea with abnormal epithelial pictures were first reported by Reifen and colleagues in 1994, under the name of "tufting enteropathy."[37] We identified nine cases of severe neonatal diarrhea, which were clearly distinguishable from MVA and resembled "tufting enteropathy."[12] Further studies of these patients allowed us to identify IED as a constitutive epithelial disorder involving both small intestine and colon.[38] A main characteristic of this disease is its clinical and histological heterogeneity and its association with malformations or other epithelial diseases.

Epidemiology

IED appears to be more common than microvillous atrophy (MVA), also known as microvillous inclusion disease (MVID), especially in Middle East, however, it remains very rare. Many cases are not yet recognized since the description of this disorder is recent. To date, no epidemiological data are available; however, the prevalence can be estimated at around 1 of 50,000 to 100,000 live births in Western Europe. The largest cohort of patients is currently being treated at the Necker-Enfants Malades Hospital in Paris, France. The prevalence is higher in countries with high degree of consanguinity. Our studies indicate that IED is frequent in patients of Arabic origin (Middle East, Turkey, and North Africa). The prevalence is also high in the island of Malta (in the Mediterranean Sea) but the phenotype appears to be milder. Indeed, one case of tufting enteropathy has had a successful pregnancy,[39] and there is evidence of amelioration of the disease with age in some young Maltese adults.

Clinical Presentation

In general, infants develop watery diarrhea within the first days after birth. It is severe in most of the cases. Stool volumes may be as high as 100 to 200 mL/kg body weight per day, with electrolyte concentrations similar to those seen in small intestinal fluid. In rare case the diarrhea may be less abundant and sometimes may mislead the diagnosis. The growth is impaired. There is no past history of hydramnios suggesting congenital chloride diarrhea or sodium malabsorption diarrhea. Most patients have consanguineous parents and/or affected siblings some of whom died during the first months of life from severe diarrhea of unknown origin.

Several cases of IED have been reported as being associated with phenotypic abnormalities, for example, Dubowitz syndrome or malformative syndrome.[40-42] Some affected children are reported to have dysmorphic facial features.[40] An association between congenital IDI and choanal atresia has been reported in four children.[41] We have observed malformations, including esophageal atresia, choanal atresia, or unperforated anus. Moreover, nonspecific punctuated keratitis, associated with abnormal conjunctival epithelium, is observed in more than 60% of patients (Figure 4A and B).[42] These associated ophthalmologic symptoms are very intriguing since it is also an epithelial disease and therefore extensive studies of conjunctival epithelium might help to elucidate the molecular mechanisms of the intestinal epithelial disease. The fact that some children have ophthalmological symptoms, keratitis and conjunctival abnormalities highlights the heterogeneity of IED (Roche et al manuscript in preparation).

Histopathological Presentation

Histological abnormalities in IED include villous atrophy, disorganization of the surface epithelium, and basement membrane abnormalities. Villous atrophy is present in all patients but variable

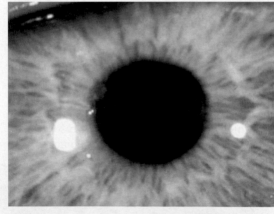

(A)

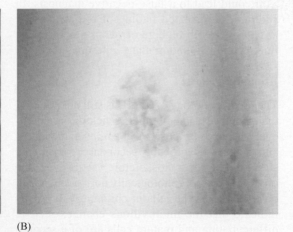

(B)

(C)

Figure 4 (A and B) Typical aspect of punctuated keratitis which is associated in about 60% of IED. (C) Typical aspect of dysplasia of the conjunctival epithelium with inflammation and reduced number of mucus cells.

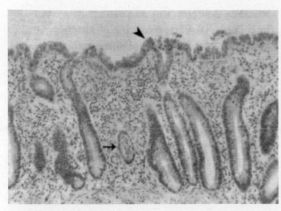
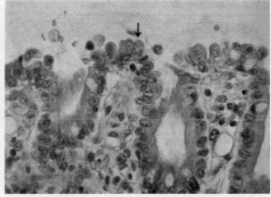

Figure 5 Typical disorganization of surface enterocytes with focal crowding forming tuft. (From reference 38.)

in severity. Repeated biopsies are required. In the typical form, abnormalities are localized mainly in the epithelium and include disorganization of surface enterocytes with focal crowding, resembling tufts (Figure 5). These characteristic "tufts" of extruding epithelium, first described by Reifen and colleagues,[37] are seen toward the villous tip and may affect up to 70% of villi. Tufts are not limited to the small intestine and also involve the colonic mucosa.[12]

Focal enterocyte crowding can also be observed in the crypt epithelium and, in addition, crypts often have an abnormal aspect: they are dilated with features of pseudo-cysts and abnormal regeneration with branching[12] (Figure 6).

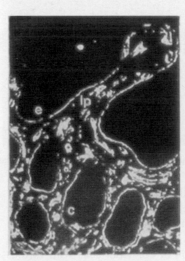

Figure 6 Intestinal epithelial dysplasia. Partial villous atrophy with crypt hyperplasia and/or pseudocystic crypt appearance, branching pictures, and disorganization of surface epithelium.

A study of biopsy specimens demonstrated that the deposition of laminin and heparan sulfate proteoglycan (HSPG) in the basement membrane was abnormal in patients with IED compared with that from patients with celiac disease or autoimmune enteropathy.[12] Relative to the controls, there was faint and irregular laminin deposition at the epithelial lamina propria interface, and the HSPG appeared large and lamellar, suggesting that abnormal development of basement membrane was at the origin of the epithelial abnormalities (Figure 7A–C). In addition, we observed an increased immunohistochemical expression of desmoglein in IED patients and ultrastructural changes in the desmosomes, which were increased in length and number[38] (Figures 8 and 9A–D).

Differential Diagnosis

Neonatal early-onset severe diarrhea may lead to the suspicion of ion transport defects. However, congenital chloride diarrhea (CLD) or congenital sodium diarrhea (CSD) can be easily distinguished from the absence of hydramnios and by blood and stool electrolytes assessment.[43–45] CLD is a rare, autosomal recessive disorder of intestinal Cl/HCO3 exchange caused by mutations in the *SLC26A3* gene and characterized by persistent Cl⁻ rich diarrhea from birth.[43–44] Patients with

CLD present with lifetime watery diarrhea with a high Cl⁻ content and low pH, causing dehydration and hypochloremic metabolic alkalosis. Chloride is low in urine and very high in stools (Cl > 150 mmol/L >sodium).

CSD is caused by defective sodium/proton exchange with only few sporadic cases reported.[45] The genetics of the disease have not been established. Patients with CSD have acidosis and hyponatremia and stools with high concentrations of HCO_3^- and sodium (150 mmol/L). Interestingly in a kindred of five CSD-affected children from a remote rural community in Austria two children presented also a choanal atresia. These children belonged to two families linked by inbreeding, strongly suggesting that CSD is transmitted as an autosomal recessive disease. Using homozygoty mapping and multipoint linkage analysis, they excluded the known sodium/proton exchangers as being causative for CSD in this large pedigree.[45]

Glucose-galactose malabsorption (GGM) is an autosomal recessive disease that presents in newborn infants as a life-threatening diarrhea.[46] The diarrhea ceases within 1 hour of removing oral intake of lactose, glucose, and galactose, but promptly returns with the introduction of one or more of the offending sugars into the diet.

IED should be suspected in neonates with early-onset intractable diarrhea persisting at bowel rest (Figure 10). Because of the early onset of diarrhea, the diagnosis of MVA may be suspected (see above). However, this is easily distinguished from IED by the characteristic PAS abnormality, increased secretory granules, and microvillous inclusions (see above). Sometimes, histopathological examination of intestinal mucosal biopsies in cases of IED do not show evidence of tufts, and the diagnosis can only be made by performing repeated intestinal biopsies. Indeed, biopsies may change from being near normal in early life (showing only signs of nonspecific villous atrophy, with or without monocellular cell infiltration of the lamina propria) to having the characteristic tufts. In addition,

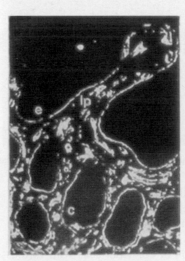
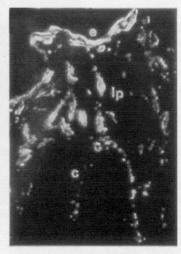
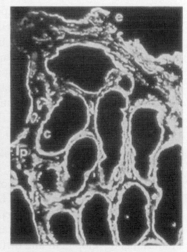

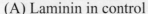

(A) Laminin in control   (B) Laminin in IED   (C) HSPD in IED

Figure 7 Normal deposition of laminin in control (A) but very feint and lamellar in IED (B) while heparan sulfate proteoglycan (HSPG) is overexpressed in the basement membrane. (C) HSBG in IED. (From reference 12.)

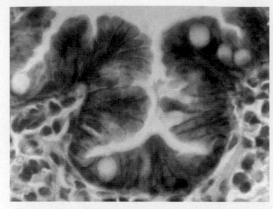

Figure 8 Intestinal epithelial dysplasia. Increased expression of desmoglein staining of the tight junction in a patient with intestinal epithelial dysplasia.

specific abnormalities of basement membrane components (integrins or desmosomes) in parts of mucosa are rare and difficult to detect in the absence of tufts.[38] In patients with neonatal diarrhea and villous atrophy, in which MVA has been ruled out, the evidence of a punctuated keratitis is very relevant for the diagnosis of IED since more than 60% of IED have this association. IED differs from the disease reported in a newborn presenting with pyloric atresia, intractable diarrhea, and severe dermatitis which was thought to be related to a congenital deficiency of $\alpha_6\beta_4$-integrin.[47]

Another difficulty is related to T-cell infiltration of the lamina propria. This is especially problematic when the tufts are missing and supports the hypothesis of an immune-related enteropathy. In a mouse model of dysfunctional E-cadherin, this primary disorder of epithelial permeability or integrity was responsible for secondary T-cell–mediated mucosal damage.[48] Murch and colleagues described these types of lesions in infants with epithelial dysplasia.[49] Despite the lack of evidence from clinical studies, increased intestinal permeability with subsequent antigen entry into the epithelium might explain immune reaction within the lamina propria. Finally, this inflammatory reaction when tufts are not identified or hard to find, often leads to the disease being treated as an immune enteropathy. In our experience, several children have been referred with the diagnosis of autoimmune enteropathy that is unresponsive to immunosuppressive treatment, and severe iatrogenic symptoms from long-term steroids treatment are evident. Repeated pathological analysis combined with ophthalmologic examination allowed us to establish the diagnosis of IED (Salomon and colleagues manuscript submitted).

Etiopathogenesis

IED has been shown to be associated with an abnormal basement membrane.[12] Basement membrane molecules are involved in epithelial mesenchymal cell interactions, which are instrumental in intestinal development and differentiation.[50–55] Alterations suggestive of abnormal cell–cell and cell–matrix interactions were seen in patients with IED without any evidence for abnormalities

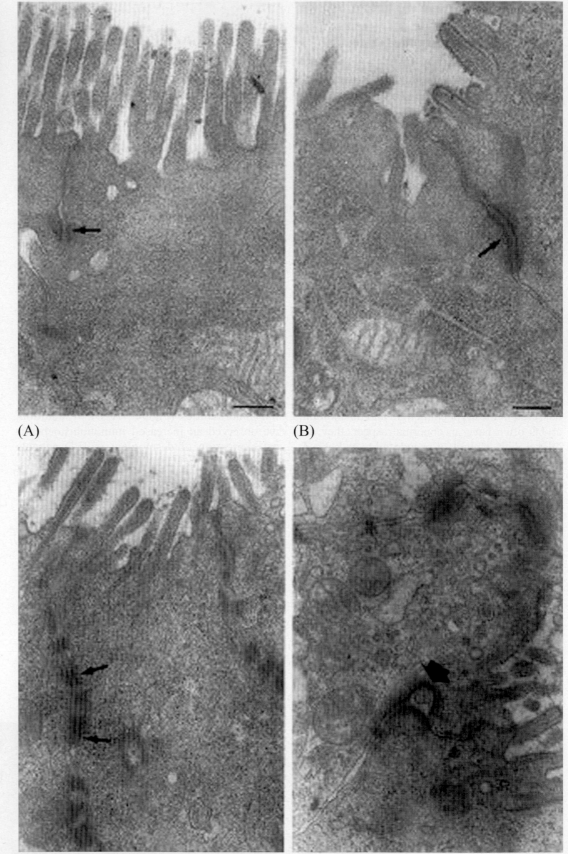

(A)

(B)

Figure 9 Different pictures showing ultrastructural changes in the desmosomes, which are increased in length and number.

in epithelial cell polarization and proliferation.[38] Alterations included an abnormal distribution of $\alpha_2\beta_1$-integrin adhesion molecules along the crypt-villous axis. The $\alpha_2\beta_1$-integrin is involved in the interaction of epithelial cells with various basement membrane components, such as laminin and collagen. To date, the pathophysiological mechanisms resulting in the increased immu-

nohistochemical expression of desmoglein and the ultrastructural changes of the desmosomes are unclear.[38] Mice in which the gene encoding the transcription factor Elf3 is disrupted have morphologic features resembling epithelial dysplasia in infants.[56] In this model, there is abnormal morphogenesis of the villi, while progenitor crypt cells appear normal. The enterocytes produce

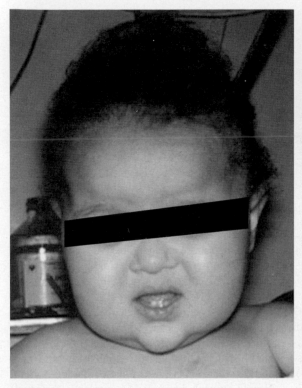

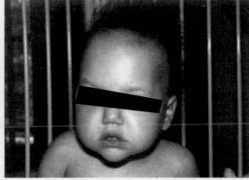

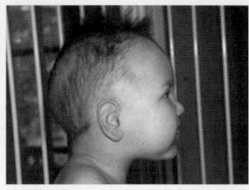

(A)   (B)

Figure 10 Typical facial dysmorphism with prominent forehead and cheeks, broad nasal root and hypertelorism. Abnormal hairs are woolly, easily removed, and poorly pigmented.

low levels of transforming growth factor-βtype 2 receptor, which induces the differentiation of immature intestinal epithelia. Both the clinical studies and the findings in experimental animal models should provide clues to the pathogenesis of these epithelial abnormalities and to the cause of the severity of this neonatal diarrhea. Tufts correspond to nonapoptotic epithelial cells at the villous tips that are no longer in contact with the basement membrane. It can be speculated that a defect in normal enterocyte apoptosis at the end of their lifespan or altered cell–cell interactions are responsible for this effect. The primary or secondary nature of the formation of tufts remains to be determined.

Management and Outcome

IDE may be life threatening since massive diarrhea leads to rapid dehydration and electrolyte imbalance with subsequent metabolic decompensation within a few days after birth. Diarrhea persists at a lower level despite bowel rest. Attempts at continuous enteral feeding (CEF) with a protein hydrolysate or amino acids based formulas worsen the diarrhea, and the newborn rapidly fail to thrive. Sometimes, patients are continued on long-term EF without diarrhea improvement and develop progressive severe protein energy malnutrition. As mentioned above, the same is true for patients treated with immunosuppressive drugs, especially steroids some time associated with cyclosporine, because of mucosal inflammation. Most of the time, this neonatal diarrhea which resists all treatments, finally requires permanent parenteral nutrition (PN). However, it seems that some infants have a milder phenotype than oth-

ers.[39] Infants with partial intestinal function and a limited amount of stool output require only partial long-term PN infusions 3 to 4 times per week. Nevertheless, careful monitoring should be performed to avoid progressive growth retardation.

In most patients, the severity of the intestinal malabsorption and diarrhea make them dependent on daily long-term PN with a subsequent risk of complications. IDE causes intestinal failure that is clearly irreversible in most patients. Liver disease may develop with subsequent end-stage liver cirrhosis in patients with intestinal failure as a consequence of both underlying digestive disease and unadapted PN. Management of patients with intestinal failure requires an early recognition of the condition and the analysis of its risk of irreversibility. Thus, in some cases, IED is an indication for intestinal transplantation (ITx)[58–61] and timing of referral is crucial.[29]

The criteria for ITx have been published in the position paper of the American Society of Transplantation[62] and continue to be debated, especially regarding vascular thrombosis and sepsis. These criteria are regarded more as guidelines than formal recommendations and must be balanced with the risks associated with ITx. For instance, in our practice only repeated life-threatening sepsis especially complicated with extensive thrombosis, may be a criterion for transplantation. The poor quality of life might serve as indication for ITx, although the usual criteria including progressive liver disease, the loss of vascular access, and recurring life-threatening sepsis have not developed. In any case, parents must be extensively informed about the risks of the procedure and about the reasons of any decision.[29]

Patients with irreversible IF and end-stage liver disease (liver cirrhosis) are candidates for a life-saving procedure such as combined liver–small bowel transplantation (LITx). Patients with severe hepatic fibrosis are more difficult to manage.[29] Repeated liver biopsies within 6 to 12 months and careful assessment for portal hypertension are necessary. In addition, it is difficult to assess the amount of functional liver tissue necessary to withstand the insult of portal diversion during the transplantation procedure. Children with severe advanced and progressive hepatic fibrosis are usually listed for LITx. However, some PN-dependent patients with advanced liver dysfunction may experience functional and biochemical liver recovery. In any case, when long-term PN is effective and well tolerated, it can be used for a prolonged period of time without intestinal transplantation. The long-term prognosis is variable. In general, management should be based on a multidisciplinary approach in centers involving pediatric gastroenterology, parenteral nutrition expertise, home parenteral nutrition program, and liver intestinal transplantation program.

Genetic Counseling

The clear association between the occurrence of IDE and the presence of parental consanguinity and/or affected siblings strongly suggests a genetic origin for this disorder. These features suggest an autosomal recessive transmission. Genetic counseling may be based on the very probable autosomal recessive mode of transmission. Since the causative gene(s) have not been yet identified, prenatal diagnosis is not possible.

SYNDROMIC DIARRHEA

Syndromic diarrhea (SD), also known as phenotypic diarrhea (PD) or tricho-hepato-enteric syndrome (THE), is a congenital enteropathy presenting with early-onset severe intractable diarrhea in SGA-born infant associated with nonspecific villous atrophy with low or without mononuclear cell infiltration of the lamina propria nor specific histological abnormalities involving the epithelium. SD is characterized by facial dysmorphism, immune disorders and in some patients early onset of severe liver cirrhosis. Two cases have been reported by Stankler and colleagues as unexplained diarrhea and failure to thrive in siblings with unusual facies and abnormal scalp hair shafts.[63] Eight cases were identified with severe diarrhea, which were clearly distinguishable from MVA and IED.[11] To date, the Necker group has reported the largest series of children presenting with the syndrome of intractable diarrhea associated with phenotypic abnormalities and immune deficiency.[11] Further case reports confirmed this new entity.[64–68] Some cases from the largest survey published in 1994 presented with early onset of severe cholestatic disease with a rapid course to cirrhosis and death.[11] A recent report including two cases with severe liver disease and the review of the published cases suggested that these patients have the same heterogeneous disease that were inappropriately separated into different entities suggesting that SD and THE are two sides of a now well-recognized disease of unclear origin.[68]

Epidemiology

SD appears much less common than MVA/MVID, or IED. Many cases are not yet recognized since the description of this disorder is recent. To date, no epidemiological data are available; however, the prevalence can be estimated at around 1 in 200,000 to 300,000 live births in Western Europe. The prevalence does not seem especially different among ethnic groups. There is a trend to a higher degree of consanguinity.

Clinical Presentation

The patients present with diarrhea starting within the first 6 months of life (≤1 month in most cases). Severe malabsorption leads to early and severe protein energy malnutrition with failure to thrive and requires PN. Diarrhea persists while on bowel rest on PN. All affected infants have several features in common. They are small for gestional age (<10° percentile). All have facial dysmorphism with prominent forehead and cheeks, broad nasal root and hypertelorism (Figure 11A and B). Most children have difficulties with fine motor movements and are mentally retarded. They have a distinct abnormality of hair that is woolly, easily removed, and poorly pigmented. Microscopic analysis of the hair shaft reveals tortuosities (pili torti), aniso- and poilkilotrichosis, tricorrhexis nodosa, and longitudinal breaks (Figure 12). Two cases were reported with tricorrhexis blastysis under scanning electron microscopy. In the same cases, biochemical analysis revealed several anomalies of the amino acid pattern, including low cystine content, although no specific biochemical profile has been established yet. Liver disease involves about half of the patients.

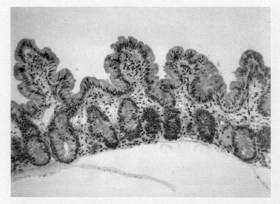

Figure 12 Small intestine biopsies of a patient with SD showing moderate villous atrophy with low degree of mononuclear cell infiltration in the lamina propria. (Courtesy of Pr Nicole Brousse Hôpital Necker, Paris, France.)

Histopathological Presentation

Small intestinal biopsies of the patients with SD show moderate or severe villous atrophy with variable mononuclear cell infiltration of the lamina propria and no epithelial abnormalities. Histologically, the lesion is nonspecific (Figure 13). Ultrastructural analysis of intestinal biopsies is limited, and no characteristic abnormalities have been identified.

In patients presenting with liver disease, pathological analysis usually shows a macronodular cirrhosis with normal extrahepatic ducts. Microscopical examination shows extensive fibrosis or cirrhosis. Perl's staining shows iron depositions involving the hepatocytes and to a lesser extent Kupfer cells. This aspect is consistent with neonatal hemochromatosis (NH) as suggested by Verloes and colleagues.[65]

Immune Profile

A functional T-cell immune deficiency with defective antibody production was first described in the original report.[11] Patients had defective antibody responses despite normal serum immunoglobulin levels, and defective antigen-specific skin tests despite positive proliferative responses in vitro. Further reports have mostly confirmed the presence of an immune dysfunction with oligoclonal hyper-IgA in some patients.[11,64,66]

Management and Outcome

Prognosis of this type of intractable diarrhea of infancy is poor since >25% of the currently reported patients died between the ages of 2 and 5 years, some of them with early onset of cirrhosis. In the largest and oldest series, five of the eight children reported died within 5 years due to sepsis or cirrhosis despite aggressive intervention.[11] More recent case reports experienced better survival with long-term PN dependency.[64-68] Indeed, in many patients, the severity of intestinal malabsorption and diarrhea make them dependent on daily long-term PN with subsequent risk of complications. However, it seems that some infants have a rather milder phenotype with partial PN dependency or require only enteral feeding. However, in spite of adequate protein energy supplies, growth velocity remains low and final stature very short. Attempts with recombinant human growth hormone in one (not reported) patient failed to improve the growth and the final stature. Moreover, patients have various degree of mental retardation.

Etiopathogenesis

Among the congenital forms of hair dysplasia, tricorrhexis nodosa (TN) is very common and can be present in several pathological conditions.[69-72] TN is the most common defect in the hair shaft, leading to hair breakage.[73] The primary abnormality is a focal loss of cuticles, causing fraying of the cortical fibers.[74] TN can occur congenitally or can be acquired from chemical or physical trauma. Congenital TN has been associated with several syndromes including arginosuccinaciduria,[75] citrullinemia,[76] Menkes syndrome,[77] Netherton disease,[78] and trichotiodystrophy.[79] SD patients have defective

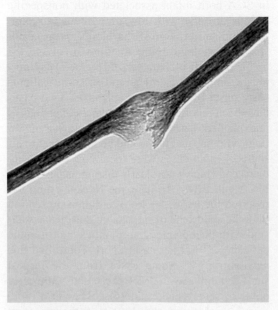

Figures 11 Microscopic analysis of the hair shaft showing tricorrhexis nodosa and longitudinal breaks.

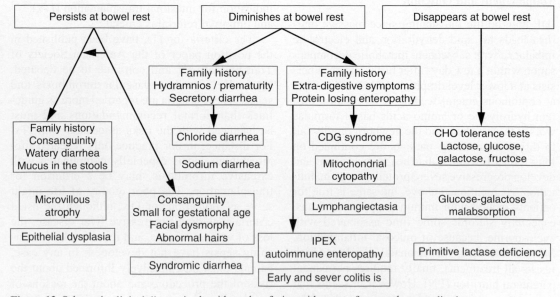

Figure 13 Schematic clinical diagnosis algorithm when facing with onset of neonatal severe diarrhea.

antibody responses despite normal serum immunoglobulin levels, and defective antigen-specific skin tests despite positive proliferative responses in vitro. The cause of this diarrhea is unknown, and the relation between low birth weight, dysmorphism, severe diarrhea, trichorrhexis, immune deficiency, and NH-like liver disease is unclear. The coexistence of morphological, trichological, and immunological abnormality with early-onset intractable diarrhea disproportionate to the mucosal architectural abnormality (consistent with a primary enterocyte abnormality) suggests either mutation within several genes, inherited together by linkage disequilibrium, or more probably interference with a higher level of control, such as a patterning gene.[80] The characteristic hair abnormalities may allow a more focused search for candidate mutations, as relatively few genes have been implicated in hair development.

Genetic Counseling

To date the genetic origin of this disorder is suspected from the frequent association of parental consanguinity and/or affected siblings. This might suggest an autosomal recessive transmission. The gene involved in this congenital inherited autosomal recessive disease is not yet identified. Ethnic origin does not appear as a characteristic of the disease.

CONCLUSIONS

The foregoing list of congenital enteropathies is not exhaustive since other forms with abnormal small bowel mucosa have been described including: mitochondrial DNA rearrangements,[81] congenital enterocyte heparan sulphate deficiency,[82] phosphomannose isomerase deficiency,[83] and carbohydrate-deficient glycoprotein syndrome with a presentation which features both hepatic and intestinal manifestations,[84] severe intractable diarrhea as the recently described congenital malabsorptive diarrhea due to a mutation in the *neurogenin-3* gene,[85] and neonatal diarrhea associated with later obesity in human proprotein convertase 1 deficiency.[86] Most of these diseases do not involve the digestive tract alone but cause intestinal failure of variable intensity. None of them are currently recognized as indication of intestinal transplantation.

REFERENCES

1. Avery GB, Villacivencio O, Lilly JR, Randolph JG. Intractable diarrhea in early infancy. Pediatrics 1968;41:712–22.
2. Ricour C, Navarro J, Frederich A, et al. La diarrhée grave rebelle du nourrisson (à propos de 84 observations). Arch Fr Pediat 1977;34:44–59.
3. Guarino A, Spagnulo MI, Russo S, et al. Etiology and risk factors of severe and protracted diarrhea. J Pediatr Gastroenterol Nutr 1995;20:173–8.
4. Catassi C, Fabiani E, Spagnuolo MI, et al. Severe and protracted diarrhea: Results of the 3-year SIGEP multicenter survey. J Pediatr Gastroenterol Nutr 1999;29:63–8.
5. Goulet O, Besnard M, Girardet JP, et al, for the French Speaking Group of Hepatology, Gastroenterology and Nutrition. Clin Nutr 1998;17:9(A).
6. Goulet O, Brousse N, Canioni D, et al. Syndrome of intractable diarrhoea with persistent villous atrophy in early childhood: A clinicopatological survey of 47 cases. J Pediatr Gastroenterol Nutr 1998;26:151–61.
7. Unsworth DJ, Walker-Smith JA. Auto-immunity in diarrheal disease. J Pediatr Gastroenterol Nutr 1985;4:375–80.
8. Phillips AD, Jenkins P, Raafat F, Walker-Smith JA. Congenital microvillous atrophy: Specific diagnostic features. Arch Dis Child 1985;60:135–40.
9. Cuenod B, Brousse N, Goulet O, et al. Classification of intractable diarrhea in infancy using clinical and immunohistological criteria. Gastroenterology 1990;99:1037–43.
10. Phillips AD, Schmitz J. Familial microvillous atrophy: A clinicopathological survey of 23 cases. J Pediatr Gastroenterol Nutr 1992;14:380–96.
11. Giraut D, Goulet O, Ledeist F, et al. Intractable diarrhea syndrome associated with phenotypic abnormalities and immune deficiency. J Pediatr 1994;125:36–42.
12. Goulet O, Kedinger M, Brousse N, et al. Intractable diarrhea of infancy: A new entity with epithelial and basement membrane abnormalities. J Pediatr 1995;127:212–9.
13. Ruemmele FM, Brousse N, Goulet O. Autoimmune enteropathy—molecular concepts. Curr Opin Gastroenterol 2004;20:587–91.
14. Davidson GP, Cutz E, Hamilton JR, Gall DG. Familial enteropathy: A syndrome of protracted diarrhea from birth, failure to thrive, and hypoplastic villous atrophy. Gastroenterology 1978;75:783–90.
15. Phillips AD, Jenkins P, Raafat F, Walker-Smith JA. Congenital microvillous atrophy: Specific diagnostic features. Arch Dis Child 1985;60:135–40.
16. Bell SW, Kerner JA Jr, Sibley RK. Microvillous inclusion disease. The importance of electron microscopy for diagnosis. Am J Surg Pathol 1991;15:1157–64.
17. Cutz E, Rhoads JM, Drumm B, et al. Microvillus inclusion disease: An inherited defect of brush-border assembly and differentiation. N Engl J Med 1989;320:646–51.
18. Youssef N, Ruemmele F, Goulet O, Patey N. CD10 expression in a case of microvillous inclusion disease Ann Pathol 2004;24:624–7.
19. Carruthers L, Dourmaskhin R, Phillips A. Disorders of the cytoskeleton of the enterocyte. Clin Gastroenterol 1986;15:05–20.
20. Groisman GM, Sabo E, Meir A, Polak-Charcon S. Enterocyte apoptosis and proliferation are increased in microvillous inclusion disease (familial microvillous atrophy). Hum Pathol 2000;31:1404–10.
21. Phillips AD, Brown A, Hicks S, et al. Acetylated sialic acid residues and blood group antigens localise within the epithelium in microvillous atrophy indicating internal accumulation of the glycocalyx. Gut 2004;53:1764–71.
22. Phillips AD, Szfranski M, Man L-Y, Wall W. Periodic acid Schiff staining abnormality in microvillous atrophy: Photometric and ultrastructural studies. J Pediatr Gastroenterol Nutr 2000;30:34–42.
23. Schmitz J, Ginies JL, Arnaud-Battandier F, et al. Congenital microvillous atrophy, a rare cause of neonatal intractable diarrhea. Pediatr Res 1982;16:1041.
24. Groisman GM, Amar M, Livne E. CD10: A valuable tool for the light microscopic diagnosis of microvillous inclusion disease (familial microvillous atrophy). Am J Surg Pathol 2002;26:902–7.
25. Michail S, Collins JF, Xu H, et al. Abnormal expression of brushborder membrane transporters in the duodenal mucosa of two patients with microvillous inclusion disease. J Pediatr Gastroenterol Nutr 1998;27:536–42.
26. Phillips A, Fransen J, Haari HP, Sterchi E. The constitutive exocytotic pathway in microvillous atrophy. J Pediatr Gastroenterol Nutr 1993;17:239–46.
27. Reinshagen K, Naim HY, Zimmer KP. Autophagocytosis of the apical membrane in microvillus inclusion disease. Gut 2002;51:514–21.
28. Croft NM, Howatson AG, Ling SC, et al. Microvillous inclusion disease: An evolving condition. J Pediatr Gastroenterol Nutr 2000;31:185–9.
29. Goulet O, Ruemmele F. Causes and management of intestinal failure. Gastroenterol 2006;130:516–28.
30. Bunn SK, Beath SV, Mckeirnan PJ, et al. Treatment of microvillous inclusion disease by intestinal transplantation. J Pediatr Gastroenterol Nutr 2000;31:176–80.
31. Herzog D, Atkison P, Grant D, et al. Combined bowel-liver transplantation in an infant with microvillous inclusion disease. J Pediatr Gastroenterol Nutr 1996;22:405–8.
32. Oliva MM, Perman JA, Saavedra JM, et al. Successful intestinal transplantation for microvillous inclusion disease. Gastroenterology 1994;106:771–4.
33. Ruemmele FM, Jan D, Lacaille F, et al. New perspectives for children with microvillous inclusion disease: Early small bowel transplantation. Transplantation 2004 15;77:1024–8.
34. Nathavitharana KA, Green NJ, Raafat F, Booth IW. Siblings with microvillous inclusion disease. Arch Dis Child 1994;71:71–3.
35. Heinz-Erian P, Schmidt H, Le Merrer M, et al. Congenital microvillous atrophy in a girl with autosomal dominant hypochondroplasia. J Pediatr Gastroenterol Nutr 1999;28:203–5.
36. Sato T, Mushiake S, Kato Y, et al. The Rab8 GTPase regulates apical protein localization in intestinal cells. Nature 2007;448:366–9.
37. Reifen RM, Cutz E, Griffiths AM, et al. Tufting enteropathy: A newly recognized clinicopathological entity associated with refractory diarrhea in infants. J Pediatr Gastroenterol Nutr 1994;18:379–85.
38. Patey N, Scoazec JY, Cuenod-Jabri B, et al. Distribution of cell adhesion molecules in infants with intestinal epithelial dysplasia (tufting enteropathy). Gastroenterology 1997;113:833–43.
39. Cameron DJ, Barnes GL. Successful pregnancy outcome in tufting enteropathy. J Pediatr Gastroenterol Nutr 2003;36:158.
40. Abely M, Hankard GF, Hugot JP, et al. Intractable infant diarrhea with epithelial dysplasia associated with polymalformation. J Pediatr Gastroenterol Nutr 1998;27:348–52.
41. Krantz M, Jansson M, Rectors S, et al. Hereditary intractable diarrhea with choanal atresia. A new familial syndrome. J Pediatr Gastroenterol Nutr 1997;24:470.
42. Djeddi D, Verkarre V, Talbotec C, et al. Tufting enteropathy and associated disorders. J Pediatr Gastroenterol Nutr 2002;34:446.
43. Hoglund P. SLC26A3 and congenital chloride diarrhoea. Novartis Found Symp 2006;273:74–86.
44. Hihnala S, Hoglund P, Lammi L, et al. Long-term clinical outcome in patients with congenital chloride diarrhea. J Pediatr Gastroenterol Nutr 2006;42:369–75.
45. Muller T, Wijmenga C, Phillips AD, et al. Congenital sodium diarrhea is an autosomal recessive disorder of sodium/proton exchange but unrelated to known candidate genes. Gastroenterology 2000;119:1506–13.
46. Wright EM, Turk E, Martin MG. Molecular basis for glucose-galactose malabsorption. Cell Biochem Biophys 2002;36:115–21.
47. Lachaux A, Bouvier R, Loras I, et al. α6β4 integrin deficiency. A new aetiology for protracted diarrhoea in infancy. J Pediatr Gastroenterol Nutr 1997;24:470.
48. Hermiston ML, Gordon JI. Inflammatory bowel disease and adenomas in mice expressing a dominant negative N-cadherin. Science 1995;270:1203–7.
49. Murch S, Graham A, Vermault A, et al. Functionnaly significant secondary inflammation occurs in a primary epithelial enteropathy. J Pediatr Gastroenterol Nutr 1997;24:467.
50. Beaulieu JF. Differential expression of the VLA family of integrins along the crypt-villus axis in the human small intestine. J Cell Sci 1992;102:427–36.
51. Simon-Assmann P, Duclos B, Orian-Rousseau V, et al. Differential expression of laminin isoforms and alpha 6-beta 4 integrin subunit in the developing human and mouse intestine. Dev Dyn 1994;201:71–85.
52. Simon-Assmann P, Bouziges F, Vigny M, Kedinger M. Origin and deposition of basement membrane heparan sulfate proteoglycan in the developing intestine. J Cell Biol 1989;109:1837–48.
53. Simo P, Simon-Assmann P, Bouziges F, et al. Changes in the expression of laminin during intestinal development. Development 1991;112:477–87.
54. Simo P, Bouziges F, Lissitzky JC, et al. Dual and asynchronous deposition of laminin chains at the epithelial-mesenchymal interface in the gut. Gastroenterology 1992;102:1835–45.
55. Simon-Assmann P, Kedinger M. Heterotypic cellular cooperation in gut morphogenesis and differentiation. Semin Cell Biol 1993;4:221–30.
56. Ng AY, Waring P, Ristevski S, et al. Inactivation of the transcription factor Elf3 in mice results in dysmorphogenesis and altered differentiation of intestinal epithelium. Gastroenterology 2002;122:1455–66.
57. Goulet O, Salomon J, Ruemmele F, et al. Intestinal epithelial dysplasia (tufting enteropathy). Orphanet J Rare Dis 2007;2:20.
58. Lacaille F, Cuenod B, Colomb V, Jan D, et al. Combined liver and small bowel transplantation in a child with epithelial dysplasia. J Pediatr Gastroenterol Nutr 1998;27:230–3.
59. Paramesh AS, Fishbein T, Tschernia A, et al. Isolated small bowel transplantation for tufting enteropathy. J Pediatr Gastroenterol Nutr 2003;36:138–40.
60. Goulet O, Sauvat F, Ruemmele F, et al. Results of the Paris program: Ten years of pediatric intestinal transplantation. Transplant Proc 2005;37:1667–70.
61. Grant D, Abu-Elmagd K, Reyes J, et al. 2003 report of the intestine transplant registry : A new era has dawned. Ann Surg 2005;241:607–13.

62. Kaufman S, Atkinson JB, Bianchi A, et al. Indications for pediatric intestinal transplantation : A position paper of the american society of transplantation. Pediatr Transpl 2001;5:80–7.

63. Stankler L, Lloyd D, Pollitt RJ, et al. Unexplained diarrhoea and failure to thrive in 2 siblings with unusual facies and abnormal scalp hair shafts: A new syndrome. Arch Dis Child 1982;57:212–6.

64. Barabino AV, Torrente F, Castellano E, et al. "Syndromic diarrhea" may have better outcome than previously reported. J Pediatr 2004;144:553–4.

65. Verloes A, Lombet J, Lambert Y et al. Tricho-hepato-enteric syndrome: Further delineation of a distinct syndrome with neonatal hemochromatosis phenotype, intractable diarrhea, and hair anomalies. Am J Med Gen 1997;68:391–5.

66. De Vries E, Visser DM, Van Dongen JJM, et al. Oligoclonal gammopathy in "phenotypic diarrhea." J Pediatr Gastroenterol Nutr 2000;30:349–50.

67. Landers MC, Schroeder TL. Intractable diarrhea of infancy with facial dysmorphism, trichorrhexis nodosa, and cirrhosis. Pediatr Dermatol. 2003;20:432–5

68. Fabre A, Andre N, Breton A, et al. Intractable diarrhea with "phenotypic anomalies" and tricho-hepato-enteric syndrome: Two names for the same disorder. Am J Med Genet A 2007;143:584–8.

69. Itin PH, Pittelkow MR. Trichothiodystrophy: Review of sulfur-deficient brittle hair syndromes and association with the ectodermal dysplasia. J Am Acad Dermatol 1990;22:705–17.

70. Happle R, Traupe H, Gröbe H, Bonsmann G. The tay syndrome (congenital ichthyosis with trichothiodystrophy). Eur J Pediatr 1984;141:147–52.

71. Stefanini M, Vermeulen W, Weeda G, et al. A new nucleotide-excision-repair gene associated with the disorder trichothiodystrophy. Am J Hum Genet 1993;53:817–21.

72. Mariani E, Facchini A, Honorati MC, et al. Immune defects in families and patients with xeroderma pigmentosum and trichothiodystrophy. Clin Exp Immunol 1992;88:376–82.

73. Whiting D. Hair shaft defect. In: Olsen EA, editor. Disorders of Hair Growth: Diagnosis and Treatment. New York: McGraw-Hill; 1994. p. 91–137.

74. Dawber RPR, Comaish S. Scanning electron microscopy of normal and abnormal hair shafts. Arch Dermatol 1970; 101:316-22.

75. Chernosky ME, Owens DW. Trichorrhesis nosoda: Clinical and investigative studies. Arch Dermato 1966;94:577–85.

76. Rauschkolb EW, Chernosky ME, Knox JM, et al. trichorrhesis nodosa—an error of amino acid metabolism? J Invest Dermatol 1967;48:260–3.

77. Danks DM, Tippet P, Zentner G. Severe neonatal citrullinemia. Arch Dis Child 1974;49:579–81.

78. Patel HP, Unis ME. Pili torti in association with citrullinia. J Am Acad Dermatol 1986;12:203–6.

79. Menkes JH. Kinky hair disease. Pediatrics 1972;50:181–3.

80. Netherton EW. A unique case of trichorrhesis nodosa "bamboo hairs." Arch Dermatol 1958;78:483–7.

81. Krafchik BR. Netherton syndrome. Pediatr Dermatol 1992; 9:158–60.

82. Gillespie JM, Marshall RC. A comparison of the proteins of normal and trichothidystrophic human hair. J Invest Dermatol 1983;80:195–202.

83. Murch SH. The molecular basis of intractable diarrhoea of infancy.Baillieres Clin Gastroenterol 1997;11:413–40.

84. Cormier-Daire V, Bonnefont JP, Rustin P, et al. Mitochondrial DNA rearrangements with onset as chronic diarrhea with villous atrophy. J Pediatr 1994;124:63–70.

85. Murch S, Winyard PJD, Koletzko S, et al. Congenital enterocyte heparan sulphate deficiency with massive albumin loss, secretory diarrhoea and malnutrition. Lancet 1996;347:1299–301.

86. Jaeken J, Matthij G, Saudubray JM, et al. Phosphomannose isomerase deficiency: A carbohydrate-deficient glycoproteins syndrome with hepatic-intestinal presentation. Am J Hum Genet 1998;62:1535–9.

87. Oren A, Houwen RH. Phosphomannoseisomerase deficiency as the cause of protein-losing enteropathy and congenital liver fibrosis. J Pediatr Gastroenterol Nutr 1999;29:231–2.

88. Wang J, Cortina G, Wu SV, et al. Mutant neurogenin-3 in congenital malabsorptive diarrhea. N Engl J Med 2006; 355:270–80.

89. Jackson RS, Creemers JWM, Farooqi IS, Raffin-Sanson M-L, et al. Small-intestinal dysfunction accompanies the complex endocrinopathy of human proprotein convertase 1 deficiency. J Clin Invest 2003;112:1551–60

Immune Enteropathies

16.1. Celiac Disease

Markku Mäki, MD, PhD

Samuel Gee accurately described the classic form of childhood celiac disease, the malabsorption syndrome in infancy, in 1888.[1] Throughout the twentieth century, celiac disease has puzzled clinicians and investigators. The major breakthrough and milestone in understanding the disease came from pioneering clinical research performed by Dr Willem Karel Dicke in the Netherlands. He discovered the harmful effect of dietary gluten in celiac disease.[2] He writes in his thesis summary that the harmful effect on patients with celiac disease is not caused by all cereals but specifically by wheat flour. Also, rye elicited or aggravated the clinical symptoms and signs, but wheat starch did not give rise to the phenomena. With construction of a peroral intestinal suction biopsy apparatus in the late 1950s, it became evident that gluten induces small intestinal villous atrophy and crypt hyperplasia. In the 1960s, it was shown that the mucosa heals on a gluten-free diet, and it became evident that gluten intolerance in celiac disease is permanent.[3] One important milestone in celiac disease clinics was the discovery of the circulating gluten-dependent autoantibodies,[4,5] the importance of which became evident only later. Celiac disease aggregation in families was a first clue to genetic susceptibility,[6] and evidence for a primary association of the disease with human leukocyte antigen (HLA)-DQ2 was shown.[7] In 1997, a new era in celiac disease clinics and research began with the discovery of transglutaminase 2 (TG-2; former tissue transglutaminase) as the autoantigen for celiac disease, the human antigen targeted by serum autoantibodies.[8] New knowledge of the disease-inducing cereal proteins, gluten, and recent discoveries in gluten-induced disease mechanisms, where both innate and adaptive immunity play a role, may also in future lead to new approaches for the treatment of celiac disease.[9–11]

DEFINITION OF CELIAC DISEASE

The synonyms in the literature for celiac disease are celiac sprue and gluten-sensitive enteropathy. Celiac disease is an autoimmune-like systemic disorder in genetically susceptible persons perpetuated by the daily ingested gluten cereals wheat, rye, and barley with manifestations in the intestine and in organs outside the gut. Today it is understood that the nature of celiac disease is much more complex than simply intestinal malabsorption, which, as such, is, in fact, no longer essential for the diagnosis.

GLUTEN: THE MAJOR ENVIRONMENTAL TRIGGER

Cereals are cultivated almost all over the world and form one important component in human nutrition. Wheat, rice, and corn are spread worldwide, and rye, barley, oat, millet, and sorghum are of importance for specific regions. Figure 1 shows the taxonomic relationship of the gluten-containing cereal grains that activate celiac disease. Wheat, rye, barley, and oat are, by definition, "gluten." Of these, the first three with excellent baking properties belong to the tribe Triticeae, whereas oat belongs to a different tribe but to the same grass subfamily as wheat, rye, barley, and rice.

Intestinal inflammation and damage in celiac disease are tightly dependent on dietary exposure to prolamins present in wheat, barley, and rye. Prolamins are characterized by their high content in glutamine (35 to 37%) and proline (17 to 23%) residues. Wheat gluten consists of a complex mixture of many gliadin and glutenin polypeptides. Gliadins are monomers, whereas glutenins form large polymeric structures. Gliadins are 250– to 300–amino acid-long polypeptides, and on the basis of their amino acid sequences, they can be subdivided into alpha-, gamma-, omega-gliadins and glutenins divided into high- (650 to 800 residues long) and low- (270 to 330 residues long) molecular-weight proteins. Furthermore, toxic prolamin peptide structures can be found in rye (secalins) and barley (hordeins),[12] which are similar to wheat gliadin peptides.[13]

T-cell stimulatory peptides, as discussed below, are also to be found in rye and barley prolamins but not in avenins from oat.[14] However, looking at the literature in a modern, evidence-based manner, only wheat has been scientifically proven to induce disease. Regarding rye and barley, the evidence is more based on consensus, and clinical research has been scarce. Rice, corn, buckwheat, millet, and sorghum are not harmful for celiac disease patients. The case of oat, which is still under debate, is discussed separately. Also, other environmental triggers may be operative, but whatever the other "secondary hits" might be, the disease responds favorably when only one trigger is removed, the dietary gluten.

Oat and Celiac Disease

Even if oat is defined as gluten, its toxicity in celiac disease was readdressed in the early 1990s.[15] When the literature was reevaluated, it was clear that earlier evidence was not thorough. Some studies were interpreted to prove that oat is harmful[16,17]; some stated that oat can be consumed by celiac disease patients without detrimental effects.[18–20] The reliability of these studies could be questioned because the evidence was based on a few patients, 1 to 12 studied cases, and none of the studies were controlled. In one study only, small intestinal biopsies had been performed.[20] In the study by Janatuinen and colleagues, oat proved to have no detrimental effect on nutritional status, laboratory values, or small intestinal mucosa in celiac disease patients in remission at 6 months, nor did it prevent the intestinal mucosa of newly diagnosed patients from healing after 1 year of treatment.[15] These results were later confirmed in other studies.[21–24] It has also been suggested that including oat can

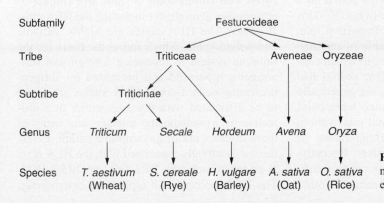

Figure 1 Taxonomy relationships of major cereal grains. (Adapted from reference 12.)

help celiac disease patients follow a strict gluten-free diet.[25,26] Dermatitis herpetiformis patients, who are thought to be very sensitive to gluten, do also seem to tolerate oat.[27,28] In the United States, Hoffenberg and colleagues first showed oat to be nonharmful for children with celiac disease.[29] In an 1-year randomized double-blind study comprising 93 children, a moderate amount of oat in a gluten-free diet did not prevent clinical or small intestinal mucosal healing or a humoral immunologic response.[30] Also, a recent 2-year controlled trial showed that oat had no detrimental effect on intestinal histology, mucosal intraepithelial inflammatory cells counts, or serology in children. In contrast, the gluten-challenge group relapsed after 3 to 12 months. Complete mucosal recovery from the disease was accomplished in all relapsed and newly detected patients on an oat-containing gluten-free diet. Long-term, up to 7 years follow-up of children consuming oat, showed that they all remained in remission.[31] Cereal toxicity studies using in vitro organ culture also point in the direction of nonharmfulness.[32,33] However, a patient intolerant to oat was identified,[34] and avenin-reactive mucosal T-cells have been detected in some patients with celiac disease.[35] It seems evident that, in rare cases, there are celiac disease patients who are intolerant to oat. They should be identified, and their diet should be designed not to contain oat. Further, oat products free of wheat and barley contamination are warranted.[36]

GENETIC FACTORS

Celiac disease is a multifactorial disease in which, in addition to environmental triggers, inherited factors confer susceptibility. A clear observable clue to genetic susceptibility is the tendency of the disease to run in families.[6] The disease prevalence among the first-degree relatives of a proband has varied from 1 to 18%, often, as a rule, at about 10%.[37] The low-prevalence figures may be due to different screening strategies or the tendency of the disease to develop late, meaning that it is found in individuals who once had been excluded for the disease.[38,39] Celiac disease is also found in healthy relatives of multiple case families.[40,41]

The concordance and discordance rates of monozygotic and dizygotic twin pairs are often compared to define the balance between environmental and genetic factors of a disease. In large celiac disease twin studies from Italy, the concordance rate of monozygotic twins above 80% compared with 20% in dizygotic twins.[42,43] This indicates that genes play a very important role. The literature is also knowledgeable of reported discordance in monozygotic twins, in which concordance has developed later.[43] One should also remember that monozygotic twins are genetically not identical. The differences come from point mutations, skewed X-chromosomal inactivation, nondisjunctions, and gene rearrangements of immunoglobulin and T-cell receptors. Recently, it was clearly shown that one identical twin may have intestinal celiac disease, whereas the other

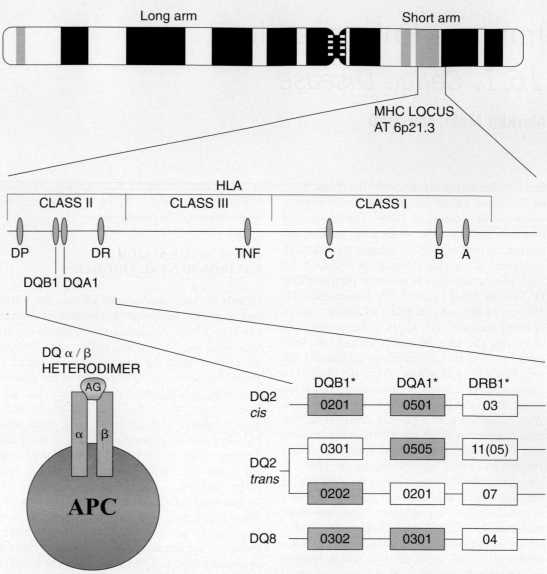

Figure 2 Human major histocompatibility complex (MHC) location in chromosome 6 short arm. In this locus, the key genetic risk factors for celiac disease and dermatitis herpetiformis, the human leukocyte antigen (HLA) class II genes DQA1*05 and DQB1*02 encoding the DQ2 alpha/beta heterodimer molecule are located. Individuals who have DR3 (the gene DRB1*03) almost always, owing to linkage disequilibrium, carry also the DQ alleles DQA1*0501 and DQB1*0201 in the *cis* position, that is, on the same chromosome. The genes encoding the DQ2 molecule may also be on different chromosomes, in *trans* position, DQA1*05 in linkage with DR5 (DRB1*11) and DQB1*02 in linkage with DR7 (DRB1*07). The genes encoding the DQ8 alpha/beta heterodimer are located in the DR4 haplotype. The HLA class II molecules are situated on antigen-presenting cells (APC), and they have a groove where the antigen (AG) peptides are presented to T helper cells.

suffers from dermatitis herpetiformis, the gluten-induced skin manifestation of the same disease.[44]

The major histocompatibility complex (MHC) on chromosome 6 short arm (Figure 2) comprises a gene cluster including the HLA class II genes. The HLA genes are highly variable and polymorphic, which forms the basis for the immune system to recognize foreign and self-antigens, processed and presented by antigen-presenting cells. Certain HLA alleles are found to be associated with diseases, either in a protective or a predisposing manner, and many of these diseases are of autoimmune nature. Celiac disease is strongly associated with the HLA class II extended haplotype DR3-DQ2 or DR5/7-DQ2. The DQ2 molecule, an alpha/beta heterodimer, is located on the surfaces of cells involved in immune responses and is encoded by the alleles DQA1*0501 and DQB1*02 (in *cis*, in which both risk alleles are located in the same chromosome in linkage with DR3, and in *trans*, in which the individual is heterozygote for DR5 and DR7) (see Figure 2). Approximately 90% of the celiac disease patients carry the DQ2 molecule, and 10% of the patients are positive for DQ8 (DR4 haplotype), in which the alpha/beta heterodimer is encoded by the genes *DQA1*0301* and *DQB1*0302*.[7,45,46] A large European multicenter study gave further evidence of the strong association to the risk alleles described above: from 1,008 celiac disease patients, 61 were identified to be negative for both DQ2 and DQ8.

Fifty-seven of these encoded half of the DQ2 heterodimer. Only 4 were found to be negative for all known risk alleles.[47] Individuals not carrying any of the risk genes have a very low probability of developing celiac disease. Clinicians may take advantage of this knowledge, and a negative test for both DQ2 and DQ8 speaks against celiac disease.[48] Also, an HLA-DQ genotyping will provide an accurate information to parents of the risk that siblings of children with celiac disease will also develop the disease.[49] On the other hand, even if most celiac disease patients carry the risk alleles, it must be borne in mind that in whites, 15 to 20% of the general population are DQ2 positive and another 20% are DQ8 positive. Owing to the extremely low DR3 gene frequencies in countries such as China and Japan and in some Black African countries, the probability of diagnosing celiac disease is very low.

HLA genes are important but not sufficient to predispose them to celiac disease. Therefore, it is probable that other genes outside the HLA region are involved in celiac disease susceptibility. Recently, autosomal genomic screenings have provided evidence of linkage of several non-HLA loci to celiac disease.[50,51] There is now strong evidence of linkage at two non-HLA regions, chromosomes 5q31–33[52] and 19p13.1.[53] The linkage to a certain chromosome region does not, however, indicate which genes might be involved. One of the future targets for celiac disease research is to identify these genes and study their role in the disease. One such gene might be the *MYO9B* gene located on chromosome 19.[54]

PATHOGENESIS

Several major hypotheses regarding the nature of the primary host defect in celiac disease have been proposed during the past decades, namely, the missing enzyme theory, the immunologic hypothesis, the membrane glycoprotein defect, and the mucosal permeability defect. When the pathogenetic mechanisms are known, it may turn out that all of the above mentioned and some so far unknown mechanisms are operative.

Today, there is strong evidence that celiac disease is a T-cell–mediated chronic inflammatory bowel disorder with an autoimmune component, clinically also with extraintestinal manifestations. There are three prominent features of celiac disease: (1) it is induced solely by an environmental trigger, the ingested cereal gluten and the

disease remission is highly dependent on a strict gluten-free diet; (2) it requires a unique genetic background for antigen presentation—expression of the HLA class II molecules DQ2 or DQ8; and (3) the ingested gluten mediates both intestinal adaptive and innate immune responses,[10,55,56] where TG-2, the autoantigen, is also targeted by specific autoantibodies.[8]

What is remarkable is the connection between these three characteristics: Partially digested gluten peptides are able to enter the lamina propria where TG-2–deamidated peptides are presented by antigen presenting cells in the context of DQ2 or DQ8 molecules to helper T-cells, resulting in activation of specific CD4+ T-cells and further release of mediators, also interferon-gamma, that ultimately lead to tissue damage. Parallel to this, B-cells receive signals and, by an unknown mechanism, turn against the self, TG-2, and start producing autoantibodies.

It had been evident for some time, that wheat-derived gliadin peptides do not bind to the HLA DQ2 and DQ8 molecule grooves, thought to be a prerequisite for antigen presentation and initiation of gluten-induced inflammatory T-cell responses. These class II molecules have a predilection to peptides having amino acids with a negative charge, missing in the gliadins. In 1998 it was shown that the autoantigen of the disease, TG-2, specifically deamidates gliadin peptides, resulting in peptides with negatively charged residues at certain anchor positions, ie, certain glutamines (Q in Figure 3) have been converted to glutamic acids,[57,58] thus enabling the peptides to bind to the class II molecule groove and further triggering T-cell responses.

A large number of immunogenic peptides are present in a variety of gluten proteins.[10,55] T-cell populations that have several distinct gluten specificities can be derived from a single patient. On the other hand, there is a hierarchy of the epitopes in that some epitopes are recognized by T-cells from almost all patients, whereas others have reactivity only in a minority of celiac disease patients.[59] One remarkable feature of T-cell–stimulating gluten regions is the high content of proline residues. It is evident that prolines play a key role in determining the structure, immunogenicity, and proteolytic resistance of immunodominant gluten peptides.

A 33-mer fragment of an alpha-gliadin is resistant to intestinal digestion (Figure 3).[9] The 33-mer fragment has turned out to be an excellent substrate of TG-2, and it has been shown

to be able to activate T-cell clones derived from celiac disease patients. It contains a cluster of partially overlapping T-cell–stimulating epitopes (oligomerized epitopes). This kind of repetitive nature of epitopes enhances their T-cell activation potential.

A crucial question in understanding the pathomechanisms of celiac disease is why only gluten, of the many food proteins, brings about such a harmful immune response. The increased level of TG-2 expression in the mucosa of celiac patients seems to be related to inflammation.[8,57] Infection and inflammation, in turn, might breach the epithelial barrier of intestine and lead to harmful influx of gluten peptides into the lamina propria. The higher concentration of gluten peptides in the lamina propria and the abundant TG-2 would promote the formation of deamidated peptides.

Recent research evidence shows that gliadin peptides also act as a trigger of an innate immune response. By using in vitro organ cultures, Maiuri and colleagues demonstrated that intestinal immune reactions in celiac disease are partly driven by the (less specific) innate immune system, which provides a quick, so-called pattern recognition response to stimuli such as viral and bacterial proteins.[60] Maiuri and colleagues' data propose that certain gluten peptides (the toxic wheat gliadin peptide 31 to 49 or 31 to 43,[13,61] Figure 3) elicit by production of the cytokine interleukin (IL)-15 an early innate immune response, which could again initiate the immunodominant peptide-driven adaptive response,[62] dependent on HLA presentation, T-cell recognition, and T-cell expansion. In overt celiac disease IL-15 activates the intraepithelial lymphocytes, the role of which, even if being one marker of untreated celiac disease, has not earlier been understood. In fact, the intraepithelial lymphocytes act as effector cells that mediate, by upregulating natural killer receptors, the destruction of enterocytes by recognition of stress signals induced by gluten.[63–65]

In active celiac disease, the level of TG-2 expression is increased: TG-2 is expressed at the epithelial brush border and extracellularly in the subepithelial region.[8,57] TG-2 is a Ca^{2+}-dependent enzyme that modifies a whole range of proteins by cross-linking, transamidating, or deamidating specific polypeptide-bound glutamines.[66] Also, the ingested gluten drives the B-cells to target the autoantigen TG-2. The role of these disease-pathognomonic TG-2 autoantibodies in the pathogenesis of celiac disease is unclear and controversial, but they might not be just bystanders, an epiphenomenon. They have been shown to inhibit the differentiation of T84 crypt-like cells in a three-dimensional tissue culture model,[67] and may play an important role in epithelial cell proliferation in celiac disease.[68] Interestingly, these autoantibodies can be found deposited in the subepithelial region of normal-appearing intestinal biopsies, targeting TG-2 even before the infiltration of T-cells into lamina propria or the onset of evident celiac disease or even before the antibodies are measurable in the sera of patients.[69–73] In

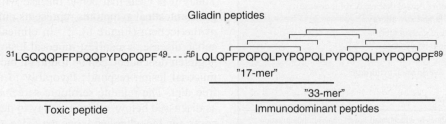

Gliadin peptides

³¹LGQQQPFPPQQPYPQPQPF⁴⁹----⁵⁶LQLQPFPQPQLPYPQPQLPYPQPQLPYPQPQPF⁸⁹

"17-mer"

"33-mer"

Toxic peptide   Immunodominant peptides

Figure 3 Amino acid sequences of part of domain I of A gliadin showing three proline- (P) and glutamine- (Q) rich peptides known to be either toxic or immunogenic for celiac disease (explained in the text). Within the immunodominant peptides, especially the 33-mer, several T-cell epitopes can be identified (oligomerized epitopes).

experimental animal models, oral administration of antigens induces systemic hyporesponsiveness, defined as oral tolerance.[74] Although it is not clear if oral tolerance operates in humans by this definition, it is obvious that the immune system of the gut tries to ensure that immune responses to food proteins are not mounted normally. Therefore, it can be envisaged that tolerance to gluten in celiac disease is either not established or is broken in early childhood. The absence of intestinal T-cell responses to gluten in nonceliacs and the preferential recognition of deamidated gluten peptides suggest that there is, in the beginning, tolerance to unmodified gluten fragments. Accordingly, deamidation and the altered affinity of modified peptides for DQ2 and DQ8 would be the key event leading to the disruption of tolerance in celiac disease patients. Another possibility is that gluten could function as an adjuvant factor in eliciting T-cell responses, or short gluten peptides might reach the underlying lamina propria of the gut at higher concentrations than do other food protein peptides.

CLINICAL DISEASE

Malabsorption Syndrome

Characteristically, celiac disease manifests during infancy and before school age. In the classic form of childhood celiac disease, symptoms and signs of malabsorption become obvious within some months of starting a gluten-containing diet. The child has chronic diarrhea or loose stools and vomiting, and the abdomen is distended (Table 1 and Figure 4). Typically, the child presents with failure to thrive, and proximal muscle wasting may be seen (see Figure 4). Young infants with a malabsorption syndrome and prolonged diarrhea, as presenting in the 1960s,[76–78] may be hypotonic and have other symptoms of severe enteropathy, for example, dehydration, hypoproteinemia, hypokalemia, hypoprothrombinemia, and hypocalcemia. Rickets may be a presenting symptom even in one-fourth of the children diagnosed for celiac disease.[79] In some communities, the delay

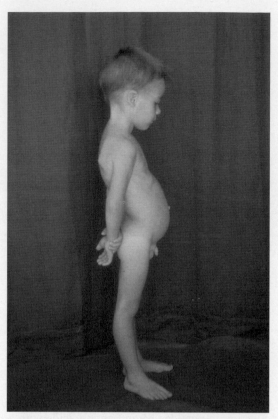

Figure 4   A 4-year-old boy with newly diagnosed celiac disease presenting with loose stools and recurrent abdominal pain. He also had growth retardation and muscle weakness. A distended abdomen is seen. (Courtesy of Dr Ilma Korponay-Szabo, Heim Pál Children's Hospital, Budapest, Hungary.)

in diagnosis might be due to the presence of other diseases clinically resembling celiac disease.[79] Table 2 lists disease conditions that may be interpreted as celiac disease also at a small intestinal mucosal level.

Presenting signs of malabsorption in celiac disease in older children may be short stature,[80–83] delayed puberty,[82] iron deficiency anemia,[82,84,85] and osteoporosis.[86] The older the child is, the more diffuse are the symptoms, and gastrointestinal symptoms may be totally missing.

Changing Clinical Features

Nowadays, celiac disease presenting with a malabsorption syndrome is an exception, not the rule, and a changing symptom pattern has been

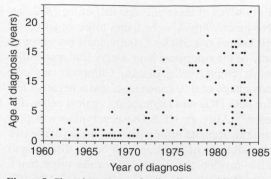

Figure 5   Changing pattern of celiac disease with decreasing numbers of cases diagnosed in young children and increasing numbers diagnosed at school age and adolescence after 1972. (Reproduced with permission from reference 82.)

experienced in most countries.[87,88] During the early 1980s, it was reported that childhood celiac disease was disappearing,[89,90] but this seemed not to be true. Rather, clinicians were experiencing a changing pattern of disease presentation with milder symptomatology and an increase in the age at diagnosis (Figure 5).[82,91] Later evidence has verified this to have been a general trend throughout Europe.[92]

One exception existed: Sweden. Ivarsson and colleagues described a countrywide epidemic of a chronic malabsorptive syndrome in infancy during a 10-year period from 1985 to 1995.[93] The annual incidence rate increased fourfold in children less than 2 years of age, when, at the same time, such cases disappeared in a neighboring country, Finland.[82,94] Before the epidemic in 1983, the recommendations for gluten introduction were changed from 4 to 6 months of age. Also, in 1983, the amount of gluten in industrially produced weaning food gruels and porridges in Sweden was doubled on average. The only difference between these two countries was the amount of gluten ingested by infants. Healthy infants in Sweden ingested two to three times more wheat protein than did infants in Finland. They also consumed 50% more than infants did in 1978, which was before the onset of increase in incidence.[94] Finnish infants again received more barley and oat. An important message here is that new authority directives or other changes within the community may change the disease panorama completely even during a short time period.

Case Finding

The observation that celiac disease exists in a completely asymptomatic form was obtained from gluten challenge[78,95] and family studies.[6,37] Today it is clear that celiac disease with typical gastrointestinal symptoms represents only the tip of the iceberg (Figure 6).[96,97] In clinically silent celiac disease, a manifest mucosal lesion, which is gluten dependent, can be found on biopsy. The mucosal lesion responds favorably to a gluten-free diet. The reliable serologic screening tools, as discussed below, allow us today to detect such cases. On the other hand, one may also argue that clinically silent celiac disease, as such, is just an undiagnosed condition.

Table 1 Data on 53 Consecutive Patients Suffering from Celiac Disease at Admission to the Children's Hospital, University of Helsinki, During the 1960s	
General data	
Number of patients	53
Age at onset of the symptoms (mo)	7.7
Gluten in the diet before the onset of symptoms (mo)	4.3
Age on admission (mo)	10.2
Symptoms	
Diarrhea or altered stools	87%
Vomiting	74%
Failure to gain weight	98%
Signs	
Weight below the 2.5 percentile	70%
Distended abdomen	64%
Adapted from Visakorpi.[75]	

Table 2   Differential Diagnosis*
Cow's milk protein intolerance
Gastroenteritis, bacteria, rotavirus
Inflammatory bowel disease (Crohn disease)
Cow's milk and soy allergy
Eosinophilic gastroenteritis
Immunodeficiency states
Giardiasis
Bacterial overgrowth syndrome
Drugs
Radiotherapy
*Disease states in which small-bowel mucosal inflammation or partial villous atrophy may occur (often not total villous atrophy with crypt hyperplasia).

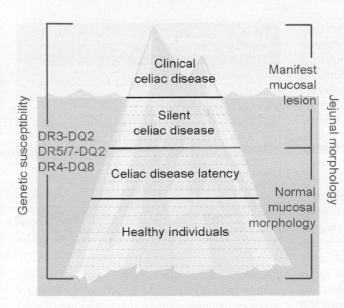

Figure 6 The iceberg of celiac disease. (Adapted with permission from reference 97.)

Celiac disease can be found in children with traditional symptoms and signs but in a very mild form (Table 3).[78] Abdominal discomfort, loose stools, flatulence problems, recurrent abdominal pain, and diagnosed lactose intolerance are conditions in which celiac disease should be sought. Arthritis and arthralgia may also be presenting symptoms in celiac disease.[98] As mentioned earlier, short stature, delayed puberty, and isolated nutritional deficiencies are already signs of malabsorption, even in cases with no gastrointestinal symptoms.

In addition to finding clinically silent celiac disease in healthy first-degree relatives of celiac disease patients,[6,37–41] the disease is highly prevalent in type 1 diabetes mellitus (2 to 12%),[99–103] in individuals with selective immunoglobulin A (IgA) deficiency (10%),[104] and in Down syndrome (10%).[105,106]

It is widely accepted that dermatitis herpetiformis is gluten induced, has the same genetic background as celiac disease,[44,46] and is a classic example of the extraintestinal manifestation of the disease.[107] Other linked disorders include permanent-tooth enamel defects,[108] central and peripheral nervous system involvement,[109,110] liver involvement,[111,112] and even autoimmune diseases in general.[113] A risk for a malignant complication of untreated celiac disease seems not to be as high as previously thought.[114]

DIAGNOSTIC CRITERIA

The gold standard for clinical diagnosis is the initially manifested small intestinal mucosal lesion, villous atrophy, together with crypt hyperplasia (Figure 7). Another characteristic is an increased density of intraepithelial lymphocytes.[115] Heavy cellular infiltrativity is not always present in untreated celiac disease. The European Society for Pediatric Gastroenterology, Hepatology and Nutrition (ESPGHAN; formerly ESPGAN) set the criteria for the diagnosis in 1970.[116] It was stated that a patient with absent or almost absent villi who shows definite improvement on a gluten-free diet cannot be designated as celiac disease before he has been proved to normalize on a dietary treatment, not only clinically but also histologically, and subsequently to relapse after reintroduction of gluten. This implies that three small intestinal biopsies should be performed. Also, a "2-year rule" was developed. It implicated that on gluten challenge, there should be a recurrence of the mucosal lesion within 2 years of gluten reintroduction. These strict criteria were later revised. However, the cornerstone remained the same, that is, in the initial biopsy, flat small intestinal mucosa should be found.[117] Neither repeated biopsy nor gluten challenge was considered mandatory in cases with full clinical remission after withdrawal of gluten from the diet. However, in uncertain cases, the old criteria may still be used, particularly when other diseases clinically complicate or resemble celiac disease (see Table 3).

Today clinicians may use new tools, serology (endomysial or TG-2 autoantibodies), and HLA-DQ typing. Positivity for the autoantibodies is an accurate indication of manifest small intestinal mucosal lesion (see below). On the other hand, negativity for the alleles encoding DQ2 and DQ8 speaks strongly against celiac disease.[48] In developing countries, the TG-2 autoantibody positivity is also highly indicative of celiac disease.[8,118] On a population-based level, the endomysial and

Table 3 Diagnostic Approach in Finding Celiac Disease in Individuals Without Clear Symptoms Suggesting Jejunal Mucosal Atrophy

Policy
High index of suspicion of celiac disease
Liberal use of serologic screening tests
Case finding in patient groups
Minor abdominal symptoms (abdominal discomfort, loose stools, recurrent abdominal pain, lactose intolerance)
Growth failure, delayed puberty, iron deficiency anemia, rickets
Other chronic or celiac disease related diseases (type 1 diabetes, thyroid disease, selective IgA deficiency)
Skin disorders, suspected dermatitis herpetiformis
Celiac-type, permanent tooth enamel defects
Joint symptoms as arthralgia, arthritis
Liver diseases
Some neurologic diseases
Down syndrome, Turner syndrome
Healthy first-degree relatives of celiac patients

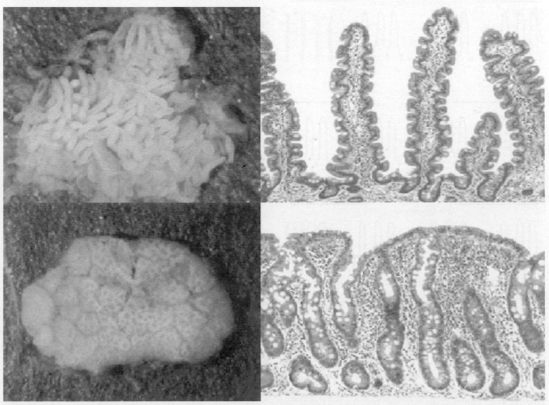

Figure 7 Dissection microscopic (*left*) (50× original magnification) and histologic sections (*right*) (hematoxylin and eoasin; 280× original magnification) of small intestinal mucosal biopsy specimen with normal mucosal morphology with high villi (*upper*) and celiac disease (*lower*) (subtotal villous atrophy with crypt hyperplasia).

TG-2 autoantibody positivity goes hand in hand with celiac disease-specific HLA-DQ markers.[119]

New Diagnostic Criteria Warranted

In celiac disease, small intestinal mucosal damage develops gradually, from normal morphology through inflammation to the so-called flat lesion (subtotal villous atrophy with crypt hyperplasia) (see Figure 7). This development is depicted in Figure 8, indicating the gradual process of mucosal deterioration, which may take years or even decades.[37–39,120–124] This means that when a child, an adult, or an elderly person on a gluten-containing diet has been shown to have a normal small intestinal mucosal morphology, even with no cellular inflammation, the disease is not excluded by conventional histology. The mucosa may deteriorate later.[125,126] A further demand on new criteria is obvious because patients suspected of having the disease, with correct HLA-DQ types but with only minor mucosal lesions and with an increased density of gamma/delta-positive intraepithelial lymphocytes, were shown to have a gluten-dependent disease and osteopenia.[127] Oral tolerance to gluten in celiac disease may be broken in some individuals only after decades. This may be due to the amount of gluten in the diet but also because other environmental factors may act as "second hits." When gluten is introduced in the infant's diet, the ingested amounts vary. Later, daily food may contain gluten from a gram to up to 15 to 30 g. With this "normal" diet, the mucosal lesion

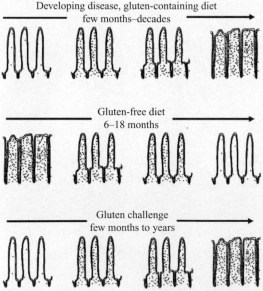

Figure 8 Schematic behavior of celiac disease small intestinal mucosa. *Upper row:* After starting a gluten-containing diet in infancy, the mucosa may deteriorate within a few months to that typical for celiac disease, villous atrophy with crypt hyperplasia. On the other hand, oral tolerance toward gluten may be kept for decades; the mucosa may be normal on morphology or show only a low-grade inflammation before deterioration. *Middle row:* The mucosa heals in 1 year on a gluten-free diet. *Lower row:* During gluten challenge, the mucosa may deteriorate within a few months, but it may also take years. The mucosal lesion in celiac disease is permanent, and a recurrence of the lesion will occur.

may manifest at any age. Celiac disease with only low-grade inflammation should be distinguished from other diseases (see Table 2). A potential new strong clinical tool may be the testing of small-bowel mucosal TG-2-targeted IgA deposits.[70–73] It can be foreseen that biopsy will not be the gold standard in the diagnosis of celiac disease in the future when the diagnostic criteria will be widened toward "celiac trait" or "genetic gluten intolerance."

When performing gluten challenge studies with "normal" food, it has become evident that the individual tolerance to gluten is variable (see Figure 8). Most individuals react with a mucosal lesion within 3 months to 2 years on gluten ingestion, but it may take even longer, up to 14 years, before the mucosa relapses. In a Finnish series of gluten challenge performed in 29 adolescents and young adults with previously confirmed and treated celiac disease, 4 girls did not relapse within 2 years, one relapse occurred after 7 years, and another relapse manifested with dermatitis herpetiformis after 14 years of gluten ingestion.[95] In the latter case, the small-bowel mucosal morphology remained normal.

SCREENING AND EPIDEMIOLOGY

Oral glucose tolerance tests, fecal fat excretion, D-xylose excretion tests, hematologic investigations, and radiologic examination of the small bowel failed to distinguish patients with suspected malabsorption from those with or without mucosal atrophy and, thus, frequently gave misleading results.[128] Guidelines for the diagnosis and treatment of celiac disease do not any more recommend these clinical malabsorption tests to be used.[88] Intestinal permeability tests are not widely used as screening methods. However, autoantibodies have been shown to be highly predictive for untreated celiac disease. When there is a suspicion of celiac disease or the antibodies are positive, small intestinal biopsy should be the first diagnostic procedure. Often serum autoantibody tests direct the patient to the invasive diagnostic test.

In the United States, the disease is rare when the criteria for diagnosis rely on classic symptoms such as diarrhea and short stature.[129] By broadening the clinical indication, however, antibody screening seems to indicate that the prevalence in the United States is similar to that in Europe.[130] This is confirmed in large-scale screening programs.[131] Screening programs within childhood populations indicate that celiac disease is heavily underdiagnosed, and serologic testing using endomysial and TG-2 autoantibodies has the potential to detect otherwise undiagnosed disease in even more than 1 in 100 individuals (Table 4).[119,132–138] However, it should be remembered that subclinical cases of celiac disease will not be detected by screening only selected groups of at-risk patients.[96,119] Early detection of the disease and subsequent dietary elimination of gluten might be an appropriate method for preventing com-

Table 4 Prevalence of Celiac Disease in Children in Various Countries

Geographic Areas	Prevalence	Study
North Africa, Saharawi people	1:18	Catassi et al[132]
Hungary	1:85	Korponay-Szabo et al[133]
Italy	1:95	Meloni et al[134]
Finland	1:99	Mäki et al[119]
Sweden	1:100	Carlsson et al[135]
The United States	1:104	Hoffenberg et al[136]
The Netherlands	1:198	Csizmadia et al[137]
Germany	1:500	Henker et al[138]

plications later in life. Today, however, we use mainly directed case finding screening. Figure 9 gives an example of the value of the use of antibody screening in one hospital: during 15 years, new cases per year have increased over 10-fold. Currently, population-based screening programs are used only in research.

Serologic Screening Tools

Serum gluten and milk antibody tests, performed with immunodiffusion techniques, were already promising in an early series of celiac disease patients.[77,78] As reviewed by Mäki, various methods have been developed to determine gliadin antibodies in serum: immunofluorescence, enzyme-linked immunosorbent assay (ELISA), diffusion-in-gel ELISA, solid-phase radioimmunoassay, and strip ELISA.[139] These antibodies have frequently been found in patients with untreated celiac disease, but the sensitivities and specificities of the tests have been unsatisfactory, and are not recommended for use any more.[88] However, gliadin antibody ELISA tests, using deamidated gliadin peptides as antigens, may turn out to be highly accurate in clinical practice.[140] The currently used autoantibody tests have been in use since 1971,[139] and by measuring the IgA class R1-type reticulin antibodies, sensitivities and specificities became high, close to 100%.[141] The endomysial autoantibody test, with

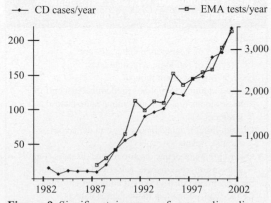

Figure 9 Significant increase of new celiac disease (CD) cases per year is obvious after starting the endomysial antibody (EMA) testing in 1987 in the Heim Pál Children's Hospital, Budapest, Hungary. (Courtesy of Dr Ilma Korponay-Szabo, Heim Pál Children's Hospital, Budapest, Hungary.)

human umbilical cord tissue as a substrate, was widely used and was standardized and ring-tested to detect untreated celiac disease.[142] Following the identification of tissue transglutaminase as the target in rodent and primate tissues for celiac disease-specific autoantibodies, a non–observer-dependent ELISA method was developed and was used to detect the antibodies.[8,143–147] Recently, a self TG-2-based rapid fingertip whole blood test proved to be as accurate as the conventional serum-based tests to detect celiac disease.[148] In contrast to conventional gliadin antibodies, the serum endomysial and TG-2 autoantibodies are genetically determined and correlate strongly with the celiac-type HLA genetics.[37,40,119]

TREATMENT

In celiac disease, a lifelong gluten-free diet is the only effective treatment. Wheat-, rye-, and barley-based products should be avoided. Even if oat, by definition, is "gluten," its prolamin avenin seems not to be disease inducing. In Finland, the United Kingdom, and other northern European countries, industrially purified wheat starch-based gluten-free flours have been accepted as part of the gluten-free diet for over 40 years. A minority of patients in Finland have been prescribed a natural gluten-free diet. On the other hand, in many countries, a zero limit is demanded, thus not allowing the use of purified wheat starch-based flours. On a long-term gluten-free diet including wheat starch-based gluten-free flours, no increased mortality, malignancies, or morbidity in the celiac disease patients over the population in general were observed.[149] On the prescribed diet, the mucosa heals and stays morphometrically normal over 10 years of flour ingestion.[150] Recently, it was concluded from a controlled study that wheat starch containing gluten-free flour products were acceptable in the gluten-free diet. No differences were observed in clinical responses; small-bowel mucosal morphology; intraepithelial T-cell densities; mucosal HLA-DR expression; serum endomysial, TG-2, or gliadin antibody levels; quality of life measurements; or bone mineral densities when compared with the group on a diet that was gluten free by nature.[151]

The daily intake of gluten by the patients can be measured. The gluten levels in the products can be determined using the new R5 ELISA method, thus allowing an estimate of even trace amounts of gluten in the gluten-free diet.[152] It should be remembered that also natural gluten-free products may contain gluten because of cross contamination. Available data suggest that a maximum gluten content for gluten-free food could be set, which protect celiac disease patients.[153] On the other hand, if compliance to any given gluten-free diet is poor, the patient may ingest daily several grams of gluten.[154]

Negative seroconversion in the celiac-type autoantibodies during treatment follow-up is a strong indicator of mucosal healing. Failure of the antibodies to decline over a period of 6 months suggests continuation of gluten intake.

FUTURE INSIGHTS

Our increasing knowledge of the molecular and cellular details of events leading to celiac disease should benefit patients. The knowledge of the harmful gluten epitopes should facilitate our ability to genetically modify these epitopes in grains without losing their baking properties. The large number of T-cell epitopes and the complexity of wheat genetics complicate manipulation of wheat to remove toxic peptides.[155] An alternative strategy might be to inhibit the deamidation process by developing TG-2–specific inhibitors.[11] However, the inhibitors should be designed to inhibit only the deamidation activity of TG-2, not the other enzymatic activities or structural properties of TG-2. One approach could be to use enzyme-supplement therapy (eg, bacterial or plant prolyl endopeptidase or other proline-specific enzymes) to destruct the proteolytically resistant proline-rich fragments of gluten proteins.[9] This approach is attractive and practical because the protease could be ingested along with a diet containing gluten. However, the enzyme should be present in large amounts, and it should work very efficiently in the correct place (upper part of small intestine) to prevent undigested peptides from activating T cells in the small intestine. Interference with the stimulation of $CD4^+$ gluten-specific T-cells, their eradication, or silencing could be another effective way to control the disease. Alternatively, blocking the peptide-binding sites of DQ2 and DQ8 HLA molecules could prevent the presentation of disease-inducing gluten fragments to T cells. One more potential strategy is blockade of signals derived from the cytokine interleukin-15 (part of innate immunity). We should not forget, however, that a gluten-exclusion diet is a safe treatment, although it is not convenient or easy to comply with. New therapeutic approaches must outweigh the current gluten-free therapy with regard to costs and safety.

REFERENCES

1. Gee S. On the coeliac affection. St Bartholomew's Hospital Reports 1888;24:17–20.
2. Dicke WK. Coeliakie [thesis]. Utrecht (the Netherlands): University of Utrecht; 1950.
3. Weijers HA, Lindqvist B, Anderson ChM, et al. Diagnostic criteria in coeliac disease. Acta Paediatr Scand 1970;59:461–3.
4. Seah PP, Fry L, Hoffbrand AV, Holborow EJ. Tissue antibodies in dermatitis herpetiformis and adult coeliac disease. Lancet 1971;i:834–6.
5. Seah PP, Fry L, Rossiter MA, et al. Anti-reticulin antibodies in childhood coeliac disease. Lancet 1971;ii:681–2.
6. MacDonald WC, Dobbins WO, Rubin CE. Studies on the familial nature of celiac sprue using biopsy of the small intestine. N Engl J Med 1965;272:448–56.
7. Sollid LM, Markussen G, Ek J, et al. Evidence for a primary association of celiac disease to a particular HLA-DQ alpha/beta heterodimer. J Exp Med 1989;169:345–50.
8. Dieterich W, Ehnis T, Bauer M, et al. Identification of tissue transglutaminase as the autoantigen of celiac disease. Nat Med 1997;3:797–801.
9. Shan L, Molberg O, Parrot I, et al. Structural basis for gluten intolerance in celiac sprue. Science 2002;297:2275–9.
10. Koning F, Schuppan D, Cerf-Bensussan N, Sollid LM. Pathomechanisms in celiac disease. Best Pract Res Clin Gastroenterol 2005;19:373–87.
11. Sollid LM, Khosla C. Future therapeutic options for celiac disease. Nat Clin Pract Gastroenterol Hepatol 2005;2:140–7.
12. Kasarda DD. Gluten and gliadin: Precipitating factors in coeliac disease. In: Mäki M, Collin P, Visakorpi JK, editors. Coeliac disease. Proceedings of the Seventh International Symposium on Coeliac Disease. Coeliac Disease Study Group. Tampere (Finland): University of Tampere; 1997. p. 195–212.
13. de Ritis G, Auricchio S, Jones HW, et al. In vitro (organ culture) studies of the toxicity of specific A-gliadin peptides in celiac disease. Gastroenterology 1988;94:41–9.
14. Vader LW, deRu A, ven der Wal Y, et al. Specificity of tissue transglutaminase explains cereal toxicity in celiac disease. J Exp Med 2002;195:643–9.
15. Janatuinen EK, Pikkarainen PH, Kemppainen TA, et al. A comparison of diets with and without oats in adults with celiac disease. N Engl J Med 1995;333:1033–7.
16. Dicke WK, Weijers HA, van de Kamer JH. Coeliac disease. II. The presence in wheat of a factor having a deleterious effect in cases of coeliac disease. Acta Paediatr 1953;42:34–42.
17. Baker PG, Read AE. Oats and barley toxicity in coeliac patients. Postgrad Med J 1976;52:264–8.
18. Moulton ALC. The place of oats in the coeliac diet. Arch Dis Child 1959;3:51–5.
19. Sheldon W. Coeliac disease. Lancet 1955;ii:1097–103.
20. Dissanayake AS, Truelove SC, Whitehead R. Lack of harmful effect of oats on small-intestinal mucosa in coeliac disease. BMJ 1974;4:189–91.
21. Srinivasan U, Leonard N, Jones E, et al. Absence of oats toxicity in adult coeliac disease. BMJ 1996;313:1300–1.
22. Srinivasan U, Jones E, Weir DG, Feighery C. Lactase enzyme, detected immunohistochemically, is lost in active celiac disease, but unaffected by oats challenge. Am J Gastroenterol 1999;94:2936–41.
23. Janatuinen EK, Kemppainen TA, Julkunen RJ, et al. No harm from five year ingestion of oats in coeliac disease. Gut 2002;50:332–5.
24. Storsrud S, Olsson M, Arvidsson Lenner R, et al. Adult coeliac patients do tolerate large amounts of oats. Eur J Clin Nutr 2003;57:163–9.
25. Storsrud S, Hulthen LR, Lennert RA. Beneficial effects of oats in the gluten-free diet of adults with special reference to nutrient status, symptoms and subjective experiences. Br J Nutr 2003;90:101–7.
26. Peräaho M, Collin P, Kaukinen K, et al. Oats can diversify a gluten-free diet in celiac disease and dermatitis herpetiformis. J Am Diet Assoc 2004;104:1148–50.
27. Hardman CM, Garioch JJ, Leonard JN. Absence of toxicity of oats in patients with dermatitis herpetiformis. N Engl J Med 1997;337:1884–7.
28. Reunala T, Collin P, Holöm K, et al. Tolerance to oats in dermatitis herpetiformis. Gut 1998;43:490–3.
29. Hoffenberg EJ, Haas J, Drescher A, et al. A trial of oats in children with newly diagnosed celiac disease. J Pediatr 2000;137:361–6.
30. Högberg L, Laurin P, Fälth-Magnusson K, et al. Oats to children with newly diagnosed coeliac disease: A randomized, double-blind study. Gut 2004;53:649–54.
31. Holm K, Mäki M, Vuolteenaho N, et al. Oats in the treatment of childhood coeliac disease: A 2-year controlled trial and a long-term clinical follow-up study. Aliment Pharmacol Ther 2006;23:1463–72.
32. Picarelli A, Di Tola M, Sabbatella L, et al. Immunologic evidence of no harmful effect of oats in celiac disease. Am J Clin Nutr 2001;74:137–40.
33. Kilmartin C, Lynch S, Abuzakouk M, et al. Avenin fails to induce a Th1 response in coeliac tissue following in vitro culture. Gut 2003;52:47–52.
34. Lundin KE, Nilsen EM, Scott HG, et al. Oats induced villous atrophy in coeliac disease. Gut 2003;52:1649–52.
35. Arentz-Hansen H, Fleckenstein B, Molberg O, et al. The molecular basis for oat intolerance in patients with celiac disease. PloS Med 2004;1:e1.
36. Thomson T. Gluten contamination of commercial oat products in the United States. N Engl J Med 2004;351:2021–2.
37. Mäki M, Holm K, Lipsanen V, et al. Serological markers and HLA genes among healthy first-degree relatives of patients with coeliac disease. Lancet 1991;338:1350–3.
38. Pittschieler K, Gentili L, Niederhofer H. Onset of coeliac disease: A prospective longitudinal study. Acta Paediatr 2003;92:1149–52.
39. Högberg L, Fälth-Magnusson K, Grodzinsky E, Stenhammar L. Familiar prevalence of coeliac disease: A twenty-year follow-up study. Scand J Gastroenterol 2003;38:61–5.
40. Mustalahti K, Sulkanen S, Holopainen S, et al. Coeliac disease among healthy members of multiple case coeliac disease families. Scand J Gastroenterol 2002;37:161–5.
41. Book L, Zone JJ, Neuhausen SL. Prevalence of celiac disease among relatives of sib pairs with celiac disease in U.S. families. Am J Gastroenterol 2003;98:377–81.

42. Greco L, Romino R, Coto I, et al. The first large population based twin study of coeliac disease. Gut 2002;50:624–8.
43. Nistico L, Fagnani C, Coto I, et al. Concordance, disease progression, and heritability of coeliac disease in Italian twins. Gut 2006;55:803–8.
44. Hervonen K, Karell K, Holopainen P, et al. Concordance of dermatitis herpetiformis and celiac disease in monozygous twins. J Invest Dermatol 2000;115:990–3.
45. Sollid LM, Thorsby E. HLA susceptibility genes in celiac disease: Genetic mapping and role in pathogenesis. Gastroenterology 1993;105:910–22.
46. Spurkland A, Ingvarsson G, Falk ES, et al. Dermatitis herpetiformis and celiac disease are both primarily associated with HLA-DQ (alpha 1*0501, beta 1*02) or the HLA-DQ (alpha 1*03, beta 1*0302) heterodimers. Tissue Antigens 1997;49:29–34.
47. Karell K, Louka AS, Moodie SJ, et al. HLA types in celiac disease patients not carrying the DQA1*05-DQB1*02 (DQ2) heterodimer: Results from the European genetics cluster on celiac disease. Hum Immunol 2003;64:469–77.
48. Kaukinen K, Partanen J, Mäki M, Collin P. HLA-DQ typing in the diagnosis of celiac disease. Am J Gastroenterol 2002;97:695–9.
49. Bourgey MM, Calcagno GG, Tunto NN, et al. HLA-related genetic risk for coeliac disease. Gut 2007;56:1054–59.
50. Zhong F, McCombs CC, Olson JM, et al. An autosomal screen for genes that predispose to celiac disease in the western counties of Ireland. Nat Genet 1996;14:329–33.
51. Greco L, Corazza G, Babron MC, et al. Genome search in celiac disease. Am J Hum Genet 1998;62:669–75.
52. Babron MC, Nilsson S, Adamovic S, et al. Meta and pooled analysis of European coeliac disease data. Eur J Hum Genet 2003;11:828–34.
53. Van Belzen MJ, Meijer JW, Sandkuijl LA, et al. A major non-HLA locus in celiac disease maps to chromosome 19. Gastroenterology 2003;125:1032–41.
54. Monsuur AJ, de Bakker PI, Alizadeh BZ, et al. Myosin IXB variant increases the risk of celiac disease and points toward a primary intestinal barrier defect. Nat Genet 2005;37:1341–4.
55. Jabri B, Sollid LM. Mechanisms of disease: Immunopathogenesis of celiac disease. Nat Clin Pract Gastroenterol Hepatol 2006;3:516–25.
56. Kagnoff MF. Celiac disease: Pathogenesis of a model immunogenetic disease. J Clin Invest 2007;117:41–9.
57. Molberg O, Macadam SN, Korner R, et al. Tissue transglutaminase selectively modifies gliadin peptides that are recognized by gut-derived T-cells. Nat Med 1998;4:713–7.
58 van de Wal Y, Kooy YMC, van Veelen P, et al. Selective deamidation by tissue transglutaminase strongly enhances gliadin-specific T cell reactivity. J Immunol 1998;161:1585–8.
59. Vader W, Kooy Y, van Veelen P, et al. The gluten response in children with celiac disease is directed toward multiple gliadin and glutenin peptides. Gastroenterology 2002;122:1729–37.
60. Maiuri L, Ciacci C, Ricciardelli I, et al. Association between innate response to gliadin and activation of pathogenic T cells in celiac disease. Lancet 2003;362:30–7.
61. Sturgess R, Day P, Ellis HJ, et al. Wheat peptide challenge in coeliac disease. Lancet 1994;343:758–61.
62. Anderson RP, Degano P, Godkin AJ, et al. In vivo antigen challenge in celiac disease identifies a single transglutaminase-modified peptide as the dominant A-gliadin T-cell epitope. Nat Med 2000;6:337–42.
63. Meresse B, Chen Z, Ciszewski C, et al. Coordinated induction by IL15 of a TCR-independent NKG2D signalling pathway converts CTL into lymphokine-activated killer cells in celiac disease. Immunity 2004;21:357–66.
64. Hüe S, Mention JJ, Monteiro RC, et al. a direct role of NKG2D/MICA interaction in villous atrophy during celiac disease. Immunity 2004;21:367–77.
65. Meresse B, Curran SA, Ciszewski C, et al. Reprogramming of CTL into natural killer-like cells in celiac disease. J Exp Med 2006;203:1343–55.
66. Lorand L, Graham RM. Transglutaminases: Crosslinking enzymes with pleiotropic functions. Nat Rev Mol Cell Biol 2003;4:140–56.
67. Halttunen T, Mäki M. Serum immunoglobulin A from patients with celiac disease inhibits human T84 intestinal crypt epithelial cell differentiation. Gastroenterology 1999;116:566–72.
68. Barone MV, Caputio I, Ribecco MT, et al. Humoral immune response to tissue transglutaminase is related to epithelial cell proliferation in celiac disease. Gastroenterology 2007; 132:1245–53.
69. Shiner M, Ballard J. antigen-antibody reactions in jejunal mucosa in childhood coeliac disease after gluten challenge. Lancet 1972;i:1202–5.
70. Korponay-Szabo IR, Halttunen T, Szalai Z, et al. In vivo targeting of intestinal and extraintestinal transglutaminase 2 by coeliac autoantibodies. Gut 2004;53:641–8.
71. Kaukinen K, Peräaho M, Collin P, et al. Small-bowel mucosal transglutaminase 2-specific IgA deposits in coeliac disease without villous atrophy: A prospective and randomized clinical study. Scand J Gastroenterol 2005;40:564–72.
72. Salmi TT, Collin P, Järvinen, et al. Immunoglobulin A autoantibodies against transglutaminase 2 in the small intestinal mucosa predict forthcoming coeliac disease. Aliment Pharmacol Ther 2006;24:541–52.
73. Salmi TT, Collin P, Korponay-Szabo IR, et al. Endomysial antibody-negative coeliac disease: Clinical characteristics and intestinal autoantibody deposits. Gut 2006;55:1746–53.
74. Weiner HL. Oral tolerance: Immune mechanisms and treatment of autoimmune diseases. Immunol Today 1997;18: 335–43.
75. Visakorpi JK. Changing features of coeliac disease. In: Mäki M, Collin P, Visakorpi JK, editors. Coeliac disease. Proceedings of the Seventh International Symposium on Coeliac Disease. Coeliac Disease Study Group. Tampere (Finland): University of Tampere; 1997. p. 1–7.
76. Visakorpi JK, Immonen P, Kuitunen P. Malabsorption syndrome in childhood. The occurrence of absorption defects and their clinical significance. Acta Paediatr Scand 1967;56:1–9.
77. Visakorpi JK, Immonen P. Intolerance to cow's milk and wheat gluten in the primary malabsorption syndrome in infancy. Acta Paediatr Scand 1967;56:49–56.
78. Visakorpi JK, Kuitunen P, Savilahti E. Frequency and nature of relapses in children suffering from the malabsorption syndrome with gluten intolerance. Acta Paediatr Scand 1970;59:481–6.
79. Rawashdeh MO, Khalil B, Raweily E. Celiac disease in Arabs. J Pediatr Gastroenterol Nutr 1996;23:415–8.
80. Verkasalo M, Kuitunen P, Leisti S, Perheentupa J. Growth failure from symptomless celiac disease. A study of 14 patients. Helv Paediatr Acta 1978;33:489–95.
81. Cacciari E, Salardi S, Volta U, et al. Can antigliadin antibody detect symptomless coeliac disease in children with short stature? Lancet 1985;i:1469–71.
82. Mäki M, Kallonen K, Lähdeaho M-L, Visakorpi JK. Changing pattern of childhood coeliac disease in Finland. Acta Paediatr Scand 1988;77:408–12.
83. Bonamico M, Scire G, Mariani P, et al. Short stature as the primary manifestation of monosymptomatic celiac disease. J Pediatr Gastroenterol Nutr 1992;14:12–6.
84. Carroccio A, Iannitto E, Cavataio E, et al. Sideropenic anemia and celiac disease: One study, two points of view. Dig Dis Sci 1998;43:673–8.
85. Demir H, Yuce A, Kocak N, et al. Celiac disease in Turkish children: Presentation of 104 cases. Pediatr Int 2000;42:483–7.
86. Mora S, Barera A, Ricotti A, et al. Reversal of low bone density with a gluten-free diet in children and adolescents with celiac disease. Am J Clin Nutr 1998;67:477–81.
87. Hill ID, Bhatnagar S, Cameron DJS, et al. Celiac disease: Working group report of the First World Congress of Pediatric Gastroenterology, Hepatology, and Nutrition. J Pediatr Gstroenterol Nutr 2002;35:S78–88.
88. Hill ID, Dirks MH, Liptak GS, et al. Guideline for the diagnosis and treatment of celiac disease in children: Recommendations of the North American Society for Pediatric Gastroenterology, Hepatology and Nutrition. J Pediatr Gastroenterol Nutr 2005;40:1–19.
89. Dossetor JF, Gibson AA, McNeish AS. Childhood coeliac disease is disappearing. Lancet 1981;i:322–3.
90. Stevens FM, Egan-Mitchell B, Cryan E, et al. Decreasing incidence of coeliac disease. Arch Dis Child 1987;62:465–8.
91. Mäki M, Holm K. Incidence and prevalence of coeliac disease in Tampere. Coeliac disease is not disappearing. Acta Paediatr Scand 1990;79:980–2.
92. Greco L, Mäki M, Di Donato F, Visakorpi JK. Epidemiology of coeliac disease in Europe and the mediterranean area. A summary report on the multicentre study by the European Society of Paediatric Gastroenterology and Nutrition. In: Auricchio S, Visakorpi JK, editors. Common food intolerances 1: Epidemiology of coeliac disease. Dyn Nutr Res 1992;2:25–44.
93. Ivarsson A, Persson LA, Nyström L, et al. Epidemic of coeliac disease in Swedish children. Acta Paediatr 2000;89:165–71.
94. Ascher H, Holm K, Kristiansson B, Mäki M. Different features of coeliac disease in two neighbouring countries. Arch Dis Child 1993;69:375–80.
95. Mäki M, Lähdeaho M-L, Hällström O, et al. Postpubertal gluten challenge in coeliac disease. Arch Dis Child 1989;64:1604–7.
96. Catassi C, Rätsch IM, Fabiani E, et al. Coeliac disease in the year 2000: Exploring the iceberg. Lancet 1994;343:200–3.
97. Mäki M, Collin P. Coeliac disease. Lancet 1997;349:1755–9.
98. Mäki M, Hällstöm O, Verronen P, et al. Reticulin antibody, arthritis, and coeliac disease in children. Lancet 1988;i:479–80.
99. Mäki M, Hällström O, Huupponen T, et al. Increased prevalence of coeliac disease in diabetes. Arch Dis Child 1984;59:739–42.
100. Holmes GK. Screening for coeliac disease in type 1 diabetes. Arch Dis Child 2002;87:495–8.
101. Baptista ML, Koda YK, Mitsunori R, et al. prevalence of celiac disease in Brazilian children and adolescents with type 1 diabetes mellitus. J Pediatr Gastroenterol Nutr 2005;41:621–4.
102. Mahmud FH, Murray JA, Kudve YC, et al. Celiac disease in type 1 diabetes mellitus in a North American community: Prevalence, serologic screening, and clinical features. Mayo Clin Proc 2005;80:1429–34.
103. Hansen D, Brock-Jacobsen B. Lund E, et al. Clinical benefit of a gluten-free diet in type 1 diabetic children with screening-detected celiac disease: A population-based screening study with 2 years' follow-up. Diabetes Care 2006;29:2452–6.
104. Korponay-Szabo IR, Dahlbom I, Laurila K, et al. Elevation of IgG antibodies against tissue transglutaminase as a diagnostic tool for coeliac disease in selective IgA deficiency. Gut 2003;52:1567–71.
105. Carlsson A, Axelsson I, Borulf S, et al. Prevalence of IgA-antigliadin antibodies and IgA-antiendomysium antibodies related to celiac disease in children with Down syndrome. Pediatrics 1998;101:272–5.
106. Book L, Hart A, Black J, et al. Prevalence and clinical characteristics of celiac disease in Down's syndrome in a US study. Am J Med Genet 2001;98:70–4.
107. Reunala T, Kosnai I, Karpati S, et al. Dermatitis herpetiformis: Jejunal findings and skin response to gluten-free diet. Arch Dis Child 1984;59:517–22.
108. Aine L, Mäki M, Collin P, Keyriläinen O. Dental enamel defects in celiac disease. J Oral Pathol Med 1990;19:241–5.
109. Gobbi G, Bouquet F, Greco L, et al. Coeliac disease, epilepsy and cerebral calcifications. Lancet 1990;340:439–43.
110. Hadjivassiliou M, Grunewald RA, Chattopadhyay AK, et al. Clinical, radiological, neurophysiological, and neuropathological characteristics of gluten ataxia. Lancet 1998;352:1582–5.
111. Volta U, De Franceschi L, Lari F, et al. Coeliac disease hidden by cryptogenic hypertransaminasaemia. Lancet 1998;352:26–9.
112. Kaukinen K, Halme L, Collin P, et al. Celiac disease in patients with severe liver disease: Gluten-free diet may reverse hepatic failure. Gastroenterology 2002;122:881–8.
113. Ventura A, Magazzu G, Greco L, et al. Duration of exposure to gluten and risk for autoimmune disorders in patients with celiac disease. Gastroenterology 1999;117:297–303.
114. Catassi C, Fabiani E, Corrao G, et al. Risk of non-Hodgkin lymphoma in celiac disease. J Am Med Assoc 2002;287:1413–9.
115. Kuitunen P, Kosnai I, Savilahti E. Morphometric study of the jejunal mucosa in various childhood enteropathies with special reference to intraepithelial lymphocytes. J Pediatr Gastroenterol Nutr 1982;1:525–31.
116. Meeuwisse GW. Diagnostic criteria in coeliac disease. Acta Paediatr Scand 1970;59:461–3.
117. Walker-Smith JA, Guandalini S, Schmitz J, et al. Revised criteria for the diagnosis of coeliac disease. Report of a working group. Arch Dis Child 1990;65:909–11.
118. Khoshoo V, Bhan MK, Unsworth DJ, et al. Anti-reticulin antibodies: Useful adjunct to histopathology in diagnosing celiac disease, especially in a developing country. J Pediatr Gastroenterol Nutr 1988;7:864–6.
119. Mäki M, Mustalahti K, Kokkonen J, et al. Prevalence of celiac disease among children in Finland. N Engl J Med 2003;348:2517–24.
120. Egan-Mitchell B, Fottrell PF, McNicholl P. Early or pre-coeliac mucosa: Development of gluten enteropathy. Gut 1981;22:65–9.
121. Mäki M, Holm K, Koskimies S, et al. Normal small bowel biopsy followed by coeliac disease. Arch Dis Child 1990;65:1137–41.
122. Mäki M, Holm K, Collin P, Savilahti E. Increase in gamma/delta T cell receptor bearing lymphocytes in normal small bowel mucosa in latent coeliac disease. Gut 1991;32:1412–4.
123. Iltanen S, Holm K, Partanen J, et al. Increased density of jejunal gammadelta+ T cells in patients having normal mucosa—marker of operative autoimmune mechanisms? Autoimmunity 1999;29:179–87.
124. Troncone R. Latent coeliac disease in Italy. The SIGEP Working Group on Latent Coeliac Disease. Italian Society for Paediatric Gastroenterology and Hepatology. Acta Paediatr 1995;84:1252–7.

125. Collin P, Helin H, Mäki M, et al. Follow-up of patients positive in reticulin and gliadin antibody tests with normal small-bowel biopsy findings. Scand J Gastroenterol 1993;28:595–8.

126. Kaukinen K, Collin P, Holm K, et al. Small-bowel mucosal inflammation in reticulin or gliadin antibody-positive patients without villous atrophy. Scand J Gastroenterol 1998;33:944–9.

127. Kaukinen K, Mäki M, Partanen J, et al. Coeliac disease without villous atrophy: Revision of criteria called for. Dig Dis Sci 2001;46:879–87.

128. Sanderson MC, Davis LR, Mowat AP. Failure of laboratory and radiological studies to predict jejunal mucosal atrophy. Arch Dis Child 1975;50:526–31.

129. Rossi TM, Albini CH, Kumar V. Incidence of celiac disease identified by the presence of serum endomysial antibodies in children with chronic diarrhea, short stature, or insulin-dependent diabetes mellitus. J Pediatr 1993;123:262–4.

130. Hill I, Fasano A, Schwartz R, et al. The prevalence of celiac disease in at-risk groups of children in the United States. J Pediatr 2000;136:86–90.

131. Fasano A, Berti I, Gerarduzzi T, et al. Prevalence of celiac disease in at-risk and not-at-risk groups in the United States: A large multicenter study. Arch Intern Med 2003;163:286–92.

132. Catassi C, Rätsch IM, Gandolfi L, et al. Why is coeliac disease endemic in the people of the Sahara? Lancet 1999;354:647–8.

133. Korponay-Szabo IR, Kovacs J, Czinner A, et al. High prevalence of silent coeliac disease in preschool children screened with IgA/IgG anti-endomysium antibodies. J Pediatr Gastroenterol Nutr 1998;28:26–30.

134. Meloni G, Dore A, Fanciulli G, et al. Subclinical coeliac disease in schoolchildren from northern Sardinia. Lancet 1999;353:37.

135. Carlsson AK, Axelsson IE, Borulf SK, et al. Serological screening for celiac disease in healthy 2.5-year-old children in Sweden. Pediatrics 2001;107:42–5.

136. Hoffenberg EJ, MacKenzie T, Barriga KJ, et al. A prospective study of the incidence of childhood celiac disease. J Pediatr 2003;143:308–14.

137. Csizmadia C, Mearin M, von Blomberg B, et al. An iceberg of childhood coeliac disease in the Netherlands. Lancet 1999;353:813–4.

138. Henker J, Lösel A, Conrad K, et al. Prävalenz der asymptomatischen Zöliakie bei Kindern und Erwachsenen in der Region Dresden. Dtsch Med Wochenschr 2002;127:1511–5.

139. Mäki M. The humoral immune system in coeliac disease. Baillieres Clin Gastroenterol 1995;9:231–49.

140. Sugai E, Vazquez H, Nachman F, et al. Accuracy of testing for antibodies to synthetic gliadin-related peptides in celiac disease. Clin Gastroenterol Hepatol 2006;4:1112–7.

141. Mäki M, Hällström O, Vesikari T, Visakorpi JK. Evaluation of a serum IgA class reticulin antibody test for the detection of childhood celiac disease. J Pediatr 1984;105:901–5.

142. Stern M. Comparative evaluation of serologic tests for celiac disease: A European initiative toward standardization. J Pediatr Gastroenterol Nutr 2000;31:513–9.

143. Korponay-Szabo IR, Sulkanen S, Halttunen T, et al. Tissue transglutaminase is the target in both rodent and primate tissues for celiac disease-specific autoantibodies. J Pediatr Gastroenterol Nutr 2000;31:520–7.

144. Korponay-Szabo IR, Laurila K, Szondy Z, et al. Missing endomysial and reticulin binding of coeliac antibodies in transglutaminase 2 knockout tissues. Gut 2003;52:199–204.

145. Dieterich W, Laag E, Schöpper H, et al. Autoantibodies to tissue transglutaminase as predictors of celiac disease. Gastroenterology 1998;115:1317–21.

146. Sulkanen S, Halttunen T, Laurila K, et al. Tissue transglutaminase autoantibody enzyme-linked immunosorbent assay in detecting celiac disease. Gastroenterology 1998;115:1322–8.

147. Sblattero D, Berti I, Trevisiol C, et al. Human recombinant tissue transglutaminase ELISA: An innovative diagnostic assay for celiac disease. Am J Gastroenterol 2000;95:1253–7.

148. Raivio T, Kaukinen K, Nemes E, et al. Self transglutaminase-based rapid coeliac disease antibody detection by a lateral flow method. Aliment Pharmacol Ther 2006;24:147–54.

149. Collin P, Reunala T, Pukkala E, et al. Coeliac disease-associated disorders and survival. Gut 1994;35:1215–8.

150. Kaukinen K, Collin P, Holm K, et al. Wheat starch-containing gluten-free flour products in the treatment of coeliac disease and dermatitis herpetiformis. A long-term follow-up study. Scand J Gastroenterol 1999;34:164–9.

151. Peräaho M, Kaukinen K, Paasikivi K, et al. Wheat-starch-based gluten-free products in the treatment of newly detected coeliac disease. Prospective and randomized study. Aliment Pharmacol Therapy 2003;17:587–94.

152. Valdés I, García E, Llorente M, Méndez E. Innovative approach to low-level gluten determination in foods using a novel sandwich enzyme-linked immunosorbent assay protocol. Eur J Gastroenterol 2003;15:465–74.

153. Hischenhuber C, Crevel R, Jarry B, et al. Review article: Safe amounts of gluten for patients with wheat allergy or coeliac disease. Aliment Pharmacol Ther 2005;23:559–75.

154. Mayer M, Greco L, Troncone R, et al. Compliance of adolescents with coeliac disease with a gluten free diet. Gut 1991;32:881–5.

155. Vader LW, Stepniak DT, Bunnik EM, et al. Characterization of cereal toxicity for celiac disease patients based on protein homology in grains. Gastroenterology 2003;125:1105–13.

16.2. Food Allergic Enteropathy

Franco Torrente, MD
Simon Murch, BSc, PhD, FRCP, FRCPCH

The best recognized intestinal manifestation of food allergy is food allergic (food-sensitive) enteropathy. The features of enteropathy may include lymphocyte and plasma cell infiltration, epithelial abnormality, or crypt hyperplastic villous atrophy, and impairing absorption. Enteropathy continues while the food remains in the diet, remitting on an exclusion diet, and usually recurring on food challenge. Diagnosis is now usually based on histological features at initial biopsy and clinical response to antigen exclusion and challenge. Clinical findings in food allergic enteropathy include abdominal distension, loose stools, micronutrient deficiency, and rarely protein-losing enteropathy. There may be other features of allergic disease, most commonly eczema. Unlike coeliac disease, food allergic enteropathies are usually transient in early life, and later challenge is usually tolerated. Cow's milk-sensitive enteropathy (CMSE) was the first recognized food allergic enteropathy and remains the most common cause.[1]

RECOGNITION OF FOOD-SENSITIVE ENTEROPATHIES

The existence of food allergic enteropathies was initially controversial and only confirmed by sequential small intestinal biopsies. Early reports demonstrated abnormal small intestinal mucosa in young children manifesting delayed clinical reactions to cow's milk.[2–4] Formal sequential biopsies during exclusion and challenge confirmed matched clinical responses and histological changes.[5,6] The reported mucosal lesion was markedly variable in severity, ranging from an almost coeliac-like flat mucosa to a mild degree of partial villous atrophy.[5–6] Disaccharidase activity was reduced in active disease,[6] and intraepithelial lymphocytes were increased.[7] These changes were maximal in the proximal small intestine and thus less extensive than in coeliac disease.[8] Similar abnormalities of the small intestinal mucosa have been reported in children with intolerance to several other proteins, including soy, wheat, oats, eggs, rice, and fish.[9–11]

CLINICAL FEATURES OF FOOD ALLERGIC ENTEROPATHY

The best-characterized syndrome is CMSE, classically presenting with chronic loose stools and failure to thrive, often beginning after an episode of gastroenteritis in a formula-fed infant.[1,12] Other clinical features include abdominal distension, perianal erythema or napkin rash (due to malabsorbed dietary carbohydrates), and dermatographia. Associated clinical features may include colic, gastroesophageal reflux, rectal bleeding, or eczema. There may be evidence of micronutrient deficiency, notably for iron and zinc.[1] Up to 40% of infants with classic CMSE also sensitize to soy, often after an initial period when it is tolerated. The great majority however settle on extensively hydrolyzed formulae.[12] Classic CMSE is usually self-limiting, with most children tolerating reintroduction at the age of 2 to 3 years.[1,12–13] By contrast, some children may have persistent low-grade symptoms for a prolonged period.[12,14–15] A proportion of children manifest additional immediate reactions to food antigens, such as rash, urticaria, angioedema, or anaphylaxis. However, many children suffer enteropathy without immediate reactions, and it is important to recognize that food allergic enteropathy often occurs in the absence of systemic signs of food allergy. Thus, skin prick tests may be negative and specific IgE undetectable.[1,12,16–17] Review of growth records in classic CMSE often shows a period of good weight gain prior to the onset of symptoms, followed by downward drift against the centiles until antigen exclusion is adequate. This presentation probably represents the loss of initially established oral tolerance.

EMERGING DISORDER OF MULTIPLE FOOD ALLERGY

By contrast to this classic presentation, there are increasing reports of early life sensitization in exclusively breast-fed infants.[16,18] In such infants, cow's milk is usually one of several antigens that induce symptoms, and many affected infants are intolerant of multiple foods. These infants have a different pattern of weight gain to classic CMSE, in that failure to thrive is seen in only about 25%, who usually show poor weight gain from birth.[19–20] For the infants with immediate reactions, diagnosis is usually straightforward as the clinical history usually indicates the causative antigens and skin prick tests are usually positive.[1,16] By contrast, those without immediate responses may present great diagnostic difficulty, particularly if weight gain is good. Recent evidence suggests that intestinal lymphoid hyperplasia may be a characteristic finding.[21–24] For these infants, it appears that oral tolerance mechanisms may not be primarily established,[17,25] causing sensitization to trace amounts of maternally ingested antigens passing into breast milk. The clinical picture in such cases may be dominated by dysmotility, with delayed gastric emptying and gastro-esophageal reflux contributing to a severe colic-like presentation with irritability.[16] Many infants have associated eczema and demonstrate napkin rash due to malabsorbed dietary sugars.[16] The histological findings are less striking than for classic CMSE (Table 1), and this can be a condition causing great diagnostic difficulty.[12]

FOOD PROTEIN–INDUCED ENTEROCOLITIS

The food protein–induced enterocolitis syndrome (FPIES) is a severe and sometimes life-threatening form of mucosal food hypersensitivity.[11,26–27] Although usually triggered by cow's milk or soy ingestion, FPIES may be induced by a variety of foods, including rice, oat, barley, vegetables, and poultry.[11] Milder symptoms may occur in breast-fed infants, triggered by milk protein in the mother's diet.[28] Most cases show negative skin-prick tests.[29] The infant usually presents with severe vomiting and diarrhea, and may become dehydrated and shocked, requiring emergency admission to hospital.[11] Some demonstrate melaena and passage of mucus per rectum, and may even undergo laparotomy if the diagnosis is not recognized.[26] Antigen withdrawal induces remission, but early challenge often induces a systemic reaction with peripheral neutrophilia. The condition may develop after an initial diagnosis of the milder cow's milk colitis, where colonic features of loose stools and rectal bleeding occur without systemic features.[1] Inadvertent antigen exposure after a period of exclusion may then precipitate the full-blown FPIES response. Tolerance is usually reestablished around 2 to 3 years for FPIES[11] and by around 1 year for cow's milk colitis.[1]

If colonoscopy is performed, macroscopic findings include loss of vascular pattern, prominent lymphoid follicles with perifollicular erythema (red halo sign), and an easily traumatized mucosa.[1] Histological changes include mononuclear cell infiltration, mucosal eosinophilia, and the presence of lymphoid follicles in most biopsies. If the ileum is visualized, lymphoid hyperplasia is usually seen. This condition may occur in older children, leading on occasion to mistaken laparotomy in the investigation of rectal bleeding.[30] A trial of cow's milk exclusion is thus recommended in all children with a history of unexplained rectal bleeding.

HISTOLOGICAL FEATURES OF FOOD PROTEIN ENTEROPATHIES

Early reports of classic CMSE lesion suggested a coeliac-like enteropathy,[5] although with current formulae mucosal damage is less striking and patchily distributed (Figure 1).[1,31–33] Typical histological findings are shown in Figures 1 and 2. If the diagnosis is being considered, at least two biopsy specimens are helpful for diagnosis, and dissecting microscopy may be helpful in detecting a patchy lesion. Increase in intraepithelial lymphocyte numbers is often focal and less than in coeliac disease.[7] Crypt cell proliferation is modestly increased in CMSE, but less than in coeliac disease.[34] Morphometry of recent cases of CMSE confirms a less severe lesion than archival biopsies from the 1980s[16] (Table 1). This causes some histopathological difficulty, as there is no international consensus in reporting of subtle lesions such as villous blunting or mild mucosal eosinophilia. One unexplained finding which may be diagnostically helpful is the accumulation of fat within the epithelium, as is also seen in postenteritis syndrome.[35] Within the lamina propria, there is often patchy increase in density of lymphocytes, and increased eosinophil accumulation may be seen (Figures 2 and 3).

In original descriptions, classic CMSE appeared to disappear by the age of 2 years, and milk challenge was then frequently successful.[1,12–13] However, there is now evidence that some children do not grow out of CMSE so soon, and an abnormal mucosa may be seen in later childhood.[14–15] Findings in older children with CMSE were endoscopically visible lymphonodular hyperplasia of the duodenal bulb, and biopsy findings of prominent lymphoid follicles without evidence of villous atrophy.[21–23] In one study, patients with definite CMSE showed increased

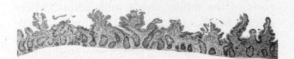

Figure 1 Low-power view of a small intestinal biopsy (fourth part of duodenum) in a child with cow's milk-sensitive enteropathy. The lesion is patchy, showing areas with preserved villous architecture and villous:crypt ratio >2, and others with villous blunting and crypt lengthening. Such patchiness is characteristic of food-sensitive enteropathy and suggests the need for taking of more than one biopsy for histological assessment. The handling of biopsies is important, and orientation under dissecting microscopy with card mounting may be helpful in optimizing biopsy orientation.

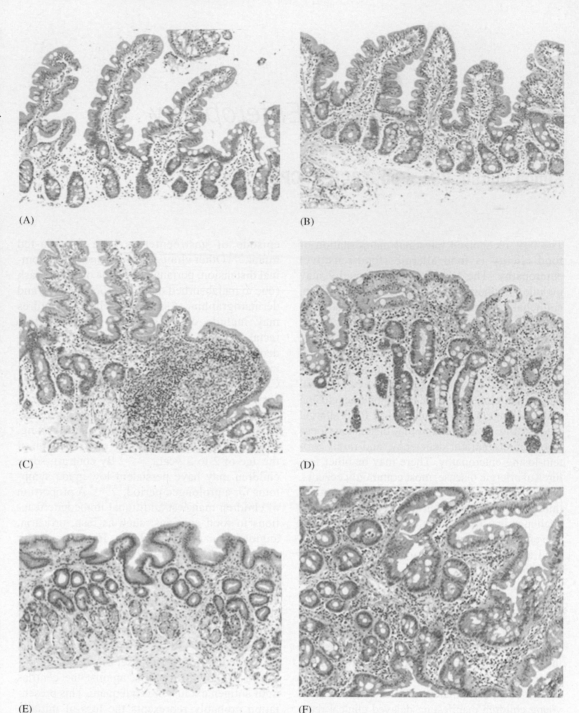

Figure 2 Subtle findings in food-sensitive enteropathy. (A) and (B) show biopsies within normal histological limits, from children with no eventual GI diagnosis. (C) shows a prominent lymphoid follicle with active germinal center in a child with cow's milk-sensitive enteropathy. Despite the recognizable villous architecture, there is evidence of some crypt lengthening. Prominent lymphoid tissue within the duodenum and terminal ileum is a recently recognized association of childhood food allergy.[21–24] By contrast, (D) shows the major disturbance of small intestinal architecture characteristic of coeliac disease, which presents little diagnostic difficulty compared to CMSE. (E) shows villous shortening in a case of cow's milk and soy-sensitive enteropathy. The prominence of Brunner's glands however suggests that the biopsy may have been taken in the first or second part of the duodenum, which may overemphasize villous shortening. Correct technique is to take biopsies in the fourth part of duodenum or the jejunum. (F) shows that although the biopsy is crosscut, there is a clear increase in the density of mononuclear cells within the duodenum in this case of CMSE.

densities of intraepithelial $\gamma\delta$ T cells,[22] although previous studies had demonstrated variability in $\gamma\delta$ IELs in CMSE,[36] suggesting that this is not a reliable marker. The consequences of T-cell activation in enteropathy include impairment of enterocyte absorptive mechanisms, such as decreased expression of lactase and other hydrolases, and an additional impairment of the small intestinal drive to pancreatic enzyme secretion[37–38]

SPECIFIC FOODS CAUSING ENTEROPATHY

Cow's Milk

Unlike human milk, cow's milk contains β-lactoglobulin, and this protein was initially implicated in the development of CMSE.[1,12–13] Allergic responses to casein may also occur, and in systemic cow's milk allergy children with IgE recognizing specific sequences of α_{S1}-casein,

Table 1 Morphometric Examination of Small Intestinal Biopsies in Food-Sensitive Enteropathy, Comparing Classic CMSE to Multiple Food Allergy

	Villous Height (μm)	Crypt Depth (μm)	Mean Villous:Crypt Ratio
Normal controls ($n = 47$)	345	164	2.1
Multiple food allergy ($n = 45$)	282	188	1.4
Classic CMSE ($n = 46$)	210	190	1.2
Coeliac disease ($n = 17$)	30	400	0.1

Adapted from Latcham et al.[16]

α_{S2}-casein, and κ-casein are less likely to outgrow their allergy.[39–40] Overall, the prognosis of the child with CMSE appears good, and the great majority outgrow their sensitization by age 3, although other allergies subsequently develop in about half the cases.[13,41]

Soy

Soy-based formulae have been used for many years as a substitute for cow's milk formulae in milk-sensitized infants, but recommendations from the American Academy of Pediatrics Committee on Nutrition[42] differ from those from the European Society for Pediatric Allergology and Clinical Immunology (ESPACI) and the European Society for Pediatric Gastroenterology, Hepatology, and Nutrition (ESPGHAN)[43] in respect of soy use. Soy-based formulae are as antigenic as cow's milk formulae[44] and cause a similar spectrum of allergic responses.[1,11] A 30 kDa soy protein may induce cross-reactivity to casein in cow's milk,[45] potentially explaining why so many cow's milk allergic children also develop soy allergy. The antigenicity of soy products varies with the method of preparation, and children may react to some soy products and not others.[46] This is important to consider if challenge testing is performed with negative response and yet symptoms suggestive of soy enteropathy continue. Skin prick testing is a poor predictor of subsequent clinical soy reactions,[47] but skin patch testing shows promise in identifying soy-sensitized children.[48]

Hydrolyzates

It is important to recognize that some children can show reactions to the trace cow's protein present in hydrolyzate formulae and thus show incomplete resolution of symptoms unless moved to an amino acid–based formula.[12,16,49–52] The clinical features tend to be less florid than induced by the unprocessed protein, and thus there is often some improvement in symptoms on commencing the hydrolyzate. Ongoing reaction to hydrolyzates may therefore be missed if the diagnosis is not considered. A recent systematic review of amino acid formulae identified a subgroup of children with hydrolyzate intolerance, showing features of early life sensitization while breast-fed and manifesting either immediate or delayed responses to multiple antigens and prominent disturbance of motility.[12] There is also evidence that a very few children may fail to settle on amino acid formulae, although this is substantially less common than hydrolyzate intolerance.[12]

Wheat Gluten

A particularly important form of food-sensitive enteropathy occurs to wheat gluten in coeliac disease. The enteropathy is quite distinct to other food-sensitive enteropathies such as CMSE and is discussed separately in Chapter 16.1, "Celiac Disease."

Multiple Food Allergy

Increasing numbers of infants and children are becoming sensitized to multiple foods, making either immediate or delayed reactions, or a combination. Many sensitize despite exclusive breast-feeding. Diets involving the elimination of single foods are usually ineffective, and many affected infants are intolerant to hydrolyzates and require amino acid formulae.[12,16,49–52] This provides a particularly challenging clinical scenario and requires experienced specialist input. The antigens most likely to provoke symptoms in the multiple food-allergic child include cow's milk, soy, wheat, egg, peanuts, tree nuts, and fish, but a variety of other food antigens have been implicated.[16,29,53] If the multiple allergic infant remains even partially breastfed, the dietary exclusions that the mother must make may have a very negative effect, and it may be necessary to discontinue breast-feeding if the mother is having to exclude more than two major foodstuffs.[54] One important clinical issue in the management of the child with multiple food allergy is the maintenance of a nutritionally adequate diet, and close liaison with an experienced dietician is mandatory. Ongoing food-sensitive enteropathy will manifest reduction in brush border disaccharidase expression due to T-cell activation,[55] causing carbohydrate malabsorption and reduced pancreatic enzyme release,[37–38] also contributing to malabsorption. In some cases, improvement in weight gain can be achieved by the temporary addition of pancreatic enzyme supplements. It is important to exclude cystic fibrosis in cases where elastase is found to be low, as both conditions can coexist. Many children with multiple food allergies do maintain normal growth and weight gain,[20] and thus the diagnosis may not be suspected if the child makes delayed non-IgE-mediated reactions only.[16,20] Unlike classic CMSE, it is unusual for an affected child to regain tolerance for cow's milk by the age of 2 years.[16,20]

IMMUNOPATHOLOGY

T-Cell Responses

Studies during serial challenges in CMSE have identified changes induced by milk, including increased CD8 IELs, increased epithelial HLA-DR expression, and activation of lamina propria CD4 cells.[10] The IELs appear to be activated, showing enhanced expression of cytotoxic markers.[56] Mucosal lymphocytes in food allergic enteropathies demonstrate increased activation, with either a T_H1 dominated or a mixed T_H1/T_H2 response.[25,57–60] Thus, T_H1 responses are not overall reduced within the mucosa or T_H2 significantly increased, in contrast to findings in peripheral blood lymphocytes from milk-allergic infants[61] or in cloned duodenal T cells.[62] T_H1 responses are also maintained within Peyer's patch lymphocytes.[63] Study of intraepithelial and lamina propria lymphocytes from children with multiple food allergies did not show T_H1 or T_H2 imbalance, but marked reduction of the T_H3 regulatory cytokine transforming growth factor-β (TGF-β).[60] Thus, while classic CMSE is an essentially T_H1-skewed mucosal lesion, infants with multiple food allergy lesions may be immunologically distinct, with reduced expression of regulatory cytokines associated with low-dose oral tolerance. Reduction of TGF-β expression has also been seen in duodenal T-cell clones from milk-allergic children[62] and in FPIES.[64]

TNF-α production is stimulated within the mucosa by milk challenge of allergic patients,[65–66] also distinct from responses seen in circulating T cells,[67] possibly reflecting its release from mucosal mast cells. Increased TNF-α responses are seen with enhanced T_H2 responses in FPIES.[68]

Mast Cells and Eosinophil Responses

One frequent association of mucosal food-allergic responses is the infiltration of both eosinophils and mast cells; both of which produce a number of proinflammatory, vasoactive, and neuroactive mediators (Figure 3). These cells have been implicated in antigen-induced dysmotility, and their products may disturb enteric neural function.[69] In response to ingested allergens, mast cell tryptase and eosinophil cationic protein (ECP) are released into the lumen and may be detected in stools.[66,70–71] In a study comparing mucosal responses in infants with enteropathy, milk intolerance was associated with increased mucosal expression of eosinophil major basic protein (MBP) and upregulation of the adhesion molecule VCAM-1.[72]

There are important differences in the time course of responses mediated by mast cells and eosinophils despite their rather similar products. Mast cells mediators are stored, preformed within intracellular granules, and released rapidly through degranulation after cross-linking of surface IgE molecules. This does not require synthesis of new protein, and thus ensures that mast cells play a predominant role in immediate mucosal responses. For eosinophils, there

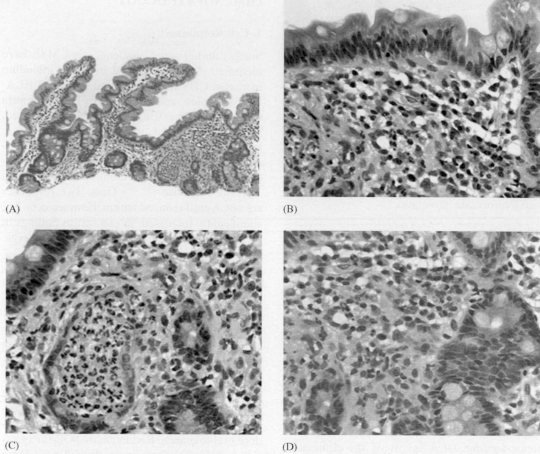

Figure 3 Eosinophil infiltrate within the mucosa in a case of food protein–induced enterocolitis. The low-power view in (A) shows preserved villous architecture in the duodenum, with a single crypt abscess. Higher-power views in (B) and (C) show the intense eosinophil infiltrate within the lamina propria. C demonstrates that the crypt abscess seen in A is in fact eosinophilic. (D) shows a sigmoid colonic biopsy from the same child, which also shows mucosal eosinophilia. This child required an amino acid formula, as he was intolerant to hydrolyzates.

is a contrasting lag period, as they need to be recruited into the tissues. Eosinophils are thus more likely to play a role in delayed responses to antigen. The three forms of response to cow's milk in sensitized infants identified by Hill and colleagues,[73] of immediate, intermediate, and delayed reactions thus correlate temporally with mast cell, eosinophil, and T-cell–mediated responses, respectively.

PATHOGENESIS OF FOOD-SENSITIVE ENTEROPATHY

T-Cell Responses

The intestine contains more T cells than any other organ. While activated mucosal T cells play a central role in inducing crypt hyperplastic villous atrophy,[74–75] several mechanisms normally prevent this occurring.[76] A tight epithelial barrier is required to prevent passage of intact macromolecules to the lamina propria. The role of the epithelium in antigen presentation and cytokine production is also important.[77–80] A direct epithelial contribution to immune tolerance was suggested by Sanderson who showed that costimulatory ligands for T-cell activation were not expressed.[79] Thus, intestinal epithelium may induce a regulatory phenotype in CD8 cells.[81] Only short-chain peptides penetrate the epithelial barrier in health,

minimizing the induction of proinflammatory T-cell responses by subepithelial antigen-presenting cells.[82] Initial sensitization may thus occur if there is epithelial leakiness, for example, with acute gastroenteritis,[1,25,83–84] where paracellular antigen presentation becomes abnormally high.[85] The subsequent immune response to penetrating antigen may contribute to maintaining epithelial hyperpermeability and thus a persistent state of increased antigen entry.[86–88]

The cytokines most implicated in increasing intestinal paracellular permeability are TNF-α and IFN-γ.[65,89–90] There is an overlap of function with the cytokines mediating oral tolerance, TGF-β and IL-10, as both oppose IFN-γ to reduce permeability,[91–92] while IFN-γ in turn blocks TGF-β signaling.[93] The relative local concentrations of IFN-γ and TGF-β or IL-10 may determine both epithelial permeability and immune tolerance.

Oral Tolerance

There has been much advance in the understanding of oral tolerance. Relevant factors include the dose of ingested antigen, as low doses invoke different responses to high doses.[17,25,94–95] Bulk dietary antigen is processed by epithelium and induces lymphocyte anergy.[79,80,96–97] By contrast, low doses of antigen are taken up by M

cells of Peyer's patches and induce regulatory lymphocytes such as TGF-β producing T$_H$3 cells.[17,25,94–95,98] Other regulatory T-cell populations include IL-10 producing T regulator 1 (Tr1) cells, and CD4+CD25+ cells.[25,80,95] Reduced CD4+CD25+ cells were identified in children with milk allergies, increasing to normal as tolerance was regained.[99] The molecule critical in the generation of regulatory lymphocytes is the transcription factor *Foxp3*, and its mutation in immunodysregulation, polyendocrinopathy, enteropathy, and X linked (IPEX) syndrome causes a severe multifocal inflammatory disease including enteropathy.[100]

In older patients a population of multiply-exposed CD4+CD25+ cells inhibit milk-allergic responses.[101] By contrast, cord blood T cells do not express mucosal homing markers[102] and show ineffective regulatory properties.[103] Thus, animals may be born with poor low-dose oral tolerance[104] and must develop this postnatally. In infants of allergic mothers, cord blood TGF-β responses to cow's milk were reduced compared to infants from nonallergic families.[105] The subsequent development of TGF-β responses appears impaired in infants with food-related enteropathies,[60,64] suggesting that a primary failure to generate low-dose oral tolerance may predispose to sensitization. Postnatal development of tolerance mechanisms is at least partly depend on responses to the enteric flora[106] and experimental blockade of innate immune responses to the flora-induced food-sensitive enteropathy.[107] It is thus notable that duodenal TGF-β producing cells are much more abundant in developing world infants, where infectious exposures are greater but food allergy is rare.[108] Such considerations raise the question of early life probiotic therapy as a possible preventative measure for intestinal food allergies.

On a worldwide basis, it is possible that food-sensitive enteropathy occurs in malnourished developing world children, as marasmic children may become milk or soy intolerant and improve on exclusion diets.[109–111] As paracellular permeability is a major determinant of mortality,[112] and progression to marasmus is characterized by reduced mucosal TGF-β expression[108]; it is possible that acquired loss of oral tolerance may occur in tropical enteropathy.

B-Cell Responses

Mucosal IgA is also important in the maintenance of tolerance to dietary antigens (Figure 4). IgA is taken up by enterocytes and directly regulates antigen ingress[113] in contrast to the stimulatory effects of IgE[87] on antigen uptake. Thus, food allergies and enteropathy are common among adults with IgA deficiency.[114] A condition of transient IgA deficiency in infants was suggested by Soothill and colleagues as a cause of allergic sensitization,[115] and low IgA is overall more predictive of infant-allergic sensitization than high IgE.[116] Normal immune development is characterized by increased mucosal

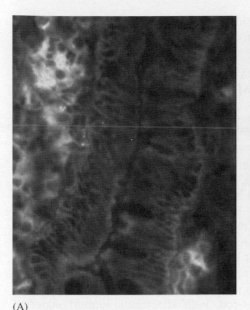 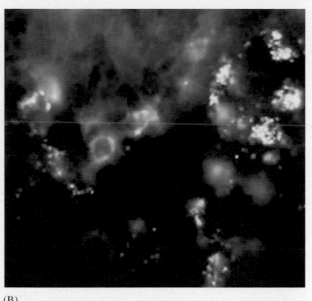

(A)   (B)

Figure 4 Immunofluorescence for IgA and IgE in a case of cow's milk-sensitive enteropathy. (A) shows detail from two adjacent villi, with the epithelium and luminal glycocalyx outlined by IgA, while strongly staining IgA plasma cells are seen in the adjacent lamina propria. (B) shows two types of IgE+ cells: round plasma cells with large unstained nuclei and homogeneously staining periphery, and intensely staining mast cells showing the characteristic granular deposition. There is evidence of some mast cell degranulation, with non-cell-associated deposition of IgE. This child had a normal total IgE, undetectable milk-specific IgE, and negative skin prick tests, demonstrating the compartmentalization of IgE responses that can occur within the intestine.[25,70,128–130]

IgA2 plasma cells[117] and acquisition of tolerance in milk-allergic patients associated with a shift to an IgA-dominated response,[118] with reduction of antigen-specific IgG4 responses.[119] Reduced mucosal IgA responses therefore predispose to development of CMSE after gastroenteritis.[120] As acquisition of IgA lineage in B cells is dependent on TGF-β, this cytokine thus plays a pivotal role in both T- and B-cell tolerance to dietary antigen.[25]

Normal infants without enteropathy often produce circulating antibodies to cows' milk proteins.[1,12–13,41] Some reports have suggested immune complex formation, complement activation, and antibody-dependent cell-mediated cytotoxicity as disease mechanisms in CMSE.[121–122] Transient IgE responses to foods are seen in normal children and are of doubtful relevance.[123] However, high-level IgE responses are usually pathological but more characteristic of systemic food allergies than enteropathy. Production of IgE is favored by the T_H2 cytokines IL-4 and IL-13[124] which share a common receptor chain (IL-4Rα). IL-4Rα signaling is a pivotal pathway in allergy, with increased signaling promoting and reduced signaling inhibiting IgE-mediated allergies.[125–127] IgE plasma cells may be generated within the mucosa without any systemic IgE responses.[128] Such locally produced IgE can be transported into the gut lumen,[128–129] where it may bind to antigen and then reenter the enterocyte with bound antigen by binding to its receptor CD23.[130] Enterocyte expression of CD23 is upregulated in food-allergic enteropathy, further promoting antigen uptake.[131] Thus, mucosal IgE responses may be elicited by dietary antigen, even if skin prick tests are negative and circulating-specific IgE undetectable.

Mast Cell and Eosinophil Responses

It is common to see focal increase of eosinophils within the mucosa in food-sensitive enteropathy. Studies by Rothenberg and colleagues have clarified the central role of the cytokine IL-5 and the chemokine eotaxin in recruiting eosinophils in mucosal allergic responses.[132–135] A particular role for eosinophils in disturbed gut motility was demonstrated by showing delayed gastric emptying of antigen-coated beads.[133] Further studies identified the esophagus as a particular target for eosinophil recruitment, both by dietary antigen and by less predictable stimuli such as inhaled aeroallergens[134] and systemic IL-5 exposure.[135] Eosinophils and mast cells may be particularly important in inducing dysmotility in food allergies, which represents an emerging area of significant clinical interest[69]

Human relevance of these findings is suggested by increased expression of IL-5 mRNA within small bowel mucosa after challenge of food-allergic patients.[136] Circulating T cells from food-allergic children produce IL-5 on challenge, unlike those from tolerant children.[67,137] Eotaxin expression is increased in the esophageal epithelium in infants with CMSE-induced gastroesophageal reflux.[138] These studies suggest IL-5 and eotaxin as potential therapeutic targets in food-allergic enteropathy.

Diagnostic Strategies for Food-Allergic Enteropathy

Several diagnostic strategies may be employed in addition to small intestinal biopsy and assessment of nutritional status as discussed earlier. The most difficult task may be to identify the causative antigen(s).

Food Challenge Testing

The core requirement for diagnosis of food allergy is response to an elimination diet with recurrence of symptoms on challenge.[139–140] Other diagnostic tests may support the diagnosis but are secondary to this. In the circumstance of allergy to a single food, complete exclusion should induce relief of all symptoms and restore normal growth if this was impaired. For secure diagnosis, the second requirement is a recurrence of symptoms on antigen challenge. In some cases parents may refuse challenge if their child has improved dramatically.

In addition to the initial diagnostic challenge, later challenges may be performed when it is likely that tolerance has been regained. This is usually after the age of 2, although later in children with multiple food allergies. ESPGHAN recommendations for investigation of possible food sensitive enteropathy included small bowel biopsy in cases of failure to thrive or diarrhea.[141] In cases of multiple food allergies, response to elimination of just one or two antigens will be incomplete, and it may be quicker to commence with a very restricted diet, which can subsequently be broadened. It may be difficult to persuade some parents to broaden the diet, if there has been a very clear clinical response, or if they have received advice from some alternative practitioners or Internet sites. In cases of exclusively non-IgE-mediated allergy, it may be difficult to obtain a clear picture of the true level of sensitization.[16,29] The associated minor immunodeficiency may increase the chance of viral infection during prolonged food challenges.[16,115] For multiple-sensitized children, it can be logistically difficult to perform lengthy blinded challenges.

Open food challenges are performed either in the outpatient clinic or in a day ward, depending on the severity and type of reaction expected.[29,142] It is mandatory to have adequate medical supervision and appropriate resuscitation facilities in cases of immediate reaction. In cases with a history of anaphylaxis, an intravenous line should be inserted. For the child who makes delayed reactions only, as in classic CMSE, challenges have to be extended over several days and are usually completed at home. In a study of 370 challenges in 242 children, 5 children demonstrated no reactions on initial hospital challenge, but then reacted on subsequent administration at home.[143] Hill and colleagues identified early reactions to milk (within 1 h), intermediate reactions (up to 1 d), and very late reactions (up to 3 d).[49,73] For the very late reactions, the cumulative intake of milk was as much as 120 mL. There are reports of even later responses to cow's milk challenge, with gastrointestinal, respiratory, or cutaneous responses beginning a week after challenge.[144] Thus, the interpretation of food challenges is by no means always straightforward, particularly in the case of non-IgE-mediated delayed symptoms. While some cases of food-sensitive enteropathy have associated immediate reactions, many do not. There is a difficult balance between missing true late responses and colluding in the overdiagnosis of food allergy.

The "gold-standard" challenge test is the double-blind placebo-controlled food challenge (DBPCFC). This is much easier for immediate reactions than delayed ones and can be quite cumbersome if several antigens need to be tested over a prolonged period. Although it may provide a degree of certainty that other challenges do not,[1,29,140,142] recent abdominal ultrasound finding of antigen-induced intestinal secretion in symptomatic patients with negative DBPCFC[145] suggests that false-negative results may sometimes occur.

Skin Prick Testing

Skin prick tests, in which cutaneous mast cell degranulation is induced by antigen, are much less useful in straightforward food-sensitive enteropathy than in immediate allergies.[16] However, for children who make immediate reactions, the size of the wheal elicited may predict positive food challenges.[146]

Skin Patch Testing

The atopy patch test may potentially offer a better insight into food-sensitive enteropathies, as the cellular mechanisms of this skin reaction are more similar to those in enteropathy. The antigen is maintained for 48 hours against the skin in a sealed patch before being removed, and the skin response studies after a further 24 hours.[48] A positive test is characterized by erythema and induration at this stage. The test appears to be mediated by a specific T-cell response to dietary antigen[147] in contrast to the simple mast cell responses in the skin prick test.

Combination of patch testing with skin prick testing or specific IgE serology may pick up food-sensitized children negative on classic testing.[148–149] Despite an apparently high sensitivity for delayed responses, the atopy patch test has not yet become widely used and remains under evaluation. There are still few data on the relevance of patch testing in food-sensitive enteropathy, in contrast to eczema, although patch testing may potentially be useful in FPIES syndrome.[150]

Specific IgE Testing

Testing of specific IgE production to individual foods can be helpful, providing results complementary to skin prick testing. For immediate allergies the information provided can be clinically predictive, although they are less useful in straightforward enteropathies. Positive predictive values of 95% were found for egg, milk, peanut, and fish reactions, at different thresholds.[151] Higher titers of specific IgE for milk, casein, or β-lactoglobulin increase the likelihood of long-lasting sensitization.[152]

Study of epitope sequences bound by food-specific IgE may give prognostic information. Binding to linear peptide sequences within the egg antigen ovomucoid was associated with long-lasting allergy, whereas binding to discontinuous sequences (only bound by IgE because of protein folding) was seen in those who outgrew allergies.[39] Thus, some children will react to raw but not cooked egg, where the tertiary sequence has been disrupted. Similarly, IgE reaction to linear sequences in α_{S1}-casein, α_{S2}-casein, and κ-casein appears to be predictive of long-lasting milk allergy.[39–40] In future, epitope sequencing may identify infants at risk of long-lasting food allergies, and thus potentially likely to benefit from immunotherapy.

In Vitro Tests

Lymphocyte function tests are a research rather than diagnostic tool, and have not proved as useful as once hoped. Analysis of cytokine production may provide one approach, particularly if surface markers of sensitized cells can be identified. Peripheral blood lymphocytes from food-allergic children produce a T_H2 response to antigen while those from healthy controls are more T_H1 skewed.[137] A promising technique, allowing recognition of antigen-specific T-cell responses, confirmed that T-cell responses to peanut in allergic children peanut were indeed skewed toward T_H2 in contrast to findings in children who had outgrown their allergies.[67] The mucosal pattern in food-sensitive enteropathy is less straightforward, and is characterized by preserved T_H1 responses, but decreased regulatory responses.[57,60,64]

MANAGEMENT OF FOOD-SENSITIVE ENTEROPATHY

Primary Prevention

It remains controversial whether food-sensitive enteropathy and other food allergies can be prevented by stringent avoidance of allergies in early life.[153] Two position statements by the American Academy of Pediatrics[42] and the European Society for Pediatric Allergology and Clinical Immunology (ESPACI) with ESPGHAN[43] differ in some important respects. Both statements suggest that primary prevention should be limited to high-risk infants only and recommend use of hypoallergenic formulae for bottle-fed high-risk infants. Neither recommends maternal exclusion diets during pregnancy, while both recommend exclusive breast-feeding. The AAP also recommends later introduction of cow's milk and eggs than the European statement.

A large study from the German Infant Nutrition Intervention (GINI) study group[154] randomly assigned 2,252 at-risk infants at birth to receive 1 of 4 blinded formulae (cow's milk-based, partially hydrolyzed whey, extensively hydrolyzed whey, or extensively hydrolyzed casein). The primary end point at 1 year was the presence of one or more of atopic dermatitis, gastrointestinal food allergy, or urticaria. The study had a high attrition rate due to exclusive breast-feeding or dropping out, but study of 945 remaining infants showed a protective effect of extensively hydrolyzed casein compared to unmodified cow's milk. Atopic dermatitis was reduced in infants fed extensively hydrolyzed casein or partially hydrolyzed whey formulae.[154]

TREATMENT OF ESTABLISHED FOOD-SENSITIVE ENTEROPATHY

For treatment of established food allergies, both AAP[42] and ESPACI/ESPGHAN[43] statements recommend complete exclusion of the causative antigen. For treatment of the milk-sensitized infant, both recommend an extensively hydrolyzed but not partially hydrolyzed formula. The AAP but not ESPACI/ESPGHAN guidelines also recommend soy as an alternative, while both recommend an amino acid formula for the infant who is intolerant to hydrolyzates. Neither recommends the use of unmodified goat's or sheep's milk. For the infant who sensitizes while breast-fed, both statements support maternal exclusion of the relevant antigen, while the AAP further recommends weaning to an extensively hydrolyzed formula or soymilk. With respect of probable food-sensitive enteropathy, both recommend extensively hydrolyzed or amino acid formulae. Thus in cases of diagnosed or probable CMSE, soymilk feeds are not recommended as an alternative.[42–43]

FUTURE POSSIBILITIES FOR FOOD-SENSITIVE ENTEROPATHY

The normal flora plays a role in the induction of tolerogenic lymphocytes and the establishment of oral tolerance.[155–156] As interaction between gut bacteria in early infancy and innate immunity may determine whether a response sufficient to tole rise occurs; probiotic organisms represent a potentially important form of immunomodulator, particularly in infancy.[157–158] In the treatment of established food-sensitive enteropathy, there may be potential benefit from supplementing dietary n-3 fatty acids, and a murine model of ovalbumin-induced enteropathy was attenuated by supplementing n-3 intake.[159] There is also murine data to suggest that the induction of regulatory lymphocytes necessary for oral tolerance may be enhanced by administration of vitamin D receptor ligands such as 1,25-dihydroxyvitamin D3.[160]

Other potentially novel therapies for food allergies include immunotherapy, which depends on increasing gradually the dose of antigen until a T_H1 response is made.[161] Future targets include small peptide vaccines, foods with altered protein sequences, DNA immunization and IgE-blocking agents. There are potentially important monoclonal antibodies, which may play a role in attenuating severe food allergies, including anti-IgE and anti-IL-5 antibodies.[162–163]

REFERENCES

1. Walker-Smith JA, Murch SH. Gastrointestinal food allergy. In: Diseases of the Small Intestine in Childhood, 4th edition. Oxford: Isis Medical Media; 1999. p. 205–34.
2. Lamy M, Nezelof C, Jos J, et al. la biopsie de la muqueuse intestinale chez enfant: Premiers résultat d'une étude des

syndromes de malabsorption. Presse Medicale 1963;71: 1267–70.

3. Kuitunen P, Visakorpi JK, Hallman N. Histopathology of duodenal mucosa in malabsorption syndrome induced by cow's milk. Ann Paediatr 1965;205:54–63.

4. Liu HY, Tsao MU, Moore B, Giday Z. Bovine milk protein-induced intestinal malabsorption of lactose and fat in infants. Gastroenterology 1968;54:27–34.

5. Kuitunen P, Rapola J, Savilahti E, Visakorpi. Response of the jejunal mucosa to cow's milk in the malabsorption syndrome with cow's milk intolerance. A light- and electron-microscopic study. Acta Paediatr Scand 1973;62:585–95.

6. Walker-Smith J, Harrison M, Kilby A, et al. Cows' milk-sensitive enteropathy. Arch Dis Child 1978;53:375–80.

7. Phillips AD, Rice SJ, France NE, Walker-Smith JA. Small intestinal lymphocyte levels in cow's milk protein intolerance. Gut 1989;20:509–12.

8. Iyngkaran N, Yadav M, Boey CG, Lam KL. Severity and extent of upper small bowel mucosal damage in cow's milk protein-sensitive enteropathy. J Pediatr Gastroenterol Nutr 1988;7:667–74.

9. Vitoria JC, Camarero C, Sojo A, et al. Enteropathy related to fish, rice, and chicken. Arch Dis Child 1982;57:44–8.

10. Nagata S, Yamashiro Y, Ohtsuka Y, et al. Quantitative analysis and immunohistochemical studies on small intestinal mucosa of food-sensitive enteropathy. J Pediatr Gastroenterol Nutr 1995;20:44–8.

11. Nowak-Wegrzyn A, Sampson HA, Wood RA, Sicherer SH. Food protein-induced enterocolitis syndrome caused by solid food proteins. Pediatrics 2003;111:829–35.

12. Hill DJ, Murch SH, Rafferty K, et al. The efficacy of amino acid-based formulas in relieving the symptoms of cow's milk allergy: A systematic review. Clin Exp Allergy 2007 (in press).

13. Host A, Jacobsen HP, Halken S, Holmenlund D. The natural history of cow's milk protein allergy intolerance. Eur J Clin Nutr 1995;49:S13–8.

14. Kokkonen J, Tikkanen S, Savilahti E. Residual intestinal disease after milk allergy in infancy. J Pediatr Gastroenterol Nutr 2001;32:156–61.

15. Kokkonen J, Haapalahti M, Laurila K, et al. Cow's milk protein-sensitive enteropathy at school age. J Pediatr 2001;139:797–803.

16. Latcham F, Merino F, Lang A, et al. A consistent pattern of minor immunodeficiency and subtle enteropathy in children with multiple food allergy. J Pediatr 2003;143:39–47.

17. Shah U, Walker WA. Pathophysiology of intestinal food allergy. Adv Pediatr 2002;49:299–316.

18. Vandenplas Y, Quenon M, Renders F, et al. Milk-sensitive eosinophilic gastroenteritis in a 10-day-old boy. Eur J Pediatr 1990;149:244–5.

19. Heine RG, Elsayed S, Hosking CS, Hill DJ. Cow's milk allergy in infancy. Curr Opin Allergy Clin Immunol 2002;2:217–25.

20. Hill DJ, Heine RG, Cameron DJ, et al. The natural history of intolerance to soy and extensively hydrolyzed formula in infants with multiple food protein intolerance. J Pediatr 1999;135:118–21.

21. Kokkonen J, Tikkanen S, Karttunen TJ, Savilahti E. A similar high level of immunoglobulin A and immunoglobulin G class milk antibodies and increment of local lymphoid tissue on the duodenal mucosa in subjects with cow's milk allergy and recurrent abdominal pains. Pediatr Allergy Immunol 2002;13:129–36.

22. Kokkonen J, Ruuska T, Karttunen TJ, Maki M. Lymphonodular hyperplasia of the terminal ileum associated with colitis shows an increase γδ+ T cell density in children. Am J Gastroenterol 2002;97:667–72.

23. Kokkonen J, Karttunen TJ. Lymphonodular hyperplasia on the mucosa of the lower gastrointestinal tract in children: An indication of enhanced immune response? J Pediatr Gastroenterol Nutr 2002;34:42–6.

24. Bellanti JA, Zeligs BJ, Malka-Rais J, Sabra A. Abnormalities of Th1 function in non-IgE food allergy, celiac disease, and ileal lymphonodular hyperplasia: A new relationship? Ann Allergy Asthma Immunol 2003;90:S84–9.

25. Murch SH. The immunologic basis for intestinal food allergy. Current Opinion Gastroenterol 2000;16:552–7.

26. Powell GK. Milk and soy-induced enterocolitis of infancy. J Pediatr 1978;93:533–60.

27. Jayasooria S, Fox A, Murch S. Don't laparotomise FPIES. Pediatric Emerg Care 2007 (in press).

28. Anveden HL, Finkel Y, Sandstedt B, Karpe B. Proctocolitis in exclusively breast-fed infants. Eur J Pediatr 1996;155:464–7.

29. Sicherer SH. Clinical aspects of gastrointestinal food allergy in childhood. Pediatrics 2003;111:1609–16.

30. Willetts IE, Dalzell M, Puntis JW, Stringer MD. Cow's milk enteropathy: Surgical pitfalls. J Pediatr Surg 1999;34:1486–8.

31. Verkasalo M, Kuitunen P, Savilahti E, Tulikainen A. Changing pattern of cow's milk intolerance. Acta Paediatr Scand 1981;70:289–95.

32. Maluenda C, Phillips AD, Briddon A, Walker-Smith JA. Quantitative analysis of small intestinal mucosa in cow's milk sensitive enteropathy. J Pediatr Gastroenterol Nutr 1984;3:349–57.

33. Manuel PD, Walker-Smith JA, France NE. Patchy enteropathy in childhood. Gut 1979;20:211–5.

34. Savidge TC, Shmakov AN, Walker-Smith JA, Phillips AD. Epithelial cell proliferation in childhood enteropathies. Gut 1996;39:185–93.

35. Variend S, Placzek M, Raafat F, Walker-Smith JA. Small intestinal mucosal fat in childhood enteropathies. J Clin Path 1984;37:373–7.

36. Spencer J, Isaacson PG, MacDonald TT, et al. Gamma/delta T cells and the diagnosis of coeliac disease. Clin Exp Immunol 1991;85:109–13.

37. Walkowiak J, Herzig KH. Fecal elastase-1 is decreased in villous atrophy regardless of the underlying disease. Eur J Clin Invest 2001;31:425–30.

38. Schappi MG, Smith VV, Cubitt D, et al. Faecal elastase 1 concentration is a marker of duodenal enteropathy. Arch Dis Child 2002;86:50–3.

39. Vila L, Beyer K, Jarvinen KM, et al. Role of conformational and linear epitopes in the achievement of tolerance in cow's milk allergy. Clin Exp Allergy 2001;31:1599–606.

40. Järvinen KM, Beyer K, Vila L, et al. B-cell epitopes as a screening instrument for persistent cow's milk allergy. J Allergy Clin Immunol 2002;110:293–7.

41. Host A. Cow's milk protein allergy and intolerance in infancy. Some clinical, epidemiological and immunological aspects. Pediatr Allergy Immunol 1994;5:S1–36.

42. American Academy of Pediatrics, Committee on Nutrition. Hypoallergenicinfant formulas. Pediatrics 2000;106:346–9.

43. Host A, Koletzko B, Dreborg S, et al. Joint Statement of the European Society for Paediatric Allergology and Clinical Immunology (ESPACI) Committee on Hypoallergenic Formulas and the European Society for Paediatric Gastroenterology, Hepatology and Nutrition (ESPGHAN) Committee on Nutrition. Arch Dis Child 1999;81:80–4.

44. Eastham EJ, Lichanco T, Pang K, Walker WA. Antigenicity of infant formulas and the induction of systemic immunological tolerance by oral feeding: Cow's milk versus soy milk. J Pediatr Gastroenterol Nutr 1982;1:23–8.

45. Rozenfeld P, Docena GH, Anon MC, Fossati CA. Detection and identification of a soy protein component that cross-reacts with caseins from cow's milk. Clin Exp Immunol 2002;130:49–58.

46. Franck P, Moneret Vautrin DA, Dousset B, et al. The allergenicity of soybean-based products is modified by food technologies. Int Arch Allergy Immunol 2002;128:212–9.

47. Roberts G, Lack G. Getting more out of your skin prick tests. Clin Exp Allergy 2000;30:1495–8.

48. Niggemann B, Reibel S, Wahn U. The atopy patch test (APT) a useful tool for the diagnosis of food allergy in children with atopic dermatitis. Allergy 2000;55:281–5.

49. Hill DJ, Cameron DJ, Francis DE, et al. Challenge confirmation of late-onset reactions to extensively hydrolyzed formulas in infants with multiple food protein intolerance. J Allergy Clin Immunol 1995;96:386–94.

50. Vanderhoof JA, Murray ND, Kaufman SS, et al. Intolerance to protein hydrolysate infant formulas: An under recognized cause of gastrointestinal symptoms in infants. J Pediatr 1997;131:741–4.

51. de Boissieu D, Dupont C. Time course of allergy to extensively hydrolyzed cow's milk proteins in infants. J Pediatr 2000;136:119–20.

52. Heine RG, Elsayed S, Hosking CS, Hill DJ. Cow's milk allergy in infancy. Curr Opin Allergy Clin Immunol 2002;2:217–25.

53. Hill DJ, Hosking CS, Heine RG. Clinical spectrum of food allergy in children in Australia and South-East Asia: Identification and targets for treatment. Ann Med 1999;31:272–81.

54. Isolauri E, Tabvanainen A, Peltola T, Arvola T. Breast-feeding of allergic infants. J Pediatr 1999;134:27–32.

55. Poley JR, Bhatia M, Welsh JD. Disaccharidase deficiency in infants with cow's milk protein intolerance. Response to treatment. Digestion 1978;17:97–107.

56. Hankard GF, Matarazzo P, Duong JP, et al. Increased TIA1-expressing intraepithelial lymphocytes in cow's milk protein intolerance. J Pediatr Gastroenterol Nutr 1997;25:79–83.

57. Hauer AC, Breese E, Walker-Smith JA, MacDonald TT. The frequency of cells secreting interferon-γ, interleukin-4, interleukin-5 and interleukin-10 in the blood and duodenal mucosa of children with cow's milk hypersensitivity. Pediatr Res 1997;42:629–38.

58. Veres G, Westerholm-Ormio M, Kokkonen J, et al. Cytokines and adhesion molecules in duodenal mucosa of chil-

dren with delayed-type food allergy. J Pediatr Gastroenterol Nutr 2003;37:27–34.

59. Pérez-Machado MA, Ashwood P, Torrente F, et al. Spontaneous T_H1 cytokine production by intraepithelial lymphocytes, but not circulating T cells, in both food-allergic and non-allergic infants. Allergy 2004;59:346–53.

60. Pérez-Machado MA, Ashwood P, Thomson MA, et al. Reduced transforming growth factor-β1 producing T cells in the duodenal mucosa of children with food allergy. Eur J Immunol 2003;33:2307–15.

61. Hill DJ, Ball G, Hoskings CS, Wood PR. γ Interferon production in cow's milk allergy. Allergy 1993;48:5–80.

62. Beyer K, Castro R, Birnbaum A, et al. Human milk-specific mucosal lymphocytes of the gastrointestinal tract display a T_H2 cytokine profile. J Allergy Clin Immunol 2002;109:707–13.

63. Nagata S, McKenzie C, Pender SL, et al. Human Peyer's patch T cells are sensitized to dietary antigen and display a Th cell type 1 cytokine profile. J Immunol 2000;165:5315–21.

64. Chung HL, Hwang JB, Park JJ, Kim SG. Expression of transforming growth factor β1, transforming growth factor type I and II receptors, and TNF-α in the mucosa of the small intestine in infants with food-protein induced enterocolitis syndrome. J Allergy Clin Immunol 2002;109:150–4.

65. Heyman M, Darmon N, Dupont C, et al. Mononuclear cells from infants allergic to cow's milk secrete tumor necrosis factor α, altering intestinal function. Gastroenterology 1994;106:1514–23.

66. Majamaa H, Miettinen A, Laine S, Isolauri E. Intestinal inflammation in children with atopic eczema: Fecal eosinophil cationic protein and tumor necrosis factor-α as non-invasive indicators of food allergy. Clin Exp Allergy 1996;26:181–7.

67. Turcanu V, Maleki SJ, Lack G. Characterization of lymphocyte responses to peanuts in normal children, peanut-allergic children, and allergic children who acquired tolerance to peanuts. J Clin Invest 2003;111:1065–72.

68. Dupont C, Heyman M. Food protein-induced enterocolitis syndrome: Laboratory perspectives. J Pediatr Gastroenterol Nutr 2000;3:S50–7.

69. Murch S. Allergy and intestinal dysmotility-evidence of genuine causal linkage. Curr Opin Gastroenterol 2006;22:664–8.

70. Kapel N, Matarazzo P, Haouchine D, et al. Fecal tumor necrosis factor α, eosinophil cationic protein and IgE levels in infants with cows milk allergy and gastrointestinal manifestations. Clin Chem Lab Med 1998;37:29–32.

71. Santos J, Bayarri C, Saperas E, et al. Characterisation of immune mediator release during the immediate response to segmental mucosal challenge in the jejunum of patients with food allergy. Gut 1999;45:553–8.

72. Chung HL, Hwang JB, Kwon YD, et al. Deposition of eosinophil-granule major basic protein and expression of intercellular adhesion molecule-1 and vascular cell adhesion molecule-1 in the mucosa of the small intestine in infants with cow's milk-sensitive enteropathy. J Allergy Clin Immunol 1999;103:1195–201.

73. Hill DJ, Firer MA, Shelton MJ, Hosking CS. Manifestations of milk allergy in infancy: Clinical and immunologic findings. J Pediatr 1986;109:270–6.

74. MacDonald TT, Spencer JM. Evidence that activated mucosal T cells play a role in the pathogenesis of enteropathy in human small intestine. J Exp Med 1988;167:1341–9.

75. Lionetti P, Breese E, Braegger CP, et al. T cell activation can induce either mucosal destruction or adaptation in cultured human fetal small intestine. Gastroenterology 1993;105:373–81.

76. Mowat AMcI. Anatomical basis of tolerance and immunity to intestinal antigens. Nature Rev Immunol 2003;3:331–41.

77. Eckmann L, Kagnoff MF, Fierer J. Epithelial cells secrete the chemokine interleukin-8 in response to bacterial entry. Infection Immun 1993;61:4569–74.

78. Walker-Smith JA, Murch SH. Enterocyte proliferation and functions. In: Diseases of the Small Intestine in Childhood, 4th edition. Oxford: Isis Medical Media; 1999. p. 29–43.

79. Sanderson IR, Ouellette AJ, Carter EA, et al. Differential regulation of B7 mRNA in enterocytes and lymphoid cells. Immunology 1993;79:434–8.

80. Mayer L. Mucosal immunity. Pediatrics 2003;111:1595–600.

81. Allez M, Brimnes J, Dotan I, Mayer L. Expansion of CD8+ T cells with regulatory function after interaction with intestinal epithelial cells. Gastroenterology 2002;123:1516–26.

82. Atisook K, Madara JL. An oligopeptide permeates intestinal tight junctions at glucose-elicited dilatations. Implications for oligopeptide absorption. Gastroenterology 1991;100:719–24.

83. Gruskay FL, Cook RE. The gastrointestinal absorption of unaltered protein in normal infants and in infants recovering from diarrhoea. Pediatrics 1955;16:763–8.

84. Keljo DF, Butler DG, Hamilton JR. Altered jejunal permeability to macromolecules during viral enteritis in the piglet. Gastroenterology 1985;88:998–1004.

85. Ford RPK, Menzies IS, Phillips AD, et al. Intestinal sugar permeability: Relationship to diarrhoeal disease and small bowel morphology. J Pediatr Gastroenterol Nutr 1985; 4:568–75.

86. Walker WA, Isselbacher KJ. Uptake and transport of macromolecules by the intestine. Possible role in clinical disorders. Gastroenterology 1974;67:531–50.

87. Bevilacqua C, Montagnac G, Benmerah A, et al. Food allergens are protected from degradation during CD23-mediated transepithelial transport. Int Arch Allergy Immunol 2004;135:108–16.

88. Dupont C, Barau E, Molkhou P, et al. Food-induced alterations of intestinal permeability in children with cow's milk-sensitive enteropathy and atopic dermatitis. J Pediatr Gastroenterol Nutr 1989;8:459–65.

89. Adams RB, Planchon SM, Roche JK. IFN-γ modulation of epithelial barrier function. Time course, reversibility, and site of cytokine binding. J Immunol 1993;150:2356–63.

90. Marano CW, Lewis SA, Garulacan LA, et al. Tumor necrosis factor-α increases sodium and chloride conductance across the tight junction of CACO-2 BBE, a human intestinal epithelial cell line. J Membr Biol 1998;161:263–74.

91. Planchon SM, Martins CA, Guerrant RL, Roche JK. Regulation of intestinal epithelial barrier function by TGF-β1. Evidence for its role in abrogating the effect of a T cell cytokine. J Immunol 1994;153:5370–9.

92. Madsen KL, Lewis SA, Tavernini MM, et al. Interleukin 10 prevents cytokine-induced disruption of T84 monolayer barrier integrity and limits chloride secretion. Gastroenterol 1997;113:151–9.

93. Ulloa L, Doody J, Massague J. Inhibition of transforming growth factor-β/SMAD signalling by the interferon-γ/STAT pathway. Nature 1999;397:710–3.

94. Weiner HL. Oral tolerance: Immune mechanisms and treatment of autoimmune diseases. Immunol Today 1997; 18:335–43.

95. Strobel S. Immunity induced after a feed of antigen during early life: Oral tolerance v. sensitisation. Proc Nutr Soc 2001;60:437–42.

96. Zimmer KP, Buning J, Weber P, et al. Modulation of antigen trafficking to MHC class II-positive late endosomes of enterocytes. Gastroenterology 2000;118:128–37.

97. Kaji T, Hachimura S, Ise W, Kaminogawa S. Proteome analysis reveals caspase activation in hyporesponsive CD4 T lymphocytes induced in vivo by the oral administration of antigen. J Biol Chem 2003;278:27836–43.

98. Groux H, Powrie F. Regulatory T cells and inflammatory bowel disease. Immunol Today 1999;20:442–6.

99. Karlsson MR, Rugtveit J, Brandtzaeg P. Allergen-responsive CD4+CD25+ regulatory T cells in children who have outgrown cow's milk allergy. J Exp Med 2004;199:1679–88.

100. Gambineri E, Torgerson TR, Ochs HD. Immune dysregulation, polyendocrinopathy, enteropathy, and X-linked inheritance (IPEX), a syndrome of systemic autoimmunity caused by mutations of FOXP3, a critical regulator of T-cell homeostasis. Curr Opin Rheumatol 2003;15:430–5.

101. Taams LS, Vukmanovic-Stejic M, Smith J, et al. Antigen-specific T cell suppression by human CD4+CD25+ regulatory T cells. Eur J Immunol 2002;32:1621–30.

102. Iellem A, Colantonio L, D'Ambrosio D. Skin-versus gut-skewed homing receptor expression and intrinsic CCR4 expression on human peripheral blood CD4+CD25+ suppressor T cells. Eur J Immunol 2003;33:1488–96.

103. Wing K, Lindgren S, Kollberg G, et al. CD4 T cell activation by myelin oligodendrocyte glycoprotein is suppressed by adult but not cord blood CD25+ T cells. Eur J Immunol 2003;33:579–87.

104. Miller A, Lider O, Abramsky O, Weiner HL. Orally administered myelin basic protein in neonates primes for immune responses and enhances experimental autoimmune encephalomyelitis in adult animals. Eur J Immunol 1994;24: 1026–32.

105. Hauer AC, Rieder M, Griessl A, et al. Cytokine production by cord blood mononuclear cells stimulated by cows milk protein in vitro: Interleukin-4 and transforming growth factor β-secreting cells detected in the CD45RO T cell population in children of atopic mothers. Clin Exp Allergy 2003;33:615–23.

106. Bedford Russell AR, Murch SH. Could peripartum antibiotics have delayed health consequences for the infant? Br J Obstetr Gynaecol 2006;113:758–65.

107. Newberry RD, Stenson WF, Lorenz RG. Cycloxygenase-2-dependent arachidonic acid metabolites are essential modulators of the immune response to dietary antigen. Nat Med 1999;5:900–6.

108. Campbell DI, Murch SH, Elia M, et al. Chronic T cell-mediated enteropathy in rural West African children: Relationship with nutritional status and small bowel function. Pediatr Res 2003;54:306–11.

109. Iyngkaran N, Yadav M, Boey CG, et al. Causative effects of cow's milk protein and soy protein on progressive small bowel mucosal damage. J Gastroenterol Hepatol 1989;4:127–36.

110. Lifshitz F, Fagundes-Neto U, Ferreira VC, et al. The response to dietary treatment of patients with chronic post-infectious diarrhea and lactose intolerance. J Am Coll Nutr 1990;9:231–40.

111. Amadi B, Mwiya M, Chomba E, et al. Improved nutritional recovery on an elemental diet in Zambian children with persistent diarrhoea and malnutrition. J Trop Pediatr 2005;51:5–10.

112. Lunn PG, Northrop-Clewes CA, Downes RM. Intestinal permeability, mucosal injury, and growth faltering in Gambian infants. Lancet 1991;338:907–10.

113. Robinson JK, Blanchard TG, Levine AD, et al. A mucosal IgA-mediated excretory immune system in vivo. J Immunol 2001;166:3688–92.

114. Klemola T, Savilahti E, Arato A, et al. Immunohistochemical findings in jejunal specimens from patients with IgA deficiency. Gut 1995;37:519–23.

115. Soothill JF, Stokes CR, Turner MW, et al. Predisposing factors and the development of reaginic allergy in infancy. Clin Allergy 1976;6:305–19.

116. Ludviksson BR, Elriksson TH, Ardal B, Sigfusson A, Valdimarsson H. Correlation between serum immunoglobulin A concentrations and allergic manifestations in infants. J Pediatr 1992;121:23–7.

117. Hacsek G, Savilahti E. Increase in density of jejunal IgA2 cells during infancy without change in IgA1 cells. J Pediatr Gastroenterol Nutr 1996;22:307–11.

118. Sletten GB, Halvorsen R, Egaas E, Halstensen TS. Casein-specific immunoglobulins in cow's milk allergic patient subgroups reveal a shift to IgA dominance in tolerant patients. Pediatr Allergy Immunol 2007;18:71–80.

119. Sletten GB, Halvorsen R, Egaas E, Halstensen TS. Changes in humoral responses to beta-lactoglobulin in tolerant patients suggest a particular role for IgG4 in delayed, non-IgE-mediated cow's milk allergy. Pediatr Allergy Immunol 2006;17:435–43.

120. Harrison BM, Kilby A, Walker-Smith JA, et al. Cows' milk protein intolerance: A possible association with gastroenteritis, lactose intolerance and IgA deficiency. BMJ 1976;i:1501–5.

121. Matthews TS, Soothill JF. Complement activation after milk feeding in children with cow's milk allergy. Lancet 1970;ii:893–7.

122. Saalman R, Dahlgren UI, Fallstrom SP, et al. ADCC-mediating capacity in children with cow's milk protein intolerance in relation to IgG subclass profile of serum antibodies to beta-lactoglobulin. Scand J Immunol 1995;42:140–6.

123. Sigurs N, Hattevig G, Kjellman B, et al. Appearance of atopic disease in relation to serum IgE antibodies in children followed from birth for 4 to 15 years. J Allergy Clin Immunol 1994;94:757–63.

124. Corry DB, Kheradmand F. Induction and regulation of the IgE response. Nature 1999;402:B18–23.

125. Hershey GK, Friedrich MF, Esswein LA, et al. The association of atopy with a gain-of-function mutation in the α subunit of the interleukin-4 receptos. New Engl J Med 1997;337:1720–5.

126. Grunewald SM, Werthmann A, Schnarr B, et al. An antagonistic IL-4 mutant prevents type I allergy in the mouse: Inhibition of the IL-4/IL-13 receptor system completely abrogates humoral immune response to allergen and development of allergic symptoms in vivo. J Immunol 1998; 160:4004–9.

127. Shimoda K, van Deursen J, Sangster MY, et al. Lack of IL-4-induced T cell response and IgE class switching in mice with disrupted Stat6 gene. Nature 1996;380:630–3.

128. Coeffier M, Lorentz A, Manns MP, Bischoff SC. Epsilon germ-line and IL-4 transcripts are expressed in human intestinal mucosa and enhanced in patients with food allergy. Allergy 2005;60:822–7.

129. Negrao-Correa D, Adams LS, Bell RG. Intestinal transport and catabolism of IgE: A major blood-independent pathway of IgE dissemination during a Trichinella spiralis infection of rats. J Immunol 1996;157:4037–44.

130. Li H, Nowak-Wegrzyn A, Charlop-Powers Z, et al. Transcytosis of IgE-antigen complexes by CD23a in human intestinal epithelial cells and its role in food allergy. Gastroenterology 2006;131:47–58.

131. Kaiserlian D, Lachaux A, Grosjean I, et al. Intestinal epithelial cells express the CD23/Fc epsilon RII molecule: Enhanced expression in enteropathies. Immunology 1993;80:90–5.

132. Hogan SP, Mishra A, Brandt EB, et al. A critical role for eotaxin in experimental oral antigen-induced eosinophilic gastrointestinal allergy. Proc Natl Acad Sci U S A 2000;97:6681–6.

133. Hogan SP, Mishra A, Brandt EB, et al. A pathological function for eotaxin and eosinophils in eosinophilic gastrointestinal inflammation. Nat Immunol 2001;2:353–60.

134. Mishra M, Hogan SP, Brandt EB, Rothenberg ME. An etiological role for aeroallergens and eosinophils in experimental esophagitis. J Clin Invest 2001;107:83–90.

135. Mishra A, Hogan SP, Brandt EB, Rothenberg ME. IL-5 promotes eosinophil trafficking to the esophagus. J Immunol 2002;168:2464–9.

136. Vandenzande LM, Wallaert B, Desreumaux P, et al. Interleukin-5 immunoreactivity and mRNA expression in gut mucosa from patients with food allergy. Clin Exp Allergy 1999;29:652–9.

137. Schade RP, Van Leperen-Van Dijk AG, Van Reijsen FC. Differences in antigen-specific T-cell responses between infants with atopic dermatitis with and without cow's milk allergy: Relevance of Th2 cytokines. J Allergy Clin Immunol 2000;106:1155–62.

138. Butt AM, Murch SH, Ng C, et al. Upregulated eotaxin expression and T cell infiltration in the basal oesophageal epithelium in cow's milk-associated reflux oesophagitis. Arch Dis Child 2002;87:124–30.

139. Sampson HA, Sicherer SH, Bimbaum AH. AGA technical review on the evaluation of food allergy in gastrointestinal disorders. American Gastroenterological Association. Gastroenterol 2001;120:1026–40.

140. Sampson HA. Use of food challenge tests in children. Lancet 2001;358:1832–3.

141. The European Society for Paediatric Gastroenterology and Nutrition Group for the diagnostic criteria for food allergy. Diagnostic criteria for food allergy with predominantly intestinal symptoms. J Pediatr Gastroenterol Nutr 1992;14:108–12.

142. Bock SA. Diagnostic evaluation. Pediatrics 2003;111: 1638–44.

143. Caffarelli C, Petroccione T. False-negative food challenges in children with suspected food allergy. Lancet 2001;358:1871–2.

144. Carroccio A, Montalto G, Custro N, et al. Evidence of very delayed clinical reactions to cow's milk in cow's milk-intolerant patients. Allergy 2000;55:574–9.

145. Arslan G, Gilja OH, Lind R, et al. Response to intestinal provocation monitored by transabdominal ultrasound in patients with food hypersensitivity. Scand J Gastroenterol 2005;40:386–94.

146. Sporik R, Hill DJ, Hosking CS. Specificity of allergen skin testing in predicting positive open food challenges to milk, egg and peanut in children. Clin Exp Allergy 2000;30: 1540–6.

147. Wistokat-Wulfing A, Schmidt P, Darsow U, et al. Atopy patch test reactions are associated with T lymphocyte-mediated allergen-specific immune responses in atopic dermatitis. Clin Exp Allergy 1999;29:513–21.

148. Isolauri E, Turjanmaa K. Combined skin prick and patch testing enhances identification of food allergy in infants with atopic dermatitis. J Allergy Clin Immunol 1996;97:9–15.

149. Stromberg L. Diagnostic accuracy of the atopy patch test and the skin-prick test for the diagnosis of food allergy in young children with atopic eczema dermatitis syndrome. Acta Paediatr 2002;91:1044–9.

150. Fogg MI, Brown-Whitehorn TA, Pawlowski NA, Spergel JM. Atopy patch test for the diagnosis of food protein-induced enterocolitis syndrome. Pediatr Allergy Immunol 2006;17:351–5.

151. Sampson HA, Ho DG. Relationship between food-specific IgE concentrations and the risk of positive food challenges in children and adolescents. J Allergy Clin Immunol 1997;100:444–51.

152. Sicherer SH, Sampson HA. Cow's milk protein-specific IgE concentrations in two age groups of milk-allergic children and in children achieving clinical tolerance. Clin Exp Allergy 1999;29:507–12.

153. Zeiger RS. Food allergen avoidance in the prevention of food allergy in infants and children. Pediatrics 2003;111:1662–71.

154. von Berg A, Koletzko S, Grubl A, et al. German Infant Nutritional Intervention Study Group. The effect of hydrolyzed cow's milk formula for allergy prevention in the first year of life: The German Infant Nutritional Intervention Study, a randomized double-blind trial. J Allergy Clin Immunol 2003;111:533–40.

155. Cebra JJ. Influences of microbiota on intestinal immune system development. Am J Clin Nutr 1999;69:1046S–51S.

156. Sudo N, Sawamura S, Tanaka K, et al. The requirement of intestinal bacterial flora for the development of an IgE

production system susceptible to oral tolerance induction. J Immunol 1997;159:1739–45.

157. Kalliomaki M, Salminen S, Arvillomi H, et al. Probiotics in primary prevention of atopic disease: A randomised placebo-controlled trial. Lancet 2001;357:1076–9.

158. Lodinova-Zadnikova R, Cukrowska B, Tlaskalova-Hogenova H. Oral administration of probiotic Escherichia coli after birth reduces frequency of allergies and repeated infections later in life (after 10 and 20 years). Int Arch Allergy Immunol 2003;131:209–11.

159. Ohtsuka Y, Yamashiro Y, Shimizu T, et al. Reducing cell membrane n-6 fatty acids attenuate mucosal damage in food-sensitive enteropathy in mice. Pediatr Res 1997;42: 835–9.

160. Adorini L, Penna G, Giarratana N, Uskokovic M. Tolerogenic dendritic cells induced by vitamin D receptor ligands enhance regulatory T cells inhibiting allograft rejection and autoimmune diseases. J Cell Biochem 2003;88:227–33.

161. Nowak-Wegrzyn A. Future approaches to food allergy. Pediatrics 2003;111:1672 80.

162. Leung DYM, Sampson HA, Yunginger JW, et al. For the TNX-901 Peanut Allergy Study Group. Effect of anti-IgE therapy in patients with peanut allergy. N Engl J Med 2003;348:986–93.

163. Stein ML, Collins MH, Villanueva JM, et al. Anti-IL-5 (mepolizumab) therapy for eosinophilic esophagitis. J Allergy Clin Immunol 2006;118:1312–9.

16.3. Autoimmune Enteropathy and IPEX Syndrome

Frank M. Ruemmele, MD, PhD

Nicole Brousse, MD, PhD

Olivier Goulet, MD, PhD

Over the past few years, major advances in the understanding of the pathophysiology of intractable diarrhea of infancy (IDI) were made allowing a new conceptual view of this heterogeneous group of different diseases (see also Chapter 15.3c, "Intractable Diarrhea of Infancy"). The term "intractable diarrhea of infancy with persistent villous atrophy" is based on the clinical observation of a diarrhea starting within the first 2 years of life, which is abundant (>100 mL/kg/d), and persists despite bowel rest along with a flat intestinal mucosa. Diarrhea rapidly becomes life threatening, and long-term total parenteral nutrition (TPN) is required. A clearly distinct presentation of IDI is in form of "autoimmune enteropathy (AIE)." The first report of AIE in the literature goes back to 1978.[1] McCarthy and colleagues reported on an adolescent boy with immunoglobulin A (IgA) deficiency who showed a severe enteropathy with total villous atrophy and circulating gut autoantibodies. The term "autoimmune enteropathy" was introduced by Unsworth and Walker-Smith for severe persistent diarrhea in the absence of immune deficiency but associated with autoimmune disorders.[2] One characteristic of AIE is the presence of specific complement-fixing circulating antibodies directed against small intestinal and colonic epithelial cells.[3] A historic keystone in the description of protracted, immune-mediated diarrhea is the report of Powell and colleagues who observed in the same family over three generations 17 boys with various autoimmune disorders.[4] Eight of them died of severe protracted diarrhea. This and other observations clearly suggest an X-linked mode of transmission.[2,5–10] We recently reported on a family over four generations with at least six affected male members and ten female carriers confirming an X-linked disorder[11] in some familial forms of AIE. There are several reports on boys with immune-mediated profuse diarrhea occurring within the first few months of life, often preceded or accompanied by insulin-dependent diabetes mellitus or other endocrinopathies, indicating rather a systemic than an isolated GI disease.[8–10] However, girls presenting with different forms of AIE were also reported,[12–14] pointing out to other than X-linked pathomechanisms.

Based on recent advances on the genetics of autoimmune enteropathy, the pathophysiology and clinical presentation, AIE can be classified into three different types: the classical form of AIE type 1, which is identical to the so-called IPEX syndrome (*i*mmune dysregulation, *p*olyendocrinopathy, *e*nteropathy, *X*-linked syndrome), type 2 as an IPEX-like form (without mutations in the FOXP3 gene) in boys and girls, and type 3 with autoimmune manifestations mainly limited to the gastrointestinal tract. AIE has clearly to be distinguished from profuse diarrhea occurring in different forms of immunodeficiency syndromes or constitutive enterocyte disorders.

DEFINITION OF AIE

The hallmark of all different forms of AIE is the occurrence of profuse diarrhea most often in the form of massive protein-losing enteropathy (potentially involving the entire GI tract), along with villous atrophy and a massive mononuclear inflammatory infiltrate of the lamina propria on duodenal/jejunal histology as well as the occurrence of antienterocyte antibodies. AIE is a typical T-cell–mediated disorders which has to be distinguished from classical immune deficiencies.

IPEX SYNDROME (AIE TYPE 1)

IPEX syndrome is a rare disorder, and clinical experience is based on a limited number of cases. To date, no estimates of incidence have been proposed. The main clinical characteristic of IPEX syndrome is the combination of early onset type 1 diabetes mellitus, severe immune-mediated enteropathy and eczema-like dermatitis (see below). IPEX is usually fatal during early infancy. Recently, with the characterization of specific mutations in the FOXP3 gene, a first clue to the understanding of this X-linked disorder was found.[15–16]

PATHOPHYSIOLOGY

Animal Model

First insight into the pathophysiology of IPEX came from scurfy mice which are a naturally occurring X-linked mutant presenting with symptoms very similar to human IPEX syndrome, ie, massive lymphoproliferation, scaly skin, diarrhea, intestinal bleeding, anemia, thrombocytopenia, and hypogonadism.[17–19] Symptoms occur only in hemizigous mutant males; female carriers are asymptomatic. In scurfy, CD4+ T cells are chronically activated and play a key role in the development of the disease.[20–21] These cells are characterized by an upregulation of the cell surface antigens CD69, CD25, CD80, and CD86, a marked hyperresponsiveness to activation via the T-cell receptor (TCR) along with a decreased requirement for costimulation through CD28. In scurfy, high levels of cytokines, such as interleukin (IL)-2, -4, -5, -10, and TNFα were produced by these cells.[20–21] The gene mutated in scurfy mice was recently identified (FOXP3) and cloned on the X chromosome.[17,22] It encodes a 48 kDa protein of the forkhead (FKH)/winged-helix transcription factor family, named scurfin.[22] This protein is expressed at low levels in CD4+ T cells with a more abundant expression in the CD4+ CD25+ T-cell subgroup. The structure of the protein suggests that it has DNA binding activity. Schubert and colleagues recently showed that scurfin acts as a repressor of transcription and regulator of T-cell activation.[23] Intact scurfin represses transcription of a reporter containing a multimeric FKH binding site. Such FKH binding sites were identified adjacent to nuclear factor of activated T cells (NFAT) regulatory sites in the promotors of IL-2 or granulocyte macrophage colony stimulating factor enhancer. This observation indicates that intact scurfy is capable to directly repress NFAT-mediated transcription of the IL-2 gene in CD4+ T cells upon activation.[23] The exact molecular mechanisms leading to scurfy are yet not fully understood. However, there is experimental evidence that the biological activity of scurfin depends on a functional FKH domain. In scurfy mice, a 2 bp insertion results in a premature stop codon leading to a loss in the C-terminal domain.[22] The loss of function of scurfin may result in abnormal (nonsuppressed) T-cell reactivity leading to an uncontrolled inflammatory reaction.

GENETIC BACKGROUND

The overwhelming clinical similarities between scurfy mice and IPEX patients led to an exhaustive genetic analysis in IPEX families. Genetic mapping in these families allowed to identify the human IPEX locus to Xp11.23-q13.3.[24–26] The gene was named FOXP3 (or JM2) and its protein product, scurfin[24] or FOXP3 protein. Wildin and colleagues recently reviewed that in 10 of 11 screened IPEX families mutations were found within the coding region potentially leading to absent FOXP3 protein or a protein product with loss of function.[27] In the eleventh family, a mutation in the 3′ untranslated region of FOXP3 was observed. Several IPEX mutations were within the winged helix domain of scurfin, altering its DNA binding capacity.[15] None of the mutations described in IPEX patients was observed in hundreds of nondisease, ethnically diverse individuals, making the possibility of gene polymorphisms unrelated to IPEX unlikely.[15] In addition, female carriers (heterozygeous for FOXP3 mutations) are completely asymptomatic[28] In some patients with typical clinical symptoms of IPEX, no mutations were found within the coding regions of FOXP3,[15–16] suggesting that regulatory or conditional mutations may occur outside FOXP3, such as described by Bennett and colleagues[29] in the polyadenylation signal following the final coding exon of FOXP3. This may result in a decreased FOXP3 mRNA expression, probably due to nonspecific degradation of the aberrant RNA. We described recently[11] an unusual deletion in an upstream, noncoding region of FOXP3 gene (exon 1/adjacent intron del(-)6247_(-)4859). This deletion impairs mRNA splicing resulting in accumulation of unspliced pre-mRNA and alternatively spliced mRNA. In addition, it is possible that other FOXP3-independent forms of IPEX or AIE occur in boys (see AIE type 2). The molecular mechanisms of these potentially FOXP3-independent forms of AIE/IPEX remain to be elucidated.

PATHOPHYSIOLOGY IN HUMANS

Autoimmunity in IPEX syndrome may be a direct consequence of a regulatory FOXP3+ T-cell defect. FOXP3 functions as transcriptional repressor within the nucleus and inhibits activation-induced IL-2 gene transcription (probably via the interference with NFAT regulatory sites). A recent precise molecular analysis[30] revealed that the majority of FOXP3 mutations in IPEX patients cluster primarily within the FKH domain and the leucine zipper. To exert its repressor functions, FOXP3 localizes to the nucleus, a process which requires a fully functional N- and C-terminal end of the FKH domain, In a second step, to become fully functional, FOXP3 homodimerizes through its leucin zipper, Therefore, mutations altering the FKH domain or leucine zipper can directly compromise these functions of the FOXP3 protein. These data indicate for the first time a molecular basis how a distinct mutation in the *FOXP3* gene interferes with its transcriptional regulatory functions.

To exert their regulatory functions, a direct cell to cell contact of CD4+CD25+ regulatory and effector T cells is necessary. To date it is believed that this direct contact allows to control and downregulate effector functions of activated T cells. Therefore, any disturbance or perturbance of this interaction is likely to cause an uncontrolled inflammatory reaction, seen in the inflammatory infiltration of various tissues, as well as the secretion of inflammatory T-cell derived cytokines. As a consequence, inflammatory lesions and tissue destruction can occur, potentially opening new antigenic structures which may give rise to the production of auto-antibodies, such as antienterocyte antibodies (see below).

Bacchetta and colleagues[31] recently observed that in some IPEX patients not only suppressor functions of regulatory T cells are compromised, but in addition, effector T cells showed clear abnormalities, indicating a more general defect of T cell. Upon CD3/CD28 stimulation effector T cells of IPEX patients produced markedly less IFNγ and IL-2 compared to healthy control T cells. Since IL-2 is a master cytokine for regulatory T-cell functions, this defect may further aggravate already insufficient regulatory T-cell controls.

Taken together autoimmune lesions in IPEX patients, as well as other forms of AIE, might be caused by a defective interaction of regulatory and effector T cells. Theoretically, this defect may affect regulation and function of regulatory T cells (primarily CD4+CD25 high FOXP+3 cells, but also other subsets of regulatory T cells could be concerned), the interaction between regulatory and effector T cells as well as the regulation and/or function of effector T cells.

CLINICAL PRESENTATION

IPEX syndrome is a systemic disorder and can be considered as a maximal form of AIE (Table 1). The major clinical symptoms are the association of a severe enteropathy with insulin-dependent diabetes mellitus along with eczema, hematological abnormalities, and eventually other endocrinopathies.[27,32–34] In many cases the onset of diabetes is prior to the first intestinal symptoms. Levy-Lahad and Wildin suggested that diabetes is the result of a complete inflammatory destruction of pancreatic islet cells.[35] Equilibration of diabetes with insulin in these patients is sometimes rather difficult.

The onset of diarrhea is often within the first 3 months of life; however, later onset was occasionally described.[6,36–37] Characteristically, diarrhea is of secretory nature and persists despite bowel rest. In our experience, stool volumes are approximately 75 to 150 mL/kg/d with sometimes mucous or blood discharge. Patients most often develop a protein losing enteropathy with a markedly increased clearance of α-1 antitrypsine and hypoalbuminemia. Severe clinical expression is most often sign of a poor prognosis. Electrolyte imbalances are secondary to diarrhea. Electrolyte correction and stabilization of IPEX patients can initially only be achieved by bowel rest and total parenteral nutrition.

Another clinical feature of a subgroup of IPEX patients is eczema (atopic dermatitis), often severe in presentation. Eczema is most often diffuse, involving the entire skin and may show follicular dermatitis. It was recently reported that eczema is present in about two-thirds of patients.[27] Further symptoms, such as thyroiditis, hematological abnormalities (Coombs-positive anemia, neutropenia,[37] and thrombocytopenia), or diffuse lymphadenopathy are markedly less frequent.[27,37] Thyroiditis most often presents in form of hypothyroidism requiring substitutive treatment. In our personal experience, hypothyroidism occurred in 2 out of 13 AIE patients followed at Necker-Enfants Malades Hospital. Renal involvement, in form of glomerulonephritis, tubulopathy, or nephrotic syndrome was also described in a subset of IPEX patients.[9,38–39] In our patients, two cases presented with biopsy-proven membranous glomerulonephritis.

Other organ systems which are occasionally involved are the liver—ranging from normal liver function to acute or chronic hepatitis,[4,7,10,40–41] as well as the lung. In three patients diffuse pulmonary interstitial lymphoid infiltrates were noted at autopsy.[3,7]

ENDOSCOPY

Upper and lower endoscopies are mandatory when AIE is suspected. The entire GI tract from the stomach to the rectum can be involved. In most cases, there is a marked discrepancy between macroscopic endoscopic and histological findings. Macroscopically, the mucosa of the stomach, duodenum, jejunum, and ileum shows only mild abnormalities that is a variable degree of enhanced mucosal granularity along with erythema. Most often, no apthes or ulcerations are observed. Macroscopic signs of small bowel mucosal atrophy are rather discrete. Colonic lesions can be more pronounced that is loss of the normal vascular pattern due to inflammatory edema, along with erythema, potentially involving the entire colonic mucosa. In addition, a marked granular aspect of the mucosa is regularly observed. These findings are most often homogenous along the entire colon and not distributed in a patchy manner with normal mucosa interposed. However, rectosigmoidal sparing can occur. Comparably to upper GI tract lesions, ulcerations are rarely observed in the colon.

Table 1 Clinical Manifestations of IPEX

Diarrhea	Atopic dermatitis
Food intolerance	Hypothyroidism
Malnutrition	Glomerulonephritis, tubulopathy
Growth retardation/failure	Hemolytic anemia, thrombocytopenia
Diabetes mellitus	Lymphadenopathy

HISTOLOGY

Obligate histological findings in IPEX are the combination of villous atrophy (moderate to severe) and a massive mucosal mononuclear cell infiltration (Figure 1). This infiltrate consists predominately of T lymphocytes and is a main feature of AIE helping to distinguish this entity from other cases of IDI related to constitutive, inherited defects of enterocytes.[42] In most cases, severe to total villous atrophy is associated with crypt hyperplasia. Total villous atrophy on duodenal biopsies can initially mislead to suspect celiac disease. However, in celiac disease, villous atrophy is associated with a striking increase in the number of intraepithelial lymphocytes.[43] In contrast, T-cell infiltration in immune-mediated enteropathy predominates in the lamina propria, with no or only moderate increase of intraepithelial lymphocytes.[44]

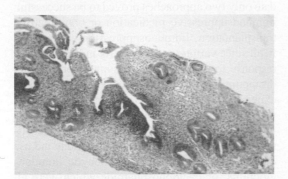

(A)

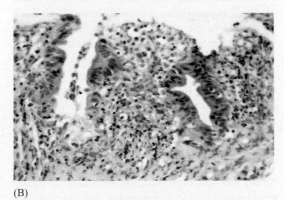

(B)

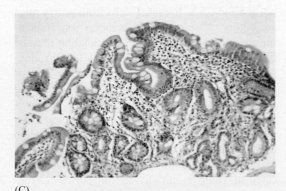

(C)

Figure 1 Duodenal biopsy of a patient with AIE type 2 showing the dense mononuclear infiltrate of the lamina propria. Note the marked villous atrophy and dedifferentiation of the intestinal epithelial cells. (A and B) At the time of diagnosis (before treatment). (C) After 4 weeks of treatment with tacrolimus, methylprednisolone, and azathioprine, the inflammatory infiltrate is markedly reduced and a normal intestinal architecture is visible.

Table 2 Laboratory Findings in IPEX

WBC	Normal, sometime eosinophilia
CD4/CD8 ratio	Normal or CD4+ slightly increased
IgG, IgA, IgM	Normal
IgE	High to extremely high
Anti-enterocyte antibodies	Present (IgG type, sometimes IgA or IgM)
Anti-colonocytes antibodies	Present (IgG type, sometimes IgA or IgM)
Anti-goblet cell antibodies	Present or absent
Anti-AIE-75 antibodies	Present or absent
Anti-GAD	Present or absent
Anti-SMA	Present or absent
Anti-DNA	Present or absent
Albumine	Always (markedly) decreased
Liver enzymes	Can be increased
α-1-Antitrypsine clearance	Pathological

Whereas in celiac disease, a marked increase in T lymphocytes expressing the T-cell receptor (TCR) of the γ/δ-type was observed,[45] in AIE, TCR expression is restricted to the α/β + subset. In some patients, villous atrophy is associated with epithelial cell death and crypt abscess formation (Figure 1B). Recent studies indicate that enterocyte cell death occurs via apoptosis, probably induced by activated cytotoxic lymphocytes. The number of goblet cells is also reduced, and in some cases, goblet cells are almost absent.[44,46]

Mononuclear cell infiltration within the lamina propria includes mainly CD4+ T lymphocytes and macrophages, with numerous cells expressing CD25. Human leukocyte antigen (HLA)–DR expression is markedly increased on crypt epithelium.[42] These inflammatory changes are largely observed in small bowel mucosa, but it can also be seen in other parts of the digestive tract, such as the stomach or colon.[40] All along the entire intestinal tract, the same type of lesions can be observed, including epithelial cell apoptosis, crypt abscess formation, and mononuclear cell infiltration of the lamina propria. Extensive digestive involvement is usually associated with a poor outcome.

LABORATORY FINDINGS

Peripheral blood lymphocyte counts are normal along with normal T- and B-cell subsets in almost all patients. In addition the CD4/CD8 ratio was also reported to be normal, except in one observation with a slightly increased CD4 count.[10] T-cell proliferation assays (mitogens and antigens) are within the low-normal range or completely normal in the vast majority of patients. Humoral immunity is normal with normal vaccination titers and normal immunoglobulin levels for IgG, IgM, and IgA. In clear contrast, IgE levels are often dramatically raised and can be considered as one diagnostic criterium of IPEX. In addition, persistent or periodic eosinophilia is also frequent, reflecting an atopic-allergic background. In fact, skin tests for immediate hypersensitivity are often pathological in IPEX.[25,42] (See Table 2.)

Autoantibodies of the antienterocyte or anticolonocyte type are present in the vast majority of IPEX patients; however, in few patients the search for classical autoantibodies was negative.[9,37,47] On the other hand, antienterocyte antibodies at very low titers and most often of nonspecific nature were also observed in other inflammatory gut conditions, such as Crohn's disease, ulcerative colitis, or cow's milk allergy.[9] In the context of IDI, the presence of antienterocyte (human duodenum and jejunum) and/or anticolonocyte antibodies of the IgG type are thus highly suggestive of AIE. Antienterocyte antibodies of the IgA or IgM type were also described in a subgroup of patients.[9] High titers and the complement-fixing ability of antienterocyte antibodies indicate a poor prognosis. Indirect immunofluorescence studies showed that these autoantibodies are directed against components of the cytoplasm of mature enterocytes, with an increasing intensity toward the villus tip. Positive staining of the intestinal brush border membrane can also be observed (Figure 2). A pathogenetic role in the onset of intestinal inflammation—as suspected in the past—is rather unlikely.[2,3,6,45–46] The occurrence of antienterocyte/anticolonocyte antibodies is rather an epiphenomenon of intestinal inflammation. A precise kinetic study showed that autoantibodies occurred after the onset of intestinal lesions.[48] Antigoblet cell antibodies are also encountered in AIE patients.[46] Another highly specific antibody often detected in IPEX and AIE patients is directed against a novel gut and kidney-specific 75 kDa antigen, named

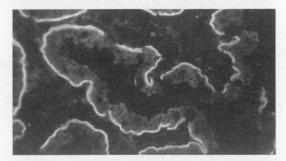

Figure 2 Immunofluorescence staining pattern of circulating antienterocyte antibodies which are directed against the brush border membrane of intestinal epithelial cells.

AIE75.[38,50] This antigen shares over 99% identity with NY-Co-38, a colon cancer–related autoantigen.[51] In IPEX a large panel of circulating autoantibodies can be found, such as antibodies against gastric parietal cells, pancreatic islets, insulin, glutamic acid decarboxylase (GAD), as well as antismooth muscle, antiendoplasmic reticulum, antireticulin and -gliadin, antiadrenal, anti-ANA, and anti-DNA antibodies. Finally, antithyreoglobulin or antimicrosomal antibodies can be seen without clinical symptoms of hypothyroidism.[3,4,13,47–49,52–54]

No particular or pathognomonic laboratory abnormality is observed in IPEX. Clinical laboratory tests are within the normal range, apart from signs of diabetes mellitus, protein-losing enteropathy, hypothyroidism, and eventually cytopenia. Electrolyte disturbances are secondary to secretory diarrhea and hypoproteinemia, and decreased albumin levels indicate the degree of protein-losing enteropathy. Abnormal biochemical liver tests (increased transaminase activity and cholestatic markers) were reported[4,7,40]; however, this can also be secondary to total parenteral nutrition.

Highly elevated stool levels for TNFα and calprotectine, as markers of intestinal mucosal inflammation, are regularly encountered in IPEX patients helping to distinguish atypical and early onset forms of AIE/IPEX from other causes of severe diarrhea.[55] With the induction of remission, these inflammatory fecal markers return to normal. A reliable marker for the degree of protein-losing enteropathy in AIE is an increased clearance of α-1-antitrypsin in the stool. Indeed, whereas normally, this clearance in the stool is less than 20 mL/d, in our IPEX patients α-1AT clearance was pathologically elevated.

AIE TYPE 2 (IPEX-LIKE WITHOUT MUTATIONS IN THE FOXP3 GENE) IN BOYS AND GIRLS

The observations of rare cases of AIE in girls[6,11–13] as well as typical IPEX presentations in boys without documented mutations or alterations of the regulation of the FOXP3 gene suggest that there might be a different non-X-linked mode of the disease. In most cases, girls present with multiple extraintestinal autoimmune manifestations, such as thyroiditis or diabetes. In the report of Mirakian and colleagues,[6] one girl presented with Still's disease, diabetes mellitus, and AIE with positive antienterocyte antibodies. Bousvaros and colleagues[11] described one girl showing typical symptoms with autoantibody-positive AIE associated with diabetes mellitus, indicating a strong autoimmune background.

If the clinical picture is that of multiple autoimmune symptoms, resembling IPEX syndrome, it is very likely that this disorder is secondary to a defect in regulatory T cells. These cells might be FOXP3+ or FOXP3– regulatory T cells. Further follow-up and detailed analyses of these patients will help to elucidate the molecular basis of these clinical descriptions.

AIE TYPE 3 (WITHOUT OR WITH FEW EXTRAINTESTINAL MANIFESTATIONS) IN BOYS AND GIRLS

Some patients were reported with symptoms exclusively limited to the GI tract in form of secretory diarrhea with positive-circulating antienterocyte/-colonocyte antibodies and positive anti-AIE-75 antibodies. In these patients, no extraintestinal manifestations were observed.[6,40] A priori, FOXP3 mutations are not a characteristic of these patients. However, in the past, mutational analyses of the FOXP3 gene were not performed; therefore, it is unclear if these children do not present with a minor or monosymptomatic form of IPEX. On the other hand, other mutations in regulatory genes controlling T-cell functions (regulatory or effector T cells, as discussed above) on the level of the intestinal mucosa are presumable. It would be interesting to elaborate, if the long-term follow-up of these patients reveals the occurrence of extraintestinal symptoms or if the disease is exclusively restricted to the GI tract.

In general, endoscopic and histological analyses are indistinguishable form IPEX syndrome, and a marked mononuclear cell infiltration of the intestinal lamina propria along with villous atrophy and epithelial cell apoptosis was described. The diagnosis of AIE type 3 is made by the presence of antienterocyte and/or anti-colonocyte antibodies along with positive anti-AIE-75 antibodies. Antienterocyte/-colonocyte antibodies fix against intracytoplasmic compounds of mature enterocytes and in some cases against intestinal brush border membrane compounds (as discussed above).

DIFFERENTIAL DIAGNOSIS

As discussed, AIE and IPEX have clearly to be distinguished from other forms of diffuse diarrhea occurring in the context of primary or secondary immunodeficiencies. Therefore, cellular and humoral immune functions have to be characterized during the initial diagnostic work-up of patients in whom IPEX is suspected. In addition, some syndromatic disorders have some overlap with IPEX; for instance, the Wiskott-Aldrich syndrome, characterized by eczema, thrombocytopenia, and autoimmunity can also present with a variable degree of enteropathy.[56] This disorder is clearly different from IPEX in that CD8+ counts are low, and signs of a combined immune defect with recurrent bacterial infections are detectable. The search for mutations in the WAS gene further helps to distinguish these disorders.[57] The so-called APECED syndrome, an acronym for autoimmune polyendocrinopathy, candidiasis, and ectodermal dystrophy[58,59] can occasionally resemble IPEX. APECED children develop diarrhea with malabsorption along with diabetes and/or hypothyroidism. However, in contrast to IPEX, symptoms occur later in life. APECED is inherited on an autosomal recessive basis, with a known mutation in the AIRE

gene.[58–59] Furthermore, Omenn syndrome is a disease which is characterized by erythrodermia with T-cell infiltration, lymphadenopathy, diarrhea with failure to thrive, and raised IgE with eosinophilia.[60] This syndrome can be easily distinguished from IPEX in that B-cell counts are low or even zero, T-cell proliferation responses are poor. Diabetes is not associated with Omenn syndrome, which is characterized by mutations in the RAG1 or RAG2 genes.[60–61]

TREATMENT AND OUTCOME

Mortality was reported to be extremely high in patients with IPEX.[62] All patients are initially dependent on parenteral nutrition. Management by TPN can be additionally complicated in patients presenting with diabetes. In the past, different treatment strategies were attempted; however, to date only two approaches proved to be successful: immunosuppressive medication or bone marrow transplantation. Immunosuppression is quite difficult since various reports clearly indicate that the response to a single immunosuppressor is rather disappointing.[4,47–49] Over the past few years, some experience was gained in treating AIE patients with steroids alone or in combination with azathioprine, cyclosporine A (CSA), or tacrolimus.[10–11,26,63–64] Other approaches include the use of immunoglobulins, antilymphocytic immunoglobulins, or cyclophosphamide which were all rather inefficient.[65] Recently, Vanderhoof and Young[66] reported the successful use of anti-TNF antibodies in the treatment of a patient with AIE. However, upon three injections, the treatment was stopped, and high-dose–steroid medication was again required to maintain remission. Therefore, no information on the long-term beneficial effect of anti-TNF treatment exists so far. Using immunosuppressive medication, a first series of patients was treated with CSA, however, only in some of them with some benefit.[62] One patient of the series of Powell and colleagues is still alive and doing well on chronic CSA medication.[4] However, many patients responded only partially or not at all to CSA. In fact, T cells from scurfy mice are highly resistant to CSA suppression, indicating that agents inhibiting TCR signaling may be of limited benefit.[21] However, with the introduction of tacrolimus, some advances in the care of AIE patients were made, significantly improving the outcome of AIE.[11,24,63–64] Chronic immunosuppression was effective in some patients, but ineffective in others. In our experience, remission can be most often induced by the combination of methylprednisolon and tacrolimus. As indicated in Table 3, initially steroid pulses (25 mg/kg) were administered at 3 consecutive days, followed by 2 mg/kg/d concomitant with tacrolimus. The doses of tacrolimus are adjusted to achieve and maintain blood levels between 8 and 12 ng/mL. To maintain remission, we use a triple therapy including azathioprine. If the response to the first steroid pulse is insufficient, a second pulse is tried. The outcome measure of immunosup-

Table 3 Necker-Enfants Malades Treatment Schema

Bowel rest and TPN	Until remission
Corticosteroids	3 pulses, eventually repeated
Tacrolimus	Blood levels 8 to 12 ng/mL
Azathioprine	2 mg/kg/d

pressive treatment and ultimate medical aim is to stop secretory diarrhea allowing to subsequently wean the child from TPN and to start normal oral or enteral nutrition. Over the last 3 years, we switched all our AIE/IPEX patients from tacrolimus to sirolimus which is markedly less toxic and theoretically interferes less with the functions of regulatory T cell.[67] Long-term follow-up data over now almost 5 years indicate that Sirolimus-based immunosuppression is efficient in maintaining long-term remission. However, further follow-up data have to show that it also is sufficient to prevent from disease progression.

Chronic immunosuppression may also increase the risk for viral, bacterial, fungal, or opportunistic infections, such as *Pneumocystis carinii* pneumonia. Therefore, we put our patients on Trimethoprin/Sulfonamid prophylaxis. A close follow-up of IPEX/AIE patients is required to avoid or at least minimize complications related to long-term immunosuppressive medication.

In our personal series, the induction of remission using this triple immunosuppression (methyprednisolone/tacrolimus/azathioprine) was successful in seven out of eight consecutive patients. In the past (before tacrolimus was available), however, all patients treated by cyclosporine A failed to come into remission and subsequently died. In the case of nonresponse to immunosuprressive drugs including tacrolimus, we now consider these patients as candidates for HLA identical allogenic bone marrow transplantation (BMT).

Since IPEX results form an absent or dysfunctional lymphocyte subset, bone marrow transplantation offers a potentially curative treatment option for boys suffering from this devastating disorder. The first successful BMT was performed in our center on a 4-month-old boy who failed to respond to tacrolimus.[33] The donor was his HLA-identical 18-year-old sister. BMT was followed by a complete remission over 2.5 years. It is important to underline that the conditioning regimen itself already controlled the disease, further confirming that IPEX is a T-cell–mediated disease.[21,33] After BMT, not only the entcropathy remained in remission but also diabetes and eczema were clinically silent. Insulin therapy could be stopped 7 days after BMT; PN was reduced 4 weeks after BMT and stopped within 6 months. Unfortunately, 29 months after BMT, the child died of a rapidly progressive hemophagocytotic syndrome which remained completely unexplained. Meanwhile, a couple more patients received BMT as ultimate treatment option for IPEX.[27] In most cases, BMT was initially successful; however, lethal, infections, fulminant graft-versus-host reactions or nonengraftment complicated the further course.

Results thus far have been mixed, but efforts are underway to optimize conditioning regimens to further improve this mode of therapy.[68–69] These cases indicate that BMT is potentially successful in otherwise treatment-resistant IPEX. Further experience with BMT has to be gained by particularly experienced teams. The role of BMT for other forms of AIE than IPEX has to be determined in the future. With the increasing understanding of the pathophysiology of IPEX and other forms of AIE, there is good hope that in the near future new immunosuppressive strategies will be available to treat these a priori T-cell–mediated autoimmune disorders.

REFERENCES

1. McCarthy DM, Katz SI, Gazze L, et al. Selective IgA deficiency associated with total villous atrophy of small intestine and an organspecific anti-epithelial cell antibody. J Immunol 1978;120:932–8.
2. Unsworth DJ, Walker-Smith JA. Auto-immunity in diarrheal disease. J Pediatr Gastroenterol Nutr 1985;4:375–80.
3. Savage MO, Mirakian R, Wozniak ER, et al. Specific autoantibodies to gut epithelium in two infants with severe protracted diarrhoea. J Pediatr Gastroenterol Nutr 1985;4:187–95.
4. Powell BR, Buist NRM, Stenzel P. An X-linked syndrome of diarrhea, polyendocrinopathy, and fatal infection in infancy. J Pediatr 1982;100:731–7.
5. Charritat IL, Polonovski C. Entéropathies auto-immunes pédiatriques avec autoanticorps anti cytoplasme entérocytaire. Ann Pediatr 1987;34:195–203.
6. Mirakian R, Richardson A, Miller P, et al. Protracted diarrhoea of infancy: Evidence in support of an autoimmune variant. BMJ 1986;293:1132–6.
7. Ellis D, Fisher SE, Smith WI, Jaffe R. Familial occurrence of renal and intestinal disease associated with tissue autoantibodies. Am J Dis Child 1982;136:323–6.
8. Kanof ME, Rance NE, Hamilton SR, et al. Congenital diarrhoea with intestinal inflammation and epithelial immaturity. J Pediatr Gastroenterol Nutr 1987;6:141–6.
9. Mitton SG, Mirakian R, Larcher VF, et al. Enteropathy and renal involvement in an infant with evidence of widespread autoimmune disturbance. J Pediatr Gastroenterol Nutr 1989;8:397–400.
10. Satake N, Nakanishi M, Okano M, et al. A Japanese family of X-linked autoimmune enteropathy with haemolytic anaemia and polyendocrinopathy. Eur J Pediatr 1993;152:313–5.
11. Torgerson TR, Moes N, Linane A, et al. A novel mutation in an upstream, non-coding region of the *FOXP3* gene leads to a variant of the IPEX syndrome with severe allergy. Gastroenterology 2007;132:1705–17.
12. Bousvaros A, Leichtner AM, Book L, et al. Treatment of pediatric autoimmune enteropathy with tacrolimus (FK506). Gastroenterology 1996;111:237–243.
13. Yamamoto H, Sugiyama K, Nomura T et al. A case of intractable diarrhea firmly suspected to have autoimmune enteropathy. Acta Paediatr Jpn 1994;36:97–103.
14. Wildin RS, Rasmdell F, Peake J, et al. X-linked neonatal diabetes mellitus, enteropathy and endocrinopathy syndrome is the human equivalent of mouse scurfy. Nat Genet 2001;27:18–20.
15. Bennett CL, Christie J, Ramsdell F, et al. The immune dysregulation, polyendocrinopathy, enteropathy X-linked syndrome (IPEX) is caused by mutations of FOXP3. Nat Genet 2001;27:20–1.
16. Lyon M, Peters J, Glenister PH, et al. The scurfy mouse mutant has previously unrecognized hemetological abnormalities and resembles Wiskott-Aldrich syndrome. PNAS 1990;87:2433–37.
17. Godfrey VL, Rouse BT, Wilkinson JE. Transplantation of T-cell mediated lymphoreticular disease from scurfy mouse. Am J Pathol 1994;145:281–6.
18. Blair PJ, Bultman SJ, Haas JC, et al. The mouse scurfy (sf) mutation is tightly linked to Gata1 and Tfe3 on the proximal X chromosome. Mamm Genoms 1994;5:652–4.
19. Kanangat S, Blair P, Reddy R, et al. Disease in the scrufy mouse is associated with overexpression of cytokine genes. Eur J Immunol 1996;26:161–5.
20. Blair PJ, Bultman SJ, Haas JC, et al. T cells are the effector cells in disease pathogenesis in the scurfy mouse. J Immunol 1994;153:3764–74.
21. Clark LB, Appleby MW, Brunkow ME, et al. Cellular and molecular characterization of the scurfy mouse mutant. J Immunol 1999;162:2546–54.
22. Brunkow ME, Jeffery EW, Hjerrild KA, et al. Disruption of a new fokhead/winged-helix protein, scurfin, results in the fatal lymphoproliferative disorder of the scurfy mouse. Nat Genet 2001;27:68–73.
23. Schubert LA, Jeffery E, Zhang Y, et al. Scurfin (FOXP3) acts as a repressor of transcription and regulates T cell activation. JBC 2001;276:37672–9.
24. Chatila TA, Blaeser F, Ho N, et al. JM2 encoding a fork head-related protein is mutated in X-linked autoimmunity-allergic dysregulation syndrome. J Clin Invest 2000;106:R75–81.
25. Bennet CL, Yoshioka R, Kiyosawa H et al. X-linked syndrome of polyendocrinoptahy, immune dysfunction and diarrhea maps to Xp 11.23-Xq13.3. Am J Hum Genet 2000;66:461–8.
26. Ferguson PJ, Blanton SH, Saulsbury FT, et al. Manifestations and linkage analysis in X-linked autoimmunity-immunodeficiency syndrome. Am J Med Genet 2000;90:390–7.
27. Wildin RS, Smyk-Oearsin S, Filipovitch AH. Clinical and molecular features of the immunodysregulation, polyendocrinopathy, enteropathy, X-linked (IPEX) syndrome. J Med Genet 2002;39:537–45.
28. Tommasini A, Ferrari S, Moratto D, et al. X-chromosome inactivation analysis in a female carrier of FOXP3 mutation. Clin Exp. Immunol 2002;130:127–30.
29. Bennett CL, Braunkow ME, Ramsdell F, et al. A rare polyadenylation signal mutation of the FOXP3 gene leads to the IPEX syndrome. Immunogenetics 2001;53:435–9.
30. Lopes JE, Torgerson TR, Schubert LA, et al. Analysis of FOXP3 reveals multiple domains required for its function as a transcriptional repressor. J Immunol 2006;177:3133–42.
31. Bacchetta R, Passerini L, Gambineri E, et al. Defective regulatory and effector T cell functions in patients with FOXP3 mutations. J Clin Invest 2006;116:1713–22.
32. Bennett CL, Ochs HD. IPEX is a unique X-linked syndrome characterized by immune dysfunction, polyendocrinopathy, enteropathy, and a variety of autoimmune phenomena. Curr Opin Pediatr 2001;13:533–8.
33. Baud O, Goulet O, Canioni D, et al. Treatment of the immune dysregulation, polyendocrinopathy, enteropathy, X-linked syndrome (IPEX) by allogenic bone marrow transplantation. N Engl J Med 2001;344:1758–62.
34. Kobayashi I, Shiari R, Yamada M, et al. Novel mutations of FOXP3 in two Japanese patients with immune dysregulation, polyendocrinopathy, enteropathy, X linked syndrome (IPEX). J Med Genet 2001;38:874–6.
35. Levy-Lahad E and Wildin RS. Neonatal diabetes mellitus, enteropathy, thrombocytopenia and endocrinopathy: Further evidence for an X-linked lethal syndrome. J Pediatr 2001;138:577–80.
36. Goulet O, Brousse N, Canioni D, et al. Syndrome of intractable diarrhoea with persistent villous atrophy in early childhood: A clinicopathological survey of 47. J Pediatr Gastroenterol Nutr 1998;26:151–61.
37. Russo PA, Brochu P, Seidman EG, Roy CC. Autoimmune enteropathy. Ped Res 1999;2:65–71.
38. Kobayashi I, Imamura K, Yamada M, et al. A 75 kDa autoantigen recognized by sera from patients with X-linked autoimmune enteropathy associated with nephropathy. Clin Exp Immunol 1998;111:527–31.
39. Colletti RB, Guillot AP, Rosen S, et al. Autoimmune enteropathy and nephropathy with circulating anti-epithelial cell antibodies. J Pediatr 1991;118:858–64.
40. Hill SM, Milla PJ, Bottazzo GF, Mirakian R. Autoimmune enteropathy and colitis: Is there a generalised autoimmune gut disorder? Gut 1991;32:36–42.
41. Lachaux A, Bouvier R, Cozzani E, et al. Familial autoimmune enteropathy with circulating anti-bullous pemphigoid antibodies and chronic autoimmune hepatitis. J Pediatr 1994;125:858–62.
42. Cuenod B, Brousse N, Goulet O, et al. Classification of intractable diarrhea in infancy using clinical and immunohistological criteria. Gastroenterology 1990;99:1037–43.
43. Kutlu T, Brousse N, Rambaud C, et al. Number of T cell receptor (TCR) αβ + but not of TCR γδ + intraepithelial lymphocytes correlate with the grade of villous atrophy in cœliac patients on a long term normal diet. Gut 1993;34:208–14.

44. Murch SH, Fertleman CR, Rodriguezs C, et al. Autoimmune enteropathy with distinct mucosal features in T cell activation deficiency: The contribution of T cells to the mucosal lesions. J Pediatr Gastroenterol Nutr 1999;28:377–9.

45. Halstensen TS, Scott H, Brantzaeg P. Intraepithelial T cells of the TcRγ/δ + CD8- and Vδ1/Øδ1 + phenotypes are increased in coeliac disease. Scand J Immunol 1989;30:665–72.

46. Moore L, Xu X, Davidson G, et al. Autoimmune enteropathy with anti-goblet cell antibody. Hum Pathol 1995;26:1162–8.

47. Jonas MM, Bell MD, Edison MS et al. Congenital diabetes mellitus and fatal secretory diarrhea in two infants. J Pediatr Gastroenterol Nutr 1991;13:415–25.

48. Walker-Smith JA, Unsworth DJ, Hutchins P, et al. Autoantibodies against gut epithelium in child with small intestinal enteropathy. Lancet 1982;i:566–7.

49. Unsworth J, Hutchings P, Mitchell J, et al. Flat small intestinal mucosa and antibodies against the gut epithelium. J Pediatr Gastroenterol Nutr 1982;1:503–13.

50. Kobayashi I, Imamura K, Kubota M, et al. Identification of an autoimmune enteropathy, related 75-kilodalton antigen. Gastroenterology 1999;117:823–30.

51. Scanlan MJ, Chen YT, Williamson B, et al. Characterization of human colon cancer antigens recognized by autologous antibodies. Int J Cancer 1998;76:652–8.

52. Sanderson IR, Phillips AD, Spencer J, Walker-Smith JA. Response of autoimmune enteropathy to cyclosporin A therapy. Gut 1991;32:1421–5.

53. Pearson RD, Swenson I, Schnek EA, et al. Fatal multisystemic disease with immune enteropathy heralded by juvenile rheumatoid arthritis. J Pediatr Gastroenterol Nutr 1989;8:259–65.

54. Savilahti E, Pelkonen R, Holmberg C, et al. Fatal unresponsive villous atrophy of the jejunum, connective tissue disease and diabetes in a girl with intestinal epithelial cell antibody. Acta Paediatr Scand 1985;74:472–6.

55. Kapel N, Roman C, Caldari D, et al. Fecal tumor necrosis factor-alpha and calprotectin as differential diagnostic markers for severe diarrhea of small infants. J Pediatr Gastroenterol Nutr. 2005;41:396–400.

56. Snapper SB, Rosen FS. The Wiskott-Aldrich syndrome protein (WASP): Roles in signaling and cytoskeletal organization. Annu Rev Immunol 1999;17:905–29.

57. Villa A, Notarangelo L, Macchi P. X-linked thrombocytopenia and Wiskott-Aldrich syndrome are allelic diseases with mutations in the WASP gene. Nat Genet 1995;9:414–7.

58. The Finnish-German APECED Consortium. An autoimmune disease APECED, caused by mutations in a novel gene featuring two PHD-type zinc-finger domains. Nat Genet 1997;17:399–403.

59. Aaltonen J, Bjores P. Cloning of the APECED gene provides new insight into human autoimmunity. Ann Med 1999;31:111–6.

60. Villa A, Santagata S, Bozzi F, et al. Omenn syndrome: A disorder of Rag1 and Rag2 genes. J Clin Immunol 1999;19:87–97.

61. Villa A, Santagata S, Bozzi F, et al. Partial V(D)J recombination activity leads to Omenn syndrome. Cell 1998;93: 885–96.

62. Seidman EG, Lacaille F, Russo P, et al. Successful treatment of autoimmune enteropathy with cyclosporine. J Ped 1990; 117:929–32.

63. Kobayashi I, Nakanishi M, Okana M, et al. Combination therapy with tacrolimus and betamethasone for a patient with X-linked auto-immune enteropathy with haemolytic anemia and polyendocrinopathy. Eur J Pediatr 1993;152:313–5.

64. Kobayashi I, Kowamura N, Okano M. A long-term survivor with the immune dysregulation, polyendocrinopathy, enteropathy, X-linked syndrome. N Engl J Med 2001;345:999–1000.

65. Finel E, Giroux JD, Metz C, et al. Diabete neonatal vrai associe a une maladie autoimmune. Arch Pediatr 1996;3:782–4.

66. Vanderhoof JA, Young RJ. Autoimmune Enteropathy in a child: Response to infliximab therapy. J Ped Gastroenterol Nutr 2002;34:312–6.

67. Bind L, Torgerson T, Perroni L, et al. Successful use of the new immune-suppressor sirolimus in IPEX (immune dysregulation, polyendocrinopathy, enteropathy, X-linked syndrome). J Pediatr 2005;147:256–9.

68. Rao A, Kamani N, Filipovich A, et al. Successful bone marrow transplantation for IPEX syndrome after reduced-intensity conditioning. Blood 2007;109:383–5.

69. Mazzolari E, Forino C, Fontana M, et al. A new case of IPEX receiving bone marrow transplantation. Bone Marrow Transplant 2005;35:1033–4.

Surgical Disorders

17.1. Intestinal Obstructions

M. Susan Moyer, MD

Brad W. Warner, MD

Intestinal obstruction in the pediatric patient may be related to a number of underlying conditions that can be intrinsic to the bowel or extraintestinal. The obstruction may be mechanical or functional, including intestinal pseudo-obstruction. These latter disorders involve neuromuscular dysfunction of the bowel and are discussed in detail elsewhere. In this chapter, the etiology and pathophysiology of mechanical intestinal obstruction will be reviewed. Further discussion will then focus on recognizing and evaluating the pediatric patient with intestinal obstruction as well as general management. Unique aspects of the approach to the neonate with intestinal obstruction will be reviewed; and finally, a few selected conditions in the pediatric patient will be highlighted.

ETIOLOGY

The list of conditions that can cause or predispose to intestinal obstruction is fairly extensive (Table 1).[1,2] Pyloric stenosis presents as gastric outlet obstruction at about 2 months of age and is the commonest cause of gastric outlet obstruction in infants. Approximately, one-third of the cases of intestinal obstruction in the neonate are secondary to intestinal atresias and stenoses, which are the most common intrinsic cause of obstruction in the newborn period. These may represent intrinsic developmental defects related to abnormal embryogenesis or to a secondary insult such as ischemia in utero.[3] Colonic atresia is rare and may be difficult to diagnose. Anorectal malformations and Hirschsprung's disease (aganglionosis) are also intrinsic intestinal conditions that cause lower gastrointestinal tract obstruction. Abnormalities of rotation and fixation during development predispose to volvulus[4] and intestinal duplications and embryonic remnants such as Meckel's diverticulum may cause extrinsic obstruction or act as the lead point for intussusceptions.[5] Crohn's disease and necrotizing enterocolitis can cause obstruction by the development of postinflammatory strictures that may involve either the small or large intestine. Colonic strictures may also be associated with ulcerative colitis. Though rare, intestinal neoplasms such as lymphoma may present with obstruction. In addition neoplasms involving other intraabdominal organs may cause extrinsic compression of the bowel lumen if large enough. Adhesions, the most common cause of obstruction in adults, are also an important extrinsic cause of obstruction in the pediatric patient with a history of abdominal surgery.

PATHOPHYSIOLOGY

The underlying pathophysiology of mechanical intestinal obstruction involves (1) bowel distension, (2) increased hydrostatic pressure with eventual third spacing of fluid into the lumen and bowel wall, (3) ischemia, and (4) bacterial overgrowth and translocation.[6] Any structural barrier to the aboral flow of gastrointestinal contents will result initially in distension of the bowel with accumulation of fluid and gas proximal the point of obstruction. The degree of distension depends largely on whether the obstruction is partial or complete and, if partial, the grade of the obstruction. Proximal (jejunal) obstruction typically results in bilious emesis with minimal abdominal distention. The dilated loops of obstructed bowel are decompressed easily by emesis. On the other hand, a more distal (ileal) bowel obstruction results in significant abdominal distention prior to the onset of emesis. Bowel distention then stimulates more fluid and electrolyte secretion as well as peristalsis. Peristalsis below the level of obstruction can result in passage of stool early on, even with a complete obstruction. In the obstructed bowel, once the hydrostatic pressure in the lumen exceeds that of the mucosal lymphatics and terminal lacteals, the lymphatic flow from the mucosa becomes obstructed and bowel wall edema develops. The combination of increasing intraluminal pressure and bowel wall lymphedema then compresses the postcapillary venules and results in progressive increase in the net filtration of fluid, electrolytes, and protein through the capillaries into the bowel wall and lumen. This third spacing in the bowel can lead to varying degrees of systemic hypovolemia and dehydration with eventual hypotension and shock if not corrected.

Anatomic Location	Causes	
	Intrinsic	Extrinsic*
Duodenum	Duodenal atresia/stenosis	Ladd's bands/midgut volvulus
	Duodenal web	Annular pancreas
	Duodenal hematoma	Preduodenal portal vein
	Intestinal duplication	Adhesions
	Pyloric stenosis	Neoplasms
		Superior mesenteric artery syndrome
Small intestine	Intestinal atresia/stenosis	Malrotation/midgut volvulus
	Crohn's disease	Meconium ileus
	Necrotizing enterocolitis	Meckel's diverticulum
	Neoplasms	Adhesions
	Intestinal duplication	Neoplasms
	Intussusception	Inguinal hernia
Large intestine	Colonic atresia	Distal intestinal obstruction syndrome (DIOS)
	Anorectal malformations	Volvulus (cecal, colonic, sigmoid)
	Hirschsprung's disease	Adhesions
	Inflammatory bowel disease	Neoplasms
	Necrotizing enterocolitis	Meconium plug syndrome
	Neonatal small left colon syndrome	
	Intestinal duplication	
	Intussusception	

Table 1 Causes of Intestinal Obstruction in Infants and Children

*Intraluminal or extraintestinal.

The elevated venous pressure in the bowel can also eventually compromise the arterial blood supply to the bowel with resulting ischemia. Ischemia may result not only from arterial occlusion in the bowel wall on the microvascular level, but also from macrovascular arterial occlusion of the mesenteric blood supply if the distended loop of bowel rotates on itself or if the mesenteric venous pressure exceeds arterial perfusion pressure.

Finally, intestinal stasis proximal to the point of obstruction predisposes to bacterial overgrowth within the bowel lumen. The normal mucosal barrier to intraluminal bacteria is compromised in intestinal obstruction by a number of factors including increased hydrostatic pressure and mucosal injury secondary to compromised blood supply. Increased translocation of bacteria to mesenteric lymph nodes has been documented in adults undergoing surgery for simple small intestinal obstruction.[7] This bacterial translocation most likely contributes to clinical sepsis and the systemic inflammatory response syndrome in some patients with intestinal obstruction.

PRESENTATION

The clinical presentation depends, in part, on the level and degree of obstruction. These factors, in turn, reflect the underlying cause of the obstruction, which varies in prevalence by age. Intestinal obstruction in the newborn occurs in approximately 1 in 2,000 live births and is most commonly related to congenital anomalies and malformations (atresia, stenoses, malrotation) or to abnormalities of intestinal contents (meconium ileus, meconium plug syndrome).[2] Prenatal obstruction is suggested by maternal polyhydramnios and signs and symptoms in the infant include vomiting which may be bilious, abdominal distension, and failure to pass meconium within the first 24 to 48 hours of life. Intestinal obstruction in the newborn will be discussed in more detail below. In older children and adolescents, symptoms include pain, which is often colicky in nature, nausea, vomiting, and obstipation. The pain may become constant in the presence of ischemia. If early in the clinical course, there may be a history of diarrhea related to diffuse stimulation of peristalsis distal to the obstruction by bowel distension.

On examination, the presence and degree of abdominal distension depend on the level and degree of obstruction and bowel sounds are usually hyperactive. With prolonged obstruction or strangulation, bowel sounds may be diminished. The abdomen is usually tender to palpation and attention should be paid to the presence of peritoneal signs. Depending on the cause of the obstruction, an abdominal mass may be palpable. A careful examination for an inguinal hernia is important as well. In general, if the obstruction is in the upper gastrointestinal tract, vomiting is prominent, occurs soon after eating and is typically bilious. Abdominal distension is not pronounced. Obstruction in the distal small bowel or colon is more likely to present with abdominal distension and vomiting may be intermittent.

The clinical setting may suggest the possibility of underlying intestinal obstruction in the presence of other consistent signs and symptoms. Examples would include patients with abdominal trauma, a history of abdominal surgery or necrotizing enterocolitis, or children and adolescents with Crohn's disease.

DIAGNOSIS

In the clinical setting in which intestinal obstruction is suspected, diagnosis is directed not only toward establishing the presence of obstruction, but determining whether the obstruction is partial or complete. If the obstruction is complete, there is a much higher risk of strangulation. Strangulation implies ischemia to the bowel and can occur in as many as 20 to 40% of cases of complete obstruction.[6] Morbidity and mortality increase significantly in the presence of strangulation compared to a simple obstruction.

Once obstruction is suspected, a plain abdominal radiograph can be very helpful in supporting the presence of obstruction. Findings include distended loops of bowel with air fluid levels and paucity of colonic air (Figure 1). A plain film may also reveal the presence of free air. Although diagnostic only 45 to 60% of the time, even in experienced hands, a plain film of the abdomen remains the cornerstone as the initial radiographic assessment in suspected obstruction.[8]

When the diagnosis of obstruction is in question, computed tomography (CT) scan of the abdomen can be very helpful. This radiographic study can not only establish the presence of obstruction, but also identify the cause, particularly if it is extrinsic to the bowel. Radiographic signs of obstruction on CT scan include (1) fluid, luminal contents and/or air filled loops of bowel proximal to the obstruction, (2) presence of a definite localized transition zone, and (3) presence of collapsed loops of small bowel or colon distal to the obstruction.[6,8,9] The use of intravenous and oral contrast, if possible, is recommended. Oral contrast can help to differentiate complete from partial obstruction and better localize the level of obstruction. There are limitations of CT scans in evaluating obstruction; however, particularly with newer multiphasic 3-D reconstruction techniques, the diagnostic accuracy of computed tomography in intestinal obstruction is excellent. (Figure 2)

Although magnetic resonance imaging (MRI) and ultrasound have been used as adjuncts in evaluating the patient with suspected obstruction, CT scans in general are faster, more readily available and less dependent on technical expertise. An upper gastrointestinal and small bowel contrast series could also identify the level of obstruction but the administration of oral contrast could be contraindicated or poorly tolerated. In addition, the CT scan is more likely to identify the underlying cause of the obstruction.[9] Exceptions to the preferred use of CT scans in obstruction are in cases of intussusception and malrotation in which ultrasound and an upper GI contrast study, respectively, are the diagnostic studies of choice. These will be discussed in more detail later in the chapter.

Discriminating Partial and Complete Obstruction

Differentiating complete from partial bowel obstruction is important for subsequent management and outcome. Clinical signs and symptoms that suggest partial obstruction include continued passage of gas or stool more than 6 to 12 hours

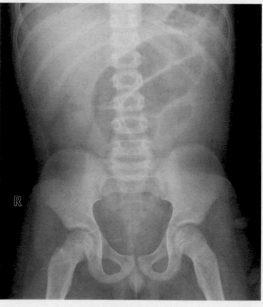
(A)

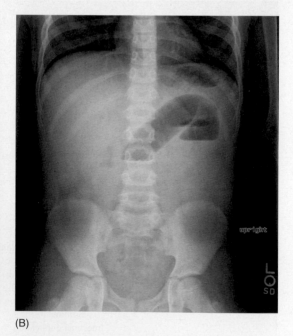
(B)

Figure 1 Plain abdominal radiographs supine (A) and upright (B) in a 10-year-old child who presented with the acute onset of nonbilious emesis and colicky abdominal pain. Dilated loops of small bowel are seen with a paucity of gas elsewhere suggestive of intestinal obstruction.

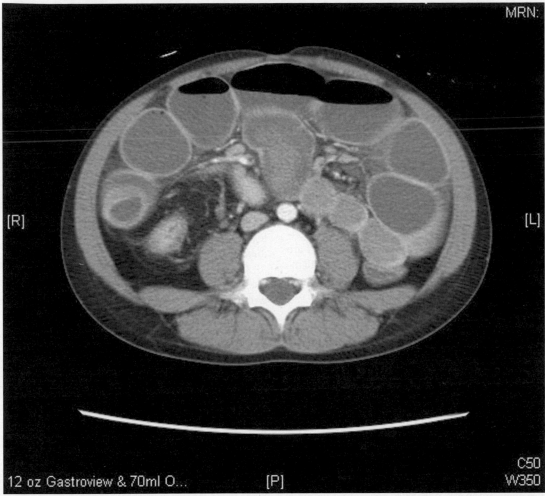

Figure 2 CT scan of the abdomen in the same 10-year-old child demonstrating a thickened and narrowed segment of distal ileum and cecum with dilation of the loops of small bowel proximal to the obstruction. The child was subsequently diagnosed with Crohn's disease and had an associated ileal structure.

after the onset of symptoms and the presence of colonic gas on abdominal films. Early complete obstruction may mimic partial, high-grade obstruction clinically and on plain films. A CT scan, particularly with oral contrast, can be very helpful in defining complete obstruction by assessing the amount of residual air and fluid in the distal bowel that is collapsed. In addition, the presence or absence of contrast in the colon can be determined on a plain film of the abdomen 12 to 24 hours after the initial study.[10]

Discriminating Simple and Strangulating Obstruction

Determining whether the circulation to the bowel has been compromised is extremely important. In adult studies, strangulation has been shown to increase mortality in obstruction from 10 to 20% and morbidity is as high as 42%.[6] Unfortunately, there are no universally reliable clinical parameters or diagnostic tests that can predict irreversible ischemia in the setting of intestinal obstruction. Clinical signs and symptoms that are concerning include continuous as opposed to colicky abdominal pain, peritoneal signs, painful abdominal mass, hematochezia, absent bowel sounds, systemic signs such as fever and tachycardia, leukocytosis, and acidosis. Once again, a CT scan may suggest strangulation by assessing

mesenteric vasculature and mucosal perfusion but, in a number of studies, has not been shown to reliably identify reversible ischemia. Some findings on CT scan that suggest strangulation include bowel wall thickening with or without a target sign, pneumatosis intestinalis, portal venous gas, mesenteric haziness, and nonenhancement after IV contrast.[6]

Reversible strangulation and bowel ischemia are almost never recognized preoperatively, in large part, because there is no reliable clinical parameter, diagnostic test, or combination of the two that predict early bowel ischemia.[6] In fact, in a prospective study of experienced clinicians, the diagnosis of nonstrangulation was incorrect

31% of the time.[11] This inability to determine the presence of ischemia with certainty continues to guide recommendations for surgical intervention in the clinical management of patients with intestinal obstruction. A composite of clinical and radiographic findings that suggest underlying bowel ischemia are listed in Table 2.

MANAGEMENT

In the vast majority of cases, general management and resuscitation supersede identifying the underlying cause. Particularly in cases of high-grade partial or complete obstruction, bowel decompression, and fluid resuscitation are paramount. Since the pathophysiology of obstruction is triggered by bowel distension, addressing this can help to reverse some of the attendant complications of obstruction including third spacing of fluid, and further obstruction and compromise of lymphatic and venous flow. This can be accomplished in most cases by placement of a large bore nasogastric tube. Fluid requirements may be significant and fluid resuscitation with isosmotic fluids such as saline or Ringer's lactate should be aggressive in order to maintain an appropriate intravascular volume. Careful monitoring of fluid status and electrolytes is recommended. The use of empiric broad-spectrum antibiotics based on the possibility of bacterial translocation in the setting of intestinal obstruction or in anticipation of surgery is common but controlled studies supporting the practice are limited.

It is generally accepted that all patients with intestinal obstruction, except in the setting of obvious septic shock, severe crampy abdominal pain, or clinical signs of peritonitis, may benefit from a period of nasogastric decompression and fluid resuscitation prior to surgery. A number of retrospective studies suggest this period of time, even in the presence of complete obstruction, is relatively safe.[6] This allows stabilization and further evaluation for the degree and/or cause of obstruction which can more specifically direct surgical management. If the obstruction is complete, early surgical intervention is advisable given the higher incidence of strangulation in this setting and the lack of reliable predictors of early ischemia. In the case of partial obstruction, a trial of nonoperative management is usually indicated with continued decompression and medical

Table 2 Signs, Symptoms, and Radiographic Findings: Suggestive of Srangulating Obstruction[6]

Signs and Symptoms	CT Scan Findings
Continuous abdominal pain	Bowel wall thickening
Fever	with or without "target sign"
Tachycardia	Pneumatosis intestinalis
Peritoneal signs	Portal venous gas
Leukocytosis	Mesenteric haziness, fluid or
Acidosis	hemorrhaging, ascites
Painful mass	Serrated "beak sign"
Absent bowel sounds	Nonenhancement with IV contrast
Hematochezia	

support as well as close monitoring for signs or symptoms of clinical deterioration.

NEONATAL INTESTINAL OBSTRUCTION

The majority of congenital causes of obstruction will present in the newborn period or during infancy. An understanding of these abnormalities and how they present will facilitate a more directed approach to diagnosis and timely management.[1,2]

Intestinal obstruction may be suspected prenatally if polyhydramnios is present and fetal ultrasound is performed. Intestinal obstruction at the time of delivery can then be anticipated and plans for delivery in the appropriate facility with access to a neonatal special care unit and pediatric surgeons can be made.

Obstructive lesions in the proximal bowel, such as atresia, stenosis, or annular pancreas, present with emesis and the dilated stomach and proximal duodenum may create the appearance a "double-bubble" on plain films of the abdomen. No further radiographic assessment may be necessary and the infant can be stabilized with nasogastric decompression and IV fluids prior to definitive surgical intervention. Lesions involving the distal small bowel and colon, may present somewhat later with signs including abdominal distension, delayed passage of meconium or obstipation and evidence of obstruction on a plain film. Again, contrast studies may be helpful including upper GI series with small bowel follow through or contrast enema. Specific evaluation and management for Hirschsprung's disease, meconium ileus, and small left colon syndrome are discussed elsewhere.

Intestinal duplications may be tubular (intramural) or cystic and present as frank mechanical obstruction or as the leading point for an intussusception. They may also present as a volvulus.[5,12] In one larger series, approximately two-thirds presented within the first 24 months of life.[12] With the more widespread use of prenatal ultrasonography, more of these infants are diagnosed prior to developing complications including obstruction.

Abnormalities of rotation associated with volvulus usually present during infancy but may present at any time in life. The presence of abnormal rotation in a patient who presents with bilious vomiting may be made by contrast studies. Surgical intervention is recommended in any infant or child who is diagnosed with malrotation since the consequences of an associated volvulus with the potential loss of small bowel secondary to ischemia is significant.

Finally, although not technically a congenital cause of obstruction, pyloric stenosis does present in the first two months of life and must be differentiated from other causes of obstruction that may present at this age. In many cases, only a high index of suspicion and careful physical examination are required to make the diagnosis. These infants present with progressive *nonbilious* emesis over the first 4 to 8 weeks of life and the hypertrophied pylorus may be palpated as a mass, or "olive," on abdominal examination. The diagnosis may be confirmed by either ultrasound or an upper gastrointestinal X-rays with contrast.

SPECIFIC CAUSES OF INTESTINAL OBSTRUCTION

Adhesions

Adhesions form following virtually any type of abdominal surgery but particularly in inflammatory conditions such as inflammatory bowel disease or appendicitis. Adhesion formation is initiated by development of a fibrin clot. The peritoneum has fibrinolytic activity by way of plasminogen activation. Inhibitors of plasminogen activation are released in the presence of ischemia or serosal damage which then decrease fibrinolytic activity and promote adhesion formation. To date, however, attempts to decrease adhesion formation pharmacologically have generally been ineffective.[6] Postoperative adhesions are the most common underlying cause of obstruction in most adult series. In a large series of pediatric patients with obstruction, postoperative adhesions were the cause in 5%.[13] Adhesive obstruction occurred within the first 2 years following surgery in 80% of children and the most commonly implicated procedures were for appendicitis and ulcerative colitis. In another series of children who had undergone a surgical procedure in the newborn period, adhesive obstruction occurred in 8% with 90% presenting within a year following the surgery.[14] Adhesive obstruction was particularly common following surgery for gastroschisis and malrotation.

In infants and children who present with symptoms and clinical and radiographic signs of obstruction and have a history of previous abdominal surgery, adhesive obstruction should be high on the differential diagnosis, particularly within the first 1 or 2 years following the procedure. The general management for intestinal obstruction should be implemented including decompression and fluid resuscitation. A CT scan may be helpful in ruling out other causes of obstruction and establishing the level and severity of obstruction. If the obstruction is partial and the patient is stable or improving, observation and medical management is indicated since the majority will resolve without surgery. In the setting of complete obstruction, where strangulation is more likely, earlier surgical intervention may be warranted. This is particularly true if there is no improvement over the first 12 hours of observation. Lysis of adhesions may be accomplished through a laparotomy or with laparoscopy. There is some evidence to suggest that the laparoscopic approach is associated with shorter hospital stay, more rapid restitution of intestinal function, and fewer complications.[15]

Superior Mesenteric Artery Syndrome

Superior mesenteric artery (SMA) syndrome is a relatively rare cause of upper gastrointestinal tract obstruction. This condition has also been called arteriomesenteric duodenal compression, duodenal ileus, the cast syndrome, and Wilkie's syndrome.[16] Obstruction of the third portion of the duodenum occurs as it courses between the superior mesenteric artery (SMA) anteriorly and the vertebral column posteriorly. Although the underlying cause is still debated, the most common contributing factor is a decrease in the angle between the SMA and the abdominal aorta. The SMA usually comes off the aorta at a 45° angle (38° to 60°). In SMA syndrome, that angle is sharply decreased to anywhere from 6° to 25°. The aortomesenteric distance is also reduced from 10 to 20 mm to about 2 to 8 mm.[17] Other potential predisposing factors include high insertion of the duodenum at the ligament of Treitz, low origin of the SMA and compression of the duodenum by peritoneal adhesions.

Clinical settings in which SMA syndrome most commonly occurs are rapid increase in height without parallel weight gain, rapid and excessive weight loss, scoliosis, spinal surgery, prolonged bed rest particularly in the supine position, and use of a body cast. In the setting of weight loss or proportionately slow weight gain, loss of the retroperitoneal fat cushion has been implicated.

In the pediatric population, this condition usually occurs in older children and adolescents. Presentation may be acute, intermittent or chronic depending on the degree of obstruction and the associated clinical condition. Symptoms of upper gastrointestinal tract obstruction predominate and include nausea, early satiety, anorexia, eructation, and postprandial epigastric abdominal pain. Emesis can be voluminous with undigested food and usually bile. Relief of symptoms may be reported when the child assumes a prone, knee-chest or left lateral, decubitus position. Physical examination usually reveals an asthenic body habitus and a succussion splash may be elicited on abdominal examination.

Plain abdominal radiographs may be normal, particularly after vomiting, or may demonstrate gastric and/or proximal duodenal dilation with retained food in the stomach. The diagnosis is usually made with an upper gastrointestinal contrast study. Partial obstruction in the third portion of the duodenum is demonstrated with dilation of the proximal duodenum. To-and-fro movement of barium proximal to the obstruction may be present and passage of the barium may be facilitated with the patient in the left lateral decubitus position. The radiographic obstruction may also be relieved by applying pressure below the umbilicus in a cephalad and dorsal direction (Hayes maneuver) which elevates the root of the small intestinal mesentery.[16] The angle of the SMA and the aortomesenteric distance may also be measured by ultrasound or CT imaging. These studies can also help to identify other extrinsic or intramural causes of duodenal obstruction. Upper endoscopy is usually recommended to identify intraluminal or mucosal causes for obstruction as well.

Initial management includes decompression with a nasogastric tube and restoration and support of hydration and electrolyte balance as clinically indicated. Nutritional rehabilitation and support may be achieved by modifying the patient's position during meals and changing eating habits to include small frequent meals of liquid supplements. Prokinetic agents such as metoclopramide may also be helpful, although these should not be used in cases of complete or near complete obstruction. If the obstruction is significant and oral intake insufficient to support weight gain, nasojejunal feedings, which bypass the obstruction, can be utilized. Rarely, total parenteral nutrition is necessary. Particularly in patients in whom weight loss, or inadequate weight gain, is the predisposing factor, restoration of an acceptable weight will result in resolution of the obstructive symptoms. In cases where conservative therapy is unsuccessful, surgical intervention may be considered. Surgical options include duodenojejunostomy or lysis of the ligament of Treitz with mobilization and repositioning of the duodenum.[18]

Intussusception

Intussusception is a condition in which a portion of the bowel telescopes onto, or invaginates into, another portion of the bowel. The intussusceptum is that portion of the bowel that is inside the other segment of bowel, the intussuscipiens. These occur most commonly in infancy and early childhood with approximately two-thirds presenting in the first year of life. In this age group they are usually idiopathic and the most common site is ileocolic or ileoileocolic. The underlying cause is thought to be related to normal intestinal lymphoid hyperplasia. In older children and adults, a pathologic leading point may be responsible for initiating the intussusception (Table 3).[19]

An increased incidence of idiopathic intussusception was noted in association with the first vaccine for rotavirus (Rotashield®), a quadrivalent human-rhesus vaccine.[20] Although the overall incidence was only about 1 in 10,000, this potentially life-threatening adverse event resulted in withdrawal of the vaccine from the market. The reason for this increased risk remains unclear but may represent a specific effect of the simian virus on the intestine in a susceptible host. The risk of intussusception related to natural rotavirus infection does not appear to be increased.[21] Large scale clinical trials of two new oral vaccines, RotaTeq® and Rotarix®, in over 130,000 infants did not show an increased risk of intussusception over that in the placebo groups.[22,23] Data derived from the placebo arms of these clinical vaccine trials,

along with other large observational studies, have added considerably to our understanding of the epidemiology of idiopathic intussusception.[21–24] It is apparent that there are population differences worldwide in the incidence of idiopathic intussusception. In addition, even though approximately two-thirds of cases of intussusception will present in the first year of life, infants less than 3 months of age are relatively spared.

Symptoms and signs at presentation in infants and children can include crampy abdominal pain, currant jelly stools, and an abdominal mass. This classic triad of clinical findings is, however, present in less than 50% of these children. Therefore, a high index of suspicion in the child with symptoms suggestive of obstruction in this age group is necessary to proceed with the appropriate diagnostic evaluation. Many will have plain abdominal radiographs as part of the initial assessment. Signs suggestive of intussusception include the meniscus sign,[25] a soft tissue mass, paucity of gas, and absence of cecal gas and stool. These signs are nonspecific and do not reliably rule in the presence of an intussusception. In children with peritoneal signs, a plain abdominal film is helpful in identifying the presence of free air that suggests a perforation, which is the major contraindication to attempting nonsurgical reduction.

Historically, the diagnostic procedure of choice has been the contrast enema. This procedure is not only diagnostic but therapeutic in the majority of cases. More recently, sonography has supplanted the contrast enema as the initial diagnostic test when intussusception is suspected and approaches 100% accuracy.[25] The characteristic sonographic appearance is a 3 to 5 cm mass, usually located on the right side of the abdomen, just below the abdominal wall. There is also a characteristic doughnut appearance with eccentric, crescent-shaped, hyperechoic mesenteric fat and associated vessels and lymph nodes that have been drawn up into the intussusception. (Figure 3). A negative ultrasound in trained hands can effectively rule out an intussusception as the cause for clinical symptoms and preclude the need for a contrast enema. Ultrasound evaluation may also identify a pathologic lead point or other intra-abdominal pathology that may mimic intussusception at presentation. Sonography may also be used to follow and verify reduction of the intussusception with a therapeutic enema. In institutions where sonography may not be readily available or, in situations where the index of suspicion is high and the ultrasound equivocal, a contrast enema with barium or air will verify the diagnosis. The diagnostic procedure then becomes therapeutic as well.

Nonsurgical reduction of intussusceptions in children is achieved in the majority of cases by a therapeutic enema using contrast (hydrostatic) or air (pneumatic).[19,26] Contraindications to attempting reduction with an enema are clinical signs of shock, peritonitis, and/or the presence of free intraperitoneal air suggesting perforation. Attempts have been made to predict the presence of bowel necrosis, and hence, a

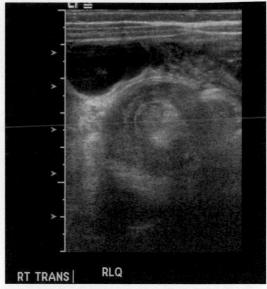

Figure 3 Ultrasound imaging of ileocolonic intussusception. The intussusception has a doughnut shaped appearance with an eccentric, crescent-shaped, hyperechoic rim.

greater risk of perforation, using specific sonographic features. These have included presence of a thick, hypoechoic rim of the intussusception, free intraperitoneal fluid, fluid trapped within the intussusception, and lack of blood flow on Doppler.[25] Because these findings have not consistently predicted either a decreased rate of reduction or increased risk of perforation, they do not preclude attempt at nonsurgical reduction. Other sonographic features such as the presence of an identified lead point or enlarged lymph nodes within the intussusception also do not reliably predict that an intussusception will not be reducible with contrast enema, although the success rate is lower.[19,25,26]

All patients should be appropriately stabilized, including fluid resuscitation, before attempting reduction of an intussusception. In the majority of infants and children, successful hydrostatic or pneumatic enema reduction may be achieved under either fluoroscopic or ultrasound guidance. Factors such as hematochezia or melena, radiographic signs of obstruction, longer duration of clinical symptoms, evidence for a pathologic lead point and younger age may decrease the success rate but do not preclude attempt at image-guided reduction.[26] Although the earliest studies used barium as the contrast, current practice favors water soluble contrast or saline when hydrostatic reduction is used. Over the past few years, pneumatic reduction has gained favor since it is easy to perform, cleaner and usually requires less radiation exposure (Figure 4). In addition, if a perforation does occur, it tends to be smaller and there is no peritoneal contamination with contrast. Review of an extensive series of intussusceptions suggests that an overall reduction rate of 80 to 95% may be achieved with either technique although large series directly comparing techniques have not been done.[26] Variability in the reduction rates reflects the population studied including criteria for exclusion from attempts at nonsurgical reduction.

Table 3 Most Common Pathologic Lead Points in Intussusception in Children*
Meckel's diverticulum
Polyps
Lymphoma
Duplication cyst
Massive lymphoid hyperplasia
Henoch-Schönlein purpura
Cystic fibrosis
Appendicitis/periappendicitis
*Compiled from six pediatric series.[25]

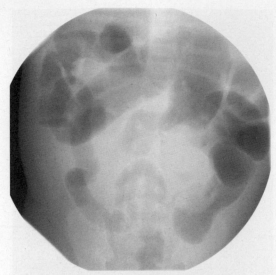

Figure 4 Air (pneumatic) enema in a child with an ileocolonic intussusception.

The major potential complication of image-guided reduction is perforation. The rate of perforation, in general, tends to be low and in most series is less than 1%, regardless of the technique used.[26] As previously mentioned, tears tend to be smaller and peritoneal irritation less of a problem with air compared to contrast enemas. Tension pneumoperitoneum with pneumatic reduction, though rare, has been reported.[27]

Complete reduction of the intussusception should be verified fluoroscopically or by ultrasound and observation for a brief period of time following reduction is recommended. Recurrence of the intussusception has been reported to occur in approximately 8 to 15% of patients regardless of the technique used and about two-thirds of these will occur within a few days of reduction.[26] A patient with a recurrent intussusception may undergo nonsurgical reduction again. The majority of patients with recurrent intussusception does not have a pathologic lead point and will not necessarily need, nor benefit from, surgical intervention.

Malrotation/Midgut Volvulus

During embryologic development of the midgut, the bowel lengthens, herniates into a U-shaped loop into the base of the umbilical cord and rotates around the SMA axis counterclockwise. It then reenters the abdomen and undergoes fixation.[4] Malrotation is defined as a failure of normal rotation of any portion of the gastrointestinal tract. It also implies abnormal fixation, which is the predisposing factor for the development of a volvulus. Peritoneal bands, or Ladd's bands, are formed as the fetus attempts to fix the malpositioned bowel. The bands course from the cecum and ascending colon to the retroperitoneum in the right upper quadrant and can cause varying degrees of duodenal obstruction themselves.

A volvulus involves twisting of the intestine around its mesenteric root causing obstruction to the bowel lumen as well as to the lymphatic and venous drainage. Eventually, the arterial supply is comprised resulting in gut ischemia and necrosis. This is a true surgical emergency and demands expeditious diagnosis and surgical intervention. Because malrotation predisposes to volvulus, when diagnosed, it is usually repaired surgically to avoid the potentially life-threatening development of a volvulus.

The incidence of malrotation is estimated to be approximately 1 in 500 live births and the majority of patients will present within the first month of life.[4] The presence of malrotation can predispose to volvulus at any point in life, although this is less likely to occur in adults.

In infancy, the most common presentation is bilious vomiting. Symptoms may be nonspecific and the presence of diarrhea does not necessarily rule out an underlying volvulus. Other associated signs and symptoms may include abdominal pain and constipation. Hematochezia occurs in approximately 10 to 15% of patients and suggests the presence of bowel ischemia. Malrotation rarely presents as an acute abdomen unless late in the clinical course. Children who present beyond infancy may have a more prolonged course with episodic symptoms of abdominal pain, vomiting, and even malabsorption and poor weight gain from chronic intermittent lymphatic obstruction. One series documented a mean delay in the diagnosis of 1.7 years.[28] Although most infants and children with malrotation have no other associated congenital abnormalities, malrotation is more common in a number of other syndromes and conditions (Table 4). The majority of patients with heterotaxy syndrome (asplenia/right isomerism and polysplenia/left isomerism) have malrotation and it is also usually present in association with congenital diaphragmatic hernia, gastroschisis, and omphalocele.

Findings on plain films of the abdomen are usually normal or nonspecific. In infants, since the obstruction is in the proximal intestine but usually distal to the ampullae of Vater, the clini-

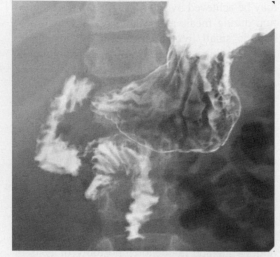

Figure 5 Upper gastrointestinal contrast radiographic study of a child with malrotation. The duodenojejunal junction does not extend sufficiently to the left of the spine and cephalad.

cal presentation may include bilious vomiting and a double-bubble sign on abdominal films, mimicking the presentation of duodenal atresia, stenosis or annular pancreas. The diagnosis is made by a contrast upper gastrointestinal series, usually with barium. In very sick infants with a concern of underlying bowel infarct or perforation, the patient should undergo expeditious surgical exploration and contrast studies are contraindicated. The duodeno-jejunal junction at the level of the ligament of Treitz, should be to the left of the left spinal pedicle (Figure 5). The radiographic signs of malrotation include (1) abnormal position of the duodeno-jejunal junction, (2) spiral or Z-shaped course of the distal duodenum and proximal jejunum, and (3) the proximal jejunum positioned in the right abdomen. The duodenum basically fails to extend sufficiently to the left of the spine and cephalad.[29]

In the presence of a volvulus, the distal duodenum and proximal jejunum course downward in the mid abdomen and may create a "corkscrew" appearance. (Figure 6) The lumen becomes narrowed and may have a "beaked" appearance at the level of obstruction. The duodenum proximal to the obstruction may be dilated. If the obstruction is complete, contrast may stop in the proximal bowel before even entering the loops involved in the volvulus.

The surgical procedure to address malrotation is termed the Ladd's procedure and includes (1) reducing the midgut volvulus if present, (2) dividing the peritoneal bands obstructing the duodenum, (3) positioning the small and large bowel in a nonrotated position, and (4) an appendectomy. Since the consequences of an acute volvulus can be so devastating, it is generally recommended that a malrotation be addressed when identified, even as an incidental radiographic finding. Two recent studies support this approach in infants and children.[30,31] A preventive Ladd's procedure in adults is somewhat more controversial since they are less likely to experience a volvulus compared to an infant or young child.[31]

Table 4 Conditions with Associated Malrotation	
Syndromes	Other Congenital GI Conditions
Heterotaxy syndrome	Congenital diaphragmatic hernia
Prune belly syndrome	Gastroschisis
Down syndrome	Omphalocele
Megacystis-microcolon-intestinal hypoperi-stalsis syndrome	Intestinal atresia
(Berdon syndrome)	Cloacal extrophy

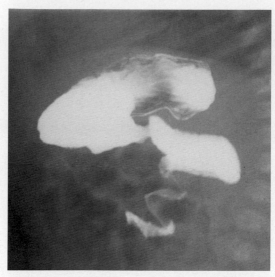

Figure 6 Upper gastrointestinal contrast radiographic study of an infant with malrotation and volvulus. "Corkscrew" appearance of the duodenum and proximal jejunum is demonstrated coursing downward in the mid abdomen.

However, if a conservative, nonsurgical approach is taken, close observation and timely evaluation at the onset of suggestive gastrointestinal symptoms are warranted.

Colonic Volvulus

Colonic volvulus in infants and children is rare. The volvulus may involve the sigmoid colon, the cecum or, occasionally, the transverse colon. In adults, common predisposing factors include chronic constipation and, in some countries, a diet that is very high in fiber and residue. Although one of the presenting symptoms in children is constipation, this may be secondary to underlying chronic recurrent volvulus rather than the cause in a significant proportion of pediatric patients. Factors that may predispose to a colonic volvulus in children include congenital elongation of the sigmoid colon, a pathologically long mesentery, a narrow-based mesocolon and abnormal fixation of the colon. Colonic volvulus is seen in certain conditions including Hirschsprung's disease, imperforate anus, and neurodevelopmental disorders including mental retardation and cerebral palsy.[32–34]

Presentation may be acute or chronic. In acute volvulus, severe colicky abdominal pain, vomiting, distension, and abdominal tenderness predominate. If there is underlying compromise of the blood supply to the involved bowel, signs and symptoms of peritonitis, intestinal ischemia, and septic shock may develop. In children with chronic recurrent volvulus, the onset and clinical course are more insidious and the diagnosis may be delayed unless the index of suspicion is high. In these patients, signs and symptoms are similar but intermittent. In one series of children with sigmoid volvulus, the most common symptoms were abdominal pain, vomiting, and constipation, and the predominant signs were abdominal distension, tenderness, and a mass.[32]

The diagnosis may be suggested on plain films of the abdomen although these studies tend to be nonspecific in children and diagnostic in less than one-third.[34] Diagnostic findings include a very dilated, twisted sigmoid loop with proximal obstruction. A barium enema may be diagnostic in about two-thirds of patients and shows a "bird's beak" configuration of the twisted colon.[32,34] The enema may also be therapeutic and was successful in 77% of children with sigmoid volvulus in one series.[32]

Contraindications to performing a contrast enema include signs and symptoms of peritonitis, cardiovascular instability or septic shock.

Prior to any intervention, the patient should be stabilized including fluid resuscitation. Nonsurgical reduction of the volvulus may be attempted by contrast enema or by sigmoidoscopy or colonoscopy as long as the child is stable and there is no evidence of peritonitis or perforation. In the latter case, immediate surgical exploration is warranted. Experience with endoscopic reduction in children is limited and this method appears to have a lower success rate than contrast enema. Regardless of the technique used for nonsurgical reduction, the recurrence rate is high and elective surgical intervention is recommended. This usually involves resection of the affected, redundant bowel or fixation of the mobile portion of the colon if the involved segment is extensive. Consideration may be given to performing a rectal biopsy to assess for Hirschsprung's disease in children with no other recognized predisposing factor.[32]

REFERENCES

1. Hajivassilou CS. Intestinal obstruction in neonatal/pediatric surgery. Semin Pediatr Surg 2003;12:241–53.
2. Shawis R, Antao B. Prenatal bowel dilatation and the subsequent postnatal management. Early Hum Develop 2006;82:297–303.
3. Dalla Vecchia LK, Grosfeld JL, West KK, et al. Intestinal atresia and stenosis: A 25-year experience with 277 cases. Arch Surg 1998;133:490–6.
4. Strouse PJ. Disorders of intestinal rotation and fixation "malrotation." Pediatr Radiol 2004;34:837–51.
5. Stern LE, Warner BW. Gastrointestinal duplications. Semin Pediatr Surg 2000;9:135–40.
6. Hayanga AJ, Bass-Wilkins K, Bulkley GB. Current management of small bowel obstruction. Adv Surg 2005;39:1–33.
7. Deitch EA. Simple intestinal obstruction causes bacterial translocation in man. Arch Surg 1989;124:699–701.
8. Maglinte DDT, Reyes BL, Harmon BH. Reliability and the role of plain film radiography and CT in the diagnosis of small bowel obstruction. Am J Roentgenol 1996;167:1451–5.
9. Maglinte DDT, Heikamp DE, Howard TJ, et al. Current concepts in imaging of small bowel obstruction. Radiol Clin North Am 2003;41:262–83.
10. Balthazar EJ. CT of small bowel obstruction. Am J Roentgenol 1994;162:255–61.
11. Sarr MG, Bulkley GB, Zuidema GD. Preoperative recognition of intestinal strangulation obstruction: Prospective evaluation of diagnostic capability. Am J Surg 1983;145:176–82.
12. Puligandla PS, Nguten LT, St-Vil D, et al. Gastrointestinal duplications. J Pediatr Surg 2003;38:740–4.
13. Janik JS, Elin SH, Filler RM, et al. An assessment of the surgical treatment of adhesive small bowel obstruction in infants and children. J Pediatr Surg 1981;16:225–35.
14. Wilkins BM, Spitz L. Incidence of postoperative adhesion obstruction following neonatal laparotomy. Br J Surg 1986;73:762–4.
15. Franklin ME, Jr, Gonzalez JJ, Jr, Miter DB, et al. Laparoscopic diagnosis and treatment of intestinal obstruction. Surg Endosc 2004;18:26–39.
16. Geer D. Superior mesenteric artery syndrome. Mil Med 1990;155:321–3.
17. Baltazar U, Dunn J, Floresguerra C, et al. Superior mesenteric artery syndrome: An uncommon cause of intestinal obstruction. South Med J 2000;93:606–8.
18. Marroud WZ. Laparoscopic management of superior mesenteric artery syndrome. Int Surg 1995;80:322–7.
19. Navarro O, Daneman A. Intussusception Part 3. Diagnosis and management of those with identifiable or predisposing cause and those that reduce spontaneously. Pediatr Radiol 2004;34:305–12.
20. Murphy TV, Gargiullo PM, Massoudi MS, et al. Intussusception among infants given an oral rotavirus vaccine. N Engl J Med 2001;344:564–72.
21. Bines JE, Liem NT, Justice FA, et al. Risk factors for intussusception in infants in Vietnam and Australia: Adenovirus implicated, but not rotavirus. J Pediatr 2006;149:452–60.
22. Vesikari T, Matson DO, Dennehy P, et al. Safety and efficacy of a pentavalent human-bovine (WC3) reassortment rotavirus vaccine. N Engl J Med 2006;354:23–33.
23. Ruiz-Palacios GM, Perez-Schael I, Velazquez FR, et al. Safety and efficacy of an attenuated vaccine against severe rotavirus gastroenteritis. N Engl J Med 2006;354:11–22.
24. O'Ryan M, Matson DO. New rotavirus vaccines: Renewed optimism. J Pediatr 2006;149:448–51.
25. Daneman A, Navarro O. Intussusception part 1. A review of diagnostic approaches. Pediatr Radiol 2004;33:79–85.
26. Daneman A, Navarro O. Intussusception part 2. An update on the evolution of management. Pediatr Radiol 2004;34:97–108.
27. Yoon CH, Kim HJ, Goo HW. Intussusception in children: US-guided pneumatic reduction initial experience. Radiology 2001;281:85–8.
28. Spigland N, Brandt ML, Yazbeck S. Malrotation presenting beyond the neonatal period. J Pediatr Surg 1990;25:1139–42.
29. Applegate KE, Anderson JM, Klatte EC. Intestinal malrotation in children: A problem-solving approach to the upper gastrointestinal series. Radiographics 2006;26:1485–500.
30. Malek MM, Burd RS. Surgical treatment of malrotation after infancy: A population-based study. J Pediatr Surg 2005;40:284–9.
31. Malek MM, Burd RS. The optimal management of malrotation diagnosed after infancy: A decision analysis. Am J Surg 2006;191:45–51.
32. Salas S, Angel CA, Salas N, et al. Sigmoid volvulus in children and adolescents. J Am Coll Surg 2000;190:717–23.
33. Ismail A. Recurrent colonic volvulus in children. J Pediatr Surg 1997;32:1739–42.
34. Samuel S, Boddy SA, Capps S. Volvulus of the transverse and sigmoid colon. Pediatr Surg Int 2000;16:522–4.

17.2. Appendicitis

Dennis P. Lund, MD

Acute appendicitis, the most common disease in children that requires emergency surgery, is also one of the most frequently misdiagnosed. More than 115 years after the description of the pathophysiology of this disease, this entity continues to befuddle clinicians and remains a continued source of considerable morbidity and occasional mortality. Why is this so? The "Holy Grail" for appendicitis—a simple and fail-safe diagnostic test—has constantly been sought by clinicians but without success.

Over 250,000 cases of acute appendicitis occur each year in the United States, and almost one-third of these occur in children. Males develop appendicitis more commonly than females (incidence ratio 1.4:1), and the peak age of appendicitis is between 10 and 14 years in boys and 15 to 19 years in girls. Approximately one-quarter of cases of acute appendicitis are perforated at the time of presentation. There remains a small but definite mortality associated with acute appendicitis, and this is usually related to delayed diagnosis or concomitant diseases. It is estimated that the lifetime risk of developing appendicitis is 8.6% for males and 6.7% for females.[1]

Accurate diagnosis of appendicitis may be very difficult. It is frequently underdiagnosed, which contributes in part to a high perforation rate. However, this disease is also frequently overdiagnosed. Most institutions will report a 10 to 20% incidence of normal, or "white," appendices having been removed when patients are explored for acute appendicitis. In fact, in most surgical training programs, it is taught that if the incidence of normal appendices is less than 10%, the rate of perforation will be unacceptably high.

Reginald Fitz first described the clinical findings of acute appendicitis in 1886. Despite the many advances of modern medicine and improvements in diagnostic accuracy with tests such as ultrasonography (US) and computed tomography (CT), there is no single test to definitively diagnose appendicitis short of pathologic examination. Accurate diagnosis of appendicitis requires clinical acumen; the practitioner must make use of skills in obtaining a thorough history and a careful physical examination—which are more difficult to obtain in children—coupled with close observation of the tempo of the disease. Since the advent of advanced imaging technology, US and CT, as well as increased pressure on clinicians to be more "productive," it seems that practitioners spend less and less time in obtaining a history and physical examination and order more tests. However, despite numerous studies touting the advantages of newer diagnostic technologies, the most accurate and cost-effective diagnostic tool to diagnose appendicitis remains for the physician to spend time performing an accurate history and physical examination.

ANATOMY AND PATHOPHYSIOLOGY

The appendix, roughly the size and shape of one's fifth finger, is a diverticulum arising from the cecum. Its length and particularly its anatomic position can be quite variable, ranging from down in the pelvis to any place on the right side of the abdomen in patients with normal intestinal rotation. Patients with appendicitis, in whom the appendix resides in a retrocecal location, can present particularly difficult diagnostic dilemmas because of the effect this may have on the presentation and location of signs and symptoms. In those who have abnormal intestinal rotation, the location may be highly variable, confusing the diagnosis even more (Figure 1).

Embryologically, the cecum is visible by the fifth gestational week as an enlargement of the hindgut, and the appendix begins to appear about the eighth week. Some villi are seen in the appendix during the fourth and fifth months, but these disappear prior to birth. Lymphatic nodules will be present by the seventh month. This lymph tissue continues to increase until puberty and then slowly recedes,[2] which may explain the age peak of appendicitis in adolescents. Despite much speculation based on comparative anatomy with other mammals, the function of the appendix in humans remains unknown.

The pathophysiologic cause of acute appendicitis is thought to be obstruction of the lumen of the appendix either by fecal matter, such as a fecalith, or by swollen lymphoid tissue. This latter cause may explain why cases of appendicitis may follow soon after a viral illness. Multiplication of bacteria in the obstructed viscus leads to swelling and invasive infection of the wall of the appendix. This initially causes activation of stretch receptors in the wall of the intestine that is perceived in the tenth thoracic (T10) dermatome, the periumbilical region. As the infection proceeds, inflammatory fluid exudes from the organ. This fluid, which contains many inflammatory mediators, travels to the parietal peritoneum adjacent to the appendix, where it causes

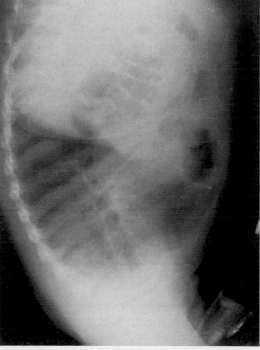

Figure 1 Posteroanterior and lateral chest radiograph from a young girl who presented with periumbilical pain that migrated to the epigastrium. She developed localized peritonitis in the epigastrium and bilious vomiting. At operation, she was found to have acute appendicitis contained within the diaphragmatic hernia of Morgagni. Note the gas-filled viscus above the diaphragm. (Courtesy of R. C. Shamberger, MD.)

stronger, localized pain in the right lower quadrant owing to irritation of the sensitive nerves of the peritoneum. It is important to remember that the peritoneal pain is due to the irritating fluid, not necessarily to direct contact of the appendix with the peritoneal surface. This phenomenon may be helpful in diagnosing unusual cases of appendicitis in which the irritating fluid may travel some distance from the infected organ.

If the inflammatory process proceeds unchecked, the appendix will usually "perforate," or begin to leak luminal fluid into the peritoneal cavity, in about 36 hours. In children, it is estimated that 20% of cases of acute appendicitis perforate within 24 hours after the beginning of symptoms and up to 80% perforate within 48 hours. Perforation may be due to gangrene of the organ as a result of thrombosis from the invasive infection, or it may be due to direct erosion of a fecalith through the infected wall of the appendix. Alternatively, the swollen organ may begin to leak owing to high pressure from fluid and gas within the obstructed, infected lumen. If inflammatory fluid seeps throughout the abdomen, generalized peritonitis ensues. However, if the infection is confined to a local area by the body's natural defense mechanisms, such as the omentum walling off the infection, localized tenderness, and a mass may be the presenting signs. When this infection is not drained in some fashion, the outcome will frequently be generalized shock and septicemia.

The bacterial floras present in acute appendicitis are those that inhabit the human colon, most of which are anaerobic. *Bacteroides fragilis, Escherichia coli, Enterococcus, Pseudomonas, Klebsiella,* and *Clostridium* species may all appear. Cultures of the peritoneum during simple appendicitis seldom yield organisms, but during the gangrenous and perforated stages of the disease, there may be a panoply of the organisms listed above.

Carcinoid tumors and parasites, particularly *Enterobius vermicularis,* or pinworm, and *Ascaris lumbricoides* may also rarely lead to obstruction of the lumen of the appendix and the development of acute appendicitis. These cases may or may not be accompanied by a history of gastrointestinal symptoms that preceded the development of the picture of appendicitis. Finally, an occasional case of appendicitis may present soon after a traumatic blow to the appendix, such as after a football injury or an automobile crash, presumably because the trauma leads to swelling of the organ with obstruction of the lumen.

DIAGNOSIS

Accuracy in assessing the time of the onset of symptoms is critical in children because of the rapid tempo of the disease, that is, roughly 36 hours to perforation from the start of the pain. The child's parents may be aware that the child awoke with pain in the night, or the child may not have eaten normally the evening before.

Questioning patients and their parents about interest in the meals that immediately preceded the presentation may help pinpoint when their child first seemed unwell. Anorexia has been described as a reliable sign of appendicitis. Unfortunately, like many of the symptoms associated with appendicitis, it may or may not be present, and up to half of patients with appendicitis may say that they are hungry.

Pain

The earliest symptom of appendicitis is usually periumbilical pain. After a few hours, the patient will frequently vomit, but the absence of vomiting does not exclude appendicitis. Many patients will progress to perforation without vomiting. Vomiting may become an important sign because it usually follows the periumbilical pain. In contrast, patients with gastroenteritis will vomit, but in these patients, the vomiting usually precedes abdominal pain. Vomiting in appendicitis is thought to be due to activation of the stretch receptors in the appendix itself; in operations done on awake, older patients under local anesthesia, traction on the bowel may induce vomiting despite complete somatic insensitivity.

After a few hours, the pain usually shifts to the right lower quadrant because of inflammatory fluid irritating the local peritoneum. This pain is stronger and overrides the periumbilical discomfort. Thus, in the classic presentation, the pain of appendicitis starts around the umbilicus and migrates to the right lower quadrant. The pain from the inflammatory fluid is quite strong. Blood or urine in the peritoneum is less painful than inflammatory fluid or pus, whereas only bile causes consistently stronger pain than does inflammatory fluid.

McBurney first noted in 1889 that in the majority of cases, the point of maximal tenderness was localized to an area two-thirds of the way from the umbilicus to the anterior iliac spine. If the pain is due to fluid, why is this pain so localized rather than spread throughout the abdomen? The answer lies in the fact that the fluid is traveling by capillary action between the thin planes that exist among coils of intestine in the unopened abdomen, and this is commonly the point where the fluid is most concentrated. Further, the inflammatory fluid becomes gradually diluted as it moves away from the point of secretion. If the appendix lies in a retrocecal location, the peritoneal irritation may not occur, and the periumbilical pain may persist and dominate. This can go on for days and may persist even after perforation. In such cases, psoas or genitofemoral nerve irritation may be the dominant complaint, and attention is often focused on the hip or other musculoskeletal area. For this reason, retrocecal appendicitis may be very difficult to diagnose.[3]

Physical Signs

The first signs of tenderness usually appear after the pain has migrated to the right lower quadrant. This may first be mild tenderness on direct palpation. It is always wise to ask the child to localize the spot of maximal tenderness for you

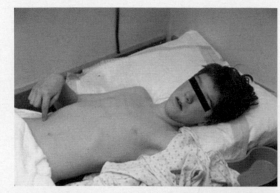

Figure 2 An 11-year-old boy with appendicitis pointing to the area of maximal pain. (Courtesy of Gary Williams, MD.)

so that this area can be examined last (Figure 2). Because children are often apprehensive about examination, making the true nature of the tenderness difficult to assess, the examiner may find the stethoscope useful for "palpation" while appearing to be listening.

The most reliable diagnostic sign of acute appendicitis is localized tenderness in the right lower quadrant. As the peritoneal irritation progresses, guarding develops (voluntary stiffening of the rectus muscle), then spasm or involuntary guarding, and, finally, rebound tenderness. Stretch receptors in the peritoneum respond to the rate of stretch, not to the direction. Rebound tenderness is elicited by the examiner pressing down slowly, holding for a few seconds while the patient accommodates, and then removing the hand rapidly. If the patient suddenly winces, this is a very reliable sign of peritoneal irritation. The patient who claims the ride into the hospital caused pain with every bump in the road is describing rebound tenderness. So, too, is the patient who winces when he coughs or has pain as he jumps off the examining table. On the other hand, the patient who willingly hops up and down on one foot seldom will have appendicitis. However, we have seen patients with a gangrenous appendix walled off by omentum who performed even the hop test satisfactorily. Again, it is important for the diagnostician to remember that no single sign, symptom, or test is diagnostic of acute appendicitis aside from examining the appendix under the microscope.

The signs of peritonitis include voluntary and involuntary guarding, direct tenderness, and rebound tenderness. These signs are due only to irritation of the anterior abdominal wall. The abdomen, however, is a six-sided cavity. Each side of the cavity has physical signs unique to it. For example, retroperitoneal irritation may generate a psoas sign or an obturator sign owing to irritation of those muscles. We have seen a case of perforated appendicitis presenting with shoulder pain when the tip of the appendix perforated into the right subphrenic space. A pelvic mass or pelvic sidewall tenderness on rectal examination may be the manifestation of an inflamed or perforated appendix in the pelvis. Performing a rectal examination on a child frequently causes discomfort, making it difficult to discern true tenderness. Asking the patient to push down as if having a bowel movement and then to relax as the finger is gently inserted causing the least discomfort.

In postpubescent and especially in sexually active girls, it may be helpful to perform a pelvic examination. This should be done carefully and thoughtfully because it may be the first pelvic examination the patient has had. The patient may have localized tenderness or a mass with appendicitis. Cervical motion tenderness, however, is not usually present with appendicitis and is more suggestive of pelvic inflammatory disease.

The overall appearance of the child with abdominal pain is important in the diagnosis of appendicitis. Frequently, the child will simply "look sick"; signs and symptoms such as flushed cheeks, listlessness, low-grade fever, and unwillingness to move often accompany appendicitis even early in its course. In contrast, the child who is happy and talkative and willing to follow commands readily probably has some other cause of the abdominal pain. Fever is not a reliable sign of appendicitis. The temperature may be slightly elevated in acute appendicitis, usually by no more than one or two degrees in the child without perforation. Complicated appendicitis—perforated or gangrenous—may have high fever associated with it, however.

Laboratory Examination

Urinalysis is probably the only important laboratory test in the diagnosis of appendicitis, and it should be used to exclude urinary tract pathology. In a boy with symptoms that are not clearly appendicitis and a urinalysis with greater than 15 white blood cells (WBCs) per high-power field, urine should be sent for Gram stain and culture. If there is evidence of a urinary tract infection, the child may be treated with intravenous antibiotics for a few hours. However, this child should still be observed closely for response to therapy. A girl with greater than 30 WBCs per high-power field can be similarly treated, but only if the urine is obtained from a midstream specimen while the labia have been spread or by bladder catheterization. Urine obtained from a collecting bag applied to the patient may have many WBCs and squamous cells from the vagina and cannot be interpreted.

An elevated WBC count is the only laboratory test that has been shown to correlate with appendicitis.[4] Despite this, the value of the WBC count is limited. Most children who have been vomiting will have an elevated WBC count. Although there may be an increase in the polymorphonuclear leukocytes, the total WBC count does not usually exceed 20,000 cells/mm³ in a patient with a nonperforated appendix. The WBC count is influenced by so many factors that it is not dependable in arriving at the diagnosis of appendicitis. It is not uncommon in a child without toxicity to see a WBC count below 5,000 cells/mm³ when the appendix is not perforated. Such children may be recovering from a

viral infection with leukopenia just prior to the onset of acute appendicitis. Indeed, such a viral episode may have led to swelling of the lymphoid tissue in the wall of the appendix and may have been the inciting factor in obstruction of the appendiceal lumen.

Experience has been reported using measurements of the C-reactive protein level. C-reactive protein is an acute-phase reactant, the concentration of which rises in whole blood within 12 hours of onset of an infection. It can be measured with a blood test. If patients have had symptoms for more than 12 hours and they have appendicitis, studies indicate that the C-reactive protein is elevated in over 85% of cases.[5] This test is not widely used because the result often takes time to obtain, but it may have benefit in excluding appendicitis in patients with symptoms of more than 1 day's duration[6]; however, this test is not specific, and any infectious or inflammatory process may be accompanied by an elevated C-reactive protein level.

In an attempt to systematize the diagnosis of appendicitis, Alvarado used a combination of signs, symptoms, and laboratory values to develop an "appendicitis score." In this score, eight variables were assessed: localized tenderness in the right lower quadrant, leukocytosis, migration of pain, WBC shift to the left, fever, nausea or vomiting, anorexia, and direct rebound tenderness. Each variable was assigned a score, and the scores were then added. In his scheme, Alvarado found excellent correlation with appendicitis in patients with higher scores.[7] Samuel applied a similar system based on signs and symptoms to children and found good statistical correlation with the presence of acute appendicitis.[8]

Radiologic Examination

Plain radiographs may be helpful if the diagnosis is in some doubt, but we do not routinely obtain films, except in infants. The most common finding on plain abdominal radiographs in the patient with appendicitis is curvature of the spine to the right. A dilated cecum containing an air–fluid level may be seen. A calcified fecalith can sometimes be seen if the films are well exposed and multiple films are obtained with the patient in different positions to portray the calcification unobscured by bony structures (Figure 3). Half the children with abdominal pain and a fecalith can be expected to have perforated appendicitis. When the appendix is perforated (especially in infants), there may be a paucity of gas in the right lower quadrant and an increase in the thickness of the lateral abdominal wall owing to soft tissue edema and evidence of free peritoneal fluid.[9] Use of routine plain radiographs is not recommended, however, because studies in adults have demonstrated no finding that correlated with appendicitis, and cost–benefit analysis showed that plain films have a very high cost-to-benefit ratio when used to diagnose this disease.[10] In the confusing case, if the diagnosis is in doubt, or the patient

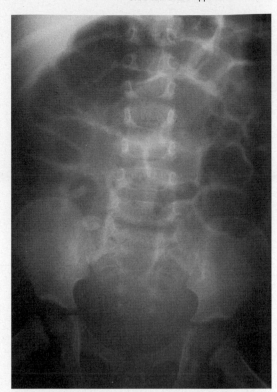

Figure 3 Plain radiograph of a teenage girl with appendicitis demonstrating a large, calcified appendicolith in the right lower quadrant. Appendicoliths are rarely this large and can be difficult to differentiate from surrounding bony structures.

has a cough or other chest findings, a chest radiograph may demonstrate a right lower lobe pneumonia that may be causing referred pain to the midabdomen.

A large amount of experience using US has been reported in the evaluation of abdominal pain in children, but the data provided by US are operator-dependent and easily misinterpreted. The normal appendix is usually not visualized on US. However, a thickened or noncompressible appendix may be seen, as well as periappendiceal fluid, a fecalith, or even a periappendiceal abscess.[11] US should be reserved for the difficult cases because it delays surgery. However, in selected cases with an experienced ultrasonographer, this test may be of value, especially in females in whom adnexal pathology may confuse the issue. In fact, in cases in which pelvic pathology is high in the differential diagnosis, US may be the most valuable test because it is better for evaluating the adnexa than is CT. Data suggest that the use of US in evaluation of difficult cases of abdominal pain changed the treatment course and increased the level of certainty of the practitioner.[12]

The data on the utility of US are quite conflicting, however. The sensitivity and specificity of US examinations for appendicitis can be quite variable. More importantly, it is not clear that use of US affects the outcome in a population of children with appendicitis, that is, it may not lower the incidence of perforation or the cost of care.[13] This test must be factored into the overall clinical picture in deciding on operative intervention, and one must remember that a negative sonogram does not exclude appendicitis.

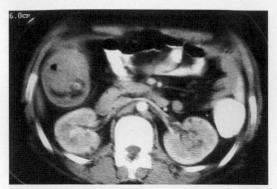

Figure 4 Computed tomographic scan showing a large periappendiceal abscess (*arrow*) containing gas. Note the contrast enhancement of the rim, which is typical with abscesses.

Use of CT in the evaluation of difficult cases of abdominal pain has also been reported extensively. The CT findings suggestive of appendicitis include appendiceal wall thickening, the presence of inflammatory changes in the periappendiceal fat, or the presence of an abscess or phlegmon (Figure 4). An appendicolith seen on a CT scan in a patient with right lower quadrant pain is also highly suggestive of appendicitis. The best results, meaning the highest specificity and accuracy, in children have come from using limited CT scanning with a thin-cut helical technique with rectal contrast. Using this technique, the sensitivity, specificity, and accuracy of the diagnosis were all reported to be 94%. This was much better than when the same group was examined with US.[14] Some of the US and CT signs of acute appendicitis are listed in Table 1. Because of the low false-negative rate with CT scanning, use of this test allows patients to be discharged home rather than admitted for observation, resulting in cost savings. However, we caution that 1 of 20 cases is still misdiagnosed, and careful follow-up of these patients is warranted, especially if they are discharged from care.[14] A follow-up telephone call the next day should reveal improvement of the patient; if this is not the case, the patient must be seen and reevaluated.

Unfortunately, it has now become common practice for CT scans to be over utilized in the evaluation of abdominal pain in children. Most scans are performed only with oral or oral and IV contrast, and often include the entire abdomen and pelvis. The contrast is frequently vomited or not allowed to percolate through the entire intestine resulting in suboptimal scans that are difficult to interpret at best, or are inaccurate at worst.

Furthermore, these scans carry with them a small but real risk of exposure to radiation that over a large population may result in an increased incidence of leukemia later in life.[15] It is wiser to use good clinical acumen, possibly with a clinical decision tool, such as that described by Kharbanda, et al, to identify those patients who would best or least benefit from advanced radiologic testing. By using a 6-part score that assigned points for nausea, focal right lower quadrant pain, migration of pain, difficulty walking, rebound or percussion tenderness, and absolute neutrophil count, the authors showed that a low score had an extremely low likelihood (>95%) of having appendicitis and therefore of not needing further imaging.[16]

Other radiologic tests, such as barium enema and intravenous pyelogram, are of little value these days because virtually all of the information that these might reveal, such as extrinsic compression of the cecum or ureteral obstruction, can be gleaned from CT scans. These tests should be reserved for selected chronic cases that present as diagnostic dilemmas.

Once again, however, it should be emphasized that obtaining a thorough history and performing a careful physical examination will accurately make the diagnosis of appendicitis in the majority of cases without radiographic testing. Use of any of the radiographic tests discussed above is not advocated unless the presentation is confusing or the diagnosis is in question.

Perforated Appendicitis

Immediately on perforation of the appendix, the child may have a period when he feels better owing to relief of the pressure that built up within the lumen of the appendix. Soon thereafter, the child will lie still, often with the right leg drawn up, and will become tachypneic. The vomiting pattern may change: although the child with early appendicitis may vomit once or twice or not at all, vomiting after perforation is more frequent, and the vomitus may contain small bowel contents from paralytic ileus. The child will be hot and dry, with temperatures of 101°F or higher. Signs of peritoneal irritation may be diffuse or localized, and a mass may be palpable. Peritoneal findings in the patient with perforation of a retrocecal appendix are more variable, and retroperitoneal signs such as the psoas or obturator signs may be more prevalent. Rectal examination may reveal lateralizing tenderness or a mass pushing on the rectum.

Many children with perforated appendicitis have what is described as "diarrhea," which leads to the erroneous diagnosis of gastroenteritis. Diarrhea accompanying perforated appendicitis is usually low-volume, irritative fluid from inflammation of the rectosigmoid colon. Peristalsis is often decreased. In contrast, gastroenteritis produces high-volume (profuse) diarrhea from the rectosigmoid, abetted by increased peristalsis.

The child who has been "sick for a week" may well have a large appendiceal abscess walled off from the peritoneal cavity. When the abscess begins to leak into the free abdominal cavity, the child shows signs of extreme toxicity, oliguria, mottling of the skin, evidence of gram-negative septicemia, and a falling platelet count. Radiographs may show signs of paralytic ileus or even partial small bowel obstruction. This is the type of patient most at risk for a disastrous outcome from appendicitis.

Diagnostic Dilemmas

Appendicitis is a common disease with many uncommon presentations. We have seen appendicitis present as an incarcerated hernia, intermittent small bowel obstruction, subphrenic abscess, and diverticulitis, just to name a few. Appendicitis must be in the differential diagnosis of any child who presents with abdominal pain. Children under the age of 2 years and obese patients, particularly perimenarchal girls, represent the most difficult diagnostic groups in our experience. Obesity interferes with the physical examination by making it difficult to elicit direct tenderness and guarding. Very young children are unable to give a history or tell where it hurts, and their parents often cannot pinpoint when the child began to feel ill. Although only 2% of children with appendicitis will be under the age of 2 years, over 70% of very young children with appendicitis will have perforated by the time of presentation.[17] Just as it was once said that if someone understood syphilis in all of its manifestations, he understood all of internal medicine, if one understands appendicitis in all of its presentations, one understands evaluation of the acute abdomen.

DIFFERENTIAL DIAGNOSIS

Gastroenteritis

This condition is the most common cause of abdominal pain in children presenting to emergency rooms. Retrocecal appendicitis can commonly be confused with gastroenteritis. Some of the signs that may help to distinguish appendicitis from gastroenteritis are listed in Table 2.[18] When there is any doubt of the diagnosis, the child should be observed closely. Gastroenteritis will usually improve gradually, whereas appendicitis will continue to get worse. It must also be remembered that the dehydrated child frequently appears quite ill and may improve dramatically simply as a result of rehydration. If improvement is seen after intravenous fluids are given, the

Table 1 Ultrasonography and Computed Tomography Criteria for Appendicitis	
Ultrasonography	Computed Tomography
Fluid-filled, noncompressible, distended tubular structure (≥6 mm)	Fluid-filled tubular structure measuring >6 mm in maximum diameter
No peristalsis in appendix	Fat stranding, abscess, or phlegmon in adjacent tissue
With or without appendicolith	With or without appendicolith
Location: anterior to psoas or retrocecal	Focal cecal apical thickening
Pericecal inflammatory changes	
Adapted from Garcia-Pena et al.[14]	

Table 2 Differential Diagnosis of Appendicitis and Gastroenteritis

Symptom	Gastroenteritis	Appendicitis
Onset of periumbilical pain	Coexistent with or after vomiting	Before vomiting
Diarrhea	High volume, frequent	Mucus or low-volume irritative type of diarrhea, infrequent
Peristalsis	High frequency, low pitch	Low frequency or absent, high pitch if paralytic ileus
Rectal tenderness	Usually absent	Usually present
Rebound tenderness or referred rebound tenderness, such as "painful ride to hospital"	Usually absent	Often present, especially in cases of perforation

Adapted from Folkman.[18]

child must still be closely examined for any signs of localized tenderness.

Of the bacterial enteritides, *Yersinia, Salmonella, Shigella,* or *Campylobacter* may present with abdominal pain. Usually, there is more than the expected amount of diarrhea, but right lower quadrant pain is common, and there may even be a shift of pain from the periumbilical region to the right lower quadrant. These patients often appear quite toxic, and leukocytosis is prominent. Cramps and high fever also are frequent, and there may be occult or frank blood in the stools, which is not usually present with appendicitis. The patient with appendicitis will rarely, if ever, thrash about in bed, but crampy, intermittent pain is frequent with gastroenteritis. If an operation is undertaken, the appendix is not inflamed. Culture of lymph nodes or stool may yield *Salmonella. Yersinia* may be diagnosed from stool cultures or serology. With Campylobacter infections, there are cramps, fever, watery diarrhea, and, frequently, blood per rectum. The diagnosis is made by culture of the organism from stool, and treatment is with oral erythromycin.

Constipation

This problem is a common cause of pain in some children, particularly in older children. The right lower quadrant pain may be intermittent, crampy, or steady, but it rarely progresses, and the pain may be perceived by the patient as quite severe. Usually, it is not possible to elicit a history of constipation. Patients will state that they have moved their bowels that day or the day before, but stool may be palpable on examination of the abdomen, or the colon may appear stool-filled on the KUB (kidney, ureter, bladder) radiograph. We see this problem most often in the heat of the summer months and in the dry winter months, when household heat is being used. At both times, chronic mild dehydration probably is a contributing factor. If there is little or no evidence of peritoneal irritation in the right lower quadrant and an abdominal film shows a colon filled with feces, it is safe to give a Fleet enema. If the symptoms disappear after a large bowel movement, the patient may be allowed to go home.

Urinary Tract Pathology

When urinary tract infection is present, the fever and leukocytosis may be increased out of proportion to the abdominal signs, in contrast to the usual signs of appendicitis. When pyelonephritis is present, there is usually flank pain and tenderness and high fever as opposed to right lower quadrant pain. If there is pyuria, the urine has been collected correctly, and the signs are not clearly consistent with appendicitis, then it is permissible to treat the patient for a few hours with intravenous antibiotics. However, if the patient does not improve rapidly, or if the diagnosis is still in doubt, we proceed with appendectomy. Crampy or intermittent severe pain in the right lower quadrant may be due to a right ureteral stone. Usually, there will be hematuria. If a stone is suspected, a CT scan without any type of contrast will be diagnostic. If this study is negative, however, and appendicitis is still in the differential diagnosis, the scan may need to be repeated with gastrointestinal and oral or, better, with rectal contrast.

Crohn's Disease

Regional enteritis usually presents with a more protracted course than appendicitis. Often the child has had bowel symptoms for months or more, including crampy abdominal pain, diarrhea, and failure to thrive. There may be a family history of inflammatory bowel disease. Occasionally, however, the presentation will be similar to that of appendicitis, and the first discovery of the disease is during appendectomy. If this is the case at operation, the bowel, usually the terminal ileum, is thickened with mesenteric fat creeping over the bowel wall. Biopsy of an ileocolic mesenteric lymph node will often show granulomas. If the cecum is uninvolved and a secure closure of the appendiceal stump can be completed, we recommend removal of the appendix. If, on the other hand, the disease involves the region of the appendix, it is safest not to proceed with appendectomy for fear of development of an enterocutaneous fistula. Primary resection of the affected bowel should not be undertaken because early disease can frequently be treated medically, and bowel resection can be delayed or avoided.

Pelvic Inflammatory Disease

Pelvic inflammatory disease in girls over 12 years is not uncommon. The onset of abdominal pain is often preceded by the menstrual period. The pain usually begins in the lower quadrants rather than in the periumbilical area, as it does in appendicitis, and frequently accompanies the onset of menses. Pain with motion of the cervix is the hallmark of pelvic inflammatory disease, and there may be bilateral adnexal tenderness. Gram stain of the purulent cervical discharge may reveal gramnegative intracellular diplococci. The sedimentation rate is greater than 15 mm/h in the majority of cases, whereas in appendicitis, the sedimentation rate is almost always normal, that is, less than or equal to 10 mm/h. If the differential diagnosis is in doubt or if the signs persist after initiation of treatment, it is wise to do an appendectomy. We have operated on young adolescents with appendicitis who were originally thought to have gonorrhea because the cervical smear revealed gram-negative diplococci. Culture in these patients showed that these were only the *saprophytic Neisseria* that may be present normally in the vagina.

Ovarian Cyst

Pathology in the ovary can mimic appendicitis. The most common cause is rupture of an ovarian cyst. The pain is usually quite abrupt in onset and begins in the right lower quadrant. There is frequently tenderness. If the girl is menstruating, the pain is often midcycle, but ovarian cysts are frequent at menarche as well. US may be helpful to delineate free fluid or other cysts in the ovary, or a recently ruptured follicular cyst may be seen. If the diagnosis is in doubt, laparoscopy may help define the pathology, but this test does not rule out appendicitis unless the appendix is fully visualized. If diagnostic laparoscopy is undertaken and the appendix is found to be normal, we usually remove it in any case. US may also suggest torsion of an ovary, usually associated with a cyst. Pain and vomiting are common with this disease as well. Ovarian torsion should be treated operatively.

Pneumonia

Right lower lobe pneumonia may refer pain to the abdomen through the tenth and eleventh thoracic nerves. A chest film, the presence of abnormal respiratory signs (flaring, grunting, tachypnea), and increased toxicity should help to confirm the diagnosis. These patients often have high fever and a cough. We occasionally see a child in whom the right lower lobe infiltrate and the fever do not improve after 2 days of antibiotic treatment, and the underlying process turns out to be a localized rupture of a high retrocecal appendix with a collection of fluid beneath the right diaphragm.

Mesenteric Adenitis

This entity is due to viral infection or other inflammation of the lymph nodes clustered in the mesentery of the terminal ileum. This diagnosis tends to be a diagnosis of exclusion and is most safely made only at laparotomy or laparoscopy. US or CT may demonstrate enlarged mesenteric lymph nodes. The clinician must be careful in this case because enlarged mesenteric lymph nodes may coexist with acute appendicitis. If, at exploration, the appendix is found to be normal, Meckel diverticulum and adnexal pathology are ruled out, and enlarged lymph nodes are found, we may biopsy the node for culture and pathologic evaluation.

Typhlitis

Patients who are severely leukopenic as a result of disease or cancer chemotherapy may develop a syndrome of severe right lower quadrant pain and tenderness. This is most likely related to invasive infection of the wall of the cecum. This usually occurs at the nadir of the leukocyte counts, and it can be confused with acute appendicitis. CT scanning may reveal a thickened, irregular cecum, and occasional pneumatosis coli. Operation in these patients has a prohibitive morbidity and mortality and is to be avoided if possible. Most patients will respond to bowel rest and high doses of intravenous broad-spectrum antibiotics.[19]

COST OF DIAGNOSTIC ERROR

The sequelae of perforation are so dangerous that if the diagnosis appears to be appendicitis, even if one is not absolutely certain, it is always preferable to remove the appendix before perforation and accept the occasional "error" of removing a normal appendix rather than waiting so long that perforation occurs. Despite improved accuracy in diagnosing this disease with modern technology, 5 to 10% of cases cannot be accurately diagnosed without an operation. Therefore, it is entirely acceptable practice for the surgeon to have occasional cases in which the appendix is found to be normal. The morbidity of a negative appendectomy should be quite small, and the alternative—a missed appendicitis leading to perforation—is quite high. If the diagnosis is doubtful, we prefer to admit the child for repeated observation by the same physician. Sending the child home to return the next day only ensures that a different physician who cannot accurately judge whether the signs have progressed will see him. The average length of hospital stay for acute appendicitis is 1 to 2 days, whereas the child with a perforated appendix will stay for as much as 10 days or more, incur much higher costs, and have greater potential for a complication or long-term sequelae.

TREATMENT

There are many possible ways to treat appendicitis, but, in general, appendectomy on the day of diagnosis is the treatment of choice. One exception to this rule is in the case of perforated appendicitis with a well-established abscess that can be drained. Even in a sick child who must be prepared with intravenous fluids, antibiotics, correction of electrolyte imbalances, and reduction of fever, we have always been able to perform the operation on the same day.

OPERATIVE TECHNIQUE

For open appendectomy, a transverse right lower quadrant muscle-splitting incision is used, more lateral than in an adult because the rectus muscle is relatively wider in a child. It is virtually always possible to remove the appendix, even in the presence of an abscess or severe perforation with peritonitis. It is safest to mobilize the cecum so that the entire appendix lies above the abdominal wall. It may be necessary to incise the lateral cecal peritoneal attachments at the white line of Toldt to do so. The mesoappendix is ligated and divided so that the appendix is completely mobilized and free at its base. A purse-string suture is placed around the base of the appendix, and the appendix is crushed and ligated with plain catgut suture near its base. The stump of the appendix is inverted while the purse-string is tied. This will give a secure closure of the stump and prevent mucocele formation because the catgut will dissolve promptly inside the lumen of the cecum. The muscle layers are closed individually, and the skin is typically closed primarily. When removing a perforated appendix, it is important not to leave behind a fecalith that may have fallen out of a perforated appendix during the procedure. This will result in later formation of an abscess.

In cases of periappendiceal abscess, we use CT- or US-guided drainage of the abscess with delayed removal of the appendix, usually about 8 weeks later. This is safe and even preferable in cases in which there is a well-defined abscess cavity. Broad-spectrum antibiotics should be given, and the patient should respond promptly to this intervention with resolution of fever and return of bowel function. This method of treatment allows the child to defervesce quickly initially without becoming too ill and has the advantage of allowing later laparoscopic appendectomy with rapid recovery. In this treatment algorithm, the appendix should be later removed because pathologic abnormalities frequently exist, and if the appendix is not removed, these patients are at risk for recurrent bouts of appendicitis.[20]

On extremely rare occasions, the appendiceal stump is so gangrenous or the cecum so edematous that the stump cannot be inverted or closed safely (Figure 5). In this situation, it is wisest to do a limited ileocecal resection with an end-to-end two-layer ileo-right colic anastomosis. We try to position the anastomosis away from the abscess cavity and separate the two with omentum. Another option if the appendix cannot be inverted but the cecum is not thickened or inflamed is to resect a small portion of the cecal wall and perform a two-layer closure. In either option, it is critical that the tissue that is closed be soft, well vascularized, and without significant inflammation. Failure to close healthy tissue without tension will result in a fecal fistula, and the patient will remain ill for a long period of time.

Considerable experience has been gained in the use of laparoscopy for appendectomy. Many surgeons now prefer laparoscopy to the open

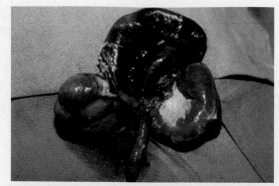

Figure 5 Gangrene of the terminal ileum secondary to perforated appendicitis with bowel obstruction. This patient was treated with ileocecectomy and primary reanastomosis. The anastomosis was placed in the right upper quadrant well away from the abscess cavity, and the patient did well.

technique for their patients, and the results are comparable to those with the open technique. Appendectomy through the laparoscope may offer the benefit of faster recovery to normal activity for older patients, but the hospital stay in uncomplicated cases is equal using both techniques. To date, operative costs associated with the laparoscopic approach still exceed those of open laparotomy, and these costs are not offset by a shorter length of hospital stay, as is usually the situation when laparoscopy is used for larger abdominal procedures. One situation in which laparoscopic appendectomy may offer an advantage is in the case of a patient—usually a teenage female—in whom there is a diagnostic dilemma, and laparoscopy offers a broader view of the abdomen and pelvis to search for other pathology.

Laparoscopic appendectomy can usually be accomplished using a three-trocar technique. Most surgeons divide the mesoappendix and the appendix with a linear stapling device, although a harmonic scalpel or another similar coagulating instrument may also be used for the mesentery. As opposed to an open technique in which the mesoappendix is typically divided first, with laparoscopy, it is often easier to divide the appendix before dividing the mesoappendix. It is very important to divide the appendix close to the cecum so that the entire viscus is removed. Cases of recurrent appendicitis have been reported when a length of appendiceal stump is left after laparoscopic appendectomy.[21]

Patients with nonperforated appendicitis receive a preoperative dose of intravenous antibiotic, usually a first- or second-generation cephalosporin, to cover skin flora and possibly some gram-negative organisms. This is continued for 24 hours if the operation reveals no evidence of perforation. Routine intraoperative cultures of the abdomen are of little value in such patients.[20]

PERFORATED APPENDICITIS

Optimal management of perforated appendicitis in the era of clinical outcome studies and managed care has been a source of some controversy,

Table 3 Protocol for Management of Perforated Appendicitis

1. Fluid resuscitation; control fever and administration of intravenous antibiotics (ampicillin 100 mg/kg/24 h, gentamicin 5 mg/kg/24 h, and clindamycin 30 mg/kg/24 h on admission, or piperacillin/tazobactam 240 mg/kg/24 h of piperacillin component, up to 18 g/24 h).
2. Explore peritoneal cavity via right lower quadrant incision.
3. Perform appendectomy in all cases.
4. Perform limited peritoneal debridement.
5. Irrigate peritoneal cavity with cephalothin solution (4 g/L).
6. Place Penrose drains in pelvis and right pericolic space, which exit through the lateral margin of the wound.
7. Close the muscle layers, scarpa fascia, and skin around the drains with absorbable sutures.
8. Encourage postoperative activity and position at will.
9. Continue parenteral antibiotics for 9, adjusting gentamicin dosage based on serum levels.
10. Remove drains slowly from the seventh to the ninth postoperative days. If the patient has been discharged for home antibiotics, he is usually seen sometime during this period in the clinic.
11. Discharge patient generally on the tenth postoperative day.

and there are probably many treatment algorithms that will successfully treat these patients. For example, the management algorithm used at Boston's Children's Hospital since 1976 is outlined in Table 3.[22] This protocol has been consistently associated with an extremely low rate of postappendicitis complications.[23] This protocol has benn modified by substituting piperacillin and tazobactam (Zosyn, Lederle Laboratories, Carolina, Puerto Rico) instead of ampicillin, gentamicin, and clindamycin. This allows simplified drug dosing and avoids the potential complications associated with gentamicin. If these children are doing clinically well, they can frequently be discharged home to finish their day intravenous antibiotic course. A prospective study of this clinical pathway again revealed an extremely low complication rate for the treatment of perforated appendicitis.[24] Duration of antibiotic therapy is an area of considerable debate among surgeons, but whatever the regimen used to treat perforated appendicitis, it should result in complication rates as low as possible, preferably no more than 5%.

The use of laparoscopy in patients with complicated appendicitis is also an area of considerable controversy among pediatric surgeons. Retrospective studies have shown a significantly higher incidence of postoperative intraabdominal abscesses in children with perforated appendicitis who were treated laparoscopically when compared with children treated by the open technique.[25,26] Other surgeons, however, argue that they see no difference between the two techniques. Virtually all these studies, however, are small, retrospective, single center or single surgeon reports. Clearly, a rigorous, large

multicenter randomized trial of open versus laparoscopic appendectomy for perforation is needed to answer this question.

COMPLICATIONS

Infections

The incidence of infectious complications in appendicitis varies with the severity of the infection at the time of surgery. Usually, the wound infection rate with simple appendicitis is quite low. In fact, the wound infection rate associated with removal of a noninflamed appendix is often higher than with simple appendicitis. The incidence of wound infections with primary closure of the wound without drains in perforated appendicitis has been reported to be quite significant, over 10%.[27] In our experience with open appendectomy in perforated appendicitis, however, with use of a drain brought through the wound, this rate can be lowered to about 1%. Primary wound closure with an absorbable suture is very much preferred by children because they strongly dislike dressing changes, suture removal, or delayed wound closures. Removal of a small Penrose drain, on the other hand, is well tolerated.

Similarly, the incidence of abdominal and pelvic abscesses after perforated appendicitis is real—1.3% in our series[28]—and is one of the most frequent and significant complications seen. Many abdominal or pelvic abscesses subside spontaneously under antibiotic therapy and probably represent a phlegmon or cellulitis with agglutinated loops of bowel rather than a true abscess. The progress of these masses can be followed by repeat rectal examinations or CT scans. If the collection does not resolve or the child remains toxic, it is necessary to drain such an abscess. With use of US and CT, it is frequently possible to drain it percutaneously, leaving a small drain in the cavity. This can usually be done with sedation and local anesthesia.

A very small number of patients who have had very severe perforated appendicitis may develop persistent feculent drainage through their wound—a fecal fistula. Virtually all will resolve with bowel rest, antibiotics, and total parenteral nutrition. One must be sure, however, that there is no cause of obstruction distal to the fistula that is preventing its closure.

Constipation

One of the most frequent reasons why a child presents for medical care soon after discharge from an appendectomy is constipation. This will be manifested by vague abdominal pain without marked tenderness or fever. This is usually due to a combination of mild dehydration as well as narcotic use. The child must be carefully evaluated for signs of early bowel obstruction or paralytic ileus secondary to infection, but most often a plain X-ray of the abdomen will reveal a large amount of stool in the colon, particularly on the right side, without other signs of obstruction. This can usually be managed with a pediatric Fleet(r) enema and vigorous oral rehydration.

Intestinal Obstruction

Paralytic ileus and fever may persist for 3 to 5 days following removal of a perforated appendix. Occasionally, this ileus is followed by a few days of normal intestinal function and then by mechanical obstruction with cramping pain. Most of these cases can be managed by nasogastric tube decompression until the inflammatory adhesions subside. Repeat laparotomy at this time is meddlesome and even dangerous unless there is evidence of strangulation or closed loop obstruction. In contrast, obstructions that occur more than 4 weeks postoperatively usually require prompt operation. This complication arises in 1 to 2% of patients with perforated appendicitis. Surgeons who are not experienced with children may be uncertain about the appropriate timing for reexploration. We saw a child who had a reexploration for intestinal obstruction 5 days after removal of a perforated appendix. No distinct point of obstruction was found at that time, but many inflammatory adhesions were present. After a number of postsurgical wound complications, the intestine began to function, but 1 month later, there was a new episode of intestinal obstruction. This was treated by a nasogastric tube, but after a few days, the child's condition deteriorated, and at operation, a loop of gangrenous bowel was found tethered by a single strong adhesive band. The initial reoperation was too early and the second too late.

Sterility

Pelvic abscess or pelvic inflammation associated with perforated appendicitis has been thought to be associated with an increased rate of infertility in female patients,[29] but the literature on this point remains quite controversial.[30] A more recent historical cohort study from Sweden found no difference in the fertility rate of women who had perforated appendicitis as young girls when compared with normal controls.[31]

Antibiotic-Associated Colitis

A few patients may develop crampy diarrhea and fever after treatment for appendicitis. A stool smear should be sent to look for leukocytes and the stool checked for Clostridium difficile. If the titer is positive, these patients will respond to orally administered vancomycin or metronidazole.

SUMMARY

Appendicitis is most noteworthy for the difficulty it presents in diagnosis. Despite tremendous progress in medical diagnostic imaging and laboratory testing, the incidence of perforation and missed diagnosis has not changed significantly over the years. Success in diagnosing appendicitis still requires a thorough history and physical examination and a complete understanding of the tempo of the disease, as well as the anatomy and pathophysiology of the pain. Finally, the practitioner must be willing to follow the patient closely over time, with frequent, even hourly, reexamination to observe the progress of the symptoms. The clinician must also recognize the difficulties inherent in diagnosing unusual cases of appendicitis, such as in very young children or in those cases in which the appendix is in a retrocecal location. In the end, successful management of this disease can lead to the ultimate satisfaction in medicine, that is, timely and complete cure of a child with a potentially life-threatening illness.

REFERENCES

1. Addis DV, Shaffer N, Fowler BS, Tauxe RV. The epidemiolgy of appendicitis and appendectomy in the United States. Am J Epidemiol 1990;132:910–25.
2. Skandalakis JE, Gray SW, editors. Embryology for Surgeons, 2nd edition. Baltimore: Williams and Wilkins; 1994. p. 2445.
3. Poole GV. Anatomic basis for delayed diagnosis of appendicitis. South Med J 1990;83:771–3.
4. Pearl RH, Hale DA, Malloy M, et al. Pediatric appendectomy. J Pediatr Surg 1995;30:178–81.
5. Albu E, Miller BM, Choi Y, et al. Diagnostic value of C-reactive protein in acute appendicitis. Dis Colon Rectum 1994;37:49–51.
6. Gronroos JM, Gronroos P. Leucocyte count and C-reactive protein in the diagnosis of acute appendicts. Br J Surg 1999;86:501–4.
7. Alvarado A. A practical score for the early diagnosis of appendicitis. Ann Emerg Med 1986;15:557–64.
8. Samuel M. Pediatric appendicitis score. J Pediatr Surg 2002;37:877–81.
9. Zona JG, Selke AC, Bellin RP. Radiologic aids in the diagnosis of appendicitis in children. South Med J 1975;68:1373–6.
10. Rao PM, Rhea JT, Rao JA, Conn AK. Plain abdominal radiography in clinically suspected appendicitis: Diagnostic yield, resource use, and comparison with CT. Am J Emerg Med 1999;17:325–8.
11. Teele RL, Share JC. Ultrasonography of Infants and Children. Philadelphia: WB Saunders; 1991. p. 346–56.
12. Carrico CW, Fenton LZ, Taylor GA, et al. Impact of sonography on the diagnosis and treatment of acute lower abdominal pain in children and young adults. Am J Radiol 1999;172:513–6.
13. Roosevelt GE, Reynolds SL. Does the use of ultrasonography improve the outcome of children with appendicitis? Acad Emerg Med 1998;5:1071–5.
14. Garcia-Pena BM, Mandl KD, Kraus SJ, et al. Ultrasonography and limited computed tomography in the diagnosis and management of appendicitis in children. JAMA 1999; 282:1041–6.
15. Brenner D, Elliston C, Hall E, et al. Estimated risks of radiation-induced fatal cancer from pediatric CT. Am J Roentgenol 2001;176:289–96.
16. Kharbanda AB, Taylor GA, Fishman SJ, et al. A clinical decision rule to identify children at low risk for appendicitis. Pediatrics 2005;116:709–16.
17. Rappaport WD, Peterson M, Stanton C. Factors responsible for the high perforation rate seen in early childhood appendicitis. Am Surgeon 1989;55:602–5.
18. Folkman MJ. Appendicitis. In: Ravitch MM, Welch KJ, Benson CD, et al, editors. Pediatric Surgery, 3rd edition. Chicago: Year Book Medical Publishers; 1979. p. 1004–9.
19. Shamberger RC, Weinstein HJ, Delorey MJ, Levey RH. The medical and surgical management of typhlitis in children with nonlymphocytic (myelogenous) leukemia. Cancer 1986;57:603–9.
20. Mazziotti MV, Marley EF, Winthrop AL, et al. Histopathologic analysis of interval appendectomy specimens: Support for the role of interval appendectomy. J Pediatr Surg 1997;32:806–9.
21. Greenberg JJ, Esposito TJ. Appendicitis after laparoscopic appendectomy: A warning. J Laparoendosc Surg 1996;6:185–7.
22. Bilik R, Bernwit C, Shandline B. Is abdominal cavity culture of any value in appendicitis? Am J Surg 1998;175:267–70.
23. Schwartz MZ, Tapper D, Solenberger RI. Management of perforated appendicitis in children. The controversy continues. Ann Surg 1983;197:407–11.
24. Fishman SJ, Pelosi L, Klavon S, O'Rourke E. Perforated appendicitis: Prospective analysis in 150 children. J Pediatr Surg 2000;35:923–6.
25. Horwitz JR, Custer MD, May BH, et al. Should laparoscopic appendectomy be avoided for complicated appendicitis in children? J Pediatr Surg 1997;32:1601–3.
26. Krisher SL, Browne A, Dibbins A, et al. Intra-abdominal abscess after laparoscopic appendectomy for perforated appendicitis. Arch Surg 2001;136:438–41.
27. Burnweit C, Bilik R, Shandling B. Primary closure of contaminated wounds in perforated appendicitis. J Pediatr Surg 1991;26:1362–5.
28. Lund DP, Murphy EA. Management of perforated appendicitis in children: A decade of aggressive treatment. J Pediatr Surg 1994;29:1130–4.
29. Mueller BA, Daling JR, Moore DE, et al. Appendectomy and the risk of tubal infertility. N Engl J Med 1986;315:1506–8.
30. Puri P, McGuinness EP, Guiney EJ. Fertility following perforated appendicitis in girls. J Pediatr Surg 1989;24:547–9.
31. Andersson R, Lambe M, Bergstrom R. Fertility patterns after appendicectomy: Historical cohort study. BMJ 1999; 318:963–7.

17.3. Pediatric Ostomy

Catherine Cord-Udy, MBBS, FRACS (Paed Surg)
Erica Thomas, RGN, RSCN, DPNS, BSc (Hons)
Sarah Hotchkin, RN
Tariq Burki, MBBS, FCPS, FRCS

A stoma can be a beneficial and life-changing surgical intervention for many chronic and acute gastrointestinal disease processes. It is a safe and effective way of diverting the fecal stream and allowing the bowel to heal while continuing enteral feeding. Indications vary depending on the age of the child, but a poorly created, poorly sited stoma can cause severe difficulties for both children and their family.

The concept of bowel decompression is as old as the fourth century BC. The first recorded formation of a colostomy on an infant was by the French surgeon Duret, in 1798,[1] when he successfully carried out the procedure on a 3-day-old infant with an imperforate anus. Although the basic principles and surgical technique have changed little over time, probably the single most significant development in pediatric stoma care has been the shift in emphasis from the earliest attempts of surgical intervention to cure or control the disease to the acknowledgment of the importance of the patient's quality of life after surgery. The identified need for education and support of the child and family before and after surgery has led to the creation of multidisciplinary teams of pediatric surgeons, pediatric stoma care nurses, dietitians, and gastroenterologists, all of whom play an important part in the rehabilitation of the child and family back into the community.

The aim of this chapter is to give an overview of the indications for stoma formation, describe the common types of stomas, and provide surgical tips for creating a good stoma and discuss the effect of diet and drugs on stomas. Practical advice will be included on coping with stomal complications and an understanding of the effect that a stoma has on both the child and the family, in particular the adolescent, who faces disturbance of body image and difficulty with emerging sexuality.

NUMBER OF PATIENTS

It is estimated that as many as 80,000 people in the United Kingdom have a stoma,[2] with only a small percentage of these being pediatric patients. Anecdotal evidence suggests that each regional center within the United Kingdom will see 40 to 100 new cases each year across the pediatric age range. The majority of stomas (76%) are formed in the first 6 weeks of life, 5% from 3 months to 1 year of age, 8% from 2 to 7 years of age, and the remaining 11% from the age of 8 to 16 years.[3]

TYPES OF STOMAS

The term stoma derives from the Greek meaning "mouth" or "opening" and is described as "an artificial opening established surgically between an organ and the exterior."[4] Stomas are described by the bowel used to create the opening and the way they are formed. Both the afferent and efferent ends of a loop of bowel may be exteriorized as a loop or a divided double barrel stoma, or the proximal bowel may be brought out as an end stoma with the distal limb oversewn and dropped back inside the abdominal cavity.

Jejunostomy

The highest-output stoma is a jejunostomy, in which the stoma is sited in the jejunum. The high fluid and electrolyte loss often prevent the establishment of enteral feeding. Trophic feeding at low volumes however may help in alleviating the cholestatic effects of parenteral nutrition.

Ileostomy

An ileostomy is a stoma formed in the ileum and can be either divided (ie, two ends spatially separated) or formed as a loop. It is our view that the bowel is not completely defunctioned by a loop because spillover of feces can occur, but it allows a release of pressure, equivalent to a blowhole.

Colostomy

A colostomy is the formation of a stoma into the colon, and it is commonly sited in either the transverse or the sigmoid colon and again can be either divided or formed as a loop. The more distal the stoma, the less of a problem occurs with sodium and fluid imbalance because of the retained length of functioning bowel.

Antegrade Colonic Enema

The antegrade colonic enema was first developed by Malone. One end of the appendix is reimplanted in a nonrefluxing manner into the cecum and the other end is brought out onto the abdominal wall as a continence stoma.[5] Surgical variations have been developed on this technique, but the basic function is to form an access port into the cecum. An alternative is the cecostomy button.[6] The procedure may be considered in children with anorectal anomalies, Hirschsprung disease, or spina bifida, or in those children with chronic idiopathic constipation as an alternative to a permanent stoma or rectal washouts. Percutaneous endoscopically placed gastrostomies (pegs) in the left colon have also been successfully used for antegrade washouts.[7]

INDICATIONS FOR STOMA FORMATION

The Neonate

An acute stoma may be necessary in the following neonatal conditions: necrotizing enterocolitis, anorectal anomalies, Hirschsprung disease, complicated meconium ileus or failure to decompress the bowel after administration of Gastrografin, some intestinal atresias, and milk curd obstruction. Acute, short-term stomas may be situated within the wound to avoid a further site or additional abdominal scars, usually without causing any significant wound-healing problem. Often the small size of the abdomen in preterm babies makes siting near the umbilicus unavoidable. The stoma is still workable and avoids a second wound. Whatever the type of stoma, there needs to be an appreciation of the fragility of the blood supply to the mesentery of the neonatal bowel, with meticulous dissection and as limited as possible devascularization of the ends of the bowel. Historically, this was why many surgeons prefer loop stomas.[8]

A neonate with gut dysmotility associated with, for example, gastroschisis or malrotation may need an end ileostomy to allow enteral nutrition to be established while the small bowel recovers function, without having to work against an ileocecal valve and unused colon. This may be required for several years and therefore should be properly sited by the stoma care nurse if possible.

The Older Child

An acute stoma in the older child may be necessary in the following conditions: trauma sustained either rectally or abdominally; some intra-abdominal catastrophes such as intussusception or volvulus associated with malrotation, in which viability of the bowel is doubtful; ulcerative colitis with toxic megacolon or intractable bleeding; perianal sepsis in the immunocompromised oncology child or those with severe neutropenic enterocolitis associated with therapy; acute abdominal abscess; or perforation in Crohn's disease.

A semiurgent stoma may be considered in the following conditions: chronic constipation, pseudo-obstruction, children with Hirschsprung disease in whom the bowel has not decompressed, and children born with anorectal anomalies who continue to have problems with constant soiling. Severe refractory ulcerative colitis will require a subtotal colectomy and formation of an end ileostomy, as may familial adenomatous polyposis[9] because of the risk of malignancy.

PREOPERATIVE CARE

Stoma Siting

It is important that, whenever practicable, patients have access to a stoma care nurse specialist for information, advice, and siting preoperatively. This is not always achievable because many stomas in children are formed as an emergency; therefore, there is little time for discussion and siting in relation to the position of the stoma, but the following principles of stoma siting should be adhered to whenever possible (Table 1).

Careful siting should involve the cooperation and consent of the patient (depending on the child's age). It is important to remember that the shape of the abdomen alters when the patient is lying, sitting, or standing and in thin or obese children. Each stoma site therefore needs to be tailored to the individual's needs, and, when possible, patients should be given the chance to familiarize themselves with the stoma bag by applying it to the site, so as to predict any potential problems with positioning. As Black noted, "There is nothing that can compensate for a badly sited stoma, achieving the correct site will have an enormous influence on the individual's postoperative rehabilitation, ability to manage his/her own care and ultimately their quality of life."[10]

Bowel Preparation

For the emergency stoma, there is no time to adequately prepare the bowel. For those children undergoing elective surgery, 24 to 48 hours of clear fluids and oral laxatives are often adequate; however, rectal washouts may be required to empty the bowel, but these should not be attempted on those at risk of perforation (eg, the immunocompromised child or the child with diffuse inflammatory bowel disease). The operative procedure is usually covered by 48 hours of intravenous broad-spectrum antibiotics.

Psychological Preparation

The majority of congenital abnormalities requiring stoma formation are not apparent until after birth, therefore allowing parents no time to prepare for the consequences of giving birth to a baby with a disability.[11] It is often difficult for parents to understand the medical terminology being presented to them. Every family will have its own means of understanding the information provided, and, wherever possible, time should be allowed for questioning, preparation, and acceptance of the need for surgery. Sometimes this is realistically impossible when faced with a sick neonate or an adolescent trauma victim.

Even in these emergency situations, parents are entitled to feel that they have adequate information about the procedure to make an informed choice about their child's care. Parenthood can be traumatic and stressful at the best of times, and the support received from staff in the initial stages can make all the difference[12] as to their acceptance of the stoma after surgery.

When stoma surgery is planned, the method of preparation used should be related to the time available and the age of the child. A number of books and dolls are available through various organizations (see contact addresses) that can allow even a young child to come to some understanding of what is about to happen. Experienced play therapists and pediatric nurses can use playacting and painting to help the child become involved in the decision-making process.[13]

Postoperatively, the older child who has suffered the consequences of inflammatory bowel disease, with pain, repeated hospitalization, polypharmacy, and exclusion from their peers, may see surgery as a relief and an opportunity to start living again. The desire for a cure often clouds many teenagers' judgment as to their true feelings about their altered body image, which tends to emerge months after surgery, when the true picture of their new life becomes apparent.

Access to the Internet can provide teenagers with information that they may feel too embarrassed to ask for (Table 2), and many self-help organizations have sites for the young adult ostomist. Approximately 20% of patients with a stoma experience clinically significant psychological symptoms postoperatively; commonly, these are anxiety and adjustment disorders.[14]

CULTURAL ISSUES

When caring for the child and family, it is important to take into account their religious, cultural, and individual needs. There may be a number of questions, such as "Is there any animal content in the makeup of the appliance being used?" According to Muslim culture, the left hand is used for cleansing and the right hand is used for eating, meeting, and greeting. This therefore requires special allowance when teaching stoma care if the left hand is the nondominant hand. The prolonged fasting during Ramadan can result in increased levels of dehydration and constipation. Children with a stoma can often be exempt from their religious duties at this time or at least be allowed some flexibility. Discussion with their religious leader can help in assistance and guidance.

COMPLICATIONS OF STOMA SURGERY: PRACTICAL ADVICE

Many of the complications listed below can be avoided by careful consideration of the site of the stoma and care being taken by the surgeon when surgically creating the stoma spout itself and its positioning in relation to the abdominal wound. Different complications can be seen at different time scales following surgery.

Avascular Necrosis

Stomas initially are often dusky and bruised in appearance, but many recover without any problems. Technical attention must be paid to preserve a good blood supply to the active stoma by not strangulating it either with a misplaced suture, closing the abdomen too tightly, or by placing the mesentery under tension. The mucus fistula can

Table 1 Areas to Avoid in Stoma Siting

Waistline
Hip bones
Previous scars
Groin area
Fat folds and bulges
Umbilicus
Under pendulous breasts
Areas of skin irritation (psoriasis, eczema, skin allergies)
Positioning of artificial limbs
Areas in which there would be difficulties if weight gain or loss occurred

Table 2 Web Organizations

Organization	Web Site
United Ostomy Association	www.uoa.org
International Ostomy Association	www.ostomyinternational.org
Wound, Ostomy and Continence Nurses Association	www.wocn.org
The Mark Allen Group Organisation (specialist stoma care nursing)	www.internurse.com/stomacare.cfm
Living with a Colostomy	www.ostomy.fsnet.co.uk
The Continence Foundation	www.continence-foundation.org.uk
The Simon Foundation for Continence	www.simonfoundation.org-html

be placed in slightly less healthy bowel, understanding that it may fibrose down, but it will preserve bowel length that would otherwise have been sacrificed in closure.

Stomas in neonates are usually covered only with a small piece of Jelonet (Smith and Nephew Healthcare Ltd, Hull, UK) and gauze to allow clear observation until the stoma becomes active. The first appliance in all age groups should always be clear-fronted and drainable with no flatus filter; this allows clear visual access and the ability to record the volume of stool passed and monitor any wind produced.

Care should be taken to protect the stoma in neonates when undergoing phototherapy because "sunburn" of the mucosa (black appearance) can result, and incubators can often dry out the stoma. Covering the stoma with Jelonet and gauze can prevent this.

Dehiscence

Complete dehiscence is when the stoma wound breaks open and a further portion of the bowel can extrude from the wound. This is unusual and requires surgical revision, and it is more likely to occur if the two stoma ends are crowded into too small a wound so that skin bridges between them fail to heal. Wound dehiscence is more likely if there is heavy soiling with fecal matter and a malnourished child or premature baby. A superficial dehiscence is more common and usually responds to topical packing, without revision being required.

Bleeding

Bleeding can be peristomal, from erosions or ulcers (usually secondary to bag placement and local trauma). Parents should be warned to expect some bleeding when the stoma is wiped clean because of surface trauma or if the infant is crying when the appliance is being changed because tension on the sutures occurs owing to the increase in intra-abdominal pressure.

Bleeding may be a symptom of the intrinsic pathology of the sick child, but it is important to beware of parastomal varices that can accompany total parenteral nutrition-induced liver failure and portal hypertension. These can bleed exsanguinating amounts of blood rapidly. Local pressure and resuscitation with comprehensive blood products can be lifesaving. Bleeding from a high jejunostomy may be gastric in origin.

Stenosis

Ischemia to the bowel end is one of the most common causes of stenosis. Closing the abdominal wall too tightly around the stoma can cause an ischemic effect and can also tighten the abdominal exit site, causing stenosis.

A narrowing of the outlet of the stoma through the abdominal wall can cause an obstruction, often with output fluctuating from little to excessive. Translocation of bacteria can occur at the site, and the patient can become toxic and unwell, often with subsequent line sepsis. If this is suspected, the stoma should be digitally probed to check its patency and may require dilation (not in the neonate), although surgical revision is usually required.

A loopogram radiologic study can show dilatation, but it is a good precaution to cover the procedure with intravenous antibiotics to avoid translocation of bacteria and septicemia.

Necrosis following an infection around the stoma can result in narrowing at the entrance, causing acute abdominal pain and no activity or difficulty in passing stool. Colostomy patients should be advised to keep the stool soft by consuming additional fluids (especially in warm weather) and avoid a high-fiber or bulky diet.

End stomas in infants and children should have a disc of fat and skin removed appropriate to the size of the bowel to avoid crowding and stenosis.

Prolapse

Prolapse of the bowel can be quite dramatic (Figure 1). This is more common with loop enterostomies, especially in the distal limb, but can occur with end stomas, especially those in a very dilated bowel as it returns to normal size. Fixing the bowel to the muscle fascia in four quadrants goes some way to preventing prolapse.

Small prolapses can be ignored if easily reduced, but an irreducible stoma needs attention to avoid bowel compromise: application of fine sugar granules followed by manual reduction or warm saline gauze and slow pressure usually achieves a result. The sugar causes a fluid shift across the bowel wall via an osmotic gradient, causing the stoma to shrink.[15]

Failure to reduce the stoma requires urgent surgical intervention and, occasionally, revision. A chronic prolapse can be encircled with a nonabsorbable suture, as in a Thiersch suture for rectal prolapse. Refashioning of the stoma is sometimes the only option, and, if required, a new site is preferable. Adolescents who have difficulty with accepting their body image because of the prolapsed stoma may request revision. If surgical revision is contemplated then thought should be given as to whether the stoma is still required and if it can be closed.

When the stoma has prolapsed, it may be difficult to apply the original size appliance; therefore, increasing the size of the aperture can sometimes prevent the stoma from suffering trauma to its edges. Many children tolerate stoma prolapse and can avoid extra surgery if it is often a cosmetic issue only and for the short term.

Retraction

Retraction of the stoma can be due to inadequate length of bowel pulled under tension, subsequent adhesions, or the disease process recurring, such as Crohn strictures. The stoma can become indrawn and flush with the skin, causing excoriation and problems with leakage. Although retraction can sometimes resolve spontaneously,

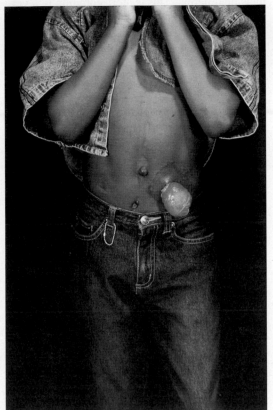

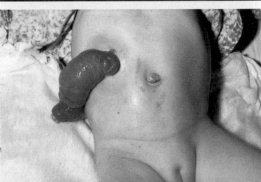

Figure 1 End sigmoid colostomy prolapse in two children.

revision may be required to make management of the stoma easier, and adequate spouting initially can make this less of a problem, even for colostomies.

Another cause can be from the child gaining a lot of weight after surgery, causing the stoma to become level with the abdominal wall; therefore, the feces has difficulty draining away from the appliance, causing pooling of stool (pancaking) under the appliance. In older children, a convex appliance can assist in pushing the stoma out and thus creating a moat effect to promote better drainage (pastes may help make the appliance stickier).

Incisional or Parastomal Hernia

This is not a big problem in young people because of the natural strength of the abdominal wall, but it may become a problem in those who have undergone repeated abdominal surgery or in those who are overweight.

The weakness in the closure of the abdominal wall adjacent to the stoma can result in an incisional hernia. This is more common in a very dilated bowel that returns to size, but it is also more frequently seen in children with Down syndrome who have required stoma formation owing to poor collagen and therefore poor healing.

If troublesome, revision may be required; otherwise, it can be ignored, although bag application can be difficult.

Intestinal Fistula

A leak of intestinal contents from a fistula adjacent to the stoma can result from an anchoring suture placed too deeply or from the disease process recurring in Crohn disease. Intra-abdominal fistulae need to be revised urgently, but a small external fistula can be of little consequence.

Mucocutaneous Separation

This results when the stoma edge comes away from the surrounding skin, leaving a shallow cavity around the stoma. It is a particular problem in neonates owing to insufficient bowel mobilization at the time of surgery, causing undue tension on the stoma sutures, which anchor it to the skin. Sore skin around the stoma can result from leakage of stool under the flange; the developing trough can be filled with hydrocolloid gel or paste to promote granulation tissue, and the appliance aperture can be cut to incorporate this.

Dehydration and Electrolyte Imbalance

Every effort should be made to site the stoma as far as practicable down the bowel, and in the immediate postoperative period, close attention to fluid balance must be maintained to avoid electrolyte imbalance. Once on a full enteral diet, the urine should be monitored to ensure that adequate total body sodium levels are maintained. Supportive parenteral nutrition or fluids may be required for some time in children with acute high-intestinal stomas. Enteral nutrition in children with jejunostomies should be given as a low continuous volume to keep the enterohepatic circulation going and decrease cholestasis; it also maintains nutrition to the enterocytes but avoids excessive fluid problems by limiting the input. Oral sodium supplements are needed almost always in children with ileostomies and even with some colostomies. The infant's or child's growth can be severely impaired by low total-body sodium.

Diversional Colitis

This can occur in the defunctioned bowel owing to stagnation of the contents and a lack of topical nutrition to the enterocytes, with the child experiencing painful discharge and bleeding. Short-chain fatty acids can be instilled into the defunctioning limb with a good result; this is usually given daily for 1 week, with the amount dependent on the length of bowel involved, and then repeated as necessary until under control.[16]

The passage of mucus from the rectum is not uncommon, with older children reporting the urge to defecate. For the occasional rectal discharge, a plain saline washout through the defunctioning stoma or rectum may alleviate the problem, although too frequent washouts can have the undesirable effect of increasing mucus production. Bleeding from the rectum may be an indication of recurrence or continuation of active inflammatory bowel disease.

Skin Problems

An atlas has been developed about abdominal stomas and their skin disorders.[17] Soreness can result from an allergic reaction or sensitivity to the adhesive part of the appliance (contact dermatitis), with the outline of the appliance clearly visible following removal. Changing the appliance used can usually resolve the problem; otherwise, barrier films or hydrocolloid dressing used under the appliance can reduce contact and therefore the likelihood of a reaction. Topical steroids should be used with extreme caution because they can result in the peristomal skin becoming very fragile. Fungal infections often respond to topical nystatin or cotrimoxazole, or a single dose of fluconazole may be required orally if severe.

Effluent dermatitis, inflammation, or excoriation caused by leakage of stool directly onto the peristomal skin is more common in ileostomy patients owing to the liquid consistency damaging the skin on contact. Gut enzymes, particularly protease and amylase found in ileostomy output, can cause fecal irritation by damaging the horny layer of the skin.[17] The cause can be simply that the shape of the stoma has changed, thus allowing fecal fluid to leak under the flange. If this occurs, barrier films can be used to protect the skin.

Poor technique in the fitting of the appliance or the changing shape of the abdomen as children grow may result in the development of troughs and ridges, which prevent the appliance from lying flat against the skin. Pastes or seals can be used to fill uneven areas, allowing the appliance a flat, even surface to which to adhere.

Wet skin under an appliance can be dried using calamine lotion, also giving a soothing effect when the area is itchy. Preexisting skin conditions such as eczema can cause reactions and itchiness from some appliances, and often trial and error is the only way to achieve a solution. The adhesive quality of the appliance can be increasedby warming the appliance either in clasped hands, leaving it on a radiator for a short period of time, or by the use of a hairdryer before sticking it to the skin.

Overfull bags can increase the likelihood of leakage because the weight of the stool pulls the flange away from the skin. Patient education should include the importance of emptying the skin before it becomes no more than two-thirds full.

Granulation tissue may be "normal" and can be controlled with topical oxytetracycline and hydrocortisone (Terra-Cortril), silver nitrate application (with caution), or the regular use of dexamethasone and framycetin ointment.

EFFECTS OF DRUGS ON STOMA OUTPUT

Drugs work in three main ways. Direct action on the gut, action via neurotransmitters, or indirect action via the other organ systems. Morphine codeine, dihydrocodeine diphenoxylate are constipating while magnesium-based antacids promote looseness as do antibiotics that can cause looseness by altering bowel flora or a by direct prokinetic effect. Cholinergic drugs increase peristaltic activity and secretory activity. Anticholinergics have a reverse effect and anticholinergic activity is part of tricyclic antidepressants and most antiemetics. Loperamide is a useful slowing agent in high-output stomas. Diuretics may cause constipation due to dehydration.[18]

CHOOSING THE RIGHT STOMA APPLIANCE

In the past decade, the choice of stoma appliances for the infant or child has increased dramatically. The following issues should be considered when offering advice to the new ostomist (Table 3):

- Stoma appliances are made either as a one-piece system, incorporating both the flange and bag (either drainable or closed), or a two-piece system with a separate flange and bag that connect together.
- One-piece drainable appliances are particularly suitable for infants and younger children who do not have a high level of output. As children grow and their diet becomes more varied, the volume of effluent increases, and with increasing levels of activity, the support and flexibility of a two-piece system may be more suitable, allowing the bag to be changed without the need of the flange to be removed.
- Bags can be drainable for high-output stomas, or if the child has difficulty in emptying the bag, a nondrainable system may be more appropriate. The size or capacity of bags can be varied depending on the activities undertaken (a larger bag may be useful overnight to decrease the need for emptying).

Table 3 Factors Influencing Choice of Stoma Appliance

Age and size of the infant/child
Type of stoma: colostomy/ileostomy
Site/position of stoma
Physical/social activities
Dexterity of the child

- To combat the effects of flatulence, "flatus filters" are available in many drainable and nondrainable appliances. These do become ineffective when wet; therefore, the outlet should be covered when bathing or swimming.
- Convexity appliances have integral convexity and help create a seal for use with retracted stomas. This system is not recommended in young children because of the risk of pressure ulcer formation, and if used long term in young children, there is also some concern about interruption of muscle growth.
- A wide range of appliances and accessories is available that will cover the individual requirements of most patients. Before finalizing any appliance orders, the opportunity to try different products should be offered because the consumer should have ultimate choice on the system used.

DISCHARGE PLANNING

As the child recovers from surgery, plans should be made for the child to return home. Teaching should involve basic stoma care, knowledge of the practical skills required to change an appliance, possible complications, and whom to reach for advice (Table 4).

Regular contact should be maintained until the family has the necessary confidence to be totally independent at home. It should be clear to the family how and where additional supplies can be obtained from community services. Ideally, home visits after discharge offer the family an opportunity to discuss issues that they may have felt unable to question while in the hospital environment. It also provides an opportunity to review bathroom facilities, which may need simple adaptation, and general storage advice for the new equipment.

EDUCATIONAL SUPPORT

Under the guidelines of The United Kingdom Education Act (1981), all children are entitled to education, and it is the duty of their local educational authority to facilitate the necessary support. The reality is that parents are often "on call" to troubleshoot any problems that occur while the child is at school. The pediatric stoma nurse can offer the child, and teachers support in terms of reintegration into the school environment and can educate teaching assistants and carers.

Most head teachers are only too willing to provide access to private toilets away from the main children's facilities, allowing the child to empty or change the appliance in private. The adolescent may have serious problems returning to school with a stoma, and avoidance behavior is common. Postoperative psychological support is often necessary to overcome this awkward period.

NUTRITIONAL CONSIDERATIONS

Concerns about eating and the associated reaction of the stoma are common among new ostomists. Initially, they are constantly aware when the stoma acts and, as a result, are cautious about eating certain foods. Flatus is produced more readily when eating pulses, baked beans, fizzy drinks, and, in some, chocolate. Eating slowly and chewing food well can reduce the amount of air swallowed.[19]

Effluent will contain more fluid when eating spicy foods, fruit, and green vegetables. Eggs, boiled rice, sweet corn, bananas, and mushrooms will thicken the stool and, in some children, lead to constipation. Foods that are known to cause problems should not be avoided, but by emptying the appliance more frequently or wearing an appliance to accommodate increased output, mealtimes should be more relaxed. It takes about 16 to 22 hours from food being swallowed to it being seen in a colostomy bag—less time with an ileostomy.

Children should be encouraged to experiment to see how their stoma reacts to different food items so that they can remain in control. A healthful balanced diet should always be encouraged. Useful tips in having a stoma can be gleaned from other patients and their families (Table 5).

TRANSITION OF CARE

The preparation to move from pediatric care to adult-based services can cause great anxiety to many families. For many parents, the security blanket of a pediatric service has enabled them to manage their children's chronic health needs and feel comfortable when attending clinic appointments. The handover of care should be planned and coordinated if possible in a combined adolescent clinic, giving the family the opportunity to meet the new team while maintaining links with the old.

REFERENCES

1. Duret C. Observations et reflexions sur une imperforation de l'anus. Recueil periodique de la Societe de Medecine de Paris; 3, 46. Reprinted in Amussat 1839. p. 88.
2. Coloplast. An Introduction to Stoma Care: A Guide for Healthcare Professionals. Peterborough, UK: Coloplast; 1999.
3. Fitzpatrick G. Stoma care in the community: A clinical resource for practitioners. Nurs Times 1999;33–56.
4. Barrett J, et al. Blackwell's Dictionary of Nursing. New York: Springer; 1994.
5. Malone PS, Ransley PG, Kiely EM. Preliminary report: The ante-grade continence enema. Lancet 1990;17:1217–8.
6. Fukunaga K, Kimura K, Lawrence JP, et al. Button device for antegrade enema in the treatment of incontinence and constipation. J Pediatr Surg 1996;31:1038–9.
7. Rawat DJ, Haddad M, Geogheagan N, et al. Percutaneous endoscopic colostomy of the left colon: A new technique for management of intractable constipation in children. Gastrointest Endosc 2004;60:39–43.
8. Bishop HC. Ileostomy and colostomy. Paediatric surgery. 4th edition.
9. Arvanitis ML, Jagelmann DG, Fazio VW, et al. Mortality in patients with familial adenomatous polyposis. Dis Colon Rectum 1990;33:639–42.
10. Black P. An Introduction to Stoma Care. Folkestone, UK: Clinical Pharmacology Research Institute; 1988.
11. Webster P. Special babies: Community outlook. Nurs Times 1985;81:19–22.
12. Stewart AJ. Mums and dads need care too: Supporting parents of babies in neonatal units. Prof Nurs 1990;5:660–5.
13. Ziegler DB, Prior MM. Preparation for surgery and adjustment to hospitalisation. Pediatr Surg Nurs 1994;29:655–69.
14. White C. Living with a Stoma: A Practical Guide to Coping with Colostomy, Ileostomy and Urostomy. London: Sheldon Press; 1997.
15. Black P. Holistic Stoma Care. London: Bailliere Tindall; 2000.
16. Vernia P, et al. Butyrate Enema Therapy Stimulates Mucosal Repair in Experimental Colitis in the Rat. Bethesda, MD: National Library of Medicine; 1995.
17. Lyon CC, Smith JA. Abdominal Stomas and Their Skin Disorders: An Atlas of Diagnosis and Management. Fredensborg: Dansac; 2001.
18. Burki T, Private dissertation on all aspects of stomas.
19. Collett K. Practical aspects of stoma management. Nurs Standard 2002;17:45–52.

Table 5 Helpful Hints from Our Patients

When gaining confidence in fitting a new bag use a mirror so that you can see what you are doing

Clean the stoma with gauze swabs because cotton wool balls can leave strands, preventing the bag from sticking

Storage of appliances should be in a cool, dry area (steamy bathrooms affect the adhesive)

Always have some bags ready cut for those emergency changes; they will always happen

It is up to you who you tell about your stoma!

To improve the stickiness of the appliance, warm it in clasped hands before applying

To enable you to see what you are doing, use a clothespeg to hold clothing out of the way

If the smell is too offensive, use scented candles in the bathroom when changing the bag

After the recovery phase of surgery, your stoma's activity will become more predictable

Often it is most active after breakfast

Beer can give you wind!

Table 4 Discharge Planning

Discharge teaching should involve
- Normal stoma function
- Preparation, application, and removal of appliance
- Skin care
- Where to obtain supplies
- Disposal of used appliances
- Exemption from prescription charges
- Recognizing complications and whom to contact for advice
- Dealing with potential problems, eg, leakage, sore skin, odor, flatus

18

Benign Perianal Lesions

Monica Langer, MD
Biren P. Modi, MD
Sidney Johnson, MD
Tom Jaksic, MD, PhD

Perianal disease in children is common and encompasses a broad spectrum of pathologic processes, including fissures, fistulae, abscesses, hemorrhoids, rectal prolapse, pilonidal sinus, and pruritus ani. Occasionally, systemic illnesses such as inflammatory bowel disease may coexist. This chapter provides a diagnostic and therapeutic guide to perianal lesions based on an understanding of the underlying anatomy and the specific pathogenesis of each entity.

ANATOMY

The diagnosis and treatment of perianal disease can be confusing if the anatomy of the pelvic floor and sphincter muscle complex is not understood. Thus, as a preface to the discussion of perianal lesions, it is useful to review the anatomy of the rectum and anus (Figure 1).

The rectum is a continuation of the sigmoid colon that starts approximately at the sacral prominence. It can be distinguished from the colon by its lack of taeniae. In their place, it has a complete covering of longitudinal muscle fibers. The luminal pattern of the rectum also differs from the colon because it has two to three lateral curves that form mucosal folds

known as the valves of Houston. The posterior rectum is free of peritoneum, and the most distal third of the rectum is devoid of peritoneum circumferentially.

The rectum terminates in the anal canal, which is composed of that portion of bowel that passes through the levator ani muscles and opens onto the anal verge. The external and internal sphincter muscles form an important continence mechanism in association with the anal canal.

The internal anal sphincter is a continuation of the circular muscle layer of the rectum. As this muscle layer enters the anal canal, it becomes thickened. Both the puborectalis muscle and external sphincter muscle then wrap the anal canal, suspending the rectum, and facilitating contraction of the anus, thereby assisting with anal continence.

On examination with anoscopy, the dentate line can be visualized marking the transition from the columnar epithelium of the rectum to the squamous epithelium of the anal canal. The dentate line is 1 to 2 cm proximal to the external orifice of the anus. The longitudinal folds of mucosa at the dentate line are known as the columns of Morgagni. The internal and external hemorrhoidal plexus of veins accomplish venous drainage of the anus and rectum.

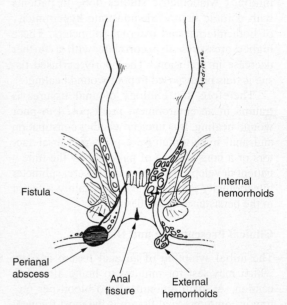

Figure 2 A diagrammatic representation of perianal lesions and their anatomic relationships is depicted in coronal section.

ANAL FISSURE

An anal fissure is a tear in the epithelium and superficial tissues of the anal canal. In children, the tear is usually linear, extending from just below the dentate line to the anal verge (Figure 2). Fissures can be classified as either acute or chronic and can be further subdivided into primary or secondary processes. When first formed, a fissure is a simple crack in the anoderm; however, with infection and poor healing, a chronic fissure can develop with a "sentinel tag" of skin, fibrotic edges, and exposure of the internal sphincter. Primary fissures are not associated with underlying systemic pathology, whereas secondary fissures are the consequence of illnesses such as Crohn's disease. Although fissures occur in all age groups, they are most common in children. The majority of anal fissures are located in the posterior midline (90%), with the next most frequent location being the anterior midline.[1]

Pathogenesis

Most cases of anal fissure are associated with constipation and they are often noted after the passage of a large, hard stool.[2] As a consequence, anal

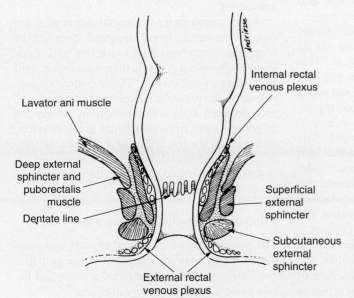

Figure 1 The anatomy of the rectum and anus is illustrated in coronal section.

fissures are thought to be traumatically induced by overstretching of the anoderm. Parents can, at times, describe which bowel movement resulted in the superficial tear of the anoderm because it is a painful event for the child. Pain with the next bowel movement leads to hesitancy and avoidance of bowel movements on the child's part. This fecal retention leads to more hardened stools and a persistent cyclic problem.

In addition to the traumatic insult to the anoderm, the pathogenesis of anal fissures appears to be closely related to two predisposing factors: hypertonicity of the anal sphincter and poor perfusion of the anoderm at the posterior midline.

Angiograms show compromised blood flow through the inferior rectal artery to the posterior midline.[3] Manometric studies done in patients with chronic fissures demonstrate hypertonicity of both internal and external sphincters. These higher pressures also correlate with a further decrease in perfusion.[4] The poorly perfused tissue is thus predisposed to poor wound healing.

Therefore, the etiology of anal fissures is trauma in an environment predisposed to poor wound healing. It is unclear whether constipation and anal hypertonicity are primary causal factors or a consequence of pain, but by the time a patient develops a symptomatic fissure, sphincter hypertonicity is present and is certainly a factor in the persistence of the fissure.

Clinical Presentation and Diagnosis

The initial symptom of an anal fissure is pain, which may last for minutes to hours after defecation. A small amount of red blood per rectum is common. Anal fissure is the most frequent cause of rectal bleeding in the first 2 years of life. The diagnosis can be made after inspection of the anal canal. If a fissure is not visualized on superficial examination, an anoscope can be helpful in identifying the lesion. Acute fissures are usually small, with no signs of chronicity. Chronic fissures are associated with hypertrophy of the anal papilla, fibrosis, or a distal skin tag. A large fissure associated with bruising (as well as other signs of injury) should raise the suspicion of child abuse. Crohn's disease and leukemic infiltration are underlying conditions that require further investigation if a fissure persists after standard treatment.

Treatment

Given the previously described etiologic factors of anal trauma, anal hypertonicity, and poor perianal perfusion, successful therapy should accomplish one or more of the following: a decrease in trauma associated with stooling, a reduction in resting anal tone, and an increase in anal blood flow.[2,5] Initially, treatment is directed at the associated constipation by the use of stool softeners, lubricants (eg, mineral oil), or fiber supplementation. Additionally, warm baths have been shown to reduce anal tone. Results from these measures are good, with a cure in over 80% of acute fissures. In children who continue to have constipation and fissures, intolerance to cow's milk may be the cause. Randomized trials substituting soy milk for a cow's milk diet resulted in improvement in over two-thirds of patients.[6,7] Topical steroid and topical or injected anesthetic have not been shown to improve healing rates.

It is important to maintain good anal hygiene in the care of fissures. Failure to adequately clean the anus after each bowel movement may result in the continued presence of fecal matter within the fissure, consequent inhibition of healing, persistent pain, and anal hypertonicity.

The treatment of chronic fissures presents a more difficult problem. A chronic fissure is defined by symptoms that persist longer than 6 weeks after treatment and the presence of fibrosis at the base of the fissure. Fortunately, this is a relatively rare problem in children. Chronic fissures are unlikely to heal with a high-fiber diet and warm baths alone. Thus, the focus of treatment must be directed at the reduction of resting anal pressure.

Nitric oxide is an agent that will lower resting anal sphincter pressure and increase anal blood flow. A 92% cure rate of chronic anal fissures in adults has been reported with the topical application of 0.2% glyceryl trinitrate ointment three times per day.[5] Randomized trials using the local application of nitric oxide donor compounds in patients with chronic fissures also report good healing rates (70 to 90%) in both adults and children and no long-term complications such as incontinence.[8–10] Recurrence rates were 32%, but 80% of these children responded to a second course of glyceryl trinitrate and no recurrences were identified beyond 1 year of follow-up.[11]

Botulinum toxin injection also reduces resting anal tone and appears to be more effective than glyceryl trinitrate. A 95% healing rate for chronic anal fissures has been reported with botulinum toxin injection.[12] However, it should be noted that in the pediatric population, botulinum toxin injection usually requires sedation or general anesthesia. Although this treatment is promising, botulinum toxin injection for chronic anal fissures has not been well studied in children.

In infants, a standard treatment for chronic fissures is gentle anal dilatation. Parents can be instructed to perform daily anal dilatations. This will help break the cycle of anal spasm and pain and thus assist wound healing. In infants and young children, anal dilatation generally has good results, and complications such as incontinence are rare.

Very infrequently, when treatment fails despite dietary regulation, hygiene, and anal dilatation, it may be necessary to operate under general anesthesia on infants with chronic fissures. This approach allows for a satisfactory examination, possible further anal dilatation, and complete excision of the chronic anal fissure.[13] In older children or young adults who require surgery, the fissure is not removed; rather, lateral internal sphincterotomy is the procedure of choice.[14] Lateral internal sphincterotomy achieves healing within several weeks. Studies comparing open versus closed lateral internal sphincterotomy show that both have excellent rates of healing (95%). Differences may exist, however, in long-term continence, with slightly better results achieved in patients undergoing closed lateral internal sphincterotomy.[15]

Special Considerations

Rarely, patients develop fissures as a consequence of systemic diseases. Fissures that result from group 0 α-hemolytic streptococcus infection have been reported. Patients may also evolve multiple, chronic, and difficult to manage fissures as an early manifestation of Crohn's disease.

PERIRECTAL ABSCESS AND FISTULA IN ANO

A perirectal abscess is a localized, purulent fluid collection in the surrounding perirectal tissues (see Figure 2). Perirectal abscesses are usually classified by their location relative to the levator and sphincteric muscles of the pelvic floor. In order of frequency, abscesses are located in the perianal, ischioanal, intersphincteric, and supralevator locations. Clinical presentation and treatment interventions vary according to site.

A fistula in ano may be the result of the spontaneous drainage of a perirectal abscess, which then forms a chronic inflammatory tract from the dentate line to the skin. The reported percentage of patients progressing from abscess to fistula varies from 20 to 80%.[16,17]

Pathogenesis

Perianal infections are often encountered in infants in diapers. Usually, there is no specific inciting event, but, occasionally, there is an accompanying diaper rash. In these cases, infection may be the result of an inward spread from the skin. Group 0 α-hemolytic streptococcal infection of the perianal tissue is also sometimes associated.

More commonly, perirectal abscesses are thought to result from abnormal columns of Morgagni. The crypts tend to trap bacteria, initiating a subsequent cryptitis that, if persistent, will become a perianal abscess. This hypothesis is supported by the presence of columnar, transitional, and stratified squamous epithelium (entrapped migratory cells from urogenital sinus development) lining the tract of a fistula in ano. In 90% of cases of perirectal abscess, the source of the abscess can be traced to an infection occurring in the crypts of Morgagni.[18]

Clinical Presentation and Diagnosis

The presentation of a perianal abscess and associated fistula may vary greatly in the pediatric population. In infants, perirectal abscess and fistula present more frequently in males.[17]

A child with a perirectal abscess will usually experience persistent rectal pain. Occasionally, diarrheal illness or anal fissure precedes the abscess. More infrequently, cryptoglandular infections are secondary to diabetes mellitus, Crohn's disease, tuberculosis, or acquired immune deficiency syndrome (AIDS).

Perirectal pain is present in 98% of patients who can communicate their discomfort. The onset can be acute and is often without history of prior perirectal pain, inflammation, or trauma. In contrast to the transient pain of an anal fissure, the pain of a perirectal abscess is constant.

The earliest sign of perianal abscess is an indurated, tender area of the perianal skin, with or without erythema, which may occur in any location around the anus. External perianal and digital rectal examinations identify the abscess in 95% of patients.[19] In children and infants who are unable to communicate, the parent will bring the child to the clinic with complaints of crying or irritability that is worse at diaper change. Examination reveals painful perirectal swelling and possibly a fever. If the abscess ruptures and progresses to a fistula, persistent drainage and recurrent abscess formation are often seen.

In children, fistula in ano usually occurs during the first year of life, when it is evident as a single cutaneous external orifice. This fistula communicates directly with the rectum at the level of the crypts of Morgagni (see Figure 2). It often passes through the lowest fibers of the internal sphincter. This type of fistula is thus termed "low" owing to its lack of compromise of the sphincter complex. Unlike a fistula in adults (in whom the internal opening of the fistula is usually posterior or midline in location with a circular tract following Goodsall law), the internal opening of a perianal fistula in children is usually located radially opposite to its external opening.

Treatment

Different treatment options exist depending on the age and presentation of the patient. In infants, neither surgery nor antibiotics may be necessary for the treatment of routine perianal abscesses.[20] The rate of progression of perianal abscesses to fistulae in ano is highly variable.[21] Many centers treat infant perianal abscesses by incision and drainage with topical anesthesia; however, a recent comparison of surgical and local care management strategies, emphasizing hygiene, and sitz baths, showed increased fistula formation in patients treated with surgical intervention (40%) compared to local care (16%).[22] This and other studies suggest that most infants with uncomplicated perianal abscesses can be managed successfully with local care with or without antibiotics.[13,22,23] In healthy infants perianal fistula also appears to follow a self-limited course and nonoperative management is safe and usually effective.[20] In the case of persistent abscesses or refractory fistula-in-ano operative management may still be necessary.

In older children, perirectal abscesses tend to extend into deeper tissues; thus, the primary treatment is surgical drainage, usually under general anesthesia. Antibiotics have no role in the primary treatment of established abscesses (although they may be useful adjuncts in complicated abscesses). In the operating room, under general anesthesia, the abscess can be drained quickly and painlessly, and a full examination is facilitated to identify concurrent abscesses or associated fistulae.

Persistence of an anal fistula beyond 1 to 3 months of conservative management is generally considered an indication for surgery for infants and children. Chronic fistulae, in addition to troubling persistent drainage, are associated with recurrent abscesses. Anal fistulae are best managed with fistulectomy (excision) or fistulotomy (opening and curetting).[24] Rarely, the use of a seton loop is necessary. This loop is placed through the fistula and slowly tightened, thus allowing for division and fibrosis of higher tracts that may encompass both sphincters. The goal of treatment of a fistula is complete eradication of the fistula with preservation of fecal continence.

Special Considerations

Recurrences of perirectal abscesses and fistulae are not uncommon, and treatment may be protracted.[21] Additionally, with recurrent perianal disease, one must always consider associated diseases. Older children with perianal abscess may have other undiagnosed medical problems, including drug-induced or autoimmune neutropenia, leukemia, human immunodeficiency virus (HIV) infection, side effects from the use of immunosuppressive drugs, diabetes mellitus, and Crohn's disease. For example, up to 15% of children with Crohn's disease present with recurrent anal fistulae. In children older than a year of age who present with an anal fistula without a history of perianal abscess, the possibility of sexual abuse should be considered.[25] Additionally, rare diseases, such as rectal duplication, may be mistaken for an anal fistula.[26] In general, with persistent and multiple fistulae, further investigation should be considered.[27]

HEMORRHOIDS

Hemorrhoids are generally classified into two subtypes, external and internal (see Figure 2). A hemorrhoid is a varicose vein from either the internal or external rectal plexus of veins. External hemorrhoids involve the skin of the anoderm external to the dentate line, and their nerve supply is cutaneously derived. Hence, newly thrombosed external hemorrhoids are associated with acute pain.

An internal hemorrhoid is also a swollen blood vessel (specifically a varicosity of the tributaries of the superior rectal vein). Internal hemorrhoids differ from external hemorrhoids in that they are located under the lining of the rectum. Patients who are suspected of having hemorrhoids should undergo a visual and digital examination to determine the type and grade of hemorrhoid. Internal hemorrhoids are graded on an ascending scale of severity from 1 to 4. With a first-degree hemorrhoid, anal cushions are present on rectal examination. Second-degree hemorrhoids may prolapse below the dentate line but reduce spontaneously. Third-degree hemorrhoids must be manually reduced. Fourth-degree hemorrhoids are irreducible.

Pathogenesis

A bout of constipation, straining, or diarrhea is often associated with a thrombosed external hemorrhoid. Chronic constipation and excessive straining are also implicated in the development of internal hemorrhoids. However, internal hemorrhoids may also be associated with chronic liver disease and portal hypertension.[28]

Clinical Presentation and Diagnosis

External hemorrhoids rarely cause symptoms. If an external hemorrhoid becomes very large, it can become difficult to clean after bowel movements. Occasionally, sudden pain occurs when a clot develops within the external hemorrhoid and it becomes thrombosed. A painful, grape-like protrusion is noted on examination. This pain usually does not persist for more than a few days because the natural history of the clot is to drain spontaneously.

In children, primary internal hemorrhoids are virtually unknown. Their presence should raise questions regarding possible portal vein obstruction leading to portal hypertension and portosystemic shunting. Internal hemorrhoids present with either a protruding rectal mass or rectal bleeding. They are a common cause of rectal bleeding in older patients, but not in children, in whom anal fissures are much more common. Internal hemorrhoids do not cause pain. Classically, they manifest in three positions around the anus: the left lateral, right posterolateral, and right anterolateral. They can enlarge to the point that they protrude out of the rectum and may have to be pushed back in after straining. In advanced cases, they protrude enough so that they cannot be pushed back inside, resulting in chronic drainage and spotting of blood.

Treatment

Generally, an external hemorrhoid does not require surgery. External hemorrhoids are of no potential danger even if left untreated because they do not develop into cancers or other serious conditions.

The thrombosed external hemorrhoid is the only hemorrhoidal condition that is actually painful and, as such, may require surgical intervention during the acute thrombotic episode. Simple incision and drainage can promptly alleviate the pain of a thrombosed external hemorrhoid.

Treatment of internal hemorrhoids can vary from simple alterations in the diet to surgical removal. Internal hemorrhoids should first be treated with stool softeners and bulk agents (eg, psyllium). This approach is generally adequate treatment for hemorrhoids of degrees 1 to 3. Fourth-degree hemorrhoids usually require surgical intervention; banding is effective. Having said this about treatment, it must be re-emphasized that primary internal hemorrhoids are so uncommon in children that their presence should raise questions as to their etiology. A full investigation is necessary prior to treatment because hemorrhoidectomy in the face of portal hypertension can cause exsanguination.

RECTAL PROLAPSE

Rectal prolapse refers to either a mucosal or full-thickness herniation of the rectum through the anus. This diagnosis can be confused with chronic prolapsed internal hemorrhoids. Because rectal prolapse is a protrusion of the entire circumference of the rectal mucosa, concentric rings of mucosa are seen on examination. In fourth-degree hemorrhoids, the protrusion occurs only in a defined sector of the anus (usually lateral).

Pathogenesis

Rectal prolapse may be attributed to various causes and should be viewed as a sign of an underlying condition rather than a specific disease in itself. Potential etiologies include increased intra-abdominal pressure, diarrheal and neoplastic diseases, malnutrition, and conditions predisposing to pelvic floor weakness (such as prior surgery).[29] The most common cause is chronic constipation that may or may not be associated with neurologic or anatomic abnormalities. Acute diarrheal disease is the next most frequent etiology, followed by cystic fibrosis. Frequently, an extensive workup fails to elucidate any underlying factor.

Clinical Presentation and Diagnosis

Rectal prolapse is not uncommon in children, occurring more often in boys than in girls and tending to appear during the period of toilet training. The condition is usually self-limited.[30] Clinically rectal prolapse usually presents as a mass protruding from the rectum, with or without associated bleeding or tenesmus.[31]

In infancy, there are two types of rectal prolapse.[32] The first is mild and intermittent; the other is more pronounced and occurs with most bowel movements over a period of several weeks or months. Patients with rectal prolapse usually present with a history of prolonged straining at defecation. Rectal prolapse may also be associated with an acute diarrheal episode, cystic fibrosis, or a neurologic or anatomic anomaly. Although seen very rarely in developed countries, severe malnutrition or parasitosis can also cause rectal prolapse.

Children with unexplained or recurrent rectal prolapse should have a sweat chloride test to rule out cystic fibrosis, although this may be unnecessary if an anatomic abnormality can be identified as a cause of rectal prolapse.[33]

Treatment

In general, the treatment of rectal prolapse is nonoperative and directed at the underlying condition predisposing the patient to prolapse. Initial management consists of manual reduction and the administration of bulk laxatives or stool softeners.

If prolapse is a persistent problem, surgical intervention may be required. Injection sclerotherapy with D50W (dextrose 50% in water) or hypertonic saline is an effective treatment with few complications.[34] Sclerotherapy can be accomplished by injecting a total of 1 cc/kg of D50W or 15% saline solution submucosally or submuscularly above the dentate line.[34,35]

More aggressive surgical efforts may be needed for prolapse that fails sclerotherapy and in children with pelvic anatomic distortion caused by previous surgery. A variety of surgical procedures have been developed to treat rectal prolapse, but there is no consensus on the operation of choice. Surgery may be relatively simple, such as encircling the anus with a suture,[36] or involve complex operations such as posterior repair and suspension,[37] transsacral rectopexy,[32] transabdominal rectopexy with resection,[38] and posterior sagittal anorectoplasty.[39] Recent series advocate for the laparoscopic treatment of rectal prolapse.[40,41] This minimally invasive technique allows for either a simple rectopexy or a more elaborate rectosigmoid resection for the treatment of prolapse. Regardless of the approach, the prognosis is generally good.

PILONIDAL DISEASE

A pilonidal abscess is an inflammatory cavity overlying the sacrococcygeal region in the midline and is often accompanied by multiple draining sinus tracts (Figure 3).

Pathogenesis

A pilonidal sinus generally begins in the natal cleft at the site of an ingrown hair follicle. It is thought that movement in the region allows hairs to get drawn into the follicle, obstruct the follicle, and cause rupture of the follicle leading to abscess and sinus formation. Disease commonly

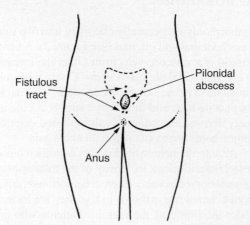

Figure 3 A pilonidal abscess and its associated tracts are shown in relation to the sacrum.

presents 1 or 2 in. above the anus and leads into a cavity underlying the skin. The result is a pilonidal cyst that may drain spontaneously. If the superficial opening of the tract is occluded, a pilonidal abscess will form.

Clinical Presentation and Diagnosis

A pilonidal abscess presents with persistent pain in the region of the sacrum accompanied by a boil located in the midline just above the anus. The diagnosis is made on physical examination that includes a rectal examination. A pilonidal abscess that drains spontaneously often results in a chronic pilonidal sinus. A pilonidal sinus tract is usually a slightly sore spot and can be a source of bloodstained or cloudy drainage that soils the underclothes.

Treatment

If a pilonidal abscess or fistula is found, the patient should be referred for surgical management. Primary treatment involves incision and drainage of any acute abscess. After resolution of the abscess, the traditional procedure of choice involves the wide excision of the underlying cyst and fistulous tracts, with the wound left to close by secondary intent.[42] More recent experience has shown that excision of the cyst and primary closure of the wound can be attempted in most cases provided that there is careful follow-up. When successful, this latter technique allows for rapid healing and less discomfort to the patient. Some have tried to improve the results of primary closure by implanting antibiotic-impregnated material, but the results are equivocal.[43] In extreme circumstances, skin or myocutaneous flaps may be necessary for coverage of the defect resulting from wide excision of a large cyst.

PRURITUS ANI

Pruritus ani simply implies persistent anal itching. It is a common skin condition and very frequently misdiagnosed as hemorrhoids. Pruritus can be grouped into either primary or secondary etiologies.

Pathogenesis

Most cases of pruritus ani are secondary in nature, with primary pruritus ani being a diagnosis of exclusion. Secondary pruritus is usually the result of chronic moisture exposure, pinworm (Enterobius vermicularis) infection, or excessive use of soaps and detergents. Caffeine intake, which reduces anal pressure, is the most common cause of pruritus ani in older subjects. Aggressive use of soaps and detergents perpetuates the problem of pruritus ani by changing cutaneous pH and stripping the natural oils of the skin.

Pinworm is a contagious intestinal parasite infestation that is common in children. It is found throughout the United States and is especially prevalent in urban areas and day-care settings. Approximately 20% of children in the United States will develop pinworm at some point in their lives. The parasite is easily spread through a fecal–oral route. The adult parasite lives in the cecum and colon and lays its eggs outside the anus during the night. In some settings, other local fungal or bacterial infections and, especially in children, scabies can also lead to pruritus ani and must be considered.[44]

Though rarer in children, other potential causes of pruritus ani include dermatologic conditions such as psoriasis, lichen planus, and seborrhea should be considered.

Clinical Presentation and Diagnosis

Patients typically present with persistent anal itching that is unrelenting. Other symptoms include irritability, sleep disturbance, decreased appetite, excoriation around the anus from constant scratching, and vaginal irritation.[45] Adults and siblings exposed to children with pinworm may also note symptoms shortly after exposure. Pinworm can be easily diagnosed by applying transparent adhesive tape to the skin around the anus before bathing or using the toilet in the morning. The tape is then transferred to a slide, where the presence of pinworm eggs may be confirmed by microscopy.

Treatment

Because most causes of anal pruritus are secondary, treatment should be directed at the underlying etiology. This is not to imply that all pruritus ani is easily treated because it can be the result of a self-perpetuating cycle. A complete anal and rectal examination should be performed to look for specific causes, especially pinworm. A thorough history of dietary and hygiene habits is also helpful.

For pinworm infestation, initial treatment consists of patient and family education about hygiene and fecal–oral spread.[46] General measures, such as hand washing, keeping fingernails short and clean, laundering all bed linens twice weekly, and cleaning toilet seats daily, can usually eliminate the problem in 1 to 2 weeks. If this fails, all family members must be treated with pyrantel pamoate, albendazole, or mebendazole.[47] To be successful, drug therapy needs to be repeated in 2 to 3 weeks.

For pruritus ani not attributable to pinworm, reassurance, patient education and follow up are key elements of treatment. Cessation of scratching, although difficult to do, can often break the itching cycle. Excessive anal hygiene habits and use of ointments, steroids, and anesthetic agents should be discouraged. Food sensitivities may exist to spices, coffee, milk, and chocolates, and patients should abstain from inciting agents. The aim of treatment is to achieve clean, dry, intact skin. In selected cases, some medications may also be of assistance, such as psyllium (promotes complete evacuation) and loperamide (increases resting anal pressure). Local care with air drying and/or cornstarch may also be of benefit.[42]

Although disturbed sphincter function has been proposed as causative (primary pruritus ani), it is an infrequent etiology. Generally, surgical intervention should be discouraged. When extensive tags or prolapsed tissue appears to contribute to poor hygiene, an operation may be considered.

REFERENCES

1. Schouten WR, Briel JW, Auwerda JJ, Boerma MO. Anal fissure: New concepts in pathogenesis and treatment. Scand J Gastroenterol Suppl 1996;218:78–81.
2. Lund JN, Scholefield JH. Aetiology and treatment of anal fissure. Br J Surg 1996;83:1335–44.
3. Klosterhalfen B, Vogel P, Rixen H, Mittermayer C. Topography of the inferior rectal artery: A possible cause of chronic, primary anal fissure. Dis Colon Rectum 1989;32:43–52.
4. Schouten WR, Briel JW, Auwerda JJ. Relationship between anal pressure and anodermal blood flow. The vascular pathogenesis of anal fissures. Dis Colon Rectum 1994;37:664–9.
5. Bacher H, Mischinger HJ, Werkgartner G, et al. Local nitroglycerin for treatment of anal fissures: An alternative to lateral sphincterotomy? Dis Colon Rectum 1997;40:840–5.
6. Andiran F, Dayi S, Mete E. Cows milk consumption in constipation and anal fissure in infants and young children. J Paediatr Child Health 2003;39:329–31.
7. Iacono G, Cavataio F, Montalto G, et al. Intolerance of cow's milk and chronic constipation in children. N Engl J Med 1998;339:1100–4.
8. Schouten WR, Briel JW, Boerma MO, et al. Pathophysiological aspects and clinical outcome of intra-anal application of isosorbide dinitrate in patients with chronic anal fissure. Gut 1996;39:465–9.
9. Sonmez K, Demirogullari B, Ekingen G, et al. Randomized, placebo-controlled treatment of anal fissure by lidocaine, EMLA, and GTN in children. J Pediatr Surg 2002;37:1313–6.
10. Tander B, Guven A, Demirbag S, et al. A prospective, randomized, double-blind, placebo-controlled trial of glyceryltrinitrate ointment in the treatment of children with anal fissure. J Pediatr Surg 1999;34:1810–2.
11. Demirbag S, Tander B, Atabek C, et al. Long-term results of topical glyceryl trinitrate ointment in children with anal fissure. Ann Trop Paediatr 2005;25:135–7.
12. Brisinda G, Maria G, Bentivoglio AR, et al. A comparison of injections of botulinum toxin and topical nitroglycerin ointment for the treatment of chronic anal fissure. N Engl J Med 1999;341:65–9.
13. Oh JT, Han A, Han SJ, et al. Fistula-in-ano in infants: Is nonoperative management effective? J Pediatr Surg 2001;36:1367–9.
14. Steele SR, Madoff RD. Systematic review: The treatment of anal fissure. Aliment Pharmacol Ther 2006;24:247–57.
15. Garcia-Aguilar J, Belmonte C, Wong WD, et al. Open vs. closed sphincterotomy for chronic anal fissure: Long-term results. Dis Colon Rectum 1996;39:440–3.
16. Macdonald A, Wilson-Storey D, Munro F. Treatment of perianal abscess and fistula-in-ano in children. Br J Surg 2003;90:220–1.
17. Piazza DJ, Radhakrishnan J. Perianal abscess and fistula-in-ano in children. Dis Colon Rectum 1990;33:1014–6.
18. Poenaru D, Yazbeck S. Anal fistula in infants: Etiology, features, management. J Pediatr Surg 1993;28:1194–5.
19. Marcus RH, Stine RJ, Cohen MA. Perirectal abscess. Ann Emerg Med 1995;25:597–603.
20. Rosen NG, Gibbs DL, Soffer SZ, et al. The nonoperative management of fistula-in-ano. J Pediatr Surg 2000;35:938–9.
21. Festen C, van Harten H. Perianal abscess and fistula-in-ano in infants. J Pediatr Surg 1998;33:711–3.
22. Christison-Lagay ER, Hall JF, Bailey K, et al. Progression of perianal abscess to fistula in infants: Implications for treatment. In: APSA 37th Annual Meeting; 2006; Hilton Head, South Carolina: American Pediatric Surgical Association; 2006. p. A38.
23. Serour F, Somekh E, Gorenstein A. Perianal abscess and fistula-in-ano in infants: A different entity? Dis Colon Rectum 2005;48:359–64.
24. Nix P, Stringer MD. Perianal sepsis in children. Br J Surg 1997;84:819–21.
25. Lahoti SL, McNeese MC, McClain N, Girardet R. Two cases of anal fistula in girls evaluated for sexual abuse. J Pediatr Surg 2002;37:132–3.
26. La Quaglia MP, Feins N, Eraklis A, Hendren WH. Rectal duplications. J Pediatr Surg 1990;25:980–4.
27. Markowitz J, Daum F, Aiges H, et al. Perianal disease in children and adolescents with Crohn's disease. Gastroenterology 1984;86:829–33.
28. Heaton ND, Davenport M, Howard ER. Symptomatic hemorrhoids and anorectal varices in children with portal hypertension. J Pediatr Surg 1992;27:833–5.
29. Siafakas C, Vottler TP, Andersen JM. Rectal prolapse in pediatrics. Clin Pediatr (Phila) 1999;38:63–72.
30. Chino ES, Thomas CG, Jr Transsacral approach to repair of rectal prolapse in children. Am Surg 1984;50:70–5.
31. Antao B, Bradley V, Roberts JP, Shawis R. Management of rectal prolapse in children. Dis Colon Rectum 2005;48:1620–5.
32. Qvist N, Rasmussen L, Klaaborg KE, et al. Rectal prolapse in infancy: Conservative versus operative treatment. J Pediatr Surg 1986;21:887–8.
33. Zempsky WT, Rosenstein BJ. The cause of rectal prolapse in children. Am J Dis Child 1988;142:338–9.
34. Chan WK, Kay SM, Laberge JM, et al. Injection sclerotherapy in the treatment of rectal prolapse in infants and children. J Pediatr Surg 1998;33:255–8.
35. Abes M, Sarihan H. Injection sclerotherapy of rectal prolapse in children with 15 percent saline solution. Eur J Pediatr Surg 2004;14:100–2.
36. Groff DB, Nagaraj HS. Rectal prolapse in infants and children. Am J Surg 1990;160:531–2.
37. Ashcraft KW, Garred JL, Holder TM, et al. Rectal prolapse: 17-year experience with the posterior repair and suspension. J Pediatr Surg 1990;25:992–4; discussion 4–5.
38. Aitola PT, Hiltunen KM, Matikainen MJ. Functional results of operative treatment of rectal prolapse over an 11-year period: Emphasis on transabdominal approach. Dis Colon Rectum 1999;42:655–60.
39. Pearl RH, Ein SH, Churchill B. Posterior sagittal anorectoplasty for pediatric recurrent rectal prolapse. J Pediatr Surg 1989;24:1100–2.
40. Rose J, Schneider C, Scheidbach H, et al. Laparoscopic treatment of rectal prolapse: Experience gained in a prospective multicenter study. Langenbecks Arch Surg 2002;387:130–7.
41. Koivusalo A, Pakarinen M, Rintala R. Laparoscopic suture rectopexy in the treatment of persisting rectal prolapse in children: A preliminary report. Surg Endosc 2006;20:960–3.
42. Billingham RP, Isler JT, Kimmins MH, et al. The diagnosis and management of common anorectal disorders. Curr Probl Surg 2004;41:586–645.
43. Holzer B, Grussner U, Bruckner B, et al. Efficacy and tolerance of a new gentamicin collagen fleece (Septocoll) after surgical treatment of a pilonidal sinus. Colorectal Dis 2003;5:222–7.
44. Zuccati G, Lotti T, Mastrolorenzo A, et al. Pruritus ani. Dermatol Ther 2005;18:355–62.
45. Ok UZ, Ertan P, Limoncu E, et al. Relationship between pinworm and urinary tract infections in young girls. Apmis 1999;107:474–6.
46. Tanowitz HB, Weiss LM, Wittner M. Diagnosis and treatment of common intestinal helminths. II: Common intestinal nematodes. Gastroenterologist 1994;2:39–49.
47. Juckett G. Common intestinal helminths. Am Fam Physician 1995;52:2039–48, 2051–2.

19

Microbial Interactions with Gut Epithelium

Eytan Wine, MD
Mauricio R. Terebiznik, PhD
Nicola L. Jones, MD, FRCPC, PhD

It is now increasingly evident that the intestinal surface provides not only the stage for nutrient digestion and absorption, and electrolyte fluid homeostasis, but also a specialized interface for constant interaction between the most abundant cells in the human body, microbes, and its largest surface area of 200 to 300 m^2 the gut epithelial lining. A multitude of murine models support the fact that the gut epithelia fulfills multiple complex roles through its interaction with the gut flora, by providing a barrier from the exterior, on the one hand, and a platform for antigen presentation and immune stimulation, on the other hand. For example, inflammatory bowel disease (IBD) mouse models lack inflammation in the absence of bacteria,[1,2] while other models show an under developed immune system when the intestinal flora is not present.[3,4] Furthermore, recent studies have highlighted the role of epithelial cells in preventing, or down regulating, proinflammatory responses to commensal bacteria (a phenomenon termed *tolerance*), while preserving their ability to detect pathogens and mount an effective defense response.[5] This point emphasizes the spectrum of relationships between microbes and the host, which can be symbiotic (where both sides benefit), commensal (where the host is not harmed), or parasitic (where only the microorganism benefits). This division is complicated by recent findings indicating that certain microbes can be commensal at times or eventually pathogenic at other times (depending on the physiological circumstances), even within the same host.[2,6] Many aspects of the multiple beneficial effects of the intestinal flora, including their trophic effects, roles in gut maturation, nutrient availability, competition for nutrients and host receptors with pathogens, barrier integrity enhancement, and contribution to defense from pathogens[7] will be discussed separately in the Chapter 19.1a, "Probiotics."

In many ways, the resident microbial flora can be considered an additional organ within the human body, with metabolic activity exceeding that of the liver, and with collective genetic material, known as *microbiome*[7] that exceeds the human genome.[8] Much of the recent advances in unraveling the complex relationships between microbes and the intestinal epithelium can be attributed to the use of novel molecular techniques and germ-free mice. The following chapter will highlight characteristics of gut–microbial interactions observed during infection with established enteropathogens,[9] the increasing data supporting the role of microbes in preserving health and homeostasis,[10] along with their putative involvement in the pathogenesis of complex diseases, such as IBD,[11] necrotizing enterocolitis (NEC),[12] cancer,[13] and even obesity.[14]

For the reader's convenience, the current concepts and recent advances in the understanding of epithelial–microbial interactions will be presented by first describing the host elements of epithelial and mucosal defenses, then outlining bacterial mechanisms of virulence, and finally, focusing on selected areas of interaction. Due to the nature of constant counterplay between both sides, reference to the interplay of mechanisms will be displayed throughout the text. This complex relationship is not simply a reflection of action and reaction, but rather represents the coevolution of a highly complex and overlapping host defense with an overwhelmingly diverse microbial virulence arsenal.

COMPONENTS OF THE MICROBIAL AND GUT EPITHELIAL INTERFACE

Host Factors

Dynamic Barrier. The main physical portion of the intestinal barrier consists of the simple, columnar, constantly renewing epithelial monolayer. These epithelial cells are polarized, with differential expression of membrane proteins on the apical and basolateral surface. The monolayer is composed of four epithelial cell lineages: enterocytes, goblet cells, enteroendocrine, and Paneth cells, all developing from the same progenitor cell, located in the base of the crypt.[15] The intercellular junctional complexes, which maintain barrier integrity, are composed of apical junctional complexes (AJC), which includes tight junctions (TJs) and adherens junctions (AJs), as well as desmosomes. TJs form a continuous fence-like ring, acting as a regulator, semipermeable to solutes and fluid, restricting free movement between the lumen and the submucosa, and also delineating apical and basolateral domains.[16] Many pathogens target proteins that form junctional complexes, as well as the cytoskeleton and the signaling pathways involved, which maintain the junctional complex, emphasizing the importance of these junctions in intestinal homeostasis, and disease prevention. Details regarding components of the AJC, its regulation, and disruption by pathogens will be presented later in this chapter (see Figure 1).

Beyond establishing a physical barrier, the epithelial lining, together with other host components, provides multiple dynamic and overlapping layers of defense.

Mucus Layer. The epithelial cell barrier is covered by a mucus coating, composed of mucins secreted by goblet cells. Mucin glycoproteins consist of a core protein surrounded by several oligosaccharides, which can bind multiple small molecules, including adhesion molecules, selectins and lectins. Membrane bound mucins, such as MUC1, MUC3A+B, MUC4, contain a short cytoplasmic tail, which is involved in cellular signaling, and may serve as an "environmental sensor."[17] For example, MUC4 serves as a ligand for the receptor tyrosine kinase ErbB2, and MUC1 binds to β-catenin, both of which are involved in cell adhesion.[18–19] Secreted mucins (eg, MUC2, MUC5B, MUC5A+C, MUC6) bind to membrane bound mucins and provide similar roles in cell adhesion. Interactions between enteropathogens and epithelial cells can alter the highly regulated mucin secretion, which may prove beneficial or harmful to the host. For example, *Listeria monocytogenes* exotoxin listeriolysin O mediates an increase in mucin exocytosis, which benefits the host by enhancing the barrier,[20] whereas in the case of *Clostridium difficile*, the A toxin inhibits mucin exocytosis, which reduces host defenses and encourages infection.[21] *Helicobacter pylori* lipopolysaccharide (LPS) is a strong stimulator of mucin production. However, mucin can inhibit the bacteria's lipid wall-forming enzyme, α-glucosyltransferase.[22] Therefore, to resist the protective effects of mucins, *H. pylori* have developed several mechanisms. For example, bacterial α-glucosyltransferase A2 interferes with gastric cell mucin synthesis,[23] a process which has also been shown to be related to endothelin-1-mediated epidermal growth factor receptor activation by *H. pylori*.[24]

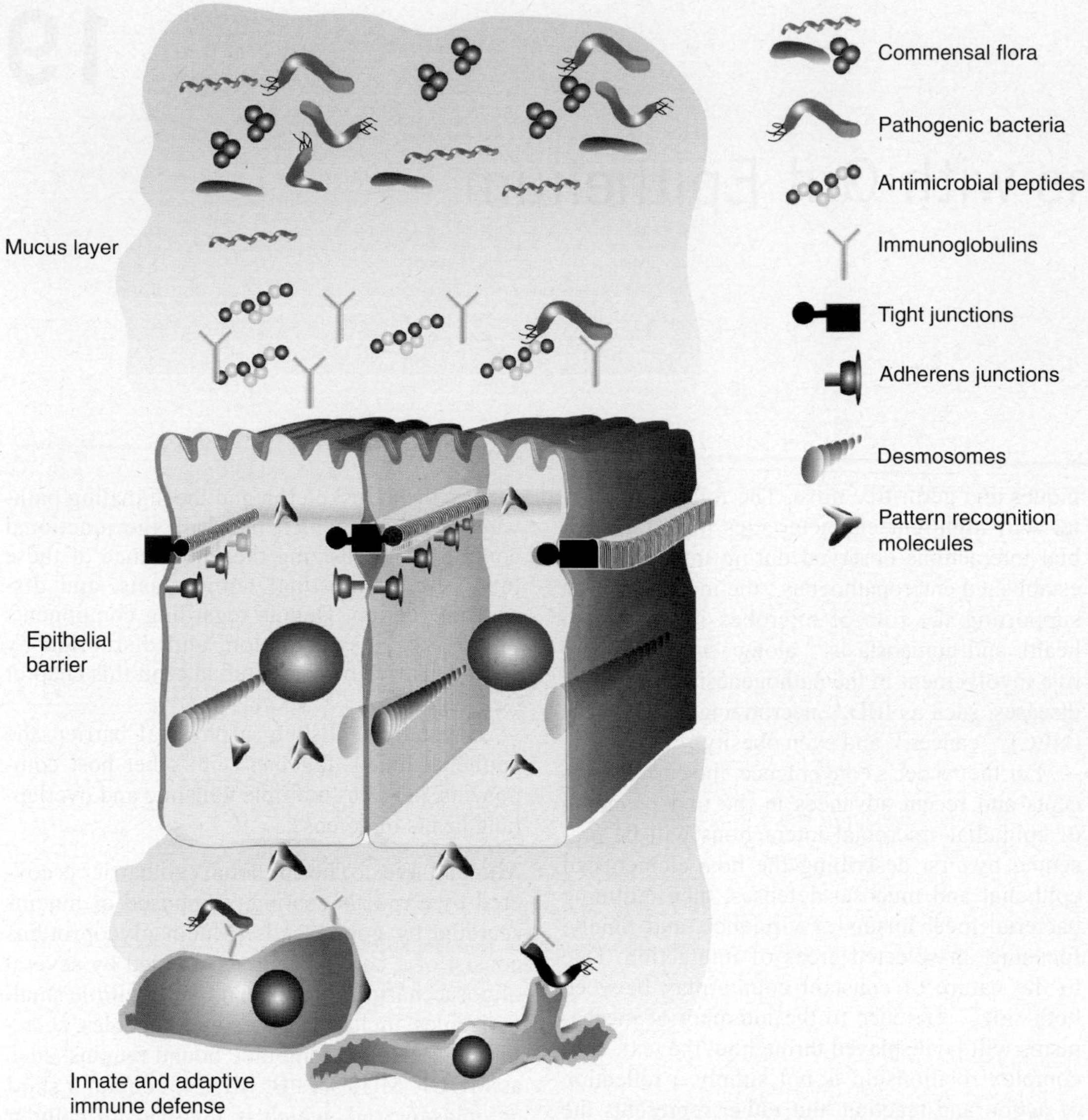

Figure 1 The multilayer physical and functional components of the intestinal mucosal barrier. A single layer of intestinal epithelial cells, bound together by rings of apical junctional complexes, provides the physical backbone for the gut mucosal barrier. The mucus layer, antimicrobial peptides, and immunoglobulin A, which are secreted by the epithelial cells, together with physical conditions (motility, sheer forces, and pH) and commensal bacteria, serve to augment the luminal components of the barrier. Epithelial cells also provide functional defense through the action of innate immune factors and inflammatory signaling cascades. The barrier is further supported by subepithelial mucosa-associated immune cells, together with endocrine, vascular, and enteral nervous system-related factors. Collectively, these features provide a dynamic, highly responsive, multilayer, and functional barrier, separating the intestinal lumen from the vulnerable submucosa.

Protection by the Intestinal Microflora. Increasing evidence points to the central role of the intestinal microflora in maintaining intestinal barrier integrity. Although this field is ever evolving, several mechanisms by which the host benefits from the presence of indigenous microbes have been described, as extensively discussed in other chapters. In the context of barrier function, one of the simple functions of the intestinal flora is to serve as a mechanical barrier of mucosa-associated microorganisms, separating potential pathogens from the host, and competing for attachment sites.[25] Furthermore, pathogenic bacteria can be deprived of essential nutrients by commensals,[26] as well as directly inhibited due to production of commensal-derived antimicrobial factors, termed bacteriocins.[27]

Antimicrobial Peptides. The intestinal lumen also contains antimicrobial factors, which are secreted by epithelial cells. Soluble immunoglobulin A (IgA), which is secreted by plasma cells and transported to the lumen by epithelial cells, exhibits antimicrobial activity, although IgA deficiency rarely results in increased susceptibility to enteric infections. Epithelial cells and circulating leukocytes of all multicellular organisms secrete two major groups of antimicrobial peptides (AMPs), defensins and cathelicidins.[28] Defensins are cationic small peptides, which disrupt bacterial membranes. Of the 6 human α-defensins (HD1 to 6 or cryptdins in mice), HD5 and HD6 are produced mainly by Paneth cells. Enteropathogens, such as *Salmonella enterica*, *Serovar typhimurium* (*S. typhimurium*), have developed methods to escape the effect of defensins, as demonstrated by this bacteria's ability to resist cryptdin-4 host defense in a murine model by use of the bacterial extracytoplasmic sigma factor sigma (E), which senses, and responds to, external stress.[29] Secretion of α-defensins by Paneth cells is dependent, in part, on nucleotide oligomerization domain

(NOD) 2/CARD15 function, as emphasized by decreased α-defensin production in Crohn's disease (CD) patients, especially those carrying NOD2 mutations.[30] Furthermore, the enhanced susceptibility of NOD2 knockout mice to oral (but not intravenous or intraperitoneal) *L. monocytogenes* infection is attributed to reduced cryptdin production.[31]

Although some of the physiologic functions of human β-defensins (hBD) still remain unclear, it appears that the role of this additional group of AMPs is to contribute to barrier function, resulting in essentially sterile crypts.[32] Only a portion of the over 30 hBD genes result in a protein product.[33] All the four defined hBDs are effective at killing a wide variety of microbes *in vitro*, although this effect is reduced at physiological salt levels.[34] The molecular basis for hBD's antimicrobial activity appears to result from the presence of six cystine residues (forming a polycationic disulfide array), which bind to the negatively charged bacterial membrane. This results in a "pore-forming" disruption of the bacterial envelope and leakage of their internal cytoplasmic content (see Figure 2).[35] hBD-1 is constitutively expressed in epithelial cells throughout the intestine, but unlike other hBDs, its expression is not upregulated by infection. Nevertheless, microbes causing intestinal disease, which are sensitive to hBD-1 *in vitro*, such as the protozoa *Cryptosporidium parvum*, downregulate hBD-1, which may support a role for this protein in barrier defense.[36] The basal levels of hBD-2, hBD-3, and hBD-4 in the intestinal epithelium are very low, but increase with specific bacterial or inflammatory stimulation, which is consistent with the protein's suggested function.[37]

Cathelicidins represent another AMP produced by epithelial cells, as well as mast cells and neutrophils.[38] The human cationic protein 18 kDa (hCAP18) is a prepropeptide, which carries the active AMP cathelicidin LL-37 in its C terminal. Site-specific hCAP18 proteolysis by neutrophil elastase results in variable antimicrobial effects.[39] Similar to defensins, cathelicidins disrupt bacterial membranes due to their amphipathic properties. In addition, cathelicidin can bind, and possibly neutralize, LPS, and plays a role in chemotaxis, angiogenesis, and other physiological processes.[39] In the intestine, propeptide hCAP18 expression is highest in surface gastric epithelial cells, as well as Brunner's glands and differentiated surface colonic cells. This "superficial" distribution of cathelicidin, which is similar to that of β-defensins, may indicate that these AMPs form a thin antimicrobial coat, lining the epithelial surface, preventing bacterial attachment, or contributing to their elimination (through their pore-forming capacity, as noted above). In support of this contention, knockout mice, lacking the murine hCAP homolog, demonstrate increased susceptibility to colonization by the mouse pathogen *Citrobacter rodentium*, with enhanced damage to the epithelial lining and dissemination of infection.[40] The function of LL-37 is further supported by inhibition of enterocyte

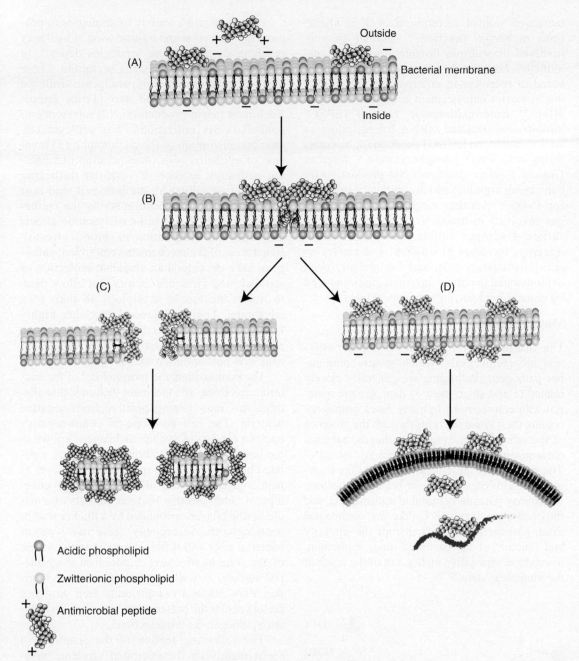

Figure 2 Mechanism of action of antimicrobial peptides. Charge-mediated association and carpeting of the bacterial membrane outer leaflet with polycationic antimicrobial peptides (A). Integration of the peptide into the bacterial membrane (B). Two possible mechanisms of antibacterial actions are suggested: formation of membrane pores and loss of membrane integrity (C) or diffusion of the antimicrobial peptide into the bacterial cytoplasm and targeting of intracellular structures (D).

structure will be provided below).[46] *S. enterica* recognizes AMPs, and responds by utilizing its PhoP/PhoQ two-component system, which leads to a decrease in the negative charge of the bacterial outer membrane and reduced binding of AMPs.[47] Similarly, Gram-positive bacteria, such as *Enterococcus faecalis*, modulate the d-alanine residues in their lipoteichoic acid, which is responsible for their bacterial cell surface negative charge, to evade AMP binding.[48] Other mechanisms of AMP resistance have been identified, including the ability of a *S. typhimurium* outer membrane protease, PtgE, to cleave α-helical cationic AMPs.[49]

Bactericidal permeability-increasing protein (BPI) is an AMP, primarily found in neutrophils and eosinophils, which was just recently described in intestinal epithelial cells.[50] The main antimicrobial functions of BPI, which are effective against Gram-negative bacteria, include inner and outer membrane interference, opsonization, and neutralization of LPS.[51] It appears that this high-affinity LPS-binding effect serves to divert LPS, and its resulting effects, from enhancing inflammation, thereby shifting the balance toward an anti-inflammatory response.[52] Such an effect may be therapeutically utilized, in theory, to modify inflammatory responses to microbes, as has been reported in a double-blind, placebo-controlled trial for meningococcal sepsis.[53]

The trefoil factors (TFFs) are secreted by epithelial cells into the lumen in response to mucosal damage, inflammation, and neoplasia, where they are considered to carry a role in repair and maintenance of mucosal integrity. This is demonstrated by increased intestinal injury in TFF-deficient mice challenged with dextran sodium sulfate.[54] Of the TFFs present in humans, TFF3 has the broadest expression.[55] It is well established that TFFs interact with mucins and modulate epithelial signaling pathways after barrier breach. Nevertheless, there are limited data concerning their interaction with bacteria, although there is some evidence to suggest that TFFs may be involved in *H. pylori* binding to the gastric mucosa.[56]

Inflammatory Response. Epithelial cells respond to the presence of pathogens by production of various inflammatory mediators. In some cases, this results in increased fluid secretion and intestinal motility, which may help in pathogen clearance by mechanical "flushing," while in many other cases the host recruits innate and adaptive inflammatory mediators and cells, ultimately contributing to pathogen clearance. In both scenarios, the downside for the host is the development of disease symptoms, and moreover, the pathogen may even benefit by increased spread to other hosts, encouraging it to induce disease.

The cytokine and chemokine responses of host cells are well documented and have been reviewed in detail elsewhere.[38,39,57] Many of these aspects, relevant to the epithelial–microbial interactions, will be presented below. As the first line of defense, epithelial cells are required to alert and attract inflammatory cells. This is mediated through

production of LL-37 by *Shigella*, coupled with the observation that in patients with shigellosis, LL-37 synthesis is blocked, but expression is restored as they recover.[41] An interesting potentially therapeutic application of this knowledge was recently demonstrated in *Shigella*-infected rabbits. The administration of the short-chain fatty acid butyrate (which is usually the product of colonic commensal bacteria and has been independently demonstrated to stimulate LL-37 production by enterocytes)[42] to infected rabbits resulted in recovery of their epithelial LL-37 levels and rapid clearance of the pathogen with recuperation of the rabbits.[43]

Lysozyme is constitutively expressed in gastric glands, Brunner's glands, and Paneth cells, where it provides additional defense against microbes after secretion into the lumen.[44] This highly cationic-charged protein hydrolyses β1-4

glycosidic bonds between *N*-acetyl glucosamine and *N*-acetyl muramic acid, which are present in bacterial cell wall peptidoglycan, causing a loss of prokaryotic cell integrity.[39] Gram-positive bacteria are more susceptible to this enzyme than Gram-negative bacteria, due to the lack of an outer membrane. *S. enterica* inhibits lysozyme production by Paneth cells in a type III secretion system-dependent fashion, thus reducing the effect of this protective layer.[45]

The innate immunity provided by these epithelial cell-secreted AMPs relies on the typical bacterial wall structure components. In order to evade the effects of these proteins, several bacteria have developed mechanisms of resistance. Gram-negative bacteria have established the ability to modify the key factors of LPS which provide targets for AMPs: the anchoring lipid A and the O antigen (details on the bacterial wall

Legend items:
- Acidic phospholipid
- Zwitterionic phospholipid
- Antimicrobial peptide

Labels: Outside, Bacterial membrane, Inside; (A), (B), (C), (D)

chemokines, which act as chemoattractants by creating a gradient of concentrations, leading host defense immune cells to the "battle zone." For example, *Campylobacter jejuni* infection results in induction of gene transcription and secretion of multiple chemokines by epithelial cells.[58]

Host cytokine responses serve to potentiate host innate immunity, facilitate inflammatory responses, and recruit and regulate adaptive immune processes. Host pattern recognition molecules (PRMs) serve as sensors of microbial motifs, termed microbe-associated molecular patterns (MAMPs).[59] Cytokines are usually produced by epithelial cells in response to activation of signal transduction pathways, leading to nuclear translocation of transcription factors, such as nuclear factor (NF)-κB. Microbes interact with these pathways in many ways, which result in induction of proinflammatory cytokines and chemokines, in some cases, or downregulation of these factors and expression of inflammatory-suppressing cytokines, in other cases. These interactions will be demonstrated throughout this chapter, and a more detailed description can be found in the chapter discussing intestinal immunity. Some of the more important pathways, which can be modified by pathogens, are demonstrated in Figure 3.

Much attention has been directed toward the role of the cyclooxygenase (Cox)-2 pathway in gastrointestinal disease.[60] Pathogenic microbes interact with this important pathway in many ways. Several invasive enteropathogens, including enteroinvasive *Escherichia coli* (EIEC) and *Salmonella dublin*, induce Cox-2-mediated prostaglandin E_2 production, resulting in activation of chloride channels and increased luminal secretion, as well as alterations in barrier function.[61] Another enzyme involved in multiple inflammatory functions, inducible nitric oxide synthase (iNOS), is activated in response to enteropathogens, resulting in barrier enhancement and a bacteriocidal effect.[62] Enteropathogenic *E. coli* (EPEC) inhibits iNOS-related mRNA transcription, as well as nitric oxide (NO) production, by interfering with iNOS phosphorylation,[63] whereas *Giardia lamblia* decreases NO production by consuming arginine, which serves as a substrate for iNOS.[64] Another small-molecular-weight gas involved in mucosal barrier is hydrogen sulfate. Hydrogen sulfate maintains mucosal integrity, increases blood flow, and carries an anti-inflammatory role, and has recently been demonstrated to reduce intestinal injury induced by nonsteroidal anti-inflammatory drugs.[65]

Microbial Factors

The vast majority of microbes within the intestine are commensals, which greatly outnumber pathogens. Pathogens are generally closely related to and share most of their genetic material with commensals. In many cases, pathogens acquire their virulence traits through the presence of specialized genetic regions within the bacterial chromosome, termed "pathogenicity islands." The presence of these genes results in the emergence of virulence factors, or bacterial effectors, which may potentially promote transmission, and thus pathogen survival. Unlike the commensal flora, pathogenic bacteria disrupt the integrity and function of the gastrointestinal epithelium, to establish replicative niches, out of the reach of the immune system.[66–69]

Pathogens use a variety of strategies to promote their survival and transmission, which may result in disease. These strategies depend, in general, on the location of the bacterium. These locations (and examples of pathogenic virulence strategies) can be divided into: (1) the intestinal lumen (toxin production); (2) adherence to epithelial cells (utilization of host cell cytoskeleton and disruption of the membrane); (3) invasion of epithelial cells (manipulation of signaling pathways, evasion of vesicular trafficking and bacterial killing by the host cell, and host cell death); (4) translocation across the epithelial layer; and (5) induction of systemic effects (through the lymphatics or blood stream). Regardless of the mechanisms employed, pathogens have developed an abundant collection of sophisticated virulence factors that allow them to divert the host's physiology to their own advantage. These virulence factors are highly host–pathogen specialized, although they share common functional and structural themes to deal with host antimicrobial defenses.

The composition and morphology of the bacterial envelope are the main features that distinguish Gram-staining positive from negative bacteria. The cell envelope of Gram-negative bacteria consists of two lipidic bilayers, known as the inner and outer membranes, which are separated by the periplasmic space and a thin layer of peptidoglycan. On the other hand, the cell envelope of Gram-positive bacteria consists of a single lipidic bilayer surrounded by a thicker wall of peptidoglycan. Accordingly, these two types of bacterial cells will differ in respect to the nature of the adhesin structures exposed on the bacterial surface, as well as in the secretion systems that allow bacteria to translocate their virulence factors across the bacterial cell envelope, to influence pathogen–host interactions.

The following section of the chapter will focus mainly on the microbial virulence arsenal involved in adhesion, invasion, and survival within the cell, as well as the host cellular counterparts involved in bacterial pathogenesis and strategies of defense, which, together, are best defined as the field of cellular microbiology.

Adhesion. Adhesion of pathogens to host tissue is the first crucial step in the establishment of infectious diseases. Attached bacteria can resist natural cleansing mechanisms of the host, and at the same time, achieve the close contact necessary to modulate host physiology. Pathogens express adhesion molecules, known as adhesins, which target and attach them selectively to tissue and cell types that express the complementary ligand or receptor. A vast number of specialized bacterial surface structures evolve to engage, secure, and promote the adhesion of bacteria to biological and inert surfaces. Examples of these are pili, adhesins, autotransporters, and fibronectin/collagen-binding proteins.[70–73]

Pili or *fimbriae* are rodlike appendage organelles that protrude out from the bacterial surface into the external milieu. Pili are assembled from

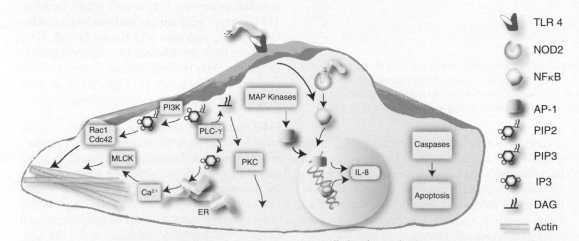

Figure 3 Selected effects of microbial enteric pathogens on host cell signal transduction cascades. Bacteria adhere to the plasma membrane of epithelial cells and induce phospholipase C (PLC)-mediated cleavage of phosphatidylinositol-4, 5-bisphosphate (PIP2) into inositol-1,4,5-triphosphate (IP3) and diacylglycerol (DAG). IP3 triggers the release of calcium from intracellular stores, which results in F-actin rearrangements, as well as activation of myosin light-chain kinase (MLCK), leading to phosphorylation of the light chain of myosin and, and ultimately to disruption of apical junction complexes. DAG activates protein kinase C (PKC), resulting in multiple secondary downstream effects. PIP2 can also be phosphorylated by phosphatidylinositol 3-kinase (PI3K) to produce phosphatidylinositol-3,4,5-trisphosphate (PIP3), which activates small GTPases, such as Rac1 and cdc42, ultimately altering actin polymerization. Mitogen-activated protein kinase (MAPK) cascades control chemokine transcription, such as interleukin-8 (IL-8), in response to various proinflammatory stimuli, such as lipopolysaccharide and tumor necrosis factor-α. Nuclear factor kappa B (NF-κB) is a transcription factor that is normally latent in the cytosol, but when activated by bacterial motifs that bind to innate immune receptors, such as TLR4 (lipopolysaccharide) and NOD2/CARD15 (peptidoglycan), moves to the nucleus, binds to DNA and initiates the production of multiple inflammatory cytokines and chemokines. Apoptosis is directly induced through activation of the caspase pathway. (Adapted from reference 9.)

the noncovalent polymerization of protein subunits called pilins. The affinity properties of pili depend on specific adhesin domains localized at the tip of its structure. During pili biogenesis, pilin protein subunits are secreted into the bacterial periplasmic space by the sec-dependent secretion machinery (see below). Pili are morphologically and functionally distinguishable, according to their biogenic mechanism. Thus, they can be categorized into three different types: P and type 1 pili that utilize the chaperon/usher pathway, type 4 pili, which are assembled by a type II secretion system, and curly pili, which are coiled surface structures generated by an extracellular nucleation/precipitation pathway.[74-77] Among these, the better studied and most relevant are P, type 1, and type 4 pili.

Once secreted to the periplasmic space type 1 and P pilin subunits associate with chaperones that prevent their incorrect aggregation, further escorting them to usher proteins localized at outer-membrane sites. At these platforms, pilins are assembled, translocated, and anchored to the bacterial surface acquiring their final quaternary structure.[78]

Type 1 pili components (fimA-fimH) are codified in the *fimH* gene cluster. A large proportion of *E. coli* strains are type 1 pilated. Indeed, 95% of *E. coli* isolates from intestinal and urinary infections, as well as most of the members of the Enterobacteriaceae family, like *Klebsiella pneumoniae*, *S. typhimurium,* and *S. enterica,* represent this pili variant.[71,79] The type 1 pili adhesin, FimH, mediates bacterial binding to mannose oligosaccharide residues exposed on the host's cell surface. Phenotypic variants of FimH adhesin have been identified according to their affinity properties. *E. coli* isolates are classified as low mannose-binding (M_1L) or high mannose-binding strains (M_1H). Adhesin affinity variants play a fundamental role in determining bacterial tissue tropism and pathology. Indeed, most of the isolates from healthy human intestine are M_1L, whereas most of the isolates from urinary track infections (uropathogenic *E. coli* (UPEC)) are M_1H. Pyelonephritis-associated (P) pilus is expressed in UPEC and will not be discussed in detail in this chapter.[80]

Type 4 pili are ubiquitous among Gram-negative bacteria, where they mediate numerous bacterial functions, including microcolony and biofilm formation, host cell adhesion, host bacterial cell signaling, horizontal gene transfer, phage attachment, and bacterial mobility. Consequently, type 4 pili are crucial for bacterial virulence, and their disruption severely abrogates pathogenicity in intestinal bacteria like *S. enterica*, *S. typhi*, EPEC, enterohemorrhagic *E. coli* (EHEC), and *Vibrio cholerae.*

One of the remarkable properties of type 4 pili is its ability to retract or elongate while remaining attached to a surface receptor. This mechanism allows bacteria to control their binding interactions with host surfaces, and to perform twitching motility; a movement modality that makes the displacement over semisolid surfaces possible, as in the case of the enterogastric epithelial mucous layer.[81,82] Twitching motility is a mechanism mediated by an ATP-dependent motor that causes association–dissociation of pilin subunits at the base of pilus structure.[83,84]

According to variations in the components of the biogenic machinery, type 4 pili can be divided into groups A or B, which show different host specificities.[85,86] Human enteropathogenic bacteria (eg, *V. cholerae*, EPEC, and *S. enterica*) are type 4b pilated. The type 4b pili from EPEC, and *V. cholerae* shows a particular morphology; it can aggregate laterally forming bundles. In EPEC, the type 4 bundling pilus (Bfp) is formed by a single pilin subunit named bundlin, which is encoded by *bfp* genes in the adherence factor plasmid (EAF). Bfp is necessary for the primary adherence of bacteria to the brush border of the intestinal epithelia and to facilitate the formation of tight microcolonies that characterize infection.[67] The *V. cholerae* type 4 pili is known as toxin-coregulated pili (TCP). TCP is essential for colonization of the human intestine and also acts as the receptor for the bacteriophage that carries the cholera toxin genes, CTX. Like Bfp, TCP promotes bacterial association, allowing the establishment of *V. cholerae* microcolonies on the intestinal epithelial cells where the bacteria secrete cholera toxin, thus causing severe diarrhea.[87] *S. typhi*'s type 4 pili are encoded by the *Pil* operon, formed by association of the pilin monomer PilS. Type 4 pili mediate the attachment of *Salmonella* to the intestinal epithelia and self-association contributing to host cell invasion and the development of enteric fever.[88]

Mono and Oligomeric Adhesins. Bacteria can produce an alternative class of adhesins, which are short-monomeric or oligomeric molecules that belong to the family of bacterial autotransporter proteins. Autotransporters are the simplest protein secretion system found in Gram-negative bacteria. They have a modular organization that includes a passenger domain that moves across the outer membrane to be presented at the bacterial surface where it can act as an adhesin. Adhesion through autotransporters can mediate bacterial autoaggregation, biofilm formation, invasive phenotype, or can bind host serum proteins, which mediate resistance to serum bactericidal activity and/or resistance to phagocytosis.[89,90]

The best characterized examples of autotransporter cell receptor pairs are BabA and SabA from the human gastric pathogen *H. pylori*. The receptors for these adhesins are the Lewis blood group antigens. BabA has affinity for Lewis b (Le^b), expressed on human red blood cells and the gastric mucosa. SabA binds sialylated sLe^X and sLe^e antigens that are normally present at very low concentration, but their expression is upregulated as a consequence of *H. pylori* infection.[91,92]

Most of the autotransporters identified so far bind extracellular matrix proteins such as collagen, fibronectin or vitronectin. Although the adhesin-binding domains for these receptors remain elusive, two putative motives have been identified: the Arg-Gly-Asp (RGD), involved in the adhesion to β-integrins, and repeated amino acid sequences, like proline-rich regions (PRR), frequently found in adhesive proteins.[89] Several autotransporters responsible for autoaggregation and biofilm formation have been characterized in *E. coli*. The autotransporters AIDA, expressed in diffuse-adhering *E. coli* (DAEC), and TibA, from enterotoxigenic *E. coli* (ETEC), are one of the few known bacterial glycosylated proteins. AIDA is responsible for the DAEC diffuse-adhering phenotype. The exact role of autotransporter glycosylation is not well understood, but in the case of AIDA it is essential for adhesion. AIDA can produce the autoproteolytic cleavage of its own passenger domain, which remains associated with the cell surface through noncovalent interaction.[93] The autotransporter Ag43 is found in all *E. coli* strains. Like type 1 pili, Ag43 synthesis is controlled by phase variation mechanisms, thus complementing pili's binding functions. Ag43 binds to β-integrins in the host's tissue, utilizing an RGD motif in its passenger domain. Importantly, Ag43 also has the ability to cross -interact with other adhesions, mediating bacterial intra- and interspecies associations, thus contributing to *E. coli* autoaggregation and biofilm formation that are fundamental for pathogenicity.[94]

A new trimeric family of autotransporters, oligomeric coiled-coil adhesins (OCA), located where the passenger domains fold as trimers, has been recently described. YadA, the *Yersinia enterocolitica* and *Y. pseudotuberculosis* protein, is the best-known example of this family. The trimerization of C-terminal subunits of YadA forms a functional pore that shows affinity to collagen and laminin, thus playing a critical role in bacterial immune resistance, autoaggregation, and invasion.[95]

Bacterial Secretion Systems. In order to secure their niche, tissue surface-attached pathogens confront numerous host barriers and defense mechanisms. To overcome host resistance, bacteria utilize a vast array of molecular tools that will hijack cellular components and pathways, deactivating cell defenses, and using host cell physiology to their own benefit. These virulence factors are either secreted by bacteria to the host cell interface, or in an even more sophisticated fashion, directly injected into the host cell cytoplasm. Secreted virulence factors are referred to as cytotoxins, while the injected ones are termed bacterial effectors. Bacteria have evolved to develop complex secretory machineries that coordinate the processing, assembly, and activation of cytotoxins and effectors, as well as the proper timing for the secretion of multiple virulence factors.

Until recently, five different secretion systems were described in Gram-negative bacteria. Types I, II, and V secretion systems are responsible for the secretion of cytotoxins to the external milieu, and types III and IV secretion system are able to inject bacterial virulence factors directly into

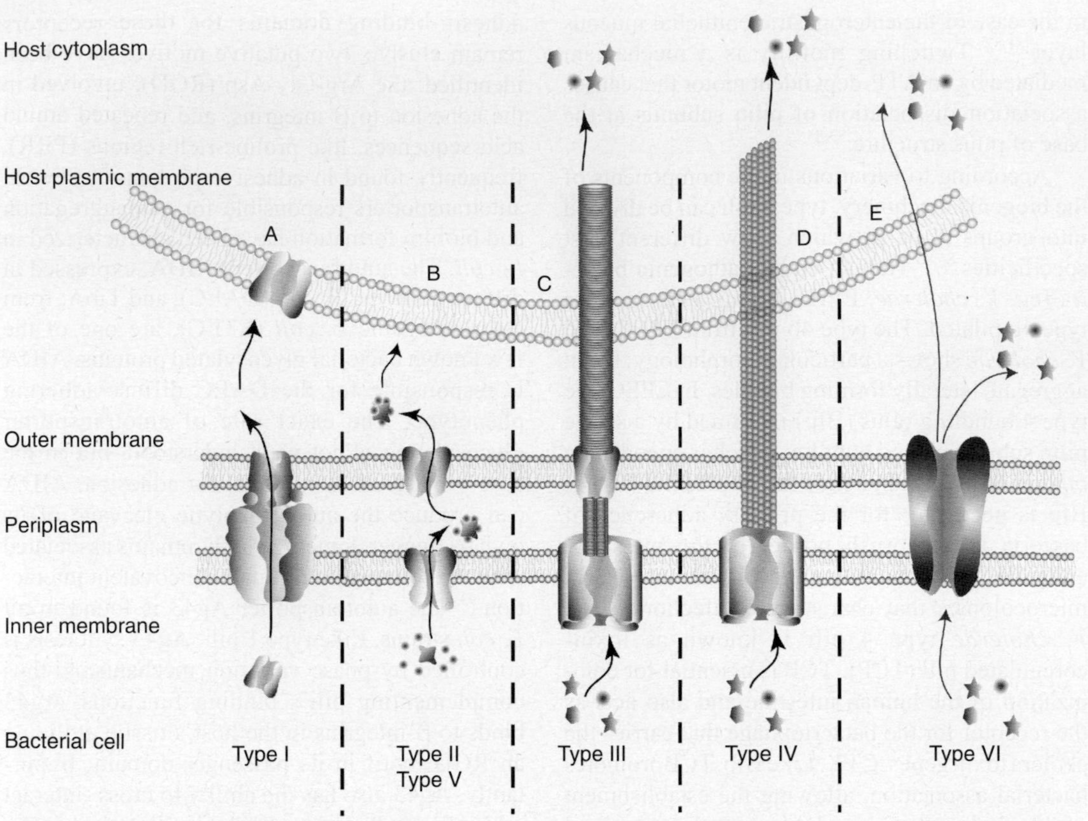

Host cytoplasm

Host plasmic membrane

A

B

C

D

E

Outer membrane

Periplasm

Inner membrane

Bacterial cell

Type I   Type II / Type V   Type III   Type IV   Type VI

Figure 4 Protein secretion systems in pathogenic bacteria. Type I secretion system depicting secretion of bacterial pore-forming toxins to the host–pathogen interface and subsequent toxin insertion through the host plasma membrane (A). The multistep secretion mechanism of bacterial toxins through type II or type V secretion systems (B). Resembling molecular needles, type III and type IV systems protrude from the bacterial cell wall complex and penetrate the host cytoplasmic membrane, injecting bacterial effector proteins directly into the mammalian cell cytoplasm (C and D). Type VI secretion system has been recently described as a mechanism capable of delivering virulence factors directly into the host cell (E). (Adapted from reference 97.)

the host cell cytoplasm. A sixth secretion system, possibly involving direct injection of cytotoxins into host cells, has been described in *V. cholera* and *Pseudomonas aeruginosa*[96,97] (see Figure 4).

Type I Secretion System. The T1SS apparatus consists of three proteins that span from the cytoplasm to the bacterial surface. These proteins include the inner-membrane ATP-binding cassette (ABC transporter), a membrane fusion protein (MFP), and an outer-membrane pore-forming protein (OMP) that are known in *E. coli* as HlyB, HlyD, and TolC, respectively.[98]

The secretion process, and sequential assembly, of T1SS components begin when a C-terminal secretion signal carried by the protein to be secreted (substrate) is recognized by T1SS cytoplasmic components. The first toxin characterized and the prototypic example of T1SS-secreted protein is HlyA, produced by UPEC. HlyA is a lipid-modified protein that inserts into the plasma membrane of eukaryotic cells, forming pores that release the cytoplasmic content. Many other similar toxins have been identified, including the bifunctional adenylcyclase hemolysin from *Bordetella pertussis*, tubulin interacting RtxA toxin from *V. cholerae*, metalloprotease of *Erwinia chrysanthemi*, leukotoxin of *Pasteurella haemolytica*, and bacteria directed toxins, like colicin V from *E. coli*.[99]

Type II Secretion System. Unlike T1SS, protein secretion by T2SS is a two-step process. At first, substrates are translocated across the inner membrane to the periplasmic space by either the generic Sec or Tat bacterial secretion system. Once in the periplasmic space, T2SS components recognize the substrate and transport it to the external media through a secretion pore in the outer membrane. Thus, T2SS structure requires cytoplasmic, inner-membrane and outer-membrane components forming a multiprotein arrangement that transverses the entire bacterial envelope. The T2SS basic structural and functional core is conserved among different bacterial genera. T2SS is utilized for protein secretion by a large number of pathogenic bacteria (eg, *Legionella pneumophila, Y. enterocolitica, V. cholerae*, EHEC, *P. aeruginosa, Burkholderia pseudomallei*). Many human diseases are mediated by the combined action of one or more T2SS-secreted cytotoxins. Well-known examples of T2SS cytotoxins are the ADP-ribosylating cholera toxin from *V. cholerae*, and the *E. coli* heat labile toxin (which will be described in detail later in this chapter), lipases from *L. pneumophila* (lysophospholipase A PlaA), and proteases like the StcE zinc metalloprotease, secreted by EHEC O157:H7.[100,101]

Type V Secretion System. T5SS is the simplest secretion machinery characterized so far in Gram-negative bacteria. T5SS-exported proteins inflict virulence by acting as adhesins, hemolysins, proteases, cytotoxins, or mediators of intracytoplasmic actin-promoted bacterial motility.

Effector Delivery. Two different bacterial apparatuses, utilized for the delivery of effectors into mammalian cells, have been described: type III and type IV secretion systems (T3SS and T4SS respectively). Both are found in different Gram-negative enteropathogenic bacteria including EPEC, EHEC, *Salmonella, Yersinia, Shigella*, and *H. pylori*. The complexity of these systems is well illustrated by the fact that T3SS and T4SS can transport virulence factors not only from the bacterial cytoplasm across the inner bacterial membrane, the peptidoglycan layer, and the outer membrane, but also directly into the mammalian cell cytoplasm by passing through the host cell plasma membrane.

Type III Secretion System. T3SS are exclusively expressed in Gram-negative bacteria and specifically utilized for the injection of bacterial virulence proteins into the host cell cytoplasm. The type and number of effectors delivered to the host cell greatly diverge between pathogenic bacteria; however, T3SS structure and composition remain highly conserved among species. Electron microscopy visualization and biochemical data indicate that TTSS is formed by three main protein structures: the needle, the inner-membrane, and the outer-membrane rings. Additionally, a fourth component, the translocon, inserts into the host cell membrane, forming a receptor pore for the needle.[102]

T3SS's needles resemble a hollow stem, or pipeline, that spans across the bacterial envelope and protrudes into the external milieu. On average, the needles are 60 to 80 nm long with an external diameter of 60 to 130 A° and an inner diameter of 20 to 30 A°. The main function of this structure is to form a channel for bacterial effector conductance from the bacteria to the host cell cytoplasm. The structure and composition of the T3SS needle are highly conserved among bacterial genera. Indeed, needle monomers from *Yersinia, Shigella*, and *Salmonella* (YscF, MxiH, and PrgI, respectively) are closely related proteins, showing 26% identity. YscP, Spa32, and InvJ tightly control the length of the needle in *Yersinia, Shigella*, and *Salmonella*, respectively. The T3SS's rings are membrane-integrated proteins, allowing the needle to traverse through the bacterial inner and outer membranes. A number of inner-membrane proteins have been found to associate with the T3SS structure. These proteins can interact with effectors at both the cytoplasm and/or the inner membrane, possibly acting as receptors for the secretion signals carried by the effector proteins. This is the case for *Yersinia*'s proteins YscV and YscU, which are integral inner-membrane proteins that bear putative cytoplasmic receptor domains for the interaction with T3SS substrates. The T3SS apparatus also associates with inner-membrane ATPase complexes that generate the energy required to drive protein secretion. Examples of ATPase complexes have been found in *Yersinia, Shigella*, and *Salmonella*. Mutations that affect the catalytic activity of the *Yersinia* ATPase, YscN, or its homologue from

Salmonella, InvC, disrupt T3SS secretion activity. The T3SS outer-membrane ring is included in the bacterial outer membrane. It is composed of secretins that form multimeric ring pore structure. Examples of T3SS secretins are *Yersinia*'s YscC and *Salmonella*'s InvG. The localization of the outer-membrane ring at the bacterial membrane is dictated by its association with small T3SS outer-membrane lipoproteins, like InvH in *Salmonella* and YscW in *Yersinia*.[102–105]

The T3SS needle passes through the host cell plasma membrane, utilizing a pore, formed by T3SS secreted proteins, known as translocons. Mutations of these proteins do not affect the secretion of T3SS proteins, but prevent translocation to the host cell. Thus, translocons are considered to be the entry portal for the translocation of effectors through the host cell membrane. Examples of translocons are *Yersinia*'s YopB and YopD, *Salmonella*'s SipB, *P. aeruginosa*'s PopB and PopD, and EPEC's EspB and EspD.[106,107]

Only a subset of the bacterial cytoplasmic proteins are secreted to the media or translocated into host cells by the T3SS. Such specificity involves the recognition of the secretion system substrates at the bacterial cytoplasm. To date, three different types of secretion signals on the effector proteins have been proposed to mediate targeting to the T3SS apparatus: the 5' region of the effector mRNA (15 initial codons), the first 20 amino acid residues at the N terminus of the effector protein, and/or a chaperone binding site, located approximately within the first 140 amino acids of the effector structure.[108,109]

Type IV Secretion System. The T4SS shows several important differences compared to the T3SS. T4SS is present in both Gram-negative and positive bacteria, and it not only secretes proteins but is also capable of exporting and importing DNA. T4SS conjugation machines translocate DNA among different bacterial species. Importantly, conjugation is of significant medical concern, since it is a mechanism for the transmission of antibiotic resistance genes between pathogenic species. Besides conjugation, some T4SS can perform the reverse operation by taking up DNA from the milieu (known as competence), which is utilized by bacteria to increase their genome plasticity.[110]

The first, and better characterized T4SS, belongs to the plant pathogen *Agrobacterium tumefaciens*, which is considered the representative functional and structural model for this secretion system. *A. tumefaciens* T4SS delivers DNA and proteins into plant cell cytoplasm, causing tumor formation (galls). T4SS play a role in delivering virulence factors into mammalian cells (eg, *B. pertussis*, *H. pylori*, *L. pneumophila*, *Brucella* ssp.). Infection with the human gastric pathogen *H. pylori* is associated with chronic gastritis, peptic ulcers, and gastric cancer. *H. pylori* pathogenic strains harbor the cag (cytotoxin-associated gene) pathogenicity island (PAI). This PAI encodes components of a T4SS and the effector CagA. CagA interferes with multiple host cell pathways, probably acting as the main determinant for gastric cancer.[111,112] Despite the functional and mechanistic resemblance between T3SS and T4SS, there is no molecular homology among the proteins that make up this system. Like T3SS, T4SS is a multistructural apparatus. T4SS is formed by a bacterial secretion channel that spans across the bacterial inner membrane, periplasm, peptidoglycan, and outer membrane, connecting to a pilus, or other surface filaments, that play a role similar to the T3SS needle. The architecture of T4SS varies significantly along bacterial genera. F pilus, the conjugative pili of Gram-negative bacteria, has an 8 to 10 nm outer diameter and a length of 2 to 20 μm, and an inner lumen 2 nm in diameter. *H. pylori* Cag PAI elaborates a considerably larger secretion apparatus. The needle portion of this structure is estimated to be 40 nm in diameter and the cross section of the sheathed structure is estimated to be 70 nm.[110] T4SS requires energy for biogenesis and function. VirB11 is an ATPase necessary for the formation of the secretion channel and/or pilus production. Homologues of VirB11 ATPase have been described in *E. coli* and *H. pylori*. In *H. pylori*, the inner-membrane ATPases HP0544 (VirB4/CagE) and HP0525 (VirB11) provide the energy for substrate translocation.[112,113]

Bacterial Colonization, Adhesion, and Invasion of Epithelial Cells. To withstand the harsh environment of the gastrointestinal lumen, bacterial pathogens have developed different strategies to manipulate host cell physiology, in order to maximize bacterial adhesion, or to induce entry into host nonphagocytic epithelial cells, thereby establishing protected niches where they can replicate and thereafter spread systemically (see Figure 5).

Platforms for Adhesion and Cell Signaling. EPEC and EHEC virulence requires adherence to intestinal epithelial cells. Thus, these bacteria have a sophisticated system to promote an intimate attachment to host cells. After a primary attachment mediated by the type 4 bundle pilus, a different adhesion molecule known as intimin mediates adhesion. Intimin does not recognize an intrinsic host cell factor, but rather a bacterial protein receptor synthesized and translocated by *E. coli* T3SS into the mammalian cell, the receptor Tir (translocated intimin receptor).[114] The binding of intimin to Tir triggers a cascade of events that change the architecture of the apical border of the epithelial cells, causing what is known as attaching and effacing lesions. These include the disruption of microvilli and the formation of host

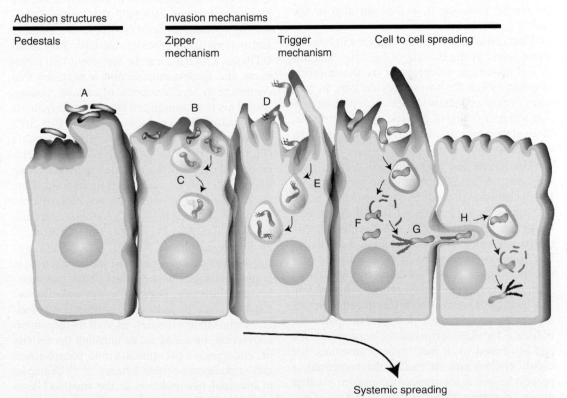

Adhesion structures | Invasion mechanisms

Pedestals | Zipper mechanism | Trigger mechanism | Cell to cell spreading

Systemic spreading

Figure 5 Host cell adhesion and invasion mechanisms utilized by enteropathogenic bacteria. EPEC and EHEC infection causes the formation of platform-like structures at the apical border of epithelial cells, known as pedestals (A), where the bacteria can tightly attach to further colonize the tissue. Enteroinvasive bacteria, such as *Yersinia* and *Listeria*, utilize the zipper mechanism to enter into epithelial cells. Bacterial virulence factors induce the formation of small host cell membrane folding rearrangements (B) that trap and engulf the bacteria into membranous compartments, which pinch off from the host plasma membrane to form an intracellular niche for the pathogen (C). *Salmonella* and *Shigella*, as well as other enteroinvasive bacteria, utilize the triggering mechanism to enter mammalian cells. This mechanism includes the induction of large host cell membrane protrusion due to the action of bacterial virulence factors (D). Massive host cell surface ruffling leads to the entrapment of pathogenic bacteria inside vacuolar compartments that eventually pinch-off from the host plasma membrane to form the pathogen's intracellular niche (E). *Listeria* and *Shigella* have the capacity to escape from the primary vacuolar compartment to the cytoplasm (F). In the host cytoplasm, these bacteria are propelled by the strength of polymerizing actin tails (G). Cytoplasmic motility allows these pathogens to invade neighboring cells (H). Intracellular bacteria can eventually bypass the epithelial barrier, causing a systemic dissemination of the infection.

cell membrane pedestal-like structures, as demonstrated in Figure 5A, which function as platforms for bacterial adhesion. Pedestals represent the consequence of host cell cytoskeletal rearrangement, which are induced upon Tir/intimin contact.

After EPEC-translocated Tir is inserted into the host cell membrane, it is phosphorylated by host kinases. Phospho-Tir mediates the recruitment of the actin polymerization proteins N-WASP and Arp2/3 at the site of bacterial attachment. In contrast, Tir from EHEC is not phosphorylated by host kinases, but instead interacts with a second bacterial protein translocated into the host cell by EHEC, EspF$_u$ that directly recruits WASP to EHEC's Tir. The activation of the host proteins WASP and Arp2/3 locally promotes abundant polymerization of actin, leading to the formation of pedestals. Thus, Tir has the ability of undermine the host's actin polymerizing machinery to create a cellular structure that favors pathogen colonization and survival. The ability of EPEC and EHEC to modulate the host cell metabolism entirely depends on the translocation Tir.[115]

Invasive Bacteria. Many enteropathogenic bacteria, including *Salmonella, Yersinia, Shigella,* and EIEC, have been described to be invasive in humans. Recent evidence supports the fact that the human pathogen *H. pylori* can also invade gastric epithelial cells.[116,117]

Host cell invasion can be triggered in two different ways: by the binding of bacterial adhesins to cell membrane receptors or by the injection of effectors into the host cell cytoplasm. In both cases, virulence factors induce actin polymerization and remodeling of the host cytoskeleton that force plasma membrane protrusions to engulf the bacterium.

The nature and extent of cell surface rearrangement differs according to the specific cellular mechanisms engaged by the bacterium. Some pathogens express adhesins that bind to host membrane proteins relevant to cell–cell and cell–matrix adhesion, such as integrins and cadherins. The cytoplasmic domains of these proteins control the strength of cell adhesion by modulating actin polymerization at the cortical cytoskeleton. The binding of bacterial adhesins to cell adhesion molecules hijacks their downstream pathway, inducing localized cytoskeletal rearrangements and associated small membrane protrusions that tightly enclose and internalize the bacterium, a process known as the zipper mechanism. Another group of pathogens utilize the T3SS to inject effectors that cause massive cytoskeletal rearrangements, producing abundant cell membrane ruffling that literally swallows the bacteria in a process that resembles macropinocytosis; this is known as the triggering mechanism.[116]

To induce changes in the host cell cytoskeleton architecture, invasive bacteria preferentially target key cellular components that control the temperospatial dynamics of actin polymerizations at the plasma membrane level. This is the case for the Rho family of small GTPases and

plasma membrane phosphoinositides. Rho small GTPases function as molecular switches alternating between active GTP-bound and inactive GDP-bound conformations. The turnover of these molecules is mainly controlled by guanine nucleotide exchange factors (GEFs), GTPase-activating proteins (GAPs), and guanine nucleotide dissociation inhibitors (GDIs). GEFs activate the small GTPases by favoring GTP binding. The inactivation is mediated by GAPs, which stimulate the GTPase activity of the molecule. GDIs control the cellular distribution of GTPases by binding inactive GTPases in the cytosol. The Rho small GTPases Rac1 and Cdc42 induce and control actin polymerization machinery by regulating the activity of the Arp2/3 complex. Arp2/3 is fundamental for the initiation of actin nucleation, branching, and actin filament bundling in various cellular processes, where movement and cell surface remodeling are necessary (ie, cell adhesion, polarization, migration, ruffling, macropinocytosis, and phagocytosis).[118,119]

The membrane lipid phosphatidylinositol (4,5)*bis*-phosphate (PI(4,5)P2) plays a crucial role in cortical actin reorganization, membrane–cytoskeleton interaction, and cell adhesion. The polar inositide head of PI(4,5)P2 allows it to interact with actin-binding proteins, promoting links between the cortical cytoskeleton and the plasma membrane. PI(4,5)P2 also acts as a scaffolding platform for actin cytoskeleton regulatory and polymerizing proteins, included Rho small GTPases. PI(4,5)P2 can be converted into membrane and cytoplasmic second messengers that contribute to several aspects of cellular metabolism. This is accomplished by phosphatidylinositol 3-kinase (PI3K) phosphorylation of PI(4,5)P2 to phosphatidylinositol(3,4,5)trisphosphate (PI(3,4,5)P3), which is involved in cell membrane and cytoskeleton remodeling by activating Rho small GTPases, and in cell survival signaling through the AKT-related pathways. PI(4,5)P2 can also be hydrolyzed to the second messengers diacylglycerol (DAG) and inositol 3-phosphate (IP3) by the enzyme phospholipase C (PLC). Pathogens subvert host cell phosphoinositide metabolism to promote changes in the cytoskeleton and membrane architecture. Bacterial toxins and effectors can hydrolyze or induce the synthesis of membrane phosphoinositoides, as well as their interconversion, by acting as, or inducing the activity of, endogenous phosphoinositide phosphatases and/or phosphoinositide kinases.[120,121] Examples of bacterial manipulation of the small GTPases and PI(4,5)P2 pathways involved in invasion will be descried below.

Invasion Zipper Mechanism. *Yersinia* and *Listeria* are well-known examples of bacteria whose invasion is mediated by the zipper mechanism, which is also the proposed mechanism for DAEC and, more recently, for *H. pylori* (see Figure 5B). At the initial phase of their infectious process, *Y. enterocolitica* and *Y. pseudotuberculosis* invade cells of the gut epithelia. These bacteria express on their surface the first

virulence factor described as responsible for inducing invasion, named invasin.[122] Invasin can bind and activate β$_1$-integrins due to its structural similarities with fibronectin, the natural ligand for this receptor. The short cytoplasmic domain of integrins functions as a scaffolding platform for signaling molecules and the actin cytoskeleton. Invasin binding to integrins triggers a signaling cascade that involves the integrin-associated focal adhesion kinase (FAK) and Src family of kinases,[123] which in turn leads to the activation of the small GTPases Rac1 and Arf6, thus inducing cytoskeletal rearrangement necessary for bacterial internalization. Activated Rac1 induces actin polymerization by means of the actin-nucleating complexes Arp2/3 and N-WASP, whereas Arf6 acts by inducing the synthesis of PI(4,5)P2, which stimulates actin polymerization at the site of bacterial attachment.[124]

L. monocytogenes is a Gram-positive pathogen that has the remarkable capacity of traversing three human tissue barriers (intestinal, blood–brain, and fetoplacental barriers) causing gastroenteritis, meningitis, or abortion.[125] Cell invasion by *L. monocytogenes* is mediated by the surface virulence proteins internalin A (InlA) and B (InlB). The host cell receptor for InlA is E-cadherin. The homophilic interaction between E-cadherin from contiguous cells is necessary for the formation and maintenance of cells adherens junctions in polarized epithelia. A leucine-rich repeat (LRR) motif in the structure of InlA mediates its interaction with E-cadherin by selectively binding a proline residue in position 16 of its structure. Importantly, proline-16 is only present in human E-cadherin. Thus, InlA exclusively targets human cells.[126] The binding of InlA to E-cadherin initiates its interaction with its downstream cellular partners, α- and β-catenins, targeting them to the bacterial contact site. Catenins, in turn, link E-cadherin to the actin cytoskeleton filaments. InlA also triggers the actin polymerization machinery, where Rac1, cortactin, and Arp2/3 are involved. Recent evidence indicates that the actin motor, unconventional myosin VIIA, generates the mechanical energy required for bringing the surface-attached *L. monocytogenes* into the cell cytoplasm.[127]

Similar to InlA, InlB specifically binds to a human cell membrane receptor, the hepatocyte growth factor (HGF) receptor (Met), via its LRR motif.[128] However, the downstream signaling induced by InlB differs from InlA. Met activation by InlB binding recruits the molecular adaptors Gab1, Cbl, and Shc, which activate PI3K. The product of PI3K activity, PI(3,4,5)P3 activates Rac1, which induces the actin cytoskeletal rearrangement necessary to sustain the formation of the zipper mechanism structures.[129,130] The binding of Met to its physiological ligand HGF causes its uptake by a clathrin-mediated endocytosis process. Surprisingly, *Listeria* can hijack the Met endocytic machinery. Indeed, activation of Met by InlB induces the internalization of *L. monocytogenes* by clathrin-mediated endocytosis. This is the first description of bacterial invasion mediated by this endocytic modality.[131]

Invasion Triggering Mechanism. *Salmonella* and *Shigella* invasion are well-studied examples of the triggering invasion mechanism (Figure 5D). *Salmonella* invasion is mediated by effectors injected into the host cell via a T3SS, which is encoded on the chromosomal pathogenicity island I (SPI-1). *Salmonella* effectors induce actin polymerization and cytoskeletal rearrangements accompanied by massive cell membrane ruffling and lamellipodia formation. Three *Salmonella* effectors, SopE, SopE$_2$, and SigD or SopB, are able to activate Rac1 and Cdc42. SopE and SopE$_2$ act like GEF factors and directly activate these small GTPases, whereas the mechanism of SopB activation is unclear and probably involves PI(3,4,5)P3 and/or the production of Ins(1,4,5,6)P4. Another group of T3SS delivered effectors, SipA and SipC, contributes to cytoskeleton remodeling by stabilizing actin filaments. SipC, a component of the T3SS needle translocon, promotes actin filament bundling, whereas SipA stabilizes actin filaments by neutralizing the actin depolymerizing factor, cofilin, as well as the actin-severing protein, gelsolin.[132–134]

To control the timing of the ruffling internalization process of *Salmonella,* some effectors can inactivate the small GTPases. In fact, the *Salmonella* effector SptP functions as a GAP for Rac1 and Cdc42. SptP GAP activity terminates the ruffling process and the uptake of bacteria, allowing the host cell to recover its normal morphology.[135] Pinching-off of *Salmonella* vacuoles occurs at the base of the ruffling membrane and is facilitated by SopB phosphatase activity. SopB shows phosphatase activity toward inositol phosphates and phosphatidyl phosphoinositides. During *Salmonella* invasion, SopB locally depletes PI(4,5)P2 at the innermost part of the ruffling membrane. The loss of PI(4,5)P2 decreases the plasma membrane–cytoskeleton interactions, facilitating the pinching off, and the biogenesis of, the nascent *Salmonella*-containing vacuole.[136] *Shigella* invasion resembles many of the aspects described for *Salmonella*. *Shigella* translocates several effectors into the host cell utilizing a T3SS apparatus encoded in a plasmid-located pathogenic island (PAI). These effectors promote cytoskeletal rearrangement and cell membrane ruffling leading to bacterial internalization. IpaB and IpaC, which are homologous to *Salmonella*'s SipB and SipC, form the translocon pore in the host cell membrane. IpaC, together with another effector, IpaA, favors the bundling of actin filaments. IpaB interacts with IpaC and binds to CD44, a host transmembrane hyaluronic receptor. Active CD44 mobilizes to lipid rafts creating signaling molecule platforms at the site of bacterial entry. Activated CD44 can recruit the cytoskeleton-associated proteins ezrin-radixin-moesin (ERM) controlling in this way actin rearrangements during *Shigella* entry.[137,138] Several *Shigella* effectors can interact with GEF proteins to activate Cdc42 and Rac1 to induce the membrane ruffling necessary for bacterial uptake. VirA can activate Rac1 by an indirect mechanism that involves the induction of microtubule depolymerization.[139] *Shigella*'s Abl/Arg tyrosine kinase phosphorylates the host adaptor molecule CrkII, which in turn mediates the activation of Cdc42/Rac1.

Shigella IpgD is the homolog of *Salmonella*'s effector SopB. Similar to SopB, IpgD dephosphorylates PI(4,5)P2, which facilitates the cytoskeletal morphological rearrangements necessary for *Shigella* invasion.[140] IpgD phosphatase activity produces PI(5)P, which has recently been shown to be a potential novel mechanism of PI3-kinase/Akt activation.[141] Thus, both phosphatases, SopB and IpgD, induce the synthesis of PI(3,4,5)P3 with possible implications on cytoskeletal rearrangement but also prompt the activation of AKT and downstream signaling for cell survival.[141–142]

Survival Mechanisms of Intracellular Bacteria. As a result of the invasion process, the internalized bacterium resides in a primary vacuole compartment, pinched off from the host plasma membrane. In order to generate their replicative niche, intracellular bacteria can remain in these vacuoles (Figure 6A to C), or, alternatively, escape to the host cell cytoplasm (Figure 6D to G). Each of these lifestyles requires different virulence factors and strategies to survive in the intracellular environment. Intracellular bacteria have reduced exposure to the host immune system but still need to avoid degradative and antimicrobial cellular mechanisms. In the case of intravacuolar bacteria, active mechanisms segregate the pathogen from the endocytic pathway. Vacuoles resulting from endocytosis or phagocytosis normally undergo a series of progressive fusion and fission events with organelles from the endocytic pathway. During this maturation process, vacuoles become acidified and fuse with late endosome and lysosomal compartments, where they acquired antimicrobial peptides and hydrolytic enzymes that can degrade internalized cargo. Intravacuolar bacteria can control the maturation of their vacuolar compartment, setting it apart from the dangerous elements of the endocytic pathway, but yet establishing complex interactions with the host cell in order to obtain the nutrients and membrane necessary to generate unique secure replicative niches.[143]

Pathogenic bacteria replicating in the host cell cytoplasm do not interact with the endocytic pathway, but instead need to actively avoid being targeted for killing by the ubiquitin-proteosome or by autophagy, as well as prevent recognition by intracellular innate immunity.[144–146] Ubiquitination is a posttranslational modification of proteins that consists of the covalent binding of one or more exposed lysine residues to the C terminus of the protein ubiquitin. Ubiquitin can form polyubiquitin chains at the surface of misfolded or defective molecules. Polyubiquitinated proteins are then recognized and degraded by the proteosome. The resultant peptide fragments can then be presented to effector T cells as part of antigens by MHC class I molecular complex, thus initiating an adaptive immune response. Growing evidence indicates that free cytoplasmic bacteria can be ubiquitinated, or associated with ubiquitinated proteins, and consequently recognized and killed by the proteosome.[146,147]

Autophagy is a highly evolutionarily conserved mechanism for the degradation of cellular components in the cytoplasm in response to nutritional deprivation or hormonal signals. During autophagy, cytoplasmic proteins and organelles are sequestered within a double membrane structure, termed the autophagosome, which ultimately fuses with lysosomes to generate a degradative compartment, the autophagolysosome, where the sequestered materials are finally degraded. The autophagy pathway participates in numerous physiological functions, including the degradation of long-lived and aggregated proteins, organelle turnover, cell detoxification, tissue remodeling, and a nonapoptotic programed cell death. Autophagy of intracellular microbes is termed xenophagy. The recently described association between the autophagy-related 16-like 1 (*ATG16L1*) gene and Crohn disease may be mediated by alterations in processing of intracellular bacteria by xenophagy.[148] Despite the fact that bacteria and viruses are susceptible to xenophagy killing, several intracellular pathogens have developed strategies to disrupt, and even utilize, this pathway for their own benefit. Indeed, it has been reported that certain types of bacteria recruit autophagosome membranes to form a protective intracellular niche.[149–151]

S. typhimurium actively maintains and selectively segregates their vacuolar niche, known as *Salmonella*-containing vacuole (SCV), from the dangerous components of the endocytic pathway.

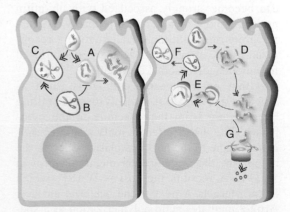

Figure 6 Intracellular survival of enteroinvasive pathogens. To survive and replicate inside host cells, enteroinvasive pathogens need to actively avoid intracellular recognition and antimicrobial systems. Pathogens that replicate inside intracellular compartments (A) need to avoid fusion of the bacterial vacuole with the lysosomal compartment (B), which bears antimicrobial agents and hydrolytic enzymes that will eliminate the bacteria (C). Intracellular pathogens that escape to, and replicate in, the host cytoplasm (D), need to actively avoid entrapment by the autophagy pathway (E), where they can be eliminated (F). Free-living cytoplasmic pathogens can be ubiquitinated and targeted for proteosome-associated destruction (G).

These actions are controlled by effectors injected into the host by a T3SS, in this case encoded by the *Salmonella* pathogenic island 2 (SPI-2), which is expressed only after entry of the bacteria into the host cells. SPI-2 independent factors that impede SCV fusion with lysosomes include the phoP/Q two-component regulatory system. The phoP/Q regulon controls expression of over 40 genes in *S. typhimurium,* many of which are important for bacterial resistance to antimicrobial peptides.[47,143] Immediately after their formation, SCVs fuse with harmless early endosomal compartments by recruiting specific elements of the host cell fusion machinery, including the phosphoinositide PI(3)P, the small GTPase Rab5, and EEA1. *Salmonella* then selectively recruit some late endosomal markers (ie, Rab7, LAMP1, LAMP2, and the vacuolar H$^+$-pump ATPase), but exclude LBPA, mannose 6-phosphate receptors, and mature lysosomal hydrolases from SCVs. At later times, 5 to 6 hours after invasion, SCVs, now located in the perinuclear area, undergo morphological changes that generate membrane tubular protrusions, known as *Salmonella*-induced filaments (Sifs). *Salmonella* start to replicate inside SCV-Sifs. The maintenance and regulation of SCV-Sifs depend on the SPI-2 effectors SifA, SopD2, SseF, SseG, and SseJ. The lack of these proteins produces replication and survival defects of *Salmonella* in macrophages (but not in epithelial cells), which correlates with reduced virulence in mouse infection models. SifA is fundamental for the integrity of Sifs replicative compartments, and its interaction with the host protein SKIP (SifA and kinesin-interacting protein) is necessary for Sifs morphogenesis.[119,143,152] Thus, the lack of SifA causes the disruption of SCV and the release of the bacteria to the host cytoplasm. It has been shown that cytoplasmic *Salmonella* can become strongly associated with ubiquitin proteins, and are, as a result, probably targeted for proteosome killing, or alternatively recognized by the autophagy machinery and targeted for autophagolysosomal degradation.[144,147]

Other enteroinvasive pathogens, such as *Shigella* and *Listeria*, avoid lysosomal killing by escaping from their vacuole to the cytoplasm. The T3SS effector IpaB mediates *Shigella* escape to the host cytoplasm. Once in the cytoplasm, the *Shigella* outer-membrane protein VirG/IcsA recruits the host N-WASP, which in turn targets Arp2/3 to the bacterial surface. Arp2/3 mediates actin polymerization at a specific pole of *Shigella*, generating a propulsive force that propels the bacterium through the cytoplasm.[153] Actin-propelled *Shigella* push forward the host plasma membrane causing the extension of membranous protrusions that penetrate into the cytoplasm of neighboring cells, eventually pinching off inside a double membrane compartment (Figure 5G). The ability to propagate from cell to cell without being exposed to the extracellular environment allows *Shigella* infection to spread while avoiding the host immune response.

Cytoplasmic bacteria are susceptible to elimination by autophagy, but *Shigella* actively evade this pathway utilizing the effector IscB.[154] Recent evidence indicates that IscB competes with the autophagic protein Atg5 for binding to the *Shigella* outer-membrane protein IpaB. In support of this, it has been demonstrated that *IscB* mutant *Shigella* bind Atg5, allowing the association of the bacteria with autophagosomes and finally its destruction in autolysosome organelles.[155]

L. monocytogenes represents another bacterium, which has adapted to survive within epithelial cells. After internalization, *Listeria* escapes from its vacuole by secreting phospholipases (PlcA and PlcB), and the pore-forming toxin listeriolysin O (LLO), thereby gaining access to the cytoplasm. Similar to *Shigella*, cytoplasmic *Listeria* polymerizes actin to propel itself through the cytoplasm and to invade neighboring cells.[125,156,157] Actin polymerization is mediated by the *Listeria* surface protein ActA. ActA fulfills this function by mimicking the eukaryotic proteins N-WASP and WAVE. The N-terminal region of ActA, necessary for actin polymerization-based motility, shows homology to the C-terminal region of WASP, which binds the actin nucleation complex Arp2/3.[158,159] A second bacterial protein that participates in motility is VASP.[160] This protein binds to ActA, recruits the actin-binding protein profilin, and causes the release of Arp2/3 from the complex. In this way, VASP modulates actin polymerization favoring the rapid elongation of straight actin filaments for bacteria propulsion. Like *Shigella*, cytoplasmic *Listeria* actively avoids elimination by the autophagy and ubiquitination pathways, but in this case utilizing an unknown mechanism.[147,161]

Although generally considered an extracellular pathogen, expanding evidence indicates that *H. pylori* also invades gastric epithelial cells.[162] Electron microscopy studies of gastric biopsy samples obtained from infected humans demonstrate the presence of *H. pylori* within gastric epithelial cells.[163,164] The ability of *H. pylori* to invade mammalian epithelial cells has been reported in gastric adenocarcinoma-derived epithelial cell lines (AGS),[165–168] and confirmed in gastric epithelial progenitor cells, in a murine model of infection.[169] Furthermore, Amieva and colleagues[167] reported that following *H. pylori* invasion of AGS cells, large vacuolar compartments are formed, where bacteria can persist for long periods of time. In addition, the authors demonstrated that *H. pylori* can egress from this compartment and infect other gastric cells.

The large bacteria-containing vacuoles in AGS cells originate through the fusion of late endocytic organelles during a process mediated by the VacA toxin-dependent retention of the small GTPase Rab7. The interactions between Rab7, and its downstream effector Rab interacting lysosomal protein (RILP), are necessary for the formation of the bacterial compartment. VacA-mediated sequestration of active Rab7 disrupts

the full maturation of vacuoles, as assessed by the lack of both colocalization with cathepsin D and degradation of internalized cargo in the *H. pylori*-containing vacuole. Thus, VacA-dependent isolation of the *H. pylori*-containing vacuole from bactericidal components of the lysosomal pathway promotes bacterial survival and contributes to the persistence of infection.[117]

Quorum Sensing. The perception of intestinal microbes as individual single cell prokaryotes, living within a highly sophisticated multicellular organism, has gradually revised with the recognition of bacterial communication and environmental sensing systems, capable of producing and responding to hormone-like chemicals. This bacterial signaling system, termed quorum sensing (QS), enables the bacterial communities to respond to their own density, and to changing environmental circumstances, by modifying their gene expression, in a similar fashion to hormones in mammals.[170] The LuxS system is central to QS, where by converting ribose homocysteine into homocysteine and 4,5-dihydrody-2, 3-pentanedione (DPD), it provides the precursor for the autoinducer-2 (AI-2).[171] AI-2 is a furanone, which can act on a variety of bacterial species, including *E. coli* and *Salmonella*, where it binds to the periplasmic receptor LsrB, causing changes in virulence gene expression.[172] LuxS is present in many commensal bacteria as well, where it is involved in producing both AI-2 and AI-3, suggesting a possible role in interspecies communication.[173]

The role of QS is well documented in EHEC. The EHEC locus of enterocyte effacement (LEE) encodes a T3SS, including the bacterial adhesin (intimin) receptor (Tir), which together promote the intimate adhesion to epithelial cells. The LEE-encoded regulator (Ler), which is encoded itself on the *LEE1* operon, activates the LEE genes. Most of the toxic effects EHEC induces are the result of Shiga toxin (Stx) types 1 and 2, whose genes are both located on a λ-like bacteriophage. Activation of this bacteriophage is triggered by bacterial cell stresses (such as disruption of DNA replication, proteins, or membranes, which can be induced by antibiotics), resulting in entry into a lytic cycle and release of Stx.[174] Both the *Stx* and *LEE* genes are sensitive to QS through the AI-3/LuxS system. Although QS is usually utilized by resident bacteria, and possibly by the host, to sense their environment, EHEC can rely on the same system as a signal, indicating the environment is appropriate for activation of virulence genes.[172]

Host involvement in QS has been suggested by recent observations. Epinephrine and norepinephrine activate the LEE genes in a way similar to LuxS.[175] These findings are supported by the inhibition of EHEC adhesion to intestinal epithelium in the presence of propranolol, a feature that may be utilized for therapeutic interventions.[176] Therefore, pathogens use the same QS tools to probe microbial and host-derived signals, representing another mode of communication between

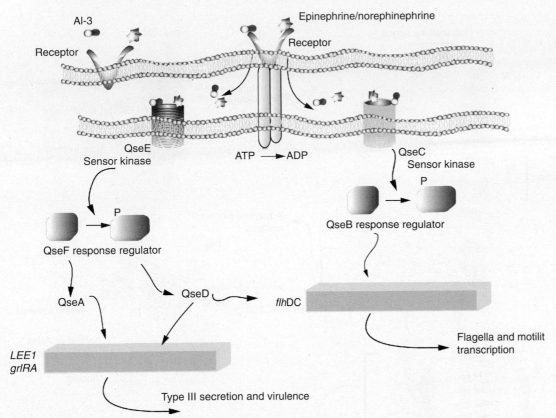

Figure 7 Qourum sensing by enterohemorrhagic *E. coli* (EHEC). Extracellular stimuli, such as the autoinducer-3 (AI-3) and epinephrine or norepinephrine, are sensed by a bacterial outer-membrane receptor. This leads to the activation of two sensor kinases, QseE and QseC. The signal is then transduced to the bacterial cytoplasm. QseE phosphorylates the response regulator QseF, eventually leading to transcription of the LEE genes by nuclear translocation of the transcription factor QseA. The *grlRA* operon, which is involved in regulating the expression of LEE genes, is also activated by QseA. Similarly, QseD is involved in modulating expression of the LEE and flagella genes. The second kinase, QseC, phosphorylates the QseB response regulator, which then binds to *flhDC* and activates expression of the genes involved in flagella activity and motility. As a result, EHEC bacteria can respond to environmental stimuli by expression of virulence genes. (Adapted from reference 172.)

these species. Recent findings indicate a complementary component to this complex, whereby the host is affected by bacterial autoinducers, resulting in modifications of cytokine production and apoptosis.[177]

PHYSIOLOGY AND PATHOPHYSIOLOGY OF HOST–MICROBE RESPONSES

Beyond the physical obstacle to pathogens that the epithelial barrier provides, several physiologic responses serve to prevent pathogenic bacteria, or their effectors, from breaching the barrier, and to respond to their presence. These functions are achieved by the presence of apical junctional complexes, secretory ability of epithelial cells (which likely serves to wash out virulence factors), recruitment of innate and adaptive immune responses, as well as other mechanisms.

Apical Junctional Complexes

Recent advances in the understanding of the apical junctional complexes (AJCs) have emphasized their importance, complexity, and vulnerability. The transmembrane proteins, which comprise the tight junctions (TJs), include occludins, claudins, junctional adhesion molecules (JAMs), and the coxsackie plaque receptor (CAR). These proteins are linked to the cytoskeleton through cytoplasmic

plaque proteins, including the PDZ domain-containing scaffolding protein, zonula occludens (ZO).[178] In adherens junctions (AJs), E-cadherin, which is mainly intracellular, but contains a transmembrane domain, is linked to proteins of the catenin family, primarily to β-catenin.[16] The actin cytoskeleton supports the junctional complexes. AJCs are highly regulated dynamic structures, involving several host cellular signaling pathways, which serve as natural targets for pathogenic virulence. Hyperphosphorylated occludin and ZO-1 have been localized to raft-like membrane microdomains (lipid rafts), and translocation of these proteins from the lipid rafts is associated with increased permeability, implicating a role in barrier.[179] By controlling the gate into the interior of the host, microbes can bypass many of the host defense mechanisms mentioned above, and as a result, traverse the monolayer via the paracellular route, disseminate, and cause disease. Defects in AJC structure and function have been implicated in IBD patients and animal models of IBD.[180] In this context, the adverse effects of microbes on junctions may offer a potential bridge connecting bacteria to IBD pathogenesis. In order to better evaluate the integrity of the AJCs, and the effects of physiology, pathogens and other stresses, *in vitro* monolayer models are tested. Infection of such polarized monolayers with pathogenic bacteria results in a decrease

in transepithelial electrical resistance (TER), reflecting increased ion flux, as well as increased permeability toward macromolecules.[181,182]

AJCs' important role in maintaining barrier integrity is displayed in multiple infection models affecting the junctions. Furthermore, murine models involving mutations in key junction proteins, such as cadherins, result in intestinal inflammation, presumably due to barrier breakdown and bacterial translocation.[183] Overall, AJC targeting can be mediated either by bacterial toxins, by direct contact of the pathogen, or by indirect effects on signaling pathways involved in host regulation of the junctions, and phosphorylation, or dephosphorylation, of junction-associated proteins. By affecting AJCs, pathogens can breakdown the intestinal barrier, resulting in enhanced fluid secretion, diarrhea, and increased transmission to other hosts.

A proportion of the common intestinal anaerobe, *Bacteroides fragilis*, secrete an enterotoxin named fragilysin, which is a zinc metalloproteinase, capable of cleaving the extracellular portion of the adherens junction protein E-cadherin, resulting in reduced TER and increased mannitol flux across the monolayer.[184,185] Interestingly, primary adult human colonic epithelial cells treated with the *B. fragilis* toxin show heterogeneity in their response,[186] suggesting a not yet identified host factor, which may be involved in permeability-related susceptibility to infection, or to IBD.[187] Recent findings implicate a host receptor to the toxin, as well as a potential additional protease-activated receptor, on the epithelial cells, as potential mediaters of *B. fragilis* toxin effects.[188] Another common cause of toxin-mediated diarrhea is *Clostridium perfringens*. The *C. perfringens* enterotoxin (CPE) is a 35 kDa toxin, which forms complexes at the host membrane, capable of binding and internalizing occludin and claudin-4, thus depleting the AJCs of these essential proteins, thereby compromising barrier integrity.[189] In contrast, another *C. perfringens* toxin, epsilon, decreases TER without binding and translocating AJC proteins. Instead, this toxin may alter the permeability by forming membrane pores.[190] *C. difficile* toxins A and B degrade actin filaments by modifying the small GTPase Rho family of proteins, which are involved in cytoskeletal regulation, resulting in redistribution of ZO-1 and occludens.[191] A recent publication focusing on the effect of the *C. sordellii* lethal toxin, which is a recognized cause of hemorrhagic enteritis, has shown a similar affect on the Rho GTPase Rac1, leading to modification in basolateral actin. This alteration in actin results in redistribution of the AJ complex of E-cadherin-catenin, causing epithelial barrier disruption.[192]

EPEC has a well-established effect on epithelial monolayer permeability and AJC protein redistribution, as shown in both *in vitro* and in vivo studies.[193,194] The T3SS effector EspF, as well as EspG and EspG2, are responsible for the effect on the junctions.[193] The precise role of EspG and EspG2 is not clear, since they do not directly alter junction proteins,[195] but rather may have an effect

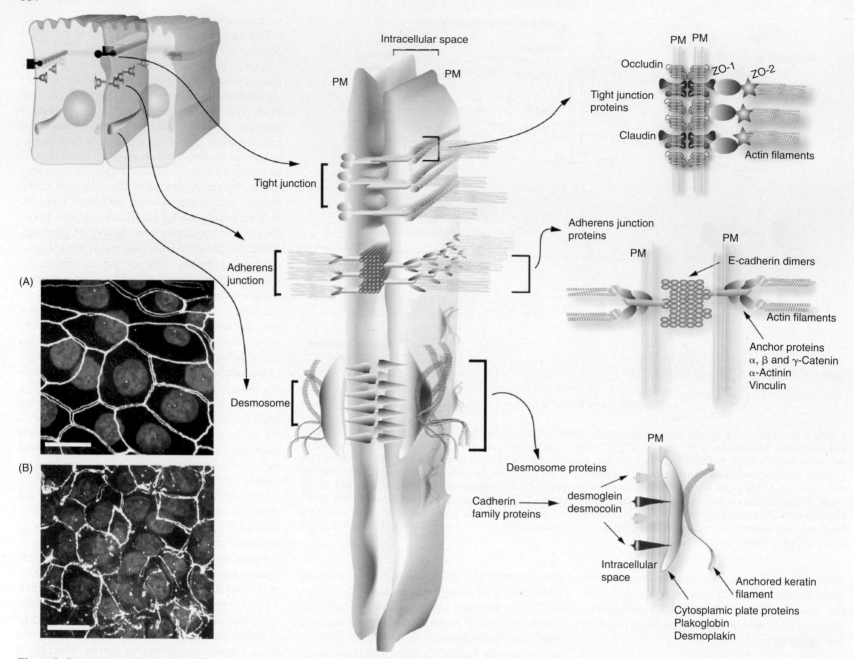

Figure 8 Components and structure of epithelial apical junction complexes and desmosomes. Apical junction complexes (AJCs) are composed of tight junctions (TJs) and adherens junctions (AJs). Desmosomes are located basal to AJCs, on the lateral borders between cells. AJCs seal the gaps between cells by forming continuous fence-like borders (A: enface confocal XY image of uninfected epithelial monolayers stained with anti-ZO-1 and DAPI, staining the nucleus). TJs are composed of transmembrane proteins (claudins and occludins), which are connected to the cytoskeleton by the adaptor proteins zonula occludens (ZO). Similarly, AJs contain the transmembrane E-cadherin, which is linked to proteins of the catenin family. Transmembrane junction proteins form a "zipper-like" interaction with similar proteins from neighboring cells, thus providing intimate adhesion. Bacterial-mediated disruption of these structures, by mechanisms presented in the text, results in loss of the normal pattern, and barrier disruption (B: EHEC-infected monolayers, demonstrating loss of ZO-1 continuity). Bar = 25 μm.

on microtubules.[196] A potential target for EPEC may be the myosin II light chain kinase (MLCK), which, when phosphorylated, increases permeability, as supported by the finding that inhibition of MLCK phosphorylation by an MLCK inhibitor restores TER of EPEC-infected monolayers.[197] Together, these pathogen-induced effects lead to alterations in junction-related protein distribution and phosphorylation, loss of protein–protein interaction, contraction of the perijunctional actinomyosin ring, and the emergence of aberrant tight junction strands,[198] all potentially contributing to the development of diarrhea. EHEC infection results in a decrease in TER as well, although this appears to be mediated through different mechanisms, which can be reversed by the effect of transforming growth factor (TGF)β.[199]

Many other bacteria induce alterations in AJCs, leading to permeability impairment. *S. typhimurium,* through *Salmonella* pathogenicity island-1 (SPI-1)-dependent type 3 secretion of several virulence factors (SopB, SopE, SopE2, and SipA), leads to disruption of tight junction structure and function.[200] *C. jejuni*-mediated barrier disruption involves phosphorylation of several junction proteins, including ERK, JNK, and p38 MAPK, as well as redistribution of lipid-raft-associated hyperphosphorylated occludin, and activation of NF-κB and AP-1 transcription pathways, although not all of these alterations have been directly connected to monolayer disruption.[201] A recent in vivo study, using the attaching-effacing (A–E) lesion inducing mouse pathogen *C. rodentium*, demonstrated alterations

in junctional protein distribution only during the phase of attachment of the enteropathogen to epithelial cells, and not during the subsequent inflammatory phase coupled with bacterial clearance, suggesting that junction disruption is mediated directly by bacterial attachment.[202] All these findings represent the diversity and complexity of the bacterial-induced, and in many cases host-mediated, changes in AJCs.

Helicobacter pylori's cag PAI codifies the cytotoxin-associated gene (*cagA*).[203] Injected CagA localizes to the host cell plasma membrane, where it is targeted for tyrosine phosphorylation by Src kinases within a repeated specific 5 amino acid EPIYA (Glu-Pro-Ile-Tyr- Ala) motif localized in the carboxy terminal region of the protein.[204] Once phosphorylated, CagA functions like an adapter protein and binds to a cytoplasmic SRC homology 2 (SH2) domain containing protein tyrosine phosphatase SHP2, activating its phosphatase activity and forming a complex that initiates mitogenic signaling, cell scattering, and elongation involving rearrangement of the F-actin cytoskeleton.[205–207] Recent evidence shows that nonphosphorylated CagA also interacts with apical junctional protein components JAM and ZO-1, forming a structural complex that alters tight junctions at sites of *H. pylori* infection.[208] In addition, expression of CagA disrupts cell polarity and cell–cell adhesion, prompting an epithelial-to-mesenchymal transition phenotype, which may contribute to its oncogenic effect.[209]

Epithelial Fluid and Electrolyte Secretion

Fluid and electrolyte homeostasis is one of the central roles of the intestinal epithelium, capable of absorbing liters of fluid from oral intake and mucosal secretions. This task is carried out by a highly regulated electrolyte transport system, coupled with the barrier provided by the epithelial lining. Enteropathogens interact with these epithelial functions by enhancing, or inhibiting, absorption and secretion, as well as modifying regulatory pathways.

Chloride is considered the key ion in transport, usually acting as the driving force for transport of other ions, such as paracellular sodium movement and subsequent water osmosis. A basolateral Na/K ATPase provides a sodium gradient, which drives chloride into the cell through the Na/K/2Cl cotransporter. The cAMP-dependent cystic fibrosis transmembrane regulator (CFTR), as well as the calcium-activated chloride channel (CaCC), which are both located apically, secrete chloride into the lumen.[210] These transporters are frequent targets for pathogens. *V. cholerae* infection typically results in dramatic secretory diarrhea, producing large amounts of fluid thorough the effects of several enterotoxins. Most of this effect results from the best known cAMP-activating enterotoxin, cholera toxin (CT), which consists of a single enzymatically active A subunit, bound to 5 identical B subunits, which are responsible for the cell surface binding. *E. coli* heat liable enterotoxins I and II (LTI&II) follow the same structural and functional pattern, although they differ in their binding to GM_1 gangliosides on the cell membrane.[211] Although it has been known for decades that CT subunit A increases intracellular cAMP, thus activating chloride secretion and causing diarrhea, gaps in understanding this process have been filled only over the last few years. GM_1 gangliosides are localized to lipid raft microdomains after CT binding, as indicated by the reversal of CT action by cholesterol chelation using β-methyl-cyclodextrin, which disrupts lipid rafts.[212] Nonclathrin-mediated endocytosis takes place, trafficking the toxin to the trans-Golgi network.[213] Retrograde transport of the CT to the endoplasmic reticulum (ER) occurs due to the presence of the KDEL sequence on the A2 subunit, which is recognized by a host shuttling protein, which is responsible for returning

lost ER proteins to the Golgi.[214] The toxin then utilizes yet another host protein, protein disulfide isomerase, to reduce disulfide bonds, thus discarding the, now unnecessary, A2 and B subunits, releasing the A subunit into the cytosol, where it is unfolded by ER chaperones.[215] The enzymatically active A subunit then irreversibly ADP-ribosylates G proteins, causing a variety of cellular reactions, including the activation of the adenylate cyclase system, and accumulation of cAMP. Activation of the cAMP-dependent protein kinase A leads to phosphorylation of serine residues on the CFTR regulatory domain, which then leads to CFTR activation, and secretory diarrhea.[211] A recent report describing the use of CFTR inhibitors to decrease CT mediated diarrhea in isolated mouse intestinal loops provides support for this complex model.[216]

Similar to cAMP, cGMP (which is the result of guanylate cyclase activity) can also cause CFTR activation. Guanylin and uroguanylin are small peptides produced by goblet cells that activate guanylate cyclase C (GC-C). Another *E. coli* enterotoxin, the heat stable toxin (ST), is structurally and functionally homologous to guanylin, and activates GC-C on the basolateral surface of epithelial cells.[217] The action of *E. coli* ST, as well as other bacterial toxins with similar effects, on GC-C has also been suggested to potentially promote resistance to colon cancer, through the apoptotic effect of cGMP elevation, although this hypothesis requires support from additional models.[218,219]

Chloride secretion, and the resulting fluid output, can also be induced by activation of the CaCC in response to increased cytosolic calcium. Many enteropathogens utilize CaCC to induce diarrhea. This is achieved by releasing calcium from intracellular stores (mitochondrial or non-mitochondrial) or by calcium transfer from the extracellular space. The regulation of calcium release from stores is mediated by several signaling pathways, including PLC-mediated inositol 3-phosphate (IP3) production (see below), which results in opening of ER calcium reservoirs and release into the cytoplasm. Several bacterial virulence factors, such as the *Yersinia enterocolitica* heat stable enterotoxin, have been shown to increase calcium levels through this pathway, resulting in diarrhea.[220]

Host factors, including hormones and inflammatory cytokines, affect electrolyte secretion in many ways, some of which can be modified by enteropathogens. Some of these factors, including prostaglandins and nitric oxide, which have been mentioned above, serve as examples of such an effect. NO-induced chloride secretion is mediated by cGMP after infection with a large variety of enteropathogens.[61] Chloride secretion is also induced by enteric nerve system stimuli, such as the neuropeptide galanin, which binds to the galanin-1 receptor (Gal-1R). Several enteropathogens, including *S. typhimurium*, *Shigella flexneri*, and pathogenic *E. coli*, induce Gal-1R expression, thereby upregulating the effect of galanin.[221] This process may be synergistically enhanced by the activation of inflammatory

cascades by these microbes, since both IL-1 and tumor necrosis factor (TNF)-α can induce galanin gene transcription, as demonstrated in cultured adrenochromaffin cells.[222]

Activation of Inflammation and Signaling Pathways

The gut epithelial layer induces a controlled and balanced inflammatory response to eliminate pathogens, while attempting to limit the destructive consequences of inflammation. Various defects in this homeostasis can result in a wide range of disorders. Therefore, from the host's perspective, the key elements ensuring health regarding inflammation are: constant surveillance, prevention, effective and appropriate initiation and recruitment, and, as is now becoming more and more evident, precise regulation, and termination of inflammation.

Many enteropathogens will benefit from avoidance of inflammation, and thus, have developed parallel mechanisms to evade or bypass recognition, and to downregulate and interfere with inflammation. In contrast, the consequences of inflammation, such as diarrhea, barrier breakdown, and colonic hyperplasia, may benefit pathogens by enhancing their colonization, survival, and spread.[223]

Thus, a large spectrum of inflammatory processes mediated by host–microbial interactions occurs. For example, commensal bacteria generally avoid induction of inflammation, and many induce an anti-inflammatory response, in order to minimize damage.[224] Some noninvasive microbes, such as *G. lamblia*, typically cause, at most, only minimal mucosal inflammation,[225] while others, represented by *C. difficile*, can induce (by toxin production) severe mucosal changes observed in biopsies, coupled with significant cytokine and chemokine responses.[226] On the other hand, adherent and invasive bacteria vary in the responses they inflict, with some mainly adherent bacteria, such as EPEC, capable of inducing severe inflammation, while other pathogens with more dominant invasive capabilities may only occasionally cause significant inflammation, like in the case of *Entamoeba histolytica* (although most invasive organisms, such as *Salmonella* and *Shigella*, induce a significant inflammatory response).[227]

The basic model for many cellular pathways includes ligands binding to receptors, which infer biochemical or conformational changes in intracellular mediators (most of which involve phosphorylation of proteins), eventually leading to nuclear translocation of a transcription factor, and expression of target genes, or modification of other cellular processes, including cell survival and death. In the case of inflammatory cascades in epithelial cells, the common initiating factor is usually the presence of a bacterial factor, or recognition of one by the host, and the common final pathway is usually the production of inflammatory cytokines and chemokines. The diversity of responses is derived from the presence of many ligands, receptors, pathways and gene products, many of which interact with each other.

Host pattern recognition molecules (PRMs) are structured to recognize microbe-associated molecular patterns (MAMPs). PRMs are located both on the plasma membrane and intracellularly. The main MAMPs recognized by membrane-bound TLRs include peptidoglycans and lipoproteins (TLR2), LPS (TLR4), and Flagellin (TLR5). Intracellular PRMs include other TLRs, such as TLR9 (recognizing unmethylated bacterial CpG DNA) and TLR7 (double-stranded RNA), as well as the NOD proteins.[59] Much attention has been directed toward these receptors, especially since polymorphisms in NOD2 (also know as CARD15), which identifies the muramyl dipeptide portion of peptidoglycan, have been linked to increased susceptibility to Crohn's disease,[228,229] and since recent findings have correlated mutations in NOD1 (CARD4), which recognizes the GlcNAc-MurNAc tripeptide motif of peptidoglycan,[230] to IBD,[231] and possibly to disease outcome of *H. pylori* infection.[232]

Upon activation of the PRMs, downstream signaling pathways are activated, resulting, in most cases, in nuclear translocation of NF-κB. This is achieved by recruitment of adaptor molecules, including MyD88. MyD88 then activates the IL-1 receptor associated kinases (IRAKs), which then (after inducing self-phosphorylation) interact with TNF receptor-associated factor 6 (TRAF6) to activate the mitogen-activated protein (MAP) kinases (see below).[233] NF-κB can also be activated by other cytokines, such as TNF-α and IL-1. This is generally achieved by phosphorylation of the inhibitory factor IκB by IκB kinase (IKK), which appears to be the common pathway of the various stimuli. This pathway is also regulated by the inhibitory effect of IRAK-M and the inhibitory Toll-interacting protein (Tollip).[233] NF-κB is involved in the transcription of multiple inflammatory mediators (including IL-1β, IL-6, IL-8, TNF, ICAM1), emphasizing its central role in intestinal inflammation.[234] Enteropathogens can induce activation of inflammatory cascades in several other ways, as will be presented in the following description of central signaling pathways, their interactions with pathogens, and the resulting effects.

Expression of PRMs in the intestinal mucosa has been tailored to accommodate the need for attenuated response of the epithelium to common bacterial stimuli under normal conditions. For example, TLR4 requires coexpression of CD14 and MD-2 in order to develop a full response to bacterial LPS. These coreceptors show low basal expression, thereby preventing overstimulation of inflammatory cytokines by resident microbes.[235] One of the suggested mechanisms by which cells respond to invasive bacteria, while remaining tolerant to commensals, may include sequestration of TLR4 in the Golgi apparatus, thus requiring internalization of LPS, or invasion, for activation to occur.[236] Of interest is the recent observation of TLR recognition of commensal bacteria by the gut epithelium, which results in production of cytoprotective factors, including IL-6 and heat-shock proteins, which help maintain intestinal homeostasis.[4] In addition, while short-term LPS stimulation of epithelial cells causes an increase in inflammation, long-term stimulation with LPS or lipoteichoic acid (LTA) results in hyporesponsiveness and tolerance, as reflected by a decrease in TLR expression and IRAK phosphorylation, possibly due to an elevation in Tollip expression.[237] A different mechanism of regulating overstimulation is the basolateral expression of LTR5 on the epithelial layer.[238] In the case of *S. typhimurium*, transcytosis of flagellin from the apical to basolateral aspect of polarized cells does not require passage of intact bacterium. This appears to be mediated by flagellin-containing vesicles, whose presence depends on the *Salmonella* pathogenicity island (SPI)-2.[239]

One of the central signaling pathways involved in many cellular processes is the MAP kinase (MAPK) pathway. This pathway includes three parallel cascades, ERK, JNK, and p38, which are all activated through the initial activation of MAPK kinase kinase (MAPKKK), which itself is activated by a receptor tyrosine kinase, through the recruitment of the active small GTPase, Ras. Some MAPKs are involved in phosphorylation of IKK, thus inducing NF-κB activation, as well as recruitment of other inflammatory reactions. For example, *S. typhimurium* activates the ERK1/2 and p38 pathways in a calcium and T3SS dependent manner, resulting in increased IL-8.[240,241] EPEC, on the other hand, activates all three MAPK cascades, leading to calcium independent IL-8 secretion and TJ disruption.[242] *H. pylori* CagA similarly induces IL-8 secretion, in an MAPK and NF-κB-dependent manner.[243]

Phospholipase Cγ (PLCγ) is a receptor-tyrosine kinase activated phosphatase, which, in turn, hydrolyzes the membrane phospholipid phosphatidylinositol-4,5-bisphosphate (PIP2) into inositol-1,4,5-triphosphate (IP3) and diacylglycerol (DAG), which are then involved in release of calcium from intracellular stores and protein kinase C (PKC) activation, respectively. PKC includes eleven known subtypes, which are divided into three types: conventional, novel, and atypical, according to the dependence of their activation on calcium and DAG. The atypical PKCζ responds to TNFα by IKK phosphorylation, as well as phosphorylation of the p65 subunit of NF-κB, which increases its binding to DNA. SipA, an *S. typhimurium* SPI-1-encoded protein, causes activation of the GTPase ARF6, which then activates phospholipase D, generating DAG, which in turn recruits PKC. This cascade of cellular responses to SipA takes place at the apical membrane, leading to the release of the "pathogen elicited epithelial derived chemoattractant" (PEEC) into the lumen, resulting in neutrophil transmigration across the epithelial monolayer, into the luminal side.[244] Recently, PKCα and PKCε have been described as mediators of activation of the Na+/H+ exchanger 2 (NHE2) in epithelial cells, in response to EPEC infection.[245]

JAK-STAT pathways can be induced by several receptor stimuli, including the proinflammatory antimicrobial mediator, interferon (IFN). IFN expression is usually induced by activation of PRRs, or other inflammatory stimuli. The three types of IFN bind to equivalent receptors, usually causing dimerization of the STAT receptors, and downstream phosphorylation of the various JAK and STAT proteins, eventually leading to modification of nuclear transcription, and, in most cases, an antimicrobial effect.[246] Bacteria, such as EHEC, have developed methods to inhibit this pathway, by specifically preventing the phosphorylation of STAT1 in response to IFNγ after contact with epithelial cells, thus debilitating the host defenses.[247]

The main potential benefits from these recent insights into the complex and interacting signaling pathways involved in enteric pathogen-induced inflammation, are the development of novel therapeutic strategies aimed at modifying these cascades. Furthermore, recent advances in the understanding of some of the mechanisms involved in IBD pathogenesis serve to emphasize the consequences of inflammatory responses to microbes. Regulation of inflammation, controlling when these pathways are turned "on" and "off," as well as alterations in signaling pathways, could be one of the primary defects in IBD, leading to uncontrolled inflammatory response to simple triggers, loss of tolerance to commensal bacteria, failure to regulate inflammation, or barrier breakdown. In addition, changes in PRM expression patterns, as reported in IBD, may result in alterations in inflammatory response and chronic immune dysregulation.[248]

FUTURE PERSPECTIVES

The main aim of this chapter is to provide a synopsis of the explosion of data in the fields of cellular microbiology, gut ecology, mucosal immunity, and other areas related to microbial–gut epithelial interactions. Advancing molecular techniques, which can be implemented utilizing *in vitro* cell cultures, animal models, and human samples, will continue to provide important insights into this complex ecosystem.

Some of the promising areas of research will most likely utilize microarray analysis of both microbial and host genes, in response to infection, which will assist in identifying candidate genes and proteins for research, and possibly, therapeutic applications. For example, microarrays of human intestinal Caco-2 cells infected with *C. jejuni* have revealed upregulation of multiple genes involved in cell growth, inflammation, cytokine production, and more.[249] The host genetic determinants affecting susceptibility, response, and outcome, have been termed "infectogenomics."[250] Studying these factors may assist in revealing differences in interspecies responses to infection (eg, why *E. coli* O157: H7 can cause severe disease in humans, while only rarely effecting cattle), as well as individual intraspecies variation (eg, the potential beneficial effect of heterozygosity for CFTR mutations regarding intestinal diarrheagenic infections).

Analysis of microbial genetic determinants of virulence (as part of a "pathogen genome project"), as well as other molecular techniques, will help overcome the disadvantages imposed by the inability to culture many of the resident microbes in the gut.

Although genetic analysis (studying DNA or mRNA) of host–microbe interactions will be most informative, other more functional methods may give a more precise cross-sectional view of this interplay. This will be achieved by methods like proteomics of the infected tissue or bacterial protein analysis, as well as proteomics of the intracellular niche. In vivo fluorescent confocal microscopy and endoscopy may be other future tools.

Development of methods to characterize the intestinal microbial flora will provide valuable information, essential for analyzing this complex ecosystem. The use of the 16S rRNA diversity, as well as other advanced molecular techniques, in order to classify the intestinal flora phylogeny, has provided researchers with insights into the vast array of microbes within the gut.[251,252] Pioneer research in this field of microbial diversity within the gut has demonstrated the extent of inter- and intraindividual variability, as well as the differences between mucosa-associated and luminal bacteria, which provide significant challenges in defining the intestinal flora of a population.[253] Attempts to define the mucosa-associated microbes in disease cohorts, such as IBD, may offer important clues regarding the role of microbes in health and disease.[254]

Use of germ-free animal models, which are then colonized in a controlled fashion by selective known microbes, have already provided important insights. In most cases, *Bacteroides thetaiotaomicron* is used as a representative of the normal flora, thus providing a model for commensal–gut interactions.[255] More complex models, including introduction of a combination of predetermined microbes, together with molecular techniques, will likely further develop our understanding of health and disease in this ecosystem.[14]

Flora-defined animal models will serve as excellent tools to investigate not only host–microbial interactions, but also the microbial–microbial interplay. This tool will serve to better define the use of probiotics. Furthermore, combining these methods with human genomic approaches may serve to predict an individual's risk of disease, and perhaps to determine the microbial profile and to choose the most appropriate beneficial regimen (including pro/prebiotics) of prevention or therapy.

REFERENCES

1. Elson CO, Cong Y, McCracken VJ, et al. Experimental models of inflammatory bowel disease reveal innate, adaptive, and regulatory mechanisms of host dialogue with the microbiota. Immunol Rev 2005;206:260–76.
2. Sartor RB. Mechanisms of disease: Pathogenesis of Crohn's disease and ulcerative colitis. Nat Clin Pract Gastroenterol Hepatol 2006;3:390–407.
3. Tlaskalova-Hogenova H, Stepankova R, Hudcovic T, et al. Commensal bacteria (normal microflora), mucosal immunity and chronic inflammatory and autoimmune diseases. Immunol Lett 2004;93:97–108.
4. Rakoff-Nahoum S, Paglino J, Eslami-Varzaneh F, et al. Recognition of commensal microflora by toll-like receptors is required for intestinal homeostasis. Cell 2004;118:229–41.
5. Kelly D, Conway S, Aminov R. Commensal gut bacteria: Mechanisms of immune modulation. Trends Immunol 2005;26:326–33.
6. Falkow S. Is persistent bacterial infection good for your health? Cell 2006;124:699–702.
7. Hooper LV, Gordon JI. Commensal host-bacterial relationships in the gut. Science 2001;292:1115–8.
8. Ley RE, Peterson DA, Gordon JI. Ecological and evolutionary forces shaping microbial diversity in the human intestine. Cell 2006;124:837–48.
9. Sherman PM, Wine E. Emerging intestinal infections. Gastroenterology and Hepatology Annual Review 2006;1:50–4.
10. Guarner F, Malagelada JR. Gut flora in health and disease. Lancet 2003;361:512–9.
11. Sartor RB. Therapeutic manipulation of the enteric microflora in inflammatory bowel diseases: Antibiotics, probiotics, and prebiotics. Gastroenterology 2004;126:1620–33.
12. Jilling T, Simon D, Lu J, et al. The roles of bacteria and TLR4 in rat and murine models of necrotizing enterocolitis. J Immunol 2006;177:3273–82.
13. Rao VP, Poutahidis T, Ge Z, et al. Innate immune inflammatory response against enteric bacteria *Helicobacter hepaticus* induces mammary adenocarcinoma in mice. Cancer Res 2006;66:7395–400.
14. Samuel BS, Gordon JI. A humanized gnotobiotic mouse model of host-archaeal-bacterial mutualism. Proc Natl Acad Sci U S A 2006;103:10011–6.
15. Moore KA, Lemischka IR. Stem cells and their niches. Science 2006;311:1880–5.
16. Laukoetter MG, Bruewer M, Nusrat A. Regulation of the intestinal epithelial barrier by the apical junctional complex. Curr Opin Gastroenterol 2006;22:85–9.
17. Lievin-Le Moal V, Servin AL. The front line of enteric host defense against unwelcome intrusion of harmful microorganisms: Mucins, antimicrobial peptides, and microbiota. Clin Microbiol Rev 2006;19:315–37.
18. Pino V, Ramsauer VP, Salas P, et al. Membrane Mucin Muc4 induces density-dependent changes in ERK activation in mammary epithelial and tumor cells: Role in reversal of contact inhibition. J Biol Chem 2006;281:29411–20.
19. Singh PK, Hollingsworth MA. Cell surface-associated mucins in signal transduction. Trends Cell Biol 2006;16:467–76.
20. Lievin-Le Moal V, Servin AL, Coconnier-Polter MH. The increase in mucin exocytosis and the upregulation of MUC genes encoding for membrane-bound mucins induced by the thiol-activated exotoxin listeriolysin O is a host cell defence response that inhibits the cell-entry of *Listeria monocytogenes*. Cell Microbiol 2005;7:1035–48.
21. Branka JE, Vallette G, Jarry A, et al. Early functional effects of *Clostridium difficile* toxin A on human colonocytes. Gastroenterology 1997;112:1887–94.
22. Lee H, Kobayashi M, Wang P, et al. Expression cloning of cholesterol alpha-glucosyltransferase, a unique enzyme that can be inhibited by natural antibiotic gastric mucin O-glycans, from *Helicobacter pylori*. Biochem Biophys Res Commun 2006;349:1235–41.
23. Slomiany BL, Slomiany A. Cytosolic phospholipase A2 activation in *Helicobacter pylori* lipopolysaccharide-induced interference with gastric mucin synthesis. IUBMB Life 2006;58:217–23.
24. Slomiany BL, Slomiany A. Up-regulation in endothelin-1 by *Helicobacter pylori* lipopolysaccharide interferes with gastric mucin synthesis via epidermal growth factor receptor transactivation. Scand J Gastroenterol 2005;40:921–28.
25. Bergonzelli GE, Granato D, Pridmore RD, et al. GroEL of *Lactobacillus johnsonii* La1 (NCC 533) is cell surface associated: Potential role in interactions with the host and the gastric pathogen *Helicobacter pylori*. Infect Immun 2006;74:425–34.
26. Schaible UE, Kaufmann SH. A nutritive view on the host-pathogen interplay. Trends Microbiol 2005;13:373–80.
27. Toshima H, Hachio M, Ikemoto Y, et al. Prevalence of enteric bacteria that inhibit growth of enterohaemorrhagic *Escherichia coli* O157 in humans. Epidemiol Infect 2006;1–8.
28. Zasloff M. Antimicrobial peptides of multicellular organisms. Nature 2002;415:389–95.
29. Crouch ML, Becker LA, Bang IS, et al. The alternative sigma factor sigma is required for resistance of *Salmonella enterica* serovar Typhimurium to anti-microbial peptides. Mol Microbiol 2005;56:789–99.
30. Wehkamp J, Salzman NH, Porter E, et al. Reduced Paneth cell alpha-defensins in ileal Crohn's disease. Proc Natl Acad Sci U S A 2005;102:18129–34.
31. Kobayashi KS, Chamaillard M, Ogura Y, et al. Nod2-dependent regulation of innate and adaptive immunity in the intestinal tract. Science 2005;307:731–4.
32. Ouellette AJ. IV. Paneth cell antimicrobial peptides and the biology of the mucosal barrier. Am J Physiol 1999;277:G257–61.
33. Pazgier M, Hoover DM, Yang D, et al. Human beta-defensins. Cell Mol Life Sci 2006;63:1294–313.
34. Huang GT, Zhang HB, Kim D, et al. A model for antimicrobial gene therapy: Demonstration of human beta-defensin 2 antimicrobial activities in vivo. Hum Gene Ther 2002;13:2017–25.
35. Brogden KA. Antimicrobial peptides. Pore formers or metabolic inhibitors in bacteria? Nat Rev Microbiol 2005;3:238–50.
36. Zaalouk TK, Bajaj-Elliott M, George JT, McDonald V. Differential regulation of beta-defensin gene expression during *Cryptosporidium parvum* infection. Infect Immun 2004;72:2772–9.
37. Zilbauer M, Dorrell N, Boughan PK, et al. Intestinal innate immunity to *Campylobacter jejuni* results in induction of bactericidal human beta-defensins 2 and 3. Infect Immun 2005;73:7281–9.
38. Eckmann L, Kagnoff MF. Intestinal mucosal responses to microbial infection. Springer Semin Immunopathol 2005;27:181–96.
39. Dommett R, Zilbauer M, George JT, Bajaj-Elliott M. Innate immune defence in the human gastrointestinal tract. Mol Immunol 2005;42:903–12.
40. Iimura M, Gallo RL, Hase K, et al. Cathelicidin mediates innate intestinal defense against colonization with epithelial adherent bacterial pathogens. J Immunol 2005;174:4901–7.
41. Islam D, Bandholtz L, Nilsson J, et al. Downregulation of bactericidal peptides in enteric infections: A novel immune escape mechanism with bacterial DNA as a potential regulator. Nat Med 2001;7:180–5.
42. Schauber J, Svanholm C, Termen S, et al. Expression of the cathelicidin LL-37 is modulated by short chain fatty acids in colonocytes: Relevance of signalling pathways. Gut 2003;52:735–41.
43. Raqib R, Sarker P, Bergman P, et al. Improved outcome in shigellosis associated with butyrate induction of an endogenous peptide antibiotic. Proc Natl Acad Sci U S A 2006;103:9178–83.
44. Wehkamp J, Chu H, Shen B, et al. Paneth cell antimicrobial peptides: Topographical distribution and quantification in human gastrointestinal tissues. FEBS Lett 2006;580:5344–50.
45. Salzman NH, Chou MM, de Jong H, et al. Enteric *Salmonella* infection inhibits Paneth cell antimicrobial peptide expression. Infect Immun 2003;71:1109–15.
46. Rosenfeld Y, Shai Y. Lipopolysaccharide (Endotoxin)-host defense antibacterial peptides interactions: Role in bacterial resistance and prevention of sepsis. Biochim Biophys Acta 2006;1758:1513–22.
47. Groisman EA, Mouslim C. Sensing by bacterial regulatory systems in host and non-host environments. Nat Rev Microbiol 2006;4:705–9.
48. Fabretti F, Theilacker C, Baldassarri L, et al. Alanine esters of enterococcal lipoteichoic acid play a role in biofilm formation and resistance to antimicrobial peptides. Infect Immun 2006;74:4164–71.
49. Guina T, Yi EC, Wang H, et al. A PhoP-regulated outer membrane protease of *Salmonella enterica* serovar typhimurium promotes resistance to alpha-helical antimicrobial peptides. J Bacteriol 2000;182:4077–86.
50. Canny G, Levy O, Furuta GT, et al. Lipid mediator-induced expression of bactericidal/ permeability-increasing protein (BPI) in human mucosal epithelia. Proc Natl Acad Sci U S A 2002;99:3902–7.
51. Canny G, Cario E, Lennartsson A, et al. Functional and biochemical characterization of epithelial bactericidal/ permeability-increasing protein. Am J Physiol Gastrointest Liver Physiol 2006;290:G557–67.
52. Levy O. A neutrophil-derived anti-infective molecule: Bactericidal/permeability-increasing protein. Antimicrob Agents Chemother 2000;44:2925–31.
53. Levin M, Quint PA, Goldstein B, et al. Recombinant bactericidal/permeability-increasing protein (rBPI21) as adjunctive treatment for children with severe meningococcal sepsis: A randomised trial. rBPI21 Meningococcal Sepsis Study Group. Lancet 2000;356:961–7.
54. Mashimo H, Wu DC, Podolsky DK, Fishman MC. Impaired defense of intestinal mucosa in mice lacking intestinal trefoil factor. Science 1996;274:262–5.
55. Hoffmann W. Trefoil factor family (TFF) peptides: Regulators of mucosal regeneration and repair, and more. Peptides 2004;25:727–30.
56. Clyne M, Dillon P, Daly S, et al. *Helicobacter pylori* interacts with the human single-domain trefoil protein TFF1. Proc Natl Acad Sci U S A 2004;101:7409–14.

57. Mumy KL, McCormick BA. Events at the host-microbial interface of the gastrointestinal tract. II. Role of the intestinal epithelium in pathogen-induced inflammation. Am J Physiol Gastrointest Liver Physiol 2005;288:G854–9.
58. Johanesen PA, Dwinell MB. Flagellin-independent regulation of chemokine host defense in *Campylobacter jejuni*-infected intestinal epithelium. Infect Immun 2006;74:3437–47.
59. Meylan E, Tschopp J, Karin M. Intracellular pattern recognition receptors in the host response. Nature 2006;442:39–44.
60. Fukata M, Chen A, Klepper A, et al. Cox-2 is regulated by Toll-like receptor-4 (TLR4) signaling: Role in proliferation and apoptosis in the intestine. Gastroenterology 2006;131:862–77.
61. Resta-Lenert S, Barrett KE. Enteroinvasive bacteria alter barrier and transport properties of human intestinal epithelium: Role of iNOS and COX-2. Gastroenterology 2002;122:1070–87.
62. Witthoft T, Eckmann L, Kim JM, Kagnoff MF. Enteroinvasive bacteria directly activate expression of iNOS and NO production in human colon epithelial cells. Am J Physiol 1998;275:G564–71.
63. Maresca M, Miller D, Quitard S, et al. Enteropathogenic *Escherichia coli* (EPEC) effector-mediated suppression of antimicrobial nitric oxide production in a small intestinal epithelial model system. Cell Microbiol 2005;7:1749–62.
64. Eckmann L, Laurent F, Langford TD, et al. Nitric oxide production by human intestinal epithelial cells and competition for arginine as potential determinants of host defense against the lumen-dwelling pathogen *Giardia lamblia*. J Immunol 2000;164:1478–87.
65. Wallace JL, Caliendo G, Santagada V, et al. Gastrointestinal safety and anti-inflammatory effects of a hydrogen sulfide-releasing diclofenac derivative in the rat. Gastroenterology 2007;132:261–71.
66. Macpherson AJ, Geuking MB, McCoy KD. Immune responses that adapt the intestinal mucosa to commensal intestinal bacteria. Immunology 2005;115:153–62.
67. Mavris M, Sansonetti P. Microbial-gut interactions in health and disease. Epithelial cell responses. Best Pract Res Clin Gastroenterol 2004;18:373–86.
68. Pizarro-Cerda J, Cossart P. Bacterial adhesion and entry into host cells. Cell 2006;124:715–27.
69. Sansonetti PJ. War and peace at mucosal surfaces. Nat Rev Immunol 2004;4:953–64.
70. Nougayrede JP, Fernandes PJ, Donnenberg MS. Adhesion of enteropathogenic *Escherichia coli* to host cells. Cell Microbiol 2003;5:359–72.
71. Sharon N. Carbohydrates as future anti-adhesion drugs for infectious diseases. Biochim Biophys Acta 2006;1760:527–37.
72. Finlay BB, Falkow S. Common themes in microbial pathogenicity revisited. Microbiol Mol Biol Rev 1997;61:136–69.
73. Telford JL, Barocchi MA, Margarit I, et al. Pili in gram-positive pathogens. Nat Rev Microbiol 2006;4:509–19.
74. Olsen A, Jonsson A, Normark S. Fibronectin binding mediated by a novel class of surface organelles on *Escherichia coli*. Nature 1989;338:652–5.
75. Thanassi DG, Saulino ET, Hultgren SJ. The chaperone/usher pathway: A major terminal branch of the general secretory pathway. Curr Opin Microbiol 1998;1:223–31.
76. Sauer FG, Barnhart M, Choudhury D, et al. Chaperone-assisted pilus assembly and bacterial attachment. Curr Opin Struct Biol 2000;10:548–56.
77. Strom MS, Lory S. Structure-function and biogenesis of the type IV pili. Annu Rev Microbiol 1993;47:565–96.
78. Wu H, Fives-Taylor PM. Molecular strategies for fimbrial expression and assembly. Crit Rev Oral Biol Med 2001;12:101–15.
79. Soto GE, Hultgren SJ. Bacterial adhesins: Common themes and variations in architecture and assembly. J Bacteriol 1999;181:1059–71.
80. Dodson KW, Pinkner JS, Rose T, et al. Structural basis of the interaction of the pyelonephritic *E. coli* adhesin to its human kidney receptor. Cell 2001;105:733–43.
81. Lory S, Strom MS. Structure-function relationship of type-IV prepilin peptidase of Pseudomonas aeruginosa—a review. Gene 1997;192:117–21.
82. Mattick JS. Type IV pili and twitching motility. Annu Rev Microbiol 2002;56:289–314.
83. Forest KT, Satyshur KA, Worzalla GA, et al. The pilus-retraction protein PilT: Ultrastructure of the biological assembly. Acta Crystallogr D Biol Crystallogr 2004;60:978–82.
84. Maier B, Koomey M, Sheetz MP. A force-dependent switch reverses type IV pilus retraction. Proc Natl Acad Sci U S A 2004;101:10961–6.
85. Craig L, Volkmann N, Arvai AS, et al. Type IV pilus structure by cryo-electron microscopy and crystallography: Implications for pilus assembly and functions. Mol Cell 2006;23:651–62.
86. Craig L, Pique ME, Tainer JA. Type IV pilus structure and bacterial pathogenicity. Nat Rev Microbiol 2004;2:363–78.
87. Butler SM, Camilli A. Going against the grain: Chemotaxis and infection in *Vibrio cholerae*. Nat Rev Microbiol 2005;3:611–20.
88. Wu HY, Zhang XL, Pan Q, Wu J. Functional selection of a type IV pili-binding peptide that specifically inhibits *Salmonella Typhi* adhesion to/invasion of human monocytic cells. Peptides 2005;26:2057–63.
89. Girard V, Mourez M. Adhesion mediated by autotransporters of Gram-negative bacteria: Structural and functional features. Res Microbiol 2006;157:407–16.
90. Henderson IR, Navarro-Garcia F, Desvaux M, et al. Type V protein secretion pathway: The autotransporter story. Microbiol Mol Biol Rev 2004;68:692–744.
91. Ilver D, Arnqvist A, Ogren J, et al. *Helicobacter pylori* adhesin binding fucosylated histo-blood group antigens revealed by retagging. Science 1998;279:373–7.
92. Mahdavi J, Sonden B, Hurtig M, et al. *Helicobacter pylori* SabA adhesin in persistent infection and chronic inflammation. Science 2002;297:573–8.
93. Charbonneau ME, Berthiaume F, Mourez M. Proteolytic processing is not essential for multiple functions of the *Escherichia coli* autotransporter adhesin involved in diffuse adherence (AIDA-I). J Bacteriol 2006;188:8504–12.
94. Owen P, Meehan M, de Loughry-Doherty H, Henderson I. Phase-variable outer membrane proteins in *Escherichia coli*. FEMS Immunol Med Microbiol 1996;16:63–76.
95. Nummelin H, Merckel MC, Leo JC, et al. The *Yersinia* adhesin YadA collagen-binding domain structure is a novel left-handed parallel beta-roll. Embo J 2004;23:701–11.
96. Schlumberger MC, Hardt WD. *Salmonella* type III secretion effectors: Pulling the host cell's strings. Curr Opin Microbiol 2006;9:46–54.
97. Yahr TL. A critical new pathway for toxin secretion? N Engl J Med 2006;355:1171–2.
98. Hanekop N, Zaitseva J, Jenewein S, et al. Molecular insights into the mechanism of ATP-hydrolysis by the NBD of the ABC-transporter HlyB. FEBS Lett 2006;580:1036–41.
99. Delepelaire P. Type I secretion in gram-negative bacteria. Biochim Biophys Acta 2004;1694:149–61.
100. Johnson TL, Abendroth J, Hol WG, Sandkvist M. Type II secretion: From structure to function. FEMS Microbiol Lett 2006;255:175–86.
101. Cianciotto NP. Type II secretion: A protein secretion system for all seasons. Trends Microbiol 2005;13:581–8.
102. Ghosh P. Process of protein transport by the type III secretion system. Microbiol Mol Biol Rev 2004;68:771–95.
103. Yip CK, Strynadka NC. New structural insights into the bacterial type III secretion system. Trends Biochem Sci 2006;31:223–30.
104. Marlovits TC, Kubori T, Lara-Tejero M, et al. Assembly of the inner rod determines needle length in the type III secretion injectisome. Nature 2006;441:637–40.
105. Marlovits TC, Kubori T, Sukhan A, et al. Structural insights into the assembly of the type III secretion needle complex. Science 2004;306:1040–2.
106. Coombes BK, Finlay BB. Insertion of the bacterial type III translocon: Not your average needle stick. Trends Microbiol 2005;13:92–5.
107. Hayward RD, Cain RJ, McGhie EJ, et al. Cholesterol binding by the bacterial type III translocon is essential for virulence effector delivery into mammalian cells. Mol Microbiol 2005;56:590–603.
108. Akeda Y, Galan JE. Chaperone release and unfolding of substrates in type III secretion. Nature 2005;437:911–5.
109. Lee SH, Galan JE. *Salmonella* type III secretion-associated chaperones confer secretion-pathway specificity. Mol Microbiol 2004;51:483–95.
110. Backert S, Meyer TF. Type IV secretion systems and their effectors in bacterial pathogenesis. Curr Opin Microbiol 2006;9:207–17.
111. Bauer B, Moese S, Bartfeld S, et al. Analysis of cell type-specific responses mediated by the type IV secretion system of *Helicobacter pylori*. Infect Immun 2005;73:4643–52.
112. Bourzac KM, Guillemin K. *Helicobacter pylori*-host cell interactions mediated by type IV secretion. Cell Microbiol 2005;7:911–9.
113. Christie PJ, Atmakuri K, Krishnamoorthy V, et al. Biogenesis, architecture, and function of bacterial type IV secretion systems. Annu Rev Microbiol 2005;59:451–85.
114. Kenny B, DeVinney R, Stein M, et al. Enteropathogenic *E. coli* (EPEC) transfers its receptor for intimate adherence into mammalian cells. Cell 1997;91:511–20.
115. Caron E, Crepin VF, Simpson N, et al. Subversion of actin dynamics by EPEC and EHEC. Curr Opin Microbiol 2006;9:40–5.
116. Cossart P, Sansonetti PJ. Bacterial invasion: The paradigms of enteroinvasive pathogens. Science 2004;304:242–8.
117. Terebiznik MR, Vazquez CL, Torbicki K, et al. *Helicobacter pylori* VacA toxin promotes bacterial intracellular survival in gastric epithelial cells. Infec Immun 2006;74:6599–6614.
118. Aktories K, Barbieri JT. Bacterial cytotoxins: Targeting eukaryotic switches. Nat Rev Microbiol 2005;3:397–410.
119. Patel JC, Rossanese OW, Galan JE. The functional interface between *Salmonella* and its host cell: Opportunities for therapeutic intervention. Trends Pharmacol Sci 2005;26:564–70.
120. Brumell JH, Grinstein S. Role of lipid-mediated signal transduction in bacterial internalization. Cell Microbiol 2003;5:287–97.
121. Hilbi H. Modulation of phosphoinositide metabolism by pathogenic bacteria. Cell Microbiol 2006;8:1697–706.
122. Isberg RR, Voorhis DL, Falkow S. Identification of invasin: A protein that allows enteric bacteria to penetrate cultured mammalian cells. Cell 1987;50:769–78.
123. Bruce-Staskal PJ, Weidow CL, Gibson JJ, Bouton AH. Cas, Fak and Pyk2 function in diverse signaling cascades to promote *Yersinia* uptake. J Cell Sci 2002;115:2689–700.
124. Wong KW, Isberg RR. Arf6 and phosphoinositol-4-phosphate-5-kinase activities permit bypass of the Rac1 requirement for beta1 integrin-mediated bacterial uptake. J Exp Med 2003;198:603–14.
125. Lecuit M. Understanding how *Listeria monocytogenes* targets and crosses host barriers. Clin Microbiol Infect 2005;11:430–6.
126. Lecuit M, Dramsi S, Gottardi C, et al. A single amino acid in E-cadherin responsible for host specificity towards the human pathogen *Listeria monocytogenes*. Embo J 1999; 18:3956–63.
127. Sousa S, Cabanes D, El-Amraoui A, et al. Unconventional myosin VIIa and vezatin, two proteins crucial for *Listeria* entry into epithelial cells. J Cell Sci 2004;117:2121–30.
128. Khelef N, Lecuit M, Bierne H, Cossart P. Species specificity of the *Listeria monocytogenes* InlB protein. Cell Microbiol 2006;8:457–70.
129. Bierne H, Miki H, Innocenti M, et al. WASP-related proteins, Abi1 and Ena/VASP are required for *Listeria* invasion induced by the Met receptor. J Cell Sci 2005;118:1537–47.
130. Hamon M, Bierne H, Cossart P. *Listeria monocytogenes*: A multifaceted model. Nat Rev Microbiol 2006;4:423–34.
131. Veiga E, Cossart P. *Listeria* hijacks the clathrin-dependent endocytic machinery to invade mammalian cells. Nat Cell Biol 2005;7:894–900.
132. Galan JE, Zhou D. Striking a balance: Modulation of the actin cytoskeleton by *Salmonella*. Proc Natl Acad Sci U S A 2000;97:8754–61.
133. McGhie EJ, Hayward RD, Koronakis V. Control of actin turnover by a *Salmonella* invasion protein. Mol Cell 2004;13:497–510.
134. Patel JC, Galan JE. Manipulation of the host actin cytoskeleton by *Salmonella*—all in the name of entry. Curr Opin Microbiol 2005;8:10–5.
135. Galan JE, Fu Y. Modulation of actin cytoskeleton by *Salmonella* GTPase activating protein SptP. Methods Enzymol 2000;325:496–504.
136. Terebiznik MR, Vieira OV, Marcus SL, et al. Elimination of host cell PtdIns(4,5)P(2) by bacterial SigD promotes membrane fission during invasion by *Salmonella*. Nat Cell Biol 2002;4:766–73.
137. Kueltzo LA, Osiecki J, Barker J, et al. Structure-function analysis of invasion plasmid antigen C (IpaC) from *Shigella flexneri*. J Biol Chem 2003;278:2792–8.
138. Lafont F, Tran Van Nhieu G, Hanada K, et al. Initial steps of *Shigella* infection depend on the cholesterol/sphingolipid raft-mediated CD44-IpaB interaction. Embo J 2002; 21:4449–57.
139. Yoshida S, Katayama E, Kuwae A, et al. *Shigella* deliver an effector protein to trigger host microtubule destabilization, which promotes Rac1 activity and efficient bacterial internalization. Embo J 2002;21:2923–35.
140. Niebuhr K, Giuriato S, Pedron T, et al. Conversion of PtdIns(4,5)P(2) into PtdIns(5)P by the *S. flexneri* effector IpgD reorganizes host cell morphology. Embo J 2002;21: 5069–78.
141. Pendaries C, Tronchere H, Arbibe L, et al. PtdIns5P activates the host cell PI3-kinase/Akt pathway during *Shigella flexneri* infection. Embo J 2006;25:1024–34.
142. Knodler LA, Finlay BB, Steele-Mortimer O. The *Salmonella* effector protein SopB protects epithelial cells from apoptosis by sustained activation of Akt. J Biol Chem 2005;280:9058–64.
143. Brumell JH, Grinstein S. *Salmonella* redirects phagosomal maturation. Curr Opin Microbiol 2004;7:78–84.
144. Birmingham CL, Smith AC, Bakowski MA, et al. Autophagy controls Salmonella infection in response to damage to

the *Salmonella*-containing vacuole. J Biol Chem 2006;281: 11374–83.

145. Colombo MI. Pathogens and autophagy: Subverting to survive. Cell Death Differ 2005;12 :1481–3.
146. Veiga E, Cossart P. Ubiquitination of intracellular bacteria: A new bacteria-sensing system? Trends Cell Biol 2005;15:2–5.
147. Perrin AJ, Jiang X, Birmingham CL, et al. Recognition of bacteria in the cytosol of mammalian cells by the ubiquitin system. Curr Biol 2004;14:806–11.
148. Hampe J, Franke A, Rosenstiel P, et al. A genome-wide association scan of nonsynonymous SNPs identifies a susceptibility variant for Crohn disease in ATG16L1. Nat Genet 2006; 39:207–11.
149. Kirkegaard K, Taylor MP, Jackson WT. Cellular autophagy: Surrender, avoidance and subversion by microorganisms. Nat Rev Microbiol 2004;2:301–14.
150. Yorimitsu T, Klionsky DJ. Autophagy: Molecular machinery for self-eating. Cell Death Differ 2005;12:1542–52.
151. Gutierrez MG, Master SS, Singh SB, et al. Autophagy is a defense mechanism inhibiting BCG and Mycobacterium tuberculosis survival in infected macrophages. Cell 2004;119:753–66.
152. Henry T, Gorvel JP, Meresse S. Molecular motors hijacking by intracellular pathogens. Cell Microbiol 2006;8:23–32.
153. Suzuki T, Sasakawa C. Molecular basis of the intracellular spreading of *Shigella*. Infect Immun 2001;69:5959–66.
154. Ogawa M, Yoshimori T, Suzuki T, et al. Escape of intracellular *Shigella* from autophagy. Science 2005;307:727–31.
155. Ogawa M, Sasakawa C. Intracellular survival of *Shigella*. Cell Microbiol 2006;8:177–84.
156. Pizarro-Cerda J, Cossart P. Subversion of cellular functions by *Listeria monocytogenes*. J Pathol 2006;208:215–23.
157. Pizarro-Cerda J, Jonquieres R, Gouin E, et al. Distinct protein patterns associated with *Listeria monocytogenes* InlA- or InlB-phagosomes. Cell Microbiol 2002;4:101–15.
158. Cicchetti G, Maurer P, Wagener P, Kocks C. Actin and phosphoinositide binding by the ActA protein of the bacterial pathogen *Listeria monocytogenes*. J Biol Chem 1999;274:33616–26.
159. Kocks C, Marchand JB, Gouin E, et al. The unrelated surface proteins ActA of *Listeria monocytogenes* and IcsA of *Shigella flexneri* are sufficient to confer actin-based motility on *Listeria* innocua and *Escherichia coli* respectively. Mol Microbiol 1995;18:413–23.
160. Samarin S, Romero S, Kocks C, et al. How VASP enhances actin-based motility. J Cell Biol 2003;163:131–42.
161. Rich KA, Burkett C, Webster P. Cytoplasmic bacteria can be targets for autophagy. Cell Microbiol 2003;5:455–68.
162. Petersen AM, Krogfelt KA. *Helicobacter pylori*: An invading microorganism? A review. FEMS Immunol Med Microbiol 2003;36:117–26.
163. Wyle FA, Tarnawski A, Schulman D, Dabros W. Evidence for gastric mucosal cell invasion by *C. pylori*: An ultrastructural study. J Clin Gastroenterol 1990;12:S92–8.
164. Dubois A. Spiral bacteria in the human stomach: The gastric helicobacters. Emerg Infect Dis 1995;1:79–85.
165. Petersen AM, Blom J, Andersen LP, Krogfelt KA. Role of strain type, AGS cells and fetal calf serum in *Helicobacter pylori* adhesion and invasion assays. FEMS Immunol Med Microbiol 2000;29:59–67.
166. Petersen AM, Sorensen K, Blom J, Krogfelt KA. Reduced intracellular survival of *Helicobacter pylori* vacA mutants in comparison with their wild-types indicates the role of VacA in pathogenesis. FEMS Immunol Med Microbiol 2001;30:103–8.
167. Amieva MR, Salama NR, Tompkins LS, Falkow S. *Helicobacter pylori* enter and survive within multivesicular vacuoles of epithelial cells. Cell Microbiol 2002;4:677–90.
168. Rittig MG, Shaw B, Letley DP, et al. *Helicobacter pylori*-induced homotypic phagosome fusion in human monocytes is independent of the bacterial vacA and cag status. Cell Microbiol 2003;5:887–99.
169. Oh JD, Karam SM, Gordon JI. Intracellular *Helicobacter pylori* in gastric epithelial progenitors. Proc Natl Acad Sci U S A 2005;102:5186–91.
170. West SA, Griffin AS, Gardner A, Diggle SP. Social evolution theory for microorganisms. Nat Rev Microbiol 2006;4:597–607.
171. Schauder S, Shokat K, Surette MG, Bassler BL. The LuxS family of bacterial autoinducers: Biosynthesis of a novel quorum-sensing signal molecule. Mol Microbiol 2001; 41:463–76.
172. Clarke MB, Sperandio V. Events at the host-microbial interface of the gastrointestinal tract III. Cell-to-cell signaling among microbial flora, host, and pathogens: There is a whole lot of talking going on. Am J Physiol Gastrointest Liver Physiol 2005;288:G1105–9.
173. Xavier KB, Bassler BL. LuxS quorum sensing: More than just a numbers game. Curr Opin Microbiol 2003;6:191–7.
174. Kaper JB, Nataro JP, Mobley HL. Pathogenic *Escherichia coli*. Nat Rev Microbiol 2004;2:123–40.
175. Walters M, Sperandio V. Autoinducer 3 and epinephrine signaling in the kinetics of locus of enterocyte effacement gene expression in enterohemorrhagic *Escherichia coli*. Infect Immun 2006;74:5445–55.
176. Chen C, Brown DR, Xie Y, et al. Catecholamines modulate *Escherichia coli* O157:H7 adherence to murine cecal mucosa. Shock 2003;20:183–8.
177. Rumbaugh KP. Convergence of hormones and autoinducers at the host/pathogen interface. Anal Bioanal Chem 2007;387:425–27.
178. Schneeberger EE, Lynch RD. The tight junction: A multifunctional complex. Am J Physiol Cell Physiol 2004;286: C1213–28.
179. Nusrat A, Parkos CA, Verkade P, et al. Tight junctions are membrane microdomains. J Cell Sci 2000;113:1771–81.
180. Bruewer M, Samarin S, Nusrat A. Inflammatory bowel disease and the apical junctional complex. Ann NY Acad Sci 2006;1072:242–52.
181. Zareie M, Riff J, Donato K, et al. Novel effects of the prototype translocating *Escherichia coli*, strain C25 on intestinal epithelial structure and barrier function. Cell Microbiol 2005;7:1782–97.
182. Guttman JA, Li Y, Wickham ME, et al. Attaching and effacing pathogen-induced tight junction disruption in vivo. Cell Microbiol 2006;8:634–45.
183. Hermiston ML, Gordon JI. Inflammatory bowel disease and adenomas in mice expressing a dominant negative N-cadherin. Science 1995;270:1203–7.
184. Obiso RJ, Jr, Bevan DR, Wilkins TD. Molecular modeling and analysis of fragilysin, the *Bacteroides fragilis* toxin. Clin Infect Dis 1997;25:S153–5.
185. Wu S, Lim KC, Huang J, et al. *Bacteroides fragilis* enterotoxin cleaves the zonula adherens protein, E-cadherin. Proc Natl Acad Sci U S A 1998;95:14979–84.
186. Sanfilippo L, Baldwin TJ, Menozzi MG, et al. Heterogeneity in responses by primary adult human colonic epithelial cells to purified enterotoxin of *Bacteroides fragilis*. Gut 1998;43:651–5.
187. Buhner S, Buning C, Genschel J, et al. Genetic basis for increased intestinal permeability in families with Crohn's disease: Role of CARD15 3020insC mutation? Gut 2006;55:342–7.
188. Wu S, Shin J, Zhang G, et al. The *Bacteroides fragilis* toxin binds to a specific intestinal epithelial cell receptor. Infect Immun 2006;74:5382–90.
189. McClane BA, Chakrabarti G. New insights into the cytotoxic mechanisms of *Clostridium perfringens* enterotoxin. Anaerobe 2004;10:107–14.
190. Petit L, Gibert M, Gourch A, et al. *Clostridium perfringens* epsilon toxin rapidly decreases membrane barrier permeability of polarized MDCK cells. Cell Microbiol 2003;5: 155–64.
191. Nusrat A, von Eichel-Streiber C, Turner JR, et al. *Clostridium difficile* toxins disrupt epithelial barrier function by altering membrane microdomain localization of tight junction proteins. Infect Immun 2001;69:1329–36.
192. Boehm C, Gibert M, Geny B, et al. Modification of epithelial cell barrier permeability and intercellular junctions by *Clostridium sordellii* lethal toxins. Cell Microbiol 2006;8:1070–85.
193. McNamara BP, Koutsouris A, O'Connell CB, et al. Translocated EspF protein from enteropathogenic *Escherichia coli* disrupts host intestinal barrier function. J Clin Invest 2001;107:621–9.
194. Shifflett DE, Clayburgh DR, Koutsouris A, et al. Enteropathogenic *E. coli* disrupts tight junction barrier function and structure in vivo. Lab Invest 2005;85:1308–24.
195. Matsuzawa T, Kuwae A, Abe A. Enteropathogenic *Escherichia coli* type III effectors EspG and EspG2 alter epithelial paracellular permeability. Infect Immun 2005;73:6283–9.
196. Tomson FL, Viswanathan VK, Kanack KJ, et al. Enteropathogenic *Escherichia coli* EspG disrupts microtubules and in conjunction with Orf3 enhances perturbation of the tight junction barrier. Mol Microbiol 2005;56:447–64.
197. Zolotarevsky Y, Hecht G, Koutsouris A, et al. A membrane-permeant peptide that inhibits MLC kinase restores barrier function in *in vitro* models of intestinal disease. Gastroenterology 2002;123:163–72.
198. Muza-Moons MM, Schneeberger EE, Hecht GA. Enteropathogenic *Escherichia coli* infection leads to appearance of aberrant tight junctions strands in the lateral membrane of intestinal epithelial cells. Cell Microbiol 2004;6:783–93.
199. Howe KL, Reardon C, Wang A, et al. Transforming growth factor-beta regulation of epithelial tight junction proteins enhances barrier function and blocks enterohemorrhagic *Escherichia coli* O157:H7-induced increased permeability. Am J Pathol 2005;167:1587–97..
200. Boyle EC, Brown NF, Finlay BB. *Salmonella enterica* serovar Typhimurium effectors SopB, SopE, SopE2 and SipA disrupt tight junction structure and function. Cell Microbiol 2006;8:1946–57.
201. Chen ML, Ge Z, Fox JG, Schauer DB. Disruption of tight junctions and induction of proinflammatory cytokine responses in colonic epithelial cells by *Campylobacter jejuni*. Infect Immun 2006;74:6581–9.
202. Guttman JA, Samji FN, Li Y, et al. Evidence that tight junctions are disrupted due to intimate bacterial contact and not inflammation during attaching and effacing pathogen infection in vivo. Infect Immun 2006;74:6075–84.
203. Odenbreit S, Puls J, Sedlmaier B, et al. Translocation of *Helicobacter pylori* CagA into gastric epithelial cells by type IV secretion. Science 2000;287:1497–500.
204. Naito M, Yamazaki T, Tsutsumi R, et al. Influence of EPIYA-repeat polymorphism on the phosphorylation-dependent biological activity of *Helicobacter pylori* CagA. Gastroenterology 2006;130:1181–90.
205. Selbach M, Moese S, Hauck CR, et al. Src is the kinase of the *Helicobacter pylori* CagA protein *in vitro* and in vivo. J Biol Chem 2002;277:6775–8.
206. Stein M, Bagnoli F, Halenbeck R, et al. c-Src/Lyn kinases activate *Helicobacter pylori* CagA through tyrosine phosphorylation of the EPIYA motifs. Mol Microbiol 2002;43:971–80.
207. Suzuki T, Matsuo K, Sawaki A, et al. Systematic review and meta-analysis: Importance of CagA status for successful eradication of *Helicobacter pylori* infection. Aliment Pharmacol Ther 2006;24:273–80.
208. Amieva MR, Vogelmann R, Covacci A, et al. Disruption of the epithelial apical-junctional complex by *Helicobacter pylori* CagA. Science 2003;300:1430–4.
209. Bagnoli F, Buti L, Tompkins L, et al. *Helicobacter pylori* CagA induces a transition from polarized to invasive phenotypes in MDCK cells. Proc Natl Acad Sci U S A 2005;102:16339–44.
210. Field M. Intestinal ion transport and the pathophysiology of diarrhea. J Clin Invest 2003;111:931–43.
211. De Haan L, Hirst TR. Cholera toxin: A paradigm for multifunctional engagement of cellular mechanisms (Review). Mol Membr Biol 2004;21:77–92.
212. Wolf AA, Fujinaga Y, Lencer WI. Uncoupling of the cholera toxin-G(M1) ganglioside receptor complex from endocytosis, retrograde Golgi trafficking, and downstream signal transduction by depletion of membrane cholesterol. J Biol Chem 2002;277:16249–56.
213. Pang H, Le PU, Nabi IR. Ganglioside GM1 levels are a determinant of the extent of caveolae/raft-dependent endocytosis of cholera toxin to the Golgi apparatus. J Cell Sci 2004;117:1421–30.
214. Majoul I, Sohn K, Wieland FT, et al. KDEL receptor (Erd2p)-mediated retrograde transport of the cholera toxin A subunit from the Golgi involves COPI, p23, and the COOH terminus of Erd2p. J Cell Biol 1998;143:601–12.
215. Tsai B, Rodighiero C, Lencer WI, Rapoport TA. Protein disulfide isomerase acts as a redox-dependent chaperone to unfold cholera toxin. Cell 2001;104:937–48.
216. Sonawane ND, Hu J, Muanprasat C, Verkman AS. Luminally active, nonabsorbable CFTR inhibitors as potential therapy to reduce intestinal fluid loss in cholera. Faseb J 2006;20:130–2.
217. Albano F, de Marco G, Canani RB, et al. Guanylin and *E. coli* heat-stable enterotoxin induce chloride secretion through direct interaction with basolateral compartment of rat and human colonic cells. Pediatr Res 2005;58:159–63.
218. Pitari GM, Zingman LV, Hodgson DM, et al. Bacterial enterotoxins are associated with resistance to colon cancer. Proc Natl Acad Sci U S A 2003;100:2695–9.
219. Pitari GM, Baksh RI, Harris DM, et al. Interruption of homologous desensitization in cyclic guanosine 3′, 5′-monophosphate signaling restores colon cancer cytostasis by bacterial enterotoxins. Cancer Res 2005;65:11129–35.
220. Saha S, Gupta DD, Chakrabarti MK. Involvement of phospholipase C in *Yersinia enterocolitica* heat stable enterotoxin (Y-STa) mediated rise in intracellular calcium level in rat intestinal epithelial cells. Toxicon 2005;45:361–7.
221. Matkowskyj KA, Danilkovich A, Marrero J, et al. Galanin-1 receptor up-regulation mediates the excess colonic fluid production caused by infection with enteric pathogens. Nat Med 2000;6:1048–51.
222. Ait-Ali D, Turquier V, Grumolato L, et al. The proinflammatory cytokines tumor necrosis factor-alpha and interleukin-1 stimulate neuropeptide gene transcription and secretion in adrenochromaffin cells via activation of extracellularly regulated kinase 1/2 and p38 protein kinases, and activator protein-1 transcription factors. Mol Endocrinol 2004;18:1721–39.
223. Klapproth JM, Sasaki M, Sherman M, et al. *Citrobacter rodentium* lifA/efa1 is essential for colonic colonization

and crypt cell hyperplasia in vivo. Infect Immun 2005;73: 1441–51.

224. O'Hara AM, O'Regan P, Fanning A, et al. Functional modulation of human intestinal epithelial cell responses by *Bifidobacterium infantis* and *Lactobacillus salivarius*. Immunology 2006;118:202–15.

225. Eckmann L, Gillin FD. Microbes and microbial toxins: Paradigms for microbial-mucosal interactions I. Pathophysiological aspects of enteric infections with the lumen-dwelling protozoan pathogen *Giardia lamblia*. Am J Physiol Gastrointest Liver Physiol 2001;280:G1–6.

226. Canny G, Drudy D, Macmathuna P, et al. Toxigenic *C. difficile* induced inflammatory marker expression by human intestinal epithelial cells is asymmetrical. Life Sci 2006;78:920–5.

227. Abd-Alla MD, Jackson TF, Rogers T, et al. Mucosal immunity to asymptomatic *Entamoeba histolytica* and *Entamoeba dispar* infection is associated with a peak intestinal anti-lectin immunoglobulin A antibody response. Infect Immun 2006;74:3897–903.

228. Hugot JP, Chamaillard M, Zouali H, et al. Association of NOD2 leucine-rich repeat variants with susceptibility to Crohn's disease. Nature 2001;411:599–603.

229. Ogura Y, Bonen DK, Inohara N, et al. A frameshift mutation in NOD2 associated with susceptibility to Crohn's disease. Nature 2001;411:603–6.

230. Girardin SE, Boneca IG, Carneiro LA, et al. Nod1 detects a unique muropeptide from gram-negative bacterial peptidoglycan. Science 2003;300:1584–7.

231. McGovern DP, Hysi P, Ahmad T, et al. Association between a complex insertion/deletion polymorphism in NOD1 (CARD4) and susceptibility to inflammatory bowel disease. Hum Mol Genet 2005;14:1245–50.

232. Rosenstiel P, Hellmig S, Hampe J, et al. Influence of polymorphisms in the NOD1/CARD4 and NOD2/CARD15 genes on the clinical outcome of *Helicobacter pylori* infection. Cell Microbiol 2006;8:1188–98.

233. Miyake K. Innate recognition of lipopolysaccharide by Toll-like receptor 4-MD-2. Trends Microbiol 2004;12:186–92.

234. Viatour P, Merville MP, Bours V, Chariot A. Phosphorylation of NF-kappaB and IkappaB proteins: Implications in cancer and inflammation. Trends Biochem Sci 2005;30:43–52.

235. Abreu MT, Vora P, Faure E, et al. Decreased expression of Toll-like receptor-4 and MD-2 correlates with intestinal epithelial cell protection against dysregulated proinflammatory gene expression in response to bacterial lipopolysaccharide. J Immunol 2001;167:1609–16.

236. Hornef MW, Normark BH, Vandewalle A, Normark S. Intracellular recognition of lipopolysaccharide by toll-like receptor 4 in intestinal epithelial cells. J Exp Med 2003;198:1225–35.

237. Otte JM, Cario E, Podolsky DK. Mechanisms of cross hyporesponsiveness to Toll-like receptor bacterial ligands in intestinal epithelial cells. Gastroenterology 2004;126:1054–70.

238. Rhee SH, Im E, Riegler M, et al. Pathophysiological role of Toll-like receptor 5 engagement by bacterial flagellin in colonic inflammation. Proc Natl Acad Sci U S A 2005;102:13610–5.

239. Lyons S, Wang L, Casanova JE, et al. *Salmonella typhimurium* transcytoses flagellin via an SPI2-mediated vesicular transport pathway. J Cell Sci 2004;117:5771–80.

240. Vitiello M, D'Isanto M, Galdiero M, et al. Interleukin-8 production by THP-1 cells stimulated by *Salmonella enterica* serovar Typhimurium porins is mediated by AP-1, NF-kappaB and MAPK pathways. Cytokine 2004;27:15–24.

241. Mynott TL, Crossett B, Prathalingam SR. Proteolytic inhibition of *Salmonella enterica* serovar typhimurium-induced activation of the mitogen-activated protein kinases ERK and JNK in cultured human intestinal cells. Infect Immun 2002;70:86–95.

242. Berkes J, Viswanathan VK, Savkovic SD, Hecht G. Intestinal epithelial responses to enteric pathogens: Effects on the tight junction barrier, ion transport, and inflammation. Gut 2003;52:439–51.

243. Kim SY, Lee YC, Kim HK, Blaser MJ. *Helicobacter pylori* CagA transfection of gastric epithelial cells induces interleukin-8. Cell Microbiol 2006;8:97–106.

244. Criss AK, Silva M, Casanova JE, McCormick BA. Regulation of *Salmonella*-induced neutrophil transmigration by epithelial ADP-ribosylation factor 6. J Biol Chem 2001;276:48431–9.

245. Hodges K, Gill R, Ramaswamy K, et al. Rapid activation of Na+/H+ exchange by EPEC is PKC mediated. Am J Physiol Gastrointest Liver Physiol 2006;291:G959–68.

246. Takaoka A, Yanai H. Interferon signalling network in innate defence. Cell Microbiol 2006;8:907–22.

247. Jandu N, Ceponis PJ, Kato S, et al. Conditioned medium from enterohemorrhagic *Escherichia coli*-infected T84 cells inhibits signal transducer and activator of transcription 1 activation by gamma interferon. Infect Immun 2006;74:1809–18.

248. Cario E, Podolsky DK. Differential alteration in intestinal epithelial cell expression of toll-like receptor 3 (TLR3) and TLR4 in inflammatory bowel disease. Infect Immun 2000;68:7010–7.

249. Rinella ES, Eversley CD, Carroll IM, et al. Human epithelial-specific response to pathogenic *Campylobacter jejuni*. FEMS Microbiol Lett 2006;262:236–43.

250. Kellam P, Weiss RA. Infectogenomics: Insights from the host genome into infectious diseases. Cell 2006;124:695–7.

251. O'Hara AM, Shanahan F. The gut flora as a forgotten organ. EMBO Rep 2006;7:688–93.

252. Zoetendal EG, Vaughan EE, de Vos WM. A microbial world within us. Mol Microbiol 2006;59:1639–50.

253. Eckburg PB, Bik EM, Bernstein CN, et al. Diversity of the human intestinal microbial flora. Science 2005;308:1635–8.

254. Conte MP, Schippa S, Zamboni I, et al. Gut-associated bacterial microbiota in paediatric patients with inflammatory bowel disease. Gut 2006;55:1760–7.

255. Bjursell MK, Martens EC, Gordon JI. Functional genomic and metabolic studies of the adaptations of a prominent adult human gut symbiont, bacteroides thet aiotaomicron, to the suckling period. J Biol Chem 2006;281:36269–79.

19.1a. Probiotics

Erika Isolauri, MD, PhD
Seppo Salminen, PhD

Probiotics are live microbial food supplements or components of bacteria that have been demonstrated to have beneficial effects on human health. Oral introduction of probiotics reinforces various lines of gut defense, including immune exclusion, immune elimination, and immune regulation. Probiotics also stimulate nonspecific host resistance to microbial pathogens and thereby aid in their eradication. Correction of the properties of unbalanced indigenous microbiota forms the rationale of probiotic therapy. The application of probiotics currently lies in reducing the risk of diseases associated with gut barrier dysfunction; the most fully documented probiotic intervention is the treatment and prevention of acute infectious diarrhea and antibiotic-associated diarrhea. Recent clinical and nutritional studies and characterization of the immunomodulatory potential of specific strains of the gut microbiota, beyond the effect on the composition of the microbiota, has led to applications not only for different infectious diarrheas, but also for allergic and inflammatory diseases.

The probiotic potential of specific strains differs; genomic understanding of different bacterial species, and even strains of the same species show that each bacterial strain is unique and has defined adherence sites, specific immunologic effects, and varied other effects induced by the local environment in the healthy versus the inflamed mucosal milieu. Current probiotic research aims at characterization of the healthy individual gut microbiota and understanding the microbe–microbe and host–microbe interactions. The goal is to use the defined microbiota both as a tool for nutritional management of specific gut-related diseases and as a source of novel microbes for future probiotic bacteriotherapy applications.

HEALTHY GUT MICROBIOTA

The human gastrointestinal tract harbors a complex collection of microorganisms, which form a typical individual microbiota for each person.[1] This specific microbiota is dependent on genetic factors and the environment. The total number of microbes in the intestinal tract is estimated to reach 10^{12} bacteria per gram of intestinal contents. Several hundred bacterial species can be identified using traditional culture methods.[1] The development of novel means of characterizing gut microbiota, in particular molecular methods, has uncovered new microbial species in intestinal mucosa and contents and it appears that more than 50% of the microbiota members remain yet-to-be cultured.[1,2]

The microbiota is metabolically active, and its composition is related to multiple disease states within the intestine and also beyond the gastrointestinal tract. Components of the human intestinal microbiota or organisms entering the intestine may, however, have both harmful and beneficial effects on human health.

The basis of healthy gut microbiota lies in early infancy and the initial process of intestinal colonization. The generation of immunophysiologic regulation in the gut depends on the establishment of an indigenous microbiota.[3-5] The microbiota of a newborn develops rapidly after birth and is initially strongly dependent on the mother's microbiota, mode of delivery, and birth environment.[6] Subsequently, feeding practices and the home environment of the child influence the composition. Major changes in composition occur during breastfeeding, weaning, and introduction of solid foods.[6,7] A recent study, evaluating a broad range of external influences to the gut microbiota composition in early infancy,[8] confirms these observations. Of 1,032 infants assessed at one month of age, those born by cesarean section showed lower numbers of bifidobacteria and *Bacteroides*, but more frequent colonization by *Clostridium difficile*, compared with vaginally delivered infants. Hospitalization and prematurity were associated with elevated *C. difficile* counts, and formula feeding with colonization by *Escherichia coli*, *C. difficile*, *Bacteroides*, and lactobacilli. Differences in culturable microbiota between vaginally born infants and infants born by caesarean section are still observed at 6 months of age.[6] Colonization, again, appeared is associated with the maturation of humoral immune mechanisms.[3] Interestingly, *Bacteroides fragilis* and, to a lesser extent, *Bifidobacterium* species are important in this respect, as infants harboring these organisms had more circulating immunoglobulin IgA- and IgM-secreting cells.

The establishment of the gut microbiota has traditionally been considered a stepwise process (Figure 1) with facultative anaerobics such as the enterobacteria, coliforms, and lactobacilli first colonizing the intestine with rapid succession by bifidobacteria and lactic acid producing bacteria.[7-10] New molecular methods indicate, however, that lactic acid–producing bacteria account for less than 1% of the total microbiota in infants, whereas bifidobacteria can range from 60 to 90% of the total fecal microbiota in breastfed infants.[2,11] Moreover, these new techniques indicate that the greatest difference in the microbiota of breastfed and formula-fed infants lies in the bifidobacterial composition of intestinal microbiota, whereas the composition of lactic acid bacteria appears to be rather similar. *Bifidobacterium breve*, *Bifidobacterium infantis*, and *Bifidobacterium longum* are frequently found in fecal samples of breastfed infants, whereas the most common lactobacilli in breastfed and formula-fed infant feces constitute *Lactobacillus acidophilus* group microorganisms such as *L. acidophilus*, *L. gasseri*, and *L. johnsonii*.[11,12]

Recently, the traditional view of maternal birth canal microbes providing the primary microbial inoculum to the child has been challenged. The fetus may well be exposed to microbiota prior to birth through contact with microbes in the amniotic fluid and umbilical cord.[13] Such exposures have been associated with preterm delivery,[14] but now also in normal, term deliveries and verified in animal studies indicating that oral probiotic intake leads to transfer of probiotic bacteria into the amniotic fluid.[13] In similar manner, exposure to mother's bacteria continues during breast-feeding after delivery (Figure 1). As breast milk is a continuous source of bacteria the result is an ongoing reinforcement of the original inoculum.[15]

The intestinal microbiota is a positive health asset, which has a significant impact on normal structural and functional development of the human mucosal immune system. The healthy microbiota induces mucosal immune responses that require precise control and also immunosensory capacity for distinguishing commensal from pathogenic bacteria. Indeed, a healthy microbiota is defined as the normal microbiota of an individual that both preserves and promotes well-being and absence of disease, especially in the intestinal tract.[16] The collective composition of the colonizing strains in infancy also provides the basis for a healthy gut microbiota later in life. In addition, the development of the disease-free state of the gut lies in host–microbe interactions in infancy.[17,18]

Strain   **Effect**   **Target**

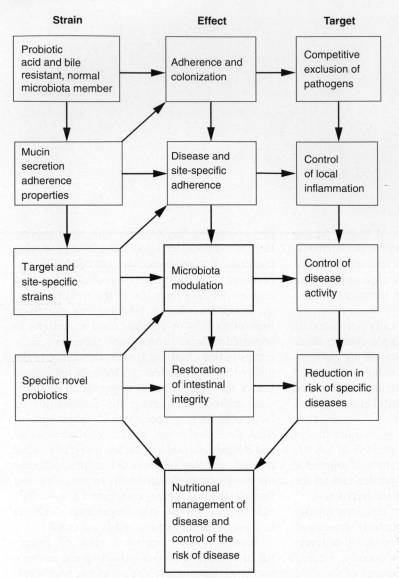

There are several mechanisms operative in the healthy intestinal epithelium which reduce inflammatory response to commensals present in the healthy intestine and ensure tolerance to indigenous gut microbiota. Especially in susceptible individuals, some microbiota components can become aberrant and contribute towards disease risk.[1,2] Inflammation is frequently accompanied by an imbalance in the intestinal microbiota. A strong inflammatory response may then be mounted against microbiota bacteria, leading to perpetuation of the mucosal inflammation and gut barrier dysfunction. (Figure 2)

This is exemplified in atopic eczema, which appears to result from an interplay between susceptibility genes, impaired barrier functions of the skin and the gut, aberrant gut microbiota, immunological dysregulation, together with bacterial and viral infections and other environmental factors. Recent reports have also revealed a possible link between intestinal microbiota and inflammatory bowel disease.[19] The most dramatic illustration of deviant host–microbe interaction occurs in preterm neonates. As a result of lower pH of the small intestine, lower mucus and proteolytic enzyme activity, decreased motility and increased intestinal permeability, the preterm is prone to

bacterial translocation at a time when both the systemic and local immune defenses are immature. Together with excessive adherence of bacteria to the immature mucosa and radically different microbiota composition in neonatal intensive care unit from that of healthy infants perpetuation of the inflammatory responses ensues.

DEFINITIONS OF PROBIOTICS

The history of probiotics dates back to ancient times, but scientific work on the health benefits was initiated by Metchnikoff early in the last century.[20] Health-promoting fermented foods have been used for the treatment and prevention of infant diarrhea in countries around the world without knowledge of the specific microbial composition of such products.[21] Beneficial bacteria in fermented foods that promote health have only more recently been called probiotics. These have been variously defined, according to their initial application, in animal feeds. For the purpose of human nutrition, a probiotic is currently defined as a live microbial food ingredient beneficial to health.[16] However, inactivated probiotic bacteria also may have beneficial health effects. The

history of the definition and the current status are presented in Table 1.[22–27]

Probiotics were initially selected to provide strains with good food-processing conditions, but, more recently, the physiologic properties of probiotics in the human intestinal tract have formed the basis for selection. These criteria have been redefined to include the healthy human intestinal or mucosal microbiota as the main source of new strains. At present, emphasis is placed on survival in the gut, acid and bile stability, temporary colonization of the mucosal surfaces in the intestinal tract, and fecal recovery of the administered probiotic to define the dosage needed for individual target uses.[28] The most frequently used genera fulfilling these criteria are lactobacilli and bifidobacteria. Currently, most probiotics have been selected from members of normal healthy adult microbiota. This practice is undergoing a rapid change as we now understand that infants and adults have different bifidobacterial species composition and activity, indicating that age and target-specific approaches need to be adopted for the selection of probiotics.

RATIONALE FOR PROBIOTIC INTERVENTION IN PEDIATRIC PRACTICE

Therapeutic and prophylactic interventions by probiotics derive from the concept of a well-functioning gut barrier and a normal balanced microbiota. In addition to its principal physiologic function, digestion and absorption of nutrients, the intestinal mucosa provides a protective interface between the internal environment and the constant challenge from antigens of the external environment, also carrying defense mechanisms against infectious and inflammatory diseases.

Gut microbiota as a component of the intestinal barrier has been considered as a physiologic blockade to foreign substances, such as antigens. One current view focuses on communication between the host and the resident commensal microbes.[27] This interaction manifests best during early infancy, when the colonization process governs the development of intestinal integrity and host immune defense mechanisms.[3–5] Conversely, the genetic background of the host and development of the immune system influence the collective composition of the intestinal microbiota.

In several gut-related inflammatory conditions, the healthy host–microbe interaction is disturbed, and inflammation is accompanied by an imbalance in the intestinal microbiota in such a way that an immune response may be generated against resident bacteria. For example, an altered gut microbiota is reported in patients with rotavirus diarrhea, inflammatory bowel diseases, rheumatoid arthritis, and allergic diseases,[28] implying that the normal gut microbiota constitutes an ecosystem responding to inflammation both in the gut and elsewhere in the human body. Normalization of the properties of an unbalanced indigenous microbiota by specific strains of the healthy gut microbiota constitutes the rationale

Figure 1 The mother-infant microbiota exchange during delivery and breast-feeding: basis for healthy microbiota development.

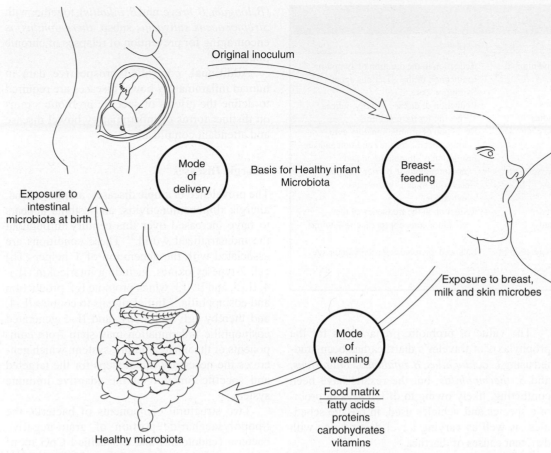

Figure 2 Local immune inflammatory reaction interferes with the intestine's barrier function. Mucosal dysfunction may lead to aberrant absorption of intraluminal antigens and to alterations in gut microbiota immunogenicity. Together these induce symptoms in child and impair growth.

for probiotic therapy. Such an approach with oral introduction of specific probiotics may halt the vicious circle in inflammation.

The probiotic effects in conditions involving impaired mucosal barrier function, particularly infectious and inflammatory diseases, lie in normalization of increased intestinal permeability and altered gut microecology, improvement of immunologic barrier functions of the intestine, and alleviation of intestinal inflammatory responses.[27,28]

Although it is well documented that balanced normal microbiota may become aberrant and immunogenic secondary to gut-related disease, it is not known whether changes in the composition of the microbiota can be a primary cause of disease. Such associations recently have been suggested in allergic disease[27] and autism.[29] Differences in the neonatal gut microbiota, in particular the balance between *Bifidobacterium* and *Clostridium* microbiota, may precede the manifestation of the atopic responder type with heightened production of antigen-specific IgE antibodies, suggesting a crucial role of the balance of the indigenous intestinal bacteria for the maturation of human immunity to a nonatopic mode.[30] These observations underline the importance of the need for precise characterization of healthy versus aberrant microbiota development and composition. This requires thorough investigation of the infant microbiota by up-to-date techniques; in particular, those based on molecular techniques including ribosomal ribonucleic acid sequencing. Indirect methods, such as fecal microbial enzyme activities,[31] may also reflect differences in microbiota development.

CLINICAL EVIDENCE OF PROBIOTIC EFFECTS IN CHILDREN

The potential health effects of normal gut microbiota must be demonstrated by well-controlled clinical and nutritional studies in human subjects.[32] To date, several clinical studies have investigated the use of probiotics, principally lactobacilli and bifidobacteria, as dietary supplements for the prevention and treatment of various gastrointestinal infectious and inflammatory conditions (Table 2).

Acute Enteritis

Currently accepted guidelines for treatment of acute diarrhea are based on correcting the dehydration by oral rehydration solutions. In addition, immediately after the completion of oral rehydration, full feedings of a previously tolerated diet can be reintroduced. Well-controlled clinical studies have shown that probiotics such as *Lactobacillus rhamnosus* GG, *Lactobacillus reuteri, Lactobacillus casei* Shirota, and *Bifidobacterium lactis* Bb12 shorten the duration of acute rotavirus diarrhea,[28] above the beneficial effect of rapid refeeding, and thus constitute safe adjunct management of the condition.

In patients hospitalized for acute rotavirus diarrhea, *L. rhamnosus* strain GG (ATCC 53103) as a fermented milk or as a freeze-dried powder reduces the duration of diarrhea, compared with the placebo group given a fermented and then pasteurized milk product.[33] This result has been confirmed in subsequent studies.[34,35] Moreover, probiotics reduce the duration of rotavirus excretion in stools.[36] A multicenter study by the European Society for Pediatric Gastroenterology, Hepatology, and Nutrition working group tested the clinical efficacy and safety of a probiotic administered in an oral rehydration solution.[37] In rotavirus diarrhea, but not in nonspecific or bacterial diarrhea, a decrease in the number of diarrhea episodes was observed. The study also confirmed the safety of administration of a probiotic in an oral rehydration solution and prevention of the evolution of rotavirus-induced diarrhea toward a protracted course. These studies have invariably evaluated patients with mild or moderate dehydration. The opposite was observed in a recent study using *Lactobacillus paracasei* strain ST11: no effect on severe rotavirus diarrhea, but significant reduction in stool output, stool frequency, and oral rehydration solution requirement in children with nonrotavirus diarrhea.[38] A recent randomized placebo-controlled study in severely dehydrated male children under 2 years of age showed no clinical benefit of supplementing oral rehydration with Lactobacillus GG.[39]

Table 1 Current Understanding and History of Probiotic Definitions	
Definition	Source
Specific bacteria in yoghurt fermentation balance intestinal microbiota	Reference 20
Substances excreted by one protozoan to stimulate the growth of another	Reference 22
Substances that have a beneficial effect on animals by contributing to the balance of the intestinal biota	Reference 23
Live microbial feed supplements that beneficially affect the host animal by improving the intestinal microbial balance	Reference 24
Mono- or mixed cultures of live microorganisms that, when applied to humans, affect beneficially the host by improving the properties of the indigenous microbiota	Reference 25
Live microbial food ingredients that are beneficial to health (efficacy and safety scientifically documented)	Reference 16
Live microbial cell preparations or components of cells that have a beneficial effect on human health	Reference 26
Specific live or inactivated microbial cultures that have documented targets in reducing the risk of human disease or in their adjunct treatment	Reference 27

Table 2 Targets of Probiotic Therapy

Effect	Method of Assessment	Outcome

Nutritional management of disease
  Diarrhea
  Allergic/inflammatory diseases
	Randomized double-blind clinical
	  studies
		Reduction in the duration of symptoms
		Eradication of the infectious agent
		Symptom score

Control of disease activity/
  reactions/relapses/inflammation
	Clinical follow-up studies
	Crossover challenge studies
	  (double blind, placebo controlled)
		Reduction of disease activity indices
		  specific for the condition
		Reduction of proinflammatory cyto
		  kines specific for the condition and site

Enhanced host defense	Intestinal permeability
	Immunomodulation in vitro/in vivo
	Gut microbiota aberrancy
		Promotion of immunologic and
		  nonimmunologic barrier function
		Generation of anti-inflammatory
		  cytokines

Reduction in risk of disease
  Diarrhea
  Allergic disease
	Randomized double-blind
	  placebo-controlled study
		Reduction in the frequency of the
		  condition after appropriate follow-up

Gut microbiota stabilization
  Regulation of bowel movement
  Comparative exclusion
	Modern techniques of evaluation of
	  the gut microecology
		Balanced microbiota appropriate for age

Probiotics, specifically *Bifidobacterium bifidum* (later renamed *B. lactis*) and *Streptococcus thermophilus* together, are also effective in the prevention of acute infantile diarrhea.[36] *Lactobacillus* GG supplementation resulted in a decrease in the incidence of diarrhea in undernourished, nonbreastfed Peruvian children followed for 15 months.[40] *Lactobacillus* GG also reduces the incidence of nosocomial diarrhea, but has no effect on the prevalence of rotavirus infection.[41] Recently, Mastretta and colleagues confirmed the result when assessing the effects of *Lactobacillus* GG and breast-feeding on nosocomial rotavirus infections in 220 hospitalized infants during one rotavirus epidemic season.[42] The frequency of nosocomial rotavirus infection was 28%. This probiotic preparation was ineffective, whereas breastfeeding was effective in reducing the risk of rotavirus infection.

The effect of probiotic therapy (see Table 2) in diarrhea has been explained by a reduction in the duration of rotavirus shedding, normalization of gut permeability caused by rotavirus infection, and an increase in IgA-secreting cells against rotavirus.[18,28] Moreover, the ability of specific probiotics to increase the expression of mucins may contribute to the barrier effect but also to inhibition of rotavirus replication.[43]

Antimicrobial treatment disturbs colonization resistance of the gut microbiota,[1] which may induce clinical symptoms, most frequently diarrhea. The incidence of diarrhea after single antimicrobial treatment and the effect of probiotics was evaluated in children with no history of antimicrobial use during the previous 3 months.[44] The frequency of diarrhea was 5% in the group given *Lactobacillus* GG and 16% in the placebo group ($p = .05$), supporting the efficacy of probiotics. *Lactobacillus* GG, compared with placebo, reduces stool frequency and increases stool consistency during antibiotic therapy in children aged 6 months to 10 years given oral antibiotics in an outpatient setting.[45] In addition, there are preliminary reports on resolution of *C. difficile* diarrhea and colitis in adults.[46]

The value of probiotic preparations for the prophylaxis of traveler's diarrhea has been studied using *L. acidophilus, B. bifidum, L. bulgaricus,* and *S. thermophilus,* but the results have been conflicting, likely owing to differences in probiotic species and vehicles used, in dosage schedules, as well as varying travel destinations with different causes of diarrhea.[16]

Inflammatory Bowel Diseases

An increasing number of clinical and experimental studies demonstrate the importance of constituents within the intestinal lumen, in particular the resident microbiota, in driving the inflammatory responses in these diseases. Intestinal microbiota appears to be responsible for deep colonic lesions and severe inflammatory response.[19] Probiotic bacteria may counteract the inflammatory process by stabilizing the gut microbial environment and the intestine's permeability barrier and by enhancing the degradation of enteral antigens and altering their immunogenicity. Another explanation for the gut-stabilizing effect could be improvement of the intestine's immunologic barrier, particularly intestinal IgA responses. Probiotic effects may also be mediated via control of the balance between pro-and anti-inflammatory cytokines.[18,28]

Preliminary reports indicate benefit in reversing some of the immunologic disturbances characteristic of Crohn's disease.[28] In addition, reductions in disease activity and increased intestinal permeability have been achieved in pediatric patients with Crohn's disease by probiotic intervention.[47] In adults operated on for the condition, however, *Lactobacillus* GG failed to prevent endoscopic recurrence during 1 year of follow-up.[48] A recent study provides evidence for treatment with a nonpathogenic *E. coli* in maintaining remission in ulcerative colitis.[49] In a clinical trial in adults, a preparation containing four strains of lactobacilli (*L. casei, L. plantarum, L. acidophilus,* and *L. delbrückii* subsp. *bulgaricus*) and three bifidobacteria strains

(*B. longum, B. breve,* and *B. infantis*), together with *Streptococcus salivarius* subsp. *thermophilus,* is encouraging for prevention of relapses of chronic pouchitis.[50]

Additional, controlled prospective data in human inflammatory bowel diseases are required to define the effects of specific probiotic strains on distinct forms of inflammatory bowel disease and attendant complications.

Allergic Diseases

The prevalence of atopic diseases, atopic eczema, allergic rhinoconjunctivitis, and asthma appears to have increased over this century throughout the industrialized world.[51] These conditions are associated with the generation of T helper (Th) cell 2-type cytokines, including interleukin (IL)-4, IL-5, and IL-13, which promote IgE production and eosinophilia.[19] Initial signals to counter IL-4, and thereby IgE and atopy, and IL-5-generated eosinophilic inflammation may stem from components of the innate immune system, which generates the necessary initial steps for the targeted and specific function of the adaptive immune system.[51]

Two structural components of bacteria, the lipopolysaccharide portion of gram-negative bacteria (endotoxin) and a specified CpG motif in bacterial deoxyribonucleic acid (DNA),[52,53] activate immunomodulatory genes via Toll-like receptors (TLR4 and TLR9, respectively) present on macrophages and dendritic and intestinal epithelial cells[54,55] and elicit an immunosuppressive effect on intestinal epithelial cells by inhibition of the transcription factor nuclear factor-κB signaling pathway.[56] Specific strains of the gut microbiota contribute to a T regulatory cell population amenable to oral tolerance induction[17] and counter allergy by the generation of IL-10 and transforming growth factor-β.[57,58] These activities are associated with suppression of proliferation of Th cells and reduced secretion of proinflammatory cytokines,[58–62] with control of IgE responses[63] and reduced allergic inflammation in the gut.[64] However, different *Lactobacillus* and *Bifidobacterium* strains appear to induce distinct, and even opposing, responses.[65,66] Thus, specific strains of the gut micobiota and probiotics may play a crucial role in determining the Th1/Th2-driving capacity of intestinal dendritic cells. In parallel, recent observations indicate that the cytokine production patterns induced by intestinal bifidobacteria are strain specific.[27] The results of clinical studies evaluating the effects of probiotics in allergic disease appear to substantiate this suggestion.

In one prospective study, the intestinal microbiota from 76 infants at high risk of atopic diseases was analyzed at 3 weeks of age by conventional bacterial cultivation and two culture-independent methods.[30] A positive skinprick reaction at 12 months was observed in 29% of the subjects. At 3 weeks of age, the bacterial cellular fatty acid profile in fecal samples differed between those infants later developing atopic sensitization and those not developing atopy. Fluorescence in situ hybridization was used to show that atopic subjects have more *Clostridium* species and fewer *Bifidobacterium* species in stools compared with nonatopic subjects.[30] Differences in the neonatal gut microbiota thus appear to precede the manifestations of atopy, suggesting a crucial role of the balance of indigenous intestinal bacteria for the maturation of human immunity to a nonatopic mode.

Improvement in the clinical course of atopic eczema and cow's milk allergy is observed in infants when given probiotic-supplemented extensively hydrolyzed formula compared with placebo-supplemented formula.[64,67] In parallel, markers of systemic[67] and intestinal[64] allergic inflammation were reduced (see Table 2). Subsequent studies in young infants as well as older children with the condition have shown similar effects.[68–70] Similar results have also been obtained in milk-hypersensitive adults.[71] In these subjects, a milk challenge in conjunction with a probiotic strain prevented the immunoinflammatory response characteristic of the response without probiotics.

The preventive potential of probiotics in atopic diseases has been demonstrated in a double-blind, placebo-controlled study.[72] Probiotics administered pre- and postnatally for 6 months to children at high risk of atopic diseases reduced the prevalence of atopic eczema to half compared with infants receiving placebo.[72] Two other reports on probiotics and allergy prevention have been successful,[73,74] but not all strains are effective as shown by the report of Taylor and coworkers on a previously uncharacterized *L. acidophilus* strain.[75] Moreover, the beneficial effect extends well beyond infancy.[76]

WHAT IS REQUIRED FOR FUTURE PROBIOTICS?

Research interest in the science of nutrition is currently directed toward improvement of defined physiologic functions beyond the nutritional impact of food, including the potential to reduce the risk of diseases. This is also the focus for probiotic research. Future probiotics must have more thoroughly defined mechanisms either to control specific physiologic processes in the evolution of disease for at-risk populations or in the dietary management of specific diseases (Figure 3).

Prerequisites for probiotic action include survival in and adhesion to specific areas of the gastrointestinal tract and competitive exclusion of pathogens or harmful antigens.[77] These processes may depend first on specific strain characteristics and secondly on the age and the immunologic state of the host. Probiotic actions may vary as they are controlled by intestinal stimuli. These include stomach enzymes, bile acids, or intestinal microbiota composition which can induce specific gene expression in the probiotic resulting in a physiologic action, such as adhesion to immune

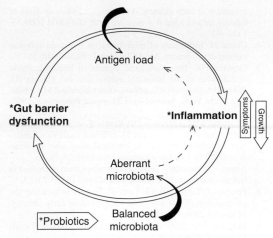

Figure 3 The selection and use of specific probiotic strains and some targets in disease risk reduction symptom management.

cells. The immunologic state of the host and the internal environment of the gut, again, can direct the probiotic response to a specific site of intestinal tract. (Table 3). Some probiotic strains adhere better to the small intestine, whereas others bind specifically to different parts of the large intestine.[78] It is likely that strains also adhere differently to healthy versus damaged mucosa.[79] It has also recently been demonstrated that strains with lower total in vitro binding capacity may still provide high competitive exclusion of pathogens or harmful bacteria,[77] indicating a need for further characterization of in vivo adhesion properties and genomic information to develop preclinical selection methodologies for candidate probiotic strains.

Genetically modified bacteria evincing improved or added functional properties may also achieve probiotic effects. These include probiotics encoding mammalian genes to produce and secrete functional anti-inflammatory cytokines, such as *L. lactis* engineered to produce IL-10 locally.[80] Other methods of probiotic modification are exposure of the microorganism to sublethal stress such as acidic conditions or

heat to improve survival in the gastrointestinal tract and tolerance to stress and thereby to furnish the organism with improved competitiveness against pathogens in the intestinal milieu.[81–83] Inactivation may also have potential in the modification of probiotics. The use of inactivated instead of viable microorganism would have merit in terms of safety, longer shelf-life, and less interaction with other components in food products.

Owing to limited availability of controlled data in humans, more research is required on the effects of specific probiotic strains, in particular when there are modifications of components of these bacteria. Probiotic effects appear to be strain specific.[65,66] Indeed, the effects of even closely related strains can be counteractive. No single probiotic strain alone can influence all of the multifactorial processes controlling the intestinal milieu. Therefore, targets of probiotic intervention should be clearly identified and effective strains and specific strain combinations must be developed with desired properties for both nutritional management and the control of human diseases (see Figure 3).

SAFETY ASPECTS OF PROBIOTIC THERAPY

Probiotic therapy forms a relatively new treatment modality for gastrointestinal disorders. The ingestion of large numbers of viable bacteria requires strict assurance of both acute and long-term safety. Probiotics currently used have been assessed as safe for use in fermented foods, but, generally, the safety assessment of microbial food supplements is not well developed.[84] The ability of probiotic strains to survive in gastric conditions and to strongly adhere to the intestinal epithelium may entail a risk of bacterial translocation,[85] bacteremia,[86] and sepsis.[87]

Reports from countries with high probiotic consumption suggest that current preparations are safe for their intended uses.[86–88] However,

Property	Target and Method
Species and strain identity, source	Molecular identification, source or origin; healthy human gut microbiota as the source
Species properties	Genomic information and properties
Resistance to pH	Model systems for gastric and bile effects
Adhesion to intestinal mucosa	Several model systems to be used (eg, cell cultures, mucus, intestinal segments); fecal recovery in human subjects
Competitive exclusion	In vitro and in vivo model systems for pathogen adherence exclusion
Immune regulation	In vitro and human studies
Generation and balance of cytokines	Cytokine profile
	Contact with immune cells
	Adhesion related to immune effects
	Improvement of gut barrier and permeability disorders
Safety	Exclusion of antibiotic resistance and virulence factors and postmarket monitoring plan
Technological properties	Stability and activity throughout the processes
Efficacy assessment	Human clinical intervention studies with final product formulations; at least two independent studies to prove efficacy in target populations and safety in all consumer groups

Table 3 Properties of Probiotics to be Assessed During the Development of New Strains and New Applications

patients with severe underlying diseases, particularly immunocompromised subjects, appear to carry an increased risk of bacteremia associated with lactic acid bacteria.[86,87] Translocation of intraluminal bacteria may be one risk factor, but recent data also suggest that some probiotic strains may directly interfere with host innate immune functions.[89]

An additional safety concern with perinatal administration of probiotics includes long-term colonization by probiotics or impairment of the natural diversity of the gut microbiota. A recent prospective study followed the symptoms and the composition of the gut microbiota in breastfed infants who received *L. rhamnosus* GG or placebo for the first 6 months of their lives.[90] The study demonstrated that the probiotic was well tolerated and did not interfere with the compositional development of the gut microbiota. Moreover, no permanent establishment of the strain, but transient colonization until the end of the period of administration, was observed.[91]

The numerous immunological properties of probiotics have also raised concern over possible effects on the growth of infants. In one short-term study, administration of probiotic bacteria in infant formula did not affect the growth of the infants.[92] Likewise, in a 4-year follow-up study, the weights and lengths of the children having received probiotic during the perinatal period remained indistinguishable from normal.[93]

Genetically modified microorganisms could be developed for use in foods. Developments in this area also may provide medical applications. However, a safety concern is the potential for the transfer of antibiotic resistance from modified organisms to gut pathogens.[94] Selection procedures have been developed to monitor the absence of antibiotic resistance thus far, specifically for *Lactococcus*.[94] The use of inactivated bacteria as probiotics has been advocated because their consumption may be safer than the use of viable bacteria.[28] In the regulatory area, specific species and strains have been given the generally recognized as safe status[95] and a qualified presumption of safety of micro-organisms in food and feed has been initiated in European Union.[96] However, information on the effects of inactivation methods on cell wall structure and composition is scarce.

To conclude, specific probiotics offer a tool for modification of the microbiota and gut barrier, and thereby the host immune defenses. The microbes used must be obtained from acceptable sources with scientifically proven safety and efficacy to guarantee their application in infectious, allergic, and inflammatory diseases.

REFERENCES

1. Guarner F, Malagelada JR. Gut flora in health and disease. Lancet 2003;361:512–9.
2. Favier C, Vaughan E, de Vos W, Akkermans A. Molecular monitoring of succession of bacterial communities in human neonates. Appl Environ Microbiol 2002;68:219–26.
3. Gronlund MM, Arvilommi H, Kero P, et al. Importance of intestinal colonisation in the maturation of humoral immunity in early infancy: A prospective follow up study of healthy infants aged 0–6 months. Arch Dis Child 2000;83: F186–92.
4. Cebra JJ. Influences of microbiota on intestinal immune system development. Am J Clin Nutr 1999;69:1046–51.
5. Gaskins HR. Immunological aspects of host/microbiota interactions at the intestinal epithelium. In: Mackie RI, White BA, Isaacson RE, editors. Gastrointestinal Microbiology. New York: International Thomson Publishing; 1997. p. 537–87.
6. Gronlund MM, Lehtonen OP, Eerola E, et al. Fecal microflora in healthy infants born by different methods of delivery: Permanent changes in intestinal flora after cesarean delivery. J Pediatr Gastroenterol Nutr 1999;28:19–25.
7. Benno Y, Mitsuoka T. Development of intestinal microflora in humans and animals. Bifidobacteria Microfi 1986;5:13–25.
8. Penders J, Thijs C, Vink C, et al. Factors influencing the composition of the intestinal microbiota in early infancy. Pediatrics 2006;118:511–21.
9. Berg RD. The indigenous gastrointestinal microflora. Trends Microbiol 1996;4:430–5.
10. Harmsen HJ, Wildeboer-Veloo AC, Raangs GC, et al. Analysis of intestinal flora development in breast-fed and formula-fed infants by using molecular identification and detection methods. J Pediatr Gastroenterol Nutr 2000;30:61–7.
11. Vaughan E, de Vries M, Zoetendal E, et al. The intestinal LABs. Anth Leeuwenh 2002;82:341–52.
12. Satokari RM, Vaughan EE, Akkermans AD, et al. Bifidobacterial diversity in human feces detected by genus-specific PCR and denaturing gradient gel electrophoresis. Appl Environ Microbiol 2001;67:504–13.
13. Jimenez E, Fernandez L, Marin ML, et al. Isolation of commensal bacteria from umbilical cord blood of healthy neonates born by cesarean section. Curr Microbiol 2005; 51:270–4.
14. Holst RM, Mattsby-Baltzer I, Wennerholm UB, et al.. Interleukin-6 and interleukin-8 in the cervical fluid in a population of swedish women in preterm labor: Relationship to microbial invasion of the amniotic fluid, intra-amniotic inflammation, and preterm delivery. Acta Obstet Gynecol Scand 2005;84:551–7.
15. Martín R, Langa S, Reviriego C, et al. Human milk is a source of lactic acid bacteria for the infant gut. J Pediatr 2003;143:754–8.
16. Salminen S, Bouley C, Boutron-Ruault MC, et al. Gastrointestinal physiology and function targets for functional food development. Br J Nutr 1998;80:147–71.
17. Sudo N, Sawamura S, Tanaka K, et al. The requirement of intestinal bacterial flora for the development of an IgE production system fully susceptible to oral tolerance induction. J Immunol 1997;159:1739–45.
18. Isolauri E, Sutas Y, Kankaanpaa P, et al. Probiotics: Effects on immunity. Am J Clin Nutr 2001;73:S444–50.
19. Guarner F, Casellas F, Borruel N, et al. Role of microecology in chronic inflammatory bowel diseases. Eur J Clin Nutr 2002;56:S34–8.
20. Metchnikoff E. Prolongation of Life. London: William Heinemann; 1907.
21. Jelliffe EF, Jelliffe DB, Feldon K, Ngokwey N. Traditional practices concerning feeding during and after diarrhoea (with special reference to acute dehydrating diarrhoea in young children). World Rev Nutr Diet 1987;53:218–95.
22. Lilly D, Stillwell E. Probiotics: Growth promoting factors produced by microorganisms. Science 1965;147:747–8.
23. Parker RB. Probiotics: The other half of the antibiotics story. Anim Nutr Health 1974;29:4–8.
24. Fuller R. Probiotic in man and animals. Appl Bacteriol 1989;66:365–78.
25. Huis in't Veld J, Havenaar R. Probiotics and health in man and animal. J Chem Technol Biotechnol 1991;51:562–7.
26. Salminen S, Ouwehand A, Benno Y, Lee YK. Probiotics: How should they be defined? Trends Food Sci Technol 1999;10:107–10.
27. Isolauri E, Rautava S, Kalliomaki M, et al. Role of probiotics in food hypersensitivity. Curr Opin Immunol Clin Allergy 2002;2:263–71.
28. Isolauri E, Kirjavainen PV, Salminen S. Probiotics: A role in the treatment of intestinal infection and inflammation? Gut 2002;50:54–9.
29. Finegold SM, Molitoris D, Song Y, et al. Gastrointestinal microflora studies in late-onset autism. Clin Infect Dis 2002;35:S6–16.
30. Kalliomaki M, Kirjavainen P, Eerola E, et al. Distinct patterns of neonatal gut microflora in infants in whom atopy was and was not developing. J Allergy Clin Immunol 2001;107:129–34.
31. Isolauri E, Kaila M, Mykkanen H, et al. Oral bacteriotherapy for viral gastroenteritis. Dig Dis Sci 1994;39:2595–600.
32. Vanderhoof JA, Young RJ. Use of probiotics in childhood gastrointestinal disorders. J Pediatr Gastroenterol Nutr 1998;27:323–32.
33. Isolauri E, Juntunen M, Rautanen T, et al. A human Lactobacillus strain (*Lactobacillus* GG) promotes recovery from acute diarrhea in children. Pediatrics 1991;88:90–7.
34. Kaila M, Isolauri E, Soppi E, et al. Enhancement of the circulating antibody secreting cell response in human diarrhea by a human *Lactobacillus* strain. Pediatr Res 1992;32:141–4.
35. Pant AR, Graham SM, Allen SJ, et al. Lactobacillus GG and acute diarrhoea in young children in the tropics. J Trop Pediatr 1996;42:162–5.
36. Saavedra JM, Bauman NA, Oung I, et al. Feeding of *Bifidobacterium bifidum* and *Streptococcus thermophilus* to infants in hospital for prevention of diarrhoea and shedding of rotavirus. Lancet 1994;344:1046–9.
37. Guandalini S, Pensabene L, Zikri MA, et al. *Lactobacillus* GG administered in oral rehydration solution to children with acute diarrhoea: A multicenter European trial. J Pediatr Gastroenterol Nutr 2000;30:54–60.
38. Sarker SA, Sultana S, Fuchs GJ, et al. *Lactobacillus paracasei* strain ST11 has no effect on rotavirus bu ameliorates the outcome of nonrotavirus diarrhea in children from Bangladesh. Pediatrics 2005;116:e221–8.
39. Costa-Ribeiro H, Ribeiro TC, Mattos AP, et al. Limitations of probiotic therapy in acute, severe dehydrating diarrhea. J Pediatr Gastroenterol Nutr 2003;36:112–5.
40. Oberhelman RA, Gilman RH, Sheen P, et al. A placebo-controlled trial of *Lactobacillus* GG to prevent diarrhea in undernourished Peruvian children. J Pediatr 1999;134:15–20.
41. Szajewska H, Kotowska M, Mrukowicz JZ, et al. Efficacy of *Lactobacillus* GG in prevention of nosocomial diarrhea in infants. J Pediatr 2001;138:361–5.
42. Mastretta E, Longo P, Laccisaglia A, et al. Effect of *Lactobacillus* GG and breast-feeding in the prevention of rotavirus nosocomial infection. J Pediatr Gastroenterol Nutr 2002;35:527–31.
43. Mack DR, Michail S, Wei S, et al. Probiotics inhibit enteropathogenic *E. coli* adherence in vitro by inducing intestinal mucin gene expression. Am J Physiol 1999;39:G941–50.
44. Arvola T, Laiho K, Torkkeli S, et al. Prophylactic *Lactobacillus* GG reduces antibiotic-associated diarrhea in children with respiratory infections: A randomized study. Pediatrics 1999;104:e64.
45. Vanderhoof JA, Whitney DB, Antonson DL, et al. *Lactobacillus* GG in the prevention of antibiotic-associated diarrhea in children. J Pediatr 1999;135:564–8.
46. Elmer GW, Surawicz CM, McFarland LV. Biotherapeutic agents. A neglected modality for the treatment and prevention of selected intestinal and vaginal infections. JAMA 1996;276:29–30.
47. Gupta P, Andrew H, Kirschner BS, Guandalini S. Is Lactobacillus GG helpful in children with Crohn's disease? Results of a preliminary, open-label study. J Pediatr Gastroenterol Nutr 2000;31:453–7.
48. Prantera C, Scribano ML, Falasco G, et al. Ineffectiveness of probiotics in preventing recurrence after curative resection for Crohn's disease: A randomised controlled trial with *Lactobacillus* GG. Gut 2002;51:405–9.
49. Rembacken BJ, Snelling AM, Hawkey PM, et al. Nonpathogenic *Escherichia coli* versus mesalazine for the treatment of ulcerative colitis: A randomised trial. Lancet 1999;354:635–9.
50. Gionchetti P, Rizzello F, Venturi A, et al. Oral bacteriotherapy as maintenance treatment in patients with chronic pouchitis: A double-blind, placebo-controlled trial. Gastroenterology 2000;119:305–9.
51. Yazdanbakhsh M, Kremsner PG, van Ree R. Allergy, parasites, and the hygiene hypothesis. Science 2002;296:490–4.
52. Hartmann G, Weiner GJ, Krieg AM. CpG DNA: A potent signal for growth, activation, and maturation of human dendritic cells. Proc Natl Acad Sci U S A 1999;96:9305–19.
53. Kranzer K, Bauer M, Lipford GB, et al. CpG-oligodeoxynucleotides enhance T-cell receptor-triggered interferon-gamma production and up-regulation of CD69 via induction of antigen-presenting cell-derived interferon type I and interleukin-12. Immunology 2000;99:170–8.
54. Cario E, Rosenberg IM, Brandwein SL, et al. Lipopolysaccharide activates distinct signaling pathways in intestinal epithelial cell lines expressing Toll-like receptors. J Immunol 2000;164:966–72.
55. Hemmi H, Takeuchi O, Kawai T, et al. A Toll-like receptor recognizes bacterial DNA. Nature 2000;408:740–5.
56. Neish AS, Gewirtz AT, Zeng H, et al. Prokaryotic regulation of epithelial responses by inhibition of IkappaB-alpha ubiquitination. Science 2000;289:1560–3.
57. Pessi T, Sutas Y, Hurme M, et al. Interleukin-10 generation in atopic children following oral Lactobacillus rhamnosus GG. Clin Exp Allergy 2000;30:1804–8.

58. Rautava S, Kalliomaki M, Isolauri E. Probiotics during pregnancy and breast-feeding might confer immunomodulatory protection against atopic disease in the infant. J Allergy Clin Immunol 2002;109:119–21.

59. Sutas Y, Soppi E, Korhonen H, et al. Suppression of lymphocyte proliferation in vitro by bovine caseins hydrolysed with *Lactobacillus* GG-derived enzymes. J Allergy Clin Immunol 1996;98:216–24.

60. Sutas Y, Hurme M, Isolauri E. Downregulation of antiCD3 antibody-induced IL-4 production by bovine caseins hydrolysed with Lactobacillus GG-derived enzymes. Scand J Immunol 1996;43:687–9.

61. Pessi T, Sutas Y, Saxelin M, et al. Antiproliferative effects of homogenates derived from five strains of candidate probiotic bacteria. Appl Environ Microb 1999;65:4725–8.

62. von der Weid T, Bulliard C, Schiffrin EJ. Induction by a lactic acid bacterium of a population of CD4+ T cells with low proliferative capacity that produce transforming growth factor beta and interleukin-10. Clin Diagn Lab Immunol 2001;8:695–701.

63. Shida K, Takahashi R, Iwadate E, et al. Lactobacillus casei strain Shirota suppresses serum immunoglobulin E and immunoglobulin G1 responses and systemic anaphylaxis in a food allergy model. Clin Exp Allergy 2002;32:563–70.

64. Majamaa H, Isolauri E. Probiotics: A novel approach in the management of food allergy. J Allergy Clin Immunol 1997;99:179–86.

65. He F, Morita H, Hashimoto H, et al. Intestinal bifidobacterium species induce varying cytokine production. J Allergy Clin Immunol 2002;109:1035–6.

66. Ibnou-Zekri N, Blum S, Schffrin EJ, von der Weid T. Divergent patterns of colonization and immune response elicited from two intestinal *Lactobacillus* strains that display similar properties in vitro. Infect Immun 2003;71:428–36.

67. Isolauri E, Arvola T, Sutas Y, et al. Probiotics in the management of atopic eczema. Clin Exp Allergy 2000;30:1605–10.

68. Rosenfeldt V, Benfeldt E, Nielsen SD, et al. Effect of probiotic Lactobacillus strains in children with atopic dermatitis. J Allergy Clin Immunol 2003;111:389–95.

69. Rosenfeldt V, Benfeldt E, Valerius N, et al. Effect of probiotics on gastrointestinal symptoms and small intestinal permeability in children with atopic dermatitis. J Pediatr 2004;145:612–6.

70. Weston S, Halbert AR, Richmond P, Prescott SL. Effect of probiotics on atopic dermatitis: A randomised controlled trial. Arch Dis Child 2005;90:892–7.

71. Pelto L, Isolauri E, Lilius EM, et al. Probiotic bacteria downregulate the milk-induced inflammatory response in milk-hypersensitive subjects but have an immunostimulatory effect in healthy subjects. Clin Exp Allergy 1998;28:1474–9.

72. Kalliomaki M, Salminen S, Kero P, et al. Probiotics in primary prevention of atopic disease: A randomised placebo-controlled trial. Lancet 2001;357:1076–9.

73. Abrahamsson TR, Jakobsson T, Bottcher MF, et al. Probiotics in prevention of IgE-associated eczema: A double-blind, randomized, placebo-controlled trial. J Allergy Clin Immunol 2007;119:1174–80

74. Kukkonen K, Savilahti E, Haahtela T, et al. Probiotics and prebiotic galacto-oligosaccharides in the prevention of allergic diseases: A randomized, double-blind, placebo-controlled trial. J Allergy Clin Immunol 2007;119:192–8.

75. Taylor AL, Dunstan JA, Prescott SL. Probiotic supplementation for the first 6 months of life fails to reduce the risk of atopic dermatitis and increases the risk of allergen sensitization in high-risk children: A randomized controlled trial. J Allergy Clin Immunol 2007;119:184–91.

76. Kalliomaki M, Salminen S, Poussa T, et al. Probiotics and prevention of atopic disease a 4-year follow-up of a randomised placebo-controlled trial. Lancet 2003:361;1869–71.

77. Lee YK, Lim CY, Teng WL, et al. Qualitative approach in the study of adhesion of lactic acid bacteria on intestinal cells and their competition with enterobacteria. Appl Environ Microbiol 2000;66:3692–7.

78. Ouwehand A, Salminen S, Tolkko S, et al. Resected human colonic tissue: A new model for characterising adhesion of lac-tic acid bacteria. Clin Diagn Labor Immunol 2002:10:184–6.

79. Mao Y, Nobaek S, Kasravi B, et al. Effects of *Lactobacillus* strains and oat bran on methotrexate-induced enterocolitis in rats. Gastroenterology 1996;111:334–44.

80. Steidler L, Hans W, Schotte L, et al. Treatment of murine colitis by *Lactococcus lactis* secreting interleukin-10. Science 2000;289:1352–5.

81. Hartke A, Bouche S, Giard JC, et al. The lactic acid stress response to *Lactococcus lactis* subsp. lactis. Curr Microbiol 1996;33:194–9.

82. Hartke A, Bouche S, Gansel X, et al. Starvation-induced stress resistance in *Lactococcus lactis* subsp. lactis IL1403. Appl Environ Microbiol 1994;60:3474–8.

83. Kets EPW, Teunissen PJM, de Bont JAM. Effect of compatible solutes on survival of lactic acid bacteria subjected to drying. Appl Environ Microbiol 1996;62:259–61.

84. Salminen S, von Wright A, Morelli L, et al. Demonstration of safety of probiotics—a review. Int J Food Microbiol 1998;44:93–106.

85. Apostolou E, Kirjavainen, Saxelin M, et al. Good adhesion properties of probiotics: A potential risk for bacteremia? FEMS Immunol Med Microbiol 2001;67:2430–5.

86. Saxelin M, Chuang NH, Chassy B, et al. Lactobacilli and bacteremia in Southern Finland. 1989–1992. Clin Infect Dis 1996;22:564–6.

87. Salminen MK, Tynkkynen S, Rautelin H, et al. Lactobacillus bacteremia during a rapid increase in probiotic use of *Lactobacillus rhamnosus* GG in Finland. Clin Infect Dis 2002;35:1155–60.

88. Sullivan A, Nord CE. Probiotic lactobacilli and bacteraemia in Stockholm. Scand J Infect Dis 2006;38:327–331.

89. Asahara T, Takahashi M, Nomoto K, et al. Assessment of safety of *Lactobacillus* strains based on resistance to host innate defense mechanisms. Clin Diagn Lab Immunol 2003;10:169–73.

90. Rinne M, Kalliomäki M, Salminen S, Isolauri E. Probiotic intervention in the first months of life: Short-term effects on gastrointestinal symptoms and long-term effects on gut microbiota. J Pediatr Gastroenterol Nutr 2006;43:200–5.

91. Gueimonde M, Kalliomäki M, Isolauri E, Salminen S. Probiotic intervention in neonates will permanent colonization ensue? J Pediatr Gastroenterol Nutr 2006;42:604–6.

92. Saavedra JM, Abi-Hanna A, Moore N, Yolken RH. Long-term consumption of infant formulas containing live probiotic bacteria: Tolerance and safety. Am J Clin Nutr 2004;79:261–267.

93. Laitinen K, Kalliomäki M, Poussa T, et al. Evaluation of diet and growth in children with and without atopic eczema: Follow-up study from birth to four years. Brit J Nutr 2005;94:565–74.

94. Salminen S, Isolauri E, von Wright A. Safety of probiotic bacteria. Rev Food Nutr Tox 2003;1:279–84.

95. U.S. Food and Drug Administration. Summary of Gras Notices. http://www.cfsan.fda.gov/~rdb/opagras.html (accessed on August 27th, 2007).

96. European Food Safety Authority. Qualified presumption of safety of micro-organisms in food and feed. http://www.efsa.europa.eu/en/science/sc_commitee/sc_consultations/sc_consultation_qps.html (accessed on August 27th, 2007).

19.1b. Prebiotics, Synbiotics, and Fermented Products

Hania Szajewska, MD

Raanan Shamir, MD

A growing understanding of the possible role of gut microbiota in health and disease has led to an interest in the development of strategies aimed at manipulating bacterial colonization. These have included the administration of probiotics (discussed in detail in Chapter 19.1a) or prebiotics or a combination of both (synbiotics).[1] This chapter was prepared following a comprehensive literature search to evaluate the available evidence of the efficacy of prebiotics, synbiotics, and fermented products principally in the pediatric population. To identify the published evidence, MEDLINE, EMBASE, the Cochrane Database of Systematic Reviews, and the Cochrane Controlled Trials Register (all up until June 2006) were searched. The search was restricted to randomized controlled trials (RCTs) or their systematic reviews or meta-analyses, using relevant keywords. The reference lists of articles identified by these strategies were also searched. Relevant key review articles published in high impact journals and book chapters, as well as position papers developed by respected scientific societies or expert groups, were considered. There was no restriction on language of publication.

After a review of definitions and properties of prebiotics, synbiotics, and fermented products with nonviable bacteria, respectively, this chapter will address different gastrointestinal entities in which prebiotics, synbiotics, or products with nonviable bacteria have been used; for each product, the chapter will provide a brief overview of its potential benefit related to its possible pathophysiological role, followed by a critical review of available published data.

PREBIOTICS DEFINITION

The term prebiotic was introduced by Gibson and Roberfroid in 1995 who defined prebiotics as "nondigestible food components that beneficially affect the host by selectively stimulating the growth and/or activity of one or a limited number of bacteria in the colon and thereby improving host health."[2] It is expected from a prebiotic product to not only get hydrolyzed by human intestinal enzymes, but that beneficial bacteria should selectively ferment it; this selective fermentation results in a beneficial effect on the health or well-being of the host.[3] Therefore, it has been suggested that one should define prebiotics as nondigestible

food ingredients that appear to be beneficial to the host mainly by selectively stimulating the growth and the activity of one or more species of "friendly" bacteria in the colon.[4] Nevertheless, as will be pointed out later, the beneficial effects of prebiotics are not limited to fermentation of these nondigestible carbohydrates. In addition, it may be advisable to define prebiotics as nondigestible or low-digestible carbohydrates,[5] since available data suggest that at least human oligosaccharides are minimally digested in the upper gastrointestinal tract[6] and enter the circulation using, depending on their characteristics, receptor mediated transcytosis and paracellular pathways.[7] Finally, to avoid the term digestion and to include fermentation, effects on the intestinal flora and possible systemic effects following intestinal uptake, it may be more appropriate to define a prebiotic as a selectively fermented ingredient that allows specific changes, both in the composition and/or activity of the intestinal microflora, that confer benefits upon the host's well-being and health.[8,9]

OLIGOSACCHARIDES IN HUMAN MILK

Oligosaccharides that are contained in human breast milk are considered the prototype of prebiotics, since they have been shown to facilitate the growth of bifidobacteria and lactobacilli in the colon of breast-fed neonates.[7,10–12] Human milk oligosaccharides comprise the third largest solid component in mature human milk after lactose and fat. In fact, there are more oligosaccharides than protein in breast milk.[13] Human milk contains more than 130 different oligosaccharides at concentrations of 15 to 23 g/L in colostrum and 8 to 12 g/L in transitional and mature milk.[14] Different concentrations have been reported mainly due to differences in measurement methods.[6] Most human milk oligosaccharides have a lactose unit at the reducing end and commonly contain variable fucose residues at the nonreducing end of the sugar. The monomers of milk oligosaccharides are D-glucose, D-galactose, N-acetylglucosamine, L-fucose, and sialic acid. The addition of L-fucose requires at least three different fucosyltransferases and is genetically determined. Close to 80% of the Caucasian population has a fucosyltransferase that is encoded by the secretor blood group type gene, whereas other fucosyltransferases are encoded by the Lewis and

related blood type genes. Therefore, the fucosylated oligosaccharides composition of human milk is linked to blood group subtype and varies in accordance with the expression of specific genetic polymorphisms.[15]

Human milk oligosaccharides are resistant to enzymatic digestion in the upper gastrointestinal tract.[16] However, as noted earlier, human milk oligosaccharides enter the circulation; oligosaccharides typical of human milk can be found in the urine of breast-fed infants, accounting for about 1% of the daily oligosaccharide intake.[6] Human milk oligosaccharides are often regarded as a model for the addition of oligosaccharides of a prebiotic nature to infant formulae or follow-on formulae; this is despite the fact that the biologic role of human milk oligosaccharides appears to be far more complex than the roles of the simple oligosaccharides presently added to formulae.[14] Due to the variety, variability, complexity, and polymorphism of their structure, it is currently not feasible to replicate the oligosaccharide component of human milk in infant and follow-on formulae.[17] This is well illustrated in a study in which banked milk samples were analyzed for oligosaccharide content.[18] In that study, moderate-to-severe diarrhea occurred less often ($p = .001$) in infants whose milk contained high levels of total 2-linked fucosyloligosaccharide, *Campylobacter*-induced diarrhea occurred less often ($p = .004$) in infants whose mother's milk contained high levels of a specific 2-linked fucosyloligosaccharide, and calicivirus diarrhea occurred less often ($p = .012$) in infants whose mother's milk contained high levels of lacto-N-difucohexaose, another 2-linked fucosyloligosaccharide. This study links oligosaccharides in human milk to the protective effects of human milk against infection. It is apparent, however, that these oligosaccharides are genetically determined and different from those found in infant formulas.

OLIGOSACCHARIDE INTAKE AND SOURCES

The average daily intake of oligosaccharides in adults varies from 1 to 4 g/d in the United States[19] to 3 to 11 g/d in Europe.[20] In the diet, the most common sources are wheat, onions, bananas, garlic, artichokes, and leeks. Prebiotic oligosaccharides can be produced by extraction from plant materials, using microbiological synthesis, enzymatic synthesis, and by enzymatic hydrolysis of polysaccharides.[9] In practice, commercial prebiotics are galactooligosaccharides and inulin-type fructans.[21] Many patents concerning prebiotic oligosaccharides have been claimed and this field is continuously increasing.[5] Therefore, it is expected that many new food items containing prebiotic oligosaccharides will be marketed. Indeed, an infant formula containing long-chain inulin (10%) and galactooligosaccharides (90%) was recently released to the market in many countries. While this formula is the only prebiotic mixture in infant nutrition that was evaluated in double-blind controlled studies (see discussion on clinical studies later in this chapter), it is important to emphasize that this oligosaccharide mixture is different from human milk oligosaccharides. Therefore, health claims made for breast milk and then attributed to oligosaccharides call for scientific confirmation of the specific product; the same is true for all future oligosaccharides that will enter the pediatric nutrition market.

MECHANISM OF ACTION

Prebiotics present in human milk, found in food, or supplemented to the diet (eg, inulin-type fructans, galactooligosaccharides) are not hydrolyzed by small intestinal enzymes; thus, they enter the colon and are fermented, resulting in a more acidic luminal pH and an increased concentration of short-chain fatty acids such as lactic, butyric, propionic, and acetic acids. This, in turn, results in increased proliferation of certain commensal bacteria, mainly but not exclusively, bifidobacteria and lactobacilli, which function as probiotics to stimulate intestinal host defenses.[22] Thus, prebiotics may be responsible indirectly for some of the beneficial effects of probiotics. In addition, the produced short-chain fatty acids provide an energy source for colonocytes as well as a stimulus for bacterial–epithelial cell "crosstalk" cellular events, eg, upregulation of toll-like receptor (TLR) expression.[23] Several studies have demonstrated the specific effect of prebiotic oligosaccharides in achieving a lower luminal pH and increased concentration of short-chain fatty acids in the colon, as well as an increased concentration of bifidobacteria and lactobacilli; however, long-term studies demonstrating a sustained effect of prebiotics are lacking. In addition, one may deduce that since prebiotics stimulate an increase in bifidobacteria and lactobacilli, the effect of this stimulation on health is similar to that observed with use of probiotics. This assumption, however, needs to be proven in clinical trials.

Prebiotics can interact with receptors on immune cells and, thus, provide direct effects that do not require the proliferation of commensal (probiotic) bacteria.[24] Along that line, Roller and colleagues have shown in rats that prebiotics, independent of their probiotic effect, can directly stimulate an upregulation of regulatory (IL-10) and protective (INF-γ) cytokines, suggesting that

prebiotics by themselves directly stimulate the mucosal immune system.[25] Furthermore, pathologic bacteria must first adhere to the mucosa and without adherence pathogens cannot act on the gut epithelium to cause disease. Specific terminal sugars on oligosaccharides (eg, fructose) can interfere with adhesins on bacteria by binding to the bacteria and preventing their attachment to the same sugar on the microvillus membrane glycoconjugates.[22] The potential to develop prebiotics with a receptor sequence with optimal antiadhesive activity to inhibit binding of enteric pathogens is discussed elsewhere (see references 9 and 26).

Prebiotic carbohydrate properties are not limited to direct and indirect immunomodulation, but also include metabolic functions such as improved mineral absorption and influence on lipid metabolism. Animal studies have shown that inulin-type fructans increase mineral absorption, especially calcium absorption[27] and bone mineralization.[28] Clinical evidence for such an effect in adolescent girls is discussed elsewhere in this chapter. Possible explanations for enhanced calcium absorption include increased absorption of calcium in the colon by scavenging unabsorbed calcium,[29] increased solubility of minerals by short-chain fatty acids in the colon, and a possible trophic effect throughout the intestine that promotes passive calcium absorption.[30] Animal studies have demonstrated that inulin-type fructans affect the metabolism of lipids, primarily by decreasing triglyceride blood levels both in the fasting and the postprandial state.[31] The effect on blood levels of cholesterol in these studies was less constant, being significant in only some of the studies. The mechanism involved may include reduced liver lipogenesis mediated by reducing the expression of the genes coding for the lipogenic enzymes, with a reduction in the number of VLDL particles. It is still unknown whether these effects are a result of intestinal or systemic processes; the interested reader can find an elaborate discussion of the various possibilities in reference 9.

PREBIOTIC OLIGOSACCHARIDES IN INFANT FORMULAE

The use of nondigestible carbohydrates (ie, oligofructosyl-saccharose and oligogalactosyl-lactose) in infant formulae and follow-on formulae has been commented on by the Committee on Nutrition of the European Society for Pediatric Gastroenterology, Hepatology, and Nutrition (ESPGHAN).[14] Below we summarize results from RCTs evaluated by the ESPGHAN Committee and trials published after the publication of the Committee report. For characteristics of these studies, see Table 1.

Effects on Stool Bifidobacterium

Several RCTs have demonstrated that supplementation of preterm or term infant formulas with the addition of 0.4, 0.8, or 1 g/dL of a mixture of 90% galactooligosaccharides (GOS) and 10%

fructooligosaccharides (FOS) compared with standard formula result in a significant increase in fecal bifidobacteria.[32–35] According to the results of one study, this effect is dose dependent, with a concentration of the GOS/FOS mixture of 0.8 g/dL of formula inducing a higher number of bifidobacteria than the concentration of 0.4 g/dL.[34] Only one RCT revealed no statistically significant differences between groups fed formula supplemented with a mixture of GOS/FOS (0.6 g/dL), formula supplemented with *Bifidobacterium animalis* strain Bb-12 (6×10^{10} CFU/L), or standard infant formula between birth and 16 weeks of age.[36] Interestingly, supplementation of infant formula with 1.5 or 3 g/L (0.15 or 0.3 g/dL) of fructooligosaccharides had a minimal effect on bifidobacteria in one study. The authors speculated that this finding, which contrasts with results from most previous studies, could indicate that the infant formula used in the control group also promoted bifidobacteria (and lactobacilli) growth.[37]

Effect on Stool Lactobacillus

Only a few studies have evaluated the effect of oligosaccharide supplementation on fecal lactobacilli; an increase in the total number of lactobacilli was demonstrated in some of them.[32–34]

Effect on Potentially Pathogenic Microflora

Three RCTs showed no effect of oligosaccharide supplementation of either GOS/FOS[32,33] or acidic oligosaccharides[38] on the number of infants with positive fecal cultures for potentially pathogenic microorganisms (*Bacteroides, E. coli, Clostridium, Enterobacter, Citrobacter, Proteus, Klebsiella,* and *Candida*). In one RCT,[33] GOS/FOS reduced the total number as well as the share of clinically relevant pathogens in the fecal flora. These findings suggest that prebiotic substances might have the capacity to protect against intestinal infections.

Effect on Stool Characteristics

Some, but not all, RCTs found that oligosaccharides softened stool consistency and increased stool frequency, with the induction of more watery stools.[32,34]

Effect on Stool pH

One RCT revealed a dose-dependent effect of a mixture of prebiotic oligosaccharides on lowering fecal pH.[34]

Effect on Growth Characteristics

Several studies have demonstrated growth characteristics. Most showed no significant group differences. In one study,[35] weight gain was greater in subjects receiving the new study formula with GOS/FOS mixture rather than the standard formula, but only in girls and only during the first 6 weeks of the 12-week study period. Head circumference was greater after 12 weeks, but again only in girls. Furthermore, the sum of skinfold

Table 1 Prebiotic Oligosaccharides in Dietetic Products for Infants: Summary of Published Randomized Controlled Trials

Study	Participants	Experimental Group	Control Group	Duration of Intervention	Effects on Stool Bifidobacterium	Effects on Stool Lactobacillus	Effect on Pathogenic Microflora	Stool Frequency	Effect on Stool Consistency	Stool pH	Anthropometric Parameters
Preterm Infants											
Boehm et al.[32]	N = 42	GOS/FOS	Placebo; BF (nonrandomized)	28 d	↑	No	NS*	Only for BF	Yes	NA	NS
Knol et al.[33]	N = 25 [Same study population]	GOS/FOS	Placebo	28 d	↑	↑	↓	NS	NA	NA	NA
Term Infants											
Moro et al.[34]	N = 90	GOS/FOS 0.4 or 0.8 g/dL	Placebo	28 d	↑Number: (dose dependent)	↑Number: (dose dependent)	NS	↑	Softer stools	↓ (dose dependent)	NS
Schmelzle et al.[35]	N = 154	GOS/FOS 0.8 g/dL*	Placebo	12 wk	↑	NA	NA	NA	NA	NA	Length NS weight gain, HC, sum of skinfolds see text
Bakker-Zierikzee et al.[36]	N = 120	GOS/FOS 6 g/L	B. animalis Bb12 6×10^10 CFU/L; IF; BF (nonrandomized)	4 mo	NS	NA	NA	NA	NA	↑ compared with standard IF and Bb-12 IF	NA
Knol et al.[101]	N = 53	GOS/FOS 0.8 g/dL	IF; BF (nonrandomized)	6 wk	↑	NA	NA	NS	NS	↓	NA
Decsi et al.[102]	N = 97	GOS/FOS 0.4 g/dL	IF; BF (nonrandomized)	12 wk	↑	NA	NA				NS
Fanaro et al.[38]	N = 46	AOS 0.2 g/dL; AOS 0.2 g/dL; + GOS/FOS 0.6 g/dL	IF+placebo	6 wk	Placebo vs AOS--NS; Placebo vs AOS+GOS/FOS p = .003; AOS vs AOS+GOS/FOS p = .0026	Significant increse in the count of lactobacilli in AOS+GOS/FOS group only	NS		Placebo vs AOS p = .0006[11]; Placebo vs AOS+GOS/FOS p = .0001; AOS + GOS FOS p = .04	Placebo vs AOS p = .003; Placebo vs AOS+GOS/FOS p < .001; AOS + GOS FOS p = .05	NS
Euler et al.[37]	N = 72; Crossover design	FOS (inulin) 1.5 g/L; FOS (inulin) 3 g/L	BF (nonrandomized)	5 wk	After 7 d: Greater in the 1.5 g/L FOS formula group than in the BF or 3 g/L FOS formula group 7 d after termination of suppl: NS	NS	Formula-fed group 100-fold greater count of bacteroides and enterococci than HM; Clostridium counts ↑ after 7 d in the 1.5 g/L FOS	3 g/L–more frequent and significantly softer stools	NA	NA	NS
Ben et al.[103]	N = 271	GOS/FOS 0.4 g/dL	IF; BF (nonrandomized); IF + GOS + BF	6 mo	↑	↑	NS (E. coli)	↑	↑	↓ Compared with nonsupplemented formula	NS

* Plus partially hydrolyzed whey protien; high–palmitic acid level; starch.

AOS acidic oligosaccharides; BF=breast feeding; FOS= fructooligosaccharides; GOS= galactooligodaccharides; HC = head circumference; IF= infant formula; NA = not assessed; NS = not significant.

measurements during the 12-week study was higher, but only in boys.

Side Effects

No adverse effects, other than the occurrence of loose stools, have been reported.

In summary, in line the summing up by the ESPGHAN Committee on Nutrition,[14] it may be concluded that currently (June, 2006) there are only limited published data on the evaluation of prebiotic substances in dietetic products for infants. No general recommendation on the use of oligosaccharide supplementation in infancy for preventive or therapeutic purposes can be made. During the time of their administration, prebiotic oligosaccharides in dietetic products have the potential to increase the total number of bifidobacteria in feces and to soften stools. The available data on oligosaccharide mixtures in infant formulae do not demonstrate adverse effects. Validated clinical outcome measures of prebiotic effects in infants should be characterized in future well-designed and carefully conducted RCTs, with relevant inclusion/exclusion criteria and adequate sample sizes. Such trials should also define the optimal quantities, types and intake durations, and safety of different oligosaccharides.

USE OF PREBIOTICS IN SOLID FOODS FOR CHILDREN

One RCT[39] conducted in 56 healthy term infants aged between 4 and 12 months evaluated the tolerance and gastrointestinal effects of an infant cereal supplemented with either 0.75 FOS per serving or placebo for 28 days. Compared with the control group, stool consistency was less often described as "hard" and more likely to be described as "soft" or "loose" in the FOS-supplemented group. The mean number of stools was 2.0 ± 0.6 per day in the FOS-supplemented group compared with 1.6 ± 0.7 per day in the control group ($p = .02$). There was no difference between the groups in crying, spitting-up, or colic. No difference in stool pH between the groups was found. There was also no significant difference in growth between the two groups. The authors concluded that FOS supplements added to cereal were well tolerated in doses of up to 3 g/d. FOS consumption led to more frequent and softer stools, without reported diarrhea; it also resulted in less-reported frequency of symptoms associated with constipation such as hard stools or days without a stool. Clinical outcomes were not reported. Limitations of this study include the use of nonvalidated tool for parental assessment of stool consistency, a small sample size, and a short follow-up period.

A more recent double-blind RCT[40] involving 35 infants aged 4 to 6 months studied the effect of adding GOS/FOS to solid foods on an increase in bifidobacteria in the intestinal microbiota. Intention-to-treat analysis revealed no significant difference between the two study groups. Only

per-protocol analysis, involving 20 children who complied with the protocol, showed that the percentage of bifidobacteria in feces increased from 43 to 57% ($p = .03$) from week 0 to week 6, but did not significantly change in the control group (36 and 32%, respectively; $p = .4$). There were no differences in stool frequency and consistency between the two groups.

USE OF PREBIOTICS FOR PEDIATRIC DISORDERS

Only a few clinical trials have reported health outcomes for children given prebiotic oligosaccharides (for characteristics of studies see Table 2).

Diarrheal Diseases

Prevention is the most important challenge posed by childhood diarrheal diseases, particularly in developing countries. In the past several years, enormous efforts have been made to develop safe and effective vaccines against enteric infections. The most recent data on rotavirus vaccines are encouraging,[41,42] but other enteric pathogens still await their turn. Children attending day care centers are also at high risk for developing intestinal and respiratory infections. The successful prevention of these infections would be beneficial to families and society. It can be hypothesized that continuous use of prebiotics might, by providing an immunologic stimulus, prove useful in preventing infectious diseases commonly encountered by young children.

In a large, well-designed study performed in Peruvian infants aged between 6 and 12 months ($n = 282$), Duggan and colleagues[43] compared an infant cereal supplemented with oligofructose (0.55 g/15 g cereal) with a nonsupplemented cereal. There was no difference in the number of diarrheal episodes (4 ± 2.9 vs 4.0 ± 3.5), episodes of severe diarrhea (1.3 ± 1.5 vs 1.1 ± 1.2), or episodes of dysentery (0.2 ± 0.6 vs 0.1 ± 0.4). No significant difference was found in the mean duration of diarrhea (10.3 ± 9.6 vs 9.8 ± 11.0 days). During a second part of the same trial involving 349 subjects, zinc (1 mg/15 g cereal) was added to both oligofructose-supplemented and control cereals.[43] Again, no significant difference was found in the number of episodes of diarrhea (3.7 ± 2.6 vs 3.7 ± 2.3), episodes of severe diarrhea (1.5 ± 1.4 vs 1.3 ± 1.3), episodes of dysentery (0.2 ± 0.4 vs 0.1 ± 0.4), or mean duration of diarrhea (10.3 ± 8.9 vs 9.5 ± 8.9 days). In both trials, postimmunization titers of the antibody to *Haemophilus influenzae type* B were similar in both groups, as was height gain (no data on weight), number of visits to the clinic, hospitalizations, and the use of antibiotics. The authors concluded that the use of cereal supplemented with this type and dose of oligosaccharide was not associated with any change in diarrhea prevalence, use of health care resource, or response to H. *influenzae* type B immunization.

Treatment of Acute Infectious Gastroenteritis

A randomized, double-blind, placebo-controlled multicenter study[44] was conducted to evaluate the efficacy and safety of administering a mixture of nondigestible carbohydrates (NDC), including soy polysaccharide 25%, α-cellulose 9%, gum arabic 19%, fructooligosaccharides 18.5%, insulin 21.5%, and resistant starch 7%, as an adjunct to oral rehydration therapy in the treatment of acute infectious diarrhea in children with mild to moderate dehydration. It was hypothesized that with the incorporation of NDC, some of them (eg, fructooligosaccharides, galactooligosaccharides, and inulin) with prebiotic effects might promote fermentation in the colon, and thus, decrease fecal volume and the duration of the diarrheal illness. One hundred forty-four boys aged between 1 and 36 months with diarrhea defined as three or more watery stools per day for >1 day but <5 days with mild or moderate dehydration (World Health Organization criteria) were randomly assigned to receive hypotonic oral rehydration solution (ORS) (Na 60 mmol/L, glucose 111 mmol/L) with or without a mixture of NDC. Intention-to-treat analysis did not show a significant difference in mean 48-hour stool volumes. The duration of diarrhea after randomization was similar in both groups (82 ± 39 hours vs 97 ± 76 hours; $p = .2$). There was no significant difference in the duration of hospital stay, and unscheduled intravenous rehydration was comparable in the two groups. No adverse effects were noted. An explanation for the negative results could originate from the type and the amount of NDC added to the ORS. An average dose of 10 to 15 g per episode in relatively mild diarrhea simply may be insufficient to achieve a shorter duration of diarrhea. Furthermore, it is possible that the timing of the intervention was inappropriate, making the addition of NDC to exclusive oral rehydration therapy an insufficient measure.

Prevention of Antibiotic-Associated Diarrhea

A common side effect of antibiotic treatment is antibiotic-associated diarrhea (AAD), defined as otherwise unexplained diarrhea that occurs in association with the administration of antibiotics.[45] AAD occurs in approximately 11 to 40% of children between the initiation of antibiotic therapy and up to 2 months after cessation of treatment.[46,47] Although no infectious agent is found in most cases, the bacterial agent commonly associated with AAD, particularly in the most severe episodes (pseudomembranous colitis), is *Clostridium difficile*.[48] Almost all antibiotics, particularly those active against anaerobes, can cause diarrhea, but the risk seems to be higher with aminopenicillins, the combination of aminopenicillins and clavulanate, cephalosporins, and clindamycin.[49,50] Preventive measures include microflora modification with probiotics and/or prebiotics. The rationale for such an approach is based on the assumption that the use of antibiotics leads to a disturbance in

Table 2 Prebiotics in Children – Summary of Randomized Controlled Trials

Study ID	Clinical Condition	Prebiotic(s)	Control	N (age)	Outcome	Effect*
Moore et al.[39]	Tolerance	FOS (0.75 mg/portion of infant cereal)	Placebo (maltodextrin)	56 (4–12 mo)	Stool consistency	↓
					Stool frequency	↑
					Crying, spitting-up, colic	NS
					Stool pH	NS
Moro et al.[60]	Prevention of atopic dermatitis in high-risk infants	GOS/FOS (with partial hydrolysate)	Placebo (with partial hydrolysate)	192 (≥ 1 atopic parent)	atopic dermatitis	RR 0.4 (0.2–0.88) NNT 8 (5–37)
Passeron et al.[58]	Treatment of atopic dermatitis	Prebiotic (lactose 0.397 g + potato strach 0.759 g) (n = 22)	Synbiotic (prebiotic + *Lactobacillus rhamnosus* Lcr35 1.2 × 10⁹ CFU (n = 17)	39 (> 2 yr)	SCORAD (SCO Ring atopic dermatitis) score	NS
Duggan et al.[43]	Prevention of diarrheal diesease	Oligofructose (0.55 g/15 g cereal)	Nonsupplemented cereal	282 (6–12 mo)	Episodes of diarrahea	NS
					Episodes of severe diarrhea	NS
					Episodes of dysentery	NS
					Duration of diarrhea	NS
					Postimmunization titers of *Haemophilus influenzae*	NS
					Gains in height, visits to clinic, hospitalizations, use of antibiotics	NS
Duggan et al.[43]	Prevention of diarrheal diesease	Oligofructose (0.55 g/15 g cereal) + Zn (1 mg/15 g cereal)	Nonsupplemented cereal	349 (6–12 mo)	Episodes of diarrhea	NS
					Episodes of severe diarrhea	NS
					Episodes of dysentery	NS
					Duration of diarrhea	NS
					Postimmunization titers of *H. influenzae*	NS
					Gains in height, visits to clinic, hospitalizations, use of antibiotics	NS
Hoekstra et al.[44]	Treatment of acute gastroenteritis	Mixture (soy polysaccharide 25%, α-cellulose 9%, gum arabic 19%, FOS 18.5%, inulin 21.5%, resistant starch 7%) with oral rehydration therapy	Placebo (cow's milk protein)	144 (1–36 mo; boys only)	Stool volume	NS
					Duration of diarrhea	NS
					Duration of hospitalization	NS
					Unscheduled intravenous rehydration	NS
Brunser et al.[57]	Prevention of antibiotic-associated diarrhea	Oligofructose + inulin (raftilose P95 and raftiline) 4.5 g/L	Placebo	140 (1–2 yr)	Diarrhea	NS
					Fecal bifidobacteria	↑
Griffin et al.[61]	Calcium bioavailability	Oligofructose (8 g/d) + inulin Oligofructose (8 g/d)	Placebo (sucrose)	59 (11–14 yr)	Ca absorption	↑
					Ca absorption	NS
Van den Heuvel et al.[62]	Calcium bioavailability	Oligofructose (15 mg/d)	Placebo (sucrose)	12 (14–16 yr, boys)	Ca absorption	↑
Abrams et al.[63]	Calcium bioavailability	Short- and long-term fructans (8 g/d)	Placebo (maltodextrin)	Young adolescents	Ca absorption	↑ (at 8 wk and 1 yr)
					Bone mineral content	↑
					Bone mineral density	↑

* The experimental (prebiotic) group compared with control group.
  FOS = fructooligosaccharides; GOS = galactooligodaccharides; NS = not significant.

the normal intestinal microflora and that this is a key factor in the pathogenesis of AAD.[51] Indeed, at least 5 systematic reviews (with or without meta-analysis) have shown that some probiotic strains are effective in preventing AAD both in adults[52–55] and in children.[56]

In contrast, there is a paucity of data on the use of prebiotics in the prevention of AAD. The only pediatric double-blind RCT[57] involved 140 children (1 to 2 years of age) who were treated with amoxicillin for acute bronchitis. This study revealed no significant difference in the frequences of diarrhea in children receiving oligofructose and inulin administered in a milk formula (4.5 g/L) for 21 days after completion of antibiotics compared with placebo (10% vs 6%, relative risk, RR 0.6, 95% confidence interval, CI 0.2 to 1.8). However, prebiotics in a milk formula increased fecal bifidobacteria early after amoxicillin treatment.

Treatment of Atopic Dermatitis

Atopic eczema is an itchy inflammatory skin condition with associated epidermal barrier dysfunction. Therapeutic options (emollients and topical steroids for mild-to-moderate eczema; topical or systemic calcineurin inhibitors, ultraviolet phototherapy, or systemic azathioprine for moderate-to-severe eczema) are relatively limited and often unsatisfactory, prompting interest in alternative treatment methods.

There has been one double-blind RCT evaluating the effect of synbiotics against prebiotics and not "normal" controls in treating atopic dermatitis.[58] The trial included 39 children, 2 years of age or older, who had a minimum score of 15 on the SCORing atopic dermatitis (SCORAD) scale. In addition to their usual diet and treatment for atopic dermatitis, children were randomized to receive *Lactobacillus rhamnosus* in a synbiotic preparation or prebiotics (lactose plus potato starch) alone, 3 times a day for 3 months. Among children receiving synbiotics, the pretreatment SCORAD score was 39.1 versus 20.7 after 3 months of treatment ($p < .0001$). Among children receiving the prebiotic alone, the pretreatment SCORAD score was 39.3 versus 24.0 after 3 months of treatment ($p < .0001$). There was no significant difference in SCORAD between the children who received synbiotics versus probiotics. In addition, no difference was found in the number of patients who reached at least 50% and 90% improvement ($p = .4$ and $p = .2$, respectively). There was also no difference in the use of topical treatments. Synbiotics and prebiotics were both well tolerated. Although the investigators demonstrated that children with moderate-to-severe atopic dermatitis have a reduction in symptoms following treatment with either prebiotics or synbiotics, these results must be confirmed against placebo and in a larger group of patients.

Prevention of Atopic Disease

The rationale for using prebiotics in the prevention of atopic disorders is based on the concept that prebiotics modify the intestinal flora of formula-fed infants towards that of breast-fed infants. The intestinal flora of atopic children has been found to differ from that of controls. Atopic subjects have more *Clostridia* and tend to have fewer bifidobacteria than nonatopic subjects.[59] Thus, there is indirect evidence that differences in the neonatal gut microflora may precede or coincide with the early development of atopy. This further suggests a crucial role for a balanced commensal gut microflora in the maturation of the early immune system.

One double-blind, randomized, placebo-controlled trial[60] investigated the effect of a prebiotic mixture (90% GOS, 10% long-chain FOS; dosage: 0.8 g/dL) on the intestinal flora and the cumulative incidence of atopic dermatitis during the first 6 months of life in infants at risk for allergy (with at least one parent with documented allergic disease confirmed by physician). Two hundred and six (79.5%) of 259 infants who were randomly assigned to receive extensively hydrolyzed whey formula supplemented either with 0.8 g GOS/FOS ($n = 102$) or maltodextrin as placebo ($n = 104$) were included in the per-protocol analysis. The frequency of atopic eczema in the experimental group was significantly reduced compared with placebo group (9.8% vs 23.1%, RR 0.42 (0.2–0.8), number needed to treat (NNT) 8 (5–31). In a subgroup of 98 infants, parents provided fresh stool samples for microbiological analysis, using plating techniques; the fecal counts of bifidobacteria were higher in the group fed the GOS/FOS formula, compared to the placebo group. By contrast, no significant difference was found for lactobacillus counts between groups. This is the first and only observation that prebiotics are able to reduce the incidence of atopic dermatitis, demonstrating the immune-modulating effect of prebiotics during the first months of life. However, these results should not influence practice until confirmed by further studies. Intention-to-treat analysis was not performed. The drop-out rate of 20% was high. In addition, the prevalence of eczema in the placebo group was relatively high (23.1%), particularly considering the fact that infants in this group received extensively hydrolyzed formula which is designed to be used as a formula to decrease allergy risk. Collectively, these findings argue for caution in applying the results of this study to current clinical practice.

Bioavailability and Absorption of Calcium

Three double-blind cross-over trials have studied the effects of administering oligosaccharides on the bioavailability and absorption of calcium in adolescents. One RCT[61] ($n = 59$) revealed that in girls at or near menarche, calcium absorption was significantly higher in a group receiving an inulin plus oligofructose (8 g/d) mixture than in the placebo group ($38.2 \pm 9.8\%$ vs $32.3 \pm 9.8\%$; $p = .01$); however, no significant difference was seen between the oligofructose without inulin group and those receiving placebo ($31.8 \pm 9.3\%$ vs $31.8 \pm 10\%$; $p = $ NS).

Another RCT[62] in 12 healthy male adolescents aged between 14 and 16 years reported that 15 grams of oligofructose per day was well tolerated and enhanced fractional calcium absorption (mean difference $\pm$ SE of difference: $10.8 \pm 5.6\%$; $p < .05$, one sided) compared with individuals receiving sucrose. No information was provided about the overall calcium balance of study subjects in either of these two RCTs. Thus, it is difficult to critically assess the degree of benefit that might be achieved for overall calcium homeostasis.

The most recent RCT[63] in young adolescents assessed the effects on calcium absorption and bone mineral accretion after 8 weeks and 1 year of supplementation with either 8 g/d of a mixed short- and long- degree of polymerization inulin-type fructan product (fructan group) or maltodextrin (control group). Bone mineral content and bone mineral density were measured before randomization and after 1 year. Calcium absorption was measured with the use of stable isotopes at baseline and at 8 weeks and 1 year after supplementation. Polymorphisms of the Fok1 vitamin D receptor gene were also determined. Daily consumption of the combination of prebiotic short and long-chain inulin-type fructans significantly increased calcium absorption and enhanced bone mineralization during pubertal growth. Effects of dietary factors on calcium absorption may be modulated by genetic factors, including specific vitamin D receptor gene polymorphisms.[30,63] The importance of this study derives from the demonstration of long lasting beneficial effects after prolonged use of prebiotics.

EFFECTS OF PREBIOTICS IN ADULTS

Several reviews of the literature are available.[64–66] In brief, a relatively small number of oligosaccharides considered as prebiotics has been evaluated. At present, there is strong evidence that administration of prebiotics results in an increase in the total number of bifidobacteria in stools.[67] Insufficient evidence is available to state whether inulin or oligofructose might have a cholesterol-lowering effect. Inulin and fructooligosaccharides have dose-related laxative effects, indicating potential for the use of these products in the treatment of constipation. A preliminary report on a small number of patients ($n = 10$ and no control group) suggests that fructooligosaccharides may have a role in the treatment of moderately active Crohn's disease. However, placebo controlled trials are required to confirm the therapeutic efficacy in this setting.[68] No beneficial effect on symptoms of irritable bowel syndrome was reported with oligofructose[69] or fructooligosaccharides.[70] The result of one RCT suggests no efficacy in the prevention of traveler's diarrhea.[71] One RCT found no effect of oligofructose in preventing AAD, whether caused by C. difficile or not.[72] Some RCTs have shown that lactulose and lactitol are superior to placebo in treating hepatic encephalopathy.[73,74] There is some evidence that prebiotic substances may enhance intestinal calcium absorption in postmenopausal women,[75] but no information is available on calcium balance and bone mineral content. Also, the effect on other minerals (Mg^{2+}, Fe^{2+}, and Zn^{2+}) is unclear.

THE ISSUE OF SAFETY OF PREBIOTICS

Prebiotics are be generally regarded as safe, although it was reported that fructans may cause dose-dependent intestinal side-effects in adults.[76]

Furthermore, the occurrence of repeated anaphylactic reactions to inulin and oligofructose was reported in one adult.[77] A study in rats showed that dietary fructooligosaccharides and lactulose improve colonization resistance against *Salmonella enteritidis;* however, in contrast to most expectations, these prebiotics concomitantly promote bacterial translocation (ie, the passage of viable bacteria from the intestinal tract through the epithelial mucosa[78]) of this invasive pathogen. No such effects were observed with resistant starch, wheat fiber, or cellulose supplementation of the diet.[79]

SYNBIOTICS

The term *synbiotic* is used *"when a product contains both probiotics and prebiotics."*[80] It has been suggested that because the word points to synergism, this term should be reserved for products in which the prebiotic compound selectively favors the probiotic compound. Applying this definition to only combinations with proven synergy would be called synbiotics. In practice, however, this term is used whenever a combination of probiotics and prebiotics is used. The rationale behind the use of prebiotics has been provided in this chapter and that of probiotics. Therefore, it is conceivable that a synergistic effect of the two categories would be beneficial for health. In this chapter, the limited literature regarding the use of synbiotics in infants and children is discussed.

EFFICACY OF SYNBIOTICS IN CHILDREN

For characteristics of studies in children see Table 3.

Prevention of Antibiotic-Associated Diarrhea

Only one RCT[81] has investigated the effect of synbiotics on AAD in 120 children aged 4 months to 15 years. In this double-blind RCT, children received antibiotics (erythromycin, other macrolides, amoxicillin + clavulanic acid) plus either 250 mg of FOS and *L. sporogenes* or placebo for 10 days. Analyses were based on intention to treat. Patients in the intervention group had a lower prevalence of diarrhea (defined as two liquid or watery stools per 24 hour) than those who received the placebo [43% vs 68%; RR 0.6 (0.4–0.9)]. For every 4 patients receiving daily synbiotics with antibiotics, one fewer would develop diarrhea (NNT 4, 95% CI 3–14). The duration of diarrhea also was reduced (0.7 vs 1.6 days; $p = .002$). Study limitations include a relatively small sample size and the use of a not widely agreed upon definition of diarrhea. Also, there was no extended period of follow-up. Without robust evidence, no recommendation can be made regarding the use of synbiotics for the prevention of AAD.

Helicobacter pylori Infection

The role of the gram-negative bacillus *Helicobacter pylori* in the pathogenesis of chronic gastritis and peptic ulcer in adults and children and as a risk factor for gastric malignancy in adults is widely accepted. Several studies have shown that various lactobacilli (eg, *L. johnsonii* La1, *L. acidophilus* CRL 639, *L. casei*) or their metabolic products can inhibit or kill *H. pylori* in vitro,[82,83] suggesting that probiotics may have a place as adjunctive treatment for *H. pylori* infection. However, evidence on the usefulness of using probiotics in the eradication of *H. pylori* is limited and questionable. In adults, there is, however, evidence that probiotics reduce the frequency and severity of adverse effects of *H. pylori* eradication regimens.[84]

Data on synbiotics for treating *H. pylori* infections are limited. There has only been one open RCT[85] evaluating whether consumption of either the combination of *Saccharomyces boulardii* plus inulin or of *L. acidophilus* LB would affect *H. pylori* eradication in the pediatric population. Two hundred and fifty-four asymptomatic children, who were positive for *H. pylori* infection by the ^{13}C urea breath test, were allocated to one of three groups: (1) an 8-day course of eradication triple therapy with lanzoprazole, amoxicillin, and clarithromycin, (2) *L. acidophilus* LB, and (3) synbiotic (*S. boulardii* plus inulin). *H. pylori* was eradicated in 66% (30/45), 12% (6/51), and 6.5% (3/46) of the children from the antibiotic group, synbiotic group, and probiotic groups, respectively ($p < .001$). There was no significant difference between the probiotic and synbiotic groups. Given the lack of benefit on *H. pylori* eradication, these data do not support the use of synbiotics alone for the treatment of *H. pylori* infection. However, *S. boulardii* plus inulin could hold promise as an adjunctive agent to triple therapy. Additional studies are needed to confirm these preliminary results.

Treatment of Atopic Dermatitis

As discussed in the prebiotic section of this chapter, there has been one double-blind RCT evaluating the beneficial effect of synbiotics compared with prebiotics in treating atopic dermatitis.[58]

Treatment of Acute Nonintestinal Bacterial Infections

There has been one open RCT[86] ($n = 129$) evaluating the beneficial effect of synbiotics in children aged between 1 and 6 years with acute infections (eg, otitis media, tonsillitis, pharyngitis, bronchitis, or mild pneumonia). All patients received antibiotic therapy. Study groups received either a nutritional supplement with synbiotics (3.5 g/L of fructooligosaccharides and 1×10^9 CFU/g of *L. acidophilus* and *Bifidobacterium* species) or without synbiotics, or a fruit-flavored drink. No significant difference was reported in the percentage of subjects without bacterial illnesses 14 days following antibiotic therapy (94.3% in the synbiotic-supplemented group vs 87.8% in the fruit-flavored drink group, and 80.6% in the nonsupplemented group). There was sig-nificantly greater increase in energy intake and weight for age in the synbiotic group compared with the fruit-flavored group following antibiotic therapy. However, the short-term benefits on body weight are not sufficient reason to recommend the use of synbiotics in the setting of acute bacterial infections.

Prevention of Acute Infections in Undernourished Children

An existing question is whether underweight children, who are at increased risk of acute infectious illnesses, could benefit from prophylaxis in the form of synbiotics. One double-blind RCT[87] addressed the effects of a synbiotic product on sickness and catch-up growth in 626 underweight children (-1SD and -3SD from the median of weight-for-height) aged between 1 and 6 years. In this study, the administration of a nutritional supplement with synbiotics (FOS 0.5 g/L and probiotic bacteria *Bifidobacterium* spp. and *L. acidophilus*, each at the level of 3×10^7 CFU/g) for 4 months did not reveal a significant difference in the incidence of sickness (including diarrhea and upper and lower respiratory tract infections), the total number of sick days, or the need for antibiotic use. The synbiotic group experienced fewer constipation days ($p = .02$), and both feeding groups experienced improved anthropometric measures over time ($p < .001$); however, there was no difference in growth rates between the experimental and control feeding groups when corrected for baseline height and weight. Thus, this RCT failed to demonstrate the efficacy of the synbiotic product. The lack of clinical benefit between groups may be potentially attributed to the benefit of nutritional supplementation overshadowing the effects of the synbiotics.

EFFECTS OF SYNBIOTICS IN ADULTS

A bifidogenic effect, defined as an increase in the size and diversity of bifidobacteria is well documented following administration of synbiotics to adults.[88] One small RCT in 18 adult patients with active ulcerative colitis demonstrated that short-term treatment with 2×10^{11} CFU of *B. longum* plus 6 g of a prebiotic fructooligosaccharide/inulin mixture decreased mucosal inflammation in adult patients with active ulcerative colitis.[89] Other clinical settings studied in RCTs that show potentially encouraging results include irritable bowel syndrome,[90] acute pancreatitis,[91,92] liver transplantation,[93] and hepatic encephalopathy.[94]

ISSUE OF SAFETY OF SYNBIOTICS

As a synbiotic is a combination of a prebiotic and probiotic, safety issues relevant to each of them also apply when the two are used together. The issue of safety of prebiotics was discussed earlier and it was concluded that they do not pose major

Table 3 Synbiotics: Summary of Randomized Controlled Trials in Children

Study ID	Experimental (Synbiotic) Group	Control Group	Design	Study Population	N (age)	Effect*
Gotteland et al.[85]	Inulin + *Saccharomyces boulardii* (n = 57)	*Lactobacillus acidophilus* LB (n = 63) OR triple eradication therapy (n = 57)	RCT, open	Asymptomatic children positive for *Helicobactor pylori* infection by ^{13}C-urea breath test	254 (8.4 ± 1.6 yr)	Significantly higher eradication rate in the triple therapy group compared with both synbiotic and probiotic groups. No significant difference in *H. pylori* eradication rate between synbiotic and probiotic groups
La Rosa et al.[81]	FOS (250 mg) + *L. sporogenes* (5.5 × 10^8 CFU) (n = 60)	Placebo (n = 60)	RCT, double-blind	Receiving antibiotic treatment	120 (4 mo–15 yr)	Reduced risk of diarrhea (RR 0.6, 95% CI 0.4–0.9; NNT 4, 95% CI 3–14)
Passeron et al.[58]	Prebiotic (lactose + potato starch) + *L. rhamnosus* Lcr35 1.2 × 10^9 CFU, for three months (n = 17)	Prebiotic (lactose + potato starch) (n = 22)	RCT, double-blind	Atopic dermatitis	48 (<2 yr)	Total SCORAD (SCORing atopic dermatitis): After 3 months, no statistical differences between the two treatment groups (p = .535), although there was statistically significant difference within the group before and after treatment. Total use of ointment: NS (p = .966). Excellent tolerance
Fisberg et al.[87]	Pediasure + FOS 0.5 g/L + *Bifidobacterium* spp., *L. acidophilus* each at the level of 3 × 10^7 CFU/g (n = 310)	Pediasure (n = 316)	RCT, double-blind	Underweight	626 (1–6 yr)	Number of sick days per month: decrease over time for both groups (p < .001). No difference between the groups. Summary of sick days per month: for both groups, trend related to baseline, p < .01. No difference between the groups. Mean normalized percentiles for weight-for-height: for both groups, trend related to baseline, p < .001. No difference between the groups.
Schrezenmeir et al.[86]	Pediasure + FOS 3.5 g/L *Bifidobacterium* spp. *L. acidophilus* 1 × 10^9 CFU/g (n = 46)	Pediasure (n = 39) OR fruit-flavored drink (n = 44)	RCT, open	Acutely ill (upper respiratory infections) children	129 (1–6 yr)	Significantly greater increase in weight for age in the synbiotic group compared with fruit-flavored group. Appetite levels: NS. Activity levels: NS. Percentage of children without relapse or new bacterial infections: NS. Lactobacillus and bifidobacterium stool content: NS (intention-to-treat analysis); greater *Lactobacillus* count analysis)

NS = not significant; RCT = randomized controlled trial.

risks. A recent review[95] concluded that probiotics are also safe for use in otherwise healthy individuals, but should be used with caution in some populations because of the risk of sepsis. Major risk factors include immune compromise, including a debilitated state or malignancy, and prematurity. Minor risk factors include the presence of a central venous catheter, an impaired intestinal epithelial barrier, (eg, diarrheal illness, intestinal inflammation), administration of the probiotic by jejunostomy, concomitant administration of broad spectrum antibiotics to which the probiotic is resistant, use of probiotics with properties of high mucosal adhesion or known pathogenicity, and cardiac valvular disease (*Lactobacillus* probiotics only). It has been suggested that the presence of a single major or more than one minor risk factor merits caution in using probiotics.

FERMENTED PRODUCTS

Definition

Fermentation products refer to the processing of food that has been fermented with lactic acid producing bacteria during the production process. Fermented milk products in infants include infant and follow-on formulas and, later in life, mainly yogurt products. The concept of formula fermentation has been accepted in the Codex Alimentarius Standard for Infant Formula[96] that lists "L(+)lactic acid-producing cultures" as permitted additives in the preparation of infant formula, with the added comment that this is "*Limited by good manufacturing practice in all types of infant formula.*" Likewise, the European Commission Directive on infant formulae and follow-on

formulae[97] permits the addition of live bacteria to infant and/or follow-on formulae for the purpose of acidification of formulas.

EFFICACY OF FERMENTED INFANT FORMULAE WITHOUT LIVE BACTERIA

Recently, the ESPGHAN Committee on Nutrition published a commentary on the use of fermented infant formulas without live bacteria, including the rationale for the use of such formulas.[98] The Committee defined fermented formulae as infant and follow-on formulae which have been fermented with lactic acid, producing bacteria during the production process, but which do not contain significant amounts of viable bacteria in the final product due to inactivation of the fermenting bacteria by homogenization, pasteurization,

Table 4 Fermented Milk Products: Summary of Randomized Controlled Trials in Children

Reference	Design	Intervention Group	Control Group	N (age)	Duration of Intervention	Main Results
Mullié et al.[99]	RCT, double-blind	FIF (*Bifidobacterium breve* C50 + *Streptococcus thermophilus*)	Standard IF (9/15)	20 (0–4 mo)	4 mo (from birth to 4 mo)	Fecal bifidobacteria level significantly higher ($p < .0499$) in the FIF group at 4 mo of age Higher antipoliovirus IgA titers ($p < .02$) after Pentacoq® vaccination in the FIF group Infants harboring *B. longum/B. infantis* exhibited higher levels of antipoliovirus IgA ($p < .002$)
Thibault et al.[100]	RCT, double-blind	FIF (*B. breve* C50 + *Str. thermophilus*) ($n = 484$)	Standard IF ($n = 484$)	971 (4–6 mo)	5 mo	No difference in incidence of diarrhea, duration of diarrheal episodes, and number of hospital admissions Reduced severity of diarrheal episodes in the FIF group Fewer cases of dehydration (2.5% vs 6.1%, $p = .01$) Fewer medical consultations (46% vs 56.6%, $p = .003$) Fewer oral rehydration solution prescriptions (41.9% vs 51.9%, $p = .003$) Fewer switches to other formulas (59.5% vs 74.9%, $p = .0001$)

Adapted from JPGN 2007; 44:392–7.

FIF = fermented infant formula; IF = infant formula; RCT = randomized controlled trial

sterilization and/or spray-drying. Potential additional properties of such formulae should result from the remaining bacterial components, such as cell membrane components or bacterial DNA, and/or from bacterial metabolites such as lactic acid and other organic acids or proteins with enzyme activity. In short, the rationale for the use of these products is that fermentation products that remain in the formula after the probiotic bacteria have been removed may have beneficial health properties.

The Committee performed a systematic review and identified only two RCTs including 988 infants that involved fermented milk products (for details see Table 4). The first double-blind placebo-controlled RCT[99] aimed to determine whether the amount of the intestinal bifidobacterial flora influences the antibody response to poliovirus vaccination in infants. Only 20 of 30 (67%) enrolled infants completed the study. From birth to 4 months, infants were given either a fermented infant formula ($n = 11$) or a standard formula ($n = 9$). Bacteria in infant stool samples were cultured monthly. Antipoliovirus IgA response to polyvalent vaccine against poliomyelitis virus, diphtheria, tetanus toxoids, *H. influenzae,* and *Bordetella pertussis* was assessed before and one month after the second vaccine injection. The mean cumulative proportion of cultivable fecal bifidobacteria detected from 1 to 4 months was higher in the fermented-formula group ($p = .05$). There was also a higher point prevalence of *B. infantis-B. longum* at 4 months in the fermented-formula group, while there were no differences at other time points or for other species. Total stool IgA contents did not differ between the study groups; however, anti-poliovirus IgA titers (U/g dry stool) were significantly higher in the fermented-formula group at 4 months (median: 1,280 and 507 U/g for the fermented-formula and placebo groups, respectively, $p < .001$). This study, performed in a small number of infants, suggests that stool excretion of anti-poliovirus IgA anti-

bodies is enhanced by a fermented infant formula. However, the clinical relevance of this finding is not known.

The second RCT[100] enrolled a total of 971 infants aged between 4 and 6 months at 94 sites in France, with the aim of assessing the effects of fermented formulae on the incidence and severity of acute diarrhea. Infants received for at least 3 months, and up to 5 months, either a fermented formula (484 infants enrolled, of which 464 completed the study) or a control formula with similar nutrient contents (484 enrolled, 449 completed). The incidence and duration of diarrheal episodes and the number of hospital admissions did not differ between the groups. However, episodes of diarrhea were less severe in the fermented-formula group in the per protocol analysis, with fewer cases of dehydration (2.5% vs 6.1%, $p = .01$), fewer medical consultations (46% vs 57%, $p = .003$), fewer ORS prescriptions (42% vs 52%, $p = .003$) and fewer switches to other formulae (60% vs 75%, $p = .0001$).

It has been shown, albeit from only one RCT, that a fermented infant formula may reduce the severity of infectious diarrhea in infants. Nevertheless, the ESPGHAN Committee on Nutrition concludes that fermented infant formulae have no clear advantage over regular infant formula.[98]

CONCLUSIONS AND FUTURE DIRECTIONS

Prebiotics, synbiotics and products with nonviable bacteria have the potential to prevent and treat many gastrointestinal disorders. Currently, the benefits are largely unproven, but there is a growing body of scientific evidence in support of such benefits. Guidance is needed as to which agent to use, timing, dosage and mode of administration. As there is still too little evidence, further studies investigating the role of prebiotics, synbiotics, and fermented products in clinical practice are required.

REFERENCES

1. Crittenden RG. Prebiotics. In: Tannock GW, editor. Probiotics: A Critical Review. Wymondham: Horizon Scientific Press; 1999. p. 141–56.
2. Gibson GR, Roberfroid MB. Dietary modulation of the human colonic microbiota. Introducing the concept of prebiotics. J Nutr 1995;125:1401–12.
3. Guarner F. Inulin and oligofructose: Impact on intestinal diseases and disorders. Br J Nutr 2005;93:S61–5.
4. Duggan C, Gannon J, Walker WA. Protective nutrients and functional foods for the gastrointestinal tract. Am J Clin Nutr 2002;75:789–808.
5. Grajek W, Olejnik A, Sip A. Probiotics, prebiotics and antioxidants as functional foods. Acta Biochem Pol 2005;52:665–71.
6. Kunz C, Rudloff S, Baier W, et al. Oligosaccharides in human milk: Structural, functional, and metabolic aspects. Ann Rev Nutr 2000;20:699–722.
7. Gnoth MJ, Rudloff S, Kunz C, Kinne RK. Investigations of the in vitro transport of human milk oligosaccharides by a Caco-2 monolayer using a novel high performance liquid chromatography-mass spectrometry technique. J Biol Chem 2001;276:34363–70.
8. Gibson GR, Probert HM, Rastall R, et al. Dietary modulation of the human colonic microbiota: Updating the concept of prebiotics. Nutr Res Rev 2004;17:257–9.
9. Roberfroid MB. Introducing inulin-type fructans. Br J Nutr 2005;93:S13–25.
10. Eshach Adiv O, Berant M, Shamir R. New supplements to infant formulas. Pediatr Endocrinol Rev 2004;2:216–24.
11. Dai D, Walker WA. Protective nutrients and bacterial colonization in the immature human gut. Adv Pediatr 1999;46:353–82.
12. Quigley EMM, Quera R. Small intestinal bacterial overgrowth: roles of antibiotics, prebiotics, and prebiotics. Gastroenterology 2006;130:S78–90.
13. Uauy R, Araya M. Novel oligosaccharides in human milk: Understanding mechanisms may lead to better prevention of enteric and other infections. J Pediatr 2004;145:283–5.
14. ESPGHAN Committee on Nutrition: Agostoni C, Axelsson I, Goulet O, et al. Prebiotic oligosaccharides in dietetic products for infants: A commentary by the ESPGHAN Committee on Nutrition. J Pediatr Gastroenterol Nutr 2004;39:465–73.
15. Newburg DS, Ruiz-Palacios GM, Altaye M, et al. Innate protection conferred by fucosylated oligosaccharides of human milk against diarrhea in breast fed infants. Glycobiology 2004;14:253–63.
16. Engfer MB, Stahl B, Finke B, et al. Human milk oligosaccharides are resistant to enzymatic hydrolysis in the upper gastrointestinal tract. Am J Clin Nutr 2000;71:1589–96.
17. Erney RM, Malone WT, Skelding MB, et al. Variability of human milk neutral oligosaccharides in a diverse population. J Pediatr Gastroenterol Nutr 2000;30:131–3.
18. Morrow AL, Ruiz-Palacios GM, Altaye M, et al. Human milk oligosaccharides are associated with protection against diarrhea in breast-fed infants. J Pediatr 2004;145:297–303.

19. Moshfegh AJ, Friday JE, Goldman JP, Ahuja JK. Presence of inulin and oligofructose in the diets of Americans. J Nutr 1999;129:1407S–11S.
20. van Loo J, Coussement P, de Leenheer L, et al. On the presence of inulin and oligofructose as natural ingredients in the western diet. Crit Rev Food Sci Nutr 1995;35:525–52.
21. Veerman-Wauters G. Application of prebiotics in infant foods. Br J Nutr 2005;93:S57–60.
22. Forchielli ML, Walker WA. The role of gut-associated lymphoid tissue and mucosal defence. Br J Nutr 2005;93: S41–8.
23. Zapolska-Downar D, Siennicka A, Kaczmarczyk M, et al. Butyrate inhibits cytokine-induced VCAM-1 and ICAM-1 expression in cultured endothelial cells: The role of NF-kappaB and PPARalpha. J Nutr Biochem 2004;15:220–8.
24. Watzl B, Girrbach S, Roller M. Inulin, oligofructose and immunomodulation. Br J Nutr 2005;93:S49–55.
25. Roller M, Rechkemmer G, Watzl B. Prebiotic inulin enriched with oligofructose in combination with the probiotics Lactobacillus rhamnosus and Bifidobacterium lactis modulates intestinal immune functions in rats. J Nutr 2004;134:153–6.
26. Gibson GR, McCartney AL, Rastall RA. Prebiotics and resistance to gastrointestinal infections. Br J Nutr 2005;93: S31–4.
27. Coudray C, Tressol JC, Gueux E, Rayssiguier Y. Effects of inulin-type fructans of different chain length and type of branching on intestinal absorption of calcium and magnesium in rats. Eur J Nutr 2003;42:91–8.
28. Roberfroid MB, Cumps J, Devogelaer JP. Dietary chicory inulin increases whole-body bone mineral density in growing male rats. J Nutr 2002;132:3599–602.
29. Mineo H, Amano M, Chui H, et al. Indigestible disaccharides open tight junctions and enhance net calcium, magnesium, and zinc absorption in isolated rat small and large intestinal epithelium. Dig Dis Sci 2004;49:122–32.
30. Abrams SA, Griffin IJ, Hawthorne KM, et al. A combination of prebiotic short-and long-chain inulin-type fructans enhances calcium absorption and bone mineralization in young adolescents. Am J Clin Nutr 2005;82:471–6.
31. Delzenne NM, Daubioul C, Neyrinck A, et al. Inulin and oligofructose modulate lipid metabolism in animals: Review of biochemical events and future prospects. Br J Nutr 2002;87: S255–9.
32. Boehm G, Lidestri M, Casetta P, et al. Supplementation of a bovine milk formula with an oligosaccharide mixture increases counts of faecal bifidobacteria in preterm infants. Arch Dis Child Fetal Neonatal Ed 2002;86:F178–81.
33. Knol J, Boehm G, Lidestri M, et al. Increase of faecal bifidobacteria due to dietary oligosaccharides induces a reduction of clinically relevant pathogen germs in the faeces of formula-fed preterm infants. Acta Paediatr Suppl 2005; 94:31–3.
34. Moro G, Minoli I, Mosca M, et al. Dosage-related bifidogenic effects of galacto-and fructooligosaccharides in formula-fed term infants. J Pediatr Gastroenterol Nutr 2002;34:291–5.
35. Schmelzle H, Wirth S, Skopnik H, et al. Randomized double-blind study of the nutritional efficacy and bifidogenicity of a new infant formula containing partially hydrolyzed protein, a high beta-palmitic acid level, and nondigestible oligosaccharides. J Pediatr Gastroenterol Nutr 2003;36:343–51.
36. Bakker-Zierikzee AM, Alles MS, Knol J, et al. Effects of infant formula containing a mixture of galacto-and fructo-oligosaccharides or viable Bifidobacterium animalis on the intestinal microflora during the first 4 months of life. Br J Nutr 2005;94:783–90.
37. Euler AR, Mitchell DK, Kline R, Pickering LK. Prebiotic effect of fructo-oligosaccharide supplemented term infant formula at two concentrations compared with unsupplemented formula and human milk. J Pediatr Gastroenterol Nutr 2005;40:157–64.
38. Fanaro S, Jelinek J, Stahl B, et al. Acidic oligosaccharides from pectin hydrolysate as new component for infant formulae: Effect on intestinal flora, stool characteristics, and pH. J Pediatr Gastroenterol Nutr 2005;41:186–90.
39. Moore N, Chao C, Yang LP, et al. Effects of fructo-oligosaccharide-supplemented infant cereal: A double-blind, randomized trial. Br J Nutr 2003;90:581–7.
40. Scholtens PA, Alles MS, Bindels JG, et al. Bifidogenic effects of solid weaning foods with added prebiotic oligosaccharides: A randomised controlled clinical trial. J Pediatr Gastroenterol Nutr 2006;42:553–9.
41. Vesikari T, Matson DO, Dennehy P, et al. Rotavirus Efficacy and Safety trial (REST) Study Team. Safety and efficacy of a pentavalent human-bovine (WC3) reassortant rotavirus vaccine. N Engl J Med 2006;354:23–33.
42. Ruiz-Palacios GM, Perez-Schael I, Velazquez FR, et al. Human Rotavirus Vaccine Study Group. Safety and efficacy of an attenuated vaccine against severe rotavirus gastroenteritis. N Engl J Med 2006;354:11–22.
43. Duggan C, Penny ME, Hibberd P, et al. Oligofructose-supplemented infant cereal: 2 randomized, blinded, community-based trials in Peruvian infants. Am J Clin Nutr 2003;77:937–42.
44. Hoekstra JH, Szajewska H, Zikri MA, et al. Oral rehydration solution containing a mixture of non-digestible carbohydrates in the treatment of acute diarrhea: A multicenter randomized placebo controlled study on behalf of the ESPGHAN working group on intestinal infections. J Pediatr Gastroenterol Nutr 2004;39:239–45.
45. Bartlett JG. Antibiotic-associated diarrhea. N Engl J Med 2002;346:334–9.
46. Turck D, Bernet JP, Marx J, et al. Incidence and risk factors of oral antibiotic-associated diarrhea in an outpatient pediatric population. J Pediatr Gastroenterol Nutr 2003;37:22–6.
47. Elstner CL, Lindsay AN, Book LS, et al. Lack of relationship of *Clostridium difficile* to antibiotic-associated diarrhea in children. Pediatr Inf Dis 1983;2:364–6.
48. Bartlett JG. Antibiotic-associated diarrhea. N Engl J Med 2002;346:334–9.
49. Barbut F, Meynard JL, Guiguet M, et al. *Clostridium difficile*-associated diarrhea in HIV infected patients: epidemiology and risk factors. J Acq Immun Def Synd 1997;16:176–81.
50. McFarland LV, Surawicz CM, Stamm WE. Risk factors for *Clostridium difficile* carriage and *C. difficile*-associated diarrhea in a cohort of hospitalized patients. J Infect Dis 1990;162:678–84.
51. Surawicz CM. Probiotics, antibiotic-associated diarrhoea and *Clostridium difficile* diarrhoea in humans. Vest Pract Res Clin Gastroenterol 2003;17:775–83.
52. D'Souza AL, Rajkumar C, Cooke J, Bulpitt CJ. Probiotics in prevention of antibiotic associated diarrhoea: Meta-analysis Br Med J 2002;324:1361–4.
53. Cremonini F, Di Caro S, Nista EC, et al. Meta-analysis: The effect of probiotic administration on antibiotic-associated diarrhoea. Aliment Pharmacol Ther 2002;16:1461–7.
54. Szajewska H, Mrukowicz J. Meta-analysis: Non-pathogenic yeast *Saccharomyces boulardii* in the prevention of antibiotic-associated diarrhea. Aliment Pharmacol Ther 2005;22:365–72.
55. Hawrelak JA, Whitten DL, Myers SP. Is *Lactobacillus rhamnosus* GG effective in preventing the onset of antibiotic-associated diarrhoea: A systematic review. Digestion 2005;72:51–6.
56. Szajewska H, Ruszczyński M, Radzikowski A. Probiotics in the prevention of antibiotic-associated diarrhea in children: A meta-analysis of randomized controlled trials. J Pediatr 2006;149:367–72.
57. Brunser O, Gotteland M, Cruchet S, et al. Effect of a milk formula with prebiotics on the intestinal microbiota of infants after an antibiotic treatment. Pediatr Res 2006;59:451–6.
58. Passeron T, Lacour JP, Fontas E, Ortonne JP. Prebiotics and synbiotics: Two promising approaches for the treatment of atopic dermatitis in children above 2 years. Allergy 2006;61:431–7.
59. Kalliomaki M, Kirjavainen P, Eerola E, et al. Distinct patterns of neonatal gut microflora in infants in whom atopy was and was not developing. J Allergy Clin Immunol 2001; 107:129–34.
60. Moro G, Arslanoglu S, Stahl B, et al. A mixture of prebiotic oligosaccahairdes reduces the incidence of atopic dermatitis during the first six months of age. Arch Dis Child 2006;91:814–9.
61. Griffin IJ, Davila PM, Abrams S.A. Non-digestible oligosaccharides and calcium absorption in girls with adequate calcium intakes. Br J Nutr 2002;87:S187–91.
62. Van den Heuvel EG, Muys T, van Dokkum W, et al. Oligofructose stimulates calcium absorption in adolescents. Am J Clin Nutr 1999;69:544–8.
63. Abrams SA, Griffin IJ, Hawthorne KM, et al. A combination of prebiotic short- and long-chain inulin-type fructans enhances calcium absorption and bone mineralization in young adolescents. Am J Clin Nutr 2005;82:471–6.
64. Conway PL. Prebiotics and human health: The state-of-the-art and future perspectives. Scand J Nutr 2001;45: 13–21.
65. Andersson H, Asp N-H, Bruce Å, et al. Health effects of probiotics and prebiotics. A literature review on human studies. Scand J Nutr 2001;45:58–75.
66. Marteau P, Boutron-Ruault MC. Nutritional advantages of probiotics and prebiotics. Br J Nutr 2002;87:S153–7.
67. Kolida S, Tuohy K, Gibson GR. Prebiotic effects of inulin and oligofructose. Br J Nutr 2002;87:S193–7.
68. Lindsay JO, Whelan K, Stagg AJ, et al. Clinical, microbiological, and immunological effects of fructo-oligosaccharide in patients with Crohn's disease. Gut 2006;55:348–55.
69. Hunter JO, Tuffnell Q, Lee AJ. Controlled trial of oligofructose in the management of irritable bowel syndrome. J Nutr 1999;129:1451S–3S.
70. Olesen M, Gudmand-Hoyer E. Efficacy, safety, and tolerability of fructooligosaccharides in the treatment of irritable bowel syndrome. Am J Clin Nutr 2000;72:1570–5.
71. Cummings JH, Christie S, Cole TJ. A study of fructo oligosaccharides in the prevention of travellers' diarrhoea. Aliment Pharmacol Ther 2001;15:1139–45.
72. Lewis S, Burmeister S, Brazier J. Effect of the prebiotic oligofructose on relapse of Clostridium difficile-associated diarrhea: A randomized, controlled study. Clin Gastroenterol Hepatol 2005;3:442–8.
73. Clausen MR, Mortensen PB. Lactulose, disaccharides and colonic flora. Clinical consequences. Drugs 1997;53: 930–42.
74. Dhiman RK, Sawhney MS, Chawla YK, et al. Efficacy of lactulose in cirrhotic patients with subclinical hepatic encephalopathy. Dig Dis Sci 2000;45:1549–52.
75. van den Heuvel EG, Schoterman MH, Muijs T. Transgalactooligosaccharides stimulate calcium absorption in postmenopausal women. J Nutr 2000;130:2938–42.
76. Anonymous. Safety evaluation of fructans. Nordic Council of Ministers, Copenhagen 2000; TemaNord 2000;523:115.
77. Gay-Crosier F, Schreiber G, Hauser C. Anaphylaxis from inulin in vegetables and processed food. N Engl J Med 2000;18:1372–3.
78. Van Leeuwen PA, Boermeester MA, Houdijk AP, et al. Clinical significance of translocation. Gut1994;35: S28–34.
79. Bovee-Oudenhoven IMJ, ten Bruggencate SJM, Lettink-Wissink MLG, et al. Dietary fructo-oligosaccharides and lactulose inhibit intestinal colonisation but stimulate translocation of salmonella in rats. Gut 2003;52:1572–8.
80. Schrezenmeir J, de Vrese M. Probiotics, prebiotics, and synbiotics-approaching a definition. Am J Clin Nutr 2001; 73:361S–4S.
81. La Rosa M, Bottaro G, Gulino N, et al. Prevention of antibiotic-associated diarrhea with Lactobacillus sporogens and fructo-oligosaccharides in children. A multicentric double-blind vs placebo study. Minerva Pediatr 2003;55:447–52.
82. Bhatia SJ, Kochar N, Abraham P, et al. *Lactobacillus acidophilus* inhibits growth of *Campylobacter pylori* in vitro. J Clin Microbiol 1989;27:2328–30.
83. Bernet MF, Brassart D, Neeser JR, et al. *Lactobacillus acidophilus* LA 1 binds to cultured human intestinal cell lines and inhibits cell attachment and cell invasion by enterovirulent bacteria. Gut 1994;35:483–9.
84. Cremonini F, Di Caro S, Covino M, et al. Effect of different probiotic preparations on anti–*Helicobacter pylori* therapy-related side effects: A parallel group, triple blind, placebo-controlled study. Am J Gastroenterol 2002;97:2744–9.
85. Gotteland M, Poliak L, Cruchet S, Brunser O. Effect of regular ingestion of *Saccharomyces boulardii* plus inulin or *Lactobacillus acidophilus* LB in children colonized by *Helicobacter pylori*. Acta Paediatr 2005;94:1747–51.
86. Schrezenmeir J, Heller K, McCue M, et al. Benefits of oral supplementation with and without synbiotics in young children with acute bacterial infections. Clinical Pediatrics 2004;43:239–49.
87. Fisberg M, Maulen-Radovan IE, Tormo R, et al. Effect of oral nutritional supplementation with and without synbiotics on sickness and catch-up growth in preschool children. Internat Pediatr 2002;17:216–22.
88. Bartosch S, Woodmansey EJ, Paterson JC, et al. Microbiological effects of consuming a synbiotic containing *Bifidobacterium bifidum*, *Bifidobacterium lactis*, and oligofructose in elderly persons,determined by real-time polymerase chain reaction and counting of viable bacteria. Clin Infect Dis 2005;40:28–37.
89. Furrie E, Macfarlane S, Kennedy A, et al. Synbiotic therapy (*Bifidobacterium longum*/synergy 1) initiates resolution of inflammation in patients with active ulcerative colitis: A randomised controlled pilot trial. Gut 2005;54:242–9.
90. Tsuchiya J, Barreto R, Okura R, et al. Single-blind follow-up study on the effectiveness of a symbiotic preparation in irritable bowel syndrome. Chin J Dig Dis 2004;5:169–74.
91. Olah A, Belagyi T, Issekutz A, et al. Randomized clinical trial of specific lactobacillus and fibre supplement to early enteral nutrition in patients with acute pancreatitis. Br J Surg 2002;89:1103–7.
92. Olah A, Belagyi T, Issekutz A, Olgyai G. Combination of early nasojejunal feeding with modern synbiotic therapy in the treatment of severe acute pancreatitis (prospective, randomized, double-blind study). Magy Seb 2005;58:173–8.
93. Rayes N, Seehofer D, Theruvath T, et al. Supply of pre- and probiotics reduces bacterial infection rates after liver transplantationa randomized, double-blind trial. Am J Transplant 2005;5:125–30.
94. Liu Q, Duan ZP, Ha da K, et al. Synbiotic modulation of gut flora: Effect on minimal hepatic encephalopathy in patients with cirrhosis. Hepatology 2004;39:1441–9.

95. Boyle RJ, Robins-Browne RM, Tang ML. Probiotic use in clinical practice: What are the risks? Am J Clin Nutr 2006;83:1256–64.

96. Codex Alimentarius Commission. Codex standard for infant formula. Codex Stan 1981;72.

97. Commission Directive of 14 May 1991 on infant formulae and follow-on formulae 91/321/EEC. Office for official publications the European Community 1991, p. 1–27.

98. ESPGHAN Committee on Nutrition. Fermented formulae without live bacteria. A commentary by the ESPGHAN Committee on Nutrition. J Pediatr Gastroenterol Nutr 2007; 44: 392–7.

99. Mullié C, Yazourh A, Thibault H, et al. Increased polio-virus-specific intestinal antibody response coincides with promotion of *Bifidobacterium longum-infantis* and *Bifidobacterium breve* in infants: A randomized, double-blind, placebo-controlled trial. Pediatr Res 2004;56:791–5.

100. Thibault H, Aubert-Jacquin C, Goulet O. Effects of long-term consumption of a fermented infant formula (with *Bifidobacterium breve c50* and *Streptococcus thermophilus* 065) on acute diarrhea in healthy infants. J Pediatr Gastroenterol Nutr 2004;39:147–52.

101. Knol J, Scholtens P, Kafka C, et al. Colon microflora in infants fed formula with galacto and fructo-oligosaccharides: More like breast-fed infants. J Pediatr Gastroenterol Nutr 2005;40:36–42.

102. Decsi T, Arato A, Balogh M, et al. Randomised placebo controlled double blind study on the effect of prebiotic oligosaccharides on intestinal flora in healthy infants. Orv Hetil 2005;146:2445–50.

103. Ben XM, Zhou XY, Zhao WH, et al. Supplementation of milk formula with galacto-oligosaccharides improves intestinal micro-flora and fermentation in term infants. Chin Med J (Engl) 2004;117:927–31.

19.1c. Antimicrobials

Michael R. Millar, MB, ChB, MD, FRCPath

Mark Wilks, BSc, Dip Bacteriol, PhD

This section deals with antibiotic modulation of the pattern of microbial colonization at a site or sites within the gastrointestinal tract. Eradication of single pathogens such as *Helicobacter pylori, Giardia lamblia,* and parasitic worms from the gastrointestinal tract by antimicrobials is covered in other sections.

The gastrointestinal tract provides the major reservoir of colonizing microorganisms. Determinants of bowel colonization are poorly understood but include mode of delivery (vaginal/cesarean), diet, health status, age, travel, and gastrointestinal physiology and pathology. The impact of the bowel flora on the human host is complex, with a wide range of metabolic, nutritional, and immunologic effects.[1] In health, the bowel flora provides many benefits for the host, including competitive exclusion of pathogens, the recovery of usable energy sources from cellulose, and production of short chain fatty acids (SCFA) such as acetate, propionate, and butyrate. SCFA, particularly butyrate, play a central role in the physiology and metabolism of the colon.[2]

The gastrointestinal microflora and interactions with the mucosa are reviewed in Chapter 19.1, "Modulation of the Intestinal Flora." Recent studies have given emphasis to the diverse metabolic capacities of the gut microbiome and the potential implications of these activities for human health and disease and for understanding individual responses to medical interventions.[3,4]

Determinants of the resistance of the microflora to perturbation are poorly understood. There is broad agreement that increasing diversity of an ecosystem promotes stability and increases the resistance to perturbation.[5,6] Administration of most antimicrobials, by a systemic route to most individuals, will lead to modulation of the bowel flora, potentially reducing bowel flora stability.[7] Conversely, microbial colonization of the gut with commensal flora benefits the host by preventing colonization or overgrowth with pathogens.[5] The concept of colonization resistance is often taken to imply that the intestinal flora, once established, is relatively static. However, molecular analysis of the bifidobacterial and lactobacillus composition of the microflora in humans suggests that this may not be so and that the pattern of bacterial flora is dynamic in healthy people, regardless of selection pressure caused by the use of antimicrobials.[8]

Gastrointestinal side effects are a common consequence of use of antimicrobials. The most frequent side effects are changes in bowel habit and overgrowth with fungi, and a large proportion of these disturbances probably result from alterations of the bowel flora.[9,10] Pseudomembranous colitis (predominantly caused by *Clostridium difficile*) is one of the most serious and feared complications associated with exposure to antibiotics. More transmissible and more virulent strains of *Clostridium difficile* have now become widespread in hospitals in North America and Europe.[11,12] However the significance of the isolation of *Clostridium difficile* or the detection of its toxins in the faeces of children is still not known.[13-15]

The clinical consequences of use of antimicrobials reflect not only modulation of the distribution of microorganisms in the gastrointestinal tract but also changes in microbial physiology and the production of microbial virulence determinants, such as lipopolysaccharide, toxins, and colonization factors.[16-20] Antimicrobials, by modifying microbial metabolic activities, can induce changes in intraluminal conditions, for example, pH, which may also have profound effects on microbial growth and physiology and modify the interaction with the host.[21] Acquisition of antibiotic resistance may be associated with changes in the production of microbial virulence or colonization factors.[22] Even a subinhibitory concentration of antibiotics can have major effects on the transcription of bacterial genes.[23,24] Antimicrobials are used in neutropenic patients both therapeutically and prophylactically. In a mouse model, administration of antibiotics (which reduced gut endotoxin levels) was associated with a reduction in cytokine-induced mobilization of stem cells suggesting a role for endotoxin in cytokine-induced stem cell mobilization.[25]

There is increasing evidence that the early pattern of colonization is an important determinant of development of the intestine.[26,27] Gram-positive bacteria, such as *Lactobacillus* spp and *Bifidobacterium* spp, may have a role in the prevention of the development of atopy, although this is still controversial.[28] Neonatal antibiotic treatment of mice leads to a long-term T helper 2 skewed immunologic response, which can be prevented by the introduction of intestinal bacteria.[29]

The effect of administration of antimicrobials in the peripartum period on the early pattern of colonization in the newborn has not been extensively studied, but there is some support for the idea that use of antibiotics in the peripartum period alters the pattern of subsequent microbial colonization and the risk of systemic infection of the newborn.[30] The effects of antibiotic treatment may be more marked in infants than in adults.[31] In a study of the fecal flora of 1- to 3-month-old infants, bifidobacteria and lactobacilli were suppressed to undetectable levels in most infants during treatment with amoxicillin, pivampicillin, cefaclor, cefadroxil, erythromycin, or cotrimoxazole.[7,32] The possible longer term effects of peripartum antimicrobial agents have recently been discussed.[33]

Antimicrobials may facilitate the acquisition of novel colonizers, a strategy that can be used to facilitate bowel colonization by probiotic strains, but can also reduce the infective inoculum of microbial pathogens.[34] Antimicrobials also provide a selection pressure for colonization or overgrowth of the gut with antimicrobial-resistant microorganisms. The density and diversity of the microflora facilitate the spread of transmissible genetic elements, hence the gastrointestinal tract can become a major reservoir for antimicrobial-resistant bacteria and resistance genes, with important consequences for both the colonized individual and others.[35]

In preterm infants cared for in a neonatal intensive care unit, use of antibiotics for suspected or proven episodes of infection encourages colonization with a limited range of antibiotic-resistant bacteria, while at the same time the opportunities are reduced for acquisition of bacteria that normally colonize healthy infants. The intestine provides a major reservoir for antibiotic-resistant bacteria, which can cause infection in the colonised infant and potentially spread to others.[36,37] The abnormal pattern of colonization has been implicated in the pathogenesis of neonatal necrotizing enterocolitis (NEC).[38] The types of antimicrobials that are used may be an important determinant of the frequency of NEC in individual units.[39]

Older infants and children nursed in intensive care units generally arrive in the unit with a complex gastrointestinal microflora but while in hospital acquire novel colonizers, which are frequently antibiotic resistant. Changes in gastrointestinal motility, use of drugs that reduce gastric acid production, and use of biomedical devices such as nasogastric tubes also contribute to modification of the gut flora in children nursed in intensive care units.

There is no agreement regarding the age at which the intestinal microflora becomes comparable to that of an adult.[40] In a recent study using both conventional and molecular methods, higher numbers of bifidobacteria and clostridial species were found in the pediatric population compared with healthy adults. Most strikingly, the carriage of Enterobacteriacae was 100-fold higher in children (16 months to 7 years) than in healthy adults (21 to 34 years).[41]

CLASSES OF ANTIBIOTIC

A wide range of antimicrobials are available, including β-lactams (cephalosporins and penicillins), related compounds such as carbapenems and monobactams, and macrolides, quinolones, aminoglycosides, tetracyclines, and peptides. Few novel classes of antimicrobial agent have been marketed over the last 10 years, and most that are currently marketed are representative of classes of antimicrobial agents that have been available for over 20 years. Newer agents with activity against resistant bacteria include an oxalidinone antibiotic (Linezolid), a glycylcycline (Tigecycline), and a cyclic lipopeptide (Daptomycin). A poorly absorbed rifamycin (Rifaximin) with broad spectrum activity may have a role in bowel flora modification particularly small intestinal overgrowth.

PENETRATION OF THE GASTROINTESTINAL TRACT BY ANTIMICROBIAL AGENTS

The main routes by which antimicrobial agents reach the lumen of the gastrointestinal tract are by oral ingestion, in bile, by transudation across the gut wall, and by rectal administration. Erythromycin, ampicillin-related drugs (including ureidopenicillins), and rifamycins are excreted in high concentrations in bile. In contrast, sulfonamides, chloramphenicol, and aminoglycosides are relatively poorly excreted in bile.

DETERMINANTS OF ANTIMICROBIAL ACTIVITY

Antimicrobial agents differ widely in the extent to which they impact on the gastrointestinal flora. Activity is dependent on a wide range of factors, including drug characteristics such as spectrum of activity, modes of administration, and routes of excretion (bile, urine) and the extent to which there is an enterobiliary circulation. Important factors specific to individuals include diet, transit time, intraluminal conditions (eg, pH, redox potential, ionic conditions, nonspecific binding to macromolecules such as proteins and mucins, presence of inhibitors, degrading enzymes, growth substrate availability, and bacterial growth phase), and bowel flora components and complexity. For example, the concentration of divalent cations, such as calcium, is an important determinant of the activity of gentamicin, iron may interfere with the activity of tetracyclines, and sulfonamides are inhibited by para-aminobenzoic acid. Some antimicrobials, such as colistin, are rapidly inactivated.[40] In addition, the pharmacokinetic and other properties of antimicrobials have been little studied in children, and there are therefore many uncertainties and assumptions made in extrapolating results from adults to children.

EFFECTS OF ANTIMICROBIAL AGENTS ON THE MICROBIAL FLORA OF THE GASTROINTESTINAL TRACT

The impact of antimicrobials on the culturable components of the oral and fecal flora has been extensively studied frequently in healthy adult volunteers.[7,41,42] On the other hand, relatively little is known about the impact of antimicrobial agents in patients with specific disease states or at less accessible sites, such as the small intestine and proximal colon. Attempts to describe the impact of antimicrobials on the flora at inaccessible sites using both in vitro continuous culture and animal models demonstrate that the fecal flora does not accurately represent changes in other parts of the gastrointestinal tract.[43]

Recent molecular studies from subjects undergoing colonoscopy confirm that whereas the fecal flora is different from that of the colon, mucosa-associated bacteria are relatively uniformly distributed along the colon.[44] There is some evidence that host-related factors are important in determining the intestinal microflora, and, as a result, attempts to modulate the gut flora in different individuals may give quite variable results.[45]

In vitro models are an attractive approach for studies of bowel flora modulation by antimicrobials but also may not accurately describe changes in vivo. For example, studies of microbial responses in models of the gastrointestinal flora in vitro have historically used planktonic (ie, free floating) populations of bacteria. In contrast, in vivo bacteria usually grow in surface-associated communities referred to as biofilms.[46] The mode of growth may prove an important element in the pathogenesis of intestinal infections.[47] Bacteria growing in biofilms show important differences from planktonic cells in metabolic activity, gene transfer, and generally show reduced susceptibility to both antimicrobial agents and host defense factors.[48-50] Swidsinski et al recently described the presence of a mucosal biofilm in >90% of patients with inflammatory bowel disease. *Bacteroides fragilis* accounted for >60% of the biofilm mass. The proportion with a mucosal biofilm and the density of biofilm when present was significantly lower in control patients. Neither 5-aminosalicylic acid or antibiotics eliminated the biofilm.[51] Antibiotics vary in their activity against biofilm bacteria, ciprofloxacin, and rifampicin are examples of antibiotics with good antibiofilm activity.

Another area of uncertainty is the impact of antimicrobials on the unculturable components of the gastrointestinal flora. Recent molecular studies suggest that 50 to 90% of the human fecal flora is unculturable using conventional techniques.[45] Current technology precludes studies of the unculturable components of the bowel flora of more than a few individuals. Accordingly, there is little information on the impact of antimicrobials on the uncultured components of the bowel flora. The use of nucleotide sequence arrays and other new techniques will facilitate further research in this area[52,53] Molecular methods have the potential to detect uncultured components of the bowel flora which may be contributing to disease, but the results must be interpreted cautiously.[54,55]

Most studies have concentrated on the impact of antimicrobials on facultative gram-positive cocci (such as staphylococci, enterococci, and streptococci), Enterobacteriaceae, anaerobic species (such as clostridia) and yeasts, and the emergence of antimicrobial resistance. For example, administration of penicillin reduces the numbers of streptococci in the mouth, whereas the numbers of Enterobacteriaceae increase. There is considerable interindividual variation in the effect of antimicrobial exposure on the microflora. In addition, antimicrobials within the same class may vary in their impact on the bowel flora.[56] The results of individual studies also will vary depending on the population studied and on the constituents of the microflora, such as the proportion of resistant components. In general, bacteria that are susceptible to the antimicrobial agent administered tend to decrease in numbers, and those that are resistant increase in numbers. Some of the effects of antimicrobial administration cannot be explained by antimicrobial susceptibility. For example, oral vancomycin reduces the numbers of *Bacteroides* spp despite poor antimicrobial activity in vitro.[57] Some antibiotics, such as macrolides, have effects on gastrointestinal motility through binding and activation of the motilin receptor, and these changes can modify the bowel flora indirectly.[58]

It is still widely assumed that there is a direct and exclusive relationship between the use of a particular antimicrobial agent and the development of resistance. This assumption underlies antibiotic use policies of clinics and hospitals and even national policies. However, it has been known for more than two decades that, at least in the case of Enterobacteriaceae, development of multidrug-resistant strains is generally not the result of accumulation of single point mutations. Instead, there is simultaneous acquisition of genetically linked resistance genes carried on transmissible genetic elements such as transposons, integrons, and plasmids.[59,60] Extensive horizontal gene transfer allows passage of resistance in the intestine between both closely related and distantly related bacteria.[61] Earlier assumptions that bacteria pay a fitness penalty in maintaining antimicrobial resistance in the absence of any selective pressure have proven to be incorrect.[62,63]

USE OF ANTIBIOTICS FOR PREVENTION OR TREATMENT OF DISEASE

Antimicrobials may be used to eradicate a specific pathogen from the gastrointestinal tract (see specific sections) or to modulate the pattern of colonization at a site or sites in the gastrointestinal tract. Antimicrobials may be prescribed for the prevention or treatment of disease and may be used as a sole treatment strategy but are also commonly used in combination with other strategies. Some classes of antimicrobial have highly selective activities, so, for example, aztreonam is active only against gram-negative bacteria, and daptomycin has specific activity against gram-positive bacteria. These agents may have a particular role in elucidating the contribution of specific elements of the bowel flora to the pathogenesis of disease.

Table 1 summarizes the activities of selective antimicrobials used for bowel flora modification. Some recently introduced antimicrobials have not been evaluated for bowel flora modulation, and some classes of agent have bowel flora activity only when administered orally or rectally, such as glycopeptides. Carbapenems do not reach high intraluminal concentrations so may have less impact on the bowel flora than antimicrobials such as cephalosporins, which have a similar spectrum of activity.

TREATMENT OF CONDITIONS ASSOCIATED WITH ABNORMAL DISTRIBUTION OF BACTERIA IN THE GASTROINTESTINAL TRACT

There is evidence that some groups of patients such as children with abnormal bowel motility or short gut following surgery may benefit from use of antimicrobials to control small bowel bacterial overgrowth.[64–67] However, there are few long-term follow-up studies of patients treated for small bowel overgrowth. Relapse of symptoms is common unless underlying defects can be corrected. Recent studies do not support the use of small bowel decontamination following liver transplant.[68,69] The use of surveillance stool cultures to guide antibiotic selection in pediatric patients after small bowel transplant was found not to be effective.[70] In a study of patients undergoing percutaneous gastrostomy feeding, staphy-

lococci, *Escherichia coli* and *Candida* spp. were only isolated from patients who had received antibiotics despite in vitro susceptibility of the isolates to the antibiotics that had been administered.[71] Antibiotics may have a role in managing small bowel overgrowth in patients with irritable bowel syndrome.[72]

Antimicrobials chosen for control of small bowel bacterial overgrowth include tetracyclines, quinolones such as ciprofloxacin, and metronidazole. Each of these classes of agent has a different spectrum of activity and produces a different range of effects on the fecal flora of healthy volunteers. There are no randomized trial data available regarding the comparative efficacy of agents used to treat and control small bowel bacterial overgrowth. Rifaximin is a newer agent which has a broad spectrum of activity and unlike tetracyclines, quinolones, and metronidazole is poorly absorbed. Rifaximin seems to be well tolerated and may have a role in control of small bowel overgrowth in patients with irritable bowel syndrome[73] and possibly in other gastrointestinal conditions.[74–77]

PROPHYLAXIS OF INFECTION IN THE IMMUNOCOMPROMISED HOST

Antifungal agents have been used to prevent fungal overgrowth of the gastrointestinal tract and thereby reduce the risk of both local and systemic fungal infections in a wide variety of groups of immunocompromised patients, such as in patients being treated for malignancies and those with human immunodeficiency virus (HIV) infection. Systemic antifungal prophylaxis probably reduces the severity of oral mucositis and the frequency of oral candidiasis in patients treated with chemotherapy for cancer.[78] Systemic antifungal prophylaxis probably also prevents invasive fungal infection in patients with neutropenia.[79] The pharmacokinetic properties and hence the correct doses have not yet been determined for many newer antifungal agents for use in children.[80] Antimicrobials also have been used to prevent

gram-negative sepsis in patients undergoing treatment for cancer, particularly hematologic malignancies.[81] However, there are concerns that this approach increases the likelihood of serious infection involving antimicrobial-resistant strains and modification in the pattern of infecting agents causing disease, with marginal benefit for patient outcomes.[82,83]

PROPHYLAXIS OF INFECTION IN THE INTENSIVE CARE UNIT

Selective decontamination of the digestive tract has been advocated as a strategy to reduce the risk of ventilator-associated pneumonia in patients undergoing intensive care. The aim of selective decontamination of the digestive tract is to reduce colonization of the upper gastrointestinal tract with aerobic gram-negative rods and Candida species. Selective decontamination of the digestive tract involves the administration of a topical antimicrobial preparation to the oropharynx, usually combined with a systemic antimicrobial agent. The use of selective decontamination of the digestive tract has been subject to a number of meta-analyses but support for the use of selective decontamination remains divided.[84] The implementation of a selective decontamination of the digestive tract strategy carries considerable costs. Between 13 and 39 patients would require selective decontamination of the digestive tract to prevent one death from ventilator-associated pneumonia.[85] The methodological quality of many studies has also been criticized.[86] Moreover, there are concerns about the long-term consequences of selective decontamination of the digestive tract on levels of antimicrobial resistance.[87,88] Given that critically ill patients are so heterogeneous and that the antibiotic treatments may be quite different (in duration, type of antibiotic, and route of administration), it is hardly surprising that no overall consensus has emerged. In the largest single trial of selective decontamination of the digestive tract (546 predominantly surgical adult patients), there was no observed increase in colonization by resistant gram-negative organisms, but there was increased colonization of all patients by ciprofloxacin-resistant coagulase-negative staphylococci and enterococci.[89] Concerns about antibiotic resistance could be reduced if oropharyngeal decontamination alone were enough to improve survival. In a recent study of oropharyngeal decontamination, the incidence of ventilator-associated pneumonia was reduced, but overall patient survival was not improved.[90] A large multicentre study in the Netherlands may resolve the issue, at least in countries in which antibiotic resistance levels are relatively low.[91]

PROPHYLAXIS AND/OR TREATMENT OF INFLAMMATORY BOWEL DISEASE

In animal models of inflammatory bowel disease, the colonizing microflora has an important etiologic role.[92] However, evidence supporting the

Table 1 Bowel Flora Activities of Selected Antimicrobials and Potential Indications for Their Use in the Prevention or Treatment of Gastrointestinal Disease

Antimicrobial Agent	Bowel Flora Activity	Potential Indications
Cephalosporin	Broad (depends on cephalosporin); generally includes gram-negative bacilli, staphylococci	Prophylaxis of infection—surgery, intensive care (selective decontamination)
Monobactam (aztreonam)	Facultative Gram-negative bacilli	Prophylaxis of gram-negative infection (necrotizing enterocolitis)
Aminoglycosides	Oral administration; gram-negative bacilli; staphylococci	Prophylaxis of infection—surgery, gut decontamination
Penicillins	Broad (depends on penicillin); penicillinase inhibitors further broaden activity (tazobactam, clavulanate)	Same as for cephalosporins
Quinolones	Gram-negative bacilli; staphylococci	Small bowel overgrowth; prophylaxis of infection—surgery, immunocompromised
Tetracyclines	Broad	Small bowel overgrowth
Metronidazole	Anaerobes	Small bowel overgrowth
Azole antifungals		Prevention of fungal infection

role of antimicrobial agents in the treatment or prevention of inflammatory bowel diseases in humans is limited.[93,94] Metronidazole, in high doses, has been shown to modify the course of Crohn's disease in some patients, such as those with perianal fistulae.[95] However, the optimal place of antimicrobials in the treatment of Crohn's disease remains controversial. Long-term use of antimicrobials is associated with the significant risk of selection of resistant bacteria, fungal overgrowth, and potentially Clostridium difficile infection, as well as drug induced side effects. There is little evidence of a role for antimicrobial agents in the control or treatment of ulcerative colitis.[96] The use of probiotics has been shown in randomized controlled triasl to benefit patients with pouchitis.[97] Antimicrobial agents also can be used to facilitate probiotic colonization, and it may be that in the future, attempts to modify the luminal flora to benefit patients with inflammatory bowel disease will use an approach in which antimicrobial agents are used to facilitate subsequent colonization with probiotics.

PROPHYLAXIS OF INFECTION ASSOCIATED WITH ABDOMINAL SURGERY

There is an extensive literature and broad agreement on the benefit of antimicrobial agents for the prophylaxis of infection associated with gastrointestinal tract surgery.[98–100] Current recommendations are that there should be a suprainhibitory concentration of appropriate antimicrobial agents present at the site of operation and at the time of bacterial contamination of the operative site. There is little evidence that extending prophylaxis beyond the period of operation is of any benefit, and it may be of harm.[101] Antimicrobial agents chosen for prophylaxis should be active against both facultative bacteria and strict anaerobes. Metronidazole alone is less effective than when it is combined with an agent active against facultative bacteria, such as a cephalosporin. However, the optimum regimen for prophylaxis in the perioperative setting has not been defined.

NEONATAL NECROTIZING ENTEROCOLITIS

Attempts to reduce the incidence of NEC by the oral administration of antibiotics have not provided conclusive results. This subject has been systematically reviewed, with the conclusion that the incidence of NEC may be reduced by the oral administration of antibiotics, but also concluding that there are concerns about the selection of antibiotic-resistant bacteria and identifying a need for further studies of sufficient size and duration to allow the risks and benefits to be assessed.[102] The antibiotics used to treat infants for episodes of suspected sepsis may also modify the bowel flora and influence the incidence of NEC.[103,104] There are no randomized comparative studies of antimicrobial efficacy in the treatment of neonatal NEC.

SHIFTING THE FLORA TO A MORE HEALTHY COMPOSITION

Recent research suggests that the pattern of bowel colonization, particularly in early life, may have an important influence on subsequent health and disease, such as on the risk of development of atopy.[105] The use of antibiotics to modulate the bowel flora of healthy individuals with a view to long-term health benefits, however, has not been systematically investigated.

It is now well established that there are major differences between the intestinal flora of formula-fed and breast milk-fed infants. These differences are particularly marked in very low birth weight infants.[106] The mode of delivery also is important, and babies born by cesarean section have a different flora, which persists at least until 6 months after birth, presumably related to the reduced exposure to the mother's bacterial flora at the time of delivery.[107]

PROBIOTICS AND ANTIMICROBIAL AGENTS

The administration of probiotics has been shown to reduce changes in the intestinal flora caused by antibiotics.[108,109] Antimicrobial agents may have a role in changing patterns of colonization to a more healthy composition and perhaps facilitate colonization of the intestinal tract by probiotic bacteria.

CONCLUSIONS

Antimicrobial agents can be used to modify the gastrointestinal flora in ways that may benefit the host, such as for prophylaxis of infection associated with gastrointestinal tract surgery. Antibiotics may also have other indirect effects on the flora that are not readily apparent. Current strategies emphasize the eradication of pathogens or suppression of flora rather than modulation to a more healthy composition. Future strategies may well see the use of antimicrobial agents to facilitate colonization of the bowel with microbes that contribute to the maintenance of health (ie, probiotics) rather than simply for the eradication or suppression of those microbes that cause disease.

REFERENCES

1. Hooper LV, Gordon JI. Commensal host-bacterial relationships in the gut. Science 2001;292:1115–8.
2. Wong JM, de Souza R, Kendall CW, et al. Colonic health: Fermentation and short chain fatty acids. J Clin Gastroenterol 2006;40:235–43.
3. Gill SR, Pop M, DeBoy RT, et al. Metagenomic analysis of the human distal gut microbiome. Science 2006;312:1355–9.
4. Clayton TA, Lindon JC, Cloarec O, et al. Pharmaco-metabonomic phenotyping and personalized drug treatment. Nature 2006;440:1073–7.
5. O'Hara AM, Shanahan F. The gut flora as a forgotten organ. EMBO Rep 2006;7:688–93.
6. Guarner F. Enteric flora in health and disease. Digestion 2006;73:5–12.
7. Sullivan A, Edlund C, Nord CE. Effect of antimicrobial agents on the ecological balance of human microflora. Lancet Infect Dis 2001;1:101–14.
8. McCartney AL, Wenzhi W, Tannock GW. Molecular analysis of the composition of the bifidobacterial and lac-

tobacillus microflora of humans. Appl Environ Microbiol 1996;62:4608–13.
9. Trenschel R, Peceny R, Runde V, et al. Fungal colonization and invasive fungal infections following allogeneic BMT using metronidazole, ciprofloxacin and fluconazole or ciprofloxacin and fluconazole as intestinal decontamination. Bone Marrow Transplant 2000;26:993–7.
10. Cotten CM, McDonald S, Stoll B, et al.The association of third-generation cephalosporin use and invasive candidiasis in extremely low birth-weight infants. Pediatrics. 2006;118:717–22.
11. Loo VG, Poirier L, Miller MA, et al A predominantly clonal multi-institutional outbreak of Clostridium difficile-associated diarrhea with high morbidity and mortality. N Engl J Med. 2005;353:2442–9.
12. McDonald LC, Killgore GE, Thompson A, et al. An epidemic, toxin gene-variant strain of Clostridium difficile. N Engl J Med. 2005;353:2433–41.
13. Enad D, Meislich D, Brodsky NL, Hurt H. The role of Clostridium difficile in childhood nosocomial diarrhea. J Perinatol 1997;17:355–9.
14. Oguz F, Uysal G, Dasdemir S, et al. Is Clostridium difficile a pathogen in the newborn intensive care unit? A prospective evaluation. Scand J Infect Dis 2001;33:731–733.
15. Wilson ME. Clostridium difficile and childhood diarrhea: Cause, consequence, or confounder.Clin Infect Dis 2006; 43:814–6.
16. Ginsburg I. Role of lipoteichoic acid in infection and inflammation. Lancet Infect Dis 2002;2:171–9.
17. Worlitzsch D, Kaygin H, Steinhuber A, et al. Effects of amoxicillin, gentamicin, and moxifloxacin on the hemolytic activity of Staphylococcus aureus in vitro and in vivo. Antimicrob Agents Chemother 2001;45:196–202.
18. Holzheimer RG, Hirte T, Reith B, et al. Different endotoxin release and IL-6 plasma levels after antibiotic administration in surgical intensive care patients. J Endotoxin Res 1996;3:261–7.
19. Kobayashi T, Tateda K, Matsumoto T, et al. Initial macrolidetreated Pseudomonas aeruginosa induces paradoxical host responses in the lungs of mice and a high mortality rate. J Antimsicrob Chemother 2002;50:59–66.
20. Tsuzuki T, Ina K, Ohta M. Clarithromycin increases the release of heat shock protein B from Helicobacter pylori. Aliment Pharmacol Ther 2002;16:217–28.
21. Qa'Dan M, Spyres LM, Ballard JD. pH-enhanced cytopathic effects of Clostridium sordellii lethal toxin. Infect Immun 2001;69:5487–93.
22. Hirakata Y, Srikumar R, Poole K, et al. Multidrug efflux systems play an important role in the invasiveness of Pseudomonas aeruginosa. J Exp Med 2002;196:109–18.
23. Goh EB, Yim G, Tsui W, et al. Transcriptional modulation of bacterial gene expression by subinhibitory concentrations of antibiotics. Proc Natl Acad Sci U S A 2002; 99:17025–30.
24. Tsui WH, Yim G, Wang HH, et al. Dual effects of MLS antibiotics: Transcriptional modulation and interactions on the ribosome. Chem Biol 2004;11:1307–16.
25. Velders GA, van Os R, Hagoort H, et al. Reduced stem cell mobilization in mice receiving antibiotic modulation of the intestinal flora: Involvement of endotoxins as cofactors in mobilization. Blood 2004;103:340–5.
26. Bry L, Falk PG, Midtvedt T, Gordon JI. A model of host-microbial interactions in an open mammalian ecosystem. Science 1996;273:1380–3.
27. Stappenbeck TS, Hooper LV, Gordon JI. Developmental regulation of intestinal angiogenesis by indigenous microbes via Paneth cells. Proc Natl Acad Sci U S A 2002;99:15451–5.
28. Williams HC. Two "positive" studies of probiotics for atopic dermatitis: or are they? Arch Dermatol 2006 ;142:1201–3.
29. Sudo N, Aiba Y, Oyama N, et al. Dietary nucleic acid and intestinal microbiota synergistically promote a shift in the Th1/Th2 balance toward Th1-skewed immunity. Int Arch Allergy Immunol 2004;135:132–5.
30. Stoll BJ, Hansen NI, Higgins RD, et al. Very low birth weight preterm infants with early onset neonatal sepsis: The predominance of Gram-negative infections continues in the National Institute of Child Health and Human Development Neonatal Research Network, 2002–2003. Pediatr Infect Dis J 2005;24:635–9.
31. Penders J, Thijs C, Vink C, et al. Factors influencing the composition of the intestinal microbiota in early infancy. Pediatrics 2006;118:511–21.
32. Bennet R, Eriksson M, Nord CE. The fecal microflora of 1-3-month-old infants during treatment with eight oral antibiotics. Infection 2002;30:158–60.
33. Bedford Russell AR, Murch SH. Could peripartum antibiotics have delayed health consequences for the infant? BJOG 2006;113:758–65.

34. Lipson A. Infecting dose of Salmonella. Lancet 1976;i:969.
35. Salyers AA, Gupta A, Wang Y.Human intestinal bacteria as reservoirs for antibiotic resistance genes. Trends Microbiol 2004 Sep;12:412–6.
36. Gupta A. Hospital-acquired infections in the neonatal intensive care unit-*Klebsiella pneumoniae*. Semin Perinatol 2002;26:340–5.
37. Singh N, Patel KM, Leger MM, et al. Risk of resistant infections with Enterobacteriaceae in hospitalized neonates. Pediatr Infect Dis J 2002;21:1029–33.
38. Hoy CM. The role of infection in necrotising enterocolitis. Rev Med Microbiol 2001;12:121–9.
39. Krediet TG, van Lelyveld N, Vijlbrief DC, et al. Microbiological factors associated with neonatal necrotizing enterocolitis: Protective effect of early antibiotic treatment. Acta Paediatr 2003;92:1180–2.
40. Fanaro S, Chierici R, Guerrini P, Vigi V. Intestinal microflora in early infancy: Composition and development. Acta Paediatr 2003;91:48–55.
41. Hopkins MJ, Sharp R, Macfarlane GT. Age and disease related changes in intestinal bacterial populations assessed by cell culture, 16S rRNA abundance, and community cellular fatty acid profiles. Gut 2001;48:198–205.
40. Veringa EM, van der Waajj D. Biological inactivation by faeces of antimicrobial drugs applicable in selective decontamination of the digestive tract. J Antimicrob Chemother 1984;14:605–12.
41. Nord CE, Heimdahl A, Kager L. Antimicrobial induced alterations of the human oropharyngeal and intestinal microflora. Scand J Infect Dis 1986;49:64–72.
42. Nord CE, Heimdahl A. Impact of orally-administered antimicrobial agents on human oropharyngeal and colonic microflora. J Antimicrob Chemother 1986;19:159–64.
43. Itoh K, Freter R. Control of *Escherichia coli* populations by a combination of indigenous clostridia and lactobacilli in gnotobiotic mice and continuous-flow cultures. Infect Immun 1989;57:559–65.
44. Zoetendal EG, von Wright A, Vilpponen-Salmela T, et al. Mucosa-associated bacteria in the human gastrointestinal tract are uniformly distributed along the colon and differ from the community recovered from feces. Appl Environ Microbiol 2002;68:3401–7.
45. Zoetendal EG, Vaughan EE, de Vos WM. A microbial world within us. Mol Microbiol 2006;59:1639–50.
46. Wilson M, Devine D, editors. Medical Implications of Biofilms. Cambridge: Cambridge University Press; 2003.
47. Donnenberg MS, Whittam TS. Pathogenesis and evolution of virulence in enteropathogenic and enterohemorrhagic *Escherichia coli*. J Clin Invest 2001;107:539–48.
48. Stewart PS, Casterton JW. Antibiotic resistance of bacteria in biofilms. Lancet 2001;358:135–8.
49. Smith AW. Biofilms and antibiotic therapy: Is there a role for combating bacterial resistance by the use of novel drug delivery systems? Adv Drug Deliv Rev 2005;57:1539–50.
50. Szomolay B, Klapper I, Dockery J, Stewart PS. Adaptive responses to antimicrobial agents in biofilms. Environ Microbiol 2005;7:1186–91.
51. Swidsinski A, Weber J, Loening-Baucke V, et al. Spatial organization and composition of the mucosal flora in patients with inflammatory bowel disease. J Clin Microbiol 2005;43:3380–9.
52. Egert M, de Graaf AA, Smidt H, et al. Beyond diversity: functional microbiomics of the human colon. Trends Microbiol 2006;14:86–91.
53. Furrie E. A molecular revolution in the study of intestinal microflora. Gut 2006;55:141–3.
54. Grahn N, Olofsson M, Ellnebo-Svedlund K, et al. Identification of mixed bacterial DNA contamination in broad-range PCR amplification of 16S rDNA V1 and V3 variable regions by pyrosequencing of cloned amplicons. FEMS Microbiol Lett 2003;219:87–91.
55. Hellmig S, Ott S, Musfeldt M, et al. Life-threatening chronic enteritis due to colonization of the small bowel with *Stenotrophomonas maltophilia*. Gastroenterology 2005;129:706–12.
56. Nord CE. Studies on the ecological impact of antibiotics. Eur J Clin Microbiol Infect Dis 1990;9:517–8.
57. Lund B, Edlund C, Barkholt L, et al. Impact on human intestinal microflora of an *Enterococcus faecium* probiotic and vancomycin. Scand J Infect Dis 2000;32:627–32.
58. Feighner SD, Tan CP, McKee KK, et al. Receptor for motilin identified in the human gastrointestinal system. Science 1999;284:2184–8.
59. Summers AO. Generally overlooked fundamentals of bacterial genetics and ecology. Clin Infect Dis 2002;34:S85–92.
60. O'Brien TF. Emergence, spread, and environmental effect of antimicrobial resistance: How use of an antimicrobial any-where can increase resistance to any antimicrobial anywhere else. Clin Infect Dis 2002;34:S78–84.
61. Salyers AA, Gupta A, Wang Y. Human intestinal bacteria as reservoirs for antibiotic resistance genes. Trends Microbiol. 2004;12:412–6.
62. Millar MR, Walsh TR, Linton CJ, et al. Carriage of antibiotic-resistant bacteria by healthy children. J Antimicrob Chemother 2001;47:605–10.
63. Andersson DI. The biological cost of mutational antibiotic resistance: Any practical conclusions? Curr Opin Microbiol 2006;9:461–5.
64. Pimentel M, Chow EJ, Lin HC. Eradication of small intestinal bacterial overgrowth reduces symptoms of irritable bowel syndrome. Am J Gastroenterol 2000;95:3503–6.
65. Attar A, Flourie B, Rambaud JC, et al. Antibiotic efficacy in small intestinal bacterial overgrowth-related chronic diarrhea: A crossover, randomized trial. Gastroenterology 1999;117:794–7.
66. Di Stefano M, Malservisi S, Veneto G, et al. Rifaximin versus chlortetracycline in the short-term treatment of small intestinal bacterial overgrowth. Aliment Pharmacol Ther 2000;14:551–6.
67. De Boissieu D, Chaussain M, Badoual J, et al. Small-bowel bacteria overgrowth in children with chronic diarrhea, abdominal pain, or both. J Pediatr 1996;128:203–7.
68. Hellinger WC, Yao JD, Alvarez S, et al. A randomized, prospective, double-blinded evaluation of selective bowel decontamination in liver transplantation. Transplantation 2002;73:1904–9.
69. Zwaveling JH, Maring JK, Klompmaker IJ, et al. Selective decontamination of the digestive tract to prevent postoperative infection: A randomized placebo-controlled trial in liver transplant patients. Crit Care Med 2002;30:1204–9.
70. John M, Gondolesi G, Herold BC, et al. Impact of surveillance stool culture guided selection of antibiotics in the management of pediatric small bowel transplant recipients. Pediatr Transplant 2006;10:198–204.
71. O'May GA, Reynolds N, Smith AR, et al. Effect of pH and antibiotics on microbial overgrowth in the stomachs and duodena of patients undergoing percutaneous endoscopic gastrostomy feeding. J Clin Microbiol 2005;43:3059–65.
72. Lin HC. Small intestinal bacterial overgrowth: A framework for understanding irritable bowel syndrome. JAMA 2004;292:2213–4.
73. Quigley EM. Germs, gas and the gut; the evolving role of the enteric flora in IBS. Am J Gastroenterol 2006;101:334–5.
74. Adachi JA, DuPont HL. Rifaximin: A novel nonabsorbed rifamycin for gastrointestinal disorders. Clin Infect Dis 2006;42:541–7.
75. Scarpignato C, Pelosini I. Experimental and clinical pharmacology of rifaximin, a gastrointestinal selective antibiotic. Digestion 2006;73:13–27.
76. Lauritano EC, Gabrielli M, Lupascu A, et al. Rifaximin dose-finding study for the treatment of small intestinal bacterial overgrowth. Aliment Pharmacol Ther 2005;22:31–5.
77. Beglinger C, Degen L. Are higher doses of rifaximin more effective for the treatment of small-intestinal bacterial overgrowth? Nat Clin Pract Gastroenterol Hepatol 2006;3:22–3.
78. Worthington HV, Clarkson JE. Prevention of oral mucositis and oral candidiasis for patients with cancer treated with chemotherapy: Cochrane Systematic Review. J Dent Educ 2002;66:903–11.
79. Bow EJ, Laverdiere M, Lussier N, et al. Antifungal prophylaxis for severely neutropenic chemotherapy recipients: A meta analysis of randomized-controlled clinical trials. Cancer 2002;94:3230–46.
80. Steinbach WJ, Benjamin DK. New antifungal agents under development in children and neonates. Curr Opin Infect Dis. 2005;18:484–9.
81. Baum HV, Franz U, Geiss HK. Prevalence of ciprofloxacin resistant *Escherichia coli* in hematological-oncologic patients. Infection 2000;28:259–60.
82. Van Belkum A, Goessens W, van der Schee C. Rapid emergence of ciprofloxacin-resistant Enterobacteriaceae containing multiple gentamicin resistance-associated integrons in a Dutch hospital. Emerg Infect Dis 2001;7:862–71.
83. Jansen J, Cromer M, Akard L, et al. Infection prevention in severely myelosuppressed patients: A comparison between ciprofloxacin and a regimen of selective antibiotic modulation of the intestinal flora. Am J Med 1994;96:335–41.
84. D'Amico R, Pifferi S, Leonetti C, et al. Effectiveness of antibiotic prophylaxis in critically ill patients: Systematic review of randomised controlled trials. BMJ 1998;316:1275–85.
85. Selective Decontamination of the Digestive Tract Triallists' Collaborative Group. Meta-analysis of randomised controlled trials of selective decontamination of the digestive tract. BMJ 1993;307:525–32.
86. van Nieuwenhoven CA, Buskens E, van Tiel FH, Bonten MJ. Relationship between methodological trial quality and the effects of selective digestive decontamination on pneumonia and mortality in critically ill patients. JAMA 2001;286:335–40.
87. Rocha LA, Martin MJ, Pita S, et al. Prevention of nosocomial infection in critically ill patients by selective decontamination of the digestive tract. Intensive Care Med 1992;18:398–404.
88. Bonten MJ, Kullberg BJ, van Dalen R, et al. Selective digestive decontamination in patients in intensive care. The Dutch Working Group on Antibiotic Policy. J Antimicrob Chemother 2000;46:351–62.
89. Krueger WA, Lenhart FP, Neeser G, et al. Influence of combined intravenous and topical antibiotic prophylaxis on the incidence of infections, organ dysfunctions, and mortality in critically ill surgical patients: A prospective, stratified, randomized, double-blind, placebo-controlled clinical trial. Am J Respir Crit Care Med 2002;166:1029–37.
90. Bergmans DC, Bonten MJ, Gaillard CA, et al. Prevention of ventilator-associated pneumonia by oral decontamination: A prospective, randomized, double-blind, placebo-controlled study. Am J Respir Crit Care Med 2001;164:382–8.
91. Bonten MJ, Krueger WA. Selective decontamination of the digestive tract: Cumulating evidence, at last? Semin Respir Crit Care Med 2006;27:18–22.
92. Seksik P, Sokol H, Lepage P, et al. Review article: The role of bacteria in onset and perpetuation of inflammatory bowel disease. Aliment Pharmacol Ther 2006;24:11–8.
93. Perencevich M, Burakoff R. Use of antibiotics in the treatment of inflammatory bowel disease. Inflamm Bowel Dis 2006;12:651–64.
94. Rufo PA, Bousvaros A. Current Therapy of Inflammatory Bowel Disease in Children. Paediatr Drugs 2006;8:279–302.
95. Sutherland L, Singleton J, Sessions J, et al. Double blind, placebo controlled trial of metronidazole in Crohn's disease. Gut 1991;32:1071–5.
96. Jani N, Regueiro MD. Medical therapy for ulcerative colitis. Gastrenterol Clin North Am 2002;31:147–66.
97. Mimura T, Rizzello F, Helwig U, et al. Once daily high dose probiotic therapy (VSL#3) for maintaining remission in recurrent or refractory pouchitis. Gut 2004;53:108–14.
98. Song F, Glenny A. Antimicrobial prophylaxis in colorectal surgery: A systematic review of randomised controlled trials. Br J Surg 1998;85:1232–41.
99. Swedish-Norwegian Consensus Group. Antibiotic prophylaxis in surgery: Summary of a Swedish-Norwegian consensus conference. Scand J Infect Dis 1998;30:547–57.
100. Antimicrobial prophylaxis in colorectal surgery. Effective Health Care Bulletins 1998;4:1–8.
101. Norrby S. Cost effective prophylaxis of surgical infections. Pharmacoeconomics 1996;10:129–39.
102. Bury RG, Tudehope D. Enteral antibiotics for preventing necrotizing enterocolitis in low birthweight or preterm infants. Cochrane Database Syst Rev 2001;(1):CD000405.
103. Millar MR, MacKay P, Levene M, et al. Enterobacteriaceae and neonatal necrotising enterocolitis. Arch Dis Child 1992;67:53–6.
104. Krediet TG, van Lelyveld N, Vijlbrief DC, et al. Microbiological factors associated with neonatal necrotizing enterocolitis: Protective effect of early antibiotic treatment. Acta Paediatr 2003;92:1180–2.
105. Hopkin JM. The rise of atopy and links to infection. Allergy 2002;57:5–9.
106. Gewolb IH, Schwalbe RS, Taciak VL, et al. Stool microflora in extremely low birthweight infants. Arch Dis Child 1999;80:F167–73.
107. Gronlund MM, Lehtonen OP, Eerola E, Kero P. Fecal microflora in healthy infants born by different methods of delivery: Permanent changes in intestinal flora after cesarean delivery. J Pediatr Gastroenterol Nutr 1999;28:19–25.
108. Madden JA,Plummer SF,Tang J, et al. Effect of probiotics on preventing disruption of the intestinal microflora following antibiotic therapy: A double-blind, placebo-controlled pilot study. Int Immunopharmacol 2005;5:1091–7.
109. Plummer SF, Garaiova I, Sarvotham T, et al. Effects of probiotics on the composition of the intestinal microbiota following antibiotic therapy. Int J Antimicrob Agents 2005;26:69–74.

19.2 Infections

19.2a. Bacterial Infections

Alessio Fasano, MD

Bacterial enteric infections exact a heavy toll on human populations, particularly among children. Despite major advance in our knowledge on the pathogenesis of enteric diseases, the number of diarrheal episodes and childhood deaths reported worldwide remains of apocalyptic dimensions.[1] The recent escalation of international terrorism is raising the risk of enteric pathogens epidemics occurring beyond the boundaries of natural endemic areas. However, bacterial genome sequencing and better understanding of the pathogenic mechanisms involved in the onset of diarrheal diseases are finally leading to preventive interventions, such as enteric vaccines,[2] which may have a significant impact on the magnitude of this human plague. This chapter reviews the major bacterial agents of infectious diarrhea (Table 1) and their interaction with the human host.

CHOLERA

Of all enteric pathogens, *Vibrio cholerae* is responsible for the most rapidly fatal diarrheal disease in humans.[3] Although cholera is rare in developed countries, it remains a major cause of diarrheal morbidity and mortality in many parts of the developing world.[4] However, with the occurrence of both natural (eg, earthquakes, tsunami) and human-generated calamities (such as ethnic wars), the spreading of cholera infection in refugee camps, where sanitary conditions resemble those in cholera-endemic areas, represents a significant threat worldwide.

Table 1 Identification of Bacterial Enteric Pathogens in Symptomatic Patients from Developing and Industrialized Countries (Percentage)

Agent	Industrialized Countries (%)	Developing Countries (%)
Vibrio cholerae	<1	0–3
Non-O1 *Vibrio species*	—	?
Salmonella	3–7	4–6
Shigella	1–3	5–9
Campylobacter	6–8	7–9
Yersinia	1–2	?
Escherichia coli	2–5	14–17
Clostridium difficile	?	?
Aeromonas, Plesiomonas, and Edwardsiella	0–2	4–5

Microbiology

Vibrio (from the Greek *comma*) *cholerae* are single, short-curved, gram-negative rods with a single long polar flagellum that confers to the microorganism the characteristic rapid linear motility that forms the basis for identification by an immobilization test.[5] Currently, 34 *Vibrio* species are recognized, a third of which are pathogenic in humans.[6] *V. cholerae* is divided into 139 serotypes on the basis of the O antigen of the cell surface polysaccharide. Work in the 1930s led to the concept that *V. cholerae* strains could be divided into two groups: those that agglutinated with antisera directed against antigens present on strains isolated from cholera patients (group O1) and other "nonagglutinating" or "noncholera" vibrios (non-O1), which were regarded primarily as nonpathogenic, environmental isolates.[6] Group O1 is further divided into two biotypes: classic and El Tor. The El Tor strains were first isolated in 1905 from returning Mecca pilgrims at the quarantine camp of El Tor in the Sinai Peninsula in Egypt.[7]

As more attention was paid to non-O1 vibrios, it became clear that they represented a heterogeneous group that includes 11 species that have been associated with human illness.[8] Until 1993, only the O1 serotype was believed to be responsible for epidemics in humans, whereas the non-O1 group was considered responsible for sporadic cases of gastroenteritis and extraintestinal infections.[9] However, a strain of *V. cholerae* non-O1 (O139 Bengal) associated with epidemic cholera appeared in southern and eastern India in October 1992 (see below).[10]

Epidemiology

V. cholerae O1 is transmitted by the fecal–oral route and is spread primarily through contaminated food and water. Since the original observation during the cholera epidemic in London in 1854,[11] water has been considered the main vehicle for cholera transmission. During the outbreak in Peru, fecal contamination of public water was identified as responsible for the majority of cases.[12]

During the past two centuries, six pandemics spread throughout the world, starting in Asia and spreading through Europe and then to the Americas.[13] The current pandemic started in 1961 from an endemic focus in Indonesia and disseminated in Southeast Asia and the Middle East, reaching Africa and Europe in 1970.[14–16]

Finally, after almost a century, *V. cholerae* made its reappearance in South America in 1991, when the pandemic developed with explosive intensity in several coastal Peruvian cities.[17] Although the classic biotype of *V. cholerae* O1 caused the fifth and sixth pandemics, the seventh pandemic was caused by the El Tor biotype.

In October 1992, a new epidemic outbreak of cholera occurred in southern and eastern India[10] and spread 3 months later in Bangladesh.[18] For the first time, a non-O1 strain (named O139 Bengal) was identified as responsible for a cholera outbreak. This strain spread faster than the *V. cholerae* O1 El Tor biotype responsible for the seventh pandemic; it appeared in Thailand in April 1993[19] and as an isolated case imported from India in the United States in February 1993.[20] These observations raised the concern that the appearance of *V. cholerae* O139 may mark the beginning of the eighth pandemic.[21]

Clinical Manifestations

The period of incubation of cholera ranges from a few hours to 5 days.[22] The vast majority of subjects infected with *V. cholerae* O1 remain asymptomatic or experience a mild disease indistinguishable from many other forms of infectious diarrhea, with a few episodes of watery stools, rare nausea or vomiting, and no significant dehydration.[23]

In cholera gravis (Figure 1), the most severe form of the disease, profuse watery diarrhea and vomiting lead to massive fluid and electrolyte loss, which can occur at a rate of 1 L/h and can reach a total volume loss during illness of 100% of body weight.[24] Cholera stools are typically described as "rice water" owing to the presence of mucus in clear stools. Diarrhea is most severe during the first 48 hours of the disease, when dehydration can reach life-threatening levels, particularly in children. Diarrhea then slowly decreases, completely resolving after 4 to 6 days.[24]

Diagnosis, Treatment, and Prevention

The stools of patients affected by acute cholera contain a large number of vibrios that can be easily identified with a simple gram stain of such stools. Direct placement of stool specimens on selective media is usually sufficient for the isolation of the microorganism. The recent spread of *V. cholerae* O139 Bengal has highlighted the need for specific tests to identify this new strain.[25]

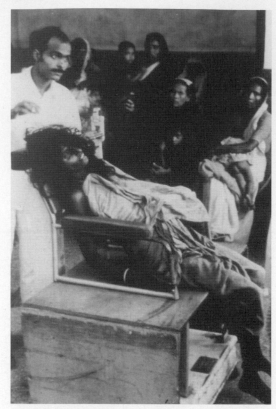

Figure 1 A case of cholera gravis in a young Bangladeshi woman.

Oral rehydration solutions are the cornerstone of cholera treatment and are typically the only necessary intervention for cholera patients. The introduction of this treatment has revolutionized the prognosis of cholera, reducing the mortality from over 50% to less than 1%.[26] If the dehydration is too severe (>10%), the mental status of the patient is affected or the presence of vomiting precludes the use of oral therapy; the use of intravenous solutions such as Ringer's lactate becomes the treatment of choice. The use of antibiotics for the treatment of cholera has limited indications. Antibiotics have been demonstrated to reduce the volume and duration of diarrhea by about half and to reduce the duration of *Vibrio* excretion to an average of 1 day.[27] Tetracycline (500 mg per dose four times/d) is the antibiotic most used; however, large outbreaks of tetracycline-resistant organisms have been reported.[28] Furazolidone (1.25 mg/kg four times/d), trimethoprim (TMP) (5 mg/kg two times/d) and sulfamethoxazole (SMX) (25 mg/kg two times/d), and erythromycin (10 mg/kg three times/d) have been suggested for children.[29]

Both killed whole cell and live attenuated cholera vaccines have been proposed as a preventive intervention for cholera.[2,30] A large double-blind field trial of the killed vaccine showed 85% efficacy for a period of 4 to 6 months, dropping to 50% over 3 years of follow-up.[31]

A locally produced killed vaccine in Vietnam provided 66% protection against El Tor cholera during an outbreak occurring 8 to 10 months after vaccination.[32] A genetically engineered attenuated cholera vaccine (CVD 103-HgR), obtained by deleting the active subunit of cholera toxin (see below) from a *V. cholerae* O1 classic biotype, was well tolerated when administered to volunteers. This vaccine elicited a high level of protection (82 to 100%) against homologous challenge with a strain of the same biotype.[33] Protection across the biotype was also observed, albeit to a lesser extent,[34] lasting for at least 6 months after a single oral dose.[35] Live attenuated *V. cholerae* O139 vaccines have been developed, with promising results.[36] Preventive and control measures prior to, and during, the cholera epidemic of 1991—to 2001 had a positive impact on the overall incidence rate of the disease and the mortality rate among children under 5 years of age in Mexico.[37] This outcome stresses the importance of coordinate public health interventions spanning multisectorial activities, involving both community participation and political leadership.

NON-O1 *VIBRIO* SPECIES

As mentioned above, non-O1 *Vibrio* species (other than O139 Bengal) that infect the gastrointestinal tract (*V. parahaemolyticus, V. fluvialis, V. mimicus, V. hollisae, V. furnissii,* and *V. vulnificus*) are responsible for sporadic cases of gastroenteritis. These vibrios have been isolated from surface water in multiple sites in North America, Europe, Asia, and Australia, and it is likely that they are present in coastal and estuarine areas throughout the world.[38] Virtually all infections by non-O1 *V. cholerae* acquired in the United States are associated with the eating of raw or undercooked shellfish.[39] Seafood is also the main vehicle of infection for sporadic non-O1 disease outside the United States; however, the transmission can also occur through other routes, including water[40] and a variety of other foods.[41] Gastroenteritis from non-O1 *V. cholerae* can range from mild illness to a profuse, watery diarrhea comparable to that seen in epidemic cholera. Diarrhea, abdominal cramps, and fever are the most common symptoms, with nausea and vomiting occurring less frequently.[39] Bloody diarrhea has been reported in 25% of cases.[39] As with *V. cholerae* O1, the mainstay of therapy for diarrheal disease is oral rehydration. In cases of septicemia (that typically occur in immunocompromised patients), supportive care and correction of shock are essential interventions associated with antibiotic treatment (tetracycline). In countries such as the United States, non-O1 infections can be prevented by not eating raw or undercooked seafood, particularly during the warm months.

SALMONELLA

For more than a century, *Salmonella* has fascinated physicians, microbiologists, epidemiologists, and geneticists by virtue of its diversity and success in nature. Non-typhi salmonellae are widely dispersed in animal hosts, including the gastrointestinal tracts of both domestic and wild mammals, as well as reptiles, birds, and insects.[42] They are effective commensals and pathogens that cause a spectrum of diseases in humans and animals.

Microbiology

Salmonella is a genus of the family of Enterobacteriaceae. These microorganisms are gram-negative, motile bacilli that can be identified on selective media because they do not ferment lactose. Based on deoxyribonucleic acid (DNA) homology and host range, *Salmonella* isolates are currently classified into two species: *S. bongor*, which includes salmonellae that infect nonhuman organisms, and *S. enterica*, which is divided into six subspecies. Most human pathogens belong to *S. enterica*, subspecies *enterica*. On the basis of somatic O-oligosaccharide cell wall antigens and flagellar H-protein antigens, over 2,300 serovars have been identified. The most commonly reported human serovar in the United States is *S. enteritidis* (formally designated *S. enterica* subspecies *enterica*, serovar enteritidis), which recently surpassed *S. typhimurium*. *S. typhi* and *S. paratyphi* A, B, and C also belong to species *S. enterica*, subspecies enterica. For clarity, only the serovar names will be used in the discussion that follows.

Epidemiology

S. typhi and S. paratyphi. *S. typhi* and *S. paratyphi* colonize only humans; therefore, disease can be acquired only through close contact with a person who has had typhoid fever or is a chronic carrier. Often acquisition of the organism occurs through the ingestion of water or food contaminated with human excrement. Typhoid fever continues to represent a global health problem, with an estimated 12.5 million cases occurring per year (excluding China) and an annual incidence of 0.5% of the world population.[43] Certain subequatorial countries report high typhoid fever mortality rates (12 to 32%) despite antibiotic treatment.[43] In these areas, typhoid fever is often endemic and typically constitutes the most important enteric disease problem among school-age children. In the United States, substantial progress has been made in the eradication of *S. typhi*. The incidence of typhoid fever decreased from 1 case per 100,000 in 1955 to 0.2 case per 100,000 in 1966 and has remained fairly stable since then.[44] These changes were clearly related to better sanitation, particularly to food-handling practices and water treatment.

Nontyphoidal *Salmonella*. In contrast to *S. typhi*, the incidence of cases of nontyphoidal *Salmonella* infections reported to the Centers for Disease Control and Prevention (CDC) increased between 1970 and 1987 from 12 to 20 per 100,000 population.[45] Because only an estimated 1 to 5% of cases are reported, it is likely that the true incidence is much higher. The incidence is greatest among children younger than 5 years of age (61.8 per 100,000), with a peak at under 1 year of age. Risk of infection and severity of disease are influenced by numerous host factors, including congenital and acquired immunodeficiency,[46] age younger than 3 months,[47] and impaired reticuloendothelial function, as is seen in patients with hemolytic anemia. Other risk factors include alterations in intestinal defenses such as achlorhydria, antacid therapy, and in situations in which there is rapid gastric emptying (neonates, postgastrectomy, and gastroenterostomy).[48] (Ingestion of antibiotics to which the organism was resistant was the most important risk factor identified in an Illinois outbreak that was traced to milk, presumably because of a diminished competition of Salmonella growth by endogenous flora.[49]) A wide range of domestic and wild animals, including poultry, swine, cattle, rodents, and reptiles, represents the typical reservoirs for nontyphoidal salmonellae.

S. enteriditis is the leading reported cause of food-borne disease outbreaks in the United States.[50] Intact and disinfected grade A eggs and egg-containing foods have been incriminated in over 80% of outbreaks with an identified vehicle.[51] The potential role of cross-contamination is exemplified in several outbreaks in which the pulp of surface-contaminated raw fruits and vegetables became inoculated during slicing.[52] Person-to-person transmission, including vertical transmission from mother to child (resulting in neonatal hematochezia),[53] is occasionally seen. Pets (chicks, ducklings, reptiles, cats, and dogs) can also be a source of Salmonella infection.[54] Approximately 80% of Salmonella isolates reported in the United States appear to be unrelated to outbreaks.[51–53]

Clinical Manifestations

Gastroenteritis. The incubation period ranges between 6 hours and 10 days (usually 6 to 48 hours).[55] The typical clinical manifestation of nontyphoidal Salmonella infection is an acute, self-limited enterocolitis sometimes accompanied by bacteremia. Diarrhea is usually watery but may contain blood, mucus, and fecal leukocytes. Associated headache, abdominal pain, and vomiting may occur. Fever is present in at least 70% of cases.[56] Most patients recover in about 1 week, but diarrhea occasionally becomes persistent.[56] Salmonella is usually detected in the stool for about 5 weeks, although approximately 5% of patients will excrete the organism for more than 1 year.[57] The reported incidence of Salmonella bacteremia is highest during the first year of life, with a peak during the first 3 months.[58] Estimates of the frequency of bacteremia in infants with S. enterocolitis (generally derived from studies of small samples of children) range from 5 to 45%.[59] In the normal host, the bacteremia is transient and usually benign.

Extraintestinal Manifestations. Severe extraintestinal infections occasionally occur, mainly in young infants or in patients with impaired immunity. These infections manifest as life-threatening sepsis or focal infections at virtually any site in the body, particularly the meninges, bones, and lungs,[60] or in areas of localized tissue pathology or anatomic abnormality. Salmonella is the most common cause of osteomyelitis in patients with sickle cell anemia.[61] Meningitis is associated with high mortality and neurologic sequelae, even with

prolonged antibiotic therapy,[62] and a high relapse rate, particularly in neonates.[63] Prolonged diarrhea, weight loss, persistent or recurrent bacteremia, and disseminated infection can develop in human immunodeficiency virus (HIV)-infected patients.[64]

Enteric Fever. Human typhoid and paratyphoid fever are severe systemic illnesses characterized by fever and gastrointestinal symptoms. Case fatality rates range from less than 1% in the United States to 10 to 30% in Africa and Asia.[58,61] The incubation period of S. typhi varies between 5 and 21 days (depending on the inoculum ingested) and may be followed by enterocolitis with diarrhea lasting several days; these symptoms typically resolve before the onset of fever. Constipation is present in 10 to 38% of patients.[65] Nonspecific symptoms such as chills, headache, cough, weakness, and muscle pain are frequent prodromes of typhoid fever. Neuropsychiatric manifestations, including psychosis and confusion (the so-called coma vigil), occur in 5 to 10% of patients with typhoid fever.[65,66] Approximately 30% of patients experience rose spots on the trunk.[67] Most symptoms resolve by the fourth week of infection without antimicrobial treatment in approximately 90% of patients who survive. Some patients improve initially only to develop high fever and increasing abdominal pain from inflammation of Peyer's patches and intestinal microperforation, followed by secondary bacteremia with normal enteric flora.

Diagnosis, Treatment, and Prevention

Nontyphoidal Salmonellosis. The diagnosis of nontyphoidal salmonellosis does not represent a major challenge because the microorganism can easily be isolated from freshly passed stools or blood culture. Antimicrobial therapy is not indicated to treat asymptomatic carriage or uncomplicated nontyphoidal Salmonella infections in the normal host. There is considerable evidence that antibiotics neither speed resolution of clinical symptoms nor eliminate fecal excretion; conversely, treatment may prolong excretion or induce relapse.[68] These observations apply to both oral and parenteral antibiotics. Although efficacy is unproven, it is common clinical practice to administer antibiotics to patients with suspected or proven salmonellosis who are at high risk of complications. This includes infants younger than 3 months; patients with hemolytic anemia, malignancy, immunodeficiency, or chronic colitis; and patients who appear "ill" or "toxic," have documented bacteremia, or have an extraintestinal focus of infection. Increasing resistance to commonly used antibiotics is seen in the United States and elsewhere, so the choice of regimens should be guided by susceptibility data. Suggested therapies include trimethoprim-sulfamethoxazole (TMP-SMX), ampicillin (10 to 20% of isolates in the United States are resistant[68]), cefotaxime, ceftriaxone, or chloramphenicol. Parenteral antibiotics should be considered for infants younger than 3 months, for children at high risk for invasive infection if they have suspected or proven sepsis, and for those who appear "ill" or "toxic" or have

a focal infection. Bacteremia is generally treated for 2 weeks, osteomyelitis for 4 to 6 weeks, and meningitis for 4 weeks.

Hygienic practices for preventing food-borne transmission are the most efficient prevention for nontyphoidal Salmonella infections because the vast majority of outbreaks and sporadic cases result from culinary practices that allow the organisms to survive and multiply in food. Parents should be instructed to avoid serving food containing raw or undercooked eggs and meat (especially poultry). Food should be thawed in the refrigerator, in the microwave, or under cold water but not at room temperature because surface bacteria begin to multiply when the outer layers warm. Eggs should be cooked until both the yolk and white are firm, and meats must reach an internal temperature of at least 74°C (165°F). Frequent hand washing is important. High-risk pets (especially chicks, ducklings, and reptiles) are not advisable for young children.

An extremely problematic situation is the management of an infected child who is attending day care. Excretion can go on for weeks and create a hardship to working parents if the child must be excluded from day care. Although the decision to admit such a child must be made in concert with day care and public health officials, it is generally recommended that the infected children be excluded from day care if they are symptomatic or if adequate hygiene cannot be ensured. There is no vaccine to prevent nontyphoidal salmonellosis.

Enteric Fever. The definitive diagnosis of enteric fever requires the isolation of S. typhi or S. paratyphi from the patient. Cultures of blood, stool, urine, rose spots, bone marrow, and gastric and enteric secretions may all be useful in establishing the diagnosis. Chloramphenicol has been the treatment of choice since its introduction, given its low costs and high efficiency after oral administration. Treatment with chloramphenicol reduced typhoid fever mortality from approximately 20 to 1% and reduced the duration of the fever from 14 to 28 days to 3 to 5 days.[69]

Currently, there are two well-tolerated and effective licensed vaccines.[70] One is based on defined subunit virulence (Vi) polysaccharide antigen and can be administered either intramuscularly or subcutaneously and the other is based on the use of live attenuated bacteria for oral administration.[70] A subunit vaccine was developed from wild-type S. typhi strain Ty2 on the basis of nondenatured purification of the Vi polysaccharide. Immunization with Vi antigen results in the induction of anti-Vi antibody titers in vaccines in endemic and nonendemic areas (a fourfold rise in anti-Vi antibodies is defined as seroconversion).[70] Ty21a is an attenuated mutant strain of S. typhi Ty2 that is safe and protective as a live oral vaccine. The TY21a strain is the active constituent of Vivotif (Berna Biotech Ltd., Switzerland), currently the only licensed live oral attenuated vaccine against typhoid fever.[70] The efficacy of Ty21a was assessed in a large number of clinical trials, with over 500,000 vaccinated adults and children. Excellent tolerability and an overall protective efficacy of 67 to 80% (applying three doses of enteric-coated capsules or a liq uid formulation) has been demonstrated for up to 7 years.[70]

SHIGELLA

Shigella dysenteriae type 1 was first isolated by Kiyoshi Shiga during a severe dysentery epidemic in Japan in 1896, when more than 90,000 cases were described with a mortality rate approaching 30%.[71] Over the subsequent 50 years, the microbiology and epidemiology of *Shigella* species were clarified, and the mechanisms whereby the microorganism causes disease have been intensively investigated.

Microbiology

Shigellae are gram-negative, non–lactose-fermenting, nonmotile bacilli of the family Enterobacteriaceae. They are classified into four species: *S. dysenteriae*, *S. flexneri*, *S. boydii*, and *S. sonnei*, also designated groups A, B, C, and D, respectively. Groups A, B, and C contain multiple serotypes, whereas group D contains only a single serotype. The predominant serogroup of *Shigella* circulating in a community appears to be related to the level of development. *S. sonnei* is the main type found in industrialized countries, whereas *S. flexneri*, followed by *S. dysenteriae*, predominates in less-developed countries.

Epidemiology

Humans are the only natural hosts for *Shigella*, and transmission is predominantly by fecal-oral contact. The low infectious inoculum (as few as 10 organisms)[72] renders *Shigella* highly contagious. Symptomatic persons with diarrhea are primarily responsible for transmission. Less commonly, transmission is related to contaminated food and water; however, the organism generally survives poorly in the environment. In certain settings where the disposal of human feces is inadequate, houseflies can serve as a mechanical vector for transmission.[73] According to a CDC report, isolation rates of *Shigella* (mostly *S. sonnei*) in the United States have gradually risen since the 1960s from 5.4 to more than 10 isolations per 100,000 population.[74] Endemic foci persist, primarily among indigent persons living in inner cities and in some Native American communities.[74] An elevated risk of shigellosis is also present in settings where hygiene is difficult to maintain, such as day-care centers,[75] in which attending children play an important role in disseminating shigellosis to others in the community.[76] In households with small children, transmission rates can exceed 50%.[77] Worldwide, the incidence of shigellosis is highest among children 1 to 4 years old, a trend also reflected in CDC surveillance data.[74] Nonetheless, *Shigella* infection is uncommon in the United States and accounts for fewer than 5% of episodes of diarrhea among children younger than 5 years of age.[78]

In developing countries, *Shigella* infections, most commonly caused by *S. flexneri*, are mainly endemics. In this setting, endemic shigellosis causes approximately 10% of all diarrheal episodes among children younger than 5 years of age.[79] It is estimated that Shigella causes 164.7 million cases of diarrhea, of which 163.2 million occur in developing countries, and 1.1 million deaths each year worldwide, mostly in developing countries.[79] One serotype of *Shigella*, *S. dysenteriae* type 1, is capable of true pandemic transmission. Pandemics of Shiga dysentery have spread across Central America, Bangladesh, South Asia, and Central and East Africa during the past 30 years[80-82] and have been particularly problematic among refugee populations.[82] In the United States, *S. dysenteriae* infection is seen exclusively among travelers returning from abroad.[79]

Clinical Manifestations

After an incubation period of 1 to 4 days, shigellosis usually begins with systemic symptoms, including fever, headache, malaise, anorexia, and occasional vomiting. Watery diarrhea typically precedes dysentery[83] and is often the sole clinical manifestation of mild infection.[84] Progression to frank dysentery may occur within hours to days, with frequent small stools containing blood and mucus accompanied by lower abdominal cramps and rectal tenesmus. Patients with severe infection may pass more than 20 dysenteric stools in 1 day. A variety of unusual extraintestinal manifestations may occur.[85] The microangiopathic hemolytic anemia that can complicate infection with organisms that produce Shiga toxin (see section "Pathogenesis") manifests itself as hemolytic uremic syndrome (HUS) in children and as thrombotic thrombocytopenic purpura in adults.[86]

Most episodes of shigellosis in otherwise healthy individuals are self-limited and resolve within 5 to 7 days without sequelae. Acute, life-threatening complications are most often seen in malnourished infants and young children living in developing countries. In the United States, *Shigella* bacteremia has been reported among HIV-infected and other immunocompromised patients.[87]

Diagnosis, Treatment, and Prevention

Shigella are extremely fastidious to culture and readily die off if the stool sample is not well handled. The best way to isolate them is to (1) obtain stool (and not rectal swab), (2) rapidly inoculate the specimens onto selective culture plates, preferably at the bedside, and (3) quickly incubate them at 37(198)°C.

Many controlled clinical trials demonstrate that appropriate antibiotics significantly decrease the duration of fever, diarrhea, intestinal protein loss, and pathogen excretion in shigellosis. Most patients in these studies were infected with either *S. flexneri* or *S. dysenteriae*. The advantages of treating *S. sonnei*, which is usually self-limited,

are less clear. Susceptible strains can be treated with ampicillin (but not amoxicillin) or TMP-SMX. With the exception of severely ill patients, therapy can be administered orally. However, since the mid-1980s, strains of *S. dysenteriae*, *S. flexneri*, and *S. sonnei* that are resistant to one or both drugs have been identified with increasing frequency in Asia, Africa, and North America,[88] dictating a more cautious approach to empiric therapy. For infections acquired in the United States and for which susceptibility is unknown, TMP-SMX is given empirically for 5 days unless resistance is suspected or proved. Fewer than 5% of domestically acquired isolates are resistant to TMP-SMX, whereas about 10% are resistant to ampicillin.[88]

Interruption of transmission by individual hygienic behavior such as hand washing is an effective way to control and prevent endemic transmission. One intensely pursued strategy for constructing modern attenuated oral vaccine candidates involves the generation of defined deletions in virulence wild-type *Shigella* genes or genes that affect the ability to survive or proliferate in vivo. Several promising deletion mutants have entered clinical trial.[30]

CAMPYLOBACTER

It is surprising that *Campylobacter* enteritis, the most common bacterial form of acute infective diarrheal disease in developed countries, was not recognized until the mid-1970s.[89] Why *Campylobacter* has been overlooked by microbiologists remains a matter for debate, but the too rigid methods of cultures and the failure to pick up ideas from the field of veterinary microbiology certainly played a role.

Microbiology

Organisms of the family Campylobacteriaceae are small, nonsporing, spiral-shaped gram-negative bacteria that exhibit rapid darting motility by means of a single flagellum at one or both ends. *Campylobacters* are largely microaerophilic, that is, they tolerate only low oxygen concentrations (5 to 10%). Molecular techniques have shown that *Campylobacter* (13 species pathogenic for humans), *Helicobacter*, *Arcobacter*, and *Wolinella* belong to a distinct phylogenetic group far removed from other gram-negative bacteria.[89] *C. jejuni* is by far the most common species isolated from patients with diarrhea in most areas (80 to 90% of infections), followed by *C. coli*.[90]

Epidemiology

Campylobacter enjoys a widespread reservoir in the intestines of both wild and domestic animals.[91] Case-control studies indicate that the vehicle for at least half of all endemic cases is poultry,[92] whereas common-source outbreaks are usually linked to consumption of unpasteurized milk[93] or contaminated water.[94] Up to 75% of raw poultry (but less than 5% of pork and beef) on sale in Western countries is contaminated with

Campylobacter.[95] As a result of its extensive animal reservoir, virtually all surface waters are contaminated with *Campylobacters*, even in remote regions.[96]

Although they share many epidemiologic features, there are important differences between *Campylobacter* and *Salmonella*. *Salmonella* is more likely to infect animals in large-scale husbandry operations and has thus become an important problem in industrialized countries. In contrast, *Campylobacter* spp. live naturally as commensals in a wide variety of animals and cause human infections globally.[97] *Campylobacter* does not multiply in food to high concentrations like *Salmonella* does; however, the inoculum required to cause infection is lower.[98] This may explain why, unlike *Salmonella*, *Campylobacter* rarely causes explosive food-borne outbreaks.

The annual incidence of *Campylobacter* infection in the United States is about 1%, making it the most frequently identified bacterial cause of diarrhea.[99] In industrialized countries with temperate climates, the peak incidence of infection occurs during the summer, and infections are more common in rural communities.[100] There is a bimodal age-specific incidence, with a principal climax during 0 to 5 years of age (highest, 12 months) and a secondary rise among young adults 15 to 29 years of age.[101] In less-developed countries, infection is hyperendemic, found in 8 to 45% of cases of diarrhea and in an equal number of asymptomatic controls during the first 5 years of life.[97]

Clinical Manifestations

After an incubation period of 3 to 6 days, *Campylobacter* enteritis begins abruptly with abdominal cramps and diarrhea.[101] Watery diarrhea often precedes the onset of blood-containing stools and is often the sole manifestation, especially among children from developing countries. However, abdominal pain may be so intense as to mimic appendicitis.[102] Diarrhea usually lasts 4 to 5 days, but in some patients, abdominal discomfort persists and brief relapses of diarrhea occur. The mean duration of fecal excretion is about 1 month in the normal host,[103] but carriage may be prolonged in patients with immunodeficiency. Neonates frequently experience milder illness, often with hematochezia in the absence of fever and diarrhea. However, severe or systemic illness may occur; *C. fetus* causes most cases of neonatal *Campylobacter* meningitis.[104]

Diagnosis, Treatment, and Prevention

A definitive diagnosis of *Campylobacter* infection can be made only by identifying the microorganism in a patient's stools. Properly taken rectal swabs are also satisfactory. The indication of antibiotic therapy for *Campylobacter* remains controversial. In some studies, early treatment shortened the course of diarrhea,[105] whereas in other studies, no clear clinical benefit was observed.[106] Given the frequent development of drug resistance,[107] it is advisable to reserve antibiotics for patients with severe illness ongoing at presentation (either dysentery or suspected *Campylobacter* infection on the basis of specific clinical or epidemiologic evidence) or if risk factors (pregnancy, systemic infection, immunosuppression) are present. Erythromycin remains the drug of choice for *Campylobacter* enteritis.[199]

Campylobacter vaccine development has proceeded cautiously because of concerns about post-exposure arthritis or Guillain-Barré syndrome. The most developed approach is to orally administer killed *Campylobacter* cells. A monovalent, formalin-inactivated *C. jejuni* whole-cell vaccine with a mucosal adjuvant has entered human trial.[30]

YERSINIA

Like *Escherichia coli* and *Salmonella*, *Yersinia* is a heterogeneous species; however, only a few pathogenic serotypes commonly cause disease in humans.

Microbiology

The genus *Yersinia*, of the family Enterobacteriaceae, contains two important human enteropathogens: *Y. enterocolitica* and *Y. pseudotuberculosis*. *Y. enterocolitica* is divided into six biotypes and more than 50 O-antigen serotypes, whereas *Y. pseudotuberculosis* contains six serotypes with four subtypes. Several other *Yersinia* species, including *Y. bercovieri*, *Y. mollaretii*, *Y. intermedia*, and *Y. rodhey*, are widespread in the environment but are rarely human pathogens. These microorganisms are non–lactose-fermenting gram-negative aerobic and facultatively anaerobic bacilli that grow better at 25°C than at 37°C.

Epidemiology

Yersinia spp. are distributed widely in the environment, with swine serving as the major reservoir for human pathogenic strains. Food-borne transmission is the suspected route for most infections, but the source is usually not identified.[108] The high infectious inoculum makes person-to-person transmission by fecal–oral spread an improbable event.[109] Most episodes of *Yersinia* gastroenteritis occur in infants and young children.[108] *Yersinia*'s preference for cool temperatures makes this pathogen more common in regions in northern latitudes, such as in Northern Europe, Scandinavia, Canada, the United States, and Japan, where it is responsible for 1 to 8% of sporadic diarrhea episodes.[110]

Clinical Manifestations

The incubation period is estimated to be 3 to 7 days. *Yersinia* enterocolitis occurs most often in children younger than 5 years of age and is characterized by watery diarrhea, usually with fever and abdominal pain.[111] The stools contain blood in 25 to 30% of patients. There may be vomiting, and approximately 20% of subjects exhibit pharyngitis that can be exudative and associated with cervical adenitis.[112] The organism can frequently be isolated from the pharyngeal exudate. Diarrhea typically lasts for 14 to 22 days, but fecal excretion may persist for 6 to 7 weeks or longer.[111] Abdominal complications may include appendicitis, diffuse ulceration of the intestine and colon, intestinal perforation, peritonitis, ileocecal intussusception, toxic megacolon, cholangitis, and mesenteric venous thrombosis.[110] The pseudoappendicitis syndrome occurs primarily in older patients and adults.[113] These patients typically present with fever and abdominal pain, with tenderness localized to the right-lower quadrant, with or without diarrhea. Computed tomography may be helpful in distinguishing true appendicitis from *Yersinia* infection.[114] Case fatality rates may reach 50%. Bacteremic spread may result in abscess formation and granulomatous lesions in the liver, spleen, lungs, kidneys, and bone and may also result in mycotic aneurysm, meningitis, and septic arthritis.[110] As with the other bacterial enteropathogens, *Y. enterocolitica* infection is associated with immunopathologic sequelae, including reactive arthritis, uveitis, Reiter's syndrome, and erythema nodosum.[110]

Diagnosis, Treatment, and Prevention

Y. enterocolitica may be isolated from stool on commonly used selective media and appears as gram-negative colonies after 48 hours of growth at 25 to 28°C. Detection of the microorganism in stool by polymerase chain reaction (PCR) methodology may represent a valid alternative.

Like *Campylobacter*, most uncomplicated cases of *Yersinia* gastroenteritis and pseudoappendicitis resolve without treatment. Therapy is reserved for patients with severe or extraintestinal infections and for immunocompromised individuals. Production of {158}-lactamases by *Y. enterocolitica* generally renders all but third-generation cephalosporins, aztreonam, and imipenem ineffective.[115] Broad-spectrum cephalosporins, often in combination with aminoglycosides, resulted in a good clinical outcome in 85% of cases of sepsis in one retrospective review.[115] The duration of therapy is generally 2 to 6 weeks, with an initial intravenous antibiotic followed by an oral agent to which the clinical isolate is sensitive. No enteric vaccines against *Y. enterocolitica* are currently available.

ESCHERICHIA COLI

An extremely heterogeneous group of microorganisms, *E. coli* encompasses almost all features of possible interactions between intestinal microflora and the host, ranging from a role of mere harmless presence to that of a highly pathogenic organism. In fact, the *E. coli* species is made up of many strains that profoundly differ from each other in terms of biologic characteristics and virulence properties.[116]

E. coli are gram-negative, lactose-fermenting motile bacilli of the family Enterobacteriaceae.

Currently, 171 somatic (O) and 56 flagellar (H) antigens are recognized. Six distinct categories of *E. coli* are currently considered enteric pathogens (based on either outbreak data or volunteer studies) (see Table 1): enteropathogenic *E. coli* (EPEC), enterotoxigenic *E. coli* (ETEC), enteroinvasive *E. coli* (EIEC), enterohemorrhagic *E. coli* (EHEC), diffusely adherent *E. coli* (DAEC), and enteroaggregative *E. coli* (EAggEC).

The diagnosis of diarrheagenic *E. coli* relies on isolation from stool and subsequent differentiation from commensal *E. coli* either by using genetic probes or by phenotypic assays. With the exception of *E. coli* O157:H7, assays for detection are not routinely available in clinical laboratories.

Enteropathogenic *E. coli*

This was the first group of *E. coli* species shown to be pathogens for humans and has been responsible for devastating outbreaks of nosocomial neonatal diarrhea and infant diarrhea in virtually every corner of the globe. Species of EPEC are distinguished from other *E. coli* species by their ability to induce a characteristic attaching and effacing lesion in the small intestinal enterocytes and by their inability to produce Shiga toxins.

Epidemiology. Between the 1940s and the 1960s, EPEC was associated with infant diarrhea in summertime and nursery outbreaks of diarrhea in the United States and other industrialized countries. Since then, it has become extremely uncommon in industrialized countries, although it is occasionally reported in child care settings.[117] However, EPEC persists as an important cause of infantile diarrhea in many developing countries.[118] In nursery outbreaks, transmission was thought to occur via the hands of caretakers and via fomites. In less-developed countries, contaminated formula and weaning foods have been incriminated.

Clinical Manifestations. Volunteer studies and epidemiologic observations suggest that the infective dose for EPEC is high ($\approx 10^9$ colony-forming units).[119] EPEC causes a self-limited watery diarrhea with a short-incubation period (6 to 48 h). There may be associated fever, abdominal cramps, and vomiting, and EPEC is a leading cause of persistent diarrhea (lasting 14 day or longer) in children in developing countries.[120]

Treatment and Prevention. Although few data exist to guide antibiotic therapy of EPEC diarrhea, administration of appropriate antibiotics seems to diminish morbidity and mortality. A 3-day course of oral, nonabsorbable antibiotics such as colistin or gentamicin (if available) has been shown to be effective.[121] Some clinicians also advocate the use of oral neomycin; however, this drug causes diarrhea in about 20% of people. In a placebo-controlled trial among Ethiopian infants with severe EPEC diarrhea, TMP-SMX and mecillinam resulted in significant clinical and bacteriologic cure rates by the third day compared with placebo.[122]

Strategies for the prevention of EPEC infection include efforts to improve social and economic conditions in developing countries, efforts to encourage breastfeeding, and prevention of nosocomial infections.

Enterotoxigenic *E. coli*

Species of ETEC are an important cause of diarrheal disease in humans and animals worldwide. The clinical importance of these microorgansims was first outlined in the 1970s by epidemiologic studies in India that identified them as a major cause of endemic diarrhea.[123] Their pathogenicity is related to the elaboration of one or more enterotoxins that are either heat stable (ST) or heat labile (LT) (see section "Pathogenesis") without invading or damaging intestinal epithelial cells.

Epidemiology. Together with *Rotavirus*, ETEC is the leading cause of dehydrating diarrheal disease among weaning infants in the developing world. These children experience two to three episodes of ETEC diarrhea in each of the first 2 years of life. This represents over 25% of all diarrheal illness[124] and results in an estimated 700,000 deaths each year.[2,125] In industrialized countries, ETEC does not contribute to endemic disease[78] but is notorious for being the leading agent of traveler's diarrhea, accounting for about half of all episodes.[126] Transmission occurs by ingestion of contaminated food and water, with peaks during the warm, wet season.

Clinical Manifestations. Like EPEC, ETEC requires a relatively high inoculum[127] and a short-incubation period (14 to 30 h). The cardinal symptom is watery diarrhea, sometimes with associated fever, abdominal cramps, and vomiting. In its most severe form, ETEC can cause cholera-like purging, even in adults. The illness is typically self-limited, lasting for less than 5 days, with few cases persisting beyond 3 weeks. Infection with ETEC has also been associated with short- and long-term adverse nutritional consequences in infants and children.

Treatment and Prevention. Most diarrheal illnesses owing to ETEC are self-limited and do not require specific antimicrobial therapy. Empiric therapy is reserved for those whose diarrhea is moderate to severe despite rehydration and supportive measures. Antibiotic regimens that have been efficacious in clinical trials, shortening the duration of illness by 1 to 2 days, include doxycycline, TMP-SMX, ciprofloxacin, quinolones, and furazolidone.[128] In the past, the drug of choice for children has been TMP-SMX; however, a large proportion of ETEC is now resistant.[129] An alternative regimen for children is furazolidone.

Prevention of ETEC infection is based on avoiding contaminated vehicles. Although antibiotics are effective as prophylactic agents, their use is not recommended. Some experts advocate the use of bismuth subsalicylate to diminish the risk of traveler's diarrhea.[130] The development

of vaccines against ETEC has received a great deal of attention because of its disease burden. Oral vaccines for ETEC are being developed by five different strategies, including killed whole cells, toxoids, purified fimbriae, living attenuated strains, and live carrier strains elaborating ETEC antigens.[2] A killed whole-cell *V. cholerae* vaccine given with cholera toxin B provided 67% protection against LT-producing ETEC diarrhea for 3 months.[2] Other new killed ETEC vaccines entered clinical trials with promising results.[131]

Enteroinvasive *E. coli*

This group consists of invasive *E. coli* species that are genetically, biochemically, and clinically nearly identical to *Shigella*. This section serves only to highlight relevant characteristics that distinguish this pathogen.

Epidemiology. Species of EIEC are endemic in developing countries, where they exhibit similar epidemiology to *Shigella* and cause an estimated 1 to 5% of diarrheal episodes among patients visiting treatment centers.[132] The occurrence of EIEC in industrialized countries is limited to rare food-borne outbreaks.[133] From volunteer studies, it appears that the infectious inoculum is higher than that required to cause shigellosis.[134]

Clinical Manifestations, Treatment, and Prevention. Like *Shigella*, EIEC can produce dysentery, but watery diarrhea is more common.[135] The rare episodes for which treatment is desired are treated with antibiotics recommended for shigellosis. The same general preventive measures used for *Shigella* infections apply to EIEC-associated diarrhea.

Enterohemorrhagic *E. coli*

These *E. coli* species produce either one or both phage-encoded potent cytotoxins termed Shiga-like toxin (SLT) I (which is neutralized by antisera to Shiga toxin produced by *S. dysenteriae* type I) or SLT II (which is not neutralized) and can cause diarrhea or HUS. *E. coli* O157:H7 is the prototypic (but not the exclusive) EHEC serotype because it is the predominant SLT-producing *E. coli*, the one most commonly associated with HUS in North America and the type most readily identified in stool specimens.[136]

Epidemiology. In 1982, a multistate outbreak of hemorrhagic colitis that was linked to the consumption of hamburgers at the same fast-food restaurant led to the identification of EHEC.[137] The causative organism was *E. coli* O157:H7, a serotype not previously recognized as a human pathogen. Soon after, Canadian investigators uncovered an association between O157:H7 and other SLT-producing strains of *E. coli* and HUS.[138] EHEC is now recognized as a global health problem; in 1996, an outbreak in Japan linked to eating radish sprouts affected over 6,000 persons.[139] One of the most severe EHEC outbreaks in the United States took place in New York State in 1999, with more than 1,000 ascertained cases,

2 HUS-related casualties, and 8 children in dialysis because of renal failure. Most of the infected individuals attended a fair whose underground water supply was contaminated by cow manure from a nearby cattle barn. EHEC-contaminated fresh spinach caused an outbreak in the United States between August 23 and September 17, 2006. According to a report from the CDC, 109 infected cases from 19 states were recorded, with 55 of these cases hospitalized, 16 suffering from HUS, and 1 casualty.

The predominant mode of transmission is ingestion of contaminated, undercooked ground beef. However, the spectrum of vehicles is widening to include raw fruits (including apple juice) and vegetables,[140] raw milk,[140] processed meats,[140] and drinking[140] or swimming[140] in contaminated water.[141] The uncooked food vehicles are usually contaminated with manure from infected animals during growth or processing. Person-to-person transmission is the mode of spread in day-care outbreaks, for which secondary transmission rates of 22% have been reported.[142]

EHEC also causes sporadic diarrhea. Isolation from stools of unselected patients is low (< 1%), but isolation from stools of patients with bloody diarrhea may be as high as 20 to 30%.[143] A national laboratory-based study demonstrated that infection is more frequent in northern states and that it peaks from June through September.[143] The highest age-specific isolation rates are in patients 5 to 9 and 50 to 59 years of age. A population-based incidence rate based on stool samples submitted to a large health maintenance organization laboratory in the state of Washington was 8 per 100,000 person-years.[144]

Clinical Manifestations. Illness with EHEC follows 3 to 9 days after ingestion of as few as 100 organisms.[145] Crampy abdominal pain and non-bloody diarrhea are the first symptoms, sometimes associated with vomiting. By the second or third day of illness, diarrhea becomes bloody in approximately 90% of cases, and abdominal pain worsens.[146] Bloody diarrhea lasts between 1 and 22 days (median 4 days). Unlike other infectious causes of bloody diarrhea, fever is usually absent or remains low grade. Younger children appear to excrete the organisms longer (median 3 weeks) than older children and adults.[147]

In outbreaks, approximately 25% of patients are hospitalized, 5 to 10% develop HUS, and 1% die.[148] Intestinal complications include rectal prolapse, appendicitis, intussusception, and pseudomembranous colitis.[136] Extraintestinal complications are rare.

The most frightening complication of EHEC infection is HUS. It is usually diagnosed 2 to 14 days after the onset of diarrhea.[138] Risk factors include young and old age, bloody diarrhea, fever, an elevated leukocyte count, and treatment with antimotility agents.[149] Two-thirds of patients who develop HUS are no longer excreting the organism at presentation.[150]

Diagnosis. The most widely accepted indication for seeking a clinical diagnosis of E. coli O157:H7 infection is a patient with bloody diarrhea, in whom an accurate diagnosis may avoid unnecessary medical procedures because a surgical abdomen (such as appendicitis or intussusception) is suspected. A multicenter study found that when the presence of fecal blood was used as the sole criterion for culturing O157 strains, only 3% of stools would be cultured to detect 63% of infections.[143] Diagnosis may also be helpful in patients with HUS or with any type of diarrhea in a contact of a patient with HUS. E. coli O157:H7 is not detected by routine stool culture. A relatively inexpensive method exploits the inability of E. coli O157 to rapidly ferment sorbitol after 24 hours of incubation on sorbitol-MacConkey agar, in contrast to approximately 90% of commensal E. coli. The "sorbitol-negative" colonies can then be screened for the presence of O157 antigen, using commercially available antisera. These strains should be considered pathogenic pending the determination of the H type in a reference laboratory.

Treatment and Prevention. Although data are not available from prospective randomized double-blind trials, there is considerable evidence to suggest that patients who receive antibiotics to which the offending E. coli O157:H7 is sensitive have either the same or a poorer outcome when compared with untreated patients.[149] Therefore, antibiotic therapy is not recommended for EHEC infection. As mentioned above, antimotility agents have been identified as a risk factor for the development of HUS and should be avoided.

Prevention of E. coli O157:H7 is a complex process. From a public health standpoint, control measures at the level of farms, slaughterhouses, and processing plants can decrease the risk of colonization of cattle and contamination of beef. Because these procedures are unlikely to achieve complete success, regulations governing proper processing and cooking of contaminated foods are also required. Advice to consumers should include recommending complete avoidance of raw foods of animal origin. Hamburger should be cooked until no pink remains and the juices are clear.

Because of the severity of the disease, there has been a recent focus on vaccine development for EHEC infection. Efforts have been concentrated on three approaches: (1) parenteral toxoids and live oral carrier strains elaborating the B subunit of Shiga toxin,[151] (2) vaccines expressing the adhesin intimin, designed to prevent intestinal colonization,[152] and (3) a bacterial ghost strategy for oral vaccine.[153]

Diffusely Adhering E. coli

Until recently, DAEC was considered a nonpathogenic E. coli because early studies failed to find an association between this microorganism and diarrheal disease.[154] However, studies performed during the past 15 years have demonstrated such an association, particularly in children older than 2 years of age.

Epidemiology. A community-based, case-control study in southern Mexico revealed that DAEC was significantly associated with diarrhea in children less than 6 years of age.[155] Prospective cohort studies in Chile, Bangladesh, and Brazil also demonstrated a diarrheagenic role for DAEC that peaked in the 48- to 60-month-age groups.[156] This microorganism was more frequently isolated from cases of prolonged diarrhea,[157] and it showed a seasonal pattern similar to that of ETEC, occurring more frequently in the warm season.[156]

Clinical Manifestations, Diagnosis, and Treatment. The gastrointestinal symptoms that characterize DAEC infection are practically indistinguishable from those caused by ETEC, with self-limiting watery diarrhea rarely associated with vomiting and abdominal pain. The diagnosis is mainly based on DNA probe technique and on the pattern of adherence of the microorganism on Hep-2 cells.[158] Given the technical challenge of both assays, their use is limited to epidemiologic surveys rather than the diagnosis of individuals.

Enteroaggregative E. coli

EAggEC are diarrheagenic E. coli defined by a characteristic aggregating pattern of adherence to Hep-2 cells and the intestinal mucosa (Figure 2). They have been particularly associated with cases of persistent diarrhea in the developing world. It has been hypothesized that the aggregating pattern of adherence may be a result of nonspecific, possibly hydrophobic, interaction; therefore, not all organisms meeting the definition of EAggEC may be pathogenic in humans. Moreover, because epidemiologic studies did not uniformly implicated EAggEC as pathogenic, some investigators in the past have questioned the virulence of all EAggEC isolates. Volunteer studies performed to address both of these questions[159] confirmed that at least some EAggEC species are genuine human pathogens but that virulence is not uniform among isolates. During the past decade, EAggEC pathogenicity has also been proven in several outbreaks.[160]

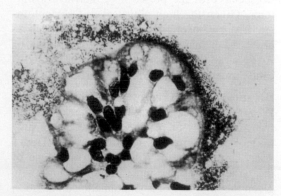

Figure 2 Histopathology of enteroggregative *Escherichia coli* (EAggEC) infection in a gnotobiotic piglet ileum. The light photomicrograph shows the aggregate pattern of adherence to the intestinal micosa that characterizes these microorganisms (hematoxylin and eosin; ×100 original magnification).

Epidemiology. From the earliest epidemiologic reports, EAggEC was most prominently associated with persistent cases of pediatric diarrhea (ie, lasting $\geq$ 14 days),[161] a condition that represents a disproportionate share of diarrheal mortality. On the Indian subcontinent, several independent studies have demonstrated the importance of EAggEC in pediatric diarrhea.[162] These studies include hospitalized patients with persistent diarrhea,[154] outpatients visiting health clinics,[162] and cases of sporadic diarrhea detected by household surveillance.[154] In Fortaleza, Brazil, Fang and colleagues demonstrated a consistent association between EAggEC and persistent diarrhea[163] in this area; EAggEC accounts for more cases of persistent diarrhea than all other causes combined.[163] EAggEC has been implicated as a cause of sporadic diarrhea in other developing countries (including Mexico, Chile, Bangladesh, Congo, and Iran), as well as in industrialized countries such as Germany and England.[160] Besides being responsible for sporadic cases of diarrhea, EAggEC has also been associated with outbreaks in UK,[164] Serbia,[165] Japan,[166] and among the US military personnel deployed in endemic areas.[167]

Clinical Manifestations. The clinical features of EAggEC diarrhea are becoming increasingly well defined in outbreaks, sporadic cases, and the volunteer model. Typically, illness is manifested by a watery, mucoid, secretory diarrheal illness with low-grade fever and little or no vomiting.[159,160] However, in epidemiologic studies, grossly bloody stools have been reported in up to one-third of patients with EAggEC diarrhea.[168] This phenomenon may well be strain dependent. In volunteers infected with EAggEC strain 042, diarrhea was mucoid, of low volume, and, notably, without occult blood or fecal leukocytes; all patients remained afebrile. In such volunteers, the incubation period of the illness ranged from 8 to 18 hours.[159]

Perhaps even more significant than the association of EAggEC with diarrhea are the data from Brazil that link EAggEC with growth retardation in infants.[168] In this study, the isolation of EAggEC from the stools of infants was associated with a low z-score for height and/or weight, irrespective of the presence of diarrheal symptoms. Given the high prevalence of asymptomatic EAggEC excretion in many areas,[160] such an observation may imply that the contribution of EAggEC to the human disease burden is significantly greater than is currently appreciated.

Diagnosis and Treatment. Colonization of EAggEC is detected by the isolation of *E. coli* from the stools of patients and the demonstration of the aggregative pattern in the Hep-2 assay. Implication of EAggEC as the cause of the patient's disease must be done cautiously, given the high rate of asymptomatic colonization in many populations.[160] If no other organism is implicated in the patient's illness and EAggEC is isolated repeatedly, then EAggEC should be considered a potential cause of the patient's illness. A DNA fragment probe has proven highly specific in the detection of EAggEC strains. A PCR assay using primers derived from the aggregative probe sequence shows similar sensitivity and specificity.[169]

The optimal management of EAggEC infection has not been studied. Acute diarrhea is apparently self-limiting; however, more persistent cases may benefit from antibiotic and/or nutritional therapy. Given the high rate of antibiotic resistance among EAggEC,[170] susceptibility testing is recommended when available.

CLOSTRIDIUM DIFFICILE

Even though *Clostridium difficile* is now recognized as the single most common cause of bacterial diarrhea in hospitalized patients, its role as a pathogen had not been established as recently as the late 1970s. *C. difficile* has the ability to become established in the gastrointestinal tract once the natural microflora has been modified by antibiotic therapy. The organism causes intestinal disease ranging from mild diarrhea to fatal pseudomembranous colitis (PMC). Although *C. difficile* is associated with almost all cases of PMC, only 25% of antibiotic-associated diarrheas are due to this pathogen.

Microbiology. *C. difficile* is a gram-positive anaerobe that forms spores, making this microorganism very difficult to remove from the hospital environment. Unlike some toxigenic clostridia, the production of spores is not associated with toxin production.

Epidemiology. *C. difficile* spreads from patient to patient[171] and tends to persist in the environment because of the formation of spores. The microorganism is not only present in the infected patient and soiled linens but can be isolated from bookshelves, curtains, and floors of rooms of infected patients, where it can persist for as long as 5 months.[171] The organism is spread primarily by health care workers; up to 60% of personnel attending patients infected with *C. difficile* in one study had the organism on their hands.[171] The isolation of *C. difficile* toxins from the feces of asymptomatic normal-term neonates and (in higher proportion) those admitted into neonatal intensive care units[172] further supports the concept of the nosocomial spreading of the infection.

Several outbreaks of *C. difficile* infection have been reported in the United States and throughout the world, and the incidence continues to rise. During the past 3 years, *C. difficile* has been more frequent, more severe, more refractory to standard therapy, and more likely to relapse.[173] This pattern is widely distributed in the United States, Canada, and Europe and is now attributed to a new strain of *C. difficile* designated BI, NAP1, or ribotype 027.[173]

Clinical Manifestations. Infections with *C. difficile* range in severity from asymptomatic forms to clinical syndromes, such as severe diarrhea, PMC, and toxic megacolon, and can even lead to death.[174] The onset of symptomatic forms usually begins several days after starting antibiotic therapy up to 2 months following cessation of treatment. Diarrhea and abdominal cramps are usually the first symptoms, followed by the development of fever and chills in severe cases.

Diagnosis and Treatment. Mild forms of colitis, with bloody stools and mucus, particularly if they are preceded by antibiotic treatment, should be considered suspicious for *C. difficile* infection. Clinical microbiologists face an array of methods and commercial tests when considering which procedure to use for the detection of *C. difficile* and its toxins. Culturing of the organism, latex agglutination, tissue culture assay, and enzyme-linked immunosorbent assay are all used as aids for the diagnosis of *C. difficile* infection.

In many instances, *C. difficile* disease is self-limiting, and the patient may respond simply to the withdrawal of the offending antibiotic. In more severe forms, particularly if complicated by PMC, antibiotic treatment with either oral vancomycin (5 to 10 mg/kg, maximum 500 mg, given every 6 hours for 7 days) or metronidazole[175] (5 to 10 mg/kg, maximum 500 mg, given every 8 hours for 7 days) is recommended. Despite pharmacologic treatment, the rate of relapse is significant (up to 40 to 50% of cases). In these complicated patients, the use of probiotics, particularly *Lactobacillus* GG and *Saccharomyces boulardii*,[176,177] has been associated with a significant eradication of *C. difficile* and a substantial decrease in the recurrence of the infection.

AEROMONAS, PLESIOMONAS, AND *EDWARDSIELLA*

This group includes microorganisms of which the existence has been known for a long time; however, only relatively recently they have been associated with human diseases.

Aeromonas

Aeromonads are gram-negative facultative anaerobic, motile bacilli. Although their association with gastroenteritis is still somewhat controversial, experimental, clinical, and epidemiologic data continue to support the evidence that at least certain strains are involved in diarrheal diseases.[178] The highest attack rate appears to be in young children, particularly those under 3 years of age. *Aeromonas* infections occur more frequently during the warm months, with an isolation rate that varies from as little as 0.7% to peaks of 50%.[179] Despite these data, a number of troubling aspects regarding the association between *Aeromonas* and diarrhea remain unresolved. In contrast to other waterborne and foodborne pathogens, no clearly defined outbreaks of diarrheal illnesses associated with the pathogen have ever been reported, even though the microorganism is often isolated from water, food, and other environmental sources.

The gastrointestinal diseases caused by *Aeromonas* cover the same spectrum of clinical manifestations secondary to other classic enteric pathogens. *Aeromonas* spp have been associated with several distinctive clinical syndromes, including watery diarrhea, dysentery, and prolonged or chronic diarrhea. Acute secretory diarrhea is the most commonly reported, with as many as 20 bowel movements a day. Abdominal pain, fever, nausea, and vomiting are common associated symptoms.[180] Although the infection is usually self-limited (<7 days in duration), dehydration or persistent diarrhea may occur in one-third of the cases. The most common *Aeromonas* species isolated in these cases is *A. caviae*. Some children with this infection experience abdominal complications secondary to their diarrheal episodes, including failure to thrive, gram-negative sepsis, and HUS.[180]

The mainstay of therapy in *Aeromonas*-associated gastroenteritis, as in any diarrheal disease, is rehydration, via either the oral or the intravenous route. The illness is usually self-limited, and previously healthy subjects who experience this form of gastroenteritis not treated with antibiotics appear to do well, with rapid resolution of the symptoms and clearance of the microorganism from the stools. TMP-SMX is considered the drug of choice for the chronic forms that seem to benefit from antibiotic treatment.[181]

Plesiomonas

Plesiomonas, originally assigned to the family Vibrionaceae but more recently reassigned to Enterobacteriaceae,[182] are gram-negative, facultative anaerobic, motile, primarily freshwater organisms, with isolation rates increasing during the warm months. Fish and shellfish, especially if associated with mud or sediment, frequently harbor plesiomonads.[183] However, the microorganism can also be isolated from the feces of asymptomatic animals, including cats and dogs.[184] Although less frequently encountered in the United States, *Plesiomonas shigelloides* is commonly isolated in other areas, particularly in Bangladesh, where this organism represents the fourth leading cause of bacterial gastroenteritis.[185] Typical symptoms of *P. shigelloides* infection include secretory or a colitis/proctitis type of diarrhea (one-third of patients experience frank bloody diarrhea), abdominal pain, nausea, vomiting, and fever. Fatal outcomes of severe gastrointestinal infections without apparent dissemination by *Plesiomonas* have also been described.[186] Quinolones and TMP-SMX are the best oral agents for the treatment of uncomplicated infections whose course seems to be shortened by antibiotic treatment.[187]

Edwardsiella

The genus *Edwardsiella* is composed of bacteria that are gram-negative, facultative anaerobic rods. *E. tarda*, the only species in this genus consistently associated with both intestinal and extraintestinal human illness, has been isolated from the feces of persons suffering from diarrheal diseases

and from fish, freshwater ecosystems, and animals that inhabit these locales, such as reptiles and amphibia. Gastroenteritis associated with *E. tarda* exists either as a benign secretory diarrhea or as a more invasive process resembling dysentery or enterocolitis. The most common symptoms include low-grade fever, vomiting, and watery stools.[188] Symptoms may be more severe (resembling PMC or invasive enterocolitis) and include cramping, abdominal pain, nausea, tenesmus, and up to 20 bowel movements per day. Occasionally, disseminated *E. tarda* infections (septicemia, hepatic abscess) can occur in subjects with liver dysfunction or iron overload conditions.[189] Ampicillin, TMP-SMX, and ciprofloxacin would all be reasonable choices for the treatment of *E. tarda* infections.

PATHOGENESIS

The distinguishing characteristics of bacteria (small size, concise deployment of genetic information, and the ability to survive in highly varied circumstances) contribute to their acclaimed virtuosic ability to adapt and learn fast in order to survive. To be a successful enteric pathogen, a bacterium must be a good colonizer, must compete for nutrients, and must be able to interact with the target eukaryotic cell to induce secretion of water and electrolytes. Because the basic metabolism of enteric pathogens and commensals is the same, it follows that pathogens must possess highly specialized attributes that enable them to activate one of the eukaryotic intracellular pathways leading to intestinal secretion.[190] This cross-communication between enteric bacteria and the intestinal host is typically activated by the elaboration of enterotoxins (Table 2) that subvert host cell signal transduction pathways, leading to the secretion of water and electrolytes and thus to diarrhea.

TOXINS THAT ACTIVATE ENTEROCYTE SIGNAL PATHWAYS

Intestinal cells operate through three main intracellular signal transduction pathways to regulate ion transport vectorially: (1) cyclic adenosine monophosphate (cAMP), (2) cyclic guanosine monophosphate (cGMP), and (3) calcium-dependent pathways (Figure 3). A fourth pathway involving cytoskeleton rearrangement has been also described (see Figure 3).

Cyclic Adenosine Monophosphate

Cholera toxin elaborated by *V. cholerae* represents the archetype of the family of cAMP-mediated toxins and is certainly the most extensively investigated. Cholera toxin is a protein with a relative molecular mass (M_r) of 84 kDa, made up of five B subunits with M_r of 10.5 kDa each and one A subunit with M_r of 27.2 kDa. The A subunit is proteolytically cleaved to yield two polypeptide chains, a 195 residue A_1 peptide of 21.8 kDa and

Table 2 Bacteria-Derived Enteric Toxins
Toxins That Activate Enterocyte Signal Pathways
Cyclic AMP
Cholera toxin
Heat-labile *Escherichia coli* enterotoxin (LT)
Salmonella enterotoxin
Pseudomonas aeruginosa enterotoxin
Shigella dysenteriae enterotoxin
Cyclic GMP
Heat-stable *Escherichia coli* enterotoxin (ST)
Yersinia enterocolitica (STI, STII)
Yersinia bercovieri enterotoxin
Heat-stable *Vibrio cholerae* non-O1 enterotoxin
Enteroaggregative *Escherichia coli* heat-stable enterotoxin (EAST 1)
Ca^{2+}
Clostridium difficile enterotoxin
Ciguatera enterotoxin
Helicobacter pylori vacuolating toxin
Vibrio parahaemolyticus thermostable direct hemolysin (TDH)
Pore-Forming Toxins
Clostridium perfringens enterotoxin (CPE)
Staphylococus aureus α-toxin
Vibrio cholerae cytolysin (CTC)
Toxins Blocking Protein Synthesis
Shigella dysenteriae Shiga toxin
EHEC Shiga-like toxin 1 (SLT1) and 2 (SLT2)
Toxins Inducing Protein Synthesis
Staphylococcus aureus enterotoxin A
Enteroggregative *Escherichia coli* (EAggEC) toxin
Toxin Affecting the Enterocyte Cytoskeleton
Clostridium difficile toxin A and B
Clostridium sordelli toxin
Clostridium botulinum C2 and C3 toxins
Escherichia coli cytotoxic necrotizing factor 1 (CNF1)
Campylobacter jejuni cytolethal distending toxin
Vibrio cholerae zonula occludens toxin (ZOT)
EAggEC plasmid-encoded protein (Pet)
Bacteroides fragilis toxin (BFT)
Vibrio parahaemolyticus thermostable direct hemolysin (TDH)
Amp = adenosine monophosphate; GMP = guanosine monophosphate.

a 45 residue A_2 peptide of 5.4 kDa.[191] As with other toxins in this group, the functions of the two subunits are specific: The B subunit serves to bind the holotoxin to the eukaryotic cell receptor, and the A subunit possesses a specific enzymatic function that acts intracellularly. The single A subunit is presumably located on the axis of the pentameric B subunit ring, with the fragment A_2 extending some distance into the central hole.[192] The cholera toxin receptor on the surface of the enterocyte is a ganglioside GM_1 that is ubiquitous in the body, being present on such diverse cell types as ovarian and neural cells as well as intestinal cells.[192] The neuraminidase produced by *V. cholerae* can increase the number of receptors by acting on higher order gangliosides to convert them to GM_1 gangliosides.[193] Reduction of the disulfide bond between A_1 and A_2 peptides on the external surface of the membrane is necessary for penetration of the A_1 peptide into the cell. The fate of the A_2 peptide is not known, but there is little evidence that it actually enters the cell. Once within the cell, the A_1 peptide activates adenylate cyclase at the basolateral membrane,

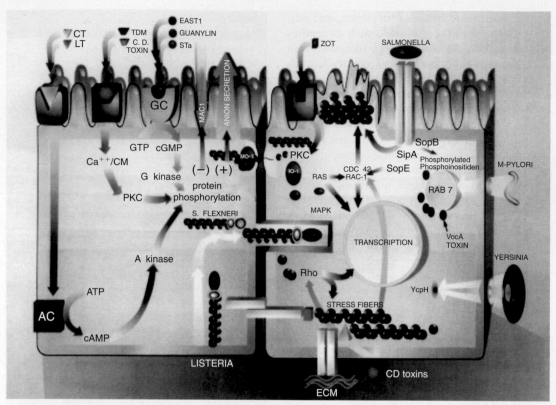

Figure 3   Enterocyte intracellular signaling leading to intestinal secretion. Four main pathways seem to be involved in the intestinal secretion of water and electrolytes: cycle adenosing monophosphate (cAMP), cyclic guanosine mon ophophosphate (xGMP), calcium (Ca), and cytoskeleton. These pathways are activated by several enteric pathogens, either directly or through the elaboration of enterotixic products. AC = adenylate cyclase' C.D. = *Clostridum difficile*' CM= calmodulin' CT= cholera toxin; EAST1 = enteroaggregativ *Escherichia coli* heat-stable toxin 1' ECM = extracellular matrix' EGF-r = epidermal growth factor receptor' GC = guanylate cyclase' LT = heat-labile enterotoxin; PKC = protein kinase C; ST_a = heat-stable toxin$_a$; TDH = thermostable direct hemolysin; ZOT = zonula occludens toxin.

where the enzyme is localized in intestinal epithelial cells. The A_1 peptide is thought to migrate to the basolateral membrane through the cytosol, although there is no convincing evidence that this actually occurs. An alternative model proposes that generation of the A_1 peptide and activation of adenylate cyclase are functionally linked to toxin endocytosis. The A_1 peptide acts as an enzyme to adenosine diphosphate ribosylate, the 157 subunit of G_s at an arginine residue. Once activated, the 157 subunit of G_s dissociates from the membrane bound subunit of G_s, leaving it free to transverse the cell and attach to the catalytic subunit of adenylate cyclase in the basolateral membrane. More recent evidence seems to suggest a different trafficking of the toxin the target enterocyte.[194] Entry is achieved by the B subunit binding to a membrane lipid that carries the toxin all the way from the plasma membrane through the trans Golgi to the endoplasmic reticulum. Once in the endoplasmic reticulum, a portion of the A subunit, the A1 chain, unfolds and separates from the B subunit to retrotranslocate to the cytosol.[194] The A1 chain then activates adenylate cyclase. The adenylate cyclase so activated induces the formation of cAMP, which then activates the catalytic unit of cAMP-dependent protein kinase (protein kinase A). Finally, the phosphorylation of membrane proteins is responsible for the transepithelial ion transport changes induced by cholera toxin. These changes consist of the inhibition of the linked sodium and chlorine absorptive process in the villous cells and the stimulation of electro-genic chlorine secretion in the crypt cells.[195] The nature of the target protein(s) phosphorylated by protein kinase A remains uncertain. One attractive candidate is the cystic fibrosis transmembrane receptor, which is a chloride channel[196] and which has multiple potential substrate sequences for protein kinase A. Unlike healthy intestinal tissue, tissues obtained from patients with cystic fibrosis do not respond to either cAMP or Ca-mediated secretagogues.[197] Heterozygotes presumably have only half of the normal number of chloride channels responsive to kinase. After infection with *V. cholerae*, the cystic fibrosis heterozygote may have less intestinal chloride secretion and, therefore, less diarrhea, suggesting a selective advantage over "normal" homozygotes in surviving cholera.

ETEC elaborate an LT (see Table 2) that closely resembles cholera toxin in structure and biochemical mode of action. Unlike cholera toxin, LT can also bind to GM_2 and asialo GM_1 gangliosides in addition to GM_1 ganglioside.[198] Toxin binding is followed by activation of the adenylate cyclase-cAMP system, resulting in water and electrolyte secretion into the lumen of the intestine, with a mechanism similar to that of cholera toxin.[199] However, whereas LT induces a mild diarrhea known as "traveler's diarrhea," cholera toxin is responsible for the severe, sometimes fatal, clinical condition typical of cholera. Rodighiero and colleagues have reported that the differential toxicity of cholera toxin and LT is related to a 10 amino acid seg-ment within the A_2 fragment of cholera toxin that confers a higher stability to the cholera toxin holotoxin during uptake and transport into intestinal epithelia.[200]

In addition to its invasiveness, *S. typhimurium* elaborates an enterotoxin, whose role in inducing diarrhea remains controversial (see Table 2).[201] Cell free lysate of *Salmonella* can cause intestinal secretion and activate intestinal epithelial cell adenylate cyclase independent of any change in inflammation.[201] How the *Salmonella* toxin activates adenylate cyclase has not been determined.

C. jejuni also produces an A–B toxin (see Table 2), whose B subunit immunologically cross-reacts with cholera toxin and ETEC LT B subunits.[202]

Cyclic Guanosine Monophosphate

Besides LT, ETEC elaborates a family of heat stable enterotoxins STs. STIp is a small peptide that stimulates guanylate cyclase (GC), causing an increased intracellular concentration of cGMP, which evokes chloride secretion and diarrhea.[190] The STIp is a typical extracellular toxin, consisting of 18 amino acid residues synthesized as a precursor protein. The precursor translocates across the inner bacterial membrane, using the general export pathway consisting of the Sec proteins.[203] The ST_a epithelial surface receptor is distinct from the cholera toxin and LT receptor and coincides with the GC activity.[204] Ileal villous epithelial cells have approximately twice as many receptors as crypt cells for the enterotoxin.[205] GC exists in two major forms, soluble and particulate. These are distinct proteins encoded by separate genes. Soluble GC is a dimeric cytosolic protein that is activated by nitric oxide.[206] Particulate GC is a family of brush border membrane glycoproteins that are activated by only two classes of substances, atrial natriuretic peptides and ST_a. In the intestine, approximately 80% of total GC is particulate.[207] So far, three different members of the particulate GC family have been cloned.[207] GC A and B are atrial natriuretic peptide receptor cyclases, whereas GC C is the specific receptor for ST_a. All three members of the GC family are proteins that span the cell membrane and contain an extracellular domain, a transmembrane domain, an intracytoplasmic domain made up of a protein kinase-like enzyme, and a catalytic domain. These proteins show minimal similarities in their extracellular domain, whereas there is a higher degree of similarity of their intracellular domains. This finding suggests that the extracellular domain represents the ligand-binding domain.[207] In addition to LT and ST exotoxins, ETEC also contains a lipopolysaccharide endotoxin. When orally administered to mice, lipopolysaccharide markedly increased the expression of the inducible nitric oxide synthase II and its effector enzyme-soluble GC in colonic cells.[208] This creates the pathophysiologic autocrine pathway, producing increased levels of cGMP and leading to hypersecretion and diarrhea.[208] Another heat-stable enterotoxin,

EAST 1, which is genetically and structurally distinct from ST, was discovered in EAggEC[209] and subsequently found in other *E. coli* belonging to several distinct diarrheagenic categories.[210] A case-control study demonstrated that 19% of children with diarrhea harbored EAST 1–positive *E. coli* in their stools compared with 3.5% of healthy individuals,[211] confirming the pathogenic role of EAST 1 in diarrheal diseases in children. Another member of the ST family has been reported by Sulakvelidze and coworkers.[212] This toxin, elaborated by *Y. bercovieri*, elicited a secretory response in both in vitro and in vivo animal models; these results were genetically and immunologically distinct from the response to *Y. enterocolitica* STI and STII.[212]

Calcium

Several toxins, including ciguatera toxin,[213] *C. difficile* toxin,[214] *Cryptosporidium* toxin,[215] and the *Helicobacter pylori*-vacuolating toxin,[216] seem to act through Ca. However, the involvement of Ca in the secretory effect of these toxins has been only indirectly demonstrated. A more definitive proof of Ca-mediated secretory effect was provided by Raimondi and colleagues.[217] Using direct intracellular (Ca$_i$) measurement, they demonstrated that the enterotoxic effect of the thermostable direct hemolysin elaborated by *V. parahaemolyticus* is mediated by Ca.[217] This toxin seems to interact with a polysialoganglioside GT1b surface receptor, whose physiologic function remains to be established.[217]

Pore-Forming Toxins

Clostridium perfrigens is a common agent of food-borne intoxication, the symptoms of which are caused by the elaboration of *C. perfrigens* enterotoxin.[218] This enterotoxin is a very hydrophobic protein that is released by bacterial lysis and subsequently binds to a brush border receptor of the host enterocyte.[218] Following this binding, *C. perfrigens* enterotoxin associates with a 70 kDa membrane protein, with subsequent formation of pores through which water, ions, nucleotides, and amino acids leak. *Staphylococcus aureus* 157 toxin also forms pores; however, its mechanism of action involves the formation of oligomers containing only toxin molecules.[218] According to Zitzer and coworkers, the *V. cholerae* cytolysin represents another prototype of pore-forming toxin.[219] The authors have demonstrated that the oligomerization of *V. cholerae* cytolysin yields a pentameric pore and has a dual specificity for both cholesterol and ceramides present in the mammalian brush border membrane of *enterocytes*.[219]

Toxins Blocking Protein Synthesis

Shiga toxin elaborated by *S. dysenteriae* represents the archetype of this family of toxins. SLT1 and -2 are related toxins elaborated by EHEC. Shiga toxin and SLTs share the AB5 structure typical of cholera toxin and LT; however, they act through a different mechanism of action. The A$_1$ subunit of Shiga toxin and SLTs binds and inactivates the 60S subunit of the host cell ribosome and, consequently, completely interrupts cell protein synthesis.[220] To induce this inhibitory effect, the toxins must interact with a glycolipid surface receptor (Gb3 receptor), whose expression in different endothelial districts varies.[221] In fact, whereas endothelial cells of large blood vessels such as the umbilical and saphenous veins produce minimal amounts of Gb3,[221] human renal[221] and intestinal[222] microvascular endothelial cells constitutively express maximal quantities of the receptor. These results provide a rationale for the targeting of the glomeruli in HUS and the endothelial cells of the colon in hemorrhagic colitis. Recent epidemiologic data suggest that the elaboration of SLTs may not be sufficient in itself to induce disease in humans. By applying a multivariate logistic regression analysis, an association between the presence of genes for intimin (a protein involved in the intimate attachment of EHEC to the host intestinal cell) and SLT2 and isolates from cases of hemorrhagic colitis and HUS have been reported.[223] Further analysis revealed an interaction between the intimin gene and the *SLT2* gene, thus supporting the hypothesis of the synergism between the adhesin intimin and SLT2.[223]

Toxins Inducing Protein Synthesis

Upregulation of protein synthesis, particularly of proinflammatory mediators, is one of the most recently described mechanisms through which bacterial toxins induce O'Brien. Nielsen and coworkers have demonstrated that staphylococcal enterotoxin A induces tyrosine phosphorylation of several host intracellular proteins, downregulation of the T-cell receptor, and production of cytokines involved in the pathogenesis of intestinal inflammatory and secretory processes.[224] Transcriptional upregulation of proinflammatory cytokines seems also to be involved in the pathogenesis of EAggEC-associated diarrhea. It has been reported that EAggEC produces a cell-free factor that upregulates interleukin-8 (IL-8) messenger ribonucleic acid in CaCo2 cells.[225] This upregulation correlates with the clinical observation that increased lactoferrin (as a marker of inflammation) and IL-8 can be found in the stools of children in Brazil with EAggEC infections.[225]

Toxins Affecting the Enterocyte Actin Cytoskeleton

(For a more complete review, see reference 226.) A growing number of toxins have been reported to act by affecting the host cell cytoskeleton. *C. difficile* has emerged as the most important pathogen causing the syndrome of antibiotic-associated colitis.[227] The virulence of this pathogen depends on its elaboration of two related toxins, TxA and TxB. These toxins are among the largest monomeric toxins described, with molecular weights of 308,000 for TxA and 270,000 for TxB. Despite the fact that TxA has traditionally been referred to as an enterotoxin and TxB as a cytotoxin,[227] they both exert a cytotoxic effect in vitro. Both TxA and TxB are glucosyltransferases and use uridine diphosphate (UDP) glucose as a substrate to inactivate, by monoglucosylation, members of the Rho family of small guanosine triphosphatases (GTPases) at Thr^{37} an amino acid residue located within the putative effector domain of the Rho proteins.[228] Rho GTPases regulate a variety of cytoskeleton-dependent cellular functions, such as cell adhesion and motility, growth factor-mediated signaling, cellular transformation, and induction of apoptosis.[229] The dramatic effects of TxA and TxB on tissues and cells, including cytoskeletal depolymerization, increased intestinal permeability and diarrhea, cellular retraction and rounding, disruption of cell adhesion and chemotaxis, and activation of apoptosis,[230] are therefore all related to the TxA- and TxB-dependent inactivation of the Rho proteins. *Clostridium sordelli* toxin also functions as a UDP glucosyltransferase and inactivates Ras, Rap, and Rac.[227] *Clostridium botulinum* C2 and C3 toxins exert their enterotoxic effect by inactivating actin and Rho, respectively.[227]

Besides the inactivation of Rho proteins, their activation is also associated with increased intestinal permeability and diarrhea. Cytotoxic necrotizing factor 1 (CNF1), a protein of approximately 115 kDa produced by pathogenic *E. coli* strains,[231] activates Rho GTPases by deamination of Gln^{62} and consequently induces polymerization of F actin.[232] When tested on CaCo2 monolayers, CNF1 reduced the monolayer resistance by 40% after 4 hours of incubation,[233] suggesting that not only depolymerization but also polymerization of actin and subsequent reorganization of the actin cytoskeleton alter the barrier function of intestinal tight junctions.

A similar mechanism was previously described for zonula occludens toxin, a toxin elaborated by *V. cholerae*.[234,235] Zonula occludens toxin is a single polypeptide chain of 44.8 kDa, encoded by the cholera toxin bacteriophage (CTXφ) present in toxigenic strains of *V. cholerae*.[236] The mechanism of action of zonula occludens toxin involves the rearrangement of the epithelial cell cytoskeleton owing to protein kinase C {157}-dependent polymerization of actin filaments strategically located to modulate intercellular tight junctions.[237] The plasmid-encoded protein (Pet) elaborated by EAggEC is a member of the autotransporter class of secreted proteins that induces contraction of the cytoskeleton and loss of the actin stress fibers when tested on either HEp-2 cells or HT29 C-cell monolayers.[238] Both the cytopathic and enterotoxic effects of Pet seem related to the serine protease activity of the toxin that elicits cytoskeletal changes without compromising cell viability.[238]

Enterotoxigenic *Bacteroides fragilis* elaborates a 20 kDa zinc-dependent metalloprotease toxin (*B. fragilis* enterotoxin) that alters tight junctions and intestinal permeability.[239] This enterotoxin specifically cleaves the extracellular domain of the zonula adherens protein E-cadherin. Its protease activity appears to be specific for E-cadherin because no proteolytic activity was detected for other cytoskeleton-associated proteins, including occludin, {158}$_1$ integrin, Zonula Occludens (ZO)1, or {157} and {158}-catenins.[239]

Clostridium perfringens type A isolates produce a 35 kDa enterotoxin (CPE) whose action involves formation of a series of complexes in mammalian plasma membranes. One such CPE-containing complex (of approximately 155 kDa) is important for the induction of plasma membrane permeability alterations, which are responsible for killing enterotoxin-treated mammalian cells.[218] Those membrane permeability changes damage the epithelium, allowing the enterotoxin to interact with the tight junction protein occludin. CPE:occludin interactions result in formation of an approximately 200 kDa CPE complex and internalization of occludin into the cytoplasm. The removal of occludin (and possibly other proteins) damages tight junctions and disrupts the normal paracellular permeability barrier of the intestinal epithelium, which may contribute to CPE-induced diarrhea.[218]

The C-terminal fragment of CPE modulates the intestinal barrier function also through its effect on the tight junction protein claudin-4. CPE Tyrosines 306, 310, and 312 are critical for the interaction of CPE with claudin-4 and for the modulation of tight junctions barrier function by CPE.[240]

Beside its Ca-mediated enterotoxic effect, mentioned above, the *V. parahaemolyticus* enterotoxin thermostable direct hemolysin also induces a significant (though reversible) decreased rate of progression through the cell cycle and morphologic changes related to the organization of the microtubular network, which appears to be the preferential cytoskeletal element involved in the cellular response to the toxin.[241]

ENTERIC BACTERIA GENOMIC REVOLUTION

Our knowledge of the complexity of the prokaryotic kingdom, including enteric pathogens, has been a dynamic process of learning that progressed hand in hand with the advent of cornerstone technologies. The microscope has been the first instrument that allowed us to appreciate the variety of microorganisms initially classified based on their appearance. Over time, disciplines such as cell and molecular biology and biochemistry significantly contributed to new discoveries in microbiology. However, the full appreciation of the extent of genetic complexity and diversity among prokaryotic organisms could not be estimated until the advent of high-throughput genome sequencing and genome annotation.[242] So far, the genomes of more than 100 bacterial species have been sequenced, including enterobacteriaceae such as *V. cholerae*, EHEC, and *S. enterica*. For several of these species, the genome sequences of both pathogenic and nonpathogenic strains have been determined, thereby launching the field of comparative bacterial genomics. This information is of crucial importance in assisting us to identify pathogenic traits and, therefore, to develop alternative strategies for the treatment of enteric bacteria-associated infections.

V. cholerae represents the typical exemplification of the genomic revolution and its possible outcomes.[243] One of the most intriguing and least understood features of *V. cholerae* is its annual epidemic profile in the Bengal region of Bangladesh and India. In this region, nearly all cases occur in synchronized, massive outbreaks toward the end of the monsoon season. Between epidemics, the microorganism resides in a stable environmental reservoir, suggesting that changes in rainfall and sunlight dictate its shift from aquatic habitat host to human pathogen. The functional annotation of *V. cholerae* genomic sequence[244] shed some light on this extraordinary adaptability to two extremely different lifestyles. The *V. cholerae* genome consists of two circular chromosomes of approximately 3 million and approximately 1 million bp, respectively that together encode almost 4,000 putative genes. The vast majority of recognizable genes for essential cell functions and pathogenicity are located on the large chromosome, whereas the small chromosome contains many genes that appear to have origins other than *V. cholerae*. This two-chromosome configuration of *V. cholerae* seems to confer to the microorganism its plasticity to adapt to climate changes and to different lifestyles. One of the most accredited hypotheses predicts that the large chromosome genes are in charge for the microorganism's adaptation to the human intestine, whereas the small chromosome genes are essential for environmental survival.[243] If this hypothesis will prove correct, it will be theoretically possible to develop strategies that will prevent *V. cholerae* to switch from environmental to human host and, consequently, its survival in the human intestine.

ENTERIC BACTERIA AND IRRITABLE BOWEL SYNDROME

Several studies have established that the prevalence of postinfective irritable bowel syndrome (PI-IBS) can affect as much as 20 to 25% of patients.[245,246] However, little is known of the pathogenesis of PI-IBS. The fact that only 25% of patients who have had infectious diarrhea develop IBS-like symptoms suggests other risk factors, including age, sex, prolonged enteric infection, and the involvement of the nervous and immune systems, are necessary for IBS symptoms to develop among patients suffering of bacterial enteritis.[245,247] Brain–gut interactions are believed to play a key role in IBS pathogenesis. Possible connections exist between enteric nerves and immune cellular components, with mast cells representing the possible connecting factor between the local immune response and the neurohormonal system during acute intestinal infection. The higher incidence of PI-IBD among patients who had longer duration infective enteri-

tis may be explained by a more severe inflammation which cause a more severe impairment of the underlining nerve fibers. The notion that PI-IBS results from an enhanced inflammatory response is further supported by Wang and colleagues that showed a higher expression of IL-1β mRNA in the intestinal mucosa in PI-IBS patients.[247] The same authors also detected an increase in the number of mast cells within the lamina propria in the terminal ileum of the IBS patients studied. The increase in number and activation of mast cells in the intestinal mucosa and release of its mediators (ie, IL-1β) could reflect enhancement of the immune response to previous inflammation in PI-IBS patients. Release of IL-1β may cause inhibition of intestinal transport of water, electrolytes, and, ultimately, diarrhea.[247] Also, IL-1β is a potent hyperalgesic agent which may be responsible for hypersensitivity to rectal stimulation in IBS.[248] An increased number of T lymphocytes in the colorectal mucosa of IBS patients has also been reported,[249] indicating persistence of the immune response in these patients. Combined, these observations suggest that activation of the mucosal immune system as an inflammatory response may play an important role in the pathogenesis of PI-IBS.

ENTERIC BACTERIA AND INFLAMMATORY BOWEL DISEASES

During the past three decades there has been an "epidemic" of inflammatory bowel diseases (IBDs), mainly affecting industrialized countries.[250] IBDs are multifactorial diseases in which the interplay between various environmental triggers and host factors (eg, polygenetic, epithelial, immune and nonimmune) play a major role in their pathogenesis. It is now generally accepted that enteric bacterial flora plays a key role in the pathogenesis of IBD. The exact mechanism by which the intestinal mucosa loses tolerance to its bacterial neighbors remains poorly defined. The role of host genetic regulation of the innate immune response in the pathogenesis of CD has been supported by the identification of mutations of the NOD2 (CARD15) intracellular pattern recognition receptors.[251] Approximately 15% of Crohn's disease cases in Western populations result from mutations in NOD2/CARD15.[251] This disease leads to defective intestinal defensin production and defective monocyte interleukin-8 response to bacterial peptidoglycan. A consequence of this defect seems to be the accumulation in tissue of macrophages containing various bacteria, perhaps particularly *E. coli*. In keeping with this observation, patients with Crohn's disease have circulating antibodies against bacterial flagellar proteins of enterobacteria and clostridia.[252]

The mucosal immune system has evolved to balance the need to respond to pathogens while maintaining active tolerance to commensal bacteria and food antigens. In IBD, this tolerance breaks down and inflammation occurs following triggering by the intestinal microbial flora.[253] Several microorganisms, such as *Mycobacterium paratuberculosis, Listeria monocytogenes, Chlamydia trachomatis, E. coli, Saccharomyces cerevisiae,* have been proposed as having a potential etiologic role. However, the association between any of the aforementioned microorganisms and the onset of IBD remains inconclusive.[253]

Mouse models of intestinal inflammation triggered by microbial infection have played a key role in understanding the mechanisms that govern the inflammatory response in the intestine and in designing new therapeutic strategies in the treatment of patients with IBD. The two common models of infectious murine colitis are infection with the murine epithelial-adherent pathogen, *Citrobacter rodentium,* and infection of streptomycin-pretreated mice with *Salmonella typhimurium.*[254]

Another interesting murine model of gut inflammation is the SAMP1/YitFc (SAMP) mouse model that develops chronic ileitis similar to human CD. These mice displayed decreased epithelial barrier resistance ex vivo and increased epithelial permeability in vivo compared to wild-type mice.[255] This permeability defect preceded the development of ileal inflammation, was present in the absence of commensal bacteria, and was accompanied by altered ileal mRNA expression of the tight junction proteins claudin-2 and occludin. Decreased barrier function suggests that defects in the epithelium may represent the primary source of SAMP ileitis susceptibility that translates in inflammation only in the presence of enteric bacteria.[255]

ENTERIC BACTERIA AND BIOTERRORISM

Recent discoveries involving bacterial genomes and virulence machinery have promoted strategies to reduce the morbidity and mortality of microbial infections. Recent progress has also been made, which has resulted in effective interventions for reducing environmental risks and preventing human-to-human transmission of infectious agents. These approaches have had a huge positive impact on childhood mortality. Both the events of September 11, 2001, and the subsequent highly publicized use of the US Postal Service to spread anthrax infection have drastically changed our sense of confidence toward the prevention and treatment of infectious diseases. It has become clear that our present disease control strategies are ineffective and possibly obsolete in dealing with bioterrorism. The standard goals of public health organizations—confinement of specific pathogens to endemic areas, eradication of microorganisms, and vaccination campaigns to eliminate specific pathogens are now undergoing a process of reprioritization in light of the new realities that we face with bioterrorism and biologic warfare. Despite the fact that hundreds of potential agents could be used in bio-

logic warfare or bioterrorism, attention has been focused on microorganisms, including anthrax and smallpox, which have the potential for aerosol dissemination.[256] It is surprising, however, that little attention has been paid so far to enteric pathogens listed in the category B agents by the CDC. Despite the fact that these microorganisms typically cause moderate morbidity and low mortality, they pose a significant risk because they are easy to produce and disseminate, they do not require complex production and stocking facilities, and they can be handled by nonprofessional personnel.[256] The threats to food and water safety represented by these agents make them an obvious choice for bioterrorism initiatives executed by terrorist groups whose level of scientific expertise may be relatively primitive. Unfortunately, deliberate contamination of food with enteric pathogens has already been perpetrated.[257] With free trade, centralized production, and wide distribution of products worldwide, the biosecurity of commercial food products is becoming a challenging task because deliberate contamination of foodstuff could present either as a slow, diffuse, and initially unremarkable increase in sporadic cases or as an explosive epidemic suddenly producing many illnesses. Among the potential enteric pathogens to be used as bioweapons, *Salmonella* serotypes need to be considered at high risk for their high rate of infectivity and their ability to survive in the environment. The bioterrorism potential of *S. typhi* was recognized in the 1970s by the World Health Organization, which assessed a potential attack on municipal water supplies with the organism.[246] *Shigella* spp. which are frequent worldwide, have a low infectious dose and cause dysentery, with severe complications and death rates of up to 20%. *S. dysenteriae* is rare in the United States, but most clinical laboratories have reference strains. *E. coli* O157:H7 causes bloody diarrhea and abdominal cramps. It is the most common cause of HUS in children, has a low infectious dose, and, therefore, is highly transmissible, and reference strains are kept by clinical laboratories.[257] The mortality rate of *V. cholerae* secondary to dehydration is limited when appropriate rehydrating therapy is enforced. However, widespread disease could overwhelm unprepared medical care facilities, and cases of severe untreated cholera have mortality rates that can reach 50%. Both cultures and purified cholera toxin are available commercially for research purposes.[256]

CONCLUSION

Despite the tremendous increase in knowledge of bacterial pathogenesis experienced during the past decade, gastrointestinal infections remain a major cause of disease and death because they are responsible for 6 to 60 billion cases of diarrhea every year and claim the life of a child every 15 seconds. Widespread travel to developing countries and the recent events of bioterrorism has brought diseases transmitted by contaminated

food and water to immunologically naive populations. These changes, along with an increased number of immunocompromised individuals and the pandemic of HIV infection, have elevated bacteria-associated diarrheal diseases to a worldwide threat. However, the widespread use of oral rehydration solutions has revolutionized the way in which this plague has being fought, and more positive results are anticipated from the development of safe enteric vaccines and a better preparedness to face possible bioterrorist attacks exploiting enteric pathogens as bioweapons.

REFERENCES

1. Harlem G. WHO report on infectious diseases: Removing the obstacle to healthy development. Brunotland, Switzerland; 1999.
2. Levine MM. Enteric infections and the vaccines to counter them: Future directions. Vaccine 2006;24:3865–73.
3. Sack DA, Sack RB, Nair GB, Siddique AK. Cholera. Lancet 2004;363:223–33.
4. Wachsmuth IK, Blake PA, Olsvik O. Vibrio cholerae and Cholera: Molecular and Perspectives, 1st edition. Washington, DC: American Society for Microbiology; 1994.
5. Benenson AS, Islam MR, Greenough WB, III. Rapid identification of Vibrio cholerae by darkfield microscopy. Bull World Health Organ 1964;30:827–31.
6. Gardner AD, Venkaraman VK. The antigens of the cholera group of vibrios. J Hyg 1935;35:262–82.
7. Gotschlich T. Vibrios choleriques isoles au compement de or. Retour du pelerinage de lannee, 1905. Report adresse au President du Conseil quarante naine d'Egypt, Alexandria. Bull Inst Louis Pasteur 1987;31:387–91.
8. Morris JG Jr, Black RE. Cholera and other vibrioses in the United States. N Engl J Med 1985;312:343–50.
9. Morris JG. Non-O group 1 *Vibrio cholerae*: A look at the epidemiology of an occasional pathogen. Epidemiol Rev 1990;12:179–91.
10. Ramamurthy T, Garg S, Sharma R, et al. Emergence of novel strain of *Vibrio cholerae* with epidemic potential in southern and eastern India. Lancet 1993;341:703–4.
11. Snow J. On the Mode of Communication of Cholera. London: John Churchill; 1849.
12. Ries AA, et al. Cholera in Piura, Peru: A modern urban epidemic. J Infect Dis 1992;166:1429–33.
13. Barua D. History of cholera. In: Barua D, Greenough WB, III, editors. Cholera. New York: Plenum Press; 1992. p. 1–36.
14. Goodgame RW, Greenough WBG, III. Cholera in Africa: A message for the west. Ann Intern Med 1975;82:101–6.
15. Baine WB, et al. Epidemiology of cholera in Italy in 1973. Lancet 1974;ii:1370–6.
16. Blakee PA, et al. Cholera in Portugal, 1974. I. Modes of transmission. Am J Epidemiol 1977;105:337–44.
17. Centers for Disease Control and Prevention. Cholera Peru, 1991. MMWR Morb Mortal Wkly Rep 1991;40:108–9.
18. Albert MJ, et al. Large outbreak of clinical cholera due to Vibrio cholerae non-O1 in Bangladesh. Lancet 1993;341:704.
19. Chongsa-nguan M, et al. *Vibrio cholerae* O139 Bengal in Bangkok. Lancet 1993;342:430–1.
20. Shimada T, et al. Outbreak of *Vibrio cholerae* non-O1 in India and Bangladesh. Lancet 1993;341:1346–7.
21. Swerdlow DL, Ries AA. *Vibrio cholerae* non-O1 the eighth pandemic, Lancet 1993;342:382–3.
22. Cash RA, et al. Response of man to infection with *Vibrio cholerae*. I. Clinical, serologic, and bacteriologic responses to a known inoculum. J Infect Dis 1974;129:45–52.
23. Rabbani GH, Greenough WB, III. Pathophysiology and clinical aspects of cholera. In: Barua D, Greenough WB, III, editors. Cholera. New York: Plenum Press; 1992. p. 209–28.
24. Hirschhorn N, et al. Decrease in net stool output in children during intestinal perfusion with glucose-containing solution. N Engl J Med 1968;279:176–81.
25. World Health Organization. Epidemic diarrhea due to *Vibrio cholerae* non-O1. Wkly Epidemiol Rec 1993;68:141–2.
26. St Louis ME, et al. Epidemic cholera in West Africa: The role of food handling and high-risk foods. Am J Epidemiol 1990;131:719–28.
27. Greenough WB, III, et al. Tetracycline in the treatment of cholera. Lancet 1964;i:355–7.

28. Glass RI, Hug I, Alim ARMA, Yunus M. Emergence of multiply antibiotic-resistant *Vibrio cholerae* in Bangladesh. J Infect Dis 1980;142:939–42.
29. World Health Organization. Guidelines for Cholera Control. Programme for Control of Diarrhoeal Disease. Geneva: World Health Organization; 1991. Publication WHO/CDD/SER/80.4 rev 2.
30. Nataro JP. Vaccines against diarrheal diseases. Semin Pediatr Infect Dis 2004;15:272–9.
31. Clemens JD, et al. Field trial of oral cholera vaccines in Bangladesh. Lancet 1986;ii:124–7.
32. Trach DD, et al. Field trial of a locally produced, killed, oral cholera vaccine in Vietnam. Lancet 1997;349:231–5.
33. Levine MM, et al. Safety, immunogenicity, and efficacy of recombinant live oral cholera vaccines, CVD103 and CVD103-HgR. Lancet 1988;ii:467–70.
34. Suharyono PM, et al. Safety and immunogenicity of single-dose live oral cholera vaccine CVD103 HgR in 59 year old Indonesian children. Lancet 1992;340:689–94.
35. Tacket CO, et al. Onset and duration of protective immunity in challenged volunteers after vaccination with live oral cholera vaccine CVD103-HgR. J Infect Dis 1992;166: 837–41.
36. Ryan ET, Calderwood SB, Qadri F. Live attenuated oral cholera vaccines. Expert Rev Vaccines. 2006;5:483–94.
37. Sepulveda J, Valdespino JL, Garcia-Garcia L. Cholera in Mexico: The paradoxical benefits of the last pandemic. Int J Infect Dis 2006;10:4–13.
38. Thompson FL, Klose KE. AVIB Group. Vibrio 2005: The First International Conference on the Biology of Vibrios. J Bacteriol 2006;188:4592–6.
39. Morris JG Jr, et al. Non-O group 1 *Vibrio cholerae* gastroenteritis in the United States. Ann Intern Med 1981;94:656–8.
40. Kamal AM. Outbreak of gastroenteritis by non-agglutinable (NAG) vibrios in the republic of the Sudan. J Egypt Public Health Assoc 1971;46:125–73.
41. Morris JG Jr. Non-O group 1 *Vibrio cholerae*: A look at the epidemiology of an occasional pathogen. Epidemiol Rev 1990;12:179–91.
42. Swaminathan B, Gerner-Smidt P, Barrett T. Focus on *Salmonella*. Foodborne Pathog Dis 2006;3:154–6.
43. Todd B. The increasing risk of *Salmonella* infections. Food industry practices, inadequate regulation, and antimicrobial resistance heighten concerns. Am J Nurs 2006;106:35–7.
44. Ryan CA, Hargrett-Bean NT, Blake PA. *Salmonella typhi* infections in the United States, 1975–1984: Increasing role of foreign travel. Rev Infect Dis 1989;11:1–8.
45. Summary of notifiable diseases, United States, 1996. MMWR Morb Mortal Wkly Rep 1997;45:1–87.
46. Celum CL, et al. Incidence of salmonellosis in patients with AIDS. J Infect Dis 1987;156:998–1002.
47. Torrey S, Fleisher G, Jaffe D. Incidence of *Salmonella* bacteremia in infants with *Salmonella* gastroenteritis. J Pediatr 1986;108:718–21.
48. Gianella RA, Broitman VI. Gastric acid barrier to ingested microorganisms in man: Studies in vivo and in vitro. Gut 1972;13:251–6.
49. Ryan CA, et al. Massive outbreak of antimicrobial-resistant salmonellosis traced to pasteurized milk. JAMA 1987;258:3269–74.
50. Centers for Disease Control and Prevention. Surveillance for foodborne-disease outbreaks, United States, 1988–1992. MMWR Morb Mortal Wkly Rep 1996;45:1S–66S.
51. Braden CR. *Salmonella enterica* serotype Enteritidis and eggs: A national epidemic in the United States. Clin Infect Dis 2006;43:512–7.
52. Tauxe RV. Emerging foodborne diseases: An evolving public health challenge. Emerg Infect Dis 1997;3:425–34.
53. Chhabra RS, Glaser JH. *Salmonella* infection presenting as hematochezia on the first day of life. Pediatrics 1994;94:739–41.
54. Woodward DL, Khakhria R, Johnson WM. Human salmonellosis associated with exotic pets. J Clin Microbiol 1997;35:2786–90.
55. Torrey S, Fleisher G, Jaffe D. Incidence of *Salmonella* bacteremia in infants with *Salmonella* gastroenteritis. J Pediatr 1986;108:718–21.
56. Khoshoo V, et al. *Salmonella typhimurium*-associated servere protracted diarrhea in infants and young children. J Pediatr Gastroenterol Nutr 1990;10:33–6.
57. Buchwald DS, Blaser MJ. A review of human salmonellosis: II. Duration of excretion following infection with nontyphi *Salmonella*. Rev Infect Dis 1984;6:345–56.
58. Blaser MJ, Feldman RA. From the Centers for Disease Control. *Salmonella* bacteremia: Reports to the Centers for Disease Control, 1968–1979. J Infect Dis 1981;143:743–6.
59. Wittler RR, Bass JW. *Nontyphoidal Salmonella* enteric infections and bacteremia. Pediatr Infect Dis J 1989;8: 364–7.
60. Ramos JM, et al. Clinical significance of primary vs. secondary bacteremia due to nontyphoid *Salmonella* in patients without AIDS. Clin Infect Dis 1994;19:777–80.
61. Wright J, Thomas P, Serjeant GR. Septicemia caused by *Salmonella* infection: An overlooked complication of sickle cell disease. J Pediatr 1997;130:394–9.
62. Huang LT, Ko SF, Lui CC. *Salmonella* meningitis: Clinical experience of third-generation cephalosporins. Acta Paediatr 1997;86:1056–8.
63. Cohen JI, Bartlett JA, Corey GR. Extra-intestinal manifestations of *Salmonella* infections. Medicine 1987;66:349–88.
64. Nelson MR, et al. *Salmonella, Campylobacter* and *Shigella* in HIV-seropositive patients. AIDS 1992;6:1495–8.
65. Butler T, Islam A, Kabir I, Jones PK. Patterns of morbidity and mortality in typhoid fever dependent on age and gender: Review of 552 hospitalized patients with diarrhea. Rev Infect Dis 1991;13:85–90.
66. Crum NF. Current trends in typhoid Fever. Curr Gastroenterol Rep 2003;5:279–86.
67. Hoffman TA, Ruiz CJ, Counts GW. Water-borne typhoid fever in Dade County, FL: Clinical and therapeutic evaluations of 105 bacteremic patients. Am J Med 1975;59:481–7.
68. Barber DA, Miller GY, McNamara PE. Models of antimicrobial resistance and foodborne illness: Examining assumptions and practical applications. J Food Prot 2003;66: 700–9.
69. Balbi HJ. Chloramphenicol: A review. Pediatr Rev 2004;25:284–8.
70. Guzman CA, Borsutzky S, Griot-Wenk M, et al. Vaccines against typhoid fever. Vaccine 2006;24:3804–11.
71. Shiga K. Ueber den Dysenteriebacillus (*Bacillus dysenteriae*). Z Bakteriol Parasit K Abt I Orig 1898;24: 817–24.
72. DuPont HL, et al. Inoculum size in shigellosis and implications for expected mode of transmission. J Infect Dis 1989;159:1126–8.
73. Cohen D, et al. Reduction of transmission of shigellosis by control of houseflies (*Musca domestica*). Lancet 1991;337:993–7.
74. Lee LA, et al. Hyperendemic shigellosis in the United States: A review of surveillance data for 1967–1988. J Infect Dis 1991;164:894–900.
75. Multiply resistant shigellosis in a day-care center, Texas. MMWR Morb Mortal Wkly Rep 1986;35:753–5.
76. Shigellosis in child day care centers, Lexington-Fayette County, Kentucky, 1991. MMWR Morb Mortal Wkly Rep 1992;41:440–2.
77. Wilson R, et al. Family illness associated with *Shigella* infection: The interrelationship of age of the index patient and the age of household members in acquisition of illness. J Infect Dis 1981;143:130–2.
78. Kotloff KL, et al. Acute diarrhea in Baltimore children attending an outpatient clinic. Pediatr Infect Dis J 1988;7:753–9.
79. Ashkenazi S. *Shigella* infections in children: New insights. Semin Pediatr Infect Dis 2004;15:246–52.
80. Talukder KA, Khajanchi BK, Dutta DK, et al. An unusual cluster of dysentery due to *Shigella* dysenteriae type 4 in Dhaka, Bangladesh. J Med Microbiol 2005;54:511–3.
81. von Seidlein L, Kim DR, Ali M, et al. A Multicentre Study of *Shigella* Diarrhoea in Six Asian Countries: Disease Burden, Clinical Manifestations, and Microbiology. PLoS Med 2006;3:e353.
82. Health status of displaced persons following civil war: Burundi, December 1993–January 1994. MMWR Morb Mortal Wkly Rep 1994;43:701–3.
83. DuPont HL, et al. The response of man to virulent *Shigella* flexneri 2a. J Infect Dis 1969;119:296–9.
84. Taylor D, et al. The role of *Shigella* spp., enteroinvasive *Escherichia* coli and other enteropathogens as causes of childhood dysentery in Thailand. J Infect Dis 1986;153:1132–8.
85. Ashkenazi S, et al. Convulsions in childhood shigellosis: Clinical and laboratory features in 153 children. Am J Dis Child 1987;141:208–10.
86. Koster F, et al. Hemolytic-uremic syndrome after shigellosis: Relation to endotoxemia and circulating immune complexes. N Engl J Med 1978;298:927–33.
87. Nelson MR, et al. *Salmonella, Campylobacter* and *Shigella* in HIV-seropositive patients. AIDS 1992;6:1495–8.
88. Centers for Disease Control and Prevention (CDC). Outbreaks of multidrug-resistant *Shigella* sonnei gastroenteritis associated with day care centers Kansas, Kentucky, and Missouri, 2005. MMWR Morb Mortal Wkly Rep 2006;55:1068–71.
89. Vandamme P, et al. Revision of *Campylobacter, Helicobacter*, and *Wolinella* taxonomy: Emendation of generic descriptions and proposal of *Arcobacter* gen. nov. Int J Syst Bacteriol 1990;41:88–103.
90. Centers for Disease Control and Prevention (CDC). Preliminary FoodNet data on the incidence of infection with pathogens transmitted commonly through food 10 States, United States, 2005. MMWR Morb Mortal Wkly Rep 2006;55:392–5.
91. Blaser MJ, Reller LB. *Campylobacter* enteritis. N Engl J Med 1981;305:1444–52.
92. Nebola M, Steinhauserova I. PFGE and PCR/RFLP typing of *Campylobacter jejuni* strains from poultry. Br Poult Sci 2006;47:456–61.
93. Wood RC, Macdonald KL, Osterholm MT. *Campylobacter* enteritis outbreaks associated with drinking raw milk during youth activities: A 10-year review of outbreaks in the United States. JAMA 1992;268:3228–30.
94. Baserisalehi M, Bahador N, Augustine SK, et al. Enhanced recovery and isolation of *Campylobacter* spp. From water using a novel device. J Appl Microbiol 2004;96:664–70.
95. Wagenaar JA, Mevius DJ, Havelaar AH. *Campylobacter* in primary animal production and control strategies to reduce the burden of human campylobacteriosis. Rev Sci Tech 2006;25:581–94.
96. Murphy C, Carroll C, Jordan KN. Environmental survival mechanisms of the foodborne pathogen *Campylobacter jejuni*. J Appl Microbiol 2006;100:623–32.
97. Black RE, et al. Incidence and etiology of infantile diarrhea and major routes of transmission in Huascar, Peru. Am J Epidemiol 1989;129:785–99.
98. Black RE, et al. Experimental *Campylobacter jejuni* infection in humans. J Infect Dis 198;157:472–9.
99. Gerner-Smidt P, Hise K, Kincaid J, et al. PulseNet USA: A five-year update. Foodborne Pathog Dis 2006;3:9–19.
100. Skirrow MB. *Campylobacter*. Lancet 1990;336:921–3.
101. Blaser MJ, et al. *Campylobacter* enteritis: Clinical and epidemiologic features. Am Intern Med 1979;91:179–85.
102. Puylaert JB, et al. Incidence and sonographic diagnosis of bacterial ileocaecitis masquerading as appendicitis. Lancet 1989;ii:84–6.
103. Kapperud G, et al. Clinical features of sporadic *Campylobacter* infections in Norway. Scand J Infect Dis 1992;24:741–9.
104. Wong SN, Tam AY, Yien KY. Campylobacter infection in the neonate: Case report and review of the literature. Pediatr Infect Dis J 1990;9:665–9.
105. Salazar-Lindo E, et al. Early treatment with erythromycin of *Campylobacter jejuni*-associated dysentery in children. J Pediatr 1986;109:355–60.
106. Williams MD, et al. Early treatment of *Campylobacter jejuni* enteritis. Antimicrob Agents Chemother 1989;33: 248–50.
107. Moore JE, Barton MD, Blair IS, et al. The epidemiology of antibiotic resistance in *Campylobacter*. Microbes Infect 2006;8:1955–66.
108. Fredriksson-Ahomaa M, Stolle A, Korkeala H. Molecular epidemiology of Yersinia enterocolitica infections. FEMS Immunol Med Microbiol 2006;47:315–29.
109. Cover TL, Aber RC. Yersinia enterocolitica. N Engl J Med 1989;321:16–24.
110. Cover TL. *Yersinia enterocolitica* and *Yersinia* pseudotuberculosis. In: Blaser MJ, et al, editors. Infections of the Gastrointestinal Tract. New York: Raven Press; 1995. p. 811–23.
111. Marks MI, et al. *Yersinia enterocolitica* gastoenteritis: A prospective study of clinical, bacteriologic and epidemiologic features. J Pediatr 1980;96:26–31.
112. Tacker CO, et al. *Yersinia enterocolitica* pharyngitis. Ann Intern Med 1983;99:40–2.
113. Hoogkamp-Korstanje JA, Stolk-Engelaar VM. *Yersinia enterocolitica* infection in children. Pediatr Infect Dis J 1995;14:771–5.
114. Rao PM, et al. Effect of computed tomography of the appendix on treatment of patients and use of hospital resources. N Engl J Med 1998;338:141–6.
115. Abdel-Haq NM, Papadopol R, Asmar BI, Brown WJ. Antibiotic susceptibilities of Yersinia enterocolitica recovered from children over a 12-year period. Int J Antimicrob Agents 2006;27:449–52.
116. Levine MM. *Escherichia coli* that cause diarrhea: Enterotoxigenic, enteropathogenic, enteroinvasive and enteroadherent. J Infect Dis 1987;155:377–89.
117. Vernacchio L, Vezina RM, Mitchell AA, et al. Diarrhea in American infants and young children in the community setting: Incidence, clinical presentation and microbiology. Pediatr Infect Dis J 2006;25:2–7.
118. Trabulsi LR, Keller R, Tardelli Gomes TA. Typical and atypical enteropathogenic *Escherichia coli*. Emerg Infect Dis 2002;8:508–13.
119. Levine MM, et al. *Escherichia coli* strains that cause diarrhoea but do not produce heat-labile or heat-stable enterotoxins and are non-invasive. Lancet 1978;i:1119–22.

120. Fagundes-Neto U, Scaletsky IC. The gut at war: The consequences of enteropathogenic *Escherichia coli* infection as a factor of diarrhea and malnutrition. Sao Paulo Med J 2000;118:21–9.

121. Nelson JD. Duration of neomycin for enteropathogenic *Escherichia coli* diarrheal disease: A comparative study of 113 cases. Pediatrics 1971;48:248–58.

122. Thoren AL. Antibiotic sensitivity of enteropathogenic *Escherichia coli* to mecillinam, trimethoprim-sulfamethoxazole and other antibiotics. Acta Pathol Microbiol Scand 1980;88:265–8.

123. Gorbach SL, Banwell JG, Chatterjee BD, et al. Acute undifferentiated human diarrhea in the tropics. Alterations in intestinal microflora. J Clin Invest 1971;50:881–9.

124. Taneja N, Rao P, Rao DS, et al. Enterotoxigenic *Escherichia coli* causing cholerogenic syndrome during an interepidemic period of cholera in North India. Jpn J Infect Dis 2006;59:245–8.

125. Walker RI. Considerations for development of whole cell bacterial vaccines to prevent diarrheal diseases in children in developing countries. Vaccine 2005;23:3369–85.

126. Al-Abri SS, Beeching NJ, Nye FJ. Traveller's diarrhoea. Lancet Infect Dis 2005;5:349–60.

127. Black RE, et al. Treatment of experimentally induced enterotoxigenic *Escherichia coli* diarrhea with trimethoprim, trimethoprim-sulfamethoxazole or placebo. Rev Infect Dis 1982;4:540–5.

128. DuPont HL, Ericsson CD. Prevention and treatment of traveler's diarrhea. N Engl J Med 1993;328:1821–7.

129. Oldfield EC, III, Wallace MR. The role of antibiotics in the treatment of infectious bacteria. Gastroenterol Clin North Am 2001;30:817–36.

130. Wolfe MD. Protection of travelers. Clin Infect Dis 1997;25:177–84.

131. Clemens J, Savarino S, Abu-Elyazeed R, et al. Development of pathogenicity driven definitions of outcomes for a field trial of a killed oral vaccine against enterotoxigenic *Escherichia coli* in Egypt: Application of an evidence-based method. J Infect Dis 2004;189:2299–307.

132. Ratchtrachenchai OA, Subpasu S, Hayashi H, Ba-Thein W. Prevalence of childhood diarrhoea ssociated *Escherichia coli* in Thailand. J Med Microbiol 2004;53:237–43.

133. Hartman AB, Essiet II, Isenbarger DW, Lindler LE. Epidemiology of tetracycline resistance determinants in *Shigella* spp. and enteroinvasive *Escherichia coli*: Characterization and dissemination of tet(A)-1. J Clin Microbiol 2003;41:1023–32.

134. DuPont HL, et al. Pathogenesis of *Escherichia coli* diarrhea. N Engl J Med 1971;285:1–9.

135. Snyder JD, et al. Outbreak of invasive *Escherichia coli* gastroenteritis on a cruise ship. Am J Trop Med Hyg 1984;33:281–4.

136. Tarr PI. *Escherichia coli* O157:H7 clinical, diagnostic and epidemiological aspects of human infection. Clin Infect Dis 1995;20:9–10.

137. Riley LW, et al. Hemorrhagic colitis associated with a rare *Escherichia coli* serotype. N Engl J Med 1983;308:681–5.

138. Karmal MA, et al. The association between idiopathic hemolytic uremic syndrome and infection by verotoxin roducing *Escherichia coli*. J Infect Dis 1985;151:775–82.

139. Isolation of *E. coli* 157:H7 from sporadic cases of hemorrhagic colitis, United States. MMWR Morb Mortal Wkly Rep 1997;46:700–4.

140. Watanabe H, Guerrant RL. Summary: Nagasaki enterohemorrhagic *Escherichia coli* meeting and workshop. J Infect Dis 1997;176:247–9.

141. Keene WE, et al. A swimming ssociated outbreak of hemorrhagic colitis caused by *Escherichia coli* O157:H7 and Shigella sonnei. N Engl J Med 1994;331:579–84.

142. Belongia EA, et al. Transmission of *Escherichia coli* O157: H7 infection in Minnesota child daycare facilities. JAMA 1993;269:883–8.

143. Slutsker L, et al. *Escherichia coli* O157:H7 diarrhea in the United States: Clinical and epidemiologic features. Ann Intern Med 1997;126:505–13.

144. Macdonald KL, et al. *Escherichia coli* O157:H7, an emerging gastrointestinal pathogen: results of a one year, prospective, population based study. JAMA 1988;59:3567–70.

145. Griffin PM, et al. Large outbreak of *Escherichia coli* O157: H7 infections in the western United States: The big picture. In: Karmali MA, Goglio AG, editors. Recent Advances in Verocytotoxin-Producing *Escherichia coli* Infection. Amsterdam: Elsevier Science BV; 1994. p. 7–12.

146. Griffen PM, et al. Illnesses associated with *Escherichia coli* O157:H7 infections: A broad clinical spectrum. Ann Intern Med 1988;109:705–12.

147. Pai CH, et al. Epidemiology of sporadic diarrhea due to verocytotoxin producing *Escherichia coli*: A two year prospective study. J Infect Dis 1988;157:1054–7.

148. Uc A, et al. Pseudomembranous colitis with *Escherichia coli* O157:H7. J Pediatr Gastroenterol Nutr 1997;24:590–3.

149. Pavia AT, et al. Hemolytic uremic syndrome during an outbreak of *Escherichia coli* O157:H7 infections in institutions for mentally retarded persons: Clinical and epidemiologic observations. J Pediatr 1990;116:544–51.

150. Tarr PI, et al. *Escherichia coli* O157:H7 and the hemolytic uremic syndrome: Importance of early cultures in establishing the etiology. J Infect Dis 1990;162:553–6.

151. Marcato P, Griener TP, Mulvey GL, Armstrong GD. Recombinant Shiga toxin B subunit keyhole limpet hemocyanin conjugate vaccine protects mice from Shigatoxemia. Infect Immun 2005;73:6523–9.

152. Butterton JR, et al. Coexpression of the B subunit of Shiga toxin 1 and EaeA from enterohemorrhagic *Escherichia coli* in *Vibrio cholerae* vaccine strains. Infect Immun 1997;65:2127–35.

153. Mayr UB, Haller C, Haidinger W, et al. Bacterial ghosts as an oral vaccine: A single dose of *Escherichia coli* O157: H7 bacterial ghosts protects mice against lethal challenge. Infect Immun 2005;73:4810–7.

154. Cravioto A, et al. Association of *Escherichia coli* Hep 2 adherence patterns with type and duration of diarrhoea. Lancet 1991;337:262–4.

155. Giron JA, et al. Diffuse adhering *Escherichia coli* (DAEC) as a putative cause of diarrhea in Mayan children in Mexico. J Infect Dis 1991;163:507–13.

156. Levine MM, et al. Epidemiologic studies of *Escherichia coli* diarrheal infections in a low socioeconomic level periurban community in Santiago, Chile. Am J Epidemiol 1993;138:849–69.

157. Baqui AH, et al. Enteropathogens associated with acute and persistent diarrhea in Bangladeshi children 5 years of age. J Infect Dis 1992;166:792–6.

158. Scaletsky IC, Fabbricotti SH, Silva SO, et al. HEp 2 adherent *Escherichia coli* strains associated with acute infantile diarrhea, Sao Paulo, Brazil. Emerg Infect Dis 2002;8:855–8.

159. Nataro JP, et al. Heterogeneity of enteroaggregative *Escherichia coli* virulence demonstrated in volunteers. J Infect Dis 1995;171:465–8.

160. Huang DB, Mohanty A, DuPont HL, et al. A review of an emerging enteric pathogen: Enteroaggregative *Escherichia coli*. J Med Microbiol 2006;55:1303–11.

161. Henry FJ, Udoy AS, Wanke CA, Aziz KMA. Epidemiology of persistent diarrhea and etiologic agents in Mirzapur, Bangladesh. Acta Paediatr Suppl 1996;381:27–31.

162. Bhatnagar S, et al. Enteroaggregative *Escherichia coli* may be a new pathogen causing acute and persistent diarrhea. Scand J Infect Dis 1993;25:579–83.

163. Fang GD, et al. Etiology and epidemiology of persistent diarrhea in northeastern Brazil: A hospital based, prospective, case-control study. J Pediatr Gastroenterol Nutr 1995;21:137–44.

164. Smith HR, Cheasty T, Rowe B. Enteroaggregative Escherichia coli and outbreaks of gastroenteritis in UK. Lancet 1997;350:814–15.

165. Cobeljic M, et al. Enteroaggregative *Escherichia coli* associated with an outbreak of diarrhoea in a neonatal nursery ward. Epidemiol Infect 1996;117:11–6.

166. Itoh Y, Nagano I, Kunishima M, Ezaki T. Laboratory investigation of enteroaggregative *Escherichia coli* O untypeable: H10 associated with a massive outbreak of gastrointestinal illness. J Clin Microbiol 1997;35:2546–50.

167. Monteville MR, Riddle MS, Baht U, et al. Incidence, etiology, and impact of diarrhea among deployed US military personnel in support of Operation Iraqi Freedom and Operation Enduring Freedom. Am J Trop Med Hyg 2006;75:762–7.

168. Steiner TS, Lima AAM, Nataro JP, Guerrant RL. Enteroaggregative *Escherichia coli* produce intestinal inflammation and growth impairment and cause interleukin-8 release from intestinal epithelial cells. J Infect Dis 1998;177:88–96.

169. Schmidt H, et al. Development of PCR for screening of enteroaggregative *Escherichia coli*. J Clin Microbiol 1995;33:701–5.

170. Vila J, Vargas M, Ruiz J, et al. Susceptibility patterns of enteroaggregative *Escherichia coli* associated with traveller's diarrhoea: Emergence of quinolone resistance. J Med Microbiol 2001;50:996–1000.

171. McFarland LV, Mulligan ME, Kwok RYY, Stamm WE. Nosocomial acquisition of *Clostridium difficile* infection. N Engl J Med 1989;320:204–10.

172. Donta ST, Myers MG. *Clostridium difficile* toxin in asymptomatic neonates. J Pediatr 1982;100:431–4.

173. Bartlett JG. Narrative review: The new epidemic of *Clostridium difficile* associated enteric disease. Ann Intern Med 2006;145:758–64.

174. Bouza E, Munoz P, Alonso R. Clinical manifestations, treatment and control of infections caused by *Clostridium difficile*. Clin Microbiol Infect 2005;11:57–64.

175. Jodlowski TZ, Oehler R, Kam LW, Melnychuk I. Emerging therapies in the treatment of *Clostridium difficile* associated disease (December). Ann Pharmacother 2006;40:2164–69.

176. McFarland IV. Meta-analysis of probiotics for the prevention of antibiotic associated diarrhea and the treatment of *Clostridium difficile* disease. Am J Gastroenterol 2006;101:812–22.

177. Katz JA. Probiotics for the prevention of antibiotic associated diarrhea and *Clostridium difficile* diarrhea. J Clin Gastroenterol 2006;40:249–55.

178. Holmber SD, Farmer JJ, III. *Aeromonas hydrophila* and *Plesiomonas shigelloides* as causes of intestinal infections. Rev Infect Dis 1984;6:633–9.

179. Pazzaglia G, et al. High frequency of coinfecting enteropathogens in Aeromonas-associated diarrhea of hospitalized Peruvian infants. J Clin Microbiol 1991;29:1151–6.

180. San Joaquin VH, Pickett DA. Aeromonas-associated gastroenteritis in children. Pediatr Infect Dis J 1988;7:53–7.

181. George WL, Nakata MM, Thompson J, White ML. *Aeromonas*-related diarrhea in adults. Arch Intern Med 1985;145:2207–11.

182. East AK, Allaway D, Collins MD. Analysis of DNA encoding 23S rRNA and 1–23S rRNA intergenic spacer regions from *Plesiomonas shigelloides*. FEMS Microbiol Lett 1992;95:57–62.

183. Miller ML, Koburger JA. Evaluation of inositol brilliant green bile salts and *Plesiomonas* agars for recovery of *Plesiomonas shigelloides* from aquatic samples in a seasonal survey of the Suwannee river estuary. J Food Protect 1986;49:274–7.

184. Miller ML, Koburger JA. *Plesiomonas shigelloides*: An opportunistic food and waterborne pathogen. J Food Protect 1985;48:449–57.

185. Khan AM, Faruque AS, Hossain MS, et al. *Plesiomonas shigelloides* associated diarrhoea in Bangladeshi children: A hospital based surveillance study. J Trop Pediatr 2004;50:354–6.

186. Sinnott IV JT, Turnquest DG, Milam MW. *Plesiomonas shigelloides* gastroenteritis. Clin Microbiol Newslett 1989;11:103–4.

187. Kain KC, Kelly MT. Clinical features, epidemiology and treatment of *Plesiomonas shigelloides* diarrhea. J Clin Microbiol 1989;27:998–1001.

188. Kourany M, Vasquez MA, Saenz R. Edwardsiellosis in man and animals in Panama: Clinical and epidemiologic characteristics. Am J Trop Med Hyg 1977;26:1183–90.

189. Wilson JP, Waterer RR, Wofford JD, Chapman SW. Serious infections with *Edwardsiella tarda*: A case report and review of the literature. Arch Intern Med 1989;149:208–10.

190. Fasano A. Cellular microbiology: Can we learn cell physiology from microorganisms? Am J Physiol 1999;276: C765–76.

191. Gill DM, Rappaport RS. Origin of the enzymatically active A1 fragment of cholera toxin. J Infect Dis 1979;139:674–80.

192. Sharmila DJ, Veluraja K. Conformations of higher gangliosides and their binding with cholera toxin investigation by molecular modeling, molecular mechanics, and molecular dynamics. J Biomol Struct Dyn 2006;23:641–56.

193. Galen J, Fasano A, Ketley J, Richardson S. The role of neuraminidase in *Vibrio cholerae* pathogenesis. Infect Immun 1992;60:406–15.

194. De Luca HE, Lencer WI. A biochemical method for tracking cholera toxin transport from plasma membrane to Golgi and endoplasmic reticulum. Methods Mol Biol 2006;341:127–39.

195. Donowitz M, Welsh MJ. Regulation of mammalian small intestinal electrolyte secretion. In: Johnson RL, editor. Physiology of the Gastrointestinal Tract. New York: Raven Press; 1987. p. 1351–88.

196. Bear CE, et al. Purification and functional reconstitution of the cystic fibrosis transmembrane conductance regulator (CFTR). Cell 1992;68:809–18.

197. Berschneider HM, et al. Altered intestinal chloride transport in cystic fibrosis. FASEB J 1988;2:2625–9.

198. Fukuta S, Twiddy EM, Magnani JL, et al. Comparison of the carbohydrate binding specificities of cholera toxin and *Escherichia coli* heat-labile enterotoxins LTH-1, Lt-la, and LT-1b. Infect Immun 1988;56:1748–53.

199. Moss J, Vaughn M. Mechanism of activation of adenylate cyclase by choleragen and *E. coli* heat-labile enterotoxin. In: Field M, Fordtran JS, Shultz GS, editors. Secretory Diarrhea. Bethesda, MD: American Physiological Society; 1980. p. 107–26.

200. Rodighiero C, Aman AT, Kenny MJ, et al. Structural basis for the differential toxicity of cholera toxin and *Escherichia coli* heat-labile enterotoxin. J Biol Chem 1999;274:3962–9.

201. Rahman H. Prevalence of enterotoxin gene (stn) among different serovars of *Salmonella*. Prevalence of enterotoxin gene (stn) among different serovars of *Salmonella*. Indian J Med Res 1999;110:43–6.

202. Ruiz-Palacios GM, Tores J, Tores NI, et al. Cholera-like enterotoxin produced by *Campylobacter jejuni*. Characterization and significance. Lancet 1983;ii:250–2.

203. Okamoto K, Takahara M. Synthesis of *Escherichia coli* heat-stable enterotoxin Stp as a pre-pro form and role of the pro sequence in secretion. J Bacteriol 1990;172:5260–5.

204. Giannella RA, Mann EA. E. coli heat-stable enterotoxin and guanylyl cyclase C: New functions and unsuspected actions. Trans Am Clin Climatol Assoc 2003;114:67–85; discussion 85–6.

205. Guandalini S, Fasano A. Acute infectious diarrhoea. In: Buts JP, Sokal EM, editors. Management of Digestive and Liver Disorders in Infants and Children. Amsterdam: Elsevier Science Publishers; 1993. p. 319–49.

206. Giannella RA, Mann EA. E. coli heat-stable enterotoxin and guanylyl cyclase C: New functions and unsuspected actions. Trans Am Clin Climatol Assoc 2003;114:67–85.

207. Garbers D. The guanylyl cyclase receptor family of guanylyl cyclases. TIPS 1991;12:116–20.

208. Closs EI, et al. Coexpression of inducible NO synthase and soluble guanylyl cyclase in colonic enterocytes: A pathophysiologic signaling pathway for the initiation of diarrhea by gram negative bacteria? FASEB J 1998;12:1643–9.

209. Savarino SJ, Fasano A, Robertson DC, Levine MM. Enteroaggregative *Escherichia coli* elaborate a heat stable enterotoxin demonstrable in an in vitro rabbit intestinal model. J Clin Invest 1991;87:1450–5.

210. Uzzau S, Fasano A. Crosstalk between enteric pathogens and the intestine. Cell Microbiol. 2000;2:83–9.

211. Vila J, et al. A case control study of diarrhoea in children caused by *Escherichia coli* producing heat stable enterotoxin (EAST 1). J Med Microbiol 1998;47:889–91.

212. Sulakvelidze A, et al. Production of enterotoxin by *Yersinia bercovieri*, a recently identified Yersinia enterocolitica like species. Infect Immun 1999;67:968–71.

213. Fasano A, Hokama Y, Russell R, Morris JG Jr. Diarrhea in ciguatera fish poisoning: Preliminary evaluation of pathophysiological mechanisms. Gastroenterology 1991;100:471–6.

214. Hughes S, et al. *Clostridium difficile* toxin induced intestinal secretion in rabbit ileum in vitro. Gut 1983;24:94–8.

215. Guarino A, et al. Enterotoxin effect of stool supernatant of *Cryptosporidium* infected calves on human jejunum. Gastroenterology 1994;106:28–34.

216. Guarino A, et al. Enterotoxic effect of the vacuolating toxin produced by *Helicobacter pylori* in CaCo2 cells. J Infect Dis 1998;178:1373–8.

217. Raimondi F, Kao JP, Fiorentini C, et al. Enterotoxicity and cytotoxicity of Vibrio parahaemolyticus thermostable direct hemolysin in in vitro systems. Infect Immun 2000;68:3180–5.

218. McClane BA, Chakrabarti G. New insights into the cytotoxic mechanisms of *Clostridium perfringens* enterotoxin. Anaerobe 2004;10:107–14.

219. Zitzer A, Zitzer O, Bhakdi S, Palmer M. Oligomerization of Vibrio cholerae cytolysin yields a pentameric pore and has a dual specificity for cholesterol and sphingolipids in the target membrane. J Biol Chem 1999;274:1375–80.

220. Karmali MA. Infection by Shiga toxin-producing *Escherichia coli*: An overview. Mol Biotechnol 2004;26:117–22.

221. Obrig TG, et al. Endothelial heterogeneity in Shiga toxin receptors and responses. J Biol Chem 1993;268:15484–8.

222. Jacewicz MS, et al. Responses of human intestinal microvascular endothelial cells to Shiga toxins 1 and 2 and pathogenesis of hemorrhagic colitis, Infect Immun 1999;67:1439–44.

223. Proulx F, Seidman EG, Karpman D. Pathogenesis of Shiga toxin-associated hemolytic uremic syndrome. Pediatr Res 2001;50:163–71.

224. O'Brien GJ, Riddell G, Elborn JS, et al. *Staphylococcus aureus* enterotoxins induce IL-8 secretion by human nasal epithelial cells. Respir Res 2006;7:115–26.

225. Steiner TS, Lima AM, Nataro JP, Guerrant RL. Enteroaggregative *Escherichia coli* produce intestinal inflammation and growth impairment and cause interleukin-8 release from intestinal epithelial cells. J Infect Dis 1998;177:88–96.

226. Fasano A, Nataro JP. Intestinal epithelial tight junctions as targets for enteric bacteria-derived toxins. Adv Drug Deliv Rev 2004;56:795–807.

227. Oldfield EC, III. *Clostridium difficile*-associated diarrhea: Resurgence with a vengeance. Rev Gastroenterol Disord 2006;6:79–96.

228. Aktories K. Bacterial toxins that target Rho proteins. J Clin Invest 1997;99:827–9.

229. Narumiya S, Yasuda S. Rho GTPases in animal cell mitosis. Curr Opin Cell Biol 2006;18:199–205.

230. Pothoulakis C. Effects of *Clostridium difficile* toxins on epithelial cell barrier. Ann NY Acad Sci 2000;915:347–56.

231. Bouquet P. The cytotoxic necrotizing factor 1 (CNF1) from *Escherichia coli*. Toxicon 2001;39:1673–80.

232. Schmidt G, et al. Gln63 of Rho is deamination by *Escherichia coli* cytotoxic necrotizing factor 1. Nature 1997;387:725–9.

233. Gerhard R, Schmidt G, Hofmann F, Aktories K. Activation of Rho GTPases by *Escherichia coli* cytotoxic necrotizing factor 1 increases intestinal permeability in CaCo2 cells. Infect Immun 1998;66:5125–31.

234. Fasano A, et al. *Vibrio cholerae* produces a second enterotoxin, which affects intestinal tight junctions. Proc Natl Acad Sci U S A 1991;88:5242–6.

235. Fasano A, et al. Zonula occludens toxin (ZOT) modulates tight junctions through protein kinase C-dependent actin reorganization, in vitro. J Clin Invest 1995;96:710–20.

236. Waldor MK, Mekalanos JJ. Lysogenic conversion by a filamentous phage encoding cholera toxin. Science 1996;272:1910–4.

237. Fasano A. Cellular microbiology: How enteric pathogens socialize with their intestinal host. J Pediatr Gastroenterol Nutr 1996;26:520–32.

238. Navarro-Garcia F, Sears C, Eslava C, et al. Cytoskeletal effects induced by Pet, the serine protease enterotoxin of enteroaggregative *Escherichia coli*. Infect Immun 1999;67:2184–92.

239. Sears CL. The toxins of Bacteroides fragilis. Toxicon 2001;39:1737–46.

240. Harada M, Kondoh M, Ebihara C, et al. Role of tyrosine residues in modulation of claudin 4 by the C-terminal fragment of *Clostridium perfringens* enterotoxin. Biochem Pharmacol 2007;73:206–14.

241. Fabbri A, et al. *Vibrio parahaemolyticus* thermostable direct hemolysin modulates cytoskeletal organization and calcium homeostasis in intestinal cultured cells. Infect Immun 1999;67:1139–48.

242. Ochman H, Bergthorsson U. Rates and patterns of chromosome evolution in enteric bacteria. Curr Opin Microbiol 1998;1:580–3.

243. Schoolnik GK, Yildiz FH. The complete genome sequence of *Vibrio cholerae*: A tale of two chromosomes and of a two lifestyles. Genome Biol 2000;1:1016.1–3.

244. Heldenberg JF, Elsen JA, Nelson WC, et al. DNA sequence of both chromosomes of the cholera pathogen Vibrio cholerae. Nature 2000;406:477–84.

245. Marshall JK, Thabane M, Garg AX, et al. Walkerton Health Study Investigators. Incidence and epidemiology of irritable bowel syndrome after a large waterborne outbreak of bacterial dysentery. Gastroenterology 2006;131:445–50.

246. Ji S, Park H, Lee D, et al. Postinfectious irritable bowel syndrome in patients with *Shigella* infection. J Gastroenterol Hepatol 2005;20:381–6.

247. Wang LH, Fang XC, Pan GZ. Bacillary dysentery as a causative factor of irritable bowel syndrome and its pathogenesis. Gut 2004;53:1096–101.

248. Ferreira SH, Lorenzetti BB, Bristow AF, et al. Interleukin-1 beta as a potent hyperalgesic agent antagonized by a tripeptide analogue. Nature 1998;334:698–700.

249. Chadwick VS, Chen WX, Shu D, et al. Activation of the mucosal immune system in irritable bowel syndrome. Gastroenterology 2002;122:1778–83.

250. Fasano A, Shea-Donohue T. Mechanisms of disease: The role of intestinal barrier function in the pathogenesis of gastrointestinal autoimmune diseases. Nat Clin Pract Gastroenterol Hepatol 2005;2:416–22.

251. Rescigno M, Nieuwenhuis EE. The role of altered microbial signaling via mutant NODs in intestinal inflammation. Curr Opin Gastroenterol 2007;23:21–6.

252. Subramanian S, Campbell BJ, Rhodes JM. Bacteria in the pathogenesis of inflammatory bowel disease. Curr Opin Infect Dis 2006;19:475–84.

253. Lakatos PL, Fischer S, Lakatos L, et al. Current concept on the pathogenesis of inflammatory bowel disease crosstalk between genetic and microbial factors: Pathogenic bacteria and altered bacterial sensing or changes in mucosal integrity take toll. World J Gastroenterol 2006;12:1829–41.

254. Eckmann L. Animal models of inflammatory bowel disease: Lessons from enteric infections. Ann NY Acad Sci 2006;1072:28–38.

255. Olson TS, Reuter BK, Scott KG, et al. The primary defect in experimental ileitis originates from a nonhematopoietic source. J Exp Med 2006;203:541–52.

256. Fasano A. Bioterrorism and biological warfare: Not only a respiratory affair. J Pediatr Gastroenterol Nutr 2003;36:305–6.

257. Sobel J, Khan AS, Swerdlow DL. Threat of a biological terrorist attack on the US food supply: The CDC perspective. Lancet 2002;359:874–80.

19.2b. Viral Infections of the Intestinal Tract

Dorsey M. Bass, MD

Although viruses had long been suspected as pathogens in acute gastroenteritis, the first report of reovirus-like particles in epithelial cells in small bowel biopsies from children with acute nonspecific diarrhea was made only 30 years ago.[1] That original discovery led to a cascade of clinical and laboratory studies that have established rotavirus as the leading cause of dehydrating acute pediatric diarrhea, which is responsible for 30 to 50% of episodes of acute gastroenteritis in children in developed countries. Now 40 to 70% of cases can be attributed to one of several pathogens, compared with only 10 to 20% in the 1970s. It is now known that astroviruses account for up to 15% of cases of acute pediatric diarrhea.[2–4] Specific types of adenoviruses account for 3 to 5% of cases.[5–6] Noroviruses, such as Norwalk and Snow Mountain agents, are also emerging as significant pediatric pathogens. Norwalk agent, one such small round virus known since 1969 to cause epidemic vomiting, can cause outbreaks of vomiting and diarrhea in children at school camps[7] as well as nosocomial infections in children's hospital wards.[8] Noroviruses are now thought to be second in frequency to rotaviruses as causative agents of acute

gastroenteritis in young children,[4] and these infections can result in children having severe episodes of gastroenteritis.[9]

None of the currently recognized intestinal viruses are "new" viruses, but are newly discovered viruses. This is illustrated by the examination of stool samples from children with acute infectious diarrhea that were stored in 1943 when Light and Hodes were searching for the elusive etiology. In 1975, after rotavirus had been discovered, Hodes tested these samples again and found rotavirus in several of them.[10] Other "novel" viruses have been described in association with acute diarrhea, but cause and effect have yet to be established for many of them. Some of these candidates are still named after the locality in which they were discovered (Breda virus) or for their appearance on electron microscopy (coronavirus) (Table 1).

Viruses also account for up to 40% of cases of severe infectious diarrhea in children in developing countries. Rotavirus is one of the single most important pathogens because of its frequency and because it is overrepresented in more severe dehydrating disease.[11] Rotavirus alone is estimated to cause 500,000 deaths per year in the developing

world.[12] Development of a rotavirus vaccine has been an objective of the World Health Organization (WHO) for many years.

Enteric viruses spread mainly by contact with feces (the fecal-oral route) or person-to-person contact. The epidemiology of rotavirus closely resembles that of childhood viruses that are spread by the respiratory route.[13] There is some evidence that transmission via contaminated water supplies may be important in developing countries.[14] Excretion after infection may be more prolonged than previously thought. PCR techniques have shown excretion of rotavirus RNA for up to 57 days after infection.[15] If this is indicative of viable virus, there are considerable implications for the management of cross-infection in day care centers and schools.

Discovery of these various enteric viruses was the result of the application of new technology, especially electron microscopy, to diarrheal disease. Most enteric viruses have proven difficult to grow in the laboratory, hence they eluded recognition by traditional tissue culture techniques. Electron microscopic identification of rotavirus has been replaced by less cumbersome enzyme immunoassay (EIA) antigen detection

Table 1 Viral Agents of Gastroenteritis

Agent	Virology	Clinical/Epidemiology	Diagnostic Tests
Group A rotavirus	80 nm, segmented ds-RNA, grow in tissue culture	Major cause of infantile dehydrating diarrhea Peak incidence in winter in temperate climate	EIA (commercial) EM PAGE RT-PCR
Astrovirus	34 nm, ssRNA, 8 human serotypes	Infant diarrhea, outbreaks in elderly, immunocompromised Peak incidence in winter in temperate climate	EIA EM RT-PCR
Calicivirus including noroviruses and sapoviruses	28 nm, ssRNA, never adapted to tissue culture	Common cause of outbreaks among adults and children, also infantile diarrhea Peak incidence in winter in temperate climate	EM RT-PCR EIA for noroviruses
Enteric adenovirus	80 nm, dsDNA, only serotypes 40 and 41 definitely associated with diarrhea	Prolonged diarrhea in infants and young children. Year-round prevalence	EIA EM
Picobirnavirus	Segmented dsRNA	? Diarrhea in immunocompromised	EM PAGE
CMV	Enveloped dsDNA	Enterocolitis in immunocompromised	Culture Serology PCR Histology
Groups B and C rotavirus	80 nm, segmented dsRNA, do not grow in tissue culture	Mostly animal pathogens with occasional human outbreaks in adults and children	EM PCR PAGE
Toroviruses	ssRNA enveloped 100 to 150 nm pleomorphic	? Infantile gastroenteritis	EM Experimental EIA

tests, which can be undertaken on large batches of stools. EIAs have been developed for group A rotaviruses, enteric adenoviruses, and astrovirus. More recently polymerase chain reaction (PCR) techniques have been emerging as important diagnostic methodology.

There is a large overlap between human and veterinary medicine in this field. Knowledge of animal enteritis viruses has often preceded their discovery in humans. Animal studies have provided much of the understanding of current pathologic and pathophysiologic sequelae of viral enteritis.

PATHOPHYSIOLOGY OF VIRAL ENTERITIS

Viruses that cause diarrhea in humans and animals generally show strong tropism for epithelial cells of the small intestine. The traditional view is that these agents cause disease by selectively destroying large numbers of mature, absorptive enterocytes via lysis and/or apoptosis leading to inadequate absorption of fluid, electrolytes, and luminal nutrients (Figure 1). In contrast to invasive bacterial pathogens, the host inflammatory response in viral enteritis is relatively mild and is not thought to contribute much to the diarrhea. Elevations of cyclic nucleotides, such as cAMP and cGMP, seen with some of the toxin-producing bacterial pathogens that stimulate chloride secretion through the CFTR channel are not observed during viral gastroenteritis.

New concepts of rotaviral pathogenesis have been evoked by the demonstration that a nonstructural rotavirus protein may function as an enterotoxin.[16] Other proposed mechanisms include neuronally mediated intestinal secretion,[17] loss of tight junctions with paracellular flux of water and electrolytes,[18] and villus tip ischemia.[19]

These comments refer to classic agents of viral enteritis such as rotavirus, astrovirus, calicivirus, and enteric adenoviruses. Viruses such as CMV, EBV, and HIV can be associated with diarrhea that is probably due to other mechanisms such as local or systemic inflammatory cytokines.

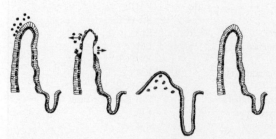

Figure 1 Traditional view of pathogenesis of viral diarrhea. (A) Mature enterocytes selectively infected. (B) Virus multiplies in enterocytes which are damaged and shed by 24 h. (C) Crypts hypertrophy by 42 h, repopulating the villi with immature enterocytes. Villi are variably stunted; mononuclear cells increase in lamina propria. Disaccharidases, glucose absorption, glucose-stimulated sodium absorption at the brush border and sodium-potassium ATPase at the basal lateral membrane are diminished. Thymidine kinase is increased. Cyclic AMP and GMP are not increased. (D) Structure and function return to normal in 7 to 14 days.

EFFECTS OF UNDERNUTRITION

The impact of viral gastroenteritis has an added dimension if the child is malnourished. While susceptibility to infection may not be greatly different, animal studies suggest that the severity of infection is greater[20] and there is evidence from both laboratory studies[21] and clinical studies in malnourished children[22] that recovery is delayed.

A detailed study of the effects of chronic protein-caloric malnutrition on small intestinal repair after acute viral enteritis was reported by Butzner and coworkers in 1985.[23] Malnourished and normally fed germ-free piglets were infected with a coronavirus called transmissible gastroenteritis virus (TGEV). In control piglets, structural changes present in the intestine at 40 hours had virtually recovered by 4 days, but changes persisted through 15 days in malnourished animals. Recovery of mucosal enzymes and glucose-stimulated sodium absorption was also delayed in malnourished piglets, suggesting that malnutrition delays intestinal repair after viral injury. This observation reinforces the need for early and effective nutritional rehabilitation during episodes of diarrhea.

Studies of rotavirus in malnourished piglets have shown that the small intestinal inflammatory response is elevated, and diarrhea persists in malnourished animals.[21] Such prolonged disease in malnourished animals is associated with local mediators or markers of intestinal inflammation. The identification of specific rotavirus-induced alterations that are responsive to malnutrition may allow determination of how macronutrients contribute to host responses to viral infection and viral clearance.

Vitamin A and zinc deficiencies are associated with diarrheal diseases in developing countries. In mouse studies, vitamin A deficiency resulted in much more severe intestinal pathology as well as impaired antibody and cell-mediated responses to rotavirus infection.[24–25] Zinc supplements have shown some efficacy in the treatment of acute watery diarrhea in the developing world.[26]

BREAST FEEDING

Breast feeding reduces the incidence of diarrheal diseases in infants, and reduces mortality in children hospitalized with diarrhea in developing countries.[27] It also reduces diarrheal disease in children who contract rotavirus as a nosocomial infection. There is some information about the influence of breast feeding on rotaviral diarrhea. A prospective study in Finland showed that if breast feeding ceased before 6 months of age, the incidence of rotavirus diarrhea between 7 and 12 months of age increased, but thereafter it was the same.[28] A study of risk factors associated with rotavirus in England found that breast feeding is protective.[29] There is also some evidence of increased risk of rotavirus diarrhea in children who continue to be breast fed after a certain age, suggesting that infection is delayed but not prevented.[30]

An interesting animal study suggested that persistent asymptomatic excretion of rotavirus by cows may protect their calves from infection, perhaps by reinforcing the immune stimulus to the cow, thus encouraging secretion of antirotavirus antibodies in the milk.[31] Thus, breast milk may be an attenuator of viral diarrheal disease, as well as providing nutritional advantages to affected infants.

IMMUNODEFICIENCY

Virus infections of the intestinal tract are common in patients with immunodeficiency. One child with severe combined immunodeficiency chronically excreted five different viruses.[32] Prolonged excretion of rotavirus may occur in such children. One group demonstrated changes in the strain of virus, suggesting that reinfection rather than prolonged infection was the problem.[33] Enteric viral infection may be seen after bone marrow transplantation[34] and as a complication of acquired immunodeficiency virus infection.[35] Cytomegalovirus is frequently associated with diarrhea in HIV-infected individuals, but the detection of other enteric viral infections varies among studies, and their role in inducing disease remains controversial. Rotavirus appears to be more invasive after liver transplantation.[36] Passive treatment with oral gamma globulin has been used in immunodeficiency[37] and as prophylaxis in premature newborn infants.[38]

ENTERIC VIRUSES THAT ARE NOT PRIMARY GUT PATHOGENS

Most viruses that traverse or even replicate within the gut cause no discernable enteric disease. Such viruses can be found in many stool samples from patients with and without symptoms of gastroenteritis. Enteroviruses such as echovirus, hepatitis A virus, coxsackie virus, and poliovirus are excellent examples of viruses that enter the host through the gut, often via M cells overlying Peyer's patches, prior to primary replication in intestinal lymphoid tissue. Other commonly identified stool viruses that do not usually cause diarrhea include nonenteric adenoviruses, reoviruses, and bacterial phages.

VIRAL GUT PATHOGENS

Rotaviruses

Epidemiology. These viruses are the single most important cause of diarrhea requiring admission to hospital during the first 6 to 24 months of life, although most infections are asymptomatic or associated with mild symptoms. Infection is common worldwide from birth to old age.[39] Every child in the world becomes infected with rotavirus, while approximately 2% of infected children are hospitalized for these infections in the United States. The attack rates for rotavirus diarrhea in children aged 6 to 24 months are 0.3 to 0.8 episode per child per year in both developing and developed countries,[40] resulting in at least 600,000 deaths annually in developing countries. The frequency and severity of rotavirus infection provide clear and compelling data for the need for an effective vaccine.[11,41]

Rotaviruses have been identified in stools from 10 to 40% of children admitted to hospital with acute diarrhea in developing countries and in 35 to 50% in developed countries. Severe infection occurs at a younger age in children in developing countries, where the majority of children admitted to hospital are 6 to 12 months old,[40] compared with 12 to 18 months for children in developed countries.[42] All children can be expected to come in contact with rotavirus by 5 years of age, and most will experience asymptomatic boosts in mucosal immunity several times each year. Rotavirus is endemic in the community, and repeated contacts maintain a high level of protection against symptomatic disease after primary infection. In temperate climates, severe rotavirus infections peak during the winter months, but some cases are seen throughout the summer. In tropical areas, seasonal variations are less pronounced.

Neonatal rotavirus infection is often asymptomatic in healthy full-term infants; presumably these infections are modified by passive immunity from placental and breast milk antibodies. Clinical observations that unique strains of rotavirus may be responsible for endemic nursery infection have been supported by RNA/RNA hybridization experiments, using nursery strains and strains from children with acute gastroenteritis.[43]

Infection in children after 3 years of age is not usually severe, but it can necessitate admission to hospital. Rotaviruses have been identified in 16% of children aged over 5 years admitted for gastroenteritis in Australia,[42] and in 5% of adults admitted to hospital in Thailand for severe diarrheal disease.

Some studies from developing countries have reported similar rates of rotavirus isolation from both controls and diarrhea patients. The balance between ingested dose of virus, mucosal immunity, breast feeding, and sensitivity of detection methods probably influence these observations.

Outbreaks of diarrhea caused by "atypical" rotaviruses have been widespread in China, where they have affected adults, children. and newborn infants.[44] These "atypical" rotaviruses lack group A–specific common antigen, but they are morphologically identical to conventional human strains. They account for 1 to 3% of cases in Finland, Mexico, and United States.[41] Overall, they account for less than 1% of all severe rotavirus disease worldwide, but if they become more common, current vaccine development strategies may need to be reconsidered. Other recent outbreaks in adults have been caused by rotavirus strains that are not the common circulating strains, suggesting that natural immunity to common strains does not always provide adequate heterotypic protection.[45]

Virology. Rotaviruses are classified as a genus within the family *Reoviridae*. The prefix rota refers to the wheel-like appearance of particles in feces seen by negative contrast electron microscopy (Figure 2). Complete particles, about 70 nm in diameter, exhibit a triple-shelled capsid (Figure 3). Incomplete double-shelled particles are common, but not infectious.

There are four major groups (A, B ,C, and D) of rotaviruses as determined by antigens on the middle layer of the viral capsid. Group A rotaviruses are responsible for the great majority of human infections. Epitopes on the outer capsid layer (VP7 and VP4) of group A rotaviruses determine the G (glycoprotein) and P (protease-sensitive) serotypes. G1, G2, G3, and G4 are the most common infecting serotypes in humans, against which current vaccines are directed. In recent years, a global increase in G9 strains has been observed.[46–47] Serotypes can be identified by enzyme immunoassay (EIA) or by PCR methods. Rotavirus strains can be further subdivided by RNA gel electrophoresis in order to follow epidemiologic patterns in a given locality. Multiple electropherotypes and serotypes exist simultaneously in most communities, but usually one or two are dominant in any 1 year in children admitted to hospital.

Pathophysiology. The traditional view of rotavirus pathophysiology is that diarrhea is a direct result of rotavirus tissue tropism. Rotavirus infects only differentiated villus enterocytes in the small intestine. Virions are ingested, activated by trypsin in the small intestine, and infect the villus enterocytes leading to their destruction and the release of thousands of progeny which are locally activated by trypsin to infect more enterocytes. The epithelium is rapidly repopulated with less differentiated enterocytes from the crypts, which lack both digestive enzymes such as lactase and mechanisms for active sodium

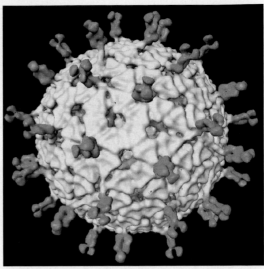

Figure 3 Three dimensional structure of rotavirus as determined by cryo-electron microscopy and image processing. Note the red, spike-like projections (VP4), which mediate cell attachment, the yellow surface consisting of the glycoprotein, VP7, which is the determinant of the G serotype. Small amounts of the inner capsid layers (blue and green) can be seen through channels that penetrate the virion core. (Courtesy of B. V. V. Prasad, Baylor College of Medicine.)

and water absorption such as sodium-potassium ATPase (Figure 4). This results in diarrhea by two mechanisms. Undigested and therefore unabsorbable carbohydrates such as lactose lead to an osmotic diarrhea, while the loss of active absorption of water in the face of intact or hypertrophied crypt secretion of chloride and water leads to a low-grade secretory diarrhea. According to this model, symptoms resolve when the new enterocytes have differentiated which may require 7 days or more in the setting of a severe primary infection.

Ball and colleagues have proposed that a rotavirus nonstructural protein, NSP4, functions as a novel viral enterotoxin. They have reported that this protein (or a derivative peptide) is capable of inducing diarrhea in susceptible suckling mice when administered by either intraluminal or intraperitoneal routes.[16] NSP4 is reported to cause chloride secretion and thus diarrhea by increasing intracellular calcium when it is either expressed intracellularly or applied externally to cells.[48] Further evidence for the role of NSP4 in the pathophysiology of rotavirus diarrhea is the fact that antibodies against NSP4 can ameliorate rotavirus diarrhea in suckling mice. It has been suggested that changes in NSP4 sequence correlate with rotavirus virulence in porcine rotavirus strains.[49] Of note, NSP4 appears to exert its chloride secretory effects through a previously unrecognized, age-dependent anion channel that is distinct from the cystic fibrosis transmembrane conductance regulator.[50] The ability of NSP4 to induce diarrhea in sucking mice has been reported for several rotavirus strains, including group C and avian rotaviruses, suggesting that structural elements of this protein, are important in enterotoxin function.[51–52] A few studies have questioned the role of NSP4 as an enterotoxin.

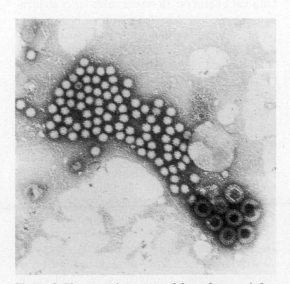

Figure 2 Electron microscopy of feces from an infant with acute diarrhea. The larger (70 nm diameter) particles are rotaviruses that have lost their electron dense core. A group of smaller unidentified virus particles is seen here in association with rotavirus.

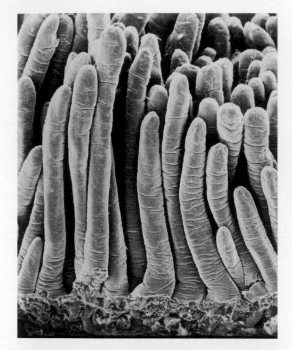

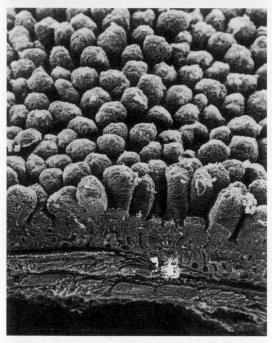

Figure 4 Scanning electron microscopic appearance of normal and rotavirus-infected calf jejunum. (A) Jejunum from a normal, conventionally reared calf, showing tall, fingerlike villi. (B) Rotavirus damaged intestine from a moribund calf. Rotavirus antigen was detected by immunoperoxidase staining of paraffin sections from adjacent tissue. Most of the epithelial cells on the surface of the stunted vill contained antigen. Note epithelial damage, decreased villous height, and increased depth of crypts. (Courtesy of Dr G. A. Hall, Institute for Animal Health, Compton, UK)

One group was unable to replicate the secretory diarrhea seen with administration of the NSP4 peptide.[53] Furthermore, although one study found a correlation of virulence with NSP4 sequence of human rotavirus strains (Kirkwood and colleagues, 1996), different studies have failed to find correlation of virulence with NSP4 sequence in other human and mouse rotavirus strains.[53–55] While this lack of correlation between NSP4 sequence may have been due to mutations in other virulence genes, the role of NSP4 as an enterotoxin in pathogenesis of rotavirus diarrhea remains an area of active investigation.

Another recent hypothesis is that modifications in intracellular tight junctions between enterocytes during rotavirus infection lead to an enhanced paracellular flux of ions and small macromolecules. Morphologic studies show alterations in components of the tight junctions during rotavirus infection. Using chamber experiments demonstrate enhanced transepithelial flux of 458 Da and 4 kDa but not 70 kDa markers in rotavirus-infected murine jejunal epithelium.[18] In another study, rotavirus NSP4 increased paracellular fluxes in vitro.[56] Recently, one of the rotavirus outer capsid proteins, VP8, has been shown to have a direct disruptive effect on tight junctions.[57]

Other possible mechanisms of diarrhea during intestinal viral infection include microischemia of villi,[19] impaired polar transport of sucrase-isomaltase and other apical proteins to the correct membrane surface,[58] cytokine generation by the epithelium or underlying mononuclear cells,[59] and neuronally mediated intestinal hypersecretion.[17] It is noteworthy that none of these proposed pathophysiologic mechanisms are mutually exclusive and the etiology of rotavirus diarrhea may well be multifactorial. Discernment of the relative contribution to disease of these mechanisms may be important in devising treatment strategies.

Recently, studies have shown that viremia occurs in both animals and humans during acute rotavirus infection.[60–64] The clinical consequences of this for most immunocompetent hosts appear to be mild but this phenomena may help explain rare cases of extraintestinal disease and disseminated infection in immunocompromised individuals. Viremia may also amplify intestinal infection since rotavirus appears to be able to infect polarized cells from either the apical or basolateral sides.[65]

Clinical Features. In severe cases, after an incubation period of 2 to 7 days, there is an abrupt onset of vomiting and fever.[66] Profuse watery diarrhea soon follows, leading to dehydration, acidosis, and electrolyte imbalance. In contrast to bacterial enterocolitis, the stool fluid does not contain blood, white cells, or mucus. Abdominal cramps are less frequent, but irritability and lethargy are often present. Respiratory symptoms have been reported in 20 to 40% of patients, but in several studies an equally high incidence has been found in controls. The temperature falls to normal quickly. Usually vomiting settles within 24 to 48 hours and diarrhea in 2 to 7 days.

Acute complications include hypernatremia or hyponatremia when water and electrolyte losses are discrepant. Febrile convulsions can occur as with any other cause of sudden high fever. Reye's syndrome, encephalitis, rectal bleeding, afebrile seizures, and intussusception have been described in association with rotavirus infection, but the evidence linking them as cause and effect is tenuous. Case reports of PCR detection of rota-virus genome in CSF are noteworthy, but their significance is not clear.[67] Raised aminoaspartate transferase levels are common in severe disease.[68] Depressed mucosal lactase activity is frequent,[69] but persisting lactose malabsorption is not common, as disaccharidase activities return to normal within a few days.

Treatment. Initial management is directed at correcting dehydration, acidosis, and electrolyte imbalance. The assessment of the degree of dehydration and treatment with oral or intravenous fluids are considered elsewhere. Early resumption of normal feeding is encouraged, especially in undernourished children, with particular emphasis on breast feeding. Breast feeding can almost always be continued, even in children with lactose malabsorption. However, in very small infants lactose malabsorption can be a serious problem, requiring lactose-free feeding for days or even weeks. These cases, although rare, should not be overlooked in the appropriate enthusiasm for continued breast feeding.

For the breast-fed infant with severe diarrhea, a combination of oral rehydration solution (ORS) and increasing volumes of breast milk can be offered. In older children early introduction of a balanced diet should be encouraged, capitalizing on the fact that temporary mucosal damage leaves a much larger reserve of maltase and isomaltase than lactase. Small amounts of fruit juices can be given, but large volumes of sucrose-containing fluids should be avoided in the acute phase, and for babies these beverages should be diluted.

Drugs are contraindicated. Antibiotics have no place in viral diarrhea. Antiperistaltic agents may lead to pooling of fluid, which is effectively removed from the circulation and yet not revealed to the observer. Complications include ileus and respiratory depression.[70–71] Antiemetics should be avoided. Vomiting is usually self-limiting, and dystonic reactions to these drugs may occur. Probiotics, such as Lactobacillus GG, have been reported to decrease the duration of diarrhea in relatively mild disease[72] but were not of significant benefit in severe disease.[73]

Prevention. Improved sanitation and hygiene are unlikely to radically alter the incidence of rotavirus diarrhea in developing countries. Such measures have proved unsuccessful in North America and Europe, where the attack rates are similar to those in less developed parts of the world. In pediatric wards, handwashing and isolation procedures may limit nosocomial outbreaks.

Breast feeding reduces the incidence of diarrheal diseases overall in the first year of life.[74] This is especially true for nonviral pathogens but is not consistent for rotavirus infection.[75] The period immediately after weaning is associated with higher risk of diarrhea in general[76] and rotavirus diarrhea in particular.[30] Breast feeding may, thus, delay rotavirus infection rather than prevent it. However, if infants are older when they contract the illness, they are likely to tolerate it better, and the many other benefits of breast feeding will not be lost.

Passive prophylaxis has been tried in special situations. Human gamma globulin, given by mouth to newborn premature infants, delays onset of viral excretion and decreases the severity of rotavirus disease.[38] Additions of bovine milk rotavirus antibody to formula given to infants protected them against symptomatic infection[77] and have been reported to hasten recovery.[78]

Vaccine Development. Because of the high morbidity and mortality of rotavirus infection in pediatric populations throughout the world, vaccine development has been a major priority. The initial vaccine prototypes have been based on animal rotavirus strains that are not virulent in humans. This approach has been termed "Jennerian" after Edward Jenner who used cowpox to immunize against smallpox in the late eighteenth century.[79] Both simian and bovine strains were employed in early trials, which were promising but failed to provide sufficient protection from rotavirus disease. A second generation of vaccines included reassortant viruses, which contained the RNA segment that encodes the viral glycoprotein for each of the four epidemiologically significant human rotavirus G types inserted in a background of the genome of an avirulent simian rotavirus.[80] A tetravalent rotavirus vaccine, Rotashield, based on such simian/human reassortant viruses was shown in major trials to provide 80 to 100% protection against dehydrating rotavirus diarrhea.[81] In 1998, the Advisory Committee on Immunization Practices (ACIP) endorsed the vaccine, and the FDA granted a license to Wyeth to produce it. Subsequently, the American Academy of Pediatrics included, for the first time, in its recommended childhood immunization schedule. Nine months later, after the administration of approximately 1.5 million doses of Rotashield, the Center for Disease Control (CDC) reported 15 cases of intussusception in infants who had received the vaccine.[82] Eleven of the intussusceptions occurred within 1 week of the first vaccine dose. Subsequent case-control and case-series investigations confirmed the temporal association and the manufacturer removed the vaccine from market.[83] Despite widespread vaccination in some states, no significant increase in intussusception was detected in ecological studies.[84] The most recent consensus of the increased attributable risk for intussusception for infants receiving Rotashield vaccine was on the order of 1 in 10,000.[81].

Currently, two other rotavirus live attenuated vaccines are available. One is a pentavalent human-bovine reassortant (Rotateq[85]) which is currently approved for use in the United States.[86] It is given as three oral doses to infants less than 6 months of age. The other vaccine, an attenuated monovalent human strain,[87] has been approved by the WHO and is given as two doses.[88] Both vaccines have undergone extensive safety testing and neither appears to induce intussusception. Both provide greater than 90% protection against severe dehydrating disease. Eventually other strategies may be employed such as noninfectious virus-like particles (VLPs) which can be produced using recombinant technology, parenteral inactivated virus vaccines, or DNA vaccines.

Astrovirus

Epidemiology. Astroviruses were first observed in 1975 by **Madeley** and **Cosgrove** using negative stain electron microscopy to examine stools obtained from children with acute enteritis.[89] Astroviruses were distinguished by their size (28 to 34 nm) and morphology containing five or six pointed stars. Because the only method of detection was electron microscopy and because the star-like morphology was variably observed, the true significance of this agent of gastroenteritis was grossly underestimated until the development of EIAs and RT-PCR assays. Astroviruses are now known to be an important cause of infantile gastroenteritis, second or third only to rotavirus in several studies.[90–93]

Astrovirus infection accounts for 7 to 15% of infantile diarrhea in a variety of settings. Most symptomatic infections occur in infants less than 1 year of age with a peak incidence in winter months in temperate climates. Transmission appears to be fecal-oral. Astrovirus is an important agent of diarrhea in the developing world,[90–92,94] in nosocomial outbreaks,[93,95] and in day-care–related diarrhea.[3] Asymptomatic infection appears to be common, particularly in day care and hospital settings. Such asymptomatic infections are important in maintaining and amplifying outbreaks. Most children have developed antibody against astrovirus by age of 5 years. Astrovirus has also been reported as an important cause of diarrhea in immunocompromised hosts such as AIDS[93,96] and bone marrow transplant patients.[97] Less common serotypes of astrovirus have been reported as responsible for outbreaks of gastroenteritis among immunocompetent military personnel[98] and nursing home residents.[99–100] Astroviruses also infect a variety of animals. To date, it appears that strains are species specific so that animal viruses are not commonly transmitted to humans.

Virology. Astroviruses have a unique genome organization, resulting in these viruses being assigned to their own viral family, *Astroviridae*. Particles consist of small (28 to 34 nm) nonenveloped capsids that consist of 2 to 3 proteins of 20 to 34 kDa mass. The genome is positive sense, single-stranded RNA containing three open reading frames that encode a viral protease, a 90 kDa capsid precursor protein, and an RNA polymerase. Infected cells contain considerable amounts of subgenomic RNA that encodes the capsid precursor. Mammalian astroviruses grow efficiently only in tissue culture in the presence of exogenous trypsin. Eight human serotypes have been identified, with serotype 1 being the most common. It is not known whether infection with one serotype confers protection against subsequent infection with other serotypes.

Pathogenesis. Knowledge of pathogenesis in humans is limited to a few observations by electron microscopy of astrovirus particles in the epithelium of a children with gastroenteritis. In one such child, villous blunting and a mild increase in mononuclear cells in the lamina propria was noted.[101] Studies in lambs have shown infection of villus tip epithelial cells, with subsequent shortening of the villi, and crypt hypertrophy.[102] Studies in calves with bovine astrovirus have shown preferential infection of M cells overlying Peyer's patches.[103] In calves astrovirus appeared to be pathogenic only as a coinfection with either Breda virus or bovine rotavirus.

Clinical Features. Astrovirus infection is associated with a moderate enteritis syndrome that is usually milder than primary rotavirus disease. The incubation period is between 1 and 4 days, probably depending on the size of the inoculum. The illness is characterized initially by low-grade fever and vomiting, followed by 3 to 4 days of watery diarrhea without blood or white blood cells. Immunocompromised hosts may experience more severe and prolonged illness. Similarly, coinfection (which is common) with rotavirus or other enteric pathogens may lead to particularly severe symptoms. Adult volunteers have very mild or no symptoms after inoculation with astrovirus.[104] Adults almost uniformly possess serum antibodies against astrovirus and astrovirus-specific T-helper cells in their small intestine.[105]

Astrovirus infection can be diagnosed by electron microscopy, EIA, or RT-PCR assay. A commercial monoclonal antibody-based diagnostic EIA kit is available in Europe but is not currently approved for use in the United States.

Treatment and Prevention. As with other viral enteritides, there is no specific treatment for astrovirus. Attention should be directed toward maintaining hydration and nutritional status. A single case report describes successful administration of intravenous immunoglobulin to an immunocompromised adult with severe astrovirus disease.[106] There are currently no active vaccine development programs.

Human Caliciviruses (Noroviruses and Sapoviruses)

Norwalk virus was observed by EM in stools from a severe outbreak of enteritis in Norwalk, Ohio, in 1972.[107] This was the first direct confirmation of a viral etiology for human gastroenteritis. Subsequent volunteer studies proved its pathogenicity. Other morphologically similar viruses were observed and named for their outbreak sites (Montgomery County, Hawaii, Snow Mountain, Sapporo, Toronto) and these viruses were often called "Norwalk-like viruses" or small round-structured viruses.

Recently, these human viruses, which cause gastroenteritis, have been reclassified as members of a distinct genus called *Noroviruses* in the *Caliciviridae* family. None of these agents have been adapted to tissue culture but the genomes of several, including the prototypic Norwalk virus, have been completely sequenced and characterized. [108]

Other human caliciviruses are classified in a separate genus called *Sapoviruses*. These viruses exhibit typical calicivirus structure when observed by electron microscopy; they cause disease primarily in young children, and they have a slightly different genome organization when compared to the noroviruses,

Epidemiology. Knowledge of the full extent of norovirus epidemiolgy remains limited because the only available diagnostic tests until quite recently were electron microscopy and immuno-electron micrscopy. These methods are not sufficiently sensitive to detect the low number of virus particles found in most diarrhea samples. Norovirus gastroenteritis is best known for explosive outbreaks of disease that affect both children and adults. Such outbreaks frequently occur in closed or semiclosed settings such as schools, camps, and cruise ships. The United States Center for Disease Control has shown that more than 95% of such outbreaks, which are not caused by conventional bacterial or parasitic pathogens, are caused by noroviruses.[109] Transmission in these outbreaks has been linked to a variety of food-stuffs including shellfish, cake icing, and lettuce (washed with contaminated water). Outbreaks are distinguished from those due to preformed toxins by the appearance of secondary cases in household contacts and the slightly longer incubation period (12 to 24 hours vs 2 to 6 hours for toxins). Vomitus has been shown to contain infectious virus and can rapidly amplify outbreaks. Noroviruses are also common nosocomial pathogens in children.[110] In addition, noroviruses are emerging as important causes of endemic childhood gastroenteritis. Like rotavirus, there appears to be an increase in the incidence of norovirus disease in winter months in temperate climates. Apoviruses cause disease in young children, but it is generally less severe than norovirus and rotavirus-induced disease.[9]

Virology. Caliciviruses are small, 28 to 34 nm, nonenveloped, positive-sense RNA viruses. Human caliciviruses are classified into several distinct genogroups within each genus and viruses in each genogroup that are genetically and serologically distinct. Despite this, there are some common epitopes among viruses in genogroups 1 and 2 of the noroviruses, and an EIA based on cross-reactive monoclonal antibodies has been developed and is commercially available in Europe.[111] The RNA genome contains three open reading frames that encode a polyprotein that makes an NTPase, viral proteinase, and RNA polymerase, the capsid protein, and a small basic protein that is found in virions. The capsid consists of 180 molecules of a single major protein and a few molecules of a minor protein. When the capsid protein is expressed in a recombinant baculovirus system, it spontaneously assembles into virus-like particles (VLPs), which have been used to create diagnostic reagents and candidate vaccines (Figure 5). The most common means of diagnosis of infections is by RT-PCR using

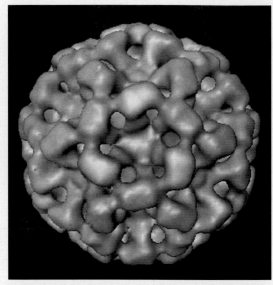

Figure 5 Three-dimensional structure of recombinant Norwalk virus-like particles generated by expression of the capsid protein in insect cells. Images were prepared by cryo-electron microscopy, followed by image processing. (Courtesy of B. V. V. Prasad, Baylor College of Medicine.)

primers, but this is not straightforward as several sets of primers or probes must be used to confirm infection. The EIA for noroviruses currently available in Europe is being evaluated for use in the United States, and other EIAs are being developed.

Pathophysiology. Human volunteer studies demonstrate villus shortening and crypt hypertrophy in the proximal duodenum associated with villus tip vacuolization and infiltration of the lamina propria with inflammatory cells.[112] Intestinal sucrase, alkaline phosphatase, and trehalase are diminished with demonstrable mild carbohydrate intolerance.[113] Mild steatorrhea is also noted. Gastric and colonic mucosas are completely normal. Delayed gastric emptying has been formally demonstrated in symptomatic volunteers and may account for the pronounced nausea and vomiting associated with this infection. Animal studies show similar histologic features. Several recent studies have suggested that specific blood group determinants may confer susceptibility or resistance to specific norovirus.[114–115]

Clinical Features. The most striking characteristics of calicivirus infections are the rapid onset of symptoms, rapid spread of disease through groups, predominance of vomiting as a symptom, and the high attack rate across all age groups. Generally, the illness is mild and self-limited to 12 to 24 hours after 1 to 2 days incubation. Attack rates are usually about 50% of exposed populations. Asymptomatic infections are common. Recent studies have shown that virus is excreted for much longer times than previously recognized. This asymptomatic shedding of virus likely contributes to virus transmission. Infantile norovirus enteritis is clinically similar to rotavirus gastroenteritis although resulting in less severe dehydration.

Treatment and Prevention. No specific treatment is available. There is evidence that protective short-term immunity to the same serotype of calicivirus develops after infection. However, this immune protection wanes fairly rapidly. Because of the economic and military liability associated with large outbreaks, there is considerable interest in finding methods of prevention. A virus-like particle vaccine is being evaluated.

Enteric Adenovirus

Adenoviruses are ubiquitous human pathogens and cause a variety of syndromes ranging from respiratory infections to hepatitis. Only 2 of more than 50 serotypes, types 40 and 41, are clearly associated with human enteritis, although a variety of serotypes may be found in stool samples. Adenovirus enteritis tends to last longer (up to 2 weeks) than disease caused by other gastroenteritis viruses.

Epidemiology. Like all of the agents of viral enteritis, enteric adenoviruses have a worldwide distribution. Most symptomatic infections occur in children less than 2 years of age. Unlike rotavirus and astrovirus, there does not seem to be a winter peak in the incidence of adenovirus enteritis. In longitudinal studies there is considerable year-to-year variation in the extent of adenovirus diarrheal disease in a given geographic area.[116] Adenovirus infections generally account for 3 to 5% of acute pediatric enteritis. Like the other agents of viral enteritis, enteric adenoviruses commonly cause asymptomatic infections, especially in day care centers.[117] Seroconversion studies suggest that enteric adenovirus infection is not as common as rotavirus infection during early childhood. Fecal shedding of adenovirus of various serotypes is common in AIDS patients, but not clearly associated with disease manifestations.[118–121] Despite the fact that up to 10^{11} virions/g stool have been reported in patients with enteric adenovirus gastroenteritis, there are fewer reports of explosive diarrhea outbreaks from enteric adenovirus than with rotavirus, calicivirus, or astrovirus.[121]

Virology. Adenoviruses are 80 nm nonenveloped particles containing a double-stranded DNA genome. Enteric adenoviruses are more fastidious in tissue culture than the other adenovirus serotypes, but can be grown on selected cell lines such as CaCo-2 cells. Diagnosis can be made by commercially available EIAs.[122]

Pathophysiology. Adenoviruses replicate in host nuclei, and intranuclear inclusions are observed in enterocyte nuclei in patients with diarrhea. There are very few systematic studies of the pathophysiology of these infections in humans or animals.

Treatment and Prevention. There is no known specific treatment although the use of ribavirin in immunocompromised patients has been reported.[123] No major efforts are underway to develop a vaccine.

OTHER RELATED PATHOGENS AND INFECTIONS

Cytomegalovirus

In the modern era of both acquired and iatrogenic immunodeficiency states, CMV has emerged with increasing frequency as an enteric pathogen. Several clinical syndromes have been described including a protein-losing gastropathy,[124] deep ulcers, which may occur anywhere in the gastrointestinal tract, and an enterocolitis endoscopically similar to Crohn's disease. Most cases occur in immunocompromised or very young patients.[125–126] Diagnosis is made by finding characteristic nuclear inclusions in mucosal biopsies or by culture of such material. Yield is much higher from the center of ulcer craters. Treatment consists of restoration of immunologic function, if possible, and the administration of ganciclovir. Selected cases may also benefit from CMV immune globulin.

Epstein-Barr Virus

In immunosuppressed, solid organ transplant patients, infection with Epstein-Barr Virus (EBV) may trigger an immunoproliferative syndrome, which may present with fever and diarrhea. Endoscopic evaluation shows nodular ulcerated lesions in the bowel that may contain many cells with EBV genome demonstrable by in situ hybridization. Treatment consists mainly of withdrawal of immunosuppression and the use of ganciclovir.

Small Round Viruses

Small round viruses (SRVs) are morphologically characterized particles observed by EM in diarrheal stools. Almost all of the previously described SRVs and "minireoviruses" are now known to be caliciviruses and astroviruses. Parvoviruses and picobirnaviruses also share this morphology. It is likely that some SRVs represent uncharacterized, novel viral agents of diarrhea, or bacterial phages.

Aichi Virus

An example of a newly described small round gastroenteritis virus is the Aichi virus. This virus was isolated in cultured cells from individuals who had gastroenteritis associated with eating oysters.[127] Aichi virus has since been detected in Pakistani children with acute enteritis children and Japanese travelers from Southeast Asia.[128] The virus contains a single-stranded RNA genome and is a new member of the *Picornaviridae* family.[129] RT-PCR assays have been developed to detect the viral genome.[130]

Picobirnavirus

These are small (35 nm) double-stranded RNA viruses with a two segment genome. They have been associated with animal diarrhea and have been found on occasion in humans with HIV infection.[131–132] Diagnosis can be made by by visualizing two distinct bands of genomic RNA on electrophorectic gels of RNA extracted from stool samples.

Parvovirus

This is a small round virus containing single-stranded DNA which causes severe diarrhea in young animals. Human diarrheal disease has not been established.

Torovirus

Large (100 to 150 nm) pleomorphic, enveloped, single-stranded RNA viruses have been associated with diarrhea in livestock. Several reports suggest they may be pathogenic in young children.[133–135]

Coronavirus

Large, enveloped ssRNA viruses related to toroviruses, coronaviruses cause severe enteritis in several species of animals and are common respiratory pathogens in humans. The pleomorphic particles have been observed in stools from infants with gastroenteritis, and from patients with tropical sprue, but their true role in human disease remains uncertain.

Measles

In the developing world, severe measles infection is often accompanied by severe diarrhea. The pathophysiology of measles gastroenteritis is not well understood although viral-mediated intestinal inflammation has been described.[136] The incidence of measles-associated diarrhea has been greatly reduced with use of the measles vaccine.

Human Immunodeficiency Virus

Even in the absence of identifiable pathogens, AIDS patients frequently develop diarrhea that is likely related to HIV infection of the intestinal mucosa. Pathology in such cases shows apoptosis and disproportionate CD4+ T-cell depletion as well demonstrable viral nucleic acid in tissue mononuclear cells.[137] It has been proposed that CD4 depletion leads to loss of epithelial integrity and subsequent microbial translocation which fuels the chronic systemic immune activation observed in progressive HIV infection.[138] The diarrhea usually responds to appropriate multiagent antiretroviral therapy.[121,139]

REFRENCES

1. Bishop RF, Davidson GP, Holmes IH, Ruck BJ. Virus particles in epithelial cells of duodenal mucosa from children with viral gastroenteritis. Lancet 1973;: p. 1281–3.
2. Dennehy PH, Nelson SM, Spangenberger S, et al. A prospective case-control study of the role of astrovirus in acute diarrhea among hospitalized young children. J infect dis 2001;184:10–5.
3. Glass RI, Noel J, Mitchell D, et al. The changing epidemiology of astrovirus-associated gastroenteritis: a review. Arch Virol Suppl 1996;12:287–300.
4. Pang XL, Joensuu J, Vesikari T. Human calicivirus-associated sporadic gastroenteritis in Finnish children less than two years of age followed prospectively during a rotavirus vaccine trial. Pediatr Infect Dis J 1999;18:420–6.
5. Kotloff KL, Losonsky GA, Morris JJ, et al. Enteric adenovirus infection and childhood diarrhea: An epidemiologic study in three clinical settings. Pediatrics 1989;84:219–25.
6. Herrmann JE, Blacklow NR, Perron HD, et al. Incidence of enteric adenoviruses among children in Thailand and the significance of these viruses in gastroenteritis. J Clin Microbiol 1988;26:1783–6.
7. Jenkins S, Horman J, Israel E, et al. An outbreak of Norwalk-related gastroenteritis at a boys' camp. Am J Dis Child 1985;139:787–9.
8. Spender Q, Lewis D, Price E. Norwalk like viruses: Study of an outbreak. Arch Dis Child 1986;61:142–7.
9. Pang XL, Honma S, Nakata S, Vesikari T. Human caliciviruses in acute gastroenteritis of young children in the community. J Infect Dis 2000;181:S288–94.
10. Hodes H. American Pediatric Society Presidential Address. Pediatr Res 1976;10:201–4.
11. Glass RI, Parashar UD. The promise of new rotavirus vaccines.[see comment][comment]. N Engl J Med 2006; 354:75–7.
12. Parashar UD, Hummelman EG, Bresee JS, et al. Global illness and deaths caused by rotavirus disease in children. Emerg Infect Diseases 2003;9:565–72.
13. Cook SM, Glass RI, LeBaron CW, Ho MS. Global seasonality of rotavirus infections. Bull World Health Organ 1990; 68:171–7.
14. Ramia S. Transmission of viral infections by the water route: Implications for developing countries. Rev Infect Dis 1985;7:180–8.
15. Richardson S, Grimwood K, Gorrell R, et al. Extended excretion of rotavirus after severe diarrhoea in young children. Lancet 1998;351:1844–8.
16. Ball JM, Tian P, Zeng CQ, et al. Age-dependent diarrhea induced by a rotaviral nonstructural glycoprotein [see comments]. Science 1996;272:101–4.
17. Lundgren O, Peregrin AT, Persson K, et al. Role of the enteric nervous system in the fluid and electrolyte secretion of rotavirus diarrhea [see comments]. Science 2000; 287:491–5.
18. Dickman KG, Hempson SJ, Anderson J, et al. Rotavirus alters paracellular permeability and energy metabolism in Caco-2 cells. Am J Physiol Gastrointest Liver Physiol 2000;279:G757–66.
19. Osborne MP, Haddon SJ, Worton KJ, et al. Rotavirus-induced changes in the microcirculation of intestinal villi of neonatal mice in relation to the induction and persistence of diarrhea [see comments]. J Pediatr Gastroenterol Nutr 1991;12:111–20.
20. Offor E, Riepenhoff TM, Ogra PL. Effect of malnutrition on rotavirus infection in suckling mice: Kinetics of early infection. Proc Soc Exp Biol Med 1985;178:85–90.
21. Zijlstra RT, Donovan SM, Odle J, et al. Protein-energy malnutrition delays small-intestinal recovery in neonatal pigs infected with rotavirus. J Nutr 1997;127:1118–27.
22. Black RE, Merson MH, Eusof A, et al. Nutritional status, body size and severity of diarrhoea associated with rotavirus or enterotoxigenic Escherichia coli. J Trop Med Hyg 1984;87:83–9.
23. Butzner J, Butler D, Miniats O, Hamilton J. Impact of chronic protein-calorie malnutrition on small intestinal repair after acute viral enteritis: A study in gnotobiotic piglets. Pediatr Res 1985;19:476–81.
24. Ahmed F, Jones DB, Jackson AA. The interaction of vitamin A deficiency and rotavirus infection in the mouse. Br J Nutr 1990;63:363–73.
25. Ahmed F, Jones DB, Jackson AA. Effect of undernutrition on the immune response to rotavirus infection in mice. Ann Nutr Metab 1990;34:21–31.
26. Bhutta ZA, Therapeutic effects of oral zinc in acute and persistent diarrhea in children in developing countries: Pooled analysis of randomized controlled trials. Am J Clin Nutr 2000;72:1516–22.
27. Sachdev H, Kumar S, Singh K, Puri R. Does breastfeeding influence mortality in children hospitalized with diarrhoea? J Trop Pediatr 1991;37:275–9.
28. Ruuska T Vesikari T. A prospective study of acute diarrhoea in Finnish children from birth to 2 1/2 years of age. Acta Paediatr Scand 1991;80:500–7.
29. Cumberland P, Hudson MJ, Rodrigues LC, et al. Study of infectious intestinal disease in England: Rates in the community, presenting to general practice, and reported to national surveillance. The Infectious Intestinal Disease Study Executive. Epidemiol Infect 2001;126:63–70.
30. Mitra AK Rabbani F. The importance of breastfeeding in minimizing mortality and morbidity from diarrhoeal diseases: The Bangladesh perspective. J Diarrhoeal Dis Res 1995;13:1–7.
31. Kodituwakku SN Harbour DA. Persistent excretion of rotavirus by pregnant cows. Vet Rec 1990;126:547–9.
32. Chrystie I, Booth I, Kidd A, et al. Multiple faecal virus excretion in immunodeficiency. Lancet 1982;1:282.

33. Eiden J, Losonsky GA, Johnson J, Yolken RH. Rotavirus RNA variation during chronic infection of immunocompromised children. Pediatr Infect Dis 1985;4:632–7.
34. Yolken R, Bishop C, Townsend T, et al. Infectious gastroenteritis in bone-marrow-transplant recipients. N Engl J Med 1982;306):1010–2.
35. Oshitani H, Kasolo FC, Mpabalwani M, et al. Association of rotavirus and human immunodeficiency virus infection in children hospitalized with acute diarrhea, Lusaka, Zambia. J Infect Dis 1994;169:897–900.
36. Fitts SW, Green M, Reyes J, et al. Clinical features of nosocomial rotavirus infection in pediatric liver transplant recipients. Clin Transplant 1995;9:201–4.
37. Losonsky GA, Johnson JP, Winkelstein JA, Yolken RH. Oral administration of human serum immunoglobulin in immunodeficient patients with viral gastroenteritis. A pharmacokinetic and functional analysis. J Clin Invest 1985; 76:2362–7.
38. Barnes G, Doyle L, Hewson P, et al. A randomised trial of oral gammaglobulin in low-birth-weight infants infected with rotavirus. Lancet 1982;1:1371–3.
39. Glass R, Bresee J, Parashar U, et al. Rotavirus vaccines at the threshold. Nature Medicine 1997;3:1324–5.
40. Bishop R, Epidemiology of diarrheal disease caused by rotavirus. In: Holmgren J, Lindeberg A, Mollby R, editors. Development of Vaccines and Drugs Against Diarrhea, 11th Nobel Conference. Lund: Student-litteratur; 1986. p. 158.
41. Barnes GL, Bishop RF, Rotavirus infection and prevention. Curr Opin Pediatr 1997;9:19–23.
42. Barnes G, Uren E, Stevens K, Bishop R. Etiology of acute gastroenteritis in hospitalized children in Melbourne, Australia, from April 1980 to March 1993. J Clin Microbiol 1998;36:133–8.
43. Flores J, Midthun K, Hoshino Y, et al. Conservation of the fourth gene among rotaviruses recovered from asymptomatic newborn infants and its possible role in attenuation. J Virol 1986;60:972–9.
44. Chen CM, Hung T, Bridger JC, McCrae MA. Chinese adult rotavirus is a group B rotavirus [letter]. Lancet 1985;2: 1123–4.
45. Griffin DD, Fletcher M, Levy ME, et al. Outbreaks of adult gastroenteritis traced to a single genotype of rotavirus. Novartis Found Symp 2001;238:153–71; discussion 171–9.
46. Griffin DD, Kirkwood CD, Parashar UD, et al. Surveillance of rotavirus strains in the United States: Identification of unusual strains. The National Rotavirus Strain Surveillance System collaborating laboratories. J Clin Microbiol 2000;38:2784–7.
47. Gentsch JR, Woods PA, Ramachandran M, et al. Review of G and P typing results from a global collection of rotavirus strains: Implications for vaccine development. J Infect Dis 1996;174:S30–6.
48. Dong Y, Zeng CQ, Ball JM, et al. The rotavirus enterotoxin NSP4 mobilizes intracellular calcium in human intestinal cells by stimulating phospholipase C-mediated inositol 1,4,5-trisphosphate production. Proc Natl Acad Sci U S A 1997;94:3960–5.
49. Zhang M, Zeng CQ, Dong Y, et al. Mutations in rotavirus nonstructural glycoprotein NSP4 are associated with altered virus virulence. J Virol 1998;72:3666–72.
50. Morris AP, Scott JK, Ball JM, et al. NSP4 elicits age-dependent diarrhea and Ca(2+)mediated I(-) influx into intestinal crypts of CF mice. Am J Physiol 1999;277:G431–44.
51. Horie Y, Nakagomi O, Koshimura Y, et al. Diarrhea induction by rotavirus NSP4 in the homologous mouse model system. Virology 1999;262:398–407.
52. Mori Y, Borgan MA, Ito N, et al. Diarrhea-inducing activity of avian rotavirus NSP4 glycoproteins, which differ greatly from mammalian rotavirus NSP4 glycoproteins in deduced amino acid sequence in suckling mice. J Virol 2002;76:5829–34.
53. Angel J, Tang B, Feng N, et al. Studies of the role for NSP4 in the pathogenesis of homologous murine rotavirus diarrhea. J Infect Dis 1998;177:455–8.
54. Ward RL, Mason BB, Bernstein DI, et al. Attenuation of a human rotavirus vaccine candidate did not correlate with mutations in the NSP4 protein gene. J Virol 1997;71: 6267–70.
55. Lee CN, Wang YL, Kao CL, et al. NSP4 gene analysis of rotaviruses recovered from infected children with and without diarrhea. J Clin Microbiol 2000;38:4471–7.
56. Tafazoli F, Zeng CQ, Estes MK, et al. NSP4 enterotoxin of rotavirus induces paracellular leakage in polarized epithelial cells. J Virol 2001;75:1540–6.
57. Nava P, Lopez S, Arias CF, et al. The rotavirus surface protein VP8 modulates the gate and fence function of tight junctions in epithelial cells. J Cell Sci 2004;117:5509–19.
58. Jourdan N, Brunet JP, Sapin C, et al. Rotavirus infection reduces sucrase-isomaltase expression in human intestinal epithelial cells by perturbing protein targeting and organization of microvillar cytoskeleton. J Virol 1998;72:7228–36.
59. Sheth R, Anderson J, Sato T, et al. Rotavirus stimulates IL-8 secretion from cultured epithelial cells. Virology 1996; 221:251–9.
60. Ray P, Fenaux M, Sharma S, et al. Quantitative evaluation of rotaviral antigenemia in children with acute rotaviral diarrhea. J Infect Dis 2006;194:588–93.
61. Azevedo MS, Yuan L, Jeong KI, et al. Viremia and nasal and rectal shedding of rotavirus in gnotobiotic pigs inoculated with Wa human rotavirus. J Virol 2005;79:5428–36.
62. Chiappini E, Azzari C, Moriondo M, et al. Viraemia is a common finding in immunocompetent children with rotavirus infection. J Med Virol 2005;76:265–7.
63. Blutt SE, Fenaux M, Warfield KL, et al. Active viremia in rotavirus-infected mice. J Virol 2006;80:6702–5.
64. Crawford SE, Patel DG, Cheng E, et al. Rotavirus viremia and extraintestinal viral infection in the neonatal rat model. J Virol 2006;80:4820–32.
65. Ciarlet M, Crawford SE, Estes MK. Differential infection of polarized epithelial cell lines by sialic acid-dependent and sialic acid-independent rotavirus strains. J Virol 2001;75:11834–50.
66. Uhnoo I, Olding SE, Kreuger A. Clinical features of acute gastroenteritis associated with rotavirus, enteric adenoviruses, and bacteria. Arch Dis Child 1986;61:732–8.
67. Makino M, Tanabe Y, Shinozaki K, et al. Haemorrhagic shock and encephalopathy associated with rotavirus infection [see comments]. Acta Paediatrica 1996;85:632–4.
68. Grimwood K, Coakley JC, Hudson IL, et al. Serum aspartate aminotransferase levels after rotavirus gastroenteritis. J Pediatr 1988;112:597–600.
69. Davidson GP, Barnes GL. Structural and functional abnormalities of the small intestine in infants and children with rotavirus enteritis. Acta Ped Scand 1979;68:181–8.
70. Karrar ZA, Abdulla MA, Moody JB, et al. Loperamide in acute diarrhoea in childhood: Results of a double blind, placebo controlled clinical trial. Ann Trop Paediatr 1987;7: 122–7.
71. WHO. The Rational Use of Drugs in the Management of Acute Diarrhea in Children. Geneva: WHO; 1990.
72. Guandalini S, Pensabene L, Zikri MA, et al. Lactobacillus GG administered in oral rehydration solution to children with acute diarrhea: A multicenter European trial. [see comments.]. J Pediatr Gastroenterol Nutr 2000;30:54–60.
73. Costa-Ribeiro H, Ribiero TC, Mattos A, et al. Limitations of probiotic therapy in acute, severe dehydrating diarrhea. J Pediatr Gastroenterol Nutr 2003;36:112–6.
74. Dewey KG, Heinig MJ, Nommsen-Rivers LA. Differences in morbidity between breast-fed and formula-fed infants. J Pediatr 1995;126:696–702.
75. Golding J, Emmett PM, Rogers IS. Gastroenteritis, diarrhoea and breast feeding. Early Hum Dev 1997;49:S83–103.
76. Fuchs SC, Victora CG, Martines J. Case-control study of risk of dehydrating diarrhoea in infants in vulnerable period after full weaning. BMJ (Clinical Research Ed.) 1996;313:391–4.
77. Turner RB, Kelsey DK. Passive immunization for prevention of rotavirus illness in healthy infants. Pediatr Infect Dis J 1993;12:718–22.
78. Sarker SA, Casswall TH, Mahalanabis D, et al. Successful treatment of rotavirus diarrhea in children with immunoglobulin from immunized bovine colostrum. Pediatr Infect Dis J 1998;17:1149–54.
79. Kapikian AZ, Flores J, Hoshino Y, et al. Rotavirus: The major etiologic agent of severe infantile diarrhea may be controllable by a "Jennerian" approach to vaccination. J Infect Dis 1986;153:815–22.
80. Kapikian AZ, Vesikari T, Ruuska T, et al. An update on the "Jennerian" and modified "Jennerian" approach to vaccination of infants and young children against rotavirus diarrhea. Adv Exp Med Biol 1992;327:59–69.
81. Kapikian AZ. A rotavirus vaccine for prevention of severe diarrhoea of infants and young children: Development, utilization and withdrawal. Novartis Found Symp 2001;238:153–71; discussion 171–9.
82. Anonymous. Intussusception among recipients of rotavirus vaccine–US, 1998-1999. Ann Pharmacother 1999;33:1020–1.
83. Murphy TV, Gargiullo PM, Massoudi MS, et al. Intussusception among infants given an oral rotavirus vaccine. [see comments.] [erratum appears in N Engl J Med 2001 May 17;344(20):1564.][Note:Livingood JR [corrected to Livengood JR]]. N Engl J Med 2001;344:564–72.
84. Simonsen L, Morens D, Elixhauser A, et al. Effect of rotavirus vaccination programme on trends in admission of infants to hospital for intussusception. [see comments.]. Lancet 2001;358:1224–9.
85. Vesikari T, Matson DO, Dennehy P, et al. Safety and efficacy of a pentavalent human-bovine (WC3) reassortant rotavirus vaccine.[see comment]. N Engl J Med 2006;354:23–33.
86. Clark HF, Offit PA, Plotkin SA, Heaton PM. The new pentavalent rotavirus vaccine composed of bovine (strain WC3) -human rotavirus reassortants. Pediatr Infect Dis J 2006;25:577–83.
87. Ruiz-Palacios GM, Perez-Schael I, Velazquez FR, et al. Safety and efficacy of an attenuated vaccine against severe rotavirus gastroenteritis.[see comment]. N Engl J Med 2006;354:11–22.
88. Bernstein DI. Live attenuated human rotavirus vaccine, Rotarix. Semin Pediatr Infect Dis 2006;17:188–94.
89. Madeley CR, Cosgrove BP. Viruses in infantile gastroenteritis. Lancet 1975;2:124.
90. Echeverria P, Hoge CW, Bodhidatta L, et al. Etiology of diarrhea in a rural community in western Thailand: Importance of enteric viruses and enterovirulent Escherichia coli. J Infect Dis 1994;169:916–9.
91. Herrmann JE, Taylor DN, Echeverria P, Blacklow NR. Astroviruses as a cause of gastroenteritis in children. N Engl J Med 1991;324:1757–60.
92. Kotloff KL, Herrmann JE, Blacklow NR, et al. The frequency of astrovirus as a cause of diarrhea in Baltimore children. Pediatr Infect Dis J 1992;11:587–9.
93. Rodriguez-Baez N, O'Brien R, Qiu SQ, Bass DM. Astrovirus, adenovirus, and rotavirus in hospitalized children: Prevalence and association with gastroenteritis. J Pediatr Gastroenterol Nutr 2002;35:64–8.
94. Maldonado Y, Cantwell M, Old M, et al. Population-based prevalence of symptomatic and asymptomatic astrovirus infection in rural Mayan infants. J Infect Dis 1998;178:334–9.
95. Shastri S, Doane AM, Gonzales J, et al. Prevalence of astroviruses in a children's hospital. J Clin Microbiol 1998;36:2571–4.
96. Grohmann GS, Glass RI, Pereira HG, et al. Enteric viruses and diarrhea in HIV-infected patients. Enteric Opportunistic Infections Working Group. N Engl J Med 1993;329:14–20.
97. Cox GJ, Matsui SM, Lo RS, et al. Etiology and outcome of diarrhea after marrow transplantation: A prospective study. Gastroenterology 1994;107:1398–407.
98. Belliot G, Laveran H, Monroe SS. Outbreak of gastroenteritis in military recruits associated with serotype 3 astrovirus infection. J Med Virol 1997;51:101–6.
99. Gray JJ, Wreghitt TG, Cubitt WD, Elliot PR. An outbreak of gastroenteritis in a home for the elderly associated with astrovirus type 1 and human calicivirus. J Med Virol 1987;23:377–81.
100. Lewis DC, Lightfoot NF, Cubitt WD, Wilson SA. Outbreaks of astrovirus type 1 and rotavirus gastroenteritis in a geriatric in-patient population. J Hosp Infect 1989;14:9–14.
101. Sebire NJ, Malone M, Shah N, et al. Pathology of astrovirus associated diarrhoea in a paediatric bone marrow transplant recipient. J Clin Pathol 2004;57:1001–3.
102. Gray EW, Angus KW, Snodgrass DR. Ultrastructure of the small intestine in astrovirus-infected lambs. J Gen Virol 1980;49:71–82.
103. Woode GN, Pohlenz JF, Gourley NE, Fagerland JA. Astrovirus and Breda virus infections of dome cell epithelium of bovine ileum. J Clin Microbiol 1984;19:623–30.
104. Kurtz JB, Lee TW, Craig JW, Reed SE. Astrovirus infection in volunteers. J Med Virol 1979;3:221–30.
105. Molberg O, Nilsen EM, Sollid LM, et al. CD4+ T cells with specific reactivity against astrovirus isolated from normal human small intestine [see comments]. Gastroenterology 1998;114:115–22.
106. Bjorkholm M, Celsing F, Runarsson G, Waldenstrom J. Successful intravenous immunoglobulin therapy for severe and persistent astrovirus gastroenteritis after fludarabine treatment in a patient with Waldenstrom's macroglobulinemia. Int J Hematol 1995;62:117–20.
107. Kapikian AZ, Wyatt RG, Dolin R, et al. Visualization by immune electron microscopy of a 27-nm particle associated with acute infectious nonbacterial gastroenteritis. J Virol 1972;10:1075–81.
108. Jiang X, Rraham DY, Wang K, Estes MK. Norwalk virus genome cloning and characterization. Science 1990;250: 1580–3.
109. Fankhauser RL, Noel JS, Monroe SS, et al. Molecular epidemiology of "Norwalk-like viruses" in outbreaks of gastroenteritis in the United States. J Infect Dis 1998;178:1571–8.
110. Spratt HC, Marks MI, Gomersall M, et al. Nosocomial infantile gastroenteritis associated with minirotavirus and calicivirus. J Pediatr 1978;93:922–6.
111. Kitamoto N, Tanaka T, Natori K, et al. Cross-reactivity among several recombinant calicivirus virus-like particles (VLPs) with monoclonal antibodies obtained from mice immunized orally with one type of VLP. J Clin Microbiol 2002;40:2459–65.
112. Agus SG, Dolin R, Wyatt RG, et al. Acute infectious nonbacterial gastroenteritis: Intestinal histopathology. Histologic and enzymatic alterations during illnes prodfuced by the Norwalk agent in man. Ann Intern Med 1973;79:18–25.

113. Schreiber DS, Blacklow NR, Trier JS. The small intestinal lesion induced by the Hawaii agent in infectious nonbacterial gastroenteritis. J. Infect. Dis 1974:705–8.

114. Atmar RL, Graham DY, Estes MK, Marionneau S. Norwalk virus binds to histo-blood group antigens present on gastroduodenal epithelial cells of secretor individuals. J Infect Dis 2002;185:1335–7.

115. Atmar RL, Marcus DM, Estes MK, Hutson AM. Norwalk virus infection and disease is associated with ABO histo-blood group type. J Virol 2003;77:405–15.

116. Brandt CD, Kim IIW, Rodriguez WJ, et al. Pediatric viral gastroenteritis during eight years of study. J Clin Microbiol 1983;18:71–8.

117. Van R, Wun CC, O'Ryan ML, et al. Outbreaks of human enteric adenovirus types 40 and 41 in Houston day care centers. J Pediatr 1992;120:516–21.

118. Khoo SH, Bailey AS, de Jong JC, Mandal BK. Adenovirus infections in human immunodeficiency virus-positive patients: Clinical features and molecular epidemiology. J Infect Dis 1995;172:629–37.

119. Dionisio D, Arista S, Vizzi E, et al. Chronic intestinal infection due to subgenus F type 40 adenovirus in a patient with AIDS. Scand J InfectDis 1997;29:305–7.

120. Durepaire N, Ranger-Rogez S, Gandji JA, et al. Enteric prevalence of adenovirus in human immunodeficiency virus seropositive patients. J Med Virol 1995;45:56–60.

121. Lew EA, Poles MA, Dieterich DT. Diarrheal diseases associated with HIV infection. Gastroenterol Clin North Am 1997;26:259–90.

122. Vizzi E, Ferraro D, Cascio A, et al. Detection of enteric adenoviruses 40 and 41 in stool specimens by monoclonal antibody-based enzyme immunoassays. Res Virol 1996;147: 333–9.

123. Kapelushnik J, Or R, Delukina M, et al. Intravenous ribavirin therapy for adenovirus gastroenteritis after bone marrow transplantation. J Pediatr Gastroenterol Nutr 1995;21: 110–2.

124. Marks MP, Lanza MV, Kahlstrom EJ, et al. Pediatric hypertrophic gastropathy. AJR. Am J Roentgenol 1986;147: 1031–4.

125. Huang YC, Lin TY, Huang CS, Hseun C. Ileal perforation caused by congenital or perinatal cytomegalovirus infection [see comments]. J Pediatr 1996;129:931–4.

126. Fox LM, Gerber MA, Penix L, et al. Intractable diarrhea from cytomegalovirus enterocolitis in an immunocompetent infant. Pediatrics 1999;103:E10.

127. Yamashita T, Kobayashi S, Sakae K, et al. Isolation of cytopathic small round viruses with BS-C-1 cells from patients with gastroenteritis. J Infect Dis 1991;164:954–7.

128. Yamashita T, Sakae K, Kobayashi EJ, et al. Isolation of cytopathic small round virus (Aichi virus) from Pakistani children and Japanese travelers from Southeast Asia. Microbiol Immunol 1995;39:433–5.

129. Yamashita T, Sakae K, Tsuzuki H, et al. Complete nucleotide sequence and genetic organization of Aichi virus, a distinct member of the Picornaviridae associated with acute gastroenteritis in humans. Uirusu 1999;49:183–91.

130. Bresee J, Jiang B, Gentsch J, et al. Application of a reverse transcription-PCR for identification and differentiation of Aichi virus, a new member of the Picornavirus family associated with gastroenteritis in humans. Novartis Found Symp 2001;238:5–19; discussion 19–25.

131. Gonzalez GG, Pujol FH, Liprandi F, et al. Prevalence of enteric viruses in human immunodeficiency virus seropositive patients in Venezuela. J Med Virol 1998;55:288–92.

132. Giordano MO, Martinez LC, Rinaldi D, et al. Detection of picobirnavirus in HIV-infected patients with diarrhea in Argentina. J Acquir Immune Defic Syndr Hum Retrovirol 1998;18:380–3.

133. Duckmanton L, Luan B, Devenish J, et al. Characterization of torovirus from human fecal specimens. Virology 1997; 239:158–68.

134. Koopmans MP, Goosen FS, Lima AA, et al. Association of torovirus with acute and persistent diarrhea in children. Pediatr Infect Dis J 1997;16:504–7.

135. Jamieson FB, Wang EE, Bain C, et al. Human torovirus: A new nosocomial gastrointestinal pathogen. J Infect Dis 1998;178:1263–9.

136. Jirapinyo P, Thakerngpol K, Chaichanwatanakul K, et al. Cytopathic effects of measles virus on the human intestinal mucosa. J pediatr gastroenterol nutr 1990;10:550–4.

137. Ullrich R, Zeitz M, Heise W, et al. Small intestinal structure and function in patients infected with human immunodeficiency virus (HIV): Evidence for HIV-induced enteropathy. Ann intern med 1989;111:15–21.

138. Brenchley JM, Price DA, Schacker TW, et al. Microbial translocation is a cause of systemic immune activation in chronic HIV infection.[see comment]. Nature Med 2006;12:1365–71.

139. Kotler DP. Characterization of intestinal disease associated with human immunodeficiency virus infection and response to antiretroviral therapy. J Infect Dis 1999;3: S454–6.

19.2c. Parasitic and Fungal Infections

Michael J. G. Farthing, DSc(Med), MD, FRCP, FMedSci
Paul Kelly, MD, FRCP
Beatrice C. Amadi, MD

Parasitic infections of the gastrointestinal (GI) tract occur in all geographic regions of the world and produce a substantial morbidity in children. Recent evidence confirms that there is increased mortality in children with some parasitic infections such as that due to *Cryptosporidium parvum,* especially when infection is associated with undernutrition and other comorbidities. Prevalence is highest in the economically deprived regions of the world, notably in the tropics. Infants and young children are particularly susceptible to *Giardia lamblia, C. parvum, Ascaris lumbricoides,* and *Trichuris trichiura.* In addition to producing GI symptoms, these parasites may impair growth and development.

There has been controversy regarding the clinical relevance of many of these common intestinal parasitic infections, which often appear to coexist with their hosts without causing significant clinical problems. However, recent studies confirm the importance of many of these infections, particularly in immunocompromised children with severe undernutrition or human immunodeficiency virus (HIV) infection.

Diagnostic tests for many GI parasites continue to be limited, usually relying on microscopic techniques and a skilled observer. Similarly, the development of new drugs for the control of these infections has been slower than that for other infectious diseases because drug development programs tend to focus on the needs of the more profitable industrialized world.

These common infections can have a major impact on child health and, therefore, need to be considered as one of the objectives of any diarrhea control and nutritional intervention program. Several GI parasites (*G. lamblia, C. parvum*) have become common in industrialized parts of the world, partly owing to increased foreign travel and immigration.

PARASITES OF THE ESOPHAGUS

Trypanosoma cruzi (South American Trypanosomiasis or Chagas Disease)

Primary infection with *T. cruzi,* a protozoan hemoflagellate, generally occurs in early childhood. The parasite is transmitted through the bite of a blood-sucking vector insect of the family Reduviidae. During the blood meal, the infective form of the parasite is deposited with the insect's feces on the skin and rubbed into the bite wound or a mucous membrane susceptible to invasion, such as the conjunctiva. The vast majority of initial illnesses pass unnoticed, but in some cases, there is marked fever, lymphadenopathy, and hepatosplenomegaly. In severe infection, there may be signs and symptoms of acute myocarditis. Death can occur as a result of this acute illness, but the individual may recover within a few weeks or months.

The development of the "megasyndromes" occurs many years later, with more than 90% of symptomatic patients being 20 or more years of age. In Brazil, achalasia and megaesophagus occur in approximately 6% of seropositive patients, whereas megacolon appears to be less common, affecting only 1%. In Argentina and Chile, however, megacolon is more common than megaesophagus.

A medical approach to the management of these conditions is usually attempted with either nifurtimox (10 mg/kg in three divided doses for at least 90 d) or benznidazole (5 to 10 mg/kg in two divided doses for 60 d).

Schistosoma mansoni

S. mansoni is a cause of esophageal varices in older children (usually over 10 yr of age), and in endemic parts of the world it is the most common cause. Although the pathology is actually due to release of eggs from adult worms resident in the mesenteric veins, the clinical manifestation (ie, the varices) is seen in the esophagus. We therefore introduce it here although the full discussion of the infection is set out in the section on colonic parasites.

PARASITES OF THE STOMACH

Anisakis anisakis

Anisakis is a nematode parasite in marine mammals and fish. Humans are incidental hosts, infected by ingestion of raw fish or poorly cooked fish, octopus and squid. It is found mainly in Japan, Holland, Scandinavia, and the Pacific Coast of South America.[1–3] Many cases have been particularly reported in Japan, where it is customary to eat raw fish, and about 20,500 cases were reported between 1980 and 1993.[4] Ninety-three percent of the cases involved the stomach and only 4.4% were intestinal disease. The growing trend of consuming raw fish is responsible for increased cases in Europe, America, and Asia. Anisakiasis is uncommon in children.

Following ingestion of contaminated food, there is usually an acute upper GI illness (usually within 6 h of ingestion of raw seafood)[5] with epigastric pain, nausea, and vomiting. The fundus of the stomach, rarely tongue, tonsil uvula, and esophagus are the usual sites of infection. The disease is also classified into gastric, intestinal, and extraintestinal (ectopic) anisakiasis. The last form is caused by larvae that penetrate into the abdominal or pleural cavity, entering abdominal or pleural organs or tissues (eg, omentum, mesentery, peritoneum, liver, pancreas, ovary lymph node, lung, and even in the subcutaneous tissue) and provoking inflammatory foci.

Intestinal anisakiasis[2] may be anywhere between the duodenum and rectum and usually developed within 2 days after infection. Symptoms usually last 1 to 5 days and then lead to ileus. At times patients may develop ascites. Patients usually have no fever but develop moderate leukocytosis and in some cases eosinophilia (4 to 41%).[3–4] Single worm infection is common, but multiple infections occur, for example, approximately 50 larvae were recovered from a Japanese patient.

Diagnosis is difficult due to the nonspecific nature of the clinical manifestations. Patients with a history of consumption of raw seafood, should be referred for endoscopy, which is both diagnostic and the mainstay of therapy. Larvae attaching to gastric mucosa and sometimes to duodenal mucosa can be identified at endoscopy and can be removed by biopsy. Recent uncontrolled reports suggest that albendazole or ivermectin,[6] and even corticosteroids,[7] may have some benefit.

PARASITES OF THE SMALL INTESTINE

A variety of protozoa and helminths may infect the small intestine (Table 1); some can simultaneously colonize the large intestine as well, notably *Cryptosporidium* species and *Strongyloides stercoralis,* the latter as part of the hyperinfection syndrome.

Table 1 Parasites of the Small Intestine

Parasite	Estimated global importance*		
	Infancy	Childhood	Adolescence
Protozoa			
Giardia intestinalis†	±	+++	+
Cryptosporidium sp.†	±	+++	+
Microsporidium sp.†	±	+	+
Isospora belli†	±	++	+
Sarcocystis sp.†	−	+	+
Cyclospora cayetanensis†	−	++	+
Nematodes			
Strongyloides stercoralis†	±	+++	+
Capillaria philippinensis†	−	++	+
Trichinella spiralis†	−	+	+
Trichostrongylus orientalis†	−	+	+
Ascaris lumbricoides	±	+++	++
Ankylostoma duodenale	±	+++	++
Necator americanus	±	+++	++
Cestodes			
Taenia saginata	−	++	++
Taenia solium	−	++	++
Hymenolepis nana	−	+	+
Trematodes			
Fasciolopis buski	−	+	+
Heterophyes heterophyes	−	+	+
Metagonimus yokogawai	−	+	+

*These are rough approximations that attempt to take into account marked geographic variations.
†Parasites that can cause diarrhea and malabsorption.

PROTOZOA

Giardia lamblia

Giardia lamblia is distributed worldwide and more common in warm climate than in cool ones.[8] It may be identified in individuals with asymptomatic colonization and can cause acute or chronic diarrheal disease. The infection is recognized more in children than in adults.[9] Giardiasis is associated with malabsorption, which may be severe, such that chronic infection in children may be associated with poor growth.

This flagellate exists as a motile trophozoite and as a cyst, the latter being the infective form of the parasite. The trophozoite has a smooth dorsal surface and a convex ventral surface occupied by the ventral disk (Figure 1). This disk consists of contractile proteins that are thought to mediate the attachment of the parasite to the intestinal epithelium. The surface membrane of *Giardia* contains a lectin that is activated by trypsin and is thought to participate in the attachment to intestinal epithelial cells.

The taxonomy of *G. lamblia* has been reported using a variety of techniques, including antigen, isoenzyme, and deoxyribonucleic acid (DNA) analyses.[8–9] These approaches have confirmed that *G. lamblia* isolates differ from one another, although the sensitivity of the techniques varies. Molecular genetic approaches show that *G. lamblia* isolates can be divided into seven assemblages, A–G, and that A and B can be subdivided into AI and AII and BI and BII.[11] Assemblages A and B can infect a wide range of animals, and there is evidence that giardiasis is frequently a zoonosis, though probably not through direct contact with animals.[12]

Epidemiology. Giardia is found in most countries of the world, and its prevalence is highest in young children in the developing world, where it may approach 30%,[13] particularly in young children. Age-specific prevalence rates increase

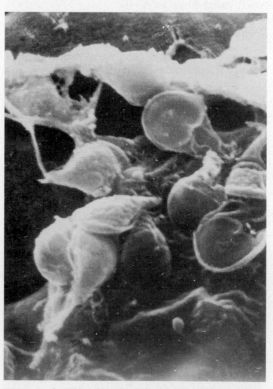

Figure 1 Scanning electron micrograph of *Giardia lamblia* trophozoites in mucus on human jejunal mucosa.

throughout infancy and childhood but approach adult levels only during adolescence.[13] Infection is transmitted by food, water, and direct person-to-person contact.

Pathophysiology. The mechanisms by which *G. lamblia* causes diarrhea and malabsorption have not been determined, and several mechanisms of pathogenesis have been put forward.[13–15]

Mucosal factors:
- Direct damage by trophozoites
  - Microvilli
  - Disaccharidases
  - Transport protein
- Parasite products
  - Proteases
  - Lectin
- Immune mediated
  - T-cell activation

Luminal factors:
- Bacterial overgrowth
- Inhibition of digestive enzymes
- Bile salt deconjugation
- Bile salt uptake by trophozoites

Jejunal morphology may be normal, although partial atrophy and even total villous atrophy are reported.[16–17] The presence of a mucosal inflammatory response, with an early increase in intraepithelial lymphocytes,[18–19] suggests that mucosal damage may be immunologically mediated. Nude mice with T-cell deficiency fail to develop significant alterations in villous architecture during experimental infection, supporting the view that activated T cells are responsible for the mucosal abnormality.[14] Steatorrhea, however, can occur in the absence of significant histopathologic abnormality, suggesting that other factors, such as bacterial overgrowth, bile salt uptake by the parasite, and inhibition of pancreatic lipase, may be additional pathogenic mechanisms.[14] It is likely that the pathophysiology of giardiasis is multifactorial.[15,20]

Evidence indicates that different *Giardia* isolates vary in virulence in experimental models of infection.[21] This relates specifically to the ability of different isolates to affect water and electrolyte absorption and to alter the expression of disaccharidases in the microvillous membrane.

Clinical Features. The most common form of giardiasis is asymptomatic carriage. Adults and children commonly harbor *Giardia* without symptoms, particularly those living in highly endemic areas in the developing countries, although it also occurs in Europe and North America. However, infection early in life is usually symptomatic. The incubation period from the time of ingestion of cysts until the onset of symptoms is 3 to 20 days, average 8 days. Acute infection often begins with watery diarrhea that persists and is associated with anorexia and abdominal distension. Other associated signs and symptoms include flatulence, abdominal cramps, malodorous, greasy stools, weight loss, and urticaria. Acute giardiasis has been well characterized in individuals traveling from areas of low to high endemicity.[8,14]

Untreated, chronic diarrhea with steatorrhea ensues, and growth may be impaired.[22] Chronic giardiasis can be associated with immunoglobulin (Ig) deficiency,[23] which may be accompanied by diffuse nodular lymphoid hyperplasia involving the small and sometimes the large intestine.[24] Fifty percent of symptomatic patients with persistent diarrhea will have biochemical evidence of fat malabsorption and possibly other nutrients, including vitamin A and vitamin B12. Secondary lactase deficiency is well recognized to occur in human giardiasis, and patients may take weeks to recover even after clearance of the parasite.

Diagnosis. Identification of *Giardia* forms by microscopy of feces, duodenal fluid, or mucosal biopsy specimens remains the "gold standard" for diagnosis.[14] However, even after examination of multiple stool specimens, only 80% of positive individuals will be diagnosed. Fresh and preserved stool samples should be examined. Motile trophozoites are best identified in a wet saline mount of fresh liquid stool obtained during the illness. Trophozoites are usually not found in semi-formed stool. Cysts are best detected in fresh stools after iodine staining or preservation in 10% buffered formalin alcohol, with subsequent trichrome or iron hematoxylin staining. Concentration techniques using formalin ether or zinc sulfate flotation may increase the yield.

Antigen-based fecal detection assays have been developed which are specific but not sensitive (none higher than 80%) and cannot be used as a substitute for careful microscopy.[25] The measurement of specific anti-*Giardia* IgG antibody has not been helpful, but there is an early IgM response in acute giardiasis that can distinguish current from past infection. Sensitive and specific IgG-based immunoassays have been developed, and some of these assays are now marketed commercially.[25–27] An immunofluorescence assay is available for detecting *Giardia* and *Cryptosporidium* species. Deoxyribonucleic acid (DNA) probes for *Giardia* species are available.

Treatment. The drugs of choice are nitroimidazole derivatives, namely metronidazole (30 mg/kg as a single dose on 3 consecutive d) or tinidazole (30 mg/kg as a single dose),[14] but recently it has emerged that nitazoxanide is as effective (100 mg bd for 3 d if age 2 to 3 yr, 200 mg bd for age 4 to 11 yr)[28]. Alternatives include mepacrine (2 mg/kg three times daily for 7 d) and furazolidone (1.25 mg/kg four times daily for 7 d). Albendazole is also effective in giardiasis (400 mg once daily for 5 to 7 d). Adverse effects with nitroimidazole derivatives include anorexia, nausea, vomiting, and peripheral neuropathy. In addition to GI side effects, mepacrine causes yellowing of the skin, sclerae, and blood dyscrasia.

Cryptosporidium Species

Cryptosporidium muris infection in the gastric mucosa of laboratory mice was first described in 1907 by Tyzzer. In 1912, Tyzzer identified a small parasite *C. parvum*, in the intestinal villi of mice, that is now recognized as a major cause of cryptosporidiosis in mammals. In 1976, the first human infection with *Cryptosporidium* was discovered in a 3-year-old immunocompromised child,[29] and since then the infection has risen to prominence due to AIDS and to some spectacularly large waterborne outbreaks. The genome of this pathogen has now been sequenced.[30] *Cryptosporidium* spp. are coccidia belonging to the subphylum sporozoa. Recently, the distinct species *C. hominis* has been recognized as a consequence of genetic studies which have established that these isolates of *Cryptosporidium* are exclusively human.[31] *Cryptosporidium* reproduces both sexually and asexually and can complete its life cycle within the host due to the generation of thin-walled oocysts which allow autoinfection. The thick-walled oocyst is the infective form which survives outside the host in cool, moist conditions. Cryptosporidiosis causes diarrhea, which can be severe but is usually self-limiting, except in immunocompromised individuals in whom chronic infection develops and can be life-threatening.

Epidemiology. *Cryptosporidium* species are found throughout the world and human infection is widespread. There is an age-related incidence and prevalence even in highly endemic areas: infection is uncommon in early infancy,[32] rises around weaning and diminishes through adolescence and into adulthood as immunity prevents infection. Even in adulthood, however, asymptomatic infection is not uncommon and as with many other infections it is apparent that immunity serves to reduce the likelihood of disease rather than the likelihood of infection. In industrialized countries, infection is much less common which leaves these populations open to waterborne outbreaks, which can be very large, and individuals are open to traveler's diarrhea when they travel to areas of higher endemicity. The protection against infection in early infancy is presumably due to breast-feeding,[32] so in endemic areas where breast-feeding is discouraged (such as in maternal HIV infection), it is likely that infection in this group will rise.

One of the strongest risk factors for cryptosporidiosis is HIV infection. Prior to highly active antiretroviral therapy (HAART), 10% or more of HIV-infected individuals could expect to become infected at some stage in their illness.[33] However, cryptosporidiosis in AIDS patients now is much less common than it was because of HAART. In sub-Saharan Africa, where the availability of HAART is more limited, cryptosporidiosis is still common, and the authors continue to see cryptosporidiosis in patients who have not started HAART and in those with failure of HAART due to resistance or noncompliance. Cryptosporidiosis remains an important infection in malnourished children.[34]

As with *Giardia*, asymptomatic carriage is well recognized (Mwiya M., personal communication). There is evidence that transmission may relate to waterborne oocyst contamination[35–36] and by direct person-to-person contact as occurs in developing countries in hospitalized children sharing cots (Mwiya M., personal communication) or day-care centers. Chlorination of water does not inactivate oocysts, so outbreaks occur when filtration systems fail. The largest of these affected over 400,000 people in Milwaukee, Wisconsin.[37] This has raised considerable concern among water supply companies around the world, including a statutory requirement to monitor water supplies for oocysts.[38]

Cryptosporidiosis is also a major case of endemic diarrhea in children among the poor of the third world. In Africa, and South and Southeast Asia, cryptosporidiosis occurs in children with and without HIV infection. In developed countries, outbreaks have originated in day care nurseries. The prevalence among children with diarrhea in developed countries ranges from 1.4% in the UK[39] to 4% in Ireland,[40] 4.6% in Switzerland,[41] and 6% in another study in the UK.[42] In underdeveloped countries, prevalence among children with diarrhea is higher, ranging from 3.4% in Myanmar[43] to 8.4% in Rwanda,[44] and 15% in Nigeria.[45] Studies from China give prevalence ranging from 1 to 13%.[46] In view of the variability in selection of children in hospitals or in the community in the quoted studies, these estimates are only approximates. In population-based studies in Lusaka, 17% of diarrhea episodes in 222 children were associated with this infection.[36] In malnourished children with persistent diarrhea admitted to the University Teaching Hospital, Lusaka, Zambia, the prevalence was 25%, and the prevalence in HIV-seropositive children was similar to that in HIV-seronegative children.[34] Cryptosporidiosis is a case-defining diagnosis for AIDS in children. It is likely that patients with AIDS-related cryptosporidiosis act as reservoirs of the parasite and transmit it to other adults and children in poor communities.

Pathophysiology. The pathophysiological processes by which this parasite produces acute watery diarrhea are unknown. The most common site of infection in persistent cases is the ileum and ileocecal region.[47] The presence of trophozoites leads to destruction of the microvilli comprising the brush border. Brush border enzymes, particularly disaccharidases, are reduced in children with cryptosporidiosis.[48] Histopathological abnormalities can be severe even when a patient does not have AIDS. AIDS patients from United States with cryptosporidiosis had jejunal mucosa that was associated with more severe enteropathy than mucosa from patients in whom no pathogen detected,[49] but this was not found in an African series.[50] Ultrastructural studies clearly show disruption of the microvillus membrane (Figure 2), particularly at the sites where the parasite is adherent to the epithelial cells. Infection is often accompanied by an inflammatory cell infiltrate in the lamina propria which may contribute to mucosal damage and dysfunction. Inflammatory mediators are likely to play a major part in the pathophysiology of cryptosporidiosis.[51]

Specific virulence factors have not been identified; however, the organism does possess an *N*-acetylgalactose-binding lectin thought to be involved in the mediation of adherence to the

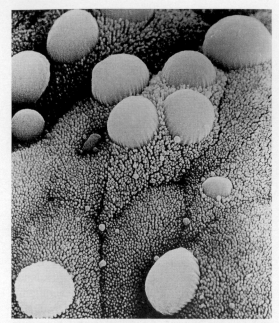

Figure 2 Scanning electron micrograph of *Cryptosporidium* species. (Courtesy of Patricia Bland and David Burden, ARFC Institute for Animal Disease Research, Compton.)

epithelial cells. In addition, a parasite phospholipase has been identified that appears to have a role in parasite invasion in vitro models.[52] Studies in experimental models indicate that impairment of water and sodium absorption is mediated, at least in part, by local production of prostaglandins in the intestinal mucosa. Intestinal perfusion studies in HIV-infected humans with cryptosporidiosis, however, failed to demonstrate any abnormality of water and electrolyte absorption in jejunum.[53] Likewise, studies in a neonatal piglet model did not show evidence of net fluid and electrolyte secretion.[54]

Clinical Features. Acute infection in an immunocompetent individual usually has an incubation period of 1 to 7 days, followed by watery diarrhea, often high volume, with or without fever, abdominal discomfort, nausea, and vomiting. The illness may resolve within 2 days or may continue for 2 to 3 weeks. As cryptosporidiosis is caused by an intracellular parasite, abnormalities of T-cell immunology seriously impair the host capacity to clear infection, leading to a persistent infection. Human immunodeficiency virus (HIV) infection and AIDS lead to a greatly increased risk of cryptosporidiosis, as do other primary or secondary immunodeficiencies. These include severe combined immunodeficiency (SCID), other T-cell deficiencies, deficiencies of mannose-binding lectin,[55] and X-linked immunodeficiency with hyperimmunoglobulin (Ig) M caused by mutations in the CD40 ligand gene.[56] Children with acute leukemia also have increased susceptibility to cryptosporidiosis.[57] The clinical picture of the infection is variable, and there is variation in disease severity even after accounting for the degree of immune deficiency by blood CD4 cell count.

There is an important interaction between cryptosporidiosis and nutritional impairment. This is true of children with and without HIV infection,[34] probably because persistent cryptosporidiosis

causes severe anorexia, and mucosal damage also leads malabsorption of micronutrients. In children, cryptosporidiosis seems to lead to an increased risk of nutritional problems. A series of studies on children living in Guinea-Bissau has revealed that children who were undernourished were not more likely to develop the infection, but children with cryptosporidiosis are more likely to go on to lose weight after the infection.[58–59] A series of Brazilian studies found that cryptosporidiosis was associated with persistent diarrhea,[60] and this is associated with nutritional shortfalls[61] and with diminished cognitive function.[62] In malnourished children with persistent diarrhea in Zambia, cryptosporidiosis was associated with considerably increased mortality independently of HIV infection.[34] Dehydration can be severe in cryptosporidiosis and is complicated in the malnourished, in whom assessment of severity of dehydration may be problematic, particularly in marasmic patients. Often the stools are acidic with positive-reducing substances, probably as a consequence of lactose intolerance which is a consequence of enteropathy due to cryptosporidiosis.

Some patients develop small bowel disease alone, while others may also have involvement of the biliary tract. A syndrome of sclerosing cholangitis, sometimes associated with cholecystitis, has been described in AIDS patients. This may be associated with cryptosporidial infection of the biliary tract, with microsporidiosis or with cytomegalovirus or it may be impossible to identify the cause. The disorder usually occurs in patients with chronic diarrhea and is associated with progressive right upper quadrant abdominal pain. Biochemical tests of hepatic damage usually show raised serum levels of alkaline phosphatase and γ-glutamyltransferase in the absence of jaundice. The definitive test is endoscopic retrograde cholangiopancreatography (ERCP) or the magnetic resonance equivalent MRCP, which shows this distortion of the biliary anatomy, with or without papillary stenosis. Cholangitis is rare now that HIV infection is treated with HAART.

Diagnosis. Cryptosporidiosis is usually diagnosed by the detection of stained oocysts in fecal smears using acid-fast methods such as modified Ziehl-Neelsen and phenol auramine. The oocysts are 4.5 to 5.0 μm in size and round or slightly oval in shape.[63] Oocysts may be concentrated beforehand by centrifugation in Sheather's sugar solution if necessary or saturated sodium chloride. Monoclonal antibodies against oocyst wall antigens have been employed in *Cryptosporidium*-specific immunofluorescence antibody tests with fecal specimens.[64] Antigen detection techniques are not yet in routine use due to low sensitivity, as with *Giardia*.[25]

Treatment. *C. parvum* has proved to be one of the most difficult protozoal infections to treat. Over 100 compounds have been tried without success.[64] Earlier hopes that spiramycin, letrazuril, and now paromomycin[65] would be effective have faded. In AIDS patients, effective antiret-

roviral therapy is a very important component of management.[66] Recent experience with HAART has had a major impact on the prevalence and severity of opportunistic infection such that cryptosporidiosis is now rarely seen in HIV-infected patients treated with this regimen. Although HAART may not completely eradicate infection, it reduces parasite numbers to such low levels that they no longer produce clinically relevant disease. However, infection may recur if HAART is discontinued and CD4 cell counts decrease. For too many of the world's AIDS patients, HAART is still inaccessible.

Nitazoxanide, a nitrothiazolyl-salicylamide derivative, is a broad-spectrum antimicrobial agent with activity against protozoa, nematodes, cestodes, trematodes, and bacteria, including *Cryptosporidium*.[67] In randomized controlled trials, nitazoxanide was found to have significant benefit in HIV-seronegative children with cryptosporidiosis in Zambia,[68] in immunocompetent adults and children in Egypt, and in AIDS patients in Mexico.[69] In December 2002, the Food and Drug Administration (FDA) approved nitazoxanide as an oral suspension to treat immunocompetent children with diarrhea caused by *Cryptosporidium*. A 3-day course is effective: children under 4 years receive 100 mg twice daily and those over 4 years 200 mg twice daily, orally. Early data indicate that HIV-positive adults or children require a longer course, but the duration is as yet uncertain. Early data suggest intriguingly that rifamycins may prevent cryptosporidiosis in AIDS patients.[70] The most important aspect of treatment is fluid and electrolyte replacement with oral rehydration solutions with continued appropriate feeding. In patients with profuse watery diarrhea, with increased frequency, intravenous therapy may be necessary. There is a chance of underreporting the frequency and amount of diarrhea since the stools at times may appear urine-like. In severely malnourished children, generally signs of dehydration may be difficult to appreciate, and hence inadequate amounts of fluids may be prescribed, leading to death due to dehydration and electrolyte imbalance. In terms of feeds, use of lactose-free feeds, particularly in children with malnutrition and persistent diarrhea may lead to reduced stool volume and better outcome (Amadi, personal communication). Antidiarrheal medications, such as opiates (morphine, codeine) and opioids (loperamide), or the somatostatin analogue octreotide also may prove useful in those patients who are intolerant or who fail to respond to HAART.

Isospora belli and *Sarcocystis* Species

Isospora belli was first described in 1915 but has received much less attention in the world literature than *Cryptosporidium* spp. It has recently attracted interest because of its importance in patients with AIDS. The infective form of the parasite is the oocyst, which releases sporozoites, leading to a small bowel infection. The parasite takes up an intracellular location and undergoes merogony and sporogony.

Epidemiology. The route of transmission is not established but fecal-oral spread seems likely. Infection is uncommon in developed countries; this is largely a tropical infection and less common in children than adults.[34]

Pathogenesis. Isosporiasis is associated with mild to a subtotal villous atrophy.[71] Inflammatory cells and eosinophils are seen in the lamina propria.

Clinical Features. As with cryptosporidiosis, isosporiasis leads to a self-limiting diarrhea in the immunocompetent, and to a chronic diarrhea in the immunocompromised. In AIDS, isosporiasis is associated with watery diarrhea, dehydration, cramping abdominal pain, nausea, and wasting.[71–72] Children can develop profuse diarrhea and go on to develop chronic malabsorptive state with steatorrhea and weight loss, though isosporiasis is less common in children than in adults with AIDS in Africa.[34,73]

Diagnosis. Stool examination using wet preparations and modified Ziehl-Neelsen acid-fast stained smears is the preferred method of diagnosis. The oocysts appear oval, larger than cryptosporidial oocysts. Some oocysts are sporulated before leaving the host and have two easily identified sporoblasts. The oocysts fluoresce with a phenol auramine stain under ultraviolet light. The parasites may also be recognized in small bowel biopsies, visible within enterocyte cytoplasmic vacuoles under electron microscopy and light microscopy.

Management. Treatment with co-trimoxazole 960 mg four times daily for 10 days eliminates parasite from stool in most cases, with an interruption in diarrhea.[72,74] This dose used for adults is doubled the usual dose, so although evidence is lacking for children, the dose used in children is also doubled. Unfortunately this is followed by relapse in 50%, usually within 12 weeks. Although retreatment is usually effective, secondary prophylaxis is necessary until immune reconstitution has been achieved with HAART. Although secondary prophylaxis requires co-trimoxazole to be given only three times per week, we believe that patients find this difficult to adhere to and we give 960 mg daily, with proportionately less for children. Pyrimethamine-sulphonamide combinations are also effective.[74] There is little information on the regimen of choice for those who are intolerant of sulphonamides.

Sarcocystis species infection, formerly known as *Isospora hominis,* is uncommon. The parasite is similar to *I. belli* in its biology,[75] but the life cycle requires alternating infection of intermediate hosts, such as cattle and pigs, and definitive hosts, such as human. In Strasbourg, France, the infection was present in 286 patients over a 5-year period, representing 0.4 to 0.2% of all stool specimens. The infection has not so far been recognized in AIDS. In some Strasbourg series, 30% of patients had peripheral eosinophilia. Biopsy specimens may show an eosinophilic infiltrate. Sporocysts are recognized in stool with the same stains as are used for isosporiasis, but the cysts are smaller.

Cyclospora cayetanensis

This organism (initially referred to as Cyanobacterium-like bodies, CLB) was first detected in travelers returning from Nepal with persistent diarrhea but subsequently has been isolated in parts of the developing world and North America; in the latter, the infection has been found in immunocompromised individual.[76–77] The infections are seasonal, with peak prevalence during the periods of high rainfall, strongly suggesting that it is waterborne. Large food-borne outbreaks have been described.[78] Diarrhea is usually prolonged, lasting approximately 7 weeks if untreated. The organism has been identified within enterocytes and is associated with varying degrees of villous atrophy.[79]

Oocysts can be identified in feces by light microscopy, and the addition of potassium dichromate induces the oocysts to sporulate. Intracellular parasites are identified in small intestinal biopsy specimens by electron microscopy. The parasite is probably under diagnosed, and its precise role as a cause of acute and chronic diarrhea worldwide needs to be established by further epidemiologic studies. The parasite can be eradicated with co-trimoxazole given in conventional doses for 7 days. This therapy eradicates more than 90% of infections; the remainder can be cured by continuing therapy for another 3 to 5 days.[77]

NEMATODES

Intestinal helminth infections significantly contribute to the burden of infections worldwide. Despite their high prevalence, the majority of infections produce few or no symptoms. Small intestinal nematodes may be considered as two groups: those that cause diarrhea and those that do not (see Table 1). Development of nematodes (roundworms) partly takes place outside the body, often in the soil, hence the description of many of them as geohelminths. In the developing countries, the frequency of infection is a general indication of the local level of development of hygiene and sanitation. These nematodes are usually found as multiple infections and measures against and treatment of one closely affect the others.

Strongyloides stercoralis

The life cycle of *S. stercoralis* is summarized in (Figure 3). Adult worms invade the intestinal mucosa (Figure 4) and produce an inflammatory response involving mononuclear cells and eosinophils. In addition, there may be varying degrees of partial villous atrophy. The adult worms of this parasite live predominantly in the duodenum and jejunum, although, occasionally, there is extensive involvement of the whole gut.

Epidemiology. *S. stercoralis* has two forms: one parasitic and the other free living. The life cycle is complex and consists of both a parasitic (homogonic) cycle and a free-living (heterogonic) cycle. Three developmental stages have been identified, the adult, rhabditiform larva, and filariform larva (infective). Man is the principal host of *Strongyloides*, but dogs, cats, chimpanzees, and other mammals can also harbor *S. stercoralis*. Larvae cannot survive in temperatures below 8°C or above 40°C or desiccation, but thrive in conditions of overcrowding on damp soil in tropical conditions. Infection is acquired from contaminated soil via free-living filariform infective larvae. There is a possibility of transmission through milk as has been demonstrated in several animal species.

S. stercoralis is distributed worldwide and endemic in tropical and subtropical regions where moist conditions and improper disposal of human waste coexist. It is also found in eastern Europe, Italy, Australia, and the southern United States. In temperate climates, it occurs sporadically in inmates of institutions, such as mental hospitals, prisons, and care homes for mentally retarded children. In immunocompetent children, strongyloidiasis remains an important cause of chronic diarrhea, cachexia, and failure to thrive. An important but rapidly diminishing groups of individuals still car-

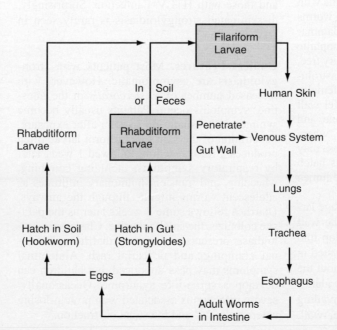

Figure 3 Life cycle of *Strongyloides stercoralis* and hookworm.

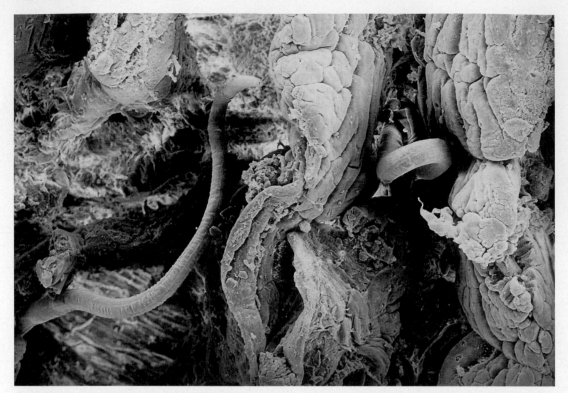

Figure 4 Scanning electron micrograph of *Strongyloides* adult worms invading intestinal mucosa. (Courtesy of Tim McHugh.)

rying this parasite are ex-servicemen who served in Southeast Asia, particularly those who were forced to work on the Thai-Burma railroad.[80–81]

Pathophysiology. Walking barefoot in contaminated soil leads to acquisition of infection. The filariform larvae enter the body through the feet by burrowing into the skin. A potent proteolytic protease secreted by the organism facilitates entry. Penetration of the skin by filariform larvae often produces a local reaction, characterized by petechial hemorrhages accompanied by intense pruritus, congestion, and edema. The larvae migrate into cutaneous blood vessels and are carried into the lungs. Once in the pulmonary capillaries, the larvae produce hemorrhages, which form the avenue for spread into the alveoli. Symptoms resembling those of bronchopneumonia with some consolidation may occur as the young worms pass through the lungs. The resulting inflammatory response is associated with an eosinophilic infiltration. Larvae migrate up the pulmonary tree, where they are swallowed, and reach the gastrointestinal system. In the intestinal crypts, the females mature and invade the tissues of the bowel wall but rarely penetrate the muscularis mucosae, and move in tissue channels beneath the villi, where the eggs are deposited. The intestinal mucosa may develop partial villous atrophy. The eggs hatch out and first-stage larvae work toward the lumen of the bowel and are passed out in feces.

Rarely, in heavy infections, the first-stage larvae develop in the intestine, bore into the wall of the duodenum and jejunum and develop into the adult stage, producing ova while encysted in the bowel. They then disseminate throughout the lymphatic system to the mesenteric lymph glands and can enter the general circulation invading the liver, lungs, kidneys, and gallbladder wall.

This is called the hyperinfection syndrome. The ileum, appendix, and colon are sites of reinvasion, and here the worms cause granulomas with a central necrotic area often containing a degenerate larva. The lungs may show abscesses, and the liver may be enlarged with small pinpoint larval granulomas. Filariform larvae gain access to the general circulation and can invade the brain, intestine, lymph glands, liver, lungs, and rarely myocardium. The pathophysiology resulting from the hyperinfection cycle, which leads to dissemination in a compromised host, is not well understood. It may occur in patients with receiving immunosuppressive therapy (particularly corticosteroids) or radiation therapy and, occasionally, in patients with debilitating disease and those with HTLV-1 infection. Surprisingly, disseminated strongyloidiasis is rarely seen in HIV infection.[82]

Clinical Features. Most patients with strongyloidiasis are asymptomatic. However, with increased number of *S. stercoralis* in the intestine, symptoms occur. Patients usually become symptomatic, usually do so soon after exposure. Penetration of the skin by filariform larvae often produces a local reaction, followed 1 week later by respiratory symptoms, including coughing, wheezing, and transient pulmonary infiltrates as adolescent worms migrate through the airways. Diarrhea follows some 2 weeks later as the parasite colonizes the small intestine. Classic strongyloidiasis presents with watery diarrhea, abdominal cramping, and urticarial rash. Abdominal symptoms may pass unnoticed, but children can develop a sprue-like syndrome. Occasionally, severe infection is associated with protein-losing enteropathy[83–84] and intestinal obstruction.[85]

The hyperinfection syndrome presents with multisystem manifestations. Bacteremia or sepsis may occur escape of enteric flora as larvae penetrate the intestinal wall. Symptoms of meningitis may occur with invasion of central nervous system, leading to headache, nausea, vomiting, nuchal rigidity, confusion, focal seizures and, in extreme cases, coma. On examination of the patients, larva currens or other urticarial rash may be seen. Lung examination may reveal scattered crackles and wheezing. Steatorrhea, hypoalbuminemia, and peripheral edema occur with prolonged malabsorption of both fat and protein. Infected children often have severe wasting with failure to thrive. Paralytic ileus is seen occasionally. Massive gastrointestinal tract bleeding, obstructive jaundice, necrotizing jejunitis, small bowel infarction, proctitis, and acute intestinal obstruction have been described.

Diagnosis. Peripheral eosinophilia (> 500 cells/ μL) is often the only abnormal laboratory test result found in patients with chronic strongyloidiasis. This probably represents an immune response to larvae migrating through the host tissues. However, this finding may be absent in the immunocompromised host. Peripheral leukocytosis may occur in the early stages of the infection. Larvae or adult females can be detected in feces, duodenal fluid, sputum, or jejunal biopsy specimens. Since female *S. stercoralis* organisms release as few as 50 eggs per day, multiple stool specimens may need to be examined to find larvae. Thus, a negative stool examination does not exclude infection.[86] Stool examination findings are negative during the early phase of infection, until the parasites reach the gut and begin to produce eggs. Serology is positive in up to 80% of patients.

Treatment. It is important to treat all persons found to harbor *Strongyloides* organisms even if they are asymptomatic, because of the risk of hyperinfection. Ivermectin as oral single dose 150 to 200 μg/kg as a single dose, repeated after 1 week or 200 μg/kg daily for 3 days is an effective intervention. Albendazole and thiabendazole are also effective, but the latter, in particular, is frequently accompanied by unwanted side effects, including nausea, anorexia, vomiting, and diarrhea

Capillaria philippinensis

Infection with this important parasite of Southeast Asia, particularly the Philippines and Thailand, results in severe diarrhea and malabsorption. Infection generally follows the ingestion of raw fish. After an incubation period of 1 to 2 months, nonspecific abdominal symptoms may be noted, followed by severe, watery diarrhea. In some cases, this progresses to intestinal malabsorption with profound weight loss. Parasite forms (ova, larvae, adult worms) are detected in stool or intestinal biopsy specimens. Infection is successfully eradicated by mebendazole and thiabendazole, provided that treatment is continued for 3 to 4 weeks. Albendazole is an effective alternative therapy.

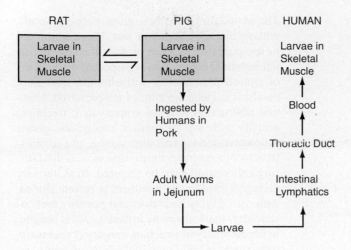

```
RAT              PIG              HUMAN

Larvae in      Larvae in       Larvae in
Skeletal   ⇌   Skeletal        Skeletal
Muscle         Muscle          Muscle
                  │               │
                  ▼               ▼
              Ingested by       Blood
              Humans in          ▲
              Pork               │
                  │          Thoracic Duct
                  ▼               ▲
              Adult Worms     Intestinal
              in Jejunum      Lymphatics
                  │               ▲
                  ▼               │
                  └──► Larvae ────┘
```

Figure 5 Life cycle of *Trichinella spiralis*.

Trichinella spiralis

Trichinella spiralis occurs worldwide in communities that eat pork.[87] It is an important infection of man in Europe and the United States; it is less important in the tropics but occurs in both East and West sub-Saharan Africa. It has been reported to cause disease and death in the Arctic, where polar explorers have died due to trichinosis. It is not a geohelminth. Unlike other nematodes, *T. spiralis* requires two hosts to complete its life-cycle (Figure 5). The female lives for 30 days and is viviparous. One female produces more than 1,500 larvae. Human infection is acquired from eating undercooked pork from infected pigs.

Pathology. The capsule of the infective larva is digested in the intestine since it is resistant to gastric juice, and the larva then penetrates the duodenal and jejunal mucosa. This penetration by the larvae induces trauma and irritation, the intensity of which depends on the number of larvae, resulting in the symptoms of the enteric phase. After 5 to 7 days, the worms mature and the females discharge larvae into the tissues, causing symptoms of the migratory or invasive stage. In striated muscle, larvae encyst, causing symptoms of encystment stage. Encystation of larvae in diaphragm, masseters, intercostals, laryngeal, tongue, and ocular muscles, leads to basophilic degeneration of the muscle fibers, followed by formation of a hyaline capsule around the larva with an inflammatory infiltrate of lymphocytes and a few eosinophils. Giant cells may be present. After 6 months calcification takes place, eventually leading to the death of the larvae.

Migration of the larvae through the brain and meninges does not lead to encystation but causes leptomeningitis, granulomatous nodules in the basal ganglia, medulla and cerebellum, and perivascular cuffing in the cortex. Larvae can be found in the cerebrospinal fluid with a raised cell count and increased protein. In the heart also, encystation does not occur, but considerable damage can occur on passage through the myocardium, with a cellular inflammatory infiltrate and necrosis followed by fibrosis of the myocardial bundles.

Clinical Features. The incubation period from eating infected meat to the development of symptoms of enteric phase is up to 7 days and for migratory phase from 7 to 21 days. Symptoms depend on the intensity of infection and the number of larvae per gram of muscle. There are three stages in the development of symptoms: enteric (invasion of intestine) phase, migration of the larvae (invasive phase), and a period of encystation in the muscles.

In the enteric phase, irritation and inflammation of the duodenum and jejunum resulting from penetration of larvae leads to nausea, vomiting, colic, and sweating, resembling an attack of acute food poisoning. There may be an erythematous rash, and in a third of cases symptoms of pneumonitis occur between the second and sixth day, lasting about 5 days.

During the migratory phase, main symptoms include, myalgia, periorbital edema, and eosinophilia. Patient experiences difficulty in mastication, breathing, and swallowing due to the involvement of the muscles, and there may be some muscular paralysis of the extremities.

There is a high-remittent fever with symptoms similar to typhoid, splinter hemorrhages under the nails and in the conjunctivae, and blood and albumin in urine. From the fourteenth day, there is hypereosinophilia which decreases after a week and persists at a lower level. Patients without eosinophilia have poor prognosis. Lymphadenopathy with parotid enlargement with or without associated splenomegaly may occur. Subphrenic, gastric, and intestinal hemorrhages may occur in severe cases.

Associated complications include pneumonitis, myocarditis, and meningoencephalitis, and focal cerebral lesions may develop. Ocular disturbances, diplopia, deafness and a syndrome resembling motor neuron disease, epileptiform attacks, and coma may occur in very heavy infections. Between the second and fifth week, sudden death from a dysrhythmia or congestive heart failure with peripheral edema may occur. Most cases recover completely but a few continue with chronic cardiac disability.

Symptoms during the encystation phase may be severe. It may be characterized by cachexia, edema, and extreme dehydration. In the second month after infection, there is decrease in muscle tenderness, fever, and itching subsides and congestive heart failure may appear. Damage to the brain may persist with protean neurological

signs which may resolve spontaneously or persist. Gram-negative septicemia from organisms introduced by the larvae, permanent hemiplegia, and Jacksonian epilepsy 10 years after an attack of trichinosis have been described.

Diagnosis. Diagnosis is confirmed by demonstrating larvae in skeletal muscle biopsy specimens by microscopy. Often there is eosinophilia and elevation of serum creatinine phosphokinase and serum glutamic oxaloacetic transaminase. Larvae have been isolated from peripheral blood in the early stages of the migration phase by mixing blood with dilute acetic acid and centrifuging.

Treatment. Treatment is directed against the larvae and the immune reaction they invoke. Mebendazole (200 mg twice a day) or thiabendazole twice a day for 10 days are both effective, although the former is better tolerated by patients.[87] In patients with disseminated severe life-threatening infections, immune response, concomitant corticosteroid (prednisolone) is recommended to minimize allergic reactions. Old calcified larvae do not need treatment.

Trichinostrongylus orientalis

Found predominantly in the Far East, this small roundworm infects those who ingest contaminated food or drink. Diarrhea occurs, but usually infection is asymptomatic. Ova can be detected in duodenal fluid or feces, and treatment is with a single dose of levamisole (2.5 mg/kg). Thiabendazole is less effective.

Ascaris lumbricoides

A. lumbricoides is the largest human intestinal nematode.[88] It is one of the most common and most widespread human infections, found worldwide, but it is most evident in the developing world, where its prevalence may exceed 90% in very deprived communities. The life cycle is summarized in Figure 6.

Epidemiology. Development of *Ascaris* eggs occurs in shady, damp soil. The eggs are resistant to recommended strengths of disinfectants and to cold, but they are killed by direct sunlight and by temperatures above 45°C. Fecal pollution of soil is important for spread of infection. Three distinct patterns in the prevalence and intensity of ascariasis have been observed in endemic areas:

- Common and constant exposure to invasive *Ascaris* eggs by dirty hands and contaminated food leading to high prevalence (>60%) in children over 2 years and lower intensity of infection in adults.
- Household or family type of transmission resulting in moderate prevalence (<50%) highest in preschool or early school ages and low values in adults.
- Focal distribution of infections related to particular housing and sanitary conditions or agricultural and behavioral practices resulting in low prevalence (<10%).

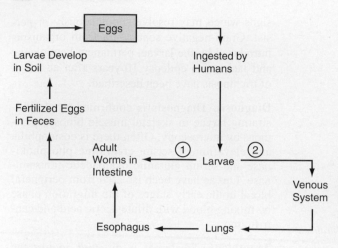

Figure 6 Life cycle of (1) *Trichuris trichiura* and *Enterobius vermicularis* and (2) *Ascaris lumbricoides*. The shaded area indicates the infective form of parasites.

Infection tends to be higher in overcrowded poorly planned underdeveloped sections of towns where hygiene is poor compared to rural areas, while in the drier areas of the tropics transmission is limited to the short-rainy season. Dung beetles, cockroaches, and animals can spread the infection widely by ingesting and excreting viable eggs. There are reports of epidemic ascariasis caused by use of raw sewage for agricultural purposes that is irrigating vegetables with wastewater. Sporadic ascariasis occurs after travel to endemic areas, consumption of imported fresh fruits and vegetables, and associated with infected immigrants. Improvement of personal hygiene, proper disposal of feces, health education, and timely treatment of infected cases are important measures for control of ascariasis.

Pathology. Infection is transmitted by fecal-oral route from ingestion of agricultural products or food contaminated with parasite eggs. Children may acquire infection when playing around the house in suitable soil. In the intestine, swallowed eggs hatch producing larvae which migrate through the blood to the pulmonary circulation. These larvae then penetrate the alveoli 1 to 2 weeks later as third-stage larvae and migrate up the tracheobronchial tree. The host swallows the larvae which develop into adult worms in the intestine. Adult worms can reach 10 to 30 cm in length. Symptoms are caused by migrating larvae and the immune reactions they elicit.

Larvae cause pulmonary symptoms as they migrate through to the intestine. Löffler's syndrome may be produced with fever, cough, sputum, asthma, eosinophilia, and radiological pulmonary infiltration.[89] In the bronchioles, fourth-stage larvae are seen associated with polymorph nuclear and eosinophilic leukocytes with scattered Charcot-Leyden crystals usually associated with lysed eosinophils.

Clinical Features. Ascariasis is common in children in whom the infection is usually asymptomatic. However, it frequently manifests by passage of the adult worm(s) in feces or through the nose or mouth. During the pulmonary phase, migrating larvae may produce coughing with sputum, wheezing, fever, and eosinophilia. In severe pulmonary infection, dyspnea, fleeting patchy pulmonary infiltrates, and rarely, hemoptysis may

be observed. *Ascaris* is one cause of eosinophilic pneumonitis.

When symptoms occur, the most common symptom is poorly localized and colicky abdominal pain. Heavy infection, particularly in children, may cause anorexia and abdominal cramps. Some evidence suggests that the parasite may impair growth and development. In younger children and those with large worm burdens, partial or total intestinal obstruction may occur. Worms may also migrate into a variety of locations, including the pancreatic and biliary systems, causing duct obstruction with jaundice and/or pancreatitis, obstruction of the appendix, volvulus, intussusception, intestinal perforation, and peritonitis.[88]

Diagnosis. Full blood count may demonstrate peripheral eosinophilia. Ova and adult worms can be detected in feces and larvae in sputum or gastric washings. A chest radiograph is indicated to demonstrate pulmonary opacities in Löffler's syndrome while ultrasound scanning, endoscopic retrograde cholangiopancreatography (ERCP), MRCP, and CT scanning are all useful in the diagnosis of biliary ascariasis.

Treatment. Available antihelminthic drugs are effective only against the adult worms. The drugs of choice is albendazole given as a single dose, children 2 to 5 years 200 mg and for older children and adults 400 mg. Mebendazole (single dose of 500 mg), levamisole (single dose of 2.5 mg/kg body weight), pyrantel pamoate (single dose of 10 mg/kg), and piperazine citrate are also effective. The dose of piperazine depends on age. For the oral suspension:

< 2 years: 600 mg three times daily (administered 4 h apart) for 1 day

2 to 8 years: 1.2 g twice daily (administered 6 h apart) for 1 day

8 to 14 years: 1.2 g three times daily (administered 4 h apart) for 1 day

> 14 years: Administer as in adults (3.5 g PO four times daily for 2 d)

For the tablets:

< 2 years: 75 mg/kg/d four times daily for 2 days (do not exceed 3.5 g/d oral suspension)

(27 kg: 2 g as a single dose

27 to 41 kg: 2 g twice daily for 1 day

> 41 kg: Administer as in adults (3.5 g four times daily for 2 days)

The above drugs are best given between meals, without any special diet or fast. There is no need to use purgatives before or after therapy. If partial intestinal obstruction is suspected on the basis of clinical presentation, antihelminths that cause paralysis (piperazine citrate) are preferred. Intestine obstruction requires conservative treatment initially with antispasmodics, analgesics, gastric decompression via nasogastric tube, and administration of intravenous fluids. However, if this fails, surgical removal may be required. In pulmonary disease, symptomatic treatment is recommended, with use of bronchodilators and possibly corticosteroids if marked airway inflammation is present. In hepatobiliary obstruction, surgery is necessary, particularly in children with high worm loads.

Hookworms: *Ankylostoma duodenale* and *Necator americanus*

Ankylostoma duodenale (old-world hookworm) is found in Africa, Asia, Australian, and parts of Southern Europe, whereas *Necator americanus* predominates in Central and South America, together with some locations in Southeast Asia, the Pacific, and Nigeria.[88] These two species of the Ancylostomatidae family are commonly infections of humans. Morphologically, the parasites are similar, with identical life cycles (see Figure 3). Adult worms attach firmly to the small intestinal mucosa by a buccal capsule consisting of tooth-like or plate-like cutting organs. It is estimated that more 500 million persons in the world are infected with these parasites.

Infection is normally acquired percutaneously from filariform (infective) larvae in the soil contaminated by human feces, or orally after ingestion of contaminated food. Other routes of infection include consumption of uncooked meat containing the larvae of *A. duodenale* and via human milk (if migrating larvae of *A. duodenale* enter the mammary gland and get excreted in milk).

Epidemiology. Man is the only reservoir of infection. Transmission of hookworm infection depends on sufficient source of infection in humans, shedding of eggs in a suitable environment for extrinsic development of the parasite, moist and warm soil to allow larvae to develop and suitable conditions for the infective larvae to penetrate the skin. Transmission is perennial in many tropical and subtropical countries, but in cooler and drier climates, transmission may take place in the warmer and wet seasons. The use of human feces for fertilizer promotes favorable conditions for infection.

Pathology. *Ankylostoma* eggs deposited in warm, moist soil take about 5 to 7 days to develop into infective larvae. Infective larvae need to infect a new host in order to survive, as they are developmentally arrested and nonfeeding. If they do not infect a new host they die, usually within 6 weeks when their metabolic reserves are exhausted. Infection occurs by ingestion of contaminated soil or via the skin when the larvae secrete a protease that facilitates boring into the skin and entry into subcutaneous tissues. The larvae migrate through the venous and lymphatic circulation into pulmonary capillaries, get into lung alveoli, and ascend the airways. Upon reaching the upper airways, the larvae are coughed up and swallowed thus getting into the gastrointestinal tract. In the proximal small intestine, larvae develop into adult, sexually mature male and female worms, which then attach to the mucosa and begin to feed. Worms mate in the small intestine where the females deposit fertilized eggs, and they appear in feces about 8 to 12 weeks after infection. Extraintestinal dormancy, lasting weeks or months, occurs in *A. duodenale*, after penetrating the skin before resuming their migration to the intestine for maturation. This explains the long occurrence of ancylostomiasis up to a year after initial exposure to the infective larvae. Adult worms digest tissue within the buccal cavity by using teeth and cutting plates, powerful esophageal muscles, and hydrolytic enzymes. At the same time, bleeding occurs from eroded capillaries in the lamina propria due to the action of a potent anticoagulant released by the worm. Every 4 to 8 hours, worms change the site of attachment, producing minute, bleeding mucosal ulcerations. The resulting chronic blood loss (estimated at 0.03 mmL/d per worm for *N. americanus* and 0.15 mL/d per worm in *A. duodenale*), depletion of iron stores, and inadequate iron intake lead to hypochromic anemia. Hookworm infection is the leading cause of iron deficiency anemia in developing countries and may affect cognitive development. Protein-losing enteropathy associated with anemia and edema is an important feature of hookworm infection. Heavy infections can cause significant protein loss as the host loses red blood cells and plasma, while adult worms secrete a potent inhibitor of digestive enzymes, which may contribute to malabsorption. In turn, malabsorption leads to hypoproteinemia which may worsen malnutrition. Studies in Puerto Rico and India[90] have demonstrated enteropathy which improves after deworming; however, this has not been confirmed from African studies.[91]

Clinical Features. Filariform larvae penetrate the skin, where a local inflammatory reaction may develop (ground itch). Pulmonary symptoms which develop after 1 to 2 weeks are less dramatic than those of *Ascaris* infections, present with a dry cough and asthmatic wheezing. Upper abdominal discomfort, mild diarrhea, and fever-associated eosinophilia usually ensue. The infection is self-limiting and symptoms gradually disappear. However, if larvae density is high, symptoms are quite alarming and steroid therapy may be needed.

The dominant response to infection is progressive iron deficiency anemia which is proportional to the worm load and the amount of iron taken in the diet. Dyspepsia may occur but diarrhea and wasting are not features. The taste may be altered resulting is some patients craving for such things as earth, mud, or lime (pica or geophagy). The stools may contain blood, and frank melena may occur in children. The occult blood test is always positive in the stools in cases where symptoms are caused by ankylostomiasis. Occasionally, heavy infection can result in protein-losing enteropathy and hypoproteinemia.

Diagnosis and Treatment. Ova and rhabditid-form larvae can be detected in stool and duodenal fluid. Treatment is aimed at eliminating the parasites and treatment of anemia, if present. Mebendazole is effective against both *A. duodenale* and *N. americanus* in a dose of 200 mg daily for 3 days. Albendazole is highly effective against both worms: 400 mg as a single dose. Levamisole (150 mg single dose orally or 2.5 mg/kg body weight) and pyrantel pamoate (10 mg/kg body weight) are also active; however, in some areas pyrantel pamoate has been found ineffective.[92]

The anemia is treated with oral iron supplements in the form of ferrous sulphate or gluconate, 200 mg three times daily and should be continued for 3 months after a normal hemoglobin level has been achieved. This will restore the iron reserves to normal. Patients presenting with severe anemia with or without heart failure require blood transfusion initially then followed by oral iron supplements.

Cestodes (Tapeworms)

Four tapeworms are common human pathogens: *Taenia saginata*, *T. solium*, *Diphyllobothrium latum*, and *Hymenolepis nana*. These flatworms are similar structurally, and their heads have suckers; *T. solium* has additional hooks. The head is joined by a short, slender neck to several segments called proglottids, which form the body of the worm. Nutrients are absorbed directly through the cuticle because these worms do not possess an intestinal tract. Tapeworms are hermaphrodites, with cross-fertilization occurring between proglottids. Adult worms reside in the intestinal tract, whereas larvae exist in tissues, particularly muscle; infection is transmitted to humans by the eating of infected tissues (Figure 7).

T. saginata (Beef Tapeworm)

The human is the definitive host and cattle are the significant intermediate hosts. The larval stage is a fluid-filled translucent bladder or cysticercus between 5 to 10 mm in diameter. The adult is a large, white tapeworm than can reach 10 m in length (more typically 2 to 5 m), with a scolex equipped with suckers but not hooks. Mature proglottides which detach from the distal end of the worm are highly motile and are the cause of symptoms as they emerge from the anus. Human infection is acquired by eating undercooked beef. Contaminated feed or grazing ground with human feces is the source of infection for cattle. Proper disposal of human feces and detection of infected meat at abattoirs are central to the prevention of transmission of infection.

Most patients infected with this tapeworm are symptom free, although mild vague abdominal discomfort and occasional diarrhea may occur. *T. saginata* carriers are often distressed by awareness of motile proglottides spontaneously emerging from the anus; they are also conspicuous in the feces because of their motility. Occasionally, adult worms obstruct the appendix or pancreatic duct, causing appendicitis and pancreatitis, respectively. Generally, infection is apparent to the host only when proglottids are identified in the feces. Segments of the worm may be vomited. Unlike in nematode infection, eosinophilia is not a feature of established *Taenia* infection.

Diagnosis is made by detection of *Taenia* eggs in feces by microscopy; however, it is difficult to identify the different species due to the similarity of all the *Taenia* ova. Species identification can be done by use of Ziehl-Neelsen staining or by the use of monoclonal antibodies or molecular techniques. It is possible to identify different species by examination for the number of uterine branches of intact proglottides.

Praziquantel given as a single dose at 10 mg/kg body weight is the treatment of choice, although niclosamide, 2 g as single-chewed dose is also effective. Infection can be avoided by thorough examination of beef for encysted larvae known as cysticerci, although freezing at (−10°C for 5 days or cooking at 57°C for several minutes destroys them.

Taenia solium (Pork Tapeworm)

The clinical features and treatment of the adult worm infection are similar to those of *T. saginata* infection. However, a serious complication occurs when autoinfection with *T. solium* larvae results in their dissemination to many sites, including skeletal muscles, brain, subcutaneous tissue, the eye, and myocardium, a condition known as cysticercosis. The cysts remain alive for many years but eventually produce a local inflammatory reaction and calcify. Cerebral involvement presents as epilepsy,

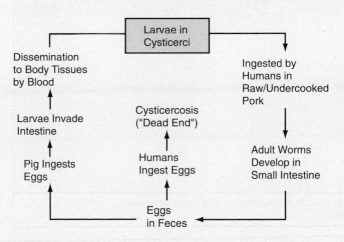

Figure 7 Life cycle of *Taenia solium* (pork tapeworm).

as a space-occupying lesion, or as focal neurologic deficits. Ocular involvement produces retinitis, uveitis, conjunctivitis, or choroidal atrophy.

Diagnosis can be established by biopsy of skin nodules, although calcified cysticerci usually can be detected radiologically. Encouraging results in the treatment of cysticercosis have been obtained with the use of praziquantel (10 mg/kg in a single dose). Surgery or photocoagulation may be required for retinal lesions.

Diphyllobothrium latum (Fish Worm)

This tapeworm is found mainly in Scandinavia, the Baltic countries, Japan, and the Swiss lakes region. Infection in humans occurs by the ingestion of raw or undercooked fish containing the infective plerocercoid form of the parasite. Infections usually asymptomatic, although there may be abdominal discomfort, vomiting, and weight loss. Occasionally, intestinal obstruction can occur. *D. latum* cleaves vitamin B12. Megaloblastic anemia owing to vitamin B12 deficiency is relatively uncommon, although it is well recognized in Finland. Diagnosis and treatment is as for other tapeworms.

Hymenolepsis nana (Dwarf Tapeworm)

This worm infects children more frequently than adults but has other natural hosts in rats and mice. Infection generally produces no symptoms, although very heavy infection may result in diarrhea and abdominal pain. Treatment is with praziquantel or niclosamide.

TREMATODES

A large number of flukes infect the biliary and intestinal tract of humans, producing a broad spectrum of disease. *Fasciola hepatica,* the largest human fluke (up to 7 cm in length), is found most often in the Far East. It attaches to the proximal small intestine, causing ulceration, bleeding, and abscesses. Although asymptomatic infection occurs, heavy parasite burdens in undernourished children result in intermittent diarrhea, abdominal pain, and protein-losing enteropathy with hypo-albuminemia, edema, and ascites. Progressive weight loss and even paralytic ileus may develop. Triclabendazole is the treatment of choice (20 mg/kg single dose, repeated if necessary), but this dose is based on doses given to adults and few trial data are available relating to children.

Clonorchis sinensis and *Opisthorchis* spp. are flukes which infect the biliary tree in South East Asia. *Heterophyes heterophyes* and *Metagonimus yokogawai* are very small flukes found in the Far East. Natural hosts include dogs, cats, foxes, humans, and other fish-eating mammals. Infection may be asymptomatic, but heavy infections produce intermittent diarrhea and abdominal discomfort. Ova can be detected in feces. Praziquantel (25 mg/kg tid for 3 days) is the treatment of choice, but again few data are available for children.

PARASITES OF THE COLON AND RECTUM

Protozoa

Entamoeba histolytica and a ciliate *Balantidium coli* are the important protozoal pathogens of the large intestine (Table 2). However, it is now clear that *C. parvum* can infect the entire small and large intestine; indeed, the first case of human infection was diagnosed by rectal biopsy. *G. lamblia* is predominantly a pathogen of the small intestine, but isolated reports in both humans and animals purport that this parasite occasionally causes colitis. Unlike *C. parvum* and *G. lamblia* which have their main impact in children, *E. histolytica* infects all age groups but has its most profound effects in adults.

Entamoeba histolytica

Fedor Löch, in St. Petersburg, Russia, first described the clinical and autopsy findings of a case of fatal dysentery and identified ameba, which he originally named *Amoeba coli*. In 1886, Kartulis in Egypt proved ameba to be the cause of intestinal and hepatic lesions in patients with diarrhea. In 1890, William Osler reported the case of a young man who contracted dysentery and developed a hepatic abscess that led to his death. One year later, Councilman and Lafleur conducted a detailed study of patients with amebic dysentery and hepatic abscess. They confirmed the pathogenic role of amebae and created the terms "amebic dysentery" and "amebic liver abscess." Walker and Sellards, in the Phillipines, definitely established the pathogenicity of *E. histolytica* by feeding cysts to volunteers. Beginning with isoenzyme analysis, then genetic analysis, a convincing body of evidence now exists that a nonpathogenic strain of *Entamoeba*, morphologically identical to *E. histolytica*, exists and this new species has now been termed *Entamoeba dispar*.[93]

Epidemiology. *Entameba histolytica* is found worldwide, but its prevalence is highest in the developing countries. Millions of people carry the parasite, with an annual mortality in the tens of thousands.[93] Amebiasis is relatively uncommon in infancy and childhood, but when infection occurs, morbidity and mortality tend to be high.

The parasite exists in two forms, the motile trophozoite and the cyst. Cysts are spread in food and water and also by person-to-person contact. Many individuals with asymptomatic carriage in fact have *E. dispar* infection, which never causes symptoms. Infection is acquired via the fecal-oral route, food and drink becoming contaminated through exposure to human feces. Food-borne outbreaks of disease occur due to unsanitary handling of food and its preparation by infected individuals. Cyst carriers constitute the main reservoir of infection. Epidemics occur when raw sewage contaminates water supplies; also the use of human feces for fertilizer is associated with high prevalence. Sexual transmission also occurs. Travelers, immigrants, immigrant workers, immmnocompromised individuals, individuals in mental institutions, prisons, and children in day care centers are recognized as high-risk group. Very young children, pregnant women, the malnourished, and individuals taking corticosteroids usually have severe infections. Patients with AIDS do not have increased risk of severe infection.

Pathogenesis. After ingestion of cysts of *E. histolytica,* there is excystation in the small bowel and invasion of the colon by the trophozoites. Incubation period of the infection ranges from 2 days to 4 months. Invasive disease begins with adherence of *E. histolytica* trophozoites to colonic mucins, epithelial cells, and leukocytes by a process which is mediated by a surface lectin. Adherence of trophozoites is followed by invasion of the colonic epithelium to produce ulcerative lesions typical of intestinal amebiasis. The capacity *E. histolytica* to kill colonic epithelial cells on contact appears to depend on a surface lectin and a range of cytotoxic proteins, including proteolytic and hydrolytic enzymes and a pore-forming protein known as amebapore.[94] Amebiasis spreads to the liver via portal blood, with trophozoites ascending the portal veins to produce liver abscesses filled with acellular proteinaceous debris. This material has the appearance of anchovy paste. The trophozoites lyse the

Table 2 Parasites of the Colon and Rectum			
	Estimated Global Importance*		
Parasite	Infancy	Childhood	Adolescence
Protozoa			
Entamoeba histolytica†	±	++	++
Balantidium coli†	−	++	+
Cryptosporidium sp.†	±	+++	++
Trypanosoma cruzi	±	++	++
Nematodes			
Trichuris trichiura	±	+++	++
Enterobius vermicularis	±	+++	++
Oesophagostomum sp.	−	+	+
Angiostrongylus costaricensis	−	+	+
Trematodes			
Schistosoma sp.†	−	+++	++

*These are rough approximations that attempt to take into account marked geographic variations.
†Parasites that can cause diarrhea and malabsorption.

hepatocytes and neutrophils which explains the paucity of inflammatory cells within the liver abscesses. The neutrophil toxins may contribute to hepatocyte necrosis. Ischemia caused by portal venous obstruction leads to occurrence of triangular areas of hepatic necrosis, with trophozoites appearing along these hepatic lesions. In severe cases, amebic trophozoites can be found in every organ of the body, including the brain, lungs, and eyes.

Clinical Features. The term amebiasis covers a wide range of clinical syndromes, from asymptomatic infection to amebic colitis and extra intestinal amebiasis, usually hepatic abscess. Most infected individuals throughout the world (80 to 90%) are asymptomatic carriers. Acute amebic dysentery produces symptoms similar to those of bacterial dysentery; in its most severe form, it may progress to colonic dilatation and severe toxemia. This progression is particularly likely to occur in pregnancy, in the puerperium, and in malnourished infants, and young children.[95]

Chronic amebic colitis begins more insidiously, with cyclic remissions during which bowel function may return to normal, or even be reduced to constipation. The pattern may mimic nonspecific inflammatory bowel disease such as Crohn's disease.[96] Constitutional upset is mild to moderate, although complications such as colonic stricture and fibrotic masses of granulation tissue (known as an ameboma) may occur.[97]

An amebic liver abscess can develop within days, months, or even years after the onset of amebic colitis, but in up to 50% of cases, there is no clear antecedent history of colonic involvement. Nonspecific symptoms, such as low-grade fever and weight loss, may begin insidiously, or there may be an acute fulminant illness with localized hepatic pain or evidence of direct extension into pleural or pericardial cavities. Distant spread to lung, brain, and kidney occurs when the abscess ruptures into a hepatic vein.

Diagnosis and Treatment. Demonstration of *E. histolytica* trophozoites and cysts in feces remains the mainstay of diagnosis. Examination of a fresh saline wet mount should reveal motile trophozoites containing ingested red blood cells. Nonpathogenic intestinal amebae are not erythrophagic. Trophozoites may be seen in rectal mucosal biopsy specimens or in slough from rectal ulcers. It is unusual to see trophozoites in pus from a liver abscess. Serology for IgG antibodies is positive in 70 to 80% of patients with amebic colitis and approaches 100% in those with amebic liver abscess.[98] The treatment of amebiasis in children is summarized in Table 3.

Balantidium coli. This protozoan is the only ciliate that produces clinically significant infection in humans; it is restricted largely to communities that live in close proximity to pigs, the preferred host.[99–100] It occurs mainly in Papua New Guinea, Philippines, and Central and South America. The cyst is the infective form, although the trophozoite can survive outside the human host for a week or more in moist conditions. Clinically, *B. coli* infection closely resembles amebiasis, and diag-

Table 3 Treatment of Amebiasis in Children

Intestina lamebiasis
  Metronidazole
  50 mg/kg daily for 10 d, followed by diloxanide furoate, 20 mg/kg daily for 10 d
Amebic liver abscess
  Metronidazole
  50 mg/kg daily for 10 d
Asymptomatic cyst passer
  Diloxanide furoate
  20 mg/kg daily for 10 d + metronidazole

nosis is made by identification of the large motile trophozoite in feces. Cysts are seen relatively rarely. Tetracycline (500 mg 4 times daily for 10 days) is the usual treatment, but the parasite is also sensitive to ampicillin, metronidazole, and paromomycin.

NEMATODES

The most common nematodes to infect the colon and rectum are *T. trichiura* (whipworm) and *Enterobius vermicularis* (threadworm). In the hyperinfection syndrome, *S. stercoralis* also colonizes the large intestine, producing ulceration and inflammatory changes after invasion and autoinfection.

Trichuris trichiura

This parasite is found worldwide, with a high prevalence in the developing world. In some particularly deprived communities, prevalence may be as high as 90%. Infection is transmitted by ingestion of ova that have matured outside the host for several weeks. Colonization involves the distal ileum and cecum, although the entire colon may be involved.

Clinical Features. Light infections are often asymptomatic, but when larger numbers of parasites are present (greater than 20,000 ova per gram of feces), diarrhea with blood and mucus is characteristic.[101] Other symptoms include abdominal pain, anorexia, weight loss, tenesmus, and rectal prolapse. Evidence suggests that within endemic areas, some children are more susceptible than others to whipworm infection. There is now persuasive evidence indicating that chronic heavy infection is an important contributor to the impairment of growth and development in young children.[102]

Diagnosis and Treatment. Typical barrel-shaped eggs can be detected in feces, and adult worms can endoscopically be seen attached to the colonic mucosa, often with the presence of ulceration and inflammatory changes. Albendazole (400 mg) or mebendazole as a single dose is now the treatment of choice, although mebendazole should not be used in children under the age of 2 years. Mebendazole and albendazole are not licensed for children under 2 years of age because few data are available on children in clinical trials, but it is probably safe in children over 12 months of age. Multiple courses may

be necessary to clear infection. Ivermectin (200 μg/kg, single dose) is also highly effective.

Enterobius vermicularis

This parasite is found worldwide, although it is more prevalent in temperate and cold climates. Children are most often infected, but infection can spread rapidly among family members, those in residential institutions, and any group living in overcrowded circumstances. Infection is spread by direct transmission of ova from person to person or indirectly, on clothing or house dust. The life cycle is summarized in Figure 6.

Anal pruritus is usually the only symptom, occurring mainly at night, when adult females lay their eggs in the perianal region. Symptoms of appendicitis may result from worms entering the lumen of the appendix. Occasionally, adult worms migrate through the intestinal wall and are found in the genital tract, peritoneum, omentum, lung, urinary tract, liver, spleen, or kidney.[103] Ova can be detected in the perianal region by applying clear adhesive tape to the perianal skin and examining this microscopically. Ova can also be found under fingernails. Adult worms may be observed directly emerging from the anal canal or on the perineal skin. Albendazole is the drug of choice (in a single oral dose of 10 to 14 mg/kg), although mebendazole, pyrantel pamoate, and piperazine are also effective. It is wise to treat the entire family and to consider a second course of treatment 2 to 4 weeks later to eradicate worms that may have matured since the first treatment.

Oesophagostomum Species

This organism infects mainly ruminants, primates, and pigs but occasionally causes human infection. The worm often penetrates the intestinal wall, resulting in multiple nodules along the intestine, some of which develop into paracolic abscesses requiring surgical drainage.

Angiostrongylus costaricensis

Infection with this nematode was first described in Costa Rican children presenting with severe pain in the right iliac fossa, fever, and anorexia.[104] An inflammatory mass involving the cecum, appendix, and terminal ileum is characteristic.[104] In its acute form, the syndrome can be confused with appendicitis. The inflammatory reaction is the result of intramural eggs that have been discharged from adult worms living in terminal mesenteric arterials. Surgical resection may be required.

TREMATODES

Schistosoma Species

Schistosomiasis is one of the most important parasitic infections worldwide, with a high morbidity and mortality. More than 200 million individuals are infected with this parasite. Five species are known to cause disease in humans: *Schistosoma mansoni* (Africa, Central and South America, the Caribbean, and the Middle East), *Schistosoma*

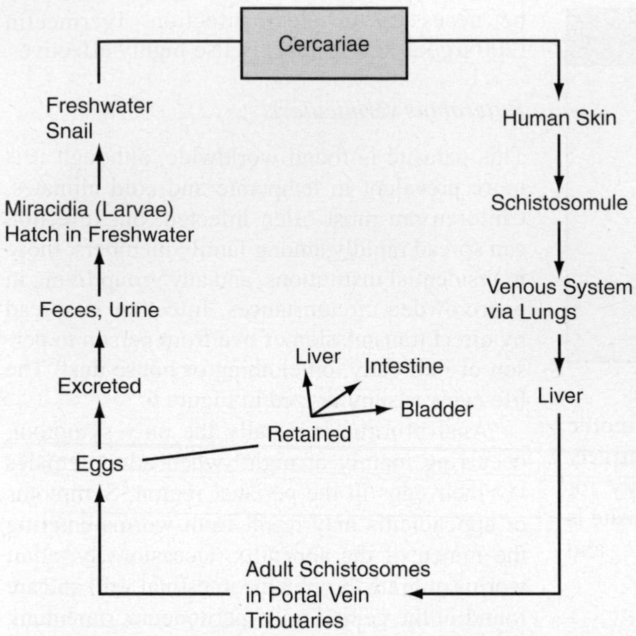

```
              ┌─────────────────┐
              │    Cercariae    │
              └─────────────────┘
   ┌──────────────────┘         └──────────────────┐
Freshwater                              Human Skin
Snail                                        │
   ↑                                         ↓
Miracidia (Larvae)                      Schistosomule
Hatch in Freshwater                          │
   ↑                                         ↓
Feces, Urine                            Venous System
   ↑                                    via Lungs
Excreted          Liver   Intestine          │
   ↑                 ↖  ↗  → Bladder          ↓
Eggs              Retained                  Liver
   │       ┌─────────┘
   │       │
   └─────→ Adult Schistosomes ←───────────────┘
           in Portal Vein
           Tributaries
```

Figure 8 Life cycle of *Schistosoma* species.

japonicum (Japan, Philippines, southeast China, and Taiwan), *Schistosoma haematobium* (Africa), *Schistosoma mekongi* (Southeast Asia), and *Schistosoma intercalatum* (Congo and Gabon). *S. haematobium* does not cause intestinal disease. Human infection is totally dependent on the intermediate host, the freshwater snail. The life cycle is summarized in Figure 8.

Clinical Features. Invasion of the skin by cercariae produces a local inflammatory response known as swimmer's itch. Within a week, there may be a generalized allergic response, with fever, urticaria, myalgia, general malaise, and associated eosinophilia. The acute phase of *S. japonicum* infection is known as Katayama fever. Hepatosplenomegaly also occurs in the early stages; in children, it is more marked in those with heavy parasite loads.[105] Intestinal symptoms of diarrhea, blood, and mucus can occur immediately but may be delayed for months or even years. Extensive colonic ulceration and polyp formation are characteristic of *S. mansoni* infections.[106] In severe cases, there may be marked iron and protein loss. Stricture formation and intestinal obstruction are characteristic, as are localized granulomatous masses within the gut wall, known as bilharziomas. *S. japonicum* can involve both small and large intestines, and infection may be more severe than that from *S. mansoni*. *S. japonicum* colitis, like extensive long-standing ulcerative colitis, has premalignant potential.[107] *S. haematobium* produces rectal inflammation and bladder involvement. The inflammatory changes in the intestine in schistosomiasis are due entirely to an intense T lymphocyte-related immune response to eggs deposited in the intestinal wall.

Diagnosis and Treatment. Characteristic ova of each species can be detected in feces or in intestinal biopsy specimens. Specific antibodies can be detected by immune assay in more than 95% of patients during the first few weeks of infection. Praziquantel given as a single dose (40 mg/kg; for *S. mansoni* 60 mg/kg in divided doses is in use by many physicians) is probably the drug of choice. Oxamniquine (20 mg/kg divided into two doses during one day) is also effective.

MICROSPORIDIA SPECIES

The Microsporidia represent a group of unicellular organisms which have always been difficult to classify. The phylum Microspora includes parasites of vertebrates and invertebrates, but recently the Microspora have been reclassified as fungi.[108–109] Although molecular analysis places them (probably) among the fungi,[109] they exhibit some sensitivity to chemotherapy with albendazole, so for the purposes of this text we place them intermediate between protozoa and fungi. In many respects, species of *Microsporidia* resemble *Cryptosporidium* in clinical features. Two species cause intestinal disease in humans: *Enterocytozoon bieneusi* and *Encephalitozoon intestinalis* (formerly *Septata intestinalis*). The clinical importance of these organisms is recognized in immunocompromised patients, particularly those with AIDS-related diarrhea.[110–111]

Microsporidia are obligate intracellular spore-forming organisms with a wide range of hosts. Infection is acquired via the spore, which after ingestion, extrudes a polar tube through which the sporoplasm is passed, infecting any enterocytes penetrated by the tube. The organism then multiplies within the infected cell by binary fission (merogony) with the meront in an intracytoplasmic position, surrounded by a simple membrane (parasitophorous vacuole). Merogony overlaps with sporogony, which leads to the development of spores. These are about 1.5×0.9 μm in size and are shed in feces.

ENTEROCYTOZOON BIENEUSI

Infection in humans had not been reported before the syndrome of AIDS-related diarrhea was recognized. The first case was reported in 1985 in an AIDS patient from France. This patient also had *Giardia* isolated from stool specimens. The parasite, in different developmental stages, was identified by electron microscopy of small intestinal biopsies. Since the first report, many cases have been identified, and Microsporidial infection is prominent among those infections to which the HIV-infected individual is susceptible.

ENCEPHALITOZOON INTESTINALIS

First named *Septata intestinalis*, this microsporidian was not recognized as a human pathogen until 1993 and reclassified in 1995.[112] Its initially reported characteristic was the ability to disseminate in AIDS patients, with renal infection predominant. It was initially named *Septata* after the characteristic septated parasitophorous vacuole (Figure 9).

Epidemiology. In developed countries, Microsporidial species were common in AIDS until the advent of HAART. They are now rarely found where HAART is freely available, but are still common in African adults[73] and children.[113] Infection has been diagnosed in immunocompromised organ transplant recipients and in one child with a congenital thymic immunodeficiency. Microsporidiosis can affect both HIV-seropositive and HIV-seronegative adults, although persistent diarrhea is more likely in patients with advanced immunodeficiency. There is evidence that microsporidiosis is a zoonosis,[108] and considerable genetic diversity among isolates from humans.[114]

Pathogenesis. The pathogenesis of infection is poorly understood, largely because of the difficulties of establishing in vitro cultures. Morphological studies of biopsies of infected small bowel reveal multiple meronts and sporonts in the host cell, often around the nucleus. Cells thus infected are apparently healthy at first, but the development of the later stages of sporogony is associated with enterocyte degeneration, vacuolation, and loss of the brush border. These cells are subsequently sloughed off into the lumen, where the spores are liberated after cytolysis. Infection of enterocytes with Microsporidia is seen only on the villi, not in the crypts. Villous atrophy occurs, possibly through increased enterocyte loss.[110] It is not known whether adjacent spread of infection occurs from cell to cell. There is no synchrony of life cycles among different organisms parasitizing the same cell.

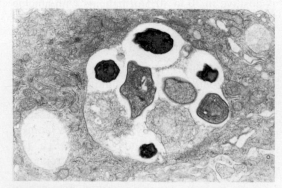

Figure 9 Electron micrograph of *Encephalitozoon intestinalis* in an intestinal biopsy from a Zambia AIDS patient.

In humans, infection appears to be confined to the small intestine, mainly from the distal duodenum to the ileum. Studies in patients have demonstrated diminished D-xylose absorption compared with patients with AIDS-related diarrhea without microsporidiosis, but serum vitamin B12 concentrations were not reduced.

Clinical Features. Clinically, infection with *E. bieneusi* resembles cryptosporidiosis, with chronic water diarrhea, anorexia, nausea, and abdominal pain. There are several reports in the literature of a sclerosing cholangitis-like syndrome[115] indistinguishable from that associated with cryptosporidiosis, but since the advent of HAART this has become rare. The biliary tract is infected by spread along the intestinal bile duct epithelium. The gall bladder can be also be infected causing acalculous cholecystitis.

Diagnosis. The original and "gold standard" technique for diagnosis is electron microscopy of small bowel biopsies. Early meronts are recognized by the paler appearance of the cytoplasm relative to that of the host cell (Figure 9). The hallmark of the late meront or sporont is the development of the characteristic electron-dense polar tube, which has about 5 to 7 coils. Other characteristics include the presence of electron-lucent inclusions (ELIs) and electron-dense discs (EDDs). Spores are identifiable by their intensely osmophilic walls. Light microscopic diagnosis of histological sections of small bowel biopsy material is possible using careful scanning of sections stained with Giemsa, Brown-Brenn, or toluidine blue (the latter is especially clear in semi-thin sections). Examination of stools with trichrome or calcafluor stains reveals 1.2 μ)m spores with characteristic equatorial banding due to the polar tube.

Treatment Albendazole[116] and fumagillin[117] are effective, though not reliably so. Albendazole inhibits microtubule formation, and thus reduces cell division and possibly polar tube action. Albendazole is more effective against *Encephalitozoon* than against *Enterocytozoon*. There are no data on doses for children.

FUNGAL INFECTIONS

A well child with intact host defense mechanisms is generally not considered to be susceptible to fungal infections of the digestive tract. As immunosuppressive therapies become more aggressive and myelotoxic regimens more effective, opportunities increase for fungi to invade and establish themselves in humans. Patients disabled from chronic malnutrition and those exposed to intense antimicrobial infection are also susceptible to these organisms. HIV infection and AIDS have produced a group of chronically immunosuppressed patients susceptible to a wide range of organisms, including fungi. The digestive tract is not a preferred site of infection in cases of disseminated fungal infection, but certain species are capable of infecting the esophagus, the stomach, or the intestine.

A consequence of modern treatment and recently evolving patterns of disease, these opportunistic infections have been recognized only in recent years. No doubt, additional GI fungal infections of significance will emerge and will be recognized in the years to come.

CANDIDIASIS

Candida species are oval cells (4 to 6 μm in size) that reproduce by budding. There are at least 80 species, of which 8, including *Candida albicans,* are of GI significance. In disseminated candidiasis, there is widespread involvement of several organs. The major risk factor leading to this serious problem is neutropenia. The liver may be involved in addition to the heart, brain, kidney, lung, spleen, and eye.[118]

Esophagitis caused by *Candida* species is seen in immunosuppressed children and in those with hematologic malignancy. In such cases, oral thrush may be seen in as few as 20% of cases.[119] Treatment with nystatin usually is effective. Ketoconazole and fluconazole also can be used, and in severe disease (particularly when oral medication cannot be taken), intravenous amphotericin B is employed.

Candida is isolated from up to 15% of gastric ulcers, but no pathogenetic role for the organism in ulcer disease has been established. *Candida* peritonitis, with infection localized usually to the peritoneum, is seen after bowel surgery and in patients undergoing chronic ambulatory peritoneal dialysis. *Candida* infection has been associated with acute watery diarrhea in newborn infants, although its causative role has not been definitely established.[120] *C. albicans* can invade the small bowel and large intestine in terminally ill patients.

ASPERGILLOSIS

The molds of the genus *Aspergillus* reproduce by means of spores that germinate, resulting in hyphae, the form in which they are associated with disease. Most cases of invasive *Aspergillus* infection are seen in severely immunocompromised patients. In about 20% of such cases of invasive infection, the small and large intestines are involved, in addition to the esophagus and stomach. Amphotericin B is the treatment of choice.

ZYGOMYCOSIS

Zygomycetes are ubiquitous agents found in organic debris, on fruit, and in soil. They grow rapidly on any carbohydrate substrate. The terms "mucormycosis" and "phycomatosis" have been used in the past for these infections. These agents can infect the subcutaneous and submucosal tissues in an immunocompetent host, but in the debilitated host, they can cause acute fulminant invasive infection.[121] Intestinal zygomycosis is encountered in severely malnourished children and sometimes as a complication of severe

chronic intestinal disease, such as amebic colitis. On occasion, the infection can occur without apparent predisposition. Treatment is with amphotericin B, in doses escalating to 1 to 1.5 mg/kg if possible; surgical debridement is also often necessary.

COCCIDIOIDOMYCOSIS

Coccidioides is a dimorphic fungus endemic in the southwest of the United States. Arthroconidia arising from mycelial growth causes infection when inhaled. Coccidioidomycosis is usually a pulmonary infection; spores can escape the chest during primary infection and with dissemination; on rare occasions, the terminal ileum and colon are involved.[122] Primary pulmonary disease is treated with fluconazole (6 to 12 mg/kg daily), but invasive disease will require amphotericin B in addition.

REFERENCES

1. Yokogawa M, Yoshimura H. Clinicopathologic studies on larval anisakiasis in Japan. Am J Trop Med Hyg 1967;16:723–8.
2. Pinkus GS, Coolidge C, Little MD. Intestinal anisakiasis: First case report from North America. Am J Med 1975;59:114–20.
3. Yoshimura K. *Angiostrongylus* (Parastrongylus) and less common nematodes. In: Cox FEG, Wakelin D, Gillespie SH, Despommier DD, editors. Topley and Wilson's Microbiology and Microbial Infections: Parasitology, 10th edition. London: Hodder Arnold; 2005. p. 802–29.
4. Ishikura H, Kikuchi K, Nagasawa K, et al. Anisakidae and anisakidosis. In: Sun T, editor. Progress in Clinical Parasitology, vol. 3. New York: Springer-Verlag; 1993. p. 43–102.
5. Deardorff TL, Kayes SG, Fukumura T. Human anisakiasis transmitted by marine food products. Hawaii Med J 1991;50:9–16.
6. Dziekonska-Rynko J, Rokicki J, Jablonowski Z. Effects of ivermectin and albendazole against *Anisakis simplex* in vitro and in guinea pigs. J Parasitol 2002;88:395–8.
7. Ramos L, Alonso C, Guilarte M, et al. *Anisakis simplex*-induced small bowel obstruction after fish ingestion: Preliminary evidence for response to parenteral corticosteroids. Clin Gastroenterol Hepatol 2005;3:667–71.
8. Garcia LS. Giardiasis. In: Cox FEG, Wakelin D, Gillespie SH, Despommier DD, editors. Topley and Wilson's Microbiology and Microbial Infections: Parasitology, 10th edition. London: Hodder Arnold; 2005. p. 241–54.
9. Farthing MJG. Host parasite interactions in human giardiasis. QJM 1989;70:191–204.
10. Carnaby S, Katelaris PH, Naeem A, Farthing MJG. Genetic heterogeneity within *Giardia lamblia* isolates demonstrated by M13 DNA fingerprinting. Infect Immun 1994;62:1875–80.
11. Bertrand I, Albertini L, Schwartzbrod J. Comparison of two target genes for detection and genotyping of *Giardia lamblia* in human feces by PCR and PCR-restriction fragment length polymorphism. J Clin Microbiol 2005;43:5940–4.
12. Hunter PR, Thompson RCA. The zoonotic transmission of *Giardia* and *Cryptosporidium*. Int J Parasitol 2005;35:1181–90.
13. Farthing MJG, Cevallos AM, Kelly P. Intestinal protozoa. In: Cook GC, Zumla A, editors. Manson's Tropical Diseases, 21st edition. London: Saunders; 2003. p. 1373–1410.
14. Farthing MJG. Giardiasis. In: Gilles HM, editor. Protozoal Disease. London: Arnold; 1999. p. 562–84.
15. Katelaris PH, Farthing MJG. Diarrhoea and malabsorption in giardiasis: A multifactorial process. Gut 1992;33:295–7.
16. Ament ME, Rubin CE. Relation of giardiasis to normal intestinal structure and function in gastrointestinal immunodeficiency syndrome. Gastroenterology 1972;62:216–26.
17. Levinson JD, Nastro LJ. Giardiasis with total villous atrophy. Gastroenterology 1978;74:271–5.
18. Wright SG, Tomkins AM. Quantification of the lymphocytic infiltrate in jejunal epithelium in giardiasis. Clin Exp Immunol 1977;29:408–12.
19. Rosekrans PCM, Lindeman J, Meijer CJLM. Quantitative histological and immuno-histochemical findings in jejunal

biopsy specimens in giardiasis. Virchows Arch [A] 1981; 393:145–518.

20. Muller N, von Allmen N. Recent insights into the mucosal reactions associated with *Giardia lamblia* infections. Int J Parasitol 2005;35:1339–47.

21. Cevallos AM, James M, Farthing MJG. Small intestinal injury in a neonatal rat model is strain dependent. Gastroenterology 1995;109:766–73.

22. Farthing MJG, Mata L, Urrutia JJ, Kronmal RA. Natural history of *Giardia* infection of infants and young children in rural Guatemala and its impact on physical growth. Am J Clin Nutr 1986;4:393–403.

23. Webster ADB. Giardiasis and immunodeficiency diseases. Trans R Soc Trop Med Hyg 1980;74:440–8.

24. Webster ADB, KenWright S, Ballard J, et al. Nodular lymphoid hyperplasia of the bowel in primary hypogammaglobulinaemia: study of in vivo and in vitro lymphocyte function. Gut 1977;18:364–72.

25. Weitzel T, Dittrich S, Mohl I, et al. Evaluation of seven commercial antigen detection tests for *Giardia* and *Cryptosporidium* in stool samples. Clin Microbiol Infect 2005;12:656–9.

26. Aldeen WE, Carroll K, Robison A, et al. Comparison of nine commercially available enzyme-linked immunosorbent assays for detection of *Giardia lamblia* in fecal specimens. J Clin Microbiol 1998;36:1338–40.

27. Fedorko DP, Williams EC, Nelson NA, et al. Performance of three enzyme immunoassays and two direct fluorescence assays for detection of *Giardia lamblia* in stool specimens preserved in ECOFIZ. J Clin Microbiol 2000;38:2781–3.

28. Ortiz JJ, Ayoub A, Gargala G, et al. Randomized clinical study of nitazoxanide compared to metronidazole in the treatment of symptomatic giardiasis in children from Northern Peru. Aliment Pharmacol Therap 2001;15:1409–15.

29. Nime FA, Kurek JD, Page DL, et al. Acute enterocolitis in a human being infected with the protozoan *Cryptosporidium*. Gastroenterology 1976;70:592–8.

30. Abrahamsen MS, Templeton TJ. Complete genome sequence of the Apicomplexan *Cryptosporidium parvum*. Science 2004;304:441–5.

31. Hunter PR, Thompson RC. The zoonotic transmission of *Giardia* and *Cryptosporidium*. Int J Parasitol 2005;35:1181–90.

32. Current WL, Garcia LS. Cryptosporidiosis. Clin Microbiol Rev 1991;4:325–58.

33. Connolly GM. Clinical aspects of cryptosporidiosis. Baill Clin Gastroenterol 1988;4:443–54.

34. Amadi BC, Kelly P, Mwiya M, et al. Intestinal and systemic infection, HIV and mortality in Zambian children with persistent diarrhoea and malnutrition. J Ped Gastroenterol Nutr 2001;32:550–4.

35. Kelly P, Nchito M, Baboo KS, et al. Cryptosporidiosis in adults in Lusaka, Zambia, and its relationship to oocyst contamination of drinking water. J Infect Dis 1997;176:1120–3.

36. Nchito M, Kelly P, Sianongo S, et al. Cryptosporidiosis in urban Zambian children: an analysis of risk factors. Am J Trop Hyg 1998;59:435–7.

37. Mac Kenzie WR, Hoxie NJ, Proctor ME, et al. A massive outbreak in Milwaukee of *Cryptosporidium* infection transmitted through the public water supply. N Engl J Med 1994;331:161–7.

38. Fairley CK, Sinclair MI, Rizak S. Monitoring not the answer to *Cryptosporidium* in water. Lancet 1999;354:967–9.

39. Hart CA, Baxby D, Blundell N. 1984 Gastroenteritis due to *Cryptosporidium:* A prospective survey in a children's hospital. J Infection 1984;9:264–70.

40. Carson JW. Changing patterns in childhood gastroenteritis. Ir Med J 1989;82:66–7.

41. Egger M, Mausezahl D, Odermatt P, et al. Symptoms and transmission of intestinal cryptosporidiosis. Arch Dis Child 1990;65:445–7.

42. Thomson MA, Benson JW, Wright PA. Two year study of *Cryptosporidium* infection. Arch Dis Child 1987;62:559–63.

43. Aye T, Moe K, Nyein MM, Swe T. Cryptosporidiosis in Myanmar infants with acute diarrhea. Southeast Asian J Trop Med Public Health 1994;25:654–6.

44. Bogaerts J, Lepage P, Rouvroy D, et al. Cryptosporidiosis in Rwanda. Clinical and epidemiological features. Ann Soc Belg Med Trop 1987;67:157–65.

45. Nwabusi C. Childhood cryptosporidiosis and intestinal parasitosis in association with diarrhoea in Kwara State, Nigeria. West Afr Med J 2001;20:165–8.

46. Zu SX, Zhu SY, Li JF. Human cryptosporidiosis in China. Trans R Soc Trop Med Hyg 1992;86:639–40.

47. Kelly P, Makumbi FA, Carnaby S, et al. Variable distribution of *Cryptosporidium parvum* in small and large intestine in AIDS revealed by polymerase chain reaction. Eur J Gastro Hepatol 1998;10:855–8.

48. Phillips AD, Thomas AG, Walker-Smith JA. *Cryptosporidium*, chronic diarrhoea and the proximal small intestinal mucosa. Gut 1992;33:1057–61.

49. Kotler DP, Francisco A, Clayton F, et al. Small intestinal injury and parasitic diseases in AIDS. Ann Int Med 1990;113:444–9.

50. Kelly P, Davies SE, Mandanda B, et al. Enteropathy in Zambians with HIV related diarrhoea: Regression modelling of potential determinants of mucosal damage. Gut 1997;41:811–6.

51. Chen X-M, Levine S, Splinter PL, et al. *Cryptosporidium parvum* activates NFκ)B in biliary epithelia preventing epithelial cell apoptosis. Gastroenterology 2001;120: 1774–83.

52. Pollok RCG, McDonald V, Kelly P, Farthing MJG. The role of *Cryptosporidium parvum*-derived phospholipase in intestinal epithelial cell invasion. Parasitol Research 2003;90:181–6.

53. Kelly P, Thillainayagam AV, Smithson J, et al. Jejunal water and electrolyte transport in human cryptosporidiosis. Dig Dis Sci 1996;41:2095–9.

54. Argenzio RA, Lecce J, Powell DW. Prostanoids inhibit intestinal NaCl absorption in experimental porcine cryptosporidiosis. Gastroenterology 1993;104:440–7.

55. Kelly P, Jack D, Naeem A, et al. Mannose Binding Lectin is a contributor to mucosal defence against *Cryptosporidium parvum* in AIDS patients. Gastroenterology 2000;119:1236–42.

56. Hayward AR, Levy J, Facchetti F, et al. Cholangiopathy and tumors of the pancreas, liver and biliary tree in boys with X-linked immunodeficiency with hyper-IgM. J Immunol 1997;158:977–83.

57. Hunter PR, Nichols G. Epidemiology and clinical features of *Cryptosporidium* infection in immunocompromised patients. Clin Microbiol Rev 2002;15:145–54.

58. Molbak K, Hojlyng N, Gottschau A, et al. Cryptosporidiosis in infancy and childhood mortality in Guinea Bissau, west Africa. BMJ 1993;307:417–20.

59. Mølbak K, Andersen M, Aaby P, et al. *Cryptosporidium* infection in infancy as a cause of malnutrition: A community study from Guinea-Bissau, West Africa. Am J Clin Nutr 1997;65:149–52.

60. Newman RD, Sears CL, Moore SR, et al. Longitudinal study of *Cryptosporidium* infection in children in Northeastern Brazil. J Infect Dis 1999;180:167–75.

61. Lima AA, Moore SR, Barboza MS, et al. Persistent diarrhea signals a critical period of increased diarrhea burdens and nutritional shortfalls: A prospective cohort study among children in Northeastern Brazil. J Infect Dis 2000;181: 1643–51.

62. Niehaus MD, Moore SR, Patrick PD, et al. Early childhood diarrhea is associated with diminished cognitive function 4 to 7 years later in children in a Northeastern Brazil shanty town. Am J Trop Med Hyg 2002;66:590–3.

63. Casemore DP, Armstrong M, Sands RL. Laboratory diagnosis of cryptosporidiosis. J Clin Pathol 1985;38:1337–41.

64. O'Donohue PJ. *Cryptosporidium* and cryptosporidiosis in man and animals. Int J Parasitol 1995;25:139–95.

65. Hewitt RG, Yiannoutsos CT, Higgs ES, et al. Paromomycin: No more effective than placebo for the treatment of cryptosporidiosis in patients with advanced HIV infection. AIDS Clinical Trial Group. Clin Infect Dis 2000;31:1084–92.

66. Miao YM, Awad El-Kariem FM, Franzen C, et al. Eradication of cryptosporidia and microsporidia following successful anti-retroviral therapy. J Acquir Immunodef Syndr 2000;25:124–9.

67. Rossignol JF. Nitazoxanide in the treatment of AIDS-related cryptosporidiosis: Results of the United States compassionate use programme in 365 patients. Aliment Pharmacol Therap 2006;24:887–94.

68. Amadi BC, Mwiya M, Musuku J, et al. Effect of nitazoxanide on morbidity and mortality in Zambian children with cryptosporidiosis: A randomised controlled trial. Lancet 2002;360:1375–80.

69. Rossignol JF, Hidalgo H, Feregrino M, et al. A double-blind placebo controlled trial of nitazoxanide in the treatment of cryptosporidial diarrhea in AIDS patients in Mexico. Trans R Soc Trop Med Hyg 1998;92:663–6.

70. Mwinga A, Hosp M, Zulu I, et al. Tuberculosis preventative treatment also prevented diarrhoea in HIV-infected patients in Zambia. AIDS 2002;16:806–8.

71. Brandborg LL, Goldberg SB, Breidenbach WC. Human coccidiosis a possible cause of malabsorption. New Engl J Med 1970;283:1306–13.

72. DeHovitz JA, Pape JW, Boncy M, Johnson WD. Clinical manifestations and therapy of *Isospora belli* infection in patients with acquired immunodeficiency syndrome. N Engl J Med 1986;315:87–90.

73. Sarfati C, Bourgeois A, Menotti J, et al. Prevalence of intestinal parasites including microsporidia in HIV-infected adults in Cameroon: A cross-sectional study. Am J Trop Med Hyg 2006;74:162–4.

74. Pape JW, Verdier R-I, Johnson WD. Treatment and prophylaxis of *Isospora belli* infection in patients with AIDS. New Engl J Med 1989;32:1044–77.

75. Sturchler D. Parasitic diseases of the small intestinal tract. In: Grey K, editor. Baillieres Clinical Gastroenterology. London: Bailliere Tindall; 1987. p. 397.

76. Ortega YR, Sterling CR, Gilman GH, et al. *Cyclospora* species: A new protozoan pathogen of humans. N Engl J Med 1993;328:1308–12.

77. Hoge CW, Schlim DR, Raja R, et al. Epidemiology of diarrhoeal illness associated with coccidian-like organism among travellers and foreign residents in Nepal. Lancet 1993;341:1175–9.

78. Ho AY, Lopez AS, Eberhart MG, et al. Outbreak of cyclosporiasis associated with imported raspberries, Philadelphia, Pennsylvania 2000. Emerg Infect Dis 2002;8:783–8.

79. Bendall RP, Lucas S, Moody A, et al. Diarrhoea associated with Cyanobacterium-like bodies: A new coccidian enteritis in man. Lancet 1993;341:590–2.

80. Gill GV, Welch E, Bailey JW, et al. Chronic *Strongyloides stercoralis* infection in former British Far East prisoners of war. QJM 2004;97:789–95.

81. Pelletier LL, Gabre-Kidan T. Chronic *Strongyloides* in Vietnam veterans. Am J Med 1985;78:139–40.

82. Viney ME, Brown M, Omoding NE, et al. Why does HIV infection not lead to disseminated strongyloidiasis? J Infect Dis 2004;190:2175–2180.

83. O'Brien W. Intestinal malabsorption in acute infection with *Strongyloides stercoralis*. Trans R Soc Trop Med Hyg 1975;69:69–77.

84. Burke JA. *Strongyloides* in childhood. Am J Dis Child 1978;132:1130–6.

85. Walker-Smith JA, McMillan B, Middleton AW, et al. *Strongyloides* causes small bowel obstruction in an aboriginal infant. Med J Aust 1969;2:1263–5.

86. Pelletier LL, Gabre-kidan T. Chronic strongyloidiasis in Vietnam veterans. Am J Med 1985;78:139–40.

87. Despommier DD. *Trichinella*. In: Cox FEG, Wakelin D, Gillespie SH, Despommier DD, editors. Topley and Wilson's Microbiology and Microbial Infections: Parasitology, 10th edition. London: Hodder Arnold; 2005. p. 757–68.

88. Holland CV. Gastrointestinal nematodes *Ascaris*, hookworm, *Trichuris* and *Enterobius*. In: Cox FEG, Wakelin D, Gillespie SH, Despommier DD, editors. Topley and Wilson's Microbiology and Microbial Infections: Parasitology, 10th edition. London: Hodder Arnold; 2005. p. 713–36.

89. Loffler P. Transient lung infiltrations with blood eosinophilia. Arch Int Allergy 1956;8:54–9.

90. Burman NN, Seghal AK, Chakravarti RN, et al. Morphological and absorption studies of small intestine in hookworm infestation (ankylostomiasis). Indian J Med Res 1970;58:317–25.

91. Gilles HM, Watson-Williams EJ, Ball PAJ. Hookworm infection and anaemia: An epidemiological, clinical and laboratory study. Q J Med 1964;331:1–24.

92. Reynoldson JA, Behnke JM, Pallant LJ, et al. Failure of pyrantel in treatment of human hookworm infections (*Ankylostoma duodenale*) in the Kimberley region of northwestern Australia. Acta Trop 1997;68:301–12.

93. Stauffer W, Ravdin JI. *Entamoeba histolytica*: An update. Curr Opin Infect Dis 2003;16:479–85.

94. Leippe A, Bruhn H, Hecht O, Grotzinger J. Ancient weapons: The three-dimensional structure of amoebapore A. Trends Parasitol 2005;21:5–7.

95. Lewis EA, Antia AU. Amoebic colitis: Review of 295 cases. Trans R Soc Trop Med Hyg 1969;63:633–638.

96. Sanderson IR, Walker-Smith JA. Indigenous amoebiasis: An important differential diagnosis of chronic inflammatory bowel disease. BMJ 1984;289:823.

97. Pittman FE, Pittman JC, El-Hashimi WK. Studies of human amebiasis. III Ameboma: A radiologic manifestation of amebic colitis. Dig Dis 1973;18:1025–31.

98. Martinez-Palomo A, Espinosa-Cantellano M. Amebiasis: *Entamoeba histolytica* infections. In: Cox FEG, Wakelin D, Gillespie SH, Despommier DDj, editors. Topley and Wilson's Microbiology and Microbial Infections: Parasitology, 10th edition. London: Hodder Arnold; 2005. p. 200–17.

99. Walzer PD, Judson FN, Murphy KB, et al. Balantidiasis outbreak in Truk. Am J Trop Med Hyg 1973;22:33–41.

100. Zaman V, Cox FEG. *Balantidium coli*. In: Cox FEG, Wakelin D, Gillespie SH, Despommier DD, editors. Topley and Wilson's Microbiology and Microbial Infections: Parasitology, 10th edition. London: Hodder Arnold; 2005. p. 275–82.

101. Gilles HM. Soil-transmitted helminthes (geohelminths). In: Cook GC, Zumla A, editors. Manson's Tropical Diseases, 21st edition. London: WB Saunders; 2003. p. 1527–60.

102. De Carneri I, Garofano M, Grass L. Investigation of the part played by *Trichuris* infections in delayed mental and physical development of children in Northern Italy. Riv Parasitol 1967;28:103–22.

103. McDonald GSA, Hourihane DO. Ectopic *Enterobius vermicularis*. Gut 1972;13:621–6.

104. Loria-Cortes R, Lobo-Sanahuja JF. Clinical abdominal angiostrongylosis: A study of 116 children with intestinal eosinophilic granuloma caused by *Angiostrongylus costaricensis*. Am J Trop Med Hyg 1980;29:538–44.

105. Strickland GT, Merritt W, El-Sahly A, Abdel-Wahab F. Clinical characteristics and response to therapy in Egyptian children heavily infected with *Schistosoma mansoni*. J Infect Dis 1982;146:20–9.

106. Smith JH, Said MN, Kelada AS. Studies on schistosomal rectal and colonic polyposis. Am J Trop Med Hyg 1977;26:80–4.

107. Chen MC, Chang PY, Chuang CY, et al. Colorectal cancer and schistosomiasis. Lancet 1981;i:971–3.

108. Didier ES, Stovall ME, Green LC, et al. Epidemiology of microsporidiosis: Sources and modes of transmission. Vet Parasitol 2004;126:145–66.

109. Fischer WM, Palmer JD. Evidence from small-subunit ribosomal RNA sequences for a fungal origin of Microsporidia. Mol Phylogenet Evol 2005;36:606–22.

110. Cali A, Owen RL. Intracellular development of *Enterocytozoon*, a unique Microsporidium found in the intestine of AIDS patients. J Protozool 1990;37:145–55.

111. Drobniewski F, Kelly P, Carew A, et al. Human microsporidiosis in African AIDS patients with chronic diarrhea. J Infect Dis 1995;171:515–6.

112. Hartskeerl RA, van Gool T, Schuitema AR, et al. Genetic and immunological characterization of the microsporidian *Septata intestinalis* Cali, Kotler and Orenstein 1993. Reclassification to *Encephulltozoon intestinalis*. Parasitology 1995;110:277–85.

113. Tumwine JK, Kekitiinwa A, Bakeera-Kitaka S, et al. Cryptosporidiosis and microsporidiosis in Ugandan children with persistent diarrhea with and without concurrent infection with the HIV virus. Am J Trop Med Hyg 2005;73:921–5.

114. Sulaiman IM, Bern C, Gilman R, et al. A molecular biologic study of *Enterocytozoon bieneusi* in HIV-infected patients in Lima, Peru. J Eukaryot Microbiol 2005;50:S591–6.

115. Sheikh RA, Prindiville TP, Yenamandra S, et al. Microsporidial AIDS cholangiopathy due to *Encephalitozoon intestinalis*: Case report and review. Am J Gastroenterol 2000; 95:2364–71.

116. Blanshard C, Ellis DS, Tovey DG, et al. Treatment of intestinal microsporidiosis with albendazole in patients with AIDS. AIDS 1992;6:311–3.

117. Molina JM, Tourneur M, Sarfati C, et al. Fumagillin treatment of intestinal microsporidiosis. New Engl J Med 2002;346:1963–9.

118. Myerwitz RL, Pazin GJ, Allen CM. Disseminated candidiasis. Changes in incidence, underlying diseases and pathology. Am J Clin Pathol 1977;68:29–38.

119. Holt H. Candida infection of the esophagus. Gut 1986;9:227–31.

120. Kumar V, Chandrasekaran R, Kumar L. Candida diarrhea. Lancet 1976;i:752.

121. Rinaldi MG. Zygomycosis. Infect Dis Clin North Am 1988;3:19–41.

122. Weisman IM, Moreno AJ, Parker AL, et al. Gastrointestinal dissemination of coccidiomycosis. Am J Gastroenterol 1986;81:589–93.

19.2d. Small Bowel Bacterial Overgrowth

Steven N. Lichtman, MD, FRCP(C)

Bacteria do not inhabit the upper small intestine and stomach in significant numbers, whereas in the colon, concentrations of 100 billion organisms/mL are the norm. Colonic microflora will proliferate in the small intestine, however, whenever intrinsic cleansing mechanisms are interrupted. Classically, colonic flora proliferate in the small intestine in areas of stasis. The clinical syndrome that results has been given a variety of names: stagnant loop, blind loop, contaminated small bowel, small bowel stasis, and small bowel bacterial overgrowth (SBBO) syndrome. In this chapter, I use the latter term, small bowel bacterial overgrowth. The characteristic features of SBBO are[1] abnormal colonization of the upper small intestine by organisms that characteristically reside in the colon,[2] steatorrhea, and[3] anemia.

NORMAL INTESTINE

At birth the intestine is sterile, but soon after parturition, orally ingested organisms begin to colonize the gut.[1] Commensal bacterial populations are not uniform in either number or type (Table 1). In the upper small intestine, aerobic bacteria typical of the oral cavity predominate. Their numbers do not exceed 10^6 organisms/mL. In the colon, strict and facultative anaerobes, adapted to growth within the fecal mass, where

bacterial metabolism quickly deprives the environment of oxygen, are most common. The total number of colonic bacteria/mL is at least 1 million times greater than that of the upper small intestine. Colonic species are listed in some detail in Table 1, but the list is, nevertheless, incomplete. There are at least 60 different bacterial species.[2] Many are present in trace numbers, but under specific circumstances, some of them, such as *Clostridium difficile,* proliferate and cause disease, such as antibiotic-associated colitis. The number of bacteria in the distal small intestine is greater than that of the proximal small bowel. Near the cecum, there may be 10^9 organisms/mL, and the composition of the microflora is similar to that of the colon.

PRESERVATION OF THE NORMAL ENVIRONMENT

The relative sterility of the small intestine depends on a number of factors (Figure 1) that act to reduce bacterial load and prevent colonization. They may be divided into nonimmune and immune categories.

NONIMMUNE ANTIBACTERIAL FACTORS

Gastric acidity acts as an initial line of defense against ingested bacteria. Gastric juice with a pH < 4.0 is bactericidal for most organisms, although not immediately. In one experiment, bacteria instilled into the normal lumen of the stomach were killed within 15 minutes, but when instilled into the achlorhydric stomach, they remained viable for at least an hour.[3] Chronic inhibition of gastric acid increases the number of gastric bacteria substantially.[4] The number of bacteria presented to the duodenum, therefore, depends on the number of organisms ingested and the length of their exposure to low pH.

Two concerns have been raised about low gastric acid and increased bacterial counts induced by the chronic use of drugs that prevent gastric acid secretion. First, N-nitroso compounds are associated with an increased incidence of gastric cancer. Second, when histamine-2 blockers were used in an intensive care unit to prevent stress ulcers, there was a twofold increased incidence of gram-negative bacteria-induced pneumonia in ventilated patients compared with those taking sucralfate, an agent that does not alter gastric pH or bacterial numbers.[5] No studies have been performed on children to determine the effects of acid suppression on SBBO. However, several studies in the elderly show that both omeprazole and ranitidine cause high duodenal bacterial counts and induce intestinal symptoms,[6-7] but this was not found in a third study.[8]

Peristaltic propagation of luminal contents in a steady distal flow toward the colon is of major importance in reducing the growth of bacteria in the proximal intestine. Interdigestive migratory motor complexes (MMCs) are especially important in this role. Bacterial populations rise within hours when the complexes are ablated pharmacologically.[9]

Pancreatic juice has antibacterial activity[10] possibly because of its proteolytic and lipolytic enzymes, although other factors, such as competitive binding and specific antibacterial activities, cannot be ruled out. Digestive secretions may help to limit bacterial growth as well. Colonization requires access to preferential growth sites in stagnant niches, such as the lumina of intestinal glands and membrane sites to which bacteria can bind. Just as importantly, it also requires a relatively large number of available bacteria to exploit these niches at any given instance. Intestinal secretions

Table 1 Commensal Enteric Flora of the Normal Intestinal Tract
Proximal small intestine
< 106 organisms/mL
Aerobic, oral flora dominate
Streptococcus, Lactobacillus, Neisseria
Distal small intestine
> 109 organisms/mL
Greater numbers of anaerobic and facultative anaerobic bacteria
Bacteroides, Escherichia coli, Bifidobacterium
Colon
109--10 organisms/mL
Anaerobic and facultative anaerobic bacteria
Bacteroides, Escherichia coli, Bifidobacterium, Clostridium

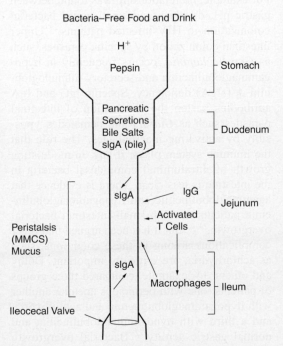

Figure 1 Prevention of small bowel bacterial overgrowth in health.

from the stomach, intestine, and pancreas are, therefore, a deterrent to growth owing to their ability to dilute the bacterial mass. Bile acids have been known to inhibit bacterial growth. Past experimental models showed that bile duct obstruction in rodents caused intestinal bacterial proliferation and oral administration of bile acids inhibited this proliferation. Inagaki and coworkers showed that bile acids activated the farnesoid X receptor (FXR) which modulates many genes, including those in intestinal epithelium. They showed that activation of FXR played an important role in preventing intestinal bacterial proliferation.[11]

Mucus is an example of an epithelial secretion with special properties that enable it to trap bacteria in an intraluminal location while moving organisms distally in bolus fashion. Mucus is composed of a variety of proteins and salts anchored within a viscous gel formed by a single carbohydrate-rich protein. About 80% of the mucus glycoprotein by weight is carbohydrate, and the protein itself is organized as a long thread of disulfide-bonded units, often amounting to a molecular weight of 5 to 10×10^7 D. These huge threads bind bacteria through specific lectin-like reactions with carbohydrate[12] by hydrophobic interactions[13] and probably also through simple trapping. The carbohydrate serves as a nutrient for some bacteria, thus attracting them to a mobile colonization site that is continuously replaced. Huge numbers of organisms (Figure 2)

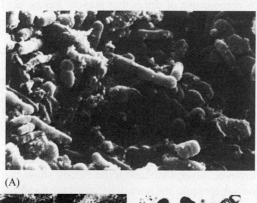

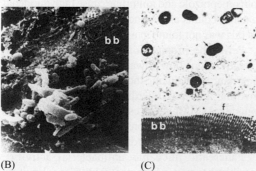

Figure 2 Association of bacteria with the mucous coat in small bowel bacterial overgrowth. (A) Scanning electron micrograph of the unwashed small intestinal surface showing bacterial rods and chains embedded in multiple layers within the surface mucous coat. (B) After gentle washing with saline, the brush border surface (bb) is exposed under strands of mucus. Bacteria remain bound to the mucous strands and not to the brush border. (C) Transmission electron microscopy of an enterocyte with a layer corresponding to surface filaments (f) on the surface of the brush border (bb). Bacteria (arrows) are confined to the mucus outside the filamentous layer.

are found in the mucus coats of the colon[14] and stagnant loops[15] whereas bacteria are relatively scarce on the underlying mucosa and glands, suggesting that mucus limits access of bacteria to the intestinal surface even in stagnant circumstances.

The ileocecal valve prevents retrograde colonization of the distal small bowel.[16] As noted in Table 1, the concentration gradient across the valve is not large, on the order of 100 times. In the absence of the valve, however, free reflux of right-sided liquid colonic content occurs, and the total load of colonic bacteria exposed to the distal small intestine increases greatly.

Bacterial load also affects intestinal colonization. Coprophagic animals, for example, harbor higher numbers of bacteria in the proximal small intestine than do humans, although colonic bacterial populations are equivalent. Poor environmental sanitation, particularly in warm climates, encourages ingestion of excessive numbers of bacteria and may increase the small intestinal bacterial count in this manner.

IMMUNE ANTIBACTERIAL FACTORS

Antibodies to indigenous intestinal bacteria develop early in life[17] and probably play an important role in controlling membrane colonization and mucosal penetration by bacteria and bacterial products. Antibodies to bacterial pilus proteins have been shown to inhibit binding to specific attachment sites on intestinal membranes.[18] Combined immunodeficiency states, notably acquired immunodeficiency syndrome (AIDS) and combined B- and T-cell immunodeficiency, predispose the upper intestine to opportunistic infestation by a variety of parasites. Surprisingly, studies of the prevalence of SBBO in patients with human immunodeficiency virus (HIV) infection yield conflicting results. For example, no relationship was found between gastric pH, diarrhea, and small bowel bacterial colonization in HIV-infected patients.[19] Upper intestinal colonization by specific parasites, such as *Giardia lamblia*, occurs frequently in hypogammaglobulinemia and secretory immunoglobulin A (sIgA) deficiency. Specific IgG and IgA antibodies hasten the elimination of intestinal parasites such as *Giardia* and nematodes[20] possibly by activating macrophages. The role that the immune system plays, if any, in modulating growth of intraluminal commensal bacteria in the intestine is less clear. There is evidence that agammaglobulinemic and hypogammaglobulinemic patients develop small intestinal bacterial overgrowth,[21–22] but it has been argued that other complications arising in these conditions, such as achlorhydria, are critically important. Dolby and others, for example, compared three groups of patients: one with pernicious anemia, another with hypogammaglobulinemia and achlorhydria, and a third with hypogammaglobulinemia and normal gastric acidity.[22] Bacterial overgrowth was found in the first two groups but not in the third. Although an impressive amount of sIgA

enters the intestinal lumen in bile, direct transmucosal secretion is also important. Upper intestinal blind loops, produced experimentally in rats, produce and secrete sIgA with specificity for the colonic-type bacteria.[23] Antibodies secreted by the mucosa may help to prevent mucosal attachment by luminal bacteria. Secretory IgA may also enhance binding of certain bacteria to mucus.[24] Recently, it has been shown that SBBO occurs in a mouse model of cystic fibrosis. SBBO induces intestinal inflammation and mucus accumulation.[25] Antibiotic treatment improves SBBO and the poor weight gain that occurs in these mice.[26] These mice also demonstrate impaired Paneth cell function which may contribute to the development of SBBO.[27]

FACTORS PREDISPOSING TO THE DEVELOPMENT OF SBBO

A large number of specific clinical entities are reported to cause SBBO. Seemingly unrelated illnesses, however, can be grouped into four categories, depending on the mechanism by which the SBBO is produced. As summarized in Table 2, these include (1) anatomic abnormalities, (2) disorders of intestinal motility, (3) lesions that increase the number of bacteria presented to the upper small intestine, and (4) deficiencies of host defense.

Anatomic lesions include diverticula (Figure 3), duplications, and mucosal strictures. These lesions each interrupt normal gut motility and thereby provide a site of relative stasis for bacterial colonization and replication. Surgical procedures such as side-to-side anastomoses,[28] jejunoileal bypass,[29] and neoreservoirs[30] (Koch pouch, ileoanal anastomosis) may create areas of poorly drained bowel and SBBO. Disruption of

Table 2 Factors Predisposing to the Development of Small Bowel Bacterial Overgrowth

Anatomic abnormalities

Diverticula, duplication

Stricture, stenosis, web

Blind loop

Motility disorders

Pseudo-obstruction

Absence of migratory motor complexes

Autonomic neuropathy (eg, diabetes mellitus)

Collagen vascular diseases (eg, scleroderma)

Excessive bacterial load

Achlorhydria

Fistula

Loss of ileocecal valve

Abnormal host defenses

Immunodeficiency

Malnutrition

Prematurity

normal intestinal motor activity causes intestinal stasis by interfering with peristaltic clearing function. Short-term disruption, such as occurs with abdominal surgery, is rarely a problem because although SBBO develops, it rapidly clears with return of motor function. Severe clinical symptoms develop when motility is adversely affected on a more long-term basis. Idiopathic intestinal pseudo-obstruction syndrome is a frequent cause of symptomatic SBBO in children. Secondary causes of a disrupted motility pattern, such as progressive systemic scleroderma and diabetes mellitus with associated autonomic neuropathy, are more frequent considerations in adults. In the elderly, otherwise isolated absence of the MMC is associated with SBBO.[31] The MMC normally has an important "housekeeper" function, helping to keep the proximal small intestine relatively sterile.[32–33] Vantrappen and colleagues showed that 5 of 18 patients with clinically documented SBBO had an absent or disordered MMC pattern.[33] These results have been confirmed and extended.[34] In addition, several studies show that SBBO is associated with delayed gastric emptying.[34–35] Because the activity of the MMC is not fully developed in the immature gut,[36] the premature infant may be at particular risk. Motor abnormalities have subsequently been shown to occur in experimentally produced SBBO[37] indicating that bacterial overgrowth can cause a motor abnormality independently and thus exacerbate the tendency to stasis.

An increased bacterial load that overwhelms the normal host defenses also can result in SBBO. Coloenteric fistulae (Crohn's disease, surgical misadventures), loss of the ileocecal valve (postresection, eg, in Crohn disease or necrotizing enterocolitis), and loss of normal gastric acid output (autoimmune gastritis, malnutrition) may all permit entry into the small intestine of

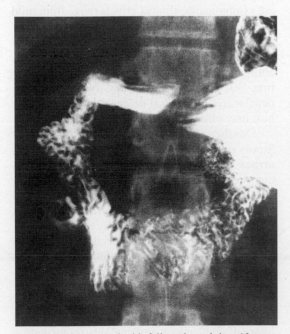

Figure 3 Barium meal with follow-through in a 13-year-old female demonstrates a diverticulum of the duodenum. (Courtesy of Dr David Stringer, Department of Radiology, The Hospital for Sick Children, Toronto.)

Table 3 Intraluminal Bacteria: Effects on the Host		
Intraluminal Effects	Mucosal Effects	Systemic Effects
Bile salt deconjugation	Disaccharidase loss	Absorption of bacterial toxins, antigens
11a-Hydroxylation	Enterocyte damage	Hepatic inflammation
Bile salt depletion		
Lipid malabsorption	Inflammation	Immune complex formation
Vitamin B12 malabsorption	Protein loss	Cutaneous vasculitis
Fermentation—short-chain fatty acids	Bleeding	Polyarthritis
Release of proteases, toxins		

abnormally large numbers of bacteria and initiate SBBO even without appreciable early stasis. Poor sanitation, particularly in the absence of a clean water supply, may also lead to the habitual ingestion of such a large oral load of bacteria that gastric acidity is overwhelmed. Abnormalities of host defense, such as, the achlorhydria associated with hypogammaglobulinemia, are frequently associated with SBBO. Protein-calorie undernutrition is associated with SBBO in children[38–39] and causes loss of gastric acidity,[40–41] decreased mucin production,[42] and impaired cellular and humoral immune function. End-stage renal failure, with creatinine above 6 mg/dL, has also been associated with SBBO.[43] SBBO is reported in patients following liver transplant.[44] Patients with chronic pancreatitis may have an increased incidence of SBBO owing to dysmotility or because of the antibacterial properties of pancreatic juices.[45]

In many clinical settings, etiologic risk factors for SBBO overlap. For example, in underdeveloped countries, it is difficult to separate the effects of an increased bacterial load owing to poor hygienic conditions from the effects of coexisting protein-calorie undernutrition. In experimental animals, using the self-filling blind loop model of SBBO, malnutrition hastens the onset of deficiencies in mucosal hydrolase activities following intestinal stasis.[46] However, in the rat model, protein-caloric deprivation without surgical intervention to induce intestinal stasis does not depress specific activities of brush border disaccharidases. Infants with short bowel syndrome frequently have associated SBBO that complicates their clinical course and medical management. In this setting, SBBO is multifactorial because it can be related to intestinal dysmotility, loss of the ileocecal valve, prior abdominal surgery, and associated malnutrition of the host. In some cases of postinfectious enteropathy, symptoms of chronic diarrhea appear to be related to associated SBBO.[47–49] Although the etiology of bacterial overgrowth in this setting is not clearly established, changes in gut motility, altered host defenses, and coexisting malnutrition each may be contributing factors. Inadequate preparation of food may also be a factor in some countries. For example, the red kidney bean contains a lectin, phytohemagglutinin, which is readily destroyed by heating but which can produce bacterial overgrowth in experimental animals when raw beans are fed to them.[50]

PATHOPHYSIOLOGY

Excessive numbers of intraluminal bacteria alter intraluminal secretions and produce metabolic products, enzymes, and toxins that damage the mucosa and are absorbed. As a consequence, they produce intraluminal, mucosal, and systemic effects (Table 3) that greatly alter the performance of their human host.

INTRALUMINAL EFFECTS

Bacteria are metabolically active organisms, and it is not surprising, therefore, that their nutritional demands conflict with those of the host when their numbers increase in a metabolically active area of the intestine. Pathologic effects are maximal when overgrowth involves the proximal small intestine. Intraluminal anaerobic bacteria, particularly fecal strains, possess enzymes that deconjugate bile salts and convert their component cholic and chenodeoxycholic acids to the secondary bile acids deoxycholate and lithocholate.[51] The net result is to lower the concentration of bile salts in the duodenum and jejunum below the critical micellar concentration (CMC).[52] Above the CMC, much of the triglyceride and cholesterol in the lumen is present in mixed micelles containing hydrolyzed lipid products (fatty acids and mono- and diglycerides) and bile salts. Below the CMC, large liquid crystalline and insoluble emulsoid forms predominate. Because pancreatic lipase is water-soluble and must operate at a lipid–water interface, the great reduction in lipid surface area has disastrous consequences for fat digestion, and malabsorption of triglyceride, fat-soluble vitamins, and other lipid molecules results. Patchy histologic abnormalities, impaired uptake of lipolytic products, and slow chylomicron transport also may contribute to fat malabsorption.[53]

Intraluminal bacteria, particularly Bacteroides species and coliforms, also use vitamin B12 and thus directly compete for dietary vitamin B12, preventing its absorption. When radioactive vitamin B12 is administered to animals or patients with SBBO, most of the radioactivity subsequently recovered from the small bowel contents is bound to enteric microorganisms.[54–55] Once bound, the vitamin is unavailable to the host unless the bacteria die. Luminal bacteria also produce inactive cobamides that are not available to the affected host.[56] Vitamin B12 malabsorption not correctable by exogenous intrinsic factor may be the most consistent feature of clinically significant SBBO.

MUCOSAL EFFECTS

Although bacteria that accumulate in SBBO do not produce classic enterotoxins,[57] they do produce enzymes[58–59] and metabolic products[60–61] that are potentially capable of injuring the mucosa. In experimental blind loops, anaerobic bacteria elaborate proteases with elastase-like properties that remove or destroy glycoprotein enzymes on the brush border surface.[58–59] As a result, mucosal disaccharidase activities are reduced.[62] Monosaccharide transport may also be impaired, reflecting damage to the microvillus plasma membrane and the toxic effects of deconjugated bile salts.[60] Impaired transport of sodium and chloride has also been demonstrated.[63] In the self-filling blind loop, bacterial overgrowth produces a relatively mild morphologic lesion. Both villus height and crypt depth are increased.[64–65] Approximately 10 to 20% of the columnar cells in the upper half of the villi are swollen and vesiculated. Apical membrane microvilli of some, but not all, enterocytes are blunted, swollen, and budded. Damaged mitochondria and endoplasmic reticulum can be found. These experimental findings are in keeping with morphologic reports in humans[66] which suggest that bacterial overgrowth causes a patchy mucosal lesion with segments of subtotal villus atrophy and a marked subepithelial inflammatory response. In infants, particularly, there is a well-established association between carbohydrate intolerance and small intestinal bacterial overgrowth. Protein loss in the intestine may be sufficiently profound in both experimental animals[67] and humans[67–68] to cause hypoproteinemia. Chronic intestinal blood loss also has been documented as a cause of anemia.[69]

Batt and colleagues described German shepherd dogs that spontaneously develop SBBO.[70] These dogs have chronic diarrhea, weight loss, vitamin B12 deficiency, increased folate, and a relative serum IgA deficiency.[71] This model of SBBO differs from that in rats and humans because aerobic bacteria play a more important role in dogs, and total bacterial numbers are generally lower. This causes different types of brush border injury because dogs with aerobic bacterial overgrowth have normal disaccharidase and aminopeptidase N activities. Ten of 17 dogs had aerobic bacterial overgrowth that induced increased γ-glutamyl transferase and decreased alkaline phosphatase.[72] Other than the relative IgA deficiency, the etiology of this spontaneously occurring SBBO is unknown. Riordan and colleagues examined the difference between overgrowth of colonic-type and oropharyngeal-type organisms and found no difference in the morphology of villus height and crypt depth.[73]

SYSTEMIC EFFECTS

Bacterial products and antigens are absorbed through the damaged mucosa, causing systemic effects. SBBO increases intestinal permeability in humans[74] and in rats causes enhanced absorption of the bacterial polymer peptidoglycan.[75]

Abnormalities in both hepatic function and liver architecture develop in the rat self-filling blindloop model of bacterial overgrowth.[76–77] Immune responses are probably responsible for complaints of arthritis and dermatitis. Circulating immune complexes containing IgG, IgA, IgM, and complement are detected during episodes of arthritis associated with SBBO caused by intestinal bypass surgery.[78–79] IgM, IgA, and C3 depositions in the reticular dermis have been demonstrated in association with necrosis of the upper dermis and adjacent vasculitis.[80–81]

Following surgical creation of jejunal self-filling blind loops, SBBO in susceptible rat strains induces hepatobiliary injury.[76] Female Lewis and male and female Wistar and Sprague-Dawley rats develop liver injury by 4 to 9, 12, and 14 weeks, respectively, but Fischer and Buffalo rats do not develop hepatobiliary injury even after 16 weeks. Total anaerobic bacteria within the loops are similar (approximately $10^{8–10}$ organisms/mL), and loop sizes are similar in each rat strain. Metronidazole and tetracycline prevent the lesions in the livers of susceptible strains.[76] Histopathology demonstrates inflammatory infiltration in the portal tracts, with bile duct proliferation and destruction, as well as fibrosis with some inflammation of the parenchyma.[76] Cholangiograms demonstrate widened extrahepatic bile ducts that are thickened and intrahepatic bile ducts that are dilated, tortuous, and irregular.[77] Taken together, these histologic and cholangiographic features resemble primary sclerosing cholangitis in humans. Further studies are required to determine the differences and similarities between SBBO-induced hepatic injury and primary sclerosing cholangitis. It should be noted that SBBO causes translocation of viable bacteria to mesenteric lymph nodes in the rat model, but its significance is unknown because translocation occurs in all rat strains and in the presence of metronidazole, tetracycline, and mutanolysin, which prevent hepatic injury.[76] Intravenous doses of lipopolysaccharide and SBBO (which increases serum lipopolysaccharide levels) worsened liver disease in rats with bile duct ligation.[82] The precise relevance of these animal models to humans remains speculative because in one study with eight adults with anaerobic colonic-type SBBO, only one patient had elevated γ-glutamyl transferase and alkaline phosphatase.[83] In additon, another group showed that only one of 22 patient with PSC had SBBO and that intestinal permeability was similar in patients with PSC compared to controls.[84]

Recently, Kaufman and colleagues showed that in patients with short bowel syndrome, SBBO causes longer total parenteral nutrition dependency and correlates with small intestinal inflammation.[85] They noted that antibiotic therapy was not always successful, resulting in the use of other therapies, including saline enemas, polyethylene glycol infusions, and probiotics.[86]

IMMUNOLOGIC EFFECTS

Rats with self-filling blind loops produce high levels of luminal sIgA specifically targeted against colonic bacteria.[23] Luminal IgA2 and IgM are increased in humans, but IgG1–4 is not.[87] C4 is also not influenced by SBBO.[88] Interleukin-6 is elevated in the lumen of patients with SBBO, but tumor necrosis factor (TNF)-α and interferon are not.[89] Interestingly, increased luminal levels of antigliadin IgA antibodies are observed in patients with SBBO.[90] Serum IgG3 levels are decreased in humans with SBBO but not other serum immunoglobulins and interleukin-2 receptor levels.[89] SBBO may reduce IgG3 in humans via an interaction with mucosa-related immunoregulatory mechanisms, a type of "tolerance."[91] In a rat model of monoarticular arthritis, the acute creation of SBBO reactivates arthritis that may be mediated by release of cytokines from the blind loop.[92] Interestingly, one study found that adults with rheumatoid arthritis have an increased incidence of SBBO.[93] In German shepherd dogs with SBBO, duodenal biopsies show increased TNF-α and transforming growth factor messenger RNA expression that decreases after antibiotic treatment.[94] A single dose of oral cholera vaccine administered to children results in less seroconversion when the children have SBBO.[95] Studies are, therefore, now showing that SBBO affects the local intestinal immune responses, which can have significant distant effects.

CLINICAL FEATURES OF SBBO

Clinical symptoms (Table 4) occur in approximately one-third of all patients.[53] In those who are symptomatic, clinical effects range from mild inconvenience to complaints that are both chronic and disabling. In general, overgrowth of bacteria in the proximal small bowel results in greater disability than overgrowth in the distal small intestine. SBBO may occur at any age, but relative deficiencies in mucosal defenses in the immature host may place the very young at increased risk.

Diarrhea is a common presenting symptom. Stools may be foul and greasy owing to steatorrhea or watery and explosive owing to maldigestion of dietary carbohydrates. In children, growth failure may be an important additional presenting clinical feature. Arrested weight velocity is usually the first feature to be noticed, but later a delay in height velocity and resultant short stature can appear. Nutritional debilitation is multifactorial. Appetite is frequently diminished. Diets may be restricted in an attempt to decrease stool frequency. Maldigestion of fat, dietary carbohydrate[60] and protein[68] and increased intestinal losses of endogenous proteins[69] also contribute.

Clinical evidence of vitamin deficiency is rarely seen. Usually, vitamin B12 deficiency is prevented in the pediatric population by adequate body stores of cobalamin. Iron deficiency anemia can occur, however, secondary to enteric iron losses.[69] Osteomalacia, rickets, and pellagra-like symptoms each have been reported as a consequence of vitamin D malabsorption[96] and vitamin B deficiency.[97] Significantly, lower bone mineral density was found in 14 adults with SBBO compared to controls,[98] but there was no correlation between bone mineral density and SBBO in 11 disabled older people.[99] Because luminal bacteria produce vitamin K and folic acid, absorption may be enhanced and serum folic acid levels were elevated in one study.[100]

Davidson and colleagues indicate that SBBO may be a cause of abdominal pain in young children owing to secondary carbohydrate intolerance.[101] De Boissieu and coworkers confirmed this observation in children under age 2 years and produced a dramatic improvement in diarrhea and abdominal pain using metronidazole and colistin.[102] However, in 8 infants, treatment with metronidazole for colic was not beneficial.[103]

The controversy of the relationship between SBBO and irritable bowel syndrome in adults continues and deserves some attention. Pimental and colleagues reported that 78% of 202 adults with irritable bowel syndrome had SBBO, and that eradication with antibiotic therapy reduced clinical symptoms.[104] A group in Italy confirmed this finding by showing retrospectively that SBBO, diagnosed using glucose breath testing, occurred in 44 of 96 adults with irritable bowel syndrome and that rifaximin helped their symptoms.[105] Others have commented that, by definition, irritable

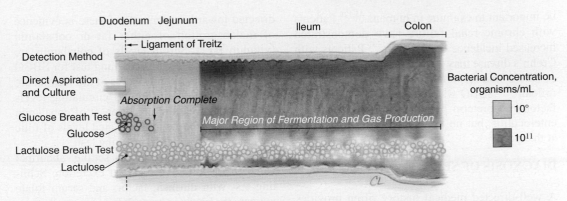

Figure 4 Regions of intestine accessible by various diagnostic methods to detect SBBO. This figure demonstrates how the classic method of duodenal aspiration and culture could yield negative results in a patient with more distal SBBO. This patient would, however, have a positive breath test for SBBO. (From Lin.[108])

bowel syndrome is not associated with underlying intestinal pathology, so these patients may not truly have irritable bowel syndrome.[106] The topic has been reviewed recently with the emphasis on the limitations of breath hydrogen testing, since several groups are unable to show SBBO using culture of duodenal fluid, yet there may be elevated breath hydrogen levels.[107] Lin's group counters these arguments by hypothesizing that the classic definition of SBBO may be too restrictive. The classic definition states that SBBO means that the numbers of bacteria are increased in the duodenum and proximal jejunum because the gold standard is duodenal fluid culture. Lin's group hypothesizes that SBBO could mean more distal increase in bacteria, say the proximal ileum and this would yield abnormal breath hydrogen testing, but normal duodenal fluid cultures Figure 4.[108] If this is true, it would indicate an important change in thinking about SBBO. Data are still conflicting, and it is possible that there is a subgroup of patients with irritable bowel syndrome who have SBBO that causes symptoms along with abnormal motility, psychosocial stresses, and/or visceral hyperalgesia.[109]

Recurrent episodes of arthralgia, nondeforming polyarthritis, tenosynovitis, and cutaneous vasculitis (the arthritis-dermatitis syndrome) occur commonly following intestinal bypass operations but also have been reported in other forms of SBBO.[80] Skin lesions are typically vesiculopustular or erythema nodosum–like. Paresthesias and Raynaud phenomenon are common. Renal damage[110] and hepatic steatosis[111] have also been reported following jejunoileal bypass surgery and could conceivably appear in other forms of SBBO. SBBO may affect drug metabolism. The half-life of antipyrine is increased by 78% in rats with SBBO.[112] Oral digoxin bioavailability is decreased owing to bacterial degradation.[113]

LIVER DISEASE AND SBBO

Many studies have reported that liver disease is associated with SBBO in humans. Dame Sheila Sherlock first described this relationship in alcoholics.[114] Subsequent studies confirmed this finding[198] and extended it to other causes of liver

disease, including viral hepatitis.[115] These studies show that the incidence of SBBO increases with the severity of liver disease and may exceed 50% in patients with Childs-Pugh Class C liver disease.[115] Data suggest that the incidence of spontaneous bacterial peritonitis (SBP) increases with SBBO, but both SBP and SBBO are more frequent as liver disease worsens.[116] Runyon and colleagues used a rat model of cirrhosis to show that increased bacterial translocation is associated with SBBO, with or without SBP.[117] They postulated that the first step toward SBP is SBBO, which causes translocation of bacteria, and then local factors (such as, ascites and ascitic complement levels) ultimately determine whether SBP will occur.[117–118] Chang and colleagues showed that risk factors for SBP in humans were lower serum C3 and C4 concentrations, lower ascitic total protein, and SBBO.[119] The incidence of SBBO in patients with SBP was 68%. Another group has confirmed these experimental studies compared with a frequency of only 17% SBBO in cirrhotics without SBP.[119] However, two other groups, although confirming that adult cirrhotics had a higher incidence of SBBO than noncirrhotics, could not correlate SBBO with SBP.[120–121] In another study of adults with cirrhosis, a 6-month treatment trial with cisapride ($n + 12$) or antibiotics (neomycin and norfloxacin; $n + 12$) enhanced small bowel motility, diminished SBBO, and was associated with slightly improved liver function.[122] This has been recently confirmed in a prospective study of 94 adults with cirrhosis and ascites.[123] Finally, as interest in nonalcoholic steatohepatitis increases,[124] Wigg and colleagues showed that patients with nonalcoholic steatohepatitis have a 50% prevalence of SBBO compared with only 22% of controls,[125] and this has been confirmed.[126] No study of SBBO in the setting of liver diseases in children has yet beenpublished.

OTHER DISEASES ASSOCIATED WITH SBBO

Patients with celiac disease may also have SBBO, especially if their symptoms do not totally improve in a gluten-free diet.[127–128] Experimental pancreatitis has been associated with SBBO and may

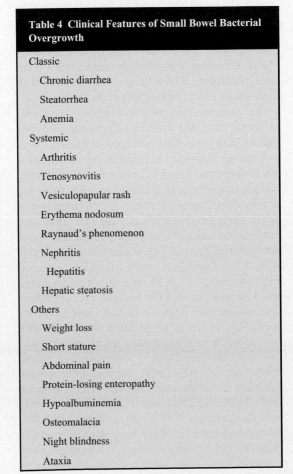

Table 4 Clinical Features of Small Bowel Bacterial Overgrowth

Classic
   Chronic diarrhea
   Steatorrhea
   Anemia
Systemic
   Arthritis
   Tenosynovitis
   Vesiculopapular rash
   Erythema nodosum
   Raynaud's phenomenon
   Nephritis
   Hepatitis
   Hepatic steatosis
Others
   Weight loss
   Short stature
   Abdominal pain
   Protein-losing enteropathy
   Hypoalbuminemia
   Osteomalacia
   Night blindness
   Ataxia

be important to examine in humans.[45,129] Patients with chronic renal failure have demonstrated increased incidence of SBBO[43,130]. Patients with Crohn's disease may have an increased incidence of SBBO that responds to metronidazole or ciprofloxin.[131] SBBO was implicated as a causative factor in a preterm piglet model of necrotizing enterocolitis, but no human studies have looked at this yet.[132]

DIAGNOSIS OF SBBO

A well-directed medical history often provides important clues to indicate that a more detailed investigation related to the possibility of underlying bacterial contamination of the small intestine is warranted. A history of previous abdominal surgery should always be sought because SBBO owing to either alterations of intestinal motility or the creation of anatomic regions of intestinal stasis can occur as a long-term adverse complication of intestinal surgery. Specific surgical procedures that affect normal nonimmunologic host defenses may also predispose the patient to SBBO. For example, interruption of the vagus nerve inhibits output of gastric acid and thereby can result in an increase in the load of viable organisms that enter into the proximal small intestine. Similarly, signs and symptoms suggestive of systemic disease—in particular, collagen vascular diseases—should be explored in a detailed history. Long-standing diabetes mellitus can result in alterations in intestinal motility owing to an autonomic neuropathy. Although not uncommon in adults, SBBO owing to autonomic dysfunction is very unusual in children with diabetes mellitus. This age-related difference may simply relate to the duration of the underlying chronic disease.

Table 5 summarizes alternatives that are useful in establishing the diagnosis of clinically significant SBBO. Evaluation should be

Table 5 Diagnostic Tests for Small Bowel Bacterial Overgrowth

Screening

Sudan stain for neutral fat

72 h fecal fat

Schilling test with intrinsic factor

Folic acid, vitamin B12

Barium meal with follow-through

Diagnostic

Invasive

Duodenal aspiration for culture (aerobic, anaerobic bacteria, and exclude known pathogens)

Deconjugated bile salts

Short-chain fatty acids

Noninvasive

Indicanuria

Serum bile acids

Breath tests

Ataxia

directed toward determining if there is evidence of malabsorption of either fat or cobalamin (vitamin B12). Serum levels of cobalamin are not, in general, a useful screening test for SBBO in children because body stores of the vitamin are sufficient to maintain normal circulating levels for at least 5 years after the onset of cobalamin malabsorption in the gut. Elevated levels of folic acid may be useful as a screening test.

In the appropriate clinical setting, abnormal values of quantitative fecal fat excretion, Schilling test with intrinsic factor, and serum folate indicate the need for more detailed investigations to establish a diagnosis of bacterial overgrowth. Although some physicians would proceed directly to an empiric course of antibiotic therapy, it should be emphasized that clinical symptoms and abnormalities in screening laboratory tests are not specific to this diagnostic consideration.

A barium meal with follow-through should be performed to document the presence of intestinal strictures, diverticula, and delayed intestinal transit. Abnormalities in the radiologic study should prompt more extensive, directed investigations. A normal barium meal study does not exclude the presence of clinically significant bacterial overgrowth in the small intestine. A biopsy of the duodenum should also be obtained because the presenting symptoms of gluten-sensitive enteropathy in children can mimic SBBO. Patchy enteropathic changes with increased numbers of inflammatory cells are typical of SBBO.

SPECIFIC DIAGNOSTIC TESTS

Quantitative culture of increased numbers of anaerobic bacteria in luminal fluid obtained from the proximal small intestine establishes the diagnosis of SBBO. The presence of more than 10^6 colony-forming units/mL of bacteria that are not typical residents of the oral cavity is an abnormal finding. Documentation of coliforms and anaerobic colonic-type bacteria is important because these bacterial species normally do not reside in the mouth or stomach and do not colonize the upper human small intestine. However, the culture of duodenal fluid as a diagnostic technique is not without its problems. Many hospitals do not have bacteriology laboratories with the ability to routinely culture fastidious strict anaerobes. Fortunately, the presence of more than 10^6 colony-forming units of facultative anaerobic bacteria, such as *Escherichia coli* strains, is relatively good evidence of associated colonization by strict anaerobic bacteria. Therefore, quantitative duodenal cultures should be performed even if one lacks anaerobic culture facilities. When culture of duodenal aspirates was compared with that of gastric aspirates and duodenal biopsies in 75 adults, duodenal aspirates proved to be significantly more sensitive.[133]

Neither duodenal aspiration nor quantitative bacterial estimation is easily performed. A great deal of investigation, therefore, has been focused

on establishing the utility of other diagnostic techniques. Two alternative tests that depend on the detection of bacterially derived products (unconjugated bile acids and short-chain fatty acids) may be performed on duodenal aspirates: (1) determination of conjugated and deconjugated bile acid profiles in duodenal fluid[134] and (2) assay of duodenal fluid for the presence of short-chain, volatile fatty acids (ie, acetic, propionic, butyric, isobutyric, valeric, and isovaleric).[135] Each test may be helpful, if decidedly abnormal, but neither has been evaluated fully nor widely performed.

Duodenal aspiration is relatively invasive, and sedation is usually required in children to permit the passage of an aspiration tube through the oral cavity into the upper small bowel. Because fluorography is often used to establish localization of the catheter tip, a small dose of radiation is frequently required. The string test is not an accurate substitute for duodenal intubation.[136] Accurate, noninvasive diagnostic methods are, therefore, an attractive alternative. Although the optimal noninvasive diagnostic probe for use in children has not yet been defined, a number of options are available. Measurement of elevated urinary indican, produced by the conversion of dietary tryptophan to indican by intraluminal bacteria, is perhaps the simplest technique. Specificity is low, however, because indicanuria is not limited to bacterial overgrowth in the small intestine.[137]

Provided that the technique is available, a relatively simple quantitative estimate of serum conjugated and free bile acids may be helpful. Total serum bile acids are often elevated in patients with SBBO, and almost all of the increase is represented by free bile acids, which are normally present in trace amounts.[138] Individual bile acid profiles show that deoxycholate is uniquely elevated, a finding that distinguishes SBBO from ileal resection, which is also associated with high-serum levels of free bile acids [138,139].

In common practice nowadays, a variety of breath tests are used as adiagnostic tools for SBBO (Table 6). Measurement of carbon 14 in expired air following oral ingestion of an appropriate substrate, which is conjugated to the radioisotope, appears to be an excellent alternative for noninvasive diagnostic purposes. ^{14}C-labeled bile acids, such as glycocholate, were the first substrates to be used.[140] Use of the substrate by luminal bacteria releases ^{14}C, which then equilibrates within the tissues of the host and is excreted from the lungs as $^{14}CO_2$ in expired air. A negative test may occur if the bacteria are not able to deconjugate bile acids.[141] In fact, several different breath tests may be required to detect SBBO because of the different metabolic capabilities of the contaminating flora.[142] False-positive results may occur in patients with mucosal inflammation affecting the distal ileum. Several reports indicate that ^{14}C-labeled D-xylose is superior to ^{14}C–bile acid as substrate.[143–144] Improvement in the ^{14}C–D-xylose breath test may be possible by incorporating transit time markers.[145] Another group

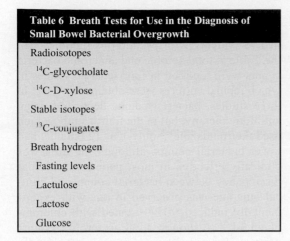

Table 6 Breath Tests for Use in the Diagnosis of Small Bowel Bacterial Overgrowth

Radioisotopes

^{14}C-glycocholate

^{14}C-D-xylose

Stable isotopes

^{13}C-conjugates

Breath hydrogen

Fasting levels

Lactulose

Lactose

Glucose

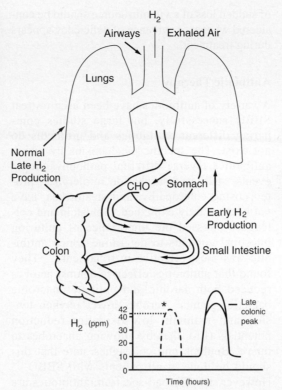

Figure 5 Conceptual framework for breath hydrogen testing. CHO denotes ingesting carbohydrate. *An early peak and an elevated baseline of hydrogen measured in expired breath samples are both suggestive of small bowel bacterial contamination.

showed that combination of the lactulose breath hydrogen test with urinary *p*-aminobenzoic acid (PABA) collection following ursodeoxycholic acid–PABA increases the chance of diagnosing SBBO.[146] Urinary cholyl-PABA excretion is a reliable test in adult patients with SBBO and correlates well with the D-xylose breath test.[147] Unfortunately, the use of ^{14}C is not satisfactory for use in diagnostics for children. Stable isotopes, such as ^{13}C substrate,[148] have been used to study children. For example, in six patients with known SBBO, 50 mg of ^{13}C-xylose produced a maximum breath ^{13}CO$_2$ with 100% sensitivity but only 67% specificity.[149]

Measurement of hydrogen (H$_2$) levels in samples of expired air provides an alternative approach that is currently applicable to the pediatric population. Mammalian cells do not produce H$_2$, whereas many prokaryotes produce it as a by-product of substrate use. The commensal colonic bacteria are generally excellent H$_2$ producers. The H$_2$ is absorbed and distributed throughout the body and is subsequently expired in the breath. Provision of a nonabsorbable sugar, such as lactulose, supplies substrate to the colonic microbial flora and results in an increase in levels of expired H$_2$.[150] If a colonic type of microflora is present in the small intestine, an early H$_2$ peak is observed following lactulose challenge (Figure 5). Absorbable carbohydrates, including lactose[151] and D-glucose[152] may also prove useful as substrates in testing for SBBO by measurement of breath H$_2$. The glucose breath hydrogen test was 44% sensitive, 80% specific and had positive predictive value of 62% in a study of 83 patients.[153]

Perman and colleagues reported that elevations in the fasting level of breath H$_2$ in children correlate with the presence of SBBO.[154] Previous meals containing nonabsorbable carbohydrates[155–156] and endogenous glycoproteins,[157] however, may elevate fasting breath H$_2$ and cause false-positive results. In children, however, a breath H$_2$ level of greater than 42 ppm was seen only in those with SBBO.[154]

Breath H$_2$ testing has shortcomings, however, which may limit its effectiveness. For instance, Douwes and colleagues reported that 9.2% of 98 healthy school-age children who were tested

were non-H$_2$ producers.[158] Children with diarrhea and low-fecal pH have an altered intestinal flora that may not yield H$_2$ in expired air samples.[159–160] Concurrent use of medications, particularly antibiotics,[161] also affects bacterial fermentation of test sugars, which can lower breath H$_2$ levels. A clear separation of "early" and "late" H$_2$ peaks following lactulose ingestion can be affected by the rate of gastric emptying and by intestinal transit time. In practice, two distinct peaks are often not documented.[162] Riordan and colleagues showed that the lactulose breath test was only 16% sensitive and 70% specific, and the double peak was frequently missing in cases of proven SBBO.[163] The same group also found that sensitivity for the rice-based breath hydrogen test was only 33% and did not provide a suitable alternative to culture of duodenal aspirates.[164] One study in adults found that a single resting breath hydrogen test was unreliable.[165] Several reports indicate that the normal microbial flora of the oral cavity also can contribute to the fermentation of carbohydrate substrates and produce modest elevations in the levels of H$_2$ in expired air.[166–167]

Breath H$_2$ tests require careful attention to technical details, which are sometimes difficult to reproduce. End-expiratory samples are most representative, but they are often difficult to obtain in toddlers and preschool-age children. Flow-through appliances that allow collection through a facemask are available and appear to be more readily tolerated.[168] Storage of collected samples in appropriate sealed containers is also critical for accurate results.[169–170] Although breath tests are

more convenient, Corazza and colleagues documented their inferiority compared to jejunal cultures; the glucose breath test yielded a sensitivity of just 62% and a specificity of only 83%.[171]

Comparative studies in adults suggest that ^{14}C–D-xylose is the most appropriate substrate for use in breath testing.[143,162] The comparative sensitivity and specificity of other noninvasive diagnostic assays that are more suitable for use in children have not been clearly defined. However, comparison of a 1 g ^{14}C–D-xylose breath test with the 50 g hydrogen glucose breath test showed that the hydrogen glucose breath test was slightly more sensitive for detecting bacterial overgrowth.[172]

TREATMENT

Correction of the Underlying Disease

As illustrated in Table 2, there are multiple causes of SBBO, some of which are potentially treatable by surgery. Reports of surgical correction include an ileal carcinoid tumor causing obstruction, a large Meckel diverticulum,[173] and an ischemic jejunal stricture following blunt trauma to the abdomen.[174] Gastrointestinal, gastrocolic, and jejunocolic fistulae and intestinal strictures that occur following radiation or surgery or in Crohn's disease are also amenable to surgery. The fact that some cases of SBBO can be cured by surgical intervention emphasizes the importance of investigating each patient carefully for such lesions.

Other cases may be improved by treatment of the primary disease, such as, by employing the use of corticosteroids in patients with symptoms of active Crohn's disease. When disordered motility is the primary problem, as in diabetes mellitus, scleroderma, and intestinal pseudo-obstruction, pharmacologic agents occasionally may prove effective. Cisapride, a prokinetic agent, can, for example, improve motility patterns in some patients with diabetic neuropathy and certain forms of intestinal pseudo-obstruction[175] but is no longer available. The long-acting somatostatin analog octreotide stimulates propagative phase 3 motor activity in the duodenum of patients with scleroderma, which can result in decreased symptoms of SBBO and reduce bacterial counts in the proximal bowel.[176] SBBO associated with scleroderma has also been treated successfully with antibiotics.[177]

Supportive Therapy

Careful attention should be given to ongoing nutritional and metabolic complications. Nutritional deficits should be anticipated and prevented by using appropriate supplements. Energy intake may be limited by anorexia, abdominal pain, and malabsorption. Easily digestible nutritional supplements, which are low in fat, may be required to maintain normal growth and development. Medium-chain triglycerides have been advocated[53] and may be helpful. In intractable situations, such as occur in the pseudo-obstruction syndromes, enteral nutrition with elemental formulae or parenteral nutrition should be employed to maintain growth. Because the course of these diseases can be unpredictable, marginal improvement may eventually allow an adequate oral intake to meet nutritional requirements.

Clinical evidence of vitamin deficiency is rare, but fat-soluble vitamin deficiencies have been reported in patients with SBBO, including a striking case of neurologic deterioration owing to vitamin E deficiency,[178] night blindness owing to vitamin A deficiency,[179] and osteomalacia owing to vitamin D deficiency.[96,180] Patients with steatorrhea should receive fat-soluble vitamins. A good rule is to follow the recommendations for cystic fibrosis.

Vitamin B12 deficiency is rare in children because of the time required to deplete body stores. It is correctable by monthly injections of cyanocobalamin. Anemia may also require treatment with supplemental iron to correct iron deficiency secondary to enteric losses.[69] Treatment with iron may unmask a coexistent and unrecognized macrocytic anemia. B vitamins, vitamin K, and folic acid are normally not depleted by bacteria, which may, indeed, add to host supplies. Tabaqchali and Pallis reported a very interesting case of nicotinamide deficiency that developed in an elderly patient with multiple jejunal diverticula, steatorrhea, and severe protein malnutrition several weeks after apparently successful treatment with protein infusions and antibiotics.[97] The sudden elimination of nicotinamide producing bacteria in the upper intestine may have precipitated pellagra. The possibility of sudden loss of a vitamin source should be considered whenever evidence of deficiency appears during treatment.

Antibiotic Therapy

A variety of antibiotics have been used to treat SBBO successfully, but large studies comparing different antibiotics and protocols do not exist. The specific mechanisms by which antibiotics reverse different pathophysiologic events, such as disaccharide intolerance, protein-losing enteropathy, and steatorrhea, have not been entirely explained. Goldstein and colleagues stressed the importance of culturing intestinal contents to determine which antibiotic was most effective in treatment.[181] They found that antibiotics effective against aerobes reduced both aerobic and obligate anaerobic bacterial counts. Aerobes lower oxygen tension and maintain low oxidation-reduction potentials (Eh), thereby allowing anaerobes to thrive. Bouhnik and colleagues state that this should be done in all patients with SBBO.[182] However, when broad-spectrum antibiotics are successful, they may work by altering the intestinal microecology to reduce the growth of a critical organism. Because no single organism is responsible for all of the abnormalities that occur in SBBO, other investigators believe that isolation of organisms and testing for antibiotic sensitivity are not necessary.

Table 7 summarizes a number of studies in which the antibiotic treatment of SBBO was evaluated by at least one objective parameter.[195-197] Antibiotics have rarely been compared for effectiveness in the same group of patients.

Barry and colleagues showed that metronidazole was superior to kanamycin when evaluated in five patients with pseudo-obstruction.[183] In the Table 7, total aerobic and anaerobic bacteria counts were reported in four separate studies in which jejunal cultures were obtained.[67,183-185] In three studies, bacterial counts decreased using antibiotic therapy, but in the fourth study, which used metronidazole[184] only 1 of 12 patients had lower bacterial counts, although the drug was clinically effective in most patients. A similar discrepancy between bacterial counts and clinical outcome was observed in rats with experimentally induced SBBO treated with chloramphenicol.[53] Although total anaerobic counts were unchanged, Bacteroides species virtually disappeared, suggesting that the effectiveness of antibiotics against that organism may be crucial. The antibiotic responses shown in Table 7 are generally consistent with the crucial role of anaerobes, particularly Bacteroides, in the pathogenesis of SBBO. Patients improve on tetracycline, metronidazole, trimethoprim-sulfamethoxazole, lincomycin, and broad-spectrum antibiotics, whereas kanamycin and neomycin, two antibiotics to which Bacteroides is generally resistant, have proven ineffective. Bacteroides also plays a crucial role in experimentally produced SBBO. Welkos and colleagues showed that kanamycin and penicillin lowered the number of aerobic bacteria in rats with self-filling blind loops but did not reverse vitamin B12 malabsorption.[186] By contrast, metronidazole greatly diminished Bacteroides counts and corrected the vitamin B12 malabsorption. Subsequently, Bacteroides species were shown to bind to intrinsic factor—vitamin B12 complex

Table 7	Results of Antibiotic Treatment of Small Bowel Bacterial Overgrowth				
Underlying Cause	Number of Cases	Symptom or Laboratory Test	Antibiotic (Number Improved)	Intestinal Bacteria (Number Reduced)	Reference
Scleroderma	4	Stool fat	Tetr (3) (Kan, Neo, Sulf—fail)	ND	195
Jejunoileal bypass	5	Diarrhea, pain	Metr (5) (Kan—fail)	Anaerobic (5); aerobic (0)	183
Billroth II	12	Diarrhea, pain, vomiting	Metr (6); cotrimoxazole (1)	Total (1/3)	184
Pseudo-obstruction	1	Indoxyl sulfate excretion	Tetr (1) (Neo—fail)	ND	196
Postanastomosis	1	Stool fat	Tetr (1)	E. coli (1)	185
Billroth II	1	51Cr clearance	Broad spectrum (2)	Aerobic (2)	67
Pelvic radiation	1	Stool fat		Anaerobic (2)	
Jejunoileal bypass	12	Liver steatosis, diarrhea	Metr: steatosis (12); diarrhea (9)	ND	111
None	9	Breath H2, abdominal pain	Linc (4); Trimeth (2); Amox (1); Flucox (1); Sulf (1)	ND	101
Malnutrition	14	Breath H2, diarrhea	Metr (11)	ND	197
Mixed	18	Breath 14CO2 (bile acid)	Tetr (12)	ND	32
Mixed	21	Breath H2, symptom score	Rifax (9/10); Chlor (2/11)	ND	188
Mixed	10	Breath H2, stool number	Norflox (9); Amox-Clav (6); Saccharo (0)	ND	189

much more avidly than to five aerobic bacteria and seven other anaerobic bacterial species.[186]

These and other studies suggest that the most appropriate therapeutic approach is to choose an antibiotic that is effective against Bacteroides, such as tetracycline, metronidazole, chloramphenicol, or lincomycin. Of these four antibiotics, metronidazole is the least likely to cause untoward side effects in children and is probably the antibiotic of choice for initiating treatment. An initial course of 2 to 4 weeks duration may be followed by clinical improvement lasting many months. If relapse occurs, a second course of the same antibiotic for a longer period (4 to 8 wk) may be tried. Relapse or persistence of steatorrhea, vitamin B12 malabsorption, or other complications may be amenable to continuous antibiotic administration, accompanied by periodic alternation with broad-spectrum antibiotics, such as trimethoprim-sulfamethoxazole or gentamicin. Chloramphenicol and lincomycin should be reserved for cases in which other antibiotics have failed.

A nonabsorbable derivative of rifamycin, rifaximin, was shown to be effective in treating SBBO.[187] Using breath hydrogen following a 50 g glucose load as an indicator of SBBO, rifaximin for 7 days normalized breath tests in 70% of subjects compared with chlortetracycline, which normalized breath tests in only 27%.[188] Rifaximin was not helpful in 14 patients with SBBO and Crohn's disease,[190] whereas metronidazole and ciprofloxin were effective.[131] In 7 patients without Crohn's disease who had blind loops, metronidazole was also shown to be more effective than rifaximin.[191] Norfloxacin and amoxicillin–clavulanic acid decreased diarrhea and improved breath hydrogen tests in a randomized crossover trial of 10 patients with SBBO.[189]

A recent case report showed that lactulose was effective in treating SBBO where broad-spectrum antibiotics had failed, perhaps by production of short-chain fatty acids and acidification of the intestinal lumen.[192]

Increasingly, probiotics are becoming a therapeutic tool for use in a variety of gastrointestinal disorders. One study failed to show improvement in 17 patients with SBBO following treatment with *Lactobacillus fermentum*.[193] In contrast, there was some success reported in 8 hemodialysis patients with SBBO by using the probiotic agent *Lactobacillus acidophilus*.[43] In another study, 22 patients with proven SBBO were treated with either a combination of *Lactobacillus casei* and *L. acidophilus* (n + 12) or placebo (n + 10).[194] Probiotic treatment improved stool frequency and glucose breath hydrogen test results but did not improve the patients' other symptoms. Use of *Saccharomyces boulardii* failed to provide clinical benefit in an open trial of 10 patients with SBBO.[189] In summary, at the end of 2006, it appears that metronidazole and tetracycline are still drugs of choice for SBBO. Rifaximin is promising but has given mixed results, and probiotics have not yet proven efficacious.

REFERENCES

1. Long SS, Swenson RM. Development of anerobic fecal flora in healthy newborn infants. J Pediatr 1977;91:298–301.
2. Drasar BS, Hill MJ. Human Intestinal Flora. London: Academic Press; 1974.
3. Giannella RA, Broitman SA, Zamcheck N. Influence of gastric acidity on bacterial and parasitic enteric infections: A perspective. Ann Intern Med 1973;78:271–6.
4. Snepar R, Poporad GA, Romano JM, et al. Effect of cimetidine and antacid on gastric microbial flora. Infect Immun 1982;36:518–24.
5. Driks MR, Craven DE, Celli BR, et al. Nosocomial pneumonia in intubated patients given sucralfate as compared with antacids or histamine type 2 blockers. The role of gastric colonization. N Engl J Med 1987;317:1376–82.
6. Pereira SP, Gainsborough N, Dowling RH. Drug-induced hypochlorhydria causes high duodenal bacterial counts in the elderly. Aliment Pharmacol Ther 1998;12:99–104.
7. Lewis SJ, Franco S, O'Keefe JD. Altered bowel function and duodenal bacterial overgrowth in patients treated with omeprazole. Aliment Pharmacol Ther 1996;10:557–61.
8. Hutchinson S, Logan R. The effect of long-term omeprazole on the glucose-hydrogen breath test in elderly patients. Age Aging 1997;26:87–9.
9. Scott LD, Cahall DL. Influence of the interdigestive myoelectric complex on enteric flora in the rat. Gastroenterology 1982;82:737–45.
10. Rubinstein E, Mark Z, Haspel J, et al. Antibacterial activity of the pancreatic fluid. Gastroenterology 1985;88:927–32.
11. Inagaki T, Moschetta A, Lee Y-K, et al. Regulation of antibacterial defense in the small intestine by the nuclear bile acid receptor. PNAS 2006;103:3920–25.
12. Drumm B, Roberton AM, Sherman PM. Inhibition of attachment of *Escherichia coli* RDEC-1 to intestinal microvillus membranes by rabbit ileal mucus and mucin in vitro. Infect Immun 1988;56:2437–42.
13. Drumm B, Neumann AW, Policova Z, Sherman PM. Bacterial cell surface hydrophobicity properties in the mediation of in vitro adhesion by the rabbit enteric pathogen *Escherichia coli* RDEC-1. J Clin Invest 1989;84:1588–94.
14. Baylis CE, Turner RJ. Examination of organisms associated with mucin in the colon by scanning electron microscopy. Micron 1982;13:35–40.
15. Sherman P, Fleming N, Forstner J, et al. Bacteria and the mucus blanket in experimental small bowel bacterial overgrowth. Am J Pathol 1987;126:527–34.
16. Griffen WO, Richardson JD, Medley ES. Prevention of small bowel contamination by the ileocecal valve. South Med J 1971;64:1056–9.
17. Crabbe PA, Bazin H, Eyssen H, Heremans JF. The normal microbial flora as a major stimulus for proliferation of plasma cells synthesizing IgA in the gut. Int Arch Allergy 1968;34:362–75.
18. Beachey EH. Bacterial adherence: Adhesin-receptor interactions mediating the attachment of bacteria to mucosal surfaces. J Infect Dis 1981;143:325–45.
19. Wilcox CM, Waites KB, Smith PD. No relationship between gastric pH, small bowel bacterial colonisation, and diarrhea in HIV-1 infected patients. Gut 1999;44:101–5.
20. Kaplan BS, Uni S, Aikawa M, Mahmoud AA. Effector mechanism of host resistance in murine giardiasis: Specific IgG and IgA cell-mediated toxicity. J Immunol 1985;134:1975–81.
21. Borriello SP, Reed PJ, Dolby JM, et al. Microbial and metabolic profile of achlorhydric stomach: Comparison of pernicious anemia and hypogammaglobulinemia. J Clin Pathol 1985;38:946–53.
22. Dolby JM, Webster AD, Borriello SP, et al. Bacterial colonization and nitrite concentration in the achlorhydric stomachs of patients with primary hypogammaglobulinemia or classical pernicious anemia. Scand J Gastroenterol 1984;19:105–10.
23. Lichtman S, Sherman P, Forstner G. Production of secretory immunoglobulin A in rat self-filling blind loops: Local sIgA immune response to luminal bacterial flora. Gastroenterology 1986;91:1495–502.
24. Magnusson KE, Stjernstrom I. Mucosal barrier mechanisms: Interplay between secretory IgA, IgG, and mucins on the surface properties and association of Salmonella with intestine and granulocytes. Immunology 1982;45:239–47.
25. De Lisle RC, Roach EA, Norkina O. Eradication of small intestinal bacterial overgrowth in the cystic fibrosis mouse reduces mucus accumulation. J Pediatr Gastroenterol Nutr 2006;42:46–52.
26. Norkina O, Burnett TG, De Lisle RC. Bacterial overgrowth in the cystic fibrosis transmembrane conductance regulator null mouse small intestine. Infect Immun 2004;72:6040–9.
27. Ouellette AJ. Paneth cell alpha-defensins:peptide mediators of innate immunity in the small intestine. Springer Semin Immunopathol 2005;27:133–46.
28. Buchnall TE, Westall C. Ileocolic blind loops following side-to-side anastomoses. J R Soc Med 1980;73:882–4.
29. Drenick EJ, Ament ME, Finegold SM, et al. Bypass enteropathy: Intestinal and systemic manifestations following small-bowel bypass. JAMA 1976;236:269–72.
30. Kelly DG, Phillips SF, Kelly KA, et al. Dysfunction of the continent ileostomy: Clinical features and bacteriology. Gut 1983;24:193–201.
31. Roberts SH, James O, Jarvis EH. Bacterial overgrowth syndrome without "blind loop": A cause for malnutrition in the elderly. Lancet 1977;ii:1193–5.
32. Sarna SK. Cyclic motor activity; migratory motor complex: 1985. Gastroenterology 1985;89:894–913.
33. Vantrappen G, Janssens J, Hellemans J, Ghoos Y. The interdigestive motor complex of normal subjects and patients with bacterial overgrowth of the small intestine. J Clin Invest 1977;59:1158–66.
34. Stotzer P-O, Bjornsson ES, Abrahamsson H. Interdigestive and postprandial motility in small-intestinal bacterial overgrowth. Scand J Gastroenterol 1996;31:875–80.
35. Stotzer P-O, Fjalling M, Gretarsdottir J, Abrahamsson H. Assessment of gastric emptying. Dig Dis Sci 1999;44:729–34.
36. Ruckebusch Y. Development of digestive motor complexes during perinatal life: Mechanism and significance. J Pediatr Gastroenterol Nutr 1986;5:523–6.
37. Justus PG, Fernandez A, Martin JL, et al. Altered myoelectric activity in the experimental blind loop syndrome. J Clin Invest 1983;72:1064–71.
38. Black RE, Brown KH, Becker S. Malnutrition is a determining factor in diarrheal duration, but not incidence, among young children in rural Bangladesh. Am J Clin Nutr 1984;39:87–94.
39. Heyworth B, Brown J. Jejunal microflora in malnourished Gambian children. Arch Dis Child 1975;50:27–33.
40. Gracey M, Culity GJ, Suharjono S. The stomach in malnutrition. Arch Dis Child 1977;52:325–7.
41. Gilman RH, Partanen R, Brown KH, et al. Decreased gastric acid secretion and bacterial colonization of the stomach in severely malnourished Bangladeshi children. Gastroenterology 1988;94:1308–14.
42. Sherman P, Forstner J, Roomi N, et al. Mucin depletion in the intestine of malnourished rats. Am J Physiol 1985;248: G418–23.
43. Simenhoff ML, Dunn SR, Zollner GP, et al. Biomodulation of the toxic and nutritional effects of small bowel bacterial over-growth in end-stage kidney disease using freeze-dried Lactobacillus acidophilus. Miner Electrolyte Metab 1996;22:92–6.
44. Mack DR, Dhawan A, Kaufman SS, et al. Small bowel bacterial overgrowth as a cause of chronic diarrhea after liver trans-plantation in children. Liv Transplant Surg 1998;4:166–9.
45. Trepsi E, Ferrieri A. Intestinal bacterial overgrowth during chronic pancreatitis. Curr Med Res Opin 1999;15:47–52.
46. Sherman P, Wesley A, Forstner G. Sequential disaccharides loss in rat intestinal blind loops: Impact of malnutrition. Am J Physiol 1985;248:G626–32.
47. Hill ID, Mann MD, Moore L, Bowie MD. Duodenal microflora in infants with acute and persistent diarrhea. Arch Dis Child 1983;58:330–4.
48. Penny ME, Harendra De Silva DG, McNeish AS. Bacterial contamination of the small intestine of infants with enteropathogenic Escherichia coli and other enteric infections: A factor in the aetiology of persistent diarrhea? BMJ 1986;292:1223–6.
49. Househam KC, Mann MD, Mitchell J, Bowie MO. Duodenal microflora of infants with acute diarrheal disease. J Pediatr Gastroenterol Nutr 1986;5:721–5.
50. Banwell JG, Boldt DH, Meyers J, Weber FL Jr. Phytohemagglutinin derived from red kidney bean (Phaseolus vulgaris): A cause for intestinal malabsorption associated with bacterial overgrowth in the rat. Gastroenterology 1983;84:506–15.
51. Hill MJ, Drasar BS. Degradation of bile salts by human intestinal bacteria. Gut 1968;9:22–7.
52. Kim YS, Spritz N, Blum M, et al. The role of altered bile acid metabolism in the steatorrhea of experimental blind loop. J Clin Invest 1966;45:956–63.
53. King CE, Toskes PP. Small intestinal bacterial overgrowth. Gastroenterology 1979;76:1035–55.
54. Schonsby H, Hofstad T. The uptake of vitamin B12 by the sediment of jejunal contents in patients with the blind-loop syndrome. Scand J Gastroenterol 1975;10:305–9.
55. Giannella RA, Broitman SA, Zamcheck N. Vitamin B12 uptake by intestinal microorganisms: mechanism and relevance to syndromes of intestinal bacterial overgrowth. J Clin Invest 1971;50:1100–7.

56. Brandt LJ, Bernstein LH, Wagle A. Production of vitamin B12 analogues in patients with small-bowel bacterial overgrowth. Ann Intern Med 1977;87:546–51.
57. Klipstein FA, Engert RF, Short HB. Enterotoxigenicity of colonising coliform bacteria in tropical sprue and blind-loop syndrome. Lancet 1978;ii:342–4.
58. Jonas A, Krishnan C, Forstner G. Pathogenesis of mucosal injury in the blind loop syndrome: Release of disaccharidases from brush border membranes by extracts of bacteria obtained from intestinal blind loops in rats. Gastroenterology 1978;75:791–5.
59. Riepe SP, Goldstein J, Alpers DH. Effect of secreted Bacteroides proteases on human intestinal brush border hydrolases. J Clin Invest 1980;66:314–22.
60. Gracey M, Burke V, Oshin A, et al. Bacteria, bile salts and intestinal monosaccharide malabsorption. Gut 1971; 12:683–92.
61. Prizont R, Whitehead JS, Kim YS. Short chain fatty acids in rats with jejunal blind loops. Gastroenterology 1975;69: 1254–65.
62. Jonas A, Flanagan PR, Forstner GG. Pathogenesis of mucosal injury in the blind loop syndrome: Brush border enzyme activity and glycoprotein degradation. J Clin Invest 1977;60:1321–30.
63. Schulke JD, Fromm M, Menge H, Rieken EO. Impaired intestinal sodium and chloride transport in the blind loop syndrome of the rat. Gastroenterology 1987;92:693–8.
64. Menge H, Kohn R, Dietermann KH, et al. Structural and functional alterations in the mucosa of self-filling intestinal blind loops in rats. Clin Sci 1979;56:121–31.
65. Toskes PP, Gianella RA, Jervis HR, et al. Small intestinal mucosal injury in the experimental blind loop syndrome. Gastroenterology 1975;68:1193–203.
66. Ament ME, Shimoda SS, Saunders DR, Rubin CE. Pathogenesis of steatorrhea in three cases of small intestinal stasis syndrome. Gastroenterology 1972;63:728–47.
67. King CE, Toskes PP. Protein-losing enteropathy in the human and experimental rat blind loop syndrome. Gastroenterology 1981;80:504–9.
68. Jones EA, Craigie A, Tavill AS, et al. Protein metabolism in the intestinal stagnant loop syndrome. Gut 1968;9:466–9.
69. Giannella RA, Toskes PP. Gastrointestinal bleeding and iron absorption in the experimental blind loop syndrome. Am J Clin Nutr 1976;29:754–7.
70. Batt RM, Carter MW, Peters TJ. Biochemical changes in the jejunal mucosa of dogs with a naturally occurring enteropathy associated with bacterial overgrowth. Gut 1984;25:816–23.
71. Whitbread TJ, Batt RM, Garthwaite G. Relative deficiency of serum IgA in the German shepherd dog: A breed abnormality. Res Vet Sci 1984;37:350–2.
72. Batt RM, McLean L. Comparison of the biochemical changes in the jejunal mucosa of dogs with aerobic and anaerobic bacterial overgrowth. Gastroenterology 1987;93:986–93.
73. Riordan SM, McIver CJ, Wakefield D, et al. Small intestinal mucosal immunity and morphometry in luminal overgrowth of indigenous gut flora. Am J Gastroenterol 2001;96:494–500.
74. Riordan SM, McIver CJ, Thomas DH, et al. Luminal bacteria and small-intestinal permeability. Scand J Gastroenterol 1997;32: 556–63.
75. Lichtman SN, Keku J, Schwab JH, Sartor RB. Evidence for peptidoglycan absorption in rats with experimental small bowel bacterial overgrowth. Infect Immun 1991;59:555–62.
76. Lichtman SN, Keku J, Schwab JH, Sartor RB. Hepatic injury associated with small bowel bacterial overgrowth in rats is prevented by metronidazole and tetracycline. Gastroenterology 1991;100:513–9.
77. Lichtman SN, Keku J, Clark RL, et al. Biliary tract disease in rats with experimental small bowel bacterial overgrowth. Hepatology 1991;13:766–72.
78. Rose E, Espinoza L, Osterland CK. Intestinal bypass arthritis: Association with circulating immune complexes and HLAB27. J Rheumatol 1977;4:129–34.
79. Clegg DO, Zone JJ, Samuelson CO, Ward JR. Circulating immune complexes containing secretory IgA in jejunoileal bypass disease. Ann Rheum Dis 1985;44:239–44.
80. Klinkhoff AV, Stein HB, Schlapper OL, Boyka WB. Postgastrectomy blind loop syndrome and the arthritis-dermatitis syndrome. Arthritis Rheum 1985;28:214–7.
81. Jorizzo JL, Apisarnthanarax P, Subrt P, et al. Bowel bypass syndrome without bowel bypass. Arch Intern Med 1983;143:457–61.
82. Mentes BB, Tatlicioglu E, Akyol G, et al. Intestinal endotoxins are co-factors of liver injury in obstructive jaundice. HPB Surg 1996;9:61–9.
83. Riordan SM, McIver CJ, Williams R. Liver damage in human small intestinal bacterial overgrowth. Am J Gastroenterol 1998;93:234–7.
84. Bjornsson E, Cederborg A, Akvist A, et al. Intestinal permeability and bacterial growth of the small bowel in patients with primary sclerosing cholangitis. Scand J Gastroenterol 2005;40:1090-4.
85. Kaufman SS, Loseke CA, Lupo JV, et al. Influence of bacterial overgrowth and intestinal inflammation in duration of parenteral nutrition in children with short bowel syndrome. J Pediatr 1997;131:356–61.
86. Vanderhoof JA, Young RJ, Murray N, Kaufman SS. Treatment strategies for small bowel bacterial overgrowth in short bowel syndrome. J Pediatr Gastroenterol Nutr 1998;27:155–60.
87. Riordan SM, McIver CJ, Wakefield D, et al. Luminal immunity in small-intestinal bacterial overgrowth and old age. Scand J Gastroenterol 1996;31:1103–9.
88. Riordan SM, McIver CJ, Thomas MC, et al. The expression of complement protein 4 and IgG3 in luminal secretions. Scand J Gastroenterol 1996;31:1098–102.
89. Riordan SM, McIver CJ, Wakefield D, et al. Mucosal cytokine production in small-intestinal bacterial overgrowth. Scand J Gastroenterol 1996;31:977–84.
90. Riordan SM, McIver CJ, Wakefield D, et al. Luminal antigliadin antibodies in small intestinal bacterial overgrowth. Am J Gastroenterol 1997;92:1335–40.
91. Riordan SM, McIver CJ, Wakefield D, et al. Serum immunoglobulin and soluble IL-2 receptor levels in small intestinal over-growth with indigenous gut flora. Dig Dis Sci 199;44:939–44.
92. Lichtman SN, Wang J, Sartor RB, et al. Reactivation of arthritis induced by small bowel bacterial overgrowth in rats: Role of cytokines, bacteria and bacterial polymers. Infect Immun 1995;63:2295–301.
93. Henriksson AEK, Blamquist L, Nord C-E, et al. Small intestinal bacterial overgrowth in patients with rheumatoid arthritis. Ann Rheum Dis 1993;52:503–10.
94. German AJ, Helps CR, Hall EJ, Day MJ. Cytokine mRNA expression from German shepherd dogs with small intestinal enteropathies. Dig Dis Sci 2000;45:7–17.
95. Lagos R, Fasano A, Wasserman SS, et al. Effect of small bowel bacterial overgrowth on the immunogenicity of single-dose live cholera vaccine CVD 103-HgR. J Infect Dis 1999;180:1709–12.
96. Schjonsby H. Osteomalacia in the stagnant loop syndrome. Acta Med Scand Suppl 1977;603:39–41.
97. Tabaqchali S, Pallis C. Reversible nicotinamide deficiency encephalopathy in a patient with jejunal diverticulosis. Gut 1970;11:1024–8.
98. Stotzer P-O, Johansson C, Mellstrom D, et al. Bone mineral density in patients with small intestinal bacterial overgrowth. Hepatogastroenterol 2003;50:1415–8.
99. Mitsui T, Shimaoka K, Takagi C, et al. Small bowel bacterial overgrowth may not affect bone mineral density in older people. Clin Nutr 2005;24:920–4.
100. Hoffbrand AV, Tabaqchali S, Mollin DL. High serum folate levels in intestinal blind-loop syndrome. Lancet 1966;i:1339–42.
101. Davidson GP, Robb TA, Kirubakaran CP. Bacterial contamination of the small intestine as an important cause of chronic diarrhea and abdominal pain: diagnosis by breath hydrogen test. Pediatrics 1984;74:229–35.
102. De Boissieu D, Chaussain M, Badoual J, et al. Small-bowel bacterial overgrowth in children with chronic diarrhea, abdominal pain, or both. J Pediatr 1996;128:203–7.
103. Hochman J, Simms C. The role of small bowel bacterial overgrowth in infantile colic. J Pediatr 2005;147:410–11.
104. Pimental M, Chow EJ, Lin HC. Eradication of small intestinal bacterial overgrowth reduces symptoms of irritable bowel syndrome. Am J Gastroenterol 2000;95:3503–6.
105. Cuoco L, Salvagnini M. Small intestine bacterial overgrowth in irritable bowel syndrome: A retrospective study of rifaximin. Minerva Gastroenterol Dietol 2006;52:89–95.
106. Cuoco L, Cammarota G, Jorizzo R, Gasbarrini G. Small intestinal bacterial overgrowth and symptoms of irritable bowel syndrome. Am J Gastroenterol 2001;96:2281–2.
107. Simren M, Stotzer P-O. Use and abuse of hydrogen breath tests. Gut 2006;55:297–3.
108. Lin HC. Small intestinal bacterial overgrowth: A framework for understanding irritable bowel syndrome. JAMA 2004;292:852–8.
109. Drossman DA. Treatment for bacterial overgrowth in the irritable bowel syndrome. Ann Intern Med 2006;145:626–7.
110. Drenick EJ, Eister J, Johnson D. Renal damage with intestinal by-pass. Ann Intern Med 1978;89:594–9.
111. Drenick EJ, Fisler J, Johnson D. Hepatic steatosis after intestinal bypass: Prevention and reversal by metronidazole, irrespective of protein-calorie malnutrition. Gastroenterology 1982;82:535–48.
112. Aarbakke J. Impaired oxidation of antipyrine in stagnant loop rats. Scand J Gastroenterol 1977;12:929–35.
113. Lindenbaum J, Rund DG, Butler VP, et al. Inactivation of digoxin by the gut flora: Reversal by antibiotic therapy. N Engl J Med 1981;305:789–94.
114. Sherlock S. Bacterial levels in cirrhosis. Clin Sci 1957; 16:35–51.
115. Yang C-Y, Chang C-S, Chen G-H. Small-intestinal bacterial over-growth in patients with liver cirrhosis, diagnosed by glucose H2 or CH4 breath tests. Scand J Gastroenterol 1998;33:867–71.
116. Guarner C, Runyon BA, Young S, et al. Intestinal bacterial over-growth and bacterial translocation in cirrhotic rats with ascites. J Hepatol 1997;26:1372–8.
117. Runyon BA, Sugano S, Kanel G, Mellencamp MA. A rodent model of cirrhosis, ascites and bacterial peritonitis. Gastroenterology 1991;100:489–93.
118. Sanchez E, Casafont F, Guerra A, et al. Role of intestinal bacterial overgrowth and intestinal motility in bacterial translocation in experimental cirrhosis. Rev Esp Enferm Dig 2005;97:805–14.
119. Chang C-S, Yang S-S, Kao C-H, et al. Small intestinal bacterial overgrowth versus antimicrobial capacity in patients with spontaneous bacterial peritonitis. Scand J Gastroenterol 2001;36:92–6.
120. Karaca C, Kaymakoglu S, Uyar A, et al. Intestinal bacterial over-growth in liver cirrhosis: is it a predisposing factor for spontaneous ascitic infection? Am J Gastroenterol 2002;97:1851.
121. Bauer TM, Steinbruckner B, Brinkmann FE, et al. Small intestinal bacterial overgrowth in patients with cirrhosis: Prevalence and relation with spontaneous bacterial peritonitis. Am J Gastroenterol 2001;96:2962–7.
122. Madrid AM, Hurtado C, Venegas M, et al. Long-term treatment with cisapride and antibiotics in liver cirrhosis: Effect on small intestinal motility, bacterial overgrowth, and liver function. Am J Gastroenterol 2001;96:1251–5.
123. Sandhu BS, Gupta R, Sharma J, et al. Norfloxacin and cisapride combination decreases the incidence of spontaneous bacterial peritonitis in cirrhotic ascites. J Gastroenterol Hepatol 2005;20:599–06.
124. Angulo P. Nonalcoholic fatty liver disease. N Engl J Med 2002;346:1221–31.
125. Wigg AJ, Roberts-Thomson IC, Dymock RB, et al. A role of small intestinal bacterial overgrowth, intestinal permeability, endotoxemia, and tumor necrosis factor in the pathogenesis of non-alcoholic steatohepatitis. Gut 2001;48:206–11.
126. Sajjad A, Motterhead M, Syn WK, et al. Ciprofloxin suppresses bacterial overgrowth, increases fasting insulin but does not correct low acylated ghrelin concentration in nonalcoholic steatohepatitis. Aliment Pharacol Ther 2005;22: 291–9.
127. Tursi A, Brandimarte G, Giorgetti G. High prevalence of small bowel bacterial overgrowth in celiac patients with persistence of gastrointestinal symptoms after gluten withdrawal. Am J Gastroenterol 2003;98:720–2.
128. Krauss N, Schuppan D. Monitoring nonresponsive patients who have celiac disease. Gastrointes Endosc Clin N Am 2006;16:317–27.
129. Felius V, Akkermans LM, Bosscha K, et al. Interdigestive small bowel motility and duodenal bacterial overgrowth in experimental acute pancreatitis. Neurogastroenterol Motil 2003;15:267–76.
130. Strid H, Simren M, Stotzer P-O, et al. Patients with chronic renal failure have abnormal small intestinal motility and a high prevalence of small intestinal bacterial overgrowth. Digestion 2003;67:129–37.
131. Castiglione F, Rispo A, Di Girolamo E, et al. Antiobiotic treatment of small bowel bacterial overgrowth in patients with Crohn's disease. Aliment Pharmacol Ther 2003;18:1107–12.
132. Sangild PT, Siggers RH, Schmidt M, Elnif J, et al. Diet- and colonization-dependent intestinal dysfunction predisposes to necrotizing enterocolitis in preterm pigs. Gastroenterol 2006;130:1776–92.
133. Stotzer PO, Brandberg A, Kilander AF. Diagnosis of small bowel bacterial overgrowth in clinical praxis: A comparison of the culture of small bowel aspirate, duodenal biopsies and gastric aspirate. Hepatogastroenterology 1998;45:1018–22.
134. Northfield TC, Drasar BS, Wright TJ. Value of small intestinal bile acid analysis in the diagnosis of the stagnant loop syndrome. Gut 1973;14:341–7.
135. Hoverstad T, Bronneklett A, Fausa O, Midtvedt T. Short-chain fatty acids in the small-bowel bacterial overgrowth syndrome. Scand J Gastroenterol 1985;20:492–9.
136. Riordan SM, McIver CJ, Duncombe VM, Bolin TD. An appraisal of a "string test" for the detection of small bowel bacterial overgrowth. J Trop Med Hyg 1995;98:117–20.
137. Aarbakke J, Schjonsby H. Value of urinary simple phenol and indican determinations in the diagnosis of the stagnant loop syndrome. Scand J Gastroenterol 1976;11:409–14.

138. Lewis B, Tabaqchali S, Panveliwalla D, et al. Serum bile-acids in the stagnant-loop syndrome. Lancet 1969;i:219–20.

139. Setchell KDR, Harrison DL, Gilbert JM, Murphy GM. Serum unconjugated bile acids: Qualitative and quantitative profiles in ileal resection and bacterial overgrowth. Clin Chim Acta 1985;152:297–306.

140. Sherr HP, Sasaki Y, Newman A, et al. Detection of bacterial deconjugation of bile acids by a convenient breath analysis technic. N Engl J Med 1971;285:656–61.

141. Shindo K, Yamazaki R, Mizuno T, et al. The deconjugation ability of bacteria isolated from the jejunal fluids in the blind loop syndrome with high 14CO2 excretion. Life Sci 1989;45.2275–83.

142. Suhr O, Danielsson A, Horstedt P, Stenling R. Bacterial contamination of the small bowel evaluated by breath tests, 75Selabelled homocholic-tauro acid, and scanning electron microscopy. Scand J Gastroenterol 1990;25:841–52.

143. King CE, Toskes PP, Guilarte TR, et al. Comparison of the one-gram D(14C)-xylose breath test to the (14C) bile acid breath test in patients with small-intestine bacterial overgrowth. Dig Dis Sci 1980;25:53–8.

144. Schneider A, Novis B, Chen V, Leichtman G. Value of the D-14C-xylose breath test in patients with intestinal bacterial over-growth. Digestion 1985;32:86–91.

145. Lewis SJ, Young G, Mann M, et al. Improvement in specificity of (14C)D-xylose breath test for bacterial overgrowth. Dig Dis Sci 1997;42:1587–92.

146. Kiss ZF, Wolfling J, Csati S, et al. The ursodeoxycholic acid-paminobenzoic acid deconjugation test, a new tool for the diagnosis of bacterial overgrowth syndrome. Eur J Gastroenterol Hepatol 1997;9:679–82.

147. Bardhan PK, Feger A, Kogon M, et al. Urinary choloyl-PABA excretion in diagnosing small intestinal bacterial over-growth. Dig Dis Sci 2000;45:474–9.

148. Klein PD, Klein ER. Application of stable isotopes to pediatric nutrition and gastroenterology: Measurement of nutrient absorption and digestion using 13C. J Pediatr Gastroenterol Nutr 1985;4:9–19.

149. Dellert SF, Nowicki MJ, Farrell MK, et al. The 13C-xylose breath test for the diagnosis of small bowel bacterial overgrowth in children. J Pediatr Gastroenterol Nutr 1997;25:153–8.

150. Rhodes JM, Middleton P, Jewell DP. The lactulose hydrogen breath test as a diagnostic test for small bowel bacterial over-growth. Scand J Gastroenterol 1979;14:333–6.

151. Nose D, Kai H, Harada T, et al. Breath hydrogen test in infants and children with blind loop syndrome. J Pediatr Gastroenterol Nutr 1984;3:364–7.

152. Kerlin P, Wong L. Breath hydrogen testing in bacterial overgrowth of the small intestine. Gastroenterology 1988;95:982–8.

153. Ghoshal UC, Ghoshal U, Das K, Misra A. Utility of hydrogen breath tests in diagnosis of small intestinal bacterial overgrowth in malabsorption syndrome and its relationship to orocecal transit time. Indian J Gastroenterol 2006: 25:6–10.

154. Perman JA, Modler S, Barr RG, Rosenthal P. Fasting breath hydrogen concentration: Normal values and clinical applications. Gastroenterology 1984;87:1358–63.

155. Hanson CF, Winterfeldt EA. Dietary fiber effects on passage rate and breath hydrogen. Am J Clin Nutr 1985;42:44–8.

156. Levitt MD, Hirsh P, Fetzer CA, et al. H2 excretion after ingestion of complex carbohydrates. Gastroenterology 1987;92:383–9.

157. Perman JA, Modler S. Glycoproteins as substrates for production of hydrogen and methane by colonic bacterial flora. Gastroenterology 1982;83:388–93.

158. Douwes AC, Schaap C, Van Der Klein-Van Moorsel JM. Hydrogen breath test in school children. Arch Dis Child 1985;60:333–7.

159. Perman JA, Modler S, Olson AC. Role of pH in production of hydrogen from carbohydrates by colonic bacterial flora. J Clin Invest 1981;67:643–50.

160. Moore D, Lichtman S, Durie P, Sherman P. Primary sucrase-isomaltase deficiency: Importance of clinical judgement. Lancet 1985;ii:164–5.

161. Rao SS, Edwards CA, Austin CJ, et al. Impaired colonic fermentation of carbohydrate after ampicillin. Gastroenterology 1988;94:928–32.

162. King CE, Toskes PP. Comparison of the 1-gram (14C) xylose, 10-gram lactulose-H2, and 80-gram glucose-H2 breath tests in patients with small intestine bacterial overgrowth. Gastroenterology 1986;91:1447–51.

163. Riordan SM, McIver CJ, Walker BM, et al. The lactulose hydrogen breath test and small intestinal bacterial overgrowth. Am J Gastroenterol 1996;91:1795–9.

164. Riordan SM, McIver CJ, Duncombe VM, et al. Evaluation of the rice breath hydrogen test for small intestinal bacterial over-growth. Am J Gastroenterol 2000;95:2858–64.

165. Riordan SM, McIver CJ, Bolin TD, Duncombe VM. Fasting breath hydrogen concentrations in gastric and small-intestinal bacterial overgrowth. Scand J Gastroenterol 1995;30:252–7.

166. Thompson DG, O'Brien DG, Hardie JM. Influence of the oropharyngeal microflora on the measurement of exhaled breath hydrogen. Gastroenterology 1986;91:853–60.

167. Mastropaolo G, Rees WDW. Evaluation of the hydrogen breath test in man: Definition and elimination of the early hydrogen peak. Gut 1987;28:721–5.

168. Tadesse K, Leung DTY, Lau S. A new method of expired gas collection for the measurement of breath hydrogen (H2) in infants and small children. Acta Paediatr Scand 1988;77:55–9.

169. Rumessen JJ, Gudmand-Hoyes E. Retention and variability of hydrogen (H2) samples stored in plastic syringes. Scand J Clin Lab Invest 1987;47:627–30.

170. Ellis CJ, Kneip J, Levitt MD. Storage of breath samples for H2 analyses. Gastroenterology 1988;94:822–4.

171. Corazza GR, Menozzi MG, Stricchi A, et al. The diagnosis of small bowel bacterial overgrowth: Reliability of jejunal culture and inadequacy of breath hydrogen testing. Gastroenterology 1990;98:302–9.

172. Stotzer P-O, Kilander AF. Comparison of the 1-gram 14C-D-xylose breath test and the 50-gram hydrogen glucose breath test for the diagnosis of small intestinal bacterial overgrowth. Digestion 2000;61:165–71.

173. Savino JA. Malabsorption secondary to Meckel's diverticulum. Am J Surg 1982;144:588–92.

174. Isaacs P, Rendall M, Hoskins EOL. Ischemic jejunal stenosis and blind loop syndrome after blunt abdominal trauma. J Clin Gastroenterol 1987;9:96–8.

175. Hyman PE, McDiarmid SV, Napolitano J, et al. Antroduodenal motility in children with chronic intestinal pseudo-obstruction. J Pediatr 1988;112:899–905.

176. Soudah HC, Hasler WL, Owyang C. Effect of octreotide on intestinal motility and bacterial overgrowth in scleroderma. N Engl J Med 1991;325:1461–7.

177. Kahn IJ, Jeffries GH, Sleisenger MH. Malabsorption in intestinal scleroderma: Correction by antibiotics. N Engl J Med 1966; 274:1339–44.

178. Brin MF, Fetell MR, Green PH, et al. Blind loop syndrome, vitamin E malabsorption, and spinocerebellar degeneration. Neurology 1985;35:338–42.

179. Levy NS, Toskes PP. Fundus albipunctatus and vitamin A deficiency. Am J Ophthalmol 1974;78:926–9.

180. Manicourt DH, Orloff S. Osteomalacia complicating a blind loop syndrome from congenital megaesophagus-megaduodenum. J Rheumatol 1979;6:57–64.

181. Goldstein F, Mandle RJ, Schaedler RW. The blind loop syndrome and its variants. Am J Gastroenterol 1973;60: 255–64.

182. Bouhnik Y, Alain S, Attar A, et al. Bacterial populations contaminating the upper gut in patients with small intestinal bacterial overgrowth syndrome. Am J Gastroenterol 1999;94:1327 31.

183. Barry RE, Chow AW, Dillesdon J. Role of intestinal microflora in colonic pseudo-obstruction complicating jejunoileal bypass. Gut 1977;18:356–9.

184. Bjorneklett A, Fausa O, Midtvedt T. Small-bowel bacterial over-growth in the postgastrectomy syndrome. Scand J Gastroenterol 1983;18:277–87.

185. Donaldson RM. Studies on the pathogenesis of steatorrhea in the blind loop syndrome. J Clin Invest 1965;44:1815–25.

186. Welkos SL, Toskes PP, Baer H. Importance of anaerobic bacteria in the cobalamin malabsorption of the experimental rat blind loop syndrome. Gastroenterology 1981;80: 313–20.

187. Corazza GR, Ventrucci M, Strocchi A, et al. Treatment of small intestine bacterial overgrowth with rifaximin, a non-absorbable rifamycin. J Int Med Res 1988;16:312–6.

188. Stefano MD, Malservisi S, Veneto G, et al. Rifaximin versus chlortetracycline in the short-term treatment of small intestinal bacterial overgrowth. Aliment Pharmacol Ther 2000;14:551–6.

189. Attar A, Flourie B, Rambaud J-C, et al. Antibiotic efficacy in small intestinal bacterial overgrowth-related chronic diarrhea: A crossover, randomized trial. Gastroenterology 1999; 117:794–7.

190. Biancone L, Vernia P, Agostini D, et al. Effect of rifaximin on intestinal bacterial overgrowth in Crohn's disease as assessed by the H2-glucose breath test. Curr Med Res Opin 2000;16:14–20.

191. Di Stefano M, Miceli E, Missanelli A, et al. Absorbable vs. non-absorbable antibiotics in the treatment of small intestine bacterial overgrowth in patients with blind-loop syndrome. Aliment Pharmacol Ther 2005;21:985–92.

192. Kurtovic J, Segal I, Riordan SM. Culture-proven small intestinal bacterial overgrowth as a cause of irritable bowel syndrome: Response to lactulose but not to broad spectrum antibiotics. J Gastroenterol 2005;40:767–8.

193. Stotzer P-O, Blomberg L, Conway PL, et al. Probiotic treatment of small intestinal bacterial overgrowth by Lactobacillus fermentum KLD. Scand J Infect Dis 1996;28:615–9.

194. Goan D, Garmendia C, Murrielo NO, et al. Effect of Lactobacillus strains on bacterial overgrowth-related chronic diarrhea. Medicina 2002;62:159–63.

195. Kahn IJ, Jeffries GH, Sleisenger MH. Malabsorption in intestinal scleroderma: Correction by antibiotics. N Engl J Med 1966;274:1339–44.

196. Pearson AJ, Brzechwa-Ajdukiewicz A, McCarthy CF. Intestinal pseudo-obstruction with bacterial overgrowth in the small intestine. Am J Dig Dis 1969;14:200–5.

197. Hammond-Gabbaden C, Heinkens GT, Jackson AA. Small bowel overgrowth in malnourished children as measured by breath hydrogen test. West Indian Med J 1985;34:48–9.

198. Gunnarsdottir SA, Sadik R, Shev S, et al. Small intestinal motility disturbances and bacterial overgrowth in patients with liver cirrhosis and portal hypertension. Am J Gastroenterol 2003;98:1362–70.

Immune and Inflammatory Disorders

20.1. Inflammation

Thomas Blanchard, PhD
Claudio Fiocchi, MD
Steven J. Czinn, MD

Inflammation is the most common type of response that the body mounts when facing an assault from the surrounding environment. This is true for all tissues, organs, and systems, but in each one of these compartments, the inflammatory response varies depending on two key factors: the nature of the inciting agent(s) and the characteristics of the microenvironment in which inflammation ensues. The gastrointestinal tract is the ultimate example of how specific cellular and functional features shape the type, degree, and duration of inflammation. In this regard, the digestive system is unique owing to several specialized features: it is permanently exposed to the external environment, is constantly stimulated by a myriad of antigens, and harbors a luxuriant mix of bacteria, fungi, and viruses making up the endogenous enteric flora. Therefore, even under completely physiologic conditions, the intestinal tract contains enormous amounts of leukocytes, which are diffusely scattered in the lamina propria and the intraepithelial compartment or are organized in the Peyer patches of the terminal ileum and the isolated lymphoid follicles of the colon.[1] Combined, they form the anatomic basis of the gut- or mucosa-associated lymphoid tissue and functionally represent a tightly controlled form of self-contained inflammation termed "physiological inflammation."[2] The latter occurs in response to stimuli coming from the luminal surface of the mucosa and is found exclusively in the gut. In fact, other body surfaces exposed to alternate external or internal environments contain comparatively minimal amounts of lymphoid cells, as found in the lungs, skin, and urinary tract. In contrast to physiologic inflammation, which is anatomically restricted, tightly controlled, beneficial, and actually indispensable to health, pathologic inflammation in the gut is an injurious process that, particularly if severe and protracted, can lead to major functional and structural changes, causing clinical symptoms and impairing the quality of life of affected individuals. Fortunately, most forms of intestinal inflammation are transient and of limited impact on the general health of the patients, as are most acute viral and bacterial infections in children. Nevertheless, there are still a considerable number of other forms of gastrointestinal inflammation that result in serious clinical manifestations, as described in other chapters of this textbook. The focus of this review is on intestinal inflammation that induces tissue damage and functional derangements.

In addition to lymphoid cells, extremely diversified and highly specialized cell types of ectodermal, mesodermal, and endodermal origin compose the intestine. These include epithelial, mesenchymal, endothelial, and nerve cells, to which the extracellular matrix (ECM) must be added in view of increasing evidence for active participation of this acellular component in both immunity and inflammation.[3] A review of intestinal inflammation includes all of the above cellular and acellular elements because of accumulating evidence that an inflammatory response is not simply the consequence of a deranged immune response but a far more complex interplay of immune and nonimmune cell interactions.[4] How such interactions take place is incompletely understood, but at least two classes of elements are involved: one is represented by an enormous variety of soluble mediators released by immune and nonimmune cells such as cytokines, eicosanoids, neuropeptides, reactive metabolites, and proteases, and the other is represented by cell adhesion molecules, structures that are primarily, although not exclusively, involved in cell-to-cell adhesion events. Combined, soluble factors and cell adhesion molecules facilitate, allow, and amplify the exchange of signaling among cells that is essential to induce and mediate inflammation. Thus, in addition to the cellular components of inflammation, soluble factors and cell adhesion molecules are included in this review.

Because intestinal inflammation encompasses numerous and diverse factors, knowledge of the exact mechanisms and sequential interactions is far from complete. To provide the reader with a reasonably comprehensive overview of intestinal inflammation, information was derived from various sources, including human (pediatric and adult) and animal studies. An inherent caveat with this approach is that most human studies are based on chronic inflammatory conditions, whereas animal studies generally use acute models of intestinal inflammation. In addition, information is complemented by data derived from in vitro studies with single or multiple cellular systems. These sources of information are used to achieve functional and conceptual integration and generate a cohe-sive view of inflammation in the gastrointestinal tract. Finally, inflammation will be discussed as a broadly applicable response, keeping in mind that, in spite of a lack of direct supporting evidence, differences may exist between how this response is mediated in children and adults.

INFLAMMATORY CELLS

Plasma Cells

Immunoglobulin-producing plasma cells, which represent terminally differentiated B-cells, are the most abundant type of lymphoid cell in the intestinal mucosa under both physiologic and inflammatory conditions. The majority of them normally produce dimeric immunoglobulin (Ig)A antibodies that are carried to the luminal surface by a well-defined transfer pathway involving a polymeric Ig receptor produced by the adjacent epithelial cells.[5] The expression of certain molecular determinants, such as the integrin $\alpha4\beta7$ on migrating B-cells (and T-cells) and of the mucosal addressin cell adhesion molecule (MAd-CAM) 1 on high endothelial venules, is believed to underlie the preferential migration of B-cells to the mucosa, but cell differentiation and the functional status probably also play an important role.[6] In fact, normal intestinal B-cells are in a higher state of activation compared with those in the peripheral circulation.[7] During inflammation, migratory patterns, cell proliferation, and state of activation are all drastically altered, resulting in major modifications in the distribution, number, class, and subclass of immunoglobulin-producing plasma cells. There is a consistent increase in IgG-secreting plasma cells that appears to be independent of the segment of the gastrointestinal tract involved, as observed in gastritis and inflammatory bowel disease.[8,9] In addition, the production of different subclasses of Igs is markedly abnormal, with predominance of IgG1- or IgG2-producing cells depending on the type of inflammatory process, as in ulcerative colitis versus Crohn's disease.[10,11] Altered proportions of monomeric (systemic) and dimeric (mucosal) IgA or IgA1 versus IgA2 also can be found.[12,13] It is still uncertain what the consequences of an increased number of B-cells in the inflamed mucosa might be because they are not, per se, pathogenic. In fact the continuous presence of large amounts of IgA in the intestinal mucus is believed to form a barrier of "natural" immunity given the broad spectrum and antigenic specificity and strong potential for cross-reactivity these antibodies possess. However, changes in IgA subclass could impair defenses against dietary and bacterial antigens, and the production of complement-fixing antibodies, primarily of the IgG1 subclass, could contribute to or amplify tissue damage, and an increase in IgE-producing cells could mediate allergic reactions, leading to the release of a vast array of inflammatory mediators.

T-Cells

The migration, distribution, and localization of T-cells in the intestinal mucosa involve some of the same molecular mechanisms used by B-cells6 and include CCR6 and CCR9 expression for homing to locally produced ligands CCL20 and CCL25 (TECK), respectively. However, these mechanisms tend to be more complex than those for B-cells and are drastically altered during inflammation. In contrast to granulocytes, whose high cell number in an inflamed tissue is directly related to an increased emigration rate, changes in T-cell number and function involve multiple abnormalities in the entry, proliferation, exit, and death in the inflamed gut.[14] Expectedly, the number and state of activation of T-cells are both increased in the inflamed intestine, but the proportions of CD4+ to CD8+ T-cells in the mucosa are usually not remarkably shifted away from the normal CD4-to-CD8 ratio, regardless of the type and location of inflammation.[15–17] This is true for T-cells infiltrating the lamina propria, which predominantly express the αβ T-cell receptor. Alterations in the composition of intraepithelial T-cells, which are predominantly CD8+ and tend to express the γδ T-cell receptor in higher proportions, are less marked in some types of inflammation, such as inflammatory bowel disease.[18] In celiac disease, on the other hand, their number can increase, as well as the type of T-cells that preferentially express the γδ T-cell receptor.[19,20]

Because T-cells control all aspects of cell-mediated immunity, their presence and abnormal state of activation suggest that they play a pivotal role in most, if not all, aspects of intestinal inflammation.[21] Their role likely includes antigen-specific responsiveness, immunoregulation, immunosuppression, cytokine production, and perhaps cytotoxic activity. With the exception of cytokine production (which is discussed in another section of this chapter), evidence that intestinal T-cells exert all other functions is still fragmentary and incomplete. Mucosal T-cells substantially differ from T-cells circulating in the periphery in regard to their intrinsic ability to respond to receptor-mediated activation. They are preferentially stimulated through the CD2 pathways, in contrast to blood T-cells that use the classic CD3 pathway for optimal activation,[22,23] an event perhaps conditioned by mucosal factors.[24] If true,

one could also expect that when the mucosa is involved by inflammation, this may also influence and modify the behavior of local T-cells. Mucosal T-cells from inflammatory bowel disease display an enhanced proliferative response to bacterial antigens in both humans and experimental models,[25–27] as small intestinal T-cells do in response to gliadin in celiac patients[28] and probably gastric T-cells to *Helicobacter pylori* antigens.[29] Additional investigation is needed, however, to understand how these antigen-specific responses may trigger the cascade of events leading to the changes recognized as hallmarks of gastrointestinal inflammation. That these events actually occur in the mucosa is suggested by experiments in which nonspecific activation of local T-cells induces an enteropathy manifested by anatomic adaptation of the mucosal architecture or even damage to the mucosa.[30,31] Additional supporting evidence comes from studies of celiac disease, in which the typical morphologic changes of flattened mucosa can be reproduced in vitro and in vivo by gliadin challenge,[32] an event associated with major histocompatibility complex (MHC) class II-restricted specific recognition of selectively modified gliadin peptides by gut mucosal T-cells.[33] Detailed knowledge of the steps leading from antigen-specific T-cell recognition to overt tissue damage is nevertheless limited. In particular, evidence for the existence of classic cytotoxic T-cells, which specifically recognize and destroy intestinal cell targets, is still missing. On the other hand, a study suggests that proteolytic injury mediated by broadly active proteases is active downstream of the T-cell activation events.[34]

The most recent type of T-cells to attract considerable attention in intestinal inflammation is regulatory T-cells (Treg). Previously called suppressor T-cells, Treg cells represent a diverse group of cells with potent immunosuppressive activity capable of controlling and preventing autoimmunity and inflammation.[35] The well-defined types are T regulator 1 (Tr1) cells, which mediate suppression primarily through the release of immunosuppressive cytokines such as interleukin (IL)-10, and CD4+CD25+ cells, which seemingly exert suppression by direct cell contact, and T helper (Th) 3 cells, which produce large amounts of transforming growth factor (TGF)-β. Tr1 and CD4+CD25+ cells have been shown to suppress intestinal inflammation in vivo in animal models of inflammatory bowel disease.[36,37] In general Tregs arise naturally as part of the immune system and play an active role in maintaining immunologic homeostasis to autoantigens and commensal organisms. The description of events that provoke the immune system to override such down-regulatory mechanisms in the gut will contribute to our understanding of the etiology of IBD.

Monocytic Cells and Toll-Like Receptors

Monocytes and macrophages are prominent inflammatory cells that, like neutrophils, lack

immunologic memory but are extremely potent in their capacity to mediate tissue damage. The normal small and large bowel contain a moderate number of resident macrophages, which are made up of heterogeneous populations of monocytic cells identifiable by morphologic characteristics and expression of specific cell surface molecules that separate them into categories with preferential antigen-presentation or scavenger activity.[38,39] Macrophages isolated from intestinal tissue carry a distinct phenotype from peripheral macrophages in that they lack several receptors that would normally favor inflammation.[40] These macrophages also tend to have a much weaker response to bacterial stimuli in vitro compared to blood monocytes. Depending on the type of inflammatory process, macrophage heterogeneity is amplified, underlying the recruitment of new cells types as well as diversification of function.[41] They undergo an enhanced respiratory burst activity with release of reactive radicals that contribute to inflammation and local tissue damage.[42] During inflammation, monocytes are actively recruited from the peripheral blood into the mucosa, where they differentiate into macrophages expressing the CD68 and L1 antigens, which differentiates them from pre-existing RFD 7+ macrophages.[43] This recently recruited subset of macrophages with monocyte-like phenotype appears to be primed for release of several proinflammatory cytokines and to have greater pathogenic potential compared with macrophages normally residing in the gut.[44] Mucosal macrophages express several costimulatory molecules, including B1 and B2, which allow them to adhere to and activate T-cells, an interaction that can further contribute to expand immune-mediated inflammation.[45]

Macrophages also express a newly described family of cell surface molecules termed pattern recognition receptors (PRRs). These PRRs recognize conserved, pathogen-associated molecular patterns (PAMPS) expressed by various microbes but not the host. One particular family of PRRs, the Toll-like receptors (TLRs), recognizes PAMPs and can influence the character of the inflammatory or immune response through synthesis of proinflammatory cytokines such as IL-1, IL-6, tumor necrosis factor (TNF)-α, and IL-12.[46,47] It has been shown that the TLRs use signaling components and engage a signaling cascade similar to the receptor for IL-1 which includes the MyD88 adaptor protein IRAK kinases, although TLR-3 and TLR-4 can induce a MyD88 independent pathway. Once a TLR recognizes the appropriate PAMP, this ultimately results in the activation of NF-κB inducing kinase and, subsequently, the phosphorylation of I-κB. Phosphorylation causes I-κB to physically dissociate from NF-κB, which is then free to translocate into the nucleus and initiate the gene transcription process that leads to the production of a variety of proinflammatory molecules.[48] Activation of NF-κB by bacterial products is not mediated exclusively by TLRs, and some members of the nucleotide-

Table 1 Toll-Like Receptors and Associated Pathogen-Associated Molecular Patterns

TLR	PAMP
TLR-1	Lipoprotein
TLR-2	Peptidogolycan, bacterial lipoprotein
TLR-3	Double-stranded RNA
TLR-4	Lipopolysaccharide
TLR-5	Flagellin
TLR-6	Lipoprotein
TLR-7	Single-stranded RNA
TLR-8	Single-stranded RNA
TLR-9	Cytosine–phosphorothioate-guanine

PAMP = pathogen-associated molecular pattern; RNA = ribonucleic acid; TLR = Toll-like receptor.

binding oligomerization domain (NOD) family of cytosolic proteins, particularly NOD1 and NOD2, also participate in the innate recognition of microorganisms and regulation of inflammatory responses.[49] They have been shown to bind to certain peptidoglycan components and specific mutations in NOD correlate with an increased risk of developing IBD.[50,51]

In humans, 11 TLRs have been described with different ligand-binding specificities, including flagellin, bacterial deoxyribonucleic acid (DNA), CpG motifs, peptidoglycan, and lipopolysaccharide (Table 1). TLRs that bind to viral or intracellular bacterial antigens tend to be expressed in the cytosol whereas TLRs that bind to surface bacterial antigens are expressed on the macrophage membrane. The binding of specific TLRs dictates the role of the macrophage in promoting the inflammatory response. TLRs also can be found on other cell types, including mast cells and dendritic cells and, to a lesser extent, epithelial cells. In the intestinal epithelium, TLRs are predominantly expressed on the basolateral surface of the cell, but apical expression of TLR-4 is up-regulated during chronic inflammation.[52,53] Some reports have demonstrated that intestinal epithelial cells from patients with Crohn's disease and ulcerative colitis expressed TLR-4, whereas intestinal epithelial cells from healthy individuals do not. TLR-3 and TLR-5 also have been identified in the small intestine.[54,55]

Other Inflammatory Leukocytes

A variety of other myeloid and lymphoid cells are found in inflamed gut, including neutrophils, eosinophils, mast cells, basophils, and dendritic cells. All of these cells are present in increased numbers in affected areas, but such an increase often represents a nonspecific response to inflammation. Less frequently, this represents a selective infiltration of cells that plays a specific role in the inflammatory reaction, such as in the case of eosinophilic gastroenteritis, allergic reactions, or helminthic infestations. Information about the contribution of these cell types is substantially less compared with what is currently known about T- and B-cells in gastrointestinal inflammation.

Polymorphonuclear neutrophils are virtually absent from the normal gut mucosa, and any increase in this cell type, no matter how minute, should raise suspicion that an inflammatory response is occurring. Because neutrophils are short-lived and quickly undergo apoptotic death once translocated into tissues, their numeric increase in the gut is exclusively due to and sustained by emigration from the circulation. This occurs through the expression of multiple adhesion molecules by the neutrophils and the mucosal microvasculature, a topic that is discussed in greater detail later in this chapter.[56] Once localized in the tissue, neutrophils mediate local injury by releasing broad-spectrum proteases and various free radicals,[57] as detailed in the section dealing with soluble mediators of inflammation.

A moderate number of eosinophils are present in the normal intestinal mucosa, whereas mast cells and basophils are less common. All of these cells are increased in number during active inflammation, as seen in inflammatory bowel disease.[58] This is a nonspecific phenomenon, except in conditions in which each cell type can predominate. For example, eosinophils dominate the inflammatory infiltrate during allergic reactions[59] and in conditions of unknown etiology such as eosinophilic gastroenteritis. Like neutrophils, eosinophils are recruited from the circulation, but once localized in the mucosa, they release mediators specifically involved in allergic and parasitic responses, such as IL-4 and IL-5. This is in contrast to mast cells, which, although also involved in similar reactions, are heterogeneous and composed of at least two well-defined populations with distinctive features: connective tissue (typical) mast cells and mucosal (atypical) mast cells.[60] Mucosal mast cells are involved in food allergy, resistance to parasites, and inflammatory bowel disease.[61] Their action is mediated by several soluble products, prominent among which is histamine, an early messenger of inflammatory and immune reactions.[62]

Dendritic cells also need to be mentioned, even though their diversity, complexity, and function in normal mucosal immunity and inflammation have just begun to be investigated. Dendritic cells represent a heterogeneous group of cells with an interdigitating morphology, which are present in low numbers in most tissues of the body and express high levels of human leukocyte antigen (HLA) class II antigens, which make them highly efficient in antigen presentation. Dendritic cells work at the host–pathogen interface to sample antigens and influence the host response to bacterial antigens.[63] They inherently populate the Peyer's patches, Mesenteric Lymph Nodes, and the lamina propria of the intestinal tract. It is not clear whether each tissue type is populated with distinct dendritic cell phenotypes but dendritic cells have been observed to span the gut epithelium and therefore are ideally suited to sample antigen from the lumen.[64] Their type and localization along the intestinal tract may provide key determinants of localized mucosal immune and inflammatory responses.[65]

ADDITIONAL CELLS INVOLVED IN INFLAMMATION

Until quite recently, mucosal inflammation was viewed as a response dominated by the action of classic immune cells, whereas all other cells had only a passive role as targets of immune cells and their products. This view is no longer tenable considering a growing body of information showing that multiple cell types display functional characteristics that make them active players in inflammation.[66] Multiple cell types composing the intestinal wall participate in inflammation, including epithelial cells, endothelial cells, nerve cells, and mesenchymal cells (fibroblasts and myofibroblasts).

Epithelial Cells

The involvement of intestinal epithelial cells in mucosal immune reactivity was initially suggested by the secretory, absorptive, and digestive adaptive changes that these cells undergo during immune and parasitic responses.[67] The identification of epithelial cell heterogeneity and the role of Paneth cell-derived defensins in innate immunity also indicate an active role of the epithelium in intestinal immunity.[68] Levels of defensin expression may vary in different types of intestinal inflammation.[69] Subsequent studies generated evidence for an active role of epithelial cells in normal mucosal immunity and inflammation. Immunohistochemistry detected MHC class II (HLA-DR) antigens on human intestinal epithelial cells,[70] and their capacity to function as antigen-presenting cells was documented in both human and animal studies.[71,72] The expression of HLA-DR antigens is enhanced during intestinal inflammation, as in inflammatory bowel disease, celiac disease, and gastritis,[73–75] indicating that it is a nonspecific response to inflammation unrelated to the type or location of disease. Enhanced expression of accessory molecules is also noted on gastric and colonic epithelial cells during inflammatory conditions, as in the case of the costimulatory molecules CD80 (B1) and CD86 (B2) in *H. pylori* gastritis and ulcerative colitis,[76,77] and intercellular adhesion molecule 1 (ICAM-1) is expressed during bacterial invasion.[78] Additional evidence for the participation of epithelial cells in inflammation comes from studies demonstrating their capacity to both produce and respond to proinflammatory and immunoregulatory cytokines[79] and to express chemokine receptors.[80] In response to bacterial invasion or inflammatory signals, intestinal epithelial cells produce a broad spectrum of bioactive molecules, including IL-1 receptor antagonist, IL-6, IL-7, IL-8, IL-15, monocyte chemotactic protein 1, granulocyte-macrophage colony-stimulating factor (GM-CSF), TNF-α, growth-regulated oncogene (GRO)-α, GRO-γ, macrophage inflammatory protein 2, nitric oxide (NO), and cyclooxygenase (COX) 2.[81–89] Some of these products act on intestinal cells, altering their function, such as the rate of proliferation and barrier function.[90–92]

The expression of various TLR molecules on intestinal epithelial cells indicates that these cells receive signals from commensal and pathogenic microbes, and mutations in NOD expressed by gut epithelial cells increases the risk of developing IDB. Finally, the normal ability to preferentially activate suppressor CD8+ T-cells appears to be shifted to stimulation of helper CD4+ T-cells in inflammatory bowel disease,[93] suggesting that epithelial cells may actually contribute to amplification or persistence of certain forms of chronic inflammation. Altogether, the number and variety of agents and functions mediated by intestinal epithelial cells combined with vigorous responses to multiple inflammatory stimuli provide irrefutable evidence of an essential role of intestinal epithelium in inflammation.

Endothelial Cells

Among the various cell types present in the intestinal wall, none is more directly involved in regulating inflammation than endothelial cells. In fact, the microvascular endothelium is a true "gatekeeper of inflammation" because translocation of leukocytes from the intravascular into the interstitial space, under both physiologic and inflammatory circumstances, is tightly controlled by the junctions between endothelial cells.[94] For translocation to occur, leukocytes must adhere to the endothelium through steps mediated by activation of both leukocytes and endothelial cells followed by the expression of adhesion molecules of the selectin, integrin, and Ig superfamily groups and their corresponding ligands in a highly orchestrated process regulated by multiple cytokines.[95] When inflammation ensues, all of these events occur at the level of the microcirculation in each specific tissue and organ.[96] This is also true for the gastrointestinal tract, in which high endothelial venules, a specialized type of endothelium, play a central role in lymphocyte migration and extravasation.[97] Among others, MAd-CAM-1 is exclusively expressed by the microvascular cells of the gut mucosa, and its level of expression is enhanced during inflammation in both human and animals.[98,99] Thus, considering the importance of the mucosal microvascular endothelium, it is not surprising that leukocyte–endothelial interactions are critical to gastrointestinal inflammation,[100] when the selectivity of lymphoid cell binding to the vascular endothelium may be lost.[101] Studies of the intestinal microvasculature in intestinal inflammation are relatively few. Nonetheless, there is good evidence that inflamed mucosal endothelial cells are in a high state of activation, as indicated by enhanced expression of HLA-DR molecules and inducible nitric oxide synthase (NOS) in areas involved by inflammatory bowel disease.[102,103] More direct evidence of the importance of the microvasculature in inflammation is provided by in vitro studies with human intestinal microvascular endothelial cells (HIMECs). When these cells are obtained from inflamed mucosa of ulcerative colitis or Crohn's disease patients, their capacity to up-regulate leukocyte adhesion is markedly increased.[104] This response is detected only when HIMECs are derived from the chronically inflamed but not the uninvolved mucosa of the same subject.[105] In addition, activated platelets interact with HIMECs via the CD40/CD40 ligand pathway and cause them to up-regulate adhesion molecule expression and chemokine production, inducing a proinflammatory response of the mucosal microvasculature.[106] These observations indicate that in the chronically inflamed intestine, the local mucosal microvascular bed undergoes important functional modifications, conditioned by prolonged exposure to a cytokine-rich milieu and other proinflammatory cellular elements, which are likely to contribute to the maintenance of the inflammatory response.

Nerve Cells

The participation of the nervous system in inflammation is well established.[107] In the gastrointestinal tract, the enteric nervous system forms a rich network of fibers regulating not only motility and secretion but also the local immune response.[108] A dramatic example of the critical role of enteric nerves on inflammation is illustrated by the development of jejunoileitis in animals whose enteric glia are specifically ablated.[109] The action of the enteric nervous system on inflammation is exerted through the release of a large number of neuropeptides that have both stimulatory and down-regulatory effects on the immune response.[110] These mediators play a modulatory role in many forms of intestinal inflammation, such as those induced by infectious agents,[111] or of idiopathic origin, such as in inflammatory bowel disease.[112] Perhaps a more important aspect of the nerve cells is to provide an anatomic basis for the effect of stressful events of life on intestinal immunity and inflammation, a connection proposed in both animal models and humans. Objective evidence supporting this connection is fairly convincing in models of experimental gut inflammation,[113] particularly with the recent demonstration that susceptibility to reactivation by stress requires CD4+ T-cells and can be adoptively transferred by these cells.[114] The link between the enteric nerves and intestinal inflammation is more tenuous in humans, in whom the negative effects of stress on the outcome of inflammatory bowel disease are still a matter of controversy.[115] Various anatomic changes of enteric nerve fibers have been documented in both Crohn's disease and ulcerative colitis,[116,117] but these are probably secondary to inflammation. Nevertheless, once established, they can alter the production and release of a variety of molecules involved in the mediation of inflammation.

Mesenchymal Cells

Mesenchymal cells have been traditionally viewed as simple structural cells, but during the last decade, abundant data demonstrate an active role of these cells in intestinal immunity and inflammation.[118] Distributed from immediately below the subepithelial basement membrane to the lamina propria, in the muscularis mucosae, submucosa, and in the muscularis propria, mesenchymal cells form a pleiotropic group of cells that respond to and secrete a large number of products that modulate the activity of surrounding epithelial and immune cells.[119] Under inflammatory conditions, mesenchymal cells display the intrinsic capacity of altering their phenotype and function evolving from pure fibroblasts to myofibroblasts, stellate cells, and muscle cells.[119,120] Resting and activated mesenchymal cells produce a variety of substances involved in inflammation, including IL-1, IL-6, TNF-α, GM-CSF, TGF-β, and prostaglandin E2 (PGE2), as well as adhesion molecules.[121,122] Through the specific action of these molecules, mesenchymal cells influence the response of epithelial cells to inflammation, such as enhancing their electrolyte secretory responses[123] or promoting wound healing by the stimulation of cell migration.[124] The recent demonstration that intestinal mesenchymal cells spontaneously express COX-2, leading to PGE2 production, has been interpreted as evidence for their contribution to the maintenance of tolerance during intestinal immune responses.[125]

On the other hand, intestinal mesenchymal cells also modulate immune function by directly and indirectly interacting with T-cells. Recent elaboration of T-cell derived IL-17 as an important promoter of inflammation implicates fibroblasts as one of the primary targets of IL-17 which then secrete chemokines that promote neutrophil recruitment and activation.[126–128] Intestinal fibroblasts bind T-cells through an ICAM-1–mediated pathway, and adherence is enhanced by proinflammatory cytokines such as IL-1, TNF-α, and interferon (IFN)-γ.[129] Intestinal smooth muscle cells can present antigens and activate T-cells in a MHC class II-dependent fashion.[130] In addition to interacting with epithelial and immune cells, intestinal mesenchymal cells also interact with the local bacterial flora, as indicated by stimulation of IL-1, IL-6, and TGF-β expression in cultured myofibroblasts and induction of fibrosis and stenosis in normal and colitic animals.[131,132] Finally, all types of intestinal mesenchymal cells are the primary source of ECM proteins, whose production is dramatically enhanced under inflammatory conditions and is responsible for fibrosis and stricture formation, a topic that is addressed in more detail in a subsequent section.

INFLAMMATORY MEDIATORS

Cytokines

Cytokines represent one of the most numerous and complex group of secreted molecules. Cytokines are involved in multiple aspects of an inflammatory response, and an extensive body of literature exists with regard to intestinal inflammation.[133–135]

Within the cytokine network, a number of properties are attributed to these proteins.[136] Pleiotropy translates the observation that a single cytokine can be synthesized by multiple cell types, induce a response in multiple target cells, and mediate a number of stimulatory or inhibitory signals within one or multiple cell types. Redundancy indicates that multiple cytokines can elicit the same biologic response, whereas cross-regulation indicates that cytokines not only directly activate immune and inflammatory cells, but this activity is, in turn, modulated by the products secreted by the cells they activate. Owing to these various properties, the classification of cytokines is often arbitrary. Cytokines can be classified according to common characteristics to facilitate understanding of the role of individual molecules in gastrointestinal inflammation. A convenient classification groups IL-2, IL-7, IL-12, and IL-18 as immunoregulatory cytokines because they play a primary role in activating, modulating, and expanding the immunoregulatory T-cell population, although they also exert activities on other immune and nonimmune cells (Table 2). Some cytokines exert both immunosuppressive and immunoregulatory functions, such as IL-4, IL-10, and IL-13 (Table 3). Other immunoregulatory and effector cytokines, including IFN-γ, GM-CSF, IL-3, IL-5, IL-9, IL-11, IL-15, and IL-17 act primarily during the effector phase of the immune response and impact on how immune and nonimmune cells function to eliminate a pathogen or perpetuate immunity and inflammation (Table 4). The last group includes the proinflammatory cytokines IL-1α, IL-1β, TNF-α, and IL-6, which are primarily produced by cells of monocytic and macrophage lineage (Table 5). Although classically categorized as a proinflammatory molecule, a number of anti-inflammatory activities have been attributed more recently to IL-6 because this molecule fails to induce activities traditionally associated with inflammation, such as enhancement of eicosanoid, NO, and metalloproteinase production and adhesion molecule expression.[137] An alternate way of classifying cytokines, which is restricted to cytokines produced by CD4+ Th cells, is following the Th1 and Th2 paradigm. According to this conceptual framework, a balance between Th1 (IL-2, IFN-γ, and TNF-α producing) and Th2 (IL-4, IL-5, IL-6, IL-10, and IL-13 producing) cytokines implies a physiologic immune response, as found in health, whereas an imbalance between Th1 and Th2 cytokines leads to conditions dominated by a delayed-type hypersensitivity/cell-mediated (Th1) or an allergic-type/antibody-mediated (Th2) pathologic response.[138]

The bulk of information on cytokine abnormalities in intestinal inflammation is based on studies of abnormalities found in human inflammatory bowel disease. The study of IL-2 has shown differential activity in Crohn disease and ulcerative colitis. Mucosal levels of IL-2 protein

and messenger ribonucleic acid (mRNA) are consistently higher than in ulcerative colitis, as are levels of the IL-2Ra chain.[139] In both adult and pediatric Crohn's disease patients, mucosal immune cells exhibit a hyper-reactivity to IL-2 when compared with cells from ulcerative colitis patients.[140,141] The Th1 disease connotation presently attributed to Crohn disease is supported by the enhanced spontaneous production of IFN-γ by

mucosal mononuclear cells.[142] In addition, both protein and mRNA for IL-12 and IL-18, cytokines essential for IFN-γ induction, are expressed at higher levels in Crohn's disease—than ulcerative colitis-affected tissues.[143–145] Low production of IL-4 by lamina propria mononuclear cells and T-cell clones of Crohn's disease patients also reinforces the concept that this is a condition with a prominent Th1-like profile.[146] The classification

Table 2 Immunoregulatory Cytokines

Cytokine	Main Cellular Source	Main Target Cell	Dominant Function
IL-2	T-cells	T-cells, all IL-2R–bearing cells	T-cell activation, proliferation, clonal expansion, and differentiation
IL-7	Stromal cells, epithelial cells	Leukocyte differentiation	T-cell proliferation and cytotoxicity
IL-12	Phagocytes, B cells, dendritic cells	T-cells	Th1 differentiation, infectious responses, induction of IFN-γ
IL-18	Macrophages, dendritic cells, epithelial cells	T-cells	IL-12–like
IL-23	Macrophages, dendritic cells	T-cells	T-cell differentiation, infectious responses, induction of IL-17

IFN = interferon; IL = interleukin; IL-2R = interleukin-2 receptor; Th = T helper.

Table 3 Immunoregulatory and Immunosuppressive Cytokines

Cytokine	Main Cellular Source	Main Target Cell	Dominant Function
IL-4	T cells, mast cells, basophils	Multiple cell types	Th2 differentiation, mediation of allergy, immunosuppression, and anti-inflammatory activity
IL-10	Monocyte, macrophages, T- and B-cells, nonimmune cells	Multiple cells	Anti-inflammatory activity and immunosuppression
IL-13	T-cells	Multiple cells (except T-cells)	IL-4–like

IL = interleukin; Th = T helper.

Table 4 Immunoregulatory and Effector Cytokines

Cytokine	Main Cellular Source	Main Target Cell	Dominant Function
IFN-γ	T-cells, natural killer cells	Most cells	Induction of MHC class II antigens, monocyte activation, Th1 differentiation, and IL-4 suppression
GM-CSF	Phagocytes, B-cells	Hematopoietic cells	Leukocyte differentiation
IL-3	Multiple cells	Hematopoietic cells	Leukocyte differentiation
IL-5	T-cells, mast cells	Eosinophils	Mediation of allergic and parasitic diseases
IL-9	Th2 cells	T-cells, mast cells	Undefined
IL-11	Hematopoietic stromal cells	Multiple cells	Stimulation of intestinal crypt cells
IL-15	Most cells	IL-2R–bearing cells	T-cell expansion, epithelial cell differentiation

GM-CSF = granulocyte-macrophage colony-stimulating factor; IFN = interferon; IL = interleukin; IL-2R = interleukin-2 receptor; MHC = major histocompatibility complex; Th = T helper.

Table 5 Proinflammatory Cytokines

Cytokine	Main Cellular Source	Main Target Cell	Dominant Function
IL-1α, IL-1β	Monocytes, macrophages	Most cells	Mediation of infectious and inflammatory responses
IL-6	Multiple cells	Most cells	Enhancement of immunoglobulin production and immunoregulation
TNF-α	Macrophages	Multiple cells	Mediation of inflammatory and cytotoxic responses
IL-17	T-cells	Multiple cells	Induce target cells to produce proinflammatory chemokines

IL = interleukin; TNF = tumor necrosis factor.

of ulcerative colitis as a Th2-like condition, however, is still in doubt. In support of this possibility are lower levels of IFN-γ produced by mucosal mononuclear cells and higher IL-5 levels in ulcerative colitis than Crohn's disease mucosa.[147,148] Little information exists on mucosal levels of IL-10 in inflammatory bowel disease,[149] probably reflecting a nonspecific response to gut inflammation. Mucosal production of IL-15, a cytokine with many of the biologic activities of IL-2, is enhanced in both forms of inflammatory bowel disease.[150]

Levels of proinflammatory cytokines are elevated in tissues involved by inflammatory bowel disease. High concentrations of IL-1α and -β are found in both Crohn's disease and ulcerative colitis,[151,152] but local effects are largely determined by the relative concentration of the natural antagonist IL-1Rα. A mucosal imbalance between IL-1Rα and IL-1 has been reported in inflammatory bowel disease, showing a relative deficiency of IL-1Rα, which could contribute to the chronicity of inflammation.[153] IL-6 is also consistently elevated in inflammatory bowel disease mucosa, where it primarily derives from macrophages and epithelial cells.[154,155] In contrast to IL-1 and IL-6, protein and mRNA levels of TNF-α have been inconsistently reported as both normal and elevated in inflammatory bowel disease. High TNF-α concentrations are found in the stools of children with Crohn's disease and ulcerative colitis,[156] and production of TNF-α is higher in cultures of Crohn's disease than in ulcerative colitis mucosal mononuclear cells.[157] In situ hybridization reveals elevated TNF-α mRNA in macrophages infiltrating inflammatory bowel disease tissues,[158] but some studies found no differences in TNF-α mRNA expression in normal and inflammatory bowel disease biopsies.[155,159]

Chemokines

Chemokines are cytokines that exhibit the ability to directionally attract leukocytes into sites of inflammation. They constitute a very large group of functionally related molecules usually divided into four families based on their content of cysteine (C) residues, which are separated by variable numbers of amino acids (X).[160] Chemokines are produced by most cells in the body, and each family displays relative selectivity in its capacity of attracting neutrophils, monocytes, macrophages, dendritic cells, T-cells, natural killer cells, eosinophils, and basophils, depending on these cells' expression of multiple chemokine receptors (Table 6). Chemokines are involved not only in the recruitment of nonspecific inflammatory cells but also in the positioning and the preferential induction of Th1 and Th2 cells, making them active participants of cell-mediated immunity and Th1 and Th2 responses.[161] Therefore, it is not surprising that chemokines play a central role in intestinal inflammation,[162] in which their levels tend to be high and correlate with the histologic grade of inflammatory activity regardless of the organ involved, as observed in

Table 6 Chemokines

Group	Main Chemokines	Main Cellular Source	Main Target Cells
C-C	MCP-1/5, MIP-1α/β, RANTES, eotaxin-1, SDF-1, IP-10	Multiple immune and nonimmune cells	Monocytes, activated T-cells, eosinophils, basophils
C	Lymphotactin, SDF-1	Multiple immune and nonimmune cells	Resting T-cells
C-X-C	IL-8, MCP-1/5, MIP-1α/β, RANTES, eotaxin-1, SDF-1, GRO-α/β/γ, IP-10, ENA-78	Multiple immune and nonimmune cells	Neutrophils, dendritic cells
C-XXX-C	IL-8, MCP-1/5, MIP-α/β, RANTES, IP-10	Multiple immune and nonimmune cells	Natural killer cells

ENA = epithelial cell-derived neutrophil-activating peptide; GRO = growth-regulated oncogene; IL = interleukin; IP = IFN-γ–inducible protein 10; MCP = monocyte chemoattractant protein; MIP = macrophage inflammatory protein; RANTES = regulated on activation normal T-cell expressed and secreted; SDF = stromal cell-derived factor.

H. pylori-induced gastritis and colitis.[163,164] In actively inflamed intestine, multiple cell types are sources of chemokines, including macrophages, T-cells, endothelial cells, and epithelial cells.[165,166] However, it is likely that most mucosal cells produce some type of chemokines, making it difficult to dissect out the relative contribution of each cell and chemokine to the initiation, amplification, and persistence of mucosal inflammation. In particular, the precise contribution of epithelial cells to chemoattraction in vivo is unclear, except for the production of the neutrophil chemokine epithelial cell-derived neutrophil activity peptide (ENA)-78 in active inflammatory bowel disease.[167] In addition to the type of chemokines produced during intestinal inflammation, it is also important to consider the expression of the various chemokine receptors by circulating and infiltrating leukocytes. This determines which cells are attracted into the mucosa and may explain the differences that exist among infiltrating cells in different types of gut inflammation and the preferential localization of particular cell subsets in distinct segments of the gut.[168,169]

GROWTH FACTORS

Intestinal inflammation has traditionally been considered as an excessively strong insult by activated immune cells and their products that ultimately results in a tissue-destructive process. An alternate and complementary view is that intestinal inflammation results from an inadequate capacity of the gut mucosa to defend itself against infectious, immune, toxic, or ischemic injuries. Because cytokines and chemokines are generally considered mediators of injury, growth factors can be considered as mediators of defense and, once damage has occurred, of remodeling and healing. Like cytokines, growth factors derive from multiple cellular sources that are primarily nonimmune, such as mesenchymal cells, and also exert a great variety of diverse functions, essential among them being the ability to induce cell proliferation.[170] In addition to proliferation, other fundamental activities include cell differentiation, cell migration, angiogenesis, and ECM deposition, all of which are necessary to wound healing and resolution of inflammation.[170] Growth factors can be divided in families, including TGF-β, epidermal growth factor (EGF) and TGF-α, insulin-like growth factors, fibroblast growth factors, hepatocyte growth factor, and trefoil factors (Table 7).

In a reductionistic model of epithelial cell wounding in vitro, TGF-β is centrally important in reconstitution of epithelial integrity by stimulating cell migration, a response that is selectively enhanced by other growth factors and cytokines including TGF-α, EGF, IL-1, and IFN-γ.[171,172] Fibroblast growth factor also

Table 7 Growth Factors

Factor	Main Target Cell	Predominant Effect
TGF-α	Nonimmune cells	Enhancement of mucus protection, cell proliferation, differentiation, and migration and deposition of extracellular matrix
TGF-β	Immune and nonimmune cells	Enhancement of cell proliferation, differentiation, and migration; deposition of extracellular matrix; mediation of immunosuppression and tolerance
EGF	Nonimmune cells	Enhancement of mucus protection, cell proliferation, differentiation, and migration and deposition of extracellular matrix
IGF	Nonimmune cells	Enhancement of cell proliferation, differentiation, and migration and deposition of extracellular matrix
FGF	Nonimmune cells	Enhancement of cell proliferation, differentiation, and migration; deposition of extracellular matrix; collagenase production; and angiogenesis
Trefoils	Epithelial cells	Enhancement of mucus protection and cell migration and inhibition of proliferation

EGF = epidermal growth factor; FGF = fibroblast growth factor; IGF = insulin-like growth factor; TGF = transforming growth factor.

promotes epithelial cell restitution.[173] A similar protective effect is exerted by TGF-α in repair of acute gastric injury in animals.[174] Keratinocyte growth factor, a member of the fibroblast growth factor family, mediates a comparable healing effect in the inflamed colonic mucosa of rats exposed to trinitrobenzenesulfonic acid.[175] Increased expression of keratinocyte growth factor in the mucosa of inflammatory bowel disease patients can be interpreted as a defense against inflammatory damage by stimulating epithelial cell proliferation and promoting healing.[176] On the other hand, other growth factors, such as insulin-like growth factor I, may be more involved in the development of fibrosis.[177] Trefoil peptides represent a different class of growth factors whose main function is to reinforce the protective action of mucus by enhancing its physical resistance to mechanical injury.[178] This concept is supported by the beneficial effect of oral trefoil peptides in ethanol- and indomethacin-induced gastric inflammation and their enhanced levels in epithelial cells overlying areas involved by active inflammatory bowel disease.[179,180]

Eicosanoids

Eicosanoids include a group of substances derived from the metabolism of arachidonic acid resulting from the breakdown of cell membrane phospholipids by the action of phospholipases. Two main classes of enzymes are involved in the metabolism of arachidonic acid: the COXs and the lipoxygenases.[181] A large spectrum of vasoactive, pro- and anti-inflammatory, and immunomodulatory activities are mediated by various eicosanoids, whose main categories include prostaglandins, thromboxanes, and leukotrienes. An extensive literature exists on the various biologic functions of these eicosanoids in the gastrointestinal tract,[181–184] and their enhanced production in mucosa affected by various forms of inflammation is well documented.[185,186] COXs exist in constitutive (COX-1) and inducible (COX-2) forms and are intimately involved in the mechanisms of cytoprotection and destruction associated with various forms of gastrointestinal inflammation.[181–184] It is firmly established that prostaglandins primarily exert a cytoprotective action, which is lost when COXs are inhibited by the action of nonsteroidal antimonocyte chemoattractant protein; MIP = macrophage inflammatory protein; RANTES = regulated on activation normal T-cell expressed and secreted; SDF = stromal cell-derived factor.

EGF = epidermal growth factor; FGF = fibroblast growth factor; IGF = insulin-like growth factor; TGF = transforming growth factor inflammatory drugs, a key step in the development of gastric ulceration.[187] This protective effect is mediated through multiple mechanisms, including stimulation of mucus and bicarbonate secretion, maintenance of mucosal blood flow, enhancement of epithelial cell resistance to cytotoxicity, inhibition of neutrophil recruitment and

Table 8 Neuropeptides		
Peptide	Main Target Cell	Predominant Effect
SP	T-cells	Modulation of proliferation, enhancement of antigen-specific responses
	B-cells	Enhancement of proliferation and antibody production
	Natural killer cells	Enhanced activity
	Macrophages	Enhancement of activity and chemotaxis
VIP	T-cells	Inhibition of proliferation, enhancement of cAMP, enhancement of IL-2 and IL-4 and inhibition of IL-5 production, modulation of homing
	B-cells	Inhibition of proliferation, modulation of antibody production
	Natural killer cells	Modulation of activity
	Macrophages	Inhibition of activity
SOM	T-cells	Modulation of proliferation, inhibition of antigen-specific responses
	B-cells	Inhibition of antibody production
	Natural killer cell	Modulation of activity
CGRP	T-cells	Inhibition of proliferation, enhancement of cAMP
	Macrophages	Inhibition of activity
	Eosinophils	Enhancement of activity

cAMP = cyclic adenosine monophosphate; CGRP = calcitonin gene-related peptide; IL = interleukin; SOM = somatostatin; SP = substance P; VIP = vasoactive intestinal polypeptide.

mast cell degranulation, and a broad immunosuppressive action (mostly by PGE2) on macrophage and T-cell responses.[181] The anti-inflammatory activity of prostaglandins has been investigated more extensively in gastric injury and less in the rest of the intestinal tract. However, it appears that prostaglandins also mediate cytoprotective and anti-inflammatory activities in the small intestine and large bowel, as indicated by their mediation of enhanced survival of crypt stem cells in a model of radiation injury,[188] and the exacerbation of experimental colitis in animals receiving a selective COX-2 inhibitor.[189] A recent report suggests that the beneficial action of prostaglandins in the intestine may be even more fundamental than previously thought. This is based on evidence showing that PGE2 produced through COX-2–dependent pathways is crucial to down-regulate physiologic immune responses to dietary antigens and, thus, maintains intestinal immune homeostasis by promoting immunologic tolerance.[190]

Leukotrienes are produced by the action of the enzyme 5-lipoxygenase, which is dependent on activation of 5-lipoxygenase activation protein. One of the main leukotrienes is LTB4, which has a potent chemotactic effect for neutrophils and, as a result, acts as a strong proinflammatory substance. LTB4 proinflammatory activity is probably exerted in both the upper and the lower gastrointestinal tract, as suggested by its elevation in the stomach of patients taking nonsteroidal anti-inflammatory drugs,[191] and in the colon of patients with inflammatory bowel disease.[192] Thromboxanes are COX-1–dependent products of platelets, and they are powerful vasoconstrictors believed to contribute to inflammation in various portions of the gastrointestinal tract, including the stomach[193] and small[194] and large bowel.[195]

Neuropeptides

Neuropeptides are small peptides released at nerve cell endings that influence the activity of immune and inflammatory cells, although many other cell types are also affected (Table 8). This effect can be stimulatory or inhibitory, depending on the type of neuropeptide and the target cells.[110] For instance, substance P tends to enhance immunity and promote inflammation, whereas vasoactive intestinal peptide (VIP) has a predominant inhibitory action on the immune response. Consequently, changes in neuropeptide levels in the intestinal mucosal can modulate immunity and alter the degree of inflammation. Loss of VIP- and somatostatin-expressing fibers and decreased VIP tissue levels are reported in active Crohn disease and ulcerative colitis,[189–198] whereas substance P levels are generally increased, particularly in ulcerative colitis.[196,199] The exact meaning of these observations to disease pathogenesis is uncertain, but the data are compatible with a decrease of inhibitory and an increase of stimulatory peptides, with a net balance in favor of a proinflammatory response. In postproctocolectomy pouchitis, both VIP and substance P are increased.[200] When gut inflammation is induced by *Clostridium difficile* toxin A, both substance P and neurotensin contribute to neurogenic inflammation.[201,202] Not only neuropeptide levels are abnormal in inflamed tissue; so are the levels of specific receptors, such as those for sub-stance P and somatostatin.[203,204] Owing to the large number and pleiotropic activities of the various neuropeptides, their overall impact on intestinal inflammation still remains to be defined but probably depends on the cause, type, and chronicity of the inflammatory process.

REACTIVE OXYGEN AND NITROGEN METABOLITES

Although a plethora of different cells and secreted products are involved in inflammation, the vast majority of them act as initiators, mediators, or amplifiers of the inflammatory process, and few directly mediate tissue damage. Among the latter are molecules classified as reactive oxygen and nitrogen metabolites, both of which are abundantly produced during gut inflammation.[205]

Table 9 Reactive Oxygen Metabolites		
Type	Name	Structure
Radicals	Superoxide anion radical	O2-
	Hydroperoxyl radical	HO2·
	Hydroxyl	OH·
	Alkoxyl radical	RO·
	Hydroperoxyl radical	ROO·
Nonradicals	Hydrogen peroxide	H2O2
	Hydroperoxide	ROOH
	Hypochlorous acid	HOCl
	N-Chloramine	RNHCl

Oxygen metabolites are highly reactive molecules that exert a direct cytotoxic effect on a broad scale by degrading amino acids, proteins, and biopolymers (eg, hyaluronic acid, mucin), oxidizing carbohydrates and sulfur-containing compounds, bleaching hemoproteins, causing lipid peroxidation, and inducing DNA strand scission.[57] Reactive oxygen metabolites are evanescent products released by activated polymorphonuclear leukocytes and include both radical and nonradical molecules (Table 9). All of them exhibit variable degrees of toxicity on multiple type cells, which explains, in addition to the release of proteolytic enzymes, the tissue-destructive capacity of neutrophils whose presence is the hallmark of inflammation.[206] The presence of neutrophils in the inflamed gut fluctuates depending on the type and phase of the disease process, but reactive oxygen metabolites are invariably produced and acquire particular importance in highly destructive conditions such as inflammatory bowel disease and necrotizing enterocolitis.[207,208] That active oxygen species are produced in heightened quantities by circulating neutrophils and monocytes of patients with intestinal inflammation is well documented,[209] but far more important is the demonstration that reactive oxygen metabolites are generated at the very sites of active inflammation, as observed in both humans and animals.[210,211]

A second group of reactive metabolites that has attracted intense attention in recent years is that of reactivenitrogen metabolites, formed by its major product NO and others resulting from its rapid oxidation, such as NO2, NO2–, N2O3, N2O4, S-nitrosothiols, and peroxynitrite (OONO–).[212] Essential to NO production are the enzymes responsible for its synthesis, NO synthesis (NOSs), which are produced by different cell types and are both constitutive or inducible.[213] NO has a broad range of activities in all tissues and organs of the body, and the gastrointestinal tract is no exception.[214] Elevated production of NO and the inducible form of NOS is extensively documented in the bowel of patients with inflammatory bowel disease and toxic megacolon,[87,215,216] as well as in various models of experimental gut inflammation.[217,218] Although there is general agreement that NO and NOS are intrinsic components of any intestinal inflammatory process, what is still unresolved is whether NO plays a protective and therefore beneficial role or whether its action is predominantly destructive and deleterious to gut tissue.[219] Examples of the noxious effects of NO are its ability to increase epithelial cell permeability and induce mucosal damage.[220,221] An explanation for the existing confusion is partly due to the multitude of actions mediated by NO but also the practical observation that the role of inducible NOS in inflammation varies in different settings and diseases, ranging from those in which the enzyme has a predominantly noxious effect to those in which it appears to benefit the host.[212] The exact roles of NO and NOS need to be better elucidated before modulation of their activity can be considered for their potentially therapeutic effects on intestinal inflammation.

PROTEOLYTIC ENZYMES

ECM-degrading proteinases (endopeptidases) include aspartic, cysteine, and serine proteinases and metalloproteinases, each of them composed of several distinct enzymes synthesized and released by both immune and nonimmune cells (Table 10). The components of the ECM, including most collagens, fibronectin, elastin, laminin, entactin, and heparan sulfate proteoglycan, are susceptible to the destructive action of these proteases. This action is counterbalanced by the protective activity of a large number of endogenous inhibitors that include a2-macroglobulin, serine protease inhibitors (serpins, kunins, and others), cysteine protease inhibitors (kininogens, stefin, cystatin, and calpastatin), and matrix metalloproteinase (MMP) inhibitors (tissue inhibitors of metalloproteinases (TIMP)-1, -2, and -3).

Matrix metalloproteinases (MMPs) are attracting increasing attention as key molecules mediating injury in most tissues because of their ability to degrade all components of the ECM.[222] This is also true in the setting of intestinal inflammation.[223] Direct evidence of ECM degradation in intestinal inflammation is relatively limited, but abnormalities of ECM glycoaminoglycans and loss of glycoaminoglycans in the subepithelial basal lamina and from vascular endothelium are detected in tissues involved by ulcerative colitis and Crohn disease.[224] In these diseases, as well as in peptic ulcers, there is an enhanced expression of the MMPs matrilysin, collagenase, and stromelysin-1,[225] suggesting a cause-and-effect relationship among inflammation, release of proteases, and tissue injury. There is also mounting evidence that the mucosal immune system can trigger events leading to MMP-dependent tissue injury. In an intestinal organ culture model, activation of lamina propria T-cells is accompanied by proteolytic degradation of ECM mediated by local release of MMPs.[226,227] These enzymes derive primarily from mucosal mesenchymal cells on stimulation by cytokines produced during the inflammatory reaction, such as TNF-α.[228] This event is inhibited by immunosuppressive cytokines, such as IL-10,[229] and exaggerated by amplifying the activity of Th1 cells with IL-12,[34] indicating that the extent of inflammatory damage is under the control of the strength and the type of ongoing immune responses. However, the degree of damage inflicted to gut tissue exposed to the action of MMPs depends not only on the absolute concentration of these proteases but also the relative proportion of MMPs and TIMPs. In inflammatory bowel disease, there is evidence for MMP overproduction, whereas the expression of TIMPs remains unaltered[230,231]; such an imbalance could well underlie the loss of mucosal integrity.

EXTRACELLULAR MATRIX

The ECM is recognized as an important player in mucosal inflammation because of its crucial role in leukocyte trafficking and activation, wound healing, and fibrosis,[232] as well as the ability to integrate (immune and nonimmune) cell-to-cell and cell-to-matrix interactions.[233] The ECM is a complex protein network secreted by various cell types and forms the intercellular space, where all cells reside.[234]

Table 10 Proteolytic Enzymes		
Enzyme	Main Source	Substrate
Aspartic proteinases	Lysosome	Collagens
Cysteine proteinases	Lysosome, cytosol	Aggrecan core protein, collagens, fibronectin, elastin
Serine proteinases	Plasma, neutrophils, fibroblasts, endothelial cells, mast cells	Collagens, fibronectin, elastin, heparan sulfate proteoglycan
Metalloproteinases		
Interstitial collagenase (MMP-1)	Fibroblasts	Aggrecan core protein, collagens, fibronectin, elastin, laminin, entactin
Gelatinase A (MMP-2)	Fibroblasts	
Stromelysin (MMP-3)	Fibroblasts	
Matrilysin (MMP-7)	Macrophages	
Neutrophil collagenase (MMP-8)	Neutrophils	
Gelatinase B (MMP-9)	Neutrophils, macrophages, fibroblasts, other mesenchymal cells	

MMP = matrix metalloproteinase.

The effects of the ECM are mediated primarily by integrins, a family of cell surface receptors that attach cells to the matrix and mediate mechanical and chemical signals from it.[235] In the gastrointestinal tract, the main components of the ECM are the basement membrane and the interstitial connective tissue matrix. The basement membrane is a specialized sheet-like ECM underlying and essential for adhesion and differentiation of epithelial and endothelial cells. It is composed of a number of multimeric glycoproteins and proteoglycans, including laminins, entactin/nidogen, type IV collagen, fibronectin, and perlecan. The interstitial connective tissue matrix serves as a working environment for all nonanchored cells and is the site of immune and inflammatory reactions. It is synthesized primarily by local mesenchymal cells and contains collagenous and noncollagenous glycoproteins such as the fibrillar collagens (collagen types I, III, and V); glycoproteins such as fibronectin, tenascin, and thrombospondin; and proteoglycans such as versican, decorin, lumican, fibromodulin; and the glycosaminoglycan hyaluronic acid.[234]

The participation of the ECM in intestinal inflammation comprises two domains. The first relates to the functional interaction of the ECM with leukocytes, resulting in the alteration of the migration, activation, and differentiation of these cells.[235] This interaction is influenced by cytokines and chemokines[233] and determines the type and strength of the resulting immune response.[3] There is a paucity of information in this area, but emerging evidence suggests that the ECM profoundly increases its capacity to adhere and retain T-cells in inflammatory bowel disease[237] and

that leukocyte–matrix interactions regulate mucosal inflammatory responses.[238] The second area of investigation is related to the quantitative and qualitative changes occurring in the intestine during inflammation. Information in this area is more abundant, although it is necessarily restricted to chronic inflammatory processes in which major structural changes are part of the natural history of the disease, as in ulcerative colitis and Crohn's disease.[239] In both forms of inflammatory bowel disease, procollagen gene transcripts are increased in sites of inflammation, but they are more abundant in the subepithelial layers in ulcerative colitis and in the deeper layers in Crohn's disease, suggesting different regulatory mechanisms in each disease.[240] The same appears to be true in collagenous colitis, in which the subepithelial basement membrane deposit of ECM stain prominently for type VI collagen and tenascin.[241] In contrast, other ECM changes are not disease specific, such as the increased expression of tenascin in colons involved by ulcerative colitis or Crohn disease.[242] Regardless of specificity, changes in ECM translate to an active process of tissue remodeling in the inflamed intestine resulting from the action of agents that both promote and hinder ECM deposition. For instance, TGF-β selectively augments collagen synthesis by intestinal smooth muscle cells,[243] a response that contributes to intestinal fibrosis. On the other hand, inflammatory mediators, such as IL-1R, promote intestinal muscle cell proliferation while concomitantly down-regulating collagen synthesis and augmenting collagenase expression.[244] In addition to classic inflammatory mediators, the local intestinal flora also appears to promote intestinal fibrosis

by directly stimulating local mesenchymal cells to secrete enhanced amounts of TGF-β, IL-1β, and IL-6.[131,132]

CELL ADHESION MOLECULES

The involvement of cell adhesion molecules in inflammation depends on the organ affected and the nature of the inflammatory stimulus. In the gastrointestinal tract,[245,246] it is modulated by cytokines, chemokines, eicosanoids, bacterial products, and complement fragments.[247] Cell adhesion molecules, which can be both cell surface bound and secreted into the intercellular space, are a large number of structurally and functionally related and unrelated molecules forming four major families: the selectin family, which is primarily responsible for leukocyte–endothelial cell interactions; the integrin family, which mediates cell–cell and cell–ECM interactions; the immunoglobulin superfamily, which mediates homophilic adhesion between an identical cell adhesion molecule on another cell; and the cadherin family, which establishes molecular links between adjacent cells (Table 11).[248] In intestinal inflammation, cell adhesion molecules of all families are involved, but perhaps the most important are those regulating the adhesion of leukocytes to the vascular endothelial cells and their subsequent translocation into the interstitial space.[56] These include ICAM-1, vascular cell adhesion molecule (VCAM)-1, platelet-endothelial cell adhesion molecule 1, and MAd-CAM-1 of the Ig superfamily; CD11/CD18, very late activation antigen (VLA)-4, and α4β7 of the integrin family; and L-, E-, and P-selectin of the selectin family (Figure 1).[249]

Table 11 Cell Adhesion Molecules

Cell Adhesion Molecule	Main Cellular Source	Main Ligand	Main Target
Selectin Family			
E-selectin	Endothelial cells	L-selectin	Neutrophils, monocytes, T-cells
L-selectin	Lymphocytes, neutrophils, monocytes	MAd-CAM-1	Mucosal HEV, endothelial cells
P-selectin	Platelets, endothelial cells	L-selectin	Neutrophils, monocytes, platelets
Integrin Family			
LFA-1 (CD11a/CD18)	All leukocytes	ICAM-1, -2, -3	Lymphoid, nonlymphoid cells
LFA-3	All cells, some T-cells	CD2	T-cells, natural killer cells
Mac-1 (CD11b/CD18)	Neutrophils, monocytes	ICAM-1 and -3, fibrinogen	Lymphoid, nonlymphoid cells, ECM
VLA-1, -2, -3	Collagen, laminin	ECM	
VLA-4	Lymphocytes, monocytes	VCAM-1, fibronectin	Endothelial cells, fibroblasts, monocytes, ECM
VLA-5	Lymphocytes, monocytes	Fibronectin	ECM
VLA-6	Lymphocytes, monocytes	Laminin	ECM
α4β7	Lymphocytes	MAd-CAM-1, fibronectin	Mucosal HEV, ECM
Immunoglobulin Superfamily			
ICAM-1 (CD54)	Lymphoid, nonlymphoid cells	LFA-1, Mac-1	Neutrophils, lymphocytes, monocytes
VCAM-1 (CD106)	Endothelial cells, fibroblasts, monocytes	VLA-4, α4β7	Neutrophils, lymphocytes, monocytes
MAd-CAM-1	Mucosal HEV	α4β7, L-selectin	Lymphocytes, monocytes, neutrophils
PECAM-1	Endothelial cells, neutrophils	PECAM-1	Endothelial cells, neutrophils
Cadherin Family			
Cadherin, α- and β-catenin	Adjacent cells	Cadherin	Same cell type
Other			
CD44 (Hermes)	Lymphoid, nonlymphoid cells	Hyaluronan, collagen	Endothelial cells, ECM

ECM = extracellular matrix; HEV = high endothelial venules; ICAM = intercellular cell adhesion molecule; LFA = leukocyte function–associated antigen; MAd-CAM = mucosal addressin cell adhesion molecule; PECAM = platelet–endothelial cell adhesion molecule; VCAM = vascular cell adhesion molecule; VLA = very late activation antigen.

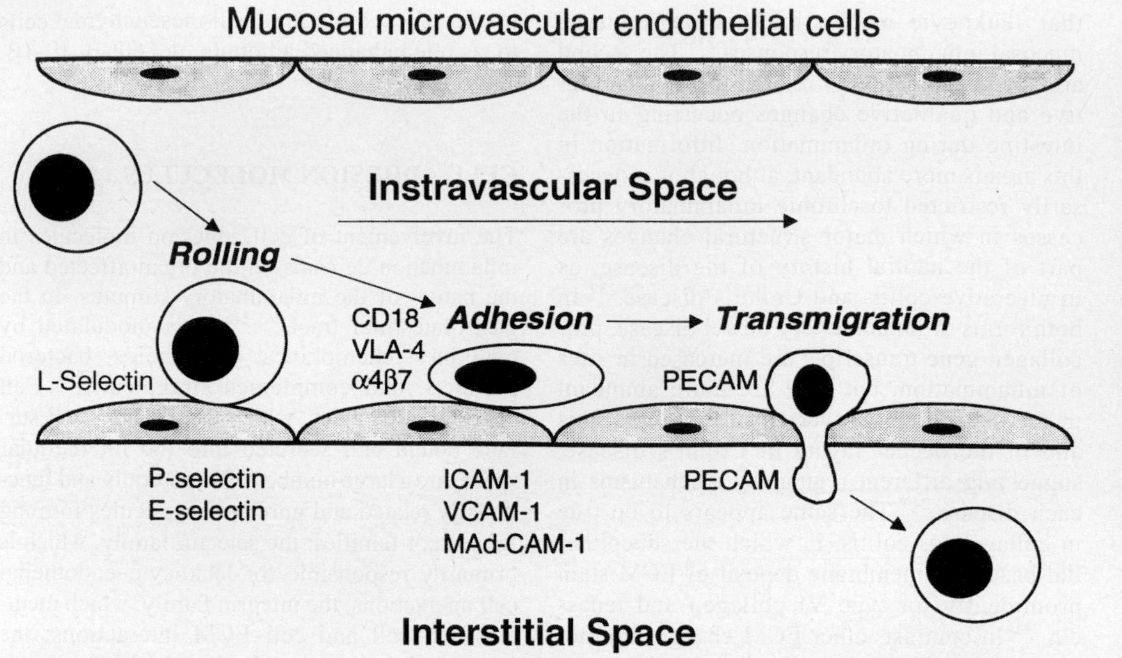

Mucosal microvascular endothelial cells

Figure 1 Major cell adhesion molecules involved in the various steps (rolling, adhesion, and transmigration) necessary to move leukocytes from the intravascular to the interstitial space. Molecules expressed by leukocytes are listed to their left, and molecules expressed by endothelial cells are listed below them. ICAM = intracellular adhesion molecule; MAd-CAM = mucosal addressin cell adhesion molecule; PECAM = platelet–endothelial cell adhesion molecule; VCAM = vascular cell adhesion molecule; VLA = very late activation antigen.

The bulk of information on the function and level of expression of cell adhesion molecules in intestinal inflammation derives from studies of chronic inflammatory processes such as inflammatory bowel disease or chronic gastritis.[98,250–253] As expected, there is an active recruitment of leukocytes by the microvascular mucosal beds in areas of active mucosal inflammation,[254] which is associated with a disruption of the normal selectivity of leukocyte–endothelial interaction.[101] This results in abnormal homing patterns of inflammatory cells to both intestinal and extraintestinal sites.[255] In addition, the level of expression of several cell adhesion molecules is increased on both leukocytes and vascular cells (CD11/CD18; VCAM-1; ICAM-1, -2, and -3; E-selectin; and VLA-4), further contributing to the inflammatory response.[98,250–253,256] Additional information derives from animal models of gastrointestinal inflammation, in which the administration of blocking antibodies confirms the importance of selected cell adhesion molecules in the mucosal inflammatory reaction. Representative examples are CD11/CD18 in rabbit gastritis,[257] ICAM-1 in rat colitis,[258] and α4β7 and VLA-4 in monkey colitis.[99,259]

CONCLUSIONS

Intestinal inflammation is a highly complex phenomenon initiated by a myriad of different triggers and involving all of the components described in this chapter. For the sake of completeness, two additional components deserve mention. One is the endogenous enteric flora, whose capacity to control the overall function of the gastrointestinal tract under physiologic

and inflammatory conditions has been underestimated.[260] The second is the phenomenon of apoptosis, which plays a central role in keeping the necessary balance between cell death and survival in the gastrointestinal tract.[261] If this balance is lost, defects of apoptosis can contribute to some forms of intestinal inflammation.[262,263] How these multiple components behave, how much each of them contributes to inflammation, and how they functionally interact among themselves will depend on the quality and quantity of the initial stimulus and the genetic makeup of the host. Together, they will ultimately determine the type, strength, and duration of the immune response and whether physiologic or pathologic inflammation will ensue (Figure 2). Each portion of the gastrointestinal tract displays specialized features that reflect adaptation to particular physiologic and metabolic requirements so that the outcome of an inflammatory process may vary in different segments of the intestine. In spite of diversity, how-ever, gut inflammation is primarily a stereotypical event mediated by common pathways of tissue injury regardless of the initiating event.[264]

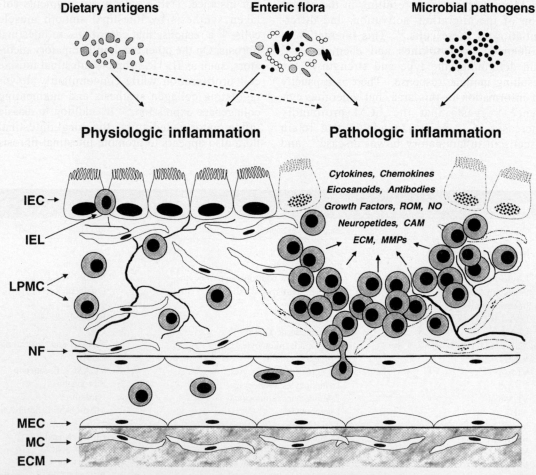

Figure 2 Key components of intestinal inflammation. In response to antigens derived from the diet and the normal enteric flora, a controlled physiologic inflammatory response is induced by the various cellular and soluble immune and nonimmune elements normally present in the intestinal mucosa. Depending on circumstances, microbial pathogens, the enteric flora, or selected dietary antigens induce a pathologic inflammatory response mediated by increased numbers of local immune and nonimmune cells and blood-derived immune cells and enhanced secretion of multiple soluble mediators. CAM = cell adhesion molecule; ECM = extracellular matrix; IEC = intestinal epithelial cells; IEL = intraepithelial lymphocytes; LPMC = lamina propria mononuclear cells; MC = mesenchymal cells; MEC = microvascular endothelial cells; MMPs = matrix metalloproteinases; NF = nerve fibers; NO = nitric oxide; ROM = reactive oxygen metabolites.

REFERENCES

1. Fiocchi C. The immunological resources of the large bowel. In: Kirsner JB, Shorter RG, editors. Diseases of the Colon, Rectum, and Anal Canal. Baltimore: Williams & Wilkins; 1988. p. 95–117.
2. Fiocchi C. The normal intestinal mucosa: A state of "controlled inflammation." In: Targan SR, Shanahan F, editors. Inflammatory Bowel Disease: Bench to Bedside. Dordrecht: Kluwer Academic Publishers; 2003. p. 101–20.
3. Lider O, Hershkovitz R, Kachalsky SG. Interactions of migrating T lymphocytes, inflammatory mediators, and the extra-cellular matrix. Crit Rev Immunol 1995;15: 271–83.
4. Fiocchi C. Intestinal inflammation: A complex interplay of immune-non immune cell interactions. Am J Physiol 1997; 273:G769–75.
5. Brandtzaeg P, Halstensen TS, Kett K, et al. Immunobiology and immunopathology of the human gut mucosa: Humoral immunity and intraepithelial lymphocytes. Gastroenterology 1989;97:1562–84.
6. Brandtzaeg P, Farstad IN, Haraldsen G. Regional specialization in the mucosal immune system: Primed cells do not always home along the same track. Immunol Today 1999;20:267–77.
7. Peters MG, Secrist H, Anders KR, et al. Normal human intestinal B lymphocytes. Increased activation compared to peripheral blood. J Clin Invest 1989;83:1827–33.
8. Valnes K, Brandtzaeg P. Subclass distribution of mucosal IgG-producing cells in gastritis. Gut 1989;30:322–6.
9. MacDermott RP, Nash GS, Bertovich MJ, et al. Alterations of IgM, IgG, and IgA synthesis and secretion by peripheral blood and intestinal mononuclear cells from patients with ulcerative colitis and Crohn's disease. Gastroenterology 1981;81:844–52.
10. Kett K, Rognum TO, Brandtzaeg P. Mucosal subclass distribution of immunoglobulin G-producing cells is different in ulcerative colitis and Crohn's disease of the colon. Gastroenterology 1987;93:919–24.
11. Scott MG, Nahm MH, Macke K, et al. Spontaneous secretion of IgG subclasses by intestinal mononuclear cells: Differences between ulcerative colitis, Crohn's disease, and controls. Clin Exp Immunol 1986;66:209–15.
12. MacDermott RP, Nash GS, Bertovich MJ, et al. Altered patterns of secretion of monomeric IgA and IgA subclass 1 by intestinal mononuclear cells in inflammatory bowel disease. Gastroenterology 1986;91:379–85.
13. Kett K, Brandtzaeg P, Fausa O. J-chain expression is more prominent in immunoglobulin A2 than in immunoglobulin A1 colonic immunocytes and is decreased in both subclasses associated with inflammatory bowel disease. Gastroenterology 1988;94:1419–25.
14. Westermann J, Bode U. Distribution of activated T cells migrating through the body: A matter of life and death. Immunol Today 1999;20:302–6.
15. Meuwissen SGM, Feltkamp-Vroom TM, DelaRiviere AB, et al. Analysis of the lympho-plasmacytic infiltrate in Crohn's disease with special reference to identification of lymphocytesubpopulations. Gut 1976;17:770–80.
16. Selby WS, Janossy G, Bofill M, Jewell DP. Intestinal lymphocyte subpopulations in inflammatory bowel disease: An analysis by immunohistological and cell isolation technique. Gut 1984;25:32–40.
17. Bamford KB, Fan X, Crowe SE, et al. Lymphocytes in the human gastric mucosa during *Helicobacter pylori* have a T helper cell 1 phenotype. Gastroenterology 1998;114: 482–92.
18. Hirata I, Berrebi G, Austin LL, et al. Immunohistological characterization of intraepithelial and lamina propria lymphocytes in control ileum and colon and in inflammatory bowel disease. Dig Dis Sci 1986;31:593–603.
19. Jenkins D, Goodall A, Scott BB. T-lymphocytes populations in normal and coeliac small intestinal mucosa defined by monoclonal antibodies. Gut 1986;27:1330–7.
20. Halstensen TS, Scott H, Brandtzaeg P. Intraepithelial T cells of the TcRy/8 CD8- and V81/J81+ phenotypes are increased in coeliac disease. Scand J Immunol 1989;30: 665–72.
21. MacDonald TT, Bajaj-Elliott M, Pender SLF. T cells orchestrate intestinal mucosal shape and integrity. Immunol Today 1999;20:505–10.
22. Qiao L, Schurmann G, Betzler M, Meuer SC. Activation and signaling status of human lamina propria T lymphocytes. Gastroenterology 1991;101:1529–36.
23. Targan SR, Deem RL, Liu M, et al. Definition of a lamina propria T cell responsive state. Enhanced cytokine responsiveness of T cells stimulated through the CD2 pathway. J Immunol 1995;154:664–75.
24. Qiao L, Schurmann G, Autschbach F, et al. Human intestinal mucosa alters T-cell reactivities. Gastroenterology 1993;105: 814–9.
25. Fiocchi C, Battisto JR, Farmer RG. Studies on isolated gut mucosal lymphocytes in inflammatory bowel disease. Detection of activated T cells and enhanced proliferation to *Staphylococcus aureus* and lipolysaccharides. Dig Dis Sci 1981;26:728–36.
26. Pirzer U, Schonhaar A, Fleischer B, et al. Reactivity of infiltrating T lymphocytes with microbial antigens in Crohn's disease. Lancet 1991;338:1238–9.
27. Cong BY, Brandwein SL, McCabe RP, et al. CD4+ T cells reactive to enteric bacterial antigens in spontaneously colitic C3H/HeJBir mice: Increased T helper cell type 1 response and ability to transfer disease. J Exp Med 1998;187: 855–64.
28. Lundin KEA, Scott H, Hansen T, et al. Gliadin-specific HLA-DQ (a1*0501,b1*0201) restricted T cells isolated from the small intestinal mucosa of celiac disease patients. J Exp Med 1993;178:187–96.
29. Karttunen R, Kartunnen T, Ekre H-PT, MacDonald TT. Interferon gamma and interleukin 4 secreting cells in the gastric antrum in *Helicobacter pylori* positive and negative gastritis. Gut 1994;36:341–5.
30. MacDonald TT, Spencer JM. Evidence that activated mucosal T cells play a role in the pathogenesis of enteropathy in human small intestine. J Exp Med 1988;167:1341–9.
31. Lionetti P, Breese E, Braegger CP, et al. T-cell activation can induce either mucosal destruction or adaptation in cultured human fetal small intestine. Gastroenterology 1993;105:373–81.
32. Godkin A, Jewel D. The pathogenesis of celiac disease. Gastroenterology 1998;115:206–10.
33. Molberg O, Macadam SN, Korner R, et al. Tissue transglutaminase selectively modifies gliadin peptides that are recognized by gut-derived T cells in celiac disease. Nat Med 1998;4:713–7.
34. Monteleone G, MacDonald TT, Wathen NC, et al. Enhancing lamina propria Th1 cell responses with interleukin 12 produces severe tissue injury. Gastroenterology 1999;117:1069–77.
35. Bach J-F. Regulatory T cells under scrutiny. Nat Rev Immunol 2003;3:189–98.
36. Groux H, O'Garra A, Bigler M, et al. A CD4+ T-cell subset inhibits antigen-specific T-cell responses and prevents colitis. Nature 1997;389:737–42.
37. Mottet C, Uhlig HH, Powrie F. Cutting edge: Cure of colitis by CD4+CD25+ regulatory T cells. J Immunol 2003;170:3939–43.
38. Selby WS, Poulter LW, Hobbs S, et al. Heterogeneity of HLA-DR positive histiocytes of human intestinal lamina propria: A combined histochemical and immunological analysis. J Clin Pathol 1983;36:379–84.
39. Allison MC, Cornwall S, Poulter LW, et al. Macrophage heterogeneity in normal colonic mucosa and in inflammatory bowel disease. Gut 1988;29:1531–8.
40. Smith PD, Ochsenbauer-Jambor C, Smythies LE. Intestinal macrophages: Unique effector cells of the innate immune system. Immunol Rev 2005;206:149–159.
41. Mahida YR, Patel S, Gionchetti P, et al. Macrophage subpopulations in lamina propria of normal and inflamed colon and terminal ileum. Gut 1989;30:826–34.
42. Mahida YR, Wu KC, Jewell DP. Respiratory burst activity of intestinal macrophages in normal and inflammatory bowel disease. Gut 1989;30:1362–70.
43. Rugtveit J, Brandtzaeg P, Halstensen TS, et al. Increased macrophage subsets in inflammatory bowel disease: Apparent recruitment from peripheral blood monocytes. Gut 1994; 35:669–74.
44. Rugtveit J, Nilsen EM, Bakka A, et al. Cytokine profiles differ in newly recruited and resident subsets of mucosal macrophages from inflammatory bowel disease. Gastroenterology 1997;112:1493–505.
45. Hara J, Ohtani H, Matsumoto T, et al. Expression of costimulatory molecules B1 anf B1 in macrophages and granulomas of Crohn's disease: Demonstration of cell-to-cell contact with T lymphocytes. Lab Invest 1997;77:175–84.
46. Imler JL, Hoffman JA. Toll receptors in innate immunity. Trends Cell Biol 2001;11:304–11.
47. Underhill DM, Ozinsky A. Toll-like receptors: Key mediators of microbe detection. Curr Opin Immunol 2002;14: 103–10.
48. Bowie A, O'Neil LA. The interleuken-1 receptor/Toll-like receptor superfamily; signal generators for pro-inflammatory interleukins and microbial products. J Leukoc Biol 2000;67:508–14.
49. Inohara N, Nunez G. NODS: Intracellular proteins involved in inflammation and apoptosis. Nat Rev Immunol 2003;3: 371–82.
50. Ogura Y, Bonen DK, Inohara N, et al. A frameshift mutation in NOD2 associated with susceptibility to Crohn's disease. Nature 2001;411:603.
51. Hugot JP, Chamaillard M, Zouali H, et al. Association of NOD2 leucine-rich repeat variants with susceptibility to Crohn's disease. Nature 2001;411:599
52. Hornef MW, Frisan T, Vanderwalle A, et al. Toll-like receptor 4 resides in the Golgi apparatus and colocalizes with internalized lipopolysaccharide in intestinal epithelial cells. J Exp Med 1995;5:559–70.
53. Cario E, Brown D, McKee M, et al. Commensal-associated molecular patterns induce selective toll-like receptor-trafficking from apical membrane to cytoplasmic compartments in polarized intestinal epithelium. Am J Pathol 2002;1:165–73.
54. Cario E, Podolsky DK. Differential alteration in intestinal epithelial cell expression of Toll-like receptor 3 (TLR3) and TLR4 in inflammatory bowel disease. Infect Immun 2000;68:7010–7.
55. Cario E, Rosenberg IM, Brandwein SL, et al. Lipopolysaccharide activates distinct signaling pathways in intestinal epithelial cell lines expressing Toll-like receptors. J Immunol 2000; 164:966–72.
56. Malik AB, Lo SK. Vascular endothelial adhesion molecules and tissue inflammation. Pharmacol Rev 1996;48:213–29.
57. Willoughby CP, Piris J, Truelove SC. Tissue eosinophils in ulcerative colitis. Scand J Gastroenterol 1979;14:395–9.
58. Sandhu IS, Grisham MB. Modulation of neutrophil function as a mode of therapy for gastrointestinal inflammation. In: Wallace JL, editor. Immunopharmacology of the Gastrointestinal Tract. San Diego: Academic Press; 1993. p. 51–67.
59. Jenkins HR, Pincott JR, Soothill JF, et al. Food allergy: The major cause of infantile colitis. Arch Dis Child 1984;59:326–9.
60. Lemanske RF, Atkins FM, Metcalfe DD. Gastrointestinal mast cells in health and disease. Part I. J Pediatr 1983;103:177–84.
61. Barrett KE, Metcalf DD. The mucosal mast cell and its role in gastrointestinal allergic disease. Clin Rev Allergy 1984;2:39–53.
62. Falus A, Meretey K. Histamine: An early messenger in inflammatory and immune reactions. Immunol Today 1992;13:154–6.
63. Kelsall BL, Biron CA, Sharma O, Kaye PM. Dendritic cells ate the host–pathogen interface. Nat Immunol 2002;3: 699–702.
64. Chieppa M, Rescigno M, Huang AY, Germain RN. Dynamic imaging of dendritic cell extension into the small bowel lumen in response to epithelial cell TLR engagement. J Exp Med 2006;203:2841–52.
65. Uhlig HH, Powrie F. Dendritic cells and the intestinal bacterial flora: A role for localized mucosal immune responses. J Clin Invest 2003;112:648–51.
66. Fiocchi C, Collins SM, James SP, et al. Immune-nonimmune cell interactions in intestinal inflammation. Inflammatory Bowel Dis 1997;3:133–41.
67. Castro GA. Immunological regulation of epithelial function. Am J Physiol 1982;243:G321–9.
68. Ouellette AJ. Paneth cells and innate immunity in the crypt microenvironment. Gastroenterology 1997;113:1779–84.
69. Wehkamp J, Harder J, Weichenthal M, et al. Inducible and constitutive P-defensins are differentially expressed in Crohn's disease and ulcerative colitis. Inflammatory Bowel Dis 2003; 9:215–23.
70. Scott H, Solheim BG, Brandtzaeg P, Thorsby E. HLA-DR-like antigens in the epithelium of human small intestine. Scand J Immunol 1980;12:77–82.
71. Bland PW, Warren LG. Antigen presentation by epithelial cells of rat small intestine. I. Kinetics, antigen specificity and blocking by anti-Ia antisera. Immunology 1986;58:1–7.
72. Mayer L, Shlien R. Evidence for function of Ia molecules on gut epithelial cells in man. J Exp Med 1987;166:1471–83.
73. Selby WS, Janossy G, Mason DY, Jewell DP. Expression of HLADR antigens by colonic epithelium in inflammatory bowel disease. Clin Exp Immunol 1983;53:614–8.
74. Arnaud-Battandier F, Cerf-Bensussan N, Amsellem R, Schmitz J. Increased HLA-DR expression by enterocytes in children with celiac disease. Gastroenterology 1986;91:1206–12.
75. Valnes K, Huitfeldt HS, Brandtzaeg P. Relation between T cell number and epithelial HLA class II expression quantified by image analysis in normal and inflamed human gastric mucosa. Gut 1990;31:647–52.
76. Ye G, Barrera C, Fan X, et al. Expression of B1 and B2 co-stimulatory molecules by human gastric epithelial cells. Potential role in CD4+ T cell activation during *Helicobacter pylori* infection. J Clin Invest 1997;99:1628–36.
77. Nakazawa A, Watanabe M, Kanai T, et al. Functional expression of costimulatory molecule CD86 on epithelial

cells in the inflamed colonic mucosa. Gastroenterology 1999;117:536–45.
78. Huang GT-J, Eckmann L, Savidge TC, Kagnoff MF. Infection of human intestinal epithelial cells with invasive bacteria upregulates apical intercellular adhesion molecule-1 (ICAM-1) expression and neutrophil adhesion. J Clin Invest 1996;98: 572–83.
79. Stadnyk AW. Cytokine production by epithelial cells. FASEB J 1994;8:1041–7.
80. Dwinell MB, Eckman L, Leopard JD, et al. Chemokine receptor expression by human intestinal epithelial cells. Gastroenterology 1999;117:359–67.
81. McGee DW, Beagley KW, Aicher WK, McGhee JR. Transforming growth factor-P and IL-1β act in synergy to enhance IL-6 secretion by the intestinal epithelial cell line, IEC-6. J Immunol 1993;151:970–8.
82. Watanabe M, Ueno Y, Yajima T, et al. Interleukin-7 is produced by human intestinal epithelial cells and regulates the proliferation of intestinal mucosal lymphocytes. J Clin Invest 1995;95:2945–53.
83. Jung HC, Eckmann L, Yang S-K, et al. A distinct array of proinflammatory cytokines is expressed in human colon epithelial cells in response to bacterial invasion. J Clin Invest 1995; 95:55–65.
84. Reinecker H-C, MacDermott RP, Mirau S, et al. Intestinal epithelial cells both express and respond to interleukin 15. Gastroenterology 1996;111:1706–13.
85. Yang S-K, Eckman L, Panja A, Kagnoff MF. Differential and regulated expression of C-X-C, C-C, and C-chemokines by human colon epithelial cells. Gastroenterology 1997;113:1214–23.
86. Castagliuolo I, Keates AC, Wang CC, et al. *Clostridium difficile* toxin A stimulates macrophage-inflammatory protein-2 production in rat intestinal epithelial cells. J Immunol 1998; 160:6039–45.
87. Singer II, Kawka DW, Scott S, et al. Expression of inducible nitric oxide synthase and nitrotyrosine in colonic epithelium in inflammatory bowel disease. Gastroenterology 1996;111: 871–85.
88. Singer II, Kawka DW, Schloemann S, et al. Cyclooxygenase 2 is induced in colonic epithelial cells in inflammatory bowel disease. Gastroenterology 1998;115:297–306.
89. Bocker U, Damiao A, Holt L, et al. Differential expression of interleukin 1 receptor antagonist isoforms in human intestinal epithelial cells. Gastroenterology 1998;115: 1426–38.
90. Kaiser GC, Polk DB. Tumor necrosis factor a regulates proliferation in a mouse intestinal cell line. Gastroenterology 1997;112:1231–40.
91. Madara JL, Stafford J. Interferon-y directly affects barrier function of cultured intestinal epithelial monolayers. J Clin Invest 1989;83:724–7.
92. Planchon S, Fiocchi C, Takafuji V, Roche JK. Transforming growth factor-β1 preserves epithelial barrier function: Identification of receptors, biochemical intermediates and cytokine antagonists. J Cell Physiol 1999;181:55–66.
93. Mayer L, Eisenhardt D. Lack of induction of suppressor T cells by intestinal epithelial cells from patients with inflammatory bowel disease. J Clin Invest 1990;86:1255–60.
94. Pober JS, Cotran RS. The role of endothelial cells in inflammation. Transplantation 1990;50:537–44.
95. Mantovani A, Bussolino F, Dejana E. Cytokine regulation of endothelial cell function. FASEB J 1992;6:2591–9.
96. Granger DN, Kubes P. The microcirculation and inflammation: Modulation of leukocyte-endothelial cell adhesion. J Leuk Biol 1994;55:662–75.
97. Girard J-P, Springer TA. High endothelial venules (HEV): Specialized endothelium for lymphocyte migration. Immunol Today 1995;16:449–57.
98. Briskin M, Winsor-Hines D, Shyjan A, et al. Human mucosal addresin cell adhesion molecule-1 is preferentially expressed in intestinal tract and associated lymphoid tissue. Am J Pathol 1997;151:97–110.
99. Hesterberg PE, Winsor-Hines D, Briskin MJ, et al. Rapid resolution of chronic colitis in the cotton-top tamarin with an anti-body to a gut-homing integrin a4P7. Gastroenterology 1996; 111:1373–80.
100. Panes J, Granger DN. Leukocyte-endothelial interactions: Molecular mechanisms and implications in gastrointestinal disease. Gastroenterology 1998;114:1066–90.
101. Salmi M, Granfors K, MacDermott RP, Jalkanen S. Aberrant binding of lamina propria lymphocytes to vascular endothelium in inflammatory bowel disease. Gastroenterology 1994;106:596–605.
102. Matsumoto T, Kitano A, Nakamura S, et al. Possible role of vascular endothelial cells in immune responses in colonic mucosa examined immunohistochemically in subjects with and with-out ulcerative colitis. Clin Exp Immunol 1989;78:424–30.
103. Iwashita E, Iwai A, Sawazaki Y, et al. Activation of microvascular endothelial cells in active ulcerative colitis and detection of inducible nitric oxide synthase. J Clin Gastroenterol 1998;27:S74–9.
104. Binion DG, West GA, Ina K, et al. Enhanced leukocyte binding by intestinal microvascular endothelial cells in inflammatory bowel disease. Gastroenterology 1997;112: 1895–907.
105. Binion DG, West GA, Volk EE, et al. Acquired increase in leukocyte binding by intestinal microvascular endothelium in inflammatory bowel disease. Lancet 1998;352:1742–6.
106. Danese S, de la Motte C, Sturm A, et al. Platelets trigger a CD40-dependent inflammatory response in the microvasculature of inflammatory bowel disease patients. Gastroenterology 2003;124:1249–64.
107. Payan D. The role of neuropeptides in inflammation. In: Gallin JI, Goldstein IM, Snyderman R, editors. Inflammation: Basic Principles and Clinical Correlates. New York: Raven; 1992. p. 177–91.
108. Collins SM. The immunomodulation of enteric neuromuscular function: Implications for motility and inflammatory disorders. Gastroenterology 1996;111:1683–99.
109. Bush TG, Savidge TC, Freeman TC, et al. Fulminant jejunoileitis following ablation of enteric glia in adult transgenic mice. Cell 1998;93:189–201.
110. Stanisz AM. Neuronal factors modulating immunity. Neuroimmunomodulation 1994;1:217–30.
111. Pothoulakis C, Castagliuolo I, LaMont JT, et al. CP-96,345, a substance P antagonist, inhibits rat intestinal responses to *Clostridium difficile* toxin A but not cholera toxin. Proc Natl Acad Sci USA 1994;91:947–51.
112. Collins SM, VanAssche G, Hogaboam C. Alterations in enteric nerve and smooth-muscle function in inflammatory bowel disease. Inflammatory Bowel Dis 1997;3:38–48.
113. Collins SM, McHugh K, Jacobson K, et al. Previous inflammation alters the response of the rat colon to stress. Gastroenterology 1996;111:1509–15.
114. Qiu BS, Vallance BA, Blennerhasset PA, Collins SM. The role of CD4+ lymphocytes in the susceptibility of mice to stress-induced reactivation of experimental colitis. Nat Med 1999;5:1178–82.
115. North CS, Clouse RE, Spitznagel EL, Alpers DH. The relation-ship of ulcerative colitis to psychiatric factors: A review of findings and methods. Am J Psychiatry 1990;147: 974–81.
116. Davis DR, Dockerty MB, Mayo CW. The myenteric plexus in regional enteritis: A study of the number of ganglion cells in the ileum in 24 cases. Surg Gynecol Obstet 1955;101:208–16.
117. Brewer DB, Thompson H, Haynes IG, Alexander-Williams J. Axonal damage in Crohn's disease is frequent, but non-specific. J Pathol 1990;161:301–11.
118. Fiocchi C. The immune system in inflammatory bowel disease. Acta Gastroenterol Belg 1997;60:156–62.
119. Powell DW, Mifflin RC, Valentich JD, et al. Myofibroblasts. II. Intestinal subepithelial myofibroblasts. Am J Physiol 1999;277:C183–210.
120. Sappino AP, Schurch W, Gabbiani G. Differentiation repertoire of fibroblastic cells: Expression of cytoskeletal proteins as marker of phenotypic modulation. Lab Invest 1990;63:144–61.
121. Pang G, Couch L, Batey R, et al. GM-CSF, IL-1a, IL-1p, IL-6, IL-8, IL-10, ICAM-1 and VCAM-1 gene expression and cytokine production in human duodenal fibroblasts stimulated by lipolysaccharide, IL-1a and TNF-a. Clin Exp Immunol 1994;96:437–43.
122. Strong SA, Pizarro TT, Klein JS, et al. Proinflammatory cytokines differentially modulate their own expression in human intestinal mucosal mesenchymal cells. Gastroenterology 1998;114:1244–56.
123. Berschneider HM, Powell DW. Fibroblasts modulate intestinal secretory responses to inflammatory mediators. J Clin Invest 1992;89:484–9.
124. McKaig BC, Makh SS, Hawkey CJ, et al. Normal human colonic subepithelial myofibroblasts enhance epithelial migration (restitution) via TGF-β3. Am J Physiol 1999;276: G1087–93.
125. Newberry RD, McDonough JS, Stenson WF, Lorenz RG. Spontaneous and continuous cyclooxygenase-2-dependent prostaglandin E2 production by stromal cells in the murine small intestine lamina propria: Directing the tone of the intestinal immune response. J Immunol 2001;166:4465–72.
126. Fossiez F, Djossou O, Chomarat P, et al. T cell interleukin-17 induces stromal cells to produce proinflammatory and hematopoietic cytokines. J Exp Med 1996;183:2593–603.
127. Harrington LE, Hatton RD, Mangan PR, et al. Interleukin 1producing CD4+ effector T cells develop via a lineage distinct form the T helper type 1 and 2 lineages. Nat Immunol 2005;6:1123–32.
128. Park H, Li Z, Yang XO, et al. A distinct lineage of CD4 T cells regulates tissue inflammation by producing interleukin 17. Nat Immunol 2005;6:1133–41.
129. Musso A, Condon TP, West GA, et al. Regulation of ICAM-1-mediated fibroblast-T-cell reciprocal interaction: Implications for modulation of gut inflammation. Gastroenterology 1999;117:546–56.
130. Hogaboam CM, Snider DP, Collins SM. Activation of T lymphocytes by syngeneic murine intestinal smooth muscle cells. Gastroenterology 1996;110:1456–66.
131. Mourelle M, Salas A, Guarnier F, et al. Stimulation of transforming growth factor β1 by enteric bacteria in the pathogenesis of rat intestinal fibrosis. Gastroenterology 1998; 114:519–26.
132. Van Tol EA, Holt L, Li FL, et al. Bacterial cell wall polymers pro-mote intestinal fibrosis by direct stimulation of myofibroblasts. Am J Physiol 1999;277:G245–55.
133. Sartor RB. Cytokines in intestinal inflammation: Pathophysiological and clinical considerations. Gastroenterology 1994; 106:533–9.
134. Fiocchi C. Cytokines in Inflammatory Bowel Disease. Austin, TX: RG Landes Company; 1996.
135. Podolsky DK, Fiocchi C. Cytokines, chemokines, growth factors, eicosanoids and other bioactive molecules in IBD. In: Kirsner JB, editor. Inflammatory Bowel Disease. Philadelphia: WB Saunders; 1999. p. 191–207.
136. Arai K, Tsuruta L, Watanabe S, Arai N. Cytokine signal net-works and a new era in biomedical research. Mol Cells 1997;7:1–12.
137. Barton BE. IL-6: Insights into novel biological activities. Clin Immunol Immunopathol 1997;85:16–20.
138. Romagnani S. Th1/Th2 cells. Inflammatory Bowel Dis 1999;5: 285–94.
139 Matsuura T, Kusugami K, Morise K, Fiocchi C. Interleukin-2 and interleukin-2 receptor in inflammatory bowel disease. In: Fiocchi C, editor. Cytokines in Inflammatory Bowel Disease. Austin, TX: RG Landes; 1996. p. 41–55.
140. Kusugami K, Youngman KR, West GA, Fiocchi C. Intestinal immune reactivity to interleukin 2 differs among Crohn's disease, ulcerative colitis and control. Gastroenterology 1989; 97:1–9.
141. Kugathasan S, Willis J, Dahms BB, et al. Intrinsic hyper-reactivity of mucosal T-cells to interleukin-2 in pediatric Crohn's disease. J Pediatr 1998;133:675–81.
142. Pallone F, Fais S, Boirivant M. The interferon system in inflammatory bowel disease. In: Fiocchi C, editor. Cytokines in Inflammatory Bowel Disease. Austin, TX: RG Landes; 1996. p. 57–67.
143. Monteleone G, Biancone L, Marasco R, et al. Interleukin 12 is expressed and actively released by Crohn's disease intestinal lamina propria mononuclear cells. Gastroenterology 1997; 112:1169–78.
144. Monteleone G, Trapasso F, Parrello T, et al. Bioactive IL-18 expression is upregulated in Crohn's disease. J Immunol 1999;163:143–7.
145. Pizarro TP, Michie MH, Bentz M, et al. IL-18, a novel immunoregulatory cytokine, is up-regulated in Crohn's disease: Expression and localization in intestinal mucosal cells. J Immunol 1999;162:6829–35.
146. West GA, Matsuura T, Levine AD, et al. Interleukin-4 in inflammatory bowel disease and mucosal immune reactivity. Gastroenterology 1996;110:1683–95.
147. Fuss IJ, Neurath M, Boirivant M, et al. Disparate CD4+ lamina propria lymphokine secretion profiles in inflammatory bowel disease. J Immunol 1996;157:1261–70.
148. Mullin GE, Maycon ZR, Braun-Elwert L, et al. Inflammatory bowel disease mucosal biopsies have specialized lymphokine mRNA profiles. Inflammatory Bowel Dis 1996;2:16–26.
149. Schreiber S, Heinig T, Thiele H-G, Raedler A. Immunoregulatory role of interleukin 10 in patients with inflammatory bowel disease. Gastroenterology 1995;108:1434–44.
150. Sakai T, Kusugami K, Nishimura H, et al. Interleukin 15 activity in the rectal mucosa of inflammatory bowel disease. Gastroenterology 1998;114:1237–43.
151. Mahida YR, Wu K, Jewell DP. Enhanced production of interleukin 1-β by mononuclear cells isolated from mucosa with active ulcerative colitis and Crohn's disease. Gut 1989;30: 835–8.
152. Youngman KR, Simon PL, West GA, et al. Localization of intestinal interleukin 1 activity, protein and gene expression to lamina propria cells. Gastroenterology 1993;104:749–58.
153. Casini-Raggi V, Kam L, Chong YJT, et al. Mucosal imbalance of interleukin-1 and interleukin-1 receptor antagonist in inflammatory bowel disease: A novel mechanism of chronic inflammation. J Immunol 1995;154:2434–40.
154. Kusugami K, Fukatsu A, Tanimoto M, et al. Elevation of interleukin-6 in inflammatory bowel disease is macrophage- and epithelial cell-dependent. Dig Dis Sci 1995;40:949–59.

155. Stevens C, Walz G, Singaram C, et al. Tumor necrosis factor-a, interleukin-1p, and interleukin-6 expression in inflammatory bowel disease. Dig Dis Sci 1992;37:818–26.

156. Braegger CP, Nicholls S, Murch SH, et al. Tumour necrosis factor alpha in stool as a marker of intestinal inflammation. Lancet 1992;339:89–91.

157. Reinecker H-C, Steffen M, Witthoeft T, et al. Enhanced secretion of tumour necrosis factor-alpha, IL-6, and IL-1β by isolated lamina propria mononuclear cells from patients with ulcerative colitis and Crohn's disease. Clin Exp Immunol 1993;94:174–81.

158. Cappello M, Keshav S, Prince C, et al. Detection of mRNA for macrophage products in inflammatory bowel disease by in situ hybridization. Gut 1992;33:1214–9.

159. Isaacs KL, Sartor RB, Haskill S. Cytokine messenger RNA pro-files in inflammatory bowel disease mucosa detected by polymerase chain reaction amplification. Gastroenterology 1992;103:1587–95.

160. Luster AD. Chemokines—Chemotactic cytokines that mediate inflammation. N Engl J Med 1998;338:436–45.

161. Sallusto F, Lanzavecchia A, MacKay CR. Chemokines and chemokine receptors in T-cell priming and Th1/Th2-mediated responses. Immunol Today 1998;19:568–74.

162. MacDermott RP, Sanderson IR, Reinecker H-C. The central role of chemokines (chemotactic cytokines) in the immunopathogenesis of ulcerative colitis and Crohn's disease. Inflammatory Bowel Dis 1998;4:54–67.

163. Ando T, Kusugami K, Ohsuga M, et al. Interleukin-8 activity correlates with histological severity in *Helicobacter pylori*-associated antral gastritis. Am J Gastroenterol 1996;91:1150–6.

164. Mazzucchelli L, Hauser C, Zgraggen K, et al. Expression of interleukin-8 gene in inflammatory bowel disease is related to the histological grade of active inflammation. Am J Pathol 1994;144:997–1007.

165. Grimm MC, Doe WF. Chemokines in inflammatory bowel disease mucosa: Expression of RANTES, macrophage inflammatory protein (MIP)-1a, MIP-1p, and y-interferon-inducible protein 10 by macrophages, lymphocytes, endothelial cells, and granulomas. Inflammatory Bowel Dis 1996;2:88–96.

166. Reinecker H-C, Loh EY, Ringler DJ, et al. Monocytechemoattractant protein 1 gene expression in intestinal epithelial cells and inflammatory bowel disease mucosa. Gastroenterology 1995;108:40–50.

167. Z'Graggen K, Walz A, Mazzucchelli L, et al. The C-X-C chemokine ENA-78 is preferentially expressed in intestinal epithelium in inflammatory bowel disease. Gastroenterology 1997;113:808–16.

168. Papadakis KA, Prehn J, Moreno ST, et al. CCR9-positive lymphocytes and thymus-expressed chemokine distinguish small bowel from colonic Crohn's disease. Gastroenterology 2001;121:246–54.

169. Yuan YH, ten Hove T, The O, et al. Chemokine receptor CXCR3 expression in inflammatory bowel disease. Inflammatory Bowel Dis 2001;7:281–6.

170. Beck PL, Podolsky DK. Growth factors in inflammatory bowel disease. Inflammatory Bowel Dis 1999;5:44–60.

171. Ciacci C, Lind SE, Podolsky DK. Transforming growth factor Q regulation of migration in wounded rat intestinal epithelial monolayers. Gastroenterology 1993;105:93–101.

172. Dignass AU, Podolsky DK. Cytokine modulation of intestinal epithelial cell restitution: Central role of transforming growth factor R. Gastroenterology 1993;105:1323–32.

173. Dignass AU, Tsunekawa S, Podolsky DK. Fibroblast growth factors modulate intestinal epithelial cell growth and migration. Gastroenterology 1994;106:1254–62.

174. Polk WH, Dempsey PJ, Russell WE, et al. Increased production of transforming growth factor a following acute gastric injury. Gastroenterology 1992;102:1467–74.

175. Zeeh JM, Procaccino F, Hoffmann P, et al. Keratinocyte growth factor ameliorates mucosal injury in an experimental model of colitis in rats. Gastroenterology 1996;110:1077–83.

176. Finch PW, Pricolo V, Wu A, Finkelstein SD. Increased expression of keratinocyte growth factor messenger RNA associated with inflammatory bowel disease. Gastroenterology 1996;110:441–51.

177. Zimmermann EM, Sartor RB, McCall RD, et al. Insulin growth factor I and interleukin 1β messenger RNA in a rat model of granulomatous enterocolitis and hepatitis. Gastroenterology 1993;105:399–409.

178. Wong WM, Poulsom R, Wright NA. Trefoil peptides. Gut 1999; 44:890–5.

179. Babyatsky MW, deBeaumont M, Thim L, Podolsky DK. Oral trefoil peptides protect against ethanol- and indomethacin-induced gastric injury in rats. Gastroenterology 1996;110:489–97.

180. Wright NA, Poulsom R, Stamp G, et al. Trefoil peptide gene expression in gastrointestinal epithelial cells in inflammatory bowel disease. Gastroenterology 1993;194:12–20.

181. Wallace JL. The arachidonic acid pathway. In: Gaginella TS, Guglietta A, editors. Drug Development: Molecular Targets for Gastrointestinal Diseases. Totowa, NJ: Humana Press; 1999. p. 1–20.

182. Eberhart CE, Dubois RN. Eicosanoids and the gastrointestinal tract. Gastroenterology 1995;109:285–301.

183. DuBois RN, Abramson SB, Crofford L, et al. Cyclooxygenase in biology and disease. FASEB J 1998;12:1063–73.

184. Wallace JL. Nonsteroidal anti-inflammatory drugs and gastroenteropathy: The second hundred years. Gastroenterology 1997;112:1000–16.

185. Boughton-Smith NK, Hawkey CJ, Whittle BJR. Biosynthesis of lipoxygenase and cyclo-oxygenase products from [14C]-arachidonic acid by human colonic mucosa. Gut 1983;24:1176–82.

186. Lauritsen K, Laursen LS, Bukhave K, Rask-Madsen J. In vivo pro-files of eicosanoids in ulcerative colitis, Crohn's colitis, and *Clostridium difficile* colitis. Gastroenterology 1988;95:11–7.

187. Vane JR. Inhibition of prostaglandin synthesis as a mechanism of action for aspirin-like drugs. Nat N Biol 1971;231:232–5.

188. Cohn SM, Schloemann S, Tessner T, et al. Crypt stem cell survival in the mouse intestinal epithelium is regulated by prostaglandins synthesized through cycooxygenase-1. J Clin Invest 1997;99:1367–79.

189. Reuter BK, Asfaha S, Buret A, et al. Exacerbation of inflammation-associated colonic injury in rat through inhibition of cyclooxygenase-2. J Clin Invest 1996;98:2076–85.

190. Newberry RD, Stenson WF, Lorenz RG. Cyclooxygenase-2-dependent arachidonic acid metabolites are essential modulators of the intestinal immune response to dietary antigen. Nat Med 1999;5:900–6.

191. Hudson N, Balsitis M, Everitt S, Hawkey CJ. Enhanced gastric mucosal leukotriene B4 synthesis in patients taking non-steroidal anti-inflammatory drugs. Gut 1993;34:742–7.

192. Sharon P, Stenson WF. Enhanced synthesis of leukotriene B4 by colonic mucosa in inflammatory bowel disease. Gastroenterology 1984;86:453–60.

193. Whittle BJR, Kauffman GL, Moncada S. Vasoconstriction with thromboxane A2 induces ulceration in the gastric mucosa. Nature 1981;292:472–74.

194. Boughton-Smith NK, Hutcheson I, Whittle BJR. Relationship between PAF-acether and thromboxane A2 biosynthesis in endotoxin-induced intestinal damage in the rat. Prostaglandins 1989;38:319–33.

195. Ligumsky M, Karmeli F, Sharon P, et al. Enhanced thromboxane A2 and prostacyclin production by cultured rectal mucosa in ulcerative colitis and its inhibition by steroids and sulfasalazine. Gastroenterology 1981;81:444–9.

196. Koch TR, Carney JA, Go VLW. Distribution and quantitation of gut neuropeptides in normal and inflammatory bowel diseases. Dig Dis Sci 1987;32:369–76.

197. Kubota Y, Petras RE, Ottaway CA, et al. Colonic vasoactive intestinal peptide nerves in inflammatory bowel disease. A digitized morphometric immunohistochemical study. Gastroenterology 1992;102:1242–51.

198. Watanabe T, Kubota Y, Sawada T, Muto T. Distribution and quantification of somatostatin in inflammatory disease. Dis Colon Rectum 1992;35:488–94.

199. Bernstein CN, Robert ME, Eysselein VE. Rectal substance P concentrations are increased in ulcerative colitis but not in Crohn's disease. Am J Gastroenterol 1993;88:908–13.

200. Keranen U, Jarvinen H, Kiviluoto T, et al. Substance P- and vasoactive intestinal polypeptide-immunoreactive innervation in normal and inflamed pouches after restorative proctocolectomy for ulcerative colitis. Dig Dis Sci 1996;41:1658–64.

201. Manyth PW, Pappas TN, Lapp JA, et al. Substance P activation of enteric neurons in response to intraluminal *Clostridium difficile* toxin A in the rat ileum. Gastroenterology 1996;111:1271–80.

202. Castagliuolo I, Wang C-C, Valenick L, et al. Neurotensin is a proinflammatory neuropeptide in colonic inflammation. J Clin Invest 1999;193:843–9.

203. Reubi JC, Mazzucchelli L, Laissue JA. Intestinal vessels express a high density of somatostatin receptors in human inflammatory bowel disease. Gastroenterology 1994;106:951–9.

204. Manyth CR, Vigna SR, Bollinger RR, et al. Differential expression of substance P receptors in patients with Crohn's disease and ulcerative colitis. Gastroenterology 1995;109:850–60.

205. Pavlick KP, Laroux FS, Fuseler J, et al. Role of reactive metabolites of oxygen and nitrogen in inflammatory bowel disease. Free Radic Biol Med 2002;33:311–22.

206. Weiss SJ. Tissue destruction by neutrophils. N Engl J Med 1989; 320:365–76.

207. Cueva JP, Hsueh W. Role of oxygen derived free radicals in platelet activating factor induced bowel necrosis. Gut 1988;29:1207–12.

208. Simmonds NJ, Rampton DS. Inflammatory bowel disease—a radical view. Gut 1993;34:865–8.

209. Kitahora T, Suzuki K, Asakura H, et al. Active oxygen species generated by monocytes and polymorphonuclear cells in Crohn's disease. Dig Dis Sci 1988;33:951–5.

210. Simmonds NJ, Allen RE, Stevens TRJ, et al. Chemiluminescence assay of mucosal reactive oxygen metabolites in inflammatory bowel disease. Gastroenterology 1992;103:186 96.

211. Keshavarzian A, Sedghi S, Kanofsky J, et al. Excessive production of reactive oxygen metabolites in inflamed colon: Analysis by chemiluminescence probe. Gastroenterology 1992;103:177–85.

212. Nathan C. Inducible nitric oxide synthase: What difference does it make? J Clin Invest 1997;100:2417–23.

213. Michel T, Feron O. Nitric oxide synthases: Which, how, and why. J Clin Invest 1997;100:2146–52.

214. Stark ME, Szurszewski JH. Role of nitric oxide in gastrointestinal and hepatic function and disease. Gastroenterology 1992;103:1928–49.

215. Lundberg JON, Lundberg JM, Alving K, Witzberg E. Nitric oxide and inflammation: The answer is blowing in the wind. Nat Med 1997;3:30–1.

216. Mourelle M, Casellas F, Guarnier F, et al. Induction of nitric oxide synthase in colonic smooth muscle from patients with toxic megacolon. Gastroenterology 1995;109:1497–502.

217. Miller MJS, Thompson JH, Zhang X-J, et al. Role of inducible nitric oxide synthase expression and peroxynitrite formation in guinea pig ileitis. Gastroenterology 1995;105:1475–83.

218. Ribbons KA, Zhang X-J, Thompson JH, et al. Potential role of nitric oxide in a model of chronic colitis in Rhesus macaques. Gastroenterology 1995;108:705–11.

219. McCafferty D-M, Mudgett JS, Swain MG, Kubes P. Inducible nitric oxide synthase plays a critical role in resolving intestinal inflammation. Gastroenterology 1997;112:1022–7.

220. Hata Y, Ota S, Hiraishi H, et al. Nitric oxide enhances cytotoxicity of cultured rabbit gastric mucosal cells induced by hydrogen peroxide. Biochem Biophys Acta 1996;1290:257–60.

221. Unno N, Menconi MJ, Smith M, et al. Hyperpermeability of intestinal epithelial monolayers is induced by NO: Effect of low extracellular pH. Am J Physiol 1997;272:G923–34.

222. Massova I, Kotra LP, Fridman R, Mobashery S. Matrix metalloproteinases: Structure, evolution, and diversification. FASEB J 1998;12:1075–95.

223. Schuppan D, Hahn EG. MMPs in the gut: Inflammation hits the matrix. Gut 2000;47:12–4.

224. Murch SH, MacDonald TT, Walker-Smith JA, et al. Disruption of sulphated glycosaminoglycans in intestinal inflammation. Lancet 1993;341:711–4.

225. Saarialho-Kere UK, Vaalama M, Puolakkainen P, et al. Enhanced expression of matrilysin, collagenase, and stromelysin-1 in gastrointestinal ulcers. Am J Pathol 1996;148:519–26.

226. Pender SLF, Lionetti P, Murch SH, et al. Proteolytic degradation of intestinal mucosal extracellular matrix following lamina propria T cell activation. Gut 1996;39:284–90.

227. Pender SLF, Tickle SP, Docherty AJP, et al. A major role for matrix metalloproteinases in T cell injury in the gut. J Immunol 1997;158:1582–90.

228. Pender SLF, Fell JME, Chamow SM, et al. A p55 TNF receptor prevents T cell-mediated intestinal injury by inhibiting matrix metalloproteinase production. J Immunol 1998;160: 4098–103.

229. Pender SLF, Breese EJ, Gunther U, et al. Suppression of T-cellmediated injury in human gut by interleukin-10: Role of matrix metalloproteinases. Gastroenterology 1998;115:573–83.

230. Heuschkel RB, MacDonald TT, Monteleone G, et al. Imbalance of stromelysin-1 and TIMP-1 in the mucosal lesions of children with inflammatory bowel disease. Gut 2000;47:57–62.

231. von Lampe B, Barthel B, Coupland SE, et al. Differential expression of matrix metalloproteinases and their inhibitors in colon mucosa of patients with inflammatory bowel disease. Gut 2000;47:63–7.

232. Raghow R. The role of extracellular matrix in postinflammatory wound healing and fibrosis. FASEB J 1994;8:823–31.

233. Smith RE, Hogaboam CM, Strieter RM, et al. Cell-to-cell and cell-to-matrix interactions mediate chemokine expression: An important component of the inflammatory lesion. J Leukoc Biol 1997;62:612–9.

234. Kreis T, Vale R. Guidebook to the extracellular matrix and adhesion proteins. New York: Oxford University Press; 1993.

235. Giancotti FG, Ruoslathi E. Integrin signaling. Science 1999; 285:1028–32.

236. Shimizu Y, Shaw S. Lymphocyte interactions with extracellular matrix. FASEB J 1991;5:2292–9.

237. Musso A, Ina K, Fiocchi C. Extracellular matrix (ECM) from inflammatory bowel disease (IBD) displays enhanced adhesiveness for T-cells. Gastroenterology 1996;110: A977.

238. Fiorucci S, Mencarelli A, Palazzetti B, et al. Importance of innate immunity and collagen binding integrin a1p1 in TNBS-induced colitis. Immunity 2002;17:769–80.

239. Lund PK, Zuniga CC. Intestinal fibrosis in human and experimental inflammatory bowel disease. Curr Opin Gastroenterol 2001;17:318–23.

240. Matthes H, Herbst H, Schuppan D, et al. Cellular localization of procollagen gene transcripts in inflammatory bowel disease. Gastroenterology 1992;102:431–42.

241. Aigner T, Neureiter D, Muller S, et al. Extracellular matrix composition and gene expression in collagenous colitis. Gastroenterology 1997;113:136–43.

242. Riedl SE, Faissner A, Schlag P, et al. Altered content and distribution of tenascin in colitis, colon adenoma, and colorectal carcinoma. Gastroenterology 1992;103:400–6.

243. Graham MF, Bryson GR, Diegelmann RF. Transforming growth factor β1 selectively augments collagen synthesis by human intestinal smooth muscle cells. Gastroenterology 1990;99: 447–53.

244. Graham MF, Willey A, Adams J, et al. Interleukin 1β down-regulates collagen and augments collagenase expression in human intestinal smooth muscle cells. Gastroenterology 1996;110:344–50.

245. Cronstein BC, Weissmann G. The adhesion molecules of inflammation. Arthritis Rheum 1993;36:147–57.

246. Kelly CP. Leukocyte adhesion in gastrointestinal inflammation. Curr Opin Gastroenterol 1993;9:962–70.

247. Albelda SM, Smith CW, Ward PA. Adhesion molecules and inflammatory injury. FASEB J 1994;8:504–12.

248. Frenette PS, Wagner DD. Adhesion molecules—part I. N Engl J Med 1996;334:1526–9.

249. Grisham MB, Granger DN. Leukocyte-endothelial cell interactions in inflammatory bowel disease. In: Kirsner JB, editor. Inflammatory Bowel Disease. Philadelphia: WB Saunders Company; 1999. p. 55–64.

250. Malizia G, Calabrese A, Cottone M, et al. Expression of leukocyte adhesion molecules by mucosal mononuclear phagocytes in inflammatory bowel disease. Gastroenterology 1991;100:150–9.

251. Koizumi M, King N, Lobb R, et al. Expression of vascular adhesion molecules in inflammatory bowel disease. Gastroenterology 1992;103:840–7.

252. Nakamura S, Ohtani H, Watanabe Y, et al. In situ expression of the cell adhesion molecules in inflammatory bowel disease. Lab Invest 1993;69:77–85.

253. Hatz RA, Rieder G, Stolte M, et al. Pattern of adhesion molecule expression on vasculature endothelium in *Helicobacter pylori*-associated antral gastritis. Gastroenterology 1997;112:1908–19.

254. Burgio VL, Fais S, Boirivant M, et al. Peripheral monocyte and naive T-cell recruitment and activation in Crohn's disease. Gastroenterology 1995;109:1029–38.

255. Salmi M, Andrew DP, Butcher EC, Jalkanen S. Dual binding capacity of mucosal immunoblasts to mucosal and synovial endothelium in humans: Dissection of the molecular mechanisms. J Exp Med 1995;181:137–49.

256. Bernstein CN, Sargent M, Gallatin WM. β2-Integrin/ICAM expression in Crohn's disease. Clin Immunol Immunopathol 1998;86:147–60.

257. Wallace JL, Arfors K-E, McKnight GW. A monoclonal antibody against the CD18 leukocyte adhesion molecule prevents indomethacin-induced gastric damage in the rabbit. Gastroenterology 1991;100:878–83.

258. Wong PY-K, Yue G, Yin K, et al. Antibodies to intercellular adhesion molecule-1 ameliorate the inflammatory response in acetic acid-induced inflammatory bowel disease. J Pharmacol Exp Ther 1995;274:475–80.

259. Podolsky DK, Lobb R, King N, et al. Attenuation of colitis in the cotton-top tamarin by anti-alpha4 integrin monoclonal anti-body. J Clin Invest 1993;92:372–80.

260. Bengmark S. Ecological control of the gastrointestinal tract. The role of probiotic flora. Gut 1998;42:2–7.

261. Ciccocioppo R, DiSabatino A, Gasbarrini G, Corazza GR. Apoptosis and gastrointestinal tract. Ital J Gastroenterol Hepatol 1999;31:162–72.

262. Boirivant M, Marini M, DiFelice G, et al. Lamina propria T cells in Crohn's disease and other gastrointestinal inflammation show defective CD2 pathway-induced apoptosis. Gastroenterology 1999;116:557–65.

263. Ina K, Ottaway CA, Musso A, et al. Crohn's disease mucosal T-cells are resistant to apoptosis. J Immunol 1999;163:1081–90.

264. Fiocchi C. From immune activation to gut tissue injury: The pieces of the puzzle are coming together. Gastroenterology 1999;117:1238–46.

20.2. Gastrointestinal Manifestations of Primary Immunodeficiency Diseases

Olivier J. Goulet , MD, PhD
Ernest G. Seidman, MD, FRCPC, FACG

The importance of the intestine as an immune barrier is highlighted by the intimate proximity of the gut associated lymphoid tissue (GALT) to the luminal surface of the gastrointestinal (GI) tract, an external environment rich in microbial pathogens and dietary antigens. Thus, it is not surprising that there is a strong clinical relationship between immunodeficiency (ID) states and significant GI disorders. IDs are usually classified as primary or secondary disorders. Acquired or secondary IDs are far more common, even among pediatric patients. Causes include malnutrition, immunosuppressive or radiation therapies, infections (human immunodeficiency virus [HIV], severe sepsis), metabolic diseases (diabetes mellitus, liver, or renal failure), loss of immunocytes and/or immunoglobulins (Igs) (via the GI tract, kidneys, or burned skin), collagen vascular diseases (such as systemic lupus erythematosis), splenectomy, and bone marrow transplantation (see Chapter 20.3, "HIV and Other Secondary Immunodeficiencies").

The past decades have seen enormous progress in the discovery of the molecular basis of primary ID, with over 120 different disorders now described.[1,2] This chapter focuses on the primary IDs which have significant GI complications. Most primary IDs are diagnosed in infants and children and, therefore, are managed by pediatricians and pediatric gastroenterologists. Advances in the treatment of these diseases have also been impressive. Antibody replacement, cytokine, and humanized anticytokine monoclonal antibodies are now available, as a result of recombinant technologies. The ability to achieve lifesaving immune reconstitution of patients with lethal severe combined immunodeficiency (SCID) has offered potential cures. Three major therapeutic approaches exist. The first is by providing life-long enzyme replacement therapy, such as for adenosinedeaminase-deficient SCID.[3] The second is gene therapy, such as reported for SCID.[4] The third and most common treatment is stem cell transplantation, administering rigorous T cell–depleted allogeneic related haploidentical bone marrow stem cells.[5] The latter two treatments are aimed at long-term cure, provided that the SCID is diagnosed before untreatable infections and complications develop. Therefore, it is imperative that pediatric gastroenterologists have a high index of suspicion for these problems in that such patients will present to them in consultation early. Rapid diagnosis and initiation of treatment are vital, now potentially allowing most pediatric patients affected by primary ID to survive into adulthood.

Primary ID may involve one or multiple components of the immune system, such as B or T cells, natural killer (NK) cells, phagocytes, complement, and/or the immune mechanisms that link these components, such as the major histocompatibility complex (MHC) I and II. Below is a brief overview of the components that participate in the host's normal intestinal immune system.

INTESTINAL MUCOSAL IMMUNE SYSTEM

The mucosal membranes that line the respiratory, digestive, and urogenital tracts, as well as the conjunctivae, ears, and ducts of exocrine glands, are constantly exposed to environmental factors. Complex protective systems have been elaborated to defend the host against pathogens, toxins, and allergens. There is a wide array of innate and specific acquired immune mechanisms that normally operate in forming a mucosal barrier to protect the host.[6,7] The fetal intestine plays an important role in the ontogeny of both the cellular and humoral immune systems. Postnatally, the human intestine develops histologic characteristics of a secondary lymphoid organ. Lymphoid follicles, germinal centers, small lymphocytes, and plasma cells are abundant. This association demonstrates the critical role of the immune system in maintaining GI homeostasis. Not only are GI abnormalities frequently encountered in patients with ID syndromes, they are also occasionally severe enough to become the patient's presenting complaint. Furthermore, primary intestinal diseases may secondarily cause substantial losses of immune system components so as to induce a secondary ID. Nonimmune host defense factors, in addition to the major contribution by the GALT, are known to play an important role in mucosal protection against the abundant, potentially noxious antigens and pathogens present in the gut lumen. These include bactericidal fluids such as gastric acidity and proteases, intestinal motility, the mucusglycocalyx, and the normal intestinal flora. These adjunctive mucosal defense mechanisms may explain why major deficiencies in either the humoral or cell-mediated immune system can exist without the presence of significant GI symptoms.

Recurrent, persistent, severe, or unusual infections are the hallmark of ID states. Chronic diarrhea, often associated with malabsorption and concomitant failure to thrive, is characteristic of several of the primary ID syndromes. Paradoxically, inflammatory and autoimmune diseases also characterize many ID syndromes.[8] As discussed below, there is also an increased incidence of malignancies in patients with certain ID states.[9]

COMPONENTS OF THE IMMUNE RESPONSE

An immune response consists of two components: a specific response to a particular antigen and a nonspecific augmentation of the effect of that response (Table 1). Specific immune responses may be classified as humoral and cellular types. Humoral responses result in the generation of antibodies reactive with a given antigen. In contrast, cell-mediated responses involve the induction of specific effector cytotoxic cells or the secretion of cytokines that can trigger an inflammatory reaction (Table 2).

Thymectomized animals, or congenitally athymic animals (including humans), have grossly impaired cell-mediated responses yet are able to generate some antibodies. In contrast, children incapable of making antibodies may be able to mount cell-mediated responses. They appear to handle many viral and fungal infections and can even reject grafts. The thymus-dependent cells (T cells) and the antibody producing lymphocytes (B cells) are the key cells involved in specific immune responses (Figure 1). The latter may be considered to involve two phases. First is the recognition phase, involving antigen-presenting cells (APCs) including macrophages, dendritic, B, and T cells that recognize the antigen as foreign. The effector phase then ensues, in which antibodies (B-cell products) and effector T cells eliminate the antigen.

Table 1 Components of the Immune Response and Typical Infections in Immunodeficiency States

	Specific Immunity			Nonspecific Immunity	
Effector mechanisms	B lymphocytes	T lymphocytes	Macrophages Polymorphonuclear leukocytes		Complement
	↓	↓	↓		↓
Defence mechanisms	Antibody	Cellular immunity	Phagocytosis		Lysis
Typical infections (when impaired)	Enteroviruses	Viruses	Bacteria		Certain viruses
	Pyogenic bacteria	Fungi	Staphylococci		Pyogenic bacteria
		Bacteria	Gram negative		*Neisseria*
			(*Klebsiella, Serratia*)		
		Protozoa	Fungi		

The nonspecific effector component of the immune response includes certain factors that can augment the effects of antibody, and some of these factors are older, in evolutionary terms, than antibody production itself. The major factors are phagocytic cells (macrophages and polymorphonuclear leukocytes), which remove antigens (including bacteria), and complement, which can either directly destroy an organism or facilitate its phagocytosis. Humoral immunity depends not only on antibody synthesis but also on effector mechanisms that eliminate antigen bound to antibody. Microorganisms coated (ie, opsonized) with IgG antibodies are readily bound and ingested by phagocytic cells. Complement-dependent lysis of bacteria needs a functioning complement pathway and a complement-fixing antibody. Thus, specific immunity requires nonspecific effector mechanisms for its efficient operation.

The primary ID syndromes[1,2] are a heterogeneous group of relatively rare diseases that result in failure to manifest an efficient immune-mediated inflammatory response, accompanied by repeated bacterial, fungal, parasitic, and viral infections of variable severity (see Table 1). An ID may involve any of the components of the immune system, as described in detail below.

CELLULAR BASIS OF THE SPECIFIC IMMUNE RESPONSE

T Cells

The progenitors of immunocompetent cells are derived from the lymphoid stem cell, whose nature still remains unclear. Within the thymus, bone marrow precursor T cells are induced to express thymus-associated surface antigens (glycoproteins) which serve as differentiation markers, as well as antigen receptors. A network of epithelial cells in the thymic cortex and in Hassall corpuscles secretes soluble thymic "factors" needed for functional T-cell maturation. Each T cell is committed to a given antigen, which it recognizes by one of two types of T-cell receptors (TCRs), depending on the cell's lineage. T cells have either TCR1, composed of γ and δ chains (determined early in ontogeny), or TCR2, another heterodimer of α and β chains. The TCR2 cells predominate in adults, although 10% of T cells in epithelial structures bear TCR1. The TCR is closely associated on the cell surface with the CD3 protein responsible for transmitting the antigen recognition signal inside the cell (transduction). Nearby accessory molecules, such as lymphocyte function antigen (LFA)-1, CD2, CD4, and CD8, are responsible for increased leukocyte adhesion. The CD4 and CD8 proteins present (predominantly) on TCR2 cells, recognize histocompatibility antigens. Class II molecules show restriction for the antigen receptor of CD4+ T cells and class I molecules for the TCR of CD8+ T cells. Lymphocytes initiate specific immune responses and possess immune memory. Some are involved in recognition, whereas others carry out effector functions. Effector T lymphocytes have several different functional activities. They may cause the death (cytotoxicity) of antigenic cells or initiate inflammation in response to an antigenic stimulus (delayed-type hypersensitivity).

Other T cells have a regulatory rather than an effector role. The T-lymphocyte subpopulations can be classified into helper (Th) and suppressor (Ts) or cytotoxic (Tc) groups. Two types of Th cells have been described, defined by their cytokine secretion patterns (see Table 2).[10,11] Th1 cells generally secrete cytokines, which activate other T cells (interleukin [IL]-2), natural and cytotoxic T cells (interferon [IFN]-γ), and other inflammatory cells (tumor necrosis factor [TNF]). Th1 cells are thus particularly effective against intracellular infections with viruses and organisms in macrophages. On the other hand, Th2 cells secrete those cytokines that activate B cells (IL-4, IL-5) or induce T cells and hematopoietic cells (IL-6) to grow and differentiate. Several other cytokines are secreted by both types of Th cells. The Th2 cells are excellent helpers for antibody production and, in the absence of Th1 cells, will induce high IgE levels owing to IL-4 production. They are well adapted for defense against parasites. Although Th1 cells can provide help for antibody production, excessive Th1 activation inhibits B-cell activation. The Th1 cells induce a strong delayed-type hypersensitivity reaction, and IgE production is inhibited at all levels of Th1 activation owing to IFN-γ production. T-cell functions of help or suppression may depend on various stimuli, resulting in different cytokines being produced, with predominantly activating or inhibitory effects. Only Th cells that have responded to antigen presented by macrophages can subsequently help B cells already committed to that antigen. The effects of Th cells are balanced by those of functional Ts cells. Such Ts cells carry the characteristic surface glycoprotein CD8.

It has recently been shown that uncommitted (naive) CD4+ T helper cells (Thp) can be induced to differentiate toward T helper 1 (Th1), Th2, Th17, and regulatory (Treg) phenotypes according to the local cytokine milieu.[12] The presence of IL-12 signaling through signal transduction and activator of transcription (STAT-4) skews toward Th1, IL-4 (signaling through STAT-6) toward Th2, transforming growth factor (TGF)-β toward Treg and IL-6 and TGF-β toward Th17. The committed cells are characterized by expression of specific transcription factors, T-β for Th1, GATA-3 for Th2, forkhead box P3 (FoxP3) for Tregs, and RORg t for Th17 cells. It has been

Table 2 Lymphocyte Subgroups, Cytokine Profiles, and Their Function

Cell Population	Cytokines	Functions
Th1	IL-2, IFN-γ, TNF	Initiation and augmentation of inflammatory reactions Enhance MHC expression
Th2	IL-3, IL-4, IL-5, IL-6, IL-10, IL-13	Enhance B-cell antibody production Inhibit Th1 cytokine production
Tc	IFN-γ	Enhance MHC expression; activation of NK cells; lysis of antigen target
Ts	Suppressor factor(s)	Suppress Th and Tc cells
B	Antibody: IgM, IgG, IgA, IgE, IgD, IL-10	Neutralization, opsonization, cell lysis Inhibit Th1 cytokine production

IFN = interferon; Ig = immunoglobulin; IL = interleukin; MHC = major histocompatibility complex; NK = natural killer; Tc = cytotoxic T cell; Th = T helper cell; TNF = tumor necrosis factor; Ts = suppressor T cell (may not be a distinct subpopulation).

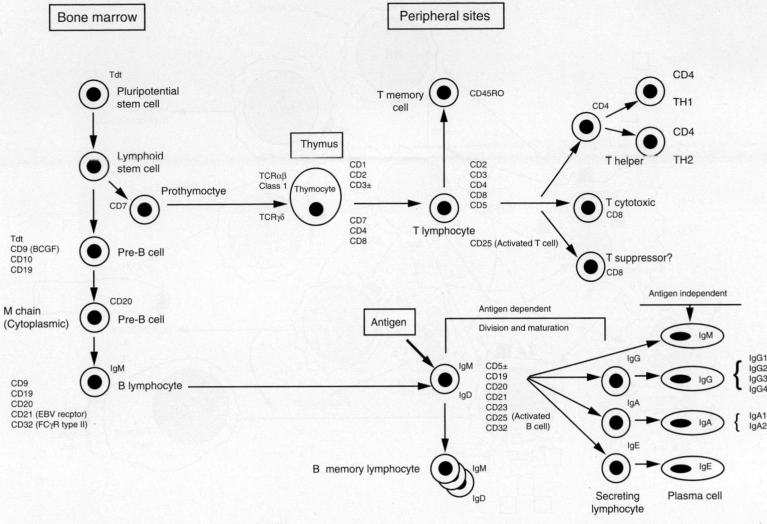

Figure 1 Maturation of T and B lymphocytes. Ig = immunoglobulin.

demonstrated that the skewing of murine Thp toward Th17 and Treg is mutually exclusive. Although human Thp can also be skewed toward Th1 and Th2 phenotypes, there is as yet no direct evidence for the existence of discrete Th17 cells in humans nor of mutually antagonistic development of Th17 cells and Tregs. There is considerable evidence, however, both in humans and in mice for the importance of IFN-γ and IL-17 in the development and progression of inflammatory and autoimmune diseases.[12] In contrast, Tregs have anti-inflammatory properties and can induce quiescence of autoimmune diseases and prolongation of transplant function. As a result, it can be proposed that skewing of responses toward Th17 or Th1 and away from Treg may be responsible for the development and/or progression of autoimmune disorders or acute transplant rejection in humans. Blocking critical cytokines in vivo, notably IL-6, may result in a shift from a Th17 toward a regulatory phenotype and induce quiescence of Autoimmune Diseases or prevent transplant rejection.[12]

Suppression by T cells is only partly understood. These cells are activated by an antigen and release factors that mediate suppression, which may be antigen specific or nonspecific. The CD8+ T cells also include Tc cells, which lyse cells infected with virus in a specific manner. The Tc cells recognize viral antigens together with MHC class I molecules. All endogenous antigens (including viral antigens) are presented in the context of MHC class I antigens. This combination probably activates CD8+ T cells and certainly provides target cells for virally induced T-cell cytotoxicity and, consequently, a potential mechanism for autoimmune damage. Cytotoxic T cells play a role in graft rejection, in which Tc cells mature and are able to lyse target cells carrying the MHC class I molecules of the stimulating cells.

Antigen-Presenting Cells

Antigen is processed by specialized cells known as APCs (Figure 2), and then carried and "presented" to lymphocytes. T cells cannot recognize antigen without such processing. Since activation of T cells is essential for most immune responses, antigen processing is a critical step. The efficiency of T-cell activation is enhanced by the secretion of cytokines such as IL-1 by APCs previously activated by antigen. The most efficient APCs are the interdigitating dendritic cells (DCs) found in T-cell regions of lymph nodes. APCs are able to move about, and increased numbers of activated DCs are found in inflamed sites such as in Crohn's disease tissue.[13] Their recruitment is due to the adhesion molecules expressed on their surface that bind to receptors in the target sites. Follicular DCs trap immune complexes that contain antigen and process and express it closely associated with MHC class II molecules on their surface. Class II molecules themselves determine the responsiveness of an individual to a particular foreign antigen because they interact with the antigen before T-cell help can be triggered. Macrophages in gut, Kupffer cells in liver, and astrocytes in brain, as well as activated B cells and intestinal epithelial cells, are also able to present antigen to T cells. Additional stimuli are provided by the binding of adhesion molecules to the cell surfaces of lymphocytes and APCs. For example, the LFA-3 on the APC binds to CD2 on Th cells, giving an additional signal for activation. Likewise, intercellular adhesion molecule (ICAM)-1 binds to LFA-1 on the T-cell surface. Other cell-to-cell interactions, such as T-cell effector with a B lymphocyte or Tc cell and its target, are also enhanced by these molecules. Following the interaction of the TCR with antigen presented in association with MHC molecules, T cells become activated to produce cytokines, such as IL-2, and to express IL-2 receptors. The subsequent interaction of IL-2 with its receptor is a critical step in immune regulation and is required for many effector and regulatory T-cell functions (see Figure 2).

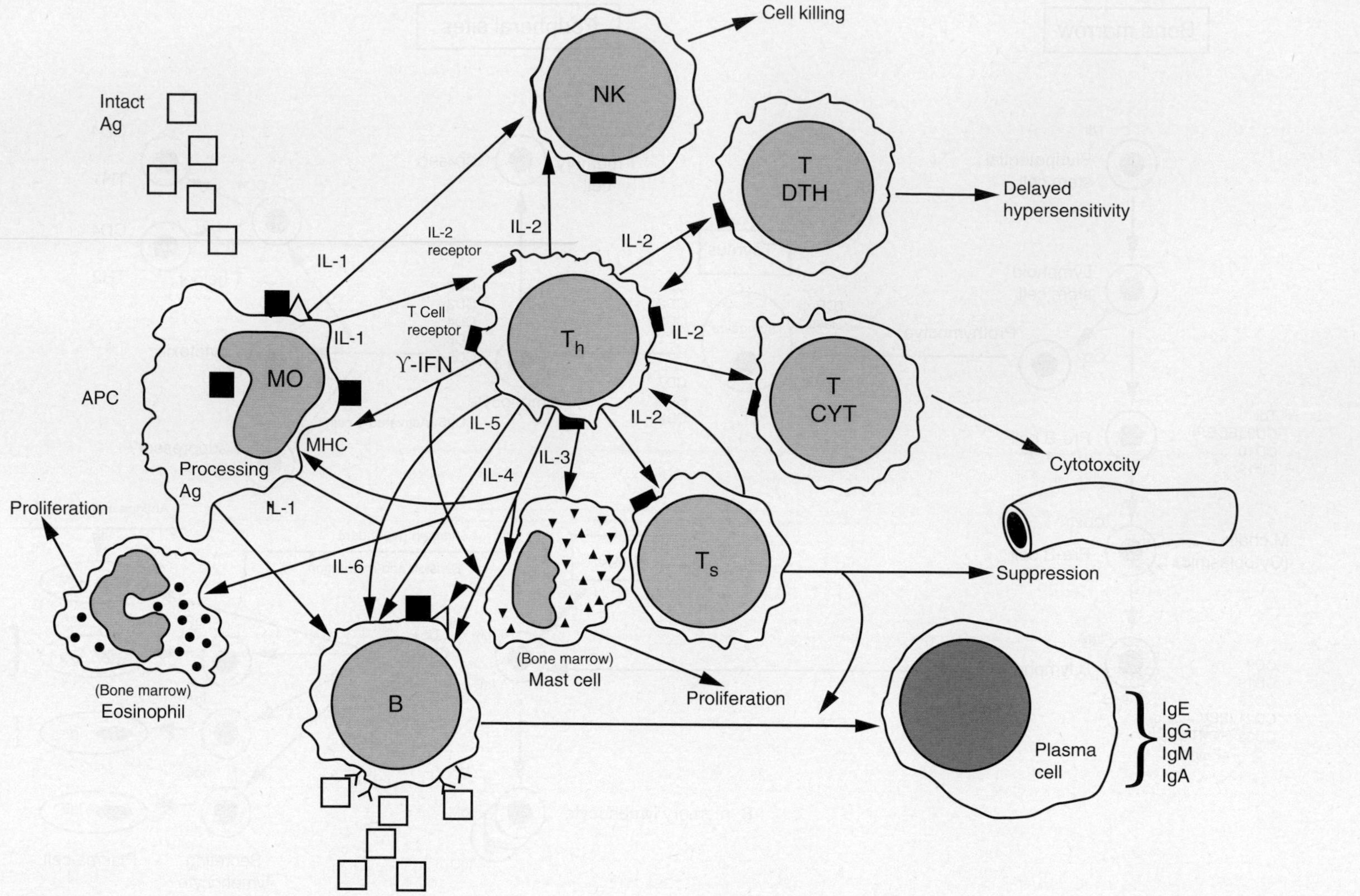

Figure 2 Cytokines and the immune response. Ag = antigen; APC = antigen-presenting cell; B = bursal cell; CYT = cytotoxicity; DTH = delayed-type hypersensitivity; IL = interleukin; γ-IFN = γ-interferon; MHC = major histocompatibility complex; Mo = macrophage; NK = natural killer cell; Th = T helper cell; TS = T suppressor cell.

B Cells

B-lymphocyte development begins within the fetal liver and subsequently proceeds in the bone marrow (see Figure 2). Precursor cells give rise to a rapidly dividing population of pre-B cells that lack Ig receptors but produce cytoplasmic heavy chains. The next differentiation stage is characterized by immature surface Ig–bearing B lymphocytes that express IgM, which are already committed to the specificity of the antibodies that they and their plasma cell progeny will secrete. Most B lymphocytes then further mature and acquire surface IgD. During subsequent development of isotype diversity, one of the subclasses of IgG (1 to 4), IgA (1 to 2), or IgE is expressed by separate subpopulations of B cells, which then lose their surface IgM and IgD (see Figure 1). The maturation sequence of B cells fits with the kinetics of an antibody response; the primary response is mainly IgM and the secondary response is predominantly IgG. During this diversification process, B lymphocytes acquire other cell-surface receptors which allow them to respond to antigens and to T-cell help by proliferation and differentiation to plasma cells. Simultaneously, a population of memory cells is produced, which expresses the same Ig receptor. This clonal expansion helps account for the increased secondary response. The initiation and completion of specific immune responses involve a complex series of genetically restricted interactions between APCs and T-cell subpopulations for cell-mediated immunity and between these cells and B cells for antibody response. The Th and Ts lymphocytes exert positive and negative regulatory effects, respectively, on B-cell responses. Similarly, B cells and antibodies can affect the activities of functionally distinct subpopulations of T cells through specific receptors. A minority of B cells can respond directly to antigens, referred to as T-independent antigens. They have repeating identical antigenic determinants and provoke predominantly IgM antibody responses. Such substances may also provoke nonspecific proliferation of other memory B cells and are therefore known as polyclonal B-cell mitogens. Such antigens include bacterial polysaccharides and endotoxin.

BASIS OF THE NONSPECIFIC IMMUNE RESPONSE

Macrophages

Macrophages and monocytes represent the mononuclear phagocytic system and are derived from bone marrow stem cells closely related to lymphocytes. Each lineage, either for lymphocytes or macrophages, has a different colony-stimulating factor. Once differentiated, functional distinctions between polymorphonuclear leukocytes, mononuclear phagocytes, and lymphocytes are evident. Most polymorphonuclear leukocytes develop in the bone marrow and emerge only when mature, whereas macrophages differentiate principally in various tissues, including the GI mucosa. Tissue macrophages are heterogeneous cells, which have as their major function the phagocytosis of invading organisms and antigens by lysosomal granules containing acid hydrolases and degradative enzymes. To be functional, macrophages must be activated by cytokines or substances that bind to their surface receptors (such as IgG:Fc receptors), or endotoxin (bacterial polysaccharides) to its receptor, or by soluble mediators such as C5a. Their activation results in release of TNF-α or IL-1, IL-6, and other cytokines (monokines), which then further amplifies the immune response and can cause further damage in already inflamed tissues (see Figure 2).

Neutrophils (Polymorphonuclear Leukocytes)

Neutrophils and macrophages constitute the main phagocytic cells. In response to chemotactic agents (anaphylotoxins, C3a, C5a), cytokines released by Th1 cells, and mast cell products (kallikrein), neutrophils migrate out of blood vessels into tissues by the expression of adhesion receptors. Organisms adhere to the surface of phagocytic cells and activate the engulfment process. They are then taken inside the cells, where they fuse with cytoplasmic granules. Neutrophils are able to kill the microorganisms and degrade the substances that they internalize. These processes occur in association with their "respiratory burst" and superoxide production.

Natural Killer Cells

NK cells are specialized lymphocytes involved in a number of important immune functions.[14] They are considered part of the innate immune system, as they do not rearrange their germline deoxyribonucleic acid (DNA) to obtain specificity. Rather, they rely upon activation by an array of receptors with distinct specificities to generate function. These include receptors that sense pathogen specific signatures or cell stress. The function of these activation systems is normally restrained by inhibitory receptors, usually recognizing MHC class-I alleles. In addition to cytotoxicity, NK cells are capable of cytokine production and costimulation of other Immune cells.[14] NK cell functions have been shown to be important for the control of numerous infections such as viruses,[14] for immunosurveillance against tumors[15] and are implicated in the pathogenesis of autoimmune disorders.[16]

Complement

The serum proteins of the complement system provide an important means of removing or destroying foreign antigens. The lysis of whole invading microorganisms and the opsonization of microorganisms and immune complexes are key functions of the complement pathway. This multicomponent-triggered enzyme cascade attracts phagocytic cells to microbes. Microorganisms coated with Ig and/or complement are more easily recognized by macrophages and more readily bound and phagocytosed through IgG:Fc and C3b receptors. All complement components are acute-phase proteins whose synthetic rates are increased by injury or infection. Most components are synthesized by hepatic macrophages. Complement activation occurs in two phases: cleavage of C3, the most abundant component, followed by activation of the "attack" or lytic sequence. The critical step is enzymatic cleavage of the C3 component by "C3 convertase." The classic and alternate pathways, both of which can generate C3 convertases in response to different stimuli (antigen-IgG, with bacterial cell wall antigens and endotoxin, respectively), achieve the cleavage of C3a. The next component (C5) is activated, yielding C5a, a potent chemotactic agent for neutrophils. The C3a and C5a components act on mast cells, inducing the release of mediators such as histamine, leukotriene B4, and TNF-α. The influx of leukocytes and increase in vascular permeability constitute major components of the acute inflammatory response. Deficiencies have been reported for every soluble complement component other than for factor B.[2,17] Autoimmune diseases such as systemic lupus erythematosis is more common in patients with partial or complete deficiency in complement components.[2] Complete deficiencies are associated with bacterial infections such as Neisseria.[17] Deficiency in C1 esterase inhibitor is associated with hereditary angioedema. A recent pediatric review[18] discusses some of the intestinal symptoms that can occur as a result of the submucosal edema.

HEMOLYMPHATIC CYCLE

Peyer patches (PPs) are intramucosal lymph nodes made of B follicles separated by T areas and topped by an area called the dome, rich in B cells, T cells, and macrophages. The dome is overlaid by a particular epithelium, deprived in the small intestine of villi and containing unusual "microfold" epithelial cells, the M cells. These cells have neither a brush border nor basement membrane. They do not synthesize the secretory component necessary for the transport of IgA. They form cytoplasmic folds into which lymphocytes and macrophages can migrate to come in close contact with the intestinal lumen. These properties enable M cells to be the elective entrance for intraluminal antigens, either soluble or particular, in their native form, as can be demonstrated by electron microscopic studies. After crossing M cells, antigens can then be trapped and digested by macrophages, which are numerous under the dome epithelium. It is likely that antigen-pulsed macrophages can then migrate into the B- and T-cell areas, where cellular interactions initiating the intestinal immune response will take place (see Figure 2). Intraluminal antigenic stimulations indeed induce proliferation of B and T cells in the B and T areas of PPs, respectively. Interestingly, 70% of B blasts differentiated in the PP microenvironment bear membrane IgA, in marked contrast with other lymphoid organs, in which such cells are in a very small minority. Hemolymphatic cycle T and B blasts are able to leave the PPs using subserosal lymphatics. They migrate toward the mesenteric lymph nodes, and then via the thoracic duct, they get into blood. Having circulated, blasts which have arisen in the PPs selectively migrate back into the intestinal mucosa. The hemolymphatic cycle thus allows dissemination of the immune response initiated at one intestinal site to the entire intestinal mucosa (Figure 3). This cycle has been well demonstrated in rodents by comparing migration patterns of blasts obtained from various lymphoid organs. During their circulation, T and B blasts undergo progressive maturation. B blasts lose their membrane IgA and acquire intracytoplasmic IgA. They transform into fully mature plasma cells when they have settled in the intestinal mucosa. Similarly, T cells stop dividing and acquire various intracytoplasmic and membrane markers, which reflect their mature and activated state.

MUCOSAL HUMORAL IMMUNITY

Secretory IgA

The mucosal surface of the GI tract normally represents an extensive and efficient barrier protecting the host internal milieu, preventing penetration by pathogenic organisms and potentially noxious luminal antigens and toxins. An important component of the host mucosal defense at the gut epithelial surface (GALT) is the presence of intestinal antibodies, most notably secretory

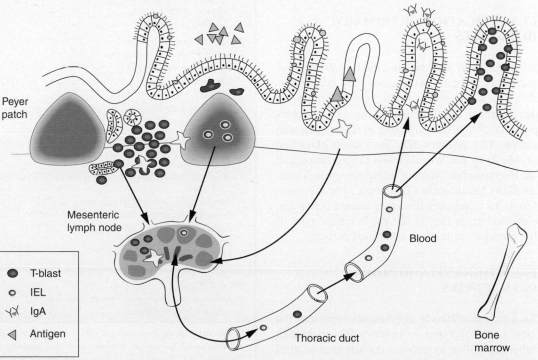

Figure 3 Hemolymphatic cycle of thymodependent T cells and IgA plasma cells. IEL = intraepithelial lymphocyte; IgA = immunoglobulin A.

IgA. A deficiency in secretory intestinal antibody may impair mucosal barrier function, resulting in increased uptake of macromolecular antigens branes, inhibiting antigen uptake or penetration by pathogens. The formation of antigen–antibody complexes on the surface of the small intestine may also facilitate the operation of other non-immunologic host defense mechanisms. Thus, under normal conditions, the mature mucosal immune system (GALT) limits antigen uptake and eliminates pathogens. These theories have been supported by studies in common variable hypogammaglobulinemia, shown to be associated with markedly increased absorption of dietary antigens.[19] An increased incidence of intestinal infections is noted in children with defects of the humoral system, such as *Campylobacter jejuni* enteritis.[20] Although symptoms were similar to those seen in normal children, the clinical course in immunodeficient patients tended to be prolonged and more often unimproved by antibiotic therapy. Chronic diarrhea is the second most common infectious complication of antibody deficiency syndromes, as detailed below.

Implication for Mucosal Immunization

The mucosal immune system is primarily protected by secretory IgA antibodies. Resident T cells produce large amounts of TGF-β, IL-4, and IL-10. These factors, also elaborated by intestinal epithelial cells, then promote the B cells to "switch" to IgA production. Site-specific vaccination by oral immunization leads to antibody production primarily in the small bowel but little in the colon. There is concomitant antibody production by the mammary and salivary glands. Intranasal immunization apparently gives rise to an antibody response in the upper airways and salivary glands, without provoking an immune response in the gut.

CLASSIFICATION OF PRIMARY ID DISEASES

ID in children may be classified as primary or secondary. Primary ID diseases may be attributable to a wide variety of inherited defects in the development and function of the various components of the host immune system, reviewed above. The primary IDs have been classified (Table 3) by the World Health Organization and the International Union of Immunological Societies PID Classification Committee.[1] The GI manifestations of primary IDs are reviewed below and classified according to the predominant type of ID: humoral, cellular, or combined defects.

PREDOMINANTLY HUMORAL DEFICIENCIES

As a group, antibody deficiencies represent the most common types of primary IDs in human subjects.[2] Often symptoms do not appear until the latter part of the first year of life, as passively acquired IgG from the mother decreases to below protective levels.[17] As with the T-cell IDs, the spectrum of antibody deficiencies is broad, ranging from the most severe type of antibody deficiency with totally absent B cells and serum Igs to patients who have a selective antibody deficiency with normal serum Ig. In addition to an increased susceptibility to infections (often respiratory with encapsulated bacteria), enteroviral

---

Table 3 Classification of Immunodeficiencies

Antibody deficiencies
- X-linked agammaglobulinemia
- Non–X-linked hyper-IgM syndrome
- Ig heavy-chain gene deletions
- κ-Chain deficiency
- Selective deficiencies of IgG or IgA subclasses or IgE class:
  - γ1 (IGHG1); γ2 (IGHG2); partial γ3 (IGHG3); γ4 (IGHG4); α1 (IGHG1); α2 (IGHG2); ε (IGHE)
- Antibody deficiency with normal Igs
- Common variable immunodeficiency
- IgA deficiency
- Transient hypogammaglobulinemia of infancy
- Autosomal recessive agammaglobulinemia

T-cell deficiencies
- Purine nucleoside phosphorylase deficiency
- CD3γ deficiency
- CD3ε deficiency
- 70 kDa Syk-family protein tyrosine kinase ZAP-70 deficiency

Combined immunodeficiencies
- Severe combined immunodeficiencies (SCIDs)
- T-B + SCID
  - X-linked γc chain deficiency
  - Autosomal recessive Jak3 deficiency
- T-B-SCID
  - RAG1 deficiency
  - RAG2 deficiency
  - Adenosine deaminase deficiency
  - Reticular dysgenesis
- Other SCIDs
  - X-linked hyper-IgM syndrome
  - CIITA, MHC-II transactivating protein deficiency
  - RFX-5, MHC-II promoter X box regulatory factor 5 deficiency
  - RFXAP, regulatory factor X-associated protein deficiency
  - TAP-2 deficiency
- Other well-defined immunodeficiency syndromes
  - Wiskott-Aldrich syndrome
  - Ataxia-telangiectasia
  - DiGeorge syndrome

Phagocytic immunodeficiencies
- Severe congenital neutropenia
- Cyclic neutropenia
- Leukocyte adhesion defect 1 (deficiency of β chain [CD18] of LFA-1, Mac-1, p150,50)
- Leukocyte adhesion defect 2 (failure to convert GDP mannose to fructose)
- Chediak-Higashi syndrome
- Specific granule deficiency
- Shwachman syndrome
- X-linked chronic granulomatous disease (CGD) (cytochrome *b* 91 kDa)
- Autosomal recessive CGD deficiency of p22phox
- Autosomal recessive CGD deficiency of p47phox
- Autosomal recessive CGD deficiency of p67phox
- Neutrophil G6PD deficiency
- Myeloperoxidase deficiency
- IFN-γ receptor deficiency

NK cell deficiencies
- Autoimmune lymphoproliferative syndrome with immunodeficiency

Familial erythrophagocytic lymphohistiocytosis types 3 & 4
Hermansky-Pudlak syndrome
Papillon-Lefevre syndrome

Complement deficiencies
- C1r
- C1s
- C4
- C2
- C3
- C3
- C5
- C6
- C7
- C8α
- C8β
- C9
- C9
- C1 inhibitor
- Factor I
- Factor H
- Factor D
- Properdin

Other primary immunodeficiency diseases
- Primary CD4 deficiency
- Primary CD7 deficiency
- IL-2 deficiency
- Multiple cytokine deficiency
- Signal transduction deficiency

Congenital or hereditary diseases associated with immunodeficiency
- Chromosomal abnormalities
  - Bloom, Seckel, Dubowitz, ICF, Turner, Nijmegen, and Down syndromes
  - Fanconi anemia
  - Abnormalities in chromosomes 1, 9, 16, and 18
- Multiorgan system abnormalities
  - Partial albinism
  - Congenital dyskeratosis
  - Cartilage hair hypoplasia
  - Agenesis of the corpus callosum
- Hereditary metabolic defects
  - Transcobalamin-2 deficiency, biotin-dependent carboxylase deficiency
  - Acrodermatitis enteropathica
  - Type I orotic aciduria, mannosidosis, methylmalonicacidemia
  - Intractable diarrhea, associated with small for gestational age facial dysmorphy, and trichorrhexis
- Hypercatabolism of Ig
  - Familial hypercatabolism of Ig
  - Intestinal lymphangiectasia
- Others
  - Chronic mucocutaneous candidiasis
  - Hypo- or asplenia
  - Graft-versus-host disease

CGD = chronic granulomatous disease; CIITA = MHC class II transactivator; GDP = guanosine diphosphate; G6PD = glucose-6-phosphate dehydrogenase; ICF = immuno-deficiency, centromere instability, and facial dysmorphism; IFN = interferon; Ig = immunoglobulin; IL = interleukin; LFA = lymphocyte function antigen; phox = phagocyte oxidase; RFX = regulatory factor X; RFXAP = regulatory factor x-associated protein; TAP-2 = antigen-peptide-transporter 2.

GI infections and a number of other disease processes (eg, autoimmunity and malignancies) can be the clinical presentation.[2,17] The availability of potent antibiotics and intravenous Ig (IVIG) infusions is the foundation of treatment for most of these patients. IVIG is contraindicated in certain diseases such as selective IgA deficiency (IgAD) and not indicated for most cases of IgG subclass deficiency.[2] Recently, molecular immunology has led to identification of the gene or genes involved in many of these antibody deficiencies.[2,7] This has led to a better elucidation of the B-cell development and differentiation pathways and a better understanding of the pathogenesis of many of these antibody deficiencies.

X-Linked Agammaglobulinemia

X-linked agammaglobulinemia (XLA), a congenital disorder first described by Bruton in 1952, is the most common (80 to 90%) congenital agammaglobulinemia.[17] Patients are typically infants or young children with recurrent, severe infections with encapsulated bacteria, once passive immunity from maternal Ig wanes. The mucous membranes are often involved (respiratory, urinary, and GI tracts). Since the discovery of the defective gene in XLA, it has been shown that a significant number of male patients with sporadic or acquired hypogammaglobulinemia actually have XLA.[21] In addition to the virtual absence of serum Igs of all classes, an inability to produce antibody after antigen stimulation characterizes XLA. In almost all the cases, circulating mature B cells are absent, and no plasma cells are detected in lymphoid tissues, including the gut.

Genetics. Mutations of the Bruton tyrosine kinase gene (*BTK*), found in many cells of hematopoiesis such as B, but not T cell precursors, disrupt intracellular signaling pathways, resulting in maturational arrest of B lymphocytes at the pre-B-cell stage. The abnormal *BTK* gene, a member of a family of proto-oncogenes that encode protein tyrosine kinases, was mapped to the proximal part of the long arm of the X chromosome. The mutation results in the inability of tyrosine kinase to function in intracellular signaling involved in the production of Igs by B cells. Hundreds of mutations in *BTK* have been identified.[2] Female carriers can be detected, and prenatal diagnosis of affected or unaffected male fetuses can be accomplished. A similar condition, likely owing to another defect, has been described in females.[22]

Pathophysiology. Cell-mediated immunity is normal, and a normal number of pre-B cells are found in the bone marrow. However, plasma cells and blood lymphocytes bearing surface Ig (CD23, CD19, and CD20) are lacking. IgG, IgA, and IgM levels are virtually absent. These patients do not demonstrate isohemagglutinins or antibody production after vaccinations.

Clinical Presentation. The afflicted infants generally remain well during the first 6 months of life by virtue of maternally transmitted Ig. The typical patient is a male presenting thereafter with severe and repeated infections due to extracellular pyogenic, often gram-positive, encapsulated organisms (such as staphylococci, pneumococci, streptococci, *Neisseria, Haemophilus,* or *Mycoplasma* species), unless given prophylactic antibiotics or IVIG therapy. The IgG, IgA, and IgM are far below the 95% confidence limits for appropriate age- and race-matched controls (usually less than 100 mg/dL total Ig). Infections often affect mucous membranes (pneumonia, gastroenteritis, otitis, urinary tract infection). Systemic infections (meningitis, septicemia), osteomyelitis, septic arthritis, cellulitis, and skin abscesses are common.[2,17] Live virus vaccines such as poliovirus can lead to viremia, CNS disease, paralysis, and death. Despite these infections, affected patients typically do not have failure to thrive unless they develop bronchiectasis or persistent enteroviral disease.[2] Polymorphonuclear functions are usually normal if IgG antibodies with intact Fc functions are provided. However, patients with this condition can have transient, persistent, or cyclic neutropenia, as BTK also is found in myeloid cell lineages.[2,23] In such cases, chronic fungal infections or *Pneumocystis carinii* pneumonia may be seen. In addition to recurrent bacterial infections, patients may have persistent viral infections, particularly with hepatitis or enteroviruses, despite normal T-cell function. From the GI point of view, the child may present with chronic diarrhea or a malabsorptive syndrome associated with a protein-losing enteropathy.[24] In general, GI manifestations are much less notable than those encountered in patients with late-onset common variable immunodeficiency (CVID), discussed below. Giardiasis, bacterial overgrowth syndrome (not correlating with diarrhea), nonspecific colitis, and chronic rotavirus infection are other well-recognized complications of XLA.[25,26] Recurrent fissuring necrosis of the small bowel resembling Crohn's disease has been described.[25] XLA has also been reported in association with growth hormone deficiency.[27] The important role of antibody in protecting against these infectious and inflammatory complications is highlighted by the favorable response of these patients to replacement therapy with IVIG.[26,28] Many patients are managed with prophylactic, long-term antibiotics.[2] However, some patients present with persistent enteroviral infections, arthritis, or cancer.[2] In particular, lymphoreticular malignancies have been reported in 6% of XLA.

AUTOSOMAL RECESSIVE AGAMMAGLOBULINEMIA

These recessive defects include μ (IgM heavy chain deficiency) deficiency, B cell linker protein deficiency, Ig-α (CD79a) deficiency, surrogate light chain (λ5 or CD179b) deficiency, and leucine-rich repeat-containing 8 gene defect.[2] They all present with clinical and immunological phenotypes that are similar to XLA, but are less common.[17]

Selective IgA Deficiency

IgAD is the most common primary ID, with an incidence of 1 in 333 to 700.[29] Most subjects are asymptomatic, although some suffer from frequent infections involving mucosal surfaces (respiratory, GI urogenital). Those with frequent infections usually have a defect in antibody responses toward polysaccharides, which is often associated with IgG2 deficiency. Some IgA-deficient patients are also prone to develop more severe ID, called common variable ID (CVID, discussed below) which is associated with decreased IgG and sometimes IgM production, as well as partial T-cell defect. In a few cases, IgAD may reveal a more severe disease such as ataxia-telangiectasia. Although the majority of patients are entirely well, the literature is replete with reports associating IgAD with many conditions, including recurrent infections and various autoimmune and atopic diseases, as well as malignancies.[2,30]

Genetics. The occurrence of IgAD is consistent with autosomal inheritance. In some families, this appears to be dominant, with variable expression. The defective expression of regulatory factors important for IgA-immunocyte differentiation has been suggested to have its origin in certain human leukocyte antigen (HLA)-gene rearrangements. Molecular genetic studies suggest that the susceptibility genes for IgAD and CVID may reside in the HLA-DQ/DR locus.[2] Normally, there is a differential distribution of IgA subclasses throughout the body (Table 4). The IgA in bone marrow plasma cells and serum is predominantly IgA1. In contrast, IgA in secretions and intestinal plasma cells contain equal amounts of IgA1 and IgA2. Most IgA-deficient patients lack both serum and secretory IgA1 and IgA2. However, in some patients with serum IgAD, IgA2-producing plasma cells may be plentiful in the bowel. An IgG subclass deficiency and IgE deficiency may also be seen in patients with "selective" IgAD, reflecting a more generalized abnormality in the terminal differentiation of B cells in such patients. This mixed defect is particularly characteristic of those patients with GI symptoms.[31] Susceptibility to infection among children with selective IgAD has been linked with associated IgG subclass 2 or 4 deficiency.[30] The identification of an IgG subclass deficiency may theoretically lead to therapeutic options in that an associated IgG subclass deficiency may benefit from replacement therapy. However, the risks of blood product administration in such patients, as mentioned above, preclude their routine use.[32]

Table 4 Secretory and Serum IgA		
Characteristics	Secretory	Serum
Molecular form	Polymeric	Monomeric
Subclasses	IgA1 = IgA2	IgA1 > IgA2
Origin	Mucosal tissues	Bone marrow
IgA deficiency	Decreased or normal IgA2	Decreased
Ig = immunoglobulin.		

Pathophysiology. The basic defect leading to selective IgAD remains unknown. Most IgA-deficient patients have immature B cells that express membrane-bound IgA, with IgM and IgD coexpression.[33] These B cells resemble those in umbilical cord blood and fail to terminally differentiate into mature IgA-secreting plasma cells, suggesting a B-cell maturation arrest.[2,33] In some patients, the defect involves the secretory component as well. Of possible etiologic and clinical importance is the presence of antibodies to IgA in the serum samples of as many as 44% of patients with selective IgAD.[34] However, it is uncertain whether these antibodies prevent development of the IgA system or whether lack of tolerance resulting from IgAD permitted the production of antibodies to exogenous determinants that are immunologically related to IgA. Patients deficient in IgA may thus have severe or even fatal anaphylactic reactions after intravenous administration of IgA-containing products.[21] For this reason, parenteral administration of blood or blood products, including serum Ig, is potentially hazardous. Only extensively washed (5) normal donor erythrocytes or blood products from other IgA-deficient individuals should be administered.

Clinical Presentation. There is an association between IgAD and a wide variety of GI disorders (Table 5). The majority of patients do not, however, suffer from significant clinical symptoms. Other host defense mechanisms likely compensate and protect the mucosal barrier, including an increase in IgG and IgM-secreting cells, and various nonimmune factors, discussed above. As would be anticipated in the deficiency of IgA, the primary Ig of mucosal secretions, there is a high rate of infection of the respiratory, GI, and urogenital tracts. Bacterial pathogens are similar to those seen in other types of antibody deficiency syndromes, with no evidence of undue susceptibility to viruses. *Giardia lamblia* infestation is a common problem in these patients. The prevalence of selective IgAD among patients with celiac and Crohn disease also appears to be significantly increased. Although there is

Table 5 Gastrointestinal Manifestations of IgA Deficiency

None
Giardia lamblia infestation (possibly recurrent)
Nodular lymphoid hyperplasia
Nonspecific enteropathy ± bacterial overgrowth ± disaccharidase deficiency
Increased incidence of circulating antibodies to food antigens
Food allergies
Gluten-sensitive enteropathy
Pernicious anemia/atrophic gastritis/increased risk of gastric cancer
Idiopathic inflammatory bowel disease (Crohn's disease, ulcerative colitis)

Ig = immunoglobulin.

an increased prevalence of both serum IgG antibodies against food antigens and circulating immune complexes in IgA-deficient patients, an association with food allergy is not clearly established.[35] As with CVID (discussed below), there is a frequent association of IgAD with collagen vascular and autoimmune diseases. Finally, an increased risk of GI malignancy has been associated with IgAD.[36]

Celiac Disease in IgAD. In addition to the high prevalence of chronic diarrhea and steatorrhea, there is a 10- to 20-fold increased incidence of celiac disease (CD) among IgA-deficient patients.[37,38] Indeed, selective IgAD and CD are frequently associated and share the ancestral haplotype HLA-8.1, which is characterized by a peculiar cytokine profile. As in nonimmunodeficient patients, the classic syndrome of chronic diarrhea, failure to thrive, and malnutrition is less common than more subtle, irritable bowel-like presentations of the disease.[39] In a prospective study of 65 consecutively diagnosed IgA-deficient children, routine jejunal biopsies revealed a diagnosis of CD in 7.7%.[37] Serum antigliadin or antiendomyseal antibodies (IgA) are often false negative. The IgG antigliadin antibodies and IgG antibodies against tissue transglutaminase are useful to screen for CD in such cases.[40] CD in the IgA-deficient patient cannot be distinguished clinically, radiologically, or by laboratory means from CD in otherwise normal individuals. The only differentiating feature is that immunohistochemical staining of small intestinal biopsies reveals a lack of IgA-producing plasma cells. Patients with IgAD may also have chronic diarrhea and villous atrophy on jejunal biopsy without a concomitant gluten-sensitive enteropathy.[41] The clinical differentiation depends on response (symptoms and biopsy) to a gluten-free diet (Figure 4). Even among treated patients on a gluten-free diet and those without CD, immunohistochemical studies have revealed a significant increase in CD25+ cells in the surface epithelium and lamina propria of jejunal biopsy specimens among individuals with IgAD.[42] The increase in CD25+ cells, along with an increase in the mitotic rate of crypt epithelial cells, was taken as evidence in favor of mucosal T-cell activation in IgA-deficient subjects.[42]

Treatment. Currently, there is no specific treatment for IgAD beyond vigorous treatment of infections with appropriate antimicrobial agents. Even if serum IgA were to be replaced, it could not be transported into external secretions because the latter is an active process involving epithelial cells and locally produced IgA. Selective IgAD contraindicates Ig administration. Only the minority of IgA-deficient patients who develop severe or frequent infections in association with IgG2 deficiency or impaired antibody response are candidates for prophylactic IVIG substitution. Ig preparations containing particularly low amounts of IgA are required to avoid adverse effects related to anti-IgA alloantibodies.

Hyper-IgM Syndrome

Genetics and Pathophysiology. The hyper-IgM syndrome is a rare, inherited ID disorder characterized by problems with Ig gene class switching, whereby B cell Ig genes cannot rearrange as the immune response progresses. B cells normally first produce IgM and IgD during a primary humoral response. This rearrangement and "class switch" from IgM to the production of IgA, IgG, and IgE is critical to host resistance to bacterial infections.[2] In X-linked hyper-IGM (XHIM) syndrome, the defective T–B cell interaction results from defects in the CD40 ligand/CD40-signaling pathway.[43,44] CD40 is a member of the TNF receptor superfamily, expressed on a wide range of cell types, including B cells, macrophages, and DCs. CD40 is a receptor for CD40 ligand, a molecule predominantly expressed by activated CD4+ T cells. CD40–CD40L interaction induces the formation of memory B lymphocytes and promotes Ig isotype switching.[45,46] XHIM syndrome is caused by mutations in the *CD40* ligand gene, whereas autosomal recessive hyper-IgM is caused by defects in the CD40-activated ribonucleic acid

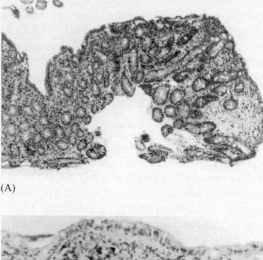

(A)

(B)

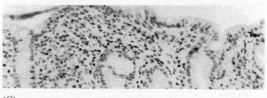

(C)

Figure 4 Gluten-sensitive enteropathy in association with autosomal recessive agammaglobulinemia. The patient was a 13-year-old female who presented with chronic diarrhea and growth failure that responded to a gluten-free diet. (A) Jejunal biopsy shows a moderate to severe villous atrophy, crypt hyperplasia, and chronic inflammatory changes. (hematoxylin phloxine saffron stain; ×120 original magnification). An abundance of immunoglobulin (Ig)M-containing plasmocytes (B) and an absence of IgA-containing plasmocytes (C) can be seen (immunoperoxidase stain; ×300 original magnification). (Courtesy of P. Russo, MD.)

(RNA)-editing enzyme, activation-induced cytidine deaminase, which is required for Ig isotype switching and somatic hypermutation in B cells.[47] This lack of interaction between T and B cells leads to unregulated production of IgM. This is accompanied by an inability to switch from IgM- to IgG- and IgA-secreting cells unless cocultured with a "switch" T-cell line or anti-CD40 plus IL-2, -4, or -10.[46]

Clinical Presentation. The clinical presentation resembles that in XLA, with recurrent pyogenic infections including otitis media, sinusitis, pneumonia, and tonsillitis in the first 2 years of life.[47] Chronic diarrhea and liver involvement are common. Both, at times, may be caused by infection with *Cryptosporidium parvum*.[48,49] Mouth or rectal ulcers, neutropenia, and *P. carinii* pneumonia are frequent presentations.[48] Unlike XLA, however, lymphoid hyperplasia is often seen in the hyper-IgM syndrome.[2] Serum IgA, IgG, and IgE levels are usually very low, whereas a markedly elevated polyclonal IgM is typically present. As with XLA, the treatment of choice is IVIG.[50] Although lymphocyte counts and in vitro proliferative response to mitogens were reported to be normal, defective response to antigens was observed.[48] Thus, additional defects of cell-mediated immunity may be presumed to be present in CD40 ligand mutations. As described with other antibody deficiencies, an association with autoimmune disorders is quite frequent. Sclerosing cholangitis requiring liver transplant has been reported in 4 of 56 cases.[50] In that series, 23% of patients with XHIM syndrome died of infections or liver disease, whereas 6% underwent bone marrow transplant.[50] Successful bone marrow transplant was reported to promote complete recovery from *C. parvum* infection with gastroenteritis and sclerosing cholangitis.[51] XHIM syndrome is thus a severe ID, with significant cellular involvement and a high mortality rate without bone marrow transplant.

Transient Hypogammaglobulinemia of Infancy

Postnatally, there is a physiologic decrease in the serum IgG concentration as maternally derived IgG is catabolized. A nadir is reached between the third and sixth months. In premature infants, the amount of transplacentally acquired Ig is considerably less; thus, serum IgG concentrations are even lower. Intrinsic Ig synthesis follows as the neonate begins to respond to antigenic stimuli, with the appearance of IgM first, followed by IgG and IgA much later. Transient hypogammaglobulinemia is primarily a deficiency of serum IgG. Normal antibody responses are demonstrable after antigenic stimulation to tetanus, polio, and pneumococcal vaccines.[40] Circulating B cells are normal in number, but the B-cell response to T cell–dependent stimulation with pokeweed mitogen is decreased, probably secondary to a lack of T-cell help.[41] Infants with this disorder usually have recurrent respiratory infections. Some may present with chronic diarrhea and malabsorption.

The disease resolves spontaneously before the age of 4 years, often between the ages of 1 and 2 years. This condition is not considered an indication for IVIG.[2]

IgG Subclass Deficiency

Patients may have deficiencies of one or more subclasses of IgG, despite normal or even elevated total serum IgG levels.[2] There is little value in measuring IgG subclasses in patients under 1 year of age owing to wide variations among normal infants.[52] Most of those with absent IgG2 are also IgA deficient,[53] whereas a minority evolve toward CVID.[54] Although many patients are asymptomatic, others resemble Ig-deficient patients. Chronic diarrhea is a common mode of presentation. Nonspecific colitis is a frequent problem among infants with IgA, IgG2, and IgG4 deficiency.[31] Some of these patients will not respond to protein and polysaccharide antigens in various vaccines, as opposed to cases of transient hypogammaglobulinemia. One study suggested that hypogammaglobulinemia may be associated with chronic intestinal pseudo-obstruction.[55] The children had a history of recurrent infections requiring gammaglobulin infusions. However, it is unclear as to whether the IDs in chronic intestinal pseudo-obstruction are primary or secondary to the intestinal problem.

Common Variable Immunodeficiency

CVID is the second most prevalent primary ID disorder but clinically the most important.[2,57] CVID is characterized by reduced serum levels of IgG, possibly low IgA, and a significant defect in antibody production upon vaccination or challenge with natural pathogens.[58] Patients are predisposed to recurrent infections of their respiratory and GI tracts. A wide spectrum of symptoms and signs affect many systems of the body. In addition to serious infection, CVID is associated with a number of comorbid disorders, including a variety of autoimmune diseases and neoplasms.[57] Many patients are diagnosed as adults, and delay in the recognition of the antibody defects is common.[58,59] A genetic mutation has been identified in only a minority of cases, as described below. CVID is a combination of humoral and cell-mediated deficiency, which explains not only why so many systems are affected but also why standard therapy in the form of IVIG is not always effective. The T-cell-mediated defects of this ID disorder are thought to be the cause of the majority of the GI disorders in CVID and not the antibody deficiency.

Genetics. The genetic basis of CVID is not known for the majority of affected individuals.[57] Inducible costimulator (*ICOS*) is a gene that codes for a T cell surface protein that interacts with the ICOS ligand on B cells.[60] Without this interaction, patients display panhypogammaglobulinemia, deficient specific antibody production, and a clinical phenotype consistent with CVID.[17] Genetic screening revealed ICOS mutations in only 9 of 226 patients with CVID.[17,60] In recent

years, monogenetic defects have been uncovered in CVID, including the ICOS, the B cell surface protein called transmembrane activator and cyclophilin ligand interactor, BAFF-R, and CD 19.[57,61] Up to 10% of CVID patients have mutations in the gene encoding transmembrane activator and cyclophilin ligand interactor.[2,60] A large proportion of CVID patients possess the same HLA haplotypes as in IgAD.[2] These two disorders have been reported in the same family.[61] In addition, certain patients with IgAD later manifest a CVID. There is also a high incidence of autoimmune disease and malignancies in both of these disorders. It has thus been suggested that IgAD and CVID may share a common genetic basis. Studies suggest that the susceptibility genes are in the class III MHC region on chromosome 6. A small number of HLA haplotypes are shared by individuals with CVID and IgAD, consistent with a common genetic basis.[61,62] However, not all members of a pedigree with these susceptibility genes will manifest an ID,[61] suggesting that environmental factors trigger the disease expression in genetically susceptible individuals.

Pathophysiology. CVID represents a heterogeneous group of familial or sporadic diseases characterized by B-cell dysfunction, low levels of serum Igs, and a failure of B cells to differentiate into mature plasma cells. The pathogenesis of CVI includes disturbances in the adaptive as well as innate immune system.[57] Although the antibody deficiencies in CVID may be as profound as those in XLA, circulating Ig-bearing B lymphocytes and lymphoid cortical follicles are present in two-thirds of cases. However, when present, B lymphocytes from CVID patients do not differentiate into Ig-producing cells or plasma cells, despite pokeweed mitogen (PWM) stimulation or coculture with normal T cells. Although T-cell subsets are usually present in normal quantities, T-cell functional abnormalities have also been described and are thought to either cause or exacerbate the B-cell defects. A decreased proliferative response to phytohemagglutinin or anti-CD3 monoclonal antibody activation has been noted, as has lower IL-2 secretion. These abnormalities are restored by addition of exogenous IL-2 or by using phorbol myristate acetate (PMA), a protein kinase activator, as a mitogen. The IL-2 receptor expression is also impaired in CVID when patients' peripheral blood mononuclear cells are incubated with anti-CD3 antibodies. However, IL-2 and IL-2 receptor messenger RNA expression by peripheral blood mononuclear cells are normal, suggesting a possible defect at the post-transcriptional level.[63] The defective IL-2 production in CVID is also reversed by normal allogeneic macrophages, reflecting a potential defect of macrophage activation in selected patients with this disorder.[63] T cells from CVID patients have been found to be deficient in a number of cytokine genes.[64] In most cases, however, the defect is intrinsic to the B cell, with abnormal terminal differentiation.[63] The pattern of expression of Ig genes after PWM stimulation varies among CVID patients, suggesting that B-cell defects may occur at different stages of maturation in such patients.

Classification. Patients with CVID are no longer classified as having a predominantly antibody- or cell-mediated immune defect. Nevertheless, such a distinction may be useful clinically. The first category is clinically similar to XLA and is characterized by low levels of IgG and of the other Ig classes. It can occur sporadically at any age, but usually later than XLA. Familial cases have been identified, primarily with autosomal recessive inheritance. The peak age at onset is in the second decade of life. Peripheral B cells do not synthesize Ig normally when stimulated by mitogens, as described above. Although CVID patients generally have a decreased number of Ig-secreting cells in GALT, this is not a consistent finding. CVID patients with predominant cellular defects may have profound deficiencies of total T cells and T-cell subsets. Despite the numeric deficiency, there is usually a normal helper (CD4) to suppressor (CD8) cell ratio, in contrast to AIDS, as described in Chapter 20.3. Peripheral lymphoid tissues are hypoplastic, with paracortical lymphocyte depletion. The thymus is typically very small, and no Hassall corpuscles or thymic epithelium is present. Thrombocytopenia and neutropenia are seen in some cases.

Clinical Presentation. There is a great deal of clinical variability in this syndrome.[2,59] Patients may present late in infancy and childhood, whereas others present earlier and are indistinguishable from those with severe combined ID syndrome (reviewed below). Children with this disorder typically present with a history of recurrent otitis media, bronchopulmonary infections, and chronic diarrhea with malabsorption.[57–59] A number of GI symptoms and signs are associated with CVID (Table 6). The majority of patients develop significant malabsorption, which is often due to giardiasis. Such patients usually have mild steatorrhea, and small bowel biopsy reveals mild to moderate villous atrophy.[65] They sometimes respond to treatment with metronidazole. There is little evidence demonstrating an increased incidence of parasites other than *Giardia* in CVID patients from industrialized countries.[49,66] Although bacterial overgrowth is commonly recognized, its presence does not correlate with achlorhydria, diarrhea, steatorrhea, lactose intolerance, vitamin B12 malabsorption, or the presence of *Giardia*. Other specific pathogens noted in CVID patients include *Rotavirus, C. jejuni,*

and *C. fetus.* In some patients with early onset of symptoms, as with SCID patients, respiratory tract infections are severe, and malnutrition is often secondary to diarrhea and malabsorption. The GI manifestations include oral, esophageal, and perianal candidiasis.

Nonspecific enterocolitis in the absence of microbial pathogens is also commonly encountered in CVID.[66] The entire small and large intestine may be involved, contributing to the chronic diarrhea and malabsorption (Figure 5). In some cases, small bowel biopsies in CVID may contain foamy histiocytes in the lamina propria, resembling Whipple disease. In others, biopsies are similar to those observed in chronic granulomatous disease (CGD), with numerous apoptotic bodies in the crypts or poorly formed granulomas, resembling Crohn's disease. Patients with CVID thus manifest a spectrum of abnormalities in the GI tract, with patterns superficially resembling graft-versus-host disease (GVHD) or inflammatory bowel disease, as well as Whipple disease or collagenous colitis.[66,67]

Gastritis may also be observed in a large number of patients with hypogammaglobulinemia and CVID. Gastritis is associated with pernicious anemia–like syndrome without antibodies

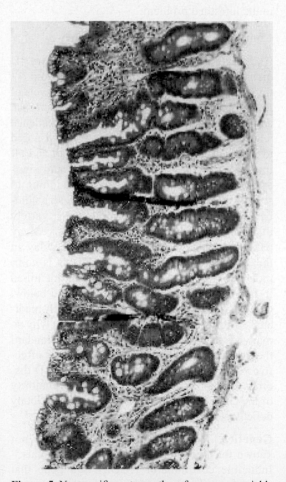

Figure 5 Nonspecific enteropathy of common variable immunodeficiency can be seen in this small bowel biopsy specimen from a 3-year-old boy with chronic diarrhea and failure to thrive who was unresponsive to a gluten-free diet or prednisone. There is irregular, partial villous atrophy with acute and chronic inflammatory cell infiltrates of the lamina propria (hematoxylin phloxine saffron stain; ×120 original magnification). (Courtesy of P. Russo, MD.)

to intrinsic factor, gastric parietal cells, or thyroglobulin.[68] Nodular lymphoid hyperplasia is often encountered in the bowels of CVID patients who do have B cells. However, nodular lymphoid hyperplasia is also seen in selective IgAD, as well as in normal individuals. Malignancy is frequent, including GI tumors and generalized bone marrow transplant can be curative in such cases.[17]

One report on eight childhood cases of CVID focused on the autoimmune manifestations that may dominate the clinical course, leading to significant morbidity and mortality.[69] These included idiopathic thrombocytopenia, autoimmune hemolytic anemia, secretory diarrhea with GI inflammation, arthritis, chronic active hepatitis, parotitis, sarcoid-like granulomatous disease, and Guillain-Barré syndrome.[8] Many patients also have lymphadenopathy, splenomegaly, growth failure, and delayed puberty, reflecting the multisystemic nature of CVID.[69] Patients who have been treated with intravenous gammaglobulin are susceptible to an aggressive progression of hepatitis C, which can respond to IFN-α therapy.[70]

The clinical and immunologic status of 248 CVID patients was reported with survival 20 years after diagnosis, being only 64% for males and 67% for females.[58] Parameters associated with mortality were lower levels of serum IgG, weaker T-cell responses to mitogens, and, particularly, a lower percentage of circulating B cells. Of interest is a report that a subset of CVID patients with excessive suppressor cell activity benefited from therapy with cimetidine.[71] This H₂-receptor antagonist reduced suppressor cell activity, presumably allowing for endogenous Ig production. Improved B-cell differentiation has also been reported with 13-*cis*-retinoic acid[72] as well as with ketoprofen,[73] the latter, however, in vitro only. Some of the changes to the adaptive immune system in CVID have been attributed to HHV8 infection, especially among the subset of patients with granulomatous disease, autoimmune manifestations, and T cell dysfunction.[57] Patients with granulomatous inflammation have a worse prognosis compared to CVID without granuloma. The optimal treatment of CVID is unclear.[74] IVIG alone reduces the frequency of infections, but may be ineffective in preventing or treating autoimmunity or the intestinal inflammation.[8] Moreover, screening for antibodies to IgA is needed, as with IgAD. Combination therapy with immunomodulators, such as azathioprine and 6-mercaptopurine, may be needed to treat the GI manifestations of CVID.[66] TNF antagonists and anti-CD20 Immunomodulators have shown some efficacy.[8] Controlled trials are needed to determine the optimal management.

Hyper-IgE Syndrome and IPEX Syndrome

Hyperimmunoglobulin E syndrome (HIES) is a primary ID characterized by the triad of markedly increased IgE (>2,000 IU/mL), recurring skin abscesses, and pneumonia with cyst or pneumatocele formation.[75] The multiple staphylococcal skin infections led to the term Job syndrome,

Table 6 Gastrointestinal Manifestations of Common Variable Immunodeficiency

Nodular lymphoid hyperplasia
Infectious enterocolitis (bacterial, viral)
Giardia lamblia infestation
Bacterial overgrowth
Nonspecific enteritis or colitis
Pernicious anemia/atrophic gastritis/gastric cancer
Gluten-sensitive enteropathy

quoting the book of Job in the Bible: "*So went Satan forth from the presence of the Lord, and smote Job with sore boils from the sole of his foot unto his crown.*" Other common manifestations include atopic skin disease, eosinophilia, skeletal abnormalities, and delayed exfoliation of primary dentition.[75] Intractable diarrhea associated with absence of islets of Langerhans and neonatal insulin-dependent diabetes mellitus was reported in the HIES.[76] Affected male infants usually die of overwhelming infection.

Although some cases of familial HIES with autosomal dominant or recessive inheritance have been reported, most cases of HIES are sporadic, and their pathogenesis has remained unknown. Recently, it was found that dominant-negative mutations in the human signal transducer and activator of transcription 3 (*STAT3*) gene result in the classical multisystem HIES.[77] Eight of 15 unrelated nonfamilial HIES patients had heterozygous STAT3 mutations, but their parents and siblings did not have the mutant STAT3 alleles, suggesting that these were de novo mutations. Five different mutations were uncovered, all of which were located in the STAT3 DNA-binding domain.[77] The patients' peripheral blood cells showed defective responses to cytokines, including IL-6 and IL-10, and the DNA-binding ability of STAT3 in these cells was greatly diminished. All five mutants were nonfunctional by themselves and showed dominant-negative effects when coexpressed with wild-type STAT3.[77] These results highlight the multiple roles played by STAT3 in humans, and underline the critical involvement of multiple cytokine pathways in the pathogenesis of HIES. Other recent studies[78] have confirmed that human mutations in the FoxP3 gene explain one of the links between primary ID and autoimmunity. The association of diabetes mellitus, severe enteropathy, and endocrinopathy involving boys has been shown to be related to mutations of the *FOXP3* gene, which is the human equivalent of mouse scurfy.[78,79] This syndrome of immune dysregulation, polyendocrinopathy, enteropathy, X-linked (IPEX) is one of a group of clinical syndromes that present with multisystemic autoimmune disease, suggesting a phenotype of immune dysregulation.[80,81] Several mutations of FOXP3 have been reported in patients with IPEX.[82,83] *FOXP3*, the gene responsible for IPEX, maps chromosome Xp11.23–Xq13.3 and encodes a putative DNA-binding protein of the forkhead family. Data indicate that the *FOXP3* gene is expressed primarily in the CD4+CD25+ regulatory T-cell subset, where it may function as a transcriptional repressor and key modulator of regulatory T-cell fate and function.[84] The gene product, scurfin, is required for the development of CD4+CD25+ T regulatory cells. In the absence of T regulatory cells, activated CD4+ T cells instigate multiorgan damage resulting in type 1 diabetes, enteropathy, eczema, hypothyroidism, and other autoimmune disorders. Clinically, IPEX manifests most commonly with severe persistent diarrhea despite complete bowel rest, early onset of insulin-dependent diabetes

mellitus, thyroid disorders, and eczema (see Chapter 16.3, "Autoimmune Enteropathy and IPEX Syndrome"). IPEX can be differentiated from other genetic immune disorders by its genetics, clinical presentation, characteristic pattern of pathology, and, except for high IgE, absence of substantial laboratory evidence of ID. Recently, a distinct familial form of IPEX syndrome was reported that combines autoimmune and allergic manifestations including severe enteropathy, food allergies, atopic dermatitis, hyper-IgE, and eosinophilia. A 1388-base pair deletion (g.del-6247_-4859) of the *FOXP3* gene encompassing a portion of an upstream noncoding exon (exon-1) and the adjacent intron (intron-1) was identified.[85] Immunosuppression, using calcineurin inhibitors (cyclosporin) or sirolimus may provide temporary benefit for some patients but does not allow complete remission.[85,86] Remission has been observed after allogeneic bone marrow transplant, but the long-term outcome is uncertain.[87,88]

CELLULAR DEFECTS

Cellular primary IDs are defined as defective T cell or NK cell function with largely normal humoral immunity.[2] IDs due primarily to phagocytic defects are grouped separately. The optimum therapy of these disorders, when severe, is to correct the cellular deficiency with a bone marrow transplant.[5]

Defects in the Interferon-γ/IL-12 Axis

IFN-γ is critically important to activate mononuclear cell cytotoxic pathways in order to control intracellular pathogens such as *Salmonella* and mycobacteria.[17] The main stimulus for IFN-γ production by T_H1 lymphocytes and NK cells is IL-12. Mutations in IL-12 (including its p40 subunit), its receptor or the IFN-γ receptor cause cellular ID.[89] The same results from defects in STAT-1, as if permits signaling via the IFN-γ receptor. Partial deficiency in these components may respond to subcutaneous IFN-γ injections.[17]

NK Cell Deficiencies

Human NK cell deficiencies can occur as part of a more pervasive ID syndrome, or rarely, in isolation (Table 3). Substantial recent progress has been made in the recognition of novel isolated NK cell deficiencies.[90] These disorders usually present clinically with recurrent sinopulmonary and/or mucocutaneous viral and bacterial infections, characteristically involving the herpesvirus family (varicella zoster virus, cytomegalovirus, herpesviruses). Another presentation is that of hemophagocytic lymphohistiocytosis (HLH), often following a viral infection.

Autoimmune Lymphoproliferative Syndrome with Immunodeficiency (Caspase 8 Deficiency)

Caspase 8 deficiency results in an autoimmune lymphoproliferative syndrome (ALPS) associated

with a combined ID. NK cells from patients with deficient caspase 8 have impaired activation receptor-Induced stimulation and NF-κB nuclear translocation.[90] In addition to Infections as a result of their combined T & B cell deficiency, affected patients experience severe mucocutaneous viral infections with members of the herpesvirus family, typical of NK cell deficiencies.

Familial Erythrophagocytic Lymphohistiocytoses

Familial erythrophagocytic lymphohistiocytosis, also called a familial form of HLH, is a clinical phenotype that results from the extraordinary immune activation typically following infection with a member of the herpesvirus family.[91] This is due to the inability to mediate cytotoxicity and eradicate the infection, leading to a lack of downregulation of the systemic inflammatory response. A similar phenotype is encountered in other disorders of cytotoxicity, including the Chekiak-Higashi syndrome due to LYST mutation (see below), Griscelli syndrome due to RAB27A mutation and X-linked lymphoproliferative (XLP) syndrome due to SH2D1A mutation.[90] Three known molecular defects can result in familial HLH (reviewed in reference 90). Familial HLH2 involves a mutation of the *PFP1* gene encoding for the pore-forming molecule perforin, involved in the intracellular traffic of NK cell lytic granules. Familial HLH3 is due to a mutation of the *UNC13* gene, encoding the Unc-13 homolog D protein, also referred to as Munc13-4. Familial HLH4 is due to a mutation of the *STX 11* gene encoding the syntaxin-11 protein. Patients typically present with hematological malignancies, HLH, and severe viral infections (Epstein-Barr virus [EBV], herpesviruses).[90]

Hermansky-Pudlak Syndrome (AP-3 Deficiency)

The Hermansky-Pudlak syndrome (HPS) is a rare autosomal recessive disorder consisting of tyrosinase-positive oculocutaneous albinism, a bleeding diathesis resulting from platelet dysfunction, and systemic complications associated with accumulation of ceroid lipofuscin.[92] The mutation associated with ID in HPS type 2 involves the *ADTB3A* gene, encoding the β chain of the adaptor protien-3 complex. Patients have defective NK cell activity and may present with HLH.[93] Notably, HPS has been associated with a Crohn's-like enterocolitis in 7% of all cases and in over 30% of patients with GI symptoms.[94,95] Typically those with HPS-1 and HPS-4 genotypes have the IBD-like illness.[96] The Crohn's-like intestinal manifestations can be severe, and has been reported to be poorly responsive to medical therapies including sulfasalazine, mesalamine, steroids, and metronidazole. Infliximab has been reported to be effective for the management of the colitis, ileitis, as well as perianal fistulae.[97] It remains contentious whether this granulomatous colitis constitutes a part of the syndrome, or rather, represents an association with Crohn's disease.

However, by accepted definition, Crohn's disease is a yet idiopathic immune-mediated chronic inflammatory bowel disorder, whereas HPS is a primary immune deficiency disorder involving NK function.

Other NK Cell Deficiency Disorders

Cathepsin C deficiency (Papillon-Lefevre syndrome) is associated with defective NK cell cytolytic activity. Affected patients have herpesvirus infections, typically including peridontitis.[90] A number of patients with NEMO deficiency due to mutation of the *IKBKG* gene have deficient NK cytotoxicity.[90] Severe CMV infection and HLH have been described early in life in this disorder.[98] Mutation of CD16, part of the FcγRIII found on NK cells is associated with an inability of NK cells to phagocytose organisms or cells coated with IgG in the absence of MHC (antibody-dependent cellular cytotoxicity). Recurrent viral infections have been observed with this NK cell defect.[90]

DEFECTS AFFECTING BOTH T AND B CELLS

Severe Combined Immunodeficiency

The SCID syndromes are hereditary primary ID disorders characterized by a profound deficiency of both T- and B-lymphocyte function. They result in the virtual absence of immune function from birth, and by the onset of severe, life-threatening infections in the first months of life.[1,2] The frequency of all types of SCID is 1 in 50,000 to 75,000. A great diversity of genetic, enzymatic, hematologic, and immunologic features (see Table 3) characterizes this large category of syndromes.[99]

Genetic Variants. The SCIDs are an ever-expanding group of primary ID with known molecular defects.[2,99] The prototypical SCID is the X-linked common γ chain deficiency (γc SCID), accounting for over half of the cases.[17] They derive from mutations in the γc chain of the receptors for the cytokines IL-2, -4, -7, -9, -15, and -21.[100] The defect leads to widespread problems in lymphocyte differentiation and cytokine signaling. In the X-linked form, the abnormal gene produces a truncated γ chain of the IL-2 receptor on T cells.[89] Affected infants have lymphopenia as well as abnormal lymphocyte proliferation to mitogenic stimuli. T cells are profoundly low, while B cell numbers are normal or even increased. However, specific antibody responses are absent and serum Ig levels are low. Among autosomal recessive cases, approximately half have a genetic deficiency in the purine degradation enzymes (see Table 3), purine nucleoside phosphorylase (PNP), or adenosine deaminase (ADA) (Figure 6).[101,102] This results in the accumulation of metabolites (deoxyguanosine triphosphate and deoxyadenosine triphosphate, respectively) toxic to lymphoid stem cells. ADA deficiency typically causes more severe

lymphopenia than other SCIDs. Janus kinase 3 is a signaling molecule associated with the common γ chain.[103] Deficiency of Janus kinase 3 results in a clinical and immunologic phenotype similar to γc SCID. CD3 is part of the T cell receptor complex that transduces the signal generated by antigen binding. Deficiency of the DC3ε or CD3γ subunits results in dysfunctional T cells, whereas CD3δ deficiency results in an SCID.[104] IL-7 receptor α is critical to T cell function and its deficiency also results in SCID. Similarly, mutations in the IL-2 receptor α chain (CD25) results in a phenotype very similar to γc SCID.[17] CD45 is a tyrosine phosphatase that regulates kinases essential to signal transmission through B and T cell antigen receptors. Its deficiency also causes SCID.[17] The winged helix nude protein is a transcriptional regulator involved in T cell development. The winged helix nude deficiency leads to an SCID with decreased CD4 cells, alopecia, and nail dystrophy. RAG1 and RAG2 encode for proteins that control somatic recombination of the T and B cell receptor genes. Mutations in the *RAG* genes that catalyze the introduction of DNA double-strand breaks have been associated with Omenn syndrome (see below). After RAG makes cuts in DNA, the protein produced from the Artemis gene is responsible for repairing the DNA. Artemis gene product deficiency results in an SCID phenotype similar to RAG deficiency (Omenn syndrome), with radiation sensitivity.[105] Reticular dysgenesis is an SCID of unknown

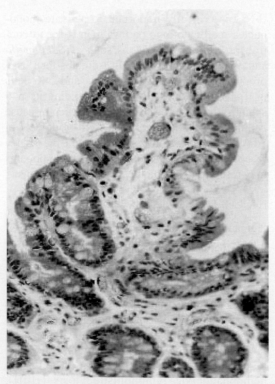

Figure 6 Intestine in severe combined immunodeficiency. The patient presented with intractable diarrhea, failure to thrive, and persistent oral candidiasis during infancy. Investigations confirmed adenosine deaminase deficiency. The jejunal and rectal biopsy specimens (not shown) demonstrate a markedly hypocellular lamina propria with absence of plasmocytes (hematoxylin phloxine saffron stain; ×300 original magnification). (Courtesy of P. Russo, MD.)

molecular etiology characterized by defective T, B, and granulocyte development, resulting in profoundly decreased T and B cells, granulocytopenia, thrombocytopenia, hypogammaglobulinemia, and deafness.[2] CD40 ligand, a protein on T helper cells, normally interacts with CD40 protein on B cells. In addition to being necessary for isotype switching, CD 40 axis is necessary for upregulating CD 80.86 costimulatory molecules, which permit T cells to become "tolerogenic." As opposed to the humoral deficiency in hyper IgM syndrome due to UNG or AICD deficiency, defects in CD40 axis result in a combined ID that is associated with malignancies (especially hepatoma) and autoimmune cytopenias.[2] Where a biochemical defect has been defined, recognition of heterozygote carriers and prenatal diagnosis become possible. For example, in ADA deficiency, measuring ADA activity in amniotic fibroblasts obtained at amniocentesis allows prenatal prediction of affected fetuses.

Clinical Presentation. The affected infant presents within the first few months of life with severe infections (often sinopulmonary and skin), chronic diarrhea with malabsorption, and failure to thrive. ADA deficiency is characterized by rib abnormalities and osteochondral dysplasia. Patients with PNP enzyme deficiency often have neurological symptoms and autoimmunity.[2] In most SCIDs, the pathogens include bacteria, viruses, mycobacteria, as well as opportunistic organisms. There may be a history of a neonatal hyperpigmented rash secondary to GVHD, resulting from transplacentally acquired maternal lymphocytes. GVHD may also occur after transfusion of nonirradiated blood products containing immunocompetent T cells or subsequent to allogenic bone marrow transplants.[2]

The SCID cases due to Omenn syndrome are associated with autoimmune features leading to squamous erythroderma with desquamation, alopecia, and intractable diarrhea.[106] Patients also have lymphoid hyperplasia and lymphadenopathy, erythroderma, and hepatosplenomegaly.[107] A lack of central tolerance contributes to the autoimmune manifestations. Cutaneous anergy and failure to reject transplants are typical, and peripheral eosinophilia is not uncommon. As noted above, this SCID syndrome is due to partial RAG1 or RAG2 deficiency.

Intractable diarrhea and recalcitrant oral and perineal thrush are common presentations. The diarrhea may begin slowly and progress to massive, watery, bloody, and mucopurulent. The pathophysiologic mechanisms underlying the intractable diarrhea remain poorly understood. These patients are extremely susceptible to viral infections and often succumb to overwhelming varicella, measles, EBV, herpes, or cytomegalovirus infection. It is worthwhile investigating stools for viral particles in these patients in that viruses—singly or in concert—may play an important role in the pathogenesis of the diarrhea. Some viral agents, such as rotavirus, adenovirus, and picornavirus, which normally cause self-limited diarrhea, may cause a chronic enteropathy in SCID. These patients are also susceptible to systemic infections caused by organisms such as *Candida albicans*, *P. carinii*, and *Listeria monocytogenes*. Enteropathogenic bacteria such as *Salmonella* and *Escherichia coli* can also cause chronic infections in these patients. Death usually occurs within the first 1 to 2 years of life unless immunologic reconstitution can be achieved, either by bone marrow transplant, enzyme replacement therapy, or gnotobiotic isolation in the absence of the above.

Histologic Features. Histologic features of the intestinal mucosa in SCID include the absence of plasma cells, blunted villi, and the presence of periodic acid–Schiff–positive macrophages in the lamina propria (see Figure 6). Most patients have a paucity of lymphoid tissue and profound lymphopenia with few mature T cells and low levels of Igs. Despite the uniformly profound lack of T- or B-cell function, many patients may have elevated percentages of B cells, such as in PNP deficiency. There is, however, marked heterogeneity among SCID patients, even in groups with similar inheritance patterns or ADA deficiency.

Management. The ultimate treatment for γc SCID and most other SCIDs is bone marrow transplantation.[3–5,108] Management involves appropriate antimicrobial therapy as well as education to avoid potentially infectious situations. Immunization with live vaccines or bacille Calmette-Guérin and conventional blood transfusions must be avoided in patients with proven or suspected defects in cellular immunity. Live vaccines can lead to disseminated infection, and blood transfusions may result in GVHD unless the blood is irradiated. IVIG does not prevent progression of disease, which is fatal by the first or second year of life if not treated.[2] Grafting of viable immunocompetent cells offers the only hope of permanent restoration of immune responsiveness. Patients with Omenn syndrome are particularly susceptible to GVHD; thus, bone marrow transplant is better performed after removal of T cells from the donor marrow using monoclonal antibodies.[88]

Enzyme replacement is beneficial to patients with ADA or PNP deficiency (see Table 3). Frozen, irradiated red blood cells may also provide a source of PNP. An ADA replacement is successful provided that a chemically modified enzyme with a prolonged in vivo life is used. Replacement of missing factors by gene transfer using a retrovirus vector is a logical approach, but has achieved only limited success. Occurrence of leukemia with such treatment has been described (K2). Both ADA and PNP deficiency forms of SCID meet the theoretic requirements for gene transfer. The gene for ADA has been identified on chromosome 20, and the DNA has been cloned. Treated patients with ADA–SCID have shown transient ADA activity in T cells and some clinical benefit. Stem cells have been transfected and reinfused to provide a renewable source of "normal" cells. Half of the ADA-deficient SCID

patients respond to transfusions of normal erythrocytes containing the enzyme. Others more severely affected also require treatment with the enzyme modified by polyethylene glycol, which prolongs its half-life. Although PEG-modified ADA can be helpful, it is not as effective as bone marrow transplantation. Some patients have been successfully treated with periodic infusions of their own T cells or umbilical cord blood cells that have been transfected with the *ADA* gene linked to a retroviral vector. Gene therapy has resulted in immune reconstitution, but leukemic complications have been reported.[109,110]

Outcome. In a series of 117 patients with SCID from 15 years ago, 22 died before transplant could be performed.[111] Among the various subtypes, infants with ADA deficiency and Omenn syndrome (large numbers of oligoclonal T cells and eosinophilia) had the highest rate of mortality before transplant could be performed. The survival rate among recipients of HLA identical bone marrow grafts was significantly higher (80%) than that among recipients of HLA haploidentical T cell–depleted bone marrow (56%).[111] Of the latter group, 35% had a persistent requirement for Ig administration after bone marrow transplant.

Major Histocompatibility Complex Class Deficiency

The MHC antigens (MHC class I or II) are of critical importance to cellular immune function. MHCs bound to processed antigen are recognized by the T cell receptor complex, allowing activation of T cells. MHC I is found on all nucleated cells and is recognized by CD8+ T cells. MHC II, present on B cells, monocytes, macrophages, and other "professional" antigen presenting cells, is recognized by CD4+ T cells. Transporter-associated protein (*TAP-1* and *TAP-2*) genes encode proteins that transport processed antigen to the MHC I complex. Mutations in TAP-1 or -2 lead to destruction of the MHC I proteins before they appear on cell surfaces, leading to a combined ID with low CD8 cells.[112] The presentation of the ID is milder than SCID and its onset is later, often in association with vasculitis.[2] A similar phenotype has been described due to tapasin gene mutations, which acts as a molecular chaperone for TAP.[113]

MHC class II deficiency is a rare primary ID disorder characterized by defects in HLA class II expression, inconsistent class I molecule expression, and a lack of cellular and humoral immune responses to foreign antigens. Mutations are of genes that code for various components (RFX5, RFXAP, RFXANK) of the multiprotein complex called RFX, which binds a promoter on the *MHC II* gene.[114] The ID is more severe than MHC Class I deficiency, and presents with very low CD4+ cell counts. Clinical onset occurs early in life, with recurrent infection and severe protracted diarrhea.[91] Small bowel biopsies show moderate to severe villous atrophy. Thymus atrophy and underdeveloped lymphoid tissue are typical. The diagnosis is usually assisted by

HLA-DR immunostaining.[115] The prognosis is poor, with death usually occurring at a mean age of 4 years. Bone marrow transplant should thus be considered early in life.

OTHER PRIMARY ID DISORDERS

IFN-γ receptor deficiency has been associated with neonatal intractable diarrhea and weight loss owing to *C. parvum*.[116] This illustrates the importance of specific cytokine deficiencies in the recovery from cryptosporidiosis and other GI disorders.

IMMUNODEFICIENCY ASSOCIATED WITH OTHER DEFECTS

Wiskott-Aldrich Syndrome

Wiskott-Aldrich syndrome is an X-linked recessive condition characterized by a triad including thrombocytopenia (small, dysfunctional platelets), severe eczema, and ID.[2,117] The ID involves an inability to respond to polysaccharide antigens, later to all antigens, and deficient cellular immunity leading to recurrent opportunistic infections. The combined ID results from mutations in the *WASP* gene that encodes a cytoskeletal adaptor protein that facilitates the branching of actin filaments.

Clinical Presentation. Patients present in the first few months of life with the above clinical picture, often accompanied by bloody diarrhea.[2,118] Although other GI complications are not prominent, malabsorption and nonspecific colitis may be encountered. The median survival has been shown to be less than 6 years, with more than 50% of patients dying of infection, 27% with hemorrhage, and 5 to 12% with tumors, almost all of which involve the lymphoreticular system.[118] In younger patients, infections are caused by pneumococci and other bacteria with polysaccharide capsules. They characteristically present with otitis media, pneumonia, meningitis, and/or sepsis. Later, infections with agents such as *P. carinii* and herpesvirus become more frequent. Such patients produce specific antibodies poorly but have normal numbers of B lymphocytes and plasma cells, along with normal or increased rates of globulin synthesis. Their T cells exhibit a progressive decrease in number and function. Patients with this defect have an impaired humoral immune response to polysaccharide antigens. Studies of Ig metabolism have shown an accelerated rate of synthesis as well as hypercatabolism of albumin, IgG, IgA, and IgM. This results in highly variable Ig concentrations, even within the same patient. The predominant pattern is a low-serum IgM, elevated IgA and IgE, and normal or slightly low IgG concentration. Lymphocyte responses to mitogens are depressed, and cutaneous anergy is frequently noted. There are low percentages of CD3 T cells, as well as CD4 and CD8 subsets. There is defective expression of the sialoglycoprotein CD43 on all leukocytes and platelets owing to its instability on cell surfaces in this syndrome. Optimal therapy requires bone marrow transplant, which appears to correct all of the problems with the exception of thrombocytopenia.

Ataxia-Telangiectasia

Ataxia-telangiectasia is a chromosomal instability disorder marked by progressive ataxia, oculocutaneous telangiectasias, and variable ID because of low IgA and IgG. This multisystem hereditary disease is associated with a complex ID, impaired organ maturation, X-ray hypersensitivity, and a high incidence of neoplasia.[119]

Pathophysiology and Genetics. The synthesis of antibodies and certain Ig subclasses appears to be disrupted owing to abnormal B-cell and Th-cell function in these patients. Individuals affected have various disorders of cell-mediated immunity, including the inability to produce antigen-specific cytotoxic lymphocytes against viral pathogens.[17] Moderately depressed proliferative responses to T- and B-cell mitogens are noted. Reduced percentages of total T cells and T cells of the helper phenotype, with normal or increased percentages of Ts cells, are found. Studies of Ig synthesis have revealed Th-cell and intrinsic B-cell defects. The thymus is very hypoplastic, with poor organization. This disease is considered a model of aberrant gene control, with persistently increased production of α-fetoprotein and carcinoembryonic antigen. However, these tests are not reliable markers of malignancy in ataxia-telangiectasia because they are elevated in the absence of cancer.[120] Cells of affected patients have an increased sensitivity to ionizing radiation, defective DNA repair, and frequent chromosomal abnormalities. Breakpoints involve the genes that code for the TCR and Ig heavy chains, thus explaining the combined T- and B-cell abnormalities. The inheritance follows an autosomal recessive pattern. The abnormal gene has been mapped to the long arm of chromosome 11 and codes for a protein with similarity to DNA-dependent protein kinases and functions in DNA repair.[2,17]

Clinical Presentation. Cerebellar ataxia becomes apparent at the time the child begins to walk, usually progressing until he or she is confined to a wheelchair, typically early in the second decade. Oculomotor abnormalities consist of nystagmus and difficulty in initiating voluntary eye movements. Oculocutaneous telangiectasia first appears as dilated venules on the conjunctiva between the ages of 3 and 6 years. Patients present with repeated sinopulmonary infections and progressive bronchiectasis (80% of cases).[119] Common viral exanthema and smallpox vaccinations have not usually resulted in untoward sequelae, although fatal varicella infection has been described. GI disease is not a characteristic feature in these patients unless secretory IgA is also deficient, reported in 50 to 80% of cases.

Outcome. The patients are at increased risk of developing malignancies, including non-Hodgkin lymphoma, lymphocytic leukemia, Hodgkin disease, and adenocarcinoma of the stomach. No satisfactory treatment has yet been found to treat this immune disorder and to prevent malignancy.

DiGeorge Syndrome

Thymic dysplasia is observed in several primary ID states, the most frequent of which is SCID (reviewed above). DiGeorge syndrome is a rare syndrome characterized by a triad including hypocalcemia, congenital heart disease, and T-cell lymphopenia from thymic hypoplasia.[121]

Pathophysiology and Genetics. Thymic dysplasia results from the failure of formation of the third and fourth pharyngeal pouches early during embryogenesis.[122] Other structures forming at the same time are also frequently affected, resulting in thymic and parathyroid gland underdevelopment, anomalies of the great vessels (right-sided aortic arch), esophageal atresia, bifid uvula, congenital heart disease (interrupted arch or truncus arteriosus, atrial and ventricular septal defects), and dysmorphic facial features (wide set eyes, low set, notched ears, mandibular hypoplasia, short upper lip philtrum). This spectrum or velocardiofacial syndrome, is usually due to deletions on chromosome 22q11.2.[17,121] Other deletions described include an area on chromosome 10p13 and mutations in the T-box-1 transcription factor.[121,123] The thymic hypoplasia or aplasia is associated with a cellular immune deficit and severe infections. A definitive diagnosis is possible using a fluorescent DNA probe on patient cells.

Clinical Presentation. Clinically, the syndrome is characterized by absent T-lymphocyte function, cardiovascular abnormalities, and hypoparathyroidism.[17,121,122] Patients present with hypocalcemic tetany early in life, congenital cardiac abnormalities, and dysmorphic features described above. Those with the complete syndrome may resemble patients with SCID in their susceptibility to infection with low-grade or opportunistic pathogens (fungi, viruses, and *P. carinii*) and to GVHD from nonirradiated blood transfusions. It has become apparent that a variable degree of hypoplasia is more frequent than total aplasia of the thymus and parathyroid glands. Some affected children may grow normally, and such patients are referred to as having partial DiGeorge syndrome. Concentrations of serum Igs are nearly normal for age, but IgA may be diminished, and IgE is sometimes elevated. The T-cell percentages are decreased, with a relative increase in the percentage of B cells. Despite low CD3+ T cells, the proportions of CD4 and CD8+ cells are usually normal. Proliferative response of lymphocytes may be absent, reduced, or normal, depending on the degree of thymic deficiency.[17] The GI manifestations in the children who survive the hypocalcemic seizures may include esophageal atresia, GI candidiasis, and intractable diarrhea.

It has recently been reported that early transplant of thymus tissue, before the development of infectious complications, can promote successful immune restitution.[124]

X-Linked Lymphoproliferative Disease

XLP syndrome is a rare, often fatal, primary ID that has profound and damaging effects on the immune system of affected children. It is a genetic disorder which requires a precise environmental factor to be clinically apparent. XLP is characterized by a dysregulated immune response to EBV infection.[104–106] In this syndrome, also known as Duncan disease or Purtilo syndrome, the affected male patient typically develops a chronic, often fatal, infectious mononucleosis, progressive hypogammaglobulinemia, aplastic anemia, or malignant B-cell lymphoma, only following EBV infection.[125–127] Although this severe susceptibility to EBV appeared to be transmitted as an X-linked recessive trait, cases have been reported in female patients.

Genetics. The defective gene in this syndrome has been identified as a signaling lymphocyte activation molecule (SLAM)-associated protein.[128–132] It is a T and NK cell–specific protein containing a single SH2 domain encoded by a gene that is defective or absent in patients with XLP syndrome. The SH2 domain of SLAM associated protein (SAP) binds with high affinity to the cytoplasmic tail of the hematopoietic cell-surface glycoprotein SLAM and five related receptors. SAP regulates signal transduction of the SLAM family receptors by recruiting SRC kinases.[130,131]

Pathophysiology. These patients generally appear to be healthy prior to EBV infection. However, immunologic studies have demonstrated elevated IgA or IgM and/or variable IgG subclass deficiencies prior to EBV infection.[133] Subsequent to EBV infection, circulating B-cell population and Igs decrease. The predominant T cell in the peripheral circulation becomes the NK cell. Subsequently, a proliferative B-cell disorder (lymphoma) may develop in approximately 35% of patients.[134,135] There is a marked impairment in the production of antibodies to the EBV nuclear antigens, whereas titers of antibodies to the viral capsid antigen are extremely variable. Antibody-dependent cell-mediated cytotoxicity against EBV-infected cells has been low in most affected individuals, and NK function is also depressed. There is also a deficiency in long-term T-cell immunity to EBV.[135] Studies of lymphocyte subpopulations have revealed elevated percentages of cells of the suppressor phenotype (CD8). Ig synthesis in response to polyclonal B-cell mitogen stimulation in vitro is markedly depressed. Thus, both EBV-specific and nonspecific immunologic abnormalities occur in these patients.

Clinical Presentation. The clinical spectrum is variable,[136] as typified by the following cases. In our experience, school-age children have presented with aplastic anemia, followed by a fulminant infectious mononucleosis with renal and hepatic failure, resulting in death within weeks. Another case presented with a history of a fever of unknown origin of several years duration. Massive hepatosplenomegaly was noted on physical examination. Liver biopsy revealed microabscesses focally without granulomas, resembling a septic hepatitis. Multiple cultures were negative for bacterial, fungal, and viral pathogens. Splenectomy revealed a lymphoproliferative disorder and erythrophagocytosis. Specific antibody titers to EBV were demonstrated to increase significantly. The patient was treated with antiviral agents but eventually died of a lymphoma. Most patients present in the preschool-age group with a severe, often fatal (80%), mononucleosis owing to severe hepatitis. The majority of those who survive the primary infection progress to a combined type of ID with hypogammaglobulinemia and/or lymphomas.

DEFECTS OF PHAGOCYTIC FUNCTION

A number of genetically determined defects affecting polymorphonuclear and/or mononuclear phagocytes have been described (see Table 3). Neutrophil function involves cell migration in response to chemotactic stimuli, adherence, endocytosis, and killing or destruction of ingested particles. Cell motility depends on the integrity of the cytoskeleton and the contractile system, whereas directional motility is adhesion molecule receptor mediated. Endocytosis depends on the expression of membrane receptors (eg, for IgG, C3b, IC3b) and on the fluidity of the membrane. Defects in intracellular killing of ingested microorganisms result from failure of the "respiratory burst," which is critical to the production of superoxide radicals, oxygen singlets, hydroxyl radicals, and hydrogen peroxide. The organisms cultured from the lesions of patients with this type of defect are generally catalase producing and typically include *Staphylococcus, E. coli,* fungi, and other opportunistic organisms. Patients with defective endocytosis and killing tend to have chronic infected granulomas, especially of the lymph nodes, liver, and lung. Patients whose neutrophils fail to adhere normally to surfaces have a biosynthetic defect of a 94 kDa glycoprotein (CD11/CD18).[137] These molecules are present on the surfaces of all leukocytes and play a critical adhesive role in cell–microbe, cell–cell, and cell–surface interactions. In a classic case, a patient with a neutrophil functional defect has had multiple invasive bacterial (especially *Pseudomonas, Serratia,* and *Staphylococcus aureus*) and fungal (*Aspergillus* and *Candida* species) infections, beginning during the first year of life. The early infections involve primarily the skin and portals of entry: impetigo, paronychia, periodontitis, sinusitis, and perirectal abscesses. Later infections involve deeper structures: lymphadenitis, pneumonia, osteomyelitis, and splenic and hepatic abscesses. Table 3 summarizes the

primary defects of phagocytic function.[3] Interestingly, several of these phagocyte disorders present with Crohn's disease–like involvement of the GI tract and perianal area, as described below.

Chronic Granulomatous Disease

CGD is an uncommon primary immune deficiency (affecting 1/200,000 newborn infants) caused by a defect in phagocyte production of oxygen metabolites, and resulting in bacterial infections produced by catalase-positive microorganisms and fungal diseases that occasionally may prove fatal. CGD is characterized by a greatly increased susceptibility to pyogenic infections with catalase-positive organisms of the respiratory tract, skin, and soft tissues.[138–141]

Genetics. CGD is caused by mutations in any one of four genes that encode the subunits of phagocyte reduced nicotinamide adenine dinucleotide phosphate (NADPH) oxidase, the enzyme that generates microbial proinflammatory oxygen radicals.[17] Of the 410 CGD mutations identified, 95% cause complete or occur in the larger of these subunits. In the majority of cases, the GP92 mutation of the phagocyte oxidase (phox) permits no cytochrome production. In a $P92_{phox}$ variant that permits low levels of superoxide production, the condition can be improved with IFN-γ. The 30% of CGD patients with the autosomal recessive disease have mutations of the smaller $P22_{phox}$ cytochrome subunit and the cytosolic $P47_{phox}$ and $P67_{phox}$ components of the total NADPH-oxidase system. Studies have revealed that recombination events between the *$P47_{phox}$* gene and its pseudogenes not only cause the absence of $P47_{phox}$ but also predict the generation of a novel fusion protein.[141]

Pathophysiology. The neutrophils of patients with CGD demonstrate normal chemotaxis, engulfment, and degranulation, but their ability to kill microorganisms is impaired owing to defective oxidative burst capacity. Neutrophils and monocytes from these patients, activated in vitro by phagocytosis with a variety of particulate and soluble stimuli, fail to consume the oxygen needed for the production of superoxide anions, hydrogen peroxide, and hydroxyl radicals. The reduced form of NADPH oxidase is found exclusively in phagocytes and is dormant unless activated. The NADPH is the physiologic electron source; a flavin and a phagocyte cytochrome *b* are also postulated to function in a short electron transport chain that transfers a single electron to molecular oxygen to form the superoxide anion. The failure to produce superoxide anions in CGD can result from abnormalities in the components of the oxidase itself, as well as in its activation pathway.

Clinical Presentation. The clinical presentation of CGD comprises recurrent infection, multifocal abscesses affecting the skin and liver, lymphadenopathy, hepatosplenomegaly, chronic lung disease, and persistent diarrhea. Patients with CGD are particularly susceptible to infections with microbes that produce catalase, allowing them

to survive destruction by endogenous peroxide. The most common pathogen is *S. aureus*. Others include gram-negative bacilli and fungi such as *Aspergillus fumigatus* and *C. albicans*. The GI tract involvement, present in the majority of cases, may be present initially and recurrently, causing substantial morbidity and mortality.[140] Steatorrhea and vitamin B_{12} malabsorption are often present. Jejunal biopsy usually reveals normal villi. However, lipid-filled pigmented foamy histiocytes are present in the lamina propria throughout the GI tract.

Diagnosis. The sine qua non for the diagnosis of CGD is the demonstration of an absent or greatly diminished respiratory burst capacity. This defect can be demonstrated by measuring superoxide (O^{2-}) production in response to both soluble (PMA) and opsonized particulate stimuli (zymosan). In the majority of cases, there is either no detectable O_2 generation or production at rates between 0.5 and 10% of controls. An alternative method for measuring respiratory burst activity is the commonly employed nitroblue tetrazolium (NBT) test. Neutrophils able to produce a normal oxidative burst reduce the NBT, causing a change in color from clear to blue. In the most common forms of CGD, no NBT reduction is observed in any of the cells. In some of the variant forms, however, a high percentage of cells may contain small amounts of formazan. The NBT test is helpful in classifying variant forms of CGD. Historically, the major classification criteria for CGD depended on the cytochrome *b* spectrum. Its determination can be accomplished using intact neutrophils or in subcellular fractions by Western blot analysis using antibodies to the two subunits of cytochrome *b*.[142]

Enterocolitis. Patients with CGD often present with an enterocolitis greatly resembling Crohn's disease.[140,143] Manifestations typically include vomiting, diarrhea, abdominal pain, weight loss, and fever. Disordered intestinal motility, ulceration, obstruction, and infection (eg, abscesses) can occur anywhere along the GI tract, from the mouth to the anus. The other similarities to Crohn's disease include physical findings (most notably perianal abscesses and fistulae), endoscopic appearance, and radiographic abnormalities. Granulomas and giant cells are found quite frequently in colonic biopsies (Figure 7). The mechanism of granuloma formation in CGD is unknown. It has been postulated that the defective respiratory burst in phagocytes results in persistent inflammation because chemoattractants are not oxidatively inactivated. Delayed clearance of microorganisms may also explain these inflammatory changes. Similar hypotheses have been proposed to explain granuloma formation in Crohn's disease. A recent study of colonic mucosal biopsies of patients with CGD showed that the inflammatory infiltrate differed from the normal controls by an increase in eosinophils and macrophages.[143] There was a paucity of neutrophils compared with ulcerative colitis. Expression of HLA-DR was increased in the epithelium and vascular endothelium compared with normal

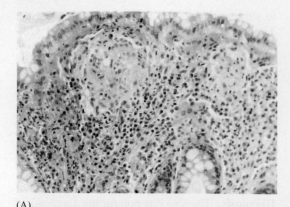

(A)

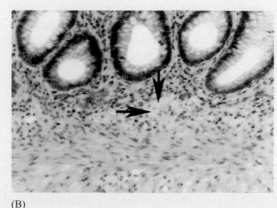

(B)

Figure 7 Long-standing colitis in a patient with chronic granulomatous disease. His severe colitis and perianal involvement resembling Crohn's disease were resistant to usual therapy (salazosulfapyridine, 5-acetylsalicylic acid, prednisone, 6-mercaptopurine) but responded to total parenteral nutrition and complete bowel rest. (A) Rectal biopsy specimen shows two granulomas in the superficial part of the mucosa and a dense chronic inflammatory reaction peripherally. (B) Foamy macrophages (*arrows*) are seen near the muscularis mucosae (hematoxylin phloxine saffron stain; ×300 original magnification). (Courtesy of P. Russo, MD.)

controls. Moreover, patterns of expression of the adhesion molecules (ICAM-1, vascular cell adhesion molecule 1, E-selectin) differed significantly in CGD from those in other inflammatory bowel disease: ICAM-1 was more strongly expressed in the lamina propria, vascular cell adhesion molecule 1 was more patchily expressed, and E-selectin was present only in the small vessels.[143]

Gastritis. In addition to frequent hepatic and perirectal abscesses, patients with CGD may develop a granulomatous narrowing of the gastric antrum, with symptoms suggestive of gastric outlet obstruction.[139–141] It is thus important to consider a diagnosis of CGD in patients presenting with an unexplained narrowing of the antrum.[144] The differential diagnosis includes pyloric stenosis, peptic ulcer disease, eosinophilic gastroenteritis, or Crohn's disease. However, histological examination of biopsies, the NBT test, and analysis of CD68-positive cells are diagnostic.

Management and Outcome. Controled studies are lacking. Management decisions depend on the extent of intestinal involvement and the presence of any complications:

- Antimicrobial therapy and drainage of abscesses lead to clinical improvement.[118] Partial loss of protein.

- The use of steroids can hasten the resolution of colitis or gastric outlet obstruction.[145]

- Sulfasalazine may be helpful to manage colonic disease.

- Malnourished patients may require enteral or parenteral nutrition (PN) support.

- The gastric outlet obstruction often can be managed medically with broad-spectrum antibiotics and continuous enteral alimentation. Nutritional support and antimicrobial agents may obviate the need for surgery, with symptomatic resolution of the obstruction after 2 to 4 months of therapy.[145]

- IFN-γ was reported to be active on CGD phagocyte superoxide generation, NADPH-

oxidase kinetics, and expression of the gene for the phagocyte cytochrome *b* heavy chain.[146] In vitro treatment with IFN-γ increased the respiratory burst activity of polymorphonuclear neutrophil (PMN) leukocytes and macrophages from patients with CGD type IA variant (X-linked; A designates a form in which phagocytes exhibit decreased but detectable superoxide production). Phagocytes from classic type I, IIA, and II CGD did not respond to IFN-γ. In vivo studies demonstrated similar responses. IFN-γ appears to upregulate expression of cytochrome *b* genes by increasing their transcription or through posttranslational stabilization of messenger RNA. These studies support the reported potential efficacy of IFN-γ in the treatment of these patients. The safety and effectiveness of long-term recombinant human IFN-γ therapy has been reported in CGD.[147] Thirty patients received recombinant IFN-γ three times weekly for an average of 2.5 years. The rate of serious infection was 0.13 per patient-year, compared with 1.10 in untreated patients.[147] Fever (23%), diarrhea (13%), and flu-like illness (13%) were the most common adverse effects of recombinant IFN-γ. No serious adverse effects or impairments in growth or development were observed.

- Recent data suggest that gene therapy might be the treatment in selected cases.[148] The recent development of advanced gene transduction protocols together with improved retroviral vectors, combined with low intensity chemotherapy conditioning, allowed partial correction of the granulocytic function with a significant clinical benefit in treated patients.

Finally, it is critically important for the clinician to consider the possibility of CGD in patients with a "Crohn-like" disease in whom a history of recurrent infections and abscesses is noted. The intestinal and perianal manifestations are remarkably similar, although the treatments differ.

Leukocyte Adhesion Molecule Deficiency 1

This immune disorder is characterized by the inability of phagocytes to adhere to vascular endothelium and migrate into tissues owing to an absence of CD11/CD18 β2 integrins on the phagocyte surface. Leukocyte adhesion molecule deficiency 1 is a rare inherited adhesion molecule disorder that is manifested by recurrent and often fatal bacterial infections.[149]

Pathophysiology. The leukocytes of affected individuals are characterized by absent or deficient expression of plasma membrane glycoproteins that are members of the leukocyte integrin family. The LFA-1 (CD11a/CD18) serves as an adhesion-promoting molecule, facilitating lymphocyte blastogenesis, cellular cytotoxicity (cytotoxic T lymphocyte, NK, and K), and lymphocyte endothelial cell adhesion. The Mac-1 (CD11b/CD18) is the receptor for C3b1 (CR3), an adhesion-promoting molecule facilitating PMN aggregation, PMN/macrophage (Mp) adhesion to substrates, and PMN/Mp chemotaxis. The P150,95 (CD11c/CD18) is a less well-defined glycoprotein that may promote adhesion of PMN and Mp to substrates and also bind C3bi.[149,150] Leukocytes in affected individuals have defective migration and adherence, resulting in an increased susceptibility to infections. There are at least two variants of CD11/CD18 leukocyte glycoprotein deficiency. The degree of CD11/CD18-deficient expression (ranging from 10% of normal to totally absent) correlates closely with the severity of the clinical manifestations and the magnitude of the in vitro cellular abnormalities. In vitro leukocyte abnormalities include a defect in adhesion by unstimulated or PMA-stimulated cells. Neutrophils fail to demonstrate aggregation in response to stimulants (eg, C5a, PMA). Impairment of directed motility is demonstrated in vitro in response to chemoattractants. A severe defect in CR3 aggregation activity is noted. The NBT for respiratory burst activity is impaired, as is secretion of granular contents by neutrophils and monocytes when induced by particulate stimuli. Lymphoid cells present a diminished blastogenic activity to mitogen (PMA). There is also impairment in cytotoxic activity mediated by T lymphocytes, NK cells, and K cells.

Clinical Presentation. Infants frequently present weeks after birth (2 to 3 weeks), with delayed umbilical cord separation and cellulitis of the umbilical stump (omphalitis). Other tissue infections such as cellulites, perirectal abscesses, and necrotizing bowel infections are characteristic. Stomatitis or pharyngitis is present in 40%, and gingivitis or periodontitis is present in 56% of patients.[150,151] The oral and perineal manifestations of this disorder may be mistaken for Crohn's disease. We have seen a patient presenting with an ischiorectal abscess and distal ileocolitis, greatly resembling Crohn's disease.[151] GI tract involvement has been reported in very few patients, including appendicitis, peritonitis, ischemic ileitis, and necrotizing enterocolitis.[150,151]

Bacterial septicemia is a common complication and may frequently be fatal. Common bacterial pathogens include *S. aureus*, group A β-hemolytic *Streptococcus*, *Proteus mirabilis*, *Pseudomonas aeruginosa*, and *E. coli*. Severe viral infections (viral meningitis or fatal enteroviral infection) and oral candidiasis have also been described.

Management and Outcome. No specific therapy has been shown to ameliorate the clinical manifestations of the disorder. Antibiotic therapy has proved to be successful in most situations, but patients have often died from bacterial sepsis. Leukocyte adhesion molecule deficiency 1 is uniformly fatal within the first 10 years of life, and bone marrow transplant is the only effective cure. It rapidly reversed the intractable Crohn-like ileocolitis in one of our young patients.[151] Because the *CD18* gene has been cloned and sequenced, this disorder is a candidate for gene therapy.[152]

OTHER DISORDERS OF NEUTROPHILS

In addition to CGD and the CD11/CD18 adhesion molecule deficiency, other hereditary errors of neutrophil number and function are notable for their association with GI manifestations. These include glycogen storage disease type 1B and the Hermansky-Pudlak syndrome. Both of these disorders are also characterized by a nonspecific colitis that resembles IBD.[92–97,153] In the former disorder, treatment with human recombinant granulocyte colony-stimulating factor has been shown to improve both the neutropenia and the colitis.[154] Finally, Shwachman syndrome is another multisystem congenital disorder associated with cyclical neutropenia. The primary GI manifestations, exocrine pancreatic insufficiency, and failure to thrive are discussed in detail elsewhere in this book.

OTHER DISORDERS AT TIMES ASSOCIATED WITH ID

A number of other clinical disorders are associated with various forms of primary ID (see Table 3). The discussion is limited to those conditions with prominent GI manifestations.

Chronic Mucocutaneous Candidiasis

Chronic mucocutaneous candidiasis is a syndrome characterized by *Candida* infection involving the esophageal and buccal mucosa, skin, and nails. It is frequently associated with an endocrinopathy (Addison disease, hypoparathyroidism, hypothyroidism) and pernicious anemia.[155] This condition may result from a variety of causes, including a primary defect in cell-mediated immunity to *Candida* (autosomal recessive). Patients may present with esophageal candidiasis in the presence or absence of oral involvement. Therefore, any patient with mucocutaneous candidiasis who has dysphagia, odynophagia, or hematemesis should be suspected of having Candida esophagitis, even if oral involvement is not evident.

These individuals are at risk for development of esophageal stricture and thus require aggressive treatment for chronic *Candida* infection. The use of antacids of H2 antagonists may worsen the esophageal involvement with *Candida* by reducing gastric acidity. Patients with familial chronic mucocutaneous candidiasis may also present with a chronic indeterminate colitis. The colitis can be unresponsive to medical management, including sulfasalazine, steroids, elemental diet, PN, thiopurine immunomodulators, and cyclosporine. In such cases, the unrelenting colitis may require colectomy. Interestingly, a parent of one such patient, also affected by chronic mucocutaneous candidiasis, also has primary biliary cirrhosis.

Autoimmune Polyendocrinopathy-Candidiasis-Ectodermal Dystrophy

This autosomal recessive disease is characterized by a variety of clinical manifestations occurring in variable combinations. Autoimmune polyendocrinopathy-candidiasis-ectodermal dystrophy (APECED) is associated with a mutation in the autoimmune regulator.[156] The polyendocrinopathy may include failure of parathyroid glands, the adrenal cortex, pancreatic beta cells with type I diabetes, gonads, gastric parietal cells, and/or thyroid gland. Other manifestations may include hepatitis, chronic mucocutaneous candidiasis, dystrophy of the dental enamel and nails, severe alopecia, vitiligo, and keratopathy.[156–159] In one series of 68 patients from 54 families, 60% initially presented with oral candidiasis, 9% with malabsorption, and 3% with keratopathy.[159] A malabsorptive syndrome has been reported in up to 24% of patients with APECED or type I polyglandular autoimmune syndrome.[160] The steatorrhea has been attributed to a number of causes. Intestinal infections (including bacterial overgrowth) may play a role, but exocrine pancreatic insufficiency is the major factor.[158,160] The malabsorptive syndrome and accompanying decreased absorption of calcium and vitamin D may aggravate the severe hypocalcemia in those patients with a polyendocrinopathy. Use of pancreatic enzymes can improve symptoms and the hypocalcemia. However, control of the various autoimmune manifestations of the disease was only achieved using cyclosporine.[158]

GRAFT-VERSUS-HOST DISEASE

Hematopoietic stem cell transplant is the treatment of choice for a number of primary ID involving cellular immunity.[5] However, GVHD has long been regarded as a serious complication of this procedure.[161,162] GVHD can present as two, but not mutually exclusive, clinical syndromes: acute GVHD and chronic GVHD. Acute GVHD is a distinctive syndrome of dermatitis, hepatitis, and enteritis occurring within 3 months of allogeneic bone marrow transplant. Although GVHD may affect any organ, intestinal GVHD is particularly important because of its frequency, severity, and impact on the general condition of

the patient. Severe diarrhea is common and usually associated with symptoms of protein-losing enteropathy. The GI tract plays a major role in the amplification of systemic disease because GI damage increases the translocation of endotoxins, which promote further inflammation and additional mucosal damage. Translocation may be complicated by septic shock and multivisceral failure. Clinical symptoms, together with timing after bone marrow transplant, facilitate the diagnosis. Techniques employed to assist in the diagnosis of acute GVHD include transabdominal ultrasonography, color Doppler imaging, and endoscopy.[163,164] Intestinal biopsies show villous atrophy, apoptotic enterocytes within glands, and lamina propria infiltration. Progressive elucidation of the mechanisms of GVHD has shown that donor T cells are critical for the induction of GVHD because depletion of T cells from bone marrow grafts effectively prevents GVHD. The standard regimen that is used to prevent GVHD classically includes cyclosporine plus short-term methotrexate.[162] Corticosteroids can be added to this regimen, but adverse effects have to be considered. Tacrolimus is a more potent alternative to cyclosporine. Mycophenolate mofetil can be used as part of a combination therapy. Systemic antibacterial therapy, including eradication of intestinal bacteria, prevents the intestinal translocation of lipopolysaccharide and avoids the subsequent increase of inflammatory cytokines.

Chronic GVHD is a more pleiotropic syndrome, involving skin, liver, lung, and intestine, suggesting a sclerodermatous-like syndrome that develops after 3 months, and includes diffuse collagen deposition resulting in fibrosis, production of autoantibodies, and ID. Digestive symptoms include nausea, vomiting, food intolerance, diarrhea, and failure to thrive. The clinical presentation and endoscopic findings are nonspecific, and there is a broad differential diagnosis, including bacterial, fungal, viral, and parasitic infections. Intestinal lesions are poorly described in the literature, primarily being described in the esophagus.[165] One study compared the histologic features of chronic GVHD and control children.[166] Chronic GVHD with intestinal involvement was usually multisystemic (88%) and proceeded by acute GVHD in 88% of cases. Histologic features from duodenal and/or colonic biopsies included (1) villous atrophy; (2) glandular lesions, mainly apoptotic with variable intensity; and (3) lamina propria infiltrates with cytotoxic T lymphocytes (CD3+, CD8+, TiA1+, granzyme B–). Differential diagnosis of GVHD includes cytomegalovirus colitis and *C. parvum* infection. In chronic GVHD, the apoptotic process could be related to Tc lymphocytes, probably with other cells, such as the enterocytes via the Fas/Fas ligand pathway. The outcome of chronic GVHD is usually severe, especially in cases of GI involvement, and requires an intensive immunosuppressive treatment that renders the host vulnerable to opportunistic infections.[162,166,167] Long-term PN is often necessary to maintain growth and nutritional status. For all of these reasons, histologic confirmation is recommended to avoid inappropriate treatment.

CONGENITAL OR HEREDITARY DISEASES ASSOCIATED WITH ID

Chediak-Higashi Syndrome

Chediak-Higashi syndrome (CHS) is a rare, autosomal recessive disorder that affects multiple systems.[168] Patients with CHS exhibit hypopigmentation of the skin, eyes and hair, prolonged bleeding times, easy bruisability, recurrent infections, abnormal NK cell function, and peripheral neuropathy. This syndrome is due to defective lysosomal granule formation in a variety of cells, resulting in phagocytic dysfunction, albinism, and neurologic impairment.[17,104] Phagocytosis occurs, but lysosomal fusion with the phagosomal membrane is deficient, with subsequent impaired bacterial killing. Morbidity results from patients succumbing to frequent bacterial infections or to an "accelerated phase" lymphoproliferation into the major organs of the body.[168] Treatment is bone marrow transplantion, which alleviates the immune problems and the accelerated phase, but does not inhibit the development of neurologic disorders that worsen with age. Positional cloning and YAC complementation resulted in the identification of the Beige and CHS1/LYST genes.[168] The gene responsible presumably functions in intracellular granule trafficking. Affected individuals suffer from pyogenic infections, which can be fatal. From the GI point of view, Crohn's disease–like bowel involvement has been observed.

Acrodermatitis Enteropathica

Metabolic or transport disorders, such as acrodermatitis enteropathica, result in hypogammaglobulinemia and abnormal cell-mediated immunity. This autosomal recessive disease,[169] characterized by an eczematous rash, alopecia, chronic diarrhea, malabsorption, and recurrent sinopulmonary infections, can be mimicked by acquired conditions, resulting in severe zinc deficiency, such as Crohn's disease and intractable diarrhea of infancy. The symptoms and immunologic abnormalities respond to zinc supplementation. Hypogammaglobulinemia may occur in some patients with more advanced disease; it is not known whether this is due to a protein-losing enteropathy or a direct effect on lymphocytic function.

Intestinal Lymphangiectasia

This intestinal disorder may be classified as ID because it is responsible for a combination of lymphopenia and hypogammaglobulinemia (IgA, IgG). Symptoms of protein-losing enteropathy suggest the diagnosis of intestinal lymphangiectasia. T lymphocytes are lost from the intestine or into chylous effusions, and this may be associated with a failure to manifest delayed-hypersensitivity skin reactions. Susceptibility to infections is variable, but rarely severe. Diagnosis requires confirmation by intestinal biopsy. Lymphangiography may show other lymphatic abnormalities in familial cases. As with other protein losing enteropathies, serum IgM tends to remain within normal limits, whereas the serum IgG and IgA levels may fall to low levels. This pattern may be seen in patients with primary hypogammaglobulinemia, although the serum IgA is usually much lower. However, it differs from that seen in the hypogammaglobulinemia secondary to lymphoproliferative disease, in which the serum IgM is usually the first Ig class to fall. There is usually a response to a fat-restricted diet and supplementation with medium-chain triglycerides. This reduces the lymphatic flow in the intestine, thus reducing the pressure driving the gut losses. Steroids are helpful when the lymphangiectasia is due to local inflammation, such as in Crohn's disease, and may also have a short-term palliative effect in malignant infiltration.

SYNDROMIC DIARRHEA ASSOCIATED WITH ID

Syndromic diarrhea, also known as phenotypic diarrhea or Tricho-hepato-enteric syndrome, is a congenital enteropathy presenting with early-onset of severe diarrhea requiring PN.[170–174] The estimated prevalence is approximately 1/300,000–400,000 live births in Western Europe. Ethnic origin does not appear characteristic for syndromic diarrhea. Patients born small for gestational age present with diarrhea starting in the first 6 months of life (less than 1 month in most cases). They have an abnormal phenotype, including facial dysmorphism with prominent forehead, broad nose, and hypertelorism, and a distinct abnormality of hair, trichorrhexis nodosa. Hairs are woolly, easily removed, and poorly pigmented. Liver disease is seen in about half of cases, with extensive fibrosis or cirrhosis.[174] There is currently no specific biochemical profile while a functional T-cell immune deficiency with defective antibody production was reported. Patients have defective antibody responses despite normal serum Ig levels and defective antigen-specific skin tests despite positive proliferative responses in vitro.[170] Microscopic analysis show twisted hair (pili torti), aniso- and poilkilotrichosis, and trichorrhexis nodosa. Histopathological analysis shows nonspecific villous atrophy with low or without mononuclear cell infiltration of the lamina propria, and no specific histological abnormalities involving the epithelium. The etiology remains unknown. The frequent association of the disorder with parental consanguinity and/or affected siblings suggests a genetic origin with an autosomal recessive transmission. Prognosis for this type of intractable diarrhea of infancy is poor. Most patients have died between the ages of 2 and 5 years, some of them with early onset of liver disease.[170,171] The cause of this diarrhea is unknown, and the relation between low birth weight, dysmorphism, severe diarrhea, trichorrhexis, and ID is unclear (see Chapter 15.3c,

"Congenital Enteropathies"). Among the congenital forms of hair dysplasia, trichorrhexis nodosa is very common and can be present in several pathologic conditions.[175,176]

Intestinal Atresia Associated with ID

Congenital intestinal atresia has been reported to be associated with ID.[177–179] The first report involved three siblings from healthy, nonconsanguineous parents, with multiple intestinal atresias.[177] One sibling had documented SCID, whereas the clinical histories of the two other siblings strongly suggested a congenital ID syndrome. All patients died before 2 years of age. One last sibling was born with the same defects and documented SCID. He survived 2.5 years with short-bowel syndrome on total PN but finally died from sepsis. This rare syndrome appears to have an autosomal recessive mode of transmission. Other cases have been reported, such as two affected siblings born 18 months apart and a third child with duodenal atresia.[179] One additional child with multiple intestinal atresias was diagnosed with ID after posttransfusion GVHD. In cases with multiple GI atresias, attention should be given to a possible associated immune disorder, and irradiation of blood products is recommended pending evaluation of immune status. Donor immune reconstitution after liver-intestine transplant was recently reported in a child with multiple intestinal atresias and SCID.[180] This child did not experience intestinal graft rejection but only a mild GVHD. It is postulate that this child engrafted a donor intestine–derived immune system and is incapable of rejecting transplanted organs.

Congenital Hypothyroidism

Bidirectional interactions between the immune and endocrine systems have been well described, particularly in relation to the growth hormone and adrenal axes. An association between congenital hypothyroidism and ID was described.[181] Severe and persistent lymphopenia was associated with bronchiectasis and chronic diarrhea. It was proposed that the prolonged thyroid hormone deficiency might be related to the impaired cellular immunity.[181] The underlying molecular mechanism is in most cases unknown, but the frequent coincidence of cardiac anomalies suggests that the thyroid morphogenetic process may depend on proper cardiovascular development. The T-box transcription factor TBX1, which is the most probable gene for the 22q11 deletion syndrome (22q11DS/DiGeorge syndrome/velo-cardio-facial syndrome), has emerged as a central player in the coordinated formation of organs and tissues derived from the pharyngeal apparatus and the adjacent secondary heart field from which the cardiac outflow tract derives.[182]

DIAGNOSIS OF PRIMARY ID

Primary ID states are relatively rare compared with those that occur secondary to various diseases or their treatment. Patients with primary ID have an increased susceptibility to infections, as well as to diverse GI problems, as reviewed above. A systematic approach to investigating children with suspected ID is necessary.[183] Early treatment may prevent otherwise inevitable and devastating complications or death. Classification into disorders of antibody production, cell-mediated immunity, combined humoral and cellular immunity, phagocytic function, and complement components facilitates an approach to diagnosis.

Clinical Analysis

In general, one should consider a possible diagnosis of primary ID on the basis of the pattern or type of infection rather than on their frequency alone. Multiple benign viral infections of the upper respiratory tract are of much less significance than a single episode of *P. carinii* pneumonia or recurrent staphylococcal and gram-negative infections. The pattern of infection may often give a clue to the component of the immune system that is most likely affected, as summarized in Table 1. Most patients with a significant ID present in the first year of life. Infants with predominantly cellular or combined defects present slightly earlier than those with humoral ID. In the latter group, maternally acquired antibodies serve to protect the child for the first 5 months or so. The age at presentation is, however, quite variable and is influenced by the timing of exposure to infectious organisms. By virtue of their associated GI manifestations, pediatric gastroenterologists are most likely to be consulted for the primary ID detailed in this chapter.

Microbiological Investigations

In patients who are febrile or severely ill, a septic workup should include blood cultures for aerobic and anaerobic bacteria, as well as fungi. Serologic testing of viral or other infections may be unreliable owing to the inability to produce specific antibodies, as discussed above. Thus, efforts should focus on attempts to isolate infectious organisms from respiratory secretions, urine, stool, blood, and cerebrospinal fluid. Polymerase chain reaction technique may be useful to enhance the sensitivity for the detection of viral genomes. Perhaps more than any other possibility, HIV infection must be extensively ruled out in cases of suspected primary ID. The immunologic and GI manifestations bear an overlap with many of the cellular immune defects described above. The diagnosis should be excluded by identification of HIV antigens and virus isolation, in addition to standard serologic methods.

Digestive and Nutritional Assessment

Patients with chronic diarrhea should have serum albumin, blood urea nitrogen, and electrolyte levels measured. If malabsorption or sinopulmonary disease is present, a sweat test and nasal ciliary biopsy should be considered to exclude cystic fibrosis and the immotile cilia syndrome, respectively. Micronutrient deficiencies of vitamins, minerals, and trace metals should be assessed in cases with malnutrition or chronic diarrhea.

Immunologic Assessment

Screening tests employed for suspected ID are summarized in Table 7. Detection of an ID requires careful assessment of the patient's ability to develop and express B-cell, T-cell, and combined B- and T-cell functions. Both the amplification of the immune response (cytokine production, complement factors) and effector mechanisms (phagocytosis and inflammatory response) require investigation. Evaluation starts with enumeration of immune cell populations. This should include T- and B-cell, granulocyte, and monocyte counts. Quantitative measurement of Ig concentrations is necessary. Serum total Ig levels lower than 2 g/L are abnormal. The humoral immune response can be examined by screening for natural antibodies to ubiquitous antigens (A and B isohemagglutinins, heteroantibodies to sheep erythrocytes, bactericidins against *E. coli*). Specific antibody response to well-tolerated active immunizations (diphtheria and tetanus toxoids, killed poliovirus antigens, and *Haemophilus* conjugates) can be analyzed. Live vaccines are prohibited. The B-cell markers (CD19, -20, and -22) can be examined by immunofluorescence and flow cytometry. T-cell function can be assessed by skin testing for delayed hypersensitivity to antigens, which generally reveals positive results in healthy individuals, such as *Candida*, *Trichophyton*, streptokinase or streptodornase, and mumps. Response to active skin sensitization may be assessed with dinitrochlorobenzene. T-cell function can also be examined by in vitro reactivity of peripheral blood mononuclear cells to phytohemagglutinin, other mitogens, and common antigens. Anti-CD3 is a good indicator of general T-lymphocyte reactivity, as is the one-way mixed lymphocyte reaction (see Table 7). Enumeration of T cells and their subsets is achieved by surface markers by flow cytometry. In vitro assays for complement components (classic and alternate pathways) can be evaluated immunochemically and functionally in those patients with relevant symptoms. Specific testing of bactericidal and other functions of polymorphs is available (see Table 7). Patients suspected of having CGD should have phagocytic function evaluated by the semiquantitative reduction of NBT dye and the stimulation of superoxide production. Additional phagocyte testing includes chemiluminescence following stimulation with PMA or dichlorofluorine, as well as by quantifying the capacity of cells to ingest and kill catalase positive microorganisms. In vitro analysis of inflammatory response capacity can be examined by measuring chemotaxis, chemokinesis, and cytokine production. Adhesion molecule expression can also be determined. Specific details are reviewed in detail elsewhere. Specific investigations that may provide clues to certain primary IDs include thrombocytopenia with small platelets in the Wiskott-Aldrich syndrome, α-fetoprotein in ataxia-telangiectasia, and a deletion on chromosome 22 in DiGeorge syndrome.

Table 7 Initial Laboratory Screening for Immunodeficiency

CBC, WBC and differential, platelets (count and size)
Serum protein electrophoresis
Chest radiography for thymic evaluation
Quantitative serum Igs
  IgG, IgM, IgA, IgE, and IgG subclasses
Flow cytometry
  Quantitation of total T cells (CD2, CD3)
  T-cell subsets (CD4, CD8)
  B cells (CDI9, CD20)
  NK cells (CD16, CD56, CD57)
  HLA-DR (to rule out bare lymphocyte syndrome)
Metabolic bursts (to rule out CGD), including NBT testing
In vitro proliferative response to mitogens (PHA, Concanavalin A) and antigens (MLR)
Isohemagglutinin titers
Antibody titers (to documented immunizations) (diphtheria, tetanus, rubella, measles)
C3, C4, CH50
If indicated
  Sweat Cl– (to rule out cystic fibrosis)
  αl-Antitrypsin
  Celiac disease screening

CBC = complete blood count; CGD = chronic granulomatous disease; HLA = human leukocyte antigen; Ig = immunoglobulin; MLR = mixed leukocyte reaction; NBT = nitroblue tetrazolium; NK = natural killer; PHA = phytohemagglutinin; WBC = white blood count.

REFERENCES

1. Notarangelo L, Casanova JL, Conley ME, et al. International Union of Immunological Societies Primary Immunodeficiency Diseases Classification Committee. Primary Immunodeficiency Diseases: An update from the International Union of Immunological Societies Primary Immunodeficiency Diseases Classification Committee Meeting in Budapest, 2005. J Allergy Clin Immunol 2006;117:883–96.
2. Kumar A, Teuber SS, Gershwin ME. Current perspectives on primary immunodeficiency diseases. Clin Dev Immunol 2006;13:223–59.
3. Hershfield M. Chaffee S, Sorensen RU. Enzyme replacement therapy with polyethylene glycol-adenosine deaminase on adenosine deaminase deficiency: Overview and case reports of three patients, including two now receiving gene therapy. Pediatr Res 1992;S42–8.
4. Cavazzana-Calvo M, Hacein-Bey S, De Saint Basile G, et al. Gene therapy of human severe combined immunodeficiency (SCID)-x1 disease. Science 2000;288:669–72.
5. Notarangelo LD, Forino C, Mazzolari E. Stem-cell transplantation in primary immunodeficiencies. Curr Opin Allergy Clin Immunol 2006;6:443–8.
6. Newberry RD, Lorenz RG. Organizing a mucosal defence. Immunol Rev 2005;206:6–21.
7. Chinien J, Finkelman F, Shearer WT. Advances in basic and clinical immunology. J Allergy Clin Immunol 2006;118:489–95.
8. Knight AK, Cunningham-Rundles C. Inflammatory and autoimmune complications of common variable immune deficiency. Autoimmun Rev 2006;5:156–9.
9. Said JW. Immunodeficiency-related Hodgkin lymphoma and its mimics. Adv Anat Pathol 2007;14:189–94.
10. Romagnani S. Regulation of the T cell response. Clin Exper Allergy 2006;36:1357–66.
11. Kutlu A, Bozkurt B, Ciftci F, Bozkanat E. Th1-Th2 interaction: Is more complex than a see-saw? Scand J Immunol 2007;65:393–5.
12. Afzali B, Lombardi G, Lechler RI, Lord GM. The role of T helper 17 (Th17) and regulatory T cells (Treg) in human organ transplantation and autoimmune disease. Clin Exp Immunol 2007;148:32–46.
13. Silva MA, López CB, Riverin F, et al. Characterization and distribution of colonic dendritic cells in Crohn's disease. Inflamm Bowel Dis. 2004;10:504–12.

14. Orange JS, Ballas ZK. Natural killer cells in human health and disease. Clin Immunol 2006;118:1–10.
15. Wu J, Lanier LL. Natural killer cells and cancer. Adv Cancer Res 2003;90:127–56.
16. French AR, Yokoyama WM. Natural killer cells and autoimmunity. Arthritis Res Ther 2004;6:8–14.
17. Bonilla FA, Geha RS. Primary immunodeficiency diseases. J Allergy Clin Immunol 2006;111:S435–41.
18. Farkas H, Varga L, Széplaki G, et al. Management of hereditary angioedema in pediatric patients. Pediatrics. 2007;120:713–22.
19. Cunningham-Rundles C, Carr RI, Good RA. Dietary protein antigenemia in humoral ID. Correlation with splenomegaly. Am J Med 1984;76:181–5.
20. Melamed I, Bujanover Y, Zakuth V, et al. *Campylobacter* enteritis in normal and immunodeficient children. Am J Dis Child 1983;137:752–3.
21. Kanegane H, Futatani T, Wang Y, et al. Clinical and mutational characteristics of X-linked agammaglobulinemia and its carrier identified by flow cytometric assessment combined with genetic analysis. J Allergy Clin Immunol 2001;108:1012–20.
22. Conley ME, Sweinberg SK. Females with a disorder phenotypically identical to X-linked gammaglobulinemia. J Clin Immunol 1992;12:139–43.
23. Cham B, Kozlowski C, Evans DIK. Neutropenia associated with primary immunodeficiency syndromes. Semin Hematol 2002;39:107–12.
24. Washington K, Stenzel TT, Buckley RH, Gottfried MR. Gastrointestinal pathology in patients with X-linked agammaglobulinemia. Am Surg Pathol 1996;20:1240–52.
25. Conley ME, Howard V. Clinical findings leading to the diagnosis of X-linked agammaglobulinemia. J Pediatr 2002;141:566–71.
26. Plebani A, Soresina A, Rondelli R, et al. Clinical, immunological, and molecular analysis in a large cohort of patients with X-linked agammaglobulinemia: An Italian multicenter study. Clin Immunol 2002;104:221–30.
27. Sitz KV, Burks AW, Williams LW, et al. Confirmation of X-linked hypogammaglobulinemia with isolated growth hormone deficiency as a disease entity. J Pediatr 1990;116:292–4.
28. Aghamohammadi A, Moin M, Farhoudi A, et al. Efficacy of intravenous immunoglobulin on the prevention of pneumonia in patients with agammaglobulinemia. FEMS Immunol Med Microbiol 2004;40:113–8.
29. Cunningham-Rundles C. Physiology of IgA and IgA deficiency. J Clin Immunol 2001;21:303–9.
30. Finocchi A, Angelini F, Chini L, et al. Evaluation of the relevance of humoral immunodeficiencies in a pediatric population affected by recurrent infections. Pediatr Allergy Immunol 2002;13:443–7.
31. Ojuawo A, St Louis D, Lindley KJ, Milla PF. Non-infective colitis in infancy: Evidence in favour of minor immunodeficiencies in its pathogenesis. Arch Dis Child 1997;76:345–8.
32. Burks AW, Sampson HA, Buckley RM. Anaphylactic reactions following gammaglobulin administration in patients with hypogammaglobulinemia: Detection of IgE antibodies to IgA. N Engl J Med 1986;314:560–4.
33. Conley ME, Cooper MD. Immature IgA B cells in IgA-deficiency patients. N Engl J Med 1981;304:475–9.
34. Ferreira A, Garcia Rodriguez MC, Lopez-Trascasa M, et al. Anti-IgA antibodies in selective IgA deficiency and primary immunodeficient patients treated with gammaglobulin. Clin Immunol Immunopathol 1988;47:199–207
35. Kowalczyk D, Baran J, Webster AD, et al. Intracellular cytokine production by Th1/Th2 lymphocytes and monocytes of children with symptomatic transient hypogammaglobulinaemia of infancy (THI) and selective IgA deficiency (SIgAD). Clin Exp Immunol 2002;127:507–12.
36. Fraser KJ, Rankin JG. Selective deficiency of IgA immunoglobulins associated with carcinoma of the stomach. Aust Ann Med 1970;19:165–7.
37. Meini A, Pillan NM, Villanacci V, et al. Prevalence and diagnosis of celiac disease in IgA-deficient children. Ann Allergy Asthma Immunol 1996;77:333–6.
38. Hill ID, et al. Guideline for the diagnosis and treatment of celiac disease in children: recommendations of the North American Society for Pediatric Gastroenterology, Hepatology and Nutrition. J Pediatr Gastroenterol Nutr 2005; 40:1–19
39. Patiroglu T, Kursad A, Kurtoglu S, Poyrazoglu H. Growth retardation in children with IgA deficiency. Pediatr Endocrinol Metab 2002;15:1035–8.
40. Korponay-Szabo IR, Dahlbom I, Laurila K, et al. Elevation of IgG antibodies against tissue transglutaminase as a diagnostic tool for coeliac disease in selective IgA deficiency. Gut 2003;52:1567–71.
41. Cataldo F, Lio D, Marino V, et al. Cytokine genotyping (TNF and IL-10) in patients with celiac disease and selective IgA deficiency. Am J Gastroenterol 2003;98:850–6.
42. Klemola T, Savilahti E, Arato A, et al. Immunohistochemical findings in jejunal specimens from patients with IgA deficiency. Gut 1995;37:519–23.
43. Fuleihan RL. The hyper IgM syndrome. Curr Allergy Asthma Rep 2001;1:445–50.
44. Gilmour KC, Walshe D, Heath S, et al. Immunological and genetic analysis of 65 patients with a clinical suspicion of X linked hyper-IgM. Mol Pathol 2003;56:256–62.
45. Bhushan A, Covey LR. CD40:CD40L interactions in X-linked hyper-IgM and non-X-linked hyper-IgM syndromes. Immunol Res 2001;24:311–24.
46. Ferrari S, Giliani S, Insalaco A, et al. Mutations of *CD40* gene cause an autosomal recessive form of immunodeficiency with hyper IgM. Proc Natl Acad Sci U S A 2001;98: 12614–9.
47. Revy P, Muto T, Levy Y, et al. Activation-induced cytidine deamidase (AID) deficiency causes the autosomal recessive form of the Hyper-IgM syndrome (HIGM-2). Cell 2000;102:565–74
48. Notarangelo LN, Duse M, Ugazio AG. Immunodeficiency with hyper IgM (HIM). Immunodefic Rev 1992;3:101–21.
49. Subauste CS. Primary Immunodeficiencies and susceptibility to parasitic Infections. Parasite Immunol 2006;28:567–75.
50. Levy J, Espanol-Boren T, Thomas C, et al. Clinical spectrum of X-linked hyper-IgM syndrome. J Pediatr 1997;131: 47–54.
51. Dimicoli S, Bensoussan D, Latger-Cannard V, et al. Complete recovery from *Cryptosporidium parvum* infection with gastroenteritis and sclerosing cholangitis after successful bone marrow transplantation in two brothers with X-linked hyper-IgM syndrome. Bone Marrow Transplant 2003;32:733–7.
52. Ballow M. Primary immunodeficiency disorders: Antibody deficiency. J Allergy Clin Immunol 2002;109:581–91.
53. Cunningham-Rundles C, Fotino M, Rosina O, Peter JB. Selective IgA deficiency, IgG subclass deficiency and the major histocompatibilty complex. Clin Immunol Immunopathol 1991;61:561–9.
54. Shackelford PG, Granoff DM, Polmar SH, et al. Subnormal serum concentrations of IgG2 in children with frequent infections associated with varied patterns of immunologic dysfunction. J Pediatr 1990;116:529–38.
55. Forchielli ML, Young MC, Flores AF, et al. Immune deficiencies in chronic intestinal pseudoobstruction. Acta Paediatr 1997;86:1077–81.
56. Abonia JP, Castells MC. Common variable immunodeficiency. Allergy Asthma Proc 2002;23:53–7.
57. Goldacker S, Warnatz K. Tackling the heterogeneity of CVID. Curr Opin Allergy Clin Immunol 2005;5:504–9.
58. Cunningham-Rundles C, Bodian C. Common variable immunodeficiency: Clinical and immunological features of 248 patients. J Appl Biomater 1999;92:34–48.
59. Cunningham-Rundles C. Common variable immunodeficiency. Curr Allergy Asthma Rep 2001;1:421–9.
60. Salzer U, Maul-Pavicic A, Cunningham-Rundles C, et al. ICOS deficincy in patients with common variable immunodeficiency. Clin Immunol 2004;113:234–40.
61. Ashman RF, Schaffer FM, Kemp JD, et al. Genetic and immunologic analysis of a family containing five patients with common variable immune deficiency or selective IgA deficiency. J Clin Immunol 1992;12:406–14.
62. Volanakis JE, Zhu ZB, Schaffer FM, et al. Major histocompatibility complex class III genes and susceptibility to immunoglobulin A deficiency and common variable immunodeficiency. J Clin Invest 1992;89:1914–22.
63. Durandy A. Terminal defect of B lymphocyte differentiation. Curr Opin Allergy Clin Immunol 2001;1:519–24
64. Sneller MC, Strober W. Abnormalities of lymphokine gene expression in patients with common variable immunodeficiency. J Immunol 1990;144:3762.
65. Luzzi G, Zullo A, Iebba F, et al. Duodenal pathology and clinical immunological implications in common variable immunodeficiency patients. Am J Gastroenterol 2003;98:118–21.
66. Kalha I, Sellin JH. Common variable immunodeficiency and the gastrointestinal tract. Curr Gastroenterol Rep 2004;6:377–83.
67. Byrne MF, Royston D, Patchett SE. Association of common variable immunodeficiency with atypical collagenous colitis. Eur J Gastroenterol Hepatol 2003;15:1051–3.
68. Twomey JJ, Jordan PH, Jr, Laughter AH, et al. The gastric disorder in immunoglobulin-deficient patients. Ann Intern Med 1970;72:499–504.
69. Conley ME, Park CL, Douglas SD. Childhood common variable ID with autoimmune disease. J Pediatr 1986;108: 915–22.
70. Wilson RA, Fischer SH, Ochs HD. Long-term interferon alpha maintenance therapy for chronic hepatitis C infection in a patient with chronic variable immune deficiency. J Clin Gastroenterol 1999;29:203–6.
71. White WB, Ballow M. Modulation of suppressor-cell activity by cimetidine in patients with common variable hypogammaglobulinemia. N Engl J Med 1985;312:198–202.
72. Adelman DC, Yen TY, Cumberland WG, et al. 13-cis Retinoic acid enhanced in vivo B lymphocyte differentiation in patients with common variable ID. J Allergy Clin Immunol 1991;88:705–12.
73. Ambrus JL, Jr, Haneiwich S, Chesky L, et al. Improved in vitro antigen-specific antibody synthesis in two patients with common variable ID taking an oral cyclooxygenase and lipoxygenase inhibitor (ketoprofen). J Allergy Clin Immunol 1991;88:775–83.
74. Sewell WA, Buckland M, Jolles SR. Therapeutic strategies in common variable immunodeficiency. Drugs 2003;63: 1359–71.
75. Grimbacher B, Schaffer AA, Holland SM, et al. Hyper-IgE syndromes. Immunol Rev 2005;203:244–50.
76. Roberts J, Searle J. Neonatal diabetes mellitus associated with severe diarrhea, hyperimmunoglobulin E syndrome, and absence of islets of Langerhans. Pediatr Pathol Lab Med 1995;15:477–83.
77. Minegishi Y, Saito M, Tsuchiya S, et al. Dominant-negative mutations in the DNA-binding domain of STAT3 cause hyper-IgE syndrome. Nature 2007;448:1058–62.
78. Chang X, Zheng P, Liu Y. FoxP3: A genetic link between immunodeficiency and autoimmune diseases. Autoimmunity Rev 2006;5:399–402.
79. Wildin RS, Ramsdell F, Peake J, et al. X-linked neonatal diabetes mellitus, enteropathy and endocrinopathy syndrome is the human equivalent of mouse scurfy. Nat Genet 2001;27:18–20.
80. Bennett CL, Ochs HD. IPEX is a unique X-linked syndrome characterized by immune dysfunction, polyendocrinopathy, enteropathy, and a variety of autoimmune phenomena. Curr Opin Pediatr 2001;13:533–8.
81. Wildin RS, Smyk-Pearson S, Filipovich AH. Clinical and molecular features of the immunodysregulation, polyendocrinopathy, enteropathy, and X-linked (IPEX) syndrome. J Med Genet 2002;39:537–45.
82. Kobayashi I, Shiari R, Yamada M, et al. Novel mutations of FOXP3 in two Japanese patients with immune dysregulation, polyendocrinopathy, enteropathy, and X-linked syndrome (IPEX). J Med Genet 2001;38:874–6.
83. Gambineri E, Torgerson TR, Ochs HD. Immune dysregulation, polyendocrinopathy, enteropathy, and X-linked inheritance (IPEX), a syndrome of systemic autoimmunity caused by mutations of FOXP3, a critical regulator of T-cell homeostasis. Curr Opin Rheumatol 2003;15: 430–5.
84. Torgerson TR, Linane A, Moes N, et al. Severe food allergy as a variant of IPEX syndrome caused by a deletion in a noncoding region of the *FOXP3* gene. Gastroenterology 2007;132:1705–17.
85. Seidman EG, Lacaille F, Russo P, et al. Successful treatment of autoimmune enteropathy with cyclosporine. J Pediatr 1990;117:929–32.
86. Bindl L, Torgerson T, Perroni L, et al. Successful use of the new immune-suppressor sirolimus in IPEX (immune dysregulation, polyendocrinopathy, enteropathy, X-linked syndrome). J Pediatr 2005;147:256–9.
87. Baud O, Goulet O, Canioni D, et al. Treatment of the immune dysregulation, polyendocrinopathy, enteropathy, and X-linked syndrome (IPEX) by allogeneic bone marrow transplantation. N Engl J Med 2001;344:1758–62.
88. Rao A, Kamani N, Filipovich A, et al. Successful bone marrow transplantation for IPEX syndrome after reduced-intensity conditioning. Blood 2007;109:383–5.
89. Noguchi M, Yi H, Rosenblatt HM, et al. Interleukin-2 receptor gamma chain mutation results in X-linked severe combined ID in humans. Cell 1993;73:147–57.
90. Orange C. Human natural killer cell deficiencies. Curr Opin Allergy Clin Immunol 2006;6:399–409.
91. Katano H, Cohen JI. Perforin and lymphohistiocytic proliferative disorders. Br J Haematol 2005;128:739–50.
92. Walker M, Payne J, Wagner B, Vora A. Hermansky-Pudlak syndrome. Br J Haematol 2007;138:671.
93. Enders A, Zieger B, Schwarz K, et al. Lethal hemophagocytic lymphohistiocytosis in Hermansky-Pudlak syndrome type II. Blood 2006;108:81–7.
94. Mahadeo R, Markowitz J, Fisher S, Daum F. Hermansky-Pudlak syndrome with granulomatous colitis in children. J Pediatr 1991;118:904–6.
95. Hazzan D, Seward S, Stock H, et al. Crohn's-like colitis, enterocolitis and perianal disease in Hermansky-Pudlak syndrome. Colorectal Dis 2006;8:539–43.

96. Anderson PD, Huizing M, Claassen DA, et al. Hermansky-Pudlak syndrome type 4 (HPS-4): Clinical and molecular characteristics. Hum Genet 2003;113:10–7.
97. Erzin Y, Cosgun S, Dobrucali A, et al. Complicated granulomatous colitis in a patient with Hermansky-Pudlak syndrome, successfully treated with infliximab. Acta Gastroenterol Belg 2006;69:213–6.
98. Schmid JM, Junge SA, Hossle JP, et al. Transient hemophagocytosis with deficient cellular cytotoxicity, monoclonal immunoglobulin M gammaopathy, increased T-cell numbers, and hypomorphic NEMO mutations. Pediatrics 2006;117:1049–56.
99. Giliani S, Mella P, Savoldi G, Mazzolari E. Cytokine-mediated signaling and early defects in lymphoid development. Curr Opin Allergy Clin Immunol 2005;5:519–24.
100. Asao H, Okuyama C, Kumaki S, et al. Cutting edge: The common gamma-chain is an indispensable subunit of the IL-21 receptor complex. J Immunol 2001;167:1–5.
101. Morgan G, Levinsky RJ, Hugh-Jones K, et al. Heterogeneity of biochemical, clinical and immunological parameters in severe combined ID due to adenosine deaminase deficiency. Clin Exp Immunol 1987;70:491–9.
102. Hirschorn R. Inherited enzyme deficiencies and ID: Adenosine deaminase (ADA) and purine nucleoside phosphorylase (PNP) deficiencies. Clin Immunol Immunopathol 1986;40:157–65.
103. Rane SG, Reddy EP. Janus kinases: Components of multiple signaling pathways. Oncogene 2000;19:5662–79.
104. Notarangelo L, Casanova JL, Fischer A, et al. Primary immunodeficiency diseases: An update. J Allergy Clin Immunol 2004;114:677–87.
105. Li L, Moshous D, Zhou Y, et al. A founder mutation in Artemis, an SNM1-like protein, causes SCID in Athabascan-speaking Native Americans. J Immunol 2002;168: 6323–9.
106. Honig H, Schwarz K. Omenn syndrome: A lack of tolerance on the background of deficient lymphocyte development and maturation. Curr Opin Rheumatol 2006;18:383–8.
107. Aleman K, Noordzij JG, de Groot R, et al. Reviewing Omenn syndrome. Eur J Pediatr 2001;160:718–25.
108. Cavazzana-Calvo, Fischer A. Gene therapy for severe combined immunodeficiency: Are we there yet? J Clin Invest 2007;117:1456–65.
109. Aiuti A. Gene therapy for adenosine–deaminase-deficient severe combined immunodeficiency. Best Pract Res Clin Haematol 2004;17:505–16.
110. Gaspar HB, Parsley KL, Howe S, et al. Gene therapy of X-linked severe combined immunodeficiency by use of a pseudotyped gammaretroviral vector. Lancet 2004;364:2181–7.
111. Stephan JL, Vlekova V, Le Deist F, et al. Severe combined ID: A retrospective single-center study of clinical presentation and outcome in 117 patients. J Pediatr 1993;123:564–72.
112. Gadola SD, Moins-Teisserenc HT, Trowsdale J, et al. TAP deficiency syndrome. Clin Exp Immunol 2000;121:173–8.
113. Yabe T, Kawamura S, Sato M, et al. A subject with a novel type I bare lymphocyte syndrome has tapasin deficiency due to deletion of 4 exons by Alumediated recombination. Blood 2002;100:1496–8.
114. Villard J, Mach B, Reith W. MHC class II deficiency: Definition of a new complementation group. Immunobiology 1997;198:264–72.
115. Canioni D, Patey N, Cuenod B, et al. Major histocompatibility complex class II deficiency needs an early diagnosis: Report of a case. Pediatr Pathol Lab Med 1997;17: 645–51.
116. Gomez Morales MA, Ausiello CM, Guarino A, et al. Severe, protracted intestinal cryptosporidiosis associated with interferon gamma deficiency: Pediatric case report. Clin Infect Dis 1996;22:848–50.
117. Oda A, Ochs HD. Wiskott-Aldrich syndrome protein and platelets. Immunol Rev 2000;178:111–7.
118. Perry GS, III, Spector BD, Schuman LM, et al. The Wiskott-Aldrich syndrome in the United States and Canada, 1892–1979. J Pediatr 1980;97:72–8.
119. Perlman S, Becker-Catania S, Gatti RA. Ataxia–telangiectasia: Diagnosis and treatment. Semin Pediatr Neurol 2003;10:173–82.
120. Swift M, Morrell D, Massey RB, Chase CL. Incidence of cancer in 161 families affected by ataxia telangicctasia. N Engl J Med 1991;325:1831–6.
121. Sullivan KE. The clinical, immunological, and molecular spectrum of chromosome 22q11.2 deletion syndrome and DiGeorge syndrome. Curr Opin Allergy Clin Immunol 2004;4:505–12.
122. DiGeorge AM. Congenital absence of the thymus and its immunologic consequences. Concurrence with congenital hypoparathyroidism. Birth Defects 1968;4:116–21.
123. Kim MS, Basson CT. Wrapping up DiGeorge syndrome in a T-box? Pediatr Res 2001;50:307–8.
124. Markert ML, Boeck A, Hale LP, et al. Transplantation of thymus tissue in complete DiGeorge syndrome. N Engl J Med 1999;341:1180–9.
125. Epstein MA. Reflections on Epstein-Barr virus: Some recently resolved old uncertainties. J Infect 2001;43:111–5.
126. Purtillo DT, Sakamoto K, Barnabei V, et al. Epstein-Barr virus induced disease in boys with the X-linked lymphoproliferative syndrome (XLP). Am J Med 1982;73:49–56.
127. Sullivan JL, Woda BA. X-linked lymphoproliferative syndrome. Immunodefic Rev 1989;1:325–47.
128. Engel P, Eck MJ, Terhorst C. The SAP and SLAM families in immune responses and X-linked lymphoproliferative disease. Nat Rev Immunol 2003;3:813–21.
129. Gilmour KC, Gaspar HB. Pathogenesis and diagnosis of X-linked lymphoproliferative disease. Exp Rev Mol Diagn 2003;3:549–61.
130. Latour S, Veillette A. Molecular and immunological basis of X-linked lymphoproliferative disease. Immunol Rev 2003;192:212–24.
131. Gaspar HB, Sharifi R, Gilmour KC, Thrasher AJ. X-linked lymphoproliferative disease: Clinical, diagnostic and molecular perspective. Br J Haematol 2002;119:585–95.
132. Sayos J, Wu C, Morra M, et al. The X-linked lymphoproliferative disease gene product SAP regulates signals induced through the co-receptor SLAM. Nature 1998;395:462–9.
133. Grierson HL, Skare J, Hawk J, et al. Immunoglobulin class and subclass deficiencies prior to Epstein-Barr virus infection in males with X-linked lymphoproliferative disease. Am J Med Genet 1991;40:294–7.
134. Purtillo DT. Abnormal lymphocyte subsets in X-linked lymphoproliferative syndrome. J Immunol 1981;127:2618–20.
135. Purtillo DT. Epstein-Barr virus-induced disease in the X-linked lymphoproliferative syndrome and related disorders. Biomed Pharmacother 1985;39:52–8.
136. Morra M, Howie D, Grande MS, et al. X-linked lymphoproliferative disease: A progressive immunodeficiency. Annu Rev Immunol 2001;19:657–82.
137. Arnaout MA. Structure and function of the leukocyte adhesion molecules CD11/CD18. Blood 1990;75:1037–50.
138. Curnutte JT. Classification of chronic granulomatous disease. Hematol Oncol Clin North Am 1988;2:241–52.
139. Dinauer MC, Orkin SH. Chronic granulomatous disease. Annu Rev Med 1992;43:117–24.
140. Barton LL, Moussa SL, Villar RG, et al. Gastrointestinal complications of chronic granulomatous disease: Case report and literature review. Clin Pediatr 1998;37:231–6.
141. Heyworth PG, Cross AR, Curnette JT. Chronic granulomatous disease. Curr Opin Immunol 2003;15:578–84.
142. Segal AW. Absence of both cytochrome b-245 subunits from neutrophils in X-linked chronic granulomatous disease. Nature 1987;326:88.
143. Schappi MG, Klein NJ, Lindley KJ, et al. The nature of colitis in chronic granulomatous disease. J Pediatr Gastroenterol Nutr 2003;36:623–31.
144. Dickerman JD, Colletti RB, Tampas JP. Gastric outlet obstruction in chronic granulomatous disease of childhood. Am J Dis Child 1986;140:567.
145. Fischer A, Segal AW, Seger R, Weening RS. The management of chronic granulomatous disease. Eur J Pediatr 1993;152:896–9.
146. Ezekowitz RAB, Orkin SH, Newburger PE. Recombinant interferon gamma augments phagocyte superoxide production and x-chronic granulomatous disease gene expression in X-linked variant chronic granulomatous disease. J Clint Invest 1987;80:1009.
147. Bemiller LS, Roberts DH, Starko KM, et al. Safety and effectiveness of long-term interferon gamma therapy in patients with chronic granulomatous disease. Blood Cells Mol Dis 1995;21:239–47.
148. Ott MG, Seger R, Stein S, et al. Advances in the treatment of chronic granulomatous disease by gene therapy. Curr Gene Ther. 2007;7:155–61.
149. Tood RF, III, Freyer DR. The CD11/CD18 leukocyte glycoprotein deficiency. Hematol Oncol Clin North Am 1988;2:13–31.
150. Anderson DC, Schnakstiec FC, Finegold MJ. The severe and moderate phenotype of heritable Mac-1, LFA-1 deficiency: Their quantitative definition and relation to leukocyte dysfunction and clinical features. J Infect Dis 1985;152:668.
151. D'Agata ID, Paradis K, Chad Z, et al. Leukocyte adhesion molecule deficiency presenting as an ileocolitis resembling Crohn's disease. Gut 1996;39:605–8.
152. Krauss JC, Ping AJ, Mayo-Bond L, et al. Complementation of genetic and functional defects in CD-18 deficient lymphocytes by retrovirus-mediated gene transfer. Am J Hum Genet 1992;50:263–70.
153. Couper R, Kapelushnik J, Griffiths AM. Neutrophil dysfunction in glycogen storage disease Ib: Association with Crohn's-like colitis. Gastroenterology 1991;100:549–54.
154. Yamaguchi T, Ihara K, Matsumoto T, et al. Inflammatory bowel disease-like colitis in glycogen storage disease type 1b. Inflamm Bowel Dis 2001;7:128–32.
155. Kirkpatrick CH. Chronic mucocutaneous candidiasis. Pediatr Inf Dis J 2001;20:197–206.
156. Villasenor J, Benoist C, Mathis D. AIRE and APECED: Molecular insights into an autoimmune disease. Immunol Rev 2005;204:156–64.
157. Ahonen P. Autoimmune polyendocrinopathy-candidiasisectodermal dystrophy (APECED): Autosomal recessive inheritance. Clin Genet 1985;27:535–42.
158. Ward L, Paquette J, Seidman E, et al. Severe autoimmune polyendocrinopathy-candidiasis-ectodermal dystrophy in an adolescent girl with a novel AIRE mutation: Response to immunosuppressive therapy. J Clin Endocrinol Metab 1999;84:844–52.
159. Ahonen P, Myllarniemi S, Sipila I, Perheentupa J. Clinical variation of autoimmune polyendocrinopathy-candidiasisectodermal dysplasia (APECED) in a series of 68 patients. N Engl J Med 1990;322:1829–36.
160. Scirè G, Magliocca FM, Cianfarani S, et al. Autoimmune polyendocrine candidiasis syndrome with associated chronic diarrhea caused by intestinal infection and pancreas insufficiency. J Pediatr Gastroenterol Nutr 1991;13: 224–7.
161. Duell T, Van Lint MT, Ljungman P, et al. Health and functional status of long-term survivors of bone marrow transplantation. Ann Intern Med 1997;126:184–92.
162. Holler E. Risk assessment in haematopoietic stem cell transplantation: GvHD prevention and treatment. Best Pract Res Clin Haematol 2007;20:281–94.
163. Klein SA, Martin H, Schreiber-Dietrich D, et al. A new approach to evaluating intestinal acute graft-versus-host disease by transabdominal sonography and colour Doppler imaging. Br J Haematol 2001;115:929–34.
164. Cruz-Crrea M, Poonwala A, Abraham SC, et al. Endoscopic findings predict the histologic diagnosis in gastrointestinal graft-versus-host disease. Endoscopy 2002;34:808–13.
165. Alpeek G, Zahurak ML, Piantadosi S, et al. Development of a prognostic model for grading graft-versus-host disease. Blood 2001;97:1219–26.
166. Patey-Mariaud de Serre N, Reijasse D, Verkarre V, et al. Chronic graft-versus-host disease: Clinical, histological and immunohistochemical analysis in 17 children. Bone Marrow Transplant 2002;29:223–30.
167. Fraser CJ, Scott Baker K. The management and outcome of chronic graft-versus-host disease. Br J Haematol. 2007;138:131–45.
168. Ward DM, Shiflett SL, Kaplan J. Chediak-Higashi syndrome: A clinical and molecular view of a rare lysosomal storage disorder. Curr Mol Med 2002;2:469–77.
169. Maverakis E, Fung MA, Lynch PJ, et al. Acrodermatitis enteropathica and an overview of zinc metabolism. J Am Acad Dermatol 2007;56:116–24.
170. Giraut D, Goulet O, Le Deist F, et al. Intractable diarrhea syndrome associated with phenotypic abnormalities and immune deficiency. J Pediatr 1994;125:36–42.
171. Vries E, Visser DM, van Dongen JJ, et al. Oligoclonal gammopathy in "phenotypic diarrhea." J Pediatr Gastroenterol Nutr 2000;30:349–50.
172. Verloes A, Lombet J, Lambert Y, et al. Tricho-hepato-enteric syndrome: Further delineation of a distinct syndrome with neonatal hemochromatosis phenotype, intractable diarrhea, and hair anomalies. Am J Med Genet 1997;68:391–5.
173. Landers MC, Schroeder TL. Intractable diarrhea of infancy with facial dysmorphism, trichorrhexis nodosa, and cirrhosis. Pediatr Dermatol 2003;20:432–5.
174. Fabre A, Andre N, Breton A, et al. Intractable diarrhea with "phenotypic anomalies" and tricho-hepato-enteric syndrome: Two names for the same disorder. Am J Med Genet A 2007;143:584–8.
175. Itin PH, Pittelkow MR. Trichothiodystrophy: Review of sulfurdeficient brittle hair syndromes and association with the ectodermal dysplasia. J Am Acad Dermatol 1990;22: 705–17.
176. Stefanini M, Vermeulen W, Weeda G, et al. A new nucleotide excision-repair gene associated with the disorder trichothiodystrophy. Am J Hum Genet 1993;53:817–21.
177. Moreno LA, Gottrand F, Turck D, et al. Severe combined immunodeficiency syndrome associated with autosomal recessive familial multiple gastrointestinal atresias: Study of a family. Am J Med Genet 1990;37:143–6.

178. Walker MW, Lovell MA, Kelly TE, et al. Multiple areas of intestinal atresia associated with immunodeficiency and posttransfusion graft-versus-host disease. J Pediatr 1993;123:93–5.

179. Moore SW, de Jongh G, Bouic P, et al. Immune deficiency in familial duodenal atresia. J Pediatr Surg 1996;31: 1733–5.

180. Gilroy RK, Coccia PF, Talmadge JE, et al. Donor immune reconstitution after liver-small bowel transplantation for multiple intestinal atresia with immunodeficiency. Blood 2004;103:171–4.

181. Pillay K. Congenital hypothyroidism and ID: Evidence for an endocrine-immune interaction. J Pediatr Endocrinol Metab 1998;11:757–61.

182. Fagman H, Liao J, Westerlund J, et al. The 22q11 deleion syndrome candidate gene Tbx1 determines thyroid size and positioning. Hum Mol Genet 2007;16: 276–85.

183. Dizon JG, Goldberg BJ, Kaplan MS. How to evaluate suspected ID. Pediatr Ann 1998;27:743–50.

20.3. HIV and Other Secondary Immunodeficiencies

Delane Shingadia, FRCPCH, MPH

Paul Kelly, MD, FRCP

Gastrointestinal symptoms are common manifestations of human immunodeficiency virus (HIV) infection in children because the digestive system represents an important point of contact with infectious organisms and an important reservoir of lymphocytes. Symptoms include diarrhea, failure to thrive, poor appetite, malabsorption, vomiting, and dysphagia. Alterations to gut morphology and function may be caused by a variety of infectious and noninfectious processes, which become increasingly severe as immunosuppression deepens. Children with HIV become susceptible to infection with opportunistic organisms and with virulent pathogens, which also infect immunocompetent children (eg, cryptosporidiosis). These virulent infections often have a worse outcome in HIV-infected children. Treatment of gastrointestinal disease in children with HIV infection may often be complex and difficult and require a multidisciplinary approach because nutritional consequences can be severe. However, recent advances in antiviral therapies have resulted in marked improvements in survival and morbidity, mainly due to preservation and improvement of immunological function. As a result, in industrialized countries there has been a decrease in the number and severity of opportunistic infections caused by enteropathogens. This chapter discusses disease of the gastrointestinal tract in children with HIV infection.

HISTORY OF HIV INFECTION

The first indication that a new disease was emerging appeared in the *Morbidity and Mortality Weekly Report* in 1981 with a report of an increase of unusual opportunistic infection in young men in San Francisco, California.[1] This report indicated that *Pneumocystis carinii* pneumonia, which until then had only been found in severely immunocompromised people undergoing chemotherapy, had been diagnosed in apparently healthy men. Further investigation revealed that this unexplained breakdown of the immune system was occurring in homosexual men who had had contact with each other. The affected individuals were found to have depletion of CD4 cells, the cells which control and direct adaptive immune responses. It was not until 1984 that the virus responsible for this immune problem was identified and called the human T lymphotropic virus type III, later renamed human immunodeficiency virus (HIV). By 1985 it was also apparent that other problems related to immunodeficiency were emerging in Africa. Molecular epidemiological analysis now suggests that HIV developed as a mutant form of simian immunodeficiency virus (SIV) which had crossed from monkeys to man several decades previously. Its successful spread in human populations is attributable to several features, including that it destroys lymphocytes and disturbs their control, thus reducing the host's potential for controlling HIV itself, its potential for sexual spread, and the fact that infected individuals apparently remain well for many years before the immune failure leads to opportunistic infections. This stage of advanced immune failure is called the acquired immune deficiency syndrome (AIDS), but it is important to emphasize that defining this stage in children is often difficult.[2]

EPIDEMIOLOGY OF HIV

Since the first descriptions of the virus in the early 1980s, HIV has been detected in every continent and has caused millions of deaths. In sub-Saharan Africa, HIV has reshaped whole populations, cutting swathes through the middle years of the population and leaving the elderly and the children. Adults in middle life constitute the most economically active sector of society, and their loss leads to breakdown of families and negative effects on development.

The impact on children is twofold.[3] First, children themselves become infected by vertical transmission from their mothers. This accounts for the great majority of HIV infection in children, although some cases arise by transmission through blood transfusion or through use of unsterile hypodermic needles. Second, children suffer through the subsequent death of their parents, and in many less developed countries there are difficulties in caring appropriately for these orphaned children. The HIV epidemic has been most severe in sub-Saharan Africa,[4–5] and it has been estimated that 90% of HIV-infected children live in Africa.[6] As HIV transmission is increasing in Asia and eastern Europe, infection in children is increasing in frequency.[5] Worldwide, 2.3 million children are estimated to be infected with HIV,[5] and many more are affected by it through illness and death of parents.

Transmission from mother to child may occur through transplacental infection, through exposure at the time of birth, or through breast-feeding. Data from several sources suggest that about 80% of all infections, at least in non-breast-feeding situations countries, occur in the last few days of pregnancy and during delivery.[7] In less-developed countries, a high proportion of infections (perhaps 40%[7]) in children are attributable to breast-feeding, implying that the gastrointestinal tract is permeable to HIV in neonates, although the precise mechanism is still to be elucidated. In Africa, the risk of mother-to-child transmission has been estimated at 25 to 45% whereas in industrialized countries the risk is probably 10 to 39%. The majority of this excess risk in Africa is probably attributable to breast-feeding in populations where breast-feeding is the norm,[7] although there is evidence that exclusive breast-feeding is less likely to be associated with transmission.[7–8] Transmission can be reduced by short-course antiretroviral therapy,[7] and currently the most widely used drug is nevirapine.[9]

HIV-1 VIROLOGY AND IMMUNOPATHOGENESIS

HIV type 1 is a retrovirus that is closely related to primate retroviruses, such as SIV, and another human lymphotropic virus, HIV-2. HIV-1 is a ribonucleic acid (RNA) virus which is composed of a cylindrical virion core, containing two copies of single-stranded RNA, together with integrase, protease, and reverse transcriptase enzymes. The core is surrounded by a spherical envelope which is also studded with glycoprotein spikes (gp120, gp41) and coreceptors (chemokine receptors) which are important for viral attachment and entry into cells. The HIV-1 genome contains structural (*gag, pol*) and viral enzyme genes together with other genes (*rev, vpr, vpu, vif,* and *nef*) that are implicated in viral replication and pathogenesis.

HIV-1 entry into cells is mediated through the attachment of virus to CD4 molecules, which are present on the surfaces of certain cells (CD4+ T cells or T-helper cells, some monocytes and macrophages).[10] The process of attachment and entry is aided by chemokine coreceptors such as CCR5 and CXCR4. Once attachment has occurred, fusion of the viral envelope and cell wall occurs with incorporation of virus into the host cell. The viral cycle begins with the generation of a deoxyribonucleic acid (DNA) transcript of viral RNA

Table 1 Age-Specific CD4+ T-Lymphocytes Count and Percentage of Total Lymphocytes

	Age <12 mo		Age 1–5 yr		Age 6–12 yr	
	μL	%	μL	%	μL	%
No suppression	≥1,500	≥25	≥1,000	≥25	≥500	≥25
Moderate suppression	750–1,499	15–24	500–999	15–24	200–499	15–24
Severe suppression	<750	<15	<500	<15	<200	<15

Modified from CDC data.[14]

genome mediated by viral reverse transcriptase. Double-stranded proviral DNA is incorporated into the host genome assisted by viral integrase. Incorporated viral DNA is then "read" as part of the process of protein synthesis within the host cell. Viral products are subsequently assembled and cleaved by viral proteases into individual virions. Viral budding occurs at the cell surface where the cell wall lipid bilayer contributes to the formation of the viral envelope together with viral envelope proteins. Budding and formation of virions often result in host cell death.

The hallmark of HIV-1 infection is the loss of cell-mediated immunity, predominantly CD4+ T cells or T-helper cells.[11] T-helper cells are key orchestrators of the immune response and responsible directly or indirectly for the induction of a wide array of immune functions. A decrease in CD4 cells results in an inverted CD4 to CD8 ratio, which usually falls to less than 1.0. The degree of immunosuppression in children with HIV is determined by the age-specific CD4 T-lymphocyte count and percentage (Table 1). T-lymphocyte function may also be impaired with loss of mitogen responses and cutaneous anergy to antigens. Cytotoxic T cell and natural killer cell function has also been shown to be diminished with HIV infection.

In addition to T-lymphocyte dysfunction, B-cell dysfunction may occur with polyclonal B-cell activation, hypergammaglobulinemia, and circulating immune complexes.[12] B-cell activation or dysregulation may actually precede CD4 depletion, with dramatic rises in immunoglobulins IgG, IgA, and IgM. Despite polyclonal activation and elevated immunoglobulins, specific antibody production is inadequate for host protection. This "functional hypogammaglobulinemia" underlies the 10- to 50-fold increase in the risk of bacteremia and bacterial infection in adults and children.[13]

Decline of T-helper cells over time results in progressive immunoparesis and subsequent risk of opportunistic infections, such as intracellular bacteria and parasitic infections. In addition to opportunistic infections, there is also an increased risk of malignancies such as non-Hodgkins lymphoma (NHL), Kaposi's sarcoma (KS), and leiomyosarcoma, although these conditions are less commonly seen in children compared with adults. Table 2 summarizes the AIDS-defining conditions.[14] Recent evidence suggests that gut-associated lymphoid tissue (GALT) is particularly severely affected during HIV infection, and may only demonstrate partial recovery if highly active antiretroviral therapy (HAART) is not initiated until late in the course of disease.[15] This may help explain why gastrointestinal infections are so important in HIV infection.

CLINICAL FEATURES IN RELATION TO PATHOLOGY

The clinical manifestations of HIV infection related to the gastrointestinal tract in children can usually be attributed to infections (opportunistic or virulent, see above) or malignancy. Because nutritional failure (failure to thrive) is so important in children, we consider this alongside the clinical features of these other processes.

INFECTIONS OF THE GASTROINTESTINAL TRACT

Infectious causes of gastrointestinal tract disease can be divided into major categories based on microbiological classification. Several different parts of the gastrointestinal tract may be affected, often simultaneously, and often multiple infectious agents may be present. Six organisms that infect the gastrointestinal tract are classified as AIDS-defining conditions including cytomegalovirus (CMV), herpes simplex virus (HSV), *Cryptosporidium* spp., *Isospora belli*, *Mycobacterium avium* complex (MAC), and *Candida* spp.[14] Many other organisms can

Table 2 AIDS-Defining Conditions

Serious bacterial infections
Candidiasis (pulmonary, esophageal)*
Coccidiomycosis
Cryptococcosis
Crytosporidiosis*
Cytomegalovirus disease*
Herpes simplex*
Histoplasmosis
HIV encephalopathy
Isosporiasis*
Kaposi's sarcoma*
Lymphoma*
Mycobacterium avium complex (disseminated/
    extrapulmonary)*
Mycobacterium tuberculosis
Pneumocystis jiroveci pneumonia
Salmonella septicemia
Toxoplasmosis (cerebral)
Wasting syndrome

*May affect the gastrointestinal tract.

produce gastrointestinal infection, and these can be broadly divided into the major classes of bacteria, viruses, fungi, and parasites. The clinical features and treatment of these infections are summarized in Table 3. Each class of infection is discussed below.

Viruses

Acute viral intestinal infections of childhood cause a similar spectrum of disease in HIV infection and are usually self-limited illnesses with no increase in severity associated with immunosuppression (eg, rotavirus[16]). Acute diarrhea is the most common presentation and can be due to any of several viral agents including rotavirus, adenovirus, astrovirus, calicivirus, and small round-structured viruses (SRSV).[16] Cytomegalovirus (CMV) is a common coinfection with HIV; however, its significance in pediatric gastrointestinal tract disease is unclear. Esophageal, hepatic, and large bowel involvement have all been described with CMV infection.[17] Herpes simplex virus has also been associated with erosive esophagitis; CMV esophagitis may look like this or may cause a solitary ulcer.

Lymphocyte populations in the gastrointestinal tract show similar depletion of CD4 lymphocytes, particularly in the lamina propria. An enteropathy, with partial villous atrophy and crypt hyperplasia, associated with HIV has also been described in the absence of opportunistic infection, but there is controversy as to whether this is due to HIV itself or to undetected opportunistic agents.[18] The consequences of this enteropathy are variable: in some instances these findings are associated with severe malabsorption, but in other cases there may be no symptoms associated with these findings.

Bacteria

Several bacterial enteric pathogens associated with acute infectious diarrhea in immunocompetent children also cause disease in HIV-infected children, notably *Campylobacter* spp., *Shigella* spp., and *Salmonella* spp.[19–20] Intestinal MAC infection, however, usually occurs in the more severely immunosuppressed children and is characterized by severe chronic diarrhea, malabsorption, and wasting. Infection with these agents is most often through contaminated food or water, contact with infected animals, or person-to-person transmission through the fecal-oral route. Infection with these enteropathogens can result in prolonged diarrhea, malnutrition, recurrence after apparently successful treatment, and extraintestinal infections.[21]

Parasites

Cryptosporidial infection is associated with protracted watery diarrhea in immunocompetent children,[22–23] and in HIV-infected children there are more severe anorexia and weight loss, and higher mortality.[24] Infection may be acquired by person-to-person contact or through

Table 3 Infections of the Gastrointestinal Tract in Children with HIV Infection

	Clinical Presentation	Treatment
Bacteria		
Shigella spp.	Acute/persistent diarrhea	Fluoroquinolone, ceftriaxone, cefotaxime
Nontyphi *Salmonella*	Acute/persistent diarrhea; septicemia	Fluoroquinolone, ceftriaxone
Campylobacter spp.	Acute/persistent diarrhea	Macrolide, fluoroquinolone
MAC	Persistent diarrhea, malabsorption	Macrolide, ethambutol, rifabutin
Viruses		
Rotavirus	Acute diarrhea	
Adenovirus	Esophagitis, colitis	Cidofovir/ribavirin
CMV	Esophagitis, perianal disease	Ganciclovir, foscarnet, cidofovir
HSV		Aciclovir
Parasites		
Cryptosporidium parvum	Acute/persistent diarrhea	Nitazoxanide*
Isospora belli	Acute/persistent diarrhea	TMP/SMX†
Giardia intestinalis	Acute/persistent diarrhea	Metronidazole, albendazole
Microsporidia	Acute/persistent diarrhea	Albendazole‡
Cyclospora cayetanensis	Acute/persistent diarrhea	TMP/SMX†
Strongyloides stercoralis	Acute/persistent diarrhea; hyperinfection syndrome	Thiabendazole, albendazole, ivermectin
Fungi		
Candida albicans	Esophagitis	Fluconazole, itraconazole, amphotericin

These anti-infective agents should be used in standard pediatric doses (see chapter 19.2c), †TMP/SMX (trimethoprim/sulphamethoxazole) for isosporiasis or cyclosporiasis when double the usual dose should be given, and ‡albendazole which should be given for 4 weeks. Only one species of microsporidian (Encephalitozoon intestinalis) is likely to respond well to albendazole, and very little information is available to confirm its efficacy in children. *Nitazoxanide has been shown to be effective in HIV seronegative children only, but there is anecdotal evidence that the same dose given for 2 to 4 weeks may be effective in this otherwise difficult to treat infection.

contaminated water supply or food. *I. belli* and *Cyclospora cayetanensis* infections may also cause a similar clinical picture, but these appear to be less common in HIV-infected children[24] than in HIV-infected adults in the same setting.[25] Acquisition of infection may take place from person-to-person or by contaminated food or water. Giardiasis may present with an acute diarrheal illness characterized by abdominal cramps and bloating or a more chronic protracted diarrheal illness leading to malabsorption and failure to thrive, but there is little evidence that giardiasis is more common or more severe in HIV infection. Again, transmission usually occurs by person-to-person transmission through the fecal-oral route or through ingestion of contaminated food or water. There is uncertainty surrounding the importance of microsporidia in HIV-related intestinal disease in children. A study in Thailand suggested that microsporidiosis was more common in HIV-related diarrhea than in HIV-unrelated diarrhea,[26] but in Uganda the prevalence of microsporidiosis was the same in children with and without diarrhea,[27] and similar observations were made in Tanzania.[28] It is important to realize that diagnosis of microsporidiosis is difficult, and no consensus yet exists as to its epidemiology.

Strongyloides stercoralis infection may be asymptomatic in HIV-infected individuals but may also cause a severe hyperinfection syndrome characterized by a Loeffler-like syndrome with eosinophilia, pulmonary infiltrates, rash, and diarrhea.[29] This is uncommon. Other helminths are not associated with disease in HIV.

Fungi

Oral thrush owing to *C. albicans* is a common presentation in children with HIV-infection, sometimes causing feeding difficulty. More troublesome symptoms of dysphagia and retrosternal chest pain are associated with *Candida* esophagitis which may be clinically indistinguishable from CMV and HSV esophagitis without endoscopic clarification.[30]

FAILURE TO THRIVE AND NUTRITIONAL PROBLEMS

Many children with HIV/AIDS experience wasting and/or failure to thrive during the course of their disease.[31] In developing countries weight loss is one of the most common presentations of HIV infection and is often associated with diarrhea.[32] The etiology of failure to thrive in this population may often be unclear and in many cases multifactorial. The most important factors include reduced oral intake, malabsorption in the gastrointestinal tract, increased energy utilization with HIV infection, and psychosocial stressors. In many instances more than one factor may be responsible but may also exacerbate other factors. Poor energy intake is an important cause of failure to thrive particularly when owing to infections of the upper gastrointestinal tract which limit oral intake, for example, esophagitis. Poor energy intake is often a consequence of anorexia related to intestinal infection. HIV encephalopathy may also cause neurological disease resulting in difficulty in swallowing or incoordination and therefore a

reduction in oral intake. More recently, newer HIV therapies have been associated with significant gastrointestinal toxicities, including severe taste aversion, which has resulted in nutritional problems in some children. Malabsorption is another important factor in children who fail to thrive, either directly owing to HIV enteropathy or secondary to enteropathogen infection (see above). Increased energy utilization may also play an important role in failure to thrive mainly through increased metabolic rate and high cellular turnover/inflammation owing to HIV infection and other coinfections; however, the exact importance of this factor has been difficulty to measure and further research is needed in this field. Psychosocial factors are important causes of failure to thrive in children with HIV infection, particularly in the setting of perinatally acquired infection where other family members may also be infected. Illness of both a child and his or her parent may have profound influences on the individual. HIV infection in this setting may also be associated with other social factors such as poverty and intravenous drug use which may impact on the HIV-infected child.

Malnutrition was a serious health problem in children in tropical populations long before the HIV pandemic, but the interaction of intestinal infection, nutritional impairment, and HIV has escalated the problem. HIV appears to induce changes in small intestinal mucosal function, and these changes are exacerbated in the presence of opportunistic infection. Whether these changes explain the increased severity of malnutrition in HIV-infected children remain to be elucidated. These children have severe malnutrition and high-mortality rates, particularly in the presence of specific infections such as cryptosporidiosis.[24] Treatment of the most severely affected children can be very challenging.

GASTROINTESTINAL MALIGNANCY

There is an increased risk for the development of malignancies in HIV infection, including KS, NHL, and leiomyosarcoma.[33] However there are clear differences between malignancies in children and adults with HIV infection. For example, Kaposi's sarcoma is relatively unusual in children and leiomyoma/myosarcoma is relatively more common.[34] All of these malignancies can affect the gastrointestinal tract and may occur without severe immunosuppression. The most common tumors seen are NHL which may affect extranodal sites such as the gastrointestinal tract, liver, and the central nervous system. NHL may behave aggressively and present with nonspecific symptoms such as weight loss, fever, and fatigue which are not dissimilar to symptoms seen with other opportunistic infections.[35] Lymphoproliferative disorders (LPDs) represent a spectrum of disease of which NHL is the most malignant and aggressive form of disease. At the benign end of the spectrum of LPD are mucosa-associated lymphoid tumors (MALTs). Several different agents have been implicated in the pathogenesis of LPD including Epstein-Barr virus and *Helicobacter pylori* infection.[36-37] MALT tumors may occur in the lung, stomach, and salivary glands and may be slow growing, indolent tumors. Kaposi's sarcoma is a hemangiosarcoma that has been associated with human herpes virus-8 (HHV-8) infection.[38] KS is reasonably uncommon in children although there has been an increased incidence in children with HIV in sub-Saharan Africa.[39] Typically, KS causes mucocutaneous lesions, including lesions in the mouth and gastrointestinal tract. Lymphadenopathic KS may also occur, affecting specific regional lymph nodes such as the inguinal areas. Less common forms of KS include visceral organ involvement such as the spleen and lungs.[40] Smooth muscle tumors (leiomyoma and leiomyosarcoma) are rare in children, although the risk is estimated to be 10,000 times higher in children with HIV infection. Smooth muscle tumors are not classified as AIDS-defining conditions (unlike NHL and KS) but are classified as Category B symptoms.[14] Epstein-Barr virus infection has been associated with smooth muscle tumors and may have a pathogenic role. After NHL, smooth muscle tumors are the second most common malignancy in children with HIV and in some surveys represents 17% of all reported tumors.[41] Leiomyosarcomas may occur in the gastrointestinal tract, spleen, retroperitoneal space, adrenal glands, and lungs.

INVESTIGATION

Children presenting with chronic gastrointestinal symptoms need to be thoroughly evaluated to determine the etiological agent and institute appropriate therapy and symptom relief. Stepwise diagnostic testing is essential to exclude common pathogens initially and search for more unusual pathogens using in some cases more invasive testing modalities. Initial investigation involves obtaining at least two stool samples for bacterial culture to exclude bacterial enteropathogens. Microscopy using specific stains (saline, iodine, trichrome, acid-fast, and fluorescein-conjugated stains) should be performed to detect specific parasites. *S. stercoralis* infection usually requires identification of the rhabditiform larvae in feces or duodenal fluid. Serodiagnosis may be less useful due to cross-reactivity with other filaria and reduced antibody responses particularly in more immunocompromised individuals. Stool samples should also be analysed by acid-fast staining to detect MAC infection. In children who have diarrhea and fever, blood for bacterial culture, mycobacterial culture and CMV culture or polymerase chain reaction (PCR) may be useful. Often repeated blood sampling may be necessary in order to identify bacteremia or viremia. If a diagnosis is not established using standard culture and microscopic techniques, then upper and lower gastrointestinal endoscopy may need to be performed to obtain biopsy specimens. This may be particularly important to detect MAC and

CMV infection because stool examination is relatively insensitive. Samples obtained by endoscopy need to be sent for histology, mycobacterial culture, and virological examination using immunohistochemistry and/or electron microscopy if available. Radiological investigations may be useful in determining the anatomical site and extent of disease. Barium swallow studies may be useful in supporting the diagnosis of *Candida* esophagitis in patients with dysphagia. Barium radiographs may also demonstrate large intestinal changes such as mucosal thickening and ulceration as seen in CMV colitis; however, endoscopic investigation may need to be performed to confirm the diagnosis. Computed tomography (CT) may be useful in demonstrating bowel wall thickening and luminal narrowing as well as intra-abdominal masses such as lymphadenopathy or malignancies. Major intra-abdominal lymphadenopathy should be investigated further and may require biopsy at laparotomy or laparoscopy to detect tuberculosis, NHL, or MAC.[42] In children from tropical populations, tuberculosis should always be considered in a child with unexplained abdominal symptoms because treatment is so dramatically successful.

MANAGEMENT

Secondary and Supportive Treatment

Treatment for children with HIV infection includes the prompt and aggressive treatment of acute infections, include opportunistic infections. These are summarized in Table 3. In children with acute diarrhea, replacement of fluid and electrolytes is initially important. Nutritional support and supplementation are frequently required, especially in children with chronic diarrhea. Enteral support should be used whenever possible, though parenteral support may sometimes be required (see Chapter XX). In children with difficult or dysfunctional swallowing, a feeding gastrostomy may be useful method of enteral support.[43]

Prophylactic therapy using sulphamethoxazole-trimethoprim (STX-TMP) is often given to prevent PCP, but it may have the desirable effect of reducing infections with *I. belli* or *C. cayetanensis*. In tropical populations, STX-TMP has been shown to reduce mortality in children with HIV.[44] Vitamin A supplementation has also marked benefits for HIV-infected and HIV-uninfected children.[45]

ANTI-HIV TREATMENT

Initial antiviral therapy for children with HIV infection involved the use of monotherapy or dual therapy with drugs such as zidovudine and didanosine that belonged to the nucleoside analogue family (see Table 4). These agents inhibit the viral enzyme reverse transcriptase and thereby reduce viral replication. Although this approach appeared to have an initial beneficial effect, it soon became

apparent that specific viral mutations developed against these drugs rendering them ineffective. Improved monitoring of HIV infection by measurement of HIV-1 viral load made it apparent that viral replication was an important prognostic marker, and complete viral suppression was a key goal in permitting immune reconstitution.[46] The development of newer antiviral agents, including the more potent protease inhibitor group, has meant that effective and prolonged viral suppression is now possible. Combination therapy or HAART has dramatically altered the outlook for many children with HIV infection who have access to this form of treatment.[47] Both mortality and morbidity have improved by HAART, and some have suggested that HIV is now another chronic treatable disease of childhood.[48] Combination therapy usually involves the use of at least three different drugs from different classes, for example, 2 NRTIs + NNRTI or PI (see Table 4 for drug classes). However, complete eradication of HIV is not possible with current drugs, and children will probably have to remain on some form of lifelong therapy. Furthermore, HAART requires high levels of compliance for sustained viral suppression and the prevention of viral resistance and treatment failure. Obstacles to long-term successful treatment and compliance include poor drug tolerability, particularly taste, and long-terms adverse effects (including abnormal lipid and glucose metabolism).[48] Despite these problems, HAART has been used effectively and safely in children in North America and Europe with dramatic improvements in long-term survival. Treatment of children in these settings has involved a multidisciplinary team, often in specialist centers that have the expertise and experience in managing the many complex physical, psychological, and social issues that affect children with HIV infection. Newer therapeutic strategies are also being developed to boost anti-HIV immune response, which may in the future give more durable immune reconstitution. Newer

---

Table 4 Classes of Antiretroviral Drugs for Children

Nucleoside analogue reverse transcriptase inhibitor (NRTI)
Zidovudine (AZT)
Didanosine (ddi)
Zalcitabine (ddC)
Lamivudine (3TC)
Stavudine (d4T)
Abacavir (ABC)

Nonnucleoside analogue reverse transcriptase inhibitor (NNRTI)
Nevirapine
Delavradine
Efavirenz

Protease inhibitor (PI)
Ritonavir
Nelfinavir
Indinavir
Saquinavir
Amprenavir
Lopinavir
Atazanavir

classes of drugs are being developed which target the entry of HIV into host cells and prevent integration of the virus into the host cell genome. These drugs are not yet in routine clinical use.

The use of HAART to treat children in resource-limited countries, which have the highest burden of HIV infection, has lagged behind their introduction for treatment of adults. However, HAART has been demonstrated to be effective and safe when used in even in the most resource-limited settings, and recent initiatives in reducing drug costs will mean that access to HAART will improve. In addition to providing affordable drugs, infrastructure development will also be necessary if treatment programes are to be successful.

Prevention of vertical HIV transmission from mother to child has been an important initiative in resource-limited countries with a high HIV burden. Uptake of antiretroviral drugs for prevention of mother-to-child transmission varies greatly. In industrialized countries uptake is high, but in developing countries remarkably heterogeneity is seen, with coverage in some countries as low as 5% and in others virtually all eligible mothers receiving appropriate treatment.[5]

OTHER SECONDARY IMMUNODEFICIENCIES

Secondary immunodeficiency may occur with a variety of different conditions (and their treatments) including hematological malignancies, transplantation, malnutrition, and autoimmune disorders, such as inflammatory bowel disease. Gastrointestinal manifestations are common in these children, with an increase in opportunistic and enteric infections, which may cause chronic, relapsing illness similar to that seen with HIV infection in children. Particularly at risk of infection due to enteric pathogens are children receiving chemotherapy for malignancies and those who are immunosuppressed following bone marrow or solid organ transplantation. In those children receiving chemotherapy, the main problems occur with neutropenia and gram-negative bacilli infection, particularly *E. coli*. In children receiving immunosuppressive therapy following transplantation, viral (CMV, adenovirus) and fungal (*Candida, Aspergillus*) infection may be particularly problematic especially when immunosuppressive therapy is maximal. In both groups of children, *Clostridium difficile* has also been recognized as a cause of pseudomembranous colitis. Antibiotic therapy is a key factor in pseudomembranous colitis, particularly through disruption of normal bowel flora and subsequent colonization with *C. difficile*. Parasitic infections, especially *Cryptosporidium* and *Strongyloides*, may be important causes of chronic diarrhea and gastrointestinal disease. Gastrointestinal syndromes associated with CMV are an increasingly important problem in bone marrow transplant recipients, causing ulceration of the esophagus, stomach, small and large bowel. Graft-versus-host disease (GVHD) is also an important cause of gastrointestinal disease in children receiving bone marrow transplantation and may be difficult to differentiate clinically from other opportunistic infections and effects of chemoradiotherapy. Acute GVHD may affect the distal small bowel and colon, presenting with profuse diarrhea, intestinal bleeding, and abdominal pain. It should also be borne in mind that any gastrointestinal problem in a child receiving corticosteroids or other immunosuppressive treatment might be related to an opportunistic infection or malignancy, and due consideration should be given to this. The approach to a child with gastrointestinal symptoms and secondary immunodeficiency will be similar to that for HIV infection where stepwise diagnostic testing is important to identify infectious agents. Endoscopy and biopsy may be required in some children, especially where GVHD is suspected. Management of these children will require treatment of infectious agent (where identified) as well as supportive treatment, particularly nutritional support.

REFERENCES

1. Kaposi's sarcoma and *Pneumocystis* pneumonia among homosexual men New York City and California. MMWR Morb Mortal Wkly Rep 1981;30:305–8.
2. Tudor-Williams G. HIV infection in developing countries. Trans Roy Soc Trop Med Hyg 2000;94:3–4.
3. Walraven G, Nicoll A, Njau M, Timaeus I. The impact of HIV-1 infection on child health in sub-Saharan Africa: The burden on the health services. Trop Med Int Health 1996; 1:3–14.
4. Buve A, Bishikwabo-Nsarhaza K, Mutangadura G. The spread and effect of HIV-1 infection in sub-Saharan Africa. Lancet 2002;359:2011–7.
5. UNAIDS. AIDS epidemic update: December 2006. http://www.unaids.org.
6. Dabis F, Ekpini ER. HIV-1/AIDS and maternal and child health in Africa. Lancet 2002;359:2097–104.
7. Kourtis AP, Lee FK, Abrams EJ, et al. Mother-to-child transmission of HIV-1: Timing and implications for prevention. Lancet Infect Dis 2006;6:726–32.
8. Coovadia HM, Rollins NC, Bland RM, et al. Mother-to-child transmission of HIV-1 infection during exclusive breastfeeding in the first 6 months of life: An intervention cohort study. Lancet 2007;369:1107–16.
9. Guay LA, Musoke P, Fleming T, et al. Intrapartum and neonatal single-dose nevirapine compared with zidovudine for prevention of mother-to-child transmission of HIV-1 in Kampala, Uganda: HIVNET 012 randomised trial. Lancet 1999;354:795–802.
10. Landau NR, Warton M, Littman DR. The envelope glycoprotein of the human immunodeficiency virus binds to the immunoglobulin-like domain of CD4. Nature 1988;334:159–62.
11. Giorgi JV, Detels R. T-cell subset alterations in HIV-infected homosexual men: NIAID Multicenter AIDS Cohort Study. Clin Immunol Immunopathol 1989;52:10–18.
12. Lane HC, Masur H, Edgar LC, et al. Abnormalities of B-cell activation and immunoregulation in patients with acquired immunodeficiency syndrome. N Engl J Med 1983;309:453–8.
13. Karstaedt A, Khoosal B, Crewe-Brown H. Pneumococcal bacteremia during a decade in children in Soweto, South Africa. Pediatr Infect Dis J 2000;19:454–7.
14. Centres for Disease Control and Prevention. 1994 revised classification system for human immunodeficiency virus infection in children less than 13 years of age. MMWR Morb Mortal Wkly Rep 1994;43:1–19.
15. Guadaloupe M, Sankaran S, George MD, et al. Viral suppression and immune restoration in the gastrointestinal mucosa of human immunodeficiency virus type 1-infected patients initiating therapy during primary or chronic infection. J Virol 2006;80:8326–47.
16. Cunliffe NA, Gondwe JS, Kirkwood CD, et al. Effect of concomitant HIV infection on presentation and outcome of rotavirus gastroenteritis in Malawian children. Lancet 2001;358:550–5.
17. Cegielski JP, Msengi AE, Miller SE. Enteric viruses associated with HIV infection in Tanzanian children with chronic diarrhea. Pediatr AIDS HIV Infect 1994;5:296–9.
18. Miller TL, Mc Quinn LB, Oran ZEJ. Endoscopy of the upper gastrointestinal tract as a diagnostic tool for children with human immunodeficiency virus infection. J Pediatr 1997;130:766–73.
19. Perlman DM, Ampel NM, Schifman RB, et al. Persistent *Campylobacter jejuni* infection in patients with human immunodeficiency virus (HIV). Ann Intern Med 1998;108: 540–6.
20. Nelson MR, Shanson DC, Hawkins DA, Gazzard BG. *Salmonella, Campylobacter* and *Shigella* in HIV-seropositive patients. AIDS 1992;6:1495–8.
21. Horsburgh CR. *Mycobacterium avium* complex infection in the acquired immunodeficiency syndrome. N Engl J Med 1991;324:1332–8.
22. Molbak K, Andersen M, Aaby P, et al. *Cryptosporidium* infection in infancy as a cause of malnutrition: A community study from Guinea-Bissau, West Africa. Am J Clin Nutr 1997;65:149–52.
23. Agnew DG, Lima AAM, Newman RC, et al. Cryptosporidiosis in northeastern Brazilian children: Association with increased diarrhoea morbidity. J Infect Dis 1998;177:754–60.
24. Amadi BC, Kelly P, Mwiya M, et al. Intestinal and systemic infection, HIV and mortality in Zambian children with persistent diarrhoea and malnutrition. J Ped Gastroenterol Nutr 2001;32:550–4.
25. Kelly P, Baboo KS, Woolf M, et al. Prevalence and aetiology of persistent diarrhoea in adults in urban Zambia. Acta Tropica 1996;61:183–90.
26. Wanachiwanawin D, Chokephaibulkit K, Lertlaituan P, et al. Intestinal microsporidiosis in HIV-infected children with diarrhea. Southeast Asian J Trop Med Publ Health 2002;33:241–5.
27. Tumwine JK, Kekitiinwa A, Nabukeera N, et al. Enterocytozoon bieneusi among children with diarrhea attending Mulago hospital in Uganda. Am J Trop Med Hyg 2002;67:299–303.
28. Cegielski JP, Ortega YR, McKee S, et al. *Cryptosporidium, Enterocytozoon,* and *Cyclospora* infections in pediatric and adult patients with diarrhea in Tanzania. Clin Infect Dis 1999;28:314–21.
29. Gompels MM, Todd J, Peters BS, et al. Disseminated *Strongyloides* in AIDS: Uncommon but important. AIDS 1991;5:329–32.
30. Chiou CC, Groll AH, Gonzales CE, et al. Esophageal candidiasis in pediatric acquired immunodeficiency syndrome: Clinical manifestation and risk factors. Pediatr Infect Dis J 2000;19:729–34.
31. Arpadi SM, Horlick MN, Wong J, et al. Body composition in prepubertal children with human immunodeficiency virus type 1 infection. Arch Pediatr Adolesc Med 1998;52: 688–93.
32. Chintu C, Dupont HC, Kaile T, et al. Human immunodeficiency virus-associated diarrhoea and wasting in Zambia; Selected risk factors and clinical associations. Am J Trop Med Hyg 1998;59:38–41.
33. Mueller BU, Pizzo PA. Malignancy in pediatric AIDS. Curr Opin Pediatr 1996;8:45–9.
34. Chadwick EG, Connor EJ, Guerra Hanson IC, et al. Tumors of smooth muscle origin in HIV-infected children. JAMA 1990;263:3182–84.
35. Granovsky M, Mueller BU. Malignancies in children with HIV infection. In: Pizzo PA, Wilfert MW, editors. Pediatric AIDS. Lippincot, Williams & Wilkins; 1994. p. 443–59.
36. Roggero E, Zucca E, Pinott G, et al. Eradication of *Helicobacter pylori* infection in primary low-grade gastric lymphoma of mucosa-associated tissue. Ann Intern Med 1995; 122:767–9.
37. Sohal EM, Carugiozoglou T, Lamy M, et al. Epstein-Barr virus serology and Epstein-Barr virus-associated lymphoproliferative disorders in pediatric liver transplant recipients. Transplantation 1993:56:1394–8.
38. Chang Y, Cesarman E, Pessin MS, et al. Identification of herpesvirus-like DNA sequences in AIDS-associated Kaposi's sarcoma. Science 1994;266:1865–9.
39. Amir H, Kaaya EE, Manji KP. Kaposi's sarcoma before and during a human immunodeficiency virus epidemic in Tanzanian children. Pediatr Infect Dis J 2001;20:518–21.
40. Ziegler JL, Katongole-Mbidde E. Kaposi's sarcoma in childhood: An analysis of 100 cases from Uganda and relationship to HIV infection. Int J Cancer 1996;65:200–3.
41. Granovsky MO, Mueller BU, Nicholson HS, et al. Cancer in human immunodeficiency virus-infected children: A case series from the Children's Cancer Group and the National Cancer Institute. J Clin Oncol 1998;16:1–8.
42. Pursner M, Haller JO, Berdon WE. Imaging features of *Mycobacterium avium* intracellulare complex (MAC) in children with AIDS. Pediatr Radiol 2000;30:426–9.

43. Henderson RA, Saavedra JM, Perman JA, et al. Effect of enteral tube feeding on growth of children with symptomatic human immunodeficiency virus infection. J Pediatr Gastroenterol Nutr 1994;18:429–34.

44. Chintu C, Bhat GJ, Walker AS, et al. Co-trimoxazole as prophylaxis against opportunistic infections in HIV-infected Zambian children (CHAP): A double-blind randomised controlled trial. Lancet 2004;364:1865–71.

45. Fawzi WW, Mbise RL, Hertzmark E, et al. A randomised trial of vitamin A supplements in relation to mortality among HIV infected and uninfected children in Tanzania. Pediatr Infect Dis J 1999;18:127–33.

46. Mofenson LM, Koreltz J, Meyer WA, et al. The relationship between serum human immunodeficiency virus type 1 (HIV-1) RNA level, CD4 lymphocyte percent and long-term mortality in HIV-1 infected children. J Infect Dis 1997;175:1029–38.

47. Resino S, Bellon JM, Sanchez-Ramon S, et al. Impact of antiretroviral protocols on dynamics of AIDS progression markers. Arch Dis Child 2002;86:119–24.

48. Gibb DM, Duong T, Tookey PA, et al. Decline in mortality, AIDS, and hospital admissions in perinatally HIV-1 infected children in the United Kingdom and Ireland. BMJ 2003;327:1019.

20.4. Necrotizing Enterocolitis

Erika C. Claud, MD

Michael S. Caplan, MD

Neonatal necrotizing enterocolitis (NEC) is an inflammatory bowel necrosis that primarily afflicts premature neonates.[1-2] Despite significant morbidity associated with this disease, the underlying pathophysiology remains poorly understood. NEC differs from other conditions in that the inherent immaturity of the premature intestine appears to be the greatest risk factor rather than any particular insult.

This chapter reviews the clinical features and pathophysiology of this disease, with particular attention to what is understood about the unique susceptibility of the preterm intestine. Although full-term infants may develop this disease, these infants generally have specific underlying risk factors for gut compromise such as birth asphyxia, polycythemia, exchange transfusion, intrauterine growth restriction, cyanotic congenital heart disease, gastroschisis, or myelomeningocele (Table 1).[3-7] In these patients, NEC often presents within the first days of life. Thus, the pathophysiology in full-term infants may be quite different from that in premature infants and is not considered further in this chapter.

CLINICAL FEATURES

NEC affects approximately 1 to 5% of all neonatal intensive care unit (NICU) admissions and 12% of premature infants <1,500 g, characteristically between 7 and 14 days of life.[8-10] Increasingly, NEC has been documented several weeks after birth, particularly in very low birth weight infants.[11] Susceptibility to NEC appears inversely related to gestational age, suggesting the role of intestinal maturation.[12-15]

Table 1 Risk Factors for Necrotizing Enterocolitis

Preterm Infant	Full-Term Infant
Prematurity—immature intestine	Birth asphyxia
Ischemia	Polycythemia
Enteral feeds	Exchange transfusion
Bacterial colonization	Intrauterine growth restriction
	Gastroschisis
	Cyanotic congenital heart disease
	Myelomeningocele

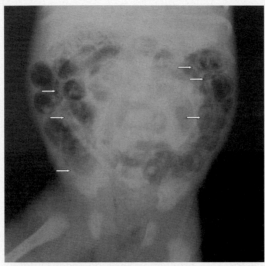

Figure 1 Abdominal radiograph depicting pneumatosis intestinalis, as indicated by arrows, in a premature infant with necrotizing enterocolitis.

NEC presents with variable symptoms, which may initially include evidence of nonspecific gastrointestinal dysfunction such as abdominal distention, feeding intolerance, and gastric aspirates with progression to bilious vomiting and hematochezia. In severe cases, pneumoperitoneum and/or systemic signs of shock and rapid death ensue.[16-17] Laboratory values are similarly nonspecific, including leukocytosis, thrombocytopenia, electrolyte imbalance, and acidosis. The only pathognomonic feature is pneumatosis intestinalis, which is detected on abdominal radiograph (Figure 1). Mortality is reported at 10 to 40% of infants with NEC. Other sequelae include stricture, short gut syndrome, abscess formation, and recurrence of disease. There does not appear to be a sex or race predilection.

Disease progression has classically been defined by the Bell's staging criteria (Table 2).[18] Stage I, or suspected NEC, is characterized by abdominal distention, increased gastric residuals, hematochezia, vomiting, lethargy, apnea, bradycardia, and hemoccult positive stools. Stage II, or definite NEC, is stage I plus pneumatosis intestinalis or portal venous air. Stage III, or advanced NEC, is progression to shock, disseminated intravascular coagulation, acidosis, thrombocytopenia, neutropenia, peritonitis, or pneumoperitoneum.

PATHOLOGY AND HISTOLOGY

NEC primarily affects the terminal ileum and proximal colon, a watershed area for the superior and inferior mesenteric arteries. Pathologic and histologic specimens have shown a combination of ischemic necrosis, acute and chronic inflammation, bacterial overgrowth, and tissue repair, suggesting that NEC is an evolving process rather than an acute event.[19-20] Specifically, surgical specimens reveal evidence of apoptosis, or programmed cell death, of enterocytes in apical villi.[21] Inflammation can be limited to the mucosa and submucosa of the intestine or progress to transmural involvement in the most severe cases. In addition, lesions may include submucosal or subserosal collections of gas, which are thought to represent bacterial fermentation of intraluminal substrates.[20]

PATHOGENESIS

Although, multiple theories have been proposed for the pathogenesis of this disease, a single explanation has eluded investigators. The primary risk factors appear to be prematurity, ischemia, enteral feeding, and bacterial colonization. The classic theory of the pathogenesis of NEC, as described by Santulli and colleagues in 1975, suggests that the disease is caused by the triad of (1) injury to the intestinal mucosa, (2) luminal bacteria, and (3) a substrate, such as formula feedings, in the bowel.[20-22] Although the pathogenesis of NEC appears to be multifactorial, the major risk factor appears to be prematurity, since more than 90% of NEC occurs in premature infants, and gestational age and birth weight correlate inversely with a higher incidence of disease.

Several factors potentially make the preterm infant more susceptible to NEC, including immature intestinal host defenses,[23-24] blood flow regulation,[25-26] bacterial colonization,[27-31] and inflammatory responses.[32-34] It is known that the fetal intestine is exposed to amniotic fluid containing hormones and peptides that may have a role in intestinal maturation. Preterm infants may not have completed this maturation process when colonized by bacteria and initially fed, potentially placing them at higher risk for NEC. At this stage, the fetal intestine is normally protected in its sterile environment and may not be prepared

Table 2 Bell's Staging Criteria

Stage	Systemic Signs	Intestinal Signs	Radiologic Signs
Stage I—suspected NEC	Temperature instability Apnea, bradycardia Lethargy	Abdominal distension Gastric residuals Vomiting Hematochezia	Normal or mild ileus
Stage II—definite NEC	Same as I	Same as I plus abdominal tenderness	Pneumatosis intestinalis or portal air
Stage III—advanced NEC	Progression to shock DIC Metabolic acidosis Thrombocytopenia Neutropenia	Peritonitis	Pneumoperitoneum

Adapted from Bell et al.[18]

to respond to the normal bacterial interactions of the extrauterine environment.

HOST DEFENSE

Several aspects of gastrointestinal host defenses are developmentally regulated, putting the premature infant at a disadvantage (Figure 2). First, there is immaturity of the intestinal physical barriers such as mucous membranes, intestinal epithelia and microvilli, epithelial tight junctions, and mucin. Animal studies have shown that pathogenic organisms adhere to and translocate across the intestine to a greater extent in immature versus mature animals. Abnormal peristaltic activity in premature infants may increase bacterial adherence, allowing for bacterial overgrowth that could increase endotoxin exposure and predispose the infant to NEC.[35–37] Cell surface glycoconjugates serve as adhesion sites for a variety of microbes, and the immature intestine has a different pattern of carbohydrate residues than the adult intestine, which could result in increased pathogen colonization in preterm infants.[38,39] Furthermore, it is known that intestinal mucus, which protects against bacterial and toxin invasion, is different in developing animals and perhaps in premature infants.[40]

There is also immaturity of the functional barrier that limits growth of bacteria that breach the physical barrier. This functional barrier is composed of immunologic host defenses and various biochemical factors. It is known that numbers of intestinal B and T lymphocytes are decreased in neonates and do not approach adult levels until 3 to 4 weeks of life. Newborns also have reduced levels of secretory immunoglobulin (Ig)A in salivary samples, presumably reflecting decreased activity in the intestine.[41–43]

Additionally, the premature infant has lower gastric acid production than do older children, and immature proteolytic enzyme activity may lead to incomplete breakdown of toxins.[41] Finally, key bacteriostatic proteins are secreted from the intestinal epithelium. Intestinal trefoil factor is one such molecule that appears to be developmentally regulated and deficient in premature infants.[44–46] Human defensins (or cryptidins) are bacteriostatic proteins synthesized and secreted from Paneth cells that protect against bacterial translocation and are also altered in premature infants and those with NEC.[47–48]

INTESTINAL BLOOD FLOW REGULATION

Early observations suggested that profound intestinal ischemia was a critical predisposing factor for NEC.[49–50] It was hypothesized that similar to the diving reflex observed in aquatic animals, in periods of stress, blood flow was diverted away from the splanchnic circulation, resulting in intestinal necrosis. Although early epidemiologic observations identified asphyxia as an important risk factor, subsequent studies have shown that the majority of NEC cases are not associated with profound impairment of intestinal perfusion.[16]

Instead, neonatal animals have differences in the intestinal microcirculation that may predispose them to NEC. Studies have shown that the newborn has compromised intestinal blood flow in response to circulatory stress. In response to hypotension, newborn animals have defective pressure/flow autoregulation, resulting in decreased intestinal oxygen delivery and reduced tissue oxygenation.[24,51–52] In addition, in the face of arterial hypoxemia, the newborn intestinal circulatory response differs from that of older animals. Although following modest hypoxemia, intestinal vasodilation and increased intestinal perfusion occur; severe hypoxemia causes vasoconstriction, intestinal ischemia, and/or hypoxia mediated at least in part by loss of nitric oxide production. Multiple chemical mediators (nitric oxide, endothelin, substance P, norepinephrine, and angiotensin) impact on intestinal vasomotor tone. In the stressed newborn, abnormal regulation of these mediators may result in compromised circulatory autoregulation, leading to perpetuation of intestinal ischemia and tissue necrosis.[53–55]

ENTERAL FEEDING

Enteral alimentation has long been considered an important risk factor for the initiation of NEC. Feeds are thought to play a major role as 90 to 95% of all infants with NEC have been enterally fed, even though the majority of fed premature infants do not develop the disease.[13] The precise relationship between enteral feedings and NEC remains poorly understood. Studies identify both the volume and rate of feeding advancement, osmolality, and substrate fermentation as important risk factors.[56–57] Preterm infants are unable to fully digest carbohydrates and proteins, leading to the production of organic acids, which may be harmful to the developing intestine.[58] Furthermore, both human studies and carefully controlled animal models show that formula-fed infants have a higher incidence of NEC than breast-fed infants.[13,31] Breast milk contains multiple bioactive factors that influence host immunity, inflammation, mucosal protection, and intestinal maturation, including secretory IgA, leukocytes, lactoferrin, lysozyme, cytokines, growth factors, enzymes, oligosaccharides, and polyunsaturated fatty acids. Specific host defense factors acquired from breast milk, such as epidermal

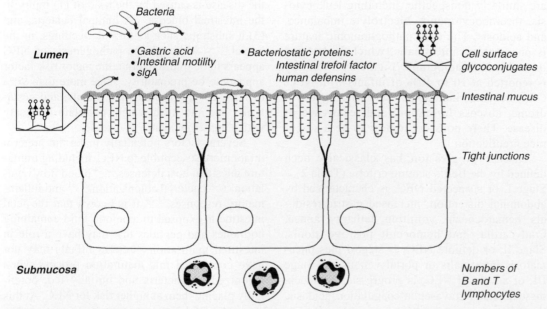

Figure 2 Aspects of immature intestinal host defense in the premature infant that may contribute to susceptibility to necrotizing enterocolitis. sIgA = secretory immunoglobulin A.

growth factor, polyunsaturated fatty acids, acetyl-hydrolase, IgA, and macrophages are effective in reducing the incidence of disease in animals, and some also have proven effective in human trials.[32,42,59–60] Many of these factors are present in amniotic fluid as well as in breast milk. Breast milk may provide for the developing intestinal ex utero in the same way that amniotic fluid supports the developing intestine in utero.

BACTERIAL COLONIZATION

Although clusters of cases of NEC have been reported, no specific organism has been linked to this disease. It is unclear whether bacteria are a primary effector of NEC or are passive participants, entering the bowel wall through a breech in the intestinal mucosal barrier. Only about 30% of infants with this disease have positive blood cultures, and, in general, consist of organisms normally present in the intestinal flora (eg, *Escherichia coli*; Klebsiella, Enterococcus, Clostridium species; and coagulase-negative Staphylococcus).[19,28,61]

Colonization of the newborn intestine is affected by the environment, variation in pH, intestinal peristalsis, bacterial opposition, and the type of enteral feeding. Before birth, the infant gut is sterile, and no cases of NEC have been described in utero, supporting the importance of bacterial colonization in the pathophysiology of the disease. The intestine is initially colonized with a complex flora that reflects maternal flora.[62–63] The preterm infant is next exposed to bacteria present in the NICU, with gut colonization frequently affected by the hospital environment, use of broad-spectrum antibiotics, interventions such as gavage feeding, opioids which slow intestinal motility, and agents which alter the gastric pH.[41,61] Although a wide range of aerobic and anaerobic flora colonizes normal infants by 10 days of age, infants in the NICU undergo delayed colonization with a more limited number of bacterial species that tend to be virulent.[9,64]

Feeding is another variable in the acquisition of intestinal flora. In breast-fed infants, Bifidobacterium is a primary organism, with Lactobacillus and Streptococcus as minor components. In formula-fed infants, similar amounts of Bacteroides and Bifidobacterium are found with minor components of the more pathogenic species, Staphylococcus, *E. coli*, and Clostridia.[63,65–68] Animal models have shown that certain bacteria, such as adherent *E. coli*, produce disease in a rabbit model of NEC, whereas nonpathogenic strains of gram-positive organisms prevent disease.[69] Furthermore, some studies suggest that early colonization by probiotics (facultative anaerobes such as Bifidobacteria and Lactobacilli) reduces the risk of NEC in both animal and human studies.[30,70–71] In preterm infants, colonization with Bifidobacterium is delayed for several weeks. Since binding of pathogenic organisms is influenced by the underlying microbial ecology through competition for binding sites or nutrients,

production of inhibiting agents, alteration in pH, and synthesis of growth factors, promotion of the growth of competitive, nonpathogenic strains of bacteria may serve to protect the premature infant from NEC.[64,69,72]

INFLAMMATORY CASCADE

Evidence from human and animal studies suggests that various perinatal insults to the immature intestinal mucosal barrier lead to a proinflammatory cascade, resulting in NEC.[31,59] Inflammation can be initiated by exogenous stimuli such as bacteria and bacterial products, including lipopolysaccharide and flagellin, as well as by endogenous inflammatory mediators such as tumor necrosis factor-α (TNF-α) and interleukin (IL)-1β.[73–77] In response to stimuli, enterocytes release proinflammatory cytokines, such as IL-6, TNF-α, and chemokines, like IL-8.[78] These stimuli have distinct interactions with the intestinal epithelium and collectively result in a propagated inflammatory response (Figure 3). Asphyxia and/or ischemia-reperfusion also activate the early mediators of inflammation in many tissues, including the intestine. Neonatal animal studies have shown that the stress of formula feeding stimulates phospholipase A2 gene expression, intestinal platelet-activating factor (PAF) production, and stimulation of apoptosis and the inflammatory response, with resulting NEC.[59–60] If counterregulatory responses to these proinflammatory events are insufficient, pathologic changes to gut mucosa then occur.

Intestinal specimens from patients with acute NEC demonstrate increased IL-1β, IL-8, and TNF-α messenger ribonucleic acid compared with controls.[79–81] Other studies document increased IL-6 levels in patients with NEC, with some studies suggesting that levels of IL-6 may correlate with the severity of disease.[28,82–83] Furthermore, patients with NEC have elevated serum PAF and TNF-α levels, but decreased acetylhydrolase

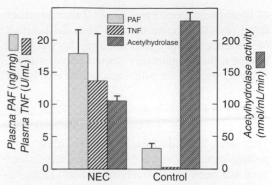

Figure 4 Plasma platelet activating factor (PAF) levels (*open bars*), plasma tumor necrosis factor (TNF) levels (*horizontally hatched bars*), and plasma acetylhydrolase activity (*vertically hatched bars*) in patients with necrotizing enterocolitis (NEC) and control subjects. Plasma PAF and TNF levels were higher in NEC patients than in control patients. Plasma acetylhydrolase activity was lower in NEC patients than in age-matched control subjects. PAF = platelet activating factor; TNF = tumor necrosis factor. (Reproduced with permission from reference 33.)

levels compared with age-matched controls (Figure 4).[33] Acetylhydrolase is a PAF breakdown enzyme; thus, higher PAF levels likely result from both decreased PAF catabolism and from increased PAF production. PAF is a potent phospholipid inflammatory mediator associated with NEC.[33,84] In rat models, PAF produces bowel necrosis similar to NEC, an effect that can be inhibited by PAF receptor antagonists.[85–86]

The balance of pro- and anti-inflammatory influences appears to be a fundamental issue. Evidence suggests that the premature neonate may be predisposed to intestinal inflammation. PAF acetylhydrolase is present in breast milk but absent in commercial formula. This finding may explain, in part, the beneficial effects of breast milk feeding. In neonatal rats, maternal milk feedings increase levels of the anti-inflammatory cytokine IL-10 and reduce the incidence of NEC, whereas in human milk specimens, a significant percentage of NEC patient pairs are deficient in this important regulatory cytokine.[87–88] Studies have also compared the proinflammatory response to lipopolysaccharide (LPS) and IL-1β in intestinal cell lines and found that IL-8 secretion is significantly higher in fetal intestinal epithelium compared with mature, adult intestine.[34] Toll-like receptors (TLRs) are a highly conserved family of pathogen associated molecular pattern (PAMP) receptors which recognize bacterial components. TLR4 specifically recognizes LPS. Interestingly, TLR4 expression decreases after birth in the intestines of healthy mother fed rat pups, but expression increases in the intestinal epithelium of formula-fed/asphyxia-stressed rat pups.[89] Nuclear factor kappaB (NF-κB) acts downstream of TLR4 to activate transcription of a wide variety of genes involved in inflammatory and immune host responses. The immature intestinal epithelium has decreased expression of the primary inhibitor of the NF-κB pathway (IκB), which is associated with increased NF-κB activation and increased transcription

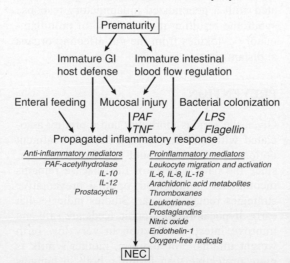

Figure 3 Potential mechanism by which risk factors for necrotizing enterocolitis (NEC) in preterm infants lead to propagation of an inflammatory response, resulting in NEC. GI = gastrointestinal; IL = interleukin; LPS = lipopolysaccharide; NEC = neonatal necrotizing enterocolitis; PAF = platelet activating factor; TNF = tumor necrosis factor.

of proinflammatory cytokines.[90] Taken together these results indicate that the neonatal balance of the inflammatory response may be weighted toward a proinflammatory response that is more likely to result in the pathologic outcome of NEC.

TREATMENT

Treatment remains focused on providing supportive care only since specific preventive steps have not been conclusively identified (Table 3). Treatment depends on prompt recognition of the disease. Therapy includes cessation of enteral feeds, nasogastric decompression, vigorous fluid resuscitation, the use of broad-spectrum antibiotics, correction of anemia and thrombocytopenia, and respiratory support as needed. Patients need to be closely monitored by clinical examination and serial abdominal radiography for evidence of disease progression and intestinal perforation. Radiographs may show nonspecific signs, such as intestinal distention and ileus, as well as pathognomonic pneumatosis intestinalis. After acute stabilization some patients can be medically managed with bowel rest and broad-spectrum antibiotics prior to the slow reintroduction of enteral feeds. Although appearing clinically to have mild or moderate disease, these patients are still at increased risk for intestinal and neurodevelopmental morbidity.[91]

Other patients progress to surgical intervention. Surgery is indicated for extraintestinal air (intestinal perforation or portal venous gas), evidence of ongoing necrosis (persistent metabolic acidosis indicating necrotic tissue, progressive shock, or persistent thrombocytopenia), abdominal wall cellulitis, or a fixed loop on serial abdominal radiographs. There are two surgical options—conventional laparotomy with resection of involved bowel or primary peritoneal drainage. Both methods have advantages but both appear to have equally poor outcomes.[92] At the time of surgery, NEC patients are often poor surgical candidates as they can be systemically ill with a sepsis-like picture, often with respiratory failure and hemodynamic instability. Primary peritoneal drainage is a minimally invasive procedure, which often can be performed at the bedside. A small abdominal incision is made and a drain placed into the peritoneal cavity in order to decompress the abdomen and drain any ascitic

fluid or spilled intestinal contents. The intent of this approach is to stabilize a patient and limit intestinal inflammation prior to a possible second-step laparotomy when the patient is better able to tolerate transfer to the operating room and the stress of a full operation. Peritoneal drainage has most commonly been used for extremely low birth weight infants in whom a laparotomy is deemed too risky. A recent multicenter, controlled clinical trial randomized preterm infants with evidence of intestinal perforation considered secondary to NEC to either laparotomy or primary peritoneal drainage.[92] This study found no short-term difference in mortality (35% for both) or rates of dependence on parenteral nutrition 90 days after operation. The authors suggest that factors prior to surgery rather than type of surgical intervention have a greater impact on outcome.[92]

OUTCOMES

Mortality from NEC has remained at 10 to 40%. In addition, there is significant intestinal morbidity including feeding difficulties, stricture formation, delayed growth, and sepsis. Infants with large intestinal resections are at risk for short gut syndrome with the associated need for long-term parenteral nutrition and risks of line sepsis, liver failure, and impaired growth. Of increasing concern are data, which demonstrate serious long-term morbidity beyond the intestinal complications. A multicenter retrospective analysis of infants <1,000 g found that patients who required surgical management of NEC have a higher frequency of periventricular leukomalacia, bronchopulmonary dysplasia, and cerebral palsy.[91] Furthermore, these infants are at significant independent risk for mental developmental index <70, psychomotor developmental index <70, and neurodevelopmental impairment.[91] The mechanisms underlying these systemic effects are unknown but may be associated with a generalized inflammatory response syndrome resulting in the release of proinflammatory cytokines from the gut affecting organs at distant sites.

PREVENTION

Given the serious morbidity and mortality associated with this disease and limited treatment options, prevention would be ideal. However, since the pathogenesis of this disease remains incompletely understood, optimal preventative strategies remain unclear. Studies indicate that early, hypocaloric, or trophic feeds are safe and improve intestinal function in very low birth weight infants.[10] In addition, mother's milk is more protective than formula, both in humans and in animal models of the disease.[13,32,93–95] The specific protective factor(s) in human milk has yet to be conclusively identified. Animal and human studies document decreased NEC in response to orally administered polyunsaturated fatty acids.[59,96] Epidermal growth factor given

with feeds decreases the incidence of NEC in an animal model and has been used intravenously to treat an older child with intestinal necrosis in one clinical case report.[32,97] Oral administration of heparin-binding epidermal growth factor[98] and antitumor necrosis factor-alpha[99] have also shown a decreased incidence of disease in animal models. Definitive clinical studies have yet to be carried out.

Halac and colleagues have shown that prenatal steroids reduce the incidence of NEC.[100] Cortisone acetate is known to accelerate maturation of the immature intestine, and studies in a rat model of NEC showed that prenatal cortisone decreases both morbidity and mortality secondary to NEC.[101] Other studies suggest the prevention of NEC by IgA–IgG feeding of low-birth-weight infants.[42]

Recent clinical trials have raised the possibility that probiotics may be beneficial in preventing NEC. Probiotics are living microorganisms in food and dietary supplements which have beneficial health effects beyond their inherent nutritive value. Bifidobacterium and Lactobacillus species are the primarily cited probiotic organisms for use in newborns. These are the same species that colonize the intestine of breast-fed infants while having delayed colonization in preterm infants. The mechanism of action is unknown, but probiotics may inhibit binding of pathogenic organisms, enhance intestinal maturation, and reduce systemic inflammation.[102] Supplementation with Bifidobacterium reduces the frequency of NEC in a rat model of the disease.[30] Several clinical studies using a variety of probiotic organisms in various patient populations and using different protocols have also demonstrated a positive effect.[70–71,103–105] The questions of which probiotic is optimal, the safety of administration of live bacteria to the immunocompromised preterm infant, the mechanism of action, and who to treat for how long remain unanswered.

Since NEC is rapidly progressive and therapeutic interventions are limited, many investigators have attempted to identify an early marker of the disease. Several studies have explored measurement of cytokine levels to determine which infants will progress to severe NEC. IL-8, IL-10, and IL-1 receptor antagonist levels each have been found to correlate with disease severity. but they are currently not used clinically.[88] A study by Rabinowitz and colleagues demonstrated that serum levels of the phospholipid platelet-activating factor correlate with NEC severity and recovery and may increase prior to the onset of clinical symptoms.[106] Other groups are currently assessing techniques to identify a unique intestinal microbial pattern or genetic predisposition that increases susceptibility for this disease.

CONCLUSION

NEC is a devastating condition without a precise known etiology. It specifically affects preterm infants and appears to be the result of an

---

Table 3 Teatment
Cessation of enteral feeds
Nasogastric decompression
Fluid resuscitation
Broad-spectrum antibiotics
Correction of anemia and thrombocytopenia
Respiratory support as needed
Careful monitoring of clinical exam
Serial abdominal radiographs
Surgical indications—extraintestinal air, ongoing necrosis, abdominal wall cellulitis, fixed loop on serial abdominal radiographs

inflammatory response to risk factors, including bacterial colonization, intestinal ischemia/hypoxia, and formula feeding. The balance of pro- and anti-inflammatory influences appears to be a fundamental factor. The premature infant differs from term infants and older patients in multiple ways, including the complex system of intestinal host defense, intestinal motility, bacterial colonization patterns, autoregulation of splanchnic blood flow, and regulation of the inflammatory cascade. Preterm infants are uniquely susceptible because of an immature immune system that is unable to sufficiently protect against pathogenic organisms. In fact, the immature enterocyte may itself increase injury by excessive cytokine production in response to gram-negative organisms. Although preventing prematurity would be the most successful approach to prevent NEC, strategies to enhance intestinal maturation and modulate inflammatory reactions should serve to decrease intestinal injury.

REFERENCES

1. Kliegman RM, Fanaroff AA. Necrotizing enterocolitis. N Engl J Med 1984;310:1093–103.
2. Caplan MS, MacKendrick W. Necrotizing enterocolitis: A review of pathogenetic mechanisms and implications for prevention. Pediatr Pathol 1993;13:357–69.
3. Bolisetty S, Lui K. Necrotizing enterocolitis in full-term neonates. J Paediatr Child Health 2001;37:413–4.
4. Lopez SL, Taeusch HW, Findlay RD, Walther FJ. Time of onset of necrotizing enterocolitis in newborn infants with known pre-natal cocaine exposure. Clin Pediatr (Phila) 1995;34:424–9.
5. Martinez-Tallo E, Claure N, Bancalari E. Necrotizing enterocolitis in full-term or near-term infants: Risk factors. Biol Neonate 1997;71:292–8.
6. Rodin AE, Nichols MM, Hsu FL. Necrotizing enterocolitis occurring in full-term neonates at birth. Arch Pathol 1973;96:335–8.
7. Wiswell TE, Robertson CF, Jones TA, Tuttle DJ. Necrotizing enterocolitis in full-term infants. A case-control study. Am J Dis Child 1988;142:532–5.
8. MacKendrick W, Caplan M. Necrotizing enterocolitis. New thoughts about pathogenesis and potential treatments. Pediatr Clin North Am 1993;40:1047–59.
9. Kosloske AM. Epidemiology of necrotizing enterocolitis. Acta Paediatr Suppl 1994;396:2–7.
10. Rayyis SF, Ambalavanan N, Wright L, Carlo WA. Randomized trial of slow versus fast feed advancements on the incidence of necrotizing enterocolitis in very low birth weight infants. J Pediatr 1999;134:293–7.
11. Lemons JA, Bauer CR, Oh W, et al. Very low birth weight out-comes of the National Institute of Child Health and Human Development Neonatal Research Network, January 1995 through December 1996. NICHD Neonatal Research Network. Pediatrics 2001;107:E1.
12. Beeby PJ, Jeffery H. Risk factors for necrotising enterocolitis: The influence of gestational age. Arch Dis Child 1992;67:432–5.
13. Lucas A, Cole TJ. Breast milk and neonatal necrotising enterocolitis. Lancet 1990;336:1519–23.
14. Ryder RW, Shelton JD, Guinan ME. Necrotizing enterocolitis: A prospective multicenter investigation. Am J Epidemiol 1980;112:113–23.
15. Uauy RD, Fanaroff AA, Korones SB, et al. Necrotizing enterocolitis in very low birth weight infants: Biodemographic and clinical correlates. National Institute of Child Health and Human Development Neonatal Research Network. J Pediatr 1991;119:630–8.
16. Walsh MC, Kliegman RM. Necrotizing enterocolitis: Treatment based on staging criteria. Pediatr Clin North Am 1986;33:179–201.
17. Faix RG, Adams JT. Neonatal necrotizing enterocolitis: Current concepts and controversies. Adv Pediatr Infect Dis 1994;9:1–36.
18. Bell MJ, Ternberg JL, Feigin RD, et al. Neonatal necrotizing enterocolitis. Therapeutic decisions based upon clinical staging. Ann Surg 1978;187:1–7.

19. Ballance WA, Dahms BB, Shenker N, Kliegman RM. Pathology of neonatal necrotizing enterocolitis: A ten-year experience. J Pediatr 1990;117:S6–13.
20. Willoughby RE, Jr, Pickering LK. Necrotizing enterocolitis and infection. Clin Perinatol 1994;21:307–15.
21. Ford H, Watkins S, Reblock K, Rowe M. The role of inflammatory cytokines and nitric oxide in the pathogenesis of necrotizing enterocolitis. J Pediatr Surg 1997;32:275–82.
22. Santulli TV, Schullinger JN, Heird WC, et al. Acute necrotizing enterocolitis in infancy: A review of 64 cases. Pediatrics 1975;55:376–87.
23. Bines JE, Walker WA. Growth factors and the development of neonatal host defense. Adv Exp Med Biol 1991;310:31–9.
24. Furlano RI, Walker WA. Immaturity of gastrointestinal host defense in newborns and gastrointestinal disease states. Adv Pediatr 1998;45:201–22.
25. Nowicki PT, Nankervis CA, Miller CE. Effects of ischemia and reperfusion on intrinsic vascular regulation in the postnatal intestinal circulation. Pediatr Res 1993;33:400–4.
26. Nowicki PT, Miller CE, Haun SE. Effects of arterial hypoxia and isoproterenol on in vitro postnatal intestinal circulation. Am J Physiol 1988;255:H1144–8.
27. Duffy LC, Zielezny MA, Carrion V, et al. Concordance of bacterial cultures with endotoxin and interleukin-6 in necrotizing enterocolitis. Dig Dis Sci 1997;42:359–65.
28. Duffy LC, Zielezny MA, Carrion V, et al. Bacterial toxins and enteral feeding of premature infants at risk for necrotizing enterocolitis. Adv Exp Med Biol 2001;501:519–27.
29. Deitch EA. Role of bacterial translocation in necrotizing enterocolitis. Acta Paediatr Suppl 1994;396:33–6.
30. Caplan MS, Miller-Catchpole R, Kaup S, et al. Bifidobacterial supplementation reduces the incidence of necrotizing enterocolitis in a neonatal rat model. Gastroenterology 1999;117:577–83.
31. Caplan MS, Hedlund E, Adler L, Hsueh W. Role of asphyxia and feeding in a neonatal rat model of necrotizing enterocolitis. Pediatr Pathol 1994;14:1017–28.
32. Dvorak B, Halpern MD, Holubec H, et al. Epidermal growth factor reduces the development of necrotizing enterocolitis in a neonatal rat model. Am J Physiol Gastrointest Liver Physiol 2002;282:G156–64.
33. Caplan MS, Sun XM, Hseuh W, Hageman JR. Role of platelet activating factor and tumor necrosis factor-alpha in neonatal necrotizing enterocolitis. J Pediatr 1990;116:960–4.
34. Nanthakumar NN, Fusunyan RD, Sanderson I, Walker WA. Inflammation in the developing human intestine: A possible pathophysiologic contribution to necrotizing enterocolitis. Proc Natl Acad Sci U S A 2000;97:6043–8.
35. Berseth CL. Gestational evolution of small intestine motility in preterm and term infants. J Pediatr 1989;115:646–51.
36. Berseth CL. Neonatal small intestinal motility: Motor responses to feeding in term and preterm infants. J Pediatr 1990;117:777–82.
37. Berseth CL. Gut motility and the pathogenesis of necrotizing enterocolitis. Clin Perinatol 1994;21:263–70.
38. Dai D, Nanthkumar NN, Newburg DS, Walker WA. Role of oligosaccharides and glycoconjugates in intestinal host defense. J Pediatr Gastroenterol Nutr 2000;30:S23–33.
39. Chu SH, Walker WA. Developmental changes in the activities of sialyl and fucosyltransferases in rat small intestine. Biochim Biophys Acta 1986;883:496–500.
40. Snyder JD, Walker WA. Structure and function of intestinal mucin: Developmental aspects. Int Arch Allergy Appl Immunol 1987;82:351–6.
41. Udall JN, Jr, Gastrointestinal host defense and necrotizing enterocolitis. J Pediatr 1990;117:S33–43.
42. Eibl MM, Wolf HM, Furnkranz H, Rosenkranz A. Prevention of necrotizing enterocolitis in low-birth-weight infants by IgAIgG feeding. N Engl J Med 1988;319:1–7.
43. Roberts SA, Freed DL. Neonatal IgA secretion enhanced by breast feeding. Lancet 1977;ii:1131.
44. Tan XD, Hsueh W, Chang H, et al. Characterization of a putative receptor for intestinal trefoil factor in rat small intestine: Identification by in situ binding and ligand blotting. Biochem Biophys Res Commun 1997;237:673–7.
45. Hoffmann W. Trefoil factors TFF (trefoil factor family) peptide-triggered signals promoting mucosal restitution. Cell Mol Life Sci 2005;62:2932–8.
46. Lin J, Holzman IR, Jiang P, Babyatsky MW. Expression of intestinal trefoil factor in developing rat intestine. Biol Neonate 1999;76:92–7.
47. Ouellette AJ. Paneth cells and innate immunity in the crypt microenvironment. Gastroenterology 1997;113:1779–84.
48. Salzman NH, Polin RA, Harris MC, et al. Enteric defensin expression in necrotizing enterocolitis. Pediatr Res 1998;44:20–6.
49. Alward CT, Hook JB, Helmrath TA, et al. Effects of asphyxia on cardiac output and organ blood flow in the newborn piglet. Pediatr Res 1978;12:824–7.

50. Touloukian RJ, Posch JN, Spencer R. The pathogenesis of ischemic gastroenterocolitis of the neonate: Selective gut mucosal ischemia in asphyxiated neonatal piglets. J Pediatr Surg 1972;7:194–205.
51. Nowicki PT, Hansen NB, Hayes JR, et al. Intestinal blood flow and O_2 uptake during hypoxemia in the newborn piglet. Am J Physiol 1986;251:G19–24.
52. Nowicki PT. Effects of sustained flow reduction on postnatal intestinal circulation. Am J Physiol 1998;275:G758–68.
53. Nankervis CA, Reber KM, Nowicki PT. Age-dependent changes in the postnatal intestinal microcirculation. Microcirculation 2001;8:377–87.
54. Reber KM, Su BY, Clark KR, et al. Developmental expression of eNOS in postnatal swine mesenteric artery. Am J Physiol Gastrointest Liver Physiol 2002;283:G1328–35.
55. Nowicki PT, Minnich LA. Effects of systemic hypotension on postnatal intestinal circulation: Role of angiotensin. Am J Physiol 1999;276:G341–52.
56. Kamitsuka MD, Horton MK, Williams MA. The incidence of necrotizing enterocolitis after introducing standardized feeding schedules for infants between 1250 and 2500 grams and less than 35 weeks of gestation. Pediatrics 2000;105:379–84.
57. Tyson JE, Kennedy KA. Minimal enteral nutrition for promoting feeding tolerance and preventing morbidity in parenterally fed infants. Cochrane Database Syst Rev 2000;CD000504.
58. Clark DA, Miller MJ. Intraluminal pathogenesis of necrotizing enterocolitis. J Pediatr 1990;117:S64–7.
59. Caplan MS, Russell T, Xiao Y, et al. Effect of polyunsaturated fatty acid (PUFA) supplementation on intestinal inflammation and necrotizing enterocolitis (NEC) in a neonatal rat model. Pediatr Res 2001;49:647–52.
60. Caplan MS, Hedlund E, Adler L, et al. The platelet-activating factor receptor antagonist WEB 2170 prevents neonatal necrotizing enterocolitis in rats. J Pediatr Gastroenterol Nutr 1997;24:296–301.
61. Hoy C, Millar MR, MacKay P, et al. Quantitative changes in faecal microflora preceding necrotising enterocolitis in premature neonates. Arch Dis Child 1990;65:1057–9.
62. Gronlund MM, Lehtonen OP, Eerola E, Kero P. Fecal microflora in healthy infants born by different methods of delivery: Permanent changes in intestinal flora after cesarean delivery. J Pediatr Gastroenterol Nutr 1999;28:19–25.
63. Harmsen HJ, Wildeboer-Veloo AC, Raangs GC, et al. Analysis of intestinal flora development in breast-fed and formula-fed infants by using molecular identification and detection methods. J Pediatr Gastroenterol Nutr 2000;30:61–7.
64. Orrhage K, Nord CE. Factors controlling the bacterial colonization of the intestine in breastfed infants. Acta Paediatr Suppl 1999;88:47–57.
65. Gewolb IH, Schwalbe RS, Taciak VL, et al. Stool microflora in extremely low birth weight infants. Arch Dis Child Fetal Neonatal Ed 1999;80:F167–73.
66. Rubaltelli FF, Biadaioli R, Pecile P, Nicoletti P. Intestinal flora in breast and bottle-fed infants. J Perinat Med 1998;26:186–91.
67. Tomkins AM, Bradley AK, Oswald S, Drasar BS. Diet and the faecal microflora of infants, children and adults in rural Nigeria and urban U.K. J Hyg (Lond) 1981;86:285–93.
68. Wold AE, Adlerberth I. Breast feeding and the intestinal microflora of the infant-implications for protection against infectious diseases. Adv Exp Med Biol 2000;478:77–93.
69. Panigrahi P, Gupta S, Gewolb IH, Morris JG, Jr. Occurrence of necrotizing enterocolitis may be dependent on patterns of bacterial adherence and intestinal colonization: Studies in Caco-2 tissue culture and weanling rabbit models. Pediatr Res 1994;36:115–21.
70. Hoyos AB. Reduced incidence of necrotizing enterocolitis associated with enteral administration of Lactobacillus acidophilus and Bifidobacterium infantis to neonates in an intensive care unit. Int J Infect Dis 1999;3:197–202.
71. Lin HC, Su BH, Chen AC, et al. Oral probiotics reduce the incidence and severity of necrotizing enterocolitis in very low birth weight infants. Pediatrics 2005;115:1–4.
72. Lodinova-Zadnikova R, Slavikova M, Tlaskalova-Hogenova H, et al. The antibody response in breast-fed and non-breast-fed infants after artificial colonization of the intestine with Escherichia coli O83. Pediatr Res 1991;29:396–9.
73. Bocker U, Schottelius A, Watson JM, et al. Cellular differentiation causes a selective down-regulation of interleukin (IL)-1betamediated NF-kappaB activation and IL-8 gene expression in intestinal epithelial cells. J Biol Chem 2000;275:12207–13.
74. Chung DH, Ethridge RT, Kim S, et al. Molecular mechanisms contributing to necrotizing enterocolitis. Ann Surg 2001;233:835–42.
75. Abreu MT, Vora P, Faure E, et al. Decreased expression of Toll-like receptor-4 and MD-2 correlates with intestinal

epithelial cell protection against dysregulated proinflammatory gene expression in response to bacterial lipopolysaccharide. J Immunol 2001;167:1609–16.

76. Eaves-Pyles T, Murthy K, Liaudet L, et al. Flagellin, a novel mediator of Salmonella-induced epithelial activation and systemic inflammation: I kappa B alpha degradation, induction of nitric oxide synthase, induction of proinflammatory mediators, and cardiovascular dysfunction. J Immunol 2001;166:1248–60.

77. Steiner TS, Nataro JP, Poteet-Smith CE, et al. Enteroaggregative *Escherichia coli* expresses a novel flagellin that causes IL-8 release from intestinal epithelial cells. J Clin Invest 2000;105:1769–77.

78. Molmenti EP, Ziambaras T, Perlmutter DH. Evidence for an acute phase response in human intestinal epithelial cells. J Biol Chem 1993;268:14116–24.

79. Nadler EP, Stanford A, Zhang XR, et al. Intestinal cytokine gene expression in infants with acute necrotizing enterocolitis: Interleukin-11 mRNA expression inversely correlates with extent of disease. J Pediatr Surg 2001;36:1122–9.

80. Tan X, Hsueh W, Gonzalez-Crussi F. Cellular localization of tumor necrosis factor (TNF)-alpha transcripts in normal bowel and in necrotizing enterocolitis. TNF gene expression by Paneth cells, intestinal eosinophils, and macrophages. Am J Pathol 1993;142:1858–65.

81. Viscardi RM, Lyon NH, Sun CC, et al. Inflammatory cytokine mRNAs in surgical specimens of necrotizing enterocolitis and normal newborn intestine. Pediatr Pathol Lab Med 1997;17:547–59.

82. Harris MC, Costarino AT, Jr, Sullivan JS, et al. Cytokine elevations in critically ill infants with sepsis and necrotizing enterocolitis. J Pediatr 1994;124:105–11.

83. Morecroft JA, Spitz L, Hamilton PA, Holmes SJ. Plasma cytokine levels in necrotizing enterocolitis. Acta Paediatr Suppl 1994;396:18–20.

84. Rabinowitz SS, Dzakpasu P, Piecuch S, et al. Platelet-activating factor in infants at risk for necrotizing enterocolitis. J Pediatr 2001;138:81–6.

85. Hsueh W, Gonzalez-Crussi F. Ischemic bowel necrosis induced by platelet-activating factor: An experimental model. Methods Achiev Exp Pathol 1988;13:208–39.

86. Hsueh W, Gonzalez-Crussi F, Arroyave JL, et al. Platelet activating factor-induced ischemic bowel necrosis: The effect of PAF antagonists. Eur J Pharmacol 1986;123:79–83.

87. Lindsay JO, Hodgson HJ. Review article: The immunoregulatory cytokine interleukin-10a therapy for Crohn's disease? Aliment Pharmacol Ther 2001;15:1709–16.

88. Edelson MB, Bagwell CE, Rozycki HJ. Circulating pro and counterinflammatory cytokine levels and severity in necrotizing enterocolitis. Pediatrics 1999;103:766–71.

89. Jilling T, Simon D, Lu J, et al. The roles of bacteria and TLR4 in rat and murine models of necrotizing enterocolitis. J Immunol 2006;177:3273–82.

90. Claud EC, Lu L, Anton PM, et al. Developmentally regulated I kappaB expression in intestinal epithelium and susceptibility to flagellin-induced inflammation. Proc Natl Acad Sci U S A 2004;101:7404–8.

91. Hintz SR, Kendrick DE, Stoll BJ, et al. Neurodevelopmental and growth outcomes of extremely low birth weight infants after necrotizing enterocolitis. Pediatrics 2005;115:696–703.

92. Moss RL, Dimmitt RA, Barnhart DC, et al. Laparotomy versus peritoneal drainage for necrotizing enterocolitis and perforation. N Engl J Med 2006;354:2225–34.

93. Hansbrough F, Priebe CJ, Jr, Falterman KW, et al. Pathogenesis of early necrotizing enterocolitis in the hypoxic neonatal dog. Am J Surg 1983;145:169–75.

94. Furukawa M, Lee EL, Johnston JM. Platelet-activating factor-induced ischemic bowel necrosis: The effect of platelet-activating factor acetylhydrolase. Pediatr Res 1993;34:237–41.

95. Moya FR, Eguchi H, Zhao B, et al. Platelet-activating factor acetylhydrolase in term and preterm human milk: A preliminary report. J Pediatr Gastroenterol Nutr 1994;19:236–9.

96. Carlson SE, Montalto MB, Ponder DL, et al. Lower incidence of necrotizing enterocolitis in infants fed a preterm formula with egg phospholipids. Pediatr Res 1998;44:491–8.

97. Sullivan PB, Brueton MJ, Tabara ZB, et al. Epidermal growth factor in necrotising enteritis. Lancet 1991;338:53–4.

98. Feng J, El-Assal ON, Besner GE. Heparin-binding epidermal growth factor-like growth factor decreases the incidence of necrotizing enterocolitis in neonatal rats. J Pediatr Surg 2006;41:144–9, discussion 144–9.

99. Halpern MD, Clark JA, Saunders TA, et al. Reduction of experimental necrotizing enterocolitis with anti TNF alpha. Am J Physiol Gastrointest Liver Physiol 2006;290:G757–64.

100. Halac E, Halac J, Begue EF, et al. Prenatal and postnatal corticosteroid therapy to prevent neonatal necrotizing enterocolitis: A controlled trial. J Pediatr 1990;117:132–8.

101. Israel EJ, Schiffrin EJ, Carter EA, et al. Prevention of necrotizing enterocolitis in the rat with prenatal cortisone. Gastroenterology 1990;99:1333–8.

102. Zhang L, Li N, des Robert C, et al. Lactobacillus rhamnosus GG decreases lipopolysaccharide-induced systemic inflammation in a gastrostomy-fed infant rat model. J Pediatr Gastroenterol Nutr 2006;42:545–52.

103. Kitajima H, Sumida Y, Tanaka R, et al. Early administration of *Bifidobacterium breve* to preterm infants: Randomised controlled trial. Arch Dis Child Fetal Neonatal Ed 1997;76:F101–7.

104. Dani C, Biadaioli R, Bertini G, et al. Probiotics feeding in prevention of urinary tract infection, bacterial sepsis and necrotizing enterocolitis in preterm infants. A prospective double-blind study. Biol Neonate 2002;82:103–8.

105. Bin-Nun A, Bromiker R, Wilschanski M, et al. Oral probiotics prevent necrotizing enterocolitis in very low birth weight neonates. J Pediatr 2005;147:192–6.

106. Rabinowitz SS, Dzakpasu P, Piecuch S, et al. Platelet-activating factor in infants at risk for necrotizing enterocolitis. J Pediatr 2001;138:81–6.

20.5. Chronic Inflammatory Bowel Disease

20.5a. Crohn's Disease

Anne M. Griffiths, MD, FRCP(C)
Jean-Pierre Hugot, MD, PhD

Crohn's disease denotes a phenotypically diverse, chronic inflammatory disorder of the gastrointestinal tract, which manifests during childhood or adolescence in up to 25% of patients. The identification of genetic determinants of susceptibility to inflammatory bowel disease (IBD), and to Crohn's disease specifically, has provided important insight into disease pathogenesis. Increasing evidence supports the contention that Crohn's disease results from genetic predisposition to interact abnormally with an environmental stimulus, which in turn leads to excessive immune activation and chronic intestinal inflammation.

In 2001, two independent groups of investigators concurrently identified nucleotide oligomerization domain 2 (NOD2), subsequently renamed caspase recruitment domain protein 15 (CARD15), as a Crohn's disease susceptibility gene.[1–2] This landmark discovery marked the first time that a gene in any complex disorder had been first localized by linkage studies[3] and then positionally cloned.[1] CARD15 participates in the innate immune system, which regulates the immediate response to microbial pathogens.[4] The recognition of CARD15 mutations in Caucasian patients with both sporadic and familial but, particularly, ileal Crohn's disease,[1,2,5] clearly linked genetic susceptibility and enteric bacteria, two factors long hypothesized as important in etiopathogenesis. The discovery of Crohn's disease-associated CARD15 polymorphisms refocused basic IBD research on the innate immune response. The role of bacteria and the mechanisms by which CARD15 polymorphisms predispose individuals to chronic intestinal inflammation continue to be elucidated. Recognizing that CARD15 variants explain only a fraction of the heritability of Crohn's disease, other susceptibility loci have been sought and intensely investigated.

Recently, a genome-wide association study has linked variants in the interleukin-23 (IL-23) receptor gene with Crohn's disease susceptibility, an observation with again major implications for our understanding of key pathways in innate and T-cell mediated chronic intestinal inflammation.[6–7] There is reason for optimism that progress in the elucidation of mechanisms will have clinical applications, both in explaining observed disease heterogeneity and in the development of novel targeted therapies.

This chapter aims to review the epidemiology, etiologic hypotheses, clinical manifestations, and current management of Crohn's disease in chil-

dren and adolescents. The emphasis will be on the exciting recent progress in understanding factors involved in disease pathogenesis and on the significant evidence-based advances in medical treatment.

EPIDEMIOLOGY

Classical epidemiologic studies characterize disease with regard to person, place, time, and associations. Hypotheses as to etiologic factors are then generated to explain observed variations in incidence.

Trends in Time

What has come to be known eponymously as Crohn's disease was first described as "regional ileitis" in 1932, although it was considered likely that the same pathologic and clinical entity had been the subject of published case reports even in the early nineteenth century.[8] The occurrence of Crohn's disease increased sharply in all age groups in most Western populations between the 1950s and 1980s. Recent longitudinal data over periods of at least 15 years have been obtained from specific geographic populations in Europe and North America.[9] From these studies, two patterns of change in incidence rates are apparent: the first is an increase followed by a plateau; the second a steady continuing increase.[9]

Increases in childhood and adolescent Crohn's disease have paralleled overall population trends. The incidence of Crohn's disease doubled among children in Wales from 1983 to 1993.[10] A threefold rise in the incidence of Crohn's disease among Scottish children between 1968 and 1983 and a continued rise at the same rate between 1981 and 1992 have been reported.[11–12]

Assessment of worldwide data demonstrates a third longitudinal pattern of IBD incidence: prolonged minimal incidence followed by a very recent increase, such as has been observed in most Asian Pacific countries including China, Korea, India, and Japan.[13] To date, this rise in incidence has been more notable for ulcerative colitis than Crohn's disease.[13]

Geographic Trends

As reviewed by Loftus, the worldwide distributions of Crohn's disease and ulcerative colitis are similar; both have historically been most prevalent in North America, Northern Europe, and in the United Kingdom.[14] Recent studies reporting the incidence of pediatric onset illness in countries where IBD is most common are summarized in Table 1.[10–12,15–19] Reported incidence rates may be significantly influenced by even slight variations in the definition of childhood, because of the steep rise in age-specific incidence during the teenage years.

Trends in Age and Gender

Peak incidences of Crohn's disease are observed in late adolescence or young adulthood.[14] There is no convincing evidence that age at onset is decreasing. The incidence of pediatric Crohn's disease generally exceeds that of pediatric ulcerative colitis, although among children very young at presentation ulcerative colitis or colonic IBD, type undefined, appears to predominate.[20–21]

Table 1 Recent Incidence Data for Inflammatory Bowel Disease in Children and Adolescents

Location (Reference)	Age Criteria	Calendar Years of Study	Incidence of Pediatric Crohn's disease (Per 100,000 Per Year)	Incidence of Pediatric Ulcerative Colitis (Per 100,000 Per Year)
Scotland[11,12]	=≤16 yr at symptom onset	1981 to 1983	2.3	1.6
		1990 to 1992	2.8	
South Glamorgan, Wales[10]	<16 yr at diagnosis	1989 to 1993	3.1 (95% CI 1.8 to 5.3)	0.7
Nord-Pas-de-Calais, France[15]	≤15 yr at diagnosis	1984 to 1989	2.1	0.5
Western Norway[17]	≤15 yr at diagnosis	1984 to 1985	2.5	4.3
Metropolitan Toronto, Canada[18]	≤17 yr at diagnosis	1991 to 1996	3.7	2.7
United Kingdom and Ireland[19]	<16 yr at diagnosis	1998 to 1999	3.0	2.2*
Copenhagen, County, Denmark[16]	<15 yr at diagnosis	1962 to 1987	0.2	2.0

*Provisionally labeled indeterminate colitis included with ulcerative colitis.

Table 2 Comparison of Demographic Data at Time of Diagnosis of Crohn's Disease

	Greater Toronto Area 1980 to 1996	United Kingdom and Ireland 1998 to 1999
Total number of children diagnosed with IBD	787	739
Crohn's disease: number (% of total)	486 (61.8)	379 (58)
Gender	62% male	62% male
Age at diagnosis (yr)	12.7 ± − 2.56 (mean ± SD)	12.9 (10.8 to 14.3) median (interquartile range: Q1 to Q3)

The Toronto, Canada, data concern children prospectively registered at the time of diagnosis in The Hospital for Sick Children pediatric IBD database. The United Kingdom and Ireland data represent the results of a 13-month surveillance of incident IBD cases (reference 19).

For Crohn's disease overall, the incidence among females exceeds that among males by 20 to 30%.[9,14] In contrast, however, studies restricted to pediatric-onset Crohn's disease document a male to female preponderance.[19–20,22] As summarized in Table 2, demographic data from a recently completed survey of new diagnoses of IBD among patients less than 16 years in the United Kingdom and Ireland are strikingly similar to relatively population-based data from the urban center of metropolitan Toronto, Canada, concerning children and adolescents diagnosed with IBD between 1980 and 1996.[19–20]

Trends Among Races and in Ethnic Groups

Individuals of Jewish descent appear particularly susceptible to IBD.[23–24] Their incidence rates for ulcerative colitis and Crohn's disease vary tremendously around the world, in parallel with but always remaining three to four times greater than the local non-Jewish population risk.[24] The persistence of increased risk across different time periods and geographical areas provides indirect evidence that there is a genetic predisposition to develop IBD.

ETIOPATHOGENESIS

It is unlikely that a simple cause and effect relation accounts for the majority of Crohn's disease. Rather, it is hypothesized that the chronic immune-mediated intestinal injury results from complex interactions between predisposing genetic factors and exogenous or endogenous triggers, likely microbial in origin.[25] The proposed multifactorial etiopathogenesis is summarized schematically in Figure 1. Impressive progress has been made in elucidating the genetic basis of Crohn's disease susceptibility, but to date the precise role played by the intestinal microflora in triggering and perpetuating chronic inflammation remains elusive.

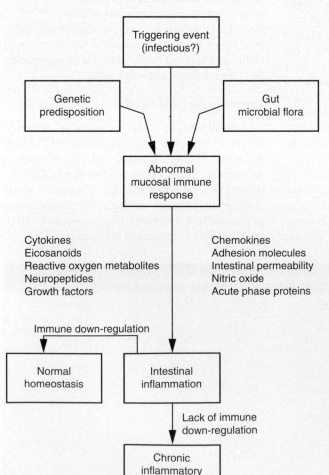

Figure 1 Multifactorial etiopathogenesis of Crohn's disease. It is postulated that in a genetically susceptible individual, interacting environmental factors and the host intestinal microbial flora, in the presence of a yet unspecified triggering event, activate an aberrant immune response, the end result of which is chronic intestinal inflammation.

GENETIC SUSCEPTIBILITY

Observations from Family Studies

The familial occurrence of Crohn's disease is well recognized.[26–28] A positive family history in a first-degree relative remains the major identified risk factor for its development. Familial aggregation could be explained by shared environmental or by genetic factors. However, the relative rarity in spouses compared to first-degree relatives and, most convincingly, data from studies comparing disease concordance in monozygotic versus dizygotic twins argue for the importance of genetic factors.[29–30]

A high (44.4 to 58%) rate of concordance for Crohn's disease among monozygotic twins versus dizygotic twins (0 to 3.8%) was reported in Swedish and Danish studies, respectively, based on unselected twin registries.[29–30] If only environmental factors were involved in Crohn's disease, the observed concordance rates between dizygotic twins and monozygotic twins would be expected to be the same. Conversely, since monozygotic twins share identical genomic material, and yet are not 100% concordant for Crohn's disease, no combination of genes is sufficient for the development of Crohn's disease. Rather, some environmental trigger is also required for the disease to be expressed.

The relative importance of genetic versus environmental factors, or heritability, is commonly expressed as λs, the prevalence in siblings divided by population prevalence.[27] For Crohn's disease, the overall λs has been calculated in several studies worldwide to range between 10 and 35.[27] Hence the relative contribution of genetic factors to the pathogenesis of Crohn's disease is greater than in schizophrenia, asthma, or hypertension, and is at least equivalent to that identified in insulin-dependent diabetes.

Familial aggregation is more common among Jewish versus non-Jewish patients.[20,31] The age-adjusted empiric risks for developing inflammatory bowel disease during a lifetime were calculated for first-degree relatives of Jewish and non-Jewish white probands with Crohn's disease in a study from southern California.[31] The age-adjusted lifetime risks for siblings of Jewish and non-Jewish probands with Crohn's disease were 16.8 and 7.0%, respectively.[31]

Crohn's disease and ulcerative colitis are observed to coexist in the same family with a frequency higher than just the cooccurrence by chance alone.[20,26–28] Nevertheless, concordance within a family for the type of inflammatory bowel disease is much more common than discordance.[20,26–28] These observations indicate that the two diseases share some but not all susceptibility genes.

Genetic factors may be particularly important in the development of early onset IBD. Polito and colleagues reported the proportion of patients with affected relatives according to the age at diagnosis in the proband.[32] Thirty percent of 177 patients diagnosed under age 20 years had a positive family history. The percentage decreased to 18% for those diagnosed between 20 and 39 years of age ($n = 311$) and to 13% among those diagnosed after age 40 years ($n = 67$).[32] Among a cohort of 770 probands with pediatric onset IBD in Toronto, Canada, 16% had a first-degree relative (parent and/or sibling) also affected.[20] Thirty percent of the Jewish children with Crohn's disease had one or more first-degree relative(s) with IBD.[20]

The number of genes, which may confer susceptibility to IBD, is still unknown. Initial segregation analyses led investigators to hypothesize that a major autosomal recessive gene may account for a proportion of the genetic predisposition to Crohn's disease.[33] It is usually accepted, however, that IBD involves multiple susceptibility loci, as well as genetic heterogeneity (whereby different genes result in a similar disease phenotype), and both gene–gene and gene–environment interactions in a complex system.[34–35]

Gene Identification Techniques

Two complementary strategies are used to search for the genetic determinants of a disease trait: genome-wide searches (by linkage studies and more recently by association studies) and candidate gene analysis.

A genome-wide linkage analysis begins with the ascertainment of numerous "sibling pair" families: two affected siblings and their parents (whether affected or not). In these families, systematic screening of the entire human genome using highly polymorphic markers consisting of di- and trinucleotide repeats provides a strategy for localizing genes without prior hypotheses about their nature. The markers have no direct relationship to disease pathogenesis, but when there is an excess of a marker allele shared among individuals with the disease, the disease gene and the marker locus are presumed to be transmitted together by virtue of being in proximity on the same chromosome.[36] Since 1996, several genome-wide linkage studies have been published, together identifying nine replicated susceptibility loci (IBD1 to IBD9) presumed to contain causal genes.[35] Whereas some loci seem specific to Crohn's disease, others are associated with IBD overall.[35]

More recently SNPs (single nucleotide polymorphisms) have been utilized in the place of microsatellite markers for the purpose of performing genome-wide association studies.[6,37–38] SNPs represent sites along the genome in which single base pair variation occurs from person to person where the least frequent allele has a frequency of 1% or greater. Many SNPs occur within genes, with some representing variations which alter gene function and, as such, may even represent the genetic lesion of interest. As many as 500,000 SNPs can be analyzed using high-throughput genotyping. This powerful approach to identifying susceptibility and disease-modifying genes is feasible because of the HapMap reference panel of common genetic variation. Among the first investigators to successfully employ this strategy in a complex disorder, two international IBD groups very recently identi-

fied associations between Crohn's disease and, respectively, the interleukin-23 receptor gene on chromosome 1p31, and a coding variant of autophagy-related 16 like-1 (ATG16L1) gene on chromosome 2q37.1.[6,37–38]

The candidate gene approach to confirmation of susceptibility genes requires determination of the frequency of different alleles at a polymorphic locus on a putative disease gene in patients versus ethnically matched controls (case-control studies). If a statistically significant difference is observed between the two groups, the allele that is more prevalent in the patient group is said to be associated with the disease. However, spurious associations may be generated by ignoring differences between the control and the disease groups that are not related to the disease. To overcome the bias of improper matching, tests that incorporate analysis of unaffected parents are used. As an example, in transmission disequilibrium testing the frequency with which an allele is transmitted from parents to affected children is compared to the theoretically expected value of 0.5. Significant departure from this expected value confirms an association between the allele and the disease. Case-control candidate gene studies and transmission disequilibrium testing using mother-father-offspring "trios" are used to test the significance of genes localized or identified by linkage or genome-wide association studies.[6,35,37–38]

Identification of CARD15/NOD2 as a Crohn's Disease Susceptibility Gene

Hugot and colleagues reported the first total genome scan in families with two or more siblings affected with Crohn's disease, and thereby identified the pericentromeric region of chromosome 16 as a possible locus of a Crohn's disease gene.[3] Linkage to this region, named IBD1, was subsequently confirmed in a multicenter replication study undertaken by the International IBD Genetics Consortium.[39] The eventual identification at this locus of NOD2, further renamed caspase recruitment domain protein 15 (CARD15), as the first Crohn's disease susceptibility gene, marked the first time a gene in any complex disorder had been first localized by linkage studies and then positionally cloned.[1,3] At the same time, Ogura and colleagues successfully used a candidate gene approach to gene identification.[2] They selected CARD15 as a potential Crohn's disease gene, based on knowledge of its role in the recognition of bacterial components, and on the gene location within the IBD1 region.

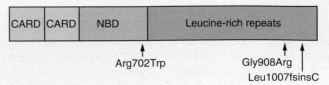

Figure 2 Structure of the NOD2/CARD15 protein. The three common Crohn's disease–associated polymorphisms are located in the leucine-rich repeat (LRR) domain. NBD = nucleotide-binding domain; CARD = caspase recruitment domain.

The 12 exon CARD15 gene encodes an intracellular protein, structurally related to the R proteins in plants, which mediate host resistance to microbial pathogens.[4] As illustrated in Figure 2, the protein product is composed of 1,040 amino acids with several functional domains: two caspase recruitment domains (CARD1 and CARD2), a nucleotide-binding domain (NBD) and a leucine-rich repeat (LRR) domain.[4] The LRR domain functions as a pattern recognition receptor for microbial components. The NBD mediates protein self-oligomerization required for activation.[4] CARDs are domains involved in apoptosis pathways and in NF-κβ activation.

Sequencing of the CARD15 gene in Crohn's disease patients revealed a cytosine insertion at position 3020 in exon 11 (Leu1007fsinsC) that gives rise to a stop codon and a truncated protein.[1–2] This frameshift mutation as well as two other common missense mutations (Arg702Trp, Gly908Arg), all within or near the LRR domain of CARD15 (Figure 2), have been highly associated with Crohn's disease, but not with ulcerative colitis.[1,2,5] This lack of association with ulcerative colitis is consistent with previous negative linkage data at the IBD1 locus.[39] Allelic frequencies for Arg702Trp, Gly908Arg, and Leu1007fsinsC are consistently higher in Caucasian Crohn's disease patients compared to controls.[41] In addition to the three major risk alleles, a number of extremely rare "private" amino acid polymorphisms, particularly within or near the LRR domain, have been defined, each present in only a few families.[1,42] These rare "private" mutations appear, nevertheless, to be similarly associated with disease pathogenesis.

While the three common Crohn's disease-associated polymorphisms are either rare or absent in Asian, Arab, and African populations, it is estimated that 27 to 38% of Caucasian patients with Crohn's disease carry one of the major risk alleles (compared to about 20% of Caucasian controls) and an additional 8 to 17% carry two copies (compared to less than 1% of controls).[41] Allele frequencies, and presumably, therefore, also the importance of CARD15 in conferring susceptibility to Crohn's disease, vary significantly even within Europe, being lower in Scandinavia and Scotland, than in central and southern parts of Europe.[35]

Several phenotypic correlations have emerged, as large patient populations have been genotyped for the Arg702Trp, Gly908Arg, and Leu1007fsinsC NOD2/CARD15 polymorphisms.[40,42–48] Firstly, CARD15 polymorphisms are associated with both sporadic and familial Crohn's disease.[1–2,5,40] Secondly, in multiple studies, a significant association has been found between ileal disease and the carriage of one or more CARD15 risk variant alleles.[40,42–48] Double-dose carriers are very uncommonly observed in colon-only Crohn's disease.[40,42,44] Patients carrying two variant alleles are characterized by a younger age at onset.[40] Finally, some studies have demonstrated an association between CARD15 risk alleles and stricturing behavior.[44–45,47,49]

The mutational spectrum of CARD15 is favorable for genetic analyses because the three major polymorphisms represent more than 80% of the variant alleles and are easily determined in laboratories involved in molecular diagnosis.[1,40] As yet, however, knowledge of CARD15 status has little role in clinical practice. The lack of any association between CARD15 polymorphisms and ulcerative colitis initially suggested that CARD15 genotyping could help to classify indeterminate colitis, but this is precluded by the low frequency of CARD15 mutations in Crohn's disease patients with a ulcerative colitis-like phenotype. To date, CARD15 status has not correlated with any treatment responsiveness, but only response to infliximab therapy has hitherto been studied.[50]

As expected for a complex genetic trait, CARD15 mutations are neither necessary nor sufficient for disease development. A recent meta-analysis calculated that the overall relative risk of developing Crohn's disease in Caucasian populations was 2.4 (95% CI 2.0 to 2.9) for carriers of one mutant allele and 17.1 (95% CI 10.7 to 27.2) for two or more mutant copies.[41] The risk varied with each mutation, with Leu1007fsinsC generally carrying the highest risk and Arg-702Trp the lowest. Given a rough prevalence of 1/1000 inhabitants in Western countries, it can be calculated that the probability of developing the disease (penetrance) is no more than .04 for the group of highest risk.[35] With such a low risk, and in the absence of any preventive action, screening of family members is not currently recommended. It has been estimated, moreover, that the three main CARD15 polymorphisms explain no more than 20% of the genetic predisposition to Crohn's disease even in Caucasians. Such observations are expected for a complex genetic disorder, where the disease results from the complex interplay between several genetic and environmental risk factors.

Other Crohn's Disease–Associated Genes

The number of individual genes, which contribute to the overall susceptibility to Crohn's disease is, as yet, unknown. One of the lessons learned from animal models is that entirely different genetic abnormalities can lead to similar clinical features of intestinal inflammation.[51] Genetic heterogeneity in Crohn's disease (the ability of different genes to result in a similar disease phenotype) could well contribute to the discrepancies observed between studies undertaken in different patient populations.[34–35] Moreover, some genes associated with a disease can modify its phenotype, but not influence susceptibility.[35] Although CARD15 remains the hitherto most important and best characterized Crohn's disease gene, several other loci have been investigated, and new technology is advancing the field rapidly.[6,37–38]

The IBD5 Locus on Chromosome 5q31

This locus was initially identified as significant by two genome-wide scans.[52–53] Subsequent analyses refined the locus to a 250 kb risk haplotype,[54] and the association of this haplotype with IBD has been widely replicated in a number of independent populations.[55–56] The IBD5 risk haplotype has been principally associated with Crohn's disease, although there have been some suggestions of a weak association with ulcerative colitis as well.[57] Phenotypically, the IBD5 locus has been associated with earlier onset disease[52] as well as perianal disease.[56]

Polymorphisms within the organic cation transporter genes (OCTN1 and OCTN2) in the region were suggested as the causative variants based on a combination of functional and genetic evidence.[58] This genetic region is particularly difficult to fine map as it contains a significant degree of linkage disequilibrium, making it difficult to discern a causative allele from a marker allele coinherited with the disease-causing allele.[54,59] Despite the efforts of several investigators, there has been an inability to replicate the findings that the OCTN1 and OCTN2 polymorphisms are independently associated with Crohn's disease. Instead, these additional studies support the possibility that the OCTN1/2 SNPs are simply part of the extended haplotype in the region.[59] OCTN1 and 2 are transporters that mediate transmembrane transport of carnitine and other organic cations. Although putative mechanisms have been suggested,[60] no direct evidence is yet available explaining the role variants in these genes could play in the pathobiology of IBD. With the uncertainty over the role of the OCTN1 and OCTN2, attention has focused on a number of additional genes, including the cytokine cluster, located within the IBD5 locus. All may be equally as likely as the OCTN genes to constitute the IBD5 causal variant.[35,59]

DLG5

The pericentromeric region of chromosome 10 was identified as a potential IBD susceptibility locus in a European genome-wide scan.[61] Stoll and colleagues then used a positional cloning approach in this region to implicate mutations of the Drosophila discs large homolog 5 (DLG5) gene in determining susceptibility to Crohn's disease, conferring a small relative risk of 1.5.[62] DLG5 is putatively involved in maintaining epithelial integrity and thus its dysfunction would be consistent with an etiologic model of impaired barrier function. Many subsequent replication studies have been undertaken with contradictory results, overall still consistent with the possibility that DLG5 has a small effect on IBD susceptibility.[35]

The MHC Region (IBD3) on Chromosome 6p

Linkage of IBD (both ulcerative colitis and Crohn's disease) to the IBD3 region on chromosome 6 has been confirmed in a variety of genome-wide scans.[63] The IBD3 region contains the major histocompatibility complex (MHC) genes (also referred to as the human leukocyte antigen or HLA complex, which is divided into regions I, II, and III). It is possible that HLA in Crohn's disease plays a greater role in determining disease phenotype, such as propensity to extraintestinal manifestations, than initial disease susceptibility.[64] Many other genes in the IBD3 region are also involved in the immune response, including tumor necrosis factor alpha (TNF-α). Associations have been found with polymorphisms in the promoter region; however, their functional significance remains unclear.

ENVIRONMENTAL INFLUENCES

Environmental factors must also be important in the development of Crohn's disease, as evidenced by the rapidly increasing incidence in recent decades,[9,13] as well as by the lack of complete concordance for disease status among monozygotic twins.[29–30] Environmental influences, if shared by family members, may also contribute to familial aggregation, as is supported by a recent analysis of birth order of affected siblings in multiplex families.[64]

The Search for a Specific Microbial Trigger

Over the past 30 years, there has been an intensive search for the antigens that trigger the immune response. The fundamental question regarding the pathogenesis of Crohn's disease has been framed as follows: does the chronic, recurring inflammatory activity reflect an appropriate response to a persistently abnormal stimulus (eg, a persistent causative agent in the intestinal lumen) or an abnormally prolonged response to a ubiquitous stimulus? Although the most widely held theory is that Crohn's disease constitutes a dysregulated immune response to common bacterial antigens, the search for specific pathogens has not been abandoned. An infectious etiology for Crohn's disease, with a direct cause-and-effect relationship between a single microorganism and inflammation in a genetically predisposed host, still remains plausible. The relationship between microbes and defined clinical entities is often ambiguous, but diseases of unknown etiology are unexpectedly proven to be infectious. The most striking example is peptic ulcer disease and *Helicobacter pylori*. A number of putative infectious agents have been proposed and discounted as etiologic factors since Crohn's disease was first identified as an entity distinct from tuberculous ileitis.

Mycobacteria

Mycobacterium paratuberculosis causes Johne's disease, an intestinal disorder in ruminants that clinically and histologically resembles Crohn's disease. Mycobacteria (named M. Linda after the patient) isolated from a Crohn's disease surgical specimen were administered orally to a young goat and caused a disease similar to Johne's disease.[66] It is quite possible, however, that this organism, although pathogenic for goats, is merely a nonpathogenic secondary agent in humans. Despite intensive efforts, *Mycobacterium* species similar or identical to *M. paratuberculosis* can be cultured from relatively few patients with Crohn's disease. Some, but not all, investigators have identified fragments of its DNA by polymerase chain reaction more commonly in Crohn's disease tissue than in tissue from patients with ulcerative colitis or controls.[67] Current evidence suggests that *M. paratuberculosis* is an environmental contaminant that preferentially invades the deeply ulcerated mucosa of Crohn's disease patients to a greater extent that controls. Results, however, do not exclude pathologic infection of a subgroup of Crohn's disease patients.

Viruses

Interest in a viral etiology of Crohn's disease was rekindled by Wakefield and others, who demonstrated evidence of persistent measles infection in foci of granulomatous vasculitis in the intestine of patients with Crohn's disease.[68] It has been proposed that measles infection early in life leads to microvascular thrombosis, multifocal gastrointestinal infarction, and eventually gross pathologic sequelae such as inflammation, fibrosis, and strictures.[69] This has been tied in with a report of a cohort effect of a measles epidemic in childhood with subsequent Crohn's disease and a striking report of three cases of serious Crohn's disease in the children of three out of four mothers affected with measles during pregnancy.[70] The same group of investigators reported that the first children participating in the measles vaccination program in the United Kingdom were more likely to subsequently develop Crohn's disease than nonvaccinated children.[71] Other investigators, however, have been unable to confirm either the epidemiologic observations or the identification of persistent measles virus infection by immunohistochemical staining of tissue from patients with Crohn's disease.[72–73]

The Role of Enteric Flora

The recognition that altered structure of the CARD15 receptor confers susceptibility to Crohn's disease, clearly links microbes to its pathogenesis.[2] Indeed, while Crohn's disease is not likely usually due to a single mucosal pathogen, several lines of evidence indicate the crucial involvement of the intestinal microflora.[74–77] Increased numbers of bacteria have been reported in both inflamed and noninflamed colonic segments in patients with Crohn's disease, compared with noninflamed and inflammatory disease controls.[74] Patients with ileal resections and a diverting ileostomy excluding the neoterminal ileum fail to develop recurrent disease until reanastomosis is performed.[75] Infusion of autologous luminal contents in excluded normal ileal loops of patients with Crohn's disease rapidly induces new inflammation, indicating that fecal component(s) may promote disease flare-up.[76] Inflammation is prevented or lessened by a germ-free environment in several knockout and transgenic animal models of inflammatory bowel disease.[77–78]

The Role of Diet

It is logical to attempt to attribute the changing incidence of gastrointestinal disorders to different dietary exposures. However, no specific dietary toxin or antigen has been incriminated. The rarity of IBD has limited traditional epidemiological methods of determining causation to case-control studies, which have failed to provide meaningful insight into disease pathogenesis. Persson and colleagues reviewed studies examining the reported preillness intake of refined sugar, cereals, fiber, and milk products in patients with Crohn's disease or ulcerative colitis compared with controls.[79] An increased intake of refined sugar before the development of symptomatic Crohn's disease has been fairly consistently reported, suggesting perhaps a modulating role, but the methodologic weaknesses of study design must be recognized. The association may represent a behavioral adaptation to rather than a cause of disease.

Nutritional factors may conceivably modulate the risk of IBD development. In a correlation study from Japan, the increasing incidence of Crohn's disease in this racially homogeneous population was shown to parallel increasing daily intake of animal protein, total fat, animal fat, especially *n*-6 polyunsaturated fatty acids (PUFAs) relative to *n*-3 PUFAs.[80] These trends indicating "Westernization" of diet in Japan were determined from sequential population surveys of dietary habits. *N*-3 PUFAs found in marine oils have an anti-inflammatory effect through modulation of proinflammatory cytokine synthesis.[81]

Risk Factors: Early Life Exposures

The finding of a birth cohort effect instead of a period effect in two independent Swedish studies indicates that events early in life influence the risk of developing inflammatory bowel disease.[82–83] Maternal or neonatal infection has been investigated as the underlying cause of this clustering phenomenon.[84] Breast-feeding in infancy may reduce the risk of developing Crohn's disease.[85]

Other Modulating Factors: Smoking

A clear dichotomy between ulcerative colitis and Crohn's disease is indicated by the opposing effect of cigarette smoking on the two disorders.[86] Smoking decreases and cessation of smoking increases the risk of developing ulcerative colitis.[86] Smoking is a risk factor for Crohn's disease with a point estimate of between 2 and 5. The risk for former smokers does not differ from the risk in people who have never smoked, indicating that smoking is not an initiator of Crohn's disease but rather a promoter. Passive exposure to smoking as well as active smoking may be influential.[87] The components of tobacco responsible for these observations are uncertain, but most attention has been focused on nicotine. Cigarette smoking has been shown to cause morphological injury to endothelial cells leading to the formation of microthrombi. Hence the increased risk of Crohn's disease among smokers has been hypothesized to relate to potentiation of multifocal gastrointestinal infarction.

Other Modulating Factors: Oral Contraceptives

Oral contraceptive use has been implicated as a risk factor for Crohn's disease, but results are not as consistent as for smoking and the risk estimates are generally lower. In some studies the increased risk has only been found in subgroups of smoking patients.[88] Oral contraceptive use may modestly increase the risk of Crohn's disease 1.5 times and 2.6 times in current smokers. It is biologically plausible that oral contraceptive use might further promote Crohn's disease through similar effects on the mesenteric vasculature.

HOST–ENVIRONMENT INTERACTIONS

The intestinal inflammation of Crohn's disease may be viewed as an exaggeration of the "physiologic" inflammatory response always present in the normal lamina propria of the intestine and colon. An enormous antigenic load is regularly presented through the lumen of the gastrointestinal tract, but an intact mucosal barrier and regulatory mechanisms normally prevent the immune and inflammatory responses important in defense against pathogenic agents from proceeding to cause tissue injury. A defect in mucosal barrier function, in antigen processing or in immunoregulation, could result in a chronic inflammatory state, lymphocyte proliferation, cytokine release, recruitment of auxiliary effectors such as neutrophils, and eventual tissue damage. Elucidation of the genetic basis of Crohn's disease has the potential to uncover the primary mechanisms underlying its development. Identification of the CARD15 polymorphisms and other more recently implicated susceptibility genes, such as ATG16L1 and IL23R, provide a tangible basis for investigating the interactions between host and environment that culminate in chronic inflammation.

Defective Mucosal Barrier

Mucosal permeability is increased in Crohn's disease, but whether the defect is primary or secondary remains controversial. Approximately 10% of asymptomatic family members of Crohn's disease patients exhibit increased permeability, and an additional subset have enhanced permeability after exposure to nonsteroidal anti-inflammatory drugs.[89–90] Whether this abnormal permeability is indicative of subclinical intestinal inflammation or represents a genetically determined predisposing factor is unclear. A recent study presented evidence that CARD15 variants could underlie the increased permeability observed in "unaffected" relatives.[91–92]

Immunoregulatory Abnormalities

In general, immune-mediated inflammation can result from activation of innate or adaptive immune responses, which are tightly linked. Adaptive immune responses are initiated when antigen is presented to a T lymphocyte by an antigen-presenting cell. The innate immune system regulates the immediate response to microbial pathogens, through "pattern recognition" receptors, that recognize bacterial products and constituents.

Defective Innate Immunity

CARD15 belongs to a family of such pattern recognition receptors located intracellularly, in contrast to toll-like receptors (TLRs) located on the cell membrane.[93] As expected for a gene involved in innate immunity, CARD15 is expressed in the monocyte–macrophage lineage (including dendritic cells) and granulocytes, cells present in Crohn's disease lesions and involved in granuloma formation. Intestinal epithelial cells, particularly Paneth cells, found in highest concentrations within the ileum, also express CARD15.

CARD15 binds muramyl dipeptide, a degradation product of bacterial peptidoglycan of both gram-negative and gram-positive bacteria.[94] As illustrated in Figure 3, stimulation of CARD15 with bacterial proteins results in activation of the nuclear factor kappa beta (NF-κβ) signaling cascade. Such activation occurs through RICK (RIP-like interacting CLARP kinase) receptor interacting protein 2 a serine/threonine kinase that phosphorylates inhibitor of NF-κβ kinase (IKK) and, therefore, allows the transport of NF-κβ to the nucleus.[95] Moreover, CARD15 may be upregulated by proinflammatory cytokines, such as tumor necrosis factor alpha (TNF–α) via an NF-κβ-binding element in its promoter region

contributing to amplification of the inflammatory process.[96]

The recognition of CARD15 as a susceptibility gene identified a primary abnormality in Crohn's disease for the first time. Precisely, how CARD15 polymorphisms confer susceptibility cannot as yet be definitively answered. The presence of caspase activation and recognition domains (CARDs) indicates that CARD15 plays a role in apoptosis. However, the Crohn's disease–associated CARD15 polymorphisms are located in the LRR domain of the gene or in its vicinity, suggesting a defect in host–bacteria interaction, as had long been hypothesized. Paneth cells synthesize and secrete several antibacterial proteins, notably the defensins, which act rapidly to kill a range of microorganisms nonspecifically. Data from Wehkamp and colleagues have shown that patients with ileal Crohn's disease have an α-defensin deficiency, which is most pronounced in those carrying the CARD15 variants.[97] Hence CARD15 mutations potentially impair ileal protection to invading bacteria as a result of impaired defensin production.

An apparent paradox, as yet incompletely explained, relates to the finding that the CARD15 Leu1007fsinsC frameshift mutation appears in functional experiments to be associated with a loss of NF-κβ activation in the presence of bacterial components.[2,98] In contrast, distinct polymorphisms in the CARD15 gene are associated with increased NF-κβ activation in Blau syndrome, another granulomatous condition.[99] Uveitis, arthritis, and skin rashes, but no digestive tract involvement, characterize this rare dominant Mendelian trait.[99] It is postulated that Blau syndrome results from basal overactivation of the CARD15 pathway, not requiring interaction with bacterial components and by direct consequence without digestive lesion.[99]

The loss of function associated with Crohn's disease–associated CARD15 polymorphisms is not as yet reconciled with the excess of NF-κβ activation observed in intestinal lesions. It is suggested that the defect in innate immunity may secondarily trigger an aberrant T-cell inflammatory response leading to abnormal cytokine pro-

duction, deregulated NF-κβ activation, and tissue damage.[51]

The Adaptive Immune Response

Until the discovery of the CARD15 gene, most investigations of the pathogenic mucosal immune response in Crohn's disease focused on the role of T cells, which are clearly important effectors. The pathophysiology of chronic intestinal inflammation from T-cell activation to tissue injury is summarized schematically in Figure 4.[293] T-cell activation occurs on presentation of antigen by a macrophage or other antigen-presenting cell to a CD4+ T cell. The antigen-specific activation of CD4+ T cells occurs through binding of the CD4 molecule to MHC class II molecules bearing processed antigen on the surface of the activated macrophage. Following activation, CD4+ T lymphocytes can differentiate into subpopulations designated T-helper 1 (Th1) cells, T-helper 17 (Th17) cells, or T-helper 2 (Th2) cells, that produce, respectively, predominantly interferon-γ interleukin (IL)-1, tumor necrosis factor (TNF-α) and IL-6 (Th-1 cytokines), IL-17 (Th-17 cytokine) or IL-4, IL-5, and IL-10 (Th-2 cytokines). Which responses predominate appears to depend on the specific costimulatory signal, the nature and concentration of the antigen, and the prevailing cytokine milieu.[51] Amplification or suppression of the inflammatory response by T cells and macrophages depends on the relative balance of proinflammatory and anti-inflammatory immunoregulatory cells and mediators.[51] Intracellular bacteria, which activate macrophages, promote Th1 cell differentiation by stimulating the synthesis of IL-12, the major Th1-inducing cytokine. The unrestrained intestinal Th1 activation in Crohn's disease appears to be due to defective regulation via regulatory T-cell populations and to T-cell resistance to normal apoptotic signals.[25,100] Recently, several studies have highlighted a central role in Crohn's disease of the IL-23 signaling pathway and activation of Th17 cells.[7] Both Th1 and Th17 cells may cause activation of a final common pathway characterized by cytokine-mediated gut destruction.[7] Th1 cytokines, such as TNF-α have many functions including induction of the expression of adhesion molecules, thereby contributing to the recruitment of monocytes, lymphocytes, and granulocytes. Cells recruited to the mucosa release a vast number of substances with nonspecific inflammatory but directly injurious properties. These include arachidonic acid metabolites (prostaglandins, thromboxane, and leukotrienes), free radicals (reactive oxygen metabolites and nitric oxide), platelet activating factor, and various proteases.

Control of Mucosal Immune Response

The mucosal immune system must tightly control the balance between responsiveness and nonresponsiveness (tolerance) to the millions of antigens continuously passing along the mucosal

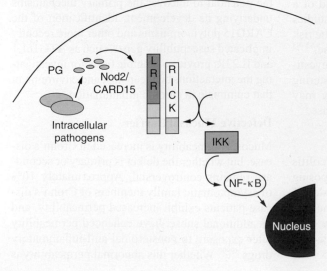

Figure 3 NOD2/CARD15 function in the innate immune response. Stimulation of NOD2/CARD15 by bacterial components, particularly peptidoglycan (PG), results in activation of the nuclear factor kappa beta (NF-κβ) signaling cascade. Such activation occurs through RICK, a serine/threonine kinase that phosphorylates IKK (inhibitor of NF-κβ kinase), thereby allowing transport of NF-κβ into the nucleus. Crohn's disease–associated polymorphisms in the NOD2/CARD15 gene are associated with a loss of NF-κβ activation in the presence of bacterial components.

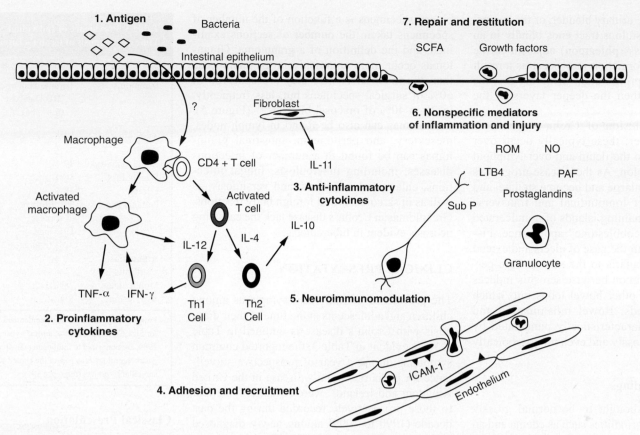

Figure 4 Proposed pathophysiology of chronic intestinal inflammation. Numbers in parentheses indicate sites for therapeutic interventions. The persistent mucosal inflammation in inflammatory bowel disease is triggered by antigen (1) believed to be bacterial in origin. Macrophages process antigen and present it in the context of HLA class II to CD4+ T cells. Upon activation, macrophages elaborate the proinflammatory cytokines (2) tumor necrosis factor-α (TNF-α) and interleukin-12 (IL-12), inducing T-helper 1 (Th1) responses. Alternatively, elaboration of interleukin-4 (IL-4) may promote differentiation toward T-helper 2 (Th2) responses and expression of the anti-inflammatory cytokine (3) interleukin-11 (IL-11). Cells are recruited from the periphery (4) via coordinated expression of integrins, chemokines, and adhesion molecules such as intercellular adhesion molecule-1(ICAM-1). Elaboration of neuropeptides, such as substance P (Sub P) may modify the local responses (5). A variety of nonspecific mediators of inflammation and injury (6) may affect tissue destruction directly. Such mediators include reactive oxygen metabolites (ROM), nitric oxide (NO), leukotriene B4 (LTB4), platelet activating factor (PAF), and prostaglandins. Finally, host responses may induce nonspecific mechanisms of restitution of the wound and repair (7). Short chain fatty acids (SCFAs) and growth factors may contribute to this process. (Modified with permission from reference 293.)

surface. The ability to distinguish between commensal and pathogenic organisms is vital to a normal mucosal immune system. Attempting to explain all the epidemiologic and pathophysiologic observations, as discussed above, it has been hypothesized that Crohn's disease may be a disorder of mucosal immune interpretation of the microbial environment[25] Genetic variants increasing susceptibility to Crohn's disease and other chronic inflammatory disorders, such as allergies and asthma, may have persisted and expanded in human populations due to a beneficial effect in mediating host–microbial interactions in an unsanitary world.[25] The survival advantage previously afforded by enhanced mucosal immune reactivity becomes a risk factor for immune-mediated disease as lifestyle and environmental conditions change.[25,101] Environmental factors, hence, may exert their influence and account for the changing incidence of Crohn's disease at the level of immune regulation rather than via a transmissible infectious agent.[25]

PATHOLOGY

Anatomic Distribution

Crohn's disease is a panenteric inflammatory process. Endoscopy with biopsies commonly identifies histologic abnormalities throughout the gastrointestinal tract. Nevertheless, classification according to the distribution of gross disease evident radiologically or macroscopically at endoscopy still guides treatment and may be useful prognostically. In comparison to the continuous distribution of ulcerative colitis, Crohn's disease is characteristically segmental with spared areas throughout the intestinal tract. The terminal ileum is the most commonly affected site.

During the most recent decade (1990 to 1999) at The Hospital for Sick Children, Toronto, Canada, 386 children and adolescents have been evaluated at initial presentation by colonoscopy and small bowel radiography. The 29% have had terminal ileal +/ cecal disease, 9% more isolated proximal (ileal or jejunal) disease, 42% ileocolonic inflammation, and 20% colon only involvement. Extent of disease was evaluated by colonoscopy and small bowel radiography. Data from 12 pediatric series as pooled by Barton and Ferguson were similar.[102] Crohn's disease was localized to the small intestine (breakdown of terminal ileum vs diffuse or more proximal small intestine not given) alone in 38%, in combination with the colon in another 38%, and the colon only in 20%. Upper endoscopy with biopsy, if routinely performed, frequently reveals at least microscopic involvement of the esophagus, stomach, or duodenum, but gastroduodenal disease is only rarely the sole or predominant site of Crohn's disease.[20,103]

The recent Montreal classification system adapted prior Vienna definitions of location. Crohn's disease is now classified based on location of macroscopic lesions as involving the ileum only (L1), colon only (L2), ileum and colon (L3). Macroscopic disease in the upper gastrointestinal tract (L4) is specified in addition L1, L2, or L3, although uncommonly may constitute the only visible involvement.[104]

Macroscopic Appearance

Gross inspection of the bowel in well-established Crohn's disease reveals marked wall thickening. Mural thickening is the result of chronic inflammation and edema in all layers and is accompanied by luminal narrowing. The mesentery is thickened and contracted and may fix the intestine in one position. Mesenteric lymph nodes are frequently enlarged. Fat extends from the mesentery and "creeps" over the serosal surface of the bowel. The unknown cause of this adiposity has recently been highlighted.[105] The transmural inflammation may cause loops of intestine to be matted together. Fistulae are thought to arise when inflammation extends through the serosa into adjacent structures, such as another loop of bowel, the urinary bladder, or the vagina. Alternatively a fistulous tract ends blindly in an inflammatory mass (phlegmon) adjacent to the bowel. Stricture formation may occur as a result of fibrous tissue proliferation involving first the submucosa and then the deeper layers of the bowel wall.

The earliest lesion of Crohn's disease is the aphthous ulcer; these typically occur over Peyer's patches in the ileum and over lymphoid follicles in the colon. As the disease progresses aphthoid ulcers enlarge and become stellate, and eventually deeper longitudinal and transverse linear ulcers. Remaining islands of nonulcerated mucosa give a "cobblestone" appearance. Fissures develop from the base of ulcers and extend through the muscularis to the serosa. Free perforation is uncommon because serositis induces the adherence of other bowel loops into which the fissure extends. Bowel inflammation and ulceration are characteristically punctuated by "skip areas" of grossly and even microscopically normal mucosa.

Microscopic Findings

Mucosa that is thought to be normal grossly often reveals abnormalities such as edema and an increase in mononuclear cell density in the lamina propria. Microscopic inflammation in such relatively uninvolved sites is often strikingly focal.[106] Even within one histologic section, inflammation may be immediately adjacent to an uninflamed microscopic "skip area." Mucosal changes may resemble ulcerative or infectious colitis with infiltration of the crypts by polymorphonuclear leukocytes (cryptitis or crypt abscesses) and distortion of crypt architecture. However, the presence of fibrosis and histiocytic proliferation in the submucosa suggests Crohn's disease. The pathologic hallmark is transmural extension to all layers of the bowel wall and adventitia.[106]

Granulomas are not always found in pathologic specimens from patients with Crohn's disease. The likelihood of finding granulomas in

biopsy specimens is a function of the number of specimens taken, the number of sections examined, and the definition of a granuloma. Granulomas occur more commonly in the submucosa than the mucosa. Hence, they are observed in 60% of surgical specimens but, less frequently, in 20 to 40% of mucosal biopsies[106] (Figure 5). Granulomas can also be found in lymph nodes, mesentery, and peritoneum. Intestinal granulomas can be found in a number of infectious diseases, including tuberculosis, fungal infections, chlamydial infections, and yersiniosis, as well as in sarcoidosis and foreign body reactions. Granulomas in Crohn's disease lack the caseating necrosis evident in tuberculosis.

CLINICAL PRESENTATION

The prevalence of individual symptoms among children and adolescents at the time of their diagnosis with Crohn's disease is outlined in Table 3. As is evident in Table 3, the reported common symptoms during a year of prospective surveillance for pediatric Crohn's disease in the United Kingdom and Ireland[19] were remarkably similar to those prospectively recorded during the past decade (1990 to 1999) among newly diagnosed children in Toronto, Canada. The mean interval between development of these presenting symptom(s) and diagnosis at The Hospital for Sick Children, Toronto, Canada, was 5.5 months. Several observations warrant emphasis.

In comparison to ulcerative colitis, the initial symptoms of Crohn's disease are more subtle and varied, in part a reflection of its diffuse and diverse anatomic localization. A careful physical examination may detect clues to underlying Crohn's disease when the presenting symptoms such as abdominal pain without other overt intestinal symptoms, isolated anemia or weight loss, do not immediately suggest inflammatory bowel disease. A plateau in linear growth, delayed pubertal development, perianal lesions, and finger clubbing are telltale signs that may be easily overlooked unless specifically sought.

Table 3 Prevalence of Individual Symptoms at the Time of Diagnosis of Crohn's Disease

Symptoms	Toronto Pediatric IBD Database (n = 386)	United Kingdom and Ireland Surveillance (n = 379)
	Patients with Each Individual Symptom (%)	
Abdominal pain	86%	72%
Diarrhea	78%	56%
Blood in the stool	49%	22%
Weight loss	80%	58%
Fevers	38%	Not stated
Perianal lesions	8% fistula or abscess	7% (fistula or abscess)
	19% tags	
	22% fissures	
Arthralgias/ arthritis	17%	8%
Mouth ulcers	28%	Not stated
Skin lesions	8%	1%

Prospectively recorded single center data from The Hospital for Sick Children, Toronto, during a year period, 1990 to 1999, are compared to multicenter data reported by pediatric gastroenterologists as part of the United Kingdom/Ireland IBD surveillance project (reference 19).

Classical Presentation

The constellation of abdominal pain, diarrhea, poor appetite, and weight loss constitutes the classical presentation of Crohn's disease in any age group. As shown in Table 4,[292] this symptom complex (with and without extraintestinal manifestations of inflammatory bowel disease) comprises the mode of presentation in nearly 80% of children and adolescents. Abdominal pain is the most common single symptom at presentation. It is often periumbilical but may localize to the right lower quadrant or diffusely to the lower abdomen with colonic disease. Diarrhea, although common, need not be present, especially when disease is confined to the small intestine. Diarrhea, especially in the absence of

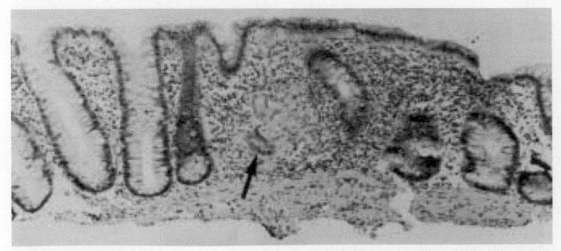

Figure 5 Colonic biopsy specimen from a child with active Crohn's disease. Notice the distortion of the crypt architecture with a prominent noncaseating granuloma and giant cells (*arrow*) amid increased acute and chronic inflammation in the lamina propria.

Table 4 Modes of Presentation of Crohn's Disease

	Number	%
Classical presentation (abdominal pain, diarrhea, weight loss + extraintestinal manifestations)	235	78.6
Growth failure predominating	10	3.3
Extraintestinal manifestations predominating	25	8.4
Arthritis 13		
Recurrent fevers 8		
Recurrent oral ulcers 1		
Oral cheilitis 1		
Pyoderma gangrenosum 1		
Recurrent acute pancreatitis 1		
Anemia (as the major complaint)	8	2.7
Perianal disease predominating	11	3.7
Anorexia, weight loss predominating	6	2.0
Laparotomy for acute abdominal pain	4	1.3
Total	299	

Data from The Hospital for Sick Children, Toronto, from 1980 to 1989.
From reference 292.

significant left-sided colonic disease, is often not grossly bloody, unless there is bleeding from a perianal fissure. The less common modes of presentation in Table 4 deserve comment because they are more likely to be associated with diagnostic confusion and delay.

Growth and Pubertal Delay

Crohn's disease may present as short stature. Impairment of linear growth and concomitant delay in sexual maturation may precede the development of intestinal symptoms and/or dominate the presentation. Impaired growth in a young adolescent becomes strikingly obvious as healthy peers experience the rapid increase in height associated with normal puberty. Affected adolescents are often normal weight for height but low height for age, that is, stunted. As will be discussed in detail later in this chapter, there is evidence that both chronic undernutrition secondary to anorexia and proinflammatory cytokines produced by the inflamed intestine contribute to the observed alterations in growth.

Perianal Disease

Perianal lesions may be the isolated presenting feature of Crohn's disease as well as an accompanying sign of other gastrointestinal symptoms. Perianal fistulae, large tags, or recurrent perianal abscesses in any child warrant investigation to exclude Crohn's disease.

Anemia

Iron deficiency anemia, unless explained by abnormal menstrual losses, reflects gastrointestinal blood loss until proven otherwise. Crohn's disease is one condition that must be included in the differential diagnosis, even if other suggestive symptoms are not readily apparent.

Weight Loss

With similar subtlety Crohn's disease can masquerade as anorexia nervosa when weight loss predominates.

EXTRAINTESTINAL MANIFESTATIONS

Inflammatory extraintestinal manifestations of Crohn's disease are more common with colonic disease than with isolated small bowel disease.[107–108] The most common target organs are the skin, joints, liver, eye, and bone.[107–108] At least one extraintestinal manifestation is seen in about 25 to 35% of adult patients with inflammatory bowel disease.[107] The prevalence would likely be higher in children if fever were included. As previously reviewed, inflammatory extraintestinal manifestations in children most often parallel the activity of intestinal inflammation, but some follow an independent course.[108] Appreciation of this relationship determines whether or not specific therapy of the extraintestinal lesion is required. Other complications, while not inflammatory themselves, result directly from the presence of diseased bowel. These include nephrolithiasis and ureteral obstruction. Growth impairment is discussed separately and in detail because of its great significance and its multifactorial pathogenesis.

JOINTS

Arthritis is less common than arthralgias, but together they constitute the most common extraintestinal manifestations of Crohn's disease (15%) in young patients.[108] As exemplified by Table 4, arthritis is the most likely of the extraintestinal manifestations to precede gastrointestinal manifestations of Crohn's disease and dominate the clinical presentation. Type I arthropathy, typically involves a few large joints, especially the knees, hips, and ankles.[109] Previously termed "colitic arthritis," the joint swelling reflects inflammatory activity in the intestine and settles without deformity as the bowel disease is treated. An association with DRB1*0103 is recognized.[64] However, peripheral arthritis of the hips or sacroiliac joints may be the first manifestation of juvenile ankylosing spondylitis, known to be associated with Crohn's disease. In this case, arthritis can be deforming and may progress independently of the bowel disease.[109] Type II arthritis, symmetrical, seronegative, small-joint arthropathy unrelated to disease activity, has been associated with HLA-B*44.[64,109]

SKIN

The commonest cutaneous manifestations (with frequencies of occurrence based on a large adult series of Crohn's disease patients) are erythema nodosum (8 to 15%) and pyoderma gangrenosum (1.3%).[107] Erythema nodosum tends to occur when the intestinal disease is active but does not necessarily indicate its severity. Pyoderma gangrenosum often runs its own course and requires specific medical treatment.

EYE

Ocular lesions appear to be less common in young patients than in adults, but acute episcleritis and uveitis, and rarely orbital myositis do occur.[107–108] Asymptomatic uveitis has been described in Crohn's disease predominantly when the colon only is involved, but there is no convincing evidence that it progresses to destructive ocular disease.[110]

HEPATOBILIARY

Primary sclerosing cholangitis (PSC) is associated most often with ulcerative colitis, but may occur also with Crohn's disease involving the colon. PSC preceded the clinical onset of the bowel disease in 50% of 17 predominantly adolescent patients (ulcerative colitis 14, Crohn's disease of colon 3) with the PSC-IBD combination identified in Toronto, Canada.[111]

PANCREAS

Acute pancreatitis may occur, albeit rarely, as an extraintestinal manifestation of either ulcerative colitis or Crohn's disease.[112] It can also be a direct complication of duodenal Crohn's disease, or PSC, or drug therapy (azathioprine, 6-mercaptopurine, and 5-aminosalicylic acid).

RENAL

Renal complications of Crohn's disease are not themselves inflammatory in nature but rather result from the presence of diseased bowel. These include ureteric obstruction and hydronephrosis from thickened, chronically inflamed bowel, and an increased incidence of urinary stones.[113] Oxalate, urate, and phosphate stones may occur. In normal persons, oxalate in the lumen is bound to calcium, and the poorly absorbed calcium oxalate is excreted in the feces. However, when the ileum is diseased or has been resected, increased luminal concentrations of malabsorbed fatty acids compete for calcium. Oxalate absorption and subsequent renal excretion are therefore increased.

VASCULAR

Hypercoagulability from thrombocytosis, hyperfibrinogenemia, elevated factor V and factor VII, and depression of antithrombin III is seen in some patients with inflammatory bowel disease.[114] Vascular complications have included deep vein thrombosis, pulmonary emboli, and cerebrovascular disease.[114]

BONE

Decreased bone density is increasingly recognized in Crohn's disease.[115] The pathogenesis is multifactorial, but a major contributory factor in children appears to be inhibition of bone formation by cytokines.[116] As recently reported, bone density was reduced to levels corresponding to < –2 SD for age and gender in 25% of newly diagnosed children with Crohn's disease prior to any corticosteroid therapy.[117] Rapid increments in bone mass are normally acquired during puberty, and peak bone mass attained is an important determinant of risk for subsequent osteoporosis in later life. Hence, childhood onset Crohn's disease, may be a particular risk factor for clinical osteoporosis in later life, although studies in adult patient cohorts have not correlated prevalence or severity of decreased bone mineral density with young age at diagnosis. Monitoring of bone densitometry and modification of other risk factors (exercise, reduction in steroid use, hormonal treatment of chronic secondary amenorrhea in adolescent girls, calcium and vitamin D

Table 5 Prevalence of Linear Growth Impairment in Pediatric Crohn's Disease

Study Details (Reference)	Time of Assessment	Patients Studied	N	Definition of Linear Growth Impairment	Percentage with Growth Impairment
Baltimore, United States (1961 to 1985)[125]	At diagnosis	Prepubertal (Tanner I or II)	50	Decrease in height velocity prior to diagnosis	88
Toronto, Canada (1980 to 1988)[122]	During follow-up	Prepubertal (Tanner I or II)	100	Height velocity < 2 SD for age for > 2 yr	49
Sweden (1983 to 1987)[123]	During follow-up	Population-based cohort < 16 yr at Dx	46	Height velocity < 2 SD for age for 1 yr	65
New York, United States (1979 to 1989)[124]	At maturity	Children in tertiary care	38	Failure to reach predicted adult height	37
Toronto, Canada (1990 to 1999)[20]	During follow-up	Prepubertal (Tanner I or II)	161	Height velocity < 2 SD for age for > 2 yr	54
United Kingdom (1998 to 1999)[19]	At diagnosis	Population-based cohort < 16 yr at Dx	338	Height SDS < −1.96	13
Israel (1991 to 2003)[126]	At diagnosis	Children in tertiary care	93	Height SDS < −2.0	20

Varying definitions and times of assessment (at the time of diagnosis and during follow-up) are applied.

supplementation) are recommended. Treatment with bisphosphonates, common among adult patients with Crohn's disease, has seldom been used in children, where decreased bone formation is often the primary mechanism leading to decreased bone mineral density.

DISEASE COMPLICATIONS

Malnutrition

At the time of first diagnosis, approximately 85% of pediatric patients with Crohn's disease have lost weight.[118] Multiple factors contribute. However, reduced intake, rather than excessive losses or increased needs, is the major cause of the caloric insufficiency. The child or adolescent may voluntarily refrain from eating to avoid aggravation of abdominal cramps and diarrhea. Moreover, disease-related anorexia may be profound. Cytokines produced by the inflamed bowel are likely responsible; for example, TNF-α has been shown to produce anorexia.

Intestinal malabsorption may factor in the equation leading to energy imbalance but is seldom a major cause. In Crohn's disease involving the ileum, the processes of fat digestion and absorption may be altered either by loss of gut surface area due to inflammation or by depletion of the circulating bile salt pool due to bile acid malabsorption in the diseased ileum or deconjugation by bacteria. In a study years ago of adults prior to intestinal resection, Filipsson and colleagues found predominantly mild steatorrhea in 24% of patients with ileal disease, 26% of those with ileocolonic involvement, and 17% of those with Crohn's colitis.[119]

Increased energy expenditure associated with active inflammation has been suggested as a further mechanism accounting for the frequency of malnutrition. In general resting energy expenditure (REE) does not differ from normal in patients with inactive disease, but can exceed predicted rates in the presence of fever and sepsis.[120] Furthermore, in comparison to comparably malnourished patients with anorexia nervosa, a lack of compensatory reduction in REE has recently been described in adolescents with Crohn's disease.[121] Reduction in REE is a normal biologic response to conserve energy. Production of inflammatory mediators may explain the lack of REE adaptation in patients with Crohn's disease and further augment the ongoing malnutrition.

Growth Impairment

Inflammatory disease occurring during early adolescence is likely to have a major impact on nutritional status and growth because of the very rapid accumulation of lean body mass that normally occurs at this time. Further, boys are more vulnerable to disturbances in growth than girls because their growth spurt comes at a later stage of normal pubertal development and is ultimately longer and greater.

Prevalence

Several studies have characterized the growth of children with Crohn's disease as treated in the 1980s and into the 1990s.[122–126] These studies are important as a benchmark of outcomes with traditional therapy. It is to be hoped that the now better understanding of the pathogenesis of growth impairment, together with the greater efficacy of immunomodulatory and emerging biologic therapies in treating intestinal inflammation, may lead to enhanced growth of young patients diagnosed in the present decade.[127]

As summarized in Table 5, the percentage of patients with Crohn's disease, whose growth is affected, varies with the definition of growth impairment and with the nature of the population under study (tertiary referral center vs population-based).[122–126] It has nevertheless been consistently observed that impairment of linear growth is common prior to recognition of Crohn's disease as well as during the subsequent years.[122–126] Height velocity is the most sensitive parameter to recognize impaired growth. It is important to obtain preillness heights, so that the impact of the inflammatory bowel disease can be fully appreciated. Mean standard deviation score (SDS) for height among 333 patients aged less than 16 years was −0.54 (95% CI −0.67 to −0.41) in the 1998 to 1999 population-based surveillance study of incident Crohn's disease in the United Kingdom[19]; evidence that growth delay prior to diagnosis still occurs and remains a challenge. The greater the height deficits at diagnosis, the greater are the demands for catch-up growth. This emphasizes the need for early recognition of Crohn's disease in young patients, and also for new approaches to optimize the catch-up growth of those diagnosed late.

Pathophysiology

As summarized in Table 6, several interrelated factors contribute to linear growth impairment in children with Crohn's disease. The fundamental mechanisms have recently been comprehensively reviewed.[128] Chronic undernutrition has long been implicated and remains an important and remediable cause of growth retardation. A simple nutritional hypothesis fails to explain all the observations related to growth patterns among children with IBD. Within the past decade, the direct growth-inhibiting effects of proinflammatory cytokines released from the inflamed intestine have been increasingly recognized.[128–130]

IGF-1, produced by the liver in response to growth hormone (GH) stimulation, is the key mediator of GH effects at the growth plate of bones. An association between impaired growth in children with Crohn's disease and low-IGF-1 levels is well recognized. Early studies emphasized the role of malnutrition in suppression of IGF-1 production. Recently, transgenic mice with defective growth were found to overexpress interleukin-6 (IL-6). Antibody to IL-6 partially

Table 6 Factors Contributing to Growth Abnormalities in Children with Crohn's Disease

Factors	Reasons
1. Cytokines produced by chronically inflamed intestine	Direct role of inflammatory cytokines in linear growth inhibition (IGF-1 inhibition; interference with kinetics of bone growth)
2. Insufficient caloric intake	Food avoidance because of exacerbation of gastrointestinal symptoms by eating; cytokine-mediated anorexia
3. Stool losses	Mucosal inflammation leading to protein-losing enteropathy; steatorrhea if extensive
4. Increased nutritional needs	Fever, chronic deficits
5. Corticosteroid treatment	Inhibition of growth hormone and insulin-like growth factor-1

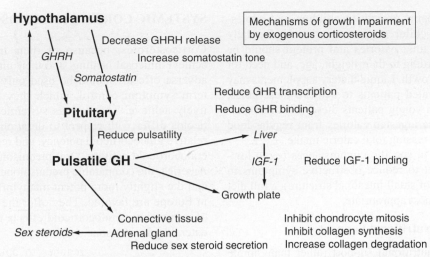

Figure 6 Exogenous corticosteroids create a state of functional growth hormone sufficiency, interfering with growth in a multiplicity of ways.

corrected the growth defect, whereas administration of IL-6 led to a decrease in IGF-1 before food intake was affected.[129] Further, IGF-1 levels were negatively correlated with IL-6 among children with juvenile rheumatoid arthritis.[129] These findings suggest that an IL-6-mediated decrease in IGF-1 production may represent a major mechanism by which chronic inflammation leads to stunting of growth.[129] The relative contributions of malnutrition and inflammation to linear growth delay were further explored by Ballinger and colleagues using a rat model of colitis.[130] Inflammatory cytokines may also inhibit linear growth through other mechanisms, including interference with growth plate kinetics.[116] Cytokines appear to impair end-organ responsiveness to circulating testosterone, thereby compounding the effects of undernutrition in delaying progression through puberty.[131]

Chronic daily corticosteroid administration augments the growth impairment associated with inflammatory disease. As depicted in Figure 6, the growth-suppressive effects of glucocorticoids are multifactorial, and include central suppression of GH release, decreased hepatic transcription of GH receptor, such that production of IGF-1 is decreased, and decreased IGF-1 binding in cartilage.[132] Hence, exogenous corticosteroids create a state of functional GH deficiency.[132]

From the foregoing discussion, it is clear that enhancement of linear growth is best achieved through control of intestinal inflammation without chronic corticosteroid therapy and assurance of adequate nutrition.

PERIANAL DISEASE

Perianal abscesses and fistulae occur in up to one-third of patients over time.[133] When skin tags and fissures are included, the prevalence of perianal disease among pediatric patients at tertiary care centers is 14 to 62%.[133] Tags and fissures are often asymptomatic, but large inflamed tags, deeper fissures, perianal fistulae, and abscesses may contribute significantly to the morbidity of Crohn's disease.

INVESTIGATION AND DIAGNOSIS

The diagnosis of Crohn's disease is made based on a compatible clinical presentation, substantiated by radiologic assessment of the small bowel, endoscopy of the ileocolon with pathologic examination of mucosal biopsies, and exclusion of other causes of chronic intestinal inflammation. *Salmonella*, *Shigella*, *Campylobacter jejuni*, enteropathogenic *Escherischia coli*, and *Clostridium difficile* infections are excluded with stool cultures. Serological techniques are important in the diagnosis of *Yersinia* infections and amebiasis. Intestinal tuberculosis and schistosomiasis should be excluded when risk factors exist.

Ultrasound has been used as a noninvasive screening test for suspected Crohn's disease. Radiology and ileocolonoscopy (with mucosal biopsies for histologic assessment) are used to define the nature and extent of intestinal inflammation and to distinguish ulcerative colitis from Crohn's disease. Differentiation of isolated colonic Crohn's disease from ulcerative colitis is made on the basis of macroscopic and microscopic criteria as discussed in the chapter. A group of pediatric IBD clinicians and pathologists have recently reviewed controversies in the diagnosis of IBD involving the colon.[134] When features of both ulcerative colitis and Crohn's disease are present, the designation of indeterminate colitis, or IBD type undefined,[102] is applied, pending clarification with time and subsequent evaluations.

Some clinicians recommend upper gastrointestinal endoscopy with biopsies as an adjunctive tool in differentiating the type of colitis, but caution must be exercised in interpreting all gastric or duodenal inflammmation as indicative of Crohn's disease.[134–135] Nonspecific histologic gastritis is common in ulcerative colitis as well as Crohn's disease; focal antral gastritis may be more specific for Crohn's disease[135]; the finding of granulomata on gastric antral biopsy may clarify a diagnosis of Crohn's disease in an otherwise indeterminate colitis.[135] Technological advances in magnetic resonance imaging or ultrasound, which allow assessment of the depth of intramural inflammation, and

videocapsule endoscopy, may provide adjunctive information facilitating differentiation of Crohn's colitis from ulcerative colitis.

Serologic Tests in the Diagnosis of IBD

Antineutrophil cytoplasmic antibodies (ANCA) and anti-*Saccharomyces cerevisiae* antibody (ASCA) have been recommended as tools to facilitate screening for IBD among children with suggestive symptoms and to differentiate ulcerative colitis from Crohn's disease.[137] However, the relatively low sensitivities of serology for Crohn's disease and ulcerative colitis argue against there being any additional value for ASCA/ANCA as routine or first-line screening tests for IBD compared to clinical acumen and the equally sensitive (albeit less specific) measurement of acute phase reactants. Moreover, the need to perform definitive radiological and endoscopic studies to guide therapy by defining the extent and nature of disease will not be averted by positive serologic tests. The working party, which drafted the Montreal phenotypic classification of IBD, concluded that the use of these markers for diagnosis is currently not justified.[136]

ASCAs are IgG and IgA antibodies that recognize mannose sequences in the cell wall of *S. cerevisiae* strain Su1. ASCA is detected in 55 to 60% of children and adults with Crohn's disease and in 5 to 10% of controls with other gastrointestinal disorders, findings indicating good specificity but relatively poor sensitivity.[138] The specificity of the antibody response makes it unlikely that the elevated titers result merely from increased intestinal permeability. It is possible that *S. cerevisiae* shares antigenic determinants with another organism of true etiopathogenetic significance in Crohn's disease. An increased prevalence in relatives is reported.[139] Whether such clustering is due to genetic or environmental factors is unknown.

ANCAs, originally described in Wegener's granulomatosis and necrotizing vasculitis, are immunoglobulin (Ig)G antibodies directed against cytoplasmic components of neutrophils. The association with IBD of a subset of ANCA with a perinuclear staining pattern on immunofluorescence studies (pANCA) was first recognized for ulcerative colitis.[140] The specificity of perinuclear staining for IBD can be confirmed by its disappearance after desoxyribonuclease (DNase) digestion of neutrophils. pANCA is considered a marker of the immunologic disturbance that underlies the development of chronic colonic inflammation.

Combined ANCA/ASCA testing has also been recommended to help differentiate Crohn's disease from ulcerative colitis. However, differentiation of Crohn's disease from ulcerative colitis is clinically problematic only when inflammation is largely confined to the colon. pANCA is positive in up to 35% of patients with colonic Crohn's disease, and ASCA is less often detected in patients with Crohn's disease confined to the colon. Hence, the utility of serology is less in the setting where it is needed most. In the one published study clearly reporting sensitivity, specificity and predictive values of combined serologic testing, the sensitivity of ASCA+ pANCA– serology for Crohn's colitis versus ulcerative colitis was only 32%.[141]

More recently, antibodies to other microbial components (anti-ompC, anti-I2, and anti-CBir1 flagellin antibodies) have been described in Crohn's disease, and associations with complicated (fistulizing or structuring) phenotypes are reported.[142] Further research in this field must include independent validation.

TREATMENT

Basic Principles Governing Treatment

The challenge in treating each child or adolescent with Crohn's disease is to employ pharmacologic, nutritional, and where appropriate surgical interventions, not only to decrease mucosal inflammation and thereby alleviate symptoms, but also to optimize growth, normalize pubertal development, facilitate normal social development, and avoid long-term disease-related complications. Growth is a measure of the success of therapy. Optimal treatment of pediatric Crohn's disease encompasses, as will be discussed in detail in subsequent sections, immunomodulatory therapy, biologic therapies, nutritional therapies, and if appropriate, resection of diseased bowel.

The natural history and severity of Crohn's disease vary greatly among patients. Increasingly, gastroenterologists are acknowledging the heterogeneity of disease and the varying treatment responsiveness of individual patients. The identification of genetic or serologic markers predictive of disease behavior, would constitute a significant advance, allowing early selection of the most appropriate treatment plan for individual patients.

Crohn's disease has traditionally been thought of as a disease characterized by exacerbations and remissions. It must be acknowledged, however, that the term "remission," as generally applied, is a clinical concept. The persistence of endoscopic and histologic lesions, despite resolution of symptoms and biochemical abnormalities with corticosteroid therapy, has been well documented.[143–144] With emerging biologic agents and optimal use of immunomodulatory drugs, healing of intestinal lesions may, however, become a more achievable goal.

NUTRITIONAL SUPPORT

Nutritional support is a vital component of the management of patients with Crohn's disease. Management goals must include correction and prevention of nutritional deficits as well as control of symptoms.

General Dietary Measures

For children and adolescents, the most important advice is to consume a diet liberal in protein with calories sufficient to maintain or restore weight and to support growth in children and adolescents. For children recommendations for daily intakes of total calories and protein should be made according to their height, age, and need for catch-up growth. Liquid dietary supplements may help motivated patients to achieve these goals, although in young patients these will often simply displace ingested calories from regular food without increasing total caloric intake.

Except in specific circumstances (eg, a low-residue diet to reduce obstructive symptoms in the setting of small intestinal stricture), a full diet for age is most appropriate.

Intensive Nutritional Support

Intensive nutritional support rather than simple dietary counseling to increase caloric intake is required when patients are significantly malnourished or when growth is retarded[145–146] Adjunctive nutritional support in these contexts may be provided by enteral nutrition using formulated food or via parenteral nutrition using a centrally placed intravenous catheter. Nocturnal nasogastric infusion of formulated food has come to constitute the preferred and more frequent approach by virtue of its lower complication rates, easier and less costly administration.[145–146]

PHARMACOLOGIC TREATMENT

Drugs constitute the mainstay of treatment of children and adolescents with Crohn's disease, although enteral nutrition using formulated food is commonly and effectively employed as an alternate primary therapy of active inflammation in some parts of the world, particularly in the United Kingdom. Table 7 summarizes validated pharmacologic options for the treatment of active inflammation and the maintenance of clinical remission based on the nature and localization of disease. Multicenter randomized controlled trials conducted predominantly among adults have helped establish the effectiveness of these therapies. For several of the commonly employed drugs, meta-analyses of individual controlled trial data have been performed. The efficacy of combination therapy (ie, more than one drug used in adjunctive fashion) has hitherto only infrequently been addressed in the clinical trial setting. Until recently, pharmacokinetic and dose-ranging studies were seldom conducted in children; many recommended dosages in Table 7 are based on extrapolation from adult studies.

The pharmacokinetics, mechanism of action, and potential adverse effects of individual drugs are discussed, and the evidence of their therapeutic efficacy critically appraised in the forthcoming sections. The challenge at the present time is to wisely employ immunomodulatory and emerging biologic therapies, with the goal of improving outcomes particularly for the subgroup of pediatric patients with otherwise chronically active, extensive, and disabling disease, formerly all too often associated with compromised growth.[122]

SYSTEMIC CORTICOSTEROIDS

Corticosteroids, because of their inability to achieve mucosal healing, and their unacceptable adverse effects, should be used only for short-term symptom control, which they can effectively achieve. The various systemic glucocorticoids differ with respect to duration of action, relative glucocorticoid potency, and relative mineralocorticoid activity. Oral prednisone in North America, the comparable prednisolone in Britain, and the slightly more potent methylprednisolone in Europe are favored. They offer the advantage of minimal mineralocorticoid effects unlike parenteral hydrocortisone.

Pharmacology and Mechanism of Action

Prednisone is a synthetic glucocorticoid of intermediate potency. It is converted to its active form, prednisolone, in the liver. Both prednisone and prednisolone are promptly and completely absorbed in most individuals. The possibility of reduced absorption in patients with active Crohn's disease of the small intestine must be borne in mind. The concept that the effects of corticosteroids at the tissue level outlast drug concentrations in serum is important to the derivation of treatment regimens. Intermittent rather than sustained high blood levels, as long as therapeutically efficacious, are preferable by virtue of causing fewer side effects.

The multifactorial mode of action of corticosteroids, while not completely understood, relates both to their inhibition of cell-mediated immunity and their anti-inflammatory effects. It has been recently demonstrated that steroids inhibit NF-κβ function, diminishing the release of inflammatory cytokines, IL-1 and IL-2.[147] Anti-inflammatory effects include decreased capillary permeability, impaired neutrophil and monocyte chemotaxis, and stabilization of lysosomal membranes. Eicosanoid production is decreased by inhibition of phospholipase, preventing arachidonic acid liberation from membranes. Additionally, steroids decrease diarrhea in inflammatory bowel disease by enhancing sodium and water absorption.

Potential Adverse Effects

The potential toxicity of systemic corticosteroids is well known and has been reviewed in the context of inflammatory bowel disease.[148] Disfigurement by acne, moon facies, hirsutism, and cutaneous striae are the most commonly observed adverse effects with treatment of acute inflammatory bowel disease and are particularly distressing to teenagers despite assurances of reversibility following drug withdrawal. Pseudotumor cerebri, steroid psychosis, and proximal myopathy are other, fortunately rare, sequelae of steroid therapy. Corticosteroid use may also contribute to renal calculi formation via hypercalciuria. Aseptic necrosis of the femoral head is one of the most serious consequences of steroid therapy and may be mistaken for inflammatory bowel disease arthropathy.

Table 7 A Summary of Evidence-Based Pharmacologic Treatment of Crohn's Disease

	Active Disease	Maintenance of Remission
Ileal or other small bowel disease		
Mild	Oral 5-ASA (50 to 100 mg/kg/d up to 4 g/d) (Pentasa or Salofalk most suitable)	(Oral 5-ASA frequently used, but RCT data combined in meta-analysis do not support a benefit when compared to placebo)
Mild or moderate	Controlled ileal release budesonide (9 mg/d) for ileal and/or right colonic inflammation	
Moderate or severe	Conventional corticosteroids (1 mg/kg/d up to 40 to 60 mg/d prednisone)	6-MP (1.5 mg/kg/d),* azathioprine (2 to 2.5 mg/kg/d),* methotrexate
Otherwise refractory and extensive	Infliximab 5 mg/kg/dose given at wk 0, 2, and 6 is customary induction regimen	Infliximab 5 mg/kg every 8 wk
Colonic disease		
Mild to moderate	Oral 5-ASA (Asacol or Dipentum most suitable)	(Oral 5-ASA or sulfasalazine frequently used, RCT data combined in meta-analysis do not support a benefit when compared to placebo)
	Sulfasalazine†	
	? 5-ASA enemas‡	
	Metronidazole (10 to 20 mg/kg/d up to 1 g daily)	
	Ciprofloxacillin (20 mg/kg/d)	
Moderate or severe	Conventional corticosteroids (1 mg/kg/d up to 40 to 60 mg/d prednisone)	6-MP (1.5 mg/kg/d)*
	Methotrexate	Azathioprine (2 to 2.5 mg/kg/d)* methotrexate
Otherwise refractory	Infliximab (dosing as above)	Infliximab (regularly scheduled infusions as above)
Perianal	Metronidazole‡ (10 to 20 mg/kg/d)	Metronidazole‡ (10 to 20 mg/kg/d)
	Ciprofloxacillin‡ (20 mg/kg/d)	Ciprofloxacillin‡ (20 mg/kg/d)
	6-MP/azathioprine*	6-MP/azathioprine*
	Methotrexate	Methotrexate
	Infliximab 5 mg/kg/dose given at wk 0, 2, 6	Infliximab regularly scheduled infusions of 5 mg/kg q 8 wk

5-ASA = 5-aminosalicylic acid; 6-MP = 6-mercaptopurine.
*Delayed onset of action.
†May have an adjunctive role with corticosteroids.
‡Not subjected to controlled clinical trial.

There are many reasons to avoid chronic corticosteroid use. Daily glucocorticoid administration suppresses insulin growth factor 1 (IGF-1) and inhibits linear growth. The effects of corticosteroids on bone are of particular concern and include both enhanced bone resorption and diminished bone formation.[162] Corticosteroids decrease calcium absorption but increase urinary calcium excretion. The secondary hyperparathyroidism is associated with osteoclastic activity. Dietary supplementation with calcium and vitamin D may be of some prophylactic benefit in reducing the rate of corticosteroid-related bone calcium loss.[162] The incidence of posterior subcapsular cataracts correlates with dose and duration of therapy. Glucocorticoids also increase intraocular pressure.

Evidence-Based Therapeutic Indications

Corticosteroids will treat moderate or severe acute exacerbations of Crohn's disease. Corticosteroid-induced clinical remission, however, is usually associated with persistence of endoscopic lesions.[143–144]

Active Disease

Steroid use in active Crohn's disease of the small intestine alone or small intestine plus colon has been validated by the National Cooperative Crohn's Disease Study (NCCDS) and the European Cooperative Crohn's Disease Study (ECCDS).[150–151] Disease confined to the colon, which, interestingly, proved relatively refractory to corticosteroid therapy in the NCCDS, benefited from combination therapy with sulphsalazine in the European study.[150–151] There are no studies directly comparing different corticosteroid-dosing regimens in adults or in children. The NCCDS titrated the dose of prednisone to the level of disease activity with a daily dose range of 0.25 to 0.75 mg/kg (maximum 60 mg). The Canadian Pediatric Crohn Disease Study employed 1 mg/kg oral prednisone (maximum 40 mg) as a once daily dose, with the option of increasing this dose briefly to 2 mg/kg/d (maximum 60 mg), if disease was refractory to the lower dose during the first 7 days of therapy. Overall 92% of children and adolescents with active Crohn's disease involving the small intestine alone or small intestine plus colon responded to this corticosteroid regimen.[152]

Maintenance of Remission

There is little justification from longitudinal placebo-controlled trials in adults for the use of low-dose corticosteroids to prevent relapse in patients with inactive Crohn's disease.[150–151] The ECCDS did suggest a benefit to continuation of low-dose prednisolone after clinical remission of Crohn's disease was induced by its use.[151] Such patients could be considered to have corticosteroid-dependent disease, as occurred in 45% of adult patients in a population-based study of outcomes in adult patients.[153] Such chronic daily corticosteroid administration is contraindicated in childhood because of the consequent inhibition of linear growth. Children with "corticosteroid-dependent" disease require alternative therapies.

CONTROLLED ILEAL RELEASE BUDESONIDE

Pharmacology and Mechanism of Action

Both therapeutic and adverse effects of glucocorticosteroids are mediated via the glucocorticosteroid receptor, which is uniform in all cells. In order to separate therapeutic from unwanted effects, glucocorticoids have been developed with high affinity for the glucocorticosteroid receptor in the intestinal mucosa (and therefore high topical anti-inflammatory potency) but a rapid transformation to inactivated metabolites by the liver following absorption (and therefore low risk of systemic effects).[154] One such compound is budesonide, which has now been formulated into orally administered delayed-release capsule preparations to facilitate delivery to the terminal ileum and proximal colon. Microgranules of the nonhalogenated glucocorticoid bound to ethylcellulose are encapsulated by Eudragit L resin and released at pH greater than 5.6 in one preparation.[155–156] Another delayed-release formulation more recently available in Europe releases budesonide at pH > 6.[157] Budesonide possesses a high topical potency, having affinity for the glucocorticosteroid receptor 15 times that of prednisolone. Rapid metabolism in the liver to compounds with vastly lower affinity for the glucocorticosteroid receptor results in systemic bioavailability of only 10% compared to 80% for prednisolone.[154]

Adverse Effects

The major promise of oral budesonide formulated for intestinal release is decreased adverse systemic effects in comparison to classical corticosteroids. In clinical trials no serious corticosteroid-related toxicity has been encountered, and the incidence of overall adverse effects has been less than with prednisolone (155–1). A dose-related biochemical impairment of adrenal function as measured by basal cortisol levels and responses to ACTH stimulation has been observed, albeit also less than with conventional oral steroids.[155,156,158]

Evidence-Based Therapeutic Indications

Active Crohn's Disease. The major clinical indication for the hitherto available oral budesonide formulations is in the treatment of Crohn's disease involving the ileum and/or right colon. In one multicenter randomized placebo-controlled trial, 8 weeks treatment of adults with 9 mg controlled ileal release (CIR) budesonide daily resulted in clinical remission in 51% of patients compared to 20% in the placebo group.[155] In a subsequent trial, the same CIR budesonide regimen induced remission in 60% of patients, as compared to 60 and 66% of adult patients treated with prednisolone.[156] In a more recently completed multicenter randomized controlled trial versus oral prednisone in children with active Crohn's disease localized to the ileum and/or right colon, 55% achieved clinical remission with CIR budesonide compared to 71% with prednisolone.[158] Taken together, the extensive randomized controlled trial data and clinical experience in adults and children suggest that response rates with CIR budesonide are intuitively less than those achieved with optimal dosing of prednisone or prednisolone. Indeed, a treatment benefit for conventional corticosteroids has been confirmed in meta-analysis.[159] Nevertheless, CIR budesonide may spare a proportion of young patients the adverse effects of short-term conventional steroids, while successfully ameliorating their Crohn's disease symptoms.[158]

Only the German Budesonide study group has studied the efficacy of an oral budesonide formulation in patients with more distal colonic disease. Comparable percentages of patients with distal colonic involvement and ileal +/− proximal colonic disease, 51% and 59% respectively, attained clinical remission in this open label study with the budesonide formulation designed for release at pH > 6.[157]

Maintenance of Remission in Crohn's Disease

Four randomized placebo-controlled studies have examined the efficacy of CIR budesonide in maintaining medically induced clinical remission.[160–163] CIR budesonide 6 mg daily in adults significantly prolonged the median duration of remission in comparison to placebo in two multicenter studies, but at one year following randomization, there was no difference in the percentage of patients remaining in continuous remission.[160–161] Two other placebo-controlled studies demonstrated a similar lack of efficacy at one year and no delay in the median time to relapse with daily doses of 6 mg or 3 mg CIR budesonide in comparison to placebo.[162–163] Long-term use to maintain remission in children must at present be considered experimental because of the marginal benefit observed among adults and the drug's hitherto unknown effect on linear growth.[164]

SULFASALAZINE AND ORAL 5-AMINOSALICYLIC ACID

Sulfasalazine and 5-aminosalicylic acid (5-ASA) have a greater role in the management of ulcerative colitis than in Crohn's disease. Indeed the multiple oral 5-aminosalicylic formulations, designed in part to extend the scope of efficacy to include active and preventive treatment of Crohn's disease, have in this respect proved disappointing.

Pharmacology and Mechanism of Action

Sulfasalazine consists of 5-aminosalicylic acid in azo bond linkage with sulfapyridine. The sulfa moiety functions primarily as a carrier facilitating delivery of the therapeutically active 5-aminosalicylic acid to the colon. There it is released from the parent molecule by bacterial cleavage of the diazo bond and acts locally in the colonic mucosa to impede the inflammatory process. The sulfapyridinesulfapyridine component is 95% absorbed and undergoes acetylation, hydroxylation, and glucuronidation in the liver. 5-Aminosalicylic acid is now recognized to modify neutrophil-mediated tissue damage through a multiplicity of actions including inhibition of leukotriene biosynthesis via the lipoxygenase pathway of arachidonic acid metabolism, interference with myeloperoxidase activity, scavenging of reactive oxygen species, and inhibition of NFκβ.[165] Even though the sulfapyridine component is therapeutically inert, there is new evidence that the complete parent molecule may act synergistically to enhance the anti-inflammatory effects of its component 5-aminosalicylic acid.[166] Recent data indicate a role for sulfasalazine, but not 5-ASA, in inducing apoptosis in T cells.[167]

5-Aminosalicylic acid ingested orally in non-protected form is rapidly absorbed in the proximal small intestine. Alternate delivery systems have been developed to facilitate transport and release of 5-aminosalicylic acid distally without the sulfa carrier. The plethora of available oral 5-aminosalicylic analogues differ importantly with respect to the mechanism and site of 5-aminosalicylic acid release.[168] The balance between release, local inactivation and local absorption determines intraluminal drug levels at specific sites.[169–170] High 5-aminosalicylic acid concentrations within the intestinal wall are thought to optimize anti-inflammatory actions.

Table 8 lists the oral 5-aminosalicylic acid preparations currently in clinical use. These analogues are best understood in three groups. Firstly, olsalazine, in which 5-aminosalicylic acid is attached to a second molecule of itself, depends, like sulfasalazine, on bacterial cleavage of the azo bond. Other azo bond derivatives are ipsalazide and balsalazide, which contain 5-aminosalicylic acid linked to an inert, unabsorbable carrier molecule. Secondly, the delayed-release preparations, known collectively as mesalazine in Europe and mesalamine in the United States, employ different acrylic-based resins, designed to break at a set pH, thereby making 5-aminosalicylic acid available to the intestinal mucosa. Finally, the timed-release formulation Pentasa contains 5-aminosalicylic acid in microgranules coated with a semipermeable membrane of ethyl cellulose. Release occurs continually but at a rate affected by pH. The predicted sites of intestinal release are given in Table 8. However, 5-aminosalicylic acid preparations that require specific alterations in pH for release may not, for example, be distributed uniformly in patients with inflammatory bowel disease, in whom the pH of luminal contents has been shown to differ from normal subjects.

Potential Adverse Effects

Potential toxicity of sulfasalazinesulfasalazine is considerable.[171] Overall 20 to 25% of patients experience adverse reactions that either limit drug dosage or preclude use entirely. Undesirable effects fall into two categories: dose-related and idiosyncratic or hypersensitivity, but the majority of both types seem attributable primarily to the therapeutically unimportant sulfapyridine component.[171] Dose-dependent adverse effects include nausea, vomiting, headaches, and mild hemolysis. The dose of sulfasalazine at which such reactions occur varies between individuals, partly reflecting acetylator status and its effect on sulfapyridine metabolism. Temporary interruption of therapy followed by a more gradual increase in dosage may avoid a recurrence of dose-dependent adverse effects. Glucose-6-phosphate dehydrogenase deficiency aggravates hemolysis and is therefore a contraindication to sulfasalazine administration. Idiosyncratic adverse reactions demand cessation of therapy rather than dose reduction. These, fortunately, are much less

Table 8 Sulfasalazine and Oral 5-Aminosalicylic Acid Analogues

Generic Name	Trade Name	Dosage Form	Release Mechanism	Site of Release
Sulfasalazine	Azulfidine	500 mg tablets	Bacterial cleavage of diazo bond	Colon
Olsalazine	Dipentum (Pharmacia)	250 mg capsules	Bacterial cleavage of diazo bond	Colon
Mesalamine	Asacol (Proctor and Gamble, United States and Canada; Tillots, United Kingdom)	400 mg tablets	PH-Dependent breakdown	Distal ileum or right colon (pH > 7.0)
Mesalamine	Salofalk (Interfalk) Claversal (Smith, Kline & French, United States) Rowasa (Reid-Rowell, United States)	250 and 500 mg tablets	PH-Dependent breakdown	From mid to small bowel distally (pH > 5.6)
Mesalamine	Pentasa (Marion, United States; Nordic, Canada; Ferring, Europe)	250 and 500 mg tablets	Timed-release	Throughout small intestine and colon

common than the dose-dependent effects and usually occur at the initiation of therapy. Fever, exanthems including Stevens-Johnson syndrome, pulmonary fibrosis, hepatotoxicity, and very rarely agranulocytosis have all been reported. A known hypersensitivity to sulphonamides is a contraindication to sulfasalazine therapy. The infrequent occurrence of exacerbation of colitic symptoms is considered related to the 5 aminosalicylic acid constituent rather than to sulfapyridine.[172] Sulfasalazine also reversibly impairs male fertility.[173] Sperm morphology and motility revert to normal after discontinuation of the drug.

Eighty to ninety percent of patients intolerant of or allergic to sulfasalazine will tolerate oral 5-aminosalicylic acid.[174] Occasionally, the same adverse hypersensitivity reaction such as fever and/or rash or exacerbation of colitic symptoms is observed.[174] The most serious idiosyncratic reactions associated with sulfasalazine (ie, agranulocytosis, pulmonary complications) have not been reported with 5-aminosalicylic acid. Sulfasalazine-related impairment of male fertility resolves with a change to 5-aminosalicylic acid. However, several case reports of acute pancreatitis in association with mesalazine formulations have been published.[175] Olsalazine, which can act as a secretagogue in the distal ileum, causes diarrhea in 10 to 15% of patients.[176]

Evidence-Based Therapeutic Indications

Active Disease. In both the National Collaborative Crohn Disease Study (NCCDS) and the European Cooperative Crohn Disease Study (ECCDS), sulfasalazine proved efficacious in treating inflammation involving the colon.[150–151] The European study suggested, furthermore, an adjunctive role in isolated colonic Crohn's disease, which is often relatively resistant to corticosteroid therapy alone.[151] Isolated ileal Crohn's disease was refractory to sulfasalazine therapy in both collaborative studies.

Timed-release and pH-dependent formulations designed to extend the scope of efficacy of 5-aminosalicylic acid have demonstrated at most modest benefit, when employed at high dosages in adults with active disease.[177] For example, in one large multicenter study 4 g of timed-release 5-aminosalicylic acid was superior to placebo, 1 and 2 g of active drug, but the mean reduction in CDAI even with the highest dosage was only 72 +/− 13 points.[177] The best reported results have been in isolated ileitis, where 4 g of a timed-release microgranular formulation achieved a mean change in CDAI of 123 at 12 weeks.[178] In keeping with these modest results, timed-release 5-ASA (4 g) induced clinical remission in significantly fewer patients (36%) than CIR budesonide (69%).[179]

If children with mildly active Crohn's disease are to be treated with 5-ASA or sulfasalazine, the choice of formulation should be made based on knowledge of the site(s) of intestinal inflammation to be targeted. Dosage of 5-ASA is extrapolated from adult studies; dose-ranging trials of efficacy specifically in children are lacking.

Maintenance of Remission

There is a paucity of data to support the efficacy of sulfasalazine in maintaining remission of quiescent Crohn's disease. Neither the NCCDS or ECCDS demonstrated a statistically significant benefit in comparison to placebo.[150–151] Efficacy of oral 5-aminosalicylic acid in maintaining remission in Crohn's disease has been observed in several individual randomized placebo-controlled trials, but initial enthusiasm has waned as additional data have been accrued. In an elegant meta-analysis Camma and colleagues combined data from 2,097 patients with medically and surgically induced remission in 15 trials, including several large studies.[180] In the setting of medically induced remission, the pooled risk difference with oral 5-aminosalicylic acid versus placebo was not significant (−4.7%, 95% CI 9.6 to 2.8%). Hence, in keeping with earlier results achieved with sulfasalazine,[150–151] randomized controlled trial data in adults do not support the use of mesalamine therapy to maintain medically induced remission in patients with inactive Crohn's disease.[180] Similarly, in a recently reported pediatric study, the 1-year remission rate with timed-release 5-aminosalicylic acid (50 mg/kg/d) initiated immediately following successful medical treatment of active disease was no different than with placebo (43 vs 37%).[181]

In the Camma meta-analysis, therapeutic effectiveness of mesalamine appeared increased in the setting of a surgically induced remission, where the pooled risk difference was −13.1% (95% CI, 0.05 to 0.21). As a measure of the efficacy of postoperative 5-aminosalicylic acid, the overall risk difference between the frequency of relapse in treated and control groups was calculated, allowing easy computation of the number of patients needing treatment to prevent one relapse.[180] Based on these data, one would need to treat eight patients following surgical resection to prevent one postoperative recurrence.[180] However, in the subsequently reported well-designed ECCDS of 318 adults, there was overall no significant difference in month clinical relapse rates with timed-release 5-aminosalicylic acid (24.5 ± 3.6%) versus placebo (31.4 ± 3.7%) begun immediately postoperatively.[182] With these additional data in the trial literature, the number needed to treat rises to 25, and it becomes hard to defend an evidence-based recommendation for routine use of oral 5-aminosalicylic acid to maintain remission following intestinal resection of all grossly diseased bowel.[183] In subgroup analysis of the ECCDS data, however, a delay in disease recrudescence was identified among patients who had undergone resection for isolated small bowel disease.[182]

ANTIBIOTICS AND PROBIOTICS

The clear implication of microbial flora in the pathophysiology of intestinal inflammation in Crohn's disease has led to a resurgence of interest in the use of antibiotics and, more recently, probiotics. Supportive data are, however, relatively scarce. Metronidazole has been the most frequently studied drug, but recently ciprofloxacin has been employed alone or in combination.

Probiotics, defined as "living organisms, which upon ingestion, exert health benefits," belong generally to a large group of bacteria that make up the natural microflora and dwell as harmless commensals. Varieties of probiotics, which have been tested in limited fashion in IBD, include *Lactobacilli, Bifidobacteria, Streptococci*, nonpathogenic strains of *E. coli*, and the yeast strain, *Saccharomyces boulardi*.

Evidence-Based Therapeutic Indications

Metronidazole is well established, albeit not by randomized controlled trial data, in the control of perianal fistulae in Crohn's disease.[184–185] In the treatment of intestinal inflammation, metronidazole was found to be at least as effective as sulfasalazine in a double-blind crossover Swedish multicenter study.[186] In a Canadian study, metronidazole was associated with a greater reduction in Crohn's disease activity than placebo, although not with a superior remission rate.[187] Two doses employed (10 mg/kg/d and 20 mg/kg/d) were comparable; the lower dose is preferred because of concerns about potential peripheral neuropathic effects with long-term use. In both studies colonic inflammation responded better than disease confined to the small intestine.[186–187] In a small randomized study of metronidazole plus ciprofloxacin versus methylprednisolone for active Crohn's disease, the clinical response rates were, respectively, 45% and 63.[188] The combination of metronidazole plus ciprofloxacin did not enhance the efficacy of CIR budesonide in active Crohn's disease involving the ileum and right colon.[189] There are supportive data for the use of metronidazole to delay recurrence after ileal resection.[190] Antimycobacterial regimens have not demonstrated benefit in comparison to placebo.[191]

The small number of inflammatory bowel disease patients, who have been treated in randomized, controlled fashion with probiotics, have to date most often had ulcerative colitis or pouchitis. Several trials examining the efficacy of different probiotic preparations in prevention of postoperative recurrence of Crohn's disease have been disappointing.[192]

Potential Adverse Effects

Metronidazole may cause a peripheral predominantly sensory neuropathy, which appears to be related to dosage and duration of therapy.[193] Clinical experience suggests that paraesthesiae always resolve, albeit at times very slowly, following discontinuation of metronidazole. Adolescents should be warned of metronidazole's disulfiram-like effect with alcohol ingestion. Another concern with long-term metronidazole therapy in young patients arises from its mutagenic and carcinogenic effects observed in laboratory animals. Ciprofloxacin has caused damage to growing bone in some laboratory animal species, but such adverse effects have not been observed in children despite substantial use in a variety of pediatric conditions.

AZATHIOPRINE AND 6-MERCATOPURINE

The immunomodulatory drugs, azathioprine and 6-mercaptopurine (6-MP), have traditionally been the first-line immunomodulatory drugs employed in the management of pediatric Crohn's disease.[194] Their delayed onset of action precludes a role for azathioprine/6-MP monotherapy in acute treatment.[194] Their importance as steroid-sparing agents in controlling intestinal inflammation and maintaining remission in children is now well established.[195]

Pharmacology and Mechanism of Action

6-MP is a purine analogue capable of interfering with endogenous purines, essential components of RNA and DNA. It has cytotoxic and immunosuppressive properties. Azathioprine was developed as a prodrug permitting liberation of 6-MP in tissues. The related structure of the two drugs leads one to anticipate similar clinical effects, but no directly comparative studies exist. There is some evidence from animal studies that azathioprine may have a better therapeutic index that is ratio of therapeutic immunosuppressive to toxic dose.[196]

As shown in Figure 7, azathioprine/6-MP undergo a series of enzymatic reactions leading to the formation of 6-thioguanine (6-TGN), which then becomes phosphorylated.[197] The precise therapeutic mechanism of action of 6-TGN or its metabolites has been uncertain. Recent work has highlighted the importance of 6-thioguanosine triphosphate in Rac1 inhibition, thereby leading indirectly to mitochondria-mediated apoptosis.[167-198] In competing enzymatic pathways, thiopurine methyltransferase (TPMT) catalyzes the formation of 6-methyl-mercaptopurine ribonucleotides (6-MMPR), metabolites that are therapeutically inactive and potentially hepatotoxic.[199]

Codominantly inherited polymorphic alleles confer high (TPMT^H) and low (TPMT^L) functional TMPT activity that potentially impact the therapeutic response to azathioprine and its toxicity.[199] Approximately 89% of the population carry two wild-type TPMT^H alleles (TPMT^H/TPMT^H) and have high TPMT activity (> 9.5 U/mL RBC); 11% are heterozygous (TPMT^H/TPMT^L) and have intermediate activity (5.0 to 9.5 U/mL RBC); and 0.3% are homozygous for the variant TPMT^L allele (TPMT^L/TPMT^L) and have low or undetectable activity (<5.0 U/mL RBC). Moreover, sulfasalazine and 5-aminosalicylic acid are recognized to inhibit TPMT activity.[199-200]

Potential Adverse Effects

Sandborn categorized the adverse effects of azathioprine and 6-MP as allergic (dose independent) or nonallergic (dose and metabolism dependent).[201] The hypersensitivity reactions, which resolve with discontinuation of therapy, include fever, pancreatitis, rash, arthralgias, nausea, vomiting, and diarrhea. Nonallergic toxicities include severe leukopenia, thrombocytopenia, infection, hepatitis, and an increased risk of neoplasia, particularly lymphoma.

Several groups have summarized the frequency of these acute and long-term unwanted complications of azathioprine or 6-MP administration. Treatment was discontinued because of an adverse effect in 17 (18%) of 95 children and adolescents,[202] a higher overall percentage than in previous adult series.[201,203] The most common hypersensitivity reaction among adults and children is pancreatitis, occuring in 3 to 4% of patients, and almost always within the first several weeks of starting therapy. Fever and gastrointestinal intolerance manifested by vomiting necessitated cessation of treatment in 4 and 3%, respectively, of pediatric patients.[202] Bone marrow toxicity may be seen shortly after therapy is begun, but also many years into therapy.[203-204] Accordingly, white blood cell counts should be monitored throughout the duration of therapy. Peripheral white blood cell counts below 2,500/mm^3 were reported in 2% of patients during more than 20 years of experience with 6-MP.[203] The British experience of 4% leukopenia with azathioprine includes 2 deaths, both related to bone marrow aplasia, among 714 patients with inflammatory bowel disease.[204] Leukopenia is partly dose-related, but individual susceptibility also varies, related in part to genetically determined differences in drug metabolism.[200]

It is standard practice in some parts of the world to determine TPMT activity and/or genotype prior to commencing azathioprine or 6-MP as a means of avoiding serious myelosuppression. It must be acknowledged, however, that observed myelosuppression is, for the majority of patients, related to factors other than low-TPMT activity.[206] Whatever the TPMT genotype, white cell counts will still need to be monitored throughout the duration of azathioprine/6-MP therapy. As an example,

Colombel and colleagues reported TPMT genotype analysis in 41 Crohn's disease patients, all of whom had experienced leukopenia (white cell count <3.0 × 10^9/L) or thrombocytopenia (platelets < 10^9/L) leading to drug withdrawal in 83% and dosage reduction in the remainder.[206] Four patients (10%) were TPMT deficient (homozygous variant allele), seven (17%) were heterozygous, but the remainder had wild-type activity (homozygous normal).[206] All four TPMT deficient patients experienced bone marrow toxicity within 1.5 months, suggesting a role for TPMT in the prediction of early myelosuppression.[206]

Infectious complications possibly attributable to or aggravated by azathioprine or 6-MP are described in overall 1 to 2% of patients.[203] One case of fatal varicella infection in a child with Crohn's disease treated with 6-MP is reported.[207] Susceptible children receiving azathioprine or 6-MP, who are exposed to chicken pox, should be given varicella zoster immune globulin within 48 hours and have immunomodulatory agents discontinued. Over time and with increased use in IBD, it has become apparent through cohort studies that AZA/6-MP use is associated with an increased risk, albeit small, of lymphoma in comparison to age-matched healthy controls.[208] Within the last year, an unexpectedly high number of young Crohn's disease patients have developed an otherwise extremely rare, and extremely aggressive hepatosplenic T-cell lymphoma (HSTCL), which affects males predominantly.[209] Each of the patients, recognized through postmarketing surveillance of infliximab, had received long-term azathioprine both prior to and concomitantly with the anti-TNF-α agent. HSTCL has been reported rarely in Crohn's disease patients treated with AZA alone.[210] Hence, the relative contributions of thiopurine immunemodulators alone, anti-TNF-α therapy alone, or combination therapy to the development of this malignancy have not been established.[209]

Evidence-Based Therapeutic Indications

A meta-analysis of placebo-controlled trials employing azathioprine (2.0 to 2.5 mg/kg/d) or 6-MP (1.5 mg/kg/d) to treat active Crohn's disease confirms the efficacy of these immunomodulatory drugs. The pooled odds ratio for response is 9.3 (95% confidence interval 7.8 to 10.8).[194] The meta-analysis demonstrated a requirement of 16 weeks to achieve therapeutic benefit. Pilot data suggesting that a large intravenous loading dose of azathioprine given at initiation of therapy might decrease the time to response were not supported in a subsequent randomized controlled trial.[211] However, the addition of azathioprine to prednisolone therapy facilitated weaning of prednisolone dosage in a placebo-controlled 8-week trial in acute Crohn's disease.[212] Duration of required therapy has always been in question. A recent randomized controlled trial in adults suggested that withdrawal of azathioprine/6-MP might be possible after 4 years of successful maintenance of remission.[213]

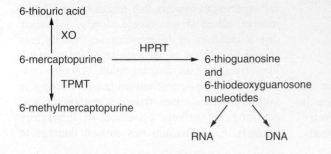

Figure 7 6-Mercaptopurine metabolism. The initial metabolism of 6-MP occurs along the competing routes catalyzed by thiopurine methyltransferase (TPMT), xanthine oxidase (XO), and hypoxanthine phosphoribosyltransferase (HPRT). Relative deficiency of TPMT or competition for XO leads to increased formation of 6-thioguanosine and 6-deoxythioguanosone nucleotides. The corporation of these nucleotides into RNA and DNA induces cytotoxicity.

Based on adult randomized controlled trial data and reported clinical experience among pediatric patients, it is reasonable to anticipate improved control of symptoms and reduced corticosteroid requirements in 60 to 70% of children and adolescents. The placebo-controlled trial of concomitant 6-MP among newly diagnosed children treated with an initial course of prednisone led the way in the trend to introduce immunomodulatory therapy early.[195] In 1 year of follow-up, children treated with 6-MP experienced fewer relapses and received a lower cumulative prednisone dosage.[195]

Direct measurement of intracellular metabolites in red blood cells is feasible and is now often recommended in order that drug dosage be adjusted on an individual basis with greater safety.[214] There are some data from the treatment of other disorders to support the concept that individualized azathioprine/6-MP dosing based on 6-TGN levels can improve response rates compared to conventional dosing regimens.[215–216] Data concerning 6-TGN levels and therapeutic response in IBD patients are, however, conflicting.[211,214,217–218] The earliest, preliminary, retrospective data were reported by Cuffari an colleagues in 1996.[217] Among 25 adolescent Crohn's disease patients treated with 6-MP, a lack of clinical response judged by high Harvey Bradshaw index (HBI) retrospectively calculated, was associated with low RBC 6-TGN levels, but a satisfactory clinical response (low HBI) was associated with a wide range of RBC 6-TGN levels.[217] Dubinsky and colleagues have published two observational studies concerning, respectively, 92 children and 62 adults, who had been receiving 6-MP or azathioprine as treatment of their Crohn's disease for at least 4 months.[214] RBC 6-TGN levels measured in these patients were found to correlate with likelihood of clinical remission, as assessed by modified Harvey Bradshaw index <5 or fistula closure, and steroid discontinuation. In the largest study to date conducted among 170 adults established on azathioprine/6-MP therapy, no difference was found between whole blood 6-TGN concentrations in patients in clinical remission compared with those with active disease.[218] Similarly in the prospective randomized controlled trial comparing an intravenous loading dose of azathioprine with standard oral dosing, there was no correlation between RBC 6-TGN concentrations and either clinical response or occurrence of leukopenia.[211]

All studies to date in Crohn's disease are observational and do not prospectively test the hypothesis that adjustment of azathioprine or 6-MP dosage to a target 6-TGN concentration will improve treatment outcomes. A double-blind multicenter trial comparing in randomized fashion azathioprine therapy at a standard 2.5 mg/kg/d dosage without subsequent metabolite monitoring versus therapy dosed according to TPMT enzyme activity and serial 6-TGN measurements is underway. At present in a patient with an unsatisfactory clinical response, determination of 6-TGN and MMPR will at least detect noncompliance and may serve to influence the next therapeutic recommendation.

METHOTREXATE

Although methotrexate has a long history of use in the treatment of juvenile idiopathic arthritis, application to the treatment of Crohn's disease has been limited. The onset of action appears more rapid than with azathioprine or 6-MP, but otherwise there are no comparative efficacy and safety data.

Mechanism of Action

Methotrexate inhibits the conversion of folic acid to its active form tetrahydrofolate, which is necessary for thymidine synthesis. Thus, methotrexate impairs DNA synthesis. Additional anti-inflammatory properties may be related to reduction in IL-1 production or induction of apoptosis of selected T-cell populations.

Potential Adverse Effects

In comparison with azathioprine and 6-MP, data establishing a safety profile for use in inflammatory bowel disease are sparse. Observed adverse effects in the published two phase multicenter trial in Crohn's disease were minor: nausea and asymptomatic increases in liver enzymes.[219–220] Hypersensitivity pneumonitis is a rare, but potentially serious complication, but has not been observed in the limited experience in Crohn's disease to date, nor reported in the much larger experience with pediatric rheumatic diseases.

Evidence-Based Therapeutic Indications

In a large placebo-controlled study that utilized intramuscular injections of methotrexate (25 mg weekly for 16 wk), 39% of patients whose Crohn's disease was persistently active despite corticosteroid therapy achieved remission with methotrexate compared to 19% with placebo.[219] Clinical improvement was seen after 6 weeks treatment. In a follow-up study, a benefit in maintaining remission in these adult patients was also observed.[220]

Eleven (78%) of 14 children and adolescents with Crohn's disease previously intolerant or refractory to azathioprine/6-mercaptopurine therapy improved with methotrexate therapy.[221] These observations have now been confirmed in a larger, multicenter, but still retrospective analysis of subcutaneous or oral methotrexate following unsuccessful thiopurine therapy.[222] There is renewed interest in methotrexate in the treatment of pediatric Crohn's disease in light of the increased recognition of the potential toxicity of long-term azathioprine/6-MP use.[208,222]

CYCLOSPORINE A/TACROLIMUS

Results from randomized controlled trials of cyclosporine in Crohn's disease have been disappointing.[223–226] In the first study conducted among adults with active corticosteroid resistant Crohn's disease, the percentage "improving" (59%) with high-dose oral cyclosporine (5 to 7.5 mg/kg/d) was greater than with placebo (32%), but the threshold level for judging clinical response was set very low.[223] A subsequent multicenter Canadian placebo-controlled study involving approximately 300 patients demonstrated no benefit from a mean of 4.8 mg/kg/d cyclosporine administered for 18 months.[224] One-third of patients had active disease and two-thirds were in remission at initial randomization. Two other multicenter trials in adults yielded essentially negative results.[225–226] Oral cyclosporine was not as effective as prednisolone in newly diagnosed children with Crohn's disease.[227] Intravenous cyclosporine was helpful in closing severe fistula in one study in adults.[228]

BIOLOGIC AGENTS: INFLIXIMAB

As the pathways involved in the pathogenesis of intestinal inflammation have been elucidated, a new class of therapeutic agents, referred to as biologics and having specific molecular targets, has been developed. These biologic therapies include cytokines, antibodies, and adhesion molecules. Infliximab, a chimeric (murine-human) monoclonal antibody directed against tumor necrosis factor alpha (TNF-α), has ushered in a new era in the management of pediatric Crohn's disease.

Pharmacology and Mechanism of Action

Infliximab is an antibody of the IgG1 isotype that binds specifically to circulating and membrane-bound TNF-α.[229] TNF-α is a key proinflammatory cytokine possessing many properties relevant to intestinal inflammation.[230] The product of activated macrophages, it is capable of activating other macrophages and priming neutrophils, inducing proteases critical to tissue destruction, enhancing chloride secretion from intestinal epithelial cells, and inducing acute phase reactants. It may also increase the expression of adhesion molecules, thereby contributing to the recruitment of monocytes, lymphocytes, and granulocytes. The expression of TNF-α is markedly increased in Crohn's disease. The efficacy of its blockade with infliximab attests to its important pathogenic role. Induction of apoptosis following binding to membrane-bound TNF-α is considered to be particularly important to efficacy of anti-TNF-α therapy in Crohn's disease.[167,231]

Evidence-Based Therapeutic Indications

In a multicenter placebo-controlled trial of three doses of infliximab in 108 adult patients with medically resistant, moderate to severe Crohn's disease, 81% of patients treated with a single infusion of 5 mg/kg were significantly improved, and 48% achieved remission by the end of 4 weeks.[229] In another placebo-controlled study of three infusions of infliximab (at 0, 2, and 6 weeks), 68% of patients with fistulous disease in the 5 mg/kg arm had at least a 50% reduction from baseline in the number of fistulae draining.[232] After a median 6 to 12 weeks, however, there is a predictable loss of infliximab-induced benefit in the treatment of inflammatory and fistulizing disease.[229–232]

The ability of repeated infusions given at 8-weekly intervals to sustain clinical response has been demonstrated in large maintenance placebo-controlled and dose-ranging studies in adults with both inflammatory (ACCENT I trial) and fistulizing disease (ACCENT II study),[233–234] and recently in children with chronically active Crohn's disease despite prior immunmodulatory therapy.[235] In comparison to 5 mg/kg, doses of 10 mg/kg were associated with longer duration of continuous clinical response in the ACCENT I trial, reflecting longer duration of detectable drug in the serum.[233] Similarly, in the pediatric trial infusions every 12 weeks were more often associated with relapse of clinical symptoms prior to the next infusion, in comparison to treatments at 8-week intervals.[235] Regularly scheduled infusions are preferable to episodic (as needed) infliximab treatment, by virtue of reduced likelihood of formation of antibodies to infliximab (ATI).[233,236] Post hoc analysis of the ACCENT I data also demonstrated greater likelihood of mucosal healing and a lower hospitalization rate with maintenance versus episodic therapy.[236]

The development of ATI is associated with a shorter duration or loss of responsiveness, as well as with an increased frequency of infusion reactions.[237] In a retrospective analysis among adults with Crohn's disease given infliximab episodically, concomitant administration of azathioprine/6-MP was associated with a lower incidence of ATI formation and of infusion reactions, as well as with prolongation of clinical response following each infusion.[237] The same benefit of concomitant methotrexate with episodic treatment has recently been reported.[238]

Although the necessity of concomitant immunemodulation with episodic therapy is undeniable, the benefit of dual therapy with regularly scheduled infusions of infliximab or other biologic agents appears much less. Among rheumatoid arthritis patients, concomitant use of methotrexate reduced the frequency of antibody formation and had an adjunctive therapeutic effect.[239] In contrast, post hoc analyses of the ACCENT I and II trials, wherein infliximab was also given by regularly scheduled infusions, do not support a significant benefit from concomitant administration of an immunemodulatory drug, either in clinical efficacy or in further prevention of ATI formation.[233,236] Children participating in the REACH multicenter pediatric study of infliximab maintenance therapy were required to receive a concomitant immunemodulatory drug.[235] However, in current clinical practice many pediatric gastroenterologists employ regularly scheduled (but not episodic) infliximab as monotherapy, weighing the small benefit of concomitant immunemodulation against the possible role of azathioprine/6-MP or combination therapy in the pathogenesis of hepatosplenic T-cell lymphoma.[209] The need for concomitant immun-emodulation (azathioprine/6-MP or methotrexate) with regularly scheduled infliximab therapy is being definitively addressed in two prospective trials in adults. Use of an intravenous corticosteroid drug at the time of infliximab infusion is another strategy to reduce ATI formation.[241]

Potential Adverse Effects

As recently and thoroughly reviewed, the adverse effects of infliximab therapy have been monitored in randomized controlled trials among Crohn's disease and rheumatoid arthritis and as a part of postmarketing surveillance.[240] These include acute infusion reactions and delayed hypersensitivity reactions.[241] The latter are characterized by malaise, fever, and muscle ache 1 to 12 days following infusion; no end-organ damage results. Infliximab may induce anti-dsDNA antibodies, which are usually low titer and very infrequently associated with clinical signs and symptoms of systemic lupus erythematosus.[240] TNF-α is an integral component of innate and adaptive immune responses, and is necessary for host defense against certain intracellular bacteria, such as *Mycobacterium tuberculosis*. It is not surprising, therefore, that infliximab treatment is associated with an increased incidence of tuberculosis, usually a consequence of reactivation of latent disease, and often presenting in disseminated form.[240,242] Screening for tuberculosis prior to initiation of infliximab therapy is mandatory. Other infections complicating infliximab therapy are much rarer, but include, for example, histoplasmosis, and Listeria meningitis.[240,243]

Clinical trial experience in adults with rheumatoid arthritis and Crohn's disease raised an initial concern about an excess of lymphoma development.[240] Occurrences of malignancy in treatment registries have not exceeded expected rates. A meta-analysis of rates of neoplasia occurring in rheumatoid arthritis patients treated with anti-TNF agents in randomized controlled trials did suggest an increased risk in comparison to control arms in those studies.[244] The recent recognition of hepatosplenic T-cell lymphoma in young patients treated with both infliximab and long-term azathioprine/6-MP has altered physician perception of the safety profile of this combination therapy.[209]

Clinical Use

Evidence-based guidelines for infliximab use among adult patients with inflammatory Crohn's disease have endorsed its use among patients refractory to or intolerant of corticosteroids and conventional immunomodulatory agents.[245] Such "step-up" recommendations constitute a balance between the often dramatic short-term efficacy and possibility of mucosal healing, and the uncertain long-term adverse effects. Infliximab has a similar role in the treatment of children and adolescents with severe disease refractory to optimally employed conventional medical therapies and not amenable to localized resection. Pediatric gastroenterologists must stay aware of evolving recommendations concerning treatment regimens, in order that efficacy be maximized and problems, including ATI formation, and lymphoma risk be minimized.[240]

Other Anti-TNF Agents

Etanercept (anti-TNF-α receptor) appears ineffective in Crohn's disease. More recently developed anti-TNF agents with efficacy in Crohn's disease include the humanized antibody, adalimumab, and the humanized pegylated antibody fragment, certolizumab.[246–248] Both are given by subcutaneous injection, adalimumab either weekly or biweekly, certulizumab once monthly, to maintain remission after initial induction regimens. Efficacy of both agents has been demonstrated in large randomized controlled trials in adults.[246–248] Both can be expected to be effective in patients who have lost response to infliximab therapy as a result of antibody formation.[249] Since these agents are humanized, antibody formation is less frequent, but still occurs at a rate dependent (as for infliximab) on the regimen of administration (regularly scheduled vs episodic) and reduced by concomitant immunemodulation. Doses in children remain to be established.

Other Biologics

Results with and IL-10 in Crohn's disease have been disappointing.[250] Diminution of active inflammation was observed with natulizimab ($\alpha_4\beta$-integrin) in a randomized controlled trial among adults.[251] However, the development of fatal multifocal leukoencephalopathy in one patient with Crohn's disease and in two patients in multiple sclerosis treated in phase II clinical trials led to a halt in further study of this agent, at least in Crohn's disease, where other options exist.

PRIMARY NUTRITIONAL THERAPY

Liquid diet therapy is an effective alternative to corticosteroids among children and adolescents with active Crohn's disease. Indeed, enteral nutrition is regarded as first line therapy for pediatric Crohn's disease in centers in the United Kingdom and is commonly employed in other parts of Europe and Canada.

ENTERAL NUTRITION IN CROHN'S DISEASE

Mechanism of Action

The mode of action of enteral nutrition as primary treatment of active Crohn's disease remains conjectural. Hypotheses have included alteration in intestinal microbial flora, elimination of dietary antigen uptake, diminution of intestinal synthesis of inflammatory mediators via reduction of dietary fat, overall nutritional repletion, or provision of important micronutrients to the diseased intestine. Effects of enteral nutrition on the gut microbial flora deserve further exploration, in light of the now well-established role of microbes in disease pathogenesis.

Evidence-Based Therapeutic Indications

Active Disease. The potential role of exclusive enteral nutrition as primary therapy of active Crohn's disease was discovered fortuitously. Patients given elemental formulae preoperatively experienced an improvement, not only in their nutritional status as intended, but also in the inflammatory activity of their disease. These observations of primary therapeutic efficacy were first confirmed in the small controlled trial conducted by O'Morain and colleagues[252] However, in the subsequent much larger ECCDS randomized trials of enteral nutrition versus corticosteroid and sulfasalazine therapy, the drug therapy proved superior to semielemental formulae containing oligopeptides as the protein source.[253, 254]

The controversy surrounding seemingly divergent outcomes has fueled several meta-analyses, each of which has concluded that there is a treatment benefit to corticosteroids in comparison to enteral nutrition.[255] Analyzing results of eight trials on an intention-to-treat basis, the pooled odds ratio for the likelihood of clinical remission with liquid diet therapy versus corticosteroids is 0.35 (95% CIs 0.23 to 0.53).[255] Furthermore, poor compliance, while contributory, does not constitute the major explanation for the lower response rates to enteral nutrition as is evident from secondary meta-analysis excluding dropouts for apparent intolerance.[255]

No controlled trials of enteral nutrition versus placebo or less effective drugs in active Crohn's disease have been conducted. However, comparison of observed response rates to exclusive liquid diet therapy (53 to 82%) with usual placebo response rates (18 to 42%) in the controlled clinical trial setting suggests that enteral nutrition is of therapeutic benefit, when tolerated, even if efficacy does not equal that of corticosteroid treatment.[255] Moreover, a reduction in gastrointestinal protein loss, a decrease in intestinal permeability, and a reduction in fecal excretion of indium-labeled leucocytes have each been demonstrated, suggesting a direct effect on intestinal inflammation.[256–257] Open trials in children have documented endoscopic healing and decreased mucosal cytokine production following exclusive enteral nutrition.[258]

Factors Influencing Efficacy

Anatomic Localization of Inflammation. Patients with Crohn's colitis are generally considered to respond less reliably to than those with ileocolitis or isolated small bowel disease.[259] Children with Crohn's disease confined to the colon were excluded from the Canadian pediatric multicenter study.[152] The results of the ECCDS did not confirm a relationship between site(s) of intestinal inflammation and outcome, but the numbers of patients with isolated colonic disease were small even in these trials.[253, 254] In one trial comparing two types of enteral nutrition, two-thirds of patients had disease confined to the colon, but excellent clinical response rates of 67 and 73% to elemental and polymeric formulae, respectively, were nevertheless observed.[260]

Formula Composition

Several clinical trials have compared the efficacy of elemental versus nonelemental formulae of varying protein and fat composition. Existing data combined in meta-analysis do not support an advantage to elemental (aminoacid based) feedings compared with more palatable polymeric formulations.[261] The importance of fat composition to efficacy is less clear, but there may be a small treatment benefit achieved by reduction in the content of total fat or n-6 PUFAs.[261–262]

Bowel Rest

When employed in the treatment of active Crohn's disease, enteral nutrition is generally combined with "bowel rest." A recent pediatric trial concluded that supplementary enteral nutrition was less effective than exclusive enteral nutrition in inducing clinical remission.[263]

Age/Disease Duration

Several small trials of enteral nutrition in children with extremely high success rates have been reported,[264] but caution is always required in drawing firm conclusions from very small studies. The Canadian Pediatric Collaborative Trial of enteral nutrition versus corticosteroids[152] employed an oligopeptide-containing liquid diet very similar in composition to that used among adults in the ECCDS.[254] These two trials included, respectively, 78 children and 107 adults. The differences in patient populations and outcomes are summarized in Table 9. It seems likely that the higher remission rate overall with enteral nutrition in the pediatric study (75%) versus the adult study (53%) reflects differences in the nature of the patients randomized rather than an inherent difference in responsiveness of childhood Crohn's disease. Indeed, the subgroup of children with disease in relapse and of longer duration had a rate of clinical response to enteral nutrition very similar to adult patients. Alternatively, it could be argued that new onset disease is more responsive to enteral nutrition, an observation that has also been made with biologic therapy.[248]

Enteral nutrition does seem to be more feasible, if not inherently more efficacious, in pediatric populations. The formula can be infused nocturnally via nasogastric tube in the home setting and not interfere with normal activities. With the support of experienced nurses and physicians, enteral nutrition is in general well accepted by young patients. There is enough evidence of its short-term efficacy in active disease to support presentation as an alternate primary treatment to all young patients, particularly with predominantly small intestinal disease, for whom corticosteroids are being considered.

Maintenance of Remission

One of the limitations of liquid diet therapy has been the observed tendency for symptoms to recur promptly following its cessation. In most studies 60 to 70% of patients experience a relapse within 12 months of stopping enteral nutrition and resuming a normal diet.[260] Chronic intermittent bowel rest with nocturnal infusion of an elemental diet 1 month out of 4 has been recommended as a means of sustaining remission.[265] The beneficial effects on disease activity and growth of such cyclical enteral nutrition were confirmed in a recent randomized controlled trial versus alternate day prednisone.[266] Phase II of the Canadian Pediatric Crohn Disease Study examined the effects of alternate day administration of 0.3 mg/kg oral prednisone on rates of clinical relapse and growth in comparison to cycles of exclusive enteral nutrition. During an month period of follow-up, the difference between the percentage of patients remaining in continuous remission with alternate day prednisone (47%) and with cyclical enteral nutrition (67%) was not statistically significant, but linear growth was significantly better among patients randomized to receive the nutritional therapy.[265] Continuation of nocturnal nasogastric feeding four to five times weekly as supplement to an unrestricted ad lib daytime diet was also associated with prolonged disease quiescence and improved growth in a historical cohort study.[146]

Another "nutritional" strategy for maintaining remission has involved the use of fish oil supplements. A placebo-controlled study employing enteric-coated fish oil capsules designed for ileal

---

Table 9 Enteral Nutrition as Primary Treatment of Active Crohn's Disease—Comparison of Two Multicenter Adult and Pediatric Controlled Trials

Study	Response	Baseline CDAI	Colon Only Involved
European Cooperative Crohn Disease Study IV[254] (n = 107)	53% to EN 85% to CS	323 (±12 SEM) 316 (±11 SEM)	22%
Canadian Pediatric Crohn Disease Study[152] (n = 78)	75% to EN 89% to CS	260 (242 to 278) 309 (282 to 335)	None*
Canadian Pediatric Crohn Disease Study subgroup with disease in relapse[152] (n = 21)	50% to EN 85% to CS)	269 (233 to 304) 292 (251 to 333)	None*

CS = corticosteroids; EN = enteral nutrition.
*Crohn's disease confined to the colon was an exclusion criterion.

release demonstrated a substantial reduction in clinical relapse rate among patients with Crohn's disease in clinical but not biochemical remission at baseline.[267] Eicosapentaenoic acid (fish oil) competes with arachidonic acid thereby reducing its metabolism to leukotriene B4, an amplifier of intestinal inflammation, by the 5-lipoxygenase pathway.

SURGICAL TREATMENT

Optimal management of young patients with inflammatory bowel disease often includes appropriate and timely referral for intestinal resection, which is increasingly performed laparoscopically.[268]

Indications for Intestinal Resection

The most common reasons for surgery include intractable symptoms despite medical therapy, intestinal complications including obstruction, intra-abdominal abscess, enterovesicular fistula, and less frequently free perforation or intractable hemorrhage. Many children have experienced growth impairment by the time resection is considered, an indication of the failure of medical treatment to adequately control intestinal inflammation.

Outcome

"To cut is not to cure."[269] Crohn's disease is a chronic panenteric inflammatory process, which cannot be eradicated by current medical therapy or by resection of gross disease. Patients who undergo ileal resection typically develop recurrent disease just proximal to the ileocolonic anastomosis, whereas the site of recurrence can be on either or both sides of the anastomosis following segmental colonic resection. Macroscopic lesions have been found in the neoterminal ileum of 72% of patients routinely colonoscoped 1 year following intestinal resection and ileocolic anastomosis.[269] However, the possibility of a significant asymptomatic interval, during which normal growth and pubertal development can resume, makes such surgery an attractive therapeutic option for young patients, despite the likelihood of eventual disease recrudescence. A substantial improvement in height velocity can be anticipated postoperatively in previously growth-impaired adolescents, provided the surgery is performed prior to or during early puberty.[270–271] The amount of catch-up growth achieved will depend on the duration of the clinical remission.

Several studies among adult patients have documented the cumulative rates of recurrence of symptomatic disease. The incidence of clinical recurrence averages about 10% per year postoperatively. Similarly, based on return of symptoms with radiological evidence of disease, the median postoperative recurrence-free interval was 5.1 years in a series of 82 children and adolescents undergoing a first resection.[270]

Factors Influencing Outcome

Risk factors for postoperative symptomatic recurrence have been examined in many studies of large cohorts of adult patients, but few reliable "prognostic factors" have been consistently identified.[272–273] The length of recurrent ileal disease appears comparable to the length of ileum inflamed preoperatively.[274] Rates of recurrence are lower after surgical resection with ileostomy than after resection with ileocolonic anastomosis.[275] The outcome after colectomy and end ileostomy for isolated Crohn's colitis is particularly good: 15% cumulative probability of symptomatic recurrence after 20 years versus 64% in patients with ileocolitis as their initial presentation in one typical study.[276] In two pediatric studies, anatomic distribution of disease was the most important factor influencing outcome.[270–271] Patients with extensive ileocolonic involvement experienced an excess of early recurrences (50% by 1 yr) in comparison to children with preoperative disease in the terminal ileum +/− right colon or in the more proximal small intestine (50% by 5 years).[270] Fistulizing and stenosing disease have been considered, respectively, poor and good prognostic factors for length of postoperative remission in adult studies.[272–273] However, children undergoing resection because of stenosing or fistulizing complications (eg, bowel obstruction or intra-abdominal abscess) had delayed recrudescence of disease in comparison to those operated upon simply for inflammatory symptoms refractory to medical therapy.[270] An early operative approach to localized disease and for complications of chronic inflammation is supported by these data.[270] The rapid return of symptoms after major resection in patients with extensive ileocolitis suggests that medical strategies should be maintained in this group.

Maintenance of disease quiescence via adjuvant pharmacologic treatment following surgery has proved as difficult as maintenance of medically induced remission. As discussed earlier in the chapter, meta-analysis of the now very large number of patients treated in randomized fashion with oral 5-aminosalicylic acid in placebo-controlled trials no longer supports its routine use following resection of all gross disease.[180,182] Patients undergoing resection of isolated ileal disease may benefit.[182] Two studies have suggested a benefit to postoperative antibiotic administration in delaying endoscopic and clinical remission, but the number of patients on whom this conclusion is currently based is small.[190] CIR budesonide administered postoperatively has not been helpful,[277] nor have probiotics.[192] Recently, published data concerning 6-MP in the maintenance of, specifically, surgically induced clinical remission do suggest a benefit.[278–279] Smoking is consistently associated with higher recurrence rates, particularly in female patients, in all studies where this variable has been examined.[280]

MANAGEMENT OF PERIANAL DISEASE

Incision and drainage is indicated for significant abscesses. Prior to the development of anti-TNF-α therapies, the first line of medical therapy for perianal fistulae, based on retrospectively reported data, was metronidazole. Eighty-three percent of adult patients with a variety of chronic perianal and rectovaginal fistulae and unhealed perineal wounds responded to 20 mg/kg/d over 2 to 4 months.[184] Subsequent follow-up for as long as 36 months indicated that, although perianal disease seldom relapsed on full-dose therapy, reduction in dose or cessation of therapy was often associated with exacerbation. Metronidazole could be successfully discontinued in only 28% of patients.[185] The place of other antibiotics in the management of perianal disease is less substantiated, but ciprofloxacin appears to offer benefit as sole or adjunctive therapy. Benefit from azathioprine or 6-mercaptopurine, methotrexate, cyclosporine A have also been observed.

As previously discussed, infliximab infused at baseline, 2 weeks and 6 weeks is highly effective in achieving reduction in drainage and clinical closure of perianal fistulae.[232] As for intestinal inflammatory disease, regularly repeated infusions may be required to sustain clinical response.[234] MRI examinations can be used to detect persistence of fistulae despite apparent clinical closure. Prior to initiating anti-TNF-α treatment for perianal disease, examination under anesthesia or magnetic resonance imaging is required in order that any abscesses be identified and properly drained, usually with a seton.[281]

CLINICAL COURSE AND PROGNOSIS

Crohn's Disease

Disease Severity. Crohn's disease is heterogeneous in nature and varying in severity. Its protean nature precludes universally applicable statements about clinical course or prognosis. As depicted in Figure 8, the spectrum of disease patterns among consecutively diagnosed prepubertal patients in Toronto, Canada, in both the past two decades were similar. In 5-year follow-up, roughly one-third have mild symptoms only and another third more troublesome exacerbations but clear-cut remissions. The remaining one-third experience chronically active steroid-dependent or steroid-refractory disease, but half of these benefit significantly from resection and then experience a sustained remission. The 36% of children diagnosed both during the 1980s and during the 1990s underwent intestinal resection by 5 years of follow-up.[122]

Disease Behavior

The Montreal Working Group (and preceding Vienna classification) categorizes Crohn's disease as penetrating/fistulizing, stenosing, or

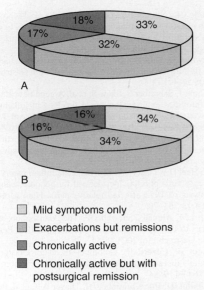

☐ Mild symptoms only
☐ Exacerbations but remissions
☐ Chronically active
☐ Chronically active but with postsurgical remission

Figure 8 Clinical course of Crohn's disease among consecutively diagnosed children at The Hospital for Sick Children, Toronto, Canada, during two decades. All children were prepubertal or in early puberty (Tanner stage 1 or 2) at the time of presentation. Patients were classified via retrospective chart review as having mild symptoms only, at least moderate exacerbations but remissions, or chronically active disease.

simply inflammatory.[104,136] The fistulizing subgroup includes any patient with enteroenteric, enterovesicular, enterocutaneous, or perianal fistula, or intra-abdominal abscess. The stenosing category includes patients with persistent abdominal pain and radiologic documentation of marked stenosis of a segment of small or large intestine. Although it has been argued that such behavior may be genetically determined, an analysis of the prevalence of each phenotype according to duration of disease suggests that stricturing and fistulizing behaviors become progressively more common over time.[282] This is in contrast to major localization of disease, which is consistent over time,[282] and appears to be genetically influenced. Nevertheless, consideration of the disease behavior at a given time may guide therapy.

Overall Mortality and Cancer Risk

A recent population-based European study, that included both pediatric onset and adult onset Crohn's disease, reported increased mortality 10 years after diagnosis compared to age- and gender-standardized mortality rates (SMR 1.85; 95% CI 1.30 to 2.55).[283] The excess mortality was mainly to gastrointestinal causes, including septic complications and cancer.[283] Persons with Crohn's colitis may be at similar risk to develop carcinoma of the colon as those with ulcerative colitis. The absolute cumulative frequency of risk for development of colorectal cancer in extensive Crohn's colitis was reported to be 8% after two decades of disease.[284] Accompanying severe perianal disease has been suggested as an additional risk factor. Colorectal carcinoma has been reported in a 21-year old diagnosed with Crohn's disease at the age of 8 years.[285]

CARING FOR THE WHOLE CHILD

The need to address the psychosocial impact of Crohn's disease on children and adolescents as well as on their families is increasingly recognized.[286] The concept of health-related quality of life (HRQOL) has been defined as the functional effect of an illness and its treatment on a patient, as perceived by the patient.[287] HRQOL is determined not only by physical well being but also by psychological state, degree of social support, effects of treatment, and complications.[286] Assessment of HRQOL provides a global measure of the patient's perceptions, illness experience, and functional status.[287] Increasingly appraisal of the impact of treatments on HRQOL is being expected in clinical trials and in health policy making.

Several recent studies have explored the concerns of young patients with inflammatory bowel disease with quite consistent findings.[287–288] Although in focus groups children initially denied that Crohn's disease interfered with their lives in any way, it became apparent that many were frustrated and angry about physical symptoms, and lack of understanding of their illness by others.[288] North American and English children shared similar concerns about body image, having to miss out on things, uncertainty about exacerbations and future health, and unpleasant treatments.[287,289] A disease-specific instrument incorporating these patient-generated concerns has been developed to facilitate assessment of the overall impact of pediatric IBD.[290] Activity indices such as the pediatric Crown's disease activity index[291] are designed to allow determination of the effects of treatment on the basic disease process, but they do not tell us how our patients are functioning day to day and how they feel about their chronic illness. Two adolescents may respond to the same physical symptoms with different outlooks and subsequent endeavors and achievements. Recognition of the disparity between activity and severity of Crohn's disease and emotional or functional disability may be facilitated by assessment of health-related quality of life.

When it is recognized that a child or adolescent needs help coping with his or her illness, it is equally important that there be effective interventions to restore emotional health and improve function. Although there are opinions and guidelines, strategies involving a multidisciplinary approach have not been subjected to scrutiny and appraisal, as have other therapies. Adolescents have a reluctance to participate in peer support groups, but whether dyadic peer support that is matching with another patient of similar or somewhat older age may be beneficial is beginning to be explored.

From the time of recognition of Crohn's disease, it is important to create an atmosphere that permits both the child and the parents to express their concerns about the physical state and the psychological aspects of the disease. As time goes by, an empathetic relationship between the medical team and the patients may enhance the likelihood of emotional expression. Support in coping with a chronic illness must be provided, but it is also important to understand and alleviate other stresses in the family environment, which may hinder coping with the illness. The overall impact of Crohn's disease on a child is the result of the complex interplay between physical, psychological, and social factors. If depression is identified, this must be dealt with psychotherapeutically by a psychiatrist or psychologist. It is important to see the child alone to make psychological communication easier. Education is vital because well-informed patients and families may be more likely to develop active coping strategies.

FINAL COMMENTS: CROHN'S DISEASE IN 2007

The past several years have witnessed exciting progress in unraveling the etiopathogenesis of Crohn's disease. The identification of the first gene conferring susceptibility was a landmark achievement in a complex disorder. The recognition of other genes determining susceptibility and influencing phenotypic expression has followed. Novel techniques allowing characterization of microbes inhabiting the gut hold promise, that the microbial trigger(s) of unrestrained inflammation in susceptible hosts will ultimately be defined. The interactions between intestinal microbial flora and the signaling pathways involved in the innate and adaptive immune response are being continually elucidated. With better understanding of these pathways have come biologic agents, which already have had a major therapeutic impact on this often disabling disease.

Although step-up versus top-down therapy can be debated, optimal management entails identification of genetic or clinical predictors of outcomes and responsiveness to treatments so that recommendations can be individualized. Pediatric gastroenterologists have become aware of the need to consistently characterize the phenotype, and as it becomes possible, the genotype, thereby establishing a framework for multicenter evaluation of emerging therapies in what is clearly a heterogeneous chronic inflammatory disorder, if not a spectrum of related but distinct Crohn's diseases.

REFERENCES

1. Hugot JP, Chamaillard M, Zouali H, et al. Association of NOD2 leucine-rich repeat variants with susceptibility to Crohn's disease. Nature 2001;411:599–603.
2. Ogura Y, Bonen DK, Inohara N, et al. A frameshift mutation in NOD2 associated with susceptibility to Crohn's disease. Nature 2001;411:537–9.
3. Hugot JP, Laurent-Puig P, Gower-Rousseau C, et al. Mapping of a susceptibility locus for Crohn's disease on chromosome 16. Nature 1996;379:821–3.
4. Ogura Y, Inohara N, Benito A, et al. Nod2, a Nod1/Apaf-1 family member that is restricted to monocytes and activates NF-kB. J Biol Chem 2001;276:4812–8.
5. Hampe J, Cuthbert A, Croucher PJ, et al. Association between insertion mutation in NOD2 gene and Crohn's disease in German and British populations. Lancet 2001;357:1925–8.

6. Duerr RH, Taylor KD, Brant SR, et al. A genome-wide association study identifies IL23R as an inflammatory bowel disease gene. Science 2006;314:1461–3.
7. Neurath MF. IL-23: A master regulator in Crohn disease. Nature Medicine 2007;13:26–8.
8. Crohn BC, Ginzburg L, Oppenheimer GD. Regional ileitis: A pathologic and clinical entity. JAMA 1932;99:1323–7.
9. Binder V. Epidemiology of IBD during the twentieth century: An integrated view. Best Pract Res Clin Gastroenterol 2004;18:463–79.
10. Cosgrove M, Al-Atia RF, Jenkins HR. The epidemiology of paediatric inflammatory bowel disease. Arch Dis Child 1996;74:460–1.
11. Barton JR, Gillon S, Ferguson A. Incidence of inflammatory bowel disease in Scottish children between 1968 and 1983: Marginal fall in ulcerative colitis, three-fold rise in Crohn's disease. Gut 1989;30:618–22.
12. Armitage E, Drummond H, Ghosh S, Ferguson A. Incidence of juvenile-onset Crohn's disease in Scotland. Lancet 1999;353:1496–7.
13. Ouyang Q, Tandon R, Goh KL, et al. The emergence of inflammatory bowel disease in the Asian Pacific region. Curr Opin Gastroenterol 2005;21:408–13.
14. Loftus EV, Jr. Clinical epidemiology of inflammatory bowel disease: Incidence, prevalence, and environmental influences. Gastroenterology 2004;126:1504–17.
15. Gottrand F, Colombel J-F, Moreno L, et al. Incidence of inflammatory bowel diseases in children in the Nor-Pas-de-Calais region. Arch Fr Pediatr 1991;48:25–8.
16. Langholz E, MunkholmP, Krasilnikoff PA, Binder V. Inflammatory bowel diseases with onset in childhood. Scand J Gastroenterol 1997;32:139–47.
17. Olafsdottir EJ, Gjermund F, Haug K. Chronic inflammatory bowel disease in children in western Norway. J Pediatr Gastroenterol Nutr 1989;8:454–8.
18. Durno C. Mode of inheritance and demographics of pediatric-onset inflammatory bowel disease. MSc Clin Epi Thesis: University of Toronto; 1999.
19. Sawczenko A, Sandhu B. Presenting features of inflammatory bowel disease in children. Arch Dis Child 2003;88:995–1000.
20. Griffiths AM. Specificities of inflammatory bowel disease in childhood. Best Pract Res Clin Gastroenterol 2004;18: 509–23.
21. Heyman MB, Kirschner BS, Gold BD, et al. Children with early-onset inflammatory bowel disease: Analysis of a pediatric IBD consortium registry. J Pediatr 2005;146:35–40.
22. Kugathasan S, Judd RH, Hoffmann RG, et al. Epidemiologic and clinical characteristics of children with newly diagnosed inflammatory bowel disease in Wisconsin: A statewide population-based study. J Pediatr 2003;143:525–31.
23. Gilat T. Inflammatory bowel disease in Jews. In: McConnel R, Rozen P, Langman M, et al, editors. The Genetics and Epidemiology of Inflammatory Bowel Disease, in Frontiers of Gastrointestinal Research. New York: Karger; 1986. p. 135–40.
24. Fireman Z, Grossman A, Lilos P, et al. Epidemiology of Crohn's disease in the Jewish population of central Israel, 1970–1980. Am J Gastroenterol 1989;84:255–8.
25. Strober W, Fuss I, Mannon P. The fundamental basis of inflammatory bowel disease. J Clin Invest 2007;117:514–21.
26. Peeters M, Nevens H, Baert F, et al. Familial aggregation in Crohn's disease: Increased age-adjusted risk and concordance in clinical characteristics. Gastroenterology 1996;111:597–603.
27. Russell RK, Satsangi J. IBD: A family affair. Best Pract Res Clin Gastroenterol 2004;18:525–39.
28. Bayless TM, Tokayer AZ, Polito JK, et al. Crohn's Disease: Concordance for site and clinical type in affected family members potential hereditary influences. Gastroenterology 1996;111:573–9.
29. Halfvarson J, Bodin L, Tysk C, et al. Inflammatory bowel disease in a Swedish twin cohort: A long-term follow-up of concordance and clinical characteristics. Gastroenterology 2003;124:1767–73.
30. Orholm M, Binder V, Sorensen TI, et al. Concordance of inflammatory bowel disease among Danish twins. Results of a nationwide study. Scand J Gastroenterol 2000;35: 1075–81.
31. Yang H, McElree C, Roth MP, et al. Familial empirical risk for inflammatory bowel disease: Differences between Jews and non-Jews. Gut 1993;34:517–24.
32. Polito, JM, Childs B, Mellits ED, et al. Crohn's disease: Influence of age at diagnosis on site and clinical type of disease. Gastroenterology 1996;111:580–6.
33. Kuster W, Pascoe L, Purmann J, et al. The genetics of Crohn's disease: Complex segregation analysis of a family study with 265 patients with Crohn disease and 5,387 relatives. Am J Med Genetics 1989;32:105–8.
34. Bonen DK, Cho JH. The genetics of inflammatory bowel disease. Gastroenterology 2003;124:521–36.
35. Gaya DR, Russell RK, Nimmo ER, Satsangi J. New genes in inflammatory bowel disease: Lessons for complex diseases. Lancet 2006;367:1271–84.
36. Glazier AM, Nadeau JH, Altman TJ. Finding genes that underlie complex traits. Science 2002;298:2345–9.
37. Hampe J, Franke A, Rosenstiel P, et al. A genome-wide association scan of nonsysnonymous SNPs identifies a susceptibility variant for Crohn disease in ATG16L1. Nat Genet 2007;39:207–11.
38. Rioux J, Xavier RJ, Taylor KD, et al. Genome-wide association study identifies new susceptibility loci for Crohn disease and implicates autophagy in disease pathogenesis. Nat Genet 2007;39:596–604.
39. The IBD International Genetics Consortium. International Collaboration Provides Convincing Linkage Replication in Complex Disease through Analysis of a Large Pooled Data Set: Crohn Disease and Chromosome 16. Am J Hum Genet 2001;68:1165–71.
40. Lesage S, Zouali H, Cézard JP, et al. CARD15/NOD2 mutational analysis and genotype-phenotype correlation in 612 patients with inflammatory bowel disease. Am J Hum Genet 2002;70:845–57.
41. Economou M, Trikalinos TA, Loizou KT, et al. Differential effects of NOD2 variants on Crohn's disease risk and phenotype in diverse populations: A metaanalysis. Am J Gastroenterol 2004;99:2393–404.
42. Ahmad T, Armuzzi A, Bunce M, et al. The molecular classification of the clinical manifestations of Crohn's Disease. Gastroenterology 2002;122:854–66.
43. Vermeire S, Wild G, Kocher K, et al. CARD15 genetic variation in a Quebec population: Prevalence, genotype-phenotype relationship, and haplotype structure. Am J Hum Genet 2002;1:74–83.
44. Brant S, Picoo MF, Achkar J-P, et al. Defining complex contributions of NOD2/CARD15 gene mutations, age at onset, and tobacco use on Crohn's disease phenotypes. Inflamm Bowel Dis 2003;9:281–9.
45. Abreu MT, Taylor KD, Lin YC, et al. Mutations in NOD2 are associated with fibrostenosing disease in patients with Crohn's disease. Gastroenterology 2002;123:679–88.
46. Hampe J, Grebe J, Nikolaus S, et al. Association of NOD2 (CARD 15) genotype with clinical course of Crohn's disease: A cohort study. Lancet 2002;359:1661–5.
47. Radlmayr M, Torok HP, Martin K, Folwaczny C. The c-insertion mutation of the NOD2 gene is associated with fistulizing and fibrostenotic phenotypes in Crohn's disease. Gastroenterology 2002;122:2091–2.
48. Cuthbert AP, Fisher SA, Mirza MM, et al. The contribution of NOD2 gene mutations to the risk and site of disease in inflammatory bowel disease. Gastroenterology 2002;122:867–74.
49. Kugathasan S, Collins N, Maresso K, et al. CARD15 gene mutations and risk for early surgery in pediatric-onset Crohn's disease. Clin Gastroenterol Hepatol 2003;2: 1003–09.
50. Mascheretti S, Hampe J, Croucher PJ, et al. Response to infliximab treatment in Crohn's diseases is not associated with mutations in the CARD15 (NOD2) gene: An analysis in 534 patients from two multicenter, prospetive GCP-level trials. Pharmacogenetics 2002;12:509–15.
51. Bouma G, Strober W. The immunologic and genetic basis of inflammatory bowel disease. Nature Reviews 2003;3: 521–55.
52. Rioux JD, Silverberg MS, Daly MJ, et al. Genomewide search in Canadian families with inflammatory bowel disease reveals two novel susceptibility loci. Am J Hum Genet 2000;66:1863–70.
53. Ma Y, Ohmen JD, Li Z, et al. A genome-wide search identifies potential new susceptibility loci for Crohn's disease. Inflamm Bowel Dis 1999;5:271–8.
54. Rioux JD, Daly MJ, Silverberg MS, et al. Genetic variation in the 5q31 cytokine gene cluster confers susceptibility to Crohn disease. Nat Genet 2001;29:223–8.
55. Negoro K, McGovern DP, Kinouchi Y, et al. Analysis of the IBD5 locus and potential gene-gene interactions in Crohn's disease. Gut 2003;52:541–6.
56. Armuzzi A, Ahmad T, Ling KL, et al. Genotype-phenotype analysis of the Crohn's disease susceptibility haplotype on chromosome 5q31. Gut 2003;52:1133–9.
57. Giallourakis C, Stoll M, Miller K, et al. IBD5 is a general risk factor for inflammatory bowel disease: Replication of association with Crohn disease and identification of a novel association with ulcerative colitis. Am J Hum Genet 2003;73:205–11.
58. Peltekova VD, Wintle RF, Rubin LA, et al. Functional variants of OCTN cation transporter genes are associated with Crohn disease. Nat Genet 2004;36:471–5.
59. Noble CL, Nimmo ER, Drummond H, et al. The contribution of OCTN1/2 variants within the IBD5 locus to disease susceptibility and severity in Crohn's disease. Gastroenterology 2005;129:1854–64.
60. Newman B, Siminovitch KA. Recent advances in the genetics of inflammatory bowel disease. Curr Opin Gastroenterol 2005;21:401–7.
61. Hampe J, Schreiber S, Shaw S, et al. A genome wide analysis provides evidence for novel linkages in inflammatory bowel disease in a large European cohort. Am J Genet 1999;64:808–16.
62. Stoll M, Corneliussen B, Costello CM, et al. Genetic variation in DLG5 is associated with inflammatory bowel disease. Nat Genet 2004;36:476–80.
63. van Heel DA, Fisher SA, Kirby A, et al. Inflammatory bowel disease susceptibility loci defined by genome scan meta-analysis of 1952 affected relative pairs. Hum Mol Genet 2004;13:763–70.
64. Yap LM, Ahmad T, Jewell DP. The contribution of HLA genes to IBD susceptibility and phenotype. Best Pract Res Clin Gastroenterol 2004;18:577–96.
65. Hugot JP, Cézard JP, Colombel JF, et al. Clustering of Crohn's disease within affected sibships. Eur J Hum Genet 2003;11:179–84.
66. Chiodini RJ, Van Kruininger HJ, Thayer WR, et al. Possible role of mycobacteria in inflammatory bowel disease. I. An unclassified *Mycobacterium* species isolated from patients with Crohn's disease. Dis Dis Sci 1984;29:1073–9.
67. Saunderson JD, Moss M, Tizard M, Hermon-Taylor J. *Mycobacterium paratuberculosis* DNA in Crohn's disease tissue. Gut 1992;33:890–6.
68. Wakefield AJ, Pittilo RM, Sim R, et al. Evidence of persistent measles virus infection in Crohn's disease. J Med Virol 1993;39:345–53.
69. Wakefield AJ, Ekbom A, Dhillon A, et al. Crohn's disease: Pathogenesis and persistent measles virus infection. Gastroenterology 1995;108:911–6.
70. Ekbom A, Zack M, Adami H. Perinatal measles infection and subsequent Crohn's disease. Lancet 1994;344:508–10.
71. Thompson NP, Pounder R, Wakefield A. Is measles vaccination a risk factor for inflammatory bowel disease? Lancet 1995;345:1071–4.
72. Feeney M, Clegg A, Winwood P, Snook J. A case-control study of measles vaccination and inflammatory bowel disease. Lancet 1997;350:764–6.
73. Haga Y, Funakoshi O, Kuroe K, et al. Absence of measles viral genomic sequence in intestinal tissues from Crohn's disease by nested polymerase chain rection. Gut 1996;38:211–5.
74. Swidinski A, Ladhoff A, Pernthaler A, et al. Mucosal flora in inflammatory bowel disease. Gastroenterology 2002;122:44–54.
75. Rutgeerts P, Geboes K, Peeters M, et al. Effect of faecal stream diversion on recurrence of Crohn's disease in the neoterminal ileum. Lancet 1991;2:771–4.
76. D'Haens G, Geboes K, Peeters M, et al. Early lesions caused by infusion of intestinal contents in excluded ileum in Crohn's disease. Gastroenterology 1998;114:262–7.
77. Ehrhardt R, Ludviksson B, Gray B, et al. Induction and prevention of colonic inflammation in IL-2-deficient mice. J Immunol 1997;158:566–73.
78. Fiocchi C. Inflammatory bowel disease: Etiology and pathogenesis. Gastroenterology 1998;115:182–205.
79. Persson P-G, Alhbom A, Hellers G. Crohn's disease and ulcerative colitis: A review of dietary studies with emphasis on methodologic aspects. Scand J Gastroenterol 1987;22:385–9.
80. Shoda R, Matsueda K, Yamato S, Umeda N. Epidemiologic analysis of Crohn's disease in Japan: Increased dietary intake of n-6 polyunsaturated fatty acids and animal protein relates to the increased incidence of Crohn's disease in Japan. Am J Clin Nutr 1996;63:741–5.
81. Blok WL, Katan MB, van der Meer JWM. Modulation of inflammation and cytokine production by dietary (n-3) fatty acids. J. Nutr 1996;126:1515–33.
82. Ekbom A, Helmick C, Zack M, Adami HO. The epidemiology of inflammatory bowel disese: A large population-based study in Sweden. Gastroenterology 1991;100:350–8.
83. Hellers G. Crohn's disease in Stockholm County 1955–1974. Acta Chi Scand 1979;490:1–84.
84. Ekbom A, Adami H, Helmick C, et al. Perinatal risk factors for inflammatory bowel disease: A case-control study. Am J Epidemiol 1990;132:1111–9.
85. Koletzko S, Sherman P, Corey M, Griffiths A. Role of infant feeding practices and the development of Crohn's disease in childhood. BMJ 1989;289:1617–8.
86. Calkins BM. A meta-analysis of the role of smoking in inflammatory bowel disease. Dig Dis Sci 1989;34:1841–54.
87. Lashner BA, Shaheen NJ, Hanauer SB, et al. Passive smoking is associated with an increased risk of developing inflam-

matory bowel disease in children. Am J Gastroenterology 1993;88:356–9.

88. Lesko SM, KaufmanD, Rosenberg L, et al. Evidence for an increased risk of Crohn's disease in oral contraceptive users. Gastroenterology 1985;89:1046–9.
89. May GR, Sutherland LR, Meddings JB. Is small intestinal permeability really increased in relatives of patients with Crohn's diseases? Gastroenterology 1993;104:1627–32.
90. Hildsen RJ, Meddings JB, Sutherland LR. Intestinal permeability changes in response to acetylsalicylic acid in relatives of patients with Crohn's disease. Gastroenterolgoy 1996;110:1395–403.
91. Buhner S, Buning C, Genschel J, et al. Genetic basis for increased intestinal permeability in families with Crohn's disease: Role of CARD15 3020insC mutation. Gut 2006;55:342–7.
92. Schreiber S. Slipping the barrier: How variants in CARD15 could alter ermeability of the intestinal wall and population health. Gut 2006;55:308–9.
93. Elson CO. Genes, microbes, and T cells-new therapeutic targets in Crohn's disease. N Engl J Med 2002;346:614–6.
94. Girardin ES, Boneca IG, Viala J, et al. NOD2 is a general sensor of peptidoglycan through muramyldipeptide (MDP) detection. J Biol Chem 2003;278:8869–72.
95. Kobayashi K, Inohara N, Hernandez LD, et al. RICK/Rip2/CARDIAK mediates signalling for receptors of the innate and adaptive immune systems. Nature 2002;416:194–9.
96. Guttierez O, Pipaon C, Inohara N, et al. Induction of NOD2 in myelomonocytic and intestinal epithelial cells via nuclear factor κβ J Biol Chem 2002;277:41701–5.
97. Wehkamp J, Harder J, Weichenthal M, et al. NOD2 (CARD15) mutations in Crohn's disease are associated with diminished mucosal alpha-defensin expression. Gut 2004;53:1658–64.
98. Chamaillard M, Philpott D, Girardin SE, et al. Gene/environment interaction modulated by allelic heterogeneity in inflammatory diseases. Proc Natl Acad Sci U S A 2003;100:3455–60.
99. Miceli-Richard C, Lesage S, Rybojad M, et al. CARD15 mutations in Blau syndrome. Nature Genet 2001;29:19–20.
100. Itoh J, Motte C de La, Strong SA, et al. Decreased Bax expression by mucosal T cells favours resistance to apoptosis in Crohn's disease. Gut 2001;49:35–41.
101. Bach J-F. The effect of infections on susceptibility to autoimmune and allergic diseases. NEJM 2002;347:911–20.
102. Barton JR, Ferguson A. Clinical features, morbidity and mortality of Scottish Children with inflammatory bowel disease. Q J Med 1990;277:423–39.
103. Lenaerts C, Roy C, Vaillancourt M, et al. High incidence of upper gastrointestinal tract involvement in children with Crohn's disease. Pediatrics 1989;83:777–81.
104. Silverberg MS, Satsangi J, Ahmad T, et al. Toward an integrated clinical, molecular and serological classification of inflammatory bowel disease: Report of a working party of the 2005 Montreal World Congress of Gastroenterology. Can J Gastroenterol 2005;19:5A–36A.
105. Peyrin-Biroulet L, Chamaillard M, Gonzalez F, et al. Mesenteric fat in Crohn's disease: A pathogenetic hallmark or an innocent bystander? Gut 2007;56:577–83.
106. Lewin KJ, Riddell RH, Weinstein WM. Inflammatory bowel diseases. In: Lewin KJ, Riddell RH, Weinstein WM, editors. Gastrointestinal Pathology and Its Clinical Implications. New York, NY: Igaku-shoin Medical Publishers; 1992. p. 858–903.
107. Greenstein AJ, Sachar DJ, Pucillo A, et al. The extraintestinal complications of Crohn's disease and ulcerative colitis: A study of 700 patients. Medicine 1979;55:410–2.
108. Hyams JS. Extraintestinal manifestations of inflammatory bowel disease in children. J Pediatr Gastro Nutr 1994;19:7–21.
109. Orchard TR, Jewell DP, Wordsworth WE. Peripheral arthropathies in inflammatory bowel disease: Their articular distribution and natural history. Gut 1998;42:387–91.
110. Hofley P, Roarty J, McGinnity G, et al. Asymptomatic uveitis in children with chronic inflammatory bowel disease. J Pediatr Gastro Nutr 1993;17:397–400.
111. Wilschanski M, Chait P, Wade JA, et al. Primary sclerosing cholangitis in 32 children: Clinical laboratory, and radiographic features, with survival analysis. Hepatology 1995;22:1415–22.
112. Keljo DJ, Sugerman KS. Pancreatitis in patients with inflammatory bowel disease. J Pediatr Gatroenterol Nutr 1997;25:108–22.
113. Clark JH, Fitzgerald JF, Bergstein JM. Nephrolithiasis in childhood inflammatory bowel disease. J Pediatr Gastroenterol Nutr 1985;4:829–34.
114. Markowitz RL, Ment LR, Gryboski JD. Cerebral thromboembolic disease in pediatric and adult inflammatory bowel disease: Case report and review of the literature. J Pediatr Gastroenterol Nutr 1989;8:413–20.
115. Gokhale R, Favus M, Karrison T, et al. Bone mineral density assessment in children with inflammatory bowel disease. Gastroenterology 1998;114:902–11.
116. Varghese S, Wyzga N, Griffiths AM, Sylvester F. Effects of serum from children with newly diagnosed Crohn disease on primary cultures of rat osteoblasts. J Pediatr Gastro Nutr 2002;35:641–8.
117. Sylvester FA, Wyzqa N, Hyams JS, et al. Natural history of bone metabolism and bone mineral density in children with inflammatory bowel disease. Inflamm Bowel Dis 2006;13:42–50.
118. Seidman E, Leleiko N, Ament M, et al. Symposium report. Nutritional issues in paediatric inflammatory bowel disease. J Pediatr Gastro Nutr 1991;12:424–38.
119. Filipsson S, Hulten L, Lindstedt G. Malabsorption of fat and vitamin B12 before and after intestinal resection for Crohn's disease. Scand J Gastro 1978;13:529–36.
120. Chan ATH, Fleming CR, O'Fallon WM, Huizenga KA. Estimated versus measured basal energy requirements in patients with Crohn's disease. Gastroenterology 1986;91:75–8.
121. Azcue M, Rashid M, Griffiths A, Pencharz P. Energy expenditure and body composition in children with Crohn's disease: Effect of enteral nutrition and prednisone treatment. Gut 1997;41:203–7.
122. Griffiths AM, Nguyen P, Smith C, et al. Growth and clinical course of children with Crohn's disease. Gut 1993;34:939–43.
123. Hildebrand H, Karlberg J, Kristiansson B. Longitudinal growth in children and adolescents with inflammatory bowel disease. J Pediatr Gastro Nutr 1994;18:165–73.
124. Markowitz J, Grancher K, Rosa J, et al. Growth failure in pediatric inflammatory bowel disease. J Ped Gastroenterol Nutr 1993;16:373–80.
125. Kanof ME, Lake AM, Bayless TM. Decreased height velocity in children and adolescents before the diagnosis of Crohn's disease. Gastroenterology 1988;95:1523–7.
126. Wine E, Reif SS, Leshinsky-Silver E, et al. Pediatric Crohn's disease and growth retardation: The role of genotype, phenotype, and disease severity. Pediatrics 2004;114:1281–6.
127. Walters TD, Gilman AR, Griffiths AM. Linear growth improves during infliximab therapy in children with chronically active severe Crohn disease. Inflamm Bowel Dis 2007;13:1–7.
128. Ballinger A. Fundamental mechanisms of growth failure in IBD. Horm Res 2002;58:7–10.
129. DeBenedetti F, Alonzi T, MorettaA, et al. Interleukin-6 causes growth impairment in transgenic mice through a decrease in insulin-growth factor I. J Clin Invest 1997;99:643–50.
130. Ballinger AB, Azooz O, El-Haj Y, et al. Growth failure occurs through a decrease in insulin-like growth factor 1 which is independent of undernutrition in a rat model of colitis. Gut 2000;46:1–6.
131. Ballinger AB, Savage MO, Sanderson IR. Delayed puberty associated with inflammatory bowel disease. Pediatric Research 2003;53:205–10.
132. Mauras N. Growth hormone therapy in the glucocorticosteroid-dependent child: Metabolic and linear growth effects. Horm Res 2001;56:13–8.
133. Palder SB, Shandling B, Bilik R, et al. Perianal complications of pediatric Crohn's disease. J Pediatr Surg 1991;26:513–5.
134. Bousvaros A, Antonioli D, Colletti R, et al. Differentiating ulcerative colitis from Crohn's disease in children and young adults. J Pediatr Gastro Nutr 2007;44:653–74.
135. Kundhal P, Stormon M, Zachos M, et al. Gastric antral biopsy in the differentiation of pediatric colitides. Am J Gastro 2003;98:557–61.
136. Satsangi J, Silverberg MS, Vermeire S, Colombel JF. The Montreal classification of IBD: Controversies, consensus and implications. Gut 2006;55:749–53.
137. Ruemmele FM, Targan S, Levy G, et al. Diagnostic accuracy of serological assays in pediatric inflammatory bowel disease. Gastroenterology 1998;115:822–9.
138. Hoffenberg EJ, Fidanza S, Sauaia A. Serologic testing for IBD. J Pediatr 1999;134:447–52.
139. Sutton CL, Yang H, Li Z, et al. Familial expression of anti-*Saccharomyces cerevisiae* mannan antibodies in affected and unaffected relatives of patients with Crohn's disease. Gut 2000;46:58–63.
140. Saxon A, Shanahan F, Landers C, et al. A distinct subset of antineutrophil cytoplasmic antibodies is associated with inflammatory bowel disease. J Allergy Clin Immunol 1990;86:202–10.
141. Quinton JF, Sendid B, Reumaux D, et al. Anti-*Saccharomyces cerevisiae* mannan antibodies combined with antineutrophil cytoplasmic autoantibodies in inflammatory bowel disease: Prevalence and diagnostic role. Gut 1998;42:788–91.
142. Mow WS, Vasilauskas EA, Lin YC, et al. Association of antibody responses to microbial antigens and complications of small bowel Crohn disease. Gastroenterology 2004;126:414–24.
143. Modigliani R, Mary J, Simon J, et al. Clinical, biological and endoscopic picture of attacks of Crohn's disease. Evaluation on prednisone. Gastroenterology 1990;98:811–6.
144. Landi B, Anh T, Cortot A, et al. Endoscopic monitoring of Crohn's disease treatment: A prospective, randomized clinical trial. Gastroenterology 1992;102:1647–53.
145. Aiges H, Markowitz J, Rosa J, Daum F. Home nocturnal supplemental nasogastric feedings in growth-retarded adolescents with Crohn's disease. Gastroenterology 1989;97:905–10.
146. Wilschanski M, Sherman P, Pencharz P, et al. Supplementary enteral nutrition maintains remission in paediatric Crohn's disease. Gut 1996;38:543–8.
147. Zimmerman MJ, Jewell DP. Cytokines and mechanisms of action of glucocorticoids and aminosalicylates in the treatment of ulcerative colitis and Crohn's disease. Aliment Pharmacol Ther 1996;10:93–8.
148. Kusunoki M, Moeslein G, Shoji Y, et al. Steroid complications in patients with ulcerative colitis. Dis Col Rectum 1992;35:1003–9.
149. Compston JE. Management of bone disease in patients on long term glucocorticoid therapy. Gut 1999;44:770–2.
150. Summers R, Switz D, Sessions J, et al. National Cooperative Crohn's Disease Study: Results of drug treatment. Gastroenterology 1979;77:847–69.
151. Malchow H, Ewe K, Brandes J, et al. European Cooperative Crohn's Disease Study: Results of drug treatment. Gastroenterology 1984;86:249–66.
152. Seidman E, Griffiths A, Jones A, et al. Semi-elemental diet versus prednisone in the treatment of acute Crohn's disease in children and adolescents. Gastroenterology 1993;104:A778.
153. Munkholm P, Langholz E, Davidson M, Binder V. Frequency of glucocorticoid resistance and dependency in Crohn's disease. Gut 1994;35:360–2.
154. Brattsand R. Overview of newer glucocorticosteroid preparations for inflammatory bowel disease. Can J Gastroenterol 1990;4:407–14.
155. Greenberg GR, Feagan BG, Martin F, et al. Oral budesonide for active Crohn's disease. Canadian Inflammatory Bowel Disease Study Group. N Engl J Med 1994;331:836–41.
156. Rutgeerts P, Lofberg R, Malchow H, et al. A comparison of budesonide with prednisolone for active Crohn's disease. N Engl J Med 1994;331:842–45.
157. Caesar I, Gross V, Roth M, et al. Treatment of active and post-active ileal and colonic Crohn's disease with oral pH-modified-release budesonide. Hepatogastroenterology 1997;44:445–51.
158. Escher JCl. Budesonide versus prednisolone for the treatment of active Crohn's disease in children: A randomised, double-blind, controlled, multicenter trial. Eur J Gastroenterol Hepatol 2004;16:47–54.
159. Papi C, Luchetti R, Gili L, et al. Budesonide in the treatment of Crohn's disease: A meta-analysis. Aliment Pharmacol Ther 2000;14:1419–28.
160. Greenberg GR, Feagan B, Martin F, et al. Oral budesonide as maintenance treatment for Crohn's disease: A placebo-controlled dose-ranging study. Gastroenterology 1996;110:45–51.
161. Lofberg R, Rutgeerts P, Malchow H, et al. Oral budesonide prolongs remission in ileocecal Crohn's disease. Gut 1996;39:82–6.
162. Ferguson A, Campieri M, Doe W, et al. Oral budesonide as maintenance therapy in Crohn's disease results of a 12-month study. Aliment Pharmacol Ther 1998;12:175–83.
163. Gross V, Andus T, Ecker KW, et al. Low dose oral pH modified release budesonide for maintenance of steroid induced remission in Crohn's disease. Gut 1998;42:493–6.
164. Kundhal P, Zachos M, Smith J, Griffiths AM. Controlled ileal release budesonide in children with Crohn's disease: Efficacy and effect on growth. J Pediatr Gastro Nutr 2001;33:75–80.
165. Gaginella TS, Walsh RE. Sulfasalazine: Multiplicity of action. Dig Dis Sci 1992;37:801–12.
166. MacDermott R. Progress in understanding the mechanisms of action of 5-aminosalicylic acid. Am J Gastroenterol 2000;95:3343–5.
167. Mudter J, Neurath MF. Apoptosis of T cells and the control of inflammatory bowel disease: Therapeutic implications. Gut 2007;56:293–303.
168. Allgayer H. Sulfasalazine and 5-ASA compounds. Gastro Clinics North America 1992;21:643–58.
169. Laursen LS, Stockholm M, Bukhave K, Lauritsen K. Disposition of 5-aminosalicylic acid by olsalazine and three mesalazine preparations in patients with ulcerative colitis: Comparison of intraluminal colonic concentrations, serum values and urinary excretion. Gut 1990;31:1271–6.

170. Rijk MCM, Van Hogezand RA, Van Schaik A, Van Tongeren JHM. Disposition of 5-aminosalicylic acid from 5-aminosalicylic acid delivering drugs during accelerated intestinal transit in healthy volunteers. Scand J Gastroenterol 1989;24:1179–85.
171. Collins JR. Adverse reactions to salicylazosulfapyridine in the treatment of ulcerative colitis. South Med J 1968;61:354–8.
172. Austin CA, Cann PA, Jones TH, et al. Exacerbation of diarrhea and pain in patients treated with 5-aminosalicylic acid for ulcerative colitis. Lancet 1984;1:917–8.
173. Birnie GG, McLeod T, Watkinson G. Incidence of sulphasalazine induced male infertility. Gut 1981;22:452–5.
174. Rao SS, Cann PA, Holdsworth CD. Clinical experience of the tolerance of mesalazine and olsalazine in patients intolerant of sulfasalazine. Scand J Gastroenterol 1987;22:332–6.
175. Sachedina B, Saibil F, Cohen LB, Whittey J. Acute pancreatitis due to 5-aminosalicylate. Ann Intern Med 1989;110:490–2.
176. Pamukcu R, Hanauer S, Chang EB. Effect of disodium azodisalicylate on electrolyte transport in rabbit ileum and colon in vitro. Gastroenterology 1988;95:975–81.
177. Singleton JW, Hanauer S, Gitnick G, et al. Mesalamine capsules for the treatment of active Crohn's disease: Results of a 16-week trial. Gastroenterology 1993;104:1293–1301.
178. Prantera C, Cottone M, Pallone F, et al. Meslamine in the treatment of mild-to-moderate active Crohn's ileitis: Results of a randomized, multicenter trial. Gastroenterology 1999;116:521–6.
179. Thomsen OO, Cortot A, Jewell D, et al. A comparison of budesonide and mesalamine for active Crohn's disease. N Engl J Med 1999;339:370–4.
180. Camma C, Giunta M, Rosselli M, Cottone M. Mesalamine in the maintenance treatment of Crohn's disease. A meta-analysis adjusted for confounding variables. Gastroenterology 1997;113:1465–73.
181. Cezard J-P, Munck A, Mouterde O, et al. Prevention of recurrence by mesalamine in pediatric Crohn's disease. A multicenter double blind trial Gastroenterology 2003;124:A379.
182. Lochs H, Mayer M, Fleig E, et al. Prophylaxis of postoperative relapse in Crohn's disease with mesalamine: European Cooperative Crohn's Disease Study VI. Gastroenterology 2000;118:264–73.
183. Sutherland LR (editorial). Mesalamine for the prevention of postoperative recurrence: Is nearly there the same as being there? Gastroenterology 2000;118:436–8.
184. Bernstein LH, Frank L, Brandt L, et al. Healing of perineal Crohn's disease with metronidazole. Gastroenterology 1979;79:357–65.
185. Brandt LJ, Bernstein L, Boley S, et al. Metronidazole therapy for perineal Crohn's disease: A follow-up study. Gastroenterology 1982;83:383–7.
186. Ursing B, Alm T, Barany F, et al. Comparative study of metronidazole and sulfasalazine for active Crohn's disease: The Cooperative Crohn's Disease Study in Sweden. II. Result. Gastroenterology 1982;83:550–62.
187. Sutherland L, Singleton J, Sessions J, et al. Double-blind, placebo-controlled trial of metronidazole in Crohn's disease. Gut 1991;32:1071–5.
188. Prantera C, Zannoni F, Scribano ML, et al. An antibiotic regimen for the treatment of active Crohns disease: A randomized, controlled clinical trial of metronidazole plus ciprofloxacin. Am J Gastro 1996;91:328–32.
189. Steinhart AH, Feagan BG, Wong CJ, et al. Combined budesonide and antibiotic therapy for active Crohn's disease: A randomized controlled trial. Gastroenterology 2002;123:33–40.
190. Rutgeerts P, Hile M, Geboes K, et al. Controlled trial of metronidazole for prevention of Crohn's recurrence after ileal resection. Gastroenterology 1995;108:1617–21.
191. Borgaonkar MR, MacIntosh DG, Fardy JM. A meta-analysis of antimycobacterial therapy for Crohn's disease. Am J Gastroenterol 2000;95:725–9.
192. Marteau P, Lemann M, Seksik P, et al. Ineffectiveness of Lactobacillus johnsonii LA1 for prophylaxis of postoperative recurrence in Crohn's disease: A randomized, double blind, placebo controlled GETAID trial. Gut 2006;55:842–7.
193. Duffy LN, Daum F, Fisher S, et al. Peripheral neuropathy in Crohn's disesae patients treated with metronidazole. Gastroenterology 1985;88:681–4.
194. Pearson DC, May GR, Fick GH, Sutherland LR. Azathioprine and 6-mercaptopurine in Crohn's disease: A meta-analysis. Ann Intern Med 1995;122:132–42.
195. Markowitz J, Grancher K, Kohn N, et al. 6-Mercaptopurine and prednisone therapy for newly diagnosed pediatric Crohn's disease: A prospective multicenter placebo-controlled clinical trial. Gastroenterology 2000;119:895–902.
196. Elion GB. The pharmacology of azathioprine. NY Acad Sci 1993;685:400–7.
197. Neurath MF, Kiesslich R, Teichgraber U, et al. 6-Thioguanosine diphosphate and triphosphate levels in red blood cells and response to azathioprine therapy in Crohn disease. Clin Gastroenterol Hepatol 2005;3:1007–14.
198. Poppe D, Tiede I, Fritz G, et al. Azathioprine suppresses ezrin-radixin-moesin-dependent T cell APC conjugation through inhibition of Vav guanosine exchange activity on Rac proteins. J Immunol 2006;176:640–51.
199. Lennard L, Van Loon JA, Weinshilboum RM. Pharmacogenetics of acute azathioprine toxicity: Relationship to thiopurine methyltransferase genetic polymorphism. Clin Pharmacol Ther 1989;46:149–54.
200. Lennard L. TPMT in the treatment of Crohn's disease with azathioprine. Gut 2002;51:143–6.
201. Sandborn WJ. A review of immune modifier therapy for inflammatory bowel disease: Azathioprine, 6-mercaptopurine, cyclosporine, and methotrexate. Am J Gastroenterol 1996;991:423–33.
202. Kirschner B. Safety of azathioprine and 6-mercaptopurine in pediatric patients with inflammatory bowel disease. Gastroenterology 1998;115:813–21.
203. Present DH, Meltzer SJ, Krumholz MP, et al. 6-Mercaptopurine in the management of inflammatory bowel disease: Short and long-term toxicity. Ann Intern Med 1989;111:641–9.
204. Connell WR, Kamm MA, Ritchie JK, Lennard-Jones JE. Bone marrow toxicity caused by azathioprine in inflammatory bowel disease: 27 years of experience. Gut 1993;34:1081–5.
205. Connell WR, Kamm MA, Dickson M, et al. Long-term neoplasia risk after azathioprine treatment in inflammatory bowel disease. Lancet 1994;343:1249–52.
206. Colombel J-F, Ferrari N, Debuysere H, et al. Genotypic analysis of thiopurine methyltransferase in patients with Crohn's disease and severe myelosuppression during azathioprine therapy. Gastroenterology 2000;118:1025–30.
207. Deutsch DE, Olson AD, Kraker S, Dickinson CJ. Overwhelming varicella pneumonia with Crohn's disease treated with 6-mercaptopurine. J Pediatr Gastro Nutr 1995;20:351–3.
208. Kandiel A, Fraser AG, Korelitz BI, et al. Increased risk of lymphoma among inflammatory bowel disease patients treated with azathioprine and 6-mercaptopurine. Gut 2005;54:1121–5.
209. Rosh JR, Gross T, Mamula P, et al. Hepatosplenic T-cell lymphoma in adolescents and young adults with Crohn disease: A cautionary tale? Inflammatory Bowel Disease 2007;13:941–946.
210. Navarro JT, Ribera JM, Mate JL, et al. Hepatosplenic T-gamma delta lymphoma in a patient with Crohn's disease treated with azathioprine. Leuk Lymphoma 2003;44:531–3.
211. Sandborn WJ, Tremaine W, Wolf D, et al. Lack of effect of intravenous administration on time to respond to azathioprine for steroid-treated Crohn's disease. North American Azathioprine Study Group. Gastroenterology 1999;117:527–35.
212. Ewe K, Press A, Singe C, et al. Azathioprine combined with prednisolone or monotherapy with prednisolone in active Crohn's disease. Gastroenterology 1993;105:367–72.
213. Holtmann MH, Krummenauer F, Claas C, et al. Long-term effectiveness of azathioprine in IBD beyond 4 years: A European multicenter study in 1176 patients. Dig Dis Sci 2006;51:1516–24.
214. Dubinsky MC, Yang HY, Hassard PV, et al. 6-MP metabolite profiles provide a biochemical explanation for 6-MP resistance in patients with inflammatory bowel disease. Gastroenterology 2002;122:904–15.
215. Bergen S, Tugstad HE, Bentdal O, et al. Monitored high-dose azathioprine treatment reduces acute rejection episodes after renal transplantation. Transplantation 1998;66:334–9.
216. Lilleyman JS, Lennard L. Mercaptopurine metabolism and the risk of relapse in childhood lymphoblastic leukemia, Lancet 1994;343:1188–90.
217. Cuffari C, Theoret Y, Latour S, Seidman G. 6-Mercaptopurine metabolism in Crohn's disease: Correlation with efficacy and toxicity. Gut 1996;39:401–6.
218. Lowry PW, Franklin CL, Weaver AL, et al. Measurement of thiopurine methyltransferase activity and azathioprine metabolites in patients with inflammatory bowel disease. Gut 2001;49:665–70.
219. Feagan BG, Rochon J, Fedorak RN, et al. Methotrexate for the treatment of Crohn's disease. N Engl J Med 1995;332:292–7.
220. Feagan BG, Fedorak RN, Irvine EF, et al. A comparison of methotrexate with placebo for the maintenance of remission in Crohn's disease. N Engl J Med 2000;342:1627–32.
221. Mack D, Young R, Kaufman S, et al. Methotrexate in patients with Crohn's disease after 6-mercaptopurine. J Pediatr 1998;132:830–5.
222. Turner D, Grossman A, Rosh J, et al. Methotrexate following unsuccessful thiopurine therapy in paediatric Crohn's disease. Gut 2007 (in press).
223. Brynskov J, Freund L, Rasmussen SN, et al. Final report on a trial of cyclosporine treatment in active chronic Crohn's disease. Scand J Gastroenterol 1991;26:689–95.
224. Feagan BG, McDonald JW, Rochon J, et al. The Canadian Crohn 's relapse prevention trial. Low dose cyclosporin A for treatment of Crohn's disease. N Engl J Med 1994;330:1846–51.
225. Jewell D, Lennard-Jones JE. Oral cyclosporine for chronic active Crohn's disease: A multicentre controlled trial. Eur J Gastroenterol Hepatol 1994;6:499–505.
226. Stange EF, Modigliani R, Pena AS, et al. European trial of cyclosporine in chronic active Crohn's disease: A 12-month study. Gastroenterology 1995;109:774–82.
227. Nicholls S, Domizio P, Williams CB, et al. Cyclosporin as initial treatment for Crohn's disease. Arch Dis Child 1994;71:243–47.
228. Present DH, Lichtiger S. Efficacy of cyclosporine in treatment of fistula of Crohn's disease. Dig Dis Sci 1994;39:374–80.
229. Targan SR, Hanauer SB, van Deventer SJ, et al. A short-term study of chimeric monoclonal antibody cA2 to tumor necrosis factor alpha for Crohn's disease. N Engl J Med 1997;337:1029–33.
230. Van Deventer SJH. Tumour necrosis factor and Crohn's disease, Gut 1997;40:443–8.
231. Van den Brande JM, Braat H, van den Brink GR, et al. Infliximab but not etanercept induces apoptosis in lamina propria T-lymphocytes from patients with Crohn's disease. Gastroenterology 2003;124:1774–85.
232. Present DH, Rutgeerts P, Targan S, et al. Infliximab for the treatment of fistulas in patients with Crohn's disease. N Engl J Med 1999;340:1398–1405.
233. Hanauer SB, Feagan BG, Lichtenstein GR, et al. Maintenance infliximab for Crohn's disease: The ACCENT I randomised trial. Lancet 2002;359:1541–9.
234. Sands BE, Anderson FH, Bernstein CN, et al. Infliximab maintenance therapy for fistulizing Crohn's disease. N Engl J Med 2004;350:876–85.
235. Hyams J, Crandall W, Kugathasan S, et al. Induction and maintenance infliximab therapy for the treatment of moderate-to-severe Crohn's disease in children. Gastroenterology 2007;132:863–7.
236. Rutgeerts P, Feagan BG, Lichtenstein GR, et al. Comparison of scheduled and episodic treatment strategies of infliximab in Crohn's disease. Gastroenterology 2004;126:402–13.
237. Baert F, Noman M, Vermeire S, et al. Influence of immunogenicity on the long-term efficacy of infliximab in Crohn's disease. N Engl J Med 2003;348:601–8.
238. Vermeire S, Noman M, van Asche G, et al. The effectiveness of concomitant immunosuppressive therapy to suppress formation of antibodies to infliximab in Crohn's disease. Gut 2007.
239. Lipsky PE, van der Heijde DM, St Clair EW, et al. Infliximab and methotrexate in the treatment of rheumatoid arthritis. Anti-tumor necrosis factor trial in rheumatoid arthritis with concomitant therapy study group. N Engl J Med 2000;343:1594–1602.
240. D'Haens G. Risks and benefits of biologic therapy for inflammatory bowel diseases. Gut 2007;56:725–32.
241. Cheifetz A, Smedley M, Martin S, et al. The incidence and management of infusion reactions in infliximab: A large center experience. Am J Gastro 2003;98:1315–24.
242. Keane J, Gershon S, Wise RP, et al. Tuberculosis associated with infliximab, a tumor necrosis factor alpha-neutralized agent. N Engl J Med 2001;345:1098–104.
243. Kamath BM, Mamula P, Baldassano RN, Markowitz JE. Listeria meningitis after treatment with infliximab. J Pediatr Gastro Nutr 2002;34:410–2.
244. Bongartz T, Sutton AJ, Sweeting MJ, et al. Anti-TNF alpha therapy in rheumatoid arthritis and the risk of serious infections and malignancy: A systematic review of randomized controlled trials. JAMA 2006;295:2275–85.
245. Pannacione R. Canadian Consensus Group on the use of infliximab in Crohn's disease. Infliximab for the treatment of Crohn's disease: Review and indications for clinical use in Canada. Can J Gastroenterol 2001;15:371–5.
246. Hanauer SB, Sandborn WJ, Rutgeerts P, et al. Human anti-tumor necrosis factor monoclonal antibody (adalimumab) in Crohn's disease: The CLASSIC-1 trial. Gastroenterology 2006;130:323–33.
247. Colombel JF, Sandborn WJ, Rutgeerts P, et al. Adalimumab for maintenance of clinical response and remission in patients with Crohn's disease: The CHARM trial. Gastroenterology 2007;132:52–65.
248. Schreiber S, Khaliq-Kareemi M, Lawrance I, et al. Certolizumab pegol, a humanised anti-TNF pegylated FAb' fragment, is safe and effective in the maintenance of response

and remission following induction in active Crohn's disease: A phase III study (PRECISE tiral). New Engl J Med 2007;357:239–250.

249. Sandborn WJ, Hanauer SB, Katz S, et al. Etanercept for active Crohn's disease: A randomized, double-blind, placebo-controlled trial. Gastroenterology 2001;121:1088–94.

250. Van Deventer SJH, Elson CO, Fedorak RN. Multiple doses of intravenous interleukin 10 in steroid-refractory Crohn's disease. Gastroenterology 1997;113:383–9.

251. Ghosh S, Goldin E, Gordon FH, et al. Natalizumab Pan European Study Group. Natalizumab for active Crohn's disease. N Engl J Med 2003;348:24 32.

252. O'Morain C, Segal AW, Levi AJ. Elemental diet as primary treatment of acute Crohn's disease. B M J 1984;288:1859–2862.

253. Malchow H, Steinhardt HJ, Lorenz-Meyer H, et al. European Cooperative Crohn's Disease Study III. Scand J Gastroenterol 1990;25:235–44.

254. Lochs H, Steinhardt HJ, Klaus-Ventz B, et al. Comparison of enteral nutrition and drug treatment in active Crohn's disease. Results of the European Cooperative Crohn's Disease Study IV. Gastroenterology 1991;101:881–8.

255. Griffiths AM, Ohlsson A, Sherman P, Sutherland LR. Meta-analysis of enteral nutrition as primary treatment of active Crohn's disease. Gastroenterology 1995;108:1056–67.

256. Teahon K, Smethurst P, Pearson M, et al. The effect of elemental diet on permeability and inflammation in Crohn's disease. Gastroenterology 1991;101:84–7.

257. Sanderson IR, Boulton P, Menzies I, Walker-Smith JA. Improvement of abnormal lactulose/rhamnose permeability in active Crohn's disease of the small bowel by an elemental diet. Gut 1987;28:1073–6.

258. Fell JME, Paintin M, Arnoud-Battandier F, et al. Resolution of mucosal inflammation and fall in IL-1 beta mRNA in active Crohn's disease in response to polymeric diet. J Pediatr Gastro Nutr 1997;24:474.

259. Afzal NA, Davies S, Paintin M, et al. Colonic Crohn's disease in children does not respond well to treatment with enteral nutrition if the ileum is not involved. Dig Dis Sci 2005;50:1471–5.

260. Rigaud D, Cosnes J, Quintrec Y, et al. Controlled trial comparing two types of enteral nutrition in treatment of active Crohn's disease. Gut 1991;32:1492–7.

261. Zachos M, Tondeur M, Griffiths AM. Enteral nutritional therapy for inducing remission in Crohn's disease. Cochrane Database of Systematic Reviews 2006.

262. Gassull MA, Fernandez-Banares F, Cabre E, et al. Fat composition may be a clue to explain the primary therapeutic effect of enteral nutrition in Crohn's disease: Results of a double blind randomized multicentre European trial. Gut 2002;51:164–8.

263. Johnson T, Macdonald S, Hill SM, et al. Treatment of active Crohn's disease in children using partial enteral nutrition with liquid formula: A randomized controlled trial. Gut 2006;55:356–361.

264. Heuschkel RB, Menache CC, Megerian JT, et al. Enteral nutrition and corticosteroids in the treatment of acute Crohn's disease in children. J Pediatr Gastro Nutr 2000;31:8–15.

265. Belli DC, Seidman E, Bouthillier L, et al. Chronic intermittent elemental diet improves growth failure in children with Crohn's disease. Gastroenterology 1988;94:603–10.

266. Seidman E, Jones A, Issenman R, Griffiths AM. Cyclical exclusive enteral nutrition versus alternate day prednisone in maintaining remission of pediatric Crohn's disease. J Pediatr Gastro Nutr 1996;23:A344.

267. Belluzzi A, Brignola C, Campieri M, et al. Effect of an enteric-coated fish-oil preparation on relapses in Crohn's disease. N Engl J Med 1996;334:1557–60.

268. Diamond IR, Langer JC. Laparoscopic-assisted versus open ileocolic resection for adolescent Crohn's disease. J Pediatr Gastro Nutr 2001;33:543–7.

269. Rutgeerts P, Geboes K, Vantrappen G, et al. Natural history of recurrent Crohn's disease at the ileocolonic anastomosis after curative surgery. Gut 1984;25:665–72.

270. Griffiths AM, Wesson D, Shandling B, et al. Factors influencing the postoperative recurrence of Crohn's disease in childhood. Gut 1991;32:491–5.

271. Davies G, Evans CM, Shand WS, Walker-Smith JA. Surgery for Crohn's disease in childhood: Influence of site of disease and operative procedure on outcome. Br J Surg 1990;77:891–4.

272. Strong SA. Prognostic parameters of Crohn's disease recurrence. In Balliere's Clinical Gastroenterology. Crohn's disease. RN Allan and MRB Keighley eds, 1998;12:167–177.

273. Sachar DB, Wolfson DM, Greenstein AJ, et al. Risk factors for postoperative recurrence of Crohn's disease. Gastroenterology 1983;85:917–21.

274. D'Haens GR, Gasparaitas AE, Hanauer SB. Duration of recurrent ileitis after ileocolonic resection correlates with presurgical extent of Crohn's disease. Gut 1995;36:715–7.

275. Ho I, Greenstein AJ, Bodian CA, Janowitz HD. Recurrence of Crohn's disease in end ileostomies. IBD 1995;1:173–8.

276. Yamamoto T, Allan RN, Keighley MRB. Audit of single stage proctocolectomy for Crohn's disease. Dis Colon Rectum 2000;43:249–56.

277. Hellers G, Cortot A, Jewell D, et al. Oral budesonide for prevention of recurrence following ileocolonic resection of Crohn's disease. A one year placebo controlled study. Gastroenterology 1999;116:294–300.

278. Hanauer S, Korelitz B, Rutgeerts P, et al. Post-operative maintenance of Crohn's disease remission with 6MP, mesalamine or placebo: A 2 year trial. Gastroenterology 2004;127:723–9.

279. Ardizzone S, Maconi G, Sampietro GM, et al. Azathioprine and mesalamine for prevention of relapse after conservative surgery for Crohn's disease. Gastroenterology 2004;127:723–9.

280. Cottone M, Rosselli M, Orlando A, et al. Smoking habits and recurrence in Crohn's disease. Gastroenterology 1994;106:643–8.

281. Topstad DR, Panaccione R, Heine JA. Combined seton placement, infliximab infusion, and maintenance immunosuppressives improve healing rate in fistulizing anorectal Crohn's disease: A single center experience. Dis Colon Rectum 2003;46:577–83.

282. Louis E, Collard A, Oger AF, et al. Behaviour of Crohn's disease according to the Vienna classification: Changing pattern over the course of the disease. Gut 2001;49:777–82.

283. Walters FL, Russel MG, Sijbrandij J, et al. Crohn's disease: Increased mortality 10 years after diagnosis in a Europewide population based cohort. Gut 2006;55:510–8.

284. Gillen CD, Walmsley RS, Prior P, et al. Ulcerative colitis and Crohn's disease: A comparison of the colorectal cancer risk in extensive colitis. Gut 1994;35:1590–2.

285. Ribeiro MB, Greenstein AJ, Sachar DB, et al. Colorectal adenocarcinoma in Crohn's disease. Ann Surg 1996;223:186–93.

286. Buller H, Thomas AG. Quality of life in childhood inflammatory bowel disease. Summary of the international meeting, Manchester, UK, 1997. J Pediatr Gastroenterol Nutr 1999;28:Supplement.

287. Griffiths AM, Nicholas D, Smith C, et al. Development of a paediatric IBD quality of life index: Dealing with differences related to age and IBD type. J Pediatric Gastro Nutr 1999;28:S1–S7.

288. Rabbett H, Elbadri A, Thwaites R, et al. Quality of life in children with Crohn's disease. J Pediatr Gastro Nutr 1996;23:528–33.

289. Thomas A, Richardson G, Griffiths A. Cross-cultural comparison of quality of life in pediatric IBD. J Pediatr Gastro Nutr 2001;32:573–8.

290. Otley A, Smith C, Nicholas D, et al. The IMPACT questionnaire: a valid measure of health-related quality of life in pediatric inflammatory bowel disease. J Pediatr Gastro Nutr 2002;35:557–63.

291. Hyams JS, Ferry GD, Mandel S, et al. Development and validation of a pediatric Crohn's disease activity index. J Pediatr Gastro Nutr 1991;12:439–47.

292. Griffiths AM. Crohn disease. In: David TJ, editor. Recent Advances in Pediatrics. Edinburgh: Churchill Livingstone; 1992. p. 145.

293. Sands BE. Novel therapies for inflammatory bowel disease. In: Lichtenstein GR, editor. Inflammatory Bowel Disease. Gastroenterology Clinics of North America, 28(2); 1999. p. 324.

20.5b. Ulcerative and Indeterminate Colitis

Nicholas M. Croft, MBBS, PhD, FRCPCH

Ulcerative and indeterminate colitis are chronic inflammatory diseases affecting the mucosa of the colon in children and adults. The following chapter will highlight important and recent advances relevant to pediatric ulcerative and indeterminate colitis.

DEFINITIONS

Diagnosis of ulcerative and indeterminate colitis are clinicopathological diagnoses relying on a combination of clinical assessment, endoscopy, and histological and radiological investigations.

Ulcerative Colitis

Ulcerative colitis (UC) (as distinct from infectious colitis) was first described in 1859 by Samuel Wilks.[1] In UC inflammation is classically limited to the large bowel and is typically continuous, starting at the rectum. Endoscopic findings include ulcers, erythema, loss of vascular pattern, friability, spontaneous bleeding, and pseudopolyps (Figure 1).[2] Histologically, inflammation is limited to the mucosa, with crypt distortion, crypt abscesses, goblet cell depletion, and rarely mucin granulomas.[2] However, with increased use of gastroscopy at the time of the initial colonoscopy, it is becoming more apparent that histological abnormalities out with the colon may be identified in 50 to 70% of cases.[3–4]

Indeterminate Colitis

The definition of indeterminate colitis (IC) has evolved over the years but there is no worldwide consensus. Most practicing pediatric gastroenterologists use this term to describe patients with chronic inflammatory bowel disease (IBD), limited to the colon, which after full investigation, including ileocolonoscopy, gastroscopy with histology, and small bowel meal and follow-through, cannot be characterized as either Crohn's disease (CD) or UC.[5] This is the definition that will apply for the remainder of this chapter.

In 2005 IBD working group of the European Society of Pediatric Gastroenterology, Hepatology, and Nutrition reported the Porto Criteria to establish uniformity in the work-up and criteria used for diagnosis of pediatric IBD.[2] These criteria include the investigations required in newly presenting patients with possible IBD, and the diagnosis of IC was applicable when having completed the diagnostic program consisting of

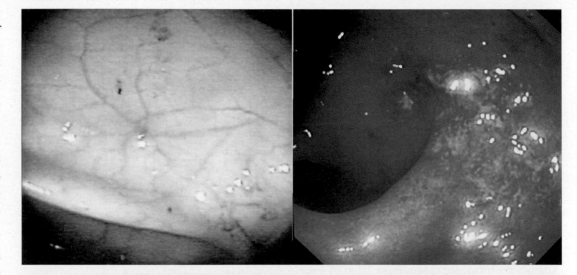

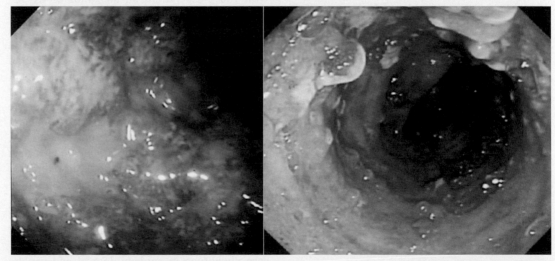

Figure 1 From clockwise from top left: normal colonic mucosa, diffuse erythematous inflamed with contact bleeding typical of ulcerative colitis, widespread inflammation with early development of pseudopolyps (indeterminate colitis), and deep ulceration seen in severe colitis.

colonoscopy with ileal intubation, upper gastrointestinal endoscopy, and contrast imaging of the small bowel one could not classify a patient with chronic IBD as having either CD or UC.

The original description of IC described the pathological features of surgical resection specimens of patients with chronic IBD, most of whom had had colectomies for fulminant disease.[6] Part of this pathological diagnosis may be based on the presence of "fissuring ulceration"; however, in one study as many as 27% of patients with severe UC were found to have this feature without any subsequent change of diagnosis to CD during extended follow-up.[7] Some pathologists

would thus suggest that IC remain a pathological diagnosis based on examination of resection specimens and not a diagnosis of exclusion based in part on mucosal biopsies. To add to the confusion, the recently published Montreal classification of IBD (an update of the earlier Vienna classifications of 1991 and 1998[8]) supports this viewpoint and created the term inflammatory bowel disease, type unclassified (IBD-U).[9] IBD-U was applied to patients with chronic IBD affecting the colon, without small bowel involvement, and no definitive histological or other evidence to favor either CD or UC.[9] For most practicing pediatric gastroenterologists, this definition applies to IC.

The inconsistency in the diagnostic label in published literature severely hampers good quality research, and it is important that the world community of pediatric (and adult) gastroenterologists and pathologists agree the definition and classifications and apply it consistently. Some believe that IC may be a specific disease phenotype (and possibly genotype); without clear and consistent case definitions it will be impossible to understand more about the disease process.

EPIDEMIOLOGY

Incidence and Prevalence

There are many studies of the incidence and prevalence of IBD; the majority are in adult practice and most are based in the developed countries of Northern Europe and North America. Estimation of the incidence and prevalence of UC/IC in pediatric patients is difficult because of variation in the definition of age limits for the pediatric population (this is particularly relevant as IBD is often diagnosed during adolescence and young adulthood), inexact and nonstandardized criteria for diagnosis, and incomplete ascertainment of cases.[10]

Adult Incidence. Unlike children, in most series of adults, UC is more common than CD. In North America the incidence ranges from 2.2 to 14.4 per 100,000 person years, with a prevalence of 37 to 246 cases per 100,000 persons.[11] This translates to 7,000 to 46,000 new cases per year and a total of 780,000 with UC. In Europe the European collaborative study on IBD (EC-IBD) estimated between 8.7 and 11.8 cases per 100,000 person years for UC (and 3.9 and 7.0 cases per 100,000 person years for CD). These data suggest up to 68,000 new cases of UC and 41,000 new cases of CD per year.[12]

Pediatric Incidence. Most studies report that up to 25% of all IBD present during childhood or adolescence.[13] There appears to be considerable uniformity in studies reporting approximately 60% of children with IBD have CD, 25 to 40% with UC, and 5 to 15% having IC.[13–15] In a prospective, population-based study in the UK and Republic of Ireland between June 1998 and July 1999, 5.2 of 100,000 children less than 16 years of age were newly diagnosed as being affected by IBD; CD (60%), UC (28%), and IC (12%).[16]

Temporal Trends of Incidence and Prevalence. While the incidence of both CD and UC has been recognized to increase, over the last 30 to 40 years there has been some leveling off in high incidence areas such as Scandinavia and Minnesota.[11] Other regions (Japan, South Korea, Singapore, northern India, and Latin America) are now reporting increasing incidence of IBD, particularly UC, with CD remaining relatively rare.[11] There is little clear data on changes of the incidence of IC largely due to not being described until 1978 and the inconsistent definition of the condition.

In children, the increase in IBD has been most marked in patients with CD. For example from 1983 to 1993, the incidence of CD in children in Wales doubled with no corresponding increase in UC.[17] CD in children also increased in Scotland between 1968 and 1983, and 1992 with a small apparent decrease in UC.[18–19] Two population-based studies report incidences of UC of 2.1 and 2.2 per 100,000 per year[20–21] with no apparent recent increase in the incidence of UC.

Geography and Race. The incidence of IBD disease of all types varies widely across different geographical areas including within countries. Overall, the diseases seem to be more common in the temporal climates and developed countries in North America and Northern Europe although at least part of this difference may be the lack of awareness and diagnostic facilities.[11,22,23]

While most data on the incidence of UC and IBD have focused on whole countries or the race of the subjects, it is becoming clearer this may not be sufficiently specific, particularly if wishing to research the genetic basis of the diseases. In the UK it has been reported that the proportion of children with UC is higher in British patients of South Asian origin (the majority of whom originated from India with large numbers from Pakistan and Bangladesh) than Caucasian.[16,24–25] However, in two centers, with 100% ascertainment, the ratios of UC/IC/CD were identical between second generation Bangladeshi/Pakistani origin and Caucasian children, whereas those of Indian origin had a higher incidence of UC (NA Afzal, personal communication, August 2006). Within Scotland, with a largely Caucasian population of about 5 million, a north–south difference in incidence has recently been reported suggesting genetic differences between the two regions.[26] Similarly, while UC is more common among Jewish than non-Jewish peoples, disease rates in people of Jewish background also vary by their geographic area of origin.[27]

These observations highlight the importance of clearly defining specific origins of the subjects within regions and countries as well as the disease phenotype in epidemiological and genetic studies of IBD.

Age. The distribution of age at onset of UC has been regarded as bimodal, with peaks occurring in the second and third decades and again in the fifth and sixth decades; however, this has not been uniformly found and may be explained by variations in diagnostic criteria and classification.[11]

Recently, a large epidemiological study of pediatric IBD, examining 1,370 subjects from six large pediatric IBD centers in North America, found that 6% of subjects presented with IBD under the age of 2 years with equal proportions having CD/UC/IC. Nine percent present between 3 to 5 years of age (47% had UC, 18% IC, and 35% CD), 47% present from 6 to 12 years, and 36% between 13 to 17 years.[14] In those over 6 years significantly more had CD (62%), compared with UC (27%) and IC (11%). Their data shown in Figure 2 suggested that UC and IC frequency remains steady from the age of about 3 years whereas CD shows a clear and dramatic increase between the ages of 6 to 12 years.

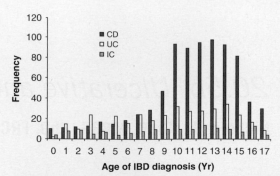

Figure 2 Age and type of IBD at presentation in an epidemiological study examining 1,370 subjects from six large pediatric IBD centers in North America.[14] (Reproduced with permission from Elsevier.)

In another series of pediatric patients, over a 10-year period, average age of presentation of UC (7.5 years) was not different to that of IC (9.5 years), both being younger than CD (12.4 years).[5]

Sex. While overall there is a slight preponderance of male children with CD for UC, the incidence appears to be equal between the sexes.[13,16]

ETIOLOGY

The etiology of IBD is not known; however, it is clear there is a strong genetic basis to the disease with as yet unidentified environmental factors. There are no data separately examining IC.

Genetics

Family Prevalence. Some of the strongest evidence that genetics may underpin part of the pathogenic processes is in epidemiological studies of families. The increased risk in family studies is significant in UC but much higher in patients with CD. In CD data suggest that early onset disease has a higher family prevalence rate and thus a stronger genetic component than late onset disease; however, this has not been demonstrated in UC.[28–29] This may be important as the phenotype of UC in children (often pancolitis) is different to adults with UC. There are no family prevalence studies focusing on IC.

First-Degree Relatives. By examining the relative risk in first-degree relatives of patients with IBD, it is essential to define the type of IBD. For probands with CD, the risk of UC is increased by 3 to 6 times compared with a 5 to 35 times increased risk of CD.[30] Equally for probands of subjects with UC, the increased risk is 6 to 16 times for UC compared with 2 or 3 times for CD. For subjects with UC, the lifetime risk (until 70 years of age) of a first-degree relative developing IBD has been estimated to be 1.6% in non-Jews and 5.2% in Jews. (For CD these figures are higher at 5 and 7.8%.)[30]

Sibling and Twin Studies. Sibling risk of UC is estimated to be 8 to 15 times increased (the equivalent figures in CD are 25 to 42); these data do not appear to be any higher than in first-degree relatives.

Incidence studies of UC in twins reveal concordance rates of 6 to 19% among monozygotic twins and 0 to 5% among dizygotic twins.[30] This difference between monozygotic and dizygotic twins is more striking in CD, with a concordance rate of 36% among monozygotic twins and 4% among dizygotic twins.[31] Although the concordance rates of disease are higher in monozygotic twins, the incomplete concordance confirms that nongenetic factors also contribute to the development of IBD.

Candidate Gene Studies

Since the development of a linkage map of the human genome, it has been possible to undertake hypothesis-free scanning of the human genome. For IBD, nine loci, termed as IBD1 to 9 have been replicated.[32] Those that have been implicated in increased susceptibility to UC (with or without CD) include IBD2 (on chromosome 12q), IBD3 (chromosome 6p), IBD5 (chromosome 5), IBD9 (chromosome 3) plus chromosome 7.[33,34]

Early linkage studies suggested an important contribution of the major histocompatibility complex (part of the IBD3 region of chromosome 6p) increasing the susceptibility to UC (and to a lesser extent CD). Candidate gene studies have strongly suggested an association between human leukocyte antigen (HLA) class II genes and IBD, and that this association is stronger in UC than in CD. Two of the reported HLA associations with UC include the serologic subtype HLA-DR2 in (Japanese subjects) and the deoxyribonucleic acid (DNA) genotypes (HLA-DRB1*1502, DRB*0103, and DRB*12).[31,34,35] The DNA genotype HLA-DRB1*0103 has also been associated with the disease phenotype of both severe extensive UC[36] and colonic CD[37] suggesting a common predisposition to colonic IBD. As pan-colitis is the more common presentation in pediatric UC, this may be of particular importance in early onset disease.

More recent genes that have been implicated (although not replicated) for both susceptibility to, and disease extent in UC include the ATP-binding cassette, subfamily B, member 1 (ABCB1) gene, also known as the multidrug resistance 1 gene (MDR1) on chromosome 7q which encodes for P-glycoprotein 170,[31,38,39] the TNF-857 on chromosome 6p (IBD3)[40] and the OCTN gene on the IBD5 region of chromosome 5q31.[41] The homozygous mutant OCTN1/2 haplotype was significantly increased in pediatric IBD (24.3% vs 16.1%, $p = .02$) and UC patients (28.2% vs 16.1%, $p = .02$) compared with controls.[42] In children the TNF-α 308 G-A promoter polymorphism of the IBD5 locus has also been implicated as important in UC.[43] No susceptibility to UC in the presence of CARD15 has been shown in children,[44–46] although there was a suggestion that CARD15 may promote the phenotype of UC presenting in children less than 6 years of age.[44]

Many other candidate genes have been implicated for IBD including genes thought to aid epithelial integrity (DLG5 on chromosome 10), and genes related to innate immunity (TLR4, TLR5, CARD4), other suspected loci (IBD2, IBD4) but have yet to be studied in any detail.[31]

Environmental Factors

It is widely believed that the pathophysiological basis of UC results from environmental factors leading to a breakdown of the regulatory restraints on the mucosal immune responses to enteric bacteria in genetically susceptible individuals. Others propose that the disease is primarily an autoimmune process. The strongest evidence for the importance of the environmental (rather than genetic) factors is the incomplete concordance for UC reported among monozygotic twins.

Multiple environmental factors have been postulated to be important, and birth cohort data suggests that early life exposure to environmental risk factors may influence the development of UC.[35,47] These include either protective factors such as breast feeding,[48] cigarette smoking,[49] and early appendectomy[50–51] or predisposing factors such as recurrent childhood infections,[52] diarrheal illness during infancy,[53] nonsteroidal anti-inflammatory drug use,[54] and stress.[55]

A recent case controlled population-based study of 282 cases of childhood onset IBD (of which 60 had UC) asked 140 questions in six areas including family history, diet including breast feeding, active/passive smoking, perinatal period, childhood infections and vaccines, home amenities, and socioeconomic status. For UC they confirmed that family history of IBD was the strongest risk factor, others being disease during pregnancy, bedroom sharing, and appendectomy as a protective factor. Neither passive smoking nor diet affected the risk.[56]

Appendectomy. Multiple studies have reported a reduced risk of UC following appendectomy at a young age.[51] In a population-based case-control study, UC was inversely related to appendectomy in those individuals who underwent surgery for inflammatory conditions (eg, appendicitis or mesenteric lymphadenitis) but not nonspecific abdominal pain before 20 years of age.[57] This suggested that the inflammatory condition leading to the appendectomy may be inversely related to the development of UC later in life.

Diet and Breast-Feeding. The intestine is exposed to numerous luminal dietary antigens; thus, a potential relationship between dietary intake, and the development of UC seems plausible. The recent case-control study reported an association with sugar-containing diet (but no other dietary issues such as the age of introducing flour, meat, and vegetables).[56] This association disappeared on multivariate analysis.

The impact of breast-feeding on the development of UC remains controversial; some published studies suggest a protective effect[48] whereas other studies show no effect.[53]

Stress. Although the early theories that UC was a psychological disorder have been discounted, up to 40% of patients report psychological stress as a potential trigger of their disease.[55] Furthermore, stress has been demonstrated to be associated with relapse in animal models of colitis,[58] and recent data in adults with UC show that acute psychological stress can lead to alterations in the systemic and mucosal inflammatory response.[59]

Smoking. The lower risk of UC among smokers has been demonstrated in multiple studies, although the potential mechanism of this association is still unknown; in vitro work suggests an inhibitory effect of nicotine on the TH2 cells that predominate in UC.[60] Limited and inconsistent data are available regarding the possible association of childhood exposure to passive smoking and the development of UC. One study demonstrated that passive smoking decreased the risk of developing UC in adulthood[61] whereas another study demonstrated an association between passive smoking and the development of both childhood UC and CD[62]; a more recent study in children does not confirm this.[56] However, another population-based study has identified smoking during early pregnancy as being protective toward the development of both UC and CD.[63]

Drugs. Nonsteroidal anti-inflammatory drug use has been suggested to precede the onset of IBD, lead to a reactivation of quiescent IBD, or exacerbate already active IBD in humans.[35] This is thought to be due to reduced mucosal protective prostanoid production due to both COX1 and COX2 inhibition.[64]

Microbial Factors. Although no specific causative infectious agent has been identified, bacterial factors are likely to play a role in the initiation or perpetuation of intestinal inflammation by serving as antigens or costimulatory factors.[65] Differences in colonic bacteria between controls and patients with CD or UC have been shown although it is not known if this is a cause or consequence of the colitis.[66]

A variety of genetic alterations in animals leads to colitis including interleukin (IL)-2, IL-10, and T-cell receptor knockout mice and HLAB27 transgenic rats. Most of these animal models do not develop colitis in germ-free environments, emphasizing the importance of bacteria in the development of colitis.

Other microbes can also have an apparently protective influence on the development of colitis. Probiotic preparations or nonpathogenic *Escherichia coli* may help maintain remission of UC.[67–69] Increasing evidence suggests that probiotic preparations may be effective for preventive and maintenance therapy for pouchitis.[70] Prebiotics or a combined approach of pre- and probiotics (known as synbiotics) are increasingly being studied with some evidence of successful prevention of relapses.[71-72]

Host and Immune Factors

Barrier Factors. Recent studies have implicated abnormalities of the epithelial barrier as a possible etiological factor in the development of UC. The passive barrier includes the mucus layer, tight junctions of the epithelial cells, and parts of the innate immune system, such as defensins and trefoil factors. The innate immune system also may recognize (and respond to) luminal antigens such as bacteria through the expression of Toll-like receptors within epithelial cells. Defects in the either passive or active epithelial barrier function could result in initiation or potentiation of mucosal inflammation by microbial antigens.[73]

The mucus layer has a high content of a glycoprotein called phosphatidyl choline (PC). Subjects with UC have been shown to have reduction of the PC content of the rectal mucus.[74] When replaced using delayed release capsules, PC may alleviate the disease.[75]

Other substances within the epithelial and mucus barrier which may play a role in the microbial responses include defensins secreted by the Paneth cells,[76-77] trefoil factors, and mucins.[78] MUC3 polymorphisms on chromosome 7q, potentially affecting the production or quality of mucins, have been implicated in UC.[79]

Another key part of the epithelial barrier are the tight junctions of the epithelial cells. In animal models genetically induced disruption of these junctions leads to intestinal inflammation.[80]

Mucosal Immune Cells. Inflammation occurs as a result of either excessive effector T-cell function or deficient regulatory T-cell function.[73] In UC, evidence suggests that an excessive T-helper (Th)2 cell response occurs rather than the Th1 cell pattern typical of CD. Although IL-4 secretion is not increased in UC, the secretion of other cytokines characteristic of a Th2 cell response, namely IL-5 and IL-13, is elevated.[81-82] Increases in the antibody formation (eg, antineutrophil cytoplasmic antibodies) and IgG1 and IgG4 more typical of Th2 responses are also found in UC and provide evidence for Th2 predominance.[73] In vitro IL-13 has been shown to impair epithelial barrier function by affecting epithelial apoptosis, tight junctions, and restitution velocity, and in vivo was secreted in larger amounts from lamina propria mononuclear cells from subjects with UC (compared with CD and controls).[83]

The data on regulatory T cells (CD4+CD25+) in patients with UC remain unclear. Increased numbers have been found in inflamed mucosa; however, in vitro these cells suppress effector T cells suggesting in vivo their suppressor effects are being overwhelmed by other cells[84] Others have found lower numbers in peripheral blood of patients with active disease and proposed this reduced number is the cause of the mucosal activity.[85]

Another group of immune cells that are increasingly thought to be central to the induction or suppression of inflammation in colitis are dendritic cells which act as regulators of immunity to pathogens, oral tolerance, and intestinal inflammation.[86] Alterations to these cells in IBD may include increased numbers and maturation, presence of activated dendritic cells, altered expression of TLR2 and 4 and differential secretion of cytokines (IL-6, IL-12 greater in CD).[86]

Once the mucosal immune system is activated, there are a number of nonspecific mediators of tissue injury produced in both CD and UC. These include eicosanoids, leukotrienes, free radicals, homocysteine, and cytokines and chemokines (such as IL-1 and TNF).[87] Matrix metalloproteinases are proteases which have the capacity to cleave components of both the extracellular matrix and chemokines, causing both mucosal degradation and recruitment of inflammatory cells.[87]

Others

Disease leading to abnormalities of the intestinal vasculature including hypercoagulability, impaired perfusion, and altered patterns of endothelial and leukocyte recruitment have been implicated in the development of all forms of IBD.[88] A protective effect of hemophilia and von-Willebrands disease has been demonstrated.[89]

PRESENTATION

History

The classical symptoms of UC and IC include the presence of chronic (more than 2 weeks) bloody diarrhea, abdominal pain, and tenesmus. The period of illness prior to presentation and diagnosis tends to be shorter (median of 3 to 4 months) compared to CD (6 months), presumably due to the anxiety provoked by the presence of bloody diarrhea.

In a 1-year national survey of newly presenting children with UC and IC respectively, the major features of the presentation were rectal blood loss (84%, 68%), diarrhea (74%, 78%), and abdominal pain (62%, 75%).[90] Weight loss was less common in UC/IC (35%/31%) than CD (58%), as were other features suggesting systemic involvement such as anorexia (6%/13% vs 25% for CD) or lethargy (12%/14% vs 27%).[90]

Quantification of Disease Severity

There are a variety of scores used in adults and children for assessing disease severity in UC; none of them have been validated in pediatric UC.

In 1955 Truelove and Witts devised their eponymous score although this was never validated in either adults or children.[91] This was later modified to a score known as the Lichtiger score (Table 1) for a pivotal study of the use of cyclosporin, with a maximum score of 21, ≥10 being severe disease activity.[92] Another score which has been widely used in clinical trials is the Mayo score.[93] This includes both clinical and endoscopic data; thus the major disadvantage of this in pediatric clinical trials is the need for sigmoidoscopic examination.[93]

In 1977 Werlin and Grand proposed and used a pediatric modification to the Truelove and Witts score in which children with severe colitis needed to have 4 out of the 5 criteria (Table 2).[212] A recent

Table 1 The Lichtiger (or Modified Truelove and Witts) Score in Pediatric Ulcerative Colitis: ≥10 Equals Severe Disease

	Score
Diarrhea	
0 to 2	0
3 to 4	1
5 to 6	2
7 to 9	3
10	4
Nocturnal diarrhea	
No/yes	0
	1
Visible blood in stools	
(% of BMs)	
0	0
<50	1
>50	2
100	3
Fecal incontinence	
No	0
Yes	1
Abdominal pain/cramps	
None	0
Mild	1
Moderate	2
Severe	3
General well-being	
Perfect	0
Very good	1
Good	2
Average	3
Poor	4
Terrible	5
Abdominal tenderness	
None	0
Mild/localized	1
Mild–moderate/diffuse	2
Severe rebound	3
Antidiarrheal drugs	
None	0
Yes	1

See text for proposed definition of response and remission.

Table 2 Werlin and Grand's Definition of Severe Colitis in UC in Children Requires Four Out of Five Following Features or the Presence of Dilatation of the Transverse Colon to > 6 cm[212]:

Features	
Bloody stools	>5 per day
Temperature	>100°F (during the first day in hospital)
Pulse	≥90 beats per minute
Anemia	Hematocrit ≤30%
Albumin	Serum albumin ≤3.0 g/dL

review proposes using the modified Truelove and Witts (Lichtiger) Score (Table 1) with additional clinical caveats for clinical assessment of children with colitis.[94] They propose that clinical response be defined as a score of <11 with a reduction in the score of ≥3 from a reduction in number of stools and/or bloody stools per day. Remission would be defined as a score of <4 with no visible blood in the stool.[94]

Examination

The physical examination of a child with UC is frequently unremarkable. Mild lower abdominal discomfort (left iliac fossa) with signs of anemia or arthritis may be present.

Where pain is more prominent, particularly if associated with systemic signs of inflammation including fever and abdominal tenderness, toxic dilatation of the colon must be suspected and occurs in about 10% of patients. This is characterized by five or more bloody stools a day, fever, tachycardia, anemia, and hypoalbuminemia. It is a life-threatening emergency and requires urgent medical intervention and close liaison with experienced surgeons.

Isolated rectal involvement is less common in children than adults and may be considered in a child who appears to be systemically well but has symptoms of tenesmus and urgency with blood and mucus mixed in with the stool. Abdominal pain or tenderness and systemic features of inflammation are less often identified in these patients.

Extraintestinal Manifestations

There are no large epidemiological studies of the incidence of extraintestinal manifestations of IBD in children. Most reports have been based on relatively small case series. During follow-up it is reported that approximately 25 to 35% of patients with IBD develop extraintestinal symptoms, the majority being arthropathy, liver abnormalities, or skin disorders.[95] Extraintestinal manifestations of IBD may or may not correlate with the activity of intestinal inflammation and can occur before, during, or after the development of gastrointestinal symptoms and may even appear after surgical removal of diseased bowel[96–98] (see Table 3).

Joints. Arthropathy occurs in approximately 20 to 25% of patients and may be a presenting manifestation in 6% of children with UC and 4% of IC (compared with 7% of CD).[99] Arthralgia without swelling is also a common symptom of pediatric IBD.

The peripheral arthritis of IBD most commonly presents as an asymmetric, nondeforming, migratory polyarthritis of one or more large joints where exacerbations of the joint disease parallels increased activity of bowel disease.[96] In a large study of adults with UC, two types of peripheral arthropathy were described[100]: a pauciarticular form with fewer than five swollen joints and a polyarticular or rheumatoid-like form with more than five joints affected. The pauciarticular form was found to be more likely

to correlate with exacerbations of bowel disease and other extraintestinal manifestation such as uveitis and erythema nodosum.[100] Axial arthropathies, ankylosing spondylitis or sacroiliitis, occur in 1 to 4% of patients and are associated with HLA-B27 positivity in most cases.[95,97]

Skin. Pyoderma gangrenosum and erythema nodosum are the two major skin manifestations associated with both UC and CD and can precede the development of bowel symptoms. Erythema nodosum occurs in 3 to 8% of subjects with IBD, more frequently in subjects with CD and usually coincides with increased bowel disease activity.[101] Pyoderma gangrenosum occurs in less than 1 to 2% of all patients with UC (although it is more commonly seen in UC than in CD) and is rarely seen in children.

Eye. Ophthalmologic abnormalities are described in approximately 1 to 3% of children with IBD and develop more commonly in patients with other extraintestinal manifestations.[95] Episcleritis and uveitis are the major ocular disorders reported, the former can present without symptoms of pain or loss of vision.[102–103] Uveitis is typically characterized by acute or subacute pain with visual blurring, photophobia, and headache and is diagnosed with a slit-lamp examination.

Liver. Transient elevations of hepatic enzymes are common in children with UC and may be related to medications, disease activity, or unrelated causes such as viral infections. Persistent

elevations suggest the presence of primary sclerosing cholangitis (PSC) or autoimmune chronic active hepatitis.

The diagnosis of PSC or autoimmune hepatitis is established through a combination of cholangiography (now largely using magnetic resonance imaging), liver biopsy, and serology.[104]

Although the chronic liver diseases are typically identified after the diagnosis of UC, they may also precede the gastrointestinal symptoms.[104–105] At diagnosis, liver disease is infrequent but more common in UC/IC (3%) compared with CD (1%).[99] In one large unit, UC has been found to be the major disorder present in patients with sclerosing cholangitis despite a much larger number of patients with CD in the clinic.[98] During follow-up, approximately 3 to 5% of children with UC develop sclerosing cholangitis and less than 1% develop chronic active hepatitis.[105]

Medical treatment has little impact on disease course, although ursodeoxycholic acid may be of some benefit and is often prescribed.[106]

Recent data have suggested a different phenotype of PSC with IBD (PSC-IBD) characterized by extensive but mild colonic disease. In this group there is thought to be an increased risk of colonic cancer as well as the increased risk of cholangiocarcinoma already known in PSC.[107–108] The possible use of 5-aminosalicylic acid (5-ASA) compounds for reducing this cancer risk has yet to be clearly established.[109]

Thromboembolic Disease. Two case-control studies have clearly demonstrated an overall increased risk of about threefold for deep vein thrombosis (DVT) or pulmonary embolism (PE) in patients with UC.[110–111] Interestingly, the greatest increased risk was in the group of patients under 40 years of age, perhaps reflecting the lower incidence of thromboembolism in the age-matched controls.[110] Thromboembolic events most commonly occur as DVTs and PEs but have been reported to involve most peripheral and central vessels. Rarely, other hematological abnormalities associated with UC occur, including immune thrombocytopenic purpura and autoimmune hemolytic anemia have been reported.

Osteopenia or Osteoporosis. Low bone mineral density (BMD) may occur in children with UC but less often than in children with CD.[112–113] Whether this is due to the treatment received or is a fundamental part of the disease process has not been clearly established although there is now evidence of reduced BMD at diagnosis for CD but not UC.[114]

Complications

A number of serious complications may occur in the course of UC. Whereas some of these, such as toxic megacolon, perforation of the colon, and hemorrhage, may occur with a severe exacerbation at any point of time, strictures and colon cancer typically happen in the setting of long-standing disease and are unusual in childhood.

Table 3 Extraintestinal Manifestations of UC/IC

Hepatobiliary	Sclerosing cholangitis
	Autoimmune hepatitis
	Transient elevations of liver enzymes
	Fatty liver disease
	Cholelithiasis
Eyes	Uveitis
	Episcleritis
	Cataracts*
Musculoskeletal	Peripheral arthropathy (pauci- or polyarticular)
	Ankylosing spondylitis
	Enthesopathy
	Osteonecrosis (avascular/ aseptic necrosis of bone or osteochondritis dissecans) *
	Osteopenia, osteoporosis*
Skin	Erthyema nodosum
	Pyoderma gangrenosum
	Alopecia
	Sweet's syndrome (acute febrile neutrophilic dermatosis)
Growth and development	Growth failure*
	Delayed puberty
Hematologic	Iron deficiency anemia
	Thromobocytosis
	Thromboembolic disease
Others	Amyloidosis
	Nephrolithiasis
	Pericarditis

*May be related to steroid use.

Toxic megacolon is a life-threatening complication of UC characterized by dilatation of the colon to greater than 5.5 cm in transverse diameter (as defined in adults) associated with systemic toxicity including fever, tachycardia, and abdominal tenderness.[115] It is important to remember that clinical signs, particularly fever and tenderness, may be masked by high-dose steroid treatment. Although reported to occur in up to 5% of UC patients over their lifetime, it is relatively rarely encountered in pediatric practice. In contrast to typical UC, in which the inflammatory changes are limited to the mucosa, the inflammation can extend into the deeper layers of the colonic wall.

Risk factors for toxic megacolon include drugs that impair motility, such as anticholinergic agents, narcotic agents prescribed for analgesia or antidiarrheal effects, or antidepressants with anticholinergic effects, and the early discontinuation or rapid tapering of steroids or 5-ASA agents.[116–117]

Various clinical criteria for the definition of severe colitis (which may lead to the need for urgent colectomy) have been defined. Most are based on the presence of frequent bloody diarrhea and systemic features of fevers and tachycardia. In children Werlin and Grand proposed that to be defined as severe colitis four of the following five criteria were required: >5 stools per day, temperature >100°F, heart rate >90 beat per minute, hematocrit <30%, and serum albumin <3 g/dL. For adults Travis proposed C-reactive protein >45 mg/L, stool frequency of 3 to 8 per day, or >8 per day on day 3.[118]

Once the disorder is recognized, management requires surgical assessment, stool bacterial culture with assay for *Clostridium difficile* toxin, establishment of fluid homeostasis, and treatment with high-dose steroids. Monitoring requires serial physical examination and periodic (every 8 to 12 hours) supine and upright radiographs to assess colonic dilatation and exclude the presence of intra-abdominal free air indicative of perforation. A nasogastric tube or, if necessary, passage of a long tube into the distal intestine may decompress the colon and minimize further fluid accumulation. "Bowel rest" has been suggested for many years; however, controlled studies have suggested that enteral feeds can be safe and may be preferable to risking the complications of parenteral nutrition.[94] Antibiotics, while normally, used have also not been confirmed to be of benefit in controlled trials.[94] Other treatments with some evidence of benefit include infliximab, cyclosporin, and tacrolimus. Patients who fail to respond to these aggressive medical measures and have persistence of toxic dilatation for longer than 48 hours, perforation, or ongoing hemorrhage may require emergency colectomy.

Cancer

There is a well-established increased risk of colorectal carcinoma in subjects with UC. A meta-analysis of 116 studies has estimated a cumulative incidence of colorectal cancer in all patients with UC of 2% at 10 years, 8% at 20 years, and 18% after 30 years of disease.[119] Risk factors that are suggested to predispose cancer include time since diagnosis, extent of disease (minimal in proctosigmoiditis, highest in pancolitis),[120] concurrent PSC,[121] family history of colorectal carcinoma,[122] the presence of backwash ileitis,[123] severity and persistence of inflammation,[124] and postinflammatory pseudopolyps.[125] Surprisingly, given that pancolitis is more common in early onset disease, childhood onset has not been consistently demonstrated to be an independent risk factor.[126]

Colonoscopic screening programs are designed to detect patients with low- or high-grade dysplasia prior to the development of cancer. Recent guidelines advise a screening colonoscopy for subjects with more than one-third of the colon affected 8 to 10 years after diagnosis when, if no dysplasia or cancer is found, surveillance should begin within 2 years.[127] The surveillance occurs every 1 to 2 years, if there are two successive negative examinations the next can be 1 to 3 years until colitis has been present for 20 years when it should be 1 to 2 years.[127] The guidelines of the British Society of Gastroenterology advise that left sided colitis the screening program can start after 15 to 20 years and the in the second decade of disease can be three yearly, third decade two yearly, and fourth decade annually.[128] There does not seem to be any good reason for surveillance to differ in patients with younger onset UC, and the higher proportion of pancolitis and longer period during which cancer may develop confirms the importance of counseling and establishing on a screening program.[129]

A Cochrane review of the efficacy of screening in subjects with IBD concludes there is no clear evidence yet that surveillance colonoscopy prolongs survival in patients with extensive colitis.[130] There is some evidence that cancers tend to be detected at an earlier stage and these patients have a correspondingly better prognosis. There is also indirect evidence that surveillance is likely to be effective at reducing the risk of death from IBD-associated colorectal cancer and that it may be acceptably cost effective.[130]

During screening colonoscopies biopsies are performed in four quadrants at 10 cm intervals from the cecum with a minimum of 33 biopsies recommended.[35] Management of dysplasia and dysplasia-associated lesion or mass requires pathologists and colonoscopists expert in colitis screening with dye spray and endoscopic mucosal resection. The American College of Gastroenterology recommends colectomy for cancer and high-grade dysplasia and dysplasia-associated lesion or mass, and low-grade dysplasia, despite the fact that some patients with low-grade dysplasia may not progress.[131] However, following advances in endoscopic mucosal resection and screening, others would suggest colectomy for cancer, visible lesions that cannot be resected endoscopically and the presence of multiple dysplasias of all grades not visible endoscopically.[132] Visible lesions where feasible may be resected using endoscopic mucosal resection, and low-grade dysplasias should undergo increased surveillance.[132]

Whether 5-ASA agents may provide a protective effect in the development of colorectal cancer in patients with UC remains controversial.[133–134] Recently, ursodeoxycholic acid has been proposed to be effective as a chemopreventive agent in patients with UC and PSC.[109,135]

DIAGNOSIS

Differential Diagnosis The diagnosis of UC is established from a detailed history, physical examination, and a combination of laboratory, radiologic, and endoscopic studies. It is important to exclude other etiologies such as infectious processes and once chronic IBD has been confirmed clarify whether it is UC/IC or CD (see Table 4).

In addition to details of the clinical presentation, the history should include family history, recent antibiotic therapy, infectious exposures, growth and sexual development, and the presence of extraintestinal manifestations of UC. Findings on physical examination may help to distinguish UC from CD; for example, pronounced growth failure or a perianal disease strongly suggests the diagnosis of CD. Pubertal status is important in order to interpret growth data.

Colonic inflammation is typically accompanied by bloody diarrhea with abdominal cramping. Painless rectal bleeding is less likely to be due to colitis and will usually be associated with

Table 4 Differential Diagnosis of Colitis in Children

Chronic idiopathic	Ulcerative colitis
	Indeterminate colitis
	Crohn's colitis
	Lymphocytic colitis
	Collagenous colitis
	Esoinophillic colitis
Infections	Bacterial: *Campylobacter, Shigella, Salmonella, enterohemorrhagic E. Coli, Yersinia, Aeromonas, Staph, Aureus, Neisseria gonorrhoea, Treponema pallidum, Mycobacterium*
	Antibiotic-associated and pseudomembranous: *Clostridium difficile* (toxin producing)
	Viral: Cytomegalovirus, herpes simplex virus, HIV
	Parasitic: *Entamoeba histolytica*
Vasculitic	Henoch-Schönlein purpura
	Hemolytic uremic syndrome
	Behcet's disease
	Churg-Strauss
	Polyarteritis nodosa
Other	Ischemic colitis
	Allergic colitis
	Hirschsprung's enterocolitis
	Graft-versus-host disease
	Necrotizing enterocolitis
	Chemotherapy or radiation-induced colitis
	Diversion colitis

normal inflammatory parameters. This may be caused by a number of other disorders in children, including polyps, vascular abnormalities, Meckel's diverticulae, intestinal duplications, surgical disorders such as intussusception and other causes of bowel ischemia. Fresh bleeding associated with hard stools would suggest the possibility of fissures secondary to constipation.

The differential diagnosis of a proven colitis depends on the age of the child at the time of evaluation. In infancy, necrotizing enterocolitis, Hirschsprung enterocolitis, and allergic colitis must be considered. In contrast, in the older child and adolescent, enteric infection and IBD are the most common diagnoses. Infection with *Salmonella*, *Shigella*, *Campylobacter*, *Yersinia*, *Aeromonas*, certain strains of *E. coli*, and *Entamoeba histolytica* may resemble UC and should be excluded. Colitis secondary to a vasculitic process may occur in children with Henoch-Schönlein purpura and hemolytic uremic syndrome and other vasculitides. The causes of colitis in children are provided in Table 4.

Laboratory Assessment. Initial laboratory assessment should include blood tests and stool cultures. A full blood count with differential may reveal a leukocytosis with or without left shift, microcytic anemia, and thrombocytosis. The presence of anemia with low mean corpuscular volume, and low iron and ferritin levels indicate an iron-deficient anemia likely to be secondary to chronic fecal blood losses. Elevated erythrocyte sedimentation rate (ESR) or C-reactive protein may indicate increased disease activity although it is important to remember that the ESR can be raised in the presence of anemia without inflammation and both may be raised in acute viral and other infections.

Children with significant mucosal inflammation may have normal laboratory test results; this is particularly true of those with distal disease. In one pediatric study, 60% of UC patients had raised CRP at diagnosis compared with 100% of CD, ESR was raised in 23% in UC and 85% for CD.[136] In another study of children 13 of 36 patients with UC (36%) had normal blood test results, including 6 of the 17 patients with severe extensive colitis.[137]

Stool cultures should be performed to detect enteric infections. Assay for both *C. difficile* toxins should be obtained in all patients in relapse, regardless of prior antibiotic treatment.[138–139]

Although insensitive and nonspecific, the presence of fecal leukocytes may suggest colitis. More recently, assays of white blood cell proteins, such as calprotectin, have been proposed as more reliable indicators of colonic inflammation and for use in monitoring the disease during follow-up.[140–142]

Serology. Perinuclear antineutrophil cytoplasmic antibodies (p-ANCAs) are seen in 60 to 80% of subjects with UC compared with 10 to 27% of those with CD and have been proposed as tools for discriminating UC from CD.[143–145]

In a study of 173 children, the detection of ANCA had a sensitivity of 57% and a specificity of 92% for UC; assay of antibodies to *saccharomyces cerevisiae* (ASCAS) yielded a sensitivity of 55% and a specificity of 95% for CD.[143] In a study of 128 pediatric patients undergoing evaluation for IBD, modified cutoff values for ASCA and ANCA increased the sensitivity for detecting IBD from 69 to 81%, but this was accompanied by an increase in false-positive rates among the children without IBD.[146] Therefore, these tests are not a substitute for the traditional evaluation to either identify or discriminate between UC/IC/CD.

While it has been hoped that serological assays may help in the classification of IC, in the small studies performed thus far this has not generally proven to be useful.[5,147] A prospective study of 97 patients with IC found that 50% were both p-ANCA and ASCA negative at diagnosis and after 6 years 66 patients remained classified as IC of which 60% still had negative serology. Additional evidence is required before the routine use of serologic testing can be endorsed in the child with suspected UC.

Endoscopic Findings

Distribution. Inflammation in UC is classically reported to be limited to the colon and rectum. In untreated UC, the distal colon is most severely affected, and the rectum is almost always involved. Inflammation is continuous, extending from the rectum proximally with varying degrees of ulceration, hemorrhage, edema, and regenerating epithelium.[148] However, there are reports of what is both histologically and clinically UC affecting the left side of the colon and the cecal area with normal mucosa in between, and might be regarded as "patchy" UC.[149]

In contrast to adult patients, who most commonly have disease confined to the left colon, only about 5 to 10% of children have isolated rectal involvement or ulcerative proctitis, 20% have left-sided disease, with pancolitis the most common pattern ranging from 43 to 90%.[20,99,150] Rectal sparing was noted in one national survey in 4% of subjects.[99]

Similarly, about 80% of patients with IC are found to have pancolitis[5,99] with rectal sparing in up to 50%.[99] For those with left-sided IC, the majority of them are reported to extend to pancolitis during follow-up.[5] Although UC is limited to the colon, "backwash ileitis" owing to nonspecific inflammation of the terminal ileum may occur in about 15% of subjects and is generally associated with pancolitis.

The presence of upper GI abnormalities in UC and IC is of major importance. Most pediatric gastroenterologists will now perform upper gastrointestinal endoscopy in addition to colonoscopy in newly presenting patients with IBD. The frequency of identifying inflammation, mostly mild, in the upper gastrointestinal tract in patients with UC ranges from 25 to 69%.[90,151] For IC there is little in the way of good quality data but a sug-

gestion of somewhere between CD and UC at about 40%.[90]

Macroscopic Features. Grossly, the colonic mucosa appears erythematous, hemorrhagic, and roughened in active disease, whereas the inactive or quiescent phase is characterized by flattening of the mucosa and effacement of the normal haustral markings. In severely active colitis in which the mucosa has been destroyed, inflammation may extend into the submucosa and occasionally down to the muscularis. Such ulcers are typically broad and shallow rather than fissuring or knife-like, as would be more typical of CD or IC. Intervening areas of regenerating granulation tissue and residual mucosa can form islands of tissue called pseudopolyps which is more often seen in UC. Thickening of the bowel wall and fibrosis are rare, although shortening of the colon and focal colonic strictures may occur in long-standing disease (see Figure 1).

Microscopic Features. The microscopic appearance of the mucosa in UC is characterized by continuous acute and chronic inflammation with diffuse mucosal infiltration by polymorphonuclear leukocytes and mononuclear cells. Features favoring a diagnosis of UC include crypt architectural distortion with branching and atrophy, severe widespread decreased crypt density, frankly villous surface, diffuse transmucosal lamina propria cell increase, and severe mucin depletion.[152] Skip lesions, well-formed granulomas, focal cryptitis, discontinuous crypt distortion, transmural inflammation, and fibrosis are regarded as being more typical of CD.[152]

IC may be diagnosed when endoscopy is equivocal and microscopy is performed upon mucosal biopsies from different segments of the colon, obtained at two sequential determinations in a patient with a history of chronic or relapsing colitis. The microscopic features of IC are proposed to include the presence of areas with minimal or moderate glandular distortion such as vertical branching of two crypts, alternating with areas with a regular epithelial pattern in conjunction with accumulation of inflammatory cells (lymphocytes and plasma cells) in the basal part of the lamina propria between the base of the crypts and the muscularis mucosa.[153] Inflammation can be minimal or intense, with or without ulcerations. The lamina propria cell infiltrate is predominantly mononuclear and usually discontinuous, but neutrophils and eosinophils can be present as well as in cryptitis. These features are comparable to those proposed in the original reports from Price in surgical resection specimens.[6] One feature that has tended to lead to a diagnosis of IC (or CD) is the presence of "fissuring ulceration"; however, one follow-up study found that during follow-up, these did not predict CD and proposed they could be normally found in severe UC. The interpretation of this is important when deciding surgical procedures such as ileal pouch anal anastomosis (IPAA) procedure.[7] A diagnosis of IC should not be based on the analysis of one single rectal biopsy.

While the above include the general descriptions of UC (and IC), there are a number of caveats that need to be recognized in specimens from the pediatric age group.[154] First is the fact that newly presenting children with UC may have patchy involvement of chronic inflammation (21%) and relative or absolute rectal sparing (26%) neither of which were found in adult subjects.[155–156] It has been proposed that these atypical features are mostly found in children presenting under 10 years of age, as they get older the features become more typical of adult.[157] Pharmacologic therapy may also significantly alter the gross and histopathologic appearance of UC by normalizing the colonic mucosa histologically or inducing patchiness or discontinuity.[158]

Capsule Endoscopy. The role of capsule endoscopy in the investigation of pediatric IBD has yet to be fully evaluated but may be of use in identifying lesions in the small intestine not detected by barium follow-through. For subject with colitis, this may help to identify small bowel disease when barium follow-through, OGD, and ileocolonoscopy have not confirmed a diagnosis of UC or CD.

Radiology. Radiological assessment of UC/IC is mainly required for the exclusion of small bowel disease using a barium follow-through, monitoring of severe colitis using plain films to look for complications such as colonic dilatation or pneumoperitoneum, or in moderately to severely ill patients ultrasound, or computed tomography may be required to identify intra-abdominal abscess formation.

Most children with IBD undergo examination of their small intestine with a barium follow-through to identify any small bowel lesions which would be suggestive of CD. The exception to this is the presence of UC-associated "backwash ileitis," which should be distinguished from terminal ileal disease of CD. The Porto criteria advise that barium meal and follow-through is not routinely required in patients with distal colonic disease, normal ileum, normal OGD, and characteristic histological features of UC.[2]

With the use of colonoscopy, barium enema now has a very limited role in the evaluation of children with UC. Doppler ultrasonography[159–160] and leukocyte-labeled scintigraphy[161] have been proposed as means of assessing the extent and activity of UC avoiding the need for total colonoscopy, especially in patients unable (due to the severity of their symptoms) or unwilling to undergo ileocolonoscopy.

TREATMENT

Medical

The broad approaches to the medical treatment of UC are the induction and then the maintenance of remission. Treatments used for induction of remission depend on the extent and severity of the relapse. For the small proportion with distal disease, topical aminosalicylate, is probably

Table 5 Broad Principles of Treatment of Ulcerative and Indeterminate Colitis		
Disease Type	Induction of Remission	Maintenance of Remission
1. Distal disease	Topical aminosalicylates (suppositories if proctitis)	Intermittent topical therapy (aminosalicylates or steroids)
	Topical corticosteroids	Oral aminosalicylates
	Oral aminosalicylate	Azathioprine/6-MP
	Oral steroids	
2. Extensive colitis	Generally oral treatment but may be combined with topical treatment with increased efficacy	
Mild to moderate	Oral aminosalicylates	Oral aminosalicylates
	Oral steroids	
Moderate to severe	Oral steroids	Oral aminosalicylates
		6-MP/azathioprine
Fulminant colitis	Intravenous steroids	Oral aminosalicylates
	Cyclosporin/tacrolimus or infliximab	6-MP/azathioprine
	Surgery	Infliximab may be considered

Adapted from Leichtner, Higuchi.[213]
6-MP = 6-mercaptopurine.

the most effective treatment although often not popular in teenagers. Careful discussion of the pros and cons of the alternatives such as oral steroids helps the individual make a reasoned choice. For more extensive but mild disease, oral aminosalicylates can be initiated although it is wise to observe them closely in case of lack of response or deterioration. For more severe extensive disease, or disease not improving with aminosalicylates, then oral steroids are indicated (see Table 5).[213]

Those with fulminant colitis require admission and joint management with surgical colleagues, intravenous fluids, and steroids. Those not responding to the above measures may require other treatments such as cyclosporin or infliximab.

For maintenance of remission aminosalicylates should be used. For those with recurrently relapsing disease, immunomodulators such as azathioprine or 6-mercaptopurine (6-MP) are often required. The role of infliximab in chronic-relapsing disease has yet to be clarified.

Aminosalicylates (sulfasalazine and 5-aminosalicylic acid (mesalamine or mesalazine)) are the most widely used treatments for mild to moderate UC although there are no high quality randomized controlled trials in children, and so recommendations are largely based on adult studies. 5-ASA is readily absorbed from the upper GI tract, so a variety of methods are used to direct the treatment to the colon. Sulfasalazine is linked by an azo bond to the sulfapyridine moiety, and this bond is cleaved by bacteria in the colon-releasing 5-ASA. Olsalazine links two molecules of 5-ASA via an azo bond; balsalazide links 5-ASA to a nonabsorbed carrier molecule. Delayed release preparations containing 5-ASA include pH-dependent release by coating the drug with eudragit (Asacol, Salofalk, Mesren, Mesasal, Claversal) or time-controlled release (microgranules coated with ethylcellulose (Pentasa)). A meta-analysis has reported the newer 5-ASA products to be generally safe[162] while SSZ has side effects in 10 to 40% of subjects.[163] Renal complications

during 5-ASA treatment have been reported to be rare and associated with severity of disease rather than dose or type of 5-ASA compound.[164] The lack of the sulfapyridine moiety is thought to explain lower incidence of side effects in the latter two treatments. A meta-analysis published as a Cochrane review reports that for the treatment of active UC, 5-ASA is superior to placebo, with a probable dose-response trend. Thus, higher doses may be of benefit in this situation. There is a trend to benefit of oral 5-ASA preparations (both in terms of efficacy and minimal side effects) over sulfasalazine. However, considering their relative costs, the authors questioned whether there was a significant clinical advantage to using the newer 5-ASA preparations in place of sulfasalazine.[165]

A recent review of treatments in IBD in children suggests a dose of 50 to 100 mg/kg/d in children for mesalamine.[166]

With respect to distal UC, topical mesalazine combined with oral 5-ASA can be effective for mild to moderate disease and is preferable to topical corticosteroids.[167] Topical mesalazine can also be used for left-sided mild to moderate CD.[167] Suppositories may be used to treat disease as far as the upper rectum; enemas/foam preparations may reach as far as the distal transverse colon.

For the maintenance of remission in UC, 5-ASA was found to be superior to placebo but slightly inferior to sulfasalazine.[168]

The choice of an appropriate oral aminosalicylate for use in children must consider ease of administration. Children who cannot swallow tablets may be able to accept suspensions of sulfasalazine, sachets of 5-ASA granules, or the content of capsules, in the form of powder or beads, when mixed in apple sauce or other foods of similar consistency.

Corticosteroids. For more severe disease or disease not responding to 5-ASA, steroids are usually indicated. These are potent anti-inflammatory compounds and have no role in the maintenance of remission.[167] Evidence for these largely come from trials reported more than 30 years ago, and placebo-controlled trials have never been performed in children.

Prednisolone (1 to 2 mg/kg/d maximum 40 mg/d) is effective in the induction of remission in moderate to severe UC/IC. This is usually given at this dose for 2 to 4 weeks by which time some improvement should have been seen and then weaned by 5 mg/d each week as the disease enters remission.[169] While AGA recommendations in adults are from 40 to 60 mg/d,[170] it has been shown in adults that adverse events were greater in those given 60 mg/d compared with 40 mg/d, without clinical benefit.[171]

Budesonide is a poorly absorbed corticosteroid with limited bioavailability and high first pass metabolism. It may be used as a topical treatment in patients with distal disease not responding to mesalazine; however, studies do not show any efficacy of oral preparations in treating UC.[167,170]

Immunosuppressants. Immunosuppressive agents are regularly used as treatments to maintain remission especially in those requiring frequent courses of steroids.

Azathioprine and 6-Mercaptopurine. 6-Mercaptopurine and azathioprine, which is converted to 6-MP in the liver, are purine analogues that inhibit RNA and DNA synthesis and downregulate cytotoxic T-cell activity and delayed hypersensitivity reactions. They are appropriate agents in cases of UC/IC refractory to or chronically dependent on steroid therapy. In children with UC, they have been estimated to induce and maintain remission in 60 to 75% of patients.[172–173] In adults two relapses in 1 year, or relapsing with 6 weeks of stopping therapy or when steroids are reduced to below 15 mg daily have been proposed as indications for immunosuppression.[167] These immunomodulatory agents can reduce disease activity and allow the withdrawal of steroid therapy in children with steroid-dependent UC; the time to clinical response is 3 to 4.5 months.[173–174]

In a study of 95 children with either CD or UC, 87% reduced their steroid use and 18% required discontinuation of the medication; the majority of side effects responded to dose reduction or improved spontaneously.[175] Side effects reported include aminotransferase elevations and hepatitis, pancreatitis, bone marrow depression, hypersensitivity reactions, and recurrent infections.[175]

Prior to initiation it has been advised to check the thiopurine methyl transferase genotype or phenotype to detect low enzyme levels (or homozygous) subjects and prevent predictable 6-MP/azathioprine toxicity.[170] Regular monitoring for complications with complete blood counts and liver function tests is advised, at least twice weekly while still adjusting the dose.[170] For a child with normal drug metabolism, the starting dose of 6-MP is 1 to 1.5 mg/kg/d as a single dose and of azathioprine is 1.5 to 2 mg/kg/d increasing to a maximum of 3 mg/kg/d. Children with intermediate levels of enzyme should be given lower doses, and homozygotes with very low levels should not receive the medication. Some clinicians have used 6-MP metabolite levels to monitor for compliance and potential toxicity and to permit safe dose adjustment in nonresponding patients[176] although the influence of 5-ASA compounds on measurement of the metabolites has recently been questioned.[177]

Given the high-relapse rate with withdrawal of 6-MP in adults with UC, the majority of children requiring azathioprine or 6-MP to suppress disease activity may require long-term maintenance therapy although one recent set of guidelines suggests the pragmatic stopping of the medication after 3 to 4 years if disease free.[167]

The evidence for lymphoma as a consequence of azathioprine therapy remains inconsistent. One meta-analysis suggested a fourfold increase in the relative risk of lymphoma.[178] A single center study over 15 years reported a slight increase in Epstein-Barr positive lymphomas with increasing usage of azathioprine or 6-MP.[179] If there is truly an increased risk, it is likely to be small however should be discussed on initiation of the treatment.[180]

Methotrexate. Although used in CD, published evidence of methotrexate for UC in children is absent,[166] and adult data do not support its use in UC.[170]

Cyclosporin/Tacrolimus. Cyclosporin and tacrolimus are inhibitors of cell-mediated immunity via the inactivation of calcineurin an intracellular mediator of production of IL-2 and IL-4.[181] In the original randomized controlled trial (RCT) of cyclosporin of 20 patients who had not responded to 7 days of steroids, 9 out of 11 who received cyclosporin responded compared with none in the control group.[92] In children there are only uncontrolled trials reporting a short-term response in about 80% of children[166] although the majority still need a colectomy within 1 year.[182] In one small study of 8 patients, adding 6-MP to the cyclosporine regimen led to long-term remission in 7 subjects.[183] A recent Cochrane review concludes the evidence for cyclosporin preventing colectomy in the medium to long-term is weak despite the short-term responses often seen.[184] Thus many use cyclosporin in the most acutely ill patients, often during their first presentation, allowing a period of remission while acclimatizing to the likely need for a colectomy in the future. A dose of 2 to 4 mg/kg/d intravenously changing to 8 mg/kg/d in two doses orally after 7 to 10 days is recommended.[166] An open label study of tacrolimus similarly demonstrated a 69% response rate; however, despite the use of azathioprine/6-MP, the majority required surgery within 1 year.[185]

Antibiotics. There are no data to support the widespread use of antibiotics in either children or adults with UC except in the situation of pouchitis.[166,186] Despite this many use antibiotics in severe colitis particularly if infection is considered to be present.[167]

Biologicals

Infliximab. The recently published ACT1 and 2 trials in adults have provided strong evidence for the use of Infliximab in moderate to severe UC resistant to standard medical treatments.[187] The doses used were 5 or 10 mg/kg given at weeks 0, 2, 6, and then 8, weekly for up to 46 weeks. The authors demonstrated a response rate of about 59 to 69% at week 8 compared with 29 to 37% for placebo. At week 54, 45% remained in remission compared with 20% of controls. However, evidence in children remains limited to retrospective open label reports with evidence of responses in up to 80% of subjects,[188] although there is a suggestion that the benefit is limited to children with acute active disease rather than those with long-term dependence on steroids.[189–190]

Other Biologicals. There are a wide range of other biologicals currently being studied with published data in adults including antiadhesion molecules such as alicaforsen (an antisense inhibitor to the adhesion molecule ICAM-1), MLN02 (a humanized antibody to alpha4beta7 integrin), visilizumab (a humanized anti-CD3 antibody), daclizumab (an IgG1 humanized anti-CD25 (IL-2Ra) antibody), basiliximab (chimeric monoclonal antibody to IL-2R), or RDP-58 (a novel drug to disrupt cell signaling at the pre-MAPK MyD88-IRAK-TRAF6 protein complex).[191] Data are awaited for pediatric patients, although one recent case series of four children with fulminant UC suggested some benefit for basiliximab.[192]

Others

Leukacytapharesis. Leukacytapharesis was first proposed about 10 years ago and has been used in a number of open label studies with apparent benefit varying from 22 to 82%. There are controlled studies underway in adults, the results of which are awaited. In one retrospective study in children, 8 of 12 improved during treatment with 4 apparently remaining in long-term remission.[193]

Probiotics. While enthusiastically promoted by many, there is little in the way of good evidence for probiotics as a treatment for UC. The strongest evidence is in adult subjects with pouchitis using a cocktail of eight bacterial strains (VSL3); however, the numerous varieties of the various probiotic strains means that positive results for one probiotic cannot be assumed for other preparations.[166]

Worms. Trichuris suis has been studied in an RCT of 54 adult patients, and improvement was found in 43% of subjects receiving the worms compared with 16.7% of placebo with no evidence of adverse events.[194] Further studies will be required to establish the efficacy of this treatment.

Others. Complementary and alternative medicines are frequently used by patients, but there is little scientific study of their worth. In one RCT there was a trend suggesting a benefit of oral aloe vera in treating UC in adults although this did not reach significance.[195] Another phase two placebo-controlled trial suggested a benefit for PC in a delayed release capsule, the principle being to replace the deficient mucus layer.[75] In this small study, improvement or remission was seen in 90% of those receiving the study compound compared with 10% of the placebo group. Phase three studies are now required to see if these impressive data can be replicated.[196]

Surgical

Although medical therapy remains the first-line treatment for UC, colectomy may be required for patients at the time of the acute presentation, with severe or medically refractory disease or as a treatment of colonic carcinoma or dysplasia. While removing the colon will cure UC, there are provisos that must be made apparent to the patient and their family. First is the possibility of the later development of CD, particularly in those patients labeled as having IC. Secondly are the significant risks of short- or long-term complications in up to 50% of the patients. Lastly is the expected change in bowel habit in subjects who undergo IPAA with a J pouch (to a mean of about 4 to 6 per day plus nighttime bowel movements) and frequent (0 to 12%) or intermittent (7 to 44%) incontinence.[197–198]

Indications for colectomy in a patient with UC include fulminant colitis or a complication of colitis, such as massive hemorrhage, perforation, stricture, or toxic megacolon; failure of medical therapy; steroid dependency; and the presence of colonic dysplasia. Retardation of growth and sexual maturation, usually associated with treatment-resistant or fulminant disease, may also prompt consideration of surgery as prepubertal children have been shown to be more likely to experience catch-up growth after colectomy than pubertal patients.[199]

With changes in medication frequency of surgery may have reduced.[200] At one center, a retrospective review of children and adolescents with UC revealed a decrease in the frequency of colectomy from 48.9% between 1955 and 1964 to 26.2% between 1965 and 1974.[201] For those presenting with mild disease, 5-year colectomy rate has been reported in 8% of patients compared with 26% in patients presenting with moderate to severe disease.[150] Another institutional review reported 22% of UC patients requiring surgery after a median of 16 months of medical treatment.[202]

Careful assessment of prior endoscopies, pathology reports, and upper gastrointestinal series with small bowel follow-through should be performed in order to exclude CD. If there is evidence suggesting the possibility of CD, the patient and family need to be informed of the potential for postoperative recurrence and the relative contraindications of ileoanal pull-through procedures. Variables that predict a poor outcome to the surgery include duration of symptoms, perianal disease, late complications, pouch fistulae, and CD (identified after pathological examination of the resected specimen).[203] Indeterminate colitis and terminal ileitis and early post-operative complications did not predict poor outcome.[203]

There are three approaches to surgery for UC/IC. The current standard surgical option for UC is colectomy with IPAA. Other options include the ileorectal anastomosis which has the advantage of not disrupting the rectal mucosa but the significant disadvantage of leaving diseased tissue which will need life-long monitoring and treatment. In children, this technique leads to intractable diarrhea in 32% requiring further surgery.[204] The third option, rarely used, involves a panproctocolectomy with formation of a permanent ileostomy.

The IPAA removes the entire colon and the rectal mucosa, with the aim of leaving the anal sphincters intact and thus preserving anorectal function. The type of pouch performed is most commonly the J pouch, which generally has better outcomes than the S pouch or straight ileoanal anastomosis.[204–205] Many centers use a two-stage approach. In the first stage, a subtotal colectomy, the removal of the distal rectal and proximal anal mucosa, and the formation of the ileal pouch are performed with a diverting loop ileostomy to allow the pouch to heal. The second stage involves closure of the loop ileostomy with restoration of fecal flow to the pouch. Others have completed the IPAA in one stage, without the loop ileostomy. Some centers, especially if the patient requires precipitous surgical intervention, perform a three-stage operative approach with a subtotal colectomy leaving a rectal stump to be treated with topical therapy.[202] At the second operation, the distal rectal and proximal anal mucosa is removed, and the ileal pouch is created. The ileostomy is reversed at the third operation.

Complications of IPAA include small bowel obstruction, pelvic sepsis, anastomotic leak, fecal incontinence, pouchitis, strictures, or fistulae and are reported in up to 50% of subjects.[198,202] In one large series of 151 children who underwent IPAA followed-up for a mean of 7.2 years, 21% suffered early complications and 45% late complications. The early complications included pelvic infections/abscess (9%), ileoanal separation (7%), small bowel obstruction (10%), and stricture (3%).[203] Nine percent had pouch failure requiring ileostomy with or without excision of the pouch, 11% had chronic pouchitis, 48% had acute simple pouchitis, and 36% had no pouchitis.[203] In one series of children aged 9 to 16 years who underwent proctocolectomy with IPAA, late complications (bowel obstruction, pouch fistula, etc) occurred in 11 of 29 (38%) and pouchitis developed in 9 of 29 (31%) of the children with UC.[198] Median follow-up was 4 years (range 6 months to 9 years).

Pouchitis, or inflammation of the newly created ileal reservoir, is the most significant chronic complication in UC patients undergoing IPAA. In adult series, approximately 15% will have recurrent pouchitis, and 5% will develop chronic pouchitis.[206] Symptoms of pouchitis include diarrhea, rectal bleeding, abdominal cramping, urgency and incontinence of stool, malaise, and fever. Patients with UC who undergo IPAA have pouchitis more commonly than patients with familial polyposis who undergo the same procedure suggesting that this complication is related to an underlying defect characterizing UC. In the large series above in children, 83% of the subjects who had chronic pouchitis or pouch failure were ultimately found to have CD compared with 3 of 127 who did not. Laboratory studies may demonstrate anemia and an elevated ESR. The definitive diagnosis is established by flexible sigmoidoscopy of the pouch with biopsies.

Metronidazole is the most commonly used antibiotic, but alternative therapies include ciprofloxacin.[167] If there is no improvement with antibiotics, other options include mesalamine enemas, steroid enemas or oral therapy with mesalamine, sulfasalazine, or steroids. Other therapies that may occasionally be effective include cyclosporin enemas, short-chain fatty acid enemas, butyrate suppositories, and glutamine suppositories. Probiotic therapy may prevent the onset of acute pouchitis after ileostomy closure and effectively maintain remission of chronic pouchitis.[167,186] A double-blind, placebo-controlled study evaluated the efficacy of a probiotic preparation, VSL#3 (containing a mixture of bifidobacteria, lactobacilli, and S. salivarius), compared with placebo for maintenance of remission of chronic pouchitis in 40 subjects.[70] Three patients (15%) in the VSL#3 group had relapses within the 9-month follow-up period compared with 20 (100%) in the placebo group.[70]

The long-term risk of development of dysplasia in ileal pouches is not known, and definitive recommendations for endoscopic screening of the pouch are not available.

PROGNOSIS

Ulcerative Colitis

Hyams and colleagues retrospective review reported that 70% of children can be expected to enter remission within 3 months of the initial diagnosis, irrespective of the severity of the initial attack.[150] About 45 to 58% remain inactive over the first year, 10% have chronic severe disease. During long-term follow-up 55% remain inactive, 40% have chronic intermittent symptoms, and 5 to 10% had continuous symptoms.[150] Colectomy is performed in 5% of all children in the first year and 19 to 23% within 5 years.[150,202,207] These figures are higher in those presenting with moderate to severe disease.

For the few presenting with proctitis, 92% are asymptomatic within 6 months, and 8% remained symptomatic despite 6 months of therapy.[208] During any subsequent yearly follow-up, interval data are similar to the subjects with extensive colitis, 55% of patients were asymptomatic, 40% had a chronic intermittent course, and <5% were continuously symptomatic despite therapy.[208]

Disease may extend proximally to the rectosigmoid in 29 to 70% of the subjects during follow-up, demonstrating the need for reassessment.[208–209]

Indeterminate Colitis

In one large northern Italian study of the 5% of adults with a presenting diagnosis of IC, 80% were reclassified as UC/CD within 8 years,[210] similarly Burakoff reported that of the 15% initially diagnosed with IC <5% remain indeterminate during follow-up, the majority being reclassified as UC.[211] For children it is reported that about 64% will be reclassified during follow-up.[153] In one recent study of 74 children labeled as having IC, 16 were reclassified to CD and 9 to UC within 2 years of follow-up. However, the group reports a higher proportion (29%) of their patients having IC than most studies and does not report the details of the investigation at diagnosis. This is a much higher rate of conversion than that seen in a population-based Swedish study of 151 children of whom only 29 were reclassified within 10 years.[200] The importance of thorough investigation at initial diagnosis with gastroscopy, ileocolonoscopy, expert histological assessment, and radiology are highlighted by these disparate data.

REFERENCES

1. Wilks S. Lectures on Pathological Anatomy. London: Ongman, Brown, Green, Longman, & Roberts; 1859.
2. IBD working group of the European Society for Paediatric Gastroenterology HaN. Inflammatory bowel disease in children and adolescents: Recommendations for diagnosis the Porto criteria. J Pediatr Gastroenterol Nutr 2005;41:1–7.
3. Abdullah BA, Gupta SK, Croffie JM, et al. The role of esophagogastroduodenoscopy in the initial evaluation of childhood inflammatory bowel disease: A 7-year study. J Pediatr Gastroenterol Nutr 2002;35:636–40.
4. Sharif F, McDermott M, Dillon M, et al. Focally enhanced gastritis in children with Crohn's disease and ulcerative colitis. Am J Gastroenterol 2002;97:1415–20.
5. Carvalho RS, Abadom V, Dilworth HP, et al. Indeterminate colitis: A significant subgroup of pediatric IBD. Inflamm Bowel Dis 2006;12:258–62.
6. Price AB. Overlap in the spectrum of non-specific inflammatory bowel disease colitis indeterminate. J Clin Pathol 1978;31:567–77.
7. Yantiss RK, Farraye FA, O'Brien MJ, et al. Prognostic significance of superficial fissuring ulceration in patients with severe indeterminate colitis. Am J Surg Pathol 2006;30:165–70.
8. Gasche C, Scholmerich J, Brynskov J, et al. A simple classification of Crohn's disease: Report of the Working Party for the World Congresses of Gastroenterology, Vienna 1998. Inflamm Bowel Dis 2000;6:8–15.
9. Satsangi J, Silverberg MS, Vermeire S, Colombel JF. The Montreal classification of inflammatory bowel disease: Controversies, consensus, and implications. Gut 2006;55:749–53.
10. Logan RF. Inflammatory bowel disease incidence: Up, down or unchanged? Gut 1998;42:309–11.
11. Loftus EV, Jr. Clinical epidemiology of inflammatory bowel disease: Incidence, prevalence, and environmental influences. Gastroenterology 2004;126:1504–17.
12. Shivananda S, Lennard-Jones J, Logan R, et al. Incidence of inflammatory bowel disease across Europe: Is there a difference between north and south? Results of the European Collaborative Study on Inflammatory Bowel Disease (EC-IBD). Gut 1996;39:690–7.
13. Griffiths AM, Griffiths AM. Specificities of inflammatory bowel disease in childhood. Baillieres Best Pract Res Clin Gastroenterology 2004;18:509–23.
14. Heyman MB, Kirschner BS, Gold BD, et al. Children with early-onset inflammatory bowel disease (IBD): Analysis of a pediatric IBD consortium registry. J Pediatr 2005;146:35–40.
15. Auvin S, Molinie F, Gower-Rousseau C, et al. Incidence, clinical presentation and location at diagnosis of pediatric inflammatory bowel disease: A prospective population-based study in northern France (1988–1999). J Pediatr Gastroenterol Nutr 2005;41:49–55.
16. Sawczenko A, Sandhu BK, Logan RF, et al. Prospective survey of childhood inflammatory bowel disease in the British Isles. Lancet 2001;357:1093–4.
17. Cosgrove M, Al-Atia RF, Jenkins HR. The epidemiology of paediatric inflammatory bowel disease. Arch Dis Child 1996;74:460–1.
18. Barton JR, Gillon S, Ferguson A. Incidence of inflammatory bowel disease in Scottish children between 1968 and 1983: Marginal fall in ulcerative colitis, three-fold rise in Crohn's disease. Gut 1989;30:618–22.
19. Armitage E, Drummond H, Ghosh S, Ferguson A. Incidence of juvenile-onset Crohn's disease in Scotland. Lancet 1999;353:1496–7.
20. Kugathasan S, Judd RH, Hoffmann RG, et al. Epidemiologic and clinical characteristics of children with newly diagnosed inflammatory bowel disease in Wisconsin: A statewide population-based study. J Pediatr 2003;143:525–31.
21. Hildebrand H, Finkel Y, Grahnquist L, et al. Changing pattern of paediatric inflammatory bowel disease in northern Stockholm 1990–2001. Gut 2003;52:1432–4.
22. Tysk C, Lindberg E, Jarnerot G, Floderus-Myrhed B. Ulcerative colitis and Crohn's disease in an unselected population of monozygotic and dizygotic twins. A study of heritability and the influence of smoking. Gut 1988;29:990–6.
23. Orholm M, Binder V, Sorensen TI, et al. Concordance of inflammatory bowel disease among Danish twins. Results of a nationwide study. Scand J Gastroenterol 2000;35:1075–81.
24. Probert CS, Jayanthi V, Hughes AO, et al. Prevalence and family risk of ulcerative colitis and Crohn's disease: An epidemiological study among Europeans and south Asians in Leicestershire. Gut 1993;34:1547–51.
25. Afzal NA, Mills S, Naik S, et al. Inflammatory bowel disease in Asian children resident in UK. J Pediatr Gastroenterol Nutr 2004;39:S305.
26. Armitage EL, Aldhous MC, Anderson N, et al. Incidence of juvenile-onset Crohn's disease in Scotland: Association with northern latitude and affluence. Gastroenterology 2004;127:1051–7.
27. Roth MP, Petersen GM, McElree C, et al. Geographic origins of Jewish patients with inflammatory bowel disease. Gastroenterology 1989;97:900–4.
28. Polito JM, Childs B, Mellits ED, et al. Crohn's disease: Influence of age at diagnosis on site and clinical type of disease. Gastroenterology 1996;111:580–6.
29. Farmer RG, Michener WM, Mortimer EA. Studies of family history among patients with inflammatory bowel disease. Clin Gastroenterol 1980;9:271–7.
30. Russell RK, Satsangi J. IBD: A family affair. Best Pract Res Clin Gastroenterol 2004;18:525–39.
31. Gaya DR, Russell RK, Nimmo ER, Satsangi J. New genes in inflammatory bowel disease: Lessons for complex diseases. Lancet 2006;367:1271–84.
32. Ahmad T, Tamboli CP, Jewell D, Colombel JF. Clinical relevance of advances in genetics and pharmacogenetics of IBD. Gastroenterology 2004;126:1533–49.
33. Satsangi J, Parkes M, Louis E, et al. Two stage genome-wide search in inflammatory bowel disease provides evidence for susceptibility loci on chromosomes 3, 7 and 12. Nat Genet 1996;14:199–202.
34. Satsangi J, Welsh KI, Bunce M, et al. Contribution of genes of the major histocompatibility complex to susceptibility and disease phenotype in inflammatory bowel disease. Lancet 1996;347:1212–7.
35. Farrell RJ, Peppercorn MA. Ulcerative colitis. Lancet 2002;359:331–40.
36. Roussomoustakaki M, Satsangi J, Welsh K, et al. Genetic markers may predict disease behavior in patients with ulcerative colitis. Gastroenterology 1997;112:1845–53.
37. Ahmad T, Armuzzi A, Bunce M, et al. The molecular classification of the clinical manifestations of Crohn's disease. Gastroenterology 2002;122:854–66.
38. Ho GT, Soranzo N, Nimmo ER, et al. ABCB1/MDR1 gene determines susceptibility and phenotype in ulcerative colitis: Discrimination of critical variants using a gene-wide haplotype tagging approach. Hum Mol Genet 2006;15:797–805.
39. Schwab M, Schaeffeler E, Marx C, et al. Association between the C3435T MDR1 gene polymorphism and susceptibility for ulcerative colitis. Gastroenterology 2003;124:26–33.
40. Tremelling M, Waller S, Bredin F, et al. Genetic variants in TNF-alpha but not DLG5 are associated with inflammatory bowel disease in a large United Kingdom cohort. Inflamm Bowel Dis 2006;12:178–84.
41. Waller S, Tremelling M, Bredin F, et al. Evidence for association of OCTN genes and IBD5 with ulcerative colitis. Gut 2006;55:809–14.
42. Russell RK, Drummond H, Nimmo E, et al. Analysis of the influence of OCTN1/2 variants within the IBD5 locus on disease susceptibility and growth parameters in early-onset inflammatory bowel disease. Gut 2006;55:1114–23.
43. Sykora J, Subrt I, Didek P, et al. Cytokine tumor necrosis factor-alpha A promoter gene polymorphism at position 308 G>A and pediatric inflammatory bowel disease: Implications in ulcerative colitis and Crohn's disease. J Pediatr Gastroenterol Nutr 2006;42:479–87.
44. Ferraris A, Torres B, Knafelz D, et al. Relationship between CARD15, SLC22A4/5, and DLG5 polymorphisms and early-onset inflammatory bowel diseases: An Italian multicentric study. Inflamm Bowel Dis 2006;12:355–61.
45. Russell RK, Drummond HE, Nimmo EE, et al. Genotype-phenotype analysis in childhood-onset Crohn's disease: NOD2/CARD15 variants consistently predict phenotypic characteristics of severe disease. Inflamm Bowel Dis 2005;11:955–64.
46. Kugathasan S, Collins N, Maresso K, et al. CARD15 gene mutations and risk for early surgery in pediatric-onset Crohn's disease. Clin Gastroenterol Hepatol 2004;2:1003–9.
47. Delco F, Sonnenberg A. Exposure to risk factors for ulcerative colitis occurs during an early period of life. Am J Gastroenterol 1999;94:679–84.
48. Corrao G, Tragnone A, Caprilli R, et al. Risk of inflammatory bowel disease attributable to smoking, oral contraception and breastfeeding in Italy: A nationwide case-control study. Cooperative Investigators of the Italian Group for the Study of the Colon and the Rectum (GISC). Int J Epidemiol 1998;27:397–404.
49. Lindberg E, Tysk C, Andersson K, Jarnerot G. Smoking and inflammatory bowel disease. A case control study. Gut 1988;29:352–7.
50. Rutgeerts P, D'Haens G, Hiele M, et al. Appendectomy protects against ulcerative colitis. Gastroenterology 1994;106:1251–3.
51. Koutroubakis IE, Vlachonikolis IG, Kouroumalis EA. Role of appendicitis and appendectomy in the pathogenesis of ulcerative colitis: A critical review. Inflamm Bowel Dis 2002;8:277–86.
52. Wurzelmann JI, Lyles CM, Sandler RS. Childhood infections and the risk of inflammatory bowel disease. Dig Dis Sci 1994;39:555–60.
53. Koletzko S, Griffiths A, Corey M, et al. Infant feeding practices and ulcerative colitis in childhood. BMJ 1991;302:1580–1.
54. Evans JM, McMahon AD, Murray FE, et al. Non-steroidal anti-inflammatory drugs are associated with emergency admission to hospital for colitis due to inflammatory bowel disease. Gut 1997;40:619–22.
55. Theis MK, Boyko EJ. Patient perceptions of causes of inflammatory bowel disease. Am J Gastroenterol 1994;89:1920.
56. Baron S, Turck D, Leplat C, et al. Environmental risk factors in paediatric inflammatory bowel diseases: A population based case control study. Gut 2005;54:357–63.
57. Andersson RE, Olaison G, Tysk C, Ekbom A. Appendectomy and protection against ulcerative colitis. N Engl J Med 2001;344:808–14.
58. Qiu BS, Vallance BA, Blennerhassett PA, Collins SM. The role of CD4+ lymphocytes in the susceptibility of mice to stress-induced reactivation of experimental colitis. Nat Med 1999;5:1178–82.
59. Mawdsley JE, Macey MG, Feakins RM, et al. The effect of acute psychologic stress on systemic and rectal mucosal measures of inflammation in ulcerative colitis. Gastroenterology 2006;131:410–9.
60. Madretsma S, Wolters LM, van Dijk JP, et al. In-vivo effect of nicotine on cytokine production by human non-adherent mononuclear cells. Eur J Gastroenterol Hepatol 1996;8:1017–20.
61. Sandler RS, Sandler DP, McDonnell CW, Wurzelmann JI. Childhood exposure to environmental tobacco smoke and the risk of ulcerative colitis. Am J Epidemiol 1992;135:603–8.
62. Lashner BA, Shaheen NJ, Hanauer SB, Kirschner BS. Passive smoking is associated with an increased risk of developing inflammatory bowel disease in children. Am J Gastroenterol 1993;88:356–9.
63. Aspberg S, Dahlquist G, Kahan T, Kallen B. Fetal and perinatal risk factors for inflammatory bowel disease. Acta Paediatr 2006;95:1001–4.
64. McCartney SA, Mitchell JA, Fairclough PD, et al. Selective COX-2 inhibitors and human inflammatory bowel disease. Aliment Pharmacol Ther 1999;13:1115–7.
65. Bruzzese E, Canani RB, De MG, Guarino A. Microflora in inflammatory bowel diseases: A pediatric perspective. J Clin Gastroenterol 2004;38:S91–S93.
66. Kleessen B, Kroesen AJ, Buhr HJ, Blaut M. Mucosal and invading bacteria in patients with inflammatory bowel disease compared with controls. Scand J Gastroenterol 2002;37:1034–41.

67. Kruis W, Schutz E, Fric P, et al. Double-blind comparison of an oral *Escherichia coli* preparation and mesalazine in maintaining remission of ulcerative colitis. Aliment Pharmacol Ther 1997;11:853–8.

68. Rembacken BJ, Snelling AM, Hawkey PM, et al. Nonpathogenic *Escherichia coli* versus mesalazine for the treatment of ulcerative colitis: A randomised trial. Lancet 1999;354:635–9.

69. Venturi A, Gionchetti P, Rizzello F, et al. Impact on the composition of the faecal flora by a new probiotic preparation: Preliminary data on maintenance treatment of patients with ulcerative colitis. Aliment Pharmacol Ther 1999;13: 1103–8.

70. Gionchetti P, Rizzello F, Helwig U, et al. Prophylaxis of pouchitis onset with probiotic therapy: A double-blind, placebo-controlled trial. Gastroenterology 2003;124:1202–9.

71. Furrie E, Macfarlane S, Kennedy A, et al. Synbiotic therapy (Bifidobacterium longum/Synergy 1) initiates resolution of inflammation in patients with active ulcerative colitis: A randomised controlled pilot trial. Gut 2005;54:242–9.

72. Haskey N, Dahl WJ. Synbiotic therapy: A promising new adjunctive therapy for ulcerative colitis. Nutr Rev 2006;64:132–8.

73. Bouma G, Strober W. The immunological and genetic basis of inflammatory bowel disease. Nat Rev Immunol 2003;3:521–33.

74. Ehehalt R, Wagenblast J, Erben G, et al. Phosphatidylcholine and lysophosphatidylcholine in intestinal mucus of ulcerative colitis patients. A quantitative approach by nano-Electrospray-tandem mass spectrometry. Scand J Gastroenterol 2004;39:737–42.

75. Stremmel W, Merle U, Zahn A, et al. Retarded release phosphatidylcholine benefits patients with chronic active ulcerative colitis. Gut 2005;54:966–71.

76. Fahlgren A, Hammarstrom S, Danielsson A, Hammarstrom ML. Beta-Defensin-3 and -4 in intestinal epithelial cells display increased mRNA expression in ulcerative colitis. Clin Exp Immunol 2004;137:379–85.

77. Wehkamp J, Harder J, Weichenthal M, et al. Inducible and constitutive beta-defensins are differentially expressed in Crohn's disease and ulcerative colitis. Inflamm Bowel Dis 2003;9:215–23.

78. Shaoul R, Okada Y, Cutz E, et al. Colonic expression of MUC2, MUC5AC, and TFF1 in inflammatory bowel disease in children. J Pediatr Gastroenterol Nutr 2004;38:488–93.

79. Kyo K, Parkes M, Takei Y, et al. Association of ulcerative colitis with rare VNTR alleles of the human intestinal mucin gene, MUC3. Hum Mol Genet 1999;8:307–11.

80. Hermiston ML, Gordon JI. Inflammatory bowel disease and adenomas in mice expressing a dominant negative N-cadherin. Science 1995;270:1203–7.

81. Fuss IJ, Neurath M, Boirivant M, et al. Disparate CD4+ lamina propria (LP) lymphokine secretion profiles in inflammatory bowel disease. Crohn's disease LP cells manifest increased secretion of IFN-gamma, whereas ulcerative colitis LP cells manifest increased secretion of IL-5. J Immunol 1996;157:1261–70.

82. Fuss IJ, Heller F, Boirivant M, et al. Nonclassical CD1d-restricted NK T cells that produce IL-13 characterize an atypical Th2 response in ulcerative colitis. J Clin Invest 2004;113:1490–7.

83. Heller F, Florian P, Bojarski C, et al. Interleukin-13 is the key effector Th2 cytokine in ulcerative colitis that affects epithelial tight junctions, apoptosis, and cell restitution. Gastroenterology 2005;129:550–64.

84. Holmen N, Lundgren A, Lundin S, et al. Functional CD4+CD25 high regulatory T cells are enriched in the colonic mucosa of patients with active ulcerative colitis and increase with disease activity. Inflamm Bowel Dis 2006;12: 447–56.

85. Takahashi M, Nakamura K, Honda K, et al. An inverse correlation of human peripheral blood regulatory T cell frequency with the disease activity of ulcerative colitis. Dig Dis Sci 2006;51:677–86.

86. Niess JH, Reinecker HC. Dendritic cells: The commanders-in-chief of mucosal immune defenses. Curr Opin Gastroenterol 2006;22:354–60.

87. Monteleone G, Fina D, Caruso R, Pallone F. New mediators of immunity and inflammation in inflammatory bowel disease. Curr Opin Gastroenterol 2006;22:361–4.

88. Hatoum OA, Binion DG. The vasculature and inflammatory bowel disease: Contribution to pathogenesis and clinical pathology. Inflamm Bowel Dis 2005;11:304–13.

89. Thompson NP, Wakefield AJ, Pounder RE. Inherited disorders of coagulation appear to protect against inflammatory bowel disease. Gastroenterology 1995;108:1011–5.

90. Sawczenko A, Lynn R, Sandhu BK. Variations in initial assessment and management of inflammatory bowel disease across Great Britain and Ireland. Arch Dis Child 2003;88:990–4.

91. Truelove SC, Witts LJ. Cortisone in ulcerative colitis: Final report on a therapeutic trial. Br Med J 1955;2:1041–8.

92. Lichtiger S, Present DH, Kornbluth A, et al. Cyclosporine in severe ulcerative colitis refractory to steroid therapy. N Engl J Med 1994330:1841–5.

93. Seo M, Okada M, Yao T, et al. Evaluation of disease activity in patients with moderately active ulcerative colitis: Comparisons between a new activity index and Truelove and Witts' classification. Am J Gastroenterol 1995;90:1759–63.

94. Kugathasan S, Dubinsky MC, Keljo D, et al. Severe colitis in children. J Pediatr Gastroenterol Nutr 2005;41:375–85.

95. Hyams JS. Extraintestinal manifestations of inflammatory bowel disease in children. J Pediatr Gastroenterol Nutr 1994;19:7–21.

96. Passo MH, Fitzgerald JF, Brandt KD. Arthritis associated with inflammatory bowel disease in children. Relationship of joint disease to activity and severity of bowel lesion. Dig Dis Sci 1986;31:492–7.

97. Lindsley CB, Schaller JG. Arthritis associated with inflammatory bowel disease in children. J Pediatr 1974;84:16–20.

98. Wilschanski M, Chait P, Wade JA, et al. Primary sclerosing cholangitis in 32 children: Clinical, laboratory, and radiographic features, with survival analysis. Hepatology 1995;22:1415–22.

99. Sawczenko A, Sandhu BK, Sawczenko A, Sandhu BK. Presenting features of inflammatory bowel disease in Great Britain and Ireland. Arch Dis Child 2003;88:995–1000.

100. Orchard TR, Wordsworth BP, Jewell DP. Peripheral arthropathies in inflammatory bowel disease: Their articular distribution and natural history. Gut 1998;42:387–91.

101. Tavarela VF. Review article: skin complications associated with inflammatory bowel disease. Aliment Pharmacol Ther 2004;20:50–3.

102. Rychwalski PJ, Cruz OA, anis-Lambreton G, et al. Asymptomatic uveitis in young people with inflammatory bowel disease. J AAPOS 1997;1:111–4.

103. Hofley P, Roarty J, McGinnity G, et al. Asymptomatic uveitis in children with chronic inflammatory bowel diseases. J Pediatr Gastroenterol Nutr 1993;17:397–400.

104. Gregorio GV, Portmann B, Karani J, et al. Autoimmune hepatitis/sclerosing cholangitis overlap syndrome in childhood: A 16-year prospective study. Hepatology 2001;33:544–53.

105. Roberts EA. Primary sclerosing cholangitis in children. J Gastroenterol Hepatol 1999;14:588–93.

106. Beuers U, Spengler U, Kruis W, et al. Ursodeoxycholic acid for treatment of primary sclerosing cholangitis: A placebo-controlled trial. Hepatology 1992;16:707–14.

107. Broome U, Lofberg R, Veress B, Eriksson LS. Primary sclerosing cholangitis and ulcerative colitis: Evidence for increased neoplastic potential. Hepatology 1995;22:1404–8.

108. Loftus EV, Jr, Harewood GC, Loftus CG, et al. PSC-IBD: A unique form of inflammatory bowel disease associated with primary sclerosing cholangitis. Gut 2005;54:91–6.

109. Tung BY, Emond MJ, Haggitt RC, et al. Ursodiol use is associated with lower prevalence of colonic neoplasia in patients with ulcerative colitis and primary sclerosing cholangitis. Ann Intern Med 2001;134:89–95.

110. Bernstein CN, Blanchard JF, Houston DS, Wajda A. The incidence of deep venous thrombosis and pulmonary embolism among patients with inflammatory bowel disease: A population-based cohort study. Thromb Haemost 2001;85:430–4.

111. Miehsler W, Reinisch W, Valic E, et al. Is inflammatory bowel disease an independent and disease specific risk factor for thromboembolism? Gut 2004;53:542–8.

112. Boot AM, Bouquet J, Krenning EP, de Muinck Keizer-Schrama SM. Bone mineral density and nutritional status in children with chronic inflammatory bowel disease. Gut 1998;42:188–94.

113. Gokhale R, Favus MJ, Karrison T, et al. Bone mineral density assessment in children with inflammatory bowel disease. Gastroenterology 1998;114:902–11.

114. Gupta A, Paski S, Issenman R, et al. Lumbar spine bone mineral density at diagnosis and during follow-up in children with IBD. J Clin Densitom 2004;7:290–5.

115. Lennard-Jones JE, Ritchie JK, Hilder W, Spicer CC. Assessment of severity in colitis: A preliminary study. Gut 1975;16:579–84.

116. Sheth SG, LaMont JT. Toxic megacolon. Lancet 1998;351: 509–13.

117. Present DH. Toxic megacolon. Med Clin North Am 1993; 77:1129–48.

118. Travis SP, Farrant JM, Ricketts C, et al. Predicting outcome in severe ulcerative colitis. Gut 1996;38:905–10.

119. Eaden JA, Abrams KR, Mayberry JF. The risk of colorectal cancer in ulcerative colitis: A meta-analysis. Gut 2001;48:526–35.

120. Langholz E, Munkholm P, Davidsen M, Binder V. Colorectal cancer risk and mortality in patients with ulcerative colitis. Gastroenterology 1992;103:1444–51.

121. Soetikno RM, Lin OS, Heidenreich PA, et al. Increased risk of colorectal neoplasia in patients with primary sclerosing cholangitis and ulcerative colitis: A meta-analysis. Gastrointest Endosc 2002;56:48–54.

122. Nuako KW, Ahlquist DA, Mahoney DW, et al. Familial predisposition for colorectal cancer in chronic ulcerative colitis: A case-control study. Gastroenterology 1998;115:1079–83.

123. Heuschen UA, Hinz U, Allemeyer EH, et al. Backwash ileitis is strongly associated with colorectal carcinoma in ulcerative colitis. Gastroenterology 2001;120:841–7.

124. Rutter MD, Saunders BP, Wilkinson KH, et al. Cancer surveillance in longstanding ulcerative colitis: Endoscopic appearances help predict cancer risk. Gut 2004;53:1813–6.

125. Velayos FS, Loftus EV, Jr, Jess T, et al. Predictive and protective factors associated with colorectal cancer in ulcerative colitis: A case-control study. Gastroenterology 2006; 130:1941–9.

126. Eaden JA, Mayberry JF. Colorectal cancer complicating ulcerative colitis: A review. Am J Gastroenterol 2000;95: 2710–9.

127. Itzkowitz SH, Present DH. Consensus conference: Colorectal cancer screening and surveillance in inflammatory bowel disease. Inflamm Bowel Dis 2005;11:314–21.

128. Eaden JA, Mayberry JF. Guidelines for screening and surveillance of asymptomatic colorectal cancer in patients with inflammatory bowel disease. Gut 2002;51:V10–12.

129. Griffiths AM, Sherman PM. Colonoscopic surveillance for cancer in ulcerative colitis: A critical review. J Pediatr Gastroenterol Nutr 1997;24:202–10.

130. Collins PD, Mpofu C, Watson AJ, Rhodes JM. Strategies for detecting colon cancer and/or dysplasia in patients with inflammatory bowel disease. Cochrane Database Syst Rev 2006;CD000279.

131. Kornbluth A, Sachar DB. Ulcerative colitis practice guidelines in adults. American College of Gastroenterology, Practice Parameters Committee. Am J Gastroenterol 1997;92:204–11.

132. Rutter MD. What to do with dysplasias, DALMs, and adenomas. In: Irving P, Rampton D, Shanahan F, editors. Clinical Dilemmas in Inflammatory Bowel Disease. Blackwell; 2006. p. 189–92.

133. Eaden J, Abrams K, Ekbom A, et al. Colorectal cancer prevention in ulcerative colitis: A case-control study. Aliment Pharmacol Ther 2000;14:145–53.

134. Pinczowski D, Ekbom A, Baron J, et al. Risk factors for colorectal cancer in patients with ulcerative colitis: A case-control study. Gastroenterology 1994;107:117–20.

135. Pardi DS, Loftus EV, Jr, Kremers WK, et al. Ursodeoxycholic acid as a chemopreventive agent in patients with ulcerative colitis and primary sclerosing cholangitis. Gastroenterology 2003;124:889–93.

136. Beattie RM, Walker-Smith JA, Murch SH. Indications for investigation of chronic gastrointestinal symptoms. Arch Dis Child 1995;73:354–5.

137. Holmquist L, Ahren C, Fallstrom SP. Relationship between results of laboratory tests and inflammatory activity assessed by colonoscopy in children and adolescents with ulcerative colitis and Crohn's colitis. J Pediatr Gastroenterol Nutr 1989;9:187–93.

138. Trnka YM, LaMont JT. Association of *Clostridium difficile* toxin with symptomatic relapse of chronic inflammatory bowel disease. Gastroenterology 1981;80:693–6.

139. Markowitz JE, Brown KA, Mamula P, et al. Failure of single-toxin assays to detect *Clostridium difficile* infection in pediatric inflammatory bowel disease. Am J Gastroenterol 2001;96:2688–90.

140. Bunn SK, Bisset WM, Main MJ, Golden BE. Fecal calprotectin as a measure of disease activity in childhood inflammatory bowel disease. J Pediatr Gastroenterol Nutr 2001;32:171–7.

141. Bunn SK, Bisset WM, Main MJ, et al. Fecal calprotectin: Validation as a noninvasive measure of bowel inflammation in childhood inflammatory bowel disease. J Pediatr Gastroenterol Nutr 2001;33:14–22.

142. Berni CR, Rapacciuolo L, Romano MT, et al. Diagnostic value of faecal calprotectin in paediatric gastroenterology clinical practice. Dig Liver Dis 2004;36:467–70.

143. Ruemmele FM, Targan SR, Levy G, et al. Diagnostic accuracy of serological assays in pediatric inflammatory bowel disease. Gastroenterology 1998;115:822–9.

144. Duerr RH, Targan SR, Landers CJ, et al. Anti-neutrophil cytoplasmic antibodies in ulcerative colitis. Comparison with other colitides/diarrheal illnesses. Gastroenterology 1991;100:1590–6.

145. Winter HS, Landers CJ, Winkelstein A, et al. Anti-neutrophil cytoplasmic antibodies in children with ulcerative colitis. J Pediatr 1994;125:707–11.

146. Dubinsky MC, Ofman JJ, Urman M, et al. Clinical utility of serodiagnostic testing in suspected pediatric inflammatory bowel disease. Am J Gastroenterol 2001;96:758–65.

147. Khan K, Schwarzenberg SJ, Sharp H, et al. Role of serology and routine laboratory tests in childhood inflammatory bowel disease. Inflamm Bowel Dis 2002;8:325–9.

148. Price AB, Morson BC. Inflammatory bowel disease: The surgical pathology of Crohn's disease and ulcerative colitis. Hum Pathol 1975;6:7–29.

149. D'Haens G, Geboes K, Peeters M, et al. Patchy cecal inflammation associated with distal ulcerative colitis: A prospective endoscopic study. Am J Gastroenterol 1997;92:1275–9.

150. Hyams JS, Davis P, Grancher K, et al. Clinical outcome of ulcerative colitis in children. J Pediatr 1996;129:81–8.

151. Tobin JM, Sinha B, Ramani P, et al. Upper gastrointestinal mucosal disease in pediatric Crohn disease and ulcerative colitis: A blinded, controlled study. J Pediatr Gastroenterol Nutr 2001;32:443–8.

152. Jenkins D, Balsitis M, Gallivan S, et al. Guidelines for the initial biopsy diagnosis of suspected chronic idiopathic inflammatory bowel disease. The British Society of Gastroenterology Initiative. J Clin Pathol 1997;50:93–105.

153. Geboes K, de HG. Indeterminate colitis. Inflamm Bowel Dis 2003;9:324–31.

154. Yantiss RK, Odze RD. Diagnostic difficulties in inflammatory bowel disease pathology. Histopathology 2006;48:116–32.

155. Glickman JN, Bousvaros A, Farraye FA, et al. Pediatric patients with untreated ulcerative colitis may present initially with unusual morphologic findings. Am J Surg Pathol 2004;28:190–7.

156. Markowitz J, Kahn E, Grancher K, et al. Atypical rectosigmoid histology in children with newly diagnosed ulcerative colitis. Am J Gastroenterol 1993;88:2034–7.

157. Robert ME, Tang L, Hao LM, et al. Patterns of inflammation in mucosal biopsies of ulcerative colitis: Perceived differences in pediatric populations are limited to children younger than 10 years. Am J Surg Pathol 2004;28:183–9.

158. Geboes K, Dalle I. Influence of treatment on morphological features of mucosal inflammation. Gut 2002;50:III37–42.

159. Maconi G, Imbesi V, Bianchi PG. Doppler ultrasound measurement of intestinal blood flow in inflammatory bowel disease. Scand J Gastroenterol 1996;31:590–3.

160. Kalantzis N, Rouvella P, Tarazis S, et al. Doppler US of superior mesenteric artery in the assessment of ulcerative colitis. A prospective study. Hepatogastroenterology 2002;49:168–71.

161. Alberini JL, Badran A, Freneaux E, et al. Technetium-99m HMPAO-labeled leukocyte imaging compared with endoscopy, ultrasonography, and contrast radiology in children with inflammatory bowel disease. J Pediatr Gastroenterol Nutr 2001;32:278–86.

162. Loftus EV, Jr, Kane SV, Bjorkman D. Systematic review: Short-term adverse effects of 5-aminosalicylic acid agents in the treatment of ulcerative colitis. Aliment Pharmacol Ther 2004;19:179–89.

163. Ransford RA, Langman MJ. Sulphasalazine and mesalazine: serious adverse reactions re-evaluated on the basis of suspected adverse reaction reports to the Committee on Safety of Medicines. Gut 2002;51:536–9.

164. Van Staa TP, Travis S, Leufkens HG, Logan RF. 5-Aminosalicylic acids and the risk of renal disease: A large British epidemiologic study. Gastroenterology 2004;126:1733–9.

165. Sutherland L, MacDonald JK. Oral 5-aminosalicylic acid for induction of remission in ulcerative colitis. Cochrane Database Syst Rev 2003:CD000543.

166. Escher JC, Taminiau JA, Nieuwenhuis EE, et al. Treatment of inflammatory bowel disease in childhood: Best available evidence. Inflamm Bowel Dis 2003;9:34–58.

167. Carter MJ, Lobo AJ, Travis SP. Guidelines for the management of inflammatory bowel disease in adults. Gut 2004;53:V1–16.

168. Sutherland L, Roth D, Beck P, et al. Oral 5-aminosalicylic acid for maintenance of remission in ulcerative colitis. Cochrane Database Syst Rev 2002:CD000544.

169. Beattie RM, Croft NM, Fell JM, et al. Inflammatory bowel disease. Arch Dis Child 2006;91:426–32.

170. Lichtenstein GR, Abreu MT, Cohen R, Tremaine W. American Gastroenterological Association Institute technical review on corticosteroids, immunomodulators, and infliximab in inflammatory bowel disease. Gastroenterology 2006;130:940–87.

171. Baron JH, Connell AM, Kanaghinis TG, et al. Out-patient treatment of ulcerative colitis. Comparison between three doses of oral prednisone. Br Med J 1962;5302:441–3.

172. Markowitz J, Grancher K, Kohn N, Daum F. Immunomodulatory therapy for pediatric inflammatory bowel disease: Changing patterns of use, 1990–2000. Am J Gastroenterol 2002;97:928–32.

173. Verhave M, Winter HS, Grand RJ. Azathioprine in the treatment of children with inflammatory bowel disease. J Pediatr 1990;117:809–14.

174. Markowitz J, Grancher K, Mandel F, Daum F. Immunosuppressive therapy in pediatric inflammatory bowel disease: Results of a survey of the North American Society for Pediatric Gastroenterology and Nutrition. Subcommittee on Immunosuppressive Use of the Pediatric IBD Collaborative Research Forum. Am J Gastroenterol 1993;88:44–8.

175. Kirschner BS. Safety of azathioprine and 6-mercaptopurine in pediatric patients with inflammatory bowel disease. Gastroenterology 1998;115:813–21.

176. Dubinsky MC. Azathioprine, 6-mercaptopurine in inflammatory bowel disease: Pharmacology, efficacy, and safety. Clin Gastroenterol Hepatol 2004;2:731–43.

177. Hande S, Wilson-Rich N, Bousvaros A, et al. 5-Aminosalicylate therapy is associated with higher 6-thioguanine levels in adults and children with inflammatory bowel disease in remission on 6-mercaptopurine or azathioprine. Inflamm Bowel Dis 2006;12:251–7.

178. Kandiel A, Fraser AG, Korelitz BI, et al. Increased risk of lymphoma among inflammatory bowel disease patients treated with azathioprine and 6-mercaptopurine. Gut 2005;54:1121–5.

179. Dayharsh GA, Loftus EV, Jr, Sandborn WJ, et al. Epstein-Barr virus-positive lymphoma in patients with inflammatory bowel disease treated with azathioprine or 6-mercaptopurine. Gastroenterology 2002;122:72–7.

180. Korelitz BI, Mirsky FJ, Fleisher MR, et al. Malignant neoplasms subsequent to treatment of inflammatory bowel disease with 6-mercaptopurine. Am J Gastroenterol 1999;94:3248–53.

181. Ho S, Clipstone N, Timmermann L, et al. The mechanism of action of cyclosporin A and FK506. Clin Immunol Immunopathol 1996;80:S40–S45.

182. Treem WR, Cohen J, Davis PM, et al. Cyclosporine for the treatment of fulminant ulcerative colitis in children. Immediate response, long-term results, and impact on surgery. Dis Colon Rectum 1995;38:474–9.

183. Ramakrishna J, Langhans N, Calenda K, et al. Combined use of cyclosporine and azathioprine or 6-mercaptopurine in pediatric inflammatory bowel disease. J Pediatr Gastroenterol Nutr 1996;22:296–302.

184. Shibolet O, Regushevskaya E, Brezis M, Soares-Weiser K. Cyclosporine A for induction of remission in severe ulcerative colitis. Cochrane Database Syst Rev 2005:CD004277.

185. Bousvaros A, Kirschner BS, Werlin SL, et al. Oral tacrolimus treatment of severe colitis in children. J Pediatr 2000;137:794–9.

186. Perencevich M, Burakoff R. Use of antibiotics in the treatment of inflammatory bowel disease. Inflamm Bowel Dis 2006;12:651–64.

187. Rutgeerts P, Sandborn WJ, Feagan BG, et al. Infliximab for induction and maintenance therapy for ulcerative colitis. N Engl J Med 2005;353:2462–76.

188. Mamula P, Markowitz JE, Cohen LJ, et al. Infliximab in pediatric ulcerative colitis: Two-year follow-up. J Pediatr Gastroenterol Nutr 2004;38:298–301.

189. Russell GH, Katz AJ. Infliximab is effective in acute but not chronic childhood ulcerative colitis. J Pediatr Gastroenterol Nutr 2004;39:166–70.

190. Eidelwein AP, Cuffari C, Abadom V, et al. Infliximab efficacy in pediatric ulcerative colitis. Inflamm Bowel Dis 2005;11:213–8.

191. Sandborn WJ, Faubion WA. Biologics in inflammatory bowel disease: How much progress have we made? Gut 2004;53:1366–73.

192. Schwarzer A, Ricciardelli I, Kirkham S, et al. Management of fulminating ulcerative colitis in childhood with chimeric anti-CD25 antibody. J Pediatr Gastroenterol Nutr 2006;42:245–8.

193. Tomomasa T, Kobayashi A, Kaneko H, et al. Granulocyte adsorptive apheresis for pediatric patients with ulcerative colitis. Dig Dis Sci 2003;48:750–4.

194. Summers RW, Elliott DE, Urban JF, Jr, et al. *Trichuris suis* therapy for active ulcerative colitis: A randomized controlled trial. Gastroenterology 2005;128:825–32.

195. Langmead L, Feakins RM, Goldthorpe S, et al. Randomized, double-blind, placebo-controlled trial of oral aloe vera gel for active ulcerative colitis. Aliment Pharmacol Ther 2004;19:739–47.

196. Croft NM. Phospholipid in UC: Novel, safe and works is it too good to be true? Gastroenterology 2006;130:1003–4.

197. Wewer V, Hesselfeldt P, Qvist N, et al. J-pouch ileoanal anastomosis in children and adolescents with ulcerative colitis: Functional outcome, satisfaction and impact on social life. J Pediatr Gastroenterol Nutr 2005;40:189–93.

198. Rintala RJ, Lindahl HG. Proctocolectomy and J-pouch ileo-anal anastomosis in children. J Pediatr Surg 2002;37:66–70.

199. Nicholls S, Vieira MC, Majrowski WH, et al. Linear growth after colectomy for ulcerative colitis in childhood. J Pediatr Gastroenterol Nutr 1995;21:82–6.

200. Lindberg E, Lindquist B, Holmquist L, Hildebrand H. Inflammatory bowel disease in children and adolescents in Sweden, 1984–1995. J Pediatr Gastroenterol Nutr 2000;30:259–64.

201. Michener WM, Farmer RG, Mortimer EA. Long-term prognosis of ulcerative colitis with onset in childhood or adolescence. J Clin Gastroenterol 1979;1:301–5.

202. Ba'ath ME, Mahmalat M, Smith NP, et al. Surgical management of inflammatory bowel disease. Arch Dis Child 2006;92:312–6.

203. Alexander F, Sarigol S, DiFiore J, et al. Fate of the pouch in 151 pediatric patients after ileal pouch anal anastomosis. J Pediatr Surg 2003;38:78–82.

204. Durno C, Sherman P, Harris K, et al. Outcome after ileoanal anastomosis in pediatric patients with ulcerative colitis. J Pediatr Gastroenterol Nutr 1998;27:501–7.

205. Rintala RJ, Lindahl H. Restorative proctocolectomy for ulcerative colitis in children is the J-pouch better than straight pull-through? J Pediatr Surg 1996;31:530–3.

206. Sandborn WJ. Pouchitis following ileal pouch-anal anastomosis: Definition, pathogenesis, and treatment. Gastroenterology 1994;107:1856–60.

207. Langholz E, Munkholm P, Krasilnikoff PA, Binder V. Inflammatory bowel diseases with onset in childhood. Clinical features, morbidity, and mortality in a regional cohort. Scand J Gastroenterol 1997;32:139–47.

208. Hyams J, Davis P, Lerer T, et al. Clinical outcome of ulcerative proctitis in children. J Pediatr Gastroenterol Nutr 1997;25:149–52.

209. Langholz E, Munkholm P, Davidsen M, et al. Changes in extent of ulcerative colitis: A study on the course and prognostic factors. Scand J Gastroenterol 1996;31:260–6.

210. Meucci G, Bortoli A, Riccioli FA, et al. Frequency and clinical evolution of indeterminate colitis: A retrospective multi-centre study in northern Italy. GSMII (Gruppo di Studio per le Malattie Infiammatorie Intestinali). Eur J Gastroenterol Hepatol 1999;11:909–13.

211. Burakoff R. Indeterminate colitis: Clinical spectrum of disease. J Clin Gastroenterol 2004;38:S41–S43.

212. Werlin SL, Grand RJ. Severe colitis in children and adolescents: Diagnosis. Course, and treatment. Gastroenterology 1977;73:828–32.

213. Leichtner AM, Higuchi S. Ulcerative colitis. In: Walker WA, Goulet O, Kleinman RE, Sherman PM, Shneider BL, Sanderson IR, editors. Pediatric Gastrointestinal Disease. Hamilton: BC Decker Inc; 2004. p. 825–49.

20.5c. Atypical Colitis and Other Inflammatory Diseases

Barbara S. Kirschner, MD, FAAP
Ranjana Gokhale, MD

This chapter describes three inflammatory disorders that are distinguishable from the chronic inflammatory bowel diseases, ulcerative colitis, Crohn's disease, and indeterminate colitis (see Chapter 20.5a, "Crohn's Disease" and Chapter 20.5b, "Ulcerative and Indeterminate Colitis"): hemolytic uremic syndrome (HUS), Henoch-Schonlein purpura (HSP), and Behcet syndrome (BS).

HEMOLYTIC UREMIC SYNDROME

HUS, first described by Gasser and colleagues in 1955, is defined as the development of microangiopathic hemolytic anemia, thrombocytopenia, and renal insufficiency in a previously healthy person.[1] It is the most common cause of acute renal failure in children. Incomplete HUS consists of acute renal failure with either hemolytic anemia or thrombocytopenia as well as *Escherichia coli* (*E. coli*) O157:H7 diarrhea with hemolytic anemia and thrombocytopenia but without renal injury. There are two major subgroups of HUS: typical HUS which generally follows an acute diarrheal illness (D+HUS) and atypical HUS which is not associated with diarrhea (D−HUS). D−HUS may be familial or sporadic and is often associated with genetic mutations in complement regulatory proteins, von Willebrand factor-cleaving protease (ADAMTS 13), infections with *Streptococcus pneumoniae*, bone marrow and renal transplantation, and chemotherapeutic agents. The two forms of HUS vary not only in etiology but age at diagnosis, risk for recurrence, and likelihood of end-stage renal disease. A prodrome of gastrointestinal (GI) symptoms averaging 3 to 16 days precedes the development of the HUS in 90 to 100% of children.[2–4]

Epidemiology

Typical Diarrhea-Associated HUS (D+HUS). Characteristically, D+HUS occurs in children less than 5 years of age.[2–4] It is endemic in Argentina, southern Africa, and the western United States, and epidemics have occurred in many other parts of the world. Between 1971 and 1980, Tarr and Hickman observed a fourfold increase in incidence in King County, Washington, from 0.63 to 2.81 cases per 100,000 children younger than 15 years.[3]

D+HUS is an infrequent sequela of *E. coli* O157:H7 infections. A report describing 350 outbreaks involving 8,598 cases noted that hospitalization occurred in 17%, HUS in 4%, and death in 0.5% of patients.[5] The routes of transmission were following: food-borne 52% (41% ground beef and 21% produce), unknown 21%, person-to-person 14%, waterborne 9%, animal contact 3%, and laboratory-related 0.3%. Neonatal presentation was reported in a day-old infant whose stool from the baby and mother were both positive for Shiga-like toxin 2.[6]

A 4-year follow-up evaluation of 951 children with acute *E. Coli* O157:H7 diarrhea showed no difference in the development of hypertension, reduced glomerular filtration rate, albumin to creatinine ratio, or microalbuminuria between asymptomatic and moderate to severely affected children. The authors recommended that only children who develop features of HUS require long-term monitoring.[7]

The epidemic form of D+HUS, occurs in the summer, is associated with the abrupt onset of diarrhea, and has a good prognosis, with an expected mortality under 6%.[2,3] A sporadic form in older children has neither seasonal influence nor obvious prodrome and has a higher mortality.[8] It is the opinion of this author that earlier reports describing siblings who developed HUS during infancy and showed a high mortality rate (68%) were probably not D+HUS but more likely had an unrecognized genetic disorder making them susceptible to D−HUS.[9–11]

Most cases of D+HUS described in the Pacific Northwest (58%) were preceded by enteric infection with Shiga toxin–producing *E. coli* (STEC) O157:H7[12]. This *E. coli* serotype has a distinct cell membrane adhesion molecule, intimin, which attaches to follicle-associated epithelium of ileal Peyer patches.[13] Over a 2-year period, the organism was isolated from the stools of nine patients with HUS in British Columbia's Children's Hospital, an incidence far in excess of the incidence in all stools submitted for routine diagnosis (1.9%).[14] In a national prospective study of postdiarrheal HUS in the United States, 80% of patients had serum samples positive for *E. coli* O157 lipopolysaccharide antibody titers.[15] This O157:H7 serotype was originally described as a cause of hemorrhagic colitis.[16] Subsequently, isolated cases of HUS were reported following outbreaks of gastroenteritis (both bloody and nonbloody) with *E. coli* O157:H7.[12,17] Among children presenting with STEC diarrhea, HUS developed in 18% of children with *E. coli* O157:H7 but none of those with the non-O157:H7 serotype.[18] Isolates of this serotype produce a toxin cytotoxic for Vero and HeLa cells in tissue culture (verocytotoxin).[14] Dissemination of *E. coli* O157:H7 has been reported to occur through contaminated food such as undercooked hamburger, unpasteurized milk, yogurt and gouda cheese, unpasteurized apple cider, and vegetables, such as raw alfalfa and radish sprouts (grown in a garden fertilized with cow manure), contaminated municipal water supplies, a recreational lake and person-to-person spread in a day-care center.[2,12,19] More recently, reports of HUS have followed trips to dairy farms (where 13% of the calves were colonized with *E. coli* O157:H7) and petting zoos (where O157 was isolated from goats and sheep).[20,21] Handwashing was protective. Thus, *E. coli* O157:H7 appears to cause a spectrum of disease, including diarrhea, hemorrhagic colitis, and HUS. The factors that determine which disease entity develops in an individual child are unknown, but environmental and genetic influences are suggested.

Non-O157:H7 STEC strains appear to account for a larger number of cases of HUS in children in Europe than in the United States. Of 394 children studied in Germany and Austria, strain frequencies were O111 43%, O26 15%, O145 9%, and O193 3%.[22] Patients with O157:H7 had bloody diarrhea more frequently and required dialysis for a longer time than non-O157:H7 patients. The authors emphasized the rising importance of recognizing non-O157:H7 serotypes in HUS. Similar findings were noted in an Australian population of 98 children with HUS.[23] Serotype O111:H- was the most common isolate, and none had O157:H7. Enteric infections with various non–*E. coli* organisms, including *Shigella*, *Salmonella*, *Campylobacter*, *Yersinia*, and enteroviruses, have also been associated with the development of HUS.[2,24]

Atypical Nondiarrhea-Associated HUS (D−HUS). Recent genetic studies have shown that mutations in complement regulatory proteins predispose patients to non-Shiga toxin-associated HUS.[25] Mutation frequencies were following: complement factor H (FH) 30.1%, membrane cofactor protein (MCP) 12.8%, and factor I (IF) 4.5%. These proteins are all involved in the regulation of the same enzyme in the alternate complement pathway, complement C3bBb convertase.[26] The mutated proteins show very low binding to surface-bound C3b thus reducing protection of red blood cells, platelets, and renal endothelium to complement activation.[27] This results in frequent recurrences of HUS often leading to renal failure. Caprioli and colleagues noted that patients with FH mutations had earlier onset of disease, higher mortality, and more failed kidney transplants than D−HUS patients without identifiable mutations.[28] Interestingly, FH mutations were both familial and sporadic D−HUS while MCP was limited to familial, and IF limited to sporadic cases.[29]

An analysis of 34 children with D−HUS was described by the British Association for Pediatric Nephrology.[30] Of the 34, 10 presented in infancy (5 with complement abnormalities, 2 following pneumococcal infections, and 2 with malignancies). There was a 2:1 excess of males and consanguinity was noted in 6 patients. The outcomes were poor: 5 died, 19 developed chronic renal failure or end-stage renal failure, and only 7 made a full recovery.

The association of D−HUS with invasive *S. pneumoniae* infections was reported in seven children, mean age 16 months, who developed HUS after pneumonia (five patients) or meningitis (two patients).[31] These children represented 23% of all HUS cases seen in Atlanta, Georgia, between 1994 and 1996. In contrast to D+HUS, which occurred between June and August, the *S. pneumoniae* HUS cases were seen year round. All seven patients required dialysis, compared with 48% of the D+HUS. This difference was not attributed to pneumococcal septic shock and disseminated intravascular coagulation because D-dimers and prothrombin time were not elevated and fibrinogen was not decreased. The authors reiterated the position of the Academy of Pediatrics that vancomycin be included in the therapy of suspected or proven invasive *S. pneumoniae* infections. A study comparing invasive pneumococcal D−HUS with D+HUS noted that the former patients were younger (22.1 vs 49 months), were more likely to require dialysis (75 vs 59%), had longer duration of hospitalization (32.2 vs 16.1 days), and needed more platelet transfusions (83 vs 47%), and red blood cell transfusions (7.8 vs 2.0).[32] Other nondiarrheal infectious agents associated with HUS are *Bordetella pertussis* and *Coxiella burnetii* (Q fever).

D−HUS has also been reported following bone marrow and renal transplantation in children. Among 293 children undergoing allogeneic bone marrow transplantation at St. Jude's Hospital, 28 (9.6%) developed HUS at a median of 171 days after transplantation.[33] Use of antithymocyte globulin and recipient CMV negativity were associated with increased risk. De novo HUS after renal transplantation has been associated with calcineuron inhibitor drugs.[34] Although most cases were associated with cyclosporine therapy, it has been suggested that tacrolimus may also induce HUS.[35] Chemotherapeutic agents including mitomycin, cisplatin, bleomycin, and gemcitabine have also been associated with the development of D−HUS.[36]

Pathogenesis

The central lesion in HUS is vascular endothelial damage. Endothelial cells show swelling and separate from the basement membrane with widening of the subendothelial space.[37] Glomerular involvement occurs in the classic form in young children, whereas arteriolar lesions with intimal and subintimal edema, proliferation, and necrosis are more common in older children.[8,37]

The precipitating cause of this vascular injury is probably the release of Shiga-like toxins (SLT-1, SLT-2, and SLT-2 variants), also called verotoxins, which damage the microvasculature of the intestinal wall, leading to hemorrhagic and ulcerative lesions.[2,16] The B subunits of the SLTs bind to high-affinity glycolipid (GB3) cell surface receptors on target organs and are internalized by endocytosis.[2] The verotoxins produced by *E. coli* O157:H7 thus cause endothelial damage and gain entrance to the circulation, leading to severe cell injury or death.[12,14,16–17] Lipopolysaccharide can also damage endothelial cells and promote thrombosis. Shiga-like toxin also induces TNF production in the kidney but not in other tissues. Proulx and colleagues observed increased circulating pro and anti-inflammatory cytokines (IL-6, IL-8, IL-10, and IL-1Ra) in children who developed HUS in contrast to normal controls and children with non−verotoxin-associated hemorrhagic colitis.[38]

In pneumococcus-induced HUS, the Thomsen-Freidenreich antigen (T antigen) present on erythrocytes, platelets, and glomerular endothelium is exposed, to which antibodies normally found in serum bind resulting in antigen−antibody activation.[39] The vascular injury induces microangiopathic hemolytic anemia, thrombocytopenia, and local deposits of fibrin microthrombi. Ischemic changes result in focal or generalized renal cortical necrosis and damage to other organs (colon, liver, myocardium, brain, pancreas, and adrenal glands).[2,37,40]

An important new area in understanding HUS concerns the role of mutations in complement regulatory proteins. This topic is discussed below in the section, "Genetic."

Genetic Aspects

Approximately 50% of patients with D−HUS have mutations in one of the complement regulatory proteins: factor H, membrane cofactor protein (MCP) or factor I. Normally, these proteins inactivate C3b by protelytic cleavage. In the case of D−HUS, the mutated proteins allow inappropriate complement activation.[41] Recent studies have identified a subset of patients with atypical HUS who have mutations in the gene coding for the soluble complement regulator factor H gene (FH1).[42] In a German series of 111 patients with atypical HUS, 14% had FH1 mutations.[43] The mutant proteins cause reduced binding of the central component C3b/C3d to heparin and endothelial cells, leading to progression of endothelial cell and microvascular damage.[44] Other mutations of the human complement regulator membrane cofactor protein were found in three families with multiple affected individuals with HUS.[45] The mutations were also associated with reduced C3b binding and diminished ability to prevent complement activation.

Clinical Manifestations

Gastrointestinal lesions occur in 90 to 100% of children with HUS. In 70 to 80%, bloody diarrhea precedes the recognition of HUS by 3 to 16 days; (2–4) other children have a prodrome of abdominal pain, nonbloody diarrhea, and/or vomiting. Resolution of the GI symptoms usually begins before the onset of renal insufficiency, with hematochezia clearing first, followed by improvement in the diarrhea and abdominal pain. However, the colitis may persist for as long as 2 months.[2] Rectal prolapse has been described in up to 10% of patients with colitis.[2] Occasionally, patients have thrombosis of vessels in the muscularis and serosa, resulting in necrosis and perforation of the colon.[46]

The endoscopic appearance of the bowel is characterized by hyperemia, edema, and petechiae, sometimes in association with ulceration.[46–47] The gross appearance may be indistinguishable from that of chronic nonspecific ulcerative colitis, but rectal biopsies in these children show only edema and submucosal hemorrhage with scant inflammation.[47] In a series of eight patients who underwent colectomy for HUS, the findings were limited to the transverse and left colon in seven, with only one patient showing involvement of the right colon.[48]

Barium enema examinations may demonstrate focal or diffuse bowel wall edema, thumbprinting, filling defects, mucosal irregularity, fine marginal spiculations, colonic spasm, or colonic dilatation (Figure 1).[45,46] Initially, the findings may mimic chronic inflammatory bowel disease until the full syndrome becomes apparent. Late complications may include colonic stricture.[49]

Hemolytic Anemia. Microangiopathic hemolytic anemia with fragmented erythrocytes occurs in all children with HUS. It usually develops suddenly within 1 to 2 days, resulting in a mean hemoglobin concentration of 6.1 g/d.[4] Several mechanisms are responsible for the anemia, including mechanical stress owing to microvascular disease, oxidative injury to red blood cells, and direct Shiga-like toxin injury.[2] Transfusions are required in 64% of children.[4] If the T antigen is detected, then washing all blood products is recommended.[50]

Thrombocytopenia. Thrombocytopenia (platelet count under 150,000/mm^3) occurs in 92% of children with HUS owing to platelet trapping within organs. As mentioned above, platelet aggregation defects may occur in the presence of normal platelet counts. Other tests of coagulation status, including prothrombin time and partial thromboplastin time, are normal.[2,4,37]

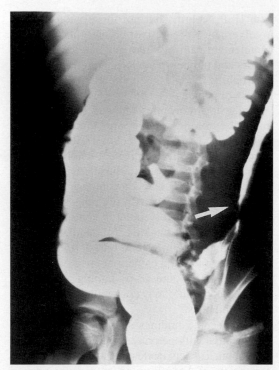

Figure 1 Barium enema in a 6-year-old child with hemolytic uremic syndrome. Extensive spasm and narrowing of the descending colon (*arrow*) are illustrated during the period of bloody diarrhea. Gastrointestinal symptoms resolved 1 week later but were followed by the onset of acute renal failure.

Renal Insufficiency. Although all children with HUS are azotemic (mean peak blood urea nitrogen of 95 mg/dL), the severity of the renal impairment is variable. Oliguria (less than 15 mL urine per kg body weight per day) and anuria (less than 25 mL urine per day) each occur in 32% of affected children.[4] In approximately 50% of cases, the anuria lasts for up to 3 days, but oliguria may persist for weeks. Among children with HUS in the Canadian Pediatric Surveillance Program, 34% required dialysis for a median of 12 days.[51] One-third of children have no documented oliguria. Hypertension, which is mild, begins early in the course of the illness in most patients, is usually labile, and is easily controlled.[2] However, some children may require peritoneal dialysis. The time for creatinine clearance to return to normal averages 3.7 months and corresponds to the duration of the preceding oliguria. Chronic renal insufficiency persists in approximately 9.5% of children.[4]

Neurologic Disease. Central nervous system (CNS) manifestations of HUS (changes in consciousness and abnormal movements, tone, and posture) are found in one-third of children usually during the acute phase of HUS.[2] The frequency of seizures has decreased with careful attention to fluid and electrolyte balance and implementation of dialysis. Serious CNS complications, such as cerebral edema or infarct leading to stroke, which are reported in up to 5% of children, may be fatal.[2]

Liver Disease. Elevations of hepatic enzymes (2- to 20-fold above normal) for serum glutamic

oxaloacetic transaminase, serum glutamic pyruvic transaminase, γ-glutamyl transpeptidase, alkaline phosphatase, and 5-nucleotidase have been observed in most patients in whom these tests were done.[46,52] This transient hepatocellular injury may be caused by focal hepatic hypoxia.

Pancreatic manifestations may manifest as pancreatitis, transient hyperglycemia, or diabetes mellitus. Elevated serum amylase and lipase levels are observed in about 20% of patients and hyperglycemia in 4 to 15%.[2] Diabetes develops in approximately 3.2% of children with D+HUS.[53] It occurs more frequently in those with severe disease (coma, seizures, or need for dialysis) and is associated with 23% mortality. Recurrence may occur up to 60 months after initial recovery so that long-term monitoring is recommended.

Myocardial dysfunction may be demonstrable to echocardiography. In this case, serum troponin I may be elevated consistent with myocardial injury.[53]

Death in children with HUS during the acute phase is most often due to CNS complications.[54] Predictive factors on admission include prodromal lethargy, oliguria or seizures, WBC >20,000 or hematocrit <23%.[55] Mortality was 4% among children listed in the Canadian Pediatric Surveillance Program.[51]

Diagnosis

HUS in childhood usually occurs in a previously healthy child who develops diarrhea (generally bloody) and abdominal pain followed by the acute onset of hemolytic anemia, thrombocytopenia, and renal insufficiency. Initially, the GI manifestations may be mimicked by intussusception, enteric infection, or inflammatory bowel disease (especially ulcerative colitis), which can be excluded by appropriate radiologic, microbiologic, and histologic studies. Typical hematologic and renal findings are discussed above.

Stool specimens should be obtained for enteric pathogens, including *E. coli* O157:H7. This serotype metabolizes sorbitol slowly; therefore, *E. coli* strains with this characteristic can be sent to specialized laboratories for confirmation. Positive results vary from 59% in Argentina to 94% of children in Montreal.[51,56] However, the yield is low if specimens are sent after the first week of diarrhrea.[2] The deoxyribonucleic acid (DNA) probes for genes associated with toxin production and polymerase chain reaction methods are being evaluated.[2]

For D−HUS, antigenic screening for factor H and factor I deficiency and detecting low levels of MCP expression by flow cytometry have been described.[41] At least 17 FH mutations have been identified in patients with D−HUS.[28] The strongest polymorphisms were 257T, 2089G, and 2881T.

Treatment

Severe GI symptoms require hospitalization and intravenous fluids during the prodromal period

prior to the development of HUS. Because *E. coli* O157:H7 is sensitive to ampicillin and amoxicillin, in the past some authors suggest treating all cases with one of these antibiotics.[14] Butler and colleagues observed that the administration of ampicillin to children with ampicillin-resistant strains of *Shigella* dysenteriae 1 was associated with a greater incidence of HUS than occurred in nonantibiotic-treated children infected with the same organism.[57] They also postulated that the risk of HUS might be reduced if children were treated early with appropriate antibiotics. Tarr and colleagues cautioned against the empiric use of antibiotics for *E. coli* O157:H7 colitis until the risks and benefits have been analyzed by controlled clinical trials.[58] These authors expressed concern that the incidence of HUS might be increased through proliferation of *E. coli* O157:H7 or the release of cytotoxins through bacterial lysis or "sublethal damage." In a prospective study of 71 children under 10 years of age with *E. coli* O157:H7 diarrhea, Wong and colleagues observed that antibiotic treatment conferred a relative risk of 14.3 when compared with children who had not received antibiotic therapy.[59] It should be noted that a meta-analysis of nine studies of whether antibiotic use increased the risk of HUS did not detect greater risk.[60] Rarely, surgical intervention may be necessitated by bowel necrosis.[46]

Primary attention should be directed toward management of fluid and electrolyte balance, renal insufficiency, hypertension, seizures, and hemolytic anemia. Siegler recommends that after correcting for necessary previous losses, fluids should be limited to ongoing loss (insensible water loss plus urine and GI output).[2] Sodium should be withheld from children with edema and hyponatremia. Similarly, potassium should not be given unless levels fall into the low normal range. Nutrition is important in these catabolic, hypoalbuminemic patients. For children with ongoing diarrhea or vomiting, transpyloric feeds or total parenteral nutrition (TPN) may be required. Peritoneal dialysis is employed as necessary in infants and preschool age children except if there is severe colitis or abdominal tenderness.[2,4,59] There is no direct evidence that anticoagulant therapy is beneficial.[9,61]

For children with severe anemia (hematocrit <15%) or those symptomatic from anemia, packed red blood cell transfusions (10 mL/kg) can be given. Those with pneumococcus-related HUS should receive blood products free of T-antigen antibody.[2] Siegler cautions against the use of platelet infusions, except for severe bleeding or those requiring invasive vascular procedures (such as TPN line placement) or surgery because exogenous platelets may provide further substrate for aggregation and microthrombus formation.[2]

Plasma transfusions, plasmapheresis (PE), or exchange transfusion has been reported to improve the anemia, thrombocytopenia, and renal insufficiency in some children with HUS and may be considered in patients demonstrating a poor response to supportive therapy.[61–64] Theoretically these modalities could remove the defective proteins associated with complement regulation in D−HUS. In a report of identical twins with D+HUS, one received PE followed by fresh frozen plasma infusions and developed renal failure. The second was subsequently treated with extended PE and has normal renal function, suggesting a possible benefit for long-term PE.[65] An anecdotal report using monoclonal antibody against the CD20 antigen (Rituximab) was beneficial in one patient with severe relapsed HUS.[66] Intravenous gammaglobulin administered to nine children did not demonstrate benefit on the duration of hemorrhagic colitis, anuria, or hospitalization when compared with nine children with HUS who did not receive this form of therapy.[67]

Hypertension usually responds to short-acting calcium channel blockers (such as nifedipine or nicardipine). Siegler recommends using either nifedipine at 0.25 to 0.5 mg/kg/dose as needed every 2 to 6 hours or nicardipine 0.5 to 1.0 mg/kg/dose every 6 to 8 hours as needed. Nicardipine can also be administered as a constant intravenous infusion of 1.0 µg/kg/min[2]. The use of dialysis has been responsible for the reduced mortality in HUS. Siegler recommends that dialysis be instituted for severe uncontrollable hyperkalemia, fluid overload associated with pulmonary edema, or severe uremic symptoms such as encephalopathy.[2] Other indications are a blood urea nitrogen over 150 mg/dL, a need for TPN when adequate fluid intake cannot be tolerated, and severe CNS dysfunction.

Renal disease may develop after years of apparent recovery. Lou-Meda and colleagues found that screening for microalbuminuria within the first 6 to 18 months after an episode of HUS was better at predicting subsequent renal disease (66.7%) versus screening for proteinuria (22%).[68] Caletti and colleagues noted that decline in renal function was less in children who received angiotensen-converting enzyme inhibitors in addition to dietary and antihypertensive therapy.[69] End-stage renal disease resulting in kidney transplantation occurs more frequently in atypical D−HUS. The European Society for Pediatric Nephrology noted that in their registry of 167 children with atypical HUS, 33 (19.7%) underwent at least one renal transplant procedure. Of these, only 18% were successful and 73% demonstrated recurrence or thrombosis. Based on this data, the authors concluded that living-related transplantation should not be performed in the D−HUS population.[70] Loirat and Niaudet compared the risk of recurrence after renal transplant among patients with D+HUS (0.8%) with D−HUS (21%).[71]

Novel approaches are being investigated which interfere with the attachment of the B subunit of vero cytotoxin to its receptor, globotriaosylceramide (Gb3) in gut epithelium although none has yet been shown to be effective in human disease. Potential agents include *Bifidobacterium longum* and Gb3 polymers which bind Shiga toxins.[72]

HENOCH-SCHONLEIN PURPURA

HSP is the most common form of systemic vasculitis in children. It primarily affects children between the ages of 1 and 15 years, with the mean age of 6 years, however, the majority of children affected are under the age of 10 years. Schonlein described an association of arthritis with purpura in 1837.[73] The clinical syndrome, subsequently extended to include abdominal pain and GI bleeding by Henoch in 1874, is characterized by urticarial or purpuric skin lesions, colicky abdominal pain, sometimes with hematochezia, arthralgias or arthritis, and hematuria, which may be accompanied by proteinuria.[74] Symptoms persist for an average of 3 weeks, although recurrences are common, occurring in 35% of patients.[75]

Epidemiology

In a recent retrospective review of 150 children with HSP followed over 5 years, most of the patients (91%) were less than 10 years of age, and two-thirds were between 3 and 6 years of age.[75] HSP occurred more commonly during the winter, fall, and spring months with few of the cases occurring during the summer (5%). A history of previous infection was noted in about two-thirds of the children, with the majority presenting with an upper respiratory illness. A slight male predominance was seen with a male-female ratio of 1.8:1 as has been noted in other studies. In children who had a recurrence of HSP, the course was milder and occurred within 12 months of the initial presentation. Nephritis, elevated erythrocyte sedimentation rate, and corticosteroid use were associated risk factors for relapse, perhaps suggesting increased risk in children with severe initial presentation of HSP. Genetic susceptibility is suggested by an analysis of DRB1 polymorphisms; increased frequencies of DRB1*01 and DRB1*11 with decreased DRB1*07 are observed in patients with HSP compared with controls.[76,77]

Pathogenesis

Although the etiology of HSP remains unknown, clinical observations suggest that infectious agents may trigger an immune response (including group A β-hemolytic streptococci, *Bartonella henselae*, *Mycoplasma*, *Yersinia*, *Legionella*, *Helicobacter pylori*, *Campylobacter jejuni*, EBV, CMV, HIV, Varicella Zoster virus, hepatitis A and B virus, and recently HPV B19). Other proposed triggers include vaccinations (MMR, pneumococcal, influenza, and hepatitis B), insect bites, or medications (including penicillins, ciprofloxacin, acetylsalicylic acid, vancomycin, levodopa, cocaine, acetylcholinesterase inhibitors, carbamazepine, and streptokinase).[75,78–82] The disease is characterized by deposition of IgA1-containing immune complexes (IgA1C) in small blood vessel walls in susceptible hosts.[77,83] IgA1C is normally cleared by the asialoglycoprotein receptor of hepatocytes, which binds the oligosaccharide chains of the IgA1 Fc fragment.[84] High levels of IgA1C are found in the circulation of patients with HSP nephritis. Abnormally glycosylated IgA1 aggregates, which may be less well cleared by hepatocytes, have been identified in patients with HSP nephritis but not those without renal involvement.[84,85] Activation of the alternate complement pathway may generate chemotactic factors and polymorphonuclear infiltration. Antineutrophilic cytoplasmic antibodies are detected in 10% of patients.[86]

Adhesion molecules induced by proinflammatory cytokines, including tumor necrosis factor-α (TNF) and interleukin 1 (IL-1), play a major role in the recruitment of neutrophils and other inflammatory cells to the site of inflammation.[87] Serum TNF levels are higher during the acute phase of HSP than during remission and in those with renal involvement in contrast to those with normal renal function. Immunohistochemical staining of skin lesions reveals intracellular TNF in the nucleated epidermal layer, with lesser amounts of IL-1 and IL-6 staining, suggesting that these cytokines may contribute to the inflammation in HSP.[88]

Microscopic findings show a leukocytoclastic vasculitis with perivascular infiltrates of polymorphonuclear leukocytes and lymphocytes, and deposition of IgA immune complexes around small blood vessels in the affected organs and the mesangial cells of the kidney. Mucosal IgA deposition can be seen in the biopsies of the duodenum in the absence of vasculitis.[89] Intimal proliferation and thrombosis have been described in cerebral vessels in children with seizures. Vasculitis results in edema and hemorrhage in various organs, including the intestine, pancreas, gallbladder, lung, myocardium, testis, and cerebral cortex.[90–92] In glomeruli, there are diffuse polymorphonuclear infiltrates or hyalinization with thickening of the basement membrane of Bowman capsule.

Clinical Manifestations

Skin Involvement. Skin lesions occur in 97 to 100% of children with HSP.[75] Usually the rash begins with an urticarial or macular eruption on the extensor surfaces of the legs, buttocks, and arms, which changes to red, palpable purpuric lesions. Involvement is usually symmetric and less common on the face and upper extremities. Children under 3 years of age may present with scalp, facial, or extremity edema, whereas older children often show petechiae, especially on the lower extremities. Prominent purpuric lesions involving the face and ears were recently described in six infants less than 1 year of age.[91]

Gastrointestinal Involvement. GI symptoms occur in 51 to 58% of children.[75,93] Colicky abdominal pain, often associated with nausea and emesis, results from submucosal edema and hemorrhage. Abdominal pain develops within 8 days of the rash in most pediatric patients, although intervals as long as 150 days between GI symptoms and skin findings have been observed.[94] Gastrointestinal symptoms may also precede the rash in some cases, and gastrointestinal symptoms have been described in the absence of rash in case reports.[95] Hypoproteinemia may develop secondary to protein-losing enteropathy. GI bleeding, either overt (melena, hematochezia, or hematemesis) or with positive stool occult blood tests occurs in 18% of children. Massive GI bleeding has been reported but is uncommon.

Children with abdominal pain frequently show tenderness to direct palpation (75%), but rebound tenderness is uncommon (9%). Rare intestinal complications include intussusception (2 to 3%), perforation, pancreatitis, and cholecystitis.[75,91–94] When intussusception develops, it is seen in children 5 to 7 years of age; early surgical intervention markedly reduces mortality. Intussusception in HSP usually originates in the ileum (90%) or jejunum (7%), and approximately 58% of cases are confined to the small bowel.[96] In contrast, most idiopathic intussusceptions are ileocolonic. In one series of children who underwent exploratory laparotomy, excessive amounts of peritoneal fluid were observed. Rarely, small bowel obstruction may develop from enteroentero fistulae or late-onset stricture formation.[97,98]

Endoscopic examination may demonstrate coalescing purpuric lesions, especially in the descending duodenum, gastritis, or punctate erythematous and ulcerative changes in the colon.[99,100] Tomomasa and colleagues described endoscopic findings in nine children with HSP.[100] No esophageal abnormalities were observed. Gastric changes in two children consisted of diffuse mucosal edema, patchy erythema, and multiple erosions. Diffuse severe erythema with erosions was noted in the duodenal bulb (two patients) and the second portion of the duodenum (three children). Rectosigmoid examination in six children demonstrated shallow ulcers in two, but studies were normal in the other four. Endoscopic biopsies revealed polymorphonuclear infiltrates in the lamina propria, predominantly around blood vessels.

Radiologic studies of the small bowel and colon show thumbprinting (Figure 2), representing

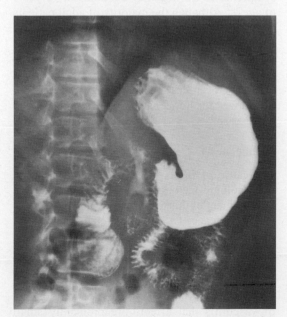

Figure 2 Upper gastrointestinal series demonstrating focally thickened folds and thumbprinting due to submucosal edema in the proximal jejunum in a 14-year-old girl with recurrent episodes of colicky abdominal pain. Four weeks later she developed typical skin lesions of Henoch-Schönlein purpura on the lower extremities.

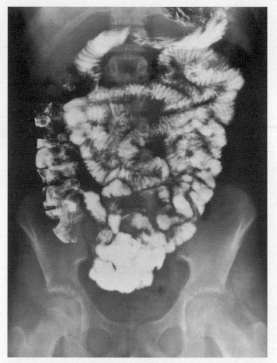

Figure 3 Upper gastrointestinal and small bowel follow-through demonstrating extensive thickening of mucosal folds in the descending duodenum and entire jejunum in a 10-year-old boy with recurrent vomiting and scattered macular erythematous lesions on the buttocks and lower extremities due to Henoch-Schönlein purpura.

submucosal edema and hemorrhage, spasm, ulceration, and pseudotumor, usually in the jejunum and ileum (Figure 3), but the colon may be affected.[101] Similar findings may be seen in lymphoproliferative disorders, other hemorrhagic conditions (hemophilia, leukemia), scleroderma, and Crohn's disease. Relapses of GI symptoms have been reported up to 7 years after the initial episode.[90]

Joint Involvement. Arthritis and arthralgias occur in 74 to 84% of children with HSP.[75] The arthritis is usually oligoarticular, transient, migratory, and nondeforming and affects large joints of the lower extremity, mainly ankles and knees. Joint involvement may be the first manifestation of HSP in 15% of patients and may precede the rash by 1 or 2 days.

Renal Manifestations. Renal involvement is seen in 20 to 54% of children with HSP at initial presentation and usually presents within 4 weeks of onset of symptoms.[75,102] The renal involvement is usually mild in children as compared to adults. Mild nephropathy was seen in 47% of cases with mild proteinuria, microscopic hematuria or both, without any evidence of renal insufficiency or changes in blood pressure. Nephrotic syndrome has been described infrequently. Muller and colleagues reported that measuring urinary tubular marker proteins (N-acetyl-P-D-glucosaminidase and (x1-microglobulin) correlated with the extent of early and late renal involvement and suggested that their use may be helpful in identifying those who will develop HSP nephritis.[103] Renal lesions are more frequent in older children than in those

less than 2 years of age. Factors associated with HSP nephritis included older age at presentation, gastrointestinal bleeding, and central nervous system involvement.[102] Serious complications include hypertension (sometimes leading to hypertensive encephalopathy) and renal failure. A review of 12 studies which included 1,133 children who were followed over 6 weeks to 36 years showed that permanent renal impairment never developed in patients with a normal urinalysis, in 1.6% with isolated urinary abnormalities and in 19.5% of patients who had nephritic or nephrotic syndrome.[104]

Renal biopsy is reserved for patients in whom the diagnosis is uncertain or who have severe renal involvement. Glomerular lesions include glomerular proliferation, crescentic glomerulonephritis, and IgA deposits in the mesangium. Autopsy studies of the kidneys demonstrate endothelial thickening, thrombosis, and medial necrosis of small renal arteries.

Hepatobiliary Involvement. Chao and colleagues described hepatobiliary involvement in 20 of 225 children with HSP.[105] Symptoms included right upper quadrant pain (80%), nausea (45%), lethargy (20%), and vomiting (15%). Laboratory tests revealed elevated alanine transaminase in 15 of 20 patients (75%) and elevated g-glutamyl transpeptidase in 6 of 20 patients (30%). Abdominal ultrasonography demonstrated hepatomegaly in 75% and gallbladder wall thickening in 25% of this group. The findings subsided within 3 to 7 days after steroid therapy. Viola and colleagues described a child with ischemic necrosis of the bile ducts (which they attributed to HSP vasculitis of the peribiliary vessels), which resulted in biliary cirrhosis and liver transplant.[106]

Scrotal Involvement. Scrotal pain and swelling from vasculitis due to HSP are the most common genital manifestations seen in 13 to 24% of boys with HSP.[107,108] Testicular pain and swelling may accompany scrotal involvement and mimic testicular torsion. High-resolution Doppler ultrasonography is useful in differentiating between the two conditions, with decrease in blood flow seen in testicular torsion as opposed to increase in blood flow in HSP, thus avoiding potential surgical intervention.

Other Presentations of HSP. Rare presentations described mainly as case reports include neurological manifestations with ataxia, owing to brainstem vasculitis, headaches, seizures, focal neurological deficits, cerebral hemorrhage, and central and peripheral neuropathy.[109,110] Neurological involvement is usually transient except in the setting of cerebral hemorrhage. Loss of vision from retinal artery occlusion, impaired lung diffusion capacity in the absence of respiratory symptoms, and pulmonary hemorrhage have also been described.[111,112]

Diagnosis

The diagnosis of HSP rests on the presence of characteristic clinical features with supporting laboratory, endoscopic, and radiologic studies as indicated. Peripheral blood counts show leukocytosis (10,000 to 20,000/mm^3) with left shift in half of the children. Erythrocyte sedimentation is elevated (greater than 20 mm/h) in 75% of children.[113] Urinalyses may not demonstrate hematuria or proteinuria until several weeks after the initial presentation. The presence of microscopic blood should be checked in stool specimens. Biopsies for histologic examination in affected organs are performed only in cases where the diagnosis is uncertain or if there is severe renal involvement.

High-frequency ultrasonography may be helpful in equivocal cases, as when abdominal pain develops prior to skin or renal involvement.[114,115] Findings of HSP include thickened bowel wall (3 to 11 mm), which may be diffuse or focal, free peritoneal fluid, impaired peristalsis of affected loops, and bowel dilatation. Serial examinations during the course of the disease can determine whether the lesions are extending or resolving and whether there is reexpansion of the small bowel lumen and reappearance of peristalsis. Complications such as intussusception and perforation can be detected by this method.

Endoscopic evaluation may be indicated to exclude other conditions if the diagnosis is unclear. Newer modalities like wireless capsule endoscopy can be used for the evaluation of gastrointestinal bleeding or severe abdominal pain in children over the age of 10 years.[116] Capsule endoscopy has also been used to evaluate need for steroids or immune suppression in children with gastrointestinal involvement.

Physicians should be aware that activation of coagulation secondary to endothelial damage may result in D-dimer concentrations more than 10 times the upper limit of normal.[117] However, in none of the 15 children were the platelet count, prothrombin time, thrombin time, protein S and C, or antithrombin 3 levels abnormal. The authors caution against interpreting the abnormal D-dimers as indicating disseminated intravascular coagulation in patients with HSP.

Management

The treatment of HSP is primarily supportive. Most patients can be managed in the ambulatory setting with attention to hydration status and pain control. Therapeutic intervention is usually directed at specific complications, such as severe abdominal pain, hypertension, renal insufficiency, and gastrointestinal or cerebral hemorrhage.

Gastrointestinal Disease. Children with severe abdominal pain should be admitted to the hospital because of the potential risk of intussusception, hemorrhage, or perforation. Supportive care with intravenous fluids and nasogastric suction is helpful in comforting severely symptomatic children. Corticosteroids used for GI manifestations of HSP are controversial.[118] A recent randomized, double-blind, placebo-controlled trial by Ronkainen and colleagues, evaluated the efficacy of early prednisone therapy in preventing renal complications and treating extrarenal and renal symptoms in 171 children with HSP. Prednisone at the dose of 1 mg/kg/d for 2 weeks, with weaning over the next 2 weeks was effective in reducing the intensity of abdominal pain and joint pain ($p = .29$, $p = .30$) in treated children as compared to placebo. Prednisone did not prevent renal involvement, but symptoms from renal involvement resolved in 61% of patients treated with prednisone as compared to 34% of patients on placebo.[119] The risk of intussusception may also be reduced in patients on early prednisone therapy.[120] However, at this time, prednisone is used only for severe involvement in patients with HSP and routine use cannot be recommended.

Intravenous immunoglobulin (IVIG) therapy has been reported to be effective in a child with massive gastrointestinal hemorrhage and may be beneficial in patients with severe GI disease or in steroid-dependent HSP.[121] Jordan suggested that glomerulonephritis may have been precipitated in one patient by this therapy.[122] In one child with severe cerebral and retinal vasculitis, intravenous pulse methylprednisolone was not effective, but plasmaphoresis led to prompt resolution of symptoms.[123] Dapsone, an antileprotic drug, was also found to be beneficial in eight patients who had severe, persistent HSP and was most efficacious for the skin manifestations of HSP.[124]

Surgical treatment is required rarely for massive gastric hemorrhage, intussusception, obstruction, intestinal perforation, or cholecystitis.[90,125] Careful and repeated physical examinations are necessary to identify early signs of these complications.

Renal Disease. Management of the renal complications of HSP will not be discussed, but, clearly, blood pressure and renal output must be carefully monitored. Urine samples should be analyzed regularly for hematuria and proteinuria. Antihypertensive medications, fluid restriction, and dialysis may be necessary.[126] Recently, the combined use of corticosteroids and azathioprine was reported to reduce the progression to chronic HSP nephritis when compared with historical controls.[127] Intravenous pulse methylprednisolone or oral prednisone followed by oral cyclophosphamide reduces proteinuria and may lessen the development of renal insufficiency.[128]

Prognosis

The long-term outcome and prognosis of HSP in children are generally excellent. Although relapses occur in 35% of children, they are usually shorter and milder than the initial episode.[75] Number of recurrences range from one to five and occur within 12 months of the initial presentation. Increased sedimentation rate, gastrointestinal disease, renal involvement, and corticosteroid use were found to be risk factors for relapse although these factors may be related to severe initial presentation of the disease.

BEHCET SYNDROME

BS is a multisystem vasculitic disorder reported first in 1937.[129] The original description included aphthous stomatitis, genital ulcers, and uveitis. Because there are no pathologic or laboratory findings that definitively establish the diagnosis, several clinical criteria have been proposed.[130,131] Although the disease affects predominantly young adults in Japan, the Mediterranean region, and the Middle East, pediatric cases have been described.[132–143] Genetic predisposition is suggested by the observation that the class I human leukocyte antigen (HLA) HLA-B51 is positive in 62.8% of patients with BS compared with 24.6% of healthy controls.[144] A positive family history is also higher in HLA-B51–positive patients (83%) versus HLA-B51–negative patients (58%). Immunologic processes are thought to be causally related to the vasculitis; thus, current forms of therapy use immunomodulatory medications. The clinical presentation of BS may closely resemble that of Crohn's disease, but the presence of genital ulcers, very severe oral ulceration, and neurologic complications aids in differentiating the two conditions.[141,145]

Epidemiologic Aspects

The prevalence of BS varies greatly among different countries. It is most common in Japan (10 per 100,000) compared with England (0.6 per 100,000) and the United States (0.3 per 100,000).[130] The incidence appears to have increased between 1958 and 1977 in Japan. Presentation prior to the onset of puberty is unusual.[146] In one series of 297 patients, only 34 had symptoms prior to 19 years of age, with the youngest being 13-year old.[146] Ammann and colleagues described six children whose onset of symptoms of BS began at 2 months to 11 years of age.[132] Although the majority of adult patients are male (70%), half of the pediatric patients are female.[132,141]

Familial cases are uncommon, but isolated instances involving parents with affected children have been described.[147] A transient form of BS may occur in neonates born to mothers with the disease.[137]

Pathogenesis

The cause of BS is unknown, but genetic and immunologic factors probably contribute to the development of this disorder. Recent studies document evidence of a Th1 dominant response in the intestinal lesions of patients with BS based on the expression by interferon gamma (IFN-γ), tumor necrosis factor (TNF-α), IL-12 mRNA, and the Th1-related chemokine receptor CCR5.[148]

The primary histopathologic lesion consists of vasculitis that affects predominantly small vessels. Initially, there is endothelial proliferation and infiltration with mononuclear cells, which is followed by a polymorphonuclear response. The same vascular lesion may occur in large veins and cause thrombophlebitis, as well as in large arteries, leading to gangrene or aneurysm formation. Studies have shown deposition of C3 and C9 in blood vessel walls and circulating immune complexes in patients with BS. In the newborn form, transient circulating IgG immune complexes and reduced total hemolytic complement were detected, suggesting transplacental passage of immune complexes or autoantibodies.[137] Additional evidence for Th1 response is supported by increases in interleukin 8, IFN-γ and IL-12 in Behcet's mucocutaneous lesions as well as an absence of Th2 cytokines, Il-4, and IL-13.[149] Gamma-delta T cells are expanded in the peripheral blood during active disease, especially CD8 and CD56 gamma-delta T-cell subsets. Elevations in IFN-γ are described in the aqueous humor of patients with Behcet's uveitis.[150]

Lehner and colleagues observed that specific HLA haplotypes are associated with some forms of BS.[151] When compared with controls, HLA-B5 occurs more frequently in patients with ocular involvement; HLA-B27 is increased in those with arthritic symptoms, and HLA-B12 correlates with mucocutaneous signs. The allele B*5101 is found in 80% of patients with BS compared with 26% in controls.[152] Additional associations with B*5101 were the development of BS at a younger age and the presence of erythema nodosum. However, there is no association between homozygosity for HLA-B51 and the severity of the course of BS.[144]

It is known that the tumor necrosis factor gene is closely linked to the HLA-B51 gene. Recently, a polymorphism at position–1031 within the TNF-α promoter region was reported to confer increased susceptibility for BS.[153]

Whole genome screening for susceptibility genes in multicase families with BS using 395 microsatellite markers showed increased linkage scores for chromosome regions 12p12–13 and 6p22–24.[154] In addition, six patients with trisomy 8 have been described with BS and myelodysplastic syndrome.[155]

Clinical Manifestations

Several classifications have been proposed to define the diagnostic criteria for BS.[130–131] These consider the major manifestations (buccal ulceration, genital ulceration, uveitis, and skin lesions) and the less frequent signs (GI lesions, thrombophlebitis, arthritis, CNS lesions, and family history).

Major Manifestations

Oral Ulcers. Painful recurrent oral ulcers are the most common feature of this disease. They persist for 7 to 14 days, subside spontaneously, and recur several days to months later. Because this finding may occur in up to 10% of the normal population, additional manifestations are necessary to establish the diagnosis of the disease.

Genital Ulcers. Ulcerations on the genitalia are reported in 93 to 98% of patients with BS.[141,156] However, the rates are lower in children at first presentation (32%).[136] Their gross appearance and clinical course are similar to those of the oral ulcers and occur equally in male and female children.

Skin Lesions. The cutaneous manifestations of the disease are varied and include folliculitis, erythema nodosum, acne, vesicles, pustules, and other nonspecific lesions.[156] The formation of a sterile pustule at the site of needle trauma (Behcetian reaction) occurs in approximately 40% of pediatric patients.[136]

Ocular Involvement. The signs of ocular disease are iritis with hypopyon and posterior uveitis. Visual impairment is usually bilateral and may result in optic nerve atrophy, glaucoma, and cataracts. This manifestation is much less common in Western countries than in Japan and Turkey, where it is a major cause of blindness. Between 21 and 47% of pediatric patients have ocular involvement.[136,141]

Minor Manifestations

Gastrointestinal Disease. The frequency of GI involvement in patients with BS varies widely in different series and perhaps in different regions. Yazici and colleagues reported that no patient had GI signs of BS in their review of 297 patients from Turkey.[146] Japanese authors have observed intestinal symptoms in at least 15% of patients with BS.[157] The frequency is higher in Japanese children with BS, with 58% having GI disease.[142] The most frequent complaints are colicky abdominal pain and nonbloody diarrhea, but vomiting, flatulence, and constipation may occur. Perianal ulceration may occur with or without concurrent genital ulceration.[134] Rare cases of esophageal involvement have been reported. GI involvement has been demonstrated by technetium 99 m leukocyte scintigraphy and follow-up by ileocolonoscopy in children with BS without GI symptoms.[138] Radiologic examinations demonstrate thickened mucosal folds, pseudopolyps, deformity of bowel loops, ulcerations, and fistulae.[158] Ulcerations are localized or diffuse, with the majority (76%) occurring in the ileocecal region.[159] Extension of the ulcers to the serosal surface may result in perforation. Recurrence is often at the site of anastomosis, and 44% of surgically treated cases require reoperation.[159] Postoperative azathioprine results in a lower reoperation rate: 7 versus 25% at 2 years and 25 versus 47% at 5 years.[160]

The typical colonoscopic findings in BS are ileocecal location (96%), solitary ulcer (67%), size greater than 1.0 cm (76%), with a mean size of 2.9 cm, and deep ulcers (80%; 62% with discreet margins).[161] The differentiation of BS from chronic nonspecific ulcerative colitis and especially Crohn's disease depends on the character of the intestinal endoscopic and radiologic findings and the associated extraintestinal manifestations. The correct extraintestinal diagnosis may be obscured by the presence of BS and ulcerative colitis or Crohn's disease in the same family.[145] Baba and colleagues noted that the ileocecal

location and the depth of the ulcers in BS distinguish this disease from chronic ulcerative colitis.[157] In comparison with Crohn's disease, there was less inflammation in the area surrounding the ulcer, and granulomas were not seen.[157,162] Enterocutaneous and rectovaginal fistulae have been reported in BS.[163] The recurrent genital ulcers and CNS signs seen in BS are rarely found in ulcerative colitis or Crohn's disease.[145]

In contrast to children with Crohn's disease, growth based on the mean height standard deviation score at the time of diagnosis is usually normal in BS: 0.38 ± 1.08 at 1 year and 0.35 at 2 years after diagnosis.[134] Body mass index is reported to be normal in children with BS. Kim and colleagues analyzed the response to medical therapy and need for surgical intervention based on the colonoscopic appearance of ulcers in 50 patients with BS.[164] The most common were volcano-type ulcers (50%), followed by aphthous ulcers (28%), and geographic ulcers (22%). Complete remission following medical therapy was better for geographic ulcers (73%) and aphthous ulcers (64%) than for the volcano type (24%). Remissions were achieved after surgical intervention in 52% of patients with volcano-type ulcers. However, recurrence rates were also higher for the volcano-type ulcers (47%) than the geographic and aphthous ulcer types (11 and 9%, respectively).

Vascular Disease. The vasculitic process described above can affect both arterial and venous systems. Small vessel disease accounts for many systemic signs, but large vessel involvement may result in severe complications. Recurrent superficial thrombophlebitis, vena cava thrombosis, and arterial occlusions leading to infarction and hemorrhage from rupture of aneurysmal dilatations have been reported. Increases in the Q–T interval, ventricular arrhythmias, and sudden death were described in 1997.[165] The pulmonary artery is most common arterial vessel to be involved in BS.[166]

Arthritis. Chronic nonmigratory seronegative pauciarticular arthritis affecting the knees, ankles, hips, elbows, and wrists occurs in up to 50% of patients with BS. The course tends to be nondestructive, with rare radiologic evidence of bone erosion, although synovial thickening and effusion may occur.[156]

Neurologic Manifestations. Headaches are reported in 37% of children with BS.[136] More severe neurologic involvement is reported in 1 to 20% of patients with BS. Episodes may be transient or progressive and include pyramidal signs, organic confusional states leading to dementia, meningoencephalitis, cranial nerve palsies, dural thrombosis, pseudotumor cerebri, seizures, and quadriparesis.[136] Neuroimaging studies may demonstrate parenchymal disease, venous sinus thrombosis or be normal. Intracranial hypertension without evidence of parenchymal involvement has been reported.[167] There may be mild pleocytosis with or without an elevation of protein in the cerebrospinal fluid, especially in those patients with parenchymal disease. Low-dose methotrexate (7.5 to 12.5 mg per week) appears to have a beneficial effect in reducing cerebrospinal fluid IL-6 levels and dementia.[168]

Diagnosis

The diagnosis depends on the presence of characteristic clinical findings.[130] The criteria of Mason and Barnes, described in 1969, include three major and two minor criteria (described under "Clinical Manifestations").[131] Subsequently, an International Study Group (ISG) recommended that the diagnosis should be based on the presence of three or more episodes of oral aphthous ulcers plus two of the following lesions: recurrent aphthous genital ulcers, uveitis or retinal vasculitis, cutaneous vasculitis, or cutaneous hyperactivity to needle prick (positive pathergy test).[130] The technique of performing the pathergy test affects the rate of positive response.[169] The positivity rate was statistically higher with nondisposable blunt needles than with disposable sharp needles. Recently, the specificity of the ISG classification compared 302 patients with BS and a control group of 438 patients with other conditions, including ulcerative colitis, Crohn's disease, and familial Mediterranean fever.[170] Of those diagnosed with BS, 98% fulfilled the ISG criteria compared with 1% of the control group.

Fujikawa and Suemitsu described 31 pediatric patients with BS and observed that the diagnosis in children may be difficult because of the long interval between disease onset and the presence of sufficient symptoms to satisfy the diagnostic criteria of BS.[133] The prevalence of oral ulcers increased from 77% in the first 6 months to 100% during the course of the illness. Similarly, genital ulcers increased from 45 to 58%, uveitis from 10 to 29%, and skin lesions from 39 to 55%. Krause and colleagues noted that the interval between the first disease sign and the full disease complex in children was 3.9 ± 3.5 years, thus emphasizing the difficulty in diagnosing BS in pediatric patients.[136]

With regard to comparisons of diagnostic tests used in patients with inflammatory bowel disease, recent reports describe prevalence values for both the three common variants of CARD15/NOD2 which predispose to Crohn's disease and anti-*Saccharomyces cerevisiae* antibody (ASCA) in patients with BS. CARD15/NOD2 polymorphisms were assessed in 374 English, Turkish, or Middle Eastern patients with BS, and no association was found.[171] In contrast, ASCA was detected in 44.3% of patients with intestinal Behcet's disease compared with 3.3% in those without intestinal involvement and was associated with a higher risk for surgery.[172]

Management

Therapeutic intervention for active disease must take into account the range and seriousness of complications as described by Yazici and colleagues.[146] Corticosteroid medications have formed the mainstay of treatment for BS.[173] Relief

of symptoms occurs initially in most patients, but recurrences are common. Topical preparations are usually effective for genital ulcers, whereas oral or intravenous administration is required for uveitis, intestinal lesions, and neurologic manifestations. A prospective randomized 2-year trial of colchicine (1 to 2 mg/kg/d) versus placebo was conducted in adults with BS.[174] There was a reduction in genital ulcers, erythema nodosum, and arthritis in the colchicine group relative to the placebo group. Colchicine use in children was described in five patients (dose: 13.5 ± 8.1 µg/kg/d increasing to 26 ± 9.2 µg/kg/d), with a response in two patients but only a partial response in three others.[134]

Immunosuppressive agents such as colchicines, azathioprine, chlorambucil (combined with prednisone 1 mg/kg/d), thalidomide (1 mg/kg dose at varying intervals of once daily to once weekly), and cyclosporine (10 mg/kg/d) have been effective in patients with severe disease who did not respond to steroids or who could not tolerate a reduction in steroid dosage.[134,173,175–179]

Yazici and colleagues and Greenwood and colleagues observed that azathioprine (2.5 mg/kg/d) was beneficial in controlling the progression of eye disease, recurrent uveitis, arthritis, the frequency of genital ulceration, reducing steroid requirement, and preventing relapse.[175,178] This finding was confirmed by Hamuryudan and colleagues, who observed significantly less deterioration in visual acuity in patients receiving azathioprine versus placebo.[176] Two children with oral, genital, and intestinal ulcerations that did not improve with steroid therapy achieved long-term control following treatment with chlorambucil.[132]

Thalidomide exerts anti-inflammatory and immunosuppressive effects, at least in part, by inhibiting TNF-α production by monocytes.[180] It also modifies the expression of TNF-α-induced adhesion molecules on endothelial cells.[181] Thalidomide has been reported to induce remission in refractory patients, including one infant who initially responded to 10 mg/kg per day for 4 weeks and subsequently relapsed but responded to 5 mg/kg daily.[140,179] Kari and colleagues reported thalidomide use for a mean duration of 2.2 years (1.3 to 4.3 years) in five children with BS who had been unresponsive to corticosteroids.[134] The dose range was very broad, varying from 0.6 to 1.1 mg/kg/d to 2.4 to 3.7 mg/kg two to three times weekly. Three achieved complete remission and two partial remission. Neuropathy developed in two children, and in one, it was irreversible after 1.3 years of treatment with 1 mg/kg/d. In some cases beginning in childhood, symptoms resolve; however, a mortality of 3% has been reported and was related to large vessel involvement.[135]

There is evidence, as discussed above, that (CD45RA+VyV82+) T cells in patients with BS produce high levels of TNF-α. Thus, it is not surprising that infliximab has been used in patients who were either: (1) refractory to corticosteroids, colchicine, thalidomide or cyclosporine,[173] or (2) chronically active and steroid-dependent,[174]

or (3) had sight-threatening panuveitis.[175] In most cases, infliximab was administered in the usual dose of 5 mg/kg. Response occurred as early as 24 hours after infusion and was followed by corticosteroid tapering and remission by 2 weeks.[173–174] In patients with panuveitis, response can be noted within 24 hours. However, repeat infusions at 6- to 8-week intervals may be necessary to maintain the remission.[182] Infliximab, Enternacept, and Adalimumab have successfully reversed severe life-threatening GI bleeding from an ileal ulcer, refractory neuro and chronic Behcets in isolated cases of BS, respectively.[183–185]

REFERENCES

1. Gasser C, Gautier E, Steck A, et al. Hemolytic-uremic syndrome: Bilateral necrosis of the renal cortex in acute acquired hemolytic anemia. Schweiz Med Wochenschr 1955;85:905–9.
2. Siegler RL. The hemolytic uremic syndrome. Pediatr Clin North Am 1995;42:1505–29.
3. Tarr PI, Hickman RO. Hemolytic uremic syndrome epidemiology: A population-based study in King County, Washington, 1971 to 1980. Pediatrics 1987;80:41–5.
4. Tune BM, Leavitt TJ, Gribble TJ. The hemolytic-uremic syndrome in California: A review of 28 nonheparinized cases with long-term follow-up. J Pediatr 1973;82:304–10.
5. Rangel JM, Sparling PH, Crowe C, et al. Epidemiology of *Escherichia coli* O157:H7 outbreaks, United States, 1982-2002. Emerg Infect Dis 2005;11:603–9.
6. Ulinski T, Lervat C, Ranchin B, et al. Neonatal hemolytic uremic syndrome after mother-to-child transmission of *Escherichia coli* O157. Pediatr Nephrol 2005;20:1334–5.
7. Garg AX, Clark WF, Salvadori M, et al. Absence of renal sequelae after childhood *Escherichia coli* O157:H7 gastroenteritis. Kidney Int 2006;70:807–12.
8. Drummond KN. Hemolytic uremic syndrome–then and now. N Engl J Med 1985;312:116–8.
9. Feldhoff C, Pistor K, Bachmann H, et al. Hemolytic uremic syndrome in 3 siblings. Clin Nephrol 1984;22:44–6.
10. Kaplan BS, Chesney RW, Drummond KN. Hemolytic uremic syndrome in families. N Engl J Med 1975;292:1090–3.
11. Kaplan BS, Drummond KN. The hemolytic-uremic syndrome is a syndrome. N Engl J Med 1978;298:964–6.
12. Neill MA, Tarr PI, Clausen CR, et al. *Escherichia coli* O157:H7 as the predominant pathogen associated with the hemolytic uremic syndrome: A prospective study in the Pacific Northwest. Pediatrics 1987;80:37–40.
13. Fitzhenry RJ, Pickard DJ, Hartland EL, et al. Intimin type influences the site of human intestinal mucosal colonisation by enterohaemorrhagic *Escherichia coli* O157:H7. Gut 2002;50:180–5.
14. Gransden WR, Damm MA, Anderson JD, et al. Further evidence associating hemolytic uremic syndrome with infection by Verotoxin-producing *Escherichia coli* O157:H7. J Infect Dis 1986;154:522–4.
15. Banatvala N, Griffin PM, Greene KD, et al. The United States National Prospective Hemolytic Uremic Syndrome Study: Microbiologic, serologic, clinical, and epidemiologic findings. J Infect Dis 2001;183:1063–70.
16. Tesh VL, O'Brien AD. Adherence and colonization mechanisms of enteropathogenic and enterohemorrhagic *Escherichia coli*. Microb Pathog 1992;12:245–54.
17. Spika JS, Parsons JE, Nordenberg D, et al. Hemolytic uremic syndrome and diarrhea associated with *Escherichia coli* O157:H7 in a day care center. J Pediatr 1986;109:287–91.
18. Klein EJ, Stapp JR, Clausen CR, et al. Shiga toxin-producing *Escherichia coli* in children with diarrhea: A prospective point-of-care study. J Pediatr 2002;141:172–7.
19. Como-Sabetti K, Reagan S, Allaire S, et al. Outbreaks of *Escherichia coli* O157:H7 infection associated with eating alfalfa sprouts—Michigan and Virginia, June-July 1997. Morb Mortal Wkly Rep 1997;46:741–4.
20. Crump JA, Sulka AC, Langer AJ, et al. An outbreak of *Escherichia coli* O157:H7 infections among visitors to a dairy farm. N Engl J Med 2002;347:555–60.
21. Heuvelink AE, van Heerwaarden C, Zwartkruis-Nahuis JT, et al. *Escherichia coli* O157 infection associated with a petting zoo. Epidemiol Infect 2002;129:295–302.
22. Gerber A, Karch H, Allerberger F, et al. Clinical course and the role of Shiga toxin-producing *Escherichia coli* infection

in the hemolytic-uremic syndrome in pediatric patients, 1997–2000, in Germany and Austria: A prospective study. J Infect Dis 2002;186:493–500.

23. Elliott EJ, Robins-Browne RM, O'Loughlin EV, et al. Nationwide study of haemolytic uraemic syndrome: Clinical, microbiological, and epidemiological features. Arch Dis Child 2001;85:125–31.

24. Koster F, Levin J, Walker L, et al. Hemolytic-uremic syndrome after shigellosis. Relation to endotoxemia and circulating immune complexes. N Engl J Med 1978;298:927–33.

25. Caprioli J, Noris M, Brioschi S, et al. Genetics of HUS: The impact of MCP, CFH, and IF mutations on clinical presentation, response to treatment, and outcome. Blood 2006;108:1267–79.

26. Zipfel PF, Misselwitz J, Licht C, Skerka C. The role of defective complement control in hemolytic uremic syndrome. Semin Thromb Hemost 2006;32:146–54.

27. Sanchez-Corral P, Perez-Caballero D, Huarte O, et al. Structural and functional characterization of factor H mutations associated with atypical hemolytic uremic syndrome. Am J Hum Genet 2002;71:1285–95.

28. Caprioli J, Castelletti F, Bucchioni S, et al. Complement factor H mutations and gene polymorphisms in haemolytic uraemic syndrome: The C-257T, the A2089G and the G2881T polymorphisms are strongly associated with the disease. Hum Mol Genet 2003;12:3385–95.

29. Dragon-Durey MA, Fremeaux-Bacchi V. Atypical haemolytic uraemic syndrome and mutations in complement regulator genes. Springer Semin Immunopathol 2005; 27:359–74.

30. Taylor CM, Chua C, Howie AJ, Risdon RA. Clinico-pathological findings in diarrhoea-negative haemolytic uraemic syndrome. Pediatr Nephrol 2004;19:419–25.

31. Cabrera GR, Fortenberry JD, Warshaw BL, et al. Hemolytic uremic syndrome associated with invasive *Streptococcus pneumoniae* infection. Pediatrics 1998;101:699–703.

32. Brandt J, Wong C, Mihm S, et al. Invasive pneumococcal disease and hemolytic uremic syndrome. Pediatrics 2002;110:371–6.

33. Hale GA, Bowman LC, Rochester RJ, et al. Hemolytic uremic syndrome after bone marrow transplantation: Clinical characteristics and outcome in children. Biol Blood Marrow Transplant 2005;11:912–20.

34. Franco A, Hernandez D, Capdevilla L, et al. De novo hemolytic-uremic syndrome/thrombotic microangiopathy in renal transplant patients receiving calcineurin inhibitors: Role of sirolimus. Transplant Proc 2003;35:1764–6.

35. Lin CC, King KL, Chao YW, et al. Tacrolimus-associated hemolytic uremic syndrome: A case analysis. J Nephrol 2003;16:580–5.

36. Saif MW, McGee PJ. Hemolytic-uremic syndrome associated with gemcitabine: A case report and review of literature. JOP 2005;6:369–74.

37. Levin M, Barratt JM. Haemolytic uraemic syndrome. Arch Dis Child 1984;59:397–400.

38. Proulx F, Turgeon JP, Litalien C, et al. Inflammatory mediators in *Escherichia coli* O157:H7 hemorrhagic colitis and hemolytic-uremic syndrome. Pediatr Infect Dis J 1998;17:899–904.

39. Huang DT, Chi H, Lee HC, et al. T-antigen activation for prediction of pneumococcus-induced hemolytic uremic syndrome and hemolytic anemia. Pediatr Infect Dis J 2006;25:608–10.

40. Upadhyaya K, Barwick K, Fishaut M, et al. The importance of nonrenal involvement in hemolytic-uremic syndrome. Pediatrics 1980;65:115–20.

41. Atkinson JP, Liszewski MK, Richards A, et al. Hemolytic uremic syndrome: An example of insufficient complement regulation on self-tissue. Ann NY Acad Sci 2005;1056:144–52.

42. Zipfel PF, Neumann HP, Jozsi M. Genetic screening in haemolytic uraemic syndrome. Curr Opin Nephrol Hypertens 2003;12:653–7.

43. Neumann HP, Salzmann M, Bohnert-Iwan B, et al. Haemolytic uraemic syndrome and mutations of the factor H gene: A registry-based study of German speaking countries. J Med Genet 2003;40:676–81.

44. Manuelian T, Hellwage J, Meri S, et al. Mutations in factor H reduce binding affinity to C3b and heparin and surface attachment to endothelial cells in hemolytic uremic syndrome. J Clin Invest 2003;111:1181–90.

45. Richards A, Kemp EJ, Liszewski MK, et al. Mutations in human complement regulator, membrane cofactor protein (CD46), predispose to development of familial hemolytic uremic syndrome. Proc Natl Acad Sci USA 2003;100:12966–71.

46. Whitington PF, Friedman AL, Chesney RW. Gastrointestinal disease in the hemolytic-uremic syndrome. Gastroenterology 1979;76:728–33.

47. Berman W, Jr, The hemolytic-uremic syndrome: Initial clinical presentation mimicking ulcerative colitis. J Pediatr 1972; 81:275–8.

48. Murray KF, Patterson K. *Escherichia coli* O157:H-induced hemolytic-uremic syndrome: Histopathologic changes in the colon over time. Pediatr Dev Pathol 2000;3:232–9.

49. Masumoto K, Nishimoto Y, Taguchi T, et al. Colonic stricture secondary to hemolytic uremic syndrome caused by *Escherichia coli* O-157. Pediatr Nephrol 2005;20:1496–9.

50. Cochran JB, Panzarino VM, Maes LY, Tecklenburg FW. Pneumococcus-induced T-antigen activation in hemolytic uremic syndrome and anemia. Pediatr Nephrol 2004;19:317–21.

51. Proulx F, Sockett P. Prospective surveillance of Canadian children with the haemolytic uraemic syndrome. Pediatr Nephrol 2005;20:786–90.

52. van Rhijn A, Donckerwolcke RA, Kuijten RH, van der Heiden C. Liver damage in the hemolytic uremic syndrome. Helv Paediatr Acta 1977;32:77–81.

53. Suri RS, Clark WF, Barrowman N, et al. Diabetes during diarrhea-associated hemolytic uremic syndrome: A systematic review and meta-analysis. Diabetes Care 2005;28:2556–62.

54. Thayu M, Chandler WL, Jelacic S, et al. Cardiac ischemia during hemolytic uremic syndrome. Pediatr Nephrol 2003;18:286–9.

55. Oakes RS, Siegler RL, McReynolds MA, et al. Predictors of fatality in postdiarrheal hemolytic uremic syndrome. Pediatrics 2006;117:1656–62.

56. Rivas M, Miliwebsky E, Chinen I, et al. Characterization and epidemiologic subtyping of Shiga toxin-producing *Escherichia coli* strains isolated from hemolytic uremic syndrome and diarrhea cases in Argentina. Foodborne Pathog Dis 2006;3:88–96.

57. Butler T, Islam MR, Azad MA, Jones PK. Risk factors for development of hemolytic uremic syndrome during shigellosis. J Pediatr 1987;110:894–7.

58. Tarr PI, Neill MA, Christie DL, Anderson DE. *Escherichia coli* O157:H7 hemorrhagic colitis. N Engl J Med 1988; 318:1697.

59. Wong CS, Jelacic S, Habeeb RL, et al. The risk of the hemolytic-uremic syndrome after antibiotic treatment of *Escherichia coli* O157:H7 infections. N Engl J Med 2000; 342:1930–6.

60. Safdar N, Said A, Gangnon RE, Maki DG. Risk of hemolytic uremic syndrome after antibiotic treatment of *Escherichia coli* O157:H7 enteritis: A meta-analysis. JAMA 2002;288:996–1001.

61. Siegler RL. Management of hemolytic-uremic syndrome. J Pediatr 1988;112:1014–20.

62. Licht C, Weyersberg A, Heinen S, et al. Successful plasma therapy for atypical hemolytic uremic syndrome caused by factor H deficiency owing to a novel mutation in the complement cofactor protein domain 15. Am J Kidney Dis 2005; 45:415–21.

63. Misiani R, Appiani AC, Edefonti A, et al. Haemolytic uraemic syndrome: Therapeutic effect of plasma infusion. Br Med J (Clin Res Ed) 1982;285:1304–6.

64. Rizzoni G, Claris-Appiani A, Edefonti A, et al. Plasma infusion for hemolytic-uremic syndrome in children: Results of a multicenter controlled trial. J Pediatr 1988;112:284–90.

65. Davin JC, Olie KH, Verlaak R, et al. Complement factor H-associated atypical hemolytic uremic syndrome in monozygotic twins: Concordant presentation, discordant response to treatment. Am J Kidney Dis 2006;47:e27–30.

66. Yassa SK, Blessios G, Marinides G, Venuto RC. Anti-CD20 monoclonal antibody (Rituximab) for life-threatening hemolytic-uremic syndrome. Clin Transplant 2005;19:423–6.

67. Robson WL, Fick GH, Jadavji T, Leung AK. The use of intravenous gammaglobulin in the treatment of typical hemolytic uremic syndrome. Pediatr Nephrol 1991;5:289–92.

68. Lou-Meda R, Oakes RS, Gilstrap JN, et al. Prognostic significance of microalbuminuria in postdiarrheal hemolytic uremic syndrome. Pediatr Nephrol 2007;22:117–20.

69. Caletti MG, Lejarraga H, Kelmansky D, Missoni M. Two different therapeutic regimes in patients with sequelae of hemolytic-uremic syndrome. Pediatr Nephrol 2004;19: 1148–52.

70. Zimmerhackl LB, Besbas N, Jungraithmayr T, et al. Epidemiology, clinical presentation, and pathophysiology of atypical and recurrent hemolytic uremic syndrome. Semin Thromb Hemost 2006;32:113–20.

71. Loirat C, Niaudet P. The risk of recurrence of hemolytic uremic syndrome after renal transplantation in children. Pediatr Nephrol 2003;18:1095–101.

72. Watanabe M, Matsuoka K, Kita E, et al. Oral therapeutic agents with highly clustered globotriose for treatment of Shiga toxigenic *Escherichia coli* infections. J Infect Dis 2004;189:360–8.

73. Schonlein J. Allgemeine und Specielle Pathologie und Therapie. Wurzburg: Herisau; 1837.

74. Henoch E. Veber ein Eigenthumliche Form von Purpura. Berl Kiln: Wochenschr; 1874.

75. Trapani S, Micheli A, Grisolia F, et al. Henoch Schonlein purpura in childhood: Epidemiological and clinical analysis of 150 cases over a 5-year period and review of literature. Semin Arthritis Rheum 2005;35:143–53.

76. Amoli MM, Thomson W, Hajeer AH, et al. HLA-DRB1*01 association with Henoch-Schonlein purpura in patients from northwest Spain. J Rheumatol 2001;28:1266–70.

77. Amoroso A, Berrino M, Canale L, et al. Immunogenetics of Henoch-Schoenlein disease. Eur J Immunogenet 1997; 24:323–33.

78. Ayoub EM, Nelson B, Shulman ST, et al. Group A streptococcal antibodies in subjects with or without rheumatic fever in areas with high or low incidences of rheumatic fever. Clin Diagn Lab Immunol 2003;10:886–90.

79. Ferguson PJ, Saulsbury FT, Dowell SF, et al. Prevalence of human parvovirus B19 infection in children with Henoch-Schonlein purpura. Arthritis Rheum 1996;39:880–1.

80. Masuda M, Nakanishi K, Yoshizawa N, et al. Group A streptococcal antigen in the glomeruli of children with Henoch-Schonlein nephritis. Am J Kidney Dis 2003;41: 366–70.

81. Novak J, Szekanecz Z, Sebesi J, et al. Elevated levels of anti-*Helicobacter pylori* antibodies in Henoch-Schonlein purpura. Autoimmunity 2003;36:307–11.

82. Sussman M, Jones JH, Almeida JD, Lachmann PJ. Deficiency of the second component of complement associated with anaphylactoid purpura and presence of mycoplasma in the serum. Clin Exp Immunol 1973;14:531–9.

83. Fauci AS, Haynes B, Katz P. The spectrum of vasculitis: Clinical, pathologic, immunologic and therapeutic considerations. Ann Intern Med 1978;89:660–76.

84. Davin JC, Weening JJ. Henoch-Schonlein purpura nephritis: An update. Eur J Pediatr 2001;160:689–95.

85. Saulsbury FT. Henoch-Schonlein purpura in children. Report of 100 patients and review of the literature. Medicine (Baltimore) 1999;78:395–409.

86. Rovel-Guitera P, Diemert MC, Charuel JL, et al. IgA antineutrophil cytoplasmic antibodies in cutaneous vasculitis. Br J Dermatol 2000;143:99–103.

87. Gattorno M, Vignola S, Barbano G, et al. Tumor necrosis factor induced adhesion molecule serum concentrations in Henoch-Schonlein purpura and pediatric systemic lupus erythematosus. J Rheumatol 2000;27:2251–5.

88. Besbas N, Saatci U, Ruacan S, et al. The role of cytokines in Henoch Schonlein purpura. Scand J Rheumatol 1997;26:456–60.

89. Kato S, Ebina K, Naganuma H, et al. Intestinal IgA deposition in Henoch-Schonlein purpura with severe gastrointestinal manifestations. Eur J Pediatr 1996;155:91–5.

90. Case records of the Massachusetts General Hospital. Weekly clinicopathological exercises. Case 14-1980. N Engl J Med 1980;302:853–8.

91. Amitai Y, Gillis D, Wasserman D, Kochman RH. Henoch-Schonlein purpura in infants. Pediatrics 1993;92:865–7.

92. Branski D, Gross V, Gross-Kieselstein E, et al. Pancreatitis as a complication of Henoch-Schonlein purpura. J Pediatr Gastroenterol Nutr 1982;1:275–6.

93. Chang WL, Yang YH, Lin YT, Chiang BL. Gastrointestinal manifestations in Henoch-Schonlein purpura: A review of 261 patients. Acta Paediatr 2004;93:1427–31.

94. Feldt RH, Stickler GB. The gastrointestinal manifestations of anaphylactoid purpura in children. Mayo Clin Proc 1962;37:465–73.

95. Gunasekaran TS, Berman J, Gonzalez M. Duodenojejunitis: Is it idiopathic or is it Henoch-Schonlein purpura without the purpura? J Pediatr Gastroenterol Nutr 2000;30:22–8.

96. Choong CK, Kimble RM, Pease P, Beasley SW. Colo-colic intussusception in Henoch-Schonlein purpura. Pediatr Surg Int 1998;14:173–4.

97. Gow KW, Murphy JJ, III, Blair GK, et al. Multiple enteroentero fistulae: An unusual complication of Henoch-Schonlein purpura. J Pediatr Surg 1996;31:809–11.

98. Lombard KA, Shah PC, Thrasher TV, Grill BB. Ileal stricture as a late complication of Henoch-Schonlein purpura. Pediatrics 1986;77:396–8.

99. Goldman LP, Lindenberg RL. Henoch-schoenlein purpura. Gastrointestinal manifestations with endoscopic correlation. Am J Gastroenterol 1981;75:357–60.

100. Tomomasa T, Hsu JY, Itoh K, Kuroume T. Endoscopic findings in pediatric patients with Henoch-Schonlein purpura and gastrointestinal symptoms. J Pediatr Gastroenterol Nutr 1987;6:725–9.

101. Rodriguez-Erdmann F, Levitan R. Gastrointestinal and roentgenological manifestations of Henoch-Schoenlein purpura. Gastroenterology 1968;54:260–4.

102. Chang WL, Yang YH, Wang LC, et al. Renal manifestations in Henoch-Schonlein purpura: A year clinical study. Pediatr Nephrol 2005;20:1269–72.

103. Muller D, Greve D, Eggert P. Early tubular proteinuria and the development of nephritis in Henoch-Schonlein purpura. Pediatr Nephrol 2000;15:85–9.

104. Narchi H. Risk of long term renal impairment and duration of follow up recommended for Henoch-Schonlein purpura with normal or minimal urinary findings: A systematic review. Arch Dis Child 2005;90:916–20.

105. Chao HC, Kong MS, Lin SJ. Hepatobiliary involvement of Henoch-Schonlein purpura in children. Acta Paediatr Taiwan 2000;41:63–8.

106. Viola S, Meyer M, Fabre M, et al. Ischemic necrosis of bile ducts complicating Schonlein-Henoch purpura. Gastroenterology 1999;117:211–4.

107. Ioannides AS, Turnock R. An audit of the management of the acute scrotum in children with Henoch-Schonlein Purpura. J R Coll Surg Edinb 2001;46:98–9.

108. Soreide K. Surgical management of nonrenal genitourinary manifestations in children with Henoch-Schonlein purpura. J Pediatr Surg 2005;40:1243–7.

109. Belman AL, Leicher CR, Moshe SL, Mezey AP. Neurologic manifestations of Schoenlein-Henoch purpura: Report of three cases and review of the literature. Pediatrics 1985;75:687–92.

110. Bulun A, Topaloglu R, Duzova A, et al. Ataxia and peripheral neuropathy: Rare manifestations in Henoch-Schonlein purpura. Pediatr Nephrol 2001;16:1139–41.

111. Besbas N, Duzova A, Topaloglu R, et al. Pulmonary haemorrhage in a 6-year-old boy with Henoch-Schonlein purpura. Clin Rheumatol 2001;20:293–6.

112. Chaussain M, de Boissieu D, Kalifa G, et al. Impairment of lung diffusion capacity in Schonlein-Henoch purpura. J Pediatr 1992;121:12–6.

113. Tramontano G, Pondrano M, Buonagura G, et al. Schonlein-Henoch syndrome. Clinico-statistical analysis of 60 cases (1978–1984). Pediatr Med Chir 1985;7:563–5.

114. Connolly B, O'Halpin D. Sonographic evaluation of the abdomen in Henoch-Schonlein purpura. Clin Radiol 1994;49:320–3.

115. Couture A, Veyrac C, Baud C, et al. Evaluation of abdominal pain in Henoch-Schonlein syndrome by high frequency ultrasound. Pediatr Radiol 1992;22:12–7.

116. Preud'Homme DL, Michail S, Hodges C, et al. Use of wireless capsule endoscopy in the management of severe Henoch-Schonlein purpura. Pediatrics 2006;118:e904–6.

117. Brendel-Muller K, Hahn A, Schneppenheim R, Santer R. Laboratory signs of activated coagulation are common in Henoch-Schonlein purpura. Pediatr Nephrol 2001;16:1084–8.

118. Haroon M. Should children with Henoch-Schonlein purpura and abdominal pain be treated with steroids? Arch Dis Child 2005;90:1196–8.

119. Ronkainen J, Koskimies O, Ala-Houhala M, et al. Early prednisone therapy in Henoch-Schonlein purpura: A randomized, double-blind, placebo-controlled trial. J Pediatr 2006;149:241–7.

120. Huber AM, King J, McLaine P, et al. A randomized, placebo-controlled trial of prednisone in early Henoch Schonlein Purpura [ISRCTN85109383]. BMC Med 2004;2:7.

121. Fagbemi AA, Torrente F, Hilson AJ, et al. Massive gastrointestinal haemorrhage in isolated intestinal Henoch-Schonlein purpura with response to intravenous immunoglobulin infusion. Eur J Pediatr 2006.

122. Jordan SC. Intravenous gamma-globulin therapy in systemic lupus erythematosus and immune complex disease. Clin Immunol Immunopathol 1989;53:S164–9.

123. Chen CL, Chiou YH, Wu CY, et al. Cerebral vasculitis in Henoch-Schonlein purpura: A case report with sequential magnetic resonance imaging changes and treated with plasmapheresis alone. Pediatr Nephrol 2000;15:276–8.

124. Iqbal H, Evans A. Dapsone therapy for Henoch-Schonlein purpura: A case series. Arch Dis Child 2005;90:985–6.

125. Katz S, Borst M, Seekri I, Grosfeld JL. Surgical evaluation of Henoch-Schonlein purpura. Experience with 110 children. Arch Surg 1991;126:849–53; discussion 853–4.

126. Andreoli SP. Chronic glomerulonephritis in childhood. Membranoproliferative glomerulonephritis, Henoch-Schonlein purpura nephritis, and IgA nephropathy. Pediatr Clin North Am 1995;42:1487–503.

127. Foster BJ, Bernard C, Drummond KN, Sharma AK. Effective therapy for severe Henoch-Schonlein purpura nephritis with prednisone and azathioprine: A clinical and histopathologic study. J Pediatr 2000;136:370–5.

128. Flynn JT, Smoyer WE, Bunchman TE, et al. Treatment of Henoch-Schonlein Purpura glomerulonephritis in children with high-dose corticosteroids plus oral cyclophosphamide. Am J Nephrol 2001;21:128–33.

129. Behcet H. Uber Rezidivierende Aphthose, durch ein Virus verursachte Geschwure am Mund, am Auge und an den Genitalien. Dermatol Wochenschr 1937;105:1152–7.

130. Criteria for diagnosis of Behcet's disease. International Study Group for Behcet's Disease. Lancet 1990;335:1078–80.

131. Mason RM, Barnes CG. Behcet's syndrome with arthritis. Ann Rheum Dis 1969;28:95–103.

132. Ammann AJ, Johnson A, Fyfe GA, et al. Behcet syndrome. J Pediatr 1985;107:41–3.

133. Fujikawa S, Suemitsu T. Behcet disease in children: A nationwide retrospective survey in Japan. Acta Paediatr Jpn 1997;39:285–9.

134. Kari JA, Shah V, Dillon MJ. Behcet's disease in UK children: Clinical features and treatment including thalidomide. Rheumatology (Oxford) 2001;40:933–8.

135. Kone-Paut I, Yurdakul S, Bahabri SA, et al. Clinical features of Behcet's disease in children: An international collaborative study of 86 cases. J Pediatr 1998;132:721–5.

136. Krause I, Uziel Y, Guedj D, et al. Childhood Behcet's disease: Clinical features and comparison with adult-onset disease. Rheumatology (Oxford) 1999;38:457–62.

137. Lewis MA, Priestley BL. Transient neonatal Behcet's disease. Arch Dis Child 1986;61:805–6.

138. Marchetti F, Trevisiol C, Ventura A. Intestinal involvement in children with Behcet's disease. Lancet 2002;359:2115.

139. Rakover Y, Adar H, Tal I, et al. Behcet disease: Long-term follow-up of three children and review of the literature. Pediatrics 1989;83:986–92.

140. Shek LP, Lee YS, Lee BW, Lehman TJ. Thalidomide responsiveness in an infant with Behcet's syndrome. Pediatrics 1999;103:1295–7.

141. Stringer DA, Cleghorn GJ, Durie PR, et al. Behcet's syndrome involving the gastrointestinal tract—a diagnostic dilemma in childhood. Pediatr Radiol 1986;16:131–4.

142. Yasui K, Komiyama A, Takabayashi Y, Fujikawa S. Behcet's disease in children. J Pediatr 1999;134:249–51.

143. Borlu M, Uksal U, Ferahbas A, Evereklioglu C. Clinical features of Behcet's disease in children. Int J Dermatol 2006;45:713–6.

144. Gul A, Uyar FA, Inanc M, et al. Lack of association of HLA-B*51 with a severe disease course in Behcet's disease. Rheumatology (Oxford) 2001;40:668–72.

145. Yim CW, White RH. Behcet's syndrome in a family with inflammatory bowel disease. Arch Intern Med 1985;145:1047–50.

146. Yazici H, Tuzun Y, Pazarli H, et al. Influence of age of onset and patient's sex on the prevalence and severity of manifestations of Behcet's syndrome. Ann Rheum Dis 1984;43:783–9.

147. Gonzalez T, Gantes M, Bustabad S. HLA haplotypes in familial Behcet's disease. J Rheumatol 1984;11:405–6.

148. Imamura Y, Kurokawa MS, Yoshikawa H, et al. Involvement of Th1 cells and heat shock protein 60 in the pathogenesis of intestinal Behcet's disease. Clin Exp Immunol 2005;139:371–8.

149. Ben Ahmed M, Houman H, Miled M, et al. Involvement of chemokines and Th1 cytokines in the pathogenesis of mucocutaneous lesions of Behcet's disease. Arthritis Rheum 2004;50:2291–5.

150. Ahn JK, Seo JM, Yu J, et al. Down-regulation of IFN-gamma-producing CD56+ T cells after combined low-dose cyclosporine/prednisone treatment in patients with Behcet's uveitis. Invest Ophthalmol Vis Sci 2005;46: 2458–64.

151. Lehner T, Batchelor JR, Challacombe SJ, Kennedy L. An immunogenetic basis for the tissue involvement in Behcet's syndrome. Immunology 1979;37:895–900.

152. Koumantaki Y, Stavropoulos C, Spyropoulou M, et al. HLA-B*5101 in Greek patients with Behcet's disease. Hum Immunol 1998;59:250–5.

153. Ahmad T, Wallace GR, James T, et al. Mapping the HLA association in Behcet's disease: A role for tumor necrosis factor polymorphisms? Arthritis Rheum 2003;48:807–13.

154. Karasneh J, Gul A, Ollier WE, et al. Whole-genome screening for susceptibility genes in multicase families with Behcet's disease. Arthritis Rheum 2005;52:1836–42.

155. Ogawa H, Kuroda T, Inada M, et al. Intestinal Behcet's disease associated with myelodysplastic syndrome with chromosomal trisomy 8—a report of two cases and a review of the literature. Hepatogastroenterology 2001;48:416–20.

156. Chajek T, Fainaru M. Behcet's disease. Report of 41 cases and a review of the literature. Medicine (Baltimore) 1975;54:179–96.

157. Baba S, Maruta M, Ando K, et al. Intestinal Behcet's disease: Report of five cases. Dis Colon Rectum 1976;19:428–40.

158. Korman U, Cantasdemir M, Kurugoglu S, et al. Enteroclysis findings of intestinal Behcet disease: A comparative study with Crohn disease. Abdom Imaging 2003;28:308–12.

159. Lee CR, Kim WH, Cho YS, et al. Colonoscopic findings in intestinal Behcet's disease. Inflamm Bowel Dis 2001;7: 243–9.

160. Choi IJ, Kim JS, Cha SD, et al. Long-term clinical course and prognostic factors in intestinal Behcet's disease. Dis Colon Rectum 2000;43:692–700.

161. Lee CR, Kim WH, Cho YS, et al. Colonoscopic findings in intestinal Behcet's disease. Inflamm Bowel Dis 2001;7:243–9.

162. Kasahara Y, Tanaka S, Nishino M, et al. Intestinal involvement in Behcet's disease: Review of 136 surgical cases in the Japanese literature. Dis Colon Rectum 1981;24:103–6.

163. Chung HJ, Goo BC, Lee JH, et al. Behcet's disease combined with various types of fistula. Yonsei Med J 2005;46:625–8.

164. Kim JS, Lim SH, Choi IJ, et al. Prediction of the clinical course of Behcet's colitis according to macroscopic classification by colonoscopy. Endoscopy 2000;32:635–40.

165. Goldeli O, Ural D, Komsuoglu B, et al. Abnormal QT dispersion in Behcet's disease. Int J Cardiol 1997;61:55–9.

166. Sarica-Kucukoglu R, Akdag-Kose A, Kayabal IM, et al. Vascular involvement in Behcet's disease: A retrospective analysis of 2319 cases. Int J Dermatol 2006;45:919–21.

167. Siva A, Kantarci OH, Saip S, et al. Behcet's disease: Diagnostic and prognostic aspects of neurological involvement. J Neurol 2001;248:95–103.

168. Hirohata S, Suda H, Hashimoto T. Low-dose weekly methotrexate for progressive neuropsychiatric manifestations in Behcet's disease. J Neurol Sci 1998;159:181–5.

169. Akmaz O, Erel A, Gurer MA. Comparison of histopathologic and clinical evaluations of pathergy test in Behcet's disease. Int J Dermatol 2000;39:121–5.

170. Tunc R, Uluhan A, Melikoglu M, et al. A reassessment of the International Study Group criteria for the diagnosis (classification) of Behcet's syndrome. Clin Exp Rheumatol 2001;19:S45–7.

171. Ahmad T, Zhang L, Gogus F, et al. CARD15 polymorphisms in Behcet's disease. Scand J Rheumatol 2005;34:233–7.

172. Choi CH, Kim TI, Kim BC, et al. Anti-*Saccharomyces cerevisiae* antibody in intestinal Behcet's disease patients: Relation to clinical course. Dis Colon Rectum 2006;49:1849–59.

173. Jorizzo JL. Behcet's disease. An update based on the 1985 International Conference in London. Arch Dermatol 1986;122:556–8.

174. Yurdakul S, Mat C, Tuzun Y, et al. A double-blind trial of colchicine in Behcet's syndrome. Arthritis Rheum 2001;44:2686–92.

175. Greenwood AJ, Stanford MR, Graham EM. The role of azathioprine in the management of retinal vasculitis. Eye 1998;12:783–8.

176. Hamuryudan V, Ozyazgan Y, Hizli N, et al. Azathioprine in Behcet's syndrome: Effects on long-term prognosis. Arthritis Rheum 1997;40:769–74.

177. Nussenblatt RB, Palestine AG, Chan CC, et al. Effectiveness of cyclosporin therapy for Behcet's disease. Arthritis Rheum 1985;28:671–9.

178. Yazici H, Pazarli H, Barnes CG, et al. A controlled trial of azathioprine in Behcet's syndrome. N Engl J Med 1990;322:281–5.

179. Yazici H, Yurdakul S, Hamuryudan V. Behcet's syndrome. Curr Opin Rheumatol 1999;11:53–7.

180. Deng L, Ding W, Granstein RD. Thalidomide inhibits tumor necrosis factor-alpha production and antigen presentation by Langerhans cells. J Invest Dermatol 2003;121:1060–5.

181. Ossandon A, Cassara EA, Priori R, Valesini G. Thalidomide: Focus on its employment in rheumatologic diseases. Clin Exp Rheumatol 2002;20:709–18.

182. Abu El-Asrar AM, Abboud EB, Aldibhi H, et al. Long-term safety and efficacy of infliximab therapy in refractory uveitis due to Behcet's disease. Int Ophthalmol 2005;26:83–92.

183. Alty JE, Monaghan TM, Bamford JM. A patient with neuro-Behcet's disease is successfully treated with etanercept: Further evidence for the value of TNF-alpha blockade. Clin Neurol Neurosurg 2007;109:279–81.

184. Ju JH, Kwok SK, Seo SH, et al. Successful treatment of life-threatening intestinal ulcer in Behcet's disease with infliximab: Rapid healing of Behcet's ulcer with infliximab. Clin Rheumatol 2007;26:1383–5.

185. van Laar JA, Missotten T, van Daele PL, et al. Adalimumab: A new modality for Behcet's disease? Ann Rheum Dis 2007;66:565–6.

20.5d. Surgical Aspects of Inflammatory Bowel Disease in Children

Jacob C. Langer, MD, FRCS(C)

Most children with inflammatory bowel disease (IBD) can be managed using a combination of nutritional and pharmacologic approaches. Initially, the goal of therapy is to bring about remission of the disease, and subsequent therapy is designed to prevent recurrence. Although historically these measures have been successful in many patients, and the continual development of newer pharmacologic agents has improved the armamentarium of the pediatric gastroenterologist, there continue to be a number of situations in which surgery may be the most appropriate course of action. The surgeon may participate in the care of these children for a number of reasons; including resection of diseased tissue, repair of narrowed or perforated intestine, bypass or defunctioning of involved bowel, drainage of abscesses, and provision of access for enteral or parenteral nutrition.

Indications for surgical management of pediatric IBD are summarized in Table 1. Although infrequent, complications such as bowel perforation, toxic megacolon, or massive bleeding are indications for emergency surgical intervention. In the majority of cases, surgery is indicated only after nonoperative management has failed, or when complications of medical management have occurred. This is particularly true in children with small bowel Crohn's disease, who are at higher risk for recurrence and further loss of bowel length.

This chapter will review the surgical management of Crohn's disease and ulcerative colitis,

and will highlight some of the special issues which these diseases pose in childhood.

PRINCIPLES OF PREOPERATIVE ASSESSMENT AND PREPARATION

Prior to considering surgery for a child with IBD, a number of steps must be taken; including confirmation of the diagnosis, staging of the disease, complete assessment of any complication that might be leading to consideration of surgery, evaluation of the surgical risk, and optimization of the patient's condition to minimize that risk. It is also important to have a series of full and complete discussions with the child and family so that they understand the risks and potential benefits of surgery.

The extent of disease should be assessed prospectively using a combination of barium studies and endoscopy. In children with colitis, it is important to differentiate between ulcerative colitis and Crohn's colitis because the surgical options differ between these two conditions. This determination is made on the basis of colonoscopic biopsies, the distribution of the disease in the colon, and the presence or absence of disease elsewhere in the gastrointestinal tract. Recent evidence suggests that the use of serological markers such as *anti-Saccharomyces cerevisiae* (ASCA) and perinuclear antinuclear cytoplasmic antibody pANCA may help to differentiate between ulcerative colitis and Crohn's disease, with particular specificity in the pediatric population,[1] although this remains controversial. Computerized tomography, ultrasonography, and magnetic resonance imaging may be very useful in evaluating the presence of inflammation or thickening, and in identifying the presence and location of fistulae or abscesses.

The goal of preoperative preparation is to achieve normal nutritional status and to minimize the dose of steroids. These steps are very important because the risk of serious complications such as anastomotic leak and sepsis are increased in patients who are malnourished or on chronic high-dose corticosteroids.[2] This is usually accomplished by using bowel rest, nutritional support, and "steroid-sparing" medical therapy. Nutritional therapy with concomitant bowel rest can be accomplished using either parenteral or enteral routes. Parenteral nutrition, although effective, is associated with significant risks from metabolic derangements, trace element deficiencies, central line complications,

and a much higher cost. For enteral nutrition, most physicians use elemental feeding through a nasogastric or gastrostomy tube. There is, however, no convincing evidence that elemental diets are better than the use of standard enteral formulae.[3] Preoperative nutritional therapy over a 4- to 6-week period is extremely effective, safe, and well tolerated.[4] The addition of immunosuppressive agents such as azathioprine, 6-mercaptopurine, cyclosporine, methotrexate, tacrolimus, or infliximab may also help to decrease or eliminate the use of steroids.[5–6]

CROHN'S DISEASE

The surgical approach to the child with Crohn's disease depends on the location of the disease and the indication for surgery.

Ileocecal Disease

Children with ileocecal disease may develop fixed fibrotic changes, local perforation, and abscess formation, or fistulization to the colon, bladder, vagina, proximal small bowel, or skin. Children may also be considered for surgery if they experience recurrent symptoms whenever the steroids are tapered, and the disease is therefore controlled only on unacceptably high doses of steroids. The decision to recommend surgery in these children may be difficult and should be made collaboratively between the family, the gastroenterologist, and the surgeon. The decision must be based on the balance of the risk of long-term high-dose steroids and the surgical risks (including infection, anastomotic leak, adhesions, and recurrent disease). Once a decision has been made, the extent of disease must be confirmed, and other studies may be done as necessary. Examples may include computerized tomography or magnetic resonance imaging to assess the possibility of local abscess or fistula formation, and renal ultrasound to look for hydronephrosis due to ureteral compression.

The surgical goal is removal of the grossly involved bowel. Although previously many surgeons did frozen sections of the resection margins to ensure that all microscopic disease had been removed, this is no longer recommended since it does not result in a lower recurrence or complication rate[7] and increases the risk of short bowel syndrome. The anastomosis can be hand-sewn or stapled, and the factors known to increase the rate of anastomotic leak include malnutrition, previous

---

Table 1 Indications for Surgical Intervention in the Management of IBD in Children

Failure of medical management
    Complications of steroid or other drug therapy
    Persistent symptoms despite maximal medical therapy

Complications
    Crohn's disease
        Perforation
        Fistula formation
        Excessive or uncontrolled bleeding
        Fibrous stricture with intestinal obstruction
        Ongoing sepsis
        Growth failure
    Ulcerative colitis
        Excessive or uncontrolled bleeding
        Toxic megacolon
        Mucosal dysplasia or fear of colon cancer

perforation or contamination, and chronic high-dose steroid administration.[2] In patients who have intra-abdominal sepsis or in whom anastomotic healing is felt to be compromised, a temporary Brooke ileostomy or a proximal defunctioning loop ileostomy should be done.

Ileocolic resection has traditionally been performed using a midline or transverse lower abdominal incision. Recently, a number of authors have described a laparoscopic-assisted approach to this procedure which results in less pain, shorter hospitalization, and an improved cosmetic appearance[8–9] (Figure 1). The laparo-

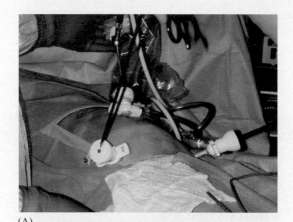

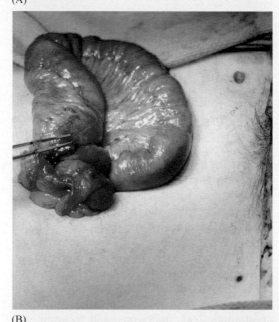

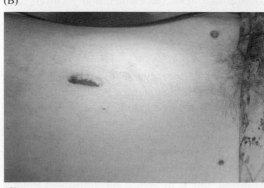

Figure 1 Laparoscopic-assisted ileocolic resection. The right colon and ileum are mobilized laparoscopically using several 3 to 5 mm ports (A), and the final resection and anastomosis are done through a small umbilical incision (B). The final incisions are shown (C).

scopic approach can be used successfully even in patients with previous intra-abdominal abscesses or fistulae. Laparoscopy may also be useful in some cases in which the diagnosis of Crohn's disease may be in doubt.

A small group of patients may present with multiple areas of symptomatic small bowel disease, with or without ileocecal involvement. Indications for surgery are similar to those mentioned above, but multiple resections would result in excessive loss of bowel length. In patients with multiple short areas of involvement, stricture-plasty has been advocated (Figure 2). The results of this procedure in both adults and children have been encouraging, with no evidence of higher rate of leak, infection, or recurrence.[10-11] Patients with ileocecal disease combined with obstructive proximal disease may require ileocolic resection and a combination of proximal resections and/or strictureplasties, and the specific operation must be individualized. The principles are to surgically treat only bowel which is thought to be causing symptoms, to do strictureplasties on short narrow areas, and to conserve small bowel length as much as possible. Like ileocolic resection, these procedures can usually be done using a laparoscopic-assisted approach.

Perianal Disease

Perianal disease can present a difficult management problem in children, since anal fistulae and abscesses are often deep and complex (Figure 3). The first order treatment should consist of metronidazole and immunosuppressive agents, which may permit healing of the fistulae without the need for surgery. True perirectal abscesses require surgical drainage, but as conservative an approach as possible should be taken because aggressive surgical treatment of deep abscesses and fistulae may lead to permanent sphincter damage. Recent evidence suggests that infliximab may be effective in healing perianal fistulae in patients with Crohn's disease,[12] but it is imperative that septic

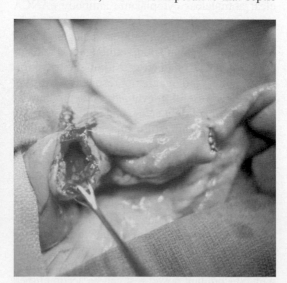

Figure 2 Strictureplasty for multiple strictures in small bowel Crohn's disease. The bowel is incised longitudinally across the stricture and then closed transversely. Strictureplasty should be performed on all strictures which cannot permit passage of a 10 cc Foley balloon.

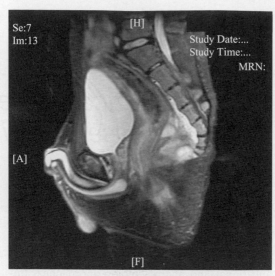

Figure 3 Magnetic resonance scan demonstrating severe perianal Crohn's disease. There are several perirectal collections (*arrows*), as well as induration and inflammatory changes in the perianal tissues.

foci be controlled first. This can often be accomplished by the use of setons, which provide constant drainage of an abscess without cutting the sphincter[13] (Figure 4).

The use of a defunctioning ileostomy for perianal disease is controversial, and in many patients the same efficacy can be achieved through the use of elemental feeding or total parenteral nutrition with bowel rest. However, a stoma may provide better control of pain and perineal excoriation because it completely diverts the fecal stream. In extremely severe cases of perianal Crohn's disease in which there has been extensive destruction of the anal sphincter, a total proctocolectomy with permanent ileostomy may be necessary.

Fistulizing Crohn's Disease

Fistulae between the small bowel or colon and the skin, intestine, bladder or vagina can often be treated medically using bowel rest, steroids, metronidazole, and immunosuppressive agents, although at least 50% of these will recur after therapy is discontinued. For cases in which medical management fails and the fistula is symptomatic, excision of the fistula with local resection of the involved bowel should be done.[14] In cases of fistulae to bladder or vagina, the defect in the normal structure can often be repaired without the need for resection. Some authors believe that fistulizing Crohn's disease is an absolute indication for surgical intervention, although improving results with newer medical approaches such as infliximab may permit some patients to avoid surgery in this setting.[15]

Gastroduodenal Disease

Although relatively common, this form of Crohn's disease can almost always be successfully managed using acid-reducing agents such as H_2 blockers or omeprazole as well as standard medical therapy for Crohn's disease. Surgery may be necessary for rare cases involving fistulae, strictures, or severe symptoms.[16]

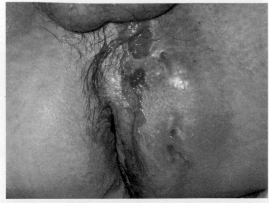

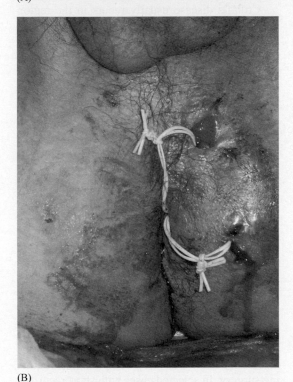

(A)

(B)

Figure 4 The use of setons for perianal Crohn's disease. The seton consists of a silastic vessel loop which is placed through the fistula from internal to external opening and tied to itself on the outside. Setons provide continuous drainage of pus so that infliximab can be used without increased risk of sepsis. The figure shows the perineum before (A) and after (B) placement of the setons.

Crohn's Colitis

Crohn's colitis often presents a complicated picture. Isolated colonic disease can usually be differentiated from ulcerative colitis by the presence of skip lesions or evidence of transmural involvement. Often both endoscopy and a barium enema are necessary because endoscopy provides mucosal detail and biopsy tissue, and the barium study permits assessment of distensability (ie, fibrosis) and fistula formation. In cases where only a small segment of colon is involved, local resection with primary anastomosis can be done. However, this approach is associated with a higher incidence of recurrence or anastomotic complications[17] (Figure 5).

Most patients have multiple areas of involvement and at least a subtotal colectomy is necessary. The options for these children are a Brooke ileostomy, an ileorectal anstomosis, or a total proctocolectomy. Sphincter-saving pouch pro-

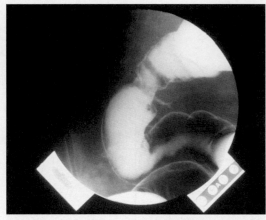

Figure 5 Child with a short segment of colonic disease, which was managed by local resection and anastomosis. The child then developed recurrent disease at the anastomosis with development of a recurrent stricture and fistula, requiring a more extensive resection.

cedures and continent ileostomies are associated with a prohibitive complication rate, and are contraindicated in the presence of Crohn's disease.[18–19] Although functional results in children are extremely good following subtotal colectomy with ileorectal anastomosis, at least 50% of these children will ultimately require a permanent ileostomy because of recurrent rectal disease.[20]

ULCERATIVE COLITIS

Emergency Management

For children with ulcerative colitis, emergent surgical intervention is carried out for life-threatening bleeding or toxic megacolon. The primary goal of surgery should be to remove the area which is bleeding or which is pathologically distended. Although a definitive procedure may be appealing, in the vast majority of emergency cases a subtotal colectomy should be performed with ileostomy and either mucous fistula or Hartmann pouch. Some authors have recommended ileostomy with "blow hole" decompression for patients with toxic megacolon as an alternative to colectomy.[21]

Nonemergency Management

Most children with ulcerative colitis consider surgery because of symptoms which are resistant to medical management or because of complications (or the fear of complications) from pharmacologic therapy. Because ulcerative colitis is a mucosal disease, surgical removal of all colonic mucosa results in cure. Options for definitive surgery include total proctocolectomy with either Brooke or continent (Kock) ileostomy, or colectomy with ileoanal anastomosis ("restorative" proctocolectomy) (Figure 6). Although the former alternatives were commonly used in the past, the need for a permanent stoma and the high complication rate of the continent ileostomy[22] has made total proctocolectomy unappealing for most children. By far the most common approach currently is subtotal (or "total abdominal") colectomy with restorative proctocolectomy, which is associated with a low

risk of complications and an excellent quality of life for most patients.

A number of controversies exist as to the best approach to restorative proctocolectomy in children. In some cases a subtotal colectomy may be performed as the primary procedure, with a reconstructive operation done in a second stage. Indications for this approach include an emergency situation, high preoperative steroid dose, poor nutrition, or concern that the diagnosis may be granulomatous colitis (Crohn's disease) rather than ulcerative colitis. If the colectomy and reconstruction are to be done simultaneously, a proximal defunctioning ileostomy is usually, but not always, placed.[23–24]

Controversy exists regarding a number of technical issues in restorative proctocolectomy, including straight ileoanal pull-through versus pouch formation, shape of pouch ("J," "S," or "W"), or stapled versus hand-sewn anastomosis. Potential advantages of the straight pull-through include a simpler procedure, lower incidence of complications, absence of postoperative pouchitis (see below), and avoidance of a defunctioning ileostomy.[25] Potential advantages of a pouch include lower stool frequency and a decreased incidence of incontinence and perianal excoriation.[26] There continue to be conflicting data with regard to this controversy.[27–29]

The use of a stapled anastomosis permits retention of a short length of transitional epithelium. This theoretically results in improved sensation with less incontinence, an advantage which is counterbalanced by the long-term risk of cancer and the need for periodic life-long surveillance using proctoscopy. Thus far, comparative studies in children have failed to document a clear advantage to either approach.[30–31]

There is also controversy around the appropriateness of restorative proctocolecomy in patients with "indeterminate" colitis. In general, it is best to start with a subtotal colectomy and ileostomy in these patients, and wait for permanent sections on the resected colon. If at that point the diagnosis of ulcerative colitis is still not certain, a pouch procedure can be safely done,[31] but the patient and family must understand that the risks of pouchitis or the ultimate development of fully blown Crohn's disease may be higher than seen with clearly defined ulcerative colitis.[32]

Both abdominal colectomy and restorative proctocolectomy have been described as laparoscopic or laparoscopic-assisted procedures (Figure 7). Advantages of this approach include less pain, shorter time to full diet, and a better cosmetic result.[33–34] In addition, since laparoscopic surgery is thought to result in a lower incidence of adhesions,[35] laparoscopic surgery will hopefully decrease the relatively high incidence of postoperative small bowel obstruction seen in patients undergoing colectomy.

COMPLICATIONS AND POSTOPERATIVE MANAGEMENT

As with any abdominal procedure, patients undergoing surgery for IBD may develop wound

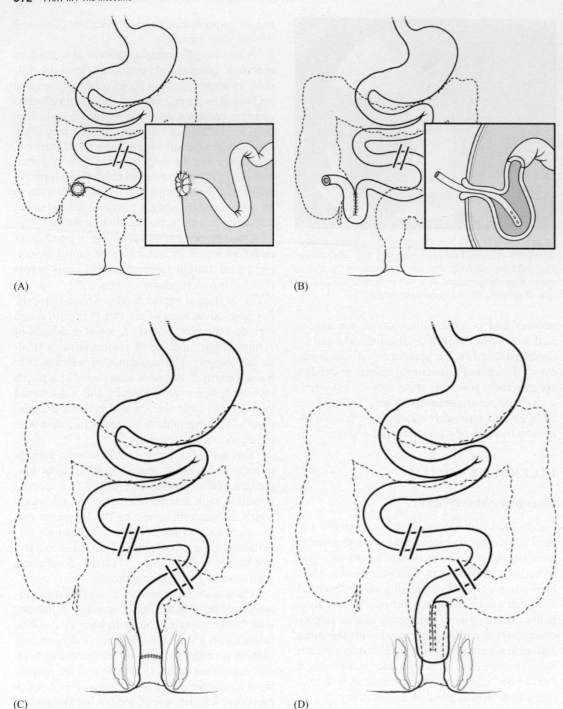

(A)

(B)

(C)

(D)

Figure 6 Options for reconstruction after colectomy for ulcerative colitis. (A) Proctocolectomy and Brooke ileostomy; (B) Proctocolectomy with continent ileostomy (Kock pouch); (C) Subtotal colectomy with straight ileoanal anastomosis; and (D) Subtotal colectomy with J pouch.

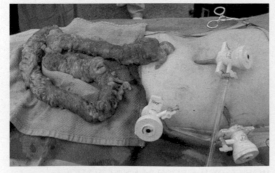

Figure 7 Laparoscopic approach to subtotal colectomy and ileostomy. The dissection is done using four port sites (one of which will become the ileostomy site), and the colon is ultimately removed through the ileostomy site.

infection, adhesions, stoma dysfunction, and ventral hernias. However, the more disturbing complications include anastomotic leak, recurrent Crohn's disease, and pouchitis.

The major risk factors for the development of an anastomotic leak are administration of steroids and nutritional status. Recent data also suggest that patients who are pANCA negative and ASCA positive are at increased risk for the development of postoperative leak and fistula after restorative proctocolectomy when compared to patients who are pANCA positive and ASCA negative.[36] A leak can be diagnosed clinically by the presence of fever, local pain and tenderness, ileus, and fluid drainage. Radiographs may demonstrate increasing free intraperitoneal air.

It is rarely necessary to do contrast studies soon after an anastomosis or pouch procedure to document a leak, and in fact such a study could potentially make matters worse. Abdominal computerized tomography or ultrasound may show free air or fluid accumulation. Treatment of documented leak usually consists of laparotomy or laparoscopy with defunctioning ileostomy. In selected cases where there is a small leak which is not accompanied by systemic sepsis and which is well localized, management with bowel rest and antibiotics may be effective. Primary revision of the anastomosis or pouch, without proximal diversion, should never be attempted.

Crohn's disease usually recurs in the region of an anastomosis and may occur weeks to many years following surgery. Early recurrence is highest in patients with active inflammation at the resection margins and patients with multiple anastomoses.[7] The risk of late recurrence is very high, especially in children, and approaches 90 to 100% in series with long-term follow-up.[37] A number of recent randomized trials in adults have demonstrated that chronic postoperative administration of 5-ASA, metronidazole, or azathioprine results in decreased recurrence rates in patients with both Crohn's colitis and ileitis.[38] Overall, patients can be given the "rule of thirds" with respect to outcome from surgery: roughly one-third will have a relatively prompt recurrence, one-third will recur 5 to 10 years before their next recurrence, and one-third will go more than 10 years or indefinitely without recurrent disease. Recurrent Crohn's disease should be approached in the same way as the initial presentation, with an attempt at medical therapy first and resection reserved for those who fail pharmacologic or who develop complications requiring surgery. In selected cases with short recurrent strictures, endoscopic balloon dilatation has been successful in avoiding an operation.[39]

Inflammation in the ileal pouch ("pouchitis") is a common complication following ileoanal pull-through for ulcerative colitis. It occurs in approximately 40% of patients, and the incidence is not influenced by type of pouch or method of anastomosis.[40] The etiology of pouchitis is unknown. Interestingly, it is never seen in patients who have had restorative proctocolectomy for familial polyposis, suggesting that the same mechanism for inflammation in ulcerative colitis may cause pouchitis.[41] Inflammation is only rarely seen in patients undergoing straight ileoanal pull-through without a pouch, suggesting that stasis within the pouch may play a role. Mucosal levels of prostaglandins and angiogenic factors are increased in the pouch, suggesting a possible etiologic role.[42] Pouchitis may be the first sign of unsuspected small bowel Crohn's disease in patients who have been initially diagnosed as ulcerative colitis or indeterminant colitis. Most patients have mild pouchitis, which can be successfully treated with metronidazole or ciprofloxacin, and some authors have also advocated the use of probiotics for the prevention and treatment of pouchitis.[43] In approximately 15% of patients, more aggressive therapy with local steroids or 5-ASA may be necessary, and in approximately 5%, the pouchitis is severe enough that the pouch must be removed. Other complications such as anastomotic stricture, perforation with pelvic sepsis or fistula formation, or poor pouch emptying may also result in loss of the pouch.[44] Successful conversion to a continent ileostomy has been reported in some patients with a failed pelvic pouch.[45]

PSYCHOSOCIAL CONSIDERATIONS

Inflammatory bowel disease presents some unique psychosocial issues in children, when compared to the same disease processes in adults. As with any chronic illness in childhood, the disease impacts not only the child, but the entire family as well. It is crucial for the attending physician and surgeon to be aware of this, and to involve the family in discussions and the decision-making process.

Most children with IBD are adolescents, and are going through a normal process developing independence from their parents and struggling with their self-image.[46] The disease may interfere with this process by imposing dependency on parents, creating self-image problems due to Cushingoid features, delay in onset of puberty, stomas, and socially isolating the child because of frequent hospitalizations, chronic pain, and diarrhea. Withdrawal from steroid medication, which often occurs during the postoperative period, commonly causes depression, which must be expected and explained to the child and family so that the feelings are not misinterpreted. It is imperative for the health-care team to be aware of and sensitive to these issues, since the mental health of the child impacts so strongly on physical recuperation.

Finally, quality of life is an important factor in the decision to perform surgery and in the assessment of postoperative results. Several quality-of-life indexes have been described for use in adults with Crohn's disease and ulcerative colitis, which may be useful for surgeons in clinical practice.[47–48] Quality-of-life issues have also been assessed in great detail for adults undergoing restorative proctocolectomy for ulcerative colitis.[49–51] However, as of yet there have been few specific attempts to measure quality of life in children and adolescents with IBD.[52–53] Despite this for many children with IBD, the decision to have an operation may revolve more around a quality-of-life issue than a medical one, and the surgeon must be patient and respectful while the child and family struggle to make these difficult choices.

THE TEAM APPROACH

The decision to operate on a child with IBD should be made by the child and family in collaboration with both the pediatric surgeon and the pediatric gastroenterologist, and with the help and support of social workers, nurse clinicians, psychologists, dieticians and other allied health professionals. It is helpful if the surgeon becomes involved in discussions with the family early in the process. This gives the surgeon the opportunity to educate the family with respect to risks and benefits of surgery, and permits a rapport to be established between the family and the surgeon. Having a surgeon consult with the family should not be considered as a "failure" on the part of the gastroenterologist. Ideally, the family should meet periodically with the team as a whole to ensure that the information being transmitted to the child, and family is consistent and clear.

REFERENCES

1. Reese GE, Constantinides VA, Simillis C, et al. Diagnostic precision of anti-*Saccharomyces cerevisiae* antibodies and perinuclear antineutrophil cytoplasmic antibodies in inflammatory bowel disease. Am J Gastroenterol 2006;101:2410–22.
2. Post P, Betzler M, von Ditfurth B, et al. Risks of intestinal anastomoses in Crohn's disease. Ann Surg 1991;213:37–42.
3. Griffiths AM, Ohlsson A, Sherman PM, Sutherland LR. Meta-analysis of enteral nutrition as a primary treatment of active Crohn's disease. Gastroenterology 1995;108:1056–67.
4. Blair GK, Yaman M, Wesson DE. Preoperative home elemental enteral nutrition in complicated Crohn's disease. J Pediatr Surg 1986;21:769–71.
5. Nguyen GC, Harris ML, Dassopoulos T. Insights in immunomodulatory therapies for ulcerative colitis and Crohn's disease. Curr Gastroenterol Rep 2006;8:499–505.
6. Greifer MK, Markowitz JF. Update in the treatment of paediatric ulcerative colitis. Expert Opin Pharmacother 2006;7:1907–18.
7. Heimann TM, Greenstein AJ, Lewis B, et al. Prediction of early symptomatic recurrence after intestinal resection in Crohn's disease. Ann Surg 1993;218:294–99.
8. Diamond IR, Langer JC. Laparoscopic-assisted vs open ileocolic resection for pediatric Crohn disease. J Pediatr Gastroent Nutr 2001;33:543–47.
9. Tilney HS, Constantinides VA, Heriot AG, et al. Comparison of laparoscopic and open ileocecal resection for Crohn's disease: A metaanalysis. Surg Endosc 2006;20:1036–44.
10. Oliva L, Wyllie R, Alexander F, et al. The results of strictureplasty in pediatric patients with multifocal Crohn's disease. J Pediatr Gastroent Nutr 1994;18:306–10.
11. Fearnhead NS, Chowdhury R, Box B, et al. Long-term follow-up of strictureplasty for Crohn's disease. Br J Surg 2006;93:475–82.
12. Bewtra M, Lichtenstein GR. Infliximab use in Crohn's disease. Expert Opin Biol Ther 2005;5:589–99.
13. Thornton M, Solomon MJ. Long-term indwelling seton for complex anal fistulas in Crohn's disease. Dis Colon Rectum 2005;48:459–63.
14. Pettit SH, Irving MH. The operative management of fistulous Crohn's disease. Surg Gynecol Obstet 1988;167:223–8.
15. Sandborn WJ, Hanauer SB. Infliximab in the treatment of Crohn's disease: A user's guide for clinicians. Am J Gastroenterol 2002;97:2962–72.
16. Yamamoto T, Bain IM, Connolly AB, Keighley MR. Gastroduodenal fistulas in Crohn's disease: Clinical features and management. Dis Colon Rectum 1998;41:1287–92.
17. Tekkis PP, Purkayastha S, Lanitis S, et al. A comparison of segmental vs subtotal/total colectomy for colonic Crohn's disease: A meta-analysis. Colorectal Dis 2006;8:82–90.
18. Martin LW. Current surgical management of patients with chronic ulcerative colitis. J Pediatr Gastroenterol Nutr 1993;17:121–31.
19. Reese GE, Lovegrove RE, Tilney HS, et al. The effect of crohn's disease on outcomes after restorative proctocolectomy. Dis Colon Rectum 2006;50:239–50
20. Goligher JC. The outcome of excisional operations for primary and recurrent Crohn's disease of the large intestine. Surg Gynecol Obstet 1979;148:1–8.
21. Fry PD, Atkinson KG. Current surgical approach to toxic megacolon. Surg, Gynecol Obst 1976;143:26–30.
22. Jarvinen HJ, Makitie A, Sivula A. Long-term results of continent ileostomy. Int J Colorectal Dis 1986;1:40–43.
23. Gorfine SR, Gelernt IM, Bauer JJ, et al. Restorative proctocolectomy without diverting ileostomy. Dis Colon Rectum 1995;38:188–94.
24. Williamson ME, Lewis WG, Sagar PM, et al. One-stage restorative proctocolectomy without temporary ileostomy for ulcerative colitis: A note of caution. Dis Colon Rectum 1997;40:1019–22.
25. Morgan RA, Manning PB, Coran AG. Experience with the straight endorectal pullthrough for the management of ulcer-

ative colitis and familial polyposis in children and adults. Ann Surg 1987;206:595–99.
26. Rintala RJ, Lindahl HG. Restorative proctocolectomy for ulcerative colitis in children—is the J-pouch better than straight pull-through? J Pediatr Surg 1996;31:530–3.
27. Fonkalsrud EW. Long-term results after colectomy and ileoanal pull-through procedure in children. Arch Surg 1996;131:881–6.
28. Coran AG. A personal experience with 100 consecutive total colectomies and straight ileoanal endorectal pull-throughs for benign disease of the colon and rectum in children and adults. Ann Surg 1990;212:242–7
29. Tilney HS, Constantinides V, Ioannides AS, et al. Pouch-anal anastomosis vs straight ileoanal anastomosis in pediatric patients: A meta-analysis. J Pediatr Surg 2006;41:1799–808.
30. Davis C, Alexander F, Lavery I, Fazio VW. Results of mucosal proctectomy versus extrarectal dissection for ulcerative colitis and familial polyposis in children and young adults. J Pediatr Surg 1994;29:305–09.
31. Alexander F, Sarigol S, Difiore J, et al. Fate of the pouch in 151 pediatric patients after ileal pouch anal anastomosis. J Pediatr Surg 2003;38:78–82.
32. Tekkis PP, Heriot AG, Smith O, et al. Long-term outcomes of restorative proctocolectomy for Crohn's disease and indeterminate colitis. Colorectal Dis 2005;7:218–23.
33. Tan JJ, Tjandra JJ. Laparoscopic surgery for ulcerative colitis—a meta-analysis. Colorectal Dis 2006;8:626–36.
34. Proctor ML, Langer JC, Gerstle JT, Kim PCW. Is laparoscopic subtotal colectomy better than open subtotal colectomy in children? J Pediatr Surg 2002;37:706–8.
35. Garrard CL, Clements RH, Nanney L, et al. Adhesion formation is reduced after laparoscopic surgery. Surg Endosc 1999;13:10–3.
36. Dendrinos KG, Becker JM, Stucchi AF, et al. Anti-*Saccharomyces cerevisiae* antibodies are associated with the development of postoperative fistulas following ileal pouch-anal anastomosis. J Gastrointest Surg 2006;10:1060–4.
37. Trnka YM, Glotzer DJ, Kasdon EJ, et al. The long-term outcome of restorative operation in Crohn's disease. Ann Surg 1982;196:345–55.
38. Sachar DB. Maintenance therapy in ulcerative colitis and Crohn's disease. J Clin Gastroenterol 1995;20:117–22.
39. Ferlitsch A, Reinisch W, Puspok A, et al. Safety and efficacy of endoscopic balloon dilation for treatment of Crohn's disease strictures. Endoscopy 2006;38:483–7.
40. Sandborn WJ. Pouchitis following ileal pouch-anal anastomosis: Definition, pathogenesis, and treatment. Gastroenterol 1994;107:1856–60.
41. Perrault J. Pouchitis in children: Therapeutic options. Curr Treat Options Gastroenterol 2002;5:389–97.
42. Romano M, Cuomo A, Tuccillo C, et al. Vascular endothelial growth factor and cyclooxygenase-2 are overexpressed in ileal pouch-anal anastomosis. Dis Colon Rectum 2007;50:650–9.
43. Ewaschuk JB, Tejpar QZ, Soo I, et al. The role of antibiotic and probiotic therapies in current and future management of inflammatory bowel disease. Curr Gastroenterol Rep 2006;8:486–98.
44. Fazio VW, Ziv Y, Church JM, et al. Ileal pouch-anal anastomoses: Complications and function in 1005 patients. Ann Surg 1995;222:120–7.
45. Ecker KW, Haberer M, Feifel G. Conversion of the failing ileoanal pouch to reservoir-ileostomy rather than to ileostomy alone. Dis Colon Rectum 1996;39:977–80.
46. Sherkin-Langer F. If This Is a Test, Have I Passed Yet? Toronto, Ontario: MacMillan; 1994.
47. Irvine EJ, Feagan B, Rochon J, et al. Quality of life: A valid and reliable measure of therapeutic efficacy in the treatment of inflammatory bowel disease. Canadian Crohn's Relapse Prevention Trial Study Group. Gastroenterology 1994;106:287–96.
48. Konig HH, Ulshofer A, Gregor M, et al. Validation of the EuroQol questionnaire in patients with inflammatory bowel disease. Eur J Gastroenterol Hepatol 2002;14:1205–15.
49. McLeod RS, Baxter NN. Quality of life of patients with inflammatory bowel disease after surgery. World J Surg 1998;22:375–81.
50. Sarigol S, Caulfield M, Wyllie R, et al. Ileal pouch-anal anastomosis in children with ulcerative colitis. Inflam Bowel Dis 1996;2:82–7.
51. Lichtenstein GR, Cohen R, Yamashita B, Diamond RH. Quality of life after proctocolectomy with ileoanal anastomosis for patients with ulcerative colitis. J Clin Gastroenterol 2006;40:669–77.
52. Griffiths AM, Nicholas D, Smith C, et al. Development of a quality-of-life index for pediatric inflammatory bowel disease: Dealing with differences related to age and IBD type. J Pediatr Gastroenterol Nutr 1999;28:S46–52.
53. Otley AR, Griffiths AM, Hale S, et al. Health-related quality of life in the first year after a diagnosis of pediatric inflammatory bowel disease. Inflamm Bowel Dis 2006;12:684–91.

20.6. Eosinophilic Gastrointestinal Diseases

Glenn T. Furuta, MD
Chris Liacouras, MD

The last decade brought a remarkable surge of interest in the eosinophil and its role in gastrointestinal disease. Multiple factors contributed to this rising interest including increasing clinical recognition of the diseases and rising prevalence of allergic intestinal diseases. Disease recognition surged due to a number of factors including heightened awareness amongst pediatric and adult providers, advocacy by parents and patient interest groups and basic, translational, and clinical research performed by multidisciplinary specialists. The atopic march that encompassed primarily lung and skin diseases seems to have continued its journey into the gastrointestinal tract; potential reasons for this expansion include the hygiene hypothesis, antiacid use, changing allergen exposure, pollution as well as recent evidence supporting global warming. Regardless of the reasons, clinicians are faced with increasing challenges to care for affected patients and researchers are challenged with attacking focused questions to improve the quality of patient care.

EOSINOPHIL LIFE CYCLE

Eosinophils are born in the bone marrow from pluripotent stem cells under the regulation of IL-3, IL-5, and GM-CSF; their biology has been reviewed completely in the recent review articles.[1,2] The development and differentiation of eosinophils is mainly governed by IL-5 as evidenced by the facts that IL-5 null mice develop significantly less eosinophilia, and transgenic IL-5 mice develop heightened eosinophilic inflammatory response. Eosinophils are also impacted by IL-4 and IL-13, two cytokines that increase eosinophil recruitment and survival thru inducing expression of eotaxin and endothelial ligands ICAM-1 and VCAM-1. Eotaxin-1, -2, and -3 are additional cytokines critical to eosinophil survival.[3] These cytokines bind to the CCR3 receptor, a seven transmembrane spanning G-protein coupled receptor expressed on eosinophils. Eotaxin is expressed in resident tissue cells such as epithelium and fibroblasts and is increased in specific disease states including inflammatory bowel disease. Murine studies suggest that eotaxin-1 is one of the critical molecules necessary for maintaining baseline levels and that it also participates in eosinophil recruitment during gastric and small intestinal inflammation.[4] When eosinophils leave the bone marrow and migrate through the vascular space, they are beckoned to the lamina propria in varying degrees during both health and disease. These findings suggest a potential impact of an anti-CCR3 antibody in certain allergic diseases.

Except for in the esophagus, eosinophils normally reside in the healthy GI tract.[5,6] Esophageal eosinophilia is always abnormal and this finding generally suggests a diagnosis of gastroesophageal reflux disease (GERD) or eosinophilic esophagitis (EE) depending upon the proper clinical setting. They are present in the healthy stomach and then gradually increase in number with a peak concentration in the cecum and ileum. During disease states, eosinophils increase and migrate into the intraepithelial spaces, lamina propria and crypts. (see Table 1).

EOSINOPHILIC ESOPHAGITIS

During the last decade, interest in EE has undergone a remarkable transformation. Once thought to be merely a clinical curiosity, an increasing body of clinical experience and research studies has now transformed EE into a well-defined clinicopathological disease. A number of factors sparked this interest including increasing incidence, improved recognition and rise in atopic diseases in general. Parallel with this surge in interest, a number of important questions have developed. What is the definition, natural history, best surveillance of the disease? What is the optimal method to care for patients; simple observation without treatment, pharmacotherapy, nutritional restriction or a treatment yet to be defined?

Definition

In an effort to address many of these questions, a multidisciplinary group of adult and pediatric gastroenterologists, allergists, immunologists, and pathologists gathered to develop recommendations for care of patients with EE at The First International Gastrointestinal Eosinophil Research Symposium at Orlando, Florida in October 2006 (http://www.naspghan.org for slide set of program). This group set forth a working definition/diagnostic criteria for EE based on the best available evidence and expert opinion. EE is a clinicopathological disease requiring clinical symptoms and isolated esophageal eosinophilia manifested by 15 or greater intraepithelial eosinophils in the most densely involved high power microscopic field (400×) (see Figure 1). GERD should be ruled out as a potential cause for esophageal eosinophilia with either a trial of proton pump inhibition or pH monitoring of the distal esophagus. Gastric and duodenal mucosal biopsies must be normal.

EE has also been termed by a number of different names including eosinophilic oesophagitis, primary eosinophilic esophagitis, allergic eosinophilic esophagitis, and idiopathic eosinophilic esophagitis. For the purposes of this chapter, the name eosinophilic esophagitis will be used.

CLINICAL PRESENTATION

Approximately 75% of all patients with EE are males with a mean age in children of 8 years. Case reports have identified patients in all continents except Africa. Noel et al estimates a disease an incidence of ~1:10,000 children per year in Ohio, United States,[7] while Straumann et al estimated an increase from 2 to 27 per 100,000 adults in Olten, Switzerland.[8]

Table 1 Differential Diagnosis for Gastrointestinal Eosinophilia	
Esophageal Eosinophilia	**Gastrointestinal Eosinophilia**
Gastroesophageal reflux disease	Inflammatory bowel disease
Crohn's disease	Food hypersensitivity
Eosinophilic esophagitis	Eosinophilic gastroenteritis
Eosinophilic gastroenteritis	Celiac disease
Connective tissue disease Hypereosinophilic syndrome Infection— Herpes virus, Candida Drug hypersensitivity response	Infection—*Anisakiasis, Helicobacter pylori, Enterobious vermicularis, Basidiobolomycosis, Schistomiasis, Toxacara canis, Ancylostoma duodenale*
	Malignancy
	Churg Strauss syndrome
	Systemic lupus erythematosis

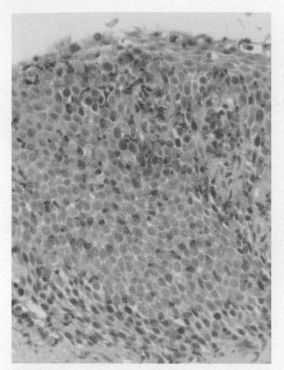

Figure 1 Photomicrograph of esophageal mucosa. Esophageal epithelium infiltrated with eosinophils and eosinophilic microabscess.

Children with EE present with at least three distinct clinical scenarios (Table 2). First, the infant or toddler may present with feeding intolerance. Second, the patients of any age may present with GERD-like symptoms that are unresponsive to acid blockade. These symptoms include vomiting, regurgitation, water brash, epigastric abdominal pain, heartburn, or chest pain. Finally, older children, teenagers, and adults may present with intermittent or chronic dysphagia or acute food impaction. Whenever a child or adult presents emergently for evaluation of a food impaction, especially if they have a history of allergic diseases or peripheral eosinophilia, strong consideration should be given to the diagnosis of EE.

Several studies have described children with EE who presented with GERD-like symptoms unresponsive to acid blockade. For instance, Kelly et al studied 10 patients, all of whom had symptoms of severe GERD, 6 of whom remained symptomatic despite fundoplication.[9] Subsequently, Orenstein performed a detailed analysis of 30 children with esophageal eosinophilia who presented with vomiting, abdominal pain, and dysphagia.[10] Many of these patients (62%) had concomitant airway symptoms including asthma, recurrent upper respiratory illnesses, and pneumonias providing support for the speculation that EE and airway diseases are related. In the largest series of patients reported to date by Liacouras, 381 children with EE were studied.[11] Of these, 312 patients had symptoms of similar to GERD while 69 presented with dysphagia.

Esophageal food impaction due to EE can occur secondary to a fixed anatomical stricture, esophageal edema or intermittent esophageal spasm (discussed further in "Pathophysiology" section). In this regard, two adult studies suggested that EE is a common etiology for esophageal food impaction. Desai et al reported that 17 of 31 adult patients presenting with an acute esophageal food impaction had >20 eosinophils per HPF.[12] Similarly, Byrne observed that a significant number of patients who presented with a food impaction eventually received the diagnosis EE.[13]

NATURAL HISTORY

To date, the only documented long-term complication associated with EE is isolated or long segment esophageal narrowing. Adult and pediatric reports have identified evidence of tissue remodeling in the form of proximal and distal esophageal strictures.[14–16] Typically, symptoms in these patients date back to childhood suggesting lesions required decades of ongoing or intermittent inflammation. Basic studies provide a link between fibrotic cascades and eosinophil-derived mediators. Eosinophils contain mediators capable of both inducing fibrotic molecules such as TGF-beta and stimulating tissue contraction such as major basic protein.[17,18] Similarly, Ngo et al suggested that eosinophil granule proteins induce intestinal epithelial contraction.[19] Aceves et al provided translational evidence supportive of a fibrotic pattern in affected children. In this study, five patients with EE and evidence of fibrosis were compared to two patients with nonfibrotic EE, seven with GERD and seven normal patients. Patients with fibrotic EE showed increased subepithelial fibrosis, TGF-beta, VCAM-1 and phospho-SMAD2/3 expression compared to GERD and normal control patients.

During the 14-year follow-up in adult patients with EE, esophageal cancer has not been reported (Straumann A, personal communication).[15,20,21]

RADIOLOGY

Radiologists were among the first to identify clinical features associated with EE (see Table 3). In 1981, Picus et al described a 16-year-old boy with an 18-month history of increasing dysphagia who also had peripheral eosinophilia.[22] His esophagram revealed an esophageal polyp and a 6 cm narrowing that spanned the proximal and middle esophagus. Histological assessment of the esophageal epithelium demonstrated large numbers of eosinophils. After 7 weeks of oral prednisone, he significantly improved however, a post-inflammatory stricture remained at the proximal end of the narrowing. Serial dilatation brought excellent results. In 1985, Feczko et al described three adults with dysphagia, allergic diseases, and eosinophilic esophageal inflammation.[23] Several long, irregular, proximal strictures, and esophageal polyps were found on a barium study. Dilatation and systemic corticosteroids successfully treated the patient's symptoms. Finally, Vitellas et al showed proximal and distal esophageal strictures in nine adults and one child. Symptom resolution occured with the use of corticosteroids.[24]

Two studies correlated endoscopic findings with radiological studies. In a retrospective study, Nurko et al observed that radiological abnormalities associated with EE may represent a transient finding rather than a fixed lesion.[25] The authors reviewed records of all children with radiographical evidence of a Schatzki ring seen over a 12-year period. Of the 18 children identified, 8 were found to have clinicopathological features of EE. Endoscopic records showed no evidence of a ring in the distal esophagus, suggesting that intermitent contraction of the distal esophagus was responsible for this radiographic finding. In 2005, Zimmerman et al characterized radiographic abnormalities in 14 patients with an average age of 41 years.[26] Symptoms ranged from dysphagia and food impaction to nonspecific symptoms of GERD. Proximal, middle, and distal strictures, sometimes segmental in distribution, were found in 10 patients. The strictures varied in length with a mean length of 5.1 cm and a maximum of 13 cm. A previously undescribed association of ringlike indentations was also visualized within the strictures. Indentations were described as multiple, closely spaced, fixed, concentric rings spanning the length of the stricture. The rings were not visualized during endoscopy in three patients again suggesting the occurrence of transient contractions. All strictures had tapered margins and 70% showed symmetric involvement. Medical treatment did not bring consistent improvement and dilatation only brought temporary relief; four patients underwent repeated dilatation. On the basis of these two studies, it is not certain whether radiological abnormalities represent esophageal remodeling secondary to chronic eosinophilic inflammation or dynamic contractions of the esophageal wall. Regardless, the radiological abnormality of esophageal narrowing, especially a proximal stricture, should raise suspicion for the diagnosis of EE.

Table 2 Symptoms Suggestive of Eosinophilic Esophagitis

Children	Adolescent and Adult
GERD symptoms unresponsive to medical/ surgical management	Dysphagia
Feeding intolerance/ difficulty Failure to thrive	Food/foreign body impaction
Food/foreign body impaction/dysphagia	GERD symptoms unresponsive to medical/ surgical management
Epigastric abdominal pain	

Table 3 Radiological Signs Associated with EE

Strictures—proximal, middle, and distal

Small caliber esophagus or longitudinal narrowing

Esophageal polyp

Esophageal diverticulum

Schatzki ring

Concentric rings

ENDOSCOPY

Early observations and clinical reports suggested that the endoscopic appearance of the esophageal mucosa of many patients with EE was normal. In fact, over a 10-year period, the endoscopic view of the esophagus was visually normal on endoscopy in over 30% of patients seen.[11] As experience has increased and photoimaging technology improved, many subtle and dramatic lesions have been associated with EE (see Table 4). Mucosal abnormalities include concentric ring formation (trachealization); longitudinal linear furrows or vertical lines of the esophageal mucosa; patches of small, white papules on the esophageal surface; and esophageal strictures. These observations emphasize the fact that close attention should be given to inspection of the esophageal mucosa and that visual findings are likely present on endoscopy in the majority of patients. Taken together, these studies and clinical experience suggests that whenever the diagnosis of EE is suspected, regardless of whether the mucosa appears normal or abnormal, esophageal biopsies should always be obtained.

One of the first mucosal abnormalities identified were whitish specks, exudates, nodules, or granular pattern originally thought to be due to an esophageal Candida infection (see Figure 2). This mucosal abnormality has been recognized as evidence of eosinophilic microabscess inflammation without evidence of Candida infection. Sundranam et al showed that the esophageal epithelium from 13 children diagnosed with EE had white specks containing between 25 to over 100 eosinophils per HPF without fungal elements.[27] Straumann et al provided further evidence that white exudates represented eosinophilic inflammation in an analysis of 30 adults with EE.[28] The density of eosinophil in biopsies obtained from white segments contained an average of 108 eosinophils per HPF whereas the nonwhite segments had an average of 14 eosinophils per HPF. The finding of white specks is not unique to EE as shown in two studies. Lim et al determined that of 153 children with eosinophilic esophageal inflammation, 92 had 15 or greater eosinophils per HPF.[29] Of these 153 children, 31 showed white lesions. Taken together with pH monitoring results, the data showed the identification of white lesions carried a sensitivity of 30% and specificity of 95% for the diagnosis of EE. Ngo et al described three patients with clinicopathological features consistent with EE which included large numbers of eosinophils

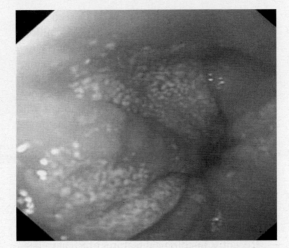

Figure 2 Endoscopic view of whitish exudates.

in the squamous epithelia; one patient had a whitish exudates.[30] After treatment with proton pump inhibition, all three resolved white exudates and eosinophilia suggesting that peptic disease was the etiological agent for the inflammatory response. Whether this finding holds true in older patients is not certain. Regardless, the finding of white material on the surface of the esophageal mucosa should invoke not only an assessment for Candida infection, but also a mucosal biopsy to investigate the possibility of the diagnosis of EE.

While no feature has been shown to be pathognomonic for EE, two lesions, the small caliber esophagus or longitudinally narrowed esophagus and the crepe paper esophagus or fragile mucosa have thus far only been reported in association with EE. Small caliber esophagus may be most apparent on a barium study in which esophageal contractions are absent and the length of the esophagus is fixed and narrowed.[20,31] Alternatively, at endoscopy, the length of the esophagus appears to be narrowed and has infrequent or diminished peristalsis. Vasilopoulos et al described five young men with dysphagia who had radiographic or endoscopic evidence of small-caliber esophagus.[32,33] Of the five, radiographic studies were interpreted as normal in two emphasizing the utility of endoscopic observations. Importantly, small caliber esophagus was suspected following dilatation with a bougie when a 17 cm longitudinal rent was found. In addition, crepe paper or fragile mucosa is most often observed following the passage of the endoscope or dilator when a longitudinal split is observed. Staumann et al described features of this finding and noted that splitting may extend from a few centimeters to nearly the entire length of the esophagus.[34] The depth of this tear is variable but typically does not appear to span the entire esophageal wall. Likely, these findings represent epithelial or subepithelial tissue remodeling but the underlying pathogenesis is unknown.

Several other endoscopic findings may also represent evidence of chronic inflammation. In addition to other causes, (congenital esophageal stricture, GERD, postsurgical scarring, and postinflammatory remodeling secondary to caus-

tic ingestions), esophageal strictures have now been strongly associated with EE; in particular, Siafakas et al and Khan et al demonstrated that when a proximal stricture is encountered, the diagnosis of EE should be strongly considered.[14,35] While these lesions are symptomatically responsive to treatment by dilatation, the underlying inflammation likely also requires therapy (see "Treatment" section). Distal esophageal rings can also be found in the association with EE, but the typical endoscopic appearance of a Schatzki ring may not be observed (see "Radiology" section).[25] Multiple concentric rings can be mistaken for either congenital esophageal rings, esophageal trachealization or feline esophagus.[36,37] Friability and ulceration, findings encountered frequently in severe GERD, are distinctly uncommon in EE. Instead, the mucosa affected by EE often reveals a whitish exudative pattern or a rubbery texture that in some patients is difficult to biopsy. What makes the mucosa transition from this appearance to the crepe paper or fragile mucosa is still not clear.

HISTOLOGY

Over the last decade, the histological pattern associated with EE continues to be the point of much discussion (see Table 5). In particular, conversations between clinician and pathologist often revolve around whether histological findings are consistent with EE or GERD. Complicating this discussion is the fact that, to date, no single histological feature is pathognomonic for EE or GERD. For instance, >15 eosinophils per high power field, eosinophilic microabscesses, superficial layering of eosinophils along the luminal epithelium, and basal cell hyperplasia have all been described in both GERD and EE, thus emphasizing the fact that the diagnosis of EE must be based on *clinical and histological* data.[30,38] If a patient has clinical symptoms, unresponsive to high dose acid blockade (or a normal pH monitoring study), and an isolated esophageal eosinophilia with >15 eosinophils per HPF one can be confident that the diagnosis of EE is correct.

At the First International Gastrointestinal Eosinophilic Research Symposium (FIGERS), a significant amount of effort was spent defining the exact number of eosinophils per HPF required to characterize EE. After much consideration of the published literature (prior to September 2006) and expert opinion, a threshold number of >15 eosinophils per HPF was chosen in order to

---

Table 4 Endoscopic Findings Associated with EE

Whitish exudates

Concentric rings, trachealization, feline esophagus

Strictures—proximal, middle, distal

Longitudinal furrows, vertical lines of the esophageal mucosa

Small caliber esophagus or longitudinal narrowing

Fragile or crepe paper mucosa, linear shearing of mucosa

Table 5 Histological Features Associated with EE

Greater than 15 eosinophils per HPF

Eosinophil microabscesses—greater than 4 eosinophils

Superficial layering of eosinophils

Severe basal zone hyperplasia

Eosinophil degranulation

Lymphocytosis—CD8+ predominant

Mast cell infiltration

identify the majority of suspected EE patients. During the course of this analysis, a large degree of variability was observed in the number of intraepithelial eosinophils used to make the diagnosis of EE. Five studies used >15 eosinophils per most densely involved HPF[20,25,39–41] and five used a mean number of >15 eosinophils from all fields.[28,42–45] In eight studies >20 eosinophils per most densely involved HPF was used as the threshold number[11,12,26,43,46–49]; two required >24 eosinophils per most densely involved HPF[50] one used a mean number from all fields[51]; and one study established a peak eosinophil count >30 eosinophils per HPF.[21] Taken together, the number 15 was chosen to increase the likelihood of identifying suspected patients again remembering that this histological data must be interpreted in the context of the clinical setting in which they were obtained.

Until the last decade, intraepithelial esophageal eosinophils were used primarily as a diagnostic criterion to make the histological diagnosis of GERD. Although a few reports identified large numbers of esophageal eosinophils in patients unresponsive to GERD treatment, it was not until 1985 when Lee et al reported a group of patients with >10 intraepithelial eosinophils per HPF who had no evidence of GERD.[52] Next, Attwood et al described a series of adults with dysphagia, normal pH monitoring of the distal esophagus, food hypersensitivity and >20 eosinophils per HPF.[48] All were treated with dilatation for symptom resolution. In 1994, Straumann et al reported very similar findings in 10 adults from Switzerland.[53] Many features such as white plaques and strictures were described in detail; in retrospect these are now readily accepted features of patients with EE but since this article was not published in English, it remains largely unrecognized.

In 1995, Kelly et al demonstrated that an amino acid based formula successfully treated 10 children with GERD symptoms who had esophageal eosinophilia and who were unresponsive to antireflux treatments consisting of pharmacotherapy and/or antireflux surgery.[9] A number of studies followed describing children and adults with dense esophageal eosinophilia (>15 to 20 per HPF), eosinophil microabscesses, superficial layering of eosinophils along the luminal surface, and marked basal zone hyperplasia. These patients had been unresponsive to acid blockade or had normal pH monitoring of the distal esophagus and were responsive to nutritional therapy or corticosteroid (systemic or topical) treatments. Ruchelli et al correlated the number of eosinophils with the likelihood of response to acid blockade.[54] When the number of intraepithelial eosinophils was greater than 7, there was an 86% predictive value for failure of acid treatment. Walsh et al compared histological findings of children whose symptoms were unresponsive to acid blockade and who had a normal pH monitoring of the distal esophagus with children with well-defined GERD.[38] Greater than 28 eosinophils per HPF, eosinophil microabscesses, and superficial layering of eosinophils

along the luminal surface were only seen in the non-GERD patients. In a study of 305 children, Steiner et al identified that patients with a low reflux index and an elevated esophageal eosinophil count likely had a nonacid cause for their inflammation.[44] In addition, the same group compared 27 children with GERD to 30 patients who had EE in order to determine if any histological features distinguished children with EE from those with GERD. Basal zone hyperplasia was significantly more severe in children with EE. Taken together, these studies show that children with symptoms intractable to GERD treatment and eosinophilic esophageal inflammation have a novel non-GERD inflammatory disease.

Recently, histological features of EE have been more closely examined in adult patients. Parfitt et al compared 157 adults with GERD or EE and showed that patients with EE were more likely to be male, present with dysphagia and display endoscopic evidence of mucosal rings.[55] Histological findings that were significantly more severe and representative of adults with EE included epithelial eosinophilia (mean = 39 HPF) basal zone hyperplasia, papillae elongation, lamina propria eosinophils, and lamina propria fibrosis. Gonsalves et al performed a retrospective study of 74 adults with EE to determine the optimal number of endoscopic mucosal biopsies to procure in order to make the diagnosis of EE.[56] Obtaining a single esophageal biopsy correlated with a sensitivity of 55% while obtaining five random esophageal biopsies increased the sensitivity to 100%. Comparisons between esophageal eosinophilia in the proximal (68 per HPF) and distal esophagus (82 per HPF) was not statistically significant.

Eosinophil degranulation represents another histologic feature that may distinguish EE from GERD. Mueller et al showed that specific immunohistochemical staining for eosinophil granule derived major basic protein (MBP) significantly enhanced the visualization of eosinophils in the mucosa of adults with EE.[57] Desai et al determined that extracellular deposition of MBP occurred significantly more in adults with EE compared to those with GERD.[12] Despite these findings, it is important to note that eosinophil degranulation can occur during biopsy procurement and processing. Lymphocyte infiltration is more significant in patients with EE compared to GERD with CD8 lymphocytes predominating.[42] As with other allergic diseases, mast cell infiltration and activation is more common in EE when compared to patients with GERD. Kirsch et al performed immunohistochemical staining on esophageal tissues from 25 children with EE, 22 with GERD, and 22 normal controls and found that patients with EE had significantly more mast cells and IgE bearing cells than in either of the other groups.[58] Interestingly, a subset of allergic patients with GERD also had increased IgE bearing cell suggesting an overlap syndrome.

The data described above are confounded by a number of technical issues that deserve comment. At FIGERS, the histopathology subcommittee determined that methodology for assessing

histopathological specimens was not standardized in studies reviewed. For instance, quantification of eosinophils per HPF reported was based on an number of factors including; numbers of HPFs counted, sizes of surface areas used for an individual HPF, and methods characterizing eosinophils. Some studies reported eosinophils in the most densely populated field, whereas others studies reported the mean number of eosinophils in five or more HPFs. Moreover, the surface areas evaluated differed by as much as threefold between different studies. Some studies included eosinophils if granules were present whereas other studies required presence of one lobe of a nucleus along with granules. In an effort to standardize diagnostic criteria and to simplify clinical assessments, the subcommittee suggested that eosinophils should be counted in the most densely populated HPF. In addition, in any research study, the surface area of the examined field should be reported as well as the criteria used for counting eosinophils.

PATHOPHYSIOLOGY

Three reports documented a familial trend for EE. Zink et al reported 17 patients from 7 families with dysphagia and gastrointestinal eosinophilia.[59] Of these, twelve patients spanning two generations were shown to have EE. Patel et al described three brothers with intermittent dysphagia and 20 to 40 eosinophils per HPF in the esophageal epithelium.[60] In a case report, Meyers documented an 80-year-old man and his 52-year-old daughter who both had dysphagia and >40 esophageal eos/HPF.[61]

Increasing clinical experience and these case descriptions suggest a familial pattern and genetic predisposition. As such, Blanchard et al hypothesized that a genetic profile existed for patients with EE.[50] Microarray analysis of esophageal tissues from patients with EE and GERD identified a unique EE gene signature with the most upregulated gene being eotaxin-3. Eotaxin-3 levels correlated with mucosal eosinophilia and a single nucleotide polymorphism suggested susceptibility to EE. The results of this study, and that of Mishra,[62] emphasizes the relevance for new therapeutic targets such as CCR-3 receptor or IL-5 antagonist, for selected patients with EE.[63]

The esophageal mucosa affected by EE has undergone further molecular characterization. Straumann et al determined that the esophageal eosinophils from EE patients expressed increased IL-4 and IL-13 compared to normal controls.[64] Gupta et al found that esophageal mRNA expression in 11 patients with EE expressed more that IFN-gamma, eotaxin-1, and IL-5 than normal children.[40]

TREATMENT

Decisions regarding the best approach to treat a disease are based on many different factors including the effectiveness of symptom control, prevention of complications, safety, compliance, treatment endpoints, and cost. Each of these areas poses problems for current treatment of EE. Effective maintenance medications have not been identified, long-term use of corticosteroid can lead to untoward side effects and compliance with severe nutritional restriction is difficult and can be costly. The question of treatment endpoints has already been addressed in research studies in which investigators typically seek normalization of esophageal eosinophilia as a marker of success. This approach raises issues for clinicians who may not decide that another endoscopy is indicated to determine histological success when a patient becomes asymptomatic. This practical approach may be reasonable but to date, knowledge regarding the long-term impact of chronic eosinophilic esophageal inflammation is not known. In particular, will strictures develop if eosinophilia persists, especially in an asymptomatic patient? Another troubling question is whether the negative aspects of chronic steroid use or nutritional restriction outweigh their benefit in children with EE who experience symptoms infrequently such as those who develop food impactions once a year and who are relatively well the rest of the time. Perhaps, detailed histories will uncover subtle symptoms suggestive of esophageal dysfunction in these patients. Assessment of patients has not been standardized, almost all treatment studies are open label format without comparison to control subjects and few natural history studies have been performed, thus making clinical decision making very difficult. Taking these factors into consideration, the approach to treatment of patients with EE should always be individualized, discussed in detail with parents and patients, and close follow-up established. Herein is a summary of the current literature focusing on available treatments followed by a brief treatment strategy.

NUTRITIONAL MANAGEMENT

Clinical observations and research studies suggest that food allergens cause eosinophilic inflammation.[4,65,66] Because of this, a number of studies have focused on the use of dietary therapy for the management of EE. Exclusive amino acid based formula diet, removal of specific foods based on allergy testing, or empirical restriction of commonly allergenic foods have all been shown to be effective in treating EE in children.

Kelly et al demonstrated the successful impact of an amino acid based diet in the treatment of EE.[9] In this study, 10 children were treated for 10 weeks with an amino acid based formula. All 10 showed clincopathological remission and redeveloped symptoms when the diet was extensively liberalized. Since then two other studies, by Markowitz and Liacouras, with a larger cohort of patients have shown that greater than 92% of children have been successfully induced and maintained with this form of treatment with symptom resolution during the first 7 to 10 days of therapy and histologic resolution within 4 weeks.[66,67] In the

past, poor compliance has stymied the oral intake of formula leading to the use of feeding tubes; the recent advances in formula development may reduce the necessity of this intervention.

Traditional methods to test for food sensitivity include RAST testing and IgE skin prick tests. Both tests have been found to be of limited value with uncertain predictive value in identifying food antigens responsible for eosinophilic esophageal inflammation.[42,66–68] An alternative method of testing, skin atopy patch tests, has been shown to be useful in identifying potential allergens.[65] Spergel et al used a combination of skin prick and skin atopy patch tests to determine food sensitivities in 146 children with EE. The results of this study showed that 77% of patients developed clinicopathological remission after removal of identified foods.

Kagalwalla et al utilized a different approach to nutritional management.[69] In this study, the six most common food allergens (eggs, soy, dairy, wheat, peanuts, fish, and shellfish), previously implicated as the cause for eosinophilic inflammation, were removed from the patient's diet without any form of allergy testing being performed. This elimination diet was compared to patients who received a strict amino acid based diet without any other added foods. Of the 35 children given the 6-food elimination diet, 74% achieved clinicopathological remission. Despite being successful, when compared to the use of a strict amino acid based formula, 88% of patients who received formula achieved remission with a significantly greater degree of esophageal eosinophilic reduction.

CORTICOSTEROIDS

In general, corticosteroids are effective in resolving clinicopathological features of EE. Potential mechanisms of action for corticosteroids impact in eosinophilic diseases include induction of eosinophil apoptosis, downregulation of chemotactic factors and inhibition of proinflammatory mediator synthesis and release. The main problems with the use of systemic corticosteroids are their detrimental side effects. An attractive alternative preparation is topical corticosteroids delivered from a metered dose inhaler (MDI) that allows the medication to be swallowed and applied to the esophageal mucosa. Since the quantity of steroid administered is significantly less than systemic steroids and the swallowed dose undergoes rapid hepatic metabolism, investigators hypothesize that the side effects should be minimal.

The positive impact of systemic steroids was shown in 1998 by Liacouras et al.[70] In 20 of 21 patients, the use of systemic corticosteroids significantly improved symptoms within 7 days. Current clinical experience suggests that when urgent symptom relief (ie, severe dysphagia leading to inability to eat or drink) is necessary, systemic corticosteroids should be considered. As discussed earlier (see "Endoscopy"

section), corticosteroids may be beneficial for patients with esophageal narrowing, but the exact patient population who will most benefit from this as opposed to esophageal dilation alone is not entirely certain.

Because of side effects associated with systemic corticosteroids, Faubion et al sought to limit steroid exposure with the use of topical fluticasone.[71] This novel method involved spraying a gavage of fluticasone from an MDI into the mouth without inhaling and without the use of a spacer. In their study, fluticasone propionate (up to 880 μg/d) or beclomethasone twice a day was prescribed to four patients with EE. All four patients demonstrated clinical improvement. Since then, four more studies have demonstrated a positive impact on clinicopathological features of EE in 47 adults and 33 children.[42,45,49,72] Pediatric studies used fluticasone propionate (220 to 440 μg twice daily) for 6 to 12 weeks. In contrast to pediatric studies, doses in adult studies ranged from 440 to 500 μg twice daily of fluticasone propionate and were administered for 4 to 6 weeks. Symptom relief was noted in all but one patient. In 2006, Konikoff et al performed a randomized double blind placebo controlled trial comparing the use of fluticasone to placebo in 36 pediatric patients.[68] The drug was given twice daily for 3 months and both the clinical and histologic response were measured. Although only 50% of the fluticasone group normalized their esophageal tissue, the trial demonstrated that the fluticasone group had significantly improved clinical symptoms as well as decreased esophageal eosinophils compared to the placebo group. In order to provide easier delivery of topical steroids to children, Aceves et al mixed a viscous preparation of budesonide.[73] Two children swallowed 500 μm of oral budesonide mixed in a sucralose suspension twice a day. Clinicopathological features normalized within 3 months of starting treatment.

Corticosteroids, whether systemic or topical, effectively resolve acute clinicopathological features of EE; however, when discontinued, EE generally recurs. Clinical experience and research studies support the fact that topical corticosteroids are the most effective pharmacologic therapy for EE. Patients should to spray the MDI in their mouth with lips sealed around the device and not eat, drink, or rinse for 30 minutes in an effort to prevent loss of the delivered dose. Because of their significant toxicity, the long-term use of systemic steroids is not recommended. On the other hand, topical corticosteroids have been utilized for a prolonged period of time in both pediatric and adult patients with EE. The main side effects reported to date have been minimal and include dry mouth epistaxis and esophageal candidiasis.

Leukotriene Receptor Antagonists

Cysteinyl leukotrienes have been theorized to participate in the esophageal inflammation and tissue eosinophilia that occurs in patients with EE. As such, two studies addressed the role of leukotriene receptor antagonists in the treatment of EE. Attwood et al treated eight adults with up to 100 mg of montelukast; seven developed clinical remission but histological sections showed no change in esophageal eosinophilia.[74] Treatment continued for 14 months and when stopped, six of eight redeveloped symptoms within 3 weeks. Reported side effects were minimal. In an effort to identify the role of leukotrienes in EE, Gupta et al measured esophageal mucosal levels of cysteinyl leukotrienes in children with EE and normal control.[75] Results demonstrated similar levels in both groups suggesting that in these patients this approach may not be effective. Additional studies examining receptor expression and alternative mechanisms will be necessary to investigate the viability of this treatment.

Cromolyn

Since mast cells are increased in tissues affected by EE, mast cell stabilizers have been used in some patients with EE. Liacouras et al treated 14 patients with 100 mg of oral cromolyn, four times daily for 1 month and found no impact on clinicopathological features.[11]

Proton Pump Inhibitors

Although gastric acid has not been shown to be the central mediator in the pathogenesis of EE, some investigators speculate on a "two-hit" hypothesis suggesting that in a allergic predispositioned host, the exposure of the esophageal epithelium to gastric acid may diminish its barrier function allowing instigating allergens to encounter the immunologically potent esophageal milieu. While this is an attractive hypothesis, clinical evidence suggests that inhibition of gastric acid production does not reduce eosinophilic inflammation.

Currently, there are two roles for PPIs in the care of patients with EE. When a child is suspected of having EE on the basis of presenting symptoms, GERD must be considered and ruled out either with pH monitoring of the distal esophagus or a trial of acid inhibition utilizing proton pump inhibitors.[30,38] If symptoms persist, a diagnostic endoscopy should be performed. Second, a subgroup of patients with well-established EE, who have achieved clinicopathological remission, may develop GERD like symptoms; ie, a patient may have both GERD and EE. In this circumstance, a PPI is often helpful in treating associated symptoms.

Esophageal Dilatation

Mechanical dilatation may be necessary for children with either isolated strictures or long segment narrowing. In fact, some patients may develop longitudinal tearing merely with the passage of the endoscope leading to improvement in symptoms (Fox V. personal communication). Dilatation as a treatment for EE has been addressed primarily in studies of adults. In Straumann's series of 11 EE patients with isolated strictures, 4 required repeat dilatation and no perforations were seen.[15] With more extensive lesions, the impact of dilatation may be more profound. Five patients with small caliber esophagus who received esophageal bougienage were reported by Vasilopoulos.[32,33] All patients were improved postdilatation, but two patients developed significant chest pain from esophageal tearing that required overnight hospitalization. Nurko et al reported that five of seven children with EE experienced complete symptom relief following dilatation.[25] Taken together, between 7 and 50% of patients require repeat dilatation suggesting ongoing inflammation or esophageal remodeling that led to severe esophageal dysfunction.

NOVEL BIOLOGICALS

Basic and translational studies provide strong support for the use of monoclonal antibodies such as anti-interleukin 5 (anti-IL-5). These molecules target the IL-5 receptors on eosinophils thus influencing their production, migration, and activation.[76] In support of this approach are murine studies in which the use of anti-IL-5 antibodies or IL-5 gene deletion inhibits esophageal eosinophilic inflammation.[62] Two clinical reports provide further evidence for a positive impact of anti-IL-5 in patients with EE. Garrett et al reported that the use of intravenous anti-IL-5 led to clinicopathological remission in an adolescent male with subsequent improvement in his severe dysphagia and esophageal eosinophilia after 3 months of treatment.[77] Recently, Stein et al utilized successive monthly infusions in four patients with clinicopathologic features of EE.[78] All four patients demonstrated significant improvement in their clinical and histologic abnormalities. The role of these biologicals in the treatment of EE awaits future definition.

TREATMENT SUMMARY

Treatment goals for patients with EE include symptom resolution and prevention of long-term complications with a minimal impact on lifestyle. To date, nutritional therapy and corticosteroids have been shown to resolve symptoms and normalize tissue eosinophilia in patients with EE. Unfortunately, the incidence of complications of EE, such as esophageal strictures and esophageal narrowing, is unknown and predictive markers are not available making decisions regarding maintenance management and monitoring difficult. In this light, using a treatment endpoint of histological remission, as in the case of previous research studies, may be the best current option in an effort to minimize chronic complications. Whether this is the best indicator for long-term outcomes is not yet known and will certainly be a question for future studies. Thus, what is a reasonable treatment strategy? At FIGERS, the following suggested approach was proposed. "Treatment should be initially aimed at improving symptoms. In those with persistent esophageal eosinophilia, the decision to advance treatment should be based upon the degree of symptoms, age of the patient, the presence of esophageal morphologic abnormalities, results of monitoring and the patient's and family's values and preferences."

EOSINOPHILIC GASTROENTERITIS

Eosinophilic gastroenteritis (EOG) is a heterogeneous group of rare diseases that are characterized by a wide variety of intestinal symptoms and histological evidence of gastrointestinal eosinophilia. Other causes of intestinal eosinophilia must have been addressed and excluded before a diagnosis of EOG can be made (see Table 1). Traditional classification strategies for EOG grouped patients in three categories: mucosal, muscular, and serial eosinophilic gastroenteritis. This schematic provides a useful clinical and pathophysiological method to think about the affected patient. Most patients with EOG have mucosal disease characterized by signs and symptoms including, but not limited to, abdominal pain and diarrhea. Abdominal pain is typically nondescript but can be severe and debilitating; in fact, patients can present with intestinal obstruction and sometimes perforation.[79,80] Patients often complain of loose nonbloody stools ranging from a one to several each day. Perplexing to these patients is the fact that their symptoms can be quite minor compared to the significantly abnormal associated laboratory abnormalities. For instance, it is not unusual to discover severe anemia and/or hypoalbuminemia in some patients.[81-84] Peripheral eosinophilia may be present[85] but if it persists despite adequate treatment, hypereosinophilic syndrome or malignancy should be investigated. Radiological findings include mucosal thickening and edema, ulcerations, and polyps.[24,86] Endoscopic views may reveal similar findings along with friability. Muscular EOG is associated with vomiting and bloating, symptoms of partial or complete intestinal obstruction.[79] Patients may have normal mucosal biopsies with the only hint of an inflammatory disease being related to peripheral eosinophilia, intestinal thickening on radiological imaging or a response to corticosteroids or dietary elimination. When performed, a full thickness biopsy reveals muscular eosinophilia. Finally, serosal EOG is extremely rare and typically presents with abdominal bloating and a fluid wave on physical examination. Analysis of the ascitic fluid reveals eosinophilia. Patients do not have associated liver disease.

Patients receiving organ transplantation are another recently described group of patients with eosinophilic gastrointestinal inflammation. Following transplant and the use of tacrolimus, patients develop severe diarrhea and significant eosinophilic inflammation of the small bowel.[87,88] To date, no studies have definitively etiologically linked inflammation and the use of this medication but an association has been made.

The pathophysiology of EOG is still unclear with clinical studies being limited to immunohistochemical descriptions. Patient's biopsies demonstrate deposition of eosinophil granule proteins and increased expression of IL-5.[89–91] Chehade identified increased mast cells in the small intestine affected by EOG in children with severe protein losing enteropathy.[83] Murine studies have identified critical roles for eotaxin-1 and Th2 lymphocytes in the pathogenesis of gastric and intestinal eosinophilic inflammation.[4,92]

To date, no standardized criteria have been developed defining histological features of EOGs. Two studies have defined normal values for the number of eosinophils in the intestinal mucosa but no specific effort has developed diagnostic guidelines. Corticosteroids form the mainstay of treatment for EOGs; because so few patients exist, controlled trials have not been performed yet.[93] Most patients quickly respond to systemic corticosteroid treatment. Topical steroids in the form of budesonide has been beneficial in one male with jejunal muscular disease who first received surgery and systemic steroids followed by budesonide[94] and another woman with mucosal duodenal and ileal disease.[81] Ketotifen, cromolyn, and montelukast have been reported to be helpful in case reports.[95–98] Newer biological agents show potential in treating EOGs; these agents include anti-IL-5 and anti-IgE antibodies.[99]

SUMMARY

The field of gastrointestinal eosinophilic diseases has made great strides during the last decade to improve the health of affected patients particularly with respect to EE. This is no longer an "emerging" disease but rather one that has become well recognized and awaits further study as to its pathogenesis, natural history, and development of suitable treatment strategy and surveillance plan[100] (see Table 6). In addition, more information will be learned about the association of eosinophils to allergic intestinal diseases and further characterization of diagnostic and histopathological features of EGIDs. Multicentered studies with collaborative efforts between pediatric and adult gastroenterologists, allergist, pathologists, and radiologists will provide answers to improve the quality of life of patients with EGIDS.

Table 6 EGID Research Areas for Multicenter, Multidisciplinary Studies

Pathogenetic mechanisms

Etiological agents

Quality of life

Diagnostic criteria

Histological characterization

Noninvasive markers

Treatment endpoints

Maintenance treatments

Natural history

Surveillance

REFERENCES

1. Hogan SP, Rothenberg ME. Eosinophil function in eosinophil-associated gastrointestinal disorders. Curr Allergy Asthma Rep 2006;6:65–71.
2. Lamouse-Smith ES, Furuta GT. Eosinophils in the gastrointestinal tract. Curr Gastroenterol Rep 2006;8:390–5.
3. Rothenberg ME. Eotaxin. An essential mediator of eosinophil trafficking into mucosal tissues. Am J Respir Cell Mol Biol 1999;21:291–5.
4. Hogan SP, Mishra A, Brandt EB, et al. A critical role for eotaxin in experimental oral antigen-induced eosinophilic gastrointestinal allergy. Proc Natl Acad Sci U S A 2000;97:6681–6.
5. Lowichik A, Weinberg A. A quantitative evaluation of mucosal eosinophils in the pediatric gastrointestinal tract. Mod Pathol 1996;9:110–4.
6. DeBrosse CW, Case JW, Putnam PE, et al. Quantity and distribution of eosinophils in the gastrointestinal tract of children. Pediatr Dev Pathol 2006;9:210–8.
7. Noel RJ, Putnam PE, Rothenberg ME. Eosinophilic esophagitis. N Engl J Med 2004;351:940–1.
8. Straumann A, Simon HU. Eosinophilic esophagitis: Escalating epidemiology? J Allergy Clin Immunol 2005;115:418–9.
9. Kelly KJ, Lazenby AJ, Rowe PC, et al. Eosinophilic esophagitis attributed to gastroesophageal reflux: Improvement with an amino acid-based formula. Gastroenterology 1995;109:1503–12.
10. Orenstein SR, Shalaby TM, Di Lorenzo C, et al. The spectrum of pediatric eosinophilic esophagitis beyond infancy: A clinical series of 30 children. Am J Gastroenterol 2000;95:1422–30.
11. Liacouras CA, Spergel JM, Ruchelli E, et al. Eosinophilic esophagitis: A 10-year experience in 381 children. Clin Gastroenterol Hepatol 2005;3:1198–206.
12. Desai TK, Stecevic V, Chang CH, et al. Association of eosinophilic inflammation with esophageal food impaction in adults. Gastrointest Endosc 2005;61:795–801.
13. Byrne KR, Panagiotakis PH, Hilden K, et al. Retrospective analysis of esophageal food impaction: Differences in etiology by age and gender. Dig Dis Sci 2007;52:717–21.
14. Khan S, Orenstein SR, Di Lorenzo C, et al. Eosinophilic esophagitis: Strictures, impactions, dysphagia. Dig Dis Sci 2003;48:22–9.
15. Straumann A, Spichtin HP, Grize L, et al. Natural history of primary eosinophilic esophagitis: A follow-up of 30 adult patients for up to 11.5 years. Gastroenterology 2003;125:1660–9.
16. Aceves SS, Newbury RO, Dohil R, et al. Esophageal remodeling in pediatric eosinophilic esophagitis. J Allergy Clin Immunol 2007;119:206–12.
17. Rochester CL, Ackerman SJ, Zheng T, Elias JA. Eosinophil-fibroblast interactions. Granule major basic protein interacts with IL-1 and transforming growth factor-beta in the stimulation of lung fibroblast IL-6-type cytokine production. J Immunol 1996;156:4449–56.
18. Levi-Schaffer F, Garbuzenko E, Rubin A, et al. Human eosinophils regulate human lung- and skin-derived fibroblast properties in vitro: A role for transforming growth factor beta (TGF-beta). Proc Natl Acad Sci U S A 1999;96:9660–5.
19. Ngo P, MacLeod R, Ramalinga P, et al. Eosinophil granule proteins stimulate intestinal epithelial cell collagen contraction via calcium-sensing receptor activation. Gastroenterology 2006;130:A89.
20. Potter JW, Saeian K, Staff D, et al. Eosinophilic esophagitis in adults: An emerging problem with unique esophageal features. Gastrointest Endosc 2004;59:355–61.
21. Croese J, Fairley SK, Masson JW, et al. Clinical and endoscopic features of eosinophilic esophagitis in adults. Gastrointest Endosc 2003;58:516–22.
22. Picus D, Frank PH. Eosinophilic esophagitis. AJR Am J Roentgenol 1981;136:1001–3.
23. Feczko P, Halpert R, Zonca M. Radiographic abnormalities in eosinophilic esophagitis. Gastrointest Radiol 1985;10:321–4.
24. Vitellas KM, Bennett WF, Bova JG, et al. Radiographic manifestations of eosinophilic gastroenteritis. Abdom Imaging 1995;20:406–13.
25. Nurko S, Teitelbaum JE, Husain K, et al. Association of Schatzki ring with eosinophilic esophagitis in children. J Pediatr Gastroenterol Nutr 2004;38:436–41.
26. Zimmerman SL, Levine MS, Rubesin SE, et al. Idiopathic eosinophilic esophagitis in adults: The ringed esophagus. Radiology 2005;236:159–65.
27. Sundaram S, Sunku B, Nelson SP, et al. Adherent white plaques: An endoscopic finding in eosinophilic esophagitis. J Pediatr Gastroenterol Nutr 2004;38:208–12.
28. Straumann A, Spichtin HP, Bucher KA, et al. Eosinophilic esophagitis: Red on microscopy, white on endoscopy. Digestion 2004;70:109–16.
29. Lim JR, Gupta SK, Croffie JM, et al. White specks in the esophageal mucosa: An endoscopic manifestation of non-reflux eosinophilic esophagitis in children. Gastrointest Endosc 2004;59:835–8.
30. Ngo P, Furuta GT, Antonioli DA, Fox VL. Eosinophils in the esophagus—peptic or allergic eosinophilic esophagitis? Case series of three patients with esophageal eosinophilia. Am J Gastroenterol 2006;101:1666–70.
31. Furuta K, Adachi K, Kowari K, et al. A Japanese case of eosinophilic esophagitis. J Gastroenterol 2006;41:706–10.
32. Vasilopoulos S, Shaker R. Defiant dysphagia; Small-caliber esophagus and refractory benign esophageal strictures. Curr Gastroenterol Rep 2001;3:225–30.
33. Vasilopoulos S, Murphy P, Auerbach A, et al. The small-caliber esophagus: An unappreciated cause of dysphagia for solids in patients with eosinophilic esophagitis. Gastrointest Endosc 2002;55:99–106.
34. Straumann A, Rossi L, Simon HU, et al. Fragility of the esophageal mucosa: A pathognomonic endoscopic sign of primary eosinophilic esophagitis? Gastrointest Endosc 2003;57:407–12.
35. Siafakas CG, Ryan CK, Brown MR, Miller TL. Multiple esophageal rings: An association with eosinophilic esophagitis: Case report and review of the literature. Am J Gastroenterol 2000;95:1572–5.
36. Morrow JB, Vargo JJ, Goldblum JR, Richter JE. The ringed esophagus: Histological features of GERD. Am J Gastroenterol 2001;96:984–9.
37. Bonis PA. Ringed esophagus: Unclear relationship to gastroesophageal reflux disease. Am J Gastroenterol 2001;96:3439; discussion 3440–1.
38. Walsh S, Antonioli D, Goldman H, et al. Allergic esophagitis in children-A clinicopathological entity. Am J Surg Pathol 1999;23:390–6.
39. Lucendo Villarin AJ, Carrion Alonso G, Navarro Sanchez M, et al. Eosinophilic esophagitis in adults, an emerging cause of dysphagia. Description of 9 cases. Rev Esp Enferm Dig 2005;97:229–39.
40. Gupta SK, Fitzgerald JF, Kondratyuk T, HogenEsch H. Cytokine expression in normal and inflamed esophageal mucosa: A study into the pathogenesis of allergic eosinophilic esophagitis. J Pediatr Gastroenterol Nutr 2006;42:22–6.
41. Fox VL, Nurko S, Teitelbaum JE, et al. High-resolution EUS in children with eosinophilic "allergic" esophagitis. Gastrointest Endosc 2003;57:30–6.
42. Teitelbaum J, Fox V, Twarog F, et al. Eosinophilic esophagitis in children: Immunopathological analysis and response to fluticasone propionate. Gastroenterology 2002;122:1216–25.
43. Steiner SJ, Kernek KM, Fitzgerald JF. Severity of basal cell hyperplasia differs in reflux versus eosinophilic esophagitis. J Pediatr Gastroenterol Nutr 2006;42:506–9.
44. Steiner SJ, Gupta SK, Croffie JM, Fitzgerald JF. Correlation between number of eosinophils and reflux index on same day esophageal biopsy and 24 hour esophageal pH monitoring. Am J Gastroenterol 2004;99:801–5.
45. Remedios M, Campbell C, Jones DM, Kerlin P. Eosinophilic esophagitis in adults: Clinical, endoscopic, histologic findings, and response to treatment with fluticasone propionate. Gastrointest Endosc 2006;63:3–12.
46. Gupta SK, Fitzgerald JF, Chong SK, et al. Vertical lines in distal esophageal mucosa (VLEM): A true endoscopic manifestation of esophagitis in children? Gastrointest Endosc 1997;45:485–9.
47. Cheung KM, Oliver MR, Cameron DJ, et al. Esophageal eosinophilia in children with dysphagia. J Pediatr Gastroenterol Nutr 2003;37:498–503.
48. Attwood S, Smyrk T, Demeester T, Jones J. Esophageal eosinophilia with dysphagia. A distinct clinicopathologic syndrome. Dig Dis Sci 1993;38:109–16.
49. Arora AS, Perrault J, Smyrk TC. Topical corticosteroid treatment of dysphagia due to eosinophilic esophagitis in adults. Mayo Clin Proc 2003;78:830–5.
50. Blanchard C, Wang N, Stringer KF, et al. Eotaxin-3 and a uniquely conserved gene-expression profile in eosinophilic esophagitis. J Clin Invest 2006;116:536–47.
51. Thompson DM, Arora AS, Romero Y, Dauer EH. Eosinophilic esophagitis: Its role in aerodigestive tract disorders. Otolaryngol Clin North Am 2006;39:205–21.
52. Lee RG. Marked eosinophilia in esophageal mucosal biopsies. Am J Surg Pathol 1985;9:475–9.
53. Straumann A, Spichtin HP, Bernoulli R, et al. [Idiopathic eosinophilic esophagitis: A frequently overlooked disease with typical clinical aspects and discrete endoscopic findings]. Schweiz Med Wochenschr 1994;124:1419–29.
54. Ruchelli E, Wenner W, Voytek T, et al. Severity of esophageal eosinophilia predicts response to conventional gastroesophageal reflux therapy. Pediatr Develop Pathol 1999;2:15–8.

55. Parfitt JR, Gregor JC, Suskin NG, et al. Eosinophilic esophagitis in adults: Distinguishing features from gastroesophageal reflux disease: A study of 41 patients. Mod Pathol 2006;19:90–6.

56. Gonsalves N, Policarpio-Nicolas M, Zhang Q, et al. Histopathologic variability and endoscopic correlates in adults with eosinophilic esophagitis. Gastrointest Endosc 2006;64:313–9.

57. Mueller S, Aigner T, Neureiter D, Stolte M. Eosinophil infiltration and degranulation in oesophageal mucosa from adult patients with eosinophilic oesophagitis: A retrospective and comparative study on pathological biopsy. J Clin Pathol 2006;59:1175–80.

58. Kirsch R, Bokhary R, Marcon MA, Cutz E. Activated mucosal mast cells differentiate eosinophilic (allergic) esophagitis from gastroesophageal reflux disease. J Pediatr Gastroenterol Nutr 2007;44:20–6.

59. Zink DA, Amin M, Gebara S, Desai TK. Familial dysphagia and eosinophilia. Gastrointest Endosc 2007;65:330–4.

60. Patel SM, Falchuk KR. Three brothers with dysphagia caused by eosinophilic esophagitis. Gastrointest Endosc 2005;61:165–7.

61. Meyer GW. Eosinophilic esophagitis in a father and a daughter. Gastrointest Endosc 2005;61:932.

62. Mishra A, Hogan SP, Brandt EB, Rothenberg ME. IL-5 promotes eosinophil trafficking to the esophagus. J Immunol 2002;168:2464–9.

63. Klion AD, Bochner BS, Gleich GJ, et al. The Hypereosinophilic Syndromes Working G. Approaches to the treatment of hypereosinophilic syndromes: A workshop summary report. J Allergy Clin Immunol 2006;117:1292–302.

64. Straumann A, Kristl J, Conus S, et al. Cytokine expression in healthy and inflamed mucosa: Probing the role of eosinophils in the digestive tract. Inflamm Bowel Dis 2005;11:720–6.

65. Spergel JM, Brown-Whitehorn T. The use of patch testing in the diagnosis of food allergy. Curr Allergy Asthma Rep 2005;5:86–90.

66. Markowitz JE, Spergel JM, Ruchelli E, Liacouras CA. Elemental diet is an effective treatment for eosinophilic esophagitis in children and adolescents. Am J Gastroenterol 2003;98:777–82.

67. Spergel JM, Beausoleil JL, Mascarenhas M, Liacouras CA. The use of skin prick tests and patch tests to identify causative foods in eosinophilic esophagitis. J Allergy Clin Immunol 2002;109:363–8.

68. Konikoff MR, Noel RJ, Blanchard C, et al. A randomized, double-blind, placebo-controlled trial of fluticasone propionate for pediatric eosinophilic esophagitis. Gastroenterology 2006;131:1381–91.

69. Kagalwalla AF, Sentongo TA, Ritz S, et al. Effect of six-food elimination diet on clinical and histologic outcomes in eosinophilic esophagitis. Clin Gastroenterol Hepatol 2006;4:1097–102.

70. Liacouras C, Wenner W, Brown K, Ruchelli E. Primary eosinophilic esophagitis in children: Successful treatment with oral corticosteroids. J Pediatr Gastroenterol Nutr 1998;26:380–5.

71. Faubion WA, Jr, Perrault J, Burgart LJ, et al. Treatment of eosinophilic esophagitis with inhaled corticosteroids. J Pediatr Gastroenterol Nutr 1998;27:90–3.

72. Noel RJ, Putnam PE, Collins MH, et al. Clinical and immunopathologic effects of swallowed fluticasone for eosinophilic esophagitis. Clin Gastroenterol Hepatol 2004;2:568–75.

73. Aceves SS, Dohil R, Newbury RO, Bastian JF. Topical viscous budesonide suspension for treatment of eosinophilic esophagitis. J Allergy Clin Immunol 2005;116:705–6.

74. Attwood SE, Lewis CJ, Bronder CS, et al. Eosinophilic oesophagitis: A novel treatment using Montelukast. Gut 2003;52:181–5.

75. Gupta SK, Peters-Golden M, Fitzgerald JF, et al. Cysteinyl leukotriene levels in esophageal mucosal biopsies of children with eosinophilic inflammation: Are they all the same? Am J Gastroenterol 2006;101:1125–8.

76. Simon D, Braathen LR, Simon HU. Anti-interleukin-5 antibody therapy in eosinophilic diseases. Pathobiology 2005;72:287–92.

77. Garrett JK, Jameson SC, Thomson B, et al. Anti-interleukin-5 (mepolizumab) therapy for hypereosinophilic syndromes. J Allergy Clin Immunol 2004;113:115–9.

78. Stein ML, Collins MH, Villanueva JM, et al. Anti-IL-5 (mepolizumab) therapy for eosinophilic esophagitis. J Allergy Clin Immunol 2006;118:1312–9.

79. Yun MY, Cho YU, Park IS, et al. Eosinophilic gastroenteritis presenting as small bowel obstruction: A case report and review of the literature. World J Gastroenterol 2007;13:1758–60.

80. Siaw EK, Sayed K, Jackson RJ. Eosinophilic gastroenteritis presenting as acute gastric perforation. J Pediatr Gastroenterol Nutr 2006;43:691–4.

81. Siewert E, Lammert F, Koppitz P, et al. Eosinophilic gastroenteritis with severe protein-losing enteropathy: Successful treatment with budesonide. Dig Liver Dis 2006;38:55–9.

82. Lima MS, dos Santos Bomfim V, Zeinad A, et al. Association of protein-losing enteropathy caused by eosinophilic gastroenteritis with essential thrombocytosis: Case report. Clinics 2006;61:271–4.

83. Chehade M, Magid MS, Mofidi S, et al. Allergic eosinophilic gastroenteritis with protein-losing enteropathy: Intestinal Pathology, Clinical Course, and Long-term Follow-up. J Pediatr Gastroenterol Nutr 2006;42:516–21.

84. Lin HH, Wu CH, Wu LS, Shyu RY. Eosinophilic gastroenteritis presenting as relapsing severe abdominal pain and enteropathy with protein loss. Emerg Med J 2005;22:834–5.

85. Mazokopakis E, Vrentzos G, Spanakis E, et al. A case of eosinophilic gastroenteritis with severe peripheral eosinophilia. Mil Med 2006;171:331–2.

86. Jimenez-Rivera C, Ngan B, Jackson R, Ahmed N. Gastric pseudopolyps in eosinophilic gastroenteritis. J Pediatr Gastroenterol Nutr 2005;40:83–6.

87. Romero R, Abramowsky CR, Pillen T, et al. Peripheral eosinophilia and eosinophilic gastroenteritis after pediatric liver transplantation. Pediatr Transplant 2003;7:484–8.

88. Saeed SA, Integlia MJ, Pleskow RG, et al. Tacrolimus-associated eosinophilic gastroenterocolitis in pediatric liver transplant recipients: role of potential food allergies in pathogenesis. Pediatr Transplant 2006;10:730–5.

89. Torpier G, COlombel JF, Mathieu-Chandelier C, et al. Eosinophilic gastroenteritis: Ultrastructural evidence for a selective release of eosinophil major basic protein. Clin Exp Immunol 1988;74:404–8.

90. Talley NJ, Kephart GM, McGovern TW, et al. Deposition of eosinophil granule major basic protein in eosinophilic gastroenteritis and celiac disease. Gastroenterol 1992;102: 137–45.

91. Kephart GM, McGovern TW, Carpenter HA, Gleich GJ. Deposition of eosinophil granule major basic protein in eosinophilic gastroenteritis and celiac disease. Gastroenterology 1992;102:137.

92. Forbes E, Smart VE, D'Aprile A, et al. T helper-2 immunity regulates bronchial hyperresponsiveness in eosinophil-associated gastrointestinal disease in mice. Gastroenterology 2004;127:105–18.

93. Chen MJ, Chu CH, Lin SC, et al. Eosinophilic gastroenteritis: Clinical experience with 15 patients. World J Gastroenterol 2003;9:2813–6.

94. Elsing C, Placke J, Gross-Weege W. Budesonide for the treatment of obstructive eosinophilic jejunitis. Z Gastroenterol 2007;45:187–9.

95. Suzuki J, Kawasaki Y, Nozawa R, et al. Oral disodium cromoglycate and ketotifen for a patient with eosinophilic gastroenteritis, food allergy and protein-losing enteropathy. Asian Pac J Allergy Immunol 2003;21:193–7.

96. Quack I, Sellin L, Buchner NJ, et al. Eosinophilic gastroenteritis in a young girl—long term remission under Montelukast. BMC Gastroenterol 2005;5:24.

97. Neustrom M, Frieson C. Treatment of eosinophilic gastroenteritis with montelukast. J Allergy Clin Immunol 1999;104:506.

98. Bolukbas FF, Bolukbas C, Uzunkoy A, et al. A dramatic response to ketotifen in a case of eosinophilic gastroenteritis mimicking abdominal emergency. Dig Dis Sci 2004;49:1782–5.

99. Kim YJ, Prussin C, Martin B, et al. Rebound eosinophilia after treatment of hypereosinophilic syndrome and eosinophilic gastroenteritis with monoclonal anti-IL-5 antibody SCH55700. J Allergy Clin Immunol 2004;114:1449–55.

100. Furuta G, Liacouras C, Collins M, et al. Eosinophilic esophagitis in children and adults: A systematic review and consensus recommendations for diagnosis and treatment. Gastroenterlogy 2007. (In press)

20.7. Peritonitis and Intra-abdominal Abscesses

David J. Hackam, MD, PhD

Ori D. Rotstein, MD

There are two major manifestations of intra-abdominal infection: (1) peritonitis and (2) abscess formation, in which infection has become walled off from the remainder of the peritoneal cavity. While peritonitis is strictly defined as inflammation of the peritoneal cavity and thus may be infectious or noninfectious in etiology, this chapter will focus on infectious causes of peritonitis, with the requisite description of circumstances where noninfectious causes may be relevant. Peritonitis may be classified as primary, secondary, or tertiary. Primary peritonitis is defined as an infection of the peritoneal cavity in which there is no obvious source, such as a perforated viscus. In secondary peritonitis, peritoneal infection and inflammation are caused by visceral disruption that is a result of an intrinsic pathological condition or of external trauma. Finally, tertiary peritonitis is used to define the presence of persistent or recurrent infection following presumed adequate treatment of secondary peritonitis. Because of their clinical importance, the management of secondary peritonitis and abscess formation will receive somewhat greater emphasis in this chapter, although both primary and secondary peritonitis will be addressed. Tertiary peritonitis has received little attention among the pediatric population and therefore will not be discussed further.

LOCAL AND SYSTEMIC RESPONSE TO BACTERIAL INFECTION IN THE PERITONEAL CAVITY

After bacterial contamination of the peritoneal cavity, a complex series of events is initiated that under ideal circumstances effects complete eradication of invading bacteria. The three major defense mechanisms are (1) mechanical clearance of bacteria via the diaphragmatic lymphatics, (2) phagocytosis and destruction of suspended or adherent bacteria by phagocytic cells, and (3) sequestration and walling off of bacteria coupled with delayed clearance by phagocytic cells. The first two mechanisms act rapidly, usually within hours. When a pure suspension of bacteria is injected into the peritoneal cavity of an experimental animal, the bacteria begin to disappear immediately, even before the influx of phagocytic cells.[1] Bacteria can be found in the mediastinum within 6 minutes and in the bloodstream within 12 minutes.[2] These observations suggest that the

first defense of the peritoneal cavity is physical removal, whereby bacteria are carried cephalad by the intraperitoneal circulation, absorbed into the diaphragmatic lymphatics, and then carried to the bloodstream. These blood-borne bacteria are presumably cleared by a variety of mechanisms, including the reticuloendothelial system of the liver. The escape of bacteria and their products from the peritoneal cavity probably contributes significantly to the development of the systemic response to peritonitis (see below).

The initial peritoneal response to bacterial contamination is characterized by hyperemia, exudation of fluid into the peritoneal cavity, and a marked influx of phagocytic cells. Resident peritoneal macrophages predominate early in the infection, but the rapid influx of neutrophils after a 2- to 4-hour delay makes them the predominant phagocytic cell in the peritoneal cavity for the first 48 to 72 hours.[3] In essence, the response mimics a typical inflammatory reaction to bacteria. The events surrounding the development of this response have not been well studied, but many can be surmised from in vitro studies or in vivo investigations of inflammation in experimental animals. For example, in experimental peritonitis, peritoneal levels of tumor necrosis factor-α (TNF-α) and interleukin-1 (IL-1) increase rapidly after the initiation of infection.[3–4] Similarly, in humans with severe intra-abdominal infection, peritoneal levels of TNF-α, IL-1, and IL-6 are higher than levels measured simultaneously in plasma.[5–6] One recent study evaluated cytokine levels in children with perforated appendicitis.[7] TNF-α and IL-10 levels are increased and reach 100- to 1,000-fold that observed in the plasma. IL-6 levels in the peritoneal exudates were also increased. Interestingly, levels of TNF-α and IL-10 remained elevated throughout the course of infection and actually persisted even after the children had recovered and systemic signs of infection had abated. Similarly, gram-negative bacterial endotoxin, a potent stimulus for production of many of these cytokines by peritoneal macrophages, is persistently elevated even after the clinical course has improved.[8] Together these findings suggest that during resolving peritonitis, compartmentalization of infection occurs with cytokines promoting local resolution of infection. Further, this localization delimits the magnitude and duration of the systemic inflammatory response. Recent studies have reported

that other cell types are important in the initiation of the local peritoneal response. Peritoneal mast cells appear to release preformed tumor necrosis factor early in the genesis of peritoneal inflammation and contribute significantly to recruiting neutrophils to the peritoneal cavity. The peritoneal mesothelial cells have also been shown to be potent producers of a range of cytokines and procoagulants. Given the strategic position of both of these cell types, their role in the initiation of the local response is undoubtedly important.[9–10] In addition, generation of other inflammatory mediator molecules, such as leukotriene B_4, platelet-activating factor, and components of the complement cascade (eg, C3a and C5a), further promotes the development of local inflammation.[11–13]

Fibrin deposition appears to play an important role in this compartmentalization of infection, not only by incorporating large numbers of bacteria within its interstices[14] but also by causing loops of intestine to adhere to each other and the omentum, thereby creating a physical barrier against dissemination. Fibrin deposition is initiated after the exudation of protein-rich fluid containing fibrinogen into the peritoneal cavity. The conversion of fibrinogen to fibrin is promoted by the release of tissue thromboplastin from both mesothelial cells and stimulated peritoneal macrophages.[15] Furthermore, a plasminogen activator, which is responsible for the activation of fibrinolytic enzymes and is normally present in the mesothelial and submesothelial cell membranes, disappears in the face of bacterial infection.[16] The effects of fibrin deposition are multiple. Early on, the sequestration of bacteria minimizes bacteremia and abrogates the systemic response. In addition, fibrin and its degradation products are potent chemoattractants and promote influx of inflammatory cells. However, the dense fibrinous exudates also provide a protected sanctuary in which bacteria may proliferate and lead to abscess formation.[17]

As proposed for the local response to infection in the peritoneal cavity, the stimulated release of products of cells of the monocyte–macrophage lineage also appears to be responsible for the characteristic septic host response observed in patients with bacterial peritonitis. Intravenous infusion of TNF into experimental animals mimics the hemodynamic alteration and lactic acidosis that follow the administration of bacterial endotoxin.[18] Both TNF and IL-1 cause fever and neutrophilia,[18–19] and IL-6 initiates the acute-phase protein response characteristic of infection.[20] In adult patients, a correlation between the magnitude of the cytokine response and outcome in infected patients has been demonstrated in several clinical studies. Higher levels of circulating TNF-α and IL-6 have been recorded in patients who later die with intra-abdominal infection.[21] Temporal analysis of this cytokine response in relation to the time of laparotomy confirms that peak TNF-α and IL-6 levels occur within 2 to 4 hours of skin incision.[22] The exaggerated cytokine response may occur as a result of mobilization of the infectious focus, with spilling of bacteria and bacterial products into the circulation. This phenomenon may account for the pronounced hemodynamic instability soon after laparotomy for intra-abdominal infection.

CONDITIONS CAUSING PERITONEAL INFLAMMATION

Table 1 lists a number of the disease processes causing peritonitis. Among these, acute appendicitis is one of the most common diagnoses requiring emergency surgery in children. Specific aspects of the diagnosis and management of appendicitis are addressed elsewhere in this volume. The spectrum of disease associated with appendicitis ranges from local acute inflammation to gangrene with or without perforation. The perforated appendix may be walled off leading to local abscess formation or alternatively may disseminate throughout the peritoneal cavity causing diffuse peritonitis. Necrotizing enterocolitis (NEC) is also a frequent cause of peritonitis leading to gastrointestinal surgical intervention in children. It also represents the most frequent and lethal cause of peritonitis in infants.[23] Over 25,000 cases of NEC are reported annually; NEC is diagnosed in between 0.9 to 2.4 per 1,000 live births, and the increase in survival rates of premature infants has led to an overall increase in the incidence of this disease.[24–25] NEC is both an acute and chronic disorder that is characterized initially by intestinal inflammation, yet may progress to intestinal necrosis with perforation in more advanced cases. In the most severe form, NEC may lead to overwhelming multisystem organ failure and death from systemic sepsis, with an overall mortality rate up to 50%.[26] Chapter 20.4, "Necrotizing Enterocolitis," is also dedicated to more detailed discussion of this entity. It is now recognized that the diagnosis of focal intestinal perforation (FIP) may be considered a separate entity, based on its preoperative findings and the fact that it has a better outcome than NEC.[26]

DIAGNOSTIC APPROACH TO PATIENTS WITH ABDOMINAL PAIN

The diagnosis of peritonitis is a clinical one, supported by the use of ancillary investigations used to define the underlying etiology. Several

Table 1 Conditions Causing Peritoneal Inflammation

Gastrointestinal in origin
Acute appendicitis
Necrotizing enterocolitis
Meckel's diverticulitis with or without rupture
Cholecystitis
Pancreatitis
Mesenteric enteritis
Intra-abdominal abscess
Visceral abscesses including liver and spleen
Spontaneous/traumatic gastrointestinal perforation
    including gastric, duodenal, small bowel, colon,
    and rectum
Meconium peritonitis
Intestinal obstruction with ischemia/necrosis including
    volvulus, intussusception
Inflammatory conditions due to vascular disease
    including Henoch-Schonlein purpura, systemic
    lupus erythematosus, sickle cell crisis
Enteric infections—bacterial, viral, parasitic
Typhlitis
Nongastrointestinal in origin
Pyelonephritis/renal colic
Pneumonia
Pelvic inflammatory disease
Endometriosis
Ovarian cyst/torsion
Testicular torsion
Other diseases mimicking peritonitis
Diabetic ketoacidosis
Addisonian crisis
Various toxins including heavy metals
Black widow spider bite

aspects of the presentation are relevant including the presence, nature and location of the abdominal pain, the presence and nature of vomiting, bowel history, associated systemic symptoms, and past medical history. Obviously, the presentation may vary somewhat based on the age of the child. For example, in the very young patient, inability to verbalize pain presents an obstacle to diagnosis and may delay treatment. The most common symptom is abdominal pain. The onset of the pain may be acute or more insidious. The pain is often steady, severe, and aggravated by movement. The patient is frequently lying still in bed, either in the fetal position or supine with knees bent and head elevated. Both these maneuvers reduce the tension on the abdominal wall and thereby alleviate abdominal discomfort. In neonates, alterations in the pitch and intensity of the cry such that it sounds more like a constant "wail" may provide an important clue to the presence of peritonitis. In toddlers, in whom the lack of cooperativeness can complicate the ability to reliably evaluate abdominal tenderness, findings such as abdominal distention, emesis, and anorexia are important coexisting features that may point to the presence of peritoneal irritation. A recent history of irritability or flexing of the hips and crying, particularly during examination may be suggestive. In the neonate, particularly in the verylow-birth weight child, systemic deterioration coupled with abdominal distension may give trigger consideration of the onset of

peritonitis, often due to necrotizing enterocolitis. Vomiting is associated with a number of surgical conditions. The frequency of the vomiting and the nature of the vomitus (eg, bile vs blood) may provide insight into the diagnosis. Bowel history including presence or absence of bloody diarrhea may provide insight into the diagnosis, especially when colitis or infectious enteritis is among the differential causes for abdominal pain. Anorexia and nausea are often accompanying symptoms. Systemic symptoms such as fever, lethargy, and associated weight loss may provide clues as to the chronicity of the problem. Queries regarding complaints such as cough, chest pain, dysuria, flank pain, and vaginal discharge may suggest non-GI etiologies for the pain. Finally, prior surgical history is critical. The sequence of events may give insight into the underlying diagnosis. Pain, then fever followed by nausea and vomiting are characteristic of appendicitis, while an onset with fever followed by diarrhea and vomiting and subsequently pain is more likely to be viral gastroenteritis.

It is critical that in all cases in which children present with bilious emesis that the diagnosis of malrotation with midgut volvulus be excluded. Failure to operatively explore such children in a timely manner will inevitably lead to intestinal necrosis and potentially to the loss of the entire midgut. The diagnosis of midgut volvulus may be ascertained on clinical grounds alone, such as in the previously well infant who suddenly develops abdominal distention and bilious emesis in the setting of systemic sepsis. In cases in which the clinical picture is less clear, an upper GI evaluation may confirm or exclude the presence of malrotation, although subtle rotational abnormalities on this evaluation may still leave significant diagnostic uncertainty. It is noteworthy that plain abdominal films may show a nonspecific bowel gas pattern, even in patients with significant volvulus, depending on the time between when the volvulus occurred and the abdominal X-ray was taken. In all cases of diagnostic uncertainty, the wisest course of action is often to proceed with abdominal exploration–either by laparotomy or laparoscopy–at which time the diagnosis can be confirmed and derotation may be performed in a timely fashion.

Abdominal examination in patients with peritonitis may be particularly challenging even in young children able to verbalize their complaints, as there is considerable anxiety surrounding the acute onset of their disease. Time spent gaining the child's (and the parents') confidence will facilitate accurate examination. In young patients, observation of their activities while in parents' arms or even without palpation may provide important clues as to the magnitude of the pain and tenderness. Physical findings vary according to the cause and the extent of the peritonitis. Children vary from being irritable to being lethargic depending on the extent of the infection. Body temperature is usually higher than 38°C (100.4°F), but in cases of severe septic shock, the patient may be hypothermic. Tachycardia and diminished pulse volume, indicative of hypovolemia, are common. Abdominal tenderness is the hallmark of peritonitis. Patients with generalized peritonitis suffer diffuse tenderness. The point of maximum tenderness frequently overlies the diseased organ. Increased abdominal tone is initially from voluntary guarding by the patient and is subsequently a result of reflex muscular spasm. The abdomen is characteristically distended, and bowel sounds are usually absent, although an occasional bowel sound may be heard. In neonates, since the abdominal musculature is still underdeveloped, the presence of abdominal wall erythema may point to the presence of an intra-abdominal septic process, such as necrotizing enterocolitis.

By contrast, localized peritonitis generally produces less intense clinical findings in the patient. The abdomen distant from the site of maximum tenderness may be soft and nontender, and bowel sounds are frequently present. Referred rebound tenderness may accurately pinpoint the site of maximal peritoneal irritation; the rectal examination, although an essential part of the physical examination, rarely pinpoints the origin of the peritonitis.

Laboratory data, particularly the presence of a leukocytosis greater than 11,000 cells/mm^3 with a shift to the left, support the clinical diagnosis of peritonitis. Leukopenia is compatible with overwhelming sepsis. Blood chemistry is generally undisturbed but in severe cases may show evidence of dehydration with elevated blood urea nitrogen levels as well as metabolic acidosis. The presence of increased amylase or lipase may indicate the presence of acute pancreatitis, or may be seen in abdominal conditions unrelated to the pancreas, such as proximal intestinal perforation or midgut volvulus. Urinalysis is essential to rule out urinary tract diseases, such as pyelonephritis and renal colic, which may mimic peritonitis. White and red blood cells are occasionally found in the urine of patients with peritonitis, but the presence of bacteria, white blood cell casts, and large numbers of erythrocytes in the urine should suggest a urinary tract source of the pain.

Plain abdominal X-rays may show evidence of ileus, with distended loops of large and small bowel, air-fluid levels, and free fluid in the peritoneal cavity. It is critical that two views of the abdomen be obtained—supine and upright. Upright films are useful for demonstrating free air under the diaphragm, an indication of a perforated viscus. The likelihood of free air on plain radiograph depends considerably on the nature of the underlying pathology. Of the common diagnoses in children, it is frequent in neonates with focal intestinal perforation or necrotizing enterocolitis, but much less common in children with appendicitis. In necrotizing enterocolitis, the finding of pneumatosis intestinalis, or portal vein gas may support the diagnosis and also serve as a differentiating feature from patients with FIP.[26] Finally, plain films may also give insight into alternate diagnoses causing abdominal pain including bowel obstruction, intussusception, and volvulus. Paracentesis may provide some clue to the nature of the underlying disease process, where recovery of intestinal contents, meconium, bile, or urine may point to a specific cause and hence direct therapy.

Imaging techniques may provide evidence of an inflammatory process within the peritoneal cavity. Ultrasonography (US) is useful in equivocal cases of right lower quadrant pain, with specificity and sensitivity of 90 and 80%, respectively, for the diagnosis of appendicitis.[27] Like ultrasonography, computed tomography is capable of detecting intraperitoneal fluid, inflammation, or infection in the viscera as well as evidence of perforation when contrast is used. A recent meta-analysis evaluated the diagnostic performance of US and CT scan in children suspected of having appendicitis. CT proved to be more sensitive and specific than US for the diagnosis of appendicitis.[28] These imaging modalities may also be valuable in the diagnosis of other nonappendiceal causes for abdominal pain.[29]

MANAGEMENT OF SECONDARY PERITONITIS

Three principles guide the treatment of secondary peritonitis: (1) the provision of adequate fluid resuscitation to restore intravascular volume, (2) the initiation of antimicrobial therapy, and (3) intervention aimed at treating the underlying pathological process and preventing subsequent infection.

Fluid Resuscitation

The combination of reduced fluid intake, vomiting, and third space fluid extravasation invariably leave the patient hypovolemic and in need of fluid resuscitation. Fluid resuscitation entails the administration of fluids and the monitoring of fluid status. The extent of these measures depends very much on the patient's premorbid status and on the underlying disease process. All patients with peritonitis have some degree of hypovolemia. Adequate volumes of fluid should therefore be administered to restore blood volume. Adequacy of resuscitation may be assessed by monitoring blood pressure, central venous pressure, and urine output. The choice of fluid used for resuscitation in critically ill patients has been the source of considerable controversy in the medical literature in both children and adults. The Pediatric Advanced Life Support Group recommends 20 mL/kg of saline or albumin fluid boluses up to 60 mL/kg until perfusion improves or overload occurs.[30] Adequate resuscitation should be assessed using clinical parameters including heart rate, blood pressure, and rapid capillary refill. A recent publication reported evidence-based clinical guidelines for treatment of neonatal and pediatric patients with hypovolemic shock by the Dutch Pediatric Society.[31] In trials considered acceptable for evaluation, crystalloid solutions were found to be equivalent to colloid choices. The authors also concluded that evidence in pediatric populations was insufficient to make firm conclusions and took into account adult studies. The authors therefore considered some of the existing adult data in making their recommendations. The SAFE Study investigators conducted a large randomized trial in adults and showed no mortality difference between 4% albumin and isotonic saline for volume restoration or maintenance.[32] One meta-analysis showed no clear mortality differences between colloid and crystalloid regimens.[33] The consensus by the multidisciplinary committee included the following recommendations: (1) In neonates and children with hypovolemia, the first choice for fluid resuscitation is isotonic saline (Grade A evidence including adult data). (2) When larger amounts of fluid are required (eg, sepsis), it is possible to use a synthetic colloid because of its longer duration in the circulation (Grade C evidence). (3) The initial fluid volume should be 10 to 20 mL/kg and repeated doses should be based on individual clinical response (Grade C evidence).

Antimicrobial Therapy

Antibiotic therapy should be initiated as soon as the clinical diagnosis of peritonitis is made, even before samples can be taken from the peritoneal cavity for aerobic and anaerobic culture. Although the initial antibiotic therapy is given on an empirical basis, the choice of antimicrobial agents should be based on the suspected offending organisms (see below) and on the ability of the antibiotics to achieve adequate levels in the peritoneal cavity. The spectrum of microorganisms inoculating the peritoneum after perforation of the gastrointestinal tract depends on the level of the perforation.[34] Upper gastrointestinal perforations usually release predominantly gram-positive organisms, which are sensitive to penicillins and cephalosporins. Patients who have been taking antacids or H$_2$-receptor blockers have greater numbers of facultative gram-negative bacilli in their stomachs before perforation.[35] Perforation of the distal small bowel or the colon results in the release of the indigenous polymicrobial flora into the peritoneal cavity. Most species are rapidly eliminated by local host defenses and in established intraperitoneal infection, only a few species remain.[36] These infections are almost always polymicrobial, containing a mixture of aerobic and anaerobic bacteria.[8,37] (see Table 2). The predictable nature of the microbial flora in these patients permits ready selection of empiric antimicrobial therapy. In neonates with focal intestinal perforation, it appears that *Candida* species and coagulase-negative staphylocci predominate over Enterobacteriaceae, microbes traditionally found in intra-abdominal infection (Table 3).[38]

A set of recommendations regarding antimicrobial use in the management of intra-abdominal infections in adults has recently been published by the Surgical Infection Society, taking into consideration the evolution of microbial flora as the complexity of the patient and infectious

Table 2 Microbial Flora of Secondary Peritonitis

Bacterial Group	Species
Gram-negative aerobic rods	E. coli*
	Klebsiella species
	Proteus species
	Pseudomonas aeruginosa
	Other
Gram-positive aerobic cocci	Enterococcus faecalis
	Beta-hemolytic streptococci
	Streptococcus pneumoniae
	Streptococcus mitis
Anaerobic bacteria	Bacteroides fragilis*
	Other Bacteroides species
	Peptococcus species
	Peptostreptococcus species

*Predominant microbes.

process progresses.[39] These guidelines were developed according to current principles of evidence-based medicine and addressed a number of issues including choice of therapy including considerations of patient factors in the selection of specific antimicrobials, duration of therapy, and switch-over to oral antibiotics. The applicability of these guidelines to the pediatric patient population remains unclear, although the frequent similarity in the microbial flora of these infections suggested their potential use in pediatric patients. The Therapeutic Agents Committee of the Surgical Infection Society has prepared an evidenced-based review of the existing literature for antimicrobial therapy in children with intra-abdominal infection.[40] At the outset, it was

Table 3 Peritoneal Isolates Recovered from Neonates with Focal Intestinal Perforation Versus Necrotizing Enterocolitis

	FIP (%)	NEC (%)
Gram positive		
Coagulase-negative staphylococci*	50	14
S. aureus	0	1
Enterococcus spp.	28	23
Streptococcus species	3	0
Diphtheroids	3	3
Gram negative		
Enterobacteriaceae*	25	75
E. coli	3	28
Klebsiella species	8	28
Enterobacter species	11	25
Citrobacter species	0	4
Proteus species	3	0
Pseudomonas species	8	1
Acinetobacter species	3	0
Anaerobes		
Bacteroides species	3	5
Clostridium species	0	1
Candida species*	44	15

Adapted from Coates et al.[38]
*Significant different between FIP and NEC.

recognized that the majority of studies addressed treatment of children with appendicitis. Accordingly, the guidelines must be extrapolated if they are to be applied to other diseases causing secondary peritonitis in children. Given that the microbiology of the majority of these pathological processes mimics that of appendicitis, these extrapolations appear justified. Exceptions will be pointed out where appropriate.

Based on the polymicrobial flora of secondary peritonitis, a rationale choice for antimicrobial therapy would consist of a single agent or a combination of agents that provide coverage for gram-negative enteric bacteria (such as Escherichia coli) and anaerobic bacteria (such as Bacteroides fragilis). There is no consensus among surgeons regarding the choice of antibiotics to be used in this setting. However, the "gold standard" for pediatric intra-abdominal infections consists of triple therapy including ampicillin, clindamycin, and gentamicin. Comparisons to this regimen, using appropriately powered prospective randomized control trials does not exist. However, a number of small trials demonstrate efficacy of monotherapy with single broad-spectrum agents including ticarcillin/clavulanate, imipenem/cilastatin, piperacillin/tazobactam as well as alternate combination therapies including cefotaxime plus metronidazole, cetriaxone plus flagyl, and ticarcillin/clavulinate plus gentamicin. None of the studies represent quality trials evaluating various choices between antimicrobial regimens. Under these circumstances, it would seem reasonable to follow the basic principle underlying selection that includes coverage for gram-negative enteric bacteria and anaerobic bacteria and then take into account local susceptibility patterns in the treating institution as well as issues of safety and cost when deciding between options of antimicrobial therapy. As noted above, the microbiology of FIP is characterized by the presence of Candida species and coagulase-negative staphylococci. Coates and colleagues recommend empiric therapy with broad-spectrum antimicrobials due to the difficulty in definitively differentiating NEC from FIP.[38] They reiterate the importance of obtaining cultures of the peritoneal fluid upon draining and adjusting therapy accordingly.

Tradition appears to dictate that antimicrobial therapy should be administered for a set period of time, usually 10 to 14 days. A retrospective review by Lelli and colleagues suggested that shortened duration of therapy for both nonperforated and perforated appendicitis did not adversely affect recovery or complications following treatment for appendicitis.[41] Hoelzer and colleagues used criteria generally applied to the adult population in treating children with appendicitis to guide discontinuation of antibiotics.[42] In this study, when a patient with complicated appendicitis was afebrile for 24 hours (temperature < 38°C), eating well and had a WBC count with ≤3% band forms, antibiotics could be safely discontinued with small risk of recurrent intra-abdominal abscess. The Surgical Infection Society (SIS) guidelines recommend discontinuation of antibiotics based

on clinical picture. Importantly, if leukocytosis or fever persists after postoperative day 7, a diligent search is initiated to locate the source of persistent sepsis. Finally, while there is strong evidence in adults that conversion from IV to oral antibiotics results in similar outcome to a full course of IV antibiotics, this has not been clearly demonstrated in children and is not yet recommended.

Operative Management of Peritonitis

Other chapters in this volume address the operative management of specific surgical problems including appendicitis and NEC. This discussion will therefore speak in broad terms regarding general approaches. The goals of operative management of peritonitis are to eliminate the source of contamination, to reduce the bacterial inoculum, and to prevent recurrent or persistent infection.

Source Control. The operative technique used to control contamination depends on the location and the nature of the pathological condition in the gastrointestinal tract.[43] In general, continued peritoneal soiling is controlled by closing, excluding, or resecting the perforated viscus. When feasible, resection of the diseased tissue appears to be the best option, preventing continued contamination from the source. For an inflammatory process where the disease is expected to progress in the absence of a frank perforation (eg, acute appendicitis or small bowel necrosis), resection is clearly preferred, because the underlying disease, if left in situ, may act as a focus of ongoing infection. Occasionally, self-limited inflammatory processes are unexpectedly discovered at laparotomy. Examples include acute Crohn's disease, an ischemic but viable loop of small intestine following release of a volvulus, and acute pancreatitis and acute diverticulitis. Under these circumstances, excision is not indicated, and treatment should address the underlying pathology.

Perforations of the stomach and duodenum are treated with debridement of the edges, closure, and an omental patch if possible. Small bowel perforations often result from obstruction secondary to atresia, volvulus, or advanced intussusception. Resection with primary anastomosis is usually performed. However, resection with exteriorization of both proximal and distal ends as stomas may be appropriate if peritoneal soiling is particularly extensive or if the viability of the intestine is uncertain. Spontaneous colon perforation may be treated with primary closure, closure with proximal diversion or resection with exteriorition.[44] The choice among these depends on the underlying disease process (eg, infectious, Hirschprung's disease), the local conditions of the peritoneal cavity, the stability of the patient, and the location in the colon. In particular, rectal perforations, which may be iatrogenic in etiology, are managed by debridement and closure when possible and proximal diversion.

Preventing Postoperative Infection. The second major goal of operative management of peritonitis is to reduce the bacterial inoculum and to prevent recurrent or persistent sepsis. At operation, gross purulent exudates should be aspirated, and loculations in the pelvis, paracolic gutters, and subphrenic regions should be gently opened and debrided. An attempt should be made to remove particulate debris, such as fecal matter or barium sulfate, if present.

Although intraoperative peritoneal lavage with warm saline has become a standard procedure during operation for peritonitis, its efficacy has not been well documented. Its major roles are to reduce the quantity of bacteria and to remove adjuvant substances. It is imperative that all fluid collections be aspirated before the abdomen is closed, as these might impair bacteria clearance and predispose to abscess formation.[45]

The addition of antibiotics and antiseptic agents to intraoperative peritoneal lavage fluid has been advocated to reduce septic complications. Older studies in adults unanimously support the use of antibiotics in lavage fluid as an effective means of reducing the septic complication rate below that achieved by systemic antibiotics alone.[46–47] This result is not surprising, given that systemically administered antibiotics achieve levels in the peritoneal fluid of patients with peritonitis that are comparable to serum levels.[48]

Other Specific Entities

Necrotizing Enterocolitis (NEC). The surgical management of NEC is addressed in Chapter 20.4, "Necrotizing Enterocolitis." The major controversy in the surgical treatment of this process centers on the relative efficacy of two different treatment strategies, namely the use of peritoneal drainage as primary therapy versus laparotomy, resection, and exterioration. A recent multicenter randomized control trial was performed in which 117 preterm infants (delivered before 34 weeks' gestation) with birth weights less than 1,500 g and perforated NEC at 15 pediatric centers were randomly assigned to undergo primary peritoneal drainage or laparotomy with bowel resection. Primary outcome was survival at 90 days, while secondary outcomes included dependence on parenteral nutrition 90 days postoperatively and length of hospital stay. The authors concluded that the type of operation performed for perforated NEC does not influence survival, dependence on parenteral nutrition, or length of hospital stay in preterm infants.[49] Further, severity of disease, gestational age, and degree of metabolic acidosis did not influence whether one treatment group was superior to another.

Meconium Peritonitis. The management approach to the patient with meconium ileus initially involves resuscitation with hypotonic saline, to correct the third space fluid losses that often results from the intestinal inflammation.[50] Plain radiographs point to the diagnosis of distal intestinal obstruction, and barium enema evaluation is then performed to exclude other diagnostic possibilities, including intestinal atresia, Hirschsprung's disease, and small left colon syndrome. Treatment strategy for meconium ileus is then guided by whether the patient has complicated or uncomplicated meconium ileus. Patients with uncomplicated meconium ileus can be treated nonoperatively. Dilute water soluble contrast is advanced through the colon under fluoroscopic control into the dilated portion of the ileum. Since these contrast agents act partially by absorbing fluid from the bowel wall into the intestinal lumen, maintaining adequate hydration of the infant during this maneuver is extremely important. The enema may be repeated at 12-hour intervals over several days until all the meconium is evacuated. Failure to reflux the contrast into the dilated portion of the ileum signifies the presence complicated meconium ileus, possibly in association with an intestinal atresia. These patients therefore warrant exploratory laparotomy, in which the goals are to relieve the intestinal obstruction. At laparotomy, irrigation of the intestinal lumen with N-acetyl cysteine (mucomyst) or saline through an enterotomy proximal to the site of obstruction may be successful. Alternatively, resection of the distended terminal ileum is performed, and the meconium pellets are flushed from the distal small bowel. At this point, an ileostomy and mucous fistula may be created from the proximal and distal ends respectively.

INTRA-ABDOMINAL ABSCESSES

Abscesses are well-defined collections of pus that are walled off from the rest of the peritoneal cavity by inflammatory adhesions, loops of intestine and their mesentery, the greater omentum, or other abdominal viscera. Abscesses may occur in the peritoneal cavity, either within or outside of abdominal viscera, as well as in the retroperitoneum.[51] Extravisceral abscesses arise in two situations: (1) after resolution of diffuse peritonitis in which a loculated area of infection persists and evolves into an abscess and (2) after perforation of a viscus or an anastomotic breakdown that is successfully walled off by peritoneal defense mechanisms. Abscesses associated with appendicitis occur in 2 to 20% of children undergoing surgery for gangrenous or perforated appendicitis.[52] Visceral abscesses are most commonly caused by hematogenous or lymphatic spread of bacteria to the organ. Retroperitoneal abscesses may be caused by several mechanisms, including perforation of the gastrointestinal tract into the retroperitoneum and hematogenous or lymphatic spread of bacteria to retroperitoneal organs, particularly the inflamed pancreas.

DIAGNOSTIC APPROACH TO INTRA-ABDOMINAL ABSCESSES

Diagnosis is based on clinical suspicion of an abscess and radiologic confirmation of this suspicion. Patients with intra-abdominal abscesses usually have local and systemic signs of inflammation. Characteristically, mild abdominal pain and localized tenderness exist in the region of the infection. Because of the presence of adherent omentum, bowel, or adjacent viscera, it is common to feel a diffuse, rather than a discrete, mass. The patient is usually febrile and anorexic and has a leukocytosis with a shift to the left. The clinical findings associated with an intra-abdominal abscess may be masked by the administration of antibiotics to the patient. However, as previously noted, in the face of antibiotic use, the presence of a fever or a leukocytosis with a band count higher than 3%, or both, is highly indicative of persistent sepsis and should lead to more intensive investigation of the patient's condition.[42,53] It is also noteworthy that infants tend not to form intra-abdominal abscesses due to the fact that their relatively thin omentum is quite inefficient at walling off infectious processes.

The armamentarium of radiologic techniques available for the diagnosis of intra-abdominal sepsis is quite extensive.[54] Plain abdominal X-rays, though rarely diagnostic, frequently point to the need for further investigation. These X-ray findings may document loculated extraluminal gas collections or mottled soft tissue masses, either of which is indicative of abscess formation. More subtle signs include the presence of a localized ileus, a pleural effusion, and atelectasis. Suspicion of an abscess, based on either clinical or basic radiologic findings, should indicate the necessity for imaging techniques to confirm the diagnosis and to pinpoint the location of the abscess.

Ultrasonography and computed tomographic scanning are clearly the examinations of choice; studies comparing the various techniques of imaging an abscess usually suggest CT scanning to be the superior modality.[55] The major advantage of CT is its ability to display, independent of the operator, both intraperitoneal and retroperitoneal structures with a high degree of resolution and accuracy. In addition, the presence of ileus, as well as of drains, dressings, or stomas, does not interfere with the performance of the test. The major disadvantages of CT scanning are its nonportability and the need for the patient to be cooperative and immobile. The accuracy of the scan is reduced in those patients whose GI tract is not opacified with contrast. Under these circumstances, the scans are limited in their ability to distinguish fluid-filled bowel loops from an abscess. Interloop abscesses, which represent approximately 4% of all abscesses, are also poorly visualized on CT scan.[54] In children an obvious effort is made to minimize radiation from CT scanning. Nevertheless, CT may be necessary to definitively localize collections for drainage.

Our general approach is to match the imaging technique to the patient. If the potential site of infection can be localized clinically, then ultrasonography is used to confirm clinical suspicions and to direct diagnostic aspiration of the collection. If the patient appears clinically septic but the site of the infection is not obvious or if the ultrasonographic examination is unsatisfactory, then we prefer to use CT scanning of the abdomen.

MANAGEMENT OF INTRA-ABDOMINAL ABSCESSES

Three basic principles guide the management of intra-abdominal abscesses: (1) general patient care, (2) antibiotic administration, and (3) drainage of the abscess.

General Patient Care

Patients with intra-abdominal abscess show a spectrum of clinical presentations: they range from the relatively well with low-grade fever and leukocytosis to those with septic shock. Clearly, the initial management of all such patients should be tailored to their clinical picture. In general, these patients have some degree of intravascular volume depletion that calls for fluid resuscitation.

Nutritional support is important in the management of patients with intra-abdominal abscess. Patients in whom abscesses develop in the postoperative period are already at a nutritional disadvantage because they have usually spent 7 to 10 days without adequate caloric intake. Historically, total parenteral nutrition has been preferred in patients with intra-abdominal infection. Recent evidence, however, suggests that nutritional supplementation by the enteral route may reduce the incidence of infectious complications, shorten hospital stay, and improve the immune status of critically ill patients.[56] In patients for whom enteral feeding is not satisfactory, parenteral nutrition should be instituted.

Antibiotics

Empiric antibiotic therapy should be directed against the microorganisms most likely to be recovered from the abscess. As for secondary peritonitis, administration of antibiotic combinations or single agents that are active against both aerobes and anaerobes is generally considered the gold standard for the management of intra-abdominal infection[52] (Table 4). The selection of antimicrobial therapy for abdominal abscesses is based on studies of patients fulfilling a broad definition of intra-abdominal infection and, in general, abscesses represent a minority of the cases studied. Therefore, the recommendations for antibiotic use are based on a heterogeneous group of diagnoses, mainly secondary peritonitis. Complex abscesses including those in patients with prolonged antibiotic use would be likely better treated with agent(s) directed against more resistant microbes including gram-negatives, coagulase-negative staphylococci, and *Candida* species, although strong evidence for this is lacking. Obviously, culture and sensitivity results, when available, should guide the focusing of antibiotic treatment. It should be emphasized that general patient care and antibiotic therapy serve primarily as adjuncts to drainage of the abscess cavity. Antibiotics alone are unlikely to be effective for numerous reasons, including poor penetration of antibiotics into the abscess center, inac-

tivation of antibiotics in the microenvironment of the infection (ie, hypoxia and acidity), and inactivity of the drug against a large bacterial inoculum. Drainage of an abscess usually reverses these adverse conditions and increases the efficacy of the antibiotics.

Drainage

Drainage, either percutaneous or surgical, is the mainstay of the management of intra-abdominal abscess. The ability to perform either technique depends on precise localization of the infection by means of CT scanning or ultrasonography.

Percutaneous drainage (PCD) has made a major contribution to the management of intra-abdominal abscess. It is the treatment of choice in the management of single, well-defined intra-abdominal abscesses in the pediatric population.[57] The management of the patient with a well-defined abscess amenable to drainage requires close collaboration between the radiologist and the surgeon. In young children, there are additional considerations. These include the need for an appropriate level of sedation, minimization of the radiation doses, equipment for monitoring hemodynamic status if the patient is septic, and measures to prevention of loss of body heat. If the patient has not improved markedly by 48 hours after initial percutaneous drainage, he or she is returned to the radiology department for a repeat CT scan. A residual abscess will be percutaneously drained at this time. Difficult locations of abscesses seem to be less of an issue. For deep pelvic abscesses, a transrectal approach or transgluteal approach may permit direct insertion of the drainage catheter.[58] An intercostal or transvisceral approach may be suitable for upper abdominal collections.

Criteria for removal of the percutaneous catheter are (1) clinical resolution of sepsis as determined by the patient's well-being, temperature, and leukocyte count, (2) minimal drainage from the catheter, and (3) radiologic evidence of resolution of the abscess on sinogram or CT scan.

The overall duration of drainage varies widely, ranging from 4 to 30 days. In general, prolonged periods of drainage are related to the presence of an enteric communication.

Successful percutaneous drainage occurs in 80 to 90% of patients. Failures may occur when drainage is performed in the early postoperative period before localization, when the abscess material is too thick for drainage (eg, pancreatic necrosis, infected hematoma, or candida abscess), when abscesses are small and multiple and, finally, when the diagnosis of abscess is erroneous (eg, an infected necrotic tumor mass). Complications occur in less than 5% of patients with major ones such as hemorrhage, enteric fistula, and empyema being extremely rare.

Improved localization techniques using either ultrasonography or CT scanning have also greatly simplified the surgical approach to the treatment of intra-abdominal abscess. Before the regular use of these techniques, a general abdominal exploration was usually performed for fear of missing multiple abscesses in the peritoneal cavity.[59] When the abscess can be located accurately by CT, a direct (often extraserous) approach to abscesses in the subphrenic, subhepatic, or pelvic region can be made, amounting to the surgical equivalent of percutaneous drainage. A general laparotomy under these circumstances is unnecessary and may lead to such complications as enteric fistula or bleeding. On the other hand, laparotomy is necessary when the abscesses are in the lesser sac or interloop or are multiple; the latter is particularly true in the early postoperative period.

No randomized, controlled studies have been performed comparing percutaneous with surgical drainage of intra-abdominal abscesses in adults. The classic mortality figure associated with surgical drainage of intra-abdominal abscesses has been in the range of 30%.[60] Studies advocating the use of percutaneous drainage have quoted mortality figures between 11 and 15%, which suggests an advantage to the approach. However, comparisons in noncontrolled studies demonstrate

Table 4 Organisms Isolated from 36 Intra-abdominal Abscesses in Children

Aerobic and Facultative Organisms	Number of Organisms Isolated	Anaerobic Organisms	Number of Organisms Isolated
Streptococcus spp. (total)	9	*Peptostreptococcus* spp.	28
Enterococcus spp.	4	*Clostridium* spp.	14
Escherichia coli	20	*Eubacterium* spp.	2
Pseudomonas aeruginosa	2	*Fusobacterium* spp.	5
Klebsiella pneumoniae	4	Pigmented *Prevotella* and *Porphyromonas* spp.	4
Proteus spp.	2	*Bacteroides* spp.	7
		Bacteroides fragilis*	14
		Bacteroides thetaiotaomicron	8
		Bacteroides vulgatus	5
		Bacteroides distasonis	2
		Bacteroides ovatus	2
Total number of anaerobic organisms and facultative organisms	41	Total number of anaerobic organisms	91

Adapted from Brook.[52]

no gross differences in mortality, although the percutaneously drained patient may stay in the hospital a shorter time.[61] The surgical patients were generally sicker, which perhaps explains this difference.[61] It is likely that the apparent improvement in survival associated with the use of percutaneous drainage is related to the use of improved imaging modalities, which can facilitate early diagnosis.

PRIMARY PERITONITIS

Primary peritonitis is defined as an infection of the peritoneal cavity in which there is no obvious source, such as a perforated viscus. It is particularly common in girls with the presumed source of infection being migration of microbes from the genitourinary tract into the peritoneal cavity via the fallopian tubes. Transmural migration of bacteria or hematogenous spread appear to be alternate origins of microbes in these cases. Children with nephrotic syndrome or postnecrotic cirrhosis appear to be at particularly high risk.[62]

Causative organisms generally fall into two categories, depending on the patient's age. In children, the usual organisms are gram-positive cocci, such as *Streptococcus pneumoniae* and group A streptococci, although gram-negative enterics such as *E. coli* are also recovered.[62–63] Anaerobes are rare, and in marked contrast to the frequency of polymicrobial infection in patients with secondary peritonitis, polymicrobial infection is present in fewer than 10% of cases. Immunocompromised patients are at risk for the development of primary peritonitis. In patients with the acquired immunodeficiency syndrome, *M. tuberculosis*, cytomegalovirus, and a variety of other opportunistic pathogens may cause primary peritonitis.[64]

Diagnostic Approach to Primary Peritonitis

In children, the clinical picture mimics that of secondary bacterial peritonitis with presenting signs and symptoms consisting of fever, nausea, vomiting, and abdominal pain. Abdominal examination reveals diffuse tenderness, rebound tenderness, guarding, and loss of bowel sounds. Primary peritonitis in patients with cirrhosis presents in a more subtle fashion. Primary peritonitis in children is infrequently diagnosed preoperatively. Children presenting to the hospital with evidence of peritonitis usually undergo laparotomy with a provisional diagnosis of acute appendicitis. The diagnosis is made after a negative laparotomy, when gram-positive organisms are cultured from the peritoneal swabs.

Management

Bacterial peritonitis caused by *S. pneumoniae* or group A streptococci should be treated with intravenous penicillin G. When other microbes, particularly gram-negative enterics, are suspected, cefotoxime or other advanced generation cephalosporins are appropriate.[65] Antimicrobial therapy should be adjusted when the results of culture and sensitivity testing become available. There is no specific indication for peritoneal dialysis in these patients, because parenterally administered antibiotics achieve adequate levels in ascitic fluid.

REFERENCES

1. Hau T, Hoffman R, Simmons RL. Mechanisms of the adjuvant effect of hemoglobin in experimental peritonitis: I. *In vivo* inhibition of peritoneal leukocytosis. Surgery 1978; 83:223–9.
2. Steinberg B. Infections of the Peritoneum. Hoeber: New York; 1944.
3. Bagby GJ, Plessala KJ, Wilson LA, et al. Divergent efficacy of antibody to tumor necrosis-alpha in intravascular and peritonitis models of sepsis. J Infect Dis 1991;163:83–8.
4. Astiz ME, Saha DC, Carpati CM, et al. Induction of endotoxin tolerance with monophosphoryl lipid A in peritonitis: Importance of localized therapy. J Lab Clin Med 1994;123:89–93.
5. Holzheimer RE, Schein M, Wittmann DH. Inflammatory response in peritoneal exudate and plasma of patients undergoing planned relaparotomy for severe secondary peritonitis. Arch Surg 1995;130:1314–9.
6. Schein M, Wittmann DH, Holzheimer R, et al. Hypothesis: Compartmentalization of cytokines in intra-abdominal infection. Surgery 1996;119:694–700.
7. Haecker FM, Fasler-Kan E, Manasse C, et al. Peritonitis in childhood: Clinical relevance of cytokines in the peritoneal exudates. Eur J Pediatr Surg 2006;16:94–9.
8. Haecker FM, Berger D, Schumacher U, et al. Peritonitis in childhood: Aspects of pathogenesis and therapy. Pediatr Surg Int 2000;16:182–188.
9. Malaviya R, Ikeda T, Ross E, et al. Mast cell modulation of neutrophil influx and bacterial clearance at sites of infection through TNF-alpha. Nature 1996;381:77–80.
10. Topley N, Brown Z, Jorres A, et al. Human peritoneal mesothelial cells synthesize interleukin-8: Synergistic induction by interleukin-1 beta and tumor necrosis factor-alpha. Am J Pathol 1993;142:1876–86.
11. Ford-Hutchinson AW. Leukotriene B$_4$ in inflammation. CRC Rev Immunol 1990;10:1.
12. Corderio RSB, Martins MA, Silva PMR. Proinflammatory activity of platelet-activating factor: Pharmacological modulation and cellular involvement. Prog Biochem Pharmacol 1988;22:156–67.
13. Mason MJ, van Epps DE. In vivo neutrophil emigration in response to interleukin-1 and tumor necrosis factor-alpha. J Leukoc Biol 989;45:62–8.
14. Dunn DL, Simmons RL. Fibrin in peritonitis: III. The mechanism of bacterial trapping by polymerizing fibrin. Surgery 1982;92:513–9.
15. Sinclair SB, Rotstein OD, Levy GA. Disparate mechanisms of induction of procoagulant activity by live and inactivated bacteria and viruses. Infect Immun 1990;58:1821–7.
16. Hau T, Payne WD, Simmons RL. Fibrinolytic activity of the peritoneum during experimental peritonitis. Surg Gynecol Obstet 1979;148:415–8.
17. Ahrenholz DH, Simmons RL. Fibrin in peritonitis: I. Beneficial and adverse effects of fibrin in experimental *E. coli* peritonitis. Surgery 1980;88:41–7.
18. Tracey KJ, Beutler B, Lowry SF, et al. Shock and tissue injury induced by recombinant human cachectin. Science 1986;234:470–4.
19. Dinarello CA. Interleukin-1. Rev Infect Dis 1984;6:51–95.
20. Castell JV, Gomez-Lechon MJ, David M, et al. Interleukin-6 is a major regulator of acute phase protein synthesis in adult human hepatocytes. FEBS Lett 1989;242:237–9.
21. Holzheimer RG, Schein M, Wittmann DH. Inflammatory response in peritoneal exudate and plasma of patients undergoing planned relaparotomy for severe secondary peritonitis. Arch Surg 1995;130:1314–9.
22. Tang G-J, Kuo C-D, Yen T, et al. Perioperative plasma concentrations of tumor necrosis factor-alpha and interleukin-6 in infected patients. Crit Care Med 1996;24:423–8.
23. Holman RC, Stoll BJ, Curns AT, et al. Necrotising enterocolitis hospitalizations among neonates in the Unites States. Paediatr Perinat Epidemiol 2006;20:498–506.
24. Hsueh W, Caplan MS, Qu XW, et al. Neonatal necrotizing enterocolitis: Clinical considerations and pathogenetic concepts. Pediatr Dev Pathol 2003;28:6–23.
25. Henry MC, Moss RL. Current issues in the management of necrotizing enterocolitis. Semin Perinatal 2004;28:221–33.
26. Blakely ML, Lally KP, McDonald S, et al. Subcommittee of the NICHD Neonatal Research Network. Postoperative outcomes of extremely low birth-weight infants with necrotizing enterocolitis or isolated intestinal perforation. Ann Surg 2005;241:984–94.
27. Abu-Yousef MM, Bleicher JJ, Maher JW, et al. High-resolution sonography of acute appendicitis. AJR Am J Roentgenol 1987;149:53–8.
28. Doria AS, Moineddin R, Kellenberger CJ, et al. US or CT for diagnosis of appendicitis in children and adults? A meta-analysis. Radiology 2006;241:83–94.
29. van Breda Vriesman AC, Puylaert JB. Mimics of appendicitis: Alternative nonsurgical diagnosis with sonography and CT. AJR Am J Roentgenol 2006;186:1103–12.
30. Paediatric Life Support Working Party of the European Resuscitation Council. Guidelines for paediatric life support. British Med J 1994;208:1349–55.
31. Boluyt N, Bollen CW, Bos AP, et al. Fluid resuscitation in neonatal and pediatric hypovolemic shock: A Dutch Pediatric Society evidence-based clinical practice guideline. Intensive Card Med 2006;32:995–1003.
32. Finfer S, Bellomo R, Boyce N, et al. A Comparison of albumin and salin for fluid resuscitation in the intensive care unit. N Engl J Med 2004;250:2247–56.
33. Choi PT, Yip G, Quinonez LG, Cook DJ. Crystalloids vs. colloids in fluid resuscitation: A systematic review. Crit Care Med 1999;27:200–10.
34. Drasar BS, Hill MJ. Human Intestinal Flora. London: Academic Press; 1974.
35. Ruddell WSJ, Axon ATR, Findlay JM, et al. Effect of cimetidine on the gastric bacterial flora. Lancet 1980;1:672.
36. Lorber B, Swenson RM. The bacteriology of intra-abdominal infections. Surg Clin North Am 1975;55:1349.
37. Mosdell DM, Morris DM, Fry DE. Peritoneal cultures and antibiotic therapy in pediatric perforated appendicitis. Am J Surg 1994;167:313–6.
38. Coates EW, Karlowicz MG, Croitoru DP, Buescher ES. Distinctive distribution of pathogens associated with peritonitis in neonates with focal intestinal perforation compared with necrotizing enterocolitis. Pediatrics 2005;116: 241–6.
39. Nadler EP, Gaines BA. The surgical infection society guidlines on antimicrobial therpay for children with appendicitis. Surg Infect 2007; in press.
40. Mazuski JE, Sawyer RG, Nathens AB, et al. The surgical infection society guildines on antimicrobial therapy for intra-abdominal infections: An executive summary. Surg Infect 2002;3:161–73.
41. Lelli JL Jr, Drongowski RA, Raviz S, et al. Historical changes in the postoperative treatment of appendicitis in children: Impact on medical outcome. J Pediatr Surg 2000; 35:239–44.
42. Hoelzer DJ, Zabel DD, Zern JT. Determining duration of antibiotics use in children with complicated appendicititis: A randomized prospective double-blinded study. Am Surg 2004;70: 858–62.
43. Nathens AB, Rotstein OD. Therapeutic options in peritonitis. Surg Clin North Am 1994;74:677–92.
44. Chang YJ, Yan DC, Kong MS, et al. Non-traumatic colon perforation in children: A 10-year review. Pediatr Surg Int 2006;22:665–9.
45. Dunn DL, Barke RA, Ahrenholz DH, et al. The adjuvant effect of peritoneal fluid in experimental peritonitis. Mechanism and clinical implications. Ann Surg 1984;199:37–43.
46. Hau T, Nishikawa R, Phangsab A. Irrigation of the peritoneal cavity and local antibiotics in the treatment of peritonitis. Surg Gynecol Obstet 1983;156:25–30.
47. Noon GP, Beall AC Jr, Jordon GL Jr, et al. Clinical evaluation of peritoneal irrigation with antibiotic solution. Surgery 1967;62:73.
48. Gerding DN, Hall WH, Schieri EA. Antibiotic concentrations in ascitic fluid of patients with ascites and bacterial peritonitis. Ann Intern Med 1977;86:708–13.
49. Moss RL, Dimmitt RA, Barnhart DC, et al. Laparotomy versus peritoneal drainage for necrotizing enterocolitis and perforation. N Engl J Med 2006;254:2225–36.
50. Rescorla FJ, Grosfeld JL. Contemporary management of meconium ileus. World J. Surg 1993;17:318–25.
51. Altemeier WA, Culbertson WR, Shook CD. Intra-abdominal abscesses. Am J Surg 1973;125:70–9.
52. Brook I. Intra-abdominal, retroperitoneal, and visceral abscess in children. Eur J Pediatr Surg 2004;14:265–73.
53. Stone HH, Bourneuf AA, Stinson LD. Reliability of criteria for predicting persistent or recurrent sepsis. Arch Surg 1985;120:17.
54. Baker ME, Blinder RA, Rice RP. Diagnostic imaging of abdominal fluid collections and abscesses. CRC Crit Rev Diagn Imaging 1986;25:233.

55. Moir C, Robins RE. Role of ultrasonography, gallium scanning, and computerized tomography in the diagnosis of intraabdominal abscess. Am J Surg 1982;143: 582–5.

56. Moore F, Feliciano D, Andrassy R, et al. Early enteral feeding, compared with parenteral, reduces postoperative septic complications: The results of a meta-analysis. Ann Surg 1992;216:172–83.

57. Gervais DA, Brown SD, Connolly SA, et al. Percutaneous imaging-guided abdominal and pelvic abscess drainage in children. Radiographics 2004;24:737–54.

58. Gervais DA, Hahn PF, O'Neill MJ, Mueller PR. CT-Guided transgluteal drainage of deep pelvic abscesses in children: Selective use as an alternative to transrectal drainage. AJR Am J Roentgenol 2000;175:1393–6.

59. Halasz NA. Subphrenic abscesses: Myths and facts. JAMA 1970;214:724–6.

60. Fry DE, Garrison RN, Heitsch RC, et al. Determinants of death in patients with intraabdominal abscess. Surgery 1980;88:517–23.

61. Olak J, Christou NV, Stein LA, et al. Operative vs percutaneous drainage of intraabdominal abscesses: Comparison of morbidity and mortality. Arch Surg 1986;121: 141–6.

62. McDougal WS, Izant RJ Jr, ,et al. Primary peritonitis in infancy and childhood. Ann Surg 1975;181:310–3.

63. Harken AH, Shochat SJ. Gram-positive peritonitis in children. Am J Surg 1973;125:769–72.

64. Wilcox CM, Forsmark CE, Darragh TM, et al. Cytomegalovirus peritonitis in a patient with the acquired immunodeficiency syndrome. Dig Dis Sci 1992;37:1288–91.

65. Sheer TA, Runyon BA. Spontaneous bacterial peritonitis. Dig Dis. 2005;23:39–46.

21

Malnutrition

Stephen John Allen, MBChB, MRCP (UK) Paeds, DTM&H, MD

The commitment to the Millennium Development Goals,[1] has brought malnutrition back in to the spotlight. Underweight in children is directly relevant to a target of MDG1 (halving between 1990 and 2015 the proportion of people who suffer from hunger—assessed by percentage of under fives who are underweight) and to reducing by two-thirds, between 1990 and 2015, the under five mortality rate (MDG 4). In fact improving nutritional status is seen as central to achieving at least 6 of the 8 MDGs[2] as well as being essential for economic development.[3]

MALNUTRITION: THE SINGLE MOST IMPORTANT RISK FACTOR FOR DISEASE

At the beginning of the third millennium, malnutrition remains closely associated with poverty[4] and is common even in politically stable regions not affected by conflict.[5,6] A recent review by UNICEF based on data available from 1996 to 2005 for 110 developing countries[7] shows that about 146 million (146 million; 10%) children under 5 are at least moderately wasted (defined as a weight for age Z [WAZ] score of <-2; WHO standards) and 2% are severely wasted (WAZ <-3). The greatest number of underweight children live in South Asia (78 million children with WAZ score <-2) with sub-Saharan Africa as the next most affected region (33 million; Figure 1).

Although the proportion of children under 5, who are underweight in developing countries, has fallen from 33% in 1990 to 28% in 2004, the improvement has not occurred in all regions (Figure 2).[2] The prevalence has fallen most sharply in Asia—mainly because of marked improvements in China. In contrast, the prevalence of underweight in countries in sub-Saharan Africa is unchanged or has even risen since 1990—and so numbers of underweight children have increased greatly in this region as a result of high population growth. The prevalence of underweight is usually twofold higher in rural than urban populations and boys and girls are equally affected except in South Asia where girls are more affected.[7]

The seminal work by Pelletier and colleagues based on calculation of attributable risk in prospective community studies[8] has been validated more recently.[9] In developing countries, over 50% of all deaths in children under 5 are attributable to malnutrition. This equates to 5.6 million of the 10.6 million deaths that occur in children each

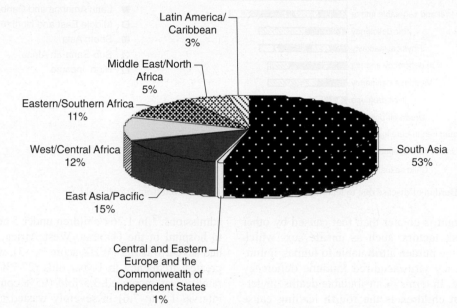

Figure 1 Where do the 146 million underweight children live? Percentage of the world's underweight children (WAZ score <-2) according to geographical region. (Adapted from reference 7.)

year. Weight for age has a direct relationship with child mortality that is independent of secular and socioeconomic factors.[10] A recent analysis of data from 2001 confirmed that underweight in children remains the single leading cause of health loss in the world today (Figure 3)[11]. Child underweight for age accounts for 8.7% of the total disease burden in people living in low and middle-income countries—mainly countries in South Asia and sub-Saharan Africa. The disease burden attributable to

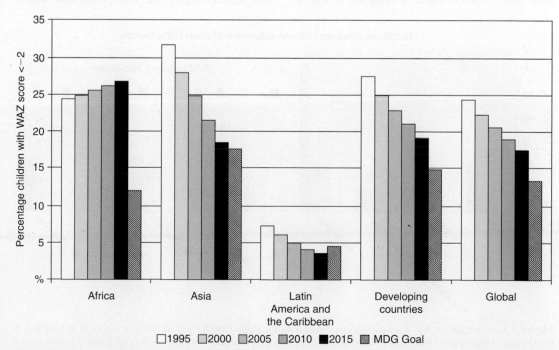

Figure 2 Current and predicted trends in underweight in children under 5 years according to geographical region. The target for percentage underweight for each region is shown. (Reproduced from reference 2.)

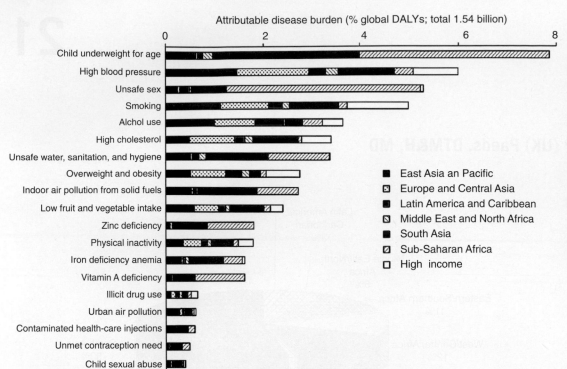

Attributable disease burden (% global DALYs; total 1.54 billion)

Figure 3 Burden of disease due to leading global risk factors. (Reproduced from reference 11.)

underweight is greater than that caused by other major risk factors, such as unsafe sex, which captures the burden attributable to human immunodeficiency virus/acquired immune deficiency syndrome. In terms of attributable deaths, underweight in children is the fourth leading cause after high blood pressure, smoking, and high cholesterol. Additional disease burdens result from specific micronutrient deficiencies (Figure 3).

Severe malnutrition is common in hospitals in economically poor countries. Among children admitted to a rural district hospital in Kenya between 1999 and 2002, 16% (1,282/8,190) had severe wasting (WHZ score ≤ -3), kwashiorkor or both. Case fatality for severely wasted children was 19.9% compared with 4.4% for all

admissions.[12] In 1,264 children under 5 admitted to hospital in the Gambia, West Africa, 13.1% had severe wasting (WHZ score < -3), with the greatest frequency in 1-year olds (27.7%). Case fatality was increased 3.5-fold (95% confidence interval 1.6 to 7.6) in severely wasted children compared with better nourished children (WHZ score > -2).[13]

The specific disease associations of malnutrition-attributable deaths have been investigated. Underweight increased susceptibility to several infections in admissions to hospitals in the Gambia.[14] In children with a primary diagnosis of malaria, severe malaria, pneumonia, meningitis, or gastroenteritis, mean WAZ score on admission was between 1.4 and 2.5 lower than that in

community controls. Weight deficits were too great to be accounted for by dehydration or anorexia during the acute illness. Overall, case fatality rose progressively with decreasing WAZ score—from 7.2% for a WAZ score > -2 to 22.7% for a WAZ score < -4—and this relationship was seen in all of these disease categories (Figure 4). Analysis of cohort and case-control studies from hospital and community settings reported that malnutrition-associated deaths occur in diarrhea, acute respiratory infections, malaria, and measles.[9,15] As well as case fatality rates for severe malnutrition of up to 60% in some settings,[16] these data highlight the fact that undernutrition is common in children with a primary diagnosis other than malnutrition. This poor nutritional status often goes unrecognized and specific nutritional support as part of inpatient management may reduce case fatality.

ALIMENTARY SYSTEM IN MALNUTRITION

The development of instruments to acquire per oral biopsies of the small intestine in the 1950s led to several classic studies of gut structure and function in malnutrition. However, marked differences in patient groups and study designs make comparisons between studies difficult. Most patients were young children (mostly aged 1 to 3 years), but the classification of malnutrition and the mix of the major types varied between studies. Classifications of nutritional deficiency are generally complicated because they combine anthropometry with clinical signs.[17] Early studies used the term "marasmus" to describe severe wasting without edema (Figure 5). Kwashiorkor was used less consistently; it denoted the presence of nutritional edema in children who were usually underweight and may, or may not, have had the classic clinical signs initially described in Ghanaian children by Williams,[18] such as dermatosis, hair changes, apathy, and irritability (Figure 6). Marasmic kwashiorkor was used for children with edema who were severely underweight. Investigations were done in children with varying severity of malnutrition ("mild" kwashiorkor) and at different stages of rehabilitation.

This terminology was summarized in the Welcome classification.[19] In a later classification, Waterlow emphasized the importance of

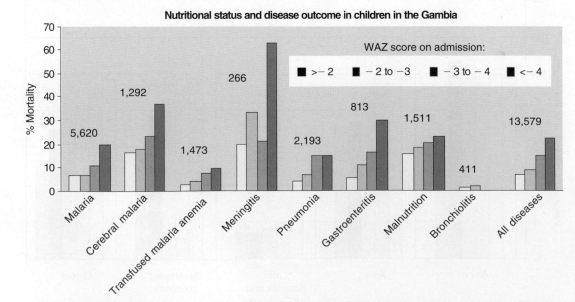

Figure 4 Low weight for age Z score was associated with increased case fatality in children admitted to hospitals in the Gambia. Underweight was common and this relationship with mortality was seen in several major diseases as well as those with a primary diagnosis of malnutrition. The number of children with each diagnosis is shown on the figure. (Adapted from reference 14.)

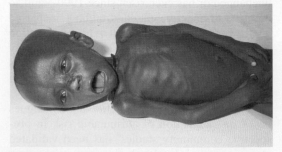

Figure 5 A severely wasted West African child who presented in 2001 with hypoglycemia, hypothermia, and dehydration. (Photograph used with permission from the carer.)

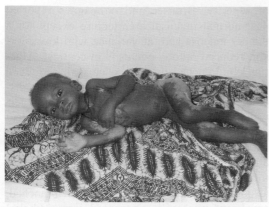

Figure 6 A West African child with marasmic-kwashiorkor who presented in 1999. (Photograph used with permission from the carer.)

distinguishing wasting, expressed as low weight for height and signifying acute malnutrition, from stunting, a sign of chronic malnutrition and reflected in low height for age.[20] In more recent studies, the term protein–energy malnutrition has been used to encompass the interrelated features of deficiency in carbohydrates, proteins, and fat, as well as vitamins, minerals, and trace elements.

Most case series report that anemia is common and serum albumin is usually low or very low. Micronutrient deficiencies were usually not assessed but will have differed between study populations. Researchers usually determined whether findings in malnourished children were abnormal by comparison with controls, but the choice of control group varied between studies. Some recruited children living in the same environment as the index cases, often hospital controls, who themselves may have had environmental enteropathy (see below) and moderate malnutrition. Others chose well-nourished local controls or even children living in developed countries.

A wide variety of acute and chronic infections are common in malnourished children and the very close synergism between malnutrition and infection has been reviewed recently by Scrimshaw.[21] A recent study of blood cultures taken from 1,093 children attending a hospital outpatient department in Kenya showed that clinically significant bacteremia was present in 8/101 (7.9%) children with WAZ score <−3 or with bilateral pedal edema compared with 14/992 (1.4%) nonseverely malnourished children (P < .001).[22] In a study of 46 malnourished children in Jamaica, 42 (91.3%) had evidence of one or more infections.[23] Acute or persistent diarrhea is extremely frequent in case series of malnourished children and many attempts have been made to identify infective causes. A wide variety of bacteria and parasites are isolated from stools, but a specific organism is not identified in many children. A further difficulty is that the detection of infections is highly dependent on the methods used, which is particularly important for gut organisms such as *Giardia lamblia*, for which routine diagnostic methods are unreliable.[24] Also, attributing pathology in the gut to specific organisms isolated from stools is complicated

because the same organisms are often isolated from healthy controls without diarrhea. It is clear that a variety of acute and chronic infections can impair linear growth by multiple mechanisms (reviewed by Stephensen 1999[25]) and that the prevention and prompt management of infection is an essential component of protecting growth.

The large mucosal surface area, with a high turnover rate, and the production of large amounts of fluids and enzymes make the gastrointestinal tract particularly susceptible to infection and nutrient deficiency. However, the specific cause(s) of gut abnormalities in malnourished children remain poorly understood. In this review, emphasis is placed on those abnormalities that may be targets for therapeutic interventions either to prevent malnutrition or to improve its outcome.

Stomach

Researchers in Egypt reported markedly prolonged gastric emptying time assessed by ultrasound after both liquid and semisolid meals in young children with marasmus, but not kwashiorkor, compared with nonmalnourished controls.[26] These findings support the need for frequent small volume feeds in malnourished children. Gastric emptying time normalized after nutritional recovery.

Gastric histology in five South African children with kwashiorkor showed variable degrees of mucosal atrophy, reduced goblet cells, and increased inflammatory infiltrate.[27] Abnormalities were still present 1 year later in one child after clinical recovery. Indonesian children with a range of nutritional deficiency showed variable degrees of gastric atrophy and chronic gastritis compared with the biopsies of healthy controls living in metropolitan Jakarta.[28]

Basal acid output was low in malnourished South African[27] and Indonesian children,[28] and 26 of 34 (76%) Bangladeshi children, mostly with marasmic kwashiorkor, had baseline hypochlorhydria.[29] Hypochlorhydria persisted despite stimulation in 4 of 20 (20%) of the South African children[27] and 8 (24%) of the Bangladeshi children.[29] Both basal and stimulated acid concentration had not improved at follow-up despite a marked increase in nutritional status and increased gastric juice volume.[29] In the South African cases, acid output increased only when clinical recovery from kwashiorkor and anemia was complete.[27] In some studies, hypochlorhydria was also common in children recruited as controls.[28,29] For example, an intubation study of Gambian infants living in rural villages reported that 4 of 29 (14%) had hypochlorhydria (gastric pH >4).[30]

Impairment of the gastric acid barrier appears to be a common finding in children living in poverty, not only those with frank malnutrition. Clearly, it is now known that *Helicobacter pylori* infection is extremely common in young children in developing countries. Infection rates often exceed 50% in children by age 5 years and 90% in adults (reviewed in reference 31). In Gambian infants, colonization determined by the urea

breath test was present in 19% at age 3 months and in 84% by 30 months[32] and acquisition of *H. pylori* was associated with hypochlorhydria, assessed noninvasively by urine acid output following a test feed.[33] This suggested that *H. pylori* may compromise the gastric acid barrier and allow bacterial contamination of the intestine. Consistent with this hypothesis, in further studies of Gambian infants, infection with *H. pylori* was associated with significantly reduced rates of weight and length gain although, in this environment at least, no weight deficit was detected at follow-up later in childhood.[34]

The Small Intestine

Prompted by the frequent occurrence of diarrhea and reports of steatorrhea, markedly reduced absorption of various nutrients has been demonstrated in malnourished children and the implications for the design of rehabilitation diets have been much debated.

Carbohydrates. Intolerance of lactose is the most consistently reported problem. Stool chromatography in 24 South African children with kwashiorkor and 3 with marasmus revealed lactose in all but 2.[35] A carbohydrate-free diet reduced stool weight and stool lactic acid content markedly in most children, including 8 children with intestinal pathogens in the stools. Reintroduction of milk increased stool output and lactic acid markedly in some children. Carbohydrate tolerance tests in a few children showed impaired lactose absorption. Lactose intolerance was also demonstrated in 14 of 17 Ethiopian boys with kwashiorkor, apparently without diarrhea[36]; in 10 South African children with kwashiorkor tested after 3 weeks of hospital treatment[37]; in 10 malnourished Jamaican infants, 4 of whom had edema but none had severe diarrhea[38]; in 9 of 100 malnourished Indian children, of whom 7 had kwashiorkor but none had enteropathogens isolated[39]; and in 21 of 43 Brazilian children with a range of nutritional deficiency.[40] Intolerant children often developed acid stools (pH <4) and abdominal symptoms during challenge tests.[39] Flat lactose tolerance tests were also common in marasmic Brazilian children.[41] Lactose maldigestion also correlated with poor growth in breastfed Gambian infants living in the community.[42]

Malabsorption of other sugars is more varied. Glucose and galactose malabsorption occurred in about half of the Ethiopian[36] and South African children.[37] All the Indian children[39] malabsorbed glucose, but only 1 of 20 Brazilian children did.[40] Sucrose malabsorption varied from 24 to 60% of cases.[36,38–40] Absorption of all sugars improved with clinical recovery. In the Jamaican series, absorption had increased after 6 to 16 weeks of treatment,[38] and all but 4 of the Indian children had normal sugar absorption after 3 months of nutritional rehabilitation.[39]

In keeping with these observations, variable deficiencies of mucosal disaccharidases have been reported. Half of a series of malnourished South African children had lactase deficiency, especially those with giardiasis, but sucrase and maltase levels were mostly normal.[43] Lactase, maltase, and sucrase activity was low in Ugandan children with mild to moderate kwashiorkor, with lower enzyme activity in those with more severe mucosal atrophy.[44] Disaccharidase deficiency persisted at 1 year after recovery. Lactose intolerance and lactase deficiency persisted in Ugandan children reassessed between 4 and 10 years after recovery from kwashiorkor.[45] However, mucosal histology was similar to that in adult hospital controls, and other disaccharidases were normal. Therefore, whether lactose intolerance was due to long-term mucosal damage or reflected the normal reduction of lactase activity with age in the population was unclear. Lactose-induced diarrhea in children with kwashiorkor did not significantly reduce absorption of nitrogen or fat, allowing continued milk feeding.[35] Despite these deficiencies in disaccharidases and carbohydrate absorption, lower intakes of sugar in milk feeds may be tolerated well without troublesome diarrhea.[37]

Nitrogen. Moderately impaired absorption of nitrogen and increased losses from the gut are related to both malnutrition and gut infection. In malnourished South African children most of whom had hookworm infection, although the proportion of nitrogen intake excreted in stools was higher than in European infants, nearly all children had adequate nitrogen retention of about 50% of dietary intake.[46] A further study confirmed high rates of nitrogen absorption in children with kwashiorkor on milk feeds.[47] In underweight Guatemalan children with edema and a heavy burden of gut pathogens,[48] markedly decreased nitrogen absorption was correlated with the degree of protein depletion as assessed by urinary creatinine-to-height ratio. Nitrogen absorption improved rapidly with clinical recovery. Four Guatemalan children with marasmic kwashiorkor studied during the late stages of recovery absorbed about 80% of ingested nitrogen, and absorption was proportional to intake, although the children remained protein depleted.[49] However, in this study, absorption fell markedly during episodes of diarrhea. A recent study showed that splanchnic glycine extraction was similar in malnourished Jamaican children with and without edema both during and after infection and also in recovery.[50]

Fat. Variable decreases in dietary fat absorption have been reported, even in children without macroscopic steatorrhea, and absorption improved slowly during recovery. Average fat absorption was 81.8% in malnourished South African children (compared with 95% in normal children),[46] and malabsorption occurred in between 30 and 100% of malnourished children from Mexico City,[51] India,[39] and Guatemala.[48] The mean increase in plasma triglycerides after an oral margarine load was significantly lower in underweight Brazilian children than in controls.[40] In the late stages of recovery from marasmic kwashiorkor, fat absorption varied from 32 to 89% in Guatemalan children[49] and improved gradually

with clinical recovery in a Mexican series.[51] Fat absorption did not appear to be affected by episodes of diarrhea.[39,49] In addition to decreased absorption, lipid catabolism, an important supply of energy, was impaired in Jamaican children with kwashiorkor.[52]

Vitamin B$_{12}$. Initial observations of markedly reduced vitamin B$_{12}$ absorption that was slow to improve with clinical recovery[48] were confirmed in a study of Guatemalan children with severe malnutrition.[53] At both admission and convalescence, absorption was reduced further in children with diarrhea. Absorption was not improved by giving intrinsic factor, suggesting mucosal dysfunction in the terminal ileum in PEM that is slow to recover, although metabolism of administered vitamin B$_{12}$ by bacteria in the upper gut is an alternative explanation.

Small Intestine—Histology

Compared with findings in developed countries, studies of kwashiorkor in Uganda,[44,54,55] Kenya,[56] South Africa,[44,57,58] and Guatemala[59] reported enteropathy in all cases with a wide range of abnormalities. Typically, the intestinal wall is thin, with a smooth, atrophic mucous membrane ("tissue paper intestine").[54] Villi tend to be convoluted and ridged rather than fingerlike. Villous atrophy reduces mucosal thickness (mean crypt-to-villus ratio 1.0; normal 0.2),[44] and there may be complete villous atrophy. The brush border is irregular and narrow and mucosal cells are irregular or cuboidal, with irregular and displaced nuclei. Intraepithelial lymphocytes are increased. There is frequent branching of crypts. The cellular infiltrate in the lamina propria is markedly increased and consists of lymphocytes, plasma cells, eosinophils, and polymorphonuclear leukocytes.

In South African children already established on a high-protein diet, accumulation of lipid droplets within epithelial cells was prominent.[57] Electron microscopy showed variable distribution of fat—as particles enclosed by smooth endoplasmic reticulum and Golgi vesicles and as chylomicrons in intercellular spaces or in vesicles within lamina propria macrophages. Mitochondria, endoplasmic reticulum, and lysosomes appeared normal. However, in another series of South African children who were studied before starting treatment, abnormalities of epithelial cells included poorly developed microvilli, sparse endoplasmic reticulum, irregular nuclei, and disorganized cytoplasmic organelles but no accumulation of lipid.[58] Crypt cells were immature with increased mitosis, suggesting a rapid turnover. These abnormalities were consistent with impaired absorptive function. Plasma cells in the lamina propria appeared inactive. The discrepancies in findings between the two studies may have been due to biopsies being taken at different stages of management.

In children with marasmus, abnormalities of mucosal architecture similar to those in kwashiorkor are seen, again with a wide range

of severity. Brunser and colleagues reported near-normal mucosal architecture except for a thinner mucosa and, at variance with kwashiorkor, reduced mitotic counts.[60] In contrast, Algerian children had thin mucosae with shortened or absent villi indistinguishable from celiac disease.[61] Studies of moderately to severely underweight Brazilian children, some with persistent diarrhea, reported variable shortening of villi from near-normal to subtotal villous atrophy, but all patients had increased inflammatory cell infiltrate.[40,41] Features on electron microscopy were also variable but included shortened, branched, or absent microvilli, increased intraepithelial lysosomes; irregular nuclei, and degenerative, detaching epithelial cells from the upper half of the villi—the latter associated with giardiasis.[41,62] Other epithelial cells had only minor abnormalities. Lamina propria plasma cells appeared inactive in about half of the patients. Barbezat and colleagues reported that mucosal atrophy in 3 South African children with marasmus was of a severity similar to that in 13 children with kwashiorkor and 1 with marasmic kwashiorkor,[43] whereas other authors consider mucosal lesions to be milder in marasmus than in kwashiorkor.[48,60]

Sullivan and colleagues performed detailed computerized image analysis of mucosal biopsies from 40 malnourished Gambian children with chronic diarrhea, mostly with marasmus and marasmic kwashiorkor.[63] Many had gut infections, especially with *G. lamblia*. The morphology of villi varied markedly from normal height to absent, but nearly all biopsies revealed crypt hypertrophy and lymphocytic infiltration of the lamina propria. Intraepithelial lymphocytes were increased, especially in the crypt epithelium. A mucosal specimen with well-preserved villi is shown in Figure 7A and an atrophic mucosa in Figure 7B. The degree of mucosal abnormality did not correlate with nutritional status or the presence of *G. lamblia* or *Strongyloides stercoralis*, but it was difficult to distinguish the effects on the mucosa of malnutrition from those of diarrhea.

In kwashiorkor, improved mucosal cell ultrastructure occurring after only 48 hours of intensive supportive treatment is consistent with a rapid increase in cell protein synthesis.[58] However, repeat biopsies following clinical recovery of kwashiorkor tend to show no or minimal improvement in mucosal appearances, even up to 1 year later.[44] Schneider and Viteri reported a progressive increase in mucosal and brush border thickness and epithelial cell height as nutritional recovery progressed, but crypt mitotic activity and the degree and composition of the cellular infiltrate in the lamina propria remained unchanged.[59]

Similarly, a common finding in studies of marasmus is the persistence of the mucosal lesion. The atrophic mucosa reported in the Algerian children persisted mostly unchanged when biopsies were repeated at 3 months despite marked clinical improvement.[61] After 3 to 4 weeks of inpatient treatment, there was little change in villous volume in the majority (16; 70%) of Gambian children in

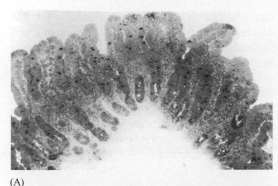

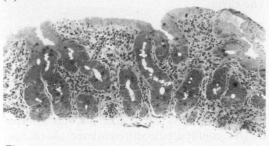

(A)

(B)

Figure 7 (A) Mucosal biopsy from a child with marasmus. The villi are well preserved but there is crypt hyperplasia and an increased inflammatory infiltrate. Dark areas at the tips of villi are fat globules. Specimen fixed in formaldehyde and stained with toluidine blue; ×100 original magnification. (Reproduced with permission from Dr P.B. Sullivan.) (B) Atrophic mucosa with intense inflammatory infiltrate and loss of surface epithelial cells in a child with marasmic-kwashiorkor. Specimen fixed in formaldehyde and stained with toluidine blue; ×100 original magnification. (Reproduced with permission from Dr P.B. Sullivan.)

whom diarrhea had resolved, weight gain was good, and mean crypt cell volume had increased.[64] Villous epithelial volume had actually decreased in three children, two of whom had failed to improve clinically. Further follow-up at 1 year after discharge in a small number of children revealed that most had diarrhea and mucosal architecture was worse than at admission. In the much longer term, between 4 and 10 years after kwashiorkor, complete recovery of the brush border and reduction in inflammatory infiltrate, at least to that seen in local controls, were observed.[45]

Given the long-term persistence of mucosal abnormalities following marasmus, it is not surprising that significant enteropathy also occurs in mildly to moderately malnourished children living in the community. Histologic evidence of this "environmental enteropathy" was found in infants with mostly mild to moderate malnutrition living in a Brazilian slum when compared with eight hospital controls from middle-class families.[65] Twenty-nine (73%) of the slum-dwellers had varying degrees of villous atrophy and increased inflammatory infiltrate in the lamina propria, with severe lesions in some children. Mucosal biopsies from stillborn fetuses in Southern India[66] and African neonates[44] had normal appearances with fingerlike villi. Therefore, environmental enteropathy appears to be an acquired lesion, the timing of its onset coinciding with weaning and possibly bacterial colonization of the upper gut (see below).

Immunohistochemistry

The mucosal inflammatory response was characterized in Gambian children with nutritional status ranging from normal to severely underweight.[67] Although most children had diarrhea, stool pathogens were infrequent. However, giardiasis may have been underestimated based on stool microscopy alone. All children were HIV antibody negative. Age-matched children living in the United Kingdom investigated for vomiting or possible enteropathy but shown to have no gastroenterologic disorder were used as controls.

All of the Gambian children, regardless of nutritional status, had increased mucosal permeability, crypt hyperplastic villous atrophy, and increased intraepithelial lymphocytes—the latter with an increased proportion of $\gamma\delta$ cells and within the range characteristic of celiac disease. There was no correlation between permeability, morphometric indices of small bowel architecture, or number of intraepithelial lymphocytes and nutritional status.

Although a wide variation was observed, compared with the UK controls, the median density of cells in the lamina propria in the Gambian children was 4 to 5 times higher for CD3+ and 15 to 30 times higher for CD25+ cells. Activation of the epithelium was evidenced by increased expression of perforin by cytotoxic lymphocytes and human leukocyte antigen (HLA)-DR by crypt cells. The numbers of B cells were increased two- to threefold compared with the UK controls, with an even greater increase in mature B cells. The density of mucosal cytokineimmunoreactive cells was greater in Gambian than in UK children for both proinflammatory (interferon [IFN]-γ and tumor necrosis factor-α) and putative regulatory (interleukin-10, transforming growth factor [TGF]-β) cytokines. However, the density of TGF-β–producing cells fell as nutritional status worsened, whereas that of proinflammatory cytokineproducing cells remained unchanged. These findings suggest a chronic cell-mediated enteropathy, similar to that in celiac disease, that did not appear to be caused by specific gut pathogens. The presence of an enteropathy in Gambian children of different nutritional states, with a shift toward greater proinflammatory responses in the most malnourished, suggests that the enteropathy of severe malnutrition may be a continuum of that seen in "tropical" or "environmental" enteropathy.

These findings in Gambian children are broadly similar to the findings of a study of Zambian and black and white South African adults investigated for dyspepsia but without other systemic or gastrointestinal illness.[68] Living conditions for the Zambians were considered to be worse than those for the South Africans. Mean body mass index and serum albumin was significantly lower in the Zambians than in the South Africans, but none were overtly malnourished. In mucosal biopsies, compared with the South Africans, the Zambians had significantly decreased villous height, increased crypt depth, and increased crypt mitotic count. Increased mucosal T-cell activation in the Zambians was evidenced by increased numbers of cells expressing CD69 and HLA-DR.

Intestinal Permeability: Severe Malnutrition

Markedly reduced absorption of D-xylose, consistent with reduced mucosal surface area, was observed in malnourished South African,[69] Indian,[39] Ethiopian,[36] Guatemalan,[48] and Brazilian[40] children. Absorption improved with clinical recovery.

Differential absorption of different-sized sugar molecules to assess simultaneously mucosal surface area and leakiness has been used extensively in studies of malnourished children in both community and hospital settings. Several studies of Gambian children have shown that decreased surface area and increased leakiness are associated with worsening nutritional status. Behrens and colleagues reported a mean ($\pm$ 2 SD) urinary lactulose-to-mannitol (L/M) ratio of 1.3 (0.2 to 13) in repeated tests done in children with marasmus compared with 0.42 (0.2 to 1.4) in well children living in an urban environment.[70] L/M ratios were even higher in 15 children with chronic diarrhea (2.85 [0.2 to 10.4]). Ratios improved with weight gain and recovery from diarrhea. In the malnourished children with persistent diarrhea reported by Sullivan and colleagues, the mean ($\pm$SD) L/M ratio on admission was 0.66 ($\pm$0.36).[71] Mannitol absorption improved slowly but progressively during treatment, suggesting some increase in mucosal surface area, but a marked increased recovery of lactulose after treatment for 3 to 4 weeks suggested persistence of abnormal mucosal leakiness.

Brewster and colleagues studied 149 Malawian children with kwashiorkor on admission and during in-patient rehabilitation, of whom one-third were likely to have had HIV infection.[72] Lactulose-to-rhamnose ratios were much higher on admission (geometric mean 0.17 [95% CI 0.15 to 0.20]) than those in hospital controls (0.07 [0.06 to 0.09]) because of decreased rhamnose absorption in the cases. Abnormal permeability was associated with oliguria, sepsis, diarrhea, wasting, young age, and death during admission. In logistic regression analysis, diarrhea and death were associated independently with both decreased absorption and increased leakiness, whereas wasting was associated with decreased absorption only. The association between increased permeability and death suggested that sepsis might have been caused by translocated bacteria from the gut. In survivors, permeability improved little despite clinical recovery and, 3 to 4 weeks later, remained higher than that of local controls, suggesting impaired intestinal cell renewal after enteric infection and malnutrition.

Permeability of the mucosa to nondegraded proteins, assessed by permeability of jejunal explants to horseradish peroxidase in Algerian children with marasmus, marasmic kwashiorkor, and kwashiorkor, was markedly increased on admission.[61] Permeability was lower during clinical recovery but remained abnormal. This finding is consistent with the increased serum antibodies to several food proteins in malnutrition, but whether immune responses to food antigens are involved in the pathogenesis of enteropathy remains unclear.[73]

Intestinal Permeability: Community Studies

In keeping with histologic evidence of enteropathy, noninvasive tests of mucosal permeability are frequently abnormal in children living in the community. D-Xylose absorption was markedly decreased in infants living in a Brazilian slum, most of whom were moderately underweight.[65] Lunn reported that the mean (SD) L/M ratio in infants living in Gambian villages was 0.38 (0.30) compared with 0.12 (0.09) in matched UK control infants.[74] Tests were repeated frequently during the first year of life in 119 infants and correlated with growth. By UK standards, L/M ratios in the Gambian infants were abnormal in 76% of tests. In regression analysis, abnormal L/M ratios accounted for about 40% of growth faltering for both weight and length gains.

A study of gut permeability in older children and adults in the Gambia showed that mannitol recovery was always at least half of expected UK values and did not improve with age.[75] However, lactulose recovery improved progressively to fall into the UK range from the age of 10 years. L/M ratios showed within-subject correlation over time, suggesting long-term persistence of enteropathy within individuals. A significant correlation between both L/M ratio and lactulose recovery and height for age Z-score was present during both childhood and adult life, suggesting that enteropathy may adversely affect growth both in childhood and during puberty.

Interventions to Improve Intestinal Permeability

The beneficial effects of vitamin A on mucosal barrier function and its effect on immune responses have been reviewed recently.[76] Encouraged by an observation in Gambian infants that mucosal integrity is least impaired at times of the year when dietary vitamin A is abundant,[77] randomized intervention studies were done in 144 hospitalized and 80 rural infants in India.[78] Infants living in the community had significantly lower L/M ratios after vitamin A supplementation (16,700 IU weekly for 8 weeks) than those receiving placebo, although the differences were small. Infants hospitalized with diarrhea or respiratory infections received 200,000 IU of vitamin A, either at admission or discharge, or placebo. The mean L/M ratio fell in all groups but was significantly lower at 10 and 30 days following discharge in the treated groups. Data on the absorption of the individual sugars were not reported.

Vitamin A supplementation during pregnancy and at delivery of HIV-positive South African mothers did not affect L/M ratios in non-HIV-infected infants.[79] However, among infants who themselves acquired HIV infection, those of supplemented mothers maintained significantly lower L/M ratios over the first 14 weeks of life compared with those of unsupplemented mothers. This effect was due to increased absorption of lactulose in the infants of the control mothers, whereas mannitol absorption in the two groups was similar. The authors concluded that the effect of vitamin A in reducing mucosal permeability may help to counter growth faltering in HIV-infected infants.

Like vitamin A, zinc is considered essential for normal immune function and protection against infections.[80] Zinc supplementation prevents episodes of diarrhea and reduces the duration and severity of acute and persistent diarrhea, with some evidence of a greater beneficial effect in malnourished children.[81,82] Roy and colleagues studied the effects of zinc supplementation (5 mg/kg/d elemental zinc for 2 weeks) on intestinal integrity in Bangladeshi children with acute and persistent diarrhea.[83] Many children had low serum vitamin A, and all received vitamin A supplements. Although mannitol absorption remained unchanged, supplementation reduced lactulose absorption in both conditions. The effects were greatest in the most undernourished children and those with hypozincemia at recruitment.

In a randomized community study of 110 Gambian children aged 0.5 to 2.3 years, zinc supplementation (70 mg twice weekly for 1.25 years) resulted in a small increase in mid-upper arm circumference but no difference in weight gain.[84] Although the mean L/M ratios were not affected by the supplement, lactulose absorption was significantly decreased in the supplemented group.

A recent study of enteral glutamine supplementation in underweight Brazilian infants managed according to WHO guidelines reported markedly improved mucosal permeability as assessed by L/M ratio.[85] However, weight gain was not significantly improved although this was only assessed after 10 days of treatment. Supplementation with both vitamin A and zinc appears to have beneficial effects on intestinal mucosa and are considered essential in the nutritional rehabilitation of severe malnutrition.[86] The role of glutamine in the management of severe malnutrition and of micronutrients in environmental enteropathy requires further study.

Large Intestine

Sigmoidoscopy in South African children with kwashiorkor showed increased vascularity of the rectal mucosa.[87] On microscopy, there was mild atrophy of epithelial cells, which had a flattened surface and displaced nuclei. Goblet cells were numerous in crypts but reduced on the luminal surface. Polymorphonuclear leukocytes were noticeable in the surface epithelium, and the number of plasma cells increased throughout the lamina propria. The numbers of lymphocytes and macrophages appeared normal. Mucosal histol-ogy returned to normal in most cases after 3 to 4 weeks of treatment, although the plasma cell infiltration persisted. In a study of 16 moderately to severely underweight Brazilian infants, colitis was present in 10, and, of these, only 6 had an enteropathogen isolated from the stools.[62] As with inflammation in the small bowel, colitis appears to be a feature of malnutrition even in the absence of gut infection and is likely to contribute to diarrhea.

The Liver

The fatty infiltration of the liver in kwashiorkor is well known. Autopsies and biopsies of 10 Ugandan children showed a progression of fatty infiltration of hepatocytes beginning at the periphery of lobules and progressing to centrolobular areas.[88] In some cases, fat infiltration was so severe that the liver appeared pale yellow and normal hepatocytes could not be differentiated on microscopy. There was moderate periportal and peripheral pericellular fibrosis and cellular infiltration in the portal areas. The infiltration was mainly of lymphocytes, but eosinophils, macrophages, and neutrophils were also present. With clinical improvement, fat retreated initially from the centrolobular region, but the fibrosis persisted. More irregular patterns of fat infiltration were seen in children with concomitant severe infection,[54] and typical cases of kwashiorkor also occurred without any fatty infiltration of the liver.[88]

Abdominal ultrasonography in Jamaican children showed that hepatic steatosis was greater in children with edematous malnutrition than in those with marasmus, but all malnourished children had more hepatic fat than healthy controls did.[89] The extent of steatosis was not correlated with liver size, and fat was slow to be mobilized from the liver during recovery. Ultrasound examinations in Indian children also confirmed the presence of liver fat in malnourished children without edema.[90] The degree of hepatic steatosis was not associated with the severity of malnutrition or serum transaminases and improved in most cases with weight gain. Compared with biopsies from recovered children, autopsy specimens obtained immediately after death in Jamaican children showed several ultrastructural abnormalities, including decreased peroxisomes, consistent with increased susceptibility to free radical damage.[91]

Impairment of hepatic synthesis in malnourished children is evident by low plasma albumin. Reduced hepatic synthesis may be an important risk factor for mortality; a prolonged prothrombin time was present in 8 of 11 Nigerian children with kwashiorkor who died compared with 4 of 29 survivors.[92] One mechanism may be through decreased production of antibacterial substances such as transferrin and fibronectin, which were reduced in Nigerian children with kwashiorkor and marasmus compared with those in well-nourished local controls.[93] Aflatoxins are found frequently in kwashiorkor, and the known effects of aflatoxins in animal models raise the possibility that they contribute to liver dysfunction in malnutrition.[94]

Pancreas and Bile Acids

The extremely high rate of protein synthesis by pancreatic acinar cells in the production of digestive enzymes makes them especially susceptible to nutritional deficiency. In keeping with a general atrophy of exocrine glands,[54] children from East and Central Africa who died with kwashiorkor had a small pancreas owing to marked atrophy of the acinar cells, which had a reduced number of enzyme secretory granules. Intercalated ducts, secreting sodium and bicarbonate-rich fluid, were relatively well preserved, but there was a generalized fibrosis.[88,54,95] Trowell and colleagues considered atrophy of the pancreatic acinar cells to be both a more constant and persistent lesion in kwashiorkor than fatty infiltration of the liver.[54] Pancreatic atrophy was common and associated with a fatty liver in Jamaican children with kwashiorkor but also occurred in marasmic children who had little liver fat.[96] Electron microscopy revealed atrophy of acinar cells with few zymogen granules and disorganization of the endoplasmic reticulum. Pancreatic fibrosis was mild in kwashiorkor and uncommon in marasmus. A further study reported ultrastructural damage of all cell types with changes in B cells, consistent with low insulin secretion.[97] Serum immunoreactive trypsinogen, a marker of either acinar cell damage or ductal obstruction, was correlated with wasting but not stunting in Aboriginal children.[98] Pancreatic atrophy appeared to improve quickly with refeeding.[54]

These histologic findings correlate well with studies of pancreatic enzyme production in severely malnourished children. Pancreatic enzymes were low in Hungarian children with nutritional edema after the siege of Budapest (c. 1944).[99] Decreased amylase, trypsin, and lipase were reported in children with severe malnutrition, some with nutritional edema, in Mexico City.[100] In kwashiorkor, amylase and lipase were markedly reduced in Ugandan children,[46] and, in addition to these enzymes, trypsin and chymotrypsin were decreased in Egyptian[101] and South Africa children.[102] Production of enzymes improved promptly and to normal levels with clinical recovery.[45,98,100,102] South African children with marasmus had decreased amylase and chymotrypsin production.[102] In this study, the volume of pancreatic juice and pH in both kwashiorkor and marasmus were variable, but average values were similar to those in better nourished local controls, suggesting less impairment of the function of pancreatic ductules.

Deficiency of conjugated bile acids was the main cause of fat maldigestion, assessed by micellar lipid content of duodenal fluid, in underweight Guatemalan children with edema.[103,104] The concentration of conjugated bile acids in the duodenum was especially low in malnourished children with diarrhea. Free bile acids were increased in both cases and controls. Lipase activity was reduced but sufficient for normal lipolytic activity ($>75 \times 10^3$ U/mL), and total pancreatic enzyme output was only mildly reduced. Micellar lipid content and lipase activity normalized with clinical recovery, and conjugated bile acids increased to levels seen in the controls, although they remained low in children with diarrhea. Free bile acids remained high during recovery, especially in children with diarrhea. Some of the cases in this study had increased bacterial colonization of the upper gut, which may have contributed to conjugated bile acid deficiency (see below).[105] Increased free bile acids have also been reported in South African children with kwashiorkor.[106]

It is clear that several factors contribute to malabsorption, and these are likely to vary in different settings. Decreased conjugated bile acids, as a consequence of bacterial colonization of the upper gut, may be more important than deficiency of pancreatic lipase in fat malabsorption in kwashiorkor. Given the marked variability in findings between studies, it is clear that dietary rehabilitation needs to be tailored to individual children, especially those with diarrhea. However, digestion and absorption of carbohydrates, nitrogen, and fat appear to be sufficient for nutritional rehabilitation.[47,51] Milk-based diets are appropriate for most children, and the WHO has produced detailed feeding guidelines.[86] Despite decreased nutrient absorption, it is important to note that diets low in protein, fat, and sodium and high in carbohydrates are recommended during initial treatment. Dietary intake is increased during the rehabilitation phase of management, a time when absorption of many nutrients is improving.

GASTROINTESTINAL FLORA

Increased numbers of a wide variety of bacteria in gastric juice have been reported in malnourished Indonesian,[107] Brazilian,[108] and Bangladeshi children.[29] Large numbers of bacteria were found in 13 children with marasmic kwashiorkor living in poor areas of Guatemala City, but 3 of 4 normal controls also had high numbers of streptococci in gastric juice.[105] Bacterial overgrowth was associated with increased gastric pH in underweight Brazilian children with chronic diarrhea (57% had pH >4), but, interestingly, hypochlorhydria was equally common in better nourished breastfed controls who did not have increased gastric microbial contamination.[108] Similarly, gram-negative bacterial colonization of gastric juice (>100 colony-forming units/mL) was associated with reduced gastric acid output and increased pH in the Bangladeshi series, but colonization was not observed in any of 20 controls despite hypochlorhydria in many.[29] This suggests that other factors, in addition to gastric pH, determine susceptibility to bacterial colonization of the stomach. In malnourished children, the numbers of microorganisms fell with clinical recovery.[105,108]

In addition to bacterial contamination, large numbers of Candida sp (up to 10^9/mL) in gastric juice were found in malnourished Australian aboriginal and Indonesian children[109] and in malnourished Guatemalan children with diarrhea.[105]

Whether yeasts contribute to the gut changes in malnutrition remains unclear.

Increased bacterial colonization of the small bowel has been reported frequently in malnourished children, and, as in gastric juice, a wide variety of organisms have been isolated. However, several authors have noted that similar bacterial colonization also occurs in children living in the same environment as malnourished children. In a series of hospitalized, underweight Brazilian children,[62] 11 of 16 had $>10^4$ bacterial colonies/mL in jejunal aspirates, including enteropathogenic strains of *Escherichia coli*, *Proteus*, *Enterobacter*, *Pseudomonas*, and *Klebsiella*. Bacterial colonization was associated with a mucus-fibrinoid pseudomembrane over the luminal surface but not with other mucosal abnormalities. In the later study of mostly moderately underweight infants living in a Brazilian slum, colonization of jejunal juice with colonic flora varied from 10^2 to 10^9 colonies/mL, with 5 of 40 children having $>10^4$/mL.[65] In the Guatemalan series,[105] apart from greater numbers of Enterobacteriaceae in the cases, bacterial colonization of the small bowel was similar in cases and controls. Between 10^3 and 10^7 bacteria/mL, mainly streptococci, were present in three of four controls. In Gambian children with a range of nutritional deficiency, 22 of 25 had $>10^5$/mL facultative anaerobes in jejunal juice, with some children having counts $>10^{10}$/mL.[110] Most children were colonized with three to four types of organisms, mainly *E. coli*, bacteroides, and enterococci, and counts were higher in those with chronic diarrhea. Although no controls were tested in this study of hospitalized children, the findings can be compared with those of a later study carried out in 37 young Gambian children living in rural villages.[30] About half of these infants had $>10^5$ organisms/mL in jejunal juice.

Omoike and Abiodun, working in Benin City, Nigeria, reported mean bacterial counts in duodenal juice ranging between 10^3 and 10^9/mL among 30 malnourished children.[111] A wide range of organisms was identified, including Enterobacteriaceae, Bacteroides, and *Candida*. In contrast to the previous studies, bacterial counts were significantly lower in 11 well-nourished hospital controls, in 2 of whom duodenal juice was sterile, who lived in the same socioeconomic environment. In underweight Australian aboriginal children with chronic diarrhea, mean small intestinal bacterial counts were 5×10^6/mL in those receiving antibiotics and 2×10^6/mL in those not receiving antibiotics compared with 2×10^3/mL in Caucasian controls.[112] Bacteria were of the oral and fecal type, but anaerobes were rarely isolated. In the Indonesian series, the mean microbial count was 7.8×10^7/mL, consisting mainly of gram-positive cocci, enterobacteria, and streptococci, with gram-negative organisms also identified in many children.[107] In the series of Australian and Indonesian children, there was marked contamination of intestinal aspirates with Candida species (10^4 to 10^8/mL) compared with Caucasian controls.[109] In the studies in Australia and Indonesia, less microbial contamination of the gut in the controls may have been explained by better living conditions in this group.

Applying molecular methods[113] to complement the findings of existing studies and better define the intestinal microflora in both malnourished and healthy children in developing countries is a priority. The marked increased bacterial contamination of the upper gut in malnourished children is likely to contribute to malabsorption, for example, through the deconjugation of bile salts. In addition, loss of immune tolerance to intestinal bacteria is implicated in the pathogenesis of the T cell–mediated enteropathy of inflammatory bowel disease.[114] More research is needed on the role of bacterial contamination of the gut in causing environmental enteropathy and the enteropathy in severely malnourished children.

MANAGEMENT OF SEVERE MALNUTRITION

Significant shortages of staff, drugs, and other resources remain common throughout the developing world.[115,116] The management of the severely malnourished child poses a huge challenge to medical staff in such settings. Detailed management guidelines based on extensive clinical experience and findings of research are widely available.[86] Emphasis is placed on a 10 step approach divided into 3 phases of care. The initial phase usually lasts 1 to 2 days and aims to stabilize the child's condition and treat complications (hypoglycemia, hypothermia, dehydration, infection). In the subsequent 2 to 6 weeks, rehabilitation is effected by increasing feeds, correcting micronutrient deficiencies, providing a stimulating environment and preparation for discharge. The third phase provides follow-up after discharge to ensure continued improvement and detect relapse early. Although these guidelines are demanding, much can be achieved by avoiding harmful practices such as using diuretics for edema, using a high-protein feed during the initial treatment phase, using IV fluids rather than reduced sodium oral rehydration fluid for dehydration and failing to provide routine broad spectrum antibiotics to all patients.

Although implementation of the WHO guidelines has been effective in reducing case fatality in many settings,[117] they have also been shown to be difficult to implement despite intensive training and ongoing support. Staff shortages, high staff turnover and shortages of feeds and essential drugs have been identified.[118,119] Given these difficulties, much attention has focused on alternative approaches to management. In particular, the management of uncomplicated severe malnutrition in the community using ready-to-use therapeutic food has produced encouraging results.[120] These are high energy foods based on cereal or peanut and enriched with micronutrients. Importantly, they do not require reconstitution with water thereby reducing bacterial contamination. The success of this approach both in emergency[121,122] and endemic[123] situations supports an update to the classification of severe

malnutrition in settings with established community programmes.[124] This allocates acutely malnourished children to one of 3 groups. Children who are clinically well, alert, and have an appetite are allocated to either moderate uncomplicated malnutrition (WHZ score ≥ -3 to < -2 and no edema) requiring outpatient supplementary feeding or severe uncomplicated malnutrition (WHZ score < -3 or edema) requiring outpatient therapeutic care. Only moderately or severely malnourished children with complications such as anorexia, severe dehydration, and infections require admission for stabilization.

The longer-term outcome after treatment of severe malnutrition is usually poor. Mortality during follow-up was 2.3% in Bangladesh,[125] 8% in Tanzania,[126] 18% in Niger,[127] 19% in Zaire,[128] 32% in the Gambia,[129] and 36% in Kenya.[130] The marked variability in the reported mortality rates may reflect differences in the adequacy of nutritional rehabilitation before discharge, the education of caregivers during admission, and the length and completeness of follow-up. Mortality may also be reduced in research studies where children are followed up frequently at home for the purposes of recording outcome. In survivors, the recurrence of wasting after discharge is variable, but stunting usually persists and morbidity is high. It is clear from these data that continuation of support and follow-up after discharge from hospital is vital. A greater emphasis on management in the community should facilitate this. WHO has already begun the process of combining both hospital and community approaches into management guidelines.[131]

PREVENTION OF MALNUTRITION

Every severely malnourished child was once moderately malnourished. Given the extreme challenge that severely malnourished children

place on understaffed and underresourced health facilities the need for prevention is obvious. A central maxim of preventive medicine, that "a large number of people exposed to a small risk may generate many more cases than a small number exposed to a high risk,"[132] is well illustrated by malnutrition. Although the risk of mortality rises progressively with worsening nutritional status, it is important to note that over 80% of malnutrition-associated deaths occur in children with mild to moderate malnutrition because these greatly outnumber severely malnourished children.[8] Therefore, attention to preventing and reversing mild and moderate malnutrition in the community is likely to be essential to improving child survival and making progress towards MDGs.

Many approaches to prevention of severe malnutrition have been tested over many years. It is clear that the effective prevention of malnutrition is likely to require multifaceted approaches that deal with several interconnected socioeconomic, public health, and disease-specific factors as summarized by Bellamy (Figure 8).[133] Recently, more attention has focused on complementary feeding in young children and the importance of including animal-source foods (reviewed by Dewey 2005[134]). Recent studies have highlighted the effectiveness of educational approaches[135,136] and also the importance of early childhood psychosocial stimulation to improve long-term nutritional and neurodevelopmental outcomes.[137]

CONCLUSIONS

Malnutrition remains a public health problem of enormous importance. In economically poor countries, growth faltering is the norm, and underweight in children is the leading global risk factor for health loss. Severe malnutrition

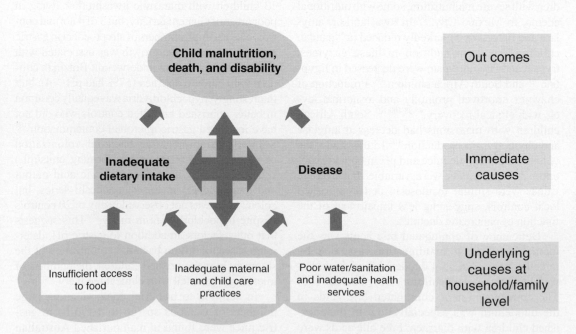

Figure 8 The vicious cycle of malnutrition, inadequate dietary intake, and disease (mostly infection) is related to underlying causes at the household and family level. (Adapted from reference 133.)

is common in children admitted to hospitals and, despite the ready availability of detailed management guidelines, case fatality remains high. Management of uncomplicated severe malnutrition in the community appears to be effective in many settings. As always, a "one size fits all" approach to management will not work and pediatricians must consider the lessons learned from both hospital and community studies to design interventions for their own situation. However, taking a broad view of malnutrition and ensuring that health staff in hospital and the community work together will result in the most effective use of limited resources.

Malnourished children have marked abnormalities of the gastrointestinal system, including a severe enteropathy in many. Translocation of bacteria from the gut through a leaky mucosa may contribute to deaths from sepsis. The persistence of the enteropathy in survivors is likely to contribute significantly to their poor longer-term outcome. The findings that the enteropathy in Gambian children with a range of nutritional status is mediated by T cells needs to be confirmed in other locations as this may present new opportunities for specific interventions. In keeping with approaches to other T-cell–mediated enteropathies, interventions to prevent or modify the gut bacterial overgrowth that is common in children in developing countries should be explored.

Epidemiological studies dictate that interventions to prevent growth faltering in "normal" children living in the community will have the greatest impact on child survival. Both histological studies of the intestinal mucosa and the measurement of mucosal permeability reveal that significant enteropathy, sufficient to impair growth, is common. This "environmental enteropathy" may be a continuum of that seen in severely malnourished children. A group of leading international experts met in Washington, DC, in 1971 under the auspices of the Committee on International Nutrition Programs and addressed a specific question: "Are there now sufficient data to justify efforts to ameliorate or prevent subclinical malabsorption as one approach to the global problem of malnutrition?"[138] This question remains unanswered. Alongside other approaches, more research is needed to assess the impact of improving environmental enteropathy on growth in children in the community as part of the new global commitment to child survival.[139]

REFERENCES

1. United Nations Millennium Development Goals. UN Web Services Section, Department of Public Information, United Nations © 2005. http://www.un.org/millenniumgoals/ (accessed Oct 22, 2006).
2. United Nations Standing Committee on Nutrition. Nutrition for improved developmental outcomes. 5th report of the world nutrition situation. Nutrition for improved developmental outcomes. Geneva: WHO, 2004. http://www.unsystem.org/scn/Publications/AnnualMeeting/SCN31/SCN5Report.pdf (accessed Oct 22, 2006).
3. World Bank 2006: Directions in Development: "Repositioning Nutrition as Central to Development. A strategy for large-scale action." http://siteresources.worldbank.org/NUTRITION/Resources/281846-1131636806329/NutritionStrategy.pdf (accessed Oct 20, 2006).
4. World Health Report; Reducing risks, promoting healthy life. Geneva: WHO; 2002.
5. Gross R, Webb P. Wasting time for wasted children: Severe child undernutrition must be resolved in nonemergency settings. Lancet 2006;367:1209–11.
6. Müller O, Becher H. Malnutrition and childhood mortality in developing countries. Lancet 2006;367:1978.
7. UNICEF 2006. Progress for children: A report card on nutrition. www.unicef.org/progressforchildren/2006n4/ (accessed Oct 19, 2006).
8. Pelletier DL. The effects of malnutrition on child mortality in developing countries. Bull World Health Organ 1995;73:443–8.
9. Caulfield LE, de Onis M, Blossner M, Black RE. Undernutrition as an underlying cause of child deaths associated with diarrhea, pneumonia and measles. Am J Clin Nutr 2004;80:193–8.
10. Pelletier DL, Frongillo EA. Changes in child survival are strongly associated with changes in malnutrition in developing countries. J Nutr 2003;133:107–19.
11. Lopez AD, Mathers CD, Ezzati M, et al. Global and regional burden of disease and risk factors, 2001: Systematic analysis of population health data. Lancet 2006;367:1747–57.
12. Berkley J, Mwangi I, Griffiths K, et al. Assessment of severe malnutrition among hospitalized children in rural Kenya: Comparison of weight for height and mid upper arm circumference. JAMA 2005;294:591–7.
13. Allen SJ, Hamer C. Improving quality of care for severe malnutrition. Lancet 2004;363:2089–90.
14. Man WD-C, Weber M, Palmer A, et al. Nutritional status of children admitted to hospital with different diseases and its relationship to outcome in The Gambia, West Africa. Trop Med Int Health 1998;3:678–86.
15. Rice AL, Sacco L, Hyder A, Black RE. Malnutrition as an under-lying cause of childhood deaths associated with infectious diseases in developing countries. Bull World Health Organ 2000;78:1207–21.
16. Schofield C, Ashworth A. Why have mortality rates for severe malnutrition remained so high? Bull World Health Organ 1996;74:223–9.
17. Neale G. Severe malnutrition in infancy and childhood. In: Preedy V, Grimble G, Watson R, editors. Nutrition in the Infant. Problems and Practical Procedures, 1st edition. London: Greenwich Medical Media Ltd; 2001. p. 11–9.
18. Williams CD. A nutritional disease of childhood associated with a maize diet. Arch Dis Child 1933;8:423–33.
19. Classification of infantile malnutrition [editorial]. Lancet 1970;ii:302–3.
20. Waterlow JC. Classification and definition of protein-calorie malnutrition. BMJ 1972;3:566–9.
21. Scrimshaw NS. Historical concepts of interactions, synergism and antagonism between nutrition and infection. J Nutr 2003;133:316S–21S.
22. Brent AJ, Ahmed I, Ndiritu M, et al. Incidence of clinically significant bacteraemia in children who present to hospital in Kenya: Community-based observational study. Lancet 2006;367:482–88.
23. Jahoor F, Badaloo A, Reid M, Forrester T. Protein kinetic differences between children with edematous and nonedematous severe childhood undernutrition in the fed and postabsorptive states. Am J Clin Nutr 2005;82:792–800.
24. Sullivan PB, Neale G, Cevallos AM, Farthing MJ. Evaluation of specific serum anti-Giardia IgM antibody response in diagnosis of giardiasis in children. Trans R Soc Trop Med Hyg 1991;85:748–9.
25. Stephensen CB. Burden of infection on growth failure. J Nutr 1999;129:534S–8S.
26. Shaaban SY, Nassar MF, Sawaby AS, et al. Ultrasonographic gastric emptying in protein energy malnutrition: Effect of type of meal and nutritional recovery. Eur J Clin Nutr 2004;58:972–8.
27. Wittman W, Hansen JDL, Browlee K. An elevation of gastric acid secretion in kwashiorkor by means of the augmented histamine test. S Afr Med J 1967;41:400–6.
28. Gracey M, Cullity GJ, Suharjono S. The stomach in malnutrition. Arch Dis Child 1977;52:325–7.
29. Gilman RH, Partanen R, Brown KH, et al. Decreased gastric acid secretion and bacterial colonisation of the stomach in severely malnourished Bangladeshi children. Gastroenterology 1988;94:1308–14.
30. Rowland MG, Cole TJ, McCollum JP. Weanling diarrhoea in The Gambia: Implications of a jejunal intubation study. Trans R Soc Trop Med Hyg 1981;75:215–8.
31. Frenck RW, Jr, Clemens J. Helicobacter in the developing world. Microbes Infect 2003;5:705–13.
32. Thomas JE, Dale A, Harding M, et al. *Helicobacter pylori* colonization in early life. Pediatr Res 1999;45:218–23.
33. Dale A, Thomas JE, Darboe MK, et al. *Helicobacter pylori,* gastric acid secretion and infant growth. J Pediatr Gastroenterol Nutr 1998;26:393–7.
34. Thomas JE, Dale A, Bunn JE, et al. Early *Helicobacter pylori* colonisation: The association with growth faltering in The Gambia. Arch Dis Child. 2004;89:1149–54.
35. Bowie MD. Effect of lactose-induced diarrhoea on absorption of nitrogen and fat. Arch Dis Child 1975;50:363–6.
36. Habte D, Hyvarinen A, Sterky G. Carbohydrate malabsorption in kwashiorkor. Ethiop Med J 1973;11:33–40.
37. Prinsloo JG, Wittmann W, Kruger H, Freier E. Lactose absorption and mucosal disaccharidases in convalescent pellagra and kwashiorkor children. Arch Dis Child 1971;46:474–8.
38. James WPT. Sugar absorption and intestinal motility in children when malnourished and after treatment. Clin Sci 1970;30: 305–18.
39. Chandra RK, Pawa RR, Ghai OP. Sugar intolerance in malnourished infants and children. BMJ 1968;4:611–3.
40. Fagundes-Neto U, Viaro T, Wehba J, et al. Tropical enteropathy (environmental enteropathy) in early childhood: A syndrome caused by contaminated environment. J Trop Pediatr 1984;30:204–9.
41. Martins Campos JV, Fagundes Neto U, Patricio FRS, et al. Jejunal mucosa in marasmic children. Clinical, pathological, and fine structural evaluation of the effect of protein energy malnutrition and environmental contamination. Am J Clin Nutr 1979;32:1575–91.
42. Northrop-Clewes CA, Lunn PG, Downes RM. Lactose maldigestion in breast-feeding Gambian infants. J Pediatr Gastroenterol Nutr 1997;24:257–63.
43. Barbezat GO, Bowie MD, Kaschula ROC, Hansen JDL. Studies on the small intestinal mucosa of children with protein-calorie malnutiriton. S Afr Med J 1967;41:1031–6.
44. Stanfield JP, Hutt MSR, Tunnicliffe R. Intestinal biopsy in kwashiorkor. Lancet 1965;ii:519–23.
45. Cook GC, Lee FD. The jejunum after kwashiorkor. Lancet 1966;ii:1263–7.
46. Holemans K, Lambrechts A. Nitrogen metabolism and fat absorption in malnutrition and in kwashiorkor. J Nutr 1955;56:477–94.
47. Hansen JDL, Schendel HE, Wilkins JA, Brock JF. Nitrogen metabolism in children with kwashiorkor receiving milk and vegetable diets. Pediatrics 1960;25:258–82.
48. Viteri FE, Flores JM, Alvarado J, Béhar M. Intestinal malabsorption in malnourished children before and during recovery. Relation between severity of protein deficiency and the malabsorption process. Dig Dis 1973;18:201–11.
49. Robinson U, Bhar M, Viteri F, et al. Protein and fat balance studies in children recovering from kwashiorkor. J Trop Pediatr 1957;2:217–23.
50. Jahoor F, Badaloo A, Reid M, Forrester T. Glycine production in severe childhood undernutrition. Am J Clin Nutr 2006;84:143–9.
51. Gómez F, Galván RR, Cravioto J, et al. Fat malabsorption in chronic severe malnutrition in children. Lancet 1956;ii:121–2.
52. Badaloo AV, Forrester T, Reid M, Jahoor F. Lipid kinetic differences between children with kwashiorkor and those with marasmus. Am J Clin Nutr 2006;83:1283–8.
53. Alvarado J, Vargas W, Daz N, Viteri FE. Vitamin B$_{12}$ absorption in protein-calorie malnourished children and during recovery: Influence of protein depletion and of diarrhea. Am J Clin Nutr 1973;26:595–9.
54. Trowell HC, Davies JNP, Dean RFA. Kwashiorkor. London: Edward Arnold; 1954. p. 149–50.
55. Banwell JG, Hutt MSR, Tunnicliffe R. Observations on jejunal biopsy in Ugandan Africans. East Afr Med J 1964;41:46–5467.
56. Burman D. The jejunal mucosa in kwashiorkor. Arch Dis Child 1965;40:526–31.
57. Theron JJ, Wittmann W, Prinsloo JG. The fine structure of the jejunum in kwashiorkor. Exp Mol Pathol 1971;14: 184–99.
58. Shiner M, Redmond AO, Hansen JD. The jejunal mucosa in protein-energy malnutrition. A clinical, histological, and ultrastructural study. Exp Mol Pathol 1973;19:61–78.
59. Schneider RE, Viteri FE. Morphological aspects of the duodenojejunal mucosa in protein-calorie malnourished children and during recovery. Am J Clin Nutr 1972;25:1092–102.
60. Brunser O, Araya M, Espinoza J. Gastrointestinal tract changes in the malnourished child. In: Suskind RM, Lewinter-Susmind L, editors. The Malnourished Child. Nestlé Nutrition Workshop Series, Volume 19. New York: Nestlé Ltd., Vevey/ Raven Press Ltd.; 1990. p. 261–76.
61. Heyman M, Boudraa G, Sarrut S, et al. Macromolecular transport in jejunal mucosa of children with severe malnutrition: A quantitative study. J Pediatr Gastroenterol Nutr 1984;3:357–63.

62. Fagundes-Neto U, De Martini-Costa S, Pedroso MZ, Scaletsky IC. Studies of the small bowel surface by scanning electron microscopy in infants with persistent diarrhea. Braz J Med Biol Res 2000;33:1437–42.

63. Sullivan PB, Marsh MN, Mirakian R, et al. Chronic diarrhea and malnutrition—histology of the small intestinal lesion. J Pediatr Gastroenterol Nutr 1991;12:195–203.

64. Sullivan PB, Mascie-Taylor CG, Lunn PG, et al. The treatment of persistent diarrhoea and malnutrition: Long-term effects of in-patient rehabilitation. Acta Paediatr 1991;80:1025–30.

65. Fagundes Neto U, Martins MC, Lima FL, et al. Asymptomatic environmental enteropathy among slum-dwelling infants. J Am Coll Nutr 1994;13:51–6.

66. Chacko CJ, Paulson KA, Mathan VI, Baker SJ. The villus architecture of the small intestine in the tropics: A necropsy study. J Pathol 1969;98:146–51.

67. Campbell DI, Murch SH, Elia M, et al. Chronic T cell-mediated enteropathy in rural West African children: Relationship with nutritional status and small bowel function. J Nutr 2003;133:1332–8.

68. Veitch AM, Kelly P, Zulu IS, et al. Tropical enteropathy: A T-cell mediated crypt hyperplastic enteropathy. Eur J Gastroenterol Hepatol 2001;13:1175–81.

69. Bowie MD, Brinkman GL, Hansen JDL. Acquired disaccharide intolerance in malnutrition. Trop Pediatr 1965;66:1083–91.

70. Behrens RH, Lunn PG, Northrop CA, et al. Factors affecting the integrity of the intestinal mucosa of Gambian children. Am J Clin Nutr 1987;45:1433–41.

71. Sullivan PB, Lunn PG, Northrop-Clewes CA, et al. Persistent diarrhoea and malnutrition—the impact of treatment on small bowel structure and permeability. J Pediatr Gastroenterol Nutr 1992;14:208–15.

72. Brewster DR, Manary MJ, Menzies IS, et al. Intestinal permeability in kwashiorkor. Arch Dis Child 1997;76:236–41.

73. Chandra RK. Food antibodies in malnutrition. Arch Dis Child 1975;50:532–4.

74. Lunn PG. Intestinal permeability, mucosal injury, and growth faltering in Gambian infants. Lancet 1991;338:907–10.

75. Campbell DI, Lunn PG, Elia M. Age-related association of small intestinal mucosal enteropathy with nutritional status in rural Gambian children. Br J Nutr 2002;88:499–505.

76. Villamor E, Fawzi WW. Effects of vitamin A supplementation on immune responses and correlation with clinical outcomes. Clin Microbiol Rev 2005;18:446–64.

77. Northrop-Clewes CA, Lunn PG, Downes RM. Seasonal fluctuations in vitamin A status and health indicators in Gambian infants [abstract]. Proc Nutr Soc 1994;53:144A.

78. Thurnham DI, Northrop-Clewes CA, McCullough FS, et al. Innate immunity, gut integrity, and vitamin A in Gambian and Indian infants. J Infect Dis 2000;182:S23–8.

79. Filteau SM, Rollins NC, Coutsoudis A, et al. The effect of ante-natal vitamin A and beta-carotene supplementation on gut integrity of infants of HIV-infected South African women. J Pediatr Gastroenterol Nutr 2001;32:464–70.

80. Black RE, Sazawal S. Zinc and childhood infectious disease morbidity and mortality. Br J Nutr 2001;85:S125–9.

81. Bhan MK, Bhandari N. The role of zinc and vitamin A in persistent diarrhea among infants and young children. J Pediatr Gastroenterol Nutr 1998;26:446–53.

82. Bhutta ZA, Bird SM, Black RE, et al. Therapeutic effects of oral zinc in acute and persistent diarrhea in children in developing countries: Pooled analysis of randomized controlled trials. Am J Clin Nutr 2000;72:1516–22.

83. Roy SK, Behrens RH, Haider R, et al. Impact of zinc supplementation on intestinal permeability in Bangladeshi children with acute diarrhoea and persistent diarrhoea syndrome. J Pediatr Gastroenterol Nutr 1992;15:289–96.

84. Bates CJ, Evans PH, Dardenne M, et al. A trial of zinc supplementation in young rural Gambian children. Br J Nutr 1993; 69:243–55.

85. Lima AA, Brito LF, Ribeiro HB, et al. Intestinal barrier function and weight gain in malnourished children taking glutamine supplemented enteral formula. J Pediatr Gastroenterol Nutr 2005;40:28–35.

86. World Health Organization. Management of severe malnutrition; a manual for physicians and other senior health workers. Geneva: World Health Organization; 1998.

87. Redmond AOB, Kaschula ROC, Freeseman C, Hansen JDL. The colon in kwashiorkor. Arch Dis Child 1971;46:470–3.

88. Davies JNP. The essential pathology of kwashiorkor. Lancet 1948;i:317–20.

89. Doherty JF, Adam EJ, Griffin GE, Golden MH. Ultrasonographic assessment of the extent of hepatic steatosis in severe malnutrition. Arch Dis Child 1992;67:1348–52.

90. Lalwani SG, Karande S, Khemani R, Jain MK. Ultrasonographic evaluation of hepatic steatosis in malnutrition. Indian Pediatr 1998;35:650–2.

91. Brooks SE, Doherty JF, Golden MH. Peroxisomes and the hepatic pathology of childhood malnutrition. West Indian Med J 1994;43:15–7.

92. Akinyinka OO, Falade AG, Ogbechie CO. Prothrombin time as an index of mortality in kwashiorkor. Ann Trop Paediatr 1990;10:85–8.

93. Akenami FO, Koskiniemi M, Siimes MA, et al. Assessment of plasma fibronectin in malnourished Nigerian children. J Pediatr Gastroenterol Nutr 1997;24:183–8.

94. Hendrickse RG. Of sick turkeys, kwashiorkor, malaria, perinatal mortality, heroin addicts and food poisoning: Research on the influence of aflatoxins on child health in the tropics. Ann Trop Med Parasitol 1997;91:787–93.

95. Thompson MD, Trowell HC. Pancreatic enzyme activity in duodenal contents of children with a type of kwashiorkor. Lancet 1952;i:1031–5.

96. Brooks SE, Golden MH. The exocrine pancreas in kwashiorkor and marasmus. Light and electron microscopy. West Indian Med J 1992;41:56–60.

97. Brooks SE, Golden MH, Payne-Robinson HM. Ultrastructure of the islets of Langerhans in protein-energy malnutrition. West Indian Med J 1993;42:101–6.

98. Cleghorn GJ, Erlich J, Bowling FG, et al. Exocrine pancreatic dysfunction in malnourished Australian aboriginal children. Med J Aust 1991;154:45–8.

99. Véghelyi PV. Pancreatic function in nutritional oedema. Lancet 1948;i:497–8.

100. Gómez F, Galván RR, Cravioto J, Frenk S. Studies on the undernourished child. XI. Enzymatic activity of the duodenal contents in children affected with third degree malnutrition. Pediatrics 1954;13:548–52.

101. Badr El-Din MK, Aboul Wafa MH. Pancreatic activity in normal and malnourished Egyptian infants. J Trop Pediatr 1957;3:17.

102. Barbezat GO, Hansen JDL. The exocrine pancreas and protein calorie malnutrition. Pediatrics 1968;42:77–92.

103. Schneider RE, Viteri FE. Luminal events of lipid absorption in protein-calorie malnourished children; relationship with nutritional recovery and diarrhea. I. Capacity of the duodenal content to achieve micellar solubilization of lipids. Am J Clin Nutr 1974;27:777–87.

104. Schneider RE, Viteri FE. Luminal events of lipid absorption in protein-calorie malnourished children; relationship with nutritional recovery and diarrhea. II. Alterations in bile acid content of duodenal aspirates. Am J Clin Nutr 1974;27:788–96.

105. Mata LJ, Jimenez F, Cordon M, et al. Gastrointestinal flora of children with protein-calorie malnutrition. Am J Clin Nutr 1972;25:118–26.

106. Redmond AO, Hansen JD, McHutchon B. Abnormal bile salt metabolism in kwashiorkor. S Afr Med J 1972;46:617–8.

107. Gracey M, Suharjono, Sunoto, Stone DE. Microbial contamination of the gut; another feature of malnutrition. Am J Clin Nutr 1973;26:1170–4.

108. Maffei HVL, Nóbrega FJ. Gastric pH and microflora of normal and diarrhoeic infants. Gut 1975;16:719–26.

109. Gracey M, Stone DE, Suharjono, Sunoto. Isolation of Candida species from the gastrointestinal tract in malnourished children. Am J Clin Nutr 1974;27:345–9.

110. Heyworth B, Brown J. Jejunal microflora in malnourished Gambian children. Arch Dis Child 1975;50:27–33.

111. Omoike IU, Abiodun PO. Upper small intestinal microflora in diarrhea and malnutrition in Nigerian children. J Pediatr Gastroenterol Nutr 1989;9:314–21.

112. Gracey M, Stone DE. Small-intestinal microflora in Australian Aboriginal children with chronic diarrhoea. Aust N Z J Med 1972;2:215–9.

113. O'Sullivan DJ. Methods for analysis of the intestinal microflora. Curr Issues Intest Microbiol 2000;1:39–50.

114. Shanahan F. Crohn's disease. Lancet 2002;359:62–9.

115. Nolan T, Angos P, Cunha AJ. Quality of hospital care for seriously ill children in less-developed countries. Lancet 2001; 357:106–110.

116. English M, Esamai F, Wasunna A, et al. Assessment of inpatient paediatric care in first referral level hospitals in 13 districts in Kenya. Lancet 2004;363:1948–53.

117. Jackson AA, Ashworth A, Khanum S. Improving child survival: Malnutrition Task Force and the paediatrician's responsibility. Arch Dis Child 2006;91:706-10.

118. Ashworth A, Chopra M, McCoy D et al. WHO guidelines for management of severe malnutrition in rural South African hospitals: Effect on case fatality and the influence of operational factors. Lancet 2004;363:1110–5.

119. Karaolis N, Jackson D, Ashworth A, et al. WHO guidelines for severe malnutrition: Are they feasible in rural African hospitals? Arch Dis Child 2007;92:198–204.

120. Collins S, Dent D, Binns P, et al. Management of severe acute malnutrition in children. Lancet 2006. Published online Sept 26, 2006. DOI:10.1016/S0140-6736(06)69443–9 (accessed Oct 20, 2006).

121. Collins S, Sadler K. Outpatient care for severely malnourished children in emergency relief programmes: A retrospective cohort study. Lancet 2002;360:1824–30.

122. Tectonidis M, Crisis in Niger—outpatient case for severe malnutrition. N Engl J Med 2006;354:224–7.

123. Ciliberto MA, Manary MJ, Ndekha MJ et al. Home-based therapy for oedematous malnutrition with ready-to-use therapeutic food. Acta Paediatr 2006;95:1012–5.

124. Collins S, Yates R. The need to update the classification of acute malnutrition. Lancet 2003;362:249.

125. Khanum S, Ashworth A, Huttly SR. Growth, morbidity, and mortality of children in Dhaka after treatment for severe malnutrition: a prospective study. Am J Clin Nutr 1998;67:940–5.

126. van Roosmalen-Wiebenga MW, Kusin JA, de With C. Nutrition rehabilitation in hospital—a waste of time and money? Evaluation of nutrition rehabilitation in a rural district hospital in South-west Tanzania. II. Long-term results. J Trop Pediatr 1987;33:24–8.

127. Pecoul B, Soutif C, Hounkpevi M, Ducos M. Efficacy of a therapeutic feeding centre evaluated during hospitalization and a follow-up period, Tahoua, Niger, 1987–1988. Ann Trop Paediatr 1992;12:47–54.

128. Hennart P, Beghin D, Bossuyt M. Long-term follow-up of severe protein-energy malnutrition in eastern Zaire. J Trop Pediatr 1987;33:10–2.

129. Winful EA. Follow-up survey of Gambian children admitted between 1995 and 1997 to the Medical Research Council Paediatric ward with malnutrition [thesis]. Liverpool (UK): Liverpool School of Tropical Medicine; 1999.

130. Reneman L, Derwig J. Long-term prospects of malnourished children after rehabilitation at the Nutrition Rehabilitation Centre of St Mary's Hospital, Mumias, Kenya. J Trop Pediatr 1997;43:293– 28.

131. WHO. Report of an informal consultation on the community-based management of severe malnutrition in children. http://www.who.int/child-adolescent-health/publications/NUTRITION/CBSM.htm (accessed Oct 19th, 2006).

132. Rose G. Sick individuals and sick populations. Int J Epidemiol 2001;30:427–32.

133. Bellamy C. The State of the World's Children 1998: Focus on Nutrition. New York: Oxford University Press for UNICEF; 1997. p. 24.

134. Dewey KG. Infant nutrition in developing countries: What works? Lancet 2005;365:1832-4.

135. Roy SK, Fuchs GJ, Mahmud Z, et al. Intensive nutrition education with or without supplementary feeding improves the nutritional status of moderately-malnourished children in Bangladesh. J Health Popul Nutr 2005;23:320–30.

136. Penny ME, Creed-Kanashiro HM, Robert RC, et al. Effectiveness of an educational intervention delivered through the health services to improve nutrition in young children: A cluster-randomised controlled trial. Lancet 2005;365:1863–72.

137. Walker SP, Chang SM, Powell CA, Grantham-McGregor SM. Effects of early childhood psychosocial stimulation and nutritional supplementation on cognition and education in growth-stunted Jamaican children: prospective cohort study. Lancet 2005;366:1804–7.

138. Rosenberg IH, Scrimshaw NS. Workshop on malabsorption and nutrition. Am J Clin Nutr 1972;25:1045–6.

139. Stoltenberg J. A new global commitment to child survival. Lancet 2006; 368:1041–44.

Intestinal Failure

22.1. Short Bowel Syndrome

Yigael Finkel, MD, PhD
Olivier Goulet, MD, PhD

INTESTINAL FAILURE

The main functions of the gastrointestinal tract of a growing child are to absorb fluid, electrolytes, and nutrients in sufficient amounts to sustain the functions and the growth of the body. "Intestinal failure" in children can be defined as the reduction of these functions in such way that absorption of fluid and nutrients for growth is inadequate and that growth can only be sustained with parenteral nutrition. Intestinal failure (IF) has many and varied causes, and may be complete or partial, acute and short lived, or chronic and permanent. The definition of IF remains a matter of debate. In times when short bowel syndrome (SBS) was the main cause of IF, the condition was defined by the length of the remaining intestine after resection. Today more definitions for IF has been suggested. They can be grouped into functional and biological definition. The functional definition presently used for epidemiological studies in children is a need for parenteral nutrition for more than 27 days (www.bifs.org). A different functional definition is based on measuring fecal energy loss of patients with short bowel syndrome.[1–2] Recently, a biological criteria for defining IF was suggested by the measurement of citrulline as the marker of small intestinal epithelial mass. Citrulline is a nonessential amino acid that is mostly produced by enterocytes, and serum citrulline levels correlate with enteral tolerance and bowel length in infants with short bowel syndrome. See also section "Arginine and Citrulline."[3–7]

EPIDEMIOLOGY

The precise epidemiology and incidence of children with IF is not known. A multicenter European survey conducted in 2001 estimated the incidence of children on home PN to be 2 to 6.8 per million population.[8]

The British Artificial Nutrition Survey registered 81 children for home PN between 1996 and 1999, giving a point prevalence of 2 children per million.[9] In Spain only 3 children below 14 years of age were registered in the national register of home parenteral nutrition (HPN) in 2002.[10] Using data from quality of life studies as a proxy, there were in 2002, 104 children below 19 years of age in France on HPN for digestive diseases and cared for by the five French HPN centers (~1.7 per million) and 21 children below the age of 16 in Sweden (~2.4 per million).[11–12] A European survey published by Pironi and colleagues provides interesting data.[13] Epidemiology of IF as estimated by candidacy for intestinal transplantation (ITx) was investigated among centers, which participated in European surveys on HPN. Candidacy was assessed by USA Medicare and American Transplantation Society criteria[14] categorized as following:

1. Life-threatening HPN complications
2. High risk of death due to the gastrointestinal disease
3. IF with high morbidity or patient HPN refusal

Physicians judged candidacy as immediate or potential. This study included 166 infants and children from seven home PN centers (France, Italy, Poland, and Spain). The main indications for HPN were SBS (52%), chronic intestinal pseudo-obstruction syndrome (CIPOS) (25%), and congenital mucosal disease (14.5%). Candidacy was considered for 57 patients (34.3%) with the following underlying disease: congenital mucosal disease (26.3%), CIPOS (26.3%), SBS (19.3%). Immediate candidacy was required for 15.8% of pediatric candidates (<50% of candidates because of HPN-related liver failure). Among the contributing countries, candidacy ranged 0.9 to 2 per million inhabitants ≤18 years.

CAUSES OF INTESTINAL FAILURE

The pathogenic causes of loss of intestinal functions can be classified into congenital and acquired with following etiological subgrouping:

- Inflammation
- Anatomic reduction of the gut, short bowel syndrome
- Neuromuscular disease involving the GI tract (see also Chapters 24.2b, "Congenital Enteropathies" and 24.2c, "Other Dysmotilites Including Chronic Intestinal Pseudo-Obstruction Syndrome")
- Congenital diseases of the intestinal epithelium (see also Chapter 15.3c, "Hirschsprung's Disease").

Intestinal Neuromuscular Motility Disorders

Total colonic aganglionosis with jejunoileal involvement is a rare form of Hirschsprung disease (HD). HD affects 1 in 5,000 newborns and is defined as an absence of ganglion cells in a variable length of distal bowel (see Chapter 24.2b, "Hirschsprung's disease"). The receptor tyrosine kinase gene *RET* is the most common gene in which a mutation may be found.[15–16] In 80% of infants, the aganglionosis is confined to the rectum and sigmoid, but it may extend to encompass the entire colon (total colonic aganglionosis) or very rarely (less than 1% of HD) affect the entire intestine. When the normal ganglionic small bowel is shorter than 50 cm, the probability for permanent PN dependency is high. Finally, total colonic aganglionosis with jejunoileal involvement is equivalent to short bowel syndrome without colon. Small bowel transplantation is the ultimate treatment, and several patients with a length of the normal bowel segment ranging from 15 to 50 cm have undergone transplantation.[17–21]

Chronic intestinal pseudo-obstruction syndrome (CIPOS) is an intestinal motility disorder in which impaired intestinal motor activity causes recurrent symptoms of intestinal obstruction in the absence of mechanical occlusion. CIPOS is a very heterogeneous condition in terms of clinical presentation, histopathological features, severity of motility disorders, and outcome (see Chapter 24.2c, "Other Dysmotilities Including Chronic Intestinal Pseudo-Obstruction Syndrome"). The condition has a very high morbidity and mortality. Careful treatment of urinary tract infections and bacterial overgrowth, decompression surgery, and judicious use of PN allows survival to adult life. Patients with the most severe form of CIPOS, whatever myopathic or neuropathic with or without urinary tract involvement, should be considered for intestinal or multivisceral transplantation.

Recent data of multivisceral transplantation in CIPOS patients, including some with associated urinary tract involvement show a 78% actuarial patient survival after 2 years. The heterogeneity of the disease and the extradigestive manifestations call for prudent ethical discussions in some cases.[2,22–30]

Congenital Enteropathies

Congenital diseases of enterocyte development such as microvillus atrophy (MVA) and intestinal epithelial dysplasia (IED) or "tufting enteropathy" cause IF. There is strong evidence that both disorders are inherited in an autosomic recessive manner. Onset of either disorders is within the first few days or weeks of life in form of severe watery diarrhea. MVA involves the intracellular pathway of brush border development and the assembly of the plasma membrane of enterocytes.[31] In contrast, IED is associated with an abnormal basement membrane structure as suggested by an abnormal $\alpha_2\beta_4$-integrin and desmoglein expression.[32,33] For both disorders, the primary defect is currently not known and genetic studies are underway; however, to date no candidate gene could be identified for either disease. Thus most patients suffering from a constitutive disorder of intestinal epithelial cells remain permanently dependent on PN and are logical candidates for intestinal transplantation. Small bowel transplantation was reported for MVA patients in variable association with liver and/or colon. The largest survey involving eight children was recently reported with 86% 1-year survival after intestinal transplantation.[34] Patients with IED underwent successfully either isolated intestinal transplantation or in combination with the liver in case of end-stage liver disease (see Chapter 15.3c, "Congenital Enteropathies").[35]

Autoimmune Enteropathy

A new well-recognized and distinct entity of severe enteropathy is in form of autoimmune enteropathy (AIE) (see Chapter 16.3, "Autoimmune Enteropathy and IPEX Syndrome"). This disorder is a cause of protracted IF which may be reversible with immunosuppression and bone marrow transplantation. One subgroup of AIE is the so-called IPEX. IPEX refers to a condition characterized by Immune dysregulation, Polyendocrinopathy, Enteropathy, and X-linkage. The syndrome has many intestinal manifestations in common with AIE, including villous atrophy with a marked infiltration into the lamina propria of activated T cells.[36-37]

SHORT BOWEL SYNDROME: DEFINITION

Short bowel syndrome (SBS) is the syndrome of intestinal dysfunction and complications following extensive resection of the small bowel.

The extent of resection results in insufficient nutritive supply requiring artificial nutrition by total or partial parenteral nutrition and/or enteral nutrition (Table 1).

CAUSES OF SHORT BOWEL SYNDROME

See Chapter 13, "Congenital Anomalies Including Hernias."

Gastroschisis

Gastroschisis is an abdominal wall defect characterized by an intact umbilical cord, evisceration of bowel through a defect in the abdominal wall, generally to the right of the cord, and with no membrane covering.

Incidence. Recent European epidemiological studies of gastroschisis show a real increase in prevalence of gastroschisis since 1980,[38] probably as a result of unknown environmental factors.[39] A regional variation within United Kingdom has been shown ranging from 1.8 to 3.2 per 10,000 registered births.[40] Recent data from the British Isles Network of Congenital Anomaly Registers (BINOCAR) show that the prevalence of gastroschisis is even higher at 4.0 per 10,000 total births for the period 2002 to 2004.[40] There has been a significant increase over the past 10 years from 2.5 to 4.4 per 10,000 total births over the period 1994 to 2003. Around 40% of babies with gastroschisis are born to mothers under the age of 20 years compared with only 9% of overall births.

Pathogenesis and Etiology. Recent theories have focused on that a dysplastic abdominal wall formation, perhaps related to a vascular abnormality, results in a thinned area of abdominal wall which ruptures because of intra-abdominal pressure.[41] Arguments for genetic factors for gastroschisis are supported by familiar incidence and selected gene polymorphism.[42] An association between maternal medication during pregnancy and an increased risk of gastroschisis is hypothesized.

Clinical Management. Prenatal diagnosis of abdominal wall defects may be easily performed. This allows one to choose delivery time and place and facilitates the preparation of the surgical team. The outcome for infants with gastroschisis seems not to be influenced by mode of delivery, according to one metanalysis.[43] However, most clinicians agree on the need for cesarean section in cases where the liver is extracorporeal.

Repair Technique. The reduction of the abdominal contents should be performed within hours after delivery to avoid fluid losses and compromise to intestinal circulation with care to avoid marked increase of abdominal pressure during reduction of the herniated viscera into the abdomen. There is no evidence either supporting, or refuting, the use of ward reduction of gastroschisis rather than performing this procedure under anesthesia in an operating room.[44] If reduction is not possible, a prosthetic silo created from silastic or Teflon is recommended.

Problems That May Lead to SBS. Survival for gastroschisis is over 85%.[45] However, feeding intolerance is highly prevalent in infants with gastroschisis due to one or a combination of factors, such as bowel hypomotility, intestinal atresia, perforation, the presence of necrotic bowel segments, and the development of volvulus. Intestinal atresia occurs in approximately 10 to 20% of infants with gastroschisis, which contributes to feeding delays, long-term parenteral nutrition, and early onset of severe liver disease.[46]

Malrotation and Midgut Volvulus

Malrotation leading to volvulus should be regarded as a surgical time bomb with early clinical signs indistinguishable from less serious disorders of intestinal obstruction in infants. It is one of the four most common conditions that lead up to intestinal failure in infants.

Incidence. The incidence of malrotation in children 1 to 18 years of age is 5.3 per million population.[47] Population-based figures for prematures and infants are unavailable.

Embryology. At the fifth gestational week the fetal small intestine forms a loop which extrudes into the umbilical cord. The fetal gut subsequently undergoes enlargement, elongation, and return of the hernial contents. The final placement of the intestine into the abdominal cavity is achieved by rotation and fixation of the fetal gut. Three steps in rotation have been identified although not fully proven and lately contested.[48]

The general belief is that separate clinical entities may arise from impairment in each of the stages, respectively. Although strict evidence is lacking, the theory of stages in gut rotation allows a comprehensible explanation of the various clinical presentations of malrotation. Failure of the first stage is seen in infants with omphalocele. Abnormality of the second stage may cause nonrotation of the gut, which is rare. The third and fourth parts of the duodenum are vertically placed along the right side of the superior mesenteric artery; the small bowel is on the right side and the colon to the left of the midline. In reversed rotation the duodenum is placed across anterior while the cecum and the colon are placed behind the superior mesenteric vessels. Malrotation occurs when the rotation is not completed and typically the cecum does not reach the right ileal fossa and is found subhepatically or in a central position in the abdomen. The

Table 1 Etiology of Short Bowel Syndrome in Children

	United States* (%) International§ (%)	Canada† (%)	France‡ (%)	(%)
Atresia	30	30	39	23
Volvulus	10	10	24	24
Gastroschisis	17	12.5	14	14
NEC	43	35	14	27

fixation of the gut may be aberrant and bands (Ladd band) may form between the duodenum and the right colon. In cases of abnormal third stage, the fixation of the midgut and cecum may be deficient.

Clinical Management. Midgut volvulus in the newborn may develop as a result of abnormal rotation but may also occur without malrotation, more often so in premature infants with lax tissue.[49] Intrauterine midgut volvulus is thought to be the cause of intestinal atresia type IIIb (see below). The symptoms of midgut volvulus are indistinguishable from other disorders with intestinal obstruction; vomiting, often bile-stained and abdominal distension in infants. Abdominal pain accompanied by bilious vomiting is more common symptom of malrotation in children >1 year of age.

Barium enema and upper gastrointestinal series, Doppler flow of the superior mesenteric vessels, and laparoscopy are used to confirm the diagnosis. The surgical management of midgut volvulus comprises expedience, detorsion of the volvulus, restoration of circulation, separation of adhesions between bowel loops, and attempts to preserve bowel length. A conservative resection of only obviously necrotic tissue is recommended and bowel with questionable viability should be left in situ for a second look 24 to 36 hours later.[50]

Intestinal Atresia

The intestinal atresias are categorized according to their localization. Duodenal lesions are classified as follows: A type I defect represents a mucosal web with normal muscular wall (most common); type II, a short fibrous cord connecting the two atretic ends of the duodenum; and type III (least common), in which there is complete separation of the atretic ends. According to the classification of jejunoileal atresias by Martin and Zerella[51] and by Grosfeld and colleagues,[52] the type I defect represents a mucosal defect with an intact mesentery, the type II defect consists of a fibrous cord connecting the atretic bowel ends, the type IIIa lesion denotes an atretic segment with a V-shaped mesenteric gap defect, while the type IIIb defect defines the apple peel deformity, in which there is a proximal jejunal atresia, and the distal bowel is supplied by a single retrograde blood vessel. In a type IV defect, multiple instances of atresias ("string of sausage" effect) are present. Atresia affecting the colon is, in most cases, a type IIIa defect, according to this classification.

Etiology. There are two major theories regarding the etiology of intestinal atresia. Tandler presented, in 1900, his theory of a lack of revacuolization of the solid cord stage of intestinal development and Louw and Barnard suggested that a late intrauterine mesenteric vascular accident is the cause of most jejunoileal and colonic atresias. Interestingly, the hypothesis on lack of revacuolization as the probable cause for most cases of duodenal atresia still persists in many review articles. Jejunoileal atresias probably occur as a result of intestinal volvulus, intussus-

ception, internal hernia, or strangulation in a tight gastroschisis or omphalocele defect. Familial instances of jejunoileal and colonic atresias have also been observed, suggesting that genetic factors may play a part in these cases.

Duodenal atresia is associated with prematurity, congenital anomalies including pancreatic anomalies, intestinal malrotation, esophageal atresia, Meckel's diverticulum, variants of imperforate anus, congenital heart disease, central nervous system lesions, renal anomalies, and, rarely, biliary tract anomalies. Down's syndrome occurs in 25 to 30% of patients.

Prenatal Diagnosis. Prenatal ultrasonography may identify the presence of maternal polyhydramnios and distension of the stomach and duodenum with swallowed amniotic fluid. These observations are often associated with a high risk of duodenal atresia. A notable number of jejunoileal and colonic atresias, however, remain undetected by prenatal ultrasonography.

Presentation. Typically, there are signs of bowel obstruction including bilious vomiting, abdominal distension, and failure to pass meconium in instances of lower obstruction. Most infants with duodenal obstruction do not have significant abdominal distension.

Clinical Management. Preoperatively, management includes a nasogastric tube to decompress the stomach, intravenous fluid resuscitation, and evaluation for associated cardiac or renal malformations. Multiple atresias or postoperative complications may lead to long-term total parenteral nutrition (TPN) and delayed or absent bowel adaptation, resulting in protracted IF.

Intestinal Atresia Associated with Immune-Deficiency

Intestinal atresia has been reported to be associated with immunodeficiency. The first report involved three siblings with multiple-level intestinal atresias. One sibling had severe combined immunodeficiency syndrome and clinical histories of the other two siblings strongly suggested a congenital immunodeficiency syndrome.[53] One report on three siblings each in two nonrelated families pointed to an association with Fanconi's anemia in three of seven pregnancies (two boys and one girl) suggesting an autosomal recessive mode of transmission. In a second family, identical multiple atresias occurred in two female siblings born 18 months apart and a third child with a duodenal stenosis. Overwhelming sepsis and a T-cell dysfunction was seen in the postoperative period, which had partially corrected by follow-up at 5 months. This rare syndrome appears to have an autosomal recessive mode of transmission.[54] In case of multiple intestinal atresias, attention should be given to possible associated immune disorder, and irradiation of blood products is recommended pending evaluation of immune system status. Donor immune reconstitution was reported in a child with multiple intestinal atresia and severe combined immu-

nodeficiency disease (SCID) who underwent liver and small bowel transplantation. The child did not experience intestinal graft rejection but only a mild graft-versus-host disease (GVHD), and it was postulated that this child engrafted a donor-derived immune system.[55]

Necrotizing Enterocolitis

Necrotizing enterocolitis (NEC) is an inflammatory bowel necrosis and a major cause of morbidity and mortality for preterm infants. 90% of NEC occurs in premature infants and the incidence of NEC is inversely correlated with gestational age and birth weight (refer to Chapter 20.4, "Necrotizing Enterocolitis").

Clinical Features. NEC presents with variable symptoms, including abdominal distension, feeding intolerance, gastric aspirates, and bilious vomiting. Local tenderness or an abdominal mass may be defined on clinical examination and progression to pneumoperitoneum and sepsis with respiratory failure, shock and death may follow.

Treatment. Therapy of NEC includes stopping feeds, nasogastric decompression, fluid and electrolyte resuscitation, broad-spectrum antibiotics, and, in selected cases, respiratory support. Severity, whether mild or critical, determines the duration of medical therapy. Parenteral antibiotics and nutrition and nil by mouth are usually prescribed for 7 to 14 days.

The indications for surgery are as follows:

1. Presence of pneumoperitoneum, indicating perforation of the intestine
2. Clinical deterioration despite maximal medical treatment
3. Abdominal mass with persistent intestinal obstruction or sepsis
4. Development of intestinal stricture

There is controversy regarding the preferred method of surgical management of NEC.[56] The options are primary peritoneal drainage or laparotomy. At laparotomy, resection of affected bowel with formation of high enterostomy or primary anastomosis of remaining gut, are well-accepted techniques. In infants suffering NEC which involves extensive inflammation of both the large and the small intestine, a proximal, diverting jejunostomy or the "clip and drop" technique have been advocated.[57] These infants will develop IF which contributes to feeding delays, long-term parenteral nutrition, and early onset of severe liver disease.

Total or Near-Total Intestinal Aganglionosis

Hirschsprung disease (HD) is a congenital disorder characterized as an interruption of the craniocaudal migration of neuroblasts and an absence of ganglionic innervation of the affected bowel causing intestinal obstruction. In 75 to 80% of the cases, the aganglionosis is confined to the rectum and sigmoid colon. Manifestation of the disease has been linked to mutations in genes that encode the crucial signals for the development of the enteric nervous system—the *RET* and *EDNRB* signaling pathways. The *Phox2b* gene is involved in neurogenesis and regulates *RET* expression in mice, in which disruption of the *Phox2b* results in an HD-like phenotype. Total or near-total aganglionosis (TAG or NTAG) is a rare form of HD, affecting less than 1% of children with HD. Recently, the concomitant existence of total bowel aganglionosis and congenital central hypoventilation syndrome in a neonate with *Phox2B* gene mutation was reported.[58]

Clinical Management. Abdominal distension and bilious vomiting within the first week of life are the main clinical features of this condition. The extent of the aganglionic segment of the small intestine and the appropriate placing of an ostomy should be guided by perioperative histopathological examinations of biopsies. In infants left with less than 50 cm of small intestine, one can presume a definite and irreversible diagnosis of IF requiring long-term parenteral nutrition. In contrast to conditions of anatomical short bowel, there is no possibility for the remnant bowel to undergo adaptation and growth allowing for intestinal independency. Myotomy–myectomy, first described by Ziegler[59] and later by Shimotake and colleagues and Saxton and colleagues,[60,19] has been suggested to improve the situation with respect to enteral nutrition in these patients. However, it has been reported that complications are the rule rather than the exception after this procedure.

Although several surgical techniques have been proposed for the use of the remnant aganglionic small bowel in total aganglionosis, at present there is no evidence to recommend any. It is rather recommended to avoid recurrent surgery for lengthening, tapering, STEP, or longitudinal myotomy. All surgical procedures that could lead to a reduction of the abdominal cavity size will thereby impair the probable intestinal transplantation procedure.

Over the last few years, the use of parenteral nutrition and new surgical techniques, including small bowel transplantation, have slightly improved the prognosis of this condition previously regarded as fatal. Aganglionosis has been estimated to account for approximately 8% of patients with a primary indication for pediatric intestinal transplantation.[61]

Therefore, an early referral to an expert unit to review the indications for small bowel transplantation is essential for the child with total aganglionosis.

CONSEQUENCES OF RESECTION OF THE SMALL INTESTINE

The more extensive the resection of the small intestine, the greater is the loss of absorptive surface area that transports nutrients, water, and electrolytes. The functional consequences of SBS depend not only on the length, surface, and site of the resected small intestine but also on the functional capacity of the remaining intestine. The cause of resection and age of the patient at the time at which surgery was carried out influence the capacity of the remnant gut function and the potential for adaptation.

Site and Extent of Intestine Removed

Jejunum. The intact jejunum absorbs a significant fraction of nutrients and fluid required by the body. However, the removal of a large segment of jejunum causes only a limited defect in the absorption of macronutrients, electrolytes, and free water because the ileum has a great capacity for adaptation and compensatory function that can take over, almost all the absorptive functions of the jejunum. The clinical experiences are that in children jejunal resections are often well tolerated.

However, the resection of the jejunum reduces the secretion of cholecystokinin and secretin leading to a decrease in biliary and exocrine pancreatic secretions which may lead in turn to a reduction in nutrient absorptive capacity. The reduced production of cholecystokinin, vasoactive intestinal peptide, gastric inhibitory peptide, and serotonin may cause gastric hypersecretion seen more frequently after jejunal resection.[62]

Ileum. The ileal epithelium is relatively impermeable in comparison with the jejunal epithelium. There is less flux of water and sodium in the ileum, and there is significant fluid reabsorption and an ability to concentrate the contents of the ileum. In cases where the ileum, or part of it, has been resected, the large input of chyme from the jejunum to the colon may exceed the capacity of the colon for handling fluid and electrolyte transport.

The ileum is the only site of active bile acid absorption from the intestine. Intestinal bile acid handling is age-dependent in experimental studies. Small amounts of bile acids are absorbed by passive diffusion in the jejunum and colon. Extensive resection of the ileum reduces the active intestinal absorption of bile acids resulting in that bile acids are left in the lumen and spill into the colon and may cause diarrhea as these bile acids are deconjugated by colonic bacteria. The deconjugated bile acids directly stimulate the colon to secrete fluid and electrolytes, causing a secretory watery diarrhea and thereby aggravating the short bowel syndrome. The secretion stimulated by bile acids causing active anion secretion in the colon acts through several mechanisms: increasing cytosolic calcium levels within colonocytes through a calcium ionophore effect; increasing prostaglandin synthesis in lamina propria cells; stimulating excitatory enteric neurons, which then stimulate active anion secretion and propulsive motor contractions; and increasing tight junction permeability to fluid and electrolytes.[63] Recent experimental studies have shown that weaning, but not adult, distal colon shows net bile acid absorption. Increased expression of the apical Na^+-dependent bile acid transporter and lipid-binding protein in weanling colon may have a relevance in enterohepatic conservation of bile acids when ileal bile acid recycling is not fully developed or theoretically when it has been resected.[64]

During intestinal adaptation, the body compensates for bile acid loss into the colon by maintaining the size of the bile acid pool through an increase in hepatic bile acid synthesis. The more extensive losses of ileum result in severe bile acid malabsorption which exceeds synthesis. The interruption of the enterohepatic circulation of bile acids by ileal resection may therefore result in a decrease of hepatic bile acid secretion and an altered composition of hepatic bile in terms of the organic components—bile acid, cholesterol, and phospholipids. A reduction in the circulating pool of bile salts follows, leading to impaired intestinal micelle formation and the spillage of fat (steatorrhea) into the colon.

The spillage of fat into the colon may lead to hydroxylation of the fat by bacteria into hydroxy fatty acids. These fatty acids have stimulatory effects on colonic net fluid and electrolyte secretion through several mechanisms involving increasing mucosal permeability and increasing propulsive motor activity. These effects are similar to those of bile acids and may be related to the detergent properties of both hydroxy fatty acids and bile acids.

The ileum is the primary site of vitamin B_{12} absorption. Malabsorption of vitamin B_{12} occurs after extensive resection of distal ileum. Removal of the ileocecal valve with an intestinal resection increases the likelihood of the development of short bowel syndrome, often in a severe form.[65] The ileocecal valve prevents the migration of luminal colonic microorganisms into the distal small bowel. Moreover, removal of ileocecal valve (ICV) may result in bacterial overgrowth within the small intestine and deconjugation of bile salts within the small intestinal lumen which in turn can result in reduced absorption of fat and fat-soluble vitamins. Deconjugated nonabsorbed bile salts spill into the colon and directly stimulate the colonic secretion of fluid and electrolytes. The bacteria use intraluminal vitamin B_{12}, limiting the availability of vitamin B_{12} for absorption.

The intact ileum markedly slows intestinal transit, and ileal resection decreases the intestinal transit time significantly. Both peptide YY and GLP-1 have been implicated as humoral mediator of the "ileal break."

Colon. The primary function of the colon is to absorb the fluid and electrolytes it receives from the ileum. There is however ample evidence that the colon acts as nutrient-salvaging organ by bacterial fermentation of malabsorbed carbohydrates to short-chain fatty acids.[1] The removal of both ileum and colon obviously drastically increases fluid loss, dehydration, volume depletion, and causes hypocalcemia, and hypomagnesemia. Preservation of the colon in cases of major small intestinal resection appears to lessen the severity of short bowel syndrome. In experimental studies, increased enterocyte expression and function of apical membrane Na/H exchangers in regions distal to the anastomosis play a role in the adaptive process after massive small bowel resection. The increased luminal Na load to distal bowel regions after proximal resection may stimulate increases in apical membrane Na/H exchangers gene transcription and protein expression.[66]

Unabsorbed bile salt and fats are deconjugated by the colonic bacteria. The deconjugated bile salts and hydroxylated fats decrease water absorption in the colon through direct stimulation of the secretion of colonic fluid and electrolytes and through osmotic effects. As free fatty acids enter the colonic lumen, they are bound to calcium leaving oxalate unbound and free to be absorbed systemically through the colonic mucosa, which causes oxalate stones in the kidneys.

INTESTINAL ADAPTATION

Definition

Intestinal adaptation is the dynamic and physiological process that can take place over a long time and that is related to functional and structural changes in the remaining intestine leading to an increased or even adequate absorption of fluid and nutrients. The ultimate adaptation is the restoration of capacities of the remaining intestine to absorb fluid, electrolytes, and nutrients in sufficient amounts to sustain the functions and the growth of the body and thus reverse from intestinal failure to adequate intestinal capacity.

Consequences of Intestinal Adaptation

Soon after resection, physiological process of adaptation of the remaining SB develops. This comprises *muscular hypertrophy* (increased bowel diameter and wall thickness) and hyperplasia of the mucosa. Mucosal *hyperplasia* is characterized by an increased number of enterocytes per unit of SB length, an increased rate of enterocyte proliferation, and an increased villous height and crypt depth (Figure 1). In animals, it was demonstrated that epithelial hyperplasia following gut resection results in increased mucosal mass, including higher mucosal wet weight, higher protein content as well as higher DNA and RNA content per unit of bowel length.[67] The

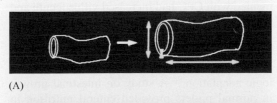
(A)

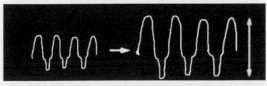
(B)

Figure 1 Schematic representation of anatomical changes during the adaptation process. (A) Intestinal hypertrophy including bowel dilatation, muscular hypertrophy, and bowel lengthening. (B) Mucosal hyperplasia including increased villous high and crypt depth.

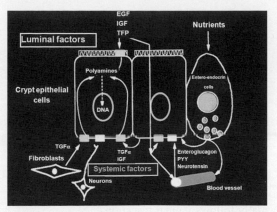

Figure 2 Systemic and luminal factors involved in the process of intestinal adaptation following extensive intestinal resection.

complex regulation of gut mucosal growth involves a multitude of factors including hormonal mediators such as glucagon-like peptide-2 (GLP-2), neurotensine, peptide YY, growth hormone, and insuline-like growth factor (Figure 2). Additionally, oral or enteral feeding stimulates the release of enterotropic hormones such as gastrin, cholecystokinin, and neurotensin, which may further improve the process of gut adaptation. Hence, intraluminal substrates and nutrients are essential for intestinal adaptation.

Factors Influencing Adaptation

Trophic Hormones

Glucagon-like Peptides. The glucagon-like peptides GLP-1 and GLP-2 are synthesized and then released from enteroendocrine cells in the small and large intestine. GLP-1 and GLP-2 modulate nutrient absorption in the intestine. GLP-1 is an incretin hormone which enhances postprandial insulin secretion. The actions of GLP-1 in healthy man include stimulation of insulin secretion in a glucose-dependent manner, suppression of glucagon, reduction in appetite and food intake, deceleration of gastric emptying.[68]

GLP-2. In 1971 an endocrine tumor in the kidney was reported in a 44-year-old woman. She had intestinal mucosal proliferation, constipation, edema, nausea, abdominal distension, and occasional vomiting. After removal of the tumor her symptom disappeared. That observation in a single patient with an "enteroglucagon"-secreting tumor of the kidney, associated with massive small bowel enlargement, provided the strong evidence of the putative role of hormonal factors as intestinotrophic factors. When the patient's renal tumor was removed, the markedly increased circulating concentrations of the glucagon-like peptide returned to normal, and her bowel anatomy was restituted.[69]

Subsequent studies showed that there is increased tissue and plasma enteroglucagon (and recently GLP-2) levels in many animal models of intestinal adaptation. Some years later several authors could establish the link between gut-derived enteroglucagons and intestinal adaptation after resection. Recent

advances have now identified GLP-2 as the main intestinal trophic agent. The peptide, consisting of 33 amino acids, results from expression of the glucagon gene in the enteroendocrine L cells of the intestinal mucosa, from where it is released mainly in response to luminal contact with unabsorbed nutrients. In addition to mucosal growth, GLP-2 enhances activities of several intestinal brush border enzymes and it delays gastric transit, thereby increasing the intestinal capacity for nutrient absorption.[70]

In experimental studies GLP-2 stimulates small bowel villous hyperplasia with increased expression of mucosal digestive enzymes.[71–72] GLP-2 enhances small intestine absorptive function in experimental as well as in clinical studies by upregulating SGLT-1 activity. Functional changes in the mucosa such as reduced serosa to mucosa Na$^+$ transport and reduced permeability were also noted. After repeated GLP-2 administration in animals, the small intestinal epithelium exhibited elongated villi due predominantly to enhanced crypt cell proliferation and decreased enterocyte apoptosis and narrower epithelial cells with longer enterocyte microvilli. The proliferative effects of GLP-2 have been demonstrated in the small bowel of mice, rats, pigs, and humans after exogenous peptide administration (Figure 3).[73–76,150]

In a study in 12 young infants with anticipated long-term TPN requirement due to short bowel syndrome or NEC plasma levels of GLP-2 level were best correlated with residual small intestinal length. GLP-2 levels were well correlated with tolerance of enteral feeds and were directly correlated with nutrient absorptive of macronutrients, however GLP-2 levels did not correlate with gestational or postnatal age.[77]

Teduglutide (ALX-0600) is a recently developed GLP-2 analog. The safety and efficacy of

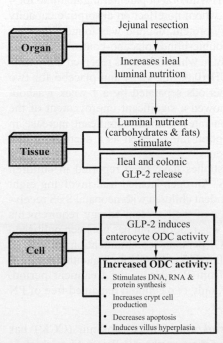

Figure 3 A proposed model for stimulation of GLP-2 production.

teduglutide were investigated in 16 adult SBS patients with and without a colon in continuity, 0.03 and 0.1 mg/kg/d, once or twice daily for 21 days. Nutrient balance studies, D-xylose tests, and intestinal mucosa biopsies were performed at baseline, on the last 3 days of treatment, and after 3 weeks of follow-up. Teduglutide increased absolute and relative wet weight absorption, urine weight, and urine sodium excretion, decreased fecal wet weight and fecal energy excretion. In SBS patients with end jejunostomy, teduglutide significantly increased villous height, crypt depth, and mitotic index; however, the improvements in intestinal absorption and decreases in fecal excretion noted after treatment had reversed after the drug-free follow-up period.[78]

Growth Hormone. Studies on the effect of recombinant human growth hormone (rhGH) on intestinal adaptation after bowel resection have shown mixed results. Animal experiments have shown evidence of mucosal cell proliferation and enhanced adaptation but also lack of response to GH. Recombinant human GH was used in adult patients with SBS in both, open and randomized, clinical trials. Several of the studies of adults have recruited mixed groups of patients regarding remnant small intestinal length and colonic length. Some studies have also combined rhGH treatment with glutamine-enriched diet and oral intake ad libitum. A study of eight adult patients found decreased percent body fat and increased body weight and lean body mass in patients with SBS, without an increase in macronutrient or fluid absorption. The positive findings were most likely a reflection of increased extracellular fluid because all eight patients developed peripheral edema on active treatment. Furthermore, the positive effect of active treatment did not appear to be sustained once discontinued.[79] Similar results were found in a study involving eight adults on long-term parenteral nutrition who received high-dose rhGH with oral or parenteral glutamine for 4 weeks in whom no effect on absorptive capacity of energy, protein, or fluid was found.[80] In contrast a double-blind, placebo-controlled, cross-over study in which 12 adults received daily low-dose rhGH (0.05 mg/kg/d) and placebo for two 3-week periods separated by a 1-week washout period showed a significant improvement of the absorption rates, without significant increase in fat absorption rate, as well as a decrease in PN requirements.[81]

Few studies have been reported in children with SBS. An open-labeled trial involving eight PN-dependent children with neonatal SBS receiving >50% of their protein energy requirements from PN was reported but has not been published (Goulet O, personal communication). Children received 0.6 IU/kg/d rhGH for 3 months. All were weaned from PN during the treatment period. However, only two children remained free of PN 1 year later.

Cholecystokinin. Cholecystokinin (CCK) has a trophic action on the small intestine which is most likely exerted by stimulating pancreatic or biliary secretions. When infused into dogs or rats maintained on total parenteral nutrition, CCK completely prevented villus hypoplasia in one study.[82] Other investigators have been unable to substantiate this effect. CCK probably has no direct trophic effect on the intestinal mucosa.

Somatostatin. The effects of somatostatin on the intestine are seemingly competing from the perspective of intestinal adaptation. Somatostatin reduces the crypt cell production rate and hyperplasia in the small intestine after resection; it also inhibits the rise in enteroglucagon levels that normally follows jejunal resection.[83]

Therefore, somatostatin may modulate mucosal cell turnover by influencing glucagon release. It increases intestinal transit time and inhibits gastric secretions. Somatostatin-induced reductions in pancreatic and biliary secretions can lead to frank fat malabsorption and steatorrhea.

Epidermal Growth Factor. Epidermal growth factor (EGF) is an important trophic peptide in the development of the intestine. Oral feeding of EGF augments gut growth and development in experimental animals, affects both the structure and the function of developing intestine and acts possibly by increasing other trophic hormones such as PYY and proglucagon-derived peptides.[84]

In clinical setting, SBS pediatric patients (<25% bowel length predicted for age) were prospectively enrolled in treatment using human recombinant EGF.[85] However, this study, involving only five patients assessed with discussable parameters, does not allow to draw any conclusion.

Insulin. Insulin given sc and po has been shown to influence intestinal structure and absorptive function.[86-87] The favorable effect of insulin is relevant and might be considered in patients on PN receiving high intravenous glucose rate that induce insulin release and relative hyperinsulinism. Interestingly, oral insulin was shown to enhance intestinal adaptation following massive resection in a rat model. This might open new perspective in clinical setting.[88]

Intraluminal Nutrients. The major mechanisms of stimuli from luminal content are direct contact with epithelial cells and stimulation of trophic gastrointestinal hormone secretion (as described above).[89-93] Most data on the effect of intraluminal nutrients in SBS derive from animal studies, while evidence-based medicine is scarce in guiding for optimal use of intraluminal nutrients in human with SBS. The clinical decisions are therefore based on a combination of physiology, animal studies, and clinical experience. Still, nobody knows exactly the best clinical management of SBS in children, and to weigh the patient's age, cause of resection and nutritional status. One of the most relevant guideline is to be as physiological as possible as the intestinal adaptation process is.

The extent to which enteral nutrients stimulate intestinal adaptation depends on the type and complexity of the nutrient administered.

Carbohydrates. Experimental studies on growth responses to disaccharides and monosaccharides in rats showed that disaccharide's infusions of the midgut stimulated mucosal growth more than monosaccharides. Mucosal adaptation was abolished when there was no hydrolysis of the disaccharide. The results suggest that the functional workload of absorbing epithelium, including the "work of hydrolysis," plays an important role in the stimulus for intestinal adaptation.[94]

Dietary Lipids. The quality of dietary lipids seems to have an effect in inducing intestinal adaptation. The addition of LCT/LCPUFAs to diets enhanced intestinal adaptation in a linear, dose-dependent manner after massive bowel resection in rats. In a subsequent study, dietary arachidonic acid seemed to facilitate the adaptation process by acting as a substrate for the synthesis of prostaglandins, and not through the derivatives of lipoxygenase such as leukotrienes or thromboxanes.[95]

In a rat model of SBS, early high fat diet increased lipid absorptive capacity of the intestine. The main mechanisms of this effect may be an acceleration of structural intestinal adaptation resulting in an increased number of enterocytes. However, this was not found at the molecular and cellular levels of fat uptake.[96] MCT lipids are not as effective as LCT in stimulating mucosal hyperplasia in an animal SBS model. The usefullness of MCT in enteral nutrition of SBS is due to rapid hydrolysis and that it may also be absorbed intact, to some extent from the stomach and duodenum.

Protein and Amino Acids. A study on the impact of colostrum protein concentrate (CPC) on intestinal adaptation after massive small bowel resection in a porcine model of infant SBS showed that animals fed polymeric infant formula alone had reduced weight gain compared with controls fed the same diet. Animals fed pig chow or polymeric infant formula supplemented with CPC grew at an equivalent rate to controls fed polymeric infant formula alone.[97] Resected animals supplemented with CPC had increased villus length and crypt depth in the remnant small intestine, and the authors conclude that CPC supplementation of polymeric infant formula resulted in normal weight gain and features of enhanced morphologic adaptation.[98] A study on intestinal growth in normal piglets provided enteral nutrition in the form of elemental nutrients or cow's milk formula showed that intestinal mucosal growth and villus morphology were similar in pigs fed elemental nutrients and cow's milk formula.[99] A novel nutrition approach in providing nutrients as nucleotide precursors showed that supplementation of oral diet pyrimidine orotate and uracil stimulated adaptive jejunal growth after massive small bowel resection in rats, and that orotate had more potent growth-stimulatory effects than uracil in this animal model.[100]

The role of dietary proteins, peptides, and amino acids have been a matter of controversy in management on SBS. Several experimental studies have been performed to answer the clinical questions regarding this problem. Hydrolyzed protein formulas (HPFs) have been evaluated by comparison with intact protein infant formula in a crossover study of 60 days duration in 10 infants with SBS.[101] No effect of formula type was observed on growth, nitrogen absorption, or mucosal permeability. In general, HPFs are lactose free and contain MCTs. Elemental aminoacid-based formula has been introduced more recently for infants suffering severe allergic diseases. It is not yet established if this type of formula may influence outcome of SBS. The beneficial effect of an elemental amino acid–based formula was reported in an open trial involving only 4 SBS patients with persistent feeding intolerance.[102] A retrospective study also found shorter duration of PN dependency with the use of an amino acid-based formula.[103] Current data are no yet sufficient for recommending such expansive formulas for infants and children with SBS.

Glutamine. Glutamine is the most abundant extracellular amino acid. It is used at high rates by the gut, liver, central nervous system, and immune cells. It is a fuel for enterocytes, colonocytes, and other rapidly dividing cells.[104] A state of relative glutamine deficiency has been postulated in humans based on the decrease in plasma glutamine in acute critical illness. In humans who have undergone intestinal resection, the turnover of glutamine is markedly diminished.[105]

Although the overall impression from small clinical studies is that glutamine appears to play an important role in maintaining the structural integrity of the small intestine at this time, no firm recommendation can be made for glutamine in enteral or parenteral nutrition for the adaptation of the remaining small intestine after resections. A small randomized and placebo controlled trial of enteral glutamine in children with gastrointestinal disease showed no effect on the duration of parenteral nutrition, tolerance of enteral feeds, or intestinal absorptive or barrier function.[106]

The conclusion from several studies in adults is that no controlled human clinical trials have thus far demonstrated that glutamate or glutamine supplementation directly enhances morphologic or functional improvement in the small intestine of patients with short bowel syndrome.[107]

Arginine and Citrulline. Arginine is a precursor for polyamines which are of importance for intestinal adaptation in SBS. Arginine is one of the most versatile amino acids in cells. It serves as a precursor for the synthesis of proteins, nitric oxide, polyamines, and proline. Arginine stimulates the secretion of hormones such as insulin, prolactin, glucagon, and growth hormone, and plays a key role in the nitrogen homeostasis modulating ureogenesis. The liver and the gut play major roles in the arginine metabolism. The arginine flux to the liver is modulated by

the intestine. On a whole-body basis, synthesis of arginine occurs principally via the intestinal–renal axis, wherein epithelial cells of the small intestine, which produce citrulline primarily from glutamine and glutamate, by two enzymes that metabolize citrulline (argininosuccinate synthetase and argininosuccinate lyase). Citrulline is extracted by the proximal tubule cells of the kidney and converted to arginine, which is returned to the circulation. Consequently, impairment of small bowel or renal function can reduce endogenous arginine synthesis, thereby increasing the dietary requirements.

Synthesis of arginine from citrulline also occurs at a low level in many other cells, and cellular capacity for arginine synthesis can be markedly increased under circumstances that also induce nitric oxide synthase (NOS). Thus, citrulline, a coproduct of the NOS-catalyzed reaction, can be recycled to arginine in a pathway known as the citrulline-NO or arginine–citrulline pathway. This is demonstrated by the fact that in many cell types, citrulline can substitute for arginine to some degree in supporting NO synthesis. This arginine-citrulline-arginine cycle can be seen as a means of protecting dietary arginine from excessive degradation in the liver especially in situations where the intake of protein is low.

In massive intestinal resection, the main site of citrulline production is greatly reduced, and hypocitrullinemia proportional to the severity of intestinal disease is observed in patients with short bowel syndrome (SBS). This observation has recently been extended to patients with celiac disease and in rejection of small bowel transplantation grafts.[5,7]

Short-Chain Fatty Acids. Short-chain fatty acids (SCFAs) are produced by bacterial fermentation of the carbohydrates and fibrous polysaccharides that spill into the colon. The principal SCFA are acetate, propionate, and butyrate. These SCFAs are absorbed by the colon and metabolized in the colonic epithelial cells as a source of fuel; carbon atoms are salvaged that would otherwise be lost.[1,108,109] It has been estimated that up to 3 kJ of energy can be absorbed each day by the adult human colon in the form of short-chain fatty acids.[110] Supplementation of an elemental diet with pectin, which is fermented to SCFA in the colon, improved adaptation of the ileum, jejunum, and colon after massive small bowel resection.[109] Experimental studies on the supplementation of parenteral nutrition by using intracecal infusion of SCFA have confirmed that supplementation reduces the mucosal atrophy and intestinal immune dysfunction following massive small bowel resection in animal models.[111–113]

In addition to their local effects, in animal studies systemic SCFA can affect the motility of both the stomach and the ileum through neuroendocrine mechanisms, likely through the expression of proglucagon and peptide YY. Furthermore, both systemic and enteral SCFA exert a trophic effect on the jejunum by increasing mucosal mass, DNA, and villus height.[111–115]

DOES WITHDRAWAL OF LUMINAL NUTRIENTS RESULT IN MUCOSAL ATROPHY?

Results from experimental studies and from human studies on the role of enteral feeding for stimulation are not congruent.[116–118] There are only few studies in humans on exclusive TPN. Jejunal biopsy specimens taken from eight normal volunteers before and after 14 days of parenteral nutrition therapy demonstrated decreased villus height, a decreased villus cell count, and increased intestinal permeability, but no changes in DNA, RNA, and protein content in comparison with controls, suggesting that the total enterocyte number did not change.[119]

A study on TPN in human adults by morphological methods of biopsies showed alterations in epithelial cell turnover and changes in expression and localization of extracellular matrix proteins, however this was not a functional study.[120] In adults who required at least 10 days of preoperative TPN before an elective laparotomy neither mucosal atrophy nor bacterial translocation was more common in parenterally fed patients compared to enterally fed controls.[121]

Eight normal volunteers received TPN for 14 days followed by 5 days of enteral refeeding with either a standard or a glutamine and arginine-supplemented formula. Endoscopic jejunal biopsies were taken before and after TPN and after enteral refeeding. TPN did not affect immunoglobulin-producing lymphocytes in the lamina propria, intestinal permeability, or bacterial translocation.[122] A similar study in seven adults before TPN, after 21 days of TPN, and after a progressive oral refeeding showed a clear-cut decrease of major enzyme activities during TPN (sucrase, maltase, lactase, glucoamylase, acid aminopeptidase, dipeptidyl peptidase) without any morphologic modifications as observed with standard histology. Electron microscopy showed a slight but significant decrease in the height of microvilli.[123] There are no similar studies in children, and we cannot conclude that depriving the short bowel intestinal lumen of enteral feeding will lead to intestinal hypoplasia or immune dysfunction.

MANAGEMENT AND OUTCOME OF CHILDREN WITH SHORT BOWEL SYNDROME

The medical management of patients with SBS aims to promote gut adaptation and to recover the intestinal functions to a level sufficient to achieve intestinal autonomy (PN weaning). The aims of the nutritional support are to provide substrates for optimal growth and development while for infants or children to stimulate oral feeding. PN is the cornerstone of management but as much nutrition as tolerated should be provided to the patient via the intestine in order to improve the physiological processes of SB adaptation and villous hyperplasia. Early use of the gastrointestinal tract especially by oral feeding (enhancement of

GI secretion, salivary EGF, gallbladder motility) is recommended.

Clinical Management of Short Bowel Syndrome

Three stages can be identified on the roadmap to intestinal independency of artificial feeding: the first is characterized by large fluid and electrolyte losses. During this stage parenteral fluid and nutrition therapy is mandatory. At this stage the nutrition support aims for adequate metabolic support and prevention of complications. Patients tend to have large-volume fluid and electrolytes secretion, losses from gastric fluid, and ostomy may be high. A tailored parenteral nutrition solution containing all appropriate fluid, electrolytes, and macro- and micronutrients for metabolic needs is recommended. Gastric hypersecretion is proportional to the extent of resection of the small intestine and H_2-blockers or proton pump inhibitors are recommended for infants and children with SBS.[124,125] Ostomy secretions should be monitored with short intervals, starting from two hourly and replaced using a separate fluid and electrolyte solution–based on actual measurement of electrolytes in the ostomy losses. Losses tend to be high in sodium content, and solutions with at least 80 to 100 meq/L of sodium are commonly needed to maintain fluid and electrolyte homeostasis. Once ostomy losses drop, fluid replacement is reduced accordingly. Separate prescriptions for parenteral nutrition and fluid replacements are important.

The second stage is characterized by the use of a combination of parenteral and enteral nutrition. The SBS is a very variable condition which can be as mild as that following terminal ileal resection to a very debilitating condition which follows total jejunoileal and colonic resection. Management and outcome varies according to the cause, the extent, and site of resection and the degree of adaptation of the remaining bowel. Patients with dilated, poorly motile segments of SB (gastroschisis, atresia, NEC) benefit from an approach aiming in reducing bowel dilatation and small intestinal bacterial overgrowth (SIBO), since they may develop rapidly severe liver disease. Adapted parenteral nutrition (PN) delivered, as soon as tolerance permits, by cyclical infusion, is mandatory. In any cases, early oral feeding (OF) should be promoted while the benefits of continuous enteral feeding should be balanced according to the workload of the technique in combination with PN, the risk of "intestinal overload" with subsequent small intestinal bacterial overgrowth and the tube feeding induced food aversion, and eating disorders. The third stage is the stage when the clinically stable child is well and growing and parenteral nutrition can be weaned off and replaced by a combination of enteral and oral feeding aiming.

Controversies in Nutritional Management of Infants with SBS

Enteral Nutrition. The type of enteral formula used and the timing of initiation of enteral feeding in the SBS pediatric patient are very important. There are controversies whether to give oral feeding or enteral, to use pump or drip feeding, whether to use polymeric, semielemental or amino acid–based formula. Besides the physiologic and nutritional perspectives of enteral feeding, there are psychological and practical problems that need to be addressed.

The preferences of the parents and also children from a young age and the quality of life of the child, the siblings and the parents must be taken into consideration as well as the medical issues.

The aim of enteral nutrition is to stimulate the adaptation and ultimately wean off from PN. The route of feeding and the type of diet need to be adapted to the child's age and general health, to the residual small bowel length and to the partially or totally present or absent colon (Table 2).

Human Milk. There are several properties of breast milk that may be beneficial for infants with SBS. Breast milk contains high levels of IgA, nucleotides, leukocytes, and other components that support the neonate's immature immune system.[126] In an animal model of SBS, colostrum protein concentration, and supplementation of polymeric infant formula resulted in normal weight gain and features of enhanced morphologic adaptation.[99] In a retrospective study of infants with SBS, the use of breast milk showed the highest correlation with shorter PN courses. This could however have been secondary to the residual small bowel length, which in this study remained a major important predictor of duration of PN.[103] It is important to stress that the high content of lactose in breast milk does not seem to be the cause of digestive intolerance.

Advancement of Enteral Nutrition. There are no controlled studies of when enteral nutrition should be started, how it should be advanced, and how problems that arise should be solved. Combined efforts by the parents, the nursing staff, experienced nurse practitioners, pediatric gastroenterologists with special interest in managing children with SBS are a prerequisite for success.

In the early stages of SBS, many children are left with an enterostomy. The placement of this stoma may have an important part in the fluid and electrolyte losses, and every effort should be made to close enterostoma. Surgical management of strictures and/or dilatation in the remaining intestine has to be emphasized to ensure maximal recovery of effective propulsive intestinal motility.

In infants and young children, advancement of enteral nutrition could be performed by either continuous or bolus feeding via a nasogastric tube (NGT). The enteral nutrition rate is gradually advanced based on several parameters. If stool losses increase by more than 50% and are greater than about 30 to 40 mL/kg/d, or stool or ostomy output is strongly positive for reducing substances, advances in enteral feeding should be withheld until these parameters improve. In patients with an intact colon, a decrease in the stool pH below 5.5 is also indicative of carbohydrate malabsorption and suggests that further advancement of enteral feedings would result in a significant increase in osmotic diarrhea. Unabsorbed enteral nutrition may act as osmotic drive, that causes diarrhea, and induces an intolerance for enteral nutrition. This could be prevented by combining oral and enteral nutrition and by using several modalities of feeding and replacing nasogastric tubes with gastrostomy in selected cases. The self-regulated feeding pattern and breastfeeding for infants should however be secured as much as possible.

Table 2 Main Characteristics of Diets for Short Bowel Patients

Breast milk
   Contains lactose
   Contains growth factors, nucleotides, long-chain fatty acids, glutamine, and other amino acids that promote intestinal adaptation
   Promote microbiota rich in *Lactobacilli* and *Bifidobacteria*
   To be used as often as possible in neonatal SBS by breast or tube feeding

Enteral formulas
   Carbohydrates
      Oligo- and polysaccharides
      Poorly tolerated by patients with limited mucosal absorptive surface area
      Broken down into small intestinal lumen in osmotically active organic acids
      Should not exceed 40% of calories, and be lactose-free in IDI patients
   Fiber supplementation
      Helpful in older children with SBS with intact colon
      Promote colonic bacterial production of short-chain fatty acids

Lipids
   Provide a dense energy source
   Long chain triglycerides
      Poorly digested in case of SIBO because of bile acids changes
   Poorly absorbed in patients with severe malabsorption
   Have trophic effects on small intestinal mucosa
   Supplementation with n-3-, n-6-FA, or PUFAs may enhance mucosal growth
   Medium cain triglycerides
      Rapidly hydrolyzed by pancreatic lipase
   Do not provides essential fatty acids
   Less dependent on an extensive absorptive surface for adequate absorption
   Water soluble and absorbed intact, directly into the portal circulation
   Appropriate for most infants with SBS
   Excessive intake can cause diarrhea
   Recommended use of formulas containing no more than 60% MCTs as fat

Nitrogen
   Hydrolyzed protein formulas (HPF)
      Used for many years
      Have changed the incidence and outcome of PDI
      No demonstrated advantages in comparison with intact protein infant formula
      Lactose free and contain MCTs
      Largely used and recommended in SBS patients
   Elemental amino acid–based formula
      Not yet established if this type of formula may influence outcome of SBS
      Do not contain MCTs
   Glutamine (Gln)
      No benefit currently demonstrated

Loss of enteral tolerance in short bowel patients should prompt a rapid search for sources of infection. For patients with indwelling lines, blood cultures should be immediately obtained. Although weaning from PN is important in the management of the short bowel pediatric patient, full enteral feedings or oral feedings can raise an increased risk for nutritional deficiencies especially at an age of rapid growth. A child with SBS who has weaned off PN may later develop a need for supplementary PN during puberty.[135]

Many children with SBS will develop oral aversions, like many other children who have been exposed to obnoxious oral stimuli (prolonged ventilation, nasogastric intubation, and airway and/or upper gastrointestinal suctioning). In order to stimulate oral feeding, solid feedings can be initiated as for healthy infants. Solid feedings can be given with a nasogastric tube in place without difficulty. This may prevent losing the "window of opportunity" to learn how to eat orally. Although the child is receiving combined PN and enteral feedings, the use of ongoing pleasant oral experiences, and if necessary speech/feeding therapy should be implemented.

Bacterial Overgrowth Is a Limiting Factor in Short Bowel Syndrome

Small bowel bacterial overgrowth (SBBO) is defined as increased bacterial content in the small intestine (see Chapter 19.2d, "Small Bowel Bacterial overgrowth").[128] Normal small bowel bacterial counts vary from 10^3 proximally to greater concentration in the ileum. A high concentration of gastric acid normally limits the number of bacteria that successfully enter the small intestine. Bacteria are subsequently eliminated from the small intestine through the combination of normal antegrade peristalsis and mucosal immune factors. In SBS, many of these factors, especially anatomy and motility, are disrupted. It is not uncommon for bacterial content of the proximal small intestine to exceed 10^5. When motility is slowed, the bowel is dilated and the ICV is absent, bacterial overgrowth is almost universally present. SBBO is a frequent complication which causes mucosal inflammation, which further may exacerbate nutrient malabsorption, deconjugate bile salts, and deplete bile salt pool with subsequent impaired micellar solubilisation resulting in steatorrhea and fat-soluble vitamins malabsorption. SBBO increases the risk of intestinal bacterial translocation. SBBO is usually associated with anorexia, vomiting, diarrhea, cramps, abdominal distension, metabolic acidosis from D-lactic acidosis, and failure to thrive. Bacterial overgrowth should be considered when a patient experiences bloating, cramps, diarrhea, or gastrointestinal blood loss in the face of seemingly adequate gut length. It is also a common cause of clinical deterioration in a previously stable patient with SBS. Screening for SBBO can often be accomplished through the use of breath hydrogen determination. Markedly elevated fasting breath hydrogen levels or a rapid rise in breath hydrogen

following oral administration of glucose (2 g/kg up to a maximum of 50 g) is suggestive of SSBO provided that the transit time through the small intestine is not so rapid as to produce immediate entry of malabsorbed glucose into the colon. Glucose is the ideal substrate for this test because it is absorbed rapidly in the small bowel and rarely makes it to the colon, where it could produce a false-positive test. Small intestinal biopsies demonstrating inflammatory changes often suggest bacterial overgrowth, especially when the small intestine is dilated, motility is poor, or a partial obstruction exists.

Two other complications of bacterial overgrowth include D-lactic acidosis and small bowel colitis. D-Lactic acidosis results because bacteria produce both D- and L-lactate, but only L-lactate is well metabolized by most humans.[129–131] Consequently, the malabsorbed carbohydrates are broken down to lactic acid by the bacteria. D-Lactate then accumulates in the bloodstream, resulting in neurologic symptoms varying from disorientation to frank coma. Bacterial overgrowth may also result in the development of colitis or ileitis, with large ulcerations.

This form of colitis occasionally responds to antimicrobial therapy. Oral metronidazole, 10 to 20 mg/kg/d, either alone or in combination with trimethoprim-sulfamethoxazole, is an effective combination. Oral gentamicin may also be used and is minimally absorbed. Probiotic therapy has been shown to reduce the risk of bacterial translocation in experimental short bowel syndrome.[132–133] However, the clinical experience

with probiotic therapy in SSBO is limited. The use of antimotility agents such as loperamide in patients with short bowel syndrome may exacerbate bacterial overgrowth and is totally contraindicated in patients whose gastrointestinal motility is already delayed.

OUTCOME OF SHORT BOWEL SYNDROME (Table 3)

Until 30 years ago, the prognosis after extensive bowel resection was poor, especially in the neonatal period. The onset of parenteral and enteral feeding in the daily practice has transformed the outcome during the past three decades.[134–138]

More than 90% of infants and children now survive after extensive small bowel resection in the neonatal period. One of the largest surveys includes 87 children who had undergone extensive neonatal small bowel resection, followed-up over a mean 15 years period. The overall survival was 89.7% depending on the date of birth. The duration of PN dependency varies according to the intestinal length and the presence of the ICV (19). All patients ($n = 9$) who remain PN dependent had less than 40 cm of small bowel and/or the absence of ICV. A group of patients ($n = 12$) with a mean small bowel length of 35 ± 19 cm, resection of the ICV in 50% of cases, and an initial period of PN 47.4 ± 23.8 months had significant decrease in height and weight gain within the 4 years after cessation of PN, requiring a new period of enteral or parenteral feeding. Finally the largest

---

Table 3 Management and Outcome of Patients with Neonatal Short Bowel Syndrome (SBS) According to Anatomical Characteristics

—SBL <40 cm without ICV and with associated partial or large colectomy
Patients need very long-term home PN, often indefinite. The indication to reduce PN is weight gain beyond the desired limit and the fact that a reduced rate of infusion does not cause electrolyte imbalance and dehydration. Patients with total colectomy or permanent proximal jejunostomy will remain indefinitely dependent on PN.

—SBL <40 cm or only duodenum with totally or largely intact colon
Patients need long-term home PN. However, many infants and children may have a degree of adaptation and require less PN and benefit from orally and/or enterally administered nutrients. Some of them may be progressively weaned from PN. Infants with duodeno-right colon anastomosis have no chance to be weaned from PN and should not receive CEF instead of oral feeding that protects liver and promotes optimal psychological behavior. These patients are at highest risk of developing D-lactic acidosis.

—SBL (40 to 100 cm) without ICV and with associated partial or large colectomy
Patients require mid-term home PN and can be fed orally immediately. Adapted CEF combined with oral feeding may help in reducing the PN duration. Bile salt–induced diarrhea may impede rapid PN weaning.

—SBL (40 to 100 cm) with preserved terminal ileum and the entire colon
Patients require very short-term PN and can be fed orally immediately. Adapted CEF in combination with oral feeding may help in reducing significantly PN duration.

—SBS with terminal ileum resection
Patients have a bile salt–induced diarrhea, and benefit from the administration of 1 to 2 g of cholestyramine three times a day to bind bile salts left unabsorbed by the resected ileum. Vitamin B_{12} plasma levels should be measured and if low supplemental B_{12} should be provided by intramuscular injection in a dose of 100 to 150 μg per mo or 1,000 μg every 6 mo.

Management and outcome varies according to anatomical factors including the remaining small bowel length (SBL), the preservation of ileum, the ileocecal valve (ICV), and the colon. Patients with dilated, poorly motile segments of SB (gastroschisis, atresia, NEC) should benefit from approach aiming in reducing bowel dilatation and small intestinal bacterial overgrowth (SIBO), since they may develop rapidly severe liver disease. Adapted parenteral nutrition (PN) delivered, as soon as tolerance permits, by cyclical infusion, is mandatory. In any cases, early oral feeding (OF) should be promoted while the benefits of continuous enteral feeding (CEF) should be balanced according to the workload of the technique in combination with PN, the risk of "intestinal overload" with subsequent SIBO, and the tube feeding–induced food aversion and eating disorders.

group (n + 57) involves patients with a mean small bowel length of 57 ± 19 cm, the presence of the ICV in 81% of cases, and a PN duration of 16.1 ± 11.4 months. By multivariate analysis, PN duration is significantly influenced by the length of residual SB and the absence of ICV. After PN weaning, they grow up normally with normal puberty and final height as expected from genetic target height. Thus, with favorable anatomic prognosis factors and short duration of initial PN, normal long-term growth may be predicted.[135] However, long-term nutritional status has to be monitored carefully.[139] However, children with negative prognostic factors such as nonadaptive remaining intestine and long-term PN dependency require careful monitoring of nutrition as well as prevention of complications associated with or due to PN. New treatment modalities to stimulate the adaptation of the remaining intestine in intestinal failure need to be developed for these children and their parents.

NONTRANSPLANT SURGERY FOR SHORT BOWEL SYNDROME

A small number of patients will acquire intestinal autonomy (PN weaning) only very slowly, if at all, because of major motility disorders or a particularly short (ultrashort) remnant small bowel without ICV. In such patients, different surgical approaches have been proposed for increasing nutrient and fluid absorption by either slowing the transit or increasing surface area. Surgical procedures aiming at slowing intestinal transit have been attempted and have been extensively reviewed while clinical results are conflicting. They include intestinal valves, reversed intestinal segments, and colon interposition. In selected patients with dilated bowel segments, longitudinal intestinal lengthening and tailoring (LILT) was first described by Bianchi and thereafter further performed by many others.[140–141] LILT has the theoretical interest of not only tapering the dilated segment but also of using the divided intestine to increase total small bowel length. Anatomical criteria have been suggested for patient selection for this procedure: (1) intestinal diameter >3 cm, (2) length of residual small bowel >40 cm, and (3) length of dilated bowel >20 cm. This procedure allows improvement in more than 50% of patients in terms of intestinal transit, stool frequency, intestinal absorption rate, weight gain, and finally PN weaning.[142] Outcome is influenced by age and clinical status, especially liver status, of the patient at time of surgery. It is yet not recommended to perform the LILT procedure in patients with severe liver disease or cirrhosis. However, this procedure may be achieved successfully following isolated liver transplantation for SBS (see below).

A new procedure called serial transverse enteroplasty (STEP) (Figure 4) was recently reported for infants and children with SBS.[143–144] The indications for STEP are SBS and bacterial overgrowth. According to the STEP

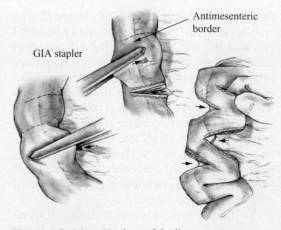

Figure 4 Serial applications of the linear stapler are used to create a zig-zag-shaped channel of lengthened small bowel. The stapler is placed perpendicular to the long axis of the bowel, so that all stapler applications are parallel to the mesenteric blood supply.

registry, 38 patients were enrolled by 19 surgery groups in United States through April 2006. Primary diagnoses were SBS (gastroschisis and intestinal atresia followed by NEC), bacterial overgrowth, and neonatal atresia with dilated proximal intestine. Mean intestinal length increased from 68 cm pre-STEP to 115 cm post-STEP and mean percent of enteral intake for the SBS group rose from 31% pre-SREP to 67% post-STEP. Intra- and postoperative complications ranged from staple line leak to bowel obstruction and late outcomes included progression to transplantation mortality due to liver failure, each in 3 children, respectively.[145]

ISOLATED LIVER TRANSPLANTATION

Some infants, especially premature babies with severe NEC or term neonates with short bowel syndrome from gastroschisis and/or extensive intestinal atresia (eg, apple peel syndrome) are at high risk of developing early end-stage liver disease because of the addition of disruption of enterohepatic cycle (ileal disease or resection) and intestinal stasis with consecutive intraluminal bacterial overgrowth and/or translocation (endotoxinemia).

These patients require liver transplantation combined with intestine or even isolated (IsLTx). Indeed in some SBS children with a length of remnant intestine theoretically sufficient to achieve PN weaning, liver disease interferes with gut adaptation and can lead to early death. The small size and poor condition of these infants means they are poor candidates for combined liver-intestine Tx, while many of them die before a combined graft is available.

The advantages of IsLTx over combined transplantation are the following: organ availability is greater, liver-reduction techniques are well established, and lower immunosuppression is required. In addition, there is greater experience in the care of children after orthotopic liver Tx. The first series of IsLTx in SBS pediatric patients was reported by Lawrence and colleagues.[146] Some isolated cases

have been reported.[147] The first larger study with a high survival rate was reported by Horslen and colleagues.[148] This survey involved 11 infants with estimated small bowel length beyond the ligament of Treitz being in the range of 25 to more than 100 cm. Some patients required intestinal lengthening procedure as described above. A recent study of 23 children with SBS and end-stage liver disease, considered to have good prognostic features for eventual full enteral adaptation, underwent isolated liver transplantation. Median age was 11 months (range, 6.5 to 48 months). Median pretransplant weight was 7.4 kg (range, 5.2 to 15 kg). All had growth retardation and advanced liver disease. Bowel length ranged from 25 to 100 cm. Some children had a liver retransplantation and whole liver, partial grafts also from living donors were used. Median follow-up was 57 months, and actuarial patient and graft survival rates at 1 year are 82 and 75% and at 5 years are 72 and 60%, respectively. Four deaths resulted from sepsis, all within 4 months of transplantation, and 1 death resulted from progressive liver failure. Out of the 17 surviving patients, 14 achieved enteral autonomy, at a median of 3 months (range, 1 to 72 months) after transplantation. Isolated liver transplantation in children with liver failure as a result of SBS, who have favorable prognostic features for full enteral adaptation, is feasible with satisfactory long-term survival.[149] However, prevention of NEC, screening for high-risk patients such as gastroschisis and prevention of IF-related liver disease might improve outcome for those patients and decrease the need for any type of liver grafting alone or in combination with small intestine.

INTESTINAL TRANSPLANTATION FOR SHORT BOWEL SYNDROME

Some patients may remain partially or almost fully dependent on PN for years or forever and are thus considered to have permanent IF.[150] The irreversibility of SBS-related IF has to be demonstrated before any referral to ITx. IF may be clearly and early considered as irreversible in patients with duodenocolic anastomosis after extensive intestinal resection for midgut volvulus or children with total aganglionosis with small bowel length less than 50 cm. These patients are potential candidates for ITx. In contrast, it can be rather difficult to confirm irreversibility of IF in SBS for which all medical and/or surgical approaches have to be tried before any decision of ITx can be taken. When long-term PN is effective and well tolerated, it can be used for a prolonged period of time without intestinal transplantation. Finally, as shown in the Pironi study, only few patients require immediate transplantation for life-threatening condition.[13] However, some patients develop complications while receiving daily long-term PN for IF. These patients can be considered as candidates for intestinal transplantation.

Extensive multidisciplinary discussion involving transplant surgeons, pediatric gastroenterologists, specialized nurses, dieticians, social workers, and psychologists is mandatory before any decision for a specific child. Assessment and decision are based on the occurrence of the complications listed in a position paper of the American Society of Transplantation.[14]

REFERENCES

1. Nordgaard I, Hansen BS, Mortensen PB. Importance of colonic support for energy absorption as small-bowel failure proceeds. Am J Clin Nutr 1996;64:222–31.
2. Jeppesen PB, Mortensen PB. Intestinal failure defined by measurements of intestinal energy and wet weight absorption. Gut 2000;46:701–6.
3. Rhoads JM, Plunkett E, Galanko J, et al. Serum citrulline levels correlate with enteral tolerance and bowel length in infants with short bowel syndrome. J Pediatr 2005;146:542–7.
4. Crenn P, Coudray-Lucas C, Thuillier F, et al. Postabsorptive plasma citrulline concentration is a marker of absorptive enterocyte mass and intestinal failure in humans. Gastroenterology 2000;119:1496–505.
5. Crenn P, Vahedi K, Lavergne-Slove A, et al. Plasma citrulline: A marker of enterocyte mass in villous atrophy-associated small bowel disease. Gastroenterology 2003;124:1210–9.
6. Jianfeng G, Weiming Z, Ning L, et al. Serum citrulline is a simple quantitative marker for small intestinal enterocytes mass and absorption function in short bowel patients. J Surg Res 2005;127:177–82.
7. Pappas PA, G Tzakis A, Gaynor JJ, et al. An analysis of the association between serum citrulline and acute rejection among 26 recipients of intestinal transplant. Am J Transplant 2004;4:1124–32.
8. Van Gossum A, Vahedi K, Abdel M, et al. Clinical, social and rehabilitation status of long-term home parenteral nutrition patients: Results of a European multicentre survey. Clin Nutr 2001;20:205–10.
9. Holden C. Review of home paediatric parenteral nutrition on the UK. Br J Nurs 2001;10:782–8.
10. Moreno JM, Planas M, Lecha M, et al. [The year 2002 national register on home-based parenteral nutrition]. Nutr Hosp 2005;20:249–53.
11. Gottrand F, Staszewski P, Colomb V, et al. Satisfaction in different life domains in children receiving home parenteral nutrition and their families. J Pediatr 2005;146:793–7.
12. Engstrom I, Bjornestam B, Finkel Y. Psychological distress associated with home parenteral nutrition in Swedish children, adolescents, and their parents: Preliminary results. J Pediatr Gastroenterol Nutr 2003;37:246–50.
13. Pironi L, Hebuterne X, Van Gossum A, et al. Candidates for intestinal transplantation: A multicenter survey in Europe. Am J Gastroenterol 2006;101:1633–43.
14. Buchman AL, Scolapio J, Fryer J. AGA technical review on short bowel syndrome and intestinal transplantation. Gastroenterology 2003;124:1111–34.
15. Doray B, Salomon R, Amiel J, et al. Mutation of the RET ligand, neurturin, supports multigenic inheritance in Hirschsprung disease. Hum Mol Genet 1998;7:1449–52.
16. Moore SW. The contribution of associated congenital anomalies in understanding Hirschsprung's disease. Pediatr Surg Int 2006;22:305–15.
17. Fortuna RS, Weber TR, Tracy TF, Jr, et al. Critical analysis of the operative treatment of Hirschsprung's disease. Arch Surg 1996;131:520–4; discussion 4–5.
18. Marty TL, Seo T, Matlak ME, et al. Gastrointestinal function after surgical correction of Hirschsprung's disease: Long-term follow-up in 135 patients. J Pediatr Surg 1995;30:655–8.
19. Saxton ML, Ein SH, Hoehner J, Kim PC. Near-total intestinal aganglionosis: Long-term follow-up of a morbid condition. J Pediatr Surg 2000;35:669–72.
20. Sharif K, Beath SV, Kelly DA, et al. New perspective for the management of near-total or total intestinal aganglionosis in infants. J Pediatr Surg 2003;38:25–8.
21. Révillon Y, Aigrain Y, Jan D, et al. Improved quality of life by combined transplantation in Hirschsprung's disease with a very long aganglionic segment. J Pediatr Surg 2003;38:422–4.
22. Faure C, Goulet O, Ategbo S, et al. Chronic intestinal pseudoobstruction syndrome: Clinical analysis, outcome, and prognosis in 105 children. French-Speaking Group of Pediatric Gastroenterology. Dig Dis Sci 1999;44:953–9.
23. Loinaz C, Mittal N, Kato T, et al. Multivisceral transplantation for pediatric intestinal pseudo-obstruction: Single center's experience of 16 cases. Transplant Proc 2004;36:312–3.
24. Masetti M, Rodriguez MM, Thompson JF, et al. Multivisceral transplantation for megacystis microcolon intestinal hypoperistalsis syndrome. Transplantation 1999;68:228–32.
25. Goulet O, Sauvat F, Jan D. Surgery for pediatric patients with chronic intestinal pseudo-obstruction syndrome. J Pediatr Gastroenterol Nutr 2005;41:S66–8.
26. Goulet O, Jobert-Giraud A, Michel JL, et al. Chronic intestinal pseudo-obstruction syndrome in pediatric patients. Eur J Pediatr Surg 1999;9:83–9.
27. Goulet O, Ruemmele F. Causes and management of intestinal failure in children. Gastroenterology 2006;130:S16–28.
28. Heneyke S, Smith VV, Spitz L, Milla PJ. Chronic intestinal pseudo-obstruction: Treatment and long term follow up of 44 patients. Arch Dis Child 1999;81:21–7.
29. Iyer K, Kaufman S, Sudan D, et al. Long-term results of intestinal transplantation for pseudo-obstruction in children. J Pediatr Surg 2001;36:174–7.
30. Vantini I, Benini L, Bonfante F, et al. Survival rate and prognostic factors in patients with intestinal failure. Dig Liver Dis 2004;36:46–55.
31. Phillips AD, Schmitz J. Familial microvillous atrophy: A clinicopathological survey of 23 cases. J Pediatr Gastroenterol Nutr 1992;14:380–96.
32. Goulet O, Kedinger M, Brousse N, et al. Intractable diarrhea of infancy with epithelial and basement membrane abnormalities. J Pediatr 1995;127:212–9.
33. Patey N, Scoazec JY, Cuenod-Jabri B, et al. Distribution of cell adhesion molecules in infants with intestinal epithelial dysplasia (tufting enteropathy). Gastroenterology 1997;113:833–43.
34. Ruemmele FM, Jan D, Lacaille F, et al. New perspectives for children with microvillous inclusion disease: Early small bowel transplantation. Transplantation 2004;77:1024–8.
35. Paramesh AS, Fishbein T, Tschernia A, et al. Isolated small bowel transplantation for tufting enteropathy. J Pediatr Gastroenterol Nutr 2003;36:138–40.
36. Kobayashi I, Shiari R, Yamada M, et al. Novel mutations of FOXP3 in two Japanese patients with immune dysregulation, polyendocrinopathy, enteropathy, X linked syndrome (IPEX). J Med Genet 2001;38:874–6.
37. Baud O, Goulet O, Canioni D, et al. Treatment of the immune dysregulation, polyendocrinopathy, enteropathy, X-linked syndrome (IPEX) by allogeneic bone marrow transplantation. N Engl J Med 2001;344:1758–62.
38. Torfs CP, Velie EM, Oechsli FW, et al. A population-based study of gastroschisis: Demographic, pregnancy, and lifestyle risk factors. Teratology 1994;50:44–53.
39. Dolk H. EUROCAT: 25 years of European surveillance of congenital anomalies. Arch Dis Child Fetal Neonatal Ed 2005;90:F355–8.
40. Rankin J, Pattenden S, Abramsky L, et al. Prevalence of congenital anomalies in five British regions, 1991–99. Arch Dis Child Fetal Neonatal Ed 2005;90:F374–9.
41. de Vries PA. The pathogenesis of gastroschisis and omphalocele. J Pediatr Surg 1980;15:245–51.
42. Torfs CP, Christianson RE, Iovannisci DM, et al. Selected gene polymorphisms and their interaction with maternal smoking, as risk factors for gastroschisis. Birth Defects Res A Clin Mol Teratol 2006;76:723–30.
43. Segel SY, Marder SJ, Parry S, Macones GA. Fetal abdominal wall defects and mode of delivery: A systematic review. Obstet Gynecol 2001;98:867–73.
44. Davies MW, Kimble RM, Woodgate PG. Ward reduction without general anaesthesia versus reduction and repair under general anaesthesia for gastroschisis in newborn infants. Cochrane Database Syst Rev 2002;(3):CD003671.
45. Snyder CL. Outcome analysis for gastroschisis. J Pediatr Surg 1999;34:1253–6.
46. Snyder CL, Miller KA, Sharp RJ, et al. Management of intestinal atresia in patients with gastroschisis. J Pediatr Surg 2001;36:1542–5.
47. Malek MM, Burd RS. Surgical treatment of malrotation after infancy: A population-based study. J Pediatr Surg 2005;40:285–9.
48. Kluth D, Kaestner M, Tibboel D, Lambrecht W. Rotation of the gut: Fact or fantasy? J Pediatr Surg 1995;30:448–53.
49. Usmani SS, Kenigsberg K. Intrauterine volvulus without malrotation. J Pediatr Surg 1991;26:1409–10.
50. Ford EG, Senac MO, Jr, Srikanth MS, Weitzman JJ. Malrotation of the intestine in children. Ann Surg 1992;215:172–8.
51. Martin LW, Zerella JT. Jejunoileal atresia: A proposed classification. J Pediatr Surg 1976;11:399–403.
52. Grosfeld JL, Ballantine TV, Shoemaker R. Operative mangement of intestinal atresia and stenosis based on pathologic findings. J Pediatr Surg 1979;14:368–75.
53. Moreno LA, Gottrand F, Turck D, et al. Severe combined immunodeficiency syndrome associated with autosomal recessive familial multiple gastrointestinal atresias: Study of a family. Am J Med Genet 1990;37:143–6.
54. Moore SW, de Jongh G, Bouic P, et al. Immune deficiency in familial duodenal atresia. J Pediatr Surg 1996;31:1733–5.
55. Gilroy RK, Coccia PF, Talmadge JE, et al. Donor immune reconstitution after liver-small bowel transplantation for multiple intestinal atresia with immunodeficiency. Blood 2004;103:1171–4.
56. Pierro A. The surgical management of necrotising enterocolitis. Early Hum Dev 2005;81:79–85.
57. Vaughan WG, Grosfeld JL, West K, et al. Avoidance of stomas and delayed anastomosis for bowel necrosis: The 'clip and drop-back' technique. J Pediatr Surg 1996;31:542–5.
58. Ou-Yang MC, Yang SN, Hsu YM, et al. Concomitant existence of total bowel aganglionosis and congenital central hypoventilation syndrome in a neonate with *PHOX2B* gene mutation. J Pediatr Surg 2007;42:e9–11.
59. Ziegler MM, Royal RE, Brandt J, et al. Extended myectomy-myotomy. A therapeutic alternative for total intestinal aganglionosis. Ann Surg 1993;218:504–9; discussion 9–11.
60. Shimotake T, Go S, Tomiyama H, et al. Proximal jejunostomy with or without myectomy-myotomy modification in five infants with total intestinal aganglionosis: An experience with surgical treatments in a single institution. J Pediatr Surg 2002;37:835–9.
61. Grant D, Abu-Elmagd K, Reyes J, et al. 2003 report of the intestine transplant registry: A new era has dawned. Ann Surg 2005;241:607–13.
62. Kajiwara T, Tamura K, Suzuki T. Follow-up study of gastrin response after resection of the jejunum and the ileum. Ann Surg 1977;186:694–9.
63. Potter GD. Bile acid diarrhea. Dig Dis 1998;16:118–24.
64. Weihrauch D, Kanchanapoo J, Ao M, et al. Weanling, but not adult, rabbit colon absorbs bile acids: Flux is linked to expression of putative bile acid transporters. Am J Physiol Gastrointest Liver Physiol 2006;290:G439–50.
65. Quiros-Tejeira RE, Ament ME, Reyen L, et al. Long-term parenteral nutritional support and intestinal adaptation in children with short bowel syndrome: A 25-year experience. J Pediatr 2004;145:157–63.
66. Musch MW, Bookstein C, Rocha F, et al. Region-specific adaptation of apical Na/H exchangers after extensive proximal small bowel resection. Am J Physiol Gastrointest Liver Physiol 2002;283:G975–85.
67. Wilmore DW. Growth factors and nutrients in the short bowel syndrome. J Parenter Enter Nutr 1999;23:117–20.
68. Holst JJ. Glucagon-like peptide-1: From extract to agent. The Claude Bernard Lecture, 2005. Diabetologia 2006;49:253–60.
69. Gleeson MH, Bloom SR, Polak JM, et al. Endocrine tumour in kidney affecting small bowel structure, motility, and absorptive function. Gut 1971;12:773–82.
70. Brubaker PL, Crivici A, Izzo A, et al. Circulating and tissue forms of the intestinal growth factor, glucagon-like peptide-2. Endocrinology 1997;138:4837–43.
71. Tsai CH, Hill M, Drucker DJ. Biological determinants of intestinotrophic properties of GLP-2 in vivo. Am J Physiol 1997;272:G662–8.
72. Tsai CH, Hill M, Asa SL, et al. Intestinal growth-promoting properties of glucagon-like peptide-2 in mice. Am J Physiol 1997;273:E77–84.
73. Kato Y, Yu D, Schwartz MZ. Glucagonlike peptide-2 enhances small intestinal absorptive function and mucosal mass in vivo. J Pediatr Surg 1999;34:18–20.
74. Cheeseman CI. Upregulation of SGLT-1 transport activity in rat jejunum induced by GLP-2 infusion in vivo. Am J Physiol 1997;273:R1965–71.
75. Cheeseman CI, Tsang R. The effect of GIP and glucagon-like peptides on intestinal basolateral membrane hexose transport. Am J Physiol 1996;271:G477–82.
76. Jeppesen PB. Glucagon-like peptide-2: Update of the recent clinical trials. Gastroenterology 2006;130:S127–31.
77. Sigalet DL, Martin G, Meddings J, et al. GLP-2 levels in infants with intestinal dysfunction. Pediatr Res 2004;56:371–6.
78. Jeppesen PB, Sanguinetti EL, Buchman A, et al. Teduglutide (ALX-0600), a dipeptidyl peptidase IV resistant glucagon-like peptide 2 analogue, improves intestinal function in short bowel syndrome patients. Gut 2005;54:1224–31.
79. Scolapio JS. Effect of growth hormone, glutamine, and diet on body composition in short bowel syndrome: A randomized, controlled study. J Parenter Enteral Nutr 1999;23:309–12; discussion 12–3.
80. Szkudlarek J, Jeppesen PB, Mortensen PB. Effect of high dose growth hormone with glutamine and no change in diet on intestinal absorption in short bowel patients: A randomised, double blind, crossover, placebo controlled study. Gut 2000;47:199–205.

81. Seguy D, Vahedi K, Kapel N, et al. Low-dose growth hormone in adult home parenteral nutrition-dependent short bowel syndrome patients: A positive study. Gastroenterology 2003;124:293–302.

82. Dowling RH, Hosomi M, Stace NH, et al. Hormones and polyamines in intestinal and pancreatic adaptation. Scand J Gastroenterol Suppl 1985;112:84–95.

83. Sagor GR, Ghatei MA, O'Shaughnessy DJ, et al. Influence of somatostatin and bombesin on plasma enteroglucagon and cell proliferation after intestinal resection in the rat. Gut 1985;26:89–94.

84. Burrin DG, Stoll B. Key nutrients and growth factors for the neonatal gastrointestinal tract. Clin Perinatol 2002;29:65–96.

85. Sigalet DL, Martin GR, Butzner JD, et al. A pilot study of the use of epidermal growth factor in pediatric short bowel syndrome. J Pediatr Surg 2005;40:763–8.

86. Sukhotnik I, Shehadeh N, Shamir R, et al. Oral insulin enhances intestinal regrowth following massive small bowel resection in rat. Dig Dis Sci 2005;50:2379–85.

87. Sukhotnik I, Mogilner J, Shamir R, et al. Effect of subcutaneous insulin on intestinal adaptation in a rat model of short bowel syndrome. Pediatr Surg Int 2005;21:132–7.

88. Shehadeh N, Sukhotnik I, Shamir R. Gastrointestinal tract as a target organ for orally administered insulin. J Pediatr Gastroenterol Nutr 2006;43:276–81.

89. Jeppesen PB, Mortensen PB. Enhancing bowel adaptation in short bowel syndrome. Curr Gastroenterol Rep 2002;4:338–47.

90. Wilmore DW. Growth factors and nutrients in the short bowel syndrome. JPEN J Parenter Enteral Nutr 1999;23:S117–20.

91. Sham J, Martin G, Meddings JB, Sigalet DL. Epidermal growth factor improves nutritional outcome in a rat model of short bowel syndrome. J Pediatr Surg 2002;37:765–9.

92. Nordgaard I, Hansen BS, Mortensen PB. Colon as a digestive organ in patients with short bowel. Lancet 1994;343:373–6.

93. Koruda MJ, Rolandelli RH, Settle RG, et al. Effect of parenteral nutrition supplemented with short-chain fatty acids on adaptation to massive small bowel resection. Gastroenterology 1988;95:715–20.

94. Weser E, Babbitt J, Hoban M, Vandeventer A. Intestinal adaptation. Different growth responses to disaccharides compared with monosaccharides in rat small bowel. Gastroenterology 1986;91:1521–7.

95. Kollman KA, Lien EL, Vanderhoof JA. Dietary lipids influence intestinal adaptation after massive bowel resection. J Pediatr Gastroenterol Nutr 1999;28:41–5.

96. Sukhotnik I, Gork AS, Chen M, et al. Effect of a high fat diet on lipid absorption and fatty acid transport in a rat model of short bowel syndrome. Pediatr Surg Int 2003;19:385–90.

97. Vanderhoof JA, Grandjean CJ, Kaufman SS, et al. Effect of high percentage medium-chain triglyceride diet on mucosal adaptation following massive bowel resection in rats. JPEN J Parenter Enteral Nutr 1984;8:685–9.

98. Nagy ES, Paris MC, Taylor RG, et al. Colostrum protein concentrate enhances intestinal adaptation after massive small bowel resection in juvenile pigs. J Pediatr Gastroenterol Nutr 2004;39:487–92.

99. Stoll B, Price PT, Reeds PJ, et al. Feeding an elemental diet vs a milk-based formula does not decrease intestinal mucosal growth in infant pigs. JPEN J Parenter Enteral Nutr 2006;30:32–9.

100. Evans ME, Tian J, Gu LH, et al. Dietary supplementation with orotate and uracil increases adaptive growth of jejunal mucosa after massive small bowel resection in rats. JPEN J Parenter Enteral Nutr 2005;29:315–20; discussion 20–1.

101. Ksiazyk J, Piena M, Kierkus J, Lyszkowska M. Hydrolyzed versus nonhydrolyzed protein diet in short bowel syndrome in children. J Pediatr Gastroenterol Nutr 2002;35:615–8.

102. Bines J, Francis D, Hill D. Reducing parenteral requirement in children with short bowel syndrome: Impact of an amino acid-based complete infant formula. J Pediatr Gastroenterol Nutr 1998;26:123–8.

103. Andorsky DJ, Lund DP, Lillehei CW, et al. Nutritional and other postoperative management of neonates with short bowel syndrome correlates with clinical outcomes. J Pediatr 2001;139:27–33.

104. Neu J, DeMarco V, Li N. Glutamine: Clinical applications and mechanisms of action. Curr Opin Clin Nutr Metab Care 2002;5:69–75.

105. Hankard R, Goulet O, Ricour C, et al. Glutamine metabolism in children with short-bowel syndrome: A stable isotope study. Pediatr Res 1994;36:202–6.

106. Duggan C, Stark AR, Auestad N, et al. Glutamine supplementation in infants with gastrointestinal disease: A randomized, placebo-controlled pilot trial. Nutrition 2004;20:752–6.

107. Alpers DH. Glutamine: Do the data support the cause for glutamine supplementation in humans? Gastroenterology 2006;130:S106–16.

108. Jeppesen PB, Mortensen PB. Colonic digestion and absorption of energy from carbohydrates and medium-chain fat in small bowel failure. JPEN J Parenter Enteral Nutr 1999;23:S101–5.

109. Koruda MJ, Rolandelli RH, Settle RG, et al. Vars award. The effect of a pectin-supplemented elemental diet on intestinal adaptation to massive small bowel resection. JPEN J Parenter Enteral Nutr 1986;10:343–50.

110. Royall D, Wolever TM, Jeejeebhoy KN. Evidence for colonic conservation of malabsorbed carbohydrate in short bowel syndrome. Am J Gastroenterol 1992;87:751–6.

111. Tappenden KA, Thomson AB, Wild GE, McBurney MI. Short-chain fatty acids increase proglucagon and ornithine decarboxylase messenger RNAs after intestinal resection in rats. JPEN J Parenter Enteral Nutr 1996;20:357–62.

112. Tappenden KA, Thomson AB, Wild GE, McBurney MI. Short-chain fatty acid-supplemented total parenteral nutrition enhances functional adaptation to intestinal resection in rats. Gastroenterology 1997;112:792–802.

113. Welters CF, Deutz NE, Dejong CH, et al. Supplementation of enteral nutrition with butyrate leads to increased portal efflux of amino acids in growing pigs with short bowel syndrome. J Pediatr Surg 1996;31:526–9.

114. Bartholome AL, Albin DM, Baker DH, et al. Supplementation of total parenteral nutrition with butyrate acutely increases structural aspects of intestinal adaptation after an 80% jejunoileal resection in neonatal piglets. JPEN J Parenter Enteral Nutr 2004;28:210–22; discussion 22–3.

115. Pratt VC, Tappenden KA, McBurney MI, Field CJ. Short-chain fatty acid-supplemented total parenteral nutrition improves nonspecific immunity after intestinal resection in rats. JPEN J Parenter Enteral Nutr 1996;20:264–71.

116. Bjornvad CR, Schmidt M, Petersen YM, et al. Preterm birth makes the immature intestine sensitive to feeding-induced intestinal atrophy. Am J Physiol Regul Integr Comp Physiol 2005;289:R1212–22.

117. Oste M, Van Ginneken CJ, Van Haver ER, et al. The intestinal trophic response to enteral food is reduced in parenterally fed preterm pigs and is associated with more nitrergic neurons. J Nutr 2005;135:2657–63.

118. Sangild PT, Petersen YM, Schmidt M, et al. Preterm birth affects the intestinal response to parenteral and enteral nutrition in newborn pigs. J Nutr 2002;132:2673–81.

119. Buchman AL, Moukarzel AA, Bhuta S, et al. Parenteral nutrition is associated with intestinal morphologic and functional changes in humans. JPEN J Parenter Enteral Nutr 1995;19:453–60.

120. Groos S, Reale E, Hunefeld G, Luciano L. Changes in epithelial cell turnover and extracellular matrix in human small intestine after TPN. J Surg Res 2003;109:74–85.

121. Sedman PC, MacFie J, Palmer MD, et al. Preoperative total parenteral nutrition is not associated with mucosal atrophy or bacterial translocation in humans. Br J Surg 1995;82:1663–7.

122. Buchman AL, Mestecky J, Moukarzel A, Ament ME. Intestinal immune function is unaffected by parenteral nutrition in man. J Am Coll Nutr 1995;14:656–61.

123. Guedon C, Schmitz J, Lerebours E, et al. Decreased brush border hydrolase activities without gross morphologic changes in human intestinal mucosa after prolonged total parenteral nutrition of adults. Gastroenterology 1986;90:373–8.

124. Hyman PE, Everett SL, Harada T. Gastric acid hypersecretion in short bowel syndrome in infants: Association with extent of resection and enteral feeding. J Pediatr Gastroenterol Nutr 1986;5:191–7.

125. DiBaise JK, Young RJ, Vanderhoof JA. Intestinal rehabilitation and the short bowel syndrome: Part 2. Am J Gastroenterol 2004;99:1823–32.

126. Xanthou M. Immune protection of human milk. Biol Neonate 1998;74:121–33.

127. Wales PW, de Silva N, Kim J, et al. Neonatal short bowel syndrome: population-based estimates of incidence and mortality rates. J Pediatr Surg 2004;39:690–95.

128. Gracey M. The contaminated small bowel syndrome: Pathogenesis, diagnosis, and treatment. Am J Clin Nutr 1979;32:234–43.

129. Gurevitch J, Sela B, Jonas A, et al. D-lactic acidosis: A treatable encephalopathy in pediatric patients. Acta Paediatr 1993;82:119–21.

130. Hudson M, Pocknee R, Mowat NA. D-lactic acidosis in short bowel syndrome—an examination of possible mechanisms. Q J Med 1990;74:157–63.

131. Mayne AJ, Handy DJ, Preece MA, et al. Dietary management of D-lactic acidosis in short bowel syndrome. Arch Dis Child 1990;65:229–31.

132. Eizaguirre I, Urkia NG, Asensio AB, et al. Probiotic supplementation reduces the risk of bacterial translocation in experimental short bowel syndrome. J Pediatr Surg 2002;37:699–702.

133. Seehofer D, Rayes N, Schiller R, et al. Probiotics partly reverse increased bacterial translocation after simultaneous liver resection and colonic anastomosis in rats. J Surg Res 2004;117:262–71.

134. Vanderhoof JA, Young RJ, Thompson JS. New and emerging therapies for short bowel syndrome in children. Paediatr Drugs 2003;5:525–31.

135. Goulet O, Baglin-Gobet S, Talbotec C, et al. Outcome and long-term growth after extensive small bowel resection in the neonatal period: A survey of 87 children. Eur J Pediatr Surg 2005;15:95–101.

136. Goulet OJ, Revillon Y, Jan D, et al. Neonatal short bowel syndrome. J Pediatr 1991;119:18–23.

137. Sondheimer JM, Cadnapaphornchai M, Sontag M, Zerbe GO. Predicting the duration of dependence on parenteral nutrition after neonatal intestinal resection. J Pediatr 1998;132:80–4.

138. Festen S, Brevoord JC, Goldhoorn GA, et al. Excellent long-term outcome for survivors of apple peel atresia. J Pediatr Surg 2002;37:61–5.

139. Gonzalez HF, Perez NB, Malpeli A, et al. Nutrition and immunological status in long-term follow up of children with short bowel syndrome. JPEN J Parenter Enteral Nutr 2005;29:186–91.

140. Bianchi A. Experience with longitudinal intestinal lengthening and tailoring. Eur J Pediatr Surg 1999;9:256–9.

141. Bianchi A. From the cradle to enteral autonomy: The role of autologous gastrointestinal reconstruction. Gastroenterology 2006;130:S138–46.

142. Thompson JS. Surgical rehabilitation of intestine in short bowel syndrome. Surgery 2004;135:465–70.

143. Kim HB, Fauza D, Garza J, et al. Serial transverse enteroplasty (STEP): A novel bowel lengthening procedure. J Pediatr Surg 2003;38:425–9.

144. Javid PJ, Kim HB, Duggan CP, Jaksic T. Serial transverse enteroplasty is associated with successful short-term outcomes in infants with short bowel syndrome. J Pediatr Surg 2005;40:1019–23; discussion 23–4.

145. Modi BP, Javid PJ, Jaksic T, et al. First report of the international serial transverse enteroplasty data registry: Indications, efficacy, and complications. J Am Coll Surg 2007;204:365–71.

146. Lawrence JP, Dunn SP, Billmire DF, et al. Isolated liver transplantation for liver failure in patients with short bowel syndrome. J Pediatr Surg 1994;29:751–3.

147. Gottrand F, Michaud L, Bonnevalle M, et al. Favorable nutritional outcome after isolated liver transplantation for liver failure in a child with short bowel syndrome. Transplantation 1999;67:632–4.

148. Horslen SP, Sudan DL, Iyer KR, et al. Isolated liver transplantation in infants with end-stage liver disease associated with short bowel syndrome. Ann Surg 2002;235:435–9.

149. Botha JF, Grant WJ, Torres C, et al. Isolated liver transplantation in infants with end-stage liver disease due to short bowel syndrome. Liver Transpl 2006;12:1062–6.

150. Goulet O, Sauvat F. Short bowel syndrome and intestinal transplantation in children. Curr Opin Clin Nutr Metab Care 2006;9:304–13.

151. Koffeman GI, van Gemert WG, George EK, Veenendaal RA. Classification, epidemiology and aetiology. Best Pract Res Clin Gastroenterol 2003;17:879–93.

22.2. Parenteral Nutrition–Associated Liver Disease

Julie E. Bines, MD, FRACP

Prue M. Pereira-Fantini, PhD

The development of parenteral nutrition (PN) in the late 1960s resulted in a marked improvement in the outcome for patients with intestinal failure.[1] Although the nutritional status of patients with intestinal failure can now be supported, long-term use of PN is associated with life threatening complications including PN-associated liver disease (PNALD). Liver dysfunction is reported to occur in 7.4 to 84% of patients receiving PN (Table 1).[2–5] In most patients, this presents as a transient abnormality in serum liver enzyme levels that return to normal with cessation of PN. Cholestasis is the most common manifestation in infants and children, whereas steatosis is more common in adults.[5,6] Children with short bowel syndrome requiring long-term PN are at increased risk for the development of complicated PNALD, and liver failure is reported in 3 to 19% of these patients.[7–9] Significant improvements in administration and solution composition over the past 10 to 15 years have led to a decrease in the incidence of PNALD from 31 to 25% in neonates receiving PN for more than 2 weeks although the mortality related to PNALD has not significantly altered.[6]

PNALD has a multifactorial etiology that reflects the underlying clinical indication for administration of PN (Table 2).[7,10,11] In particular, the role of sepsis in the early development of PNALD has been the focus of a number of studies as PNALD is associated with intraluminal bacteria overgrowth and recurrent episodes of catheter related sepsis.[7,12,13]

CLINICAL SPECTRUM OF HEPATOBILIARY DYSFUNCTION IN PATIENTS RECEIVING PN

Histopathology

Few studies have described the evolution of PNALD; however, case reports and case series

Table 1 Spectrum of Hepatobiliary Dysfunction in Patients Receiving Parenteral Nutrition

Abnormal liver function tests
Steatosis
Cholestasis
Cirrhosis
Liver failure
Hepatocellular carcinomas
Acalculous cholecystitis
Biliary sludge
Cholelithiasis, cholecystitis

Table 2 Factors Associated With Development of Parenteral Nutrition Associated Liver Disease

Patient factors
Low birth weight
Prematurity
Male sex
Preexisting liver disease

Disease factors
Primary disease etiology
Length of residual small intestine
Dysmotility in remaining segment of small intestinal
Residual intestinal disease (ie, Crohn's disease)
Length of time with diverting ileostomy or colostomy
Small intestinal bacterial overgrowth
Sepsis
Type of microorganism
Source of infection

Nutritional factors
Lack of enteral feeding
Undigested nutrients and bacterial overgrowth
Proportion of enteral calories
Formula composition
Duration of parenteral nutrition administration
Overfeeding
Glucose excess
Specific amino acid excess/deficiency
Lipid excess
Accumulation of phytosterols
Specific micronutrient excess/deficiency

do provide evidence for a histological progression of liver damage influenced by the duration of PN therapy (Figure 1). Within the first 2 weeks following initiation of PN therapy, steatosis within the liver may be observed. This is characterized by diffuse macrovesicular and microvesicular fat accumulation. Cholestasis follows characterized by Kupffer cell hyperplasia, bile duct plugging, and extramedullary hematopoiesis within the centrilobular region (Figure 2B and C).[14] Mild to moderate periportal inflammation is observed. This is usually a lymphocytic infiltrate, although neutrophils and eosinophils may also be present. With disease progression, hepatocytes become ballooned with lipofuscin granules identified in the periportal region. Kupffer cells are hyperplastic and may also have lipofuscin granules. The lobular architecture becomes disordered with periportal fibrosis observed in most patients (Figure 2D). Bile duct proliferation and, less commonly, bridging fibrosis may occur (Figure 2A). In infants, extramedullary hematopoiesis is common. If PN

administration continues, steatosis and extramedullary hematopoiesis tend to improve, but cholestasis, fibrosis, and progression to cirrhosis can occur.[15] If PN therapy is ceased before the development of cirrhosis, many of the histological features of liver disease improve.[15] The estimated time from onset of long-term PN to the development of moderate fibrosis (<50% portal spaces involved) in children with short bowel syndrome is reported to be about 40 months.[15] Following the development of fibrosis, there is often a more rapid progression to cirrhosis (mean duration 14 months). Hepatocellular carcinoma was reported in a 6-month-old infant dependent on long-term PN.[16]

Abnormal Liver Function Tests

In most patients, PNALD presents as a transient elevation in serum hepatic aminotransferase concentration[17] with an early increase in the serum bilirubin concentration of preterm infants[14] during the first 1 to 3 weeks of PN. These return to normal with cessation of PN. High concentrations of serum direct bilirubin correlate with serum alkaline phosphatase and transaminase concentrations and the number of deaths after 28 days of PN treatment is significantly increased in infants with higher direct bilirubin and transaminase concentrations.[18]

Hepatic Steatosis

Hepatic steatosis is the most common manifestation of PNALD in adults and is characterized by infiltration of lipid or glycogen within hepa-

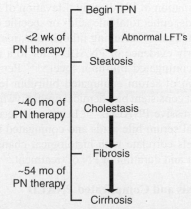

Figure 1 Time course of parenteral nutrition–associated liver disease.

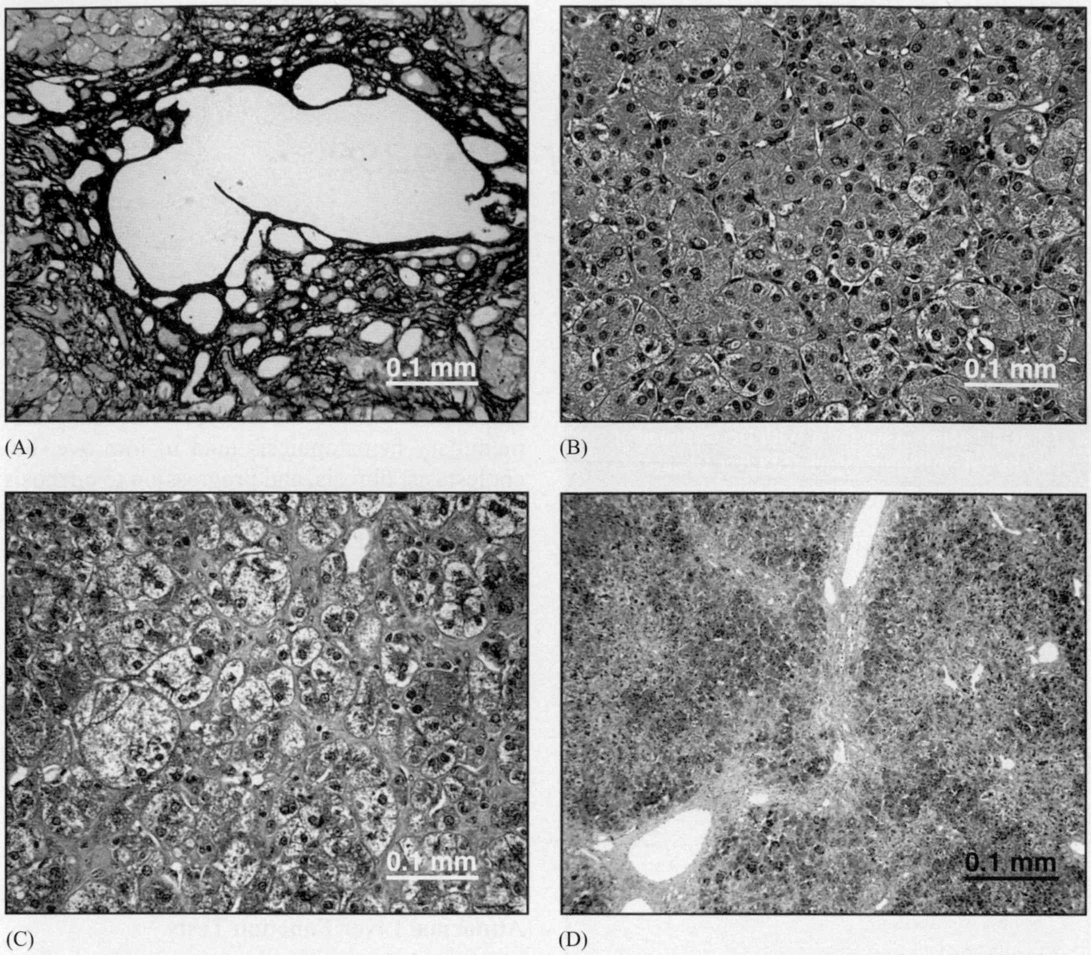

Figure 2 Histological aspects of parenteral nutrition associated liver disease (PNALD) may include (A) bile duct proliferation, (B) swollen liver cells/cholestasis, (C) hepatocyte ballooning, and (D) periportal and bridging fibrosis.

tocytes.[19,20] It often occurs in association with excessive parenteral carbohydrate intake and may resolve when parenteral carbohydrate intake is reduced.[20] Hepatic steatosis clinically presents as hepatomegaly associated with a mild to moderate increase in serum aminotransferase levels.[5]

Chronic Cholestasis

Chronic cholestasis is the primary manifestation of PNALD in infants and children and in adults with intestinal failure[5,7,21] and is the precursor of complicated PNALD and liver failure.[21–23] Cholestasis is usually defined as a serum conjugated bilirubin level of >1.5 mg/dL or 40% total bilirubin concentration. In infants, serum bilirubin levels may begin to rise as early as 1 to 2 weeks after initiation of PN therapy. Elevation of serum bile acids, either total bile acids or specific cholic acid conjugates, including lithocholate, may provide early evidence of PNALD prior to a rise in serum conjugated bilirubin level.[24,25] Persistent elevation of serum conjugated bilirubin level is the most consistent biochemical predictive marker of progressive PNALD.[11,26] In animals receiving PN, total serum bile acids and conjugated bilirubin levels correlate with histological changes in the liver and duration of PN of treatment.[27]

Cirrhosis and Complicated PNALD

With progression of disease, the serum alkaline phosphatase gradually increases. However, this may be difficult to interpret in infants and children because the bone isoenzyme may also be elevated due to bone disease. Serum alkaline phosphatase may also be decreased by zinc deficiency. Levels of serum transaminases and alkaline phosphatase do not correlate with the severity of liver histology in PNALD.[27] Serum γ-glutamyl transpeptidase or 5'-nucleotidase may also be elevated but provide no significant diagnostic benefit over serum bilirubin concentration alone in infants.[11,26] Reduced serum albumin levels are associated with increased mortality in patients with PNALD.[5] However, in patients with excessive protein loss or severe protein–energy malnutrition, hypoalbuminemia and hypoproteinemia may reflect nutritional deficit and not liver dysfunction. Similarly, nutritional vitamin K deficiency may also result in a prolonged prothrombin time.

Biliary Tract Abnormalities

Biliary sludge and/or cholelithiasis occur in 12 to 40% of children receiving long-term PN.[28,29] These may occur as a result of gallbladder hypomotility, changes in the composition of bile, or altered enterohepatic circulation of bile acids. The risk of cholelithiasis is increased in children with ileal resection, ileal disease, or hemolytic anemia or in those receiving furosemide therapy. Biliary stones usually consist of both cholesterol and pigment. Acalculous cholecystitis is associated with high morbidity and mortality.[30]

RISK FACTORS FOR THE DEVELOPMENT OF PNALD

Patient Related Factors

Birth Weight/Gestational Age. Low birth weight is a key predisposing factor for the development of PNALD.[10,18,31] PNALD was reported in 50% of infants with a birth weight <1,000 g compared with 7% of infants weighing >1,500 g at birth (Figure 3). Almost two-thirds of all infants weighing less than 2,000 g at birth develop cholestasis after 2 weeks of PN therapy.[31] Gestational age has also been identified as an independent factor for the development of PNALD in some but not all studies.[10,31–33] The increased incidence of PNALD observed in premature infants is thought to reflect the immaturity of hepatic function and the enterohepatic circulation of bile acids.[31,34–36] Normal enterohepatic circulation requires that bile acids are delivered to the intestinal lumen, reabsorbed, and then returned to the hepatocyte for recirculation. However, neonates have reduced hepatic uptake, bile acid synthesis, and the volume of the total bile salt pool is also reduced.[34–37] In addition, premature infants exhibited reduced intraluminal concentration and reabsorption of bile acids, and may have reduced hepatic sulfation, all of which may place them at increased risk of hepatic injury due to toxic bile acids.[38,39]

Gender. An association between male sex and the development of PNALD was recently reported.[12] The investigators postulate that a genetic and/or hormonal effect on immune function predisposes males to infection and PNALD.

Preexisting Illness. Preexisting liver disease or a PN-independent risk factor for liver disease is associated with an increased incidence of PNALD.[21]

Disease Related Factors

Gastrointestinal Disease. Massive small bowel resection is an important risk factor for the development of PNALD in children and adults.[7,21] PN-associated cholestasis is reported in 30 to 60% of children with short bowel syndrome.[8,9] Residual small intestinal length was identified as the only independent predictor of peak serum bilirubin level in infants and children with PN-associated

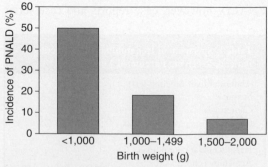

Figure 3 Relationship between the incidence of parenteral nutrition–associated liver disease (PNALD) and low birth weight. (Adapted from reference 31.)

cholestasis.[40] Seventy percent of infants with <50 cm of residual small intestine and all adults with entire small intestinal resection developed PN-associated cholestasis.[21,41,42]

A link between gastroschisis and PNALD has been reported.[7] Infants with gastroschisis frequently develop intestinal obstruction in utero and, following surgery, there is a high rate of dilatation and dysmotility of the proximal intestine. A study of 9,547 neonatal intensive care unit patients suggested gastroschisis predisposed infants to a higher risk of developing PNALD.[18]

Dysmotility following bowel resection results in stasis of luminal contents and the establishment of large numbers of strict anaerobes and facultative organisms that are normally confined to the lower small bowel and colon. Providing enteral nutrients in excess of absorptive capacity of the remaining gut further promotes bacterial overgrowth.[11] These bacteria produce lipopolysaccharide endotoxin and peptidoglycan-polysaccharide complexes that are thought to egress from gut to liver via the postulated sequence of mucosal injury, increased mucosal permeability, and lymphatic and/or mesenteric venous translocation.[11] Once in the liver, gut-derived bacterial toxins may exert deleterious effects.[11] Patients with short bowel syndrome may be particularly susceptible to translocation because of the loss of gut associated lymphoid tissue that normally acts as a microbial barrier in the intact gastrointestinal tract.[43]

The approach to surgical management of short bowel syndrome in the neonatal period may influence the development of progression of PNALD. Although emphasis is placed on retaining the maximal length of intestine, there is a risk of enhancing exposure of the liver to intestinally derived endotoxin from retained ischemic bowel.[11] Absence of disease in the remaining small intestine is associated with improved survival in patients receiving home PN for intestinal failure.[21] The number of operations and the length of time with a diverting ileostomy or colostomy have been identified as risk factors for the development of PNALD.[23,40] Conversely, the absence of the ileocecal valve does not appear to predispose patients to PNALD.[40]

Sepsis. Recurrent sepsis is an important risk factor for the development of PNALD, and is associated with cholestasis in infants receiving PN and in infants who have never received PN.[6,13,14,23,31,44,45] PNALD is more common in neonates who have recurrent episodes of sepsis irrespective of whether this is related to central line infections or bacterial translocation from bacterial overgrowth.[13,44,46–48] In a review of eight fatal cases of progressive liver failure in surgical neonates, the development of hepatic failure was closely related to septic episodes and/or peritonitis.[49]

Cholestasis occurred in 26% of 152 neonates who developed an infection while receiving short-term PN.[13] In contrast, cholestasis was not observed in any patient who did not develop an infection.[13] A close association between invasive bacterial or fungal infection and the onset of jaundice in neonates with short bowel syndrome has been observed.[7] Infection occurred before the onset of jaundice in 90% of infants and occurred earlier in cholestatic patients compared with noncholestatic patients (Figure 4).[7] Cholestatic patients had more episodes of infection in the first 6 months of life, although the total number of episodes was the same in both groups. Importantly, once established, cholestasis did not resolve with antibiotic therapy and continued to rise, either progressing to hepatic failure or gradually resolving.[5] These data suggest that early exposure to infection is important in the development of PNALD in infants with short bowel syndrome, in whom the liver is immature and susceptible to cholestatic injury and potentially further affected by PN administration.[7]

Cholestasis occurs more commonly after gram-negative bacterial infections (in particular *Escherichia. coli*).[50] In patients with a normal gastrointestinal tract, cholestasis during an episode of gram-negative sepsis is usually transient.[11] However, in patients with short bowel syndrome, episodes of gram-negative sepsis have been closely linked to the development of PN-associated cholestasis and progressive PNALD.[7,11,21] Lipopolysaccharide and peptidoglycan-polysaccharide endotoxins produced by gram-negative and gram-positive bacteria promote the release of tumor necrosis factor (TNF)-alpha and interleukin-2 from Kupffer cells in rats, resulting in hepatic inflammation and fibrosis.[51] The potential role of TNF in the pathogenesis of PNALD has been a recent focus of interest.[52,53] The administration of antibodies to TNF to PN-treated rats results in an improvement in PNALD.[53] In rats with PNALD, the administration of polymyxin B, an antibiotic aimed at gram-negative bacteria, blocks endotoxin activity and TNF production and results in an improvement in steatosis.[54]

Bacterial Overgrowth. Small bowel bacterial overgrowth is a frequent complication of functional and mechanical disorders of the small intestine. Small bowel bacterial overgrowth is identified more frequently in patients with an absence of the ileocecal valve, in the presence of a dysmotile or dilated small bowel segment, or in the presence of a tight anastomotic stricture.[55] Following small bowel resection, the residual small intestine becomes dilated and intestinal transit is slowed in an attempt to compensate for loss of bowel length. This may result in intestinal stasis and predisposes short bowel patients to the proliferation of strict anaerobic and facultative anaerobic bacteria within the small intestine. Bacterial overgrowth is often associated with anorexia, vomiting, diarrhea, cramps, abdominal distension, metabolic acidosis from D-lactic acidosis, and failure to thrive.[56] Hepatic dysfunction as a direct result of bacterial overgrowth, bacterial translocation, or endotoxemia has never been proven in humans; however small bowel bacterial overgrowth is associated with mucosal inflammation, which may in turn further exacerbate nutrient malabsorption, deconjugate bile salts, deplete the bile salt pool,[56] and alter mucosal integrity thereby increasing the risk of bacterial translocation.

Altered Bile Salt Metabolism

Bacterial overgrowth of the small intestine induces intraluminal deconjugation of bile salts and increases production of potentially toxic bile acids such as lithocholic acid.[57,58] Patients with PNALD have increased serum and bile concentration of lithocholic acid.[24,59] Lithocholic acid impairs bile flow and, in animals, is associated with hepatic injury similar to the histologic changes observed in patients with PNALD.[49,59]

Nutrition Related Factors

Lack of Enteral Nutrition. PNALD occurs more frequently in those children who are unable to tolerate any enteral feeding compared with those who receive some enteral nutrition.[11,40,44] Enteral feeding induces hormonal stimulation of bile flow, gallbladder emptying, and hepatobiliary development.[60] Serum cholecystokinin, glucagon, enteroglucagon, gastrin, motilin, gastric inhibitory polypeptide, and secretin levels differ markedly between infants who are enterally fed compared with infants receiving PN.[60] In animals with PNALD, treatment with cholecystokinin-octapeptide resulted in decreased periportal inflammation and fibrosis but no improvement

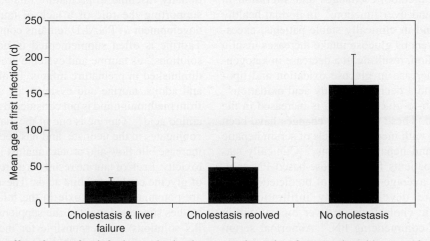

Figure 4 The effect of age at first infection on the development and severity of parenteral nutrition–associated cholestasis in neonates with intestinal resection. (Adapted from reference 7.)

in bile flow, bile acid secretion, or hepatocellular injury.[61] Human studies suggest that cholecystokinin (or cholecystokinin-octapeptide) may improve the conjugated hyperbilirubinemia associated with PNALD provided that liver failure is not established.[62,63]

Luminal nutrients aid in the maintenance of gut mucosal barrier function. In the absence of enteral nutrition, the intestine undergoes atrophy, which may increase the risk of bacterial translocation and portal sepsis.[64] In the absence of enteral feeding, intestinal motility and the enterohepatic circulation of bile acids are decreased.[65] These factors may contribute to hepatocyte stress and injury.

Composition of Enteral Nutrition. In neonates with short bowel syndrome, there is a significant relationship between the proportion of calories received enterally at 6 and 12 weeks and subsequent weaning from PN therapy.[7,40] The composition of the enteral feed may also contribute to the development of PNALD. Breast milk or amino acid formulas are associated with greater success at weaning from PN in children with short bowel syndrome.[40,41] Formula composition and excess enteral macronutrients may increase the risk of bacterial overgrowth. Mice fed a commercial liquid enteral formula had a higher rate of bacterial overgrowth and bacterial translocation compared with control animals fed chow.[66]

Duration of Parenteral Nutrition Administration. There is a direct relationship between the duration of PN administration and the prevalence of PNALD in premature infants.[31] In surgical neonates, the incidence of cholestasis is reported to increase from 35% after 2 weeks of PN therapy to 75% after 90 days and 100% after 180 days of therapy.[50] The incidence of cholestasis is higher in infants commencing PN at an earlier age and in infants who have had a delay in the introduction of enteral feeds.[23] Chronic cholestasis developed in 65% of adults receiving PN for a median of 6 months.[21] Complicated PNALD developed in 50% of adults after receiving PN for 6 years.[21]

Overfeeding with Parenteral Nutrition. Total caloric and carbohydrate overfeeding is associated with metabolic changes and alteration in bile flow and liver function.[67] In normal healthy subjects and in clinically stable patients, excessive intravenous glucose intake increases insulin concentration, resulting in a decrease in ketogenesis, an increase in glucose oxidation and lipogenesis, and a decrease in fatty acid oxidation.[68] The insulin-to-glucagon ratio is increased in the portal vein. These metabolic changes have been associated with increased levels of serum hepatic enzymes and hepatic steatosis.[68] Clinically stable adult patients fed a glucose-based PN solution to an average of 177% of predicted energy expenditure developed fatty infiltration and intrahepatic cholestasis on liver biopsy within 5 days of commencing PN.[68] Abnormal serum tests of liver function were detected by 14 days in 83% of patients, with abnormalities occurring in

proportion to the increase in carbohydrate load.[67] Repeat liver biopsy at day 21 showed bile duct proliferation, canalicular bile plugs, centrilobular cholestasis with accumulation of bile pigment within hepatocytes, and periportal inflammation.[67] Similar abnormalities have been observed in stable infants receiving glucose-based PN.[69]

Acute metabolic stress may exacerbate the impact of carbohydrate overfeeding on hepatic morphology and function. Lipolysis and fatty acid oxidation increase relative to glucose oxidation owing to the action of counter-regulatory hormones and resulting in insulin resistance.[70] In the presence of excessive glucose administration, serum glucose and insulin concentrations are elevated.[70] These factors may increase the risk for hepatic injury. Pyruvate dehydrogenase is a rate-limiting step in glucose oxidation; however, during sepsis, the activity of this enzyme may be inhibited.[71] Increased glucose load during a period of inhibition of this enzyme may further add to hepatocyte injury during stress.[71] Overfeeding during a stress-free period is reported to diminish the hepatic response to subsequent injury, in particular sepsis.[72] In addition, bacterial translocation from the gut is increased during periods of nonprotein overfeeding in animals.[73]

Nutrient Deficiencies of PN Solutions. Carnitine deficiency may occur during long-term PN as it is absent from many commercially available amino acid solutions. Carnitine is synthesized from methionine and lysine; however, in infants, this conversion may be limited owing to immature metabolic pathways.[74] Carnitine is essential for the transport of long chain fatty acids across the inner mitochondrial membrane for oxidation.[14] Carnitine deficiency is associated with hepatic steatosis[75] and plasma total and free carnitine concentrations are decreased in patients who receive long-term PN.[76,77] However, these low levels of carnitine were not observed to have identifiable clinical consequences[78,79] and intravenous carnitine supplementation has not consistently resulted in improved serum and hepatic carnitine levels or features of PNALD.[80,81]

Owing to the immaturity of amino acid metabolic pathways, some amino acids become conditionally essential in premature infants. Evidence supporting the role of a lack of taurine in the development of PNALD remains controversial.[82] Taurine is often supplemented in neonatal PN solutions[14] as taurine and cysteine production are diminished in premature infants. In older infants and adults, taurine and cysteine are synthesized from methionine and is not considered an essential amino acid.[83] Taurine is one of the main bile acid conjugates in the neonate, and has been shown to increase bile flow and protect against lithocholate toxicity. Lack of taurine results in a predominance of glycine conjugated bile acids. These bile acids are potentially hepatotoxic in the infant.[82] Early studies suggested that taurine supplementation of PN solutions was responsible for the decreased incidence of neonatal PNALD,[84] although this has not been confirmed by more recent studies.

Choline is usually absent from commercially available PN solutions. Plasma-free choline is low in more than 90% of patients who require long-term PN.[85,86] Choline deficiency is associated with hepatic steatosis due to very low-density lipoprotein synthesis. In clinical trials of choline supplementation resolution of hepatic steatosis has been observed and abnormalities in serum aminotransferase levels significantly improved.[87,88] Although choline deficiency appears to be associated with PN-associated hepatic steatosis, it is not clear if the deficiency alone is sufficient to result in the development of fibrosis, cirrhosis, and hepatic failure.[14]

Toxic Components of PN Solutions. Overfeeding patients with intravenous carbohydrate or lipid may be associated with hepatic steatosis and/or cholestasis.[14] Glucose infusion has been associated with hepatic steatosis.[10,57] Bile flow is reduced during glucose infusion in animal studies.[89,90] Preterm infants require approximately 4 to 8 mg/kg/min of glucose to suppress hepatic glucose oxidation; however, infusions should not exceed 12.6 mg/kg/min because excess exogenous glucose that is not oxidized may be converted to glycogen or fat in the liver.[91]

Lipid overload in infants following dose of >2.5 to 3.0 g/kg/d is associated with the development of cholestasis, hypoxia, thrombocytopenia, disseminated intravascular coagulation, and death.[92,93] Some commercially available lipid emulsions contain large concentrations of phytosterols and it is hypothesized that phytosterols can accumulate and contribute to cholestatic liver disease and other complications of PN.[93] If incompletely metabolized by the liver, the phytosterols can accumulate in the macrophages of hepatic sinusoids and disrupt normal macrophage function.[94] The development of PN-associated phytosterolemia appears to correlate with the onset and severity of PNALD and with the dose of commercial lipid emulsion used, however, a causal relationship has not been established.[14] No specific correlation with hepatic abnormalities in humans has been demonstrated and reduction of the volume of lipid infusion is not invariably associated with improvement or resolution of liver abnormalities.[93]

Lipid emulsions containing cottonseed oil were associated with the development of cholestasis and liver damage[95]; however, these solutions are no longer in use. Long-chain triglyceride lipid emulsions are a rich source of linoleic acid that promote the synthesis of leukotriene B4, a proinflammatory cytokine, and may contribute to an increased inflammatory response to cytokines.[96] Commercially available long-chain triglyceride lipid emulsions were not thought to cause PNALD if administered in doses of 1 to 2 g per kilogram body weight per day.[32,95,96] However, in intestinal failure patients receiving home PN, cholestasis and complicated PNALD were associated with a dose of lipid emulsion ≥1 g/kg/d.[21]

Amino acid infusions have been associated with cholestatic liver disease in both human and animal studies.[32,67] A more rapid rise and higher bilirubin concentration were reported in premature infants receiving 3.6 g amino acids/kg/d compared with infants receiving 2.5 g amino acids per kilogram body weight per day.[32] Individual amino acids have been implicated in the development of PN-associated cholestasis.[10,57] This may reflect immaturity of amino acid metabolism, resulting in an excess of precursor amino acids or a defect in the synthesis of amino acids or proteins. Serum methionine levels are increased in some infants receiving PN owing to a block in the transsulfuration pathway, remethylation of homocystine, or impaired oxidation of sulfur-containing amino acids.[97] Hepatocellular injury observed in neonatal rats receiving infusions of methionine was prevented by supplementation with arginine and glycine.[98,99] Increased cystine has been related to cholestasis and morphologic alterations, including bile duct proliferation, periportal necrosis, portal fibrosis, and inflammation of portal triads.[100] Increased homocystine causes hepatocellular injury and iron deposition in animal studies.[101] Photooxidation of amino acid solutions may result in production of hepatotoxic metabolites.[102] The extent of cholestasis was dependent on the dose of tryptophan and degree of light protection in newborn rats receiving an intraperitoneal amino acid solution.[102]

Manganese toxicity has been identified in patients receiving long-term PN therapy.[103,104] In a study of 57 children receiving long-term PN, 79% of patients had whole-blood manganese concentrations above the reference range.[104] Children with impaired liver function had the highest manganese levels, and there was a significant correlation between whole-blood manganese levels, aspartate aminotransferase ($r = .63$, $p < .001$), and total plasma bilirubin ($r = .64$, $p < .001$).[104] Of these children 11 (11/57) had both hypermagnesemia and cholestasis, and 4 died. In the seven survivors, whole-blood manganese concentrations declined in response to withdrawal of manganese supplementation.[104] Since manganese excretion is via the biliary tract, manganese retention may occur following a decrease in biliary flow. Monitoring of manganese levels is recommended in patients on long-term PN therapy and in patients with PNALD.

MANAGEMENT OF ESTABLISHED PNALD

Cessation of parenteral nutrition is the most effective therapy for the management of PNALD.[5,15,16,105] However, this may not be possible in some patients, and treatment is aimed at minimizing the impact of parenteral nutrition on the liver. This includes the identification of individual risk factors and the development of a multidirected strategy to reduce the adverse impact on the liver. Meehan and Georgeson reported that liver failure in long-term PN patients could be prevented by a combination of taurine, prevention and aggressive treatment of sepsis, strict catheter care, early parenteral nutrition cycling, "appropriate" enteral feeding, and inhibition of bacterial translocation.[106] The timing of the progression of liver disease is critical in planning which patients may benefit from isolated liver or small bowel or combined liver–small bowel transplant.[5,11,26] In the absence of liver and or small bowel transplant, PNALD can be fatal.[7]

Enteral Feeding

For patients who are unable to discontinue PN, small volumes of enteral nutrition have been shown to reduce the progression of PNALD.[10,107] Minimal or "trophic" enteral feeding encourages normal biliary dynamics and is associated with gallbladder contraction, improved bile flow, increased gastrin and glucagon secretion, a reduction in intestinal stasis, and bacterial overgrowth.[5,107] Supplementation of enteral feeds with fish oil rich in omega-3 long-chain polyunsaturated fatty acids has been advocated in an attempt to limit exposure to omega-6 polyunsaturated long-chain fatty acids.[108] Excess omega-6 polyunsaturated long-chain fatty acids have been linked to hepatic inflammation. Supplementation of feeds with omega-3 long-chain polyunsaturated fatty acids and/or antioxidants (vitamins C and E, N-acetylcysteine) has been proposed as a treatment strategy for the prevention of PNALD.[109]

Pharmacological Management

A number of pharmacologic agents have been proposed for the prevention and treatment of PNALD. Nonsteroidal anti-inflammatory drugs, including acetylsalicylic acid, have been shown to be beneficial in the prevention of PNALD in animal studies.[110,111] Cholecystokinin-octapeptide and the cholecystokinin analog, Ceruletide stimulate gallbladder contraction and prevent the development of biliary sludge and cholelithiasis in patients receiving PN.[61,62] The use of these agents in the prevention and treatment of PNALD is encouraging but warrants further clinical investigation.

Ursodeoxycholic acid improves bile flow and reduces serum and liver bilirubin concentrations in piglets with PNALD.[112] In humans, treatment with ursodeoxycholic acid has been associated with a reduction in markers of liver dysfunction, including serum γ-glutamyltransferase, aspartate transaminase, alanine transaminase, alkaline phosphatase, and/or serum bilirubin concentration.[113] A rebound increase in serum γ-glutamyltransferase, alkaline phosphatase, and alanine transaminase concentration was observed in children in whom ursodeoxycholic acid was discontinued in the presence of ongoing PN administration.[113] These patients responded to reintroduction of ursodeoxycholic acid therapy. This raises the question of whether ursodeoxycholic acid reduces serum markers of liver dysfunction in PNALD but does not influence the progression of liver disease. Enteral administration of tauro-ursodeoxycholic acid was not found to be effective in the prevention of PNALD in neonates.[81]

Other pharmacologic agents, including antibiotics, cholestyramine, rifampin, and phenobarbital, have been studied in the context of management of PNALD.[114] Surgical approaches aimed at improving bile flow, including biliary irrigation, have also been associated with improvement in PNALD in some patients.[115,116]

Modification to Parenteral Nutrition Solution and Administration

Modification of the macronutrient concentrations and balancing their composition in the PN solution is recommended in patients with established PNALD. Energy should be provided to meet individual needs for growth and activity however infants receiving energy at 110 kcal/kg/d or greater had a higher incidence of cholestasis compared with infants receiving a lower energy intake.[4] Glucose infusions should be limited to less than or equal to 15 g/kg/d or 12.6 mg/kg/min in premature infants.[91]

Recommendations for intravenous amino acid intakes for premature infants are generally aimed at providing between 2 and 3 g/kg/d.[91] Specialized pediatric amino acid solutions have been developed with the goal of limiting the complications of amino acid imbalance owing to immature metabolism in the premature and young infant. However, the efficacy of these solutions in preventing or minimizing PNALD has not yet been established.[117,118] Supplementation of PN solutions with taurine has not been shown to reduce serum hepatic enzyme, bilirubin, or bile acid concentrations in premature infants receiving short-term PN.[80,82,119] Intravenous glutamine supplementation has been shown to improve gut barrier integrity, although its role in the prevention and treatment of PNALD in infants and children requires further study.[120]

Soybean-based lipid emulsions, in particular, those composed mainly of omega-6 fatty acids and phytosterols are postulated to have deleterious effect on biliary secretion.[1] Animal studies have shown that intravenous fish oil emulsions that are high in eicosapentaenoic and docosahexaenoic acids, do not impair bile flow and may minimize fat accumulation in comparison to soybean oil fat emulsions.[121] In a recent report by Gura and colleagues,[1] the use of a fat emulsion consisting of fish oils was shown to reverse severe PN-associated cholestasis in two infants within 8 weeks of initiation of therapy. However, randomized controlled trials in a larger cohort are necessary to support its wide spread use. Current evidence suggests that in infants and children, lipid emulsions should be limited to <3 g/kg/d and less than 60% of total daily energy.[32,122] Lipid doses of >1 g/kg/d were associated with cholestasis and complicated liver disease in adults with intestinal failure receiving home PN. However, this has not yet been confirmed in children.[21] In vitro studies suggest that exposure of lipid emulsion to ultraviolet light results in the production of potentially toxic hydroperoxidases.[123] Therefore, lipid emulsions should be protected from ultraviolet light, particularly during phototherapy. The addition of fat-soluble vitamins to the lipid emulsion may provide some protection from this effect.[124]

In the presence of progressive cholestasis and cirrhosis, modification of the micronutrient composition of the PN solution may include the removal of copper and manganese.[23] This underscores the importance of routine monitoring of micronutrient status in patients receiving long-term PN. Cycling of PN for up to 12 h/d may help in limiting the progression of PNALD in patients requiring long-term PN.[125,126]

Liver Small Bowel Transplant

Most children requiring long-term PN have underlying intestinal disease, either short bowel syndrome or severe intestinal dysfunction. If transition to full enteral nutrition cannot be achieved and PN cannot be discontinued, PNALD may progress to overt liver failure.[5] Liver failure may have deleterious effects on the physiological process of small bowel adaptation.

The size and instability of infants with liver failure secondary to SBS can render these patients poor candidates for combined liver and intestinal transplant. However, isolated liver transplant in patients with severe liver disease may provide time to allow intestinal adaptation. Isolated liver transplants have the advantage of greater organ availability, established liver reduction techniques, and less required immunosuppression. However, as the fate of the transplanted liver is dependent on the ability to establish enteral feeding, isolated liver transplant is contraindicated in children with ultra short bowel (residual bowel length of less than 25 cm), children with an underlying primary motility, or a mucosal gastrointestinal disorder. Results from studies to date have shown isolated liver transplantation in pediatric SBS patients is highly successful in a selected population. In initial studies by Lawerence and colleagues,[127] four of the five pediatric patients receiving an isolated liver transplant were alive 4 to 9 months after transplant, and 3 had successfully progressed to enteral feeding. Similarly in a larger study by Horslen and colleagues,[128] of 11 SBS patients who underwent liver transplant, eight patients were alive for 15 to 66 months after transplant and only two remain on partial PN with increasing enteral tolerance.

Isolated small bowel transplant prior to progression to severe liver disease is a therapeutic option for patients with intestinal failure and reversible liver disease whereas combined liver–small bowel transplant is indicated for patients with irreversible intestinal failure and PN-associated liver failure. Current data suggests that isolated small bowel transplantation is as successful as combined small bowel and liver transplantation,[129] however in patients with moderate to severe liver disease, a liver and small bowel transplant is recommended.[130] To assess all potential options for therapy it is recommended that referral to a transplant center is made before the liver disease becomes irreversible.[11,26,114,131] Elevation of the total serum bilirubin level of >3 mg/dL for over 3 months in a PN-dependent infant and/or early clinical features of progressive liver disease, including mild splenomegaly, dilatation of abdominal wall veins, and a deteriorating platelet count, are clinical indications for referral.[11,26] Serum hepatic or biliary enzyme levels provide no additional predictive benefit in patients with PNALD.[11] Hypoalbuminemia, coagulopathy, and hypoglycemia during cycling of PN are markers of hepatic synthetic dysfunction. These are considered late features of liver disease and are associated with a poor prognosis.[11] In the setting of progressive PNALD and portal hypertension, severe bleeding may occur from stomas in patients with short bowel syndrome.

CONCLUSION

Infants and children receiving PN are at risk of developing PNALD. No single factor has been shown to be responsible for the development of this potentially fatal complication. Current evidence suggests that the developing liver is particularly sensitive to injury resulting from a range of factors, such as infection and intestinal stasis. Discontinuation of PN is the most effective treatment, but this cannot be achieved in patients with intestinal failure. Treatment strategies that include the identification of risk factors and the development of a multidirected approach to the prevention and treatment of PNALD are required. Although new pharmacologic and surgical approaches have been reported, the risks and benefits of these therapies still need to be assessed in randomized prospective controlled trials. Isolated small bowel or liver transplantation, or combined liver–small bowel transplant provide therapeutic options for long-term parenteral nutrition-dependent patients with PNALD with short bowel syndrome or severe intestinal dysfunction.

REFERENCES

1. Gura KM, Duggan CP, Collier SB, et al. Reversal of parenteral nutrition-associated liver disease in two infants with short bowel syndrome using parenteral fish oil: Implications for future management. Pediatrics 2006;118:e197–201.
2. Bell RL, Ferry GD, Smith EO, et al. Total parenteral nutrition-related cholestasis in infants. JPEN J Parenter Enteral Nutr 1986;10:356–9.
3. Cohen C, Olsen MM. Pediatric total parenteral nutrition. Liver histopathology. Arch Pathol Lab Med 1981;105:152–6.
4. Kubota A, Okada A, Nezu R, et al. Hyperbilirubinemia in neonates associated with total parenteral nutrition. JPEN J Parenter Enteral Nutr 1988;12:602–6.
5. Kelly DA. Liver complications of pediatric parenteral nutrition-epidemiology. Nutrition 1998;14:153–7.
6. Kubota A, Yonekura T, Hoki M, et al. Total parenteral nutrition-associated intrahepatic cholestasis in infants: 25 years' experience. J Pediatr Surg 2000;35:1049–51.
7. Sondheimer JM, Asturias E, Cadnapaphornchai M. Infection and cholestasis in neonates with intestinal resection and long-term parenteral nutrition. J Pediatr Gastroenterol Nutr 1998;27:131–7.
8. Merritt RJ. Cholestasis associated with total parenteral nutrition. J Pediatr Gastroenterol Nutr 1986;5:9–22.
9. Caniano DA, Starr J, Ginn-Pease ME. Extensive short-bowel syndrome in neonates: Outcome in the 1980s. Surgery 1989;105:119–24.
10. Galea MH, Holliday H, Carachi R, Kapila L. Short-bowel syndrome: A collective review. J Pediatr Surg 1992;27:592–6.
11. Kaufman SS. Prevention of parenteral nutrition-associated liver disease in children. Pediatr Transplant 2002;6:37–42.
12. Albers MJ, de Gast-Bakker DA, van Dam NA, et al. Male sex predisposes the newborn surgical patient to parenteral nutrition-associated cholestasis and to sepsis. Arch Surg 2002;137:789–93.
13. Wolf A, Pohlandt F. Bacterial infection: The main cause of acute cholestasis in newborn infants receiving short-term parenteral nutrition. J Pediatr Gastroenterol Nutr 1989;8:297–303.
14. Buchman AL, Iyer K, Fryer J. Parenteral nutrition-associated liver disease and the role for isolated intestine and intestine/liver transplantation. Hepatology 2006;43:9–19.
15. Dahms BB, Halpin TC, Jr. Serial liver biopsies in parenteral nutrition-associated cholestasis of early infancy. Gastroenterology 1981;81:136–44.
16. Patterson K, Kapur SP, Chandra RS. Hepatocellular carcinoma in a noncirrhotic infant after prolonged parenteral nutrition. J Pediatr 1985;106:797–800.
17. Grant JP, Cox CE, Kleinman LM, et al. Serum hepatic enzyme and bilirubin elevations during parenteral nutrition. Surg Gynecol Obstet 1977;145:573–80.
18. Christensen RD, Henry E, Wiedmeier SE, et al. Identifying patients, on the first day of life, at high-risk of developing parenteral nutrition-associated liver disease. J Perinatol 2007.
19. Zaman N, Tam YK, Jewell LD, Coutts RT. Effects of intravenous lipid as a source of energy in parenteral nutrition associated hepatic dysfunction and lidocaine elimination: A study using isolated rat liver perfusion. Biopharm Drug Dispos 1997;18:803–19.
20. Tulikoura I, Huikuri K. Morphological fatty changes and function of the liver, serum free fatty acids, and triglycerides during parenteral nutrition. Scand J Gastroenterol 1982;17:177–85.
21. Cavicchi M, Beau P, Crenn P, et al. Prevalence of liver disease and contributing factors in patients receiving home parenteral nutrition for permanent intestinal failure. Ann Intern Med 2000;132:525–32.
22. Pierro A, van Saene HK, Donnell SC, et al. Microbial translocation in neonates and infants receiving long-term parenteral nutrition. Arch Surg 1996;131:176–9.
23. Drongowski RA, Coran AG. An analysis of factors contributing to the development of total parenteral nutrition-induced cholestasis. JPEN J Parenter Enteral Nutr 1989;13:586–9.
24. Farrell MK, Balistreri WF, Suchy FJ. Serum-sulfated lithocholate as an indicator of cholestasis during parenteral nutrition in infants and children. JPEN J Parenter Enteral Nutr 1982;6:30–3.
25. Kaplowitz N, Kok E, Javitt NB. Postprandial serum bile acid for the detection of hepatobiliary disease. JAMA 1973;225:292–3.
26. Bueno J, Ohwada S, Kocoshis S, et al. Factors impacting the survival of children with intestinal failure referred for intestinal transplantation. J Pediatr Surg 1999;34:27–32; discussion 32–3.
27. Demircan M, Ergun O, Avanoglu S, et al. Determination of serum bile acids routinely may prevent delay in diagnosis of total parenteral nutrition-induced cholestasis. J Pediatr Surg 1999;34:565–7.
28. Roslyn JJ, Berquist WE, Pitt HA, et al. Increased risk of gallstones in children receiving total parenteral nutrition. Pediatrics 1983;71:784–9.
29. King DR, Ginn-Pease ME, Lloyd TV, et al. Parenteral nutrition with associated cholelithiasis: Another iatrogenic disease of infants and children. J Pediatr Surg 1987;22: 593–6.
30. Petersen SR, Sheldon GF. Acute acalculous cholecystitis: A complication of hyperalimentation. Am J Surg 1979;138:814–7.
31. Beale EF, Nelson RM, Bucciarelli RL, et al. Intrahepatic cholestasis associated with parenteral nutrition in premature infants. Pediatrics 1979;64:342–7.
32. Vileisis RA, Inwood RJ, Hunt CE. Prospective controlled study of parenteral nutrition-associated cholestatic jaundice: Effect of protein intake. J Pediatr 1980;96:893–7.
33. Pereira GR, Sherman MS, DiGiacomo J, et al. Hyperalimentation-induced cholestasis. Increased incidence and severity in premature infants. Am J Dis Child 1981;135:842–5.
34. Balistreri WF, Heubi JE, Suchy FJ. Immaturity of the enterohepatic circulation in early life: Factors predisposing to "physiologic" maldigestion and cholestasis. J Pediatr Gastroenterol Nutr 1983;2:346–54.
35. Back P, Walter K. Developmental pattern of bile acid metabolism as revealed by bile acid analysis of meconium. Gastroenterology 1980;78:671–6.
36. Lester R, St Pyrek J, Little JM, Adcock EW. Diversity of bile acids in the fetus and newborn infant. J Pediatr Gastroenterol Nutr 1983;2:355–64.

37. Little JM, Richey JE, Van Thiel DH, Lester R. Taurocholate pool size and distribution in the fetal rat. J Clin Invest 1979;63:1042–9.

38. Watkins JB, Szczepanik P, Gould JB, et al. Bile salt metabolism in the human premature infant. Preliminary observations of pool size and synthesis rate following prenatal administration of dexamethasone and phenobarbital. Gastroenterology 1975;69:706–13.

39. de Belle RC, Vaupshas V, Vitullo BB, et al. Intestinal absorption of bile salts: Immature development in the neonate. J Pediatr 1979;94:472–6.

40. Andorsky DJ, Lund DP, Lillehei CW, et al. Nutritional and other postoperative management of neonates with short bowel syndrome correlates with clinical outcomes. J Pediatr 2001;139:27–33.

41. Ito Y, Shils ME. Liver dysfunction associated with long-term total parenteral nutrition in patients with massive bowel resection. JPEN J Parenter Enteral Nutr 1991;15:271–6.

42. Teitelbaum DH, Drongowski R, Spivak D. Rapid development of hyperbilirubinemia in infants with the short bowel syndrome as a correlate to mortality: Possible indication for early small bowel transplantation. Transplant Proc 1996;28:2699–700.

43. Bianchi A. Longitudinal intestinal lengthening and tailoring: Results in 20 children. J R Soc Med 1997;90:429–32.

44. Beath SV, Davies P, Papadopoulou A, et al. Parenteral nutrition-related cholestasis in postsurgical neonates: Multivariate analysis of risk factors. J Pediatr Surg 1996;31:604–6.

45. Hamilton JR, Sass-Kortsak A. Jaundice associated with severe bacterial infection in young infants. J Pediatr 1963;63:121–32.

46. Heine RG, Bines JE. New approaches to parenteral nutrition in infants and children. J Paediatr Child Health 2002;38:433–7.

47. Candusso M, Faraguna D, Sperli D, Dodaro N. Outcome and quality of life in paediatric home parenteral nutrition. Curr Opin Clin Nutr Metab Care 2002;5:309–14.

48. Bueno J, Guiterrez J, Mazariegos GV, et al. Analysis of patients with longitudinal intestinal lengthening procedure referred for intestinal transplantation. J Pediatr Surg 2001;36:178–83.

49. Hodes JE, Grosfeld JL, Weber TR, et al. Hepatic failure in infants on total parenteral nutrition (TPN): Clinical and histopathologic observations. J Pediatr Surg 1982;17:463–8.

50. Ginn-Pease ME, Pantalos D, King DR. TPN-associated hyperbilirubinemia: A common problem in newborn surgical patients. J Pediatr Surg 1985;20:436–9.

51. Lichtman SN, Wang J, Schwab JH, Lemasters JJ. Comparison of peptidoglycan-polysaccharide and lipopolysaccharide stimulation of Kupffer cells to produce tumor necrosis factor and interleukin-1. Hepatology 1994;19:1013–22.

52. Jones A, Selby PJ, Viner C, et al. Tumour necrosis factor, cholestatic jaundice, and chronic liver disease. Gut 1990;31:938–9.

53. Pappo I, Bercovier H, Berry E, et al. Antitumor necrosis factor antibodies reduce hepatic steatosis during total parenteral nutrition and bowel rest in the rat. JPEN J Parenter Enteral Nutr 1995;19:80–2.

54. Pappo I, Bercovier H, Berry EM, et al. Polymyxin B reduces total parenteral nutrition-associated hepatic steatosis by its antibacterial activity and by blocking deleterious effects of lipopolysaccharide. JPEN J Parenter Enteral Nutr 1992;16:529–32.

55. Goulet O, Ruemmele F, Lacaille F, Colomb V. Irreversible intestinal failure. J Pediatr Gastroenterol Nutr 2004;38:250–69.

56. Goulet O, Ruemmele F. Causes and management of intestinal failure in children. Gastroenterology 2006;130:S16–28.

57. Btaiche IF, Khalidi N. Parenteral nutrition-associated liver complications in children. Pharmacotherapy 2002;22:188–211.

58. Hofmann AF. Defective biliary secretion during total parenteral nutrition: Probable mechanisms and possible solutions. J Pediatr Gastroenterol Nutr 1995;20:376–90.

59. Fouin-Fortunet H, Le Quernec L, Erlinger S, et al. Hepatic alterations during total parenteral nutrition in patients with inflammatory bowel disease: A possible consequence of lithocholate toxicity. Gastroenterology 1982;82:932–7.

60. Lucas A, Bloom SR, Aynsley-Green A. Metabolic and endocrine consequences of depriving preterm infants of enteral nutrition. Acta Paediatr Scand 1983;72:245–9.

61. Curran TJ, Uzoaru I, Das JB, et al. The effect of cholecystokinin-octapeptide on the hepatobiliary dysfunction caused by total parenteral nutrition. J Pediatr Surg 1995;30:242–6; discussion 246–7.

62. Teitelbaum DH, Han-Markey T, Schumacher RE. Treatment of parenteral nutrition-associated cholestasis with cholecystokinin-octapeptide. J Pediatr Surg 1995;30:1082–5.

63. Rintala RJ, Lindahl H, Pohjavuori M. Total parenteral nutrition-associated cholestasis in surgical neonates may be reversed by intravenous cholecystokinin: A preliminary report. J Pediatr Surg 1995;30:827–30.

64. Johnson LR, Copeland EM, Dudrick SJ, et al. Structural and hormonal alterations in the gastrointestinal tract of parenterally fed rats. Gastroenterology 1975;68:1177–83.

65. Levinson S, Bhasker M, Gibson TR, et al. Comparison of intraluminal and intravenous mediators of colonic response to eating. Dig Dis Sci 1985;30:33–9.

66. Haskel Y, Udassin R, Freund HR, et al. Liquid enteral diets induce bacterial translocation by increasing cecal flora without changing intestinal motility. JPEN J Parenter Enteral Nutr 2001;25:60–4.

67. Lowry SF, Goodgame JT, Jr, et al. Effect of chronic protein malnutrition on host-tumor composition and growth. J Surg Res 1979;26:79–86.

68. Nussbaum M, Fischer J. Pathogenesis of hepatic steatosis during total parenteral nutrition. In: Nyhus L, editor. Surgery Annual. Norwalk: Appleton and Lange; 1991. p. 1–11.

69. Das JB, Cosentino CM, Levy MF, et al. Early hepatobiliary dysfunction during total parenteral nutrition: An experimental study. J Pediatr Surg 1993;28:14–8.

70. Bursztein S, Elwyn DH, Askanazi J. Energy metabolism and indirect calorimetry in critically ill and injured patients. Acute Care 1988;14-15:91–110.

71. Vary TC, Siegel JH, Nakatani T, et al. Effect of sepsis on activity of pyruvate dehydrogenase complex in skeletal muscle and liver. Am J Physiol 1986;250:E634–40.

72. Yamazaki K, Maiz A, Moldawer LL, et al. Complications associated with the overfeeding of infected animals. J Surg Res 1986;40:152–8.

73. Yamanouchi T, Suita S, Masumoto K. Nonprotein energy overloading induces bacterial translocation during total parenteral nutrition in newborn rabbits. Nutrition 1998;14:443–7.

74. Schiff D, Chan G, Seccombe D, Hahn P. Plasma carnitine levels during intravenous feeding of the neonate. J Pediatr 1979;95:1043–6.

75. Karpati G, Carpenter S, Engel AG, et al. The syndrome of systemic carnitine deficiency. Clinical, morphologic, biochemical, and pathophysiologic features. Neurology 1975;25:16–24.

76. Dahlstrom KA, Ament ME, Moukarzel A, et al. Low blood and plasma carnitine levels in children receiving long-term parenteral nutrition. J Pediatr Gastroenterol Nutr 1990;11:375–9.

77. Moukarzel AA, Dahlstrom KA, Buchman AL, Ament ME. Carnitine status of children receiving long-term total parenteral nutrition: A longitudinal prospective study. J Pediatr 1992;120:759–62.

78. Bowyer BA, Fleming CR, Ludwig J, et al. Does long-term home parenteral nutrition in adult patients cause chronic liver disease? JPEN J Parenter Enteral Nutr 1985;9:11–7.

79. Bonner CM, DeBrie KL, Hug G, et al. Effects of parenteral L-carnitine supplementation on fat metabolism and nutrition in premature neonates. J Pediatr 1995;126:287–92.

80. Cooke RJ, Whitington PF, Kelts D. Effect of taurine supplementation on hepatic function during short-term parenteral nutrition in the premature infant. J Pediatr Gastroenterol Nutr 1984;3:234–8.

81. Heubi JE, Wiechmann DA, Creutzinger V, et al. Tauroursodeoxycholic acid (TUDCA) in the prevention of total parenteral nutrition-associated liver disease. J Pediatr 2002;141:237–42.

82. Howard D, Thompson DF. Taurine: An essential amino acid to prevent cholestasis in neonates? Ann Pharmacother 1992;26:1390–2.

83. Zlotkin SH, Anderson GH. The development of cystathionase activity during the first year of life. Pediatr Res 1982;16:65–8.

84. Okamoto E, Rassin DK, Zucker CL, et al. Role of taurine in feeding the low-birth-weight infant. J Pediatr 1984;104:936–40.

85. Buchman AL, Moukarzel A, Jenden DJ, et al. Low plasma free choline is prevalent in patients receiving long term parenteral nutrition and is associated with hepatic aminotransferase abnormalities. Clin Nutr 1993;12:33–7.

86. Sheard NF, Tayek JA, Bistrian BR, et al. Plasma choline concentration in humans fed parenterally. Am J Clin Nutr 1986;43:219–24.

87. Buchman AL, Dubin M, Jenden D, et al. Lecithin increases plasma free choline and decreases hepatic steatosis in long-term total parenteral nutrition patients. Gastroenterology 1992;102:1363–70.

88. Buchman AL, Dubin MD, Moukarzel AA, . Choline deficiency: A cause of hepatic steatosis during parenteral nutrition that can be reversed with intravenous choline supplementation. Hepatology 1995;22:1399–403.

89. Zahavi I, Shaffer EA, Gall DG. Total parenteral nutrition-associated cholestasis: acute studies in infant and adult rabbits. J Pediatr Gastroenterol Nutr 1985;4:622–7.

90. Mashima Y. Effect of calorie overload on puppy livers during parenteral nutrition. JPEN J Parenter Enteral Nutr 1979;3:139–45.

91. Kien C. Nutritional Needs of the Preterm Infant: Scientific Basis and Practical Guidelines. Baltimore: Williams and Wilkins; 1993.

92. Salvian AJ, Allardyce DB. Impaired bilirubin secretion during total parenteral nutrition. J Surg Res 1980;28:547–55.

93. Clayton PT, Bowron A, Mills KA, et al. Phytosterolemia in children with parenteral nutrition-associated cholestatic liver disease. Gastroenterology 1993;105:1806–13.

94. Cukier C, Waitzberg DL, Logullo AF, et al. Lipid and lipid-free total parenteral nutrition: Differential effects on macrophage phagocytosis in rats. Nutrition 1999;15:885–9.

95. Hakansson I. Experience in long-term studies on nine intravenous fat emulsions in dogs. Nutr Dieta Eur Rev Nutr Diet 1968;10:54–76.

96. Jeppesen PB, Hoy CE, Mortensen PB. Differences in essential fatty acid requirements by enteral and parenteral routes of administration in patients with fat malabsorption. Am J Clin Nutr 1999;70:78–84.

97. Zarif MA, Pildes RS, Szanto PB, Vidyasagar D. Cholestasis associated with administration of L-amino acids and dextrose solutions. Biol Neonate 1976;29:66–76.

98. Stekol JA, Szaran J. Pathological effects of excessive methionine in the diet of growing rats. J Nutr 1962;77:81–90.

99. Klavins JV, Peacocke IL. Pathology of amino acid excess. 3. Effects of administration of excessive amounts of sulphur-containing amino acids: Methionine with equimolar amounts of glycine and arginine. Br J Exp Pathol 1964;45:533–47.

100. Klavins JV. Pathology of amino acid excess. I. Effects of administration of excessive amounts of sulphur containing amino acids: Homocystine. Br J Exp Pathol 1963;44:507–15.

101. Klavins JV. Pathology of amino acid excess. Ii. Effects of administration of excessive amounts of sulphur containing amino acids: L-Cystine. Br J Exp Pathol 1963;44:516–9.

102. Merritt RJ, Sinatra FR, Henton D, Neustein H. Cholestatic effect of intraperitoneal administration of tryptophan to suckling rat pups. Pediatr Res 1984;18:904–7.

103. Reynolds AP, Kiely E, Meadows N. Manganese in long term paediatric parenteral nutrition. Arch Dis Child 1994;71:527–8.

104. Fell JM, Reynolds AP, Meadows N, et al. Manganese toxicity in children receiving long-term parenteral nutrition. Lancet 1996;347:1218–21.

105. Moss RL, Amii LA. New approaches to understanding the etiology and treatment of total parenteral nutrition-associated cholestasis. Semin Pediatr Surg 1999;8:140–7.

106. Meehan JJ, Georgeson KE. Prevention of liver failure in parenteral nutrition-dependent children with short bowel syndrome. J Pediatr Surg 1997;32:473–5.

107. Berseth CL. Minimal enteral feedings. Clin Perinatol 1995;22:195–205.

108. Chan S, McCowen KC, Bistrian BR, et al. Incidence, prognosis, and etiology of end-stage liver disease in patients receiving home total parenteral nutrition. Surgery 1999;126:28–34.

109. Will Y, Fischer KA, Horton RA, et al. gamma-glutamyltranspeptidase-deficient knockout mice as a model to study the relationship between glutathione status, mitochondrial function, and cellular function. Hepatology 2000;32:740–9.

110. Nussinovitch M, Zahavi I, Marcus H, et al. The choleretic effect of nonsteroidal anti-inflammatory drugs in total parenteral nutrition-associated cholestasis. Isr J Med Sci 1996;32:1262–4.

111. Demircan M, Uguralp S, Mutus M, et al. The effects of acetylsalicylic acid, interferon-alpha, and vitamin E on prevention of parenteral nutrition-associated cholestasis: An experimental study. J Pediatr Gastroenterol Nutr 1999;28:291–5.

112. Duerksen DR, Van Aerde JE, Gramlich L, et al. Intravenous ursodeoxycholic acid reduces cholestasis in parenterally fed newborn piglets. Gastroenterology 1996;111:1111–7.

113. Spagnuolo MI, Iorio R, Vegnente A, Guarino A. Ursodeoxycholic acid for treatment of cholestasis in children on long-term total parenteral nutrition: a pilot study. Gastroenterology 1996;111:716–9.

114. Goulet O, Lacaille F, Jan D, Ricour C. Intestinal transplantation: indications, results and strategy. Curr Opin Clin Nutr Metab Care 2000;3:329–38.

115. Rintala R, Lindahl H, Pohjavuori M, et al. Surgical treatment of intractable cholestasis associated with total parenteral nutrition in premature infants. J Pediatr Surg 1993;28:716–9.

116. Cooper A, Ross AJ, III, O'Neill JA, Jr, et al. Resolution of intractable cholestasis associated with total parenteral nutrition following biliary irrigation. J Pediatr Surg 1985;20:772–4.

117. Forchielli ML, Gura KM, Sandler R, Lo C. Aminosyn PF or trophamine: Which provides more protection from cholestasis associated with total parenteral nutrition? J Pediatr Gastroenterol Nutr 1995;21:374–82.

118. Coran AG, Drongowski RA. Studies on the toxicity and efficacy of a new amino acid solution in pediatric parenteral nutrition. JPEN J Parenter Enteral Nutr 1987;11:368–77.

119. Heird WC, Dell RB, Helms RA, et al. Amino acid mixture designed to maintain normal plasma amino acid patterns in infants and children requiring parenteral nutrition. Pediatrics 1987;80:401–8.

120. Souba WW, Klimberg VS, Plumley DA, et al. The role of glutamine in maintaining a healthy gut and supporting the metabolic response to injury and infection. J Surg Res 1990;48:383–91.

121. Alwayn IP, Gura K, Nose V, et al. Omega-3 fatty acid supplementation prevents hepatic steatosis in a murine model of nonalcoholic fatty liver disease. Pediatr Res 2005;57:445–52.

122. Cohen IT, Dahms B, Hays DM. Peripheral total parenteral nutrition employing a lipid emulsion (Intralipid): Complications encountered in pediatric patients. J Pediatr Surg 1977;12:837–45.

123. Neuzil J, Darlow BA, Inder TE, et al. Oxidation of parenteral lipid emulsion by ambient and phototherapy lights: Potential toxicity of routine parenteral feeding. J Pediatr 1995;126:785–90.

124. Silvers KM, Darlow BA, Winterbourn CC. Lipid peroxide and hydrogen peroxide formation in parenteral nutrition solutions containing multivitamins. JPEN J Parenter Enteral Nutr 2001;25:14–7.

125. Hwang TL, Lue MC, Chen LL. Early use of cyclic TPN prevents further deterioration of liver functions for the TPN patients with impaired liver function. Hepatogastroenterology 2000;47:1347–50.

126. Maini B, Blackburn GL, Bistrian BR, et al. Cyclic hyperalimentation: An optimal technique for preservation of visceral protein. J Surg Res 1976;20:515–25.

127. Lawrence JP, Dunn SP, Billmire DF, et al. Isolated liver transplantation for liver failure in patients with short bowel syndrome. J Pediatr Surg 1994;29:751–3.

128. Horslen SP, Sudan DL, Iyer KR, et al. Isolated liver transplantation in infants with end-stage liver disease associated with short bowel syndrome. Ann Surg 2002;235:435–9.

129. Registry IT. Intestinal Transplant Registry. www.intestinaltransplant.org.

130. Gupte GL, Beath SV, Kelly DA, et al. Current issues in the management of intestinal failure. Arch Dis Child 2006;91:259–64.

131. Kaufman SS, Atkinson JB, Bianchi A, et al. Indications for pediatric intestinal transplantation: A position paper of the American Society of Transplantation. Pediatr Transplant 2001;5:80–7.

22.3. Small Intestinal Transplantation

Stuart S. Kaufman, MD

Cal S. Matsumoto, MD

Thomas M. Fishbein, MD

Replacement of the small intestine with or without other parts of the digestive system such as the stomach, liver, pancreas, and colon represents the ultimate treatment for *intestinal failure*, the state of permanent dependence on parenteral nutrition for support of life with an anatomically or functionally inadequate gastrointestinal tract.[1] Intestinal transplantation was performed in humans as an experimental, end-of-life procedure in the 1960s but was consistently unsuccessful at that time on account of the failure of the then available immunosuppressive agents to prevent severe allograft rejection.[2] Interest in intestinal transplantation faded over the next two to three decades, which were without meaningful improvements in the immunosuppressive armamentarium, when parenteral nutrition became increasingly available for use in the home setting. Interest in intestinal transplantation returned during the late 1980s and early 1990s as limitations of extended parenteral nutrition therapy for intestinal failure became increasingly apparent and as immunosuppressive agents with markedly increased efficacy, specifically the calcineurin inhibitors cyclosporine and later tacrolimus, became available for clinical use.[2,3] Despite improved immunosuppressive therapy, morbidity and mortality were considerable during the first decade of clinical intestinal transplantation, because rates of severe allograft rejection and secondary postoperative sepsis and multiorgan failure remained high. The frequently desperately ill state of patients undergoing transplant, the scarcity of suitable allografts, the highly immunogenic yet nonsterile nature of the intestine itself, and the limitations of available laboratory and imaging methods contributed to poor outcomes during these early years. In fact, 5-year patient survival through the 1990s was no greater than 50%, rendering outcomes in intestinal transplantation markedly inferior to contemporaneous outcomes following most other solid-organ transplants.[4] Subsequent refinements in patient selection, operative techniques, immunosuppressive therapy, and postoperative rehabilitation comprehensively managed by integrated teams of transplant surgeons, physicians, nurses, dieticians, social workers, and others have substantially improved results. The current approach to intestinal transplantation summarized in this chapter describes the sum of these efforts to date.

THE ROLE OF INTESTINAL TRANSPLANTATION IN MANAGEMENT OF INTESTINAL FAILURE

Intestinal transplantation has not superseded extended parenteral nutrition as the primary therapeutic modality for intestinal failure in infants and children. Rather, pediatric patients with intestinal failure are candidates for intestinal transplantation only if they are either failing or can be reasonably predicted to fail parenteral nutrition therapy. There are at least two reasons for the continued secondary role of intestinal transplantation in the management of pediatric intestinal failure. First, there is often considerable uncertainty, particularly in infants following major intestinal resection, whether true intestinal failure, that is, unequivocally permanent parenteral nutrition, is present.[5] In fact, about 55 to 80% of infants who are committed to parenteral nutrition because of intestinal resection in the neonatal period have transient intestinal insufficiency rather than intestinal failure and eventually adapt to full enteral feeding.[6–10] Second, survival following intestinal transplantation has historically been no better than long-term survival of pediatric intestinal failure patients receiving parenteral nutrition.[4,6,11] Currently, 3-year survival following isolated intestinal transplantation has increased to approximately 85%, and survival following small intestinal transplantation combined with transplantation of other organs such as the liver approximates 70%.[12,13] Moreover, recent data indicate that the annual cost associated with successful transplantation is less than that of home parenteral nutrition by 1 to 3 years following surgery.[14,15] These trends suggest that intestinal transplantation may eventually replace extended parenteral nutrition therapy as the most appropriate therapeutic option for pediatric patients with intestinal failure.[2] However, the continued challenges of intestinal transplantation continue to make an initial trial of potentially indefinite parenteral nutrition, the preferred approach in most circumstances.[15,16]

INDICATIONS FOR INTESTINAL TRANSPLANTATION

Etiologies of intestinal failure that lead to intestinal transplantation and their frequencies in children are shown in Table 1. Life-threatening complications of intestinal failure and parenteral nutrition therapy that indicate intestinal transplantation are summarized in Table 2. These complications include (1) progressive, parenteral nutrition-associated liver disease, in this context more appropriately designated intestinal failure-associated liver disease,[17] (2) loss of central venous access required to deliver parenteral nutrition, (3) recurring life-threatening infection, and (4) intra-abdominal neoplasia that requires visceral exenteration to obtain a reasonable chance of cure.[18]

Intestinal Failure-Associated Liver Disease

Progressive, life-threatening intestinal failure-associated liver disease (IFALD) is the most common indication for intestinal transplantation in the pediatric age group, presumably because the infant liver is more vulnerable to the deleterious effects of intestinal failure and parenteral nutrition therapy than the mature organ. The rapid progression of IFALD in younger patients is emphasized by the fact that one-half of intestinal transplants performed in infants and children include a liver transplant compared to only one-quarter of intestinal transplants performed in adults.[4] Similarly, whereas about one-half of all intestinal transplants are now performed in adults (Figure 1A), the majority of intestinal transplants that include a liver allograft are performed in children less than 5 years of age

Table 1 Indications for Intestinal Transplantation in Children Based on Diagnosis.	
Anatomic: 62%	Congenital anomaly: 50%
	Gastroschisis: 21%
	Volvulus: 17%
	Intestinal atresia: 8%
	Other short bowel: 4%
	Necrotizing enterocolitis: 12%
Functional: 28%	Chronic enteropathy: 10%
	Microvillus inclusion disease: 6%
	Other enteropathy: 4%
	Dysmotility: 18%
	Pseudo-obstruction: 9%
	Aganglionosis: 7%
	Other dysmotility: 2%
Tumor: 1%	
Retransplant: 8%	

Adapted from R. Smith, http://www.intestinaltransplant.org/.

Table 2 Indications for Intestinal Transplantation Evaluation

Liver disease with portal hypertension
    Total serum bilirubin ≥6 mg/dL
    Platelet count ≤150,000/μL
        or
Loss of half of standard central venous access sites
    Infant 2/4 (jugular, subclavian)
    All others: 3/6 (jugular, subclavian, femoral)
        or
Recurrent life-threatening infection related to:
    Central venous catheter
    Diseased remnant gastrointestinal tract
        or
Total intestinal loss
    Congenital malformation
    Necrotizing enterocolitis
    Vascular accident
    Nonmetastatic tumor

Adapted from Kaufman et al.[18]

Table 3 Kaplan-Meier Waiting Times for an Intestinal Transplant Based on Age in the United States: 2001 to 2002

Age (yr)	Median Waiting Time (d)
<1	438
1 to 5	185
6 to 10	270
11 to 17	335

Source: UNOS reports; http://www.optn.org/latestData/rptStrat.asp. Based on OPTN data as of June 2, 2006.

Table 4 Risk Factors for Permanent Parenteral Nutrition and Liver Failure

Anatomic short-bowel syndrome
  Infants
    Less than 40 cm of remnant small bowel *without* ileocecal valve
    Less than 20 cm of remnant small bowel *with* ileocecal valve
  Older patients
    Less than 65 cm of remnant small bowel *without* ileocecal valve
    Less than 30 cm of remnant small bowel *with* ileocecal valve
Functional intestinal failure
  Chronic intestinal pseudo-obstruction syndromes with continuous parenteral nutrition
  Congenital secretory diarrhea syndromes, eg, microvillus inclusion disease

(Figure 1B). The incidence of death from liver failure and its complications in infants receiving parenteral nutrition due to gastrointestinal tract disease is approximately 5 to 25%, most commonly occurring between ages 8 to 18 months.[6,8–11,19] The comparatively young age at death requires early recognition of potentially progressive liver disease, because the waiting period for matching with an intestinal allograft during infancy commonly exceeds 1 year in the United States, particularly when a liver allograft is simultaneously required (Table 3). The scarcity of donor organs contributes to the death of approximately 35 to 40% of patients waiting for a combined intestinal and liver transplant.[20] The precise cause or causes of IFALD remains unknown. Postulated etiologies include hepatotoxic components of parenteral nutrition such as intravenous lipid emulsions, absence of essential hepatotrophic nutrients such as choline, and protracted exposure to hepatic toxins emanating from an abnormal gut lumen, particularly bacterial endotoxins and other substances of microbial origin.[17] Most relevant to discussion of intestinal transplantation is the generally accepted principle that enteral nutrition is essential for prevention of IFALD.

There are essentially three groups of patients who should be considered for intestinal transplantation because of IFALD. The first group consists of those patients who have lost virtually the entire small intestine or who have certain forms of functional intestinal failure, particularly intestinal pseudo-obstruction of neonatal onset, for example, megacystis-microcolon-intestinal hypoperistalsis syndrome, and congenital enterocyte disorders, in particular, microvillus inclusion disease and tufting enteropathy. The risk of progressive IFALD is consistently very high in this group, presumably because of the unremitting nature of parenteral nutrition dependence and consistent intolerance to even small quantities of enteral feeding. These patients should be referred for intestinal transplantation immediately after diagnosis and/or postoperative stabilization.[21–26] Risk factors for permanent, total parenteral nutrition, and liver failure are summarized in Table 4.

The second group consists of those patients with short bowel sufficient to predict permanent parenteral nutrition (Table 4), but who tolerate enough enteral feeding to retard or prevent development of IFALD for an extended period. These patients should be considered for intestinal transplantation at the first clinical indication of progressive liver disease. Also in this group are patients with milder forms of pseudo-obstruction, with intermittent and/or less than complete requirements for parenteral nutrition support, many of whom will also eventually develop chronic liver disease.

The third group of potential candidates for intestinal transplantation comprises those patients with short-bowel syndrome and evidence of IFALD but who retain enough remnant intestine to predict complete adaptation to enteral feeding. The prognosis of IFALD and the decision to refer for transplant is most difficult in this group, because stabilization if not resolution of IFALD frequently depends on the rate at which parenteral nutrition can be replaced with enteral nutrients while preserving appropriate growth; this process is not always predictable or entirely within the control of care providers. Prolonged underutilization of the gastrointestinal tract for any reason may commit a patient to transplantation that might not otherwise have been necessary. Factors that influence the rate of parenteral nutrition withdrawal and progression of IFALD include severity of, and recovery from, the original surgical illness and occurrence of other medical complications that can interfere with feeding, including repeated infection. Prediction of liver recovery while patients continue to receive parenteral nutrition is further complicated by the fact that no specific percentage of enteral caloric intake has been shown to prevent or reverse established IFALD,[29] presumably because protection of the liver afforded by enteral nutrition is most likely not based on the relative or absolute quantity of calories delivered into the gastrointestinal tract but, rather, on the amount of nutrients actually absorbed by the gastrointestinal tract and processed by the liver.

Only limited evidence is available to guide the clinician in considering intestinal transplantation because of persistent or apparently worsening IFALD despite an underlying potential for intestinal adaptation. The combination of cholestasis indicated by hyperbilirubinemia and portal hypertension indicated by splenomegaly and thrombocytopenia are probably the most important predictors of eventual liver failure based on the following observations: elevation

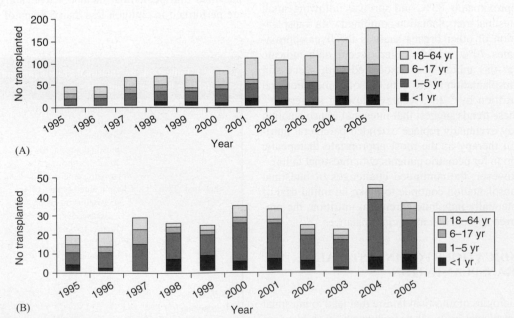

Figure 1 Annual intestinal (A) and liver/intestinal (B) transplants in the United States based on recipient age. (Source: UNOS reports; http://www.optn.org/latestData/rptStrat.asp. Based on OPTN data as of June 2, 2006.)

of total serum bilirubin concentration to around 12 mg/dL or above in patients referred for transplantation has been associated with death within 6 months,[30] and a fall in the platelet count below 100,000/μL indicates 1- and 2-year actuarial survivals of only 30% and 15%, respectively.[31] In light of long waits for transplantation following listing, referral must be made early enough to provide a reasonable opportunity for organ matching, while not unnecessarily referring patients for intestinal transplantation who have mild and self-limited cholestasis. Reconciling these objectives, the following referral criteria have been recommended by the intestinal transplant community: a total serum bilirubin concentration consistently of about 6 mg/dL and a platelet count that has fallen to 150,000 to 200,000/μL despite aggressive enteral nutrition.[18] These values are usually found by the age of 6 months in patients with intestinal failure of neonatal onset (Table 2). Some patients who meet these criteria will recover from IFALD if complete adaptation is achieved. Because hepatic recovery is generally apparent before successful donor organ procurement, referral for transplantation may be justified before permanence of parenteral nutrition and irreversibility of existing liver disease have been established unequivocally.

One obstacle to early consideration of patients for transplantation is that their appearance differs from that of patients with advanced liver disease who usually appear quite unwell. Infants with IFALD may only demonstrate jaundice and abdominal distention, as parenteral nutrition prevents malnutrition. Furthermore, hepatocellular synthetic function is less consistently impaired than bile flow early in the course of IFALD. Other than thrombocytopenia secondary to marked splenomegaly, the only other consistent sign of portal hypertension accompanying IFALD is bleeding from the mucocutaneous interface of abdominal wall stomas, which usually indicates very advanced liver disease. In contrast with end-stage liver disease associated with a normal gastrointestinal tract, large esophagogastric varices and hemodynamically significant ascites are unusual with end-stage IFALD, probably because of the marked reduction in superior mesenteric vein blood flow associated with absence of all or most of the midgut.[3,32]

Loss of Central Venous Access

Patients with intestinal failure who have not developed progressive IFALD remain at risk of death as a result of technical complications of parenteral nutrition delivery. The most obvious challenge is maintenance of indefinite central venous catheterization, since venous thrombosis is closely associated with catheter-related blood stream infection, a common occurrence in patients with intestinal failure.[33] Coincidental genetic thrombophilia may increase the cumulative risk of venous occlusion.[34] Four central venous access sites are routinely available in infants, the two internal jugular and two subclavian veins. In older patients, central access via the femoral veins is generally

feasible. The degree of lost venous access that defines parenteral nutrition failure is influenced by two principles from the perspective of intestinal transplantation. First, morbidity and mortality of transplant candidates and recipients increase when central venous catheter placement is inordinately difficult.[35] Second, central venous access may be needed for a prolonged period after transplant, up to several weeks to months. For these reasons, the prevailing philosophy of most transplant centers is, somewhat arbitrarily, that *loss of half of all central venous access sites in the setting of permanent parenteral nutrition* despite optimal catheter care provided by a center with expertise in intestinal rehabilitation is sufficient to recommend intestinal transplantation.[18] Determining patency of central venous access generally requires venography; ultrasonography is less sensitive.[36] Magnetic resonance imaging has largely replaced conventional fluoroscopy for this purpose.

Recurring, Life-Threatening Blood Stream or Metastatic Infection

The position of the American Society of Transplantation is that repeated life-threatening infection, both within the bloodstream or elsewhere, in the setting of protracted central vein catheterization despite presumably optimal management by an intestinal rehabilitation center justifies consideration of intestinal transplantation.[18] The source of infection in affected patients is rarely known with certainly but potentially results from repeated external catheter contamination and vascular seeding from a chronically ischemic, inflamed, and/or dysmotile bowel.[37,38] The total number of infections, sites of infection distant from the blood stream, or specific infective agents that are necessary to meet this indication for intestinal transplantation remains undefined. Occurrence of spleen or brain abscess and endocarditis are probably appropriate indications for transplant once infection has been eradicated. It is also highly desirable that patients with recurring infections be considered for transplantation before they are colonized with highly resistant bacteria such as extended spectrum beta-lactamase–producing coliforms and vancomycin-resistant enterococci, because these pathogens are often extremely difficult to manage successfully in immunosuppressed patients, particularly those with poor vascular access. In practice, recurring infection is rarely the sole indicator of parenteral nutrition failure; rather, recurring infection typically coexists with, and accelerates the tempo of, progressive liver failure and declining vascular access in vicious cycle.

Intra-Abdominal Neoplastic Disease

There are isolated reports of intra-abdominal congenital malformations for which cure may require near-complete bowel resection, resulting in a greatly increased risk of secondary liver failure.[39] More commonly, this situation arises in adolescent patients with familial adenomatous polyposis and colectomy who have developed extensive intra-abdominal and pelvic desmoid

tumors.[40] Immediate referral for intestinal transplantation is justified in these patients, because absence of the alimentary tract beyond the esophagus or stomach is not only a major risk for liver failure but also for repeated life-threatening fluid and electrolyte imbalances. In contrast with intestinal transplantation for desmoid tumors that are only locally invasive, transplantation for intra-abdominal neoplasms that have produced distant metastases is contraindicated.

EVALUATION FOR TRANSPLANT

The decision to list a patient for intestinal transplantation is based on several factors that include (1) a clear and convincing indication for the operation based on the foregoing considerations, (2) absence of contraindicating comorbid disorders, and (3) establishing that the intended recipient's family has or shall have a social support structure that shall permit them to deliver appropriate postoperative care.

Confirmation of an Indication for Intestinal Transplant

In most cases, need for intestinal transplantation is obvious based on an unequivocal diagnosis of anatomic or functional intestinal failure that predicts little or no tolerance of enteral nutrition and high risk of rapidly progressive IFALD or future inability to deliver parenteral nutrition. On other occasions, need for intestinal transplant may be uncertain at referral. Useful testing may include endoscopic biopsy, as demonstration of a relatively atrophic mucosa despite enteral nutrition implies a low probability for additional rehabilitation, particularly if functional studies such as plasma citrulline concentration are not encouraging.[41] Conversely, contrast radiography of the upper and lower gastrointestinal tracts may reveal new or evolving stricture, stenosis, or dysfunctional segments that indicate intestinal reconstruction, stoma closure, or related procedures rather than immediate listing for transplant.[42,43]

Isolated intestinal versus Combined liver and Intestinal Transplantation

Isolated intestinal transplantation may be indicated to interdict progressive IFALD at a mild, reversible stage. The usual clinical scenario is an increasing total serum bilirubin concentration that remains less than 10 mg/dL, mild splenomegaly, and a platelet count in the low–normal range,[44] whereas the combination of severe hepatosplenomegaly, hyperbilirubinemia that often exceeds 10 mg/dL, and thrombocytopenia not attributable to recent infection, with or without recurring gastrointestinal tract hemorrhage and coagulopathy indicate inclusion of liver in the proposed transplant. When severity of liver disease is ambiguous based on clinical and laboratory data, biopsy may discriminate mild from advanced and irreversible disease. Historically, fully established cirrhosis or extensive, that is grade 3, bridging fibrosis indicates liver (and intestinal) transplantation, while purely portal fibrosis (grade 1) or portal plus mild bridging fibrosis (grade 2) supports isolated intestinal transplantation.[45] In practice, liver biopsy has a limited role in decision making, because initially mild IFALD often worsens dramatically during the usually prolonged wait for an allograft. Regression of fibrosis after isolated intestinal transplant is inconsistent.[46] A risk of isolated intestinal transplant in the setting of moderate-to-severe liver disease is precipitation of early postoperative hepatic decompensation.

There remains some uncertainty concerning the role of isolated liver transplantation for pediatric patients partially dependent on parenteral nutrition with impending hepatic decompensation; some may have the potential to end parenteral nutrition following restoration of normal liver function. Clinical experience suggests that reasonable criteria for, and optimal outcome from, isolated liver transplantation consist of tolerance of a minimum of 50% of necessary calories via the gastrointestinal tract at evaluation and sufficient intestinal length to predict little or no parenteral nutrient requirement after transplant.[47]

Inclusion of Additional Organs in the Transplant

A "multivisceral transplant" includes *stomach, duodenum, and pancreas* with a small intestinal transplant. Multivisceral transplantation is most often performed in infants and children because of profound gastroduodenal dysmotility that has often produced historically greater intolerance of oral or gastric than jejunal feeding. Foregut disease may be primary as in chronic idiopathic intestinal pseudo-obstruction or secondary to extensive neonatal necrotizing enterocolitis and congenital anomalies; desmoid tumors involving the foregut in patients with familial adenomatous polyposis are also in this category.[48] Assessment may include contrast fluoroscopy of the upper gastrointestinal tract, nuclear gastroduodenal imaging, and, in ambiguous cases, antroduodenal manometry. Patients with desmoid tumors may benefit from evaluation at a transplant center at initial diagnosis in order to coordinate tumor and bowel resection with transplantation.[40] Because presence of the colon in continuity with small bowel substantially improves body fluid and electrolyte conservation, *colon* transplantation is highly desirable for patients lacking both functional small and large intestine, including those with long-segment Hirschsprung's disease, intestinal pseudo-obstruction, and familial adenomatous polyposis.[49] Although initial results of colonic transplantation were disappointing, current experience indicates that the colon can be included in a composite allograft with no additional morbidity.[50]

Venous Access

During the transplant evaluation, a plan for maintaining adequate central venous access in the perioperative period can be formulated that may include dilatation and stenting of partially thrombosed vessels.[35] Rarely, inability to guarantee adequate venous access contraindicates intestinal transplantation.

Assessment of Comorbid Disorders

Cardiac Function. Formal cardiac evaluation is generally indicated for all intestinal transplant candidates in light of the potential for structural cardiovascular disease associated with protracted central venous catheterization and for subtle congenital anomalies, presence of which may be overshadowed by intestinal failure. When congenital or acquired cardiovascular disease necessitates surgical intervention, the transplant and cardiovascular teams must jointly determine whether repair should be attempted before or after the transplant.

Pulmonary Function. A history of chronic respiratory disease is relatively common in pediatric candidates for intestinal transplantation owing to the frequency of extreme prematurity associated with necrotizing enterocolitis. Most relevant to transplant surgery is past or current oxygen dependence. A history of lung disease before transplant is likely to prolong mechanical ventilation after transplant significantly and to increase the probability of tracheostomy. X-rays or computed tomography of the chest are generally indicated at evaluation as well as echocardiography to assess secondary right ventricular hypertrophy and pulmonary hypertension. Pulmonary function tests may be useful if available. Sustained oxygen dependence (room air saturation <92 to 93%) is probably the most common reason to decline transplant.

Renal Function. Intestinal failure predisposes to renal insufficiency.[51] Contributory factors include repeated exposure to nephrotoxic drugs, for example, aminoglycoside antibiotics, chronic underhydration, and conjugated hyperbilirubinemia in patients with IFALD.[52] Significant urinary tract dilatation and renal dysfunction are common features of some intestinal dysmotility syndromes such as megacystis-microcolon-hypoperistalsis syndrome. Assessment of renal function during evaluation is essential, because pre-existing renal impairment complicates perioperative fluid management and amplifies the nephrotoxic effects of numerous essential drugs, notably tacrolimus. Ultrasound or computed tomography of the kidneys is an essential part of evaluation to detect renal atrophy, nephrocalcinosis, or hydronephrosis. Since plasma urea nitrogen and creatinine concentrations are relatively insensitive measures of renal function, nuclear renal imaging may be useful. Markedly impaired renal function may require formulation of alternative immunosuppressive and infection prophylaxis strategies or concurrent kidney transplantation.[26]

Neurodevelopmental Function. Concerns about intellectual functioning most commonly arise in infants with intestinal failure that results from necrotizing enterocolitis associated with extreme prematurity. Less often, neuromuscular and developmental disabilities may be severe enough to contraindicate intestinal transplantation, including syndromic Hirschsprung's disease and mitochondrial diseases such as mitochondrial neurogastrointestinal encephalomyopathy (MNGIE) syndrome.[53,54] In the absence of precise guidelines that define the magnitude of disability that should contraindicate transplant, most centers follow the dictum that the patient should be functional enough, both at referral and for the foreseeable future, obviously to obtain improved life quality from the operation.[5] Developmental assessment is useful for all pediatric intestinal transplant candidates. Testing of visual acuity and hearing is important before transplant to guide future rehabilitation. Additional studies such as magnetic resonance imaging of the brain are obtained in selected individuals based on history and examination.

Psychosocial Status. Care of the pediatric intestinal transplant recipient following hospital discharge to home is complicated and demanding, initially exceeding the challenge of caring for the patient with intestinal failure. The transplant center is obliged to estimate the ability of a patient's family to deliver adequate posttransplant care, to initiate supportive or corrective interventions in concert with the referring center where possible, and potentially to deny transplantation if a family provides clear and ongoing indications that it is not likely to be able to deliver adequate care and if alternate care arrangements cannot be made in conjunction with social service agencies. The key predictor of successful family care after transplant is successful family care before referral. Events that cast doubt about a family's willingness or ability to care for an intestinal transplant recipient include a history of delayed hospital discharge due to an inadequate home environment, reliance on professional home health providers to perform basic tasks such as connecting and disconnecting parenteral nutrition infusions, and previous involvement of child protective agencies.

Infection and Immune Status. As with transplantation of other organs, the frequency of, and dangers posed by, opportunistic infections after intestinal transplantation require determination of susceptibility to primary infection and reactivation of latent infection with agents that include but are not limited to herpes simplex virus,[55] varicella zoster,[56] cytomegalovirus (CMV),[57] Epstein–Barr virus (EBV),[58] hepatitis C virus,[59] and Toxoplasma gondii.[60] Serological testing may not accurately indicate disease susceptibility in candidates less than 1 year of age on account of persisting maternal antibodies. A negative test for human immunodeficiency virus is generally mandatory before listing. The not infrequent necessity of transplantation under the age of 1 year undermines completion of pretransplant immunization against agents that include hepatitis A virus and varicella.[61] Some transplant centers also perform an initial screen for anti-HLA antibodies, production of which is promoted by frequent blood transfusions that are common with advanced IFALD. Because a high titer of anti-

HLA antibodies has been associated with adverse outcomes in intestinal transplantation,[62] depletion of these antibodies before transplant may be considered during evaluation.[63,64]

Intestinal Transplantation Versus Rehabilitation Versus Continued Parenteral Nutrition Therapy

Pediatric patients who are referred to an intestinal transplant center and are candidates for the procedure are placed on a national wait list for organ matching (the United Network for Organ Sharing or "UNOS" in the United States). Thereafter, approximately one-third to two-thirds of listed patients will match with an appropriate allograft.[65–67] Approximately 25 to 50% of all patients listed for intestinal transplant die while on the wait list, usually those patients in need of a liver as well as intestinal allograft who have succumbed to septic complications of liver failure. Approximately 10% of patients are either not listed for transplant or removed from the list for several possible reasons, including apparent resolution or stabilization of IFALD with continued partial parenteral nutrition, successful rehabilitation despite early onset of IFALD and initially poor enteral feeding tolerance, and, rarely, a parental decision to decline transplantation.[68] Pediatric patients with intestinal failure are increasingly receiving medical care at regional centers that provide comprehensive parenteral nutrition, rehabilitation including nontransplant corrective surgery, and transplant services when indicated. The purported benefit of this approach is the ability to transition patients from one pathway to another seamlessly as dictated by changing medical conditions and guided by the experience and expertise of the center in several distinct but inter-related disciplines.[65–67,69]

EVALUATION OF THE INTESTINAL TRANSPLANT DONOR

Criteria for judging the suitability of potential intestinal allografts are similar to those employed in transplantation of other solid organs. Items of particular importance in intestinal transplantation include the following.

Major Blood Group Matching

ABO-identical donor and recipient blood types are preferred. However, transplantation of an ABO-compatible allograft is acceptable for critically ill patients needing a combined liver and intestinal transplant, because inclusion of liver in a composite allograft may reduce the potential for antibody-mediated rejection and hemolytic reactions. Nonidentical ABO-compatible donor–recipients matches are generally discouraged in isolated intestinal transplantation.[70,71]

Donor Size Review

Selecting an intestinal allograft of appropriate size is essential for successful transplantation.

An allograft that is oversized for the recipient abdominal cavity may preclude tension-free, primary abdominal closure that is required for adequate allograft perfusion. The ideal donor-to-recipient body–weight ratio is only about 50 to 67% for recipients with short-bowel syndrome on account of the reduction in abdominal cavity volume, referred to as "loss of domain," resulting from intestinal loss.[77] Even massive hepatosplenomegaly associated with severe IFALD only partially compensates for intestinal loss.

Donor History Review

Once donor major blood group and size are deemed acceptable, the transplant team considers premorbid and in-hospital donor history. A history of inflammatory bowel disease, failure to thrive potentially referable to the gastrointestinal tract, feeding intolerance, suspected inborn errors of metabolism, and previous gastrointestinal operations are associated with poor intestinal allograft quality as is recent abdominal trauma; transplantation of intestine procured from these patients is generally avoided. In the case of trauma, abdominal computed tomography is essential to screen for visceral injury. Recent apparently infectious enteritis or respiratory tract disease involving either the potential donor or the close family members may also preclude acceptance for transplantation because of the risk of infecting the recipient. Hemodynamic stability of the donating individual before and after death minimizes the risk of allograft ischemia that is also associated with poor transplant outcome. Potential donors with a history of cardiac arrest, hypotension, or substantial catecholamine requirement before procurement are generally avoided as are those with symptoms suggestive of ischemic enteropathy such as ileus or hematochezia. Conversely, a history of enteral feeding tolerance just prior to death and the absence of ileus thereafter suggest preserved postmortem alimentary tract integrity and suitability for grafting.

Lymphocytotoxic Crossmatching

Testing recipient serum against donor lymphocytes before surgery is often performed, because a positive crossmatch that identifies preformed, anti-HLA antibodies in the recipient against donor T lymphocytes may be associated with increased incidence and severity of acute rejection, particularly when liver is not included in the composite allograft. These antibodies may be removed or inactivated before, during, and/or after transplantation using methods that include intravenous immunoglobulin therapy and plasmapheresis.[63]

SURGERY OF THE INTESTINAL TRANSPLANT RECIPIENT

Establishment of Adequate Vascular Access

The potential for hemodynamic instability associated with massive blood loss, particularly in recipients who are in liver failure, demands capacious intravenous access. Obtaining adequate

vascular access for an intestinal transplant may be extremely challenging when loss of access is the indication for the operation. As many patients have thrombosis of both the inferior and the superior vena cava, interventional radiological placement of translumbar, azygous, or transhepatic lines before transplantation or intraoperative placement of retrohepatic vena caval lines or other techniques may be required.[73]

Recipient Surgical Technique: Isolated Intestinal Transplantation

There are two technical options in isolated intestinal transplantation based on whether allograft venous outflow is directed to the native portal venous system, that is, mesenteric vascular reconstruction, or shunted to the inferior vena cava, that is, systemic vascular reconstruction (Figure 2). The underlying recipient intestinal disease, severity of IFALD, and recipient venous anatomy determine which of the two reconstruction methods are utilized, as the choice has no impact on nutritional outcome.[1,74–76] *Mesenteric vascular reconstruction* is generally appropriate for isolated intestinal transplant recipients with congenital secretory diarrhea syndromes and pseudo-obstruction, in whom presence of all or most native small intestine preserves mesenteric vasculature. Mesenteric reconstruction is also required when thrombosis of the recipient inferior vena cava secondary to previous catheterization precludes systemic vascular reconstruction. In contrast with functional intestinal failure, most patients with short-bowel syndrome require *systemic vascular reconstruction*, because loss of

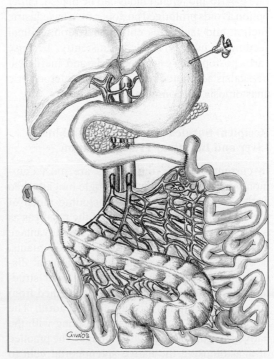

Figure 2 Isolated intestinal transplant using systemic vascular reconstruction (inferior vena cava) with short extension vascular grafts. Allograft is in color, native viscera are shaded. Proximal and distal enteric continuity are obtained with a jejunojejunostomy and distal chimney ileocolostomy, respectively.

all or most of the midgut produces an undersized recipient portal venous system that cannot accommodate the high-volume mesenteric venous outflow emanating from an intact midgut, that is, the allograft. Hepatic fibrosis, albeit insufficient to justify concurrent liver transplantation, also contraindicates mesenteric vascular reconstruction, not only because of the risk of inducing hepatic decompensation, but also because secondary portal hypertension may lead to acute intestinal allograft congestion and necrosis.[77] Arterial flow to the isolated intestinal allograft is established directly from the recipient infrarenal aorta; the technical challenge is obtaining a tension-free anastomosis under the weight of bowel that avoids the sequence of arterial traction, thrombosis, and necrosis of the allograft. Another key technical objective essential to good, early allograft function is ligation of tissues around the base of the mesentery in order to prevent posttransplant chylous ascites.[78]

Allograft continuity with remnant native gut is usually established proximally beyond the native ligament of Treitz. However, a native-to-recipient duodenojejunostomy can be performed if native jejunum is inadequate. Distal continuity is routinely established in conjunction with formation of an ileostomy that provides access for surveillance endoscopy. A twin lumen, that is, loop, ileostomy may be constructed, the efferent limb of which is anastomosed to the native left colon. Alternatively, a single lumen "chimney" ileostomy with internal end-to-side anastomosis to native colon may be performed. The transplant is completed with placement of one or more abdominal drains plus tubes for intestinal lumen access; a combined gastrojejunal tube or separate gastric and jejunal tubes can be placed; either option avoids prolonged postoperative nasogastric suction and facilitates enteral nutrition. Jejunal feeding is usually needed transiently, because early postoperative gastroparesis and inefficient peristalsis across the native-to-graft enteroenteric anastomosis are common.[79,80]

Recipient Surgical Technique: Combined Liver and Intestinal Transplantation

In current practice, the organs are most commonly implanted en bloc as a single unit attached at the porta hepatis, thereby including much of the donor duodenum and head of the pancreas as a composite allograft (Figure 3). The advantage of the en bloc technique, particularly for infants, is that it avoids biliary and hepatic arterial dissection that can easily injure small hilar structures.[81–83] Arterial blood flow is established from either the infrarenal or supraceliac aorta. The native spleen is usually preserved along with the native foregut and requires drainage. The practice of anastomosing the native splenoportal vein to the allograft portal vein has been superseded by routine construction of a native-to-native portocaval shunt.[84,85] Cholecystectomy is routine, and enteral continuity is accomplished in the same manner as in isolated intestinal transplantation.

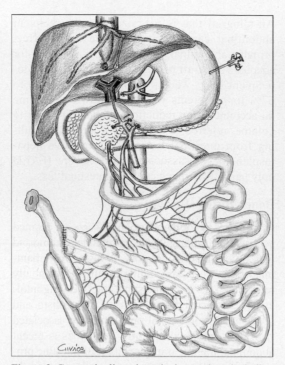

Figure 3 Composite liver–intestinal transplant, including duodenum and head of pancreas. Allograft is in color, native viscera are shaded. Gastrointestinal reconstruction as shown in Figure 2. Native portocaval shunt, which is deep to the porta hepatis, is not shown.

Recipient Surgical Technique: Multivisceral Transplantation

Multivisceral intestinal transplantation differs from combined liver and intestinal transplantation in that the entire splanchnic circulation is removed as a consequence of resection of the pancreas, spleen, stomach, root of the intestinal mesentery, and, often, the liver, obviating the need for a native-to-native portosystemic shunt (Figure 3). Allograft hepatic veins are anastomosed to the recipient inferior vena cava, and the allograft celiac and superior mesenteric arteries may be anastomosed to their corresponding recipient vessels. Alternatively, arterial flow to the allograft may be accomplished with a single anastomosis of donor infrarenal aorta to the infrarenal aorta of the recipient. Gut lumen continuity may be established proximally with anastomosis of the native esophagus to the cardia of the gastric allograft, although proximal gastrogastric anastomosis may reduce the risk of anastomotic leak.[86] Pyloroplasty promotes emptying of the denervated stomach. Gastric decompression is mandatory, usually with a combined gastrojejunal tube that allows early feeding into the graft jejunum. Distal enteral continuity is reestablished with ileostomy construction and colon anastomosis as described above (Figure 4).

MANAGEMENT FOLLOWING INTESTINAL TRANSPLANTATION

Postoperative Management

Patients undergoing isolated intestinal transplantation are generally not critically ill at the time of surgery, and the early postoperative course is

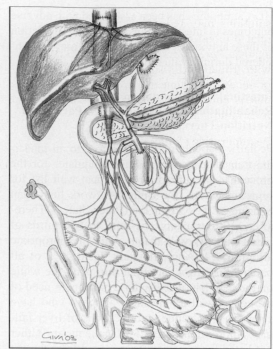

Figure 4 Multivisceral transplant with "piggyback" hepatic venous drainage to native inferior vena cava and an inflow conduit from the recipient infrarenal aorta. A gastrogastric anastomosis and standard distal reconstruction (see Figure 2) are employed. A pyloroplasty facilitates gastric drainage.

similar to that following any major abdominal operation. Extubation is usually accomplished within 24 to 48 hours. In contrast, recovery following a combined liver and intestinal transplant is often prolonged, since the operation has taken place in the setting of preoperative liver as well as intestinal failure that typically includes renal insufficiency, fluid overload, infection, and protracted hemodynamic stress; mechanical ventilation may be required for several weeks. In all intestinal transplant variants, marked intraabdominal third space fluid losses are typical and require aggressive fluid resuscitation within the first 24 to 36 postoperative hours. The challenge in the intensive care unit is to maintain hemodynamic stability and fluid balance in a way that optimizes allograft and renal perfusion but avoids persistent and frank pulmonary fluid overload that prolongs mechanical ventilation. Blood flow to the allograft may be assessed by frequent Doppler ultrasound of the ileostomy at the bedside, whereas overlying bowel gas limits the utility of transabdominal ultrasonongraphy. The intestinal vasculature is sensitive to vasoconstricting agents, particularly alpha-adrenergic agonists that should be avoided.

Routine posttransplant medical therapy typically includes a proton pump inhibitor to forestall development of acute gastric mucosal erosive hemorrhage.[87] Broad-spectrum prophylactic antibacterial and antifungal therapy is maintained for several days to a few weeks after transplant; endoscopic confirmation of allograft mucosal integrity and initial tolerance of enteral nutrition may serve as thresholds for discontinuation. Increasing use of antibiotic and ethanol lock solutions may reduce occurrence of catheter-related blood stream infections.[88,89] Prophylaxis against *Pneumocystis carinii* is accomplished with trimethoprim-sulfamethoxazole or, in the presence of continued bone marrow suppression that is common in patients with pretransplant liver failure, intravenous pentamidine.

Postoperative Complications

Important early postoperative problems directly related to surgery, summarized in Table 5, are similar to those that can follow major abdominal surgery in any chronically ill patient but are influenced by two factors unique to intestinal transplantation: placement into the abdominal cavity of a nonsterile organ(s) and coincident initiation of massive immunosuppressive therapy. Major concerns include spontaneous, that is, nonperforating peritonitis, abdominal/pelvic abscess, perforation with secondary peritonitis, pleural effusion, hemorrhage, chylous ascites, and bowel obstruction. Computerized tomography of the abdomen and pelvis using gastrojejunal and intravenous contrast, and also the chest as appropriate, is generally indicated when there is a possibility of surgical complication. Spontaneous peritonitis and infected fluid collections often occur 1 to 2 weeks after transplant, that is, after initiation of feeding and removal of abdominal drains. Symptoms and signs are usually subtle, presumably as a consequence of concurrent immunosuppressive therapy, and may include minimal abdominal wall tenderness or guarding, abdominal wall erythema, stoma breakdown or wound dehiscence, elevation of baseline body temperature often insufficient to constitute a true fever, and a mild increase in heart or respiratory rate. An increase in the absolute neutrophil count with bandemia and feeding intolerance are inconsistent. Suspected peritonitis without a discrete fluid collection demonstrated by body imaging commonly requires surgical exploration to establish the diagnosis and to ascertain if there has been vascular compromise of the allograft associated with arterial or venous thrombosis or perforation. Spontaneous bowel perforation is uncommon but most often occurs in the proximal jejunal allograft or distal native small bowel remnant. Perforation may also be precipitated by mural compression from the tip of an appropriately positioned gastrojejunal feeding tube. Disproportionately

greater ischemia–reperfusion injury in the upper bowel may explain this tendency. Diagnosis of perforation can be challenging, as symptoms and signs of perforation may be minimal and plain X-rays insensitive; computerized tomography is most useful.

When imaging demonstrates one or more fluid collections that may be infected, guided percutaneous drainage and antibiotic therapy based on culture results often obviates the need for surgical exploration. The majority of postoperative infections are bacterial.[90,91] A single species of virtually any class including coliforms, pseudomonads, staphylococci, or enterococci is usually cultured in the setting of nonperforating peritonitis.[92] Candida species may be documented as well, usually later in the postoperative course. Transient pleural effusion is common early after intestinal transplantation, usually an expression of body fluid overload in the setting of assisted ventilation and deep sedation. Clinical suspicion of infected pleural fluid requires drainage with culture; confirmed infection within the left pleural space is especially common following multivisceral transplantation, possibly because this procedure includes splenectomy.

Postoperative bleeding may be intraluminal in origin, generally at a bowel anastomosis. Bleeding into the abdomen is most often observed in the early postoperative period following a liver and intestinal transplant and is first suggested by appearance of fresh blood in an abdominal drain. Torrential bleeding from a discrete vessel may be the culprit and require surgical exploration. Alternatively, coagulopathic postoperative bleeding is often transient and typically responds to transfusion alone. Chylous ascites is most often avoidable with appropriate surgical technique and early avoidance of an enteral diet rich in long-chain triglycerides. The abdominal drain is usually left in place until enteral feeding tolerance has been established (see below). In contrast with other surgical complications that are generally early postoperative occurrences, mechanical bowel obstruction generally occurs late in intestinal transplantation. Rare causes of early obstruction include ileostomy kink and adhesive attachment of the stomach or proximal small bowel allograft to the liver surface.[93] Most commonly, late obstruction results from generalized or focal stricture or stenosis associated with severe acute or chronic allograft rejection (see below). Simple adhesions may also produce late obstruction sporadically, particularly in the vicinity of the allograft to native enterocolonic anastomosis.

Enteral Nutrition

In the absence of significant postoperative cardiopulmonary instability or surgical complications that require abdominal exploration, ileus generally resolves within 3 to 5 days at which time enteral feeding, generally with an amino acid or peptide formula, is introduced and increased gradually thereafter. Formulas with reduced long-chain triglyceride content or

enriched with medium-chain triglycerides are often used, since lymphatic drainage cannot be established surgically, for example, Vivonex RTF or Peptinex.[94] Parenteral nutrition, which is usually reintroduced 2 or 3 days postoperatively, is tapered as enteral feeding is increased. Intestinal allograft transit is generally rapid, which has been attributed to allograft denervation that removes the inhibitory influence of the central nervous system on bowel motility.[79] Antiperistaltic agents such as loperamide (Imodium), alone or in combination with diphenoxylate-atropine (Lomotil), are almost always necessary to reduce stoma effluent volume, generally to less than 30 to 40 mL/kg/d, in order to permit gradual reduction in intravenous fluid therapy.[95] Side effects of these agents that include abdominal distention, vomiting, and lethargy are rare, even in small infants. In the absence of allograft dysfunction that is mainly due to rejection, respiratory instability, or sepsis, total caloric needs can usually be delivered entirely through the allograft within 4 weeks.

The objective of intestinal transplantation is acquisition or restoration of the ability to consume an unrestricted or minimally restricted, age-appropriate diet. Within certain limitations, this objective eventually can be met in most patients. Continued tolerance of enteral feeding is also a practical, ongoing test of allograft function. Once total enteral nutrition has been established with an amino acid or peptide formula, a polymeric formula or mixed diet may be substituted, and improving gastric emptying usually permits transition from jejunal to gastric or oral feeding. Infants who have eaten little or nothing by mouth prior to intestinal transplantation tend to remain dependent on formula feeding delivered by tube for several years. Extensive occupational therapy may be necessary to teach these children to eat. Retroperitoneal lymphatic drainage develops by 4 to 6 weeks after transplant, improving tolerance of a regular diet or standard formula.[94] However, fried foods often continue to produce diarrhea that is only partially responsive to antiperistaltic drugs even when allograft histology is normal. High osmolality, sugary fluids also often increase stool output dramatically in intestinal transplant recipients of all ages. In many patients, this phenomenon may improve or resolve over time. Experience has demonstrated that when the diet is nutritionally complete and allograft function is good, vitamin and mineral supplementation is not routinely necessary with the specific exception of iron. It is unclear whether high iron requirements are due to frequent blood sampling, occult bleeding from an otherwise intact allograft, or poor iron absorption.

Immunosuppressive Therapy

Although there are many variations in immunosuppressive practices among transplant centers, there are also numerous areas of consensus, including (1) the need for allograft lymphocyte

Table 5 Surgical Complications Following Intestinal Transplantation	
Type	Incidence (%)
Reoperation for any reason	58–68
Bacteremia	29–93
Abdominal/pelvic abscess	4–27
Chylous ascites	12
Bowel obstruction	12
Perforation	12
Hemorrhage	7
Thrombosis	5
Spontaneous peritonitis	4–6

depletion before implantation, (2) the benefit of antibody induction for the recipient, and (3) the continued suitability of the calcineurin-inhibitor tacrolimus (Prograf)-based immunosuppression in most instances. Allograft lymphocyte depletion is most commonly accomplished by treatment of the donating individual with antilymphocyte globulin, usually Thymoglobulin, before removal of the bowel.[15] Tacrolimus dose and frequency of administration are based on achieving a whole blood trough concentration initially of around 15 to 25 µg/L. Induction antibody therapy for the recipient generally employs either a lymphocyte-depleting agent such as Thymoglobulin or alem-tuzumab (Campath) or an agent that inhibits activated IL-2 receptor, either daclizumab (Zenapax) or basiliximab (Simulect).[4] Intravenous corticosteroids as methylprednisolone are given in high dose for several days, later replaced by prednisone or prednisolone.

In the absence of allograft rejection, both corticosteroids and tacrolimus are gradually reduced during the first posttransplant year by 50 to 75%.[80] Some programs favor steroid discontinuation if allograft rejection has been absent or infrequent for an extended period, while others favor minimal or no maintenance steroid therapy from the beginning when Thymoglobulin is used for initial induction.[96] Because of the side effects and limitations of prolonged, high-dose tacrolimus therapy in preventing allograft rejection, another immunosuppressive agent is often added. The rationale is that low doses of two drugs, with or without corticosteroids, are both safer and more efficacious than a high dose of a single agent. Sirolimus, also known as rapamycin (Rapamune), is usually favored based on established efficacy and bioavailability.[97]

Surveillance of the Allograft

Protocol endoscopy of the allograft is an essential component of intestinal transplant care, given the absence of a sensitive and specific blood or other noninvasive indicator of incipient or established allograft rejection.[80] The intent of endoscopic surveillance is detection of rejection while still histologically mild, asymptomatic or minimally symptomatic, and presumably reversible with only modest intensification of immunosuppressive therapy. Surveillance endoscopy is generally done once or twice weekly for the first few postoperative weeks and then at least biweekly to monthly for several months thereafter.

Endoscopy is typically performed via the ileostomy; findings are usually representative of the entire allograft.[98] Ileoscopy in infants and children generally utilizes a gastroscope inserted 5 to 20 cm into the allograft. Two to four specimens are taken for histology and an additional specimen often for viral culture. Use of 1.8 mm forceps may be preferable because of the increased risk of intramural and luminal hemorrhage from the allograft compared to native small bowel, even when blood coagulation is normal. If the native colon is anastomosed to the ileal allograft within a short distance from the exterior, inspection and biopsy of the colon is helpful for detection of opportunistic infection and, much less often, graft-versus-host disease. Endoscopy of the proximal, that is, duodenojejunal, side of the allograft is generally performed when new symptoms are present that are not adequately explained by ileoscopy findings, when ileoscopy findings are ambiguous, or when determination of the extent of an abnormality such as allograft rejection will influence therapy. If the upper native to graft anastomosis is located distal to the native duodenum, intubation of the allograft may be facilitated if an infant gastroscope can be passed through the gastrostomy orifice.

Adverse Immunological Events

Immune-mediated intestinal allograft injury is complex and remains incompletely understood. Several types of injury and their putative mechanisms have been described. Most probably results primarily from activation of recipient cell-mediated immunity; the role of host antibody-mediated events is less certain.[62,99] Including liver in the composite allograft appears to reduce frequency and severity of intestinal rejection.[2] Mechanisms by which the liver allograft could increase tolerance of the bowel allograft by the recipient immune system remain obscure. Including a liver allograft may reduce perioperative ischemia–reperfusion injury of the bowel, thereby reducing its immunogenicity.[100,101] The liver allograft may also promote clearance of sensitized recipient lymphocytes. These events may depend on maintenance of physiological perfusion of the liver by en bloc implantation of the composite allograft.[102] Alternatively, results reported by the Miami group indicate a reduced propensity for severe rejection and a corresponding survival benefit from multivisceral transplantation irrespective of whether the composite allograft includes liver, presumably owing to removal of the spleen during the procedure.[103]

Acute intestinal allograft rejection by the host is relatively well defined clinically and histologically.[104] This form of allograft injury is most common within the first few months after transplant. When corticosteroids and calcineurin inhibitors, tacrolimus and before that, cyclosporine, were the only drugs available for maintenance, immunosuppressive therapy and antibody induction was not routinely employed, prevalence of acute allograft rejection was high, at least 80 to 90%, and death was common.[3] Recently, prevalence of allograft rejection has fallen significantly, as low as 20 to 40%, and is now only rarely severely enough to result in allograft loss and/or death of the patient.[103] The immunopathological process is roughly the reverse of intestinal graft-versus-host disease following bone marrow or stem cell transplantation, and clinical features are similar. Clinical stages of acute intestinal allograft rejection are summarized in Table 6, and the consensus microscopic grading system for acute intestinal allograft rejection is summarized in greater detail in Table 7.[105] In general, light microscopy demonstrates early changes of acute rejection before standard endoscopy. Zoom endoscopy may permit visual recognition of pathological findings simultaneously with the microscopic, although the large caliber of currently available zoom endoscopes typically precludes their use in infants and small children.[106] The earliest (zoom) endoscopic features of *mild allograft rejection* are mild and focal widening and erythema of the crypts. At this stage, standard endoscopy generally reveals no abnormalities. Contemporaneous pinch biopsies reveal increased crypt enterocyte apoptosis along with a mild increase in lympho-

Table 6 Clinical Sequence of Acute Allograft Rejection

	Symptoms	Endoscopy	Biopsy	Treatment
Indeterminate	• None	• None	• Minimal chronic inflammation • Rare apoptosis	• None
Mild	• None, or • Mildly increased stoma output	• None, or • Crypt widening and erythema (zoom endoscopy)	• Common apoptosis (>6/high power field) • Mild chronic inflammation • Intact villi • Intact crypts	• Pulsed steroids for 2 to 3 d • Higher tacrolimus level
Moderate	• Markedly increased stoma output • Vomiting	• Focal ulceration • Erythema and villus atrophy	• Apoptotic crypt destruction • Severe chronic inflammation	• Sustained pulsed steroids • Higher tacrolimus level • Antilymphocyte globulin
Severe	• Bloody stoma output • Systemic inflammatory response • Abdominal pain	• Confluent ulceration • Exfoliated mucosa	• Granulation tissue • Little or no recognizable mucosa	• Sustained pulsed steroids • Antilymphocyte globulin

Table 7 Consensus Grading System for Acute Intestinal Allograft Rejection

Indeterminate for acute cellular rejection
- Minor focal epithelial injury with minimal chronic inflammation
- Fewer than 6 apoptotic bodies per 10 crypt cross-sections

Mild acute cellular rejection
- Mild crypt injury with mucin depletion, hyperplasia, and unequivocally increased crypt enterocyte apoptosis = greater than 6 apoptotic bodies per 10 crypt cross-sections
- Mild-to-moderate mixed chronic inflammatory infiltrate
- Mild villus blunting and distortion

Moderate acute cellular rejection
- Multiple apoptotic bodies per crypt (confluent apoptosis) producing focal crypt destruction
- Moderate-to-severe mixed chronic inflammatory infiltrate
- Villus blunting, edema, and focal erosion

Severe acute cellular rejection
- Severe mucosal injury with focal to extensive crypt loss resulting in less prominent crypt apoptosis than in milder rejection grades.
- Severe mixed chronic and acute inflammation
- Extensive villus epithelial erosion or ulceration with granulation tissue replacing recognizable mucosa

Adapted from Kato et al.[103]

cytes, plasma cells, and eosinophils in adjacent lamina propria (Figure 5A). These lesions may be generalized or focal with intervening areas of entirely normal mucosa. Symptoms are often absent at this stage.

Undetected and/or untreated, mild rejection progresses to *moderate acute rejection*, as increased apoptotic crypt destruction is accompanied by flattening and widening of villi and a denser, mixed chronic inflammatory cell infiltrate in the lamina propria. Focal villus erosion may be present. Standard endoscopy often demonstrates mild erythema and focal erosion that can be easily missed (Figure 5B). At this stage, ileostomy (or rectal) output predictably increases, often markedly, over baseline, but frank hematochezia is usually absent. Bilious emesis is common, however, which probably results from reduced motility and increased enterocyte fluid secretion that accompanies the inflammation.

Severe acute allograft rejection supervenes when progressive crypt destruction and intense inflammation that includes a polymorphonuclear leukocyte infiltrate produces deep ulceration with areas of granulation tissue completely devoid of crypts. More extensive ulceration leads to mucosa–submucosa separation that results in a characteristic peeling or exfoliation of the mucosa, either regionally or throughout the entire allograft (Figure 5C). Mucosal exfoliation exposes large areas of submucosa to the gut lumen that fills with plugs of compressed necrotic mucosa (Figure 5D). Ileostomy output that contains mucosal plugs also usually contains visible blood. Progression to severe acute rejection is

almost always accompanied by hypoalbuminemia and occasionally by fever and leukocytosis with left shift. Patients with severe, acute allograft rejection experience profound abdominal pain that is likely the result of peritonitis associated with inflammation of allograft serosa and mesentery. Abdominal distention resulting from dilatation and mural edema of the allograft is typical. Intestinal rejection can vary in severity between different regions of the allograft and also within individual loops of bowel in the same region, both in visual and microscopic appearance.[93,98] In practice, classification of rejection tends to be based on appearance of the most severely affected portion of the allograft, particularly as relates to treatment.

Successful *treatment of acute allograft rejection* depends on early diagnosis. For mild histological rejection associated with few if any symptoms or visual endoscopic changes, several intravenous boluses of methylprednisolone may resolve inflammation and clear apoptosis, after which the trough tacrolimus level is often elevated by 33 to 50%. When visible endoscopic abnormalities are associated with moderately or severely abnormal histology, early administration of the most potent antilymphocyte antibody preparations available, most commonly Thymoglobulin, is much more likely to be required to restore the allograft to normal. Antitumor necrosis factor-alpha therapy (infliximab) has also been used in treatment of severe, acute intestinal allograft rejection, although its precise role in relation to conventional therapy remains ill-defined.[107] Exfoliating allograft rejection is often refractory to all forms of intervention, and mortality resulting from this complication continues to be very high.[108] In contrast, occurrence of mild or moderate rejection does not appear directly to affect patient survival.[103]

Less well defined in intestinal transplantation is *chronic allograft rejection*. The hallmark of chronic rejection of any transplanted organ is obliterative endarteriopathy, a myointimal hyperplasia that, in the intestinal allograft, affects submucosal and mesenteric arteries. The outcome is progressive intestinal ischemia, fibrosis, stricture, and eventual allograft loss.[93] It is gener-

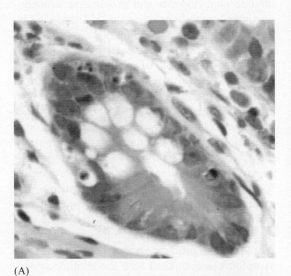

(A)

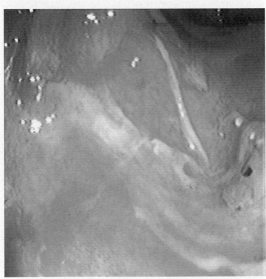

(C)

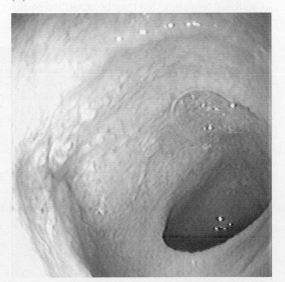

(B)

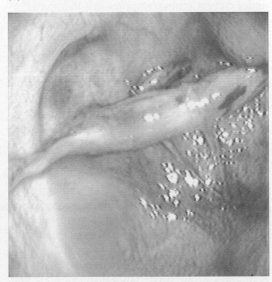

(D)

Figure 5 Endoscopic features of allograft rejection. (A) Photomicrograph of allograft mucosal biopsy demonstrating increased numbers of crypt enterocyte apoptotic bodies (arrows) (hematoxylin and eosin stain; original magnification ×400). (B) Moderate rejection with focal erosion. (C) Severe rejection with early mucosal exfoliation. (D) Exfoliative rejection with plug of necrotic mucosa in lumen.

ally recognized no earlier than 6 to 12 months after transplant. Although cell-mediated rather than antibody-mediated events are thought to predominate in chronic intestinal rejection,[62] it does not generally respond to heightened conventional immunosuppressive therapy. Chronic rejection may present acutely with symptoms of obstruction related to focal allograft stenosis and stricture, sometimes producing perforation and fistula. More commonly, chronic rejection develops surreptitiously with gradually worsening diarrhea, malabsorption, and weight loss absent any evidence of protracted intestinal infection. Occasionally, episodes of superimposed acute rejection unresponsive to heightened immunosuppressive therapy may suggest the cause. Diagnosis of chronic rejection is often difficult, because endoscopy may be normal or demonstrate only subjective changes of tortuosity and reduced mural compliance accompanied by nonspecific inflammatory change. Chronic allograft rejection may also be suggested by radiological imaging of the allograft that reveals focal or more generalized dilatation and stricture. Confirmation generally requires full-thickness allograft biopsy or explantation and indicates retransplantation with interval resumption of parenteral nutrition. Ulceration of terminal ileal mucosa or allograft to native colonic anastomosis may be accompanied by extensive mesenteritis and mesenteric fibrosis in the absence of pathognomonic obliterative endarteriopathy, but whether these findings represent a variant form of chronic allograft rejection or a different immunological or nonimmunological disorder remains controversial.[109–112] In the presence of focal or multiple allograft ulcerations, opportunistic infection with agents such as CMV, EBV, and Mycobacterial species must always be excluded[113] (see below).

Stomach and colon rejection may develop when these organs are part of the allograft but occur less commonly and with lesser severity than concomitant rejection of the small bowel under current immunosuppressive therapies.[98,114] Similarly, *rejection of the liver* component of a composite allograft in the absence of any indication of intestinal allograft rejection is unusual, simply because aggregate immunosuppressive therapy that successfully protects the bowel from rejection is much greater than usually required for the liver.[115] However, periodic self-limited elevation of serum aminotransferase and cholestatic enzyme levels occurs in over half of recipients of a multivisceral transplant that includes a liver allograft and at least one-quarter of recipients of an isolated intestinal allograft.[116] Parenteral nutrition appears to be responsible in many cases; hepatotoxic drugs also probably contribute, but there is no definable cause in at least one-half of occurrences.

Early results of experimental intestinal transplantation using small laboratory animals suggested that *graft-versus-host disease* would constitute a major impediment in clinical practice. These concerns have proven to be unwarranted, as clinically apparent graft-versus-host disease

is uncommon in human intestinal transplantation with a reported incidence of around 5%, presumably because the magnitude of immunosuppression required to prevent allograft rejection is sufficient to eliminate offending immunocompetent cells from the allograft in most circumstances.[3] Incidence may be increased in multivisceral as compared to isolated intestinal or combined liver and intestinal transplantation.[103] Involvement of the native remnant gastrointestinal tract and skin are most common. Colonic graft-versus-host disease may present with blood-streaked diarrhea. Graft-versus-host disease arising within the esophagus is suggested by a new refusal to swallow or chest pain, although viral or fungal infection of the esophagus more commonly causes these symptoms.[117] Ulceration within the buccal cavity may also be present. Endoscopy and biopsy confirm the diagnosis, demonstrating focal or extensive mucosal exfoliation in native gut in advanced cases that appears similar to severe rejection of the allograft. An erythematous, maculopapular, and desquamating skin rash concentrated in the extremities and skin folds suggests cutaneous graft-versus-host disease.[118] Other manifestations include pancytopenia and progressive bronchopneumonia with hypoxemia and infiltrates but no evidence of an infectious etiology.[119,120]

Dietary protein hypersensitivities, particularly to cow milk but also other common allergens, are relatively frequent following intestinal transplantation in infants and young children with an incidence of at least 10%.[121] A similar phenomenon occurs following isolated liver transplantation.[122] Several factors may contribute to the occurrence of food allergies following solid-organ transplantation, including the propensity for tacrolimus to increase intestinal mucosa permeability and, presumably, dietary protein antigen uptake. Enhanced food antigen contact with the immature immune system may be inherently more prone to produce an aberrant response with symptoms as compared with the immune system of adults, a tendency that may be amplified by the

immunomodulatory properties of tacrolimus.[123] Transplantation of the intestine per se probably independently increases mucosal permeability to food antigens,[79] although an increased incidence of food allergies in intestinal transplant as compared to pediatric liver transplant recipients has not been proven. Symptoms include chronic diarrhea and weight loss as well as urticaria, hives, and pruritis.[121] As in recipients of an isolated liver allograft,[122] eosinophilic enterocolitis may be demonstrable that may suggest allograft rejection, but involvement of both allograft and native bowel points to the correct etiology. Diagnostic testing for specific food allergens is often unrevealing.

NONIMMUNE COMPLICATIONS OF INTESTINAL TRANSPLANTATION

Allograft-Specific Infection

Viral infections, particularly those that involve the allograft, are the greatest source of morbidity in pediatric intestinal transplantation not directly connected with rejection. The most important agents are summarized in Table 8. What distinguishes viral infection in highly immunosuppressed intestinal transplant patients is the severity and often protracted nature of symptoms rather than prevalence of infection, which is probably no greater than in the general pediatric population. Viruses that infect the gastrointestinal tract fall into two categories, those that have little or no affinity for other tissues, for example, rotavirus, and those that commonly infect and produce disease elsewhere. Within the gastrointestinal tract, pathogens have particular affinity for engrafted tissue, presumably because the recipient immune system mounts a less efficient response in sites bearing HLA-dissimilar antigens.[124]

Although intestine-specific viruses are a major source of morbidity based on severity and duration of diarrhea, they do not produce severe and/or permanent allograft injury that threatens

Table 8 Viral Infections Commonly Involving the Intestinal Allograft

	Symptoms	Other Sites	Diagnosis
Enterotropic			
Rotavirus	• Osmotic diarrhea • Secretory diarrhea (rare)	• ? Liver	• Stool enzyme immunoassay
Calicivirus (norovirus)	• Secretory diarrhea	• ? Liver	• Stool (or biopsy) RNA PCR
Systemic			
Cytomegalorvirus	• Osmotic or bloody diarrhea • Sepsis syndrome	• Lungs • Liver • Eyes	• Histology/immunochemistry • Tissue culture • Blood DNA PCR
Epstein–Barr virus	• Bloody diarrhea • Bowel obstruction • Sepsis syndrome	• Head and neck • Chest • Abdomen • Pelvis • Subcutaneous	• Histology/immunochemistry • Body imaging • Blood DNA PCR
Adenovirus	• Osmotic diarrhea • Secretory diarrhea (rare) • Sepsis syndrome	• Upper respiratory tract • Lower respiratory tract • Liver	• Histology/immunochemistry • Tissue culture • Stool enzyme immunoassay • Blood DNA PCR

allograft destruction or death of the patient.[124] The most important enterotropic viruses described in intestinal transplantation include the rotaviruses and caliciviruses, the most important members of which are the *Noroviruses*.[125] Although other agents such as astroviruses have been described in immunosuppressed populations,[126] they have yet to be reported following intestinal transplantation. Symptoms are similar irrespective of the particular responsible agent, consisting primarily of an abrupt onset of profuse, often secretory, watery diarrhea. Hematochezia is virtually never present, whereas fever and vomiting are inconsistent, mainly at the outset of symptoms. Although potentially a feature of any viral enteropathy, extraordinarily high stoma output that exceeds 100 mL/kg/d is especially characteristic of calicivirus enteritis.[125] Histological features of acute viral enteritis are similar irrespective of cause and include villus atrophy and a mixed acute and chronic inflammatory infiltrate in the lamina propria. Increased crypt apoptosis is also common to a degree that can simulate allograft rejection. However, calicivirus enteritis can often be distinguished from allograft rejection by certain unique features not characteristic of rejection that include flattening and pseudostratification of villus enterocytes, apoptosis of villus in addition to crypt enterocytes, and also apoptosis of macrophages in villus lamina propria (Figure 6).

Accurate diagnosis of viral enteritis is important for several reasons. First, evidence of a viral etiology for increased stoma or stool output reduces the probability of allograft rejection and emphasizes the importance of reducing immunosuppressive therapy to clear the infection. Second, a positive viral diagnosis in the setting of severe secretory diarrhea suggests that duration of feeding intolerance shall be lengthy, up to several weeks, which implies that a period of parenteral nutrition will be required. Third, at least in the case of rotavirus, intravenous immunoglobulin therapy delivered via the gastrointestinal tract might be indicated, although no data have been presented that show efficacy in the intestinal transplant recipient population. Timely and accurate viral diagnosis often represents a challenge for the clinician. Although PCR methodology provides greater sensitivity, fecal enzyme immunoassay for antigen is adequate in clinical practice for rotavirus.[124,127] The standard method for diagnosis of calicivirus enteritis is demonstration of virus-specific RNA in stool or intestinal biopsy material based on reverse transcription and PCR amplification of genomic sequences, as currently available enzyme immunoassays lack sensitivity.[128] Historically performed primarily by state and other governmental health agencies, commercial PCR testing has recently become available (Focus Diagnostics Inc., Cypress, CA, USA).

Allograft Infection with Systemic Viruses

The three most important agents in this category affecting pediatric intestinal transplant recipients

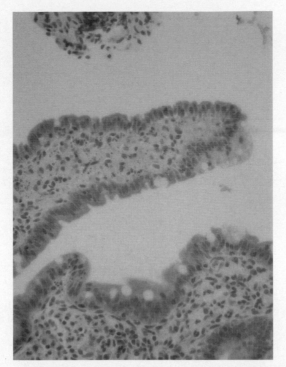

Figure 6 Photomicrograph of allograft mucosa with enteritis, positive for calicivirus RNA. Note reduction in villus goblet cells, disarray of villus enterocytes, and increased numbers of villus enterocyte and lamina propria apoptotic bodies (hematoxylin and eosin stain; original magnification ×400).

are CMV, EBV, and adenovirus. Theses viruses are important causes of allograft loss or patient death, not only because of the potential magnitude of allograft injury, but also because of their propensity to damage other vital organs including the liver, respiratory tract, and central nervous system. With all of these agents, however, the intestinal allograft is often the first apparent site of disease.

The highest risk scenario for acquiring CMV infection in solid-organ transplantation is that of a latently infected, that is, seropositive, allograft being placed into a CMV-naive, that is, seronegative, recipient.[129] Conversely, the cohort at lowest risk for acquisition of CMV disease is the group of seronegative recipients of seronegative allografts.[130] In practice, CMV-immune status of donor and recipient do not substantially influence patient management, which includes routine posttransplant monitoring for viremia and prophylaxis against primary infection or reactivation for all patients.[79,131] Either an antigen assay, for example, pp65, or DNA detection can be used for surveillance, at weekly to biweekly intervals for the first several postoperative months and less frequently thereafter. There is no consensus concerning optimal type and duration of posttransplant prophylaxis; intravenous ganciclovir, enteral ganciclovir or valganciclovir, and CMV immune globulin are routinely administered in varying combinations, usually for 3 to 12 months.

Following cessation of anti–CMV prophylaxis, detection of new viremia generally prompts resumption of therapy preemptively. The choice of therapy, usually either intravenous ganciclo-

vir or oral valganciclovir, is usually made based on the intensity of prevailing immunosuppressive therapy, magnitude of the viremia (or rate of rise on repetitive and quantitative sampling), and on simultaneous appearance of symptoms suggestive of early tissue invasion; more threatening infection favors the intravenous route. The objective of preemptive therapy is to suppress new or reactivated viral proliferation before deep tissue invasion occurs. Because the intestinal allograft is often the initial target of invasion, it should be assessed with pan-endoscopy if there is any possibility of invasive disease; wireless capsule endoscopy may supplement conventional endoscopy for this task. Incidence of CMV disease in pediatric intestinal transplantation is currently about 5%.[96] Surveillance monitoring of blood for CMV and preemptive treatment of confirmed viremia may fail; CMV disease, particularly enteritis, may appear without warning as the interval between onset of viremia and local tissue invasion may be short. A key diagnostic feature of CMV enteritis is the often bloody quality of diarrhea that results from deep allograft ulceration associated with infection of vascular endothelium and local tissue ischemia[132] (Figure 7). Spontaneous perforation can occur. Appearance of nuclear and cytoplasmic CMV inclusion bodies in infected endothelial and other lamina propria cells is characteristic; enterocytes are generally spared. Development of invasive CMV disease in native tissues including remnant native alimentary tract is inconsistent. Invasive CMV disease generally requires intravenous ganciclovir therapy. In addition, immunosuppressive therapy is usually reduced, since invasive disease implies excess immune suppression. Emergence of ganciclovir-resistant CMV is an increasing problem in solid-organ transplantation and requires use of alternatives, particularly foscarnet and cidofovir.[133,134]

EBV infection is important, because it can lead to development of posttransplant lymphoproliferative disease (PTLPD). PTLPD is a single or multifocal proliferation of EBV-transformed B lymphocytes that is made possible by depletion

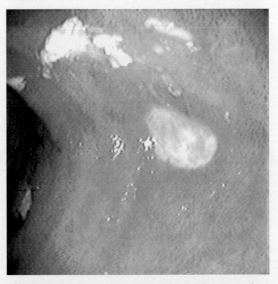

Figure 7 Severe CMV allograft enteritis. Note deep ulceration and surrounding erythema.

of EBV-specific T lymphocytes as a result of immunosuppressive therapy. In the past, when most intestinal transplant recipients experienced at least one episode of allograft rejection and received numerous courses of high-dose intravenous corticosteroids, incidence of PTLPD was extraordinarily high in comparison with other solid-organ transplants, around 30%.[78] Presently, incidence of PTLPD in intestinal transplantation is about 5 to 10%,[4,96,103] the decline resulting not only from a reduced prevalence of severe allograft rejection, but also widespread availability of EBV surveillance methods based on detection of viral genomes in peripheral blood.[135] Like blood testing for CMV, the objective of EBV surveillance is to detect and respond to a new or worsening viremia before symptoms of invasive EBV disease or transition to PTLPD develop. Although EBV-seronegative recipients of a seropositive allograft may be at greatest risk of developing PTLPD, recipients who are EBV seropositive before transplant are also at significant risk.[58] Surveillance for PTLPD may fail, because it occasionally develops in the allograft or elsewhere with no or minimal viremia.[136]

Initial symptoms of EBV infection not necessarily complicated by PTLPD are nonspecific and include fever, rash, and neutropenia. Any indication of rapidly increasing lymphoid mass effect, either in natural sites such as the tonsils and adenoids, atypical locations such as the lungs, or in the native remnant gut or allograft must be assumed to be PTLPD until proven otherwise, whether or not viremia is present. Gastrointestinal PTLPD appears as intramural masses of variable size, single, or clustered. They generally have a central umbilication, with or without overlying mucosal ulceration (Figure 8A) and, like CMV infection in the gastrointestinal tract, can produce bleeding or perforation (Figure 8B). Asymptomatic gastrointestinal PTLPD may be detected during protocol endoscopic surveillance for allograft rejection or during endoscopy indicated by partial intestinal obstruction, feeding intolerance, bleeding, and fever of obscure cause. Standard initial response to asymptomatic viremia includes preemptive reduction of immunosuppression and resumption of ganciclovir therapy, although efficacy of antiviral therapy for EBV in solid-organ transplantation remains controversial.[135,137] The greater propensity for the intestinal allograft to be rejected compared to the isolated liver allograft severely constrains reducing immunosuppression, which has traditionally served as the impetus for a more aggressive approach to treatment of PTLPD in intestinal transplant recipients utilizing chemotherapy, often based on cyclophosphamide.[138] Recently, recognition of the safety and efficacy of monoclonal anti–B lymphocyte antibody therapy (rituximab, Rituxan) has made this agent a practical alternative to immediate chemotherapy, as overall response approximates 50 to 70%.[139–142]

Adenovirus is a common pathogen in infants and young children but not older patients following intestinal transplantation, incidence

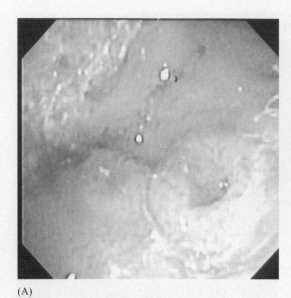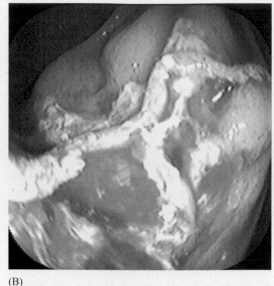

(A)   (B)

Figure 8 Gastrointestinal EBV-associated posttransplant lymphoproliferative disease. (A) Note protruberant intramural masses with central umbilication. (B) Note large, ulcerated and hemorrhagic mass.

of infection being as high as around 20%.[143,144] Although capable of infecting numerous organs that include lungs and liver, the main site of adenovirus infection is the intestinal allograft itself. As with CMV and EBV, allograft infection with adenovirus can probably be acquired in several ways. Latent infection may be present within the recipient before transplant or introduced to the recipient by latent infection of the allograft, later activating in either situation under the influence of immunosuppressive therapy. Alternatively, adenovirus can produce primary infection at any time after transplant. Like the enterotropic viruses, the primary site of infection is the population of villus enterocytes, where tissue invasion can be identified by characteristic intranuclear inclusions.[145] Recently, adenovirus infection of lamina propria stromal cells has also been shown.[146] Infection progresses to invasive intestinal disease in about half of cases. Fever commonly accompanies or precedes gastrointestinal symptoms, although severity of diarrhea is often less than observed with calicivirus or rotavirus enteritis. The endoscopic appearance of adenovirus enteritis in intestinal transplantation is that of either normal or variably erythematous mucosa with scant thin exudates.[145] Ulceration and bleeding are uncommon, and native bowel is usually spared. Usual duration of symptoms is about 1 to 2 weeks, and temporary reduction in immunosuppression appears to promote viral clearance. The risk of death from adenovirus relates primarily to the risk of systemic infection and multiple-organ involvement, which is partly related to intensity of recent immunosuppressive therapy, particularly corticosteroids.[143] Cidofovir has been increasingly employed for treatment of severe local or systemic disease, although unequivocal proof of efficacy has yet to be presented.[147,148]

Other Morbidities

Additional challenges, encountered to variable degrees in all pediatric solid-organ transplant recipients, include the potential for diabetes mellitus, hypertension, hyperlipidemia, drug-induced renal insufficiency, late malignancy, impaired linear growth, developmental delay, and impaired socialization. These complications and their etiologies are summarized in Table 9. In general, the better the function of the allograft and the lesser the immunosuppression needed, the lower the probability that these complications shall occur and/or the faster they shall resolve after transplant. Although posttransplant diabetes requires indefinite insulin therapy in some patients, most episodes of glucose intolerance are confined to periods of intensified corticosteroid therapy for rejection. The risk of end-stage kidney disease that requires dialysis or transplantation following liver transplantation of adult patients is thought to be about 8% after 10 years,

Table 9 Other Posttransplant Morbidities

Problem	Etiology
Diabetes mellitus	Corticosteroid therapy, tacrolimus, genetic predisposition
Progressive renal insufficiency	Tacrolimus ± sirolimus therapy
Hypertension	Corticosteroid therapy, tacrolimus, renal insufficiency
Hyperlipidemias (hypertriglyceridemia, hypercholesterolemia)	Corticosteroid therapy, sirolimus
Impaired growth	Corticosteroid therapy, poor allograft function/ chronic rejection
Developmental delay	Disabling and protracted intestinal (± liver) failure before transplant, prolonged perioperative recovery, poor allograft function/chronic rejection
Late malignancy	Cumulative immunosuppression

largely due to calcineurin inhibitor toxicity.[149] Whether this is a reasonable estimate for pediatric patients following intestinal transplantation is unclear at present. This risk has emphasized the importance of ongoing reappraisal of immunosuppressive therapy relative to the perceived risk of rejection; minimization of immunosuppression is the objective whenever possible. Hyperlipidemia is occasionally sufficiently severe and prolonged to justify statin or fibrate therapy, usually in the setting of chronic renal insufficiency, recurring rejection, and intense corticosteroid therapy. Although risks associated with opportunistic infection have been most heavily emphasized, long-standing suppression of the immune system also impairs neoplasm surveillance, producing a long-term risk of nonlymphoid as well as hematological malignancies that include adenocarcinoma and skin cancer.[150]

Growth and Development after Intestinal Transplantation

There is relatively little information available concerning body size at the time of intestinal or combined liver and intestinal transplantation because of heretofore limited opportunities for long-term follow-up. The value of reported data over time may be suspect, given the rapid evolution of clinical practices, including nutrition support and immunosuppressive therapy, and of clinical outcomes, including occurrence of allograft rejection. Nonetheless, some generalizations apply. Impaired linear growth is typically present at transplant, reported mean height Z-scores ranging between −2.8 and −1.8.[151–153] It is intuitive that growth should be more impaired in patients with both liver and intestinal failure compared to those with intestinal failure alone,[154] although this supposition remains unproven.[155] Presumably because patients awaiting intestinal transplantation are supported with parenteral nutrition by definition, impairments in weight at transplant are usually somewhat less profound than impairments in height; reported weight Z-scores ranging between −2.6 and −1.0.[151–153]

Patients who obtain good allograft function within a few months after transplant that permits ending of parenteral nutrition and who continue to require little or no supplemental intravenous fluids during subsequent years have demonstrated significant growth improvements in some studies[151,152] but not in others.[153,156] Selection bias may be operative, because the most striking improvements in growth occur in those patients with the most severe initial impairment, viz. height Z-scores < −2.0;[155] in one such a group, average height Z-scores increased from −4.71 at transplant to −3.59 at 1 year and −2.43 at 2 years after surgery.[103] Even when significantly improved linear growth following intestinal transplantation has been documented, eventual attainment of average to above-average body size is uncommon. Acute allograft rejection (as compared to chronic rejection) does not appear to interfere significantly with growth.[151,155]

Quality of Life after Intestinal Transplantation

Improved allograft and patient survival following intestinal transplantation in recent years has increased interest in long-term physical and psychosocial outcomes, since the ultimate objective of intestinal transplantation is rehabilitation of the patient that includes reintegration into society. Relatively little information is available concerning quality of life after intestinal transplantation in either children or adults. A return to work or school is now achieved in most patients despite rehospitalizations that are particularly frequent during the first few years after transplant.[14,157] Common sense dictates that patients and their parents should perceive improved life quality following intestinal transplantation, with or without concurrent liver transplantation, when good allograft function permits early ending of parenteral nutrition, at least some tolerance of foods by mouth, and elimination of the illnesses including recurrent infections, pain-producing procedures, and repeated hospitalizations that had originally indicated transplantation. A positive relationship between allograft function and patient perception of posttransplant life quality has, in fact, been demonstrated in adults.[158] Similarly, preadolescent patients with good allograft function have self-perceptions of physical and emotional well being that are similar to those of healthy children.[159] In contrast, parents of intestinal transplant recipients tend to perceive the functioning of their children as inferior to normal children, particularly in general and physical health and participation in family activities. Parent evaluations of their children also seem to be inferior to patients' personal assessments, perhaps reflecting an inherently greater adaptive potential of children and the relatively greater anxieties of parents.

Coordination of Care after Intestinal Transplantation

Following discharge to ambulatory status, most transplant centers insist that patients remain in their care for periods that vary from several weeks to months, since an experienced transplant center is best equipped to manage complications that remains frequent during the first several posttransplant months. These complications include episodes of fever, increased stoma output or other indications of rejection, opportunistic infection, electrolyte disturbances, and marked fluctuations in blood immunosuppressive drug concentrations. A period of relative clinical stability enables patients to return to home to the care of referring physicians or others who shall assume responsibility for digestive care. The relatively greater and more prolonged medical fragility of intestinal transplant recipients compared to other solid-organ transplant recipients requires maintenance of a close working relationship between the transplant center and referring physicians. This dictum is particularly apt for patients who live most distant from the transplant center.

There are no formal guidelines that govern how an intestinal transplant team should maintain collaboration with local physicians. Procedures will undoubtedly continue to vary based on the established practices of transplant teams, the individual interests and knowledge bases of local physicians, and ability of patients and their families to return to the transplant center for periodic follow-up. In general, most transplant centers expect to determine the immunosuppressive therapy including targeted blood levels when applicable. Surveillance endoscopy practices vary; colonoscopy, upper endoscopy, or both, is often recommended annually indefinitely and can usually be performed by the local gastroenterologist. Well patients generally undergo blood testing, including chemistries, hemograms, PCR monitoring, and immunosuppressive levels monthly to bimonthly; most transplant centers prefer to receive these data along with local physicians. Decisions concerning nutrition support, monitoring of growth and development, and management of ancillary medical problems such as glucose intolerance, renal insufficiency, and hypertension are generally made locally, the transplant center serving as consultant. Acute illness that requires hospitalization does not necessarily require transfer to the transplant center, particularly if the reason is not directly related to the transplant and if alteration of immunosuppressive therapy does not appear to be warranted. Conversely, transfer back to the transplant center is generally appropriate when there are indications of serious allograft dysfunction, for example, markedly increased fecal volume over several days without definable cause or lower gastrointestinal bleeding that suggests rejection or invasive opportunistic infection. Serious opportunistic infection elsewhere, for example, the lower respiratory tract, may also warrant transfer in the event that major reductions in immunosuppressive therapy are required.

Allograft Loss and Long-Term Outcomes of Intestinal Transplantation

Within the first posttransplant year, refractory acute rejection that requires allograft removal is the most common cause of transplant failure either that requires retransplantation (usually for the isolated intestinal transplant recipient) or results in death of the patient (usually a combined liver and intestinal or multivisceral transplant recipient). Similarly, the most common later cause of allograft loss or death is chronic allograft rejection, with or without superimposed acute rejection.[93] In all, refractory acute or chronic rejection is responsible for about one-third of postintestinal transplant deaths. Opportunistic infection not directly related to rejection is the cause of death of an additional third, and various miscellaneous causes are responsible for the remainder.[103] Severe opportunistic infections that may or may not be precipitated by intensified immunosuppressive therapy for treatment of severe rejection is most common within the first

6 months after transplantation, when immunosuppressive therapy is usually maximal but remains a risk at any time after transplant.

As noted, historical 3-year patient survival following isolated intestinal transplantation has historically exceeded survival following transplantation that includes the liver, 85 versus 70%. Superior early survival of isolated intestinal transplant recipients is undoubtedly due to performance of a less complex operation in patients without advanced liver disease.[12,13,100,160] In fact, being at home before surgery is independently associated with superior posttransplant survival compared to being in the hospital, 74 versus 59%.[4,90] Conversely, isolated intestinal transplant recipients have historically accounted for a disproportionately greater share of late allograft loss and patient mortality, likely reflecting the increased risk of chronic rejection of the isolated intestinal allograft beyond the first few years after transplant.[98,103,110] However, historical 5- and 10-year survival statistics may have little relevance to current transplant efforts,[4] because reduced early acute allograft rejection that owes to more efficacious immunosuppression may reduce late allograft loss in all types of intestinal recipients. In that event, recipients of an isolated intestinal transplant shall likely obtain the highest extended posttransplant survival rates in the future.

CONCLUSION

Intestinal transplantation represents the ultimate treatment of intestinal failure. It has not supplanted extended parenteral nutrition as the primary therapy for affected pediatric patients in light of its enormous complexities and hazards.[68,161] In the future, improving outcomes may lead to consideration of parenteral nutrition simply as a bridge to transplantation rather than a primary therapeutic modality, which is increasingly the case in adult medicine.[158] Indications for transplantation and the organs to be included in the operation require careful consideration. Intestinal transplantation may not be appropriate for all pediatric patients and their families. Families and health-care providers must recognize that, as with any solid-organ transplant, intestinal transplantation does not represent a cure in the conventional sense but, rather, is intended to convert a fatal disorder into a manageable challenge of daily living. Because long-term success in intestinal transplantation requires appropriate management of immunosuppressive therapy, nutrition, fluid and electrolyte balance, and surveillance for and treatment of allograft rejection and infection, families and health-care providers must be prepared to commit an enormous amount of physical and intellectual energy to the process indefinitely.

REFERENCES

1. Reyes J, Mazariegos GV, Bond GM, et al. Pediatric intestinal transplantation: Historical notes, principles and controversies. Pediatr Transplant 2002;6:193–207.
2. Middleton SV, Jamieson NV. The current status of small bowel transplantation in the UK and internationally. Gut 2005;54:1650–7.
3. Abu-Elmagd K, Reyes J, Bond G, et al. Clinical intestinal transplantation: A decade of experience at a single center. Ann Surg 2001;234:404–17.
4. Grant D, Abu-Elmagd K, Reyes J, et al. 2003 Report of the intestine transplant registry. Ann Surg 2005;241:607–13.
5. Goulet O, Sauvat F. Short bowel syndrome and intestinal transplantation in children. Curr Opin Clin Nutr Metab Care 2006;9:304–13.
6. Quiros-Tejeira RE, Ament ME, Reyen L, et al. Long-term parenteral nutritional support and intestinal adaptation in children with short bowel syndrome: A 25-year experience. J Pediatr 2004;145:157–63.
7. Goulet O, Baglin-Gobet S, Talbotec C, et al. Outcome and long-term growth after extensive small bowel resection in the neonatal period: A survey of 87 children. Eur J Pediatr Surg 2005;15:95–101.
8. Spencer AU, Neaga A, West B, et al. Pediatric short bowel syndrome: Redefining predictors of success. Ann Surg 2005;242:403–9.
9. Andorsky DJ, Lund DP, Lillehei CW, et al. Nutritional and other postoperative management of neonates with short bowel syndrome correlates with clinical outcomes. J Pediatr 2001;139:27–33.
10. Sondheimer JM, Cadnapaphornchai M, Sontag M, Zerbe GO. Predicting the duration of dependence on parenteral nutrition after neonatal intestinal resection. J Pediatr 1998;132:80–4.
11. Wales PW, de Silva N, Kim JH, et al. Neonatal short bowel syndrome: A cohort study. J Pediatr Surg 2005;40:755–62.
12. Fishbein TM, Matsumoto CS. Intestinal replacement therapy: Timing and indications for referral of patients to an intestinal rehabilitation and transplant program. Gastroenterology 2006;130:S147–51.
13. Farmer DG, McDiarmid SV, Edelstein S, et al. Improved outcome after intestinal transplantation at a single institution over 12 years. Transplant Proc 2004;36:303–4.
14. Sudan D. Cost and quality of life after intestinal transplantation. Gastroenterology 2006;130:S158–62.
15. Abu-Elmagd KM. Intestinal transplantation for short bowel syndrome and gastrointestinal failure: Current consensus, rewarding outcomes, and practical guidelines. Gastroenterology 2006;130:S132–7.
16. O'Keefe SJ. Candidacy for intestinal transplantation. Am J Gastroenterol 2006;101:1644–6.
17. Kelly DA. Intestinal failure-associated liver disease: What do we know? Gastroenterology 2006;130:S70–7.
18. Kaufman SS, Atkinson JB, Bianchi A, et al. Indications for pediatric intestinal transplantation: A position paper of the American Society of Transplantation. Pediatr Transplant 2001;5:80–7.
19. Kaufman SS, Loseke CA, Lupo JV, et al. Influence of bacterial overgrowth and intestinal inflammation on duration of parenteral nutrition in children with short bowel syndrome. J Pediatr 1997;131:356–61.
20. Fryer J, Pellar S, Ormond D, et al. Mortality in candidates waiting for combined liver–intestine transplants exceeds that for other candidates waiting for liver transplants. Liver Transpl 2003;9:748–53.
21. Hancock BJ, Wiseman NE. Lethal short-bowel syndrome. J Pediatr Surg 1990;25:1131–4.
22. Kurkchubasche AG, Rowe MI, Smith SD. Adaptation in short-bowel syndrome: reassessing old limits. J Pediatr Surg 1993;28:1069–71.
23. Mousa H, Hyman PE, Cocjin J, et al. Long-term outcome of congenital intestinal pseudoobstruction. Dig Dis Sci 2002;47:2298–305.
24. Ruemmele FM, Jan D, Lacaille F, et al. New perspectives for children with microvillous inclusion disease: Early small bowel transplantation. Transplantation 2004;77:1024–8.
25. Paramesh AS, Fishbein T, Tschernia A, et al. Isolated small bowel transplantation for tufting enteropathy. J Pediatr Gastroenterol Nutr 2003;36:138–40.
26. Loinaz C, Rodriguez MM, Kato T, et al. Intestinal and multivisceral transplantation in children with severe gastrointestinal dysmotility. J Pediatr Surg 2005;40:1598–604.
27. Galea MH, et al[s3]. Short-bowel syndrome: A collective review. J Pediatr Surg 1992;5:592–6
28. Messing B, et al. Long-term survival and parenteral nutrition dependence in adult patients with the short bowel syndrome. Gastroenterology 1999;117:1043–50.
29. Javid PJ, Collier S, Richardson D, et al. The role of enteral nutrition in the reversal of parenteral nutrition-associated liver dysfunction in infants. J Pediatr Surg 2005;40:1015–8.
30. Beath SV, Booth IW, Murphy MS, et al. Nutritional care and candidates for small bowel transplantation. Arch Dis Child 1995;73:348–50.
31. Bueno J, Ohwada S, Kocoshis S, et al. Factors impacting the survival of children with intestinal failure referred for intestinal transplantation. J Pediatr Surg 1999;34:27–33.
32. Kato T, Mittal N, Nishida S, et al. The role of intestinal transplantation in the management of babies with extensive gut resections. J Pediatr Surg 2003;38:145–9.
33. Timsit JF, Farkas JC, Boyer JM, et al. Central vein catheter-related thrombosis in intensive care patients: Incidence, risks factors, and relationship with catheter-related sepsis. Chest 1998;114:207–13.
34. Nowak-Göttl U, Dübbers A, Kececioglu D, et al. Factor V Leiden, protein C, and lipoprotein (a) in catheter-related thrombosis in childhood: A prospective study. J Pediatr 1997;131:608–12.
35. Rodrigues AF, van Mourik IDM, Sharif K, et al. Management of end-stage central venous access in children referred for possible small bowel transplantation. J Pediatr Gastroenterol Nutr 2006;42:427–33.
36. Shankar KR, Abernethy LJ, Das KS, et al. Magnetic resonance venography in assessing venous patency after multiple venous catheters. J Pediatr Surg 2002;37:175–9.
37. Costa SF, Miceli MH, Anaissie EJ. Mucosa or skin as source of coagulase-negative staphylococcal bacteraemia? Lancet Infect Dis 2004;4:278–86.
38. Pierro A, van Saene HK, Donnell SC, et al. Microbial translocation in neonates and infants receiving long-term parenteral nutrition. Arch Surg 1996;131:176–9.
39. Steyaert H, Guitard J, Moscovici J, et al. Abdominal cystic lymphangioma in children: Benign lesions that can have a proliferative course. J Pediatr Surg 1996;31:677–80.
40. Moon JI, Selvaggi G, Nishida S, et al. Intestinal transplantation for the treatment of neoplastic disease. J Surg Oncol 2005;92:284–91.
41. Rhoads JM, Plunkett E, Galanko J, et al. Serum citrulline levels correlate with enteral tolerance and bowel length in infants with short bowel syndrome. J Pediatr 2005;146:542–7.
42. Javid PJ, Kim HB, Duggan CP, Jaksic T. Serial transverse enteroplasty is associated with successful short-term outcomes in infants with short bowel syndrome. J Pediatr Surg 2005;40:1019–24.
43. Iyer KR, Horslen S, Torres C, et al. Functional liver recovery parallels autologous gut salvage in short bowel syndrome. J Pediatr Surg 2004;39:340–4.
44. Sudan DL, Kaufman SS, Shaw BW, Jr, et al. Isolated intestinal transplantation for intestinal failure. Am J Gastroenterol 2000;95:1506–15.
45. Beath SV, Needham SJ, Kelly DA, et al. Clinical features and prognosis of children assessed for isolated small bowel or combined small bowel and liver transplantation. J Pediatr Surg 1997;32:459–61.
46. Hasegawa T, Sasaki T, Kimura T, et al. Effects of isolated small bowel transplantation on liver dysfunction caused by intestinal failure and long-term total parenteral nutrition. Pediatr Transplant 2002;6:235–9.
47. Botha JF, Grant WJ, Torres C, et al. Isolated liver transplantation in infants with end-stage liver disease due to short bowel syndrome. Liver Transpl 2006;12:1062–6.
48. Goulet O, Sauvat F, Jan D. Surgery for pediatric patients with chronic intestinal pseudo-obstruction syndrome. J Pediatr Gastroenterol Nutr 2005;41:S66–8.
49. Goulet O, Auber F, Fourcade L, et al. Intestinal transplantation including the colon in children. Transplant Proc 2002;34:1885–6.
50. Yann R, Yves A, Dominique J, et al. Improved quality of life by combined transplantation in Hirschsprung's disease with a very long aganglionic segment. J Pediatr Surg 2003;38:422–4.
51. Lauverjat M, Hadj Aissa A, Vanhems P, et al. Chronic dehydration may impair renal function in patients with chronic intestinal failure on long-term parenteral nutrition. Clin Nutr 2006;25:75–81.
52. Buyukgebiz B, Arslan N, Ozturk Y, et al. Complication of short bowel syndrome: An infant with short bowel syndrome developing ammonium acid urate urolithiasis. Pediatr Int 2003;45:208–9.
53. Masumoto K, Arima T, Izaki T, et al. Ondine's curse associated with Hirschsprung disease and ganglioneuroblastoma. J Pediatr Gastroenterol Nutr 2002;34:83–6.
54. Nishino I, Spinazzola A, Papadimitriou A, et al. Mitochondrial neurogastrointestinal encephalomyopathy: An autosomal recessive disorder due to thymidine phosphorylase mutations. Ann Neurol 2000;47:792–800.
55. Delis S, Kato T, Ruiz P, et al. Herpes simplex colitis in a child with combined liver and small bowel transplant. Pediatr Transplant 2001;5:374–7.
56. Weinberg A, Horslen SP, Kaufman SS, et al. Safety and immunogenicity of varicella-zoster virus vaccine in pediatric liver and intestine transplant recipients. Am J Transplant 2006;6:565–8.

57. Burroughs M, Sobanjo A, Florman S, et al. Cytomegalovirus matching does not predict symptomatic disease in intestinal transplantation. Transplant Proc 2002;34:946–7.
58. Allen UD, Farkas G, Hebert D, et al. Risk factors for post-transplant lymphoproliferative disorder in pediatric patients: A case–control study. Pediatr Transplant 2005;9:450–5.
59. Tsamandas AC, Furukawa H, Abu-Elmagd K, et al. Liver allograft pathology in liver/small bowel or multivisceral recipients. Mod Pathol 1996;9:767–73.
60. Campbell AL, Goldberg CL, Magid MS, et al. First case of toxoplasmosis following small bowel transplantation and systematic review of tissue-invasive toxoplasmosis following noncardiac solid organ transplantation. Transplantation 2006;81:408-17.
61. Campbell AL, Herold BC. Immunization of pediatric solid-organ transplantation candidates: Immunizations in transplant candidates. Pediatr Transplant 2005;9:652–61.
62. Wu T, Abu-Elmagd K, Bond G, Demetris AJ. A clinicopathologic study of isolated intestinal allografts with preformed IgG lymphocytotoxic antibodies. Hum Pathol 2004;35:1332–9.
63. Tschernia A, LeLeiko NS, Grima K, et al. Anti-HLA antibody removal by extracorporeal immunoadsorption in two hyperimmunized pediatric patients awaiting hepatointestinal transplantation. Transplant Proc 2002;34:900–1.
64. Glotz D, Antoine C, Julia P, et al. Desensitization and subsequent kidney transplantation of patients using intravenous immunoglobulins (IVIg). Am J Transplant. 2002;2:758–60.
65. Fishbein TM, Schiano T, LeLeiko N, et al. An integrated approach to intestinal failure: Results of a new program with total parenteral nutrition, bowel rehabilitation, and transplantation. J Gastrointest Surg 2002;6:554–62.
66. Sudan D, DiBaise J, Torres C, et al. A multidisciplinary approach to the treatment of intestinal failure. J Gastrointest Surg 2005;9:165–76.
67. Gupte GL, Beath SV, Protheroe S, et al. Improved outcome of referrals for intestinal transplantation in the UK. Arch Dis Child 2007;92:147–52.
68. Gupte GL, Beath SV, Kelly DA, et al. Current issues in the management of intestinal failure. Arch Dis Child 2006;91:259–64.
69. Koehler AN, Yaworski JA, Gardner M, et al. Coordinated interdisciplinary management of pediatric intestinal failure: A 2-year review. J Pediatr Surg 2000;35:380–5.
70. Panaro F, DeChristopher PJ, Rondelli D, et al. Severe hemolytic anemia due to passenger lymphocytes after living-related bowel transplant. Clin Transplant 2004;18:332–5.
71. Sindhi R, Landmark J, Shaw B, et al. Combined liver/small bowel transplantation using a blood group compatible but nonidentical donor. Transplantation 1996;61:1782–3.
72. Kato T, Ruiz P, Thompson J, et al. Intestinal and multivisceral transplantation. World J Surg 2002;26:226–7.
73. Mims TT, Fishbein TM, Feierman DE. Management of a small bowel transplant with complicated central venous access in a patient with asymptomatic superior and inferior vena cava obstruction. Transplant Proc 2004;36:388–91.
74. Fishbein TM, Kaufman SS, Florman SS, et al. Isolated intestinal transplantation: Proof of clinical efficacy. Transplantation 2003;76:636–40.
75. Shaffer D, Diflo T, Love W, et al. Immunological and metabolic effects of caval versus portal drainage in small bowel transplantation. Surgery 1988;104:518–24.
76. Berney T, Kato T, Nishida S, et al. Portal versus systemic venous drainage of small bowel allografts: Comparative assessment of survival, function, rejection and bacterial translocation. J Am Coll Surg 2002;195:804–13.
77. Fishbein T, Schiano T, Jaffe D, et al. Isolated intestinal transplantation in adults with nonreconstructible GI tracts. Transplant Proc 2000;32:1231-2.
78. Reyes J, Bueno J, Kocoshis S, et al. Current status of intestinal transplantation in children. J Pediatr Surg 1998;33:243–54.
79. Pakarinen MP, Halttunen J. The physiology of the transplanted small bowel: An overview with insight into graft function. Scand J Gastroenterol 2000;35:561–77.
80. Horslen SP. Optimal management of the post-intestinal transplant patient. Gastroenterology 2006;130:S163–9.
81. Sudan D, Iyer K, Deroover A, et al. A new technique for combined liver/small intestinal transplantation. Transplantation 2001;72:1846–8.
82. Bueno J, Abu-Elmagd K, Mazariegos G, et al. Composite liver-small bowel allografts with preservation of donor duodenum and hepatic biliary system in children. J Pediatr Surg 2000; 35:2:291–6.
83. Kato T, Romero R, Verzaro R, et al. Inclusion of entire pancreas in the composite liver and intestinal graft in pediatric intestinal transplantation. Pediatr Transpl 1999;3:210–4.
84. Grant D, Wall W, Mimeault R, et al. Successful small bowel/liver transplantation. Lancet 1990;335:181–4.
85. Starzl T, Rowe M, Todo S, et al. Transplantation of multiple abdominal viscera. JAMA 1989;261:1449–57.
86. Kato T, Tzakis A, Selvaggi G, et al. Surgical techniques used in intestinal transplantation. Current Opin Organ Transpl 2004;9:207–13.
87. Kaufman SS, Lyden ER, Brown CR, et al. Omeprozole therapy in pediatric patients after liver and intestinal transplantation. J Pediatr Gastroenterol Nutr 2002;34:194–8.
88. Onland W, Shin CE, Fustar S, et al. Ethanol-lock technique for persistent bacteremia of long-term intravascular devices in pediatric patients. Arch Pediatr Adolesc Med 2006;160:1049–53.
89. Onder AM, Kato T, Simon N, et al. Prevention of catheter-related bacteremia in pediatric intestinal transplantation/short gut syndrome children with long-term central venous catheters. Pediatr Transplant 2007;11:87–93.
90. Sauvat F, Dupic L, Caldari D, et al. Factors influencing outcome after intestinal transplantation in children. Transplant Proc 2006;38:1689–91.
91. Guaraldi G, Cocchi S, Codeluppi M, et al. Outcome, incidence, and timing of infectious complications in small bowel and multivisceral organ transplantation patients. Transplantation 2005;80:1742–8.
92. Loinaz C, Kato T, Nishida S, et al. Bacterial infections after intestine and multivisceral transplantation. Transplant Proc 2003;35:1929–30.
93. Noguchi Si S, Reyes J, Mazariegos GV, et al. Pediatric intestinal transplantation: The resected allograft. Pediatr Dev Pathol 2002;5:3–21.
94. Kaufman SS, Lyden ER, Brown CR, et al. Disaccharidase activities and fat assimilation in pediatric patients after intestinal transplantation. Transplantation 2000;69:362–5.
95. Huighebaert S, Awouters F, Tytgat GN. Racecadotril versus loperamide: Antidiarrheal research revisited. Dig Dis Sci 2003;48:239–50.
96. Bond GJ, Mazariegos GV, Sindhi R, et al. Evolutionary experience with immunosuppression in pediatric intestinal transplantation. J Pediatr Surg 2005;40:274–9.
97. Gupta P, Kaufman S, Fishbein TM. Sirolimus for solid organ transplantation in children. Pediatr Transplant 2005;9:269–76.
98. Sigurdsson L, Reyes J, Todo S, et al. Anatomic variability of rejection in intestinal allografts after pediatric intestinal transplantation. J Pediatr Gastroenterol Nutr. 1998;27:403–6.
99. Zeevi A, Britz JA, Bentlejewski CA, et al. Monitoring immune function during tacrolimus tapering in small bowel transplant recipients. Transpl Immunol 2005;15:17–24.
100. Jugie M, Canioni D, Le Bihan C, et al. Study of the impact of liver transplantation on the outcome of intestinal grafts in children. Transplantation 2006;81:992–7.
101. Martins PN, Chandraker A, Tullius SG. Modifying graft immunogenicity and immune response prior to transplantation: Potential clinical applications of donor and graft treatment. Transpl Int 2006;19:351–9.
102. Meyer D, Otto C, Rummel C, et al. "Tolerogenic effect" of the liver for a small bowel allograft. Transpl Int 2000; 13:S123–6.
103. Kato T, Tzakis AG, Selvaggi G, et al. Intestinal and multivisceral transplantation in children. Ann Surg 2006;243: 756–64.
104. White FV, Reyes J, Jaffe R, Yunis EJ. Pathology of intestinal transplantation in children. Am J Surg Pathol 1995; 19:687–98.
105. Ruiz P, Bagni A, Brown R, et al. Histological criteria for the identification of acute cellular rejection in human small bowel allografts: Results of the pathology workshop at the VIII International Small Bowel Transplant Symposium. Transplant Proc 2004;36:335–7.
106. Sasaki T, Hasegawa T, Nakai H, et al. Zoom endoscopic evaluation of rejection in living-related small bowel transplantation. Transplantation 2002;73:560–4.
107. Pascher A, Klupp J, Langrehr JM, et al. Anti-TNF-alpha therapy for acute rejection in intestinal transplantation. Transplant Proc 2005;37:1635–6.
108. Ishii T, Mazariegos GV, Bueno J, et al. Exfoliative rejection after intestinal transplantation in children. Pediatr Transplant 2003;7:185–91.
109. Ruiz P, Suarez M, Nishida S, et al. Sclerosing mesenteritis in small bowel transplantation: Possible manifestation of acute vascular rejection. Transplant Proc 2003;35:3057–60.
110. Iyer KR, Srinath C, Horslen S, et al. Late graft loss and long-term outcome after isolated intestinal transplantation in children. J Pediatr Surg 2002;37:151–4.
111. Turner D, Martin S, Ngan BY, et al. Anastomotic ulceration following small bowel transplantation. Am J Transplant 2006;6:236–40.
112. Macedo C, Sindhi R, Mazariegos GV, et al. Sclerosing peritonitis after intestinal transplantation in children. Pediatr Transplant 2005;9:187–91.
113. Sarkar S, Selvaggi G, Mittal N, et al. Gastrointestinal tract ulcers in pediatric intestinal transplantation patients: Etiology and management. Pediatr Transplant 2006;10:162–7.
114. Takahashi H, Selvaggi G, Nishida S, et al. Organ-specific differences in acute rejection intensity in a multivisceral transplant. Transplantation 2006;81:297–9.
115. Lacaille F, Canioni D, Fournet JC, et al. Centrilobular necrosis in children after combined liver and small bowel transplantation. Transplantation 2002;73:252–7.
116. Ueno T, Kato T, Gaynor J, et al. Temporary elevation of serum transaminases after pediatric intestinal transplantation: Incidence and clinical correlation in multivisceral transplant vs isolated intestinal transplant. Transplant Proc 2006;38:1765 7.
117. Forrest G. Gastrointestinal infections in immunocompromised hosts. Curr Opin Gastroenterol 2004;20:16–21.
118. Mazariegos GV, Abu-Elmagd K, Jaffe R, et al. Graft versus host disease in intestinal transplantation. Am J Transplant 2004;4:1459–65.
119. Kohli-Seth R, Killu C, Amolat MJ, et al. Bronchiolitis obliterans organizing pneumonia after orthotopic liver transplantation. Liver Transpl 2004;10:456–9.
120. Assi MA, Pulido JS, Peters SG, et al. Graft-vs.-host disease in lung and other solid organ transplant recipients. Clin Transplant 2007;21:1–6.
121. Chehade M, Nowak-Wegrzyn A, Kaufman SS, et al. De novo food allergy after intestinal transplantation: a report of three cases. J Pediatr Gastroenterol Nutr 2004;38:545–7.
122. Saeed SA, Integlia MJ, Pleskow RG, et al. Tacrolimus-associated eosinophilic gastroenterocolitis in pediatric liver transplant recipients: Role of potential food allergies in pathogenesis. Pediatr Transplant 2006;10:730–5.
123. Boyle RJ, Hardikar W, Tang ML. The development of food allergy after liver transplantation. Liver Transpl 2005;11:326–30.
124. Ziring D, Tran R, Edelstein S, et al. Infectious enteritis after intestinal transplantation: Incidence, timing, and outcome. Transplantation 2005;79:702–9.
125. Kaufman SS, Chatterjee NK, Fuschino ME, et al. Characteristics of human calicivirus enteritis in intestinal transplant recipients. J Pediatr Gastroenterol Nutr 2005;40:328–33.
126. Sebire NJ, Malone M, Shah N, et al. Pathology of astrovirus associated diarrhoea in a paediatric bone marrow transplant recipient. J Clin Pathol 2004;57:1001–3.
127. Richardson S, Grimwood K, Gorrell R, et al. Extended excretion of rotavirus after severe diarrhoea in young children. Lancet 1998;351:1844–8.
128. Gonzalez GG, Liprandi F, Ludert JE. Evaluation of a commercial enzyme immunoassay for the detection of norovirus antigen in fecal samples from children with sporadic acute gastroenteritis. J Virol Methods 2006;136:289–291.
129. Freeman RB, Paya C, Pescovitz MD, et al. Risk factors for cytomegalovirus viremia and disease developing after prophylaxis in high-risk solid-organ transplant recipients. Transplantation 2004;78:1765–73.
130. Bueno J, Green M, Kocoshis S, et al. Cytomegalovirus infection after intestinal transplantation in children. Clin Infect Dis 1997;25:1078–83.
131. Pascher A, Klupp J, Schulz RJ, et al. CMV, EBV, HHV6, and HHV7 infections after intestinal transplantation without specific antiviral prophylaxis. Transplant Proc 2004;36:381–2.
132. Omori K, Hasegawa K, Ogawa M, et al. Small-bowel hemorrhage caused by cytomegalovirus vasculitis following fulminant hepatitis. J Gastroenterol. 2002;37:954–60.
133. Nogueira E, Ozaki KS, Tomiyama H, et al. The emergence of cytomegalovirus resistance to ganciclovir therapy in kidney transplant recipients. Int Immunopharmacol 2006;6:2031–7.
134. Biron KK. Antiviral drugs for cytomegalovirus diseases. Antiviral Res 2006;71:154–63.
135. Humar A, Hebert D, Davies HD, et al. A randomized trial of ganciclovir versus ganciclovir plus immune globulin for prophylaxis against Epstein–Barr virus related post-transplant lymphoproliferative disorder. Transplantation 2006;81:856–61.
136. Axelrod DA, Holmes R, Thomas SE, Magee JC. Limitations of EBV-PCR monitoring to detect EBV associated post-transplant lymphoproliferative disorder. Pediatr Transplant 2003;7:223–7.
137. Funch DP, Walker AM, Schneider G, et al. Ganciclovir and acyclovir reduce the risk of post-transplant lymphoproliferative disorder in renal transplant recipients. Am J Transplant 2005;5:2894–900.
138. Gross TG, Bucuvalas JC, Park JR, et al. Low-dose chemotherapy for Epstein–Barr virus-positive post-transplantation lymphoproliferative disease in children after solid organ transplantation. J Clin Oncol 2005;23:6481–8.
139. Elstrom RL, Andreadis C, Aqui NA, et al. Treatment of PTLD with rituximab or chemotherapy. Am J Transplant 2006;6:569–76.
140. Codeluppi M, Cocchi S, Guaraldi G, et al. Rituximab as treatment of posttransplant lymphoproliferative disorder in patients

who underwent small bowel/multivisceral transplantation: report of three cases. Transplant Proc 2005;37:2634–5.

141. Oertel SH, Verschuuren E, Reinke P, et al. Effect of anti-CD 20 antibody rituximab in patients with post-transplant lymphoproliferative disorder (PTLD). Am J Transplant 2005;5:2901–6.

142. Blaes AH, Peterson BA, Bartlett N, et al. Rituximab therapy is effective for posttransplant lymphoproliferative disorders after solid organ transplantation: Results of a phase II trial. Cancer 2005;104:1661–7.

143. Hoffman JA. Adenoviral disease in pediatric solid organ transplant recipients. Pediatr Transplant 2006;10:17–25.

144. McLaughlin GE, Delis S, Kashimawo L, et al. Adenovirus infection in pediatric liver and intestinal transplant recipients: Utility of DNA detection by PCR. Am J Transplant 2003;3:224–8.

145. Pinchoff RJ, Kaufman SS, Magid MS, et al. Adenovirus infection in pediatric small bowel transplantation recipients. Transplantation 2003;76:183–9.

146. Ozolek JA, Cieply K, Walpusk J, et al. Adenovirus infection within stromal cells in a pediatric small bowel allograft. Pediatr Dev Pathol 2006;9:321–7.

147. Ison MG. Adenovirus infections in transplant recipients. Clin Infect Dis 2006;43:331–339.

148. Neofytos D, Ojha A, Mookerjee B, et al. Treatment of adenovirus disease in stem cell transplant recipients with cidofovir. Biol Blood Marrow Transplant 2007;13:74–81.

149. Wilkinson A, Pham PT. Kidney dysfunction in the recipients of liver transplants. Liver Transpl 2005;11:S47–51.

150. Abu-Elmagd KM, Zak M, Stamos JM, et al. De novo malignancies after intestinal and multivisceral transplantation. Transplantation 2004;77:1719–25.

151. Encinas JL, Luis A, Avila LF, et al. Nutritional status after intestinal transplantation in children. Eur J Pediatr Surg 2006;16:403–6.

152. Venick RS, Farmer DG, Saikali D, et al. Nutritional outcomes following pediatric intestinal transplantation. Transplant Proc 2006;38:1718–9.

153. Iyer K, Horslen S, Iverson A, et al. Nutritional outcome and growth of children after intestinal transplantation. J Pediatr Surg 2002;37:464–6.

154. Bartosh SM, Thomas SE, Sutton MM, et al. Linear growth after pediatric liver transplantation. J Pediatr 1999;135:624–31.

155. Ueno T, Kato T, Revas K, et al. Growth after intestinal transplant in children. Transplant Proc 2006;38:1702–4.

156. Nucci AM, Barksdale EM, Beserock N, et al. Long-term nutritional outcome after pediatric intestinal transplantation. J Pediatr Surg 2002;37:460–3.

157. Sudan DL, Iverson A, Weseman RA, et al. Assessment of function, growth and development, and long-term quality of life after small bowel transplantation. Transplant Proc 2000;32:1211–2.

158. O'Keefe SJ, Emerling M, Koritsky D, et al. Nutrition and quality of life following small intestinal transplantation. Am J Gastroenterol 2007;102:1093–100.

159. Sudan D, Horslen S, Botha J, et al. Quality of life after pediatric intestinal transplantation: The perception of pediatric recipients and their parents. Am J Transplant 2004;4:407–13.

160. López-Santamaría M, Gámez M, Murcia J, et al. Intestinal transplantation in children: Differences between isolated intestinal and composite grafts. Transplant Proc 2005;37:4087–8.

161. Goulet O, Ruemmele F. Causes and management of intestinal failure in children. Gastroenterology 2006;130: S16–28.

Intestinal Tumors

23.1. Intestinal Polyps and Polyposis

Jean-François Mougenot, MD
Sylviane Olschwang, MD, PhD
Michel Peuchmaur, MD, PhD

Polyps refer to any mass projecting into the lumen of the gastrointestinal tract. However, when one refers to intestinal polyps, one usually thinks of an epithelial lesion. Histologically, epithelial polyps may be divided into two major groups: neoplastic and nonneoplastic. Neoplastic polyps include benign adenomas and malignant carcinomas. Nonneoplastic types include hamartomas as juvenile polyps, hyperplastic polyps, and inflammatory polyps. However, the term "polyp" encompasses many gastrointestinal lesions (Table 1) as submucosal lesions that also may impart a polypoid appearance to the overlying mucosa.

Occasionally, polyps in children may occur in the context of a genetic gastrointestinal polyposis disorder characterized by the presence of multiple polyps throughout the gastrointestinal tract, their histopathology, their heritability within a family, and an increase in the lifetime risk of cancer in the gastrointestinal tract and other organs. Two major categories of polyposis are recognized: adenomatous polyposis syndromes and hamartomatous polyposis syndromes (Table 2).

COLONIC POLYPS

Juvenile Polyps

Solitary polyps of the large intestine are common during childhood, usually presenting with painless rectal bleeding. These lesions, known

Table 1 Classification of Colorectal Polyps
Epithelial polyps
Adenomas
Hyperplastic polyps
Juvenile polyps
Peutz-Jeghers polyps
Nonepithelial polyps
Submucosal leiomyoma
Lymphoïd polyps
Paraganglioma
Carcinoïd tumor
Submucosal lipoma
Submucosal neurofibroma
Submucosal schwannoma
Ganglioneuroma

Table 2 Classification of Polyposis Syndromes
Adenomatous polyposis syndromes
Familial adenomatous polyposis (FAP)
Gardner syndrome
Turcot syndrome
MYH-associated polyposis
Hamartomatous polyposis syndromes
Juvenile polyposis
Bannayan-Riley-Ruvalcaba syndrome
Cowden syndrome
Peutz-Jeghers syndrome
Mixed polyposis syndrome
Hyperplastic polyposis

as juvenile polyps, are benign and carry no long-term risk of neoplasia.

Frequency

Juvenile polyps, single or multiple (<5), are the most frequent type of gastrointestinal polypoid lesion encountered in pediatric practice (97% of colonic polyps in our personal registry).[1] However, the true incidence of polyps in childhood remains unknown. Most often, juvenile polyps are diagnosed in the first decade of life.[1–3] The peak incidence occurs between 2 and 6 years of life.[1,2,4] Polyps are rare in the first year of life and much less common in children older than 10 years of age. In all studies, a male preponderance is noted.[1,2,4] All ethnic groups can be affected.[1]

Pathology

The various appellations given to juvenile polyps reflect some of the areas of uncertainty about the current understanding of the pathogenesis of these lesions: juvenile retention polyp, juvenile inflammatory polyp, and juvenile hamartomatous polyp.

Grossly, juvenile polyps usually have a smooth, bright red, friable surface that bleeds easily when traumatized. Initially sessile, 90% of juvenile polyps appear pedunculated, spherical, and mushroom-like and are attached to the colonic mucosa with a narrow stalk (Figure 1). These lesions measure 1 to 2 cm in average diameter—rarely 2 to 4 cm. The length of the

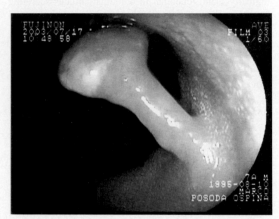

Figure 1 Pedunculated solitary juvenile polyp with a smooth, bright red, friable surface.

stalk varies from 0.5 to 1.5 cm. The base of insertion is always broader than the distal extremity. The stalk has the same color as the colonic mucosa. The colonic chicken skin mucosa, characterized by a pale yellow, speckled pattern of the colonic mucosa, resulting from lipid accumulation in lamina propria macrophages, is observed only on larger juvenile polyps in the rectosigmoid colon, most concentrated at the base of the stalk and extending to the surrounding mucosa.[2] A cut section of polyps demonstrates numerous large cystic spaces of variable size, filled with a grayish or yellowish mucus surrounded by reddish stroma—hence the term "retention" polyp.

Microscopically, juvenile polyps have a characteristic Swiss cheese appearance created by dilated mucinous lakes widely separated by abundant stroma (Figure 2). The lamina propria is infiltrated by numerous inflammatory cells, consisting of neutrophils, eosinophils, lymphocytes, plasma cells, and histiocytes with, in some cases, lymphoid follicles. In contrast to the hamartomatous polyps of Peutz-Jeghers syndrome (PJS), smooth muscle cells are not present in the stroma.[1,2,4] However, bands of smooth muscle associated with mucosal blood vessels, serrated or stellate glands with epithelial infolding, and osseous metaplasia are occasionally seen. A single layer of cytologically bland, cuboidal to columnar, mucus-secreting epithelium lines the glands. Paneth cells are present but sparse. Some glands, filled with mucus, become cystically

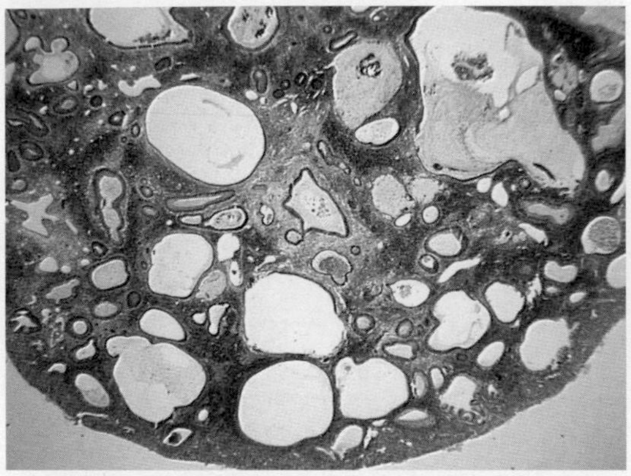

Figure 2 Juvenile polyp. Light microscopy: Swiss cheese appearance created by dilated mucinous lakes widely separated by abundant stroma. Lamina propria infiltrated by numerous inflammatory cells. A single layer of cytologically bland, cuboidal to columnar, mucus-secreting epithelium lines the glands. Hematoxylin and eosin; ×75 original magnification.

dilated. Epithelial cells demonstrate no atypia. Focal ulceration and hemorrhage may be seen.

Etiology

The etiology of the common juvenile polyp is unknown. If the usual mutations found in preneoplastic or neoplastic lesions are not found,[3] gene mutations implicated in juvenile polyposis (see "Hamartomatous Polyposis Syndromes") have been identified in solitary juvenile polyps but not in the somatic cells of patients.

Clinical Features

Intermittent painless rectal bleeding is the most common presentation. Rectal bleeding occurs during defecation. Major rectal bleeding responsible for acute anemia is a rare event, likely the result of autoamputation of pedunculated polyps. However, iron deficiency anemia is found in as many as one-third of cases.[2] Rectal bleeding is recurrent, present for over 3 months in 55% of cases.[1] Additional manifestations are unusual, including colicky abdominal pain, diarrhea with mucus, autoamputation with spontaneous extrusion, prolapse of rectal polyp, and prolapse of rectum.[1,4] Colocolic intussusception rarely occurs.

Diagnosis

By anorectal examination, lower rectal polyps are felt as firm, moderately mobile, pedunculated masses. Colonoscopy is the procedure of choice for diagnosis of colorectal polyps of all sizes. It allows resection of most polyps.[1,2,4,5] Endoscopic evaluation of the colon requires cleansing. The most effective preparations appear to be polyethylene glycol (PEG) electrolyte lavage solution, PEG alone, and Fleet Phosphosoda oral laxative used only in patients older than 12 years.[6] Although juvenile polyps may be distributed throughout the colorectum, they have a distal predominance within the rectosigmoid (70%).[1,2,5] They are more often single (73%) than multiple.[1,2,4] Because juvenile polyps are often found in the rectosigmoid but also in the proximal colon,

in front of recurrent painless rectal bleeding, and without anoperineal lesions, the preferred method for diagnosis and treatment is pancolonoscopy under anesthesia followed by snare polypectomy. Finding a polyp in the rectum does not relieve the endoscopist from the responsibility of pancolonoscopy to identify and remove additional lesions.

Treatment

Polypectomy is performed in a medicosurgical environment under anesthesia. Cold forceps resection is feasible only for tiny (1 to 2 mm) colorectal polyps. Removal with hot biopsy forceps can be used for polyps less than or equal to 4 mm in size. However, the hot biopsy forceps technique anecdotally has been associated with an unexpected high rate of perforation and delayed postpolypectomy hemorrhage. Moreover, the use of hot biopsy forceps in the right colon is five times more likely to result in complication than their use in the left colon.[5] So, the monopolar hot biopsy forceps has severe risks and has no indication in this context. An alternative is to guillotine small polyps using a snare without an electric current. Tiny snares have greatly facilitated the use of snares for removal of small sessile polyps.[7] Polyps 5 mm or larger in size should generally be removed using monopolar snare cautery. Application of detachable snare loops (Endoloop, Olympus, Tokyo, Japan) to a very large stalk (>10 mm) of pedunculated polyps has reduced the risk of delayed hemorrhage.[5,7] Immediate hemorrhage from pedunculated polyps can be managed by grasping the residual polyp stalk and holding it with a snare or by application of either a detachable snare or metallic clips (Endoclips, Olympus).[7] A 1:10,000 solution of epinephrine can be injected into the bleeding site to promote hemostasis. To stop more severe bleeding, an argon plasma coagulator may be useful. Postpolypectomy perforation (Table 3) occurs more frequently in children than in adults.[1,5,7] More than 200 procedures are reported for an endoscopist to be technically competent, and a higher complication rate appears to occur in an examiner's first 50 procedures.[5,7] Resected polyps or multiple polyp fragments are collected for histopathologic examination by suction into a trap if they are small or by using a Roth basket, and, if unsuccessful, soon after colonoscopy by colorectal enema. Although the risk of development of malignancy in a solitary polyp is very small, such polyps should be removed, even when discovered incidentally. It is important to emphasize that polyp histology

cannot be predicted by gross appearance alone. Forceps biopsies performed through the endoscope only have a yield of correct histologic diagnosis in 75% of patients.[5]

In general, juvenile polyps do not tend to recur. However, in a large pediatric retrospective serie, recurrence was observed in 4%.[1] The risk of malignant change for a solitary juvenile polyp is almost negligible. There are only eight cases of patients developing neoplasia in the literature.[8] In addition, a review of 82 patients with a solitary juvenile polyp showed no increased risk for colorectal cancer or of dying as result of the polyp.[9] So, if a polyp is found to be solitary after full colonoscopy and if there is no relevant family history, endoscopic polypectomy is sufficient treatment. Parents must be aware that juvenile polyps may be the first feature of juvenile polyposis. If fresh symptoms arise, the child should be reinvestigated. However, when there is a positive family history or when multiple juvenile polyps are found, the possibility of juvenile polyposis syndrome (JPS) is raised. Multiple juvenile polyps are associated with a risk of colon neoplasia,[8] but the precise number that statistically increases cancer risk is unknown. Three or more juvenile polyps or any number of polyps occurring in the context of a family of juvenile polyposis or colon cancer have been proposed as a criterion for a risk of colon cancer.[8]

Serrated and Hyperplastic Polyps

Colorectal serrated polyps characterized by a sawtooth architectural pattern include the classical hyperplastic polyps and the much rare traditional serrated adenomas (Figure 3), mixed polyps and sessile serrated adenomas (Table 4).[10–12]

Hyperplastic polyps rarely occur in children: 3% in our personal series of single and multiple polyps.[1] They appear as single or multiple dewdrop mucosal elevations with a smooth convex surface, arising on the mucosal crest, usually less than 5 mm, and mainly in the rectosigmoid. These small lesions are asymptomatic. When a small polyp (<5 mm) is encountered during flexible sigmoidoscopy, it should be biopsied to ascertain whether it represents a true hyperplastic polyp or an adenoma. A hyperplastic polyp is not, by itself, an indication for further colonoscopy or follow-up in childhood.

The recently described sessile serrated adenomas need to be thoroughly investigated by gastroenterologists and pathologists.[13,14] Certain serrated polyps, very rarely observed in childhood, can progress to cancer and the molecular phenotype of different subtypes introduces the concept of "serrated neoplastic pathway" in the development of colorectal cancer (Table 4).[11,12]

Isolated Adenomas

Whereas in adult patients, the relationship between adenomatous polyps and adenocarcinomas has been extensively studied, isolated adenomas are extremely rare in pediatric practice. Knox et al and Rodesch et al, as reported in Mougenot et al,[1]

Table 3 Complications of Colonoscopic Polypectomy		
Retrospective Studies in Children	Hemorrhage	Perforation
Williams et al (1982)	0/81 (0%)	4/81 patients (5%)
Mougenot et al (1996)	1/340 patients (0.29%)	3/340 patients (0.88%)

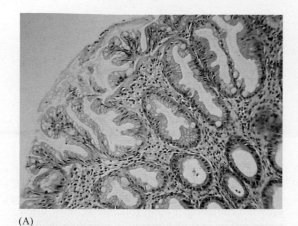

(A)

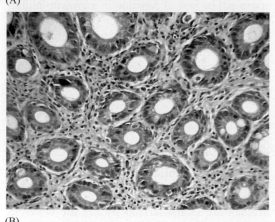

(B)

Figure 3 Low-power photomicrograph of a serrated adenoma showing a saw-toothed surface and stellate luminal profiles (A). However, the nuclei are mildly pseudostratified (B). Hematoxylin and eosin; ×250 original magnifications.

did not observe such adenomas in patients younger than 15 years. One to three cases have been reported in a series of, respectively, 50, 77, and 129 consecutive patients with polyps.[1]

Pathology. Adenomas are neoplastic epithelial polyps. All adenomas feature dysplastic aspects, that is, cellular atypia, increased mitotic activity, and nuclear hyperchromatism owing to abnormal cellular differentiation and renewal. The dysplasia can be graded as low (Figure 4) or high grade (Figure 5). In high-grade dysplasia, the nuclear abnormalities are marked, and the nuclei are stratified with nucleoli and uneven coarse chromatin. When cells appear overtly malignant but confined within the basement membrane, the lesion can be designated as carcinoma in situ. In practice, the term "high-grade dysplasia" encompasses severe dysplasia and carcinoma in situ. If the malignant cells extend beyond the basement membrane into the lamina propria, the diagnosis of intramucosal carcinoma must be used. In the colon, lymphatics extend only in the submucosa, which explains the absence of a risk of metastasis associated with high-grade dysplasia or intramucosal carcinoma. Invasive adenocarcinoma is defined by extension of malignant cells through the muscularis mucosa into the submucosa.

Two overall glandular patterns are separated: tubular with an organized glandular pattern (Figure 6) and villous with a frond-like pattern that is more likely present in large adenomas and is associated with a greater risk of high-grade dysplasia and invasive cancer, independent of polyp size. Adenomas demonstrating more than 75% tubular elements are called tubular adenomas. Those demonstrating more than 75% villous elements are called villous adenomas, and those with less than 75% of each are designated tubulovillous adenomas.

Adenomas originate through the process of gene mutation. Sporadic adenomas begin most commonly with somatic mutations in both alleles of the adenomatous polyposis coli gene (see section "Familial Adenomatous Polyposis"). Subsequent accumulation of additional mutations results in the development of

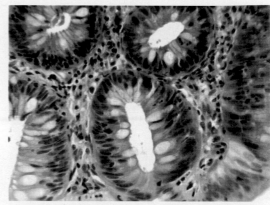

Figure 4 Colonic adenomatous polyp showing low-grade dysplasia with nuclear abnormalities, consisting of elongated, crowded, cigar-shaped nuclei. Hematoxylin and eosin; ×500 original magnification.

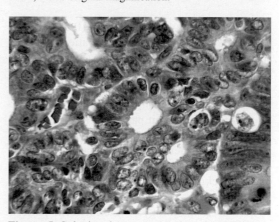

Figure 5 Colonic adenomatous polyp showing high-grade dysplasia with loss of goblet cell vacuoles, pleomorphic nuclei, prominent nucleoli, and an increased nuclear-cytoplasmic ratio. Hematoxylin and eosin; ×500 original magnification.

cancer. Most adenomas do not develop sufficient mutations to generate into cancer. Development of cancer requires an average time of 7 to 10 years.

Table 4 Features of Serrated Polyp Subtypes

Polyp Name	Alternative Terminology	Morphology and Significance	Molecular Features
Serrated polyp	Various	General term for all colorectal polyp with glandular serration	
Hyperplastic polyp, goblet type	Type 1 hyperplastic polyp	Subtype of hyperplastic polyp with conspicuous goblet cells and showing the least morphologic deviation from normal; described as goblet-cell rich type. Found predominantly in the distal colon	Frequent *K-ras* mutation (54%)
Hyperplastic polyp, microvesicular type	Type 2 hyperplastic polyp	Variant of hyperplastic polyp in which columnar cells have mucin-filled vesicles within the apical cytoplasm and goblet cells are relatively inconspicuous	Frequent *BRAF* mutations (76%) and CIMP (CpG island methylator phenotype) (68%)
Sessile serrated adenoma (SSA)	Sessile serrated polyp, serrated polyp with atypical proliferation	Advanced type of serrated polyp with abnormalities of architecture and proliferation but lacking the classic features of epithelial dysplasia	Frequent *BRAF* mutations (75–82%) and CIMP (92%)
Mixed serrated polyp (MP)	Admixed polyp	Rare serrated polyp that includes two separate components One component is usually nondysplastic (usually SSA) whereas the second dysplastic component is either traditional adenoma or serrated adenoma. Polyps with mixtures of adenoma and SA have also been described as mixed polyps	Frequent BRAF mutation, especially when SSA forms part of the lesion (89%)
Serrated adenoma (SA)	a – Mixed hyperplastic adenomatous polyp, b – Atypical hyperplastic polyp, c – Traditional SA	Relatively rare neoplastic polyp having a serrated architecture reminiscent of hyperplastic polyp but with unequivocal traditional adenomatous dysplasia.	Marked molecular heterogeneity. Overlapping molecular pathways. May have either *K-ras* or *BRAF* mutation or features of the adenoma–carcinoma pathway

Adapted from Young, Jass.[11]

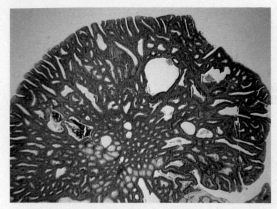

Figure 6 Low-magnification micrograph of a typical colonic tubular adenoma. Hematoxylin and eosin; ×75 original magnification.

Endoscopy. Only dye spraying (0.5% indigo carmine solution or initial application of 1.5% acetic acid with or without subsequent indigo carmin dye) in combination with high-resolution endoscopy offers the opportunity to distinguish adenomas from hyperplastic polyps in real time by analysis of their pit pattern.[15] The pit pattern is classified into six groups (Table 5). Hyperplastic polyps demonstrate the normal honeycomb (type I) or evenly dotted pattern (type II) of the background colonic mucosa. All other patterns on the surface of the polyp favor an adenomatous histology.[16] A cribriform pattern is commonly evident in adenomas when visualized with high-resolution endoscopes and chromoendoscopy with magnification.[17] If lesions show the following pit patterns, type IIIS, type IIIL, type IV, and type VN, they are suitable for endoscopic treatments.[5,18] In the examination of colonic lesions the NBI system (Olympus) or the FICE system, a computed virtual chromoendoscopy (Fujinon) provides imaging features additional to those of conventional videoendoscopy and chromoendoscopy.[19]

Pediatric Management. If an adenoma histopathologic diagnosis is made for an isolated or small number of polyps in a child or an adolescent, the following recommendations should be considered: (1) looking for a history of familial adenomatous polyposis (FAP), although a family history may be absent in sporadic forms of this disease; (2) searching for a history of familial colorectal cancer; and (3) employing postpolypectomy surveillance colonoscopy as proposed for adults by the Agency for Health Care Policy and Research Consortium (Table 6).[20]

Table 5 Pit Pattern Classification

Type	Pit Pattern
Type I	Round pits
Type II	Stellar or papillary pits
Type IIIS	Small tubular or roundish pits
Type IIIL	Large tubular or roundish pits
Type IV	Sulcus-, branch-, or gyrus-like pits
Type V	Irregular (type VI) or nonstructural (type VN) pits

Table 6 Postpolypectomy Surveillance Colonoscopy Recommendations of the Agency for Health Care Policy and Research Consortium

Findings at Index Examination	Surveillance
Single tubular adenoma	5 years
Multiple adenomas or villous histology	3 years
Numerous adenomas	Consider 1 year
Large sessile adenomas	3–6 months to examine the site

Adapted from Winawer et al.[20]

Polyps and Ureterosigmoidostomy

After ureterosigmoidostomy, adenomas and colorectal cancer near, or distal to, the stoma have been observed in at least 29% of patients. The delay varies from 2 to 38 years after surgery: 20 years for the development of adenoma and 28 years for arising colorectal cancer. Juvenile polyps also have been seen at sites of previous surgery, including ureterosigmoidostomy. A colonoscopy follow-up at regular intervals is indicated in such cases.

Inflammatory Polyps

Inflammatory polyps arise during the healing phase of severe colitis, following full-thickness ulceration. These polyps, which have no intrinsic neoplastic potential, may mimic a neoplastic mass in diseased colon (Ulcerative colitis and Crohn colitis). Because patients with these diseases are at increased risk for developing colon cancer, careful examination of these lesions has to be considered.[21,22]

POLYPOSIS SYNDROMES

Recently, major progress has been made in understanding the molecular pathogenesis of polyposis syndromes (Table 7).[23–28] A gastrointestinal polyp results from a defect in the highly regulated counterbalance of cellular growth promotion and cellular growth inhibition. This may be the result of either aberrant gain of function in a growth-promoting protein (oncogene, most often activated) or loss of function in a growth-inhibiting protein (tumor suppressor gene, most often inactivated). In the genetic gastrointestinal polyposis syndromes, a germline inactivating mutation of a tumor suppressor gene is the crucial event. Loss of normal growth regulation results from an eventual somatic mutation of the normal allele. Progression of the polyp to gastrointestinal cancer requires further acquisition of additional genetic defects.

Inherited Adenomatous Polyposis Syndromes

The inherited adenomatous polyposis syndromes are characterized by (1) the development of a large number of adenomas in the colorectum and (2) extracolonic features (ie, gastroduodenal polyps, desmoid tumors, osteomas of the mandible, skull, and long bones, and congenital hypertrophy of the retinal pigment epithelium (CHRPE)). FAP is the most common polyposis syndrome in children. It is

Table 7 Polyposis Syndromes Affecting Children

	Gene	Clinical Feature	Cancer Risk
Adenomatous syndromes			
Familial adenomatous polyposis MIM 175100	APC	GI polyposis, CHRPE	Colon 100%, periampullary, thyroid, hepatoblastoma, other
Gardner syndrome	APC	Colon adenomas, desmoids, dental anomalies, osteomas, epidermal cysts	As for FAP above
Attenuated FAP	APC	Reduced adenomas number	Colon
Turcot syndrome: type II (BTPS) MIM 276300	APC	GI adenomas, CNS tumors	Colon, brain
Hamartomatous syndromes			
Peutz-Jeghers syndrome MIM 175200	LKB1/STK11	GI hamartomas, mucocutaneous pigmentation	GI tract, pancreas, ovary, breast, cervix, testicle
Juvenile polyposis MIM 174900, 601299	SMAD4, BMPR1A	Colon/stomach hamartomas, congenital heart disease, cleft lip/palatine, malrotation	Colon, stomach, duodenum, pancreas
PTEN harmatoma tumor syndromes			
Cowden syndrome MIM 158350	PTEN	GI hamartomas, macrocephaly, mucocutaneous pigmentation, thyroid disease, fibrocystic breast disease, endometrial fibroids, urinary/uterine abnormalities	Breast, thyroid, skin
Bannayan-Riley-Ruvalcaba syndrome MIM 601728	PTEN	GI hamartomas, macrocephaly, speckled penis	Breast, thyroid

CHRPE = congenital hypertrophy of the retinal pigment epithelium; CNS = central nervous system; FAP = familial adenomatous polyposis; GI = gastrointestinal.

also known as familial polyposis for patients without extracolonic manifestations or Gardner syndrome for patients with extracolonic manifestations. Identification of the adenomatous polyposis coli (*APC*) gene as the gene mutated in the germline deoxyribonucleic acid (DNA) of patients affected by FAP has been a major development in understanding the pathogenesis of colorectal cancer[23–25] and has allowed proper classification of Gardner syndrome, attenuated FAP (AFAP), and some cases of Turcot syndrome as variants of classic FAP coli (Mendelian Inheritance in Man [MIM] 175100). *MYH*-associated polyposis (MAP), a recently described autosomal-recessive syndrome is also characterized by adenomatous polyps.[29–31]

Familial Adenomatous Polyposis

FAP is characterized by the progressive development of hundreds to thousands of adenomatous polyps in the large intestine (Figure 7).[32,33] The disease begins in younger patients with a small number of tiny polyps less than 5 mm (Figure 8).[32] Half of FAP gene carriers will have polyps at colonoscopy by approximately age 15 years. The number of polyps increases progressively, with all of the colonic length being covered by countless adenomas. In all cases, the vast majority of polyps are less than 10 mm (Figure 9).

At histologic examination, all varieties of adenomatous polyps may be seen, including tubular, tubulovillous, and villous adenomas. In addition, light microscopy reveals numerous microscopic

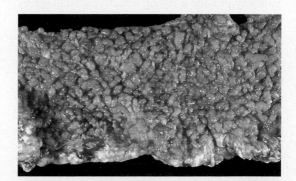

Figure 7 Familial adenomatous polyposis. Macroscopic aspect of resected colon with multiple adenomatous polyps carpeting the colonic surface.

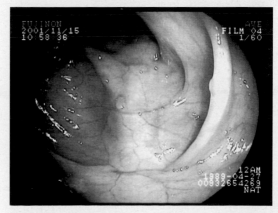

Figure 8 Familial adenomatous polyposis. Tiny colonic adenomatous polyps less than 3 mm.

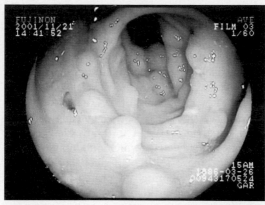

Figure 9 Familial adenomatous polyposis. Multiple adenomatous colonic polyps less than 10 mm.

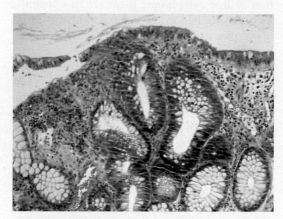

Figure 10 Familial adenomatous polyposis. Light microscopy reveals microscopic adenomas in a few crypts showing reduction of goblet cell vacuoles and crowded nuclei. Hematoxylin and eosin; ×250 original magnification.

adenomas, the smallest of which may involve a single colonic crypt (Figure 10). The dysplasia exhibited by all adenomas is now categorized as low (mild and moderate dysplasia) or high grade (severe dysplasia and carcinoma in situ).

The lifetime risk for colorectal neoplasia is 100%. Although the mean ages for adenoma and colon cancer development in FAP are 16 and 39 years, respectively, reports exist of colon cancer in children as young as 5 years of age, with an estimated incidence of one case younger than 20 years per 157 families.[31] Colorectal cancers in FAP have the same localization as sporadic cancer, but in 26 to 50% they are multiple and synchronous.[33]

Recently, attention has been paid to adenoma variants such as serrated adenomas, flat adenomas, and foci of aberrant crypts. Endoscopic/histopathologic correlations focusing on the differentiation of neoplastic from nonneoplastic lesions and identification of early malignant transformation have been supported in adult FAP by using new high-resolution videoendoscopes combined with optical zoom and dye spraying to define the mucosal pit pattern.[15–19]

Genetics

APC Gene and FAP-Associated Germline Mutations

Germline Mutations in the *APC* Gene. Germline mutations in the *APC* gene on chromosome 5q21[23,24] are responsible for FAP, an autosomal dominant disease. Its prevalence is estimated at 1 in 5,000 to 10,000.[33] Somatic APC mutations are found in the vast majority of sporadic colorectal cancers regardless of the histologic stage, which places APC at the very start of the adenoma–carcinoma sequence in humans.

APC Gene. The *APC* gene, a tumor suppressor gene, includes 21 exons contained within a 98 kb locus. The largest, exon 15, comprises more than 75% of the 8,535 basepairs of the coding sequence (Figure 11) and is the target of most germline mutations in FAP patients. The *APC* gene encodes a large protein consisting of 2,843 amino acids with a predicted molecular weight of greater than 309,000 kDa. Studies indicate that APC participates in a variety of cellular functions, including proliferation, differentiation, apoptosis, adhesion, migration, and chromosomal segregation.[34]

Mutation Penetrance. More than 825 germline mutations have been reported to the *APC* mutation database.[35] Most FAP patients carry germline mutations scattered in the 5′ half of the *APC* gene. Two codons, 1061 and 1309, are mutational hotspots and account for approximately 11 and 17% of all germline mutations. An accumulation of mutations is observed from codon 1250 to 1464, in a region called the "mutation cluster region" (MCR).[33] About 95% of *APC* germline mutations

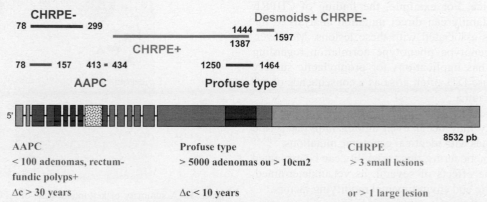

Figure 11 APC protein domains and familial adenomatous polyposis phenotype association with germline mutation position. AAPC = attenuated adenomatous polyposis coli; CHRPE = congenital hypertrophy of the retinal pigmented epithelium.

are either nonsense (28%) or truncating frameshift (67%) mutations, which result in truncated gene products without the C-terminus.[35] In 30 to 50% of patients with the FAP or AFAP phenotype, no germline *APC* mutations is detected.[36,37] In 10 to 15% of mutation-negative patients with the classical phenotype, large genomic deletions were detected. These deletions were not found in AFAP patients.[38,39]

The heterogeneity of the spectrum of *APC* germline mutations and the phenotypic variability observed among FAP families have allowed the establishment of genotype–phenotype correlations at this locus.[33] Germline mutations between codons 168 and 1680 are associated with classic FAP, whereas germline mutations between codons 1250 and 1464, especially around codon 1300, are associated with the highest number of polyps, thousands rather than hundreds of colorectal adenomas with an earlier onset of the disease.[33] The expression of some extracolonic features correlates with specific *APC* germline mutations. CHRPE is associated with germline mutations between codons 457 to 1444[33,40] but is also occasionally described in patients with germline mutations in exon 9.[33] Mutations downstream of codon 1444 correlate with the highest frequency of mandibular osteomas and desmoid tumors (DTs).[41] Upper gastrointesinal tumors cannot be attributed to a definite APC gene region.

Attenuated adenomatous polyposis coli (AAPC) is characterized by multiple adenomas, late onset of carcinoma, and, frequently, the absence of extracolonic features.[42,43] This phenotype is associated with germline mutations occurring in the 5′ (codons 78 to 157) and 3′ (approximately codons 1581 to 2843) regions of the *APC* gene and in exon 9.[43] The penetrance of AAPC, although lower than that of FAP, might still be high. An attenuated phenotype has also been reported in some families with large deletion within the APC.[44] Some mutations associated with AAPC lead to an unstable messenger ribonucleic acid (mRNA) or protein. Other mutations in alternatively spliced exons, such as those in exon 9, result in splicing out of at least some mRNA species, without modifying the reading frame.[45]

The established genotype–phenotype correlations might have implications for clinical practice. For example, the finding of CHPRE in a family can direct mutation analysis to the exons associated with these lesions. Moreover, the genotype–phenotype correlation regarding DTs has implications for prophylactic surgery because DTs often arise as a consequence of tissue trauma.[33]

Nevertheless, considerable phenotypic variability may occur even among individuals and families with identical genotypic mutations.[33,43,46] In genetic terms, this variability can be explained by the effects of several, as yet undetermined, genetic and environmental modifying factors.

APC Functional Domains. The large APC protein comprises several functional domains. Heptad repeats at the amino-terminal end mediate APC homodimer formation.[24,47] Amino acids 453 to 767 show some homology to the central repeat region of the *Drosophila* segment polarity protein armadillo, which controls cell adhesion and motility via modulation of the actin cytoskeleton. A summary of key interactions of APC and β-catenin in the cell, including the Wnt-1 signaling pathway, where binding of Wnt-1 to the frizzled receptor activates disheveled, which inhibits glycogen synthase kinase (GSK) 3β phosphorylation of β-catenin, preventing its proteosomal degradation, is shown in Figure 12. This leads to the dissociation of the complex formed by axin/conductin, APC, and GSK, resulting in the accumulation of free cytoplasmic β-catenin. β-Catenin is then translocated to the nucleus, where it forms a complex with T-cell factors (Tcfs), resulting in the activation of gene transcription, including the proto-oncogenes cyclin D1 and c-myc and subsequent cell proliferation. Mutations in *APC* have the same effect as Wnt signaling in destabilizing the axin–APC–GSK complex. Also shown in Figure 12 are the interactions of APC with the microtubule and actin cytoskeleton and the interaction of β-catenin with the E-cadherin cell adhesion system and Tcf transcription factor. Interspersed between these motifs are three SAMP (serine–alanine–methionine–proline) repeats that mediate axin binding. APC mediates microtubule binding when transiently overexpressed in epithelial cells and triggers tubulin polymerization in vitro. Further signals are present in the β-catenin and microtubule binding domains, which are thought to mediate nuclear localization and export of APC.[48] The C-terminus of APC (residues 2560 to 2843) interacts with the microtubule associated protein EB1 and also binds hDLG (human homolog of the *Drosophila* disks large tumor suppressor protein) and the protein tyrosine phosphatase PTP-BL.[49]

Recent studies have shown that the C-terminus of APC is involved in chromosomal stability at mitosis.[50] APC localizes at the kinetochore of metaphase chromosomes, and this location is likely to be dependent on the interaction between APC and EB1. On the one hand, loss of the former function will lead to nondysjunction and tetraploidy; on the other hand, defects of the latter result in mitotic cells with multipolar spindles that exert multidirectional forces on the kinetochore, resulting in chromosomal breakage and fragmentation.

APC protein shows a diffuse cytoplasmic distribution, accumulating along lateral margins or subapical regions of certain cells, in particular surface cells. However, epithelial cells of the same lineage may show striking differences in the subcellular localization of the APC protein. For example, enterocytes at the base of intestinal crypts are almost always APC negative, whereas expression increases toward the upper third of the crypt and the luminal surface, where all cells are positive. In addition, enterocytes on the luminal surface show accumulation of the APC protein along their apical surfaces. The expression of APC thus seems to increase with enterocyte maturation during the migration of cells from the crypt base to the luminal surface.[47]

Model of Carcinogenesis. A general picture is emerging from the analysis of the essential roles of the Wnt signal transduction pathway in providing selective advantage to the nascent tumor cell and in exerting genetic instability to ensure both tumor progression and malignant transformation: the *APC* gene, because it encompasses both functions, plays a central initiating and promoting role in colorectal cancer.[50] Its inactivation and the resulting constitutive activation of the Wnt pathway provide a strong selective advantage by affecting cell proliferation, migration, apoptosis, and, possibly, differentiation of the intestinal stem cell. Subsequently, other synergistic mutational events may allow the mutant APC to induce chromosomal instability and accelerate tumor progression along the adenoma–carcinoma sequence.

Based on the above considerations, APC has been proposed to have a rate-limiting role

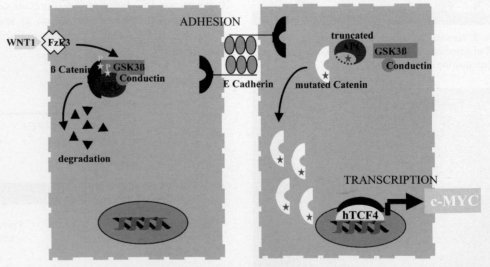

Figure 12 A summary of key interactions of APC and β-catenin in the cell, including the Wnt-1 signaling pathway to the frizzled receptor activates disheveled, which inhibits glycogen synthase kinase 3 β phosphorylation of β-catenin, preventing its proteosomal degradation. Also shown is the interaction of β-catenin with the E-cadherin cell adhesion system and T-cell factor transcription factor.

in tumor initiation and progression.[51] Loss of β-catenin regulation by APC provides the intestinal cell with a selective advantage and allows the initial clonal expansion. At this stage, chromosomal instability caused by loss of the C-terminus functional motifs of APC is latent owing to surveillance by the cell cycle and mitotic checkpoint machinery. The early activation of the oncogenes *K-ras* (by point mutation) and *c-myc* (as a downstream target of the Wnt pathway) will synergize with APC in triggering chromosomal instability and the subsequent allelic imbalances at chromosomes 17p and 18q. Additional synergisms between APC and other tumor suppressor genes in eliciting aneuploidy and chromosomal instability will progressively lead to malignant transformation and metastasis.

Clinical Features

Colorectal Adenomatous Polyps. FAP is clinically characterized by the occurrence of hundreds to thousands of colorectal adenomatous polyps at an early age and the inevitable development of colon cancer unless colectomy is performed.[52] Accounting for 1% of all colorectal cancer patients, FAP affects both genders equally and has a worldwide distribution. The average age at diagnosis ranges from 34 to 43 years; the average age at colorectal cancer diagnosis is 39 years (34 years in the profuse phenotype, compared to 42 years in the intermediate type).[40,52] Seventy to eighty of tumors occur on the left side of the colon.[52]

In pediatric practice, FAP is recognized through family screening. Rarely, rectal bleeding can reveal a sporadic or a familial case.

Extracolonic Manifestations. In addition to polyposis coli, patients with FAP can develop a variety of benign extracolonic manifestations and, infrequently, other cancers, as shown in Table 8.[33,35,41–43,52–55]

Extracolonic Adenomas. Fundic gland polyps (FGPs), the most common type of gastric polyp to occur in FAP patients, are observed at pediatric age (Figure 13), in contrast to antral adenomas.[57] Twenty five per cent of FGPS in FAP patients show foveolar dysplasia; 51% demonstrate an inactivating somatic *APC* gene alteration.

Subtle flat adenomas can be detected in the duodenum of children with FAP at the same time as colonic adenomas. In adults with FAP, duodenal adenomatous polyps have an average incidence of 61% (Figures 14 and 15).[55] The relative risk of duodenal cancer and periampullary malignancy is enhanced. At least 1% will develop duodenal cancer, diagnosed at an average age of 47 years. Spigelman and colleagues have elaborated a staging of duodenal polyposis that may help to assess the risk of malignant transformation (Table 9).[58]

Other Manifestations. The extra intestinal manifestations of FAP, first attributed to Gardner syndrome, are listed in Table 8. Some of these manifestations may contribute to identify at-risk individuals.

Mandibular osteomas are sought by orthopantomography.[59]

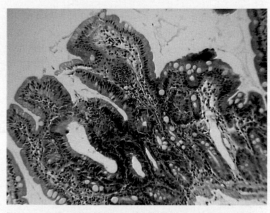

Figure 15 Familial adenomatous polyposis. Light microscopic aspect of duodenal adenomas. Hematoxylin and eosin; ×250 original magnification.

Congenital hypertrophy of the retinal pigment epithelium, defined as multiple and bilateral pigmented ocular fundus lesions, is found with increased frequency in some FAP kindreds (Figure 16).[60] It has been identified in infants as young as 3 months old. This abnormality, which generally does not affect vision, is a reliable early marker for gene carriage in FAP and its absence indicates lack of carriage in families affected with CHRPE.[60]

DTs may dramatically complicate the course of FAP and represent, since the widespread acceptance of prophylactic colectomy, a major cause of death.[61] The lifetime cumulative risk of developing DT is approximately 15 to 21%,[62] with a 1.5 female to male ratio, mainly during the third decade of life.[63] The risk is 2.5-fold greater in first-degree relatives of FAP patients with DT

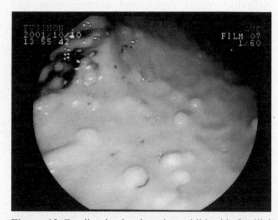

Figure 13 Fundic gland polyps in a child with familial adenomatous polyposis.

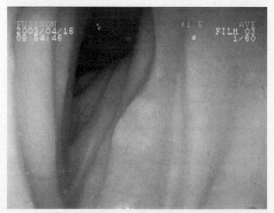

Figure 14 Familial adenomatous polyposis. Tiny, flat, superficially spreading duodenal adenomas.

Table 9 Stages of Severity in Duodenal Polyposis

	Grade (Points)		
	1	2	3
No of polyps	1–4	5–20	>20
Size of polyps (mm)	1–4	5–10	>10
Histology	Tubular	Tubulovillous	Villous
Dysplasia	Mild	Moderate	Severe

Stage 0: 0 point; Stage I: 1–4 points; Stage II: 5–6 points;
Stage III: 7–8 points; Stage IV: 9–12 points.
Adapted from Spigelman et al.[58]

Table 8 Extracolonic Features in FAP

Cancers (Lifetime Risk)	Others Lesions
Duodenal (1 to 5%)	CHRPE
Pancreatic (2%)	Nasopharyngeal angiofibromas
Thyroid (2%)	Osteomas
Brain (medulloblastoma) (<1%)	Radiopaque jaw lesions
Hepatoblastoma (0.7% of children <5-year old)	Dental abnormalities
	Lipomas, fibromas, epidermoid cysts
	Desmoid tumors
	Gastric adenomas/fundic gland polyps
	Duodenal, jejunal, ileal adenomas

CHRPE = congenital hypertrophy of the retinal pigment epithelium; FAP = familial adenomatous polyposis.
Adapted from reference 56.

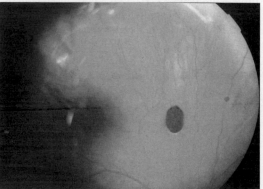

Figure 16 Congenital hypertrophy of the retinal pigmented epithelium.

than FAP patients in general. Eighty percent of DTs occur after prophylactic colectomy within 5 years on average. They consist in desmoplastic mesenteric infiltration or progressively growing masses within the mesentery, retroperitoneum, and abdominal wall. They do not metastasize but are prone to local invasion, causing small bowel obstruction, hydronephrosis, vascular obstruction, and bowel perforation. Their usual development after surgical trauma and their high potentiality of recurrence must be taken into account in therapeutic indications.

Hepatoblastomas occur in 1.6% of children born to a parent with FAP, a relative risk approximately 850-fold greater than the general population, leading some experts to recommend annual serum α-fetoprotein determination and hepatic ultrasonography in at-risk children between 0 and 6 years of age.[53,63] All six children with the FAP mutation who recovered from the hepatoblastoma have developed colorectal adenomatous polyposis.[53]

Thyroid cancer can occur in PAF, especially in females in the third decade. It is reasonable to include a thyroid palpation in the physical exam.[64]

Other Variants of FAP

Other variants of FAP include attenuated familial adenomatous polyposis (AFAP),[65] Turcot syndrome, defined as typical FAP together with central nervous system malignancies, in particular medulloblastoma and hereditary desmoid disease.

Attenuated FAP. The clinical characteristics of AFAP include oligopolyposis, usually less than 100 colorectal adenomas at presentation, which are mostly right-sided, a delayed onset of polyps (mean age of 44 years) and cancer (mean age of 56 years) with colorectal cancer occurring on average more than 12 years later than in classic FAP.[65] Total colonoscopy should be considered in families with an atypical form of polyposis because adenomas may be located in the proximal part of the colon. In such families, the endoscopic examinations may be started at a later age (18 to 20 years).[46] The adenomas have a flat rather than a polypoid aspect, leading to the initial description as "hereditary flat adenoma syndrome."[65] This condition should not be confused with hereditary nonpolyposis colorectal cancer.[66] In patients with AFAP, FGPs and duodenal adenomas are more prominent than colonic polyps.[57] Recently, Attard and colleagues described the first pediatric patient with AFAP diagnosed at age 9 in the setting of a strong family history of gastric carcinoma who had multiple FGPs with severe dysplastic changes requiring prophylactic gastrectomy at age 11.[67]

Turcot Syndrome. Turcot syndrome, or brain tumor polyposis syndrome is characterized by multiple colonic adenomas associated with a primary brain tumor of various histopathologic types.[54,68] Molecular genetic studies have established a new classification of Turcot syndrome kindreds into two groups according to the type of brain tumor and the

genetic defect.[54] The more common group (Turcot syndrome type II) has germline mutations of the *APC* gene and medulloblastoma, which precedes the diagnosis of polyposis in some cases.[68] The other group with the family originally described by Turcot (Turcot syndrome type I) includes patients with glioblastomas and germline mutations in DNA base mismatch repair genes also implicated in hereditary nonpolyposis colon cancer.[54]

Hereditary Desmoid Disease. In 1996, Eccles et al, coined the term "hereditary desmoid disease" (HDD) to describe a family with multiple desmoid tumors inherited across three generations at sites unusual for FAP-related desmoids (paraspinal muscles, breast, occiput, arms, and lower limbs).[69] Affected kindreds lacked colonic adenomas, except for one patient who had a palpable rectal mass, and another who had <50 adenomatous polyps. HDD inheritance was autosomal dominant, with 100% penetrance. All patients had truncating frameshift mutations at codon 1924 of the *APC* gene.

Diagnosis

The diagnosis of classical FAP among individuals with a family history is confirmed by the presence of 100 or more adenomatous polyps on colonoscopic examination.[33] Adults with attenuated FAP exhibit fewer than 100 colorectal adenomas, whereas those with hereditary nonpolyposis colorectal cancer usually exhibit only a few colorectal adenomas, generally localized in the right colon.[70,71] However, in children, the finding of even one adenomatous polyp should alert the pediatrician to the possibility of a FAP (Figure 17). Additionally, in at-risk individuals, the presence of more than three pigmented ocular fundic lesions on ophthalmologic examination confirms the diagnosis of FAP.[60]

To differentiate FAP from the other polyposis syndromes and from nodular lymphoid hyperplasia or hyperplastic polyps, which may mimic FAP endoscopically, histology is the key. The diagnosis can be confirmed by mutation analysis. The simultaneous inheritance of both a germline frame shift mutation in the *APC* gene and a germline splice-site mutation in the *MLH1* gene was

recently described in a 10-year-old boy with rapidly progressive FAP.[72]

Screening

An *APC* gene mutation can be identified in 90% of classical FAP families. The integration of genetic testing (Table 10) into clinical practice provides multiple benefits with earlier detection of lesions and prevention of cancer, removal of patient uncertainty, and elimination of unnecessary screening.[73] In the setting of a known mutation in a family, genetic testing of relatives can discriminate between affected and unaffected individuals with a high degree of certainty. Nevertheless, inappropriate use of genetic testing has the potential to misinform affected patients with false-negative results. Written informed consent for genetic testing must be obtained from the patient and/or parents.[74] Taking into account that 1% of the FAP patients will develop colorectal cancer between ages 15 and 20 years, genetic testing can be proposed at 10 to 12 years of age.[75,76] Genetic diagnosis can be usually achieved by detection of *APC* mutations in DNA from peripheral blood lymphocytes using a commercially available protein truncation assay or by direct DNA sequencing or it can require genetic tests for identification of intragenetic deletions.[76,77] A child found to be mutation negative in a family with an identified mutant *APC* allele has the same colorectal cancer risk as the general population.

If the pedigree mutation is not found or if informative genetic testing cannot be done, all first-degree family members should undergo endoscopic screening.[20,46,77] Formal recommendations exist for surveillance (Table 11) of at-risk individuals.[20] In addition, upper endoscopy for surveillance of the stomach, duodenum, and periampullary region is recommended with front-viewing and side-viewing endoscopes.[78,79] Owing to the increased risk of hepatoblastoma in patients with FAP, screening with α-fetoprotein levels and ultrasound imaging of the liver may be prudent in the children of affected parents from infancy to 7 years of age.[53]

Prenatal Diagnosis and Preimplantation Diagnosis in FAP

In a high proportion of cases, prenatal diagnosis of FAP can be performed using linkage or mutational analysis.[80] In some countries, preimplantation diagnosis (PGD) is an alternative to prenatal diagnosis for couples at risk of having offspring affected with this genetic condition, a disorder that does not affect the child at the time of birth.[80]

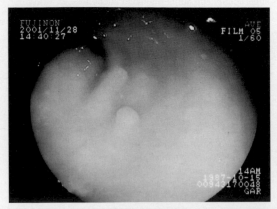

Figure 17 One or two adenomatous polyps at pancolonoscopy may be the early alert leading to the diagnosis of familial adenomatous polyposis in a child.

Table 10 Indications for *APC* Gene Screening

> 100 colorectal adenomas
  First-degree relatives of patients with FAP
> 20 cumulative colorectal adenomas
  First-degree relatives of patients with attenuated FAP

Table 11 Screening/Surveillance Guidelines in FAP Patients

At-risk individuals	
Genotyping	*APC* gene mutation (+): flexible colonoscopy annually starting at age 10 to 12
	APC gene mutation (−): flexible sigmoidoscopy at age 25
If genotype not available:	Flexible sigmoidoscopy or colonoscopy annually starting at age 10 to 12, then 2 years starting at age 35, then as per the guidelines for average-risk individuals starting at age 50
Affected individuals	Upper gastrointestinal surveillance every 3 to 4 years, and annually if upper tract polyps
	If retained rectum or J-pouch, flexible sigmoidoscopy every 6 months or 1 to 2 years respectively
	Annual physical exam and routine blood tests

Treatment

Colonic Polyposis

Colectomy. Colectomy is the recommended treatment for FAP patients to eliminate the risk of colorectal cancer. Timing and extent of surgery, that is, subtotal colectomy with ileorectal anastomosis (IRA) versus proctocolectomy and ileal-pouch-anal anastomosis (IPAA), have been widely debated.[46] In children and adolescents, surgery can usually be safely postponed for several years, while continuing with annual colonoscopy, until an appropriate psychological age is reached where colectomy can be accepted.[52]

IRA. Some argues that the risk of dying from rectal cancer after an IRA is only 2% after a 15-year follow-up, making it an acceptable primary treatment option for FAP patients and laparoscopic colectomy with IRA has proven to be a safe and minimally invasive treatment option for selected patients.[81] After IRA, close endoscopic surveillance of the remaining rectum every 6 months is mandatory, for recurrent adenomas or cancer.[82]

IPAA. IPAA includes total colectomy, proctectomy, endoanal mucosectomy, and handsewn ileal J-pouch-anal anastomosis.[82] IPAA has various disadvantages: (1) a risk of severe postoperative complications necessitating removal of the pouch and construction of an ileostomy (<5%); (2) a worse functional outcome compared with that of IRA, although the quality of life after IRA and IPAA seemed to be the same[83]; (3) a pouch failure in 7.7% of FAP patients over a 2-year follow-up period, mostly due to ischemia and pelvic sepsis[84]; (4) a pouchitis in 11% of FAP patients[85]; (5) a 46% drop of the fecondity of women with FAP after IPAA compared to the preoperative level, while this fact was not observed after IRA.[86]

IPAA versus IRA. If FAP has a clinical expression during childhood and adolescence, the decision of an IPAA seems to be the best surgical option because the remaining risk of developing rectal cancer increases over time, and a secondary proctectomy is needed in approximately half of the cases because of uncontrollable polyposis.[82] Management of young patients is summarized in Figure 18. After IPAA, the risk of developing one or more adenomas in the ileal pouch at 5, 10, and 15 years is 7, 35, and 75, respectively.[88] There is

also a substantial risk for the development of polyps at the anastomotic site of 8% at 3.5 years and 18% at 7 years, even if this risk can be partially reduced by handsewn anastomosis with mucosectomy.[89] All FAP patients who undergo an IPAA procedure, irrespective of the applied surgical technique, should have endoscopic IPAA surveillance at regular intervals of at least once a year.[88,89]

Only patients with a few rectal polyps from families with a similar mild phenotype might be selected for IRA. The results of molecular genetic testing might be used to identify such patients.

Nonselective or Selective Cyclooxygenase-2 Inhibitors. Several studies have shown that treatment of FAP patients with a nonselective or selective cyclooxygenase-2 inhibitor (eg, sulindac or celecoxib, respectively) leads to reduction in the number and size of the colonic and rectal adenomas in both short- and long-term studies.[90,91] However, administration of sulindac for primary chemoprevention of FAP failed to prevent the development of adenomatous polyposis in gene mutation carriers,[92] and rectal cancer has been reported after prolonged sulindac chemoprevention.[91] Moreover, recent reports of increased cardiovascular and thrombotic events with COX-2 inhibitors in adenoma chemoprevention trials are cause for concern.[93,94]

Duodenal Polyposis. The therapeutic challenge of duodenal polyposis arises in adulthood. Chemoprevention by Celecoxib has been proposed.[95]

Endoscopic procedures have limitations.[96] In severe cases the only treatment may be prophylactic pylorus-preserving pancreaticoduodenectomy.[97]

Abdominal DTs. In FAP families with associated DTs, this specific risk has to be taken into account in surgical management. Timing for surgery as late as possible, at least in patients with a smaller number of polyps and an expected later onset of disease, and performing the colectomy procedure in one stage must be considered. In such families, we prefer to perform an IPAA procedure as the initial prophylactic colorectal procedure because conversion of an IRA to an IPAA may be precluded by mesenteric DTs. Before surgery, abdominal computed tomography is performed in clinically indicated cases and in cases with a family history of desmoid disease. Nonsteroidal antiinflammatory drugs (usually sulindac) and antioestrogens (tamoxifen or toremifene) are considered first-line therapies for Dts.[98]

Multiple Colorectal Adenoma Syndromes

Multiple colorectal adenomas indicate the presence of 3 to 100 colonic adenomas. In patients with oligopolyposis the chance of having a germline mutation in *APC* or *MYH*, a base excision repair gene, is approximately 35 to 40%.

MYH Associated Polyposis

Recently, another polyposis-causing gene was detected on chromosome 1p33-34, the *MYH* gene.[29] Mutations in this gene are associated with a recessively inherited form of colonic polyposis. The two most common mutations are Y165C and G382D. *APC* mutations are detected in approximately 60 to 90% of classic FAP patients and in 10 to 30% of AFAP patients; *MYH* mutations are likely to account for about 10% and 20 to 25% of patients in these groups, respectively.[80] No patients with bi-allelic *MYH* mutations had profuse polyposis. CHRPE and duodenal polyps have both been reported in individuals with bi-allelic *MYH* mutations.[99] By contrast, desmoid tumors have not been noted. The youngest case identified among a group of 25 patients with bi-allelic mutations of the

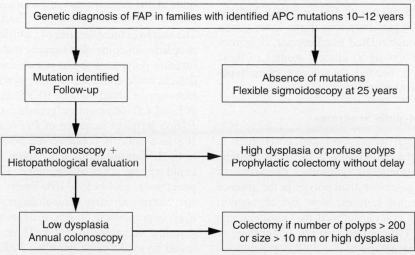

Figure 18 Management of at-risk familial adenomatous polyposis (FAP) patients in childhood and adolescence. (Adapted from reference 87.)

MYH gene was a 13-year-old male who developed gastric cancer at age 17.[100] The youngest MAP patient with colorectal carcinoma reported is a 21-year-old female with 36 colonic polyps.[80] Currently, genetic analysis of *MYH* should be offered to patients younger than 18 years with a phenotype resembling FAP or AFAP when no *APC* mutation is identified and no obvious vertical transmission of the disease is observed.[20] Predictive genetic testing should be offered to siblings of patients found to have bi-allelic mutations to assess the need for endoscopic surveillance beginning at 21 years of age. *MYH* testing also may be useful for patients with young-onset colorectal cancer in the absence of polyps when the tumor does not exhibit genetic defect in the DNA mismatch repair pathway. The clinical management of patients with bi-allelic mutations in *MYH* should be the same as for individuals with classic FAP.

Hamartomatous Polyposis Syndromes

Hamartomatous polyposis syndromes are characterized by an overgrowth of cells or tissues native to the area in which they normally occur, ie, mesenchymal, stromal, endodermal, and ectodermal elements.[101] This overgrowth of cells or tissues, at least initially, has no presumed neoplastic potential. However, several of these syndromes are associated with an increased lifetime risk of both intestinal and extraintestinal malignancies. Hamartomatous polyposis syndromes include juvenile polyposis syndrome (JPS), Cowden disease (CD), Bannayan-Riley-Ruvalcaba syndrome (BRRS), or Ruvalcaba-Myhre-Smith syndrome (RMSS), and Peutz-Jeghers syndrome (PJS).[101–103] In JPS, polyps involving the gastrointestinal tract are the major manifestation of the disease. In contrast, for the other syndromes, they are a component among a variety of extraintestinal features.[102] The mechanism of inheritance for all of these syndromes is autosomal dominant with variable penetrance. A significant number of patients have no family history and have sporadic disease due to de novo gene mutations. Thus, the diagnosis of these syndromes remains primarily a clinical process. Furthermore, it must be emphasized that, in children, it may be difficult to distinguish patients with JPS and those with CD or BRRS because extraintestinal manifestations in the latter conditions are an age-related phenomenon. Rigorous long-term follow-up in clinical studies of these syndromes is needed to achieve phenotype-genotype correlations.

Juvenile Polyposis Syndrome

First described by McColl and colleagues in 1964 (in reference 101) JPS is the most common of the hamartomatous syndromes characterized by multiple gastrointestinal polyps in the absence of extraintestinal features. Most authors support the diagnosis criteria outlined by Giardiello and colleagues.[8] These criteria include either three or more juvenile polyps of the colon or polyposis involving the entire gastrointestinal tract or any number of polyps in a proband with a known family history of juvenile polyps. JPS is inherited in an autosomal dominant manner with variable penetrance, with approximately 25% of cases having a family history of juvenile polyposis.[101–103]

Presentation. In children, JPS is always symptomatic. Symptoms include rectal bleeding, rectal prolapse, cramping abdominal pain, and intussusception. Most cases of JPS come to medical attention between 2 and 12 years of age, although rare cases of failure to thrive, anemia, and severe hypoalbuminemia resulting from a protein-losing enteropathy have been described in infants.[104] Polyps vary in number from 3 to 200 and show great variation in size and configuration. In most cases, juvenile polyps are found only in the colon.[101–103] In a review of 272 cases by Hofting and colleagues, the most frequently affected site was the colorectum (98%), followed by the stomach (14%), jejunum and ileum (15%), and duodenum (2.3%).[105] When polyps are numerous, follow-up should include serum albumin and α_1-antitrypsin fecal clearance. There is an association with congenital birth defects in 15% of cases, including malrotation of the midgut, genitourinary defects, and cardiac defects. The majority of congenital defects have been reported in individuals with the nonfamilial variant of the disease.[101] JPS may also co-occur with hereditary hemorrhagic telangectasia (Osler–Weber–Rendu syndrome).[101]

Pathology. The typical gastrointestinal polyp in JPS has the same histopathologic aspects as solitary juvenile polyp. In contrast to the polyps of PJS, muscle fibers are not present in the stroma.

Molecular Genetics

JPS and the SMAD Pathway. There is evidence of genetic heterogeneity in JPS. Hereditary juvenile polyposis is not linked to APC. Subsets of JPS families have mutations in the tumor suppressor gene phosphatase and tensin homolog (PTEN 601728) located at chromosome 10q23.3.[106] PTEN is a ubiquitously expressed dual-specificity phosphatase that acts as a tumor suppressor and is mutated in several sporadic tumor types.[26] Mutations in this gene are also important in a subset of familial thyroid carcinoma, CD, and BRRS.[25,107] The shared clinical features of CD/BRRS and JPS, coupled with coincident somatic mutation data in juvenile polyps, raise the possibility that PTEN defects could cause all of these syndromes.[108,109] However, if about 60% of BRRS and more than 80% of CD demonstrate germline mutations in *PTEN*, germline mutation of *PTEN* as a cause of JPS in a child is controversial because extraintestinal manifestations that would exclude JPS could appear after adolescence, CD having a penetrance well below 10% under 15 years of age, altering an early clinical diagnosis.[110] Moreover, a proportion of JPS patients do not have germline mutations in *PTEN*. Three groups have found no evidence of germline *PTEN* mutations in 21 JPS families and 16 sporadic cases.[111,112] In a recent review of PTEN, JPS is not considered a so-called PTEN hamartoma-tumor syndrome (PHTS).[110] In summary, the association of germline *PTEN* mutations as a cause for JPS is not yet clearly substantiated. Nevertheless, Huang and colleagues identified a germline mutation of *PTEN* in a family in which identical twin 6-year-old girls were diagnosed with JPS.[113] Their 55-year-old father lacked manifestations of CD or BRRS and had the same mutation in *PTEN*.

Recently, constitutional mutations in *MADH4* (mothers against decapentaplegic homolog 4, also known as *SMAD4*), located at chromosome 18q21,[27,114,115] and bone morphogenetic receptor 1A (*BMPR1A*), located on chromosome 10q22.3, were shown to cause JPS.[27,114–117] *SMAD4* mutations seem to be the most relevant mutations in JPS patients without stigmata of other polyposis syndromes and account for approximately 50% of the reported familial cases of the syndrome.[27] These genes, which code for proteins involved in transforming growth factor-β (TGF-β) signal transduction, are mutated in a number of gastrointestinal cancers. Other members of the SMAD family (SMAD1, -2, -3, or -5) are not involved in the pathogenesis of JPS. No consistent mutations of the deleted in colon cancer gene (*DCC*), which is located at the same locus as *SMAD4*, have been found.[101] BMPR1A and its receptors belong to the TGF-β superfamily, and the recent finding of four JPS kindreds with *BMPR1A* mutations further supports the importance of TGF-β superfamily mutations in JPS.[116] Friedl et al observed that patients with a mutation in the *MADH4* gene were more likely to be affected with massive gastric polyposis than those with a mutation in the *BMPR1A* gene.[115] Sayed et al confirmed this observation.[114]

SMAD proteins transduce signals from TGF-β ligands that regulate cell proliferation, differentiation, and death through activation of receptor serine/threonine kinases.[118] Thus, TGF-β is a potent immunosuppressor, and perturbation of TGF-β signaling is linked to autoimmunity, inflammation, and cancer. Activated SMADs regulate transcription of target genes, including cell-cycle inhibitors such as p21, which mediate the antiproliferative response and partially explain the tumor suppressive action of the TGF-β pathway. At late stages of tumor progression, TGF-β promotes tumorigenesis via suppression of the immune system and changes in cell differentiation of epithelial tumor cells. Phosphorylation of receptor-activated SMADs (R-SMADs) leads to formation of complexes with the common mediator SMAD (Co-SMAD), which are imported to the nucleus. Nuclear SMAD oligomers bind to DNA and associate with transcription factors to regulate the expression of target genes. Alternatively, nuclear R-SMADs associate with ubiquitin ligases and promote degradation of transcriptional repressors, thus facilitating target gene regulation by TGF-β. SMADs themselves can also become ubiquitinated and are degraded by proteasomes. Finally, the inhibitory SMADs (I-SMADs) block phosphorylation of R-SMADs by the receptors and promote ubiquitination and degradation of receptor complexes, thus inhibiting signaling.[118] Multiple somatic genetic alterations, including *APC*, *MMR*, and *K-ras* mutations, seem to play a role in the neoplastic transformation of juvenile polyps coli.

Neoplastic Risk. In a large retrospective review from St Mark's Polyposis Registry published in 1988, 1,032 juvenile polyps from 87 patients were examined.[119] Pathologic specimens were available for reevaluation from 80 patients. Twenty-two percent of the patients subsequently developed colorectal cancer. The mean age at the time of diagnosis was 34 years. Some patients also developed upper gastrointestinal malignancies.[120] In 1993, Hofting and colleagues found 48 cases of gastrointestinal cancer (18%) among 272 patients with JPS.[105] In 1995, Desai and colleagues re-evaluated the data from the St Mark's Polyposis Registry and estimated that the projected incidence of colorectal cancer alone by the age of 60 was approximately 68%.[121] The incidence of gastric adenocarcinomas is 21% in JPS patients who have gastric polyps.[8]

Management and Surveillance. Recommendations for endoscopic screening and treatment in patients with JPS are summarized in Figure 19.[102] The proband also should undergo upper gastrointestinal endoscopic screening. It is not clear whether upper and lower endoscopic surveillance is adequate to prevent malignancy. If surgery becomes mandatory, the extent of rectal polyposis is a major consideration in determining the modality of colectomy. There are insufficient data to justify prophylactic coloproctectomy or colectomy solely for the risk of colorectal carcinoma.[122] The therapeutic role of cyclooxygenase inhibitors in pediatric JPS is also unclear.

In three of eight JPS families, polyps were identified in asymptomatic first-degree relatives.[122] Accordingly, first-degree relatives of patients with JPS should be screened by upper and lower endoscopy starting at 12 years of age, even when the subject is asymptomatic. Howe and colleagues recommend incorporating genetic testing into the screening algorithm.[26] However, given the presumed genetic heterogeneity of this syndrome, failure to show a mutation in *SMAD4* or *BMPR1A* does not support lengthening the surveillance interval in asymptomatic first-degree relatives.[27]

Juvenile Polyposis of the Stomach. Juvenile polyposis involving the stomach without intestinal polyps at initial presentation, first described by Watanabe and colleagues in 12 patients aged 10 to 63 years, (4 of them younger than 20 years) may be regarded as a clinical entity separate from generalized gastrointestinal polyposis.[123] Anemia (89%) and hypoproteinemia with most patients requiring gastrectomy (67%) are the most striking clinical features. Three subjects developed gastric cancer from 32 to 65 years.

Phosphatase and Tensin Homolog Hamartoma-Tumor Syndromes (PHTS)

PHTS. PHTS, that is CD[124] and BRRS,[109,125] is a rare autosomal disorder characterized by multiple phenotypic abnormalities and hamartomas in the intestine and other tissues. Recent nomenclature favors the term "PHTS" because germline mutations in the *PTEN* gene account for up to 80% of cases of CD and 60% of BRRS patients.[110] Clinical differences are likely caused by allelic variations.[109,117] PTEN is a major dual lipid and protein phosphatase that signals apoptosis and mediates cellular growth arrest by inhibition of phosphoinositol-3-kinase.[110] Furthermore, the protein phosphatase, with the ability to dephosphorylate both serine and threonine residues, regulates cell survival pathways, such as the mitogen-activated kinase (MAPK) pathway.

Cowden Disease (CD). CD (MIM 1583350) is an autosomal dominant condition characterized by multiple hamartomas that affect derivates of all three germ layers with an increased risk of neoplasia affecting breast (36% of the patients), thyroid (10%), and endometrium.[110,124] The diagnostic criteria for CD have been revised recently (Table 12).[125] Ninety percent of patients present with dermatologic manifestations among which tricholemmomas are very suggestive of CD. Progressive macrocephaly is frequently observed.[125] CD in concert with cerebellar gangliocytomatosis is referred to as the Lhermitte-Duclos syndrome. Only 35 to 40% of patients who meet the diagnosis criteria for CD have symptomatic gastrointestinal polyposis. Polyps can be typical juvenile polyps or hyperplastic polyps. It is noteworthy that CD has a great variation in expression and carries an age-related penetrance (10% below age 15 years, 90% at age 20 years).

Gastrointestinal polyposis should be addressed by endoscopic surveillance. Although no definite increased risk of colorectal carcinoma has been documented, the true risk may be unrecognized because of the rarity of the syndrome. Screening for breast and thyroid malignancies should begin in the teenage years.[124]

Germline mutations in *PTEN* have been found in 80% of probands with CD, especially in exons 5, 7, and 8, when operational criteria (International Cowden Consortium) are applied to the diagnosis of CD (see Table 12).[124] The majority of CD cases appear to be isolated; 10 to 50% are familial.

Bannayan–Riley–Ruvalcaba Syndrome. Hamartomatous polyposis is also seen as a component of BRRS (also Bannayan-Zonana syndrome, Riley-Smith syndrome, and Ruvalcaba-Myhre-Smith syndrome. OMIM 153480) associated with macrocephaly, a speckled penis, delayed

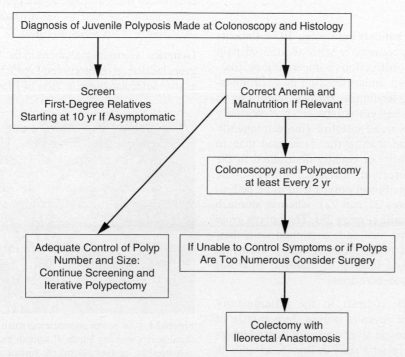

Figure 19 Management and surveillance in young patients with juvenile polyposis syndrome. (Adapted from reference 87.)

Table 12 International Cowden Consortium Operational Diagnostic Criteria

Pathognomonic criteria (mucocutaneous lesions)
Facial trichilemmomas
Acral keratoses
Papillomatous papules
Mucosal lesions

Major criteria
Breast carcinoma
Thyroid carcinoma (nonmedullary), especially follicular thyroid carcinoma
Macrocephaly (megalencephaly)
Lhermitte–Duclos disease (LDD)
Endometrial carcinoma

Minor criteria
Other thyroid lesions (eg, adenoma or multinodular goiter)
Mental retardation
Gastrointestinal hamartomas
Fibrocystic disease of the breast
Lipomas
Fibromas
Genito–urinary tumors (eg, renal cell carcinoma or uterine fibroids) or malformation

development in childhood, lipomatosis, and hemangiomatosis. Intestinal polyposis affects up to 45% of these patients.[101] Sixty percent of patients with BRRS have germline *PTEN* mutations.[124] Zhou et al demonstrated that a significant portion of patients have germline deletions of the *PTEN* gene.[117] The mutational spectra of BRRS and CD seem to overlap. For some authors, there is a higher frequency of breast tumors, fibroadenomas, and lipomas among the mutation-positive group of patients with BRRS who meet published diagnosis criteria than among the 40% of mutation-negative patients. It is not known if genes other than *PTEN* may also be responsible for BRRS.[126]

Infantile Gastrointestinal Juvenile Polyposis. Recently four cases of infantile gastrointestinal juvenile polyposis have been related to heterozygous de novo germline deletion of varying lengths encompassing the two contiguous genes, *PTEN* and *BMPRIA*.[127] This entity is characterized by its very early manifestations, generalized polyposis with recurrent gastrointestinal bleeding, exsudative enteropathy, and inanition, in the absence of family history. Profuse polyps develop from the stomach to the rectum. The digestive disease is always associated with macrocephaly present at birth and facial dysmorphy. Hemangiomas, lipomas, and speckled penis may occur. The severity of bleeding and exsudative enteropathy led to colectomy in three cases at age 10, 17 months, and 8 years. Adenomatous polyps in stomach, duodenum and proximal jejunum with low- or high-grade dysplasia have been proved at 4 and 14 years, respectively. The severity of the disease could reflect a cooperation between the two implicated tumor suppressor genes.

Peutz-Jeghers Syndrome

PJS (MIM 1752001) is another hamartomatous gastrointestinal polyposis syndrome associated with a risk of gastrointestinal and extraintestinal cancers. The incidence of PJS is estimated as 1 in 120,000 births. Mucocutaneous melanin deposition, recognized by early investigators,[128] is a hallmark for this syndrome resulting from mutations of the *LKB1/STK11* gene, located on chromosome 19p 13.3.[28,128–131]

Clinical Manifestations. Skin pigmentation (Figure 20) consists of small (1 to 5 mm) pigmented macules, primarily clustered around the mouth, eyes, and nostrils and sometimes also the perianal area.[128,129] The buccal mucosa is also affected. These pigmented lesions occur before gastrointestinal polyps but are rarely observed during early infancy. The cutaneous pigment pattern often fades after puberty, but buccal mucosa lesions tend to persist.[129] PJS is a clinically heterogeneous disorder, and cases of individuals from Peutz-Jeghers kindreds having pigmentation without polyposis, and the converse, have been reported.[129]

One-third of PJS patients will experience symptoms during the first decade of life, and

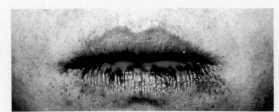

Figure 20 Mucocutaneous buccal melanin pigmentation in a patient with Peutz-Jeghers syndrome.

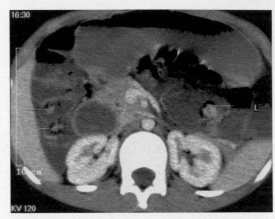

Figure 21 Peutz-Jeghers syndrome: abdominal pelvic computed tomographic scan showing jejunal polyps.

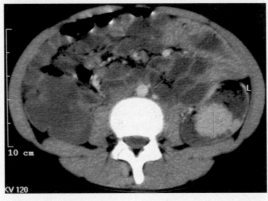

Figure 22 Peutz-Jeghers syndrome: abdominal pelvic computed tomographic scan showing a very large colonic polyp at the splenic flexure.

50 to 60% of patients before age 20.[132] Patients present most commonly with abdominal pain secondary to obstruction or impending obstruction with polyp intussusception or gastrointestinal bleeding leading to anemia. According to series, Peutz-Jeghers polyps are preferentially located in the small intestine (more frequently in the jejunum than in the ileum and than in the duodenum)[132] or equally distributed in the stomach, colorectum, and small bowel.[129] The small and large bowel polyps tend to be pedunculated (Figures 21 and 22), whereas stomach polyps are sessile (Figure 23). The polyps grow to a very large size and, combined with their pedunculated aspect, can result in recurrent intussusception, leading to multiple laparotomies and bowel resections.[129]

Pathology. In contrast to the inflammatory appearance of juvenile polyps, hyperplasia of the smooth muscle layer occurs in Peutz-Jeghers polyps. Hyperplastic smooth muscle extends in a tree-like manner toward the epithelial layer

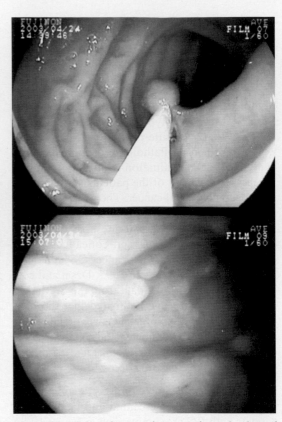

Figure 23 Peutz-Jeghers syndrome: endoscopic view of sessile and pedunculated stomach polyps from the same patient as in Figures 20 and 21.

(Figure 24). The extensive dilation of cystic-filled spaces, pathognomonic for the juvenile polyp, is not seen in PJS. Invagination of the epithelium will result in islands of epithelial cells trapped within the underlying smooth muscle, resulting in "epithelial cell misplacement" in the absence of cellular atypia and an increased mitotic rate.[129] Histologic evidence of hamartomatous–adenomatous–carcinomatous evolution has been demonstrated for stomach, small bowel, and colorectal polyps in PJS.[133,134] In addition, there is evidence that PJS patients are prone to develop adenomatous as well as hamartomatous polyps, particularly in the large intestine.[133,134]

Genetics. Germline mutations in the *STK11/LKB1* gene, located on chromosome 19p13.3, are reported as the molecular cause in 70% of PJS families and

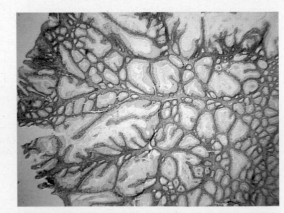

Figure 24 Low-power photomicrograph of Peutz-Jeghers rectal polyp showing bands of smooth muscle extending in a tree-like manner toward the epithelial layer. Hematoxylin and eosin; ×75 original magnification.

50% of sporadic PJS patients.[28,130,131,133,134] The gene is divided into nine exons that encode a 433 amino acid protein containing a serine/threonine kinase domain, a nuclear localization signal in its N-terminus domain, and a prenylation consensus sequence in its C-terminus.[135–137] The protein is located in the nucleus of cells but is also detected in the cytoplasm and at cell membranes. LKB1 is widely expressed during embryonic development. Immunostaining of the small intestine reveals that LKB1 is expressed in two distinct topographic regions: the crypts that contain rapidly dividing stem cells and the top of the villi, where cells undergo apoptosis. It has been proposed to act as a tumor suppressor. LKB1 is also involved in p53-mediated apoptosis. LKB1 phosphorylates p53 at low levels, which might be required for p53 activation. LKB1 also controls cell proliferation. It interacts with the chromatin remodeling protein brahma-related gene-1 (*BRG1*) and with the cell-cycle regulatory proteins LKB1-interacting protein 1 (LIP1) and WAF1.

The *LKB1* mutations (truncated protein with incomplete catalytic domains) lead to loss in kinase activity, whereas other cancer susceptibility syndromes are associated with activation of kinase activity. Allelic imbalance has previously been reported in a number of PJS polyps and found in a colonic adenoma from a PJS patient, strongly suggesting the existence of a hamartoma–carcinoma sequence in tumorigenesis.[133]

There is marked inter- and intrafamily phenotypic variability of expression in Peutz-Jeghers kindreds. The availability of predictive genetic testing may have some value but cannot determine the likely severity of the phenotype.[129] Moreover, not all PJS patients have demonstrable mutations in the *LBK1/STK11* gene.[28,129,138,139] However, if the gene mutation is known for previous affected cases in the family, it might have a role in presymptomatic testing for family members without pigmentation.

Cancer Risk. The risk of developing malignancy, both in the gastrointestinal tract and at extraintestinal sites, is increased in adults with PJS.[129,134] Moreover, malignancy can evolve as early as childhood and adolescence.[132] In a recent meta-analysis of 210 PJS patients, the relative risk of stomach, small bowel, and large bowel cancer developing in PJS male patients was estimated at 235, 279, and 98, respectively, compared with that in the general population.[140] In a series of 222 Japanese patients, with 28 cases of digestive malignancy, 3 teenagers with advanced gastric cancer were included.[141] Of 70 patients under 16 years identified by a literature search, 5 had tumors, 2 of which were adenocarcinomas (1 gastric, 1 jejunal).[132] The risk of developing pancreatic cancer in PJS is estimated to be increased 100-fold.[140] The most common cancers associated with *STK11* germline mutations in the context of PSJ were gastrointestinal in origin and the risk for the cancers at ages 30, 40, 50, and 60 years was 1, 10, 18, and 42%, respectively. In women, the risk for breast cancer was substantially increased.[142]

Gonadal tumors have been reported at an increased frequency in females and occasionally in male patients with PJS.[129] Ovarian sex cord tumors with annular tubules (SCTAT), usually found in young adult women, may cause sexual precocity in young girls.[129] Analogous tumors have been identified in male patients, referred to as either large cells calcifying Sertoli cell tumors or as testicular tumors resembling SCTAT.[143] The clinical presentation is gynecomastia and rapid growth with advanced bone age in prepubescent boys.[143] Although often bilateral and multifocal, SCTATs usually have a benign course in the setting of PJS. Other neoplasms of the genital tract have been described in PJS females, but the major risk is breast cancer.

Diagnosis. According to Giardiello et al[140] a definite diagnosis is made in the presence of histopathologically confirmed hamartomatous polyps and at least two of the following clinical criteria: (1) family history, (2) mucocutaneous hyperpigmentation, and (3) small bowel polyposis.[144] Genetic testing may then be used. For patients without a family history of PJS, definitive diagnosis depends upon the presence of two or more histologically verified PJ-type polyps. For patients with a first-degree relative with PJS, the presence of hyperpigmentation is sufficient for presumptive diagnosis. The true incidence of a solitary hamartomatous polyp, particularly in the duodenum, without the true PJS is not currently known.[145]

Clinical Management The gastrointestinal polyposis of PJS carries the dual risk of repeated resections for infarction secondary to intussusception and malignancy. More than three-quarters with PJS had one or more laparotomies owing to the recurrence or progression of polyps.[146] This high reoperation rate might be reduced in skilled hands by removal of other polyps through upper and lower endoscopy and double balloon enteroscopy or intraoperative enteroscopy.[147] Intraoperative small bowel endoscopy identifies 38% more polyps at laparotomy compared with external palpation and small bowel transillumination.[147]

Children with well-defined mucocutaneous pigmentation should be enrolled into a screening program, as outlined in Table 13. For children who are asymptomatic with small polyps (ie, <1 cm in size), parents should be counseled about the risk of intussusception. If the child later develops relevant symptoms, a therapeutic approach is started.[146,147] Every 2 years, the symptomatic PJS patient should have upper and lower endoscopies with polypectomy[147] and some form of examination of the small bowel, such as barium study or capsule enteroscopy. Ingesting the capsule on the same day as routine gastroscopy and colonoscopy may be considered.[148,149] In adults, capsule endoscopy is able to detect a higher number of relevant small-intestinal polyps, but is a less reliable technique for the analysis of very large polyps.[148,149] Confirmatory barium follow-through, magnetic resonance enteroclysis or multidetector row CT enterography should be considered before significant management decisions. The size of the polyps and their location influence the clinical management (Figure 25). Patients with symptomatic midgut polyps greater than 1.5 cm in the jejunoileum should be referred for double balloon enteroscopy or laparotomy with intraoperative endoscopy. During laparotomy, the surgeon can assist in telescoping the endoscope over the entire small intestine. A noncrushing clamp can be placed over the cecum to prevent large bowel distention.[146] Smaller polyps can be removed by an electrocautery snare. Larger, broad-based polyps will require an enterotomy. If needed, a sterile endoscope can also be advanced through the enterotomy site to aid endoscopic examination of the entire small bowel followed by snare resection of polyps. Extensive small bowel surgical resection should not be undertaken in order to preserve gut function and limit the risk of short-bowel syndrome.

Hereditary Mixed Polyposis Syndrome

Hereditary mixed polyposis syndrome (MIM 601228) is characterized by atypical juvenile polyps, with mixed features of hamartomas and adenomas located in the colon with the risk of subsequent colorectal cancer. The known HMPS kindreds are all of Ashkenazy Jewish origin. The locus initially attributed to chromosome 6q16, maps to a minimal region of 15q13–q14.[149]

Table 13 Surveillance Guidelines for Peutz-Jeghers Syndrome

Site	Procedure	Onset (Years)	Interval (Years)
Stomach	Upper endoscopy	10	2
Small bowel	Small bowel follow-through or capsule endoscopy	10	2*
Colon	Pancolonoscopy	10	2*
Breast	Breast examination	25	1
	Mammography	25	2–3
Testicle	Testicular examination	10	1
Ovary	Uterus Pelvic examination	20	1
	Pelvic ultrasonography	12	1
Pancreas	Abdominal ultrasonography or endoscopic ultrasonography (if available)	30	1–2

*May consider lengthening interval based on clinical history.

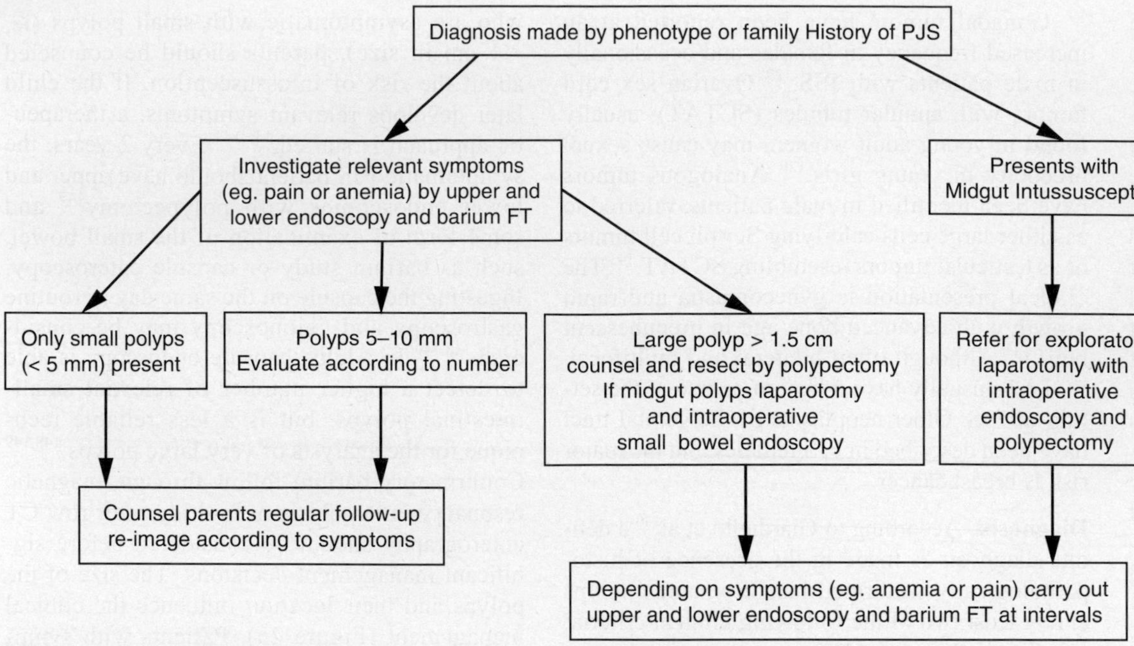

Figure 25 Management and surveillance in patients with Peutz-Jeghers syndrome (PJS). FT = follow-through. (Adapted from reference 87.)

Bourneville Tuberous Sclerosis

Tuberous sclerosis is a dominantly inherited disease with a variable penetrance characterized by the classic triad of mental retardation, epilepsy, and adenoma sebaceum in the presence of hamartomatous lesions. Mutations have been identified in two genes: tuberous sclerosis locus 1 (*TSC1*) and tuberous sclerosis locus 2 (*TSC2*). Hamartomatous polyps resembling Peutz-Jeghers polyps diagnosed at a mean age of 12 years, as well as adenomatous polyps diagnosed at a mean age of 45 years, may occur and are often located within the distal 25 cm of the colon. An invasive adenocarcinoma was reported in a 17-year-old girl in association with adenomatous polyps throughout the proximal and distal colon without a family history of colorectal neoplasia.[150]

Hyperplastic Polyposis Coli Syndrome

Hyperplastic polyposis coli syndrome (HPCS) is an uncommon condition. Diagnosis criteria are (1) the presence of at least 30 colonic hyperplastic polyps, or (2) the presence of 5 hyperplastic polyps (2–10 mm) above the sigmoid, or (3) the presence of hyperplastic polyps in a proband with a first-degree relative affected with hyperplastic polyposis.[14,151] In four of the 29 reports (14%) of the literature, HPCS occurred among young patients (11 to 29 years of age).[151] Keljo et al described a rectal cancer developing in an 11-year-old girl with hyperplastic polyposis.[152]

REFERENCES

1. Mougenot JF, Baldassarre LMN, Mashako GC, et al. Polypes recto-coliques de l'enfant. Analyse de 183 cas. Arch Fr Pediatr 1989;48:245–8.
2. Nowicki MJ, Subramony C, Bishop PR, Parker PH. Colonic chicken skin mucosa: Association with juvenile polyps in children. Am J Gastroenterol 2001;96:788–92.
3. Wu T, Rezai B, Rashid A, et al. Genetic alterations and epithelial dysplasia in juvenile polyposis syndrome and sporadic juvenile polyps. Am J Pathol 1997;150:939–47.
4. Hoffenberg EJ, Sauaia A, Maltzman T, et al. Symptomatic colonic polyps in childhood: Not so benign. J Pediatr Gastroenterol Nutr 1999;28:175–81.
5. Mougenot JF, Vargas J. Colonoscopic polypectomy and endoscopic mucosal resection. In: Winter H, Murphy S, Mougenot JF, Cadranel S, editors. Pediatric Gastrointestinal Endoscopy: Textbook and Atlas. Hamilton: BC Deker; 2006. p. 161–79.
6. Rex DK. Colonoscopy. Gastrointest Endosc Clin N Am 2000; 10:135–60.
7. Waye JD. New methods of polypectomy. Gastrointest Endosc Clin N Am 1997;7:413–65.
8. Giardiello FM, Hamilton SR, Kern SE, et al. Colorectal neoplasia in juvenile polyposis or juvenile polyps. Arch Dis Child 1991;66:971–5.
9. Nugent KP, Talbot IC, Hodgson SV, et al. Solitary juvenile polyps: Not a marker for subsequent malignancy. Gastroenterology 1993;105:698–700.
10. Buecher B, Bezieau S, Dufilhol C, et al. Les polypes festonnés colorectaux: une entité revisitée. Gastroenterol Clin Biol 2007;31:139–54.
11. Young J, Jass RJ. The case of a genetic predisposition to serrated neoplasia in the colorectum: Hypothesis and review of the litterature. Cancer Epidemiol Biomarkers Prev 2006;15:1778–84.
12. Lauwers GY, Chung DC. The serrated polyp comes to age. Gastroenterology 2006; 131:1631–4.
13. Jaramillo E, Tamura S, Mitomi H. Endoscopic appearance of serrated adenomas in the colon. Endoscopy 2005;37:254–60.
14. Torlakovic E, Snover DC. Sessile serrated adenoma: A brief history and current status. Crit Rev Oncogen 2006;121:27–39.
15. Togashi K, Hewett DG, Whitaker DA, et al. The use of acetic acid in magnification chromocolonoscopy for pit pattern analysis of small polyps. Endoscopy 2006;38:613–6.
16. Rubio CA, Jaramillo E, Lindblom A, Fogt F. Classification of colorectal polyps: Guidelines for the endoscopist. Endoscopy 2002;34:226–36.
17. Fu KI, Sano Y, Kato S, et al. Chromoendoscopy using indigo dye spraying with magnifying observation is the most reliable method for differential diagnosis between non-neoplastic and neoplastic colorectal lesions: A prospective study. Endoscopy 2004;36:1089–93.
18. Fleischer DE. Chromoendoscopy and magnification endoscopy in the colon. Gastrointest Endosc 1999;50: 704–6.
19. Machida H, Sano Y, Hamamoto Y, et al. Narrow-band imaging in the diagnosis of colorectal mucosal lesions: A pilot study. Endoscopy 2004;36:1094–8.
20. Winawer S, Fletcher R, Rex D, et al. (U.S. Multisociety Task Force on Colorectal Cancer). Colorectal cancer screening and surveillance: Clinical guidelines and rationale—Update based on new evidence. Gastroenterology 2003;124:544–60.
21. Jess T, Loftus EV, Jr, Velayos FS, et al. Risk of intestinal cancer in inflammatory bowel disease: A population-based study from Olmsted County, Minnesota. Gastroenterology 2006;130:1039–46.
22. Rutter MD, Saunders BP, Wilkinson KH, et al. Thirty-year analysis of a colonoscopic surveillance program for neoplasia in ulcerative colitis. Gastroenterology 2006; 130:1030–8.
23. Bodmer WF, Bailey CJ, Bussey HJR, et al. Localization of the gene for familial adenomatous polyposis on chromosome 5. Nature 1987;328:614–6.
24. Kinzler KW, Nilbert MC, Su LK, et al. Identification of FAP locus genes from chromosome 5q21. Science 1991;253:661–5.
25. Groden J, Thliveris A, Samowitz W, et al. Identification and characterization of the familial adenomatous polyposis coli gene. Cell 1991;66:589–600.
26. Liaw D, Marsh DJ, Li J, et al. Germ-line mutations of the PTEN gene in Cowden's disease, an inherited breast and thyroid cancer syndrome. Nat Genet 1997;16:64–7.
27. Howe JR, Roth S, Ringold JC, et al. Mutations in the SMAD4/DPC4 gene in the juvenile polyposis. Science 1998;280:1086–8.
28. Hemminki A, Markie D, Tomlinson I, et al. A serine/threonine kinase gene defective in Peutz-Jeghers syndrome. Nature 1998;391:184–7.
29. Al Tassan N, Chmiel NH, Maynard J, et al. Inherited variants of *MYH* associated with somatic G:C T:A mutations in colorectal tumors. Nat Genet 2002;30:227–32.
30. Jones S, Emmerson P, Maynard J, et al. Biallelic germline mutations in *MYH* predispose to multiple colorectal adenoma and somatic G:C T:A mutations. Hum Mol Genet 2002;11:2961–7.
31. Sieber OM, Lipton L, Crabtree M, et al. Multiple colorectal adenomas, classic adenomatous polyposis, and germ-line mutations in *MYH*. N Engl J Med 2003;348: 791–9.
32. Church JM, McGannon E, Burke C, Clark B. Teenagers with familial adenomatous polyposis. What is their risk for colorectal cancer? Dis Colon Rectum 2002;45:887–9.
33. Nieuwenhuis MH, Vasen HFA. Correlations between mutation site in APC and phenotype of familial adenomatous polyposis (FAP): A review. Crit Rev Oncol/Hematol 2007;61:153–61.
34. van Hes JH, Giles RH, Clevers HC. The many faces of the tumor suppressor gene APC. Exp Cell Res 2001;264:126–34.
35. Beroud C, Soussi T. APC gene: Database of germline and somatic mutations in human tumors and cell lines. Nucl Acids Res 1996;24:121–4.
36. Bertario L, Russo A, Sala P, et al. Multiple approach to the exploration of genotype–phenotype corelations in familial adenomatous polyposis. J. Clin Oncol 2003; 21:1698–707.
37. Moisio A-L, Järvinen H, Peltomäki P. Genetic and clinical characterisation of familial adenomatous polyposis: A population based study. Gut 2002;50:845–50.
38. Sieber OM, Lamlum H, Crabtree MD, et al. Whole-gene APC deletion cause classical familial adenomatous polyposis, but not attenuated polyposis or multiple colorectal adenomas. Proc Natl Acad Sci USA 2002;99:2954–8.
39. Michils G, Tejpar S, Thoelen R, et al. Large deletions of the APC gene in 15% of mutation-negative patients with classical polyposis (FAP): A Belgian study. Hum Mut 2005; 25:125–34.
40. Giardiello FM, Petersen GM, Piantadosi S, et al. APC gene mutations and extraintestinal phenotype of familial polyposis. Gut 1997;62:1290–301.

41. Caspari R, Olschwang S, Friedl W, et al. Familial adenomatous polyposis: Desmoid tumors and lack of ophthalmic lesions (CHRPE) associated with APC mutations beyond codon 1444. Hum Mol Genet 1995;4:337–40.
42. Giardello FM, Brensinger JD, Luce MC, et al. Phenotypic expression of disease in families that have mutations in the 5′ region of the adenomatous polyposis coli gene. Ann Intern Med 1997;126:514–9.
43. Soravia C, Berk T, Madlensky L, et al. Genotype–phenotype correlations in attenuated adenomatous polyposis coli. Am J Hum Genet 1998;62:1290–301.
44. Hodgson SV, Fagg NL, Talbot IC, Wikinson M. Deletions of the entire APC gene are associated with sessile colonic adenomas. J Med Genet 1994;31:426.
45. Young J, Simms LA, Tarish J, et al. A family with attenuated familial adenomatous polyposis due to a mutation in the alternatively spliced region of APC exon 9. Hum Mutat 1998;11:450–5.
46. Vasen HFA. Clinical diagnosis and management of hereditary colorectal cancer. J Clin Oncol 2000;21s:81–92.
47. Sieber OM, Tomlinson JP, Lamlum H. The adenomatous polyposis coli (APC) tumor suppresor—Genetics, function and disease. Mol Biol Today 2000;6:462–9.
48. Rosin-Arbesfeld R, Townsley F, Benz M. The APC tumour suppressor has a nuclear export function. Nature 2000;406:1009–12.
49. Erdmann KS, Kuhlmann J, Lesmann V, et al. The adenomatous polyposis coli-protein (APC) interacts with the protein tyrosine phosphatase PTP-BL via an alternatively spliced PDZ domain. Oncogene 2000;19:3894–901.
50. Yiang VW. APC as a checkpoint gene: The beginning or the end? Gastroenterology 2002;123:935–9.
51. Fodde R, Smits R, Clevers H. APC, signal transduction and genetic instability in colorectal cancer. Nat Rev Cancer 2001;1:55–67.
52. Galiatsatos P, Foulkes WD. Familial adenomatous polyposis. Am J Gastroenterol 2006;101:385–98.
53. Giardello FM, Petersen GM, Brensinger JD, et al. Hepatoblastoma and APC gene mutation in familial adenomatous polyposis. Gut 1996;39:867–9.
54. Hamilton SR, Liu B, Parsons RD, et al. The molecular basis of Turcot syndrome. N Engl J Med 1995;332:839–47.
55. Kashiwagi H, Spigelman AD. Gastroduodenal lesions in familial adenomatous polyposis. Surg Today 2000;30: 675–82.
56. Cruz-Correa M, Giardiello FM. Diagnosis and management of hereditary colon cancer. Gastroenterol Clin N Am 2002;31:53–49.
57. Burt RW. Gastric fundic gland polyps. Gastroenterology 2003;125:1462–9.
58. Spigelman AD, Williams CB, Talbot IC, et al. Upper gastrointestinal cancer in patients with familial adenomatous polyposis. Lancet 1989;ii:783–5.
59. Offerhaus JA, Levin LS, Giardiello FM, et al. Occult radio-opaque jaw lesions in familial adenomatous polyposis coli and hereditary non polyposis coli cancer. Gastroenterology 1987;93:490–7.
60. Traboulsi EI, Apostolides J, Giardiello FM, et al. Pigmented ocular fundus lesions and APC mutations in familial adenomatous polyposis. Ophthalmic Genet 1996;17:167–74.
61. Soravia Cl, Berk T, McLeod RS, Cohen Z. Desmoid disease in patients with familial adenomatous polyposis. Dis Colon Rectum 2000;43:363–9.
62. Strut NJH, Gallagher MXC, Bassett P, et al. Evidence for genetic predisposition to desmoid tumors in familial adenomatous polyposis independent of the germline mutation. Gut 2004;53:1832–6.
63. King JE, Dozois RR, Lindor NM, Alqhuist DA. Care of patients and their families with familial adenomatous polyposis. Mayo Clin Proc 2000;75:57–67.
64. Bülow C, Bülow S, Leeds Castle Polyposis Group. Is screening for thyroid carcinoma indicated in familial adenomatous polyposis? Int J Colorectal Dis 1997;12:240–2.
65. Lynch HT, Smyrk T, McGinn T, et al. Attenuated familial adenomatous polyposis (AFAP): A phenotypically and genotypically distinctive variant of FAP. Cancer 1995;76:2427–33.
66. Gruber SB. New developments in Lynch syndrome (Hereditary Nonpolyposis Colorectal Cancer) and mismatch repair gene testing. Gastroenterology 2006;130:577–87.
67. Attard TM, Giardiello FM, Pedram A, Cuffari C. Fundic gland polyposis with high-grade dysplasia in a child with attenuated familial adenomatous polyposis and familial gastric cancer. J Pediatr Gastroenterol Nutr 2001;32: 215–8.
68. Mori T, Nagase H, Horii A, et al. Germline and somatic mutations of the APC gene in patients with Turcot syndrome and analysis of APC mutations in brain tumors. Genes Chromosomes Cancer 1994;9:168–72.
69. Eccles DM, Van der Luijt R, Breukel C, et al. Hereditary desmoid disease due to a frameshift mutation at codon 1924 of the APC gene. Am J Hum Genet. 1996;59:1193–201.
70. Chung DC, Rustgi AK. The hereditary nonpolyposis colorectal cancer syndrome: Genetics and clinical implications. Ann Intern Med 2003;138: 560–70.
71. Muller A, Giuffre G, Edmonston TB, et al. Challenges and pitfalls in HNPCC screening by microsatellite analysis and immunohistochemistry. J Mol Diagn 2004;6:308–15.
72. Scheenstra R, Rijcken FEM, Koornstra JJ, et al. Rapidly progressive adenomatous polyposis in a patient with germline mutations in both the APC and MLH1 genes: The worst of two worlds. Gut 2003;52:898–9.
73. Bülow S. Results of national registration of familial adenomatous polyposis. Gut 2003;52:742–6.
74. Giardiello FM, Brensinger JD, Petersen G. American Gastroenterological Association. Medical position statement: Hereditary colorectal cancer and genetic testing. Gastroenterology 2001;121:195–7.
75. Grady WM. Genetic testing for high-risk colon cancer patients. Gastroenterology 2003;124:1574–94.
76. Burt R, Neklason DW. Genetic testing for inherited colon cancer. Gastroenterology 2005;128:1696–716.
77. Su LK, Kohlmann W, Ward PA, Lynch PM. Different familial adenomatous polyposis phenotypes resulting from deletions of the entire *APC* exon 15. Hum Genet 2002;111:88–95.
78. Bülow S, Björk J, Christensen IJ, et al. Duodenal adenomatosis in familial adenomatous polyposis. The DAF study group. Gut 2004; 53:381–6.
79. Morpugo E, Vitale G, Galandiuk S, et al. Clinical characteristics of familial adenomatous polyposis and management of duodenal adenomas. J Gastrointest Surg 2004;8:559–64.
80. Durno CA, Gallinger S. Genetic predisposition to colorectal cancer: New pieces in the pediatric puzzle. J Pediatr Gastroenterol Nutr 2006;43:5–15.
81. Mison JW, Ludwig KA, Church JM, et al. Laparoscopic total abdominal colectomy with ileorectal anastomosis for familial adenomatous polyposis. Dis Colon Rectum 1997;40:675–8.
82. Kartheuser A, Stangherlin P, Brandt D, et al. Restorative proctocolectomy and ileal pouch-anal anastomosis for familial adenomatous polyposis revisited. Familial Cancer 2006;5:241–60.
83. van Duijvendijk P, Slors JF, Taat CW, et al. Quality of life after total colectomy with ileorectal anastomosis or proctocolectomy and ileo pouch-anal anastomosis for familial adenomatous polyposis. Br J Surg 2000;87:590–6.
84. Körgsen S, Keighley MRB. Causes of failure and life expancy of the ileoanal pouch. Int J Colorect Dis 1997; 12:4–8.
85. Barton JG, Paden MA, Lane M, et al. Comparison of postoperative outcomes in ulcerative colitis and familial polyposis patients after ileoanal pouch operations. Am J Surg 2001;182:616–20.
86. Olsen KO, Juul S, Bülow S, et al. Female fecundity before and after operation for familial adenomatous polyposis. Br J Surg 2003;90:227–31.
87. Hyer W, Beveridge I, Domizio P, Phillips R. Clinical management and genetics of gastrointestinal polyps in children. J Pediatr Gastroenterol Nutr 2000;31:469–79.
88. Parc YR, Olschwang S, Desaint B, et al. Familal adenomatous polyposis: Prevalence of adenomas in the ileal pouch after restorative proctocolectomy. Ann Surg 2001;233: 360–4.
89. van Duijvendijk P, Vasen HFA, Bertario L, et al. Cumulative risk of developing polyps or malignancy at the ileal pouch-anal anastomosis in patients with familial adenomatous polyposis. J Gastrointest Surg 1999;3:325–30.
90. Steinbach G, Lynch PM, Phillips RK, et al. The effect of celecoxib, a cyclooxygenase-2 inhibitor in familial adenomatous polyposis. N Engl J Med 2000;342:1946–52.
91. Cruz-Correa M, Hylind LM, Romans KE, et al. Long-term treatment with sulindac in familial adenomatous polyposis: A prospective cohort study. Gastroenterology 2002;122:641–5.
92. Yang VW, Casero RA, Geiman DE, et al. Primary prevention of familial adenomatous polyposis: Stratification of clinical response to sulindac by mucosal prostanoid levels. N Engl J Med 2002;346:1054–9.
93. Bresalier RS, Sandler RS, Quan H, et al. Cardiovascular events associated with rofecoxib in a colorectal adenoma chemoprevention trial. N Engl J Med 2005;352:1092–102.
94. Solomon SD, McMurray JJ, Pfeffer MA, et al. Cardiovascular risk associated with celecoxib in a clinical trial for colorectal adenoma prevention. N Engl J Med 2005;352:1071–80.
95. Phillips RK, Wallace MH, Lynch PM, et al. A randomised, double blind, placebo controlled study of celecoxib, a selective cyclooxygenase 2 inhibitor, on duodenal polypsis in familial polyposis. Gut 2002;50:857–60.
96. Cheng CL, Sherman S, Fogel EL, et al. Endoscopic snare papillectomy for tumors of the duodenal papillae. Gastrointest Endosc 2004;60:757–64.
97. De Vos tot Nederveen Cappel WH, Järvinen HJ, Björk J, et al. Worldwide survey among polyposis registries of surgical management of severe duodenal adenomatosis in familial adenomatous polyposis. Br J Surg 2003;90:705–10.
98. Sturt NJH, Clark SK. Current ideas in desmoid tumours. Familial Cancer 2006;5:275–85.
99. Sieber OM, Lipton L, Crabtree M, et al. Multiple colorectal adenomas, classic adenomatous polyposis, and germline mutations in MYH. N Engl J Med 2003; 348: 791–9.
100. Samson JR, Dolwani S, Jones S, et al. Autosomal recessive colorectal adenomatous polyposis due to inherited mutations of MYH. Lancet 2003;362;39–41.
101. Screibman IA, Baker M, Amos C, McGarrity TJ. The hamartomatous polyposis syndromes: A clinical and molecular review. Am J Gastroenterol 2005;100:476–90.
102. Carethers JM. Hamartomatous poyposis syndromes: Genetic pathways. Curr Opin Gastroentrol 2002;18:60–67.
103. Wirtzfeld DA, Petrelli NJ, Rodriguez-Bigas MA. Hamartomatous polyposis syndromes: Molecular genetics, neoplastic risk, and surveillance recommendations. Ann Surg Oncol 2001;8:319–27.
104. Sachatello CR, Hahn IS, Carrington CB. Juvenile gastrointestinal polyposis in a female infant: Report of a case and review of the literature of a recently recognized syndrome. Surgery 1974;74:107–14.
105. Hofting I, Pott G, Schrameyer B, Stolte M. Familiare juvenile polyposis mit vorwiegender Magenbeteiligung. Z Gastroenterol 1993;31:480–3.
106. Lynch ED, Ostermeyer EA, Lee MK, et al. Inherited mutations in PTEN that are associated with breast cancer, Cowden disease, and juvenile polyposis. Am J Hum Genet 1997;61:1254–60.
107. Dahia PLM, Marsh DJ, Zheng Z, et al. Somatic deletions and mutations in the Cowden disease gene, PTEN, in sporadic thyroid tumors. Cancer Res 1997;57:4710–3.
108. Olschwang S, Serova-Sinilnikova OM, Lenoir GM, Giles T. PTEN-germline mutations in juvenile polyposis coli. Nat Genet 1998;18:12–4.
109. Arch EM, Goodman BK, Van Wesep RA, et al. Deletion of PTEN in a patient with Bannayan–Riley–Ruvalcaba syndrome suggests allelism with Cowden disease. Am J Med Genet 1997;71:489–93.
110. Waite KA, Eng C. Protein PTEN: Form and function. Am J Hum Genet 2002;70:829–44.
111. Howe JR, Ringold JC, Summers RW, et al. A gene for familial juvenile polyposis maps to chromosome 18q21.1. Am J Hum Genet 1998;62:1129–36.
112. Marsh DJ, Roth S, Lunetta KL, et al. Exclusion of PTEN and 10q22-24 as the susceptibility locus for juvenile polyposis syndrome. Cancer Res 1997;57:5017–21.
113. Huang SC, Chen CR, Lavine JE, et al. Genetic heterogeneity in familial juvenile polyposis. Cancer Res 2000;60:6882–5.
114. Sayed MG, Ahmed AF, Ringold R, et al. Germline SMAD4 or BMPR1A mutations and phenotype of juvenile polyposis. Ann Surg Oncol 2002;9:901–6.
115. Friedl W, Uhlhaas S, Schulmann K, et al. Juvenile polyposis: Massive gastric polyposis is more common in MADH4 mutation carriers than in BMPR1A mutation carriers. Hum Genet 2002;111:108–11.
116. Howe JR, Bair JL, Sayed MG, et al. Germline mutations of the gene encoding bone morphogenetic protein receptor 1A in juvenile polyposis. Nat Genet 2001;28:184–7.
117. Zhou X, Woodford-Richens K, Lehtonen R, et al. Germline mutations in BMPR1A/ALK3 cause a subset of cases of juvenile polyposis syndrome and of Cowden and Bannayan–Riley–Ruvalcaba syndromes. Am J Hum Genet 2001;69:704–11.
118. Moustakas A, Souchelnytskyi S, Heldin CH. Smad regulation in TGF-beta signal transduction. J Cell Sci 2001;114:4359–69.
119. Jass JR, Williams CB, Bussey HJR, Morson BC. Juvenile polyposis: A precancerous condition. Histopathology 1988;13:619–30.
120. Coburn MC, Pricolo VE, DeLuca FG, Bland KI. Malignant potential in intestinal juvenile polyposis syndromes. Ann Surg Oncol 1995;2:386–91.
121. Desai DC, Neale KF, Talbot IC, et al. Juvenile polyposis. Br J Surg 1995;82:14–7.
122. Giardello FM, Hamilton SR, Kern SE, et al. Colorectal neoplasia in juvenile polyposis or juvenile polyps. Arch Dis Child 1991;66:971–5.
123. Hizawa K, Iida M, Yao T, et al. Juvenile polyposis of the stomach: Clinicopathological features and its malignant potential. J Clin Pathol 1997;50:771–4.
124. Eng C. PTEN: One gene, many syndromes. Hum Mutat 2003;22:183–98.

125. Marsh DJ, Dahia PLM, Zheng Z, et al. Germline mutations in PTEN are present in Bannayan–Zonana syndrome. Nat Genet 1997;16:333–4.

126. Carethers JM, Furnari FB, Zigman AF, et al. Absence of PTEN/MMAC1 germ-line mutations in sporadic Bannayan–Riley–Ruvalcaba syndrome. Cancer Res 1998;58:2724–6.

127. Delnatte C, Sanlaville D, Mougenot JF, et al. Contiguous gene deletion within chromosome arm 10q is associated with juvenile polyposis of infancy, reflecting cooperation between the BMPR1A and PTEN tumor-suppressor genes. Am J Hum Genet 2006;78:1066–74.

128. Westerman AM, Entius MM, de Baar E et al. Peutz-Jeghers syndrome: 78 year follow-up of the original family. Lancet 1999;353:1211–5.

129. McGarrity T, Kulin H, Zaino R. Clinical reviews: Peutz-Jeghers syndrome. Am J Gastroenterol 2000;95:596–604.

130. Jenne DE, Reimann H, Nezu J, et al. Peutz-Jeghers syndrome is caused by mutations in a novel serine threonine kinase. Nat Genet 1998;18:38–43.

131. Hemminki A. The molecular basis and clinical aspects of Peutz-Jeghers syndrome. Cell Mol Life Sci 1999;55:356–60.

132. Tovar JA, Eizaguirre I, Albert A, et al. Peutz-Jeghers syndrome in children: Report of two cases and review of the literature. J Pediatr Surg 1983;18:1–6.

133. Wang ZJ, Ellis I, Zauber P. Allelic imbalance at the LKB1 (STK11) locus on 19p13.3 in hamartomas, adenomas and carcinomas from patients with Peutz-Jeghers syndrome provides evidence for a hamartoma–adenoma–carcinoma sequence. J Pathol 1999;188:613–7.

134. Lim W, Hearle N, Shah B, et al. Further observations on LKB1/STK1 status and cancer risk in Peutz-Jeghers syndrome. Br J Cancer 2003;89:308–13.

135. Yoo LI, Chung DC, Yuan J. LKB1—A master tumour suppressor of the small intestine and beyond. Nat Rev 2002;2:529–35.

136. Boudeau J, Sapkota G, Alesi DR. LKB1, a protein kinase regulating cell proliferation and polarity. FEBS Lett 2003;546:159–65.

137. Marignani PA. LKB1, the multiasking tumour suppressor kinase. J Clin Pathol 2005;58:15–9.

138. Olschwang S, Markie D, Seal S, et al. Peutz-Jeghers disease: Most, but not all, families are compatible with linkage to 19p13.3. J Med Genet 1998;35:42–4.

139. Olschwang S, Boisson C, Thomas G. Peutz-Jeghers families unlinked to STK11/LKB1 gene mutations are highly predisposed to primitive biliary adenocarcinoma. J Med Genet 2001;38:356–60.

140. Giardiello FM, Brensinger JD, Tersmette AC, et al. Very high risk of cancer in familial Peutz-Jeghers syndrome. Gastroenterology 2000;119:1447–53.

141. Hizawa K, Iida M, Matsumoto T, et al. Neoplastic transformation arising in Peutz-Jeghers polyposis. Dis Colon Rectum 1993;36:953–7.

142. Lim W, Olschwang S, Keller JJ et al. Relative frequency and morphology of cancers in STK11 mutations cancers. Gastroenterology 2004;126:1788–94.

143. Young S, Gooneratne S, Straus FH, et al. Feminizing Sertoli cell tumors in boys with Peutz-Jeghers syndrome. Am J Surg Pathol 1995;19:50–8.

144. Kitaoka F, Shiogama T, Mizutani A, et al. A solitary Peutz-Jeghers-type hamartomatous polyp in the duodenum: A case report including results of mutational analysis. Digestion 2004;69:79–82.

145. Spigelman AD, Arese P, Phillips RKS. Polyposis: The Peutz-Jeghers syndrome. Br J Surg 1995;82:1311–4.

146. Pennazio M, Rossini FP. Small bowel polyps in Peutz-Jeghers syndrome: Management by combined push enteroscopy and intraoperative endoscopy. Gastrointest Endosc 2000;51:304–8.

147. Brown G, Fraser C, Schofield G, et al. Videocapsule endoscopy in Peutz-Jeghers syndrome: A blinded comparison with barium follow-through for detection of small polyps. Endoscopy 2006;38:385–90.

148. Caspari R, von Falkenhausen M, Krautmacher C, et al. Comparison of capsule endoscopy and magnetic imaging for the detection of polyps of the small intestine in patients with familial adenomatous polyposis or with Peutz-Jeghers syndrome. Endoscopy 2004;36:1054–9.

149. Jaeger EE, Woodford-Richens KL, Lockett M, et al. An ancestral Ashkenazi haplotype at the HMPS/CRAC1 locus on 15q13-q14 is associated with hereditary mixed polyposis syndrome. Am J Hum Genewt 2003;72:1261–7.

150. Digoy GP, Tibayan F, Young H, Edelstein PJ. Adenocarcinoma of the rectum with associated colorectal adenomatous polyps in tuberous sclerosis. Pediatr Surg 2000;35:526–7.

151. Rubio CA, Stemme S, Jaramillo E, Lindblom A. Hyperplastic polyposis coli syndrome and colorectal carcinoma. Endoscopy 2006;28:266–70.

152. Keljo, DJ, Weinberg AG, Winick N, Tomlinson G. Rectal cancer in an 11-year-old girl with hyperplastic polyposis. J Pedriat Gastroenterol Nutr 1999;28:327–32.

23.2. Other Neoplasms

Kamran Badizadegan, MD

Intestinal neoplasms collectively represent a significant fraction of gastrointestinal diseases in all age groups. While malignant intestinal tumors are a leading cause of cancer morbidity and mortality in adults, malignant tumors of the intestines constitute only a small fraction (<2%) of all childhood malignancies.[1] In spite of this relatively low prevalence, children are affected by a diverse group of benign and malignant intestinal neoplasms, the recognition of which is essential in proper diagnosis and management. In fact, the relative rarity of intestinal tumors in children makes their timely and appropriate diagnosis somewhat more challenging than in adults.

Throughout this volume, various chapters are dedicated to discussion of gastrointestinal neoplasms. The present chapter complements the preceding discussion of intestinal epithelial polyps and polyposis syndromes (see Chapter 23.1, "Intestinal Polyps and Polyposis"), while neoplasms of the esophagus and stomach are separately discussed in Chapter 10, "Esophageal and Gastric Neoplasms." Rather than provide an encyclopedic discussion of all potential neoplasms, this chapter will highlight the most important issues related to pathology, pathophysiology, and clinical behavior of the most significant lesions. In particular, unique pediatric aspects of epithelial neoplasms, lymphoproliferative disorders, and mesenchymal tumors are discussed. These tumors constitute the bulk of malignant or otherwise clinically significant intestinal neoplasms, and approach to their diagnosis and management will also provide a general approach for management of other less common lesions.

EPITHELIAL NEOPLASMS

Colorectal Carcinoma (CRC)

Benign and premalignant epithelial polyps and polyposis syndromes were discussed in the preceding chapter. Malignant epithelial neoplasms of the gastrointestinal tract are generally rare and constitute only an estimated 1% of all malignant pediatric tumors. Among this group, colorectal adenocarcinoma is only second to primary hepatocellular tumors in prevalence.[2,3] Other intestinal tumors of epithelial origin, excluding low-grade endocrine tumors (carcinoid tumors), are virtually unheard of, and their diagnosis should be made with extreme caution.

Epidemiology and Clinical Features. The estimated incidence rate of colorectal adenocarcinoma is 1 in 10 million for all individuals younger than 20 years of age.[4,5] CRC can present at any age and rare cases are reported as early as the first year of life.[6,7] Nevertheless, most reported cases appear to present in the second decade of life, specially in the early teens. Pediatric CRC may present in any anatomic location. The relative predilection for the left colon seen in the adult population appears to be lacking by most accounts,[2,3,8–11] although some reported series of pediatric CRC show a clear preference for the rectosigmoid location.[12]

Presenting symptoms are often nonspecific and range from abdominal pain to rectal bleeding and intestinal obstruction. As in any other intestinal mass lesion, clinical signs, and symptoms are more closely related to location, size, and extent of the tumor, rather than the specific underlying phenotype. Pediatric CRCs are said to have a worse prognosis than their adult counterpart,[8] but studies that are adequately matched for disease stage at presentation, tumor subtype, and clinical management are lacking. Therefore, it is unclear whether the often cited conclusion about the poor prognosis in pediatric CRC is a true biological behavior or a reflection of other factors such as aggressive tumor phenotype or a delay in diagnosis resulting in a more advanced stage at presentation.

Pathology and Pathophysiology. Although CRC in children has many pathological similarities to adult CRC, some notable difference emerge. Perhaps the most striking of these differences is the incidence of mucinous phenotype in the pediatric population.

Mucinous adenocarcinomas are defined as colorectal adenocarcinomas in which greater than 50% of the tumor mass consists of extracellular pools of mucin containing free-floating malignant cells, singly or in small clusters (Figure 1).[13] Individual signet-ring cells are often present in mucin pools of the mucinous adenocarcinoma, although if they are present in large numbers

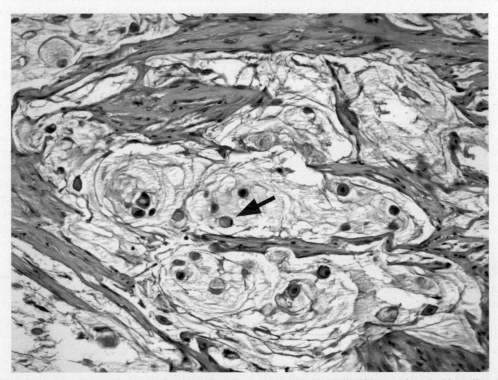

Figure 1 Mucinous adenocarcinoma of the cecum from a teenage child with medical history of atypical juvenile polyposis. Relatively acellular pools of mucin are surrounded by desmoplastic connective tissue. Rare signet-ring cell (*arrow*) are identifiable within the pools of mucin.

(representing greater than 50% of the tumor cellularity), it is recommended to further subclassify the tumor as a signet-ring cell adenocarcinoma.[13] Mucinous and signet-ring cell adenocarcinoma are relatively uncommon in adults, representing approximately 10% of all cases.[14] In contrast, the majority of reported pediatric CRCs show a mucinous phenotype, with or without a prominent signet-ring cell component. The reported incidence of this phenotype in pediatric series ranges from 50 to 90% of cases, making this the predominant CRC subtype in individuals under the age of 20 years.[3,11,12,15,16]

The biological basis of the high prevalence of mucinous tumors in children is not entirely clear. Mucinous tumors have a somewhat distinct molecular pathology that may be linked to their high prevalence in children. In contrast to nonmucinous colorectal neoplasms, defects in DNA mismatch repair genes with high microsatellite instability (MSI) are more common in mucinous tumors.[17,18] Conversely, the subgroup of mucinous tumors that show high MSI are more likely to present in younger patients.[19] Unfortunately, however, mucinous phenotype and signet-ring cells are generally not a specific marker of microsatellite instability,[18] making it difficult to draw definitive conclusions. Specific studies of molecular pathological data in children with CRC are needed to determine the significance of these observations.

The potential association between CRC and DNA mismatch repair in children warrants clinical and pathological investigation of the affected children for hereditary nonpolyposis colorectal cancer syndrome (HNPCC). HNPCC, also known as Lynch syndrome, is clinically characterized by early onset of colorectal neoplasms and an increased lifetime risk of malignant tumors in various extraintestinal sites including—but not limited to—the endometrium, urinary tract, and the ovaries.[20] HNPCC is associated with mutations in DNA mismatch repair genes *MLH1*, *MSH2*, *MSH6*, and *PMS2*, and is clinically diagnosed based on the age of onset and family characteristics as defined in the revised Amsterdam criteria.[21] However, the sensitivity of clinical criteria for identification of HNPCC in patients with colorectal cancer is less than ideal,[20,22] making a tissue-based diagnosis highly preferable. Methodologies for tissue-based algorithms for the diagnosis of HNPCC are well defined and must be considered in any child or young adult who presents with colorectal carcinoma.[23,24]

In addition to its clinical importance for surveillance and follow-up, testing for MSI has become an increasingly important component of therapeutic decision making and assessment of response to treatment in CRC patients. Independent of tumor stage at presentation, CRC patients with high MSI appear to have a more favorable prognosis than those without.[25] Furthermore, patients with high MSI appear not to benefit from standard adjuvant chemotherapy.[25,26] Collectively, these observations make it critical to establish the MSI status of all pediatric patients with CRC, especially those presenting with mucinous phenotype.

Clinical Management. Recognition of the possibility that CRCs occur with a measurable frequency in children is the most important step toward a timely diagnosis. Diagnostic workup of CRC is no different than that of any other mass lesion in the intestinal tract. Endoscopic surveillance with biopsy is an essential step, with the understanding that sigmoidoscopy may not be an adequate screening method because many pediatric lesions arise in the proximal colon. In patients with documented CRC, imaging modalities such as computed tomography, magnetic resonance imaging, and positron emission tomography are required in evaluating the extent of the disease and in identification of potential distant metastases.[27–29]

Evidence-based recommendations for treatment of pediatric CRCs are lacking, and treatment options are generally based on adult studies. Standard treatment for patients with localized colorectal cancer is surgical resection of the primary tumor and regional lymph nodes. Laparoscopic-assisted colectomy is an acceptable alternative to open colectomy in patients who meet the surgical criteria for laparoscopic resection.[30] Laparoscopic resection, however, does not appear to provide long-term quality-of-life benefits in comparison with open colectomy.[31]

Regardless of the method of resection, pathological staging of the extent of tumor invasion and the lymph node status are among the most important determinants of management and prognosis. Although the modification of Dukes' original staging method by Astler and Coller is the most commonly used pathological staging system,[32] it is recommended that all newly diagnosed cases be staged according to the TNM staging criteria.[33] TNM staging not only provides a unified basis for development of a much-needed cross-institutional database of pediatric CRC, but is also the basis for essentially all new adjuvant therapies and outcome analyses.

Adjuvant chemotherapy and chemotherapy for treatment of advanced or metastatic disease provide clinical benefit in selected patients, although most patients require individual evaluation for determination of the potential benefits (if any), combination of agents, dosage, and duration of treatment. At the present, the American Society of Clinical Oncology does not support routine use of adjuvant chemotherapy for patients with stage II colon cancer.[34] However, the recommendations allow considering the use of adjuvant chemotherapy in stage II patients who deemed to be at high risk. Although specific guidelines for defining "high risk" are lacking, several histological features such as pathological stage T4 lesion, perforated tumors, or poorly differentiated neoplasms may be considered to be high-risk compared to other stage II cancers. In addition, patients with pathological stage T3, in whom the number of lymph nodes examined at the time of resection is deemed to be too small, may be regarded as understaged and therefore of higher risk. Precise recommendations for an adequate number of lymph nodes are lacking, but it has been recommended that a minimum of 13 lymph nodes should be examined to label a T3 colon cancer as definitely node negative.[35]

In contrast to stage II lesions, the benefit of adjuvant chemotherapy in patients with stage III colon cancer is well established. Essentially all accepted therapeutic regimens include fluorouracil alone or in combination with one or more agents such as leucovorin or levamisole. A detailed discussion of these regimens is beyond the scope of this chapter, but outstanding and up-to-date reviews are available in the form of Gastrointestinal Cancer Evidence-based Series and Practice Guidelines.[36] It must be emphasized, however, that essentially all accepted treatment guidelines are based on adult clinical trials and specific pediatric guidelines are lacking.

Radiation therapy has a significant role in management of selected CRC patients who have low rectal cancers. Based on a meta-analysis of 15 published clinical trials, Cancer Care Ontario Practice Guideline Initiative recommends that patients with resected stage II or III rectal cancer be offered adjuvant therapy with the combination of radiation and chemotherapy.[37] Furthermore, there is increasing evidence that preoperative radiotherapy, alone or in combination with chemotherapy, improves survival and surgical outcome in patients with low rectal cancer.[38,39] Again, specific information about children are lacking. In one recent series, two children with unresectable lesions (location not specified) and planned preoperative radiation therapy were successfully converted to resectable lesions.[3] In the same study, three additional children who received radiation for symptomatic relief and/or local control did not appear to benefit from the procedure.

Small Intestinal Adenocarcinoma

Pediatric small intestinal adenocarcinoma is exceedingly rare, and only isolated cases have been reported.[40–44] Documentation of a small intestinal adenocarcinoma in a child must prompt investigation for an underlying risk factor such as familial adenomatous polyposis or Peutz-Jeghers syndrome, although many of the reported cases do not indicate a specific risk factor. Chronic inflammatory bowel disease (Crohn's disease and ulcerative colitis) is a known risk factor for neoplastic progress in the general population, and children with longstanding disease may be at risk of malignancy in early adult life.[45] Although routine screening for small intestinal malignancies is not practical, unexplained gastrointestinal blood loss or symptoms of small intestinal obstruction must include a differential diagnosis of a small intestinal tumor. In addition to traditional imaging modalities, capsule endoscopy may aid in the diagnosis.[46] A definitive diagnosis of malignancy, however, would require tissue sampling and histopathological examination.

Endocrine Tumors

Endocrine cell tumors of the small and large intestine include a diverse group of neoplasms ranging from benign carcinoid tumors to highly malignant small-cell carcinomas. Intestinal endocrine cell tumors in children, however, are almost always low-grade carcinoid tumors.

Epidemiology and Clinical Features. Analysis of thousands of cases from the Surveillance, Epidemiology, and End Results (SEER) program of the National Cancer Institute has resulted in significant epidemiological characterization of carcinoid tumors in the general population.[47,48] Comparable data about the incidence and behavior of carcinoid tumors in children are lacking. Based on the analysis of more than 10,000 cases, gastrointestinal carcinoids appear to account for nearly two-thirds of all carcinoid tumors.[47] Among this group, tumors are nearly equally distributed between the small intestine (44%) and the colon (44%), with ileal (23%) and rectosigmoid (24%) tumors accounting for the majority of all cases.[47] Appendiceal tumors, which in earlier studies accounted for up to half of all gastrointestinal carcinoids,[49] represent only 7.4% of the cases collected under SEER.[47] Incidental or causative association with acute appendicitis in children, however, has resulted in a pediatric literature that is almost exclusively based on carcinoids of the appendix. Appendiceal carcinoids are found in as many as 1.4% of all resected specimens,[50–52] either in the form of an incidental tumor at the tip of the appendix (Figure 2A) or as a partially obstructing mass, presumably contributing to the presentation of appendicitis itself. Carcinoid tumors outside of the appendix are rarely encountered in the pediatric population, although two widely metastatic pediatric carcinoids were described in the ileum and the transverse colon, respectively.[53] Rarely, carcinoid tumors may also be seen in Meckel's diverticulum or intestinal duplications.[54,55]

Pathology and Pathophysiology. Carcinoid tumors arise from any of the endocrine cells of the gastrointestinal mucosa, and can be morphologically subdivided based on the type and content of cytoplasmic granules. The vast majority of pediatric intestinal carcinoids, however, arise from the enterochromaffin (EC) cells and do not generally require further subclassification. Morphologically, carcinoid tumors are nodular, infiltrative masses with ill-defined borders. In spite of their highly infiltrative microscopic appearance (Figure 2B), carcinoid tumors are often benign, specially when small (less than 1 cm in diameter). Pathological diagnosis is straightforward with the typical appearance of polygonal cells with round to oval nuclei, finely dispersed chromatin, and trabecular or insular growth pattern (Figure 2B). Mitoses are rare and nuclear atypia is virtually absent in classical cases. Immunohistochemical staining for chromogranin, synaptophysin, or other endocrine markers is generally not required, but may be used to confirm diagnoses in questionable cases.

Although carcinoid tumors can potentially secrete functional (bioactive) peptides with physiological consequences ("carcinoid syndrome"), the vast majority of carcinoid tumors are nonfunctional and are found incidentally. This is particularly true of the appendiceal carcinoids, which comprise the most frequently encountered carcinoid tumor in the pediatric population. Ileal and rectosigmoid carcinoids, which are often seen as submucosal nodules and account for a significant portion of adult intestinal carcinoids, are not typically encountered in children.

Clinical Management. Although rare metastatic cases are reported,[48,53,56,57] deaths associated with the carcinoid tumors are exceedingly rare.[53] In the vast majority of cases in which the tumor is small and localized, no specific additional treatment is needed for completely excised tumors. In cases with suspicion of residual tumor or with wide tumor spread beyond the muscularis propria, additional local resection may be considered on a case-by-case basis. In general, local resection appears to be an adequate clinical goal for pediatric carcinoids regardless of size or extent of

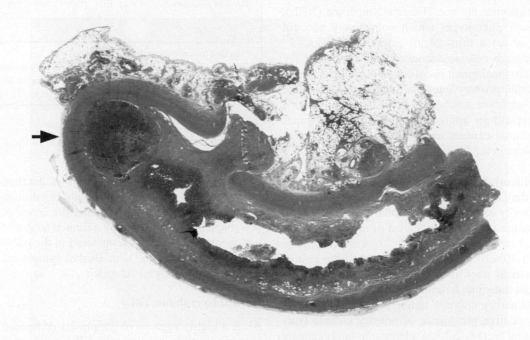

(A)

(B)

Figure 2 Classic presentation of a small carcinoid tumor at the tip (A, *arrow*) of an incidentally resected appendix. Tumor is confined to the appendix and no significant invasion into the wall is present. High-power microscopic view of a hematoxylin and eosin stained section (B) shows islands of round, uniform cells infiltrating the muscular wall of the appendix. Nuclear texture shows the characteristic finely dispersed chromatin pattern, which is commonly described as a "salt-and-pepper" appearance.

invasion.[51,58,59] Adjuvant chemotherapy has been tried in rare widely metastatic cases with questionable benefit.[53,57]

LYMPHOID NEOPLASMS (LYMPHOMAS)

Lymphomas are a clinically and pathologically heterogeneous group of neoplasms characterized by the clonal proliferation of lymphocytes. Although most lymphomas arise from the lymph nodes, primary extranodal lymphomas are seen in a variety of soft tissues including the gastrointestinal tract. The vast majority of primary intestinal lymphomas are non-Hodgkin lymphoma (NHL), B cell phenotype, which collectively account for about a third of all extranodal NHLs.[60–62] Although colonic adenocarcinoma is by far the leading malignant neoplasm of the intestinal tract overall, primary intestinal lymphomas constitute a significant number of small intestinal tumors, representing approximately 18% of all small intestinal cancers and nearly a third of all ileal tumors in the United States.[63]

Epidemiology and Clinical Features. While epithelial neoplasms constitute the overwhelming majority of malignant intestinal tumors in adults, lymphomas dominate the list of malignant intestinal tumors in children,[64,65] representing more than 70% of all malignant tumors of the gastrointestinal tract in some pediatric centers.[1] In the small intestine, lymphomas appear to be the predominant malignant tumor of childhood, while the relative prevalence of primary colonic lymphoma (versus colonic adenocarcinoma) appears to vary from study to study.[1,64] Stomach is one of the most common sites for extranodal NHL in adults, while colon and small intestine are the most common sites for primary extranodal NHL in children, collectively accounting for nearly half of all extranodal NHLs in this cohort.[66]

Involvement of the gastrointestinal tract with Hodgkin's disease is extremely rare, and seen almost exclusively in the upper gastrointestinal tract and in association with advanced stage, multifocal disease. Among the non-Hodgkin lymphomas, small noncleaved lymphoma of the Burkitt's type (Burkitt lymphoma) accounts for the majority of pediatric intestinal lymphomas, representing more than 75% of all cases.[66] However, the pathological spectrum of pediatric gastrointestinal lymphoma shows marked geographical variation due to different risk factors and predisposing condition in different parts of the world. For instance, Burkitt lymphoma is endemic in equatorial Africa, representing nearly half of all childhood cancers in this region.[67] Two widespread human pathogens, the Epstein-Barr virus (EBV) and the *Plasmodium falciparum*, are thought to be responsible for the pathogenesis of this disease in Africa.[68] Similarly, Immunoproliferative Small Intestinal Disease, also known as Mediterranean lymphoma, is characteristically seen in the Mediterranean basin, the Middle East, and North Africa, and is thought to be associated with poor living conditions in these regions of the world.[69,70]

Pathology and Pathophysiology. A detailed description of the pathology and pathophysiology of intestinal lymphomas is beyond the scope of this chapter. Fortunately, only a limited subset of lymphomas is typically encountered in the intestinal tract of children, with Burkitt lymphoma representing the largest subgroup.

Burkitt Lymphoma (BL)

BL is a highly aggressive lymphoma composed of monomorphic, medium-sized B lymphocytes with a characteristic immunophenotype and a strikingly high proliferation rate (Table 1). BL often presents at extranodal sites, and can occur anywhere in the gastrointestinal tract. Nevertheless, the terminal ileum and the ileocecal region are the most common sites of origin, where the tumor is often identified as a submucosal and/or mural lesion presenting with obstruction or intussusception (Figure 3). This is particularly true of the nonendemic (sporadic) BL, in which the majority of tumors present as abdominal masses,[71,72] with the ileocecal region representing the most frequent site of involvement.[73] Diagnostic workup consists of imaging and endoscopic studies where the often rapidly growing mass lesion is readily identifiable. Endoscopic biopsy may be used to confirm the diagnosis, although given the submucosal/intramural growth pattern, superficial biopsies may only show nonspecific mucosal damage or contain inadequate diagnostic tissue.

The pathophysiology of BL is dependent on the clinical circumstances and the underlying risk factors. In particular, three somewhat distinct groups of tumor including endemic and sporadic types, as well as BL associated with immunodeficiency are recognized (Table 1). In endemic BL, which occurs primarily in equatorial Africa and Papua New Guinea, the EBV genome is present in the majority of neoplastic cells. Furthermore, development of lymphoma follows a long period of polyclonal B-cell activation secondary to

Table 1 Characteristics of Common Burkitt Lymphoma Subtypes*

	Endemic	Sporadic	Immunodeficiency-associated
Geographic predisposition	Equatorial Africa, Papua New Guinea	US, Europe	Worldwide
Incidence rate in geographic hot spots	1–20 per 100,000	1 per 10,000,000	Variable
Age distribution	2–14yr	All ages	All ages
EBV association	>90%	<20%	<40%
Ig-myc translocation[†‡]	>95%	>95%	>95%
Immunophenotype	CD10+ BCL6+ BCL2−	CD10+ BCL6+ BCL2−	CD10+ BCL6+ BCL2−
Proliferation index (fraction Ki-67+)[‡]	>95%	>95%	>95%
Possible cofactors	EBV, malaria, and other chronic infections	EBV infection	HIV infection Congenital immunodeficiency EBV infection and/or reactivation

*Modified from references 68 and 94.

[†]*Ig-myc* translocation denotes translocation between c-*myc* and one of the immunoglobulin (Ig) gene loci encoding Ig heavy or light chains.

[‡]Tissue confirmation of these features is required to distinguish BL from diffuse large B cell lymphoma that can clinically and pathologically mimic BL.

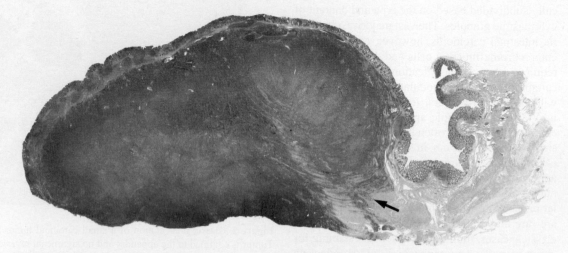

Figure 3 Burkitt lymphoma presenting as a large, obstructing polypoid lesion at the ileocecal valve of an 8-year-old. Although some intramucosal tumor is present (best seen in the upper left region of the surface mucosa), the bulk of the tumor is submucosal and there is diffuse infiltration into the muscularis propria (*arrow*).

multiple bacterial, viral, and parasitic infections, the most important of which is *P. falciparum,* the agent of malaria.[68] In contrast, the frequency of EBV association in sporadic BL, which is the common form of the disease in the United States and Europe, is less than 20%. Similarly, in immunodeficiency-associated BL, the EBV infection rate is less than 40%, suggesting a secondary or cofactor role for EBV in the pathogenesis of these cases. Common to all BL subtypes, however, are genetic abnormalities involving the c-*myc* protooncogene. Classically, this genetic aberration involves a translocation between the immunoglobulin heavy chain (IgH) enhancer on chromosome 14q and the c-*myc* gene on chromosome 8q, resulting in the cytogenetically identifiable t(8; 14)(q24; q32) translocation that is a diagnostic hallmark of BL. Collectively, these findings suggest that chronic B cell stimulation increases the probability of oncogenic events, and that B cell infection by oncogenic viruses such as EBV further increases the risk of malignant transformation in the at-risk population of B lymphocytes.

Regardless of its pathogenesis, BL is an aggressive B-cell lymphoma with a rapid clinical course that can be fatal within months. Nevertheless, with timely diagnosis and the use of aggressive chemotherapy regimens that often include methotrexate and cytarabine, cure rates for sporadic Burkitt's lymphoma approach 90% in children and 70% in adults.[74]

Immunoproliferative Small Intestinal Disease (IPSID)

IPSID is a distinct small intestinal lymphoproliferative disease with a high prevalence in young individuals in endemic areas (see below). IPSID was first recognized as a cluster of small intestinal lymphomas in the Mediterranean region (hence the name "Mediterranean Lymphoma") in patients presenting with diarrhea and malabsorption syndrome.[75–77] Identification of the key role of plasma cells in this disease with their characteristic production of an abnormal (truncated) immunoglobulin A heavy chain with no associated light chain resulted in the alternative designation of alpha chain disease.[78,79] The disease was subsequently renamed as IPSID and formally defined as an extranodal marginal zone B cell lymphoma of mucosa-associated lymphoid tissue (MALT lymphoma).[80]

IPSID is nearly endémic in the underdeveloped or underprivileged regions of the Mediterranean basin, the Middle East and the Far East.[69,70,81] IPSID is uncommon in other parts of the world, although sporadic cases can be seen in many locations, especially in immigrants from endemic countries. Most patients with IPSID are between the ages of 10 to 35 years and live in poor living conditions. Weight loss, intermittent diarrhea, and colicky abdominal pain are the most common presenting symptoms. More advanced disease may be associated with significant malabsorption and intestinal obstruction due to a lymphomatous mass effect. Anemia and clubbing of the fingers

are seen in more than half of the reported cases, and laboratory studies often confirm the presence of alpha heavy chain protein. Radiological findings are nonspecific in early disease, but will show evidence of luminal and mural small intestinal disease in more advanced cases. The clinical differential diagnosis often includes Celiac disease, gastrointestinal infections, and other forms of lymphoma. Upper gastrointestinal endoscopy typically shows thickening, erythema, and nodularity of the small intestinal mucosa. Endoscopy with mucosal biopsy is the diagnostic procedure of choice.

Pathology and Pathophysiology. IPSID is a MALT lymphoma characterized by infiltration of the small intestinal mucosa with a neoplastic population of marginal zone B cells. Lesional cells have small to medium-sized, slightly irregular nuclei with dispersed chromatin and inconspicuous nucleoli, resembling normal centrocytes. Cytoplasm is abundant and pale, leading to a monocytoid appearance. Plasmacytic differentiation is often prominent, and large cells resembling centroblasts or immunoblasts are often present. The glandular epithelium is usually invaded and damaged by the neoplastic cells, resulting in the characteristic lymphoepithelial lesion. The disease can cause a spectrum of histopathological changes, ranging from a seemingly benign intramucosal lymphoid infiltrate to transformation into diffuse large B-cell lymphoma. Lymphoid infiltration of the mucosa and the associated epithelial damage that result in clinical manifestation of malabsorption and protein-losing enteropathy.

The mechanisms of disease development and progression in IPSID are at not fully understood. As is the case with most B-cell lymphomas, chronic antigenic stimulation of an at-risk population of lymphocytes is likely the inciting event in clonal selection of neoplastic cells. With progression of disease and accumulation of more and more genetic abnormalities, the clonal population becomes independent of stimulatory signals, resulting in a self-sustaining lymphoproliferative disease.

Several agents have been suspected of providing the chronic antigenic stimulation required for development of IPSID, but unlike the association between *Helicobacter pylori* and gastric MALT lymphoma, no definite infectious agent responsible for development of IPSID has been identified. Lecuit and colleagues demonstrated the presence of *Campylobacter jejuni* in the intestinal biopsies of a patient with IPSID and documented a dramatic clinical response to antibiotic treatment, suggesting a causative association.[69] In the same study, retrospective analysis of archival biopsy specimens from an additional six patients with IPSID identified *Campylobacter* species in four, providing further support for a possible link. In addition to possible environmental cofactors, a genetic predisposition to IPSID has been suggested based on disease association with human leukocyte antigens (HLAs) AW19, A9, and B12;

blood group B; development of disease in relatives living apart from each other; and other clinical observations.[82–85] Future studies, however, are needed to determine if the association between *C. jejuni* and IPSID is a causative association, and if the genetic/familial associations are indeed related to an independent genetic predisposition for the disease.

Clinical Management. Spontaneous remissions may occur in early stage disease if the environmental stimuli are removed, but established disease with significant clinical symptoms requires specific treatment. Treatment options are largely based on the experience with gastric MALT lymphomas and the possible association of IPSID with a bacterial infection. A prospective study of 21 Tunisian patients with IPSID, including 6 early stage disease confined to the intestinal wall, 2 intermediate and 13 advanced stage disease with mass lesion, showed an overall remission rate of 90 ± 12% at 2 years and 67 ± 25% at 3 years.[86] The 6 patients with early-stage disease responded well to antibiotics (tetracycline or metronidazole and ampicillin/tetracycline), while the remaining 15 patients received anthracycline-based combination chemotherapy. A more recent series from Turkey showed that tetracycline alone in 7 early-stage patients resulted in 71% complete remission rate and 43% 5-year disease-free survival.[87] Eleven of the other 16 patients with intermediate or advanced disease achieved complete remission only after chemotherapy with COPP (cyclophosphamide, vincristine, procarbazine, and prednisone) followed by tetracycline treatment. The overall 5-year survival for the entire cohort was 70%, and the 5-year disease-free survival for patients in complete remission was 75%.

Intestinal T Cell Lymphoma

T cell lymphomas of the intestinal tract are uncommon (less than 5% of all gastrointestinal lymphomas), but they represent a clinically significant disease because of their strong association with Celiac disease.[88] Enteropathy-associated T cell lymphoma (EATL) is an intestinal T-cell lymphoma in patients with known or concomitantly diagnosed Celiac disease. With an annual incidence rate of 0.5 to 1 per million people in Western countries, EATL is a relatively rare cancer, but it accounts for approximately 35% of all small intestinal lymphomas in this population. Although a rare case of lymphoma in a 10-year-old child with Celiac disease has been reported,[89] EATL appears to peak in the late adult life, and there is no measurable association between Celiac disease and incidence of lymphoma in children.[90,91]

Large Cell Lymphomas

Large cell lymphomas are a somewhat diverse group of lymphoid neoplasms with variable morphology and clinical presentation, that collectively account for a significant number of the non-Burkitt, non-Hodgkin lymphomas of the gastrointestinal tract in children.[92] Among the various subtypes, diffuse large B-cell lymphoma (DLBCL) is the most likely subtype to involve the intestinal tract in children. DLBCL is characterized by a diffuse proliferation of large neoplastic B cells that often destroys the underlying architecture of the site of involvement. Nevertheless, rare unusual presentations such as colonic polypoid lesions have been described in children.[93] Cytologically, the neoplastic cells are divided into various morphological variants including centroblastic, immunoblastic, T-cell/histiocytic rich, and anaplastic. In addition to expression of one or more B cell markers, neoplastic cells are often characterized by immunohistochemical expression of BCL6, BCL2, and CD10. Given the overlapping histopathological features with Burkitt Lymphoma, it is of utmost importance to definitively distinguish DLBCL from BL in order to develop an adequate treatment plan.[94] In histologically difficult cases, cytogenetic analysis of the tissue for translocations involving c-*myc*, *BCL2*, and *BCL6* genes may be the only definitive way to distinguish DLBCL from BL.[95,96]

MESENCHYMAL TUMORS

Gastrointestinal Stromal Tumors (GISTs)

Although the full spectrum of mesenchymal tumors may be occasionally encountered, GISTs represent the most significant primary mesenchymal tumors encountered in the gastrointestinal tract of adults and children alike. Pediatric GISTs are nevertheless rare and a significant number of them occur in the stomach (see Chapter 10, "Esophageal and Gastric Neoplasms"). However, as highlighted below, intestinal stromal tumors that do occur in children raise unique pathophysiological and medical issues that are the primary focus of this discussion.

Epidemiology and Clinical Features. As is commonly the case with primary gastrointestinal neoplasms, GISTs are characteristically tumors of the adult life.[97,98] Nevertheless, there has been an increasing recognition and awareness of this entity in children.[99–101] Combined with previous case reports and small series, recent cohort studies have provided new insights on pediatric gastrointestinal stromal tumors.

In slightly more than two decades of experience at the Memorial Sloan-Kettering Cancer Center (from 1982 to 2003), only 5 of 350 patients diagnosed with GIST were less than 18 years of age.[99] Interestingly, all five were girls between the ages of 10 and 15 years who had a primary gastric tumor with aggressive behavior as defined by clinical features (liver/peritoneal metastases or recurrence) or pathological criteria as defined by Fletcher and colleagues.[102] These demographics are somewhat distinct from the experience at St. Jude's Hospital, where 7 children with GISTs were treated in a 40-year period between 1962 and 2002.[101] In this cohort, the male to female

ratio was 3:4, and only 2 of 7 GISTs were primary gastric. Colonic and small intestinal tumors represented two patients each, and one additional child was reported to have an abdominal wall primary. This discrepancy is likely explained by the fact that the average age of the four children with intestinal GIST in the St. Jude's experience was only 5 years, while the youngest patient in the cohort reported from the Memorial Sloan-Kettering was 10 years of age. Collectively, these observations suggest that intestinal GISTs may be more common in the first decade of life, while gastric GISTs predominate in the second decade of life, a features that is also common to the adults.[98]

Pathology and Pathophysiology. Based on ultrastructural features, functional studies and the characteristic expression of receptor tyrosine kinases, the interstitial cells of Cajal appear to be the cell or origin for all GISTs.[103–105] GISTs are pathologically defined as primary mesenchymal tumors of the gastrointestinal tract with activating mutations in the receptor tyrosine kinase *KIT* or the closely related kinase, platelet-derived growth factor receptor, alpha polypeptide (*PDGFRA*).[106,107] Activation of these receptor tyrosine kinases leads to downstream signal transduction through the PI3K-AKT, MAP-kinase and JAK-STAT3 signaling cascades. This molecular pathway is at the heart of chemotherapeutic targeting of the common subset of GISTs (those with *KIT* mutations) using the tyrosine kinase inhibitor imatinib, resulting in a clinical benefit in a significant number of patients with aggressive disease.[108]

Morphologically, GISTs are a somewhat variable group of tumors with spindle and/or epithelioid phenotype and varying minor patterns of differentiation.[102,109] Immunohistochemical expression of *KIT* (also known as CD117) has become the hallmark of tissue diagnosis for GISTs harboring a mutation in *KIT*.[97,110] CD117-negative GISTs are rare and require molecular analysis for mutations in *KIT* and PDGFRA to establish a definitive diagnosis.[111,112] Rarely, GISTs may be primary to the mesentery or other anatomic locations where interstitial cells of Cajal or related neural pacemaker cells may be anatomically located.

Multifocal and Familial Tumors. Although stromal tumors are often sporadic, the presence of multifocal GIST must alert to the possibility of a syndromic disease such familial GIST syndrome, Carney's triad, or neurofibromatosis type 1 (NF1). Patients with familial GIST syndrome harbor germline gain-of-function mutations in *KIT* or *PDGFRA*, both of which predispose the patient to diffuse hyperplasia of interstitial cells of Cajal and multifocal development of GISTs.[113–115]

The molecular association between GISTs and Carney's triad is less well defined. Careny's triad was first described in 1977 as the heritable association between gastric leiomyosarcoma, functioning extraadrenal paraganglioma and

pulmonary chondroma,[116] with the subsequent recognition that an association between gastric sarcoma and paraganglioma alone may represent a distinct familial syndrome.[117,118] Over the years, however, it has become more and more apparent that the gastrointestinal tumors of Carney's triad or and its variants are indeed pathologically classifiable as GISTs or a distinct subset often diagnosed as gastrointestinal autonomic nerve tumor or GANT.[117–120] Gastrointestinal tumors in these patients are not limited to the stomach, and small intestinal stromal tumors have been described.[119] These unique associations between GISTs, paragangliomas, and other potential tumors described in patients with Carney's triad offer unique opportunities for future research in the molecular association between these entities.

Finally, there is a well-described association between NF1 and solitary or multiple GISTs, the vast majority of which appear to be small intestinal in origin (Figure 4).[121,122] NF1-associated GISTs typically express CD117 by immunohistochemical analysis, but unlike sporadic GISTs no *KIT* or *PDGFRA* mutations are detected in these tumors.[121–123] These observations suggest an alternative and yet poorly understood molecular pathway for the development of intestinal stromal tumors in patients with NF1. New insights into this unique pathway were provided by Maertens and colleagues who recently demonstrated that the molecular event underlying GIST development in NF1 patients is a somatic inactivation of the wild-type *NF1* (neurofibromin) gene allele leading to hyperactivation of the downstream signaling pathways that are common to pathogenesis of all GISTs.[124] Future studies on pathophysiology of NF1-associated stromal tumors will undoubtedly shed more light on pathological differences between intestinal and gastric GISTs in children and adults.

Clinical Management. Complete surgical resection is the primary treatment goal for solitary GISTs or multifocal disease amenable to complete surgical resection. Treatment with imatinib may be clinically effective in metastatic disease, specially in patients with documented *KIT* mutations.[108] Specific recommendations for treatment of children with imatinib are lacking. In a recent series reported by Prakash and colleagues, two of five children were treated with imatinib.[99] One child with extensive liver and intra-abdominal recurrence was treated for 4 months without response and died soon thereafter. A second child with intra-abdominal recurrence had stable disease 12 months after the start of imatinib therapy.

Smooth Muscle Neoplasms

Smooth muscle tumors of the gastrointestinal tract are far less common in the small and large intestine than the proximal gut, specially the esophagus (see Chapter 10, "Esophageal and Gastric Neoplasms"). Solitary leiomyomas and diffuse leiomyomatosis are characteristically seen in the esophagus, while leiomyomas of the

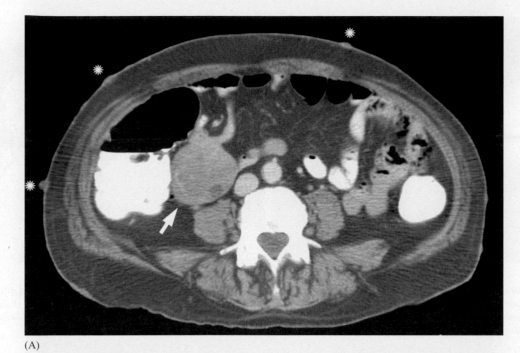

(A)

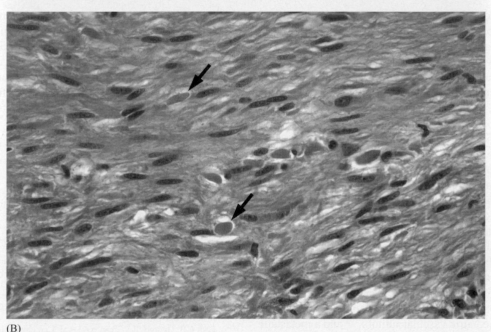

(B)

Figure 4 A young adult with neurofibromatosis type 1 (NF1) presenting with multiple small intestinal tumors. Abdominal CT scan (A) shows a well-circumscribed mass adjacent to loops of bowel (*white arrow*), as well as several small cutaneous nodules consistent with neurofibromas (*asterisks*). Hematoxylin and eosin stained microscopic section of the abdominal mass (B) shows a low-grade spindle cell tumor with prominent skeinoid fibers (*black arrows*), characteristic of NF1-associated small intestinal GISTs.

intestinal tract are only rarely reported.[125–130] In addition, many of the reported cases fail to definitely distinguish Leiomyoma from GIST, making a conclusive analysis of this literature difficult. Nevertheless, given the occasional presence of submucosal leiomyomas in the general population, it is not unexpected to encounter an occasional submucosal leiomyoma in the intestinal tract of children. More important than an incidental leiomyoma, however, is identification of a malignant smooth muscle tumor or leiomyosarcoma.

Intestinal leiomyosarcoma is a rare pediatric tumor, accounting for an estimated 0.3% of all neoplasms in children younger than 15 years of age.[131] Furthermore, nearly half of pediatric intestinal leiomyosarcomas are diagnosed in the neonatal period or during infancy.[132,133] Intestinal tumors often arise from the smooth muscle of the muscularis propria, and are locally invasive. In advanced disease, distant metastases to lung and liver are more typical than local lymph node metastases, although metastatic disease at the time of presentation is unusual in the pediatric population in general.[132,133] Clinically, children often present with bleeding, obstruction, intussusceptions or perforation, and there seems to be a slight female predominance.[132–134] Pediatric intestinal leiomyosarcomas can arise anywhere in the small intestine, colon or rectum, although there appears to be a slight preference for the distal small intestine.[132,135] In contrast to adult

patients in whom intussusception is associated with smooth muscle tumors in nearly a third of all cases, intussusception due to leiomyosarcoma is rare in infancy and childhood.[134] Pediatric leiomyosarcomas show other distinct clinical and pathological behavior compared to adults. While leiomyosarcoma represents less than 2% of all adult gastrointestinal malignancies, nearly 20% of all small intestinal malignancies in some pediatric centers were diagnosed as leiomyosarcoma.[136] In addition, leiomyosarcomas of infancy appear to have a relatively favorable prognosis even when the histological appearance is suggestive of an aggressive tumor, suggesting that adjuvant therapy may be unnecessary when tumors are completely excised.[135,137] In spite of this survival advantage for infantile case, which is likely due to a higher complete resection rate compared with other cohorts, the overall prognosis for long-term survival appears to be similar in pediatric and adult patients, with 5-year survival between 40 and 50%.[134]

Immunodeficiency-Associated Smooth Muscle Neoplasms

Although smooth muscle tumors are rare in the general pediatric population, there is a strong association between immunodeficiency, specially acquired immunodeficiency syndrome (AIDS) secondary to human immunodeficiency virus (HIV) infection, and the development of smooth muscle tumors. In a retrospective survey of 64 HIV-positive children followed by the Children's Cancer Group and the National Cancer Institute between 1982 and 1997, smooth muscle tumors were identified in 11 children (17%), second only to non-Hodgkin lymphoma, which was diagnosed in 42 children (65%).[138] The gastrointestinal tract is a common site of tumor development in HIV-positive children, although tumors can arise in almost any location and may be multiple.[139–142] An unusual feature of the immunodeficiency-associated smooth muscle tumors is a nearly uniform expression of the EBV in neoplastic cells.[141,142] In particular, the presence of clonal EBV in the lesion indicates that infection occurs at an early stage of tumor development and suggests that EBV has a causal role in the pathogenesis of smooth muscle tumors in immunodeficient children.[142] Immunodeficiency may facilitate EBV infection or reactivation, but the precise role of HIV coinfection in the pathogenesis of leiomyosarcomas is not fully understood. Similar tumors have been seen in children and adults with immunodeficiency secondary to organ transplantation and in children with congenital immunodeficiency, suggesting that HIV infection may not be an absolute requirement for the development of EBV-associated smooth muscle tumors.[143–149]

Neural Tumors

Primary neural tumors of the gastrointestinal tract include benign Schwannomas/neuromas, neurofibromas, ganglioneuromas, and granular cells tumors, as well as malignant peripheral nerve sheath neoplasms. Among this group, ganglioneuromas are the only category that may be encountered as polypoid lesions in the intestinal tract of children with any measurable frequency.

Intestinal ganglioneuromas consist of a mixed proliferation of ganglion cells and various glial elements in a background of irregularly distorted glandular architecture. Sessile or pedunculated polyps may occur anywhere in the intestinal tract, and may be solitary (ganglioneuroma), multiple (ganglioneuromatous polyposis), or diffuse throughout the gastrointestinal tract (diffuse ganglioneuromatosis). In a review of their 50-year experience at the Armed Forces Institute of Pathology, Shekitka and Sobin measured frequencies of 65, 16, and 19% for each of these classes of ganglioneuromas, respectively.[150] Furthermore, in 16 of 24 patients with isolated ganglioneuromas for whom follow-up was available (average follow-up of 8-years), none developed polyposis or showed evidence of a syndromic association, suggesting that isolated ganglioneuromas are most likely an incidental finding.

In contrast to solitary ganglioneuromas, the presence of multiple polyps or diffuse ganglioneuromatosis must alert to the presence of an underlying syndrome or familial disease.[150–156] Although multiple associated syndromes including multiple endocrine neoplasia, type 2B (MEN2B), neurofibromatosis, type 1 (NF1), juvenile polyposis, and Cowden's syndrome have been described, specific pathological or molecular data linking morphological features with each syndrome are lacking.

Pediatric intestinal neurofibromas and Schwannomas are less common than ganglioneuromas, but may occasionally be seen in isolation or in association with an underlying syndrome. Neurofibromas consist of a proliferation of bland spindle cells with a usually prominent collagenous stroma, and may be difficult to distinguish from GISTs, specially given the increased incidence of GISTs in patients with NF1. Nevertheless, presence of a plexiform neurofibroma or multiple neurofibromas must raise the possibility of underlying NF1.[156–160] Intestinal Schwannomas constitute less than 3% of all small and large intestinal tumors,[161,162] and are rarely, if ever, seen in children.

Vascular Tumors

Benign vascular tumors, hemangiomas, and lymphangiomas, will occasionally present as mass lesions in the gastrointestinal tract of children (Figure 5). Vascular tumors account for nearly a quarter of all pediatric soft tissue masses, although the vast majority of the lesions occur in the soft tissues of the head and neck, extremities, or the trunk.[163] Various forms of hemangioma account for more than half of these lesions, while lymphangiomas constitute the bulk of the remaining cases. Multifocal cases occasionally occur, and borderline or frankly malignant cases are exceedingly rare.[163]

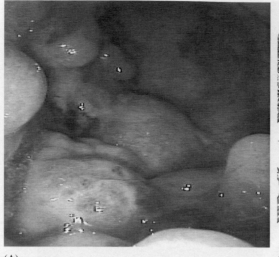
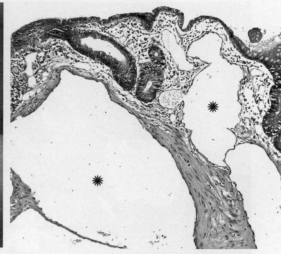

(A)   (B)

Figure 5 As seen in this endoscopic image of a colonic lymphangioma (A), vascular lesions of the intestinal tract often present as irregular submucosal nodules with superficial erosions that predispose the patient to chronic blood loss. Histological features are characteristically that of thin-walled, dilated vascular channel (B, *asterisks*) which disrupt the normal architecture of the mucosa (B), submucosa or the wall.

Hemangiomas consist of a benign proliferation of capillaries and/or other small blood vessels, and constitute the most common tumor of infancy in the Western population.[164,165] Hemangiomas of the intestinal tract are rare, but may present in any location, either in an isolated form,[166–172] or in association with a systemic vascular disease.[173–177] Clinical presentations vary depending on the size, distribution and precise location of the tumor, but gastrointestinal bleeding and intussusception appear to be the most common presenting symptoms. Significant progress has been made in understanding the pathophysiology and management of pediatric hemangiomas,[178,179] although specific data related to the intestinal lesions is lacking.

Malignant vascular tumors of gastrointestinal tract in childhood are exceedingly rare. Coffin and Dehner describe 3 angiosarcomas and 1 Kaposi sarcoma (KS) in their experience with 228 pediatric vascular tumors,[163] and a metastatic colonic angiosarcoma was reported by Smith and colleagues.[180] Pediatric intestinal KS is often associated with immunosuppression and EBV infection, with the bulk of reported cases found in renal transplant recipients.[181–183]

Tumors of lymphatic origin (lymphangiomas) may be seen anywhere in the gastrointestinal tract, although they are classically found in the mesenteric soft tissues of the small and large intestine.[184–186] Although lymphangiomas are benign lesions, they can lead to intestinal obstruction or intussusception, requiring surgical intervention.

SUMMARY

Pediatric intestinal neoplasms are generally uncommon, but they constitute a diverse and challenging group of benign and malignant lesions. Proper diagnosis and management of these lesions often requires a multidisciplinary clinical approach with an understanding of molecular genetics and the underlying pathophysiology.

Clinical recommendations for treatment of malignant lesions are often based on adult studies, making dedicated pediatric trials in the future a much-desired necessity. Furthermore, the close interrelations between pediatric intestinal tumors and many prominent genetic disorders make future basic research in this field an exciting opportunity for translation from bench to bedside.

REFERENCES

1. Bethel CA, Bhattacharyya N, Hutchinson C, et al. Alimentary tract malignancies in children. J Pediatr Surg 1997;32:1004–8; discussion 1008–9.
2. Sessions RT, Riddell DH, Kaplan HJ, Foster JH. Carcinoma of the colon in the first two decades of life. Ann Surg 1965;162:279–84.
3. Rao BN, Pratt CB, Fleming ID, et al. Colon carcinoma in children and adolescents. A review of 30 cases. Cancer 1985;55:1322–6.
4. Young JL, Jr, Percy CL, Asire AJ, et al. Cancer incidence and mortality in the United States, 1973–77. Natl Cancer Inst Monogr 1981:1–187.
5. Pratt CB, George SL, Green AA, et al. Carcinomas in children. Clinical and demographic characteristics. Cancer 1988;61:1046–50.
6. Anfeld F. Casuistik der congenitalen neoplasm. Arch Gynaekol. 1980;16:135–7.
7. Kern WH, White WC. Adenocarcinoma of the colon in a 9-month-old infant; Report of a case. Cancer 1958;11:855–7.
8. Brown RA, Rode H, Millar AJ, et al. Colorectal carcinoma in children. J Pediatr Surg 1992;27:919–21.
9. Angel CA, Pratt CB, Rao BN, et al. Carcinoembryonic antigen and carbohydrate 19–9 antigen as markers for colorectal carcinoma in children and adolescents. Cancer 1992;69:1487–91.
10. Andersson A, Bergdahl L. Carcinoma of the colon in children: A report of six new cases and a review of the literature. J Pediatr Surg 1976;11:967–71.
11. Middelkamp JN, Haffner H. Carcinoma of the Colon in Children. Pediatrics 1963;32:558–71.
12. Karnak I, Ciftci AO, Senocak ME, Buyukpamukcu N. Colorectal carcinoma in children. J Pediatr Surg 1999;34:1499–504.
13. Hamilton SR, Vogelstein B, Kudo S, et al. Carcinoma of the colon and rectum. In: Hamilton SR, Aaltonen LA, editors. World Health Organization Classification of Tumours: Pathology and Genetics of Tumours of the Digestive System. Lyon, France: IARC Press; 2000. p. 105–19.
14. Symonds DA, Vickery AL. Mucinous carcinoma of the colon and rectum. Cancer 1976;37:1891–900.
15. Odone V, Chang L, Caces J, et al. The natural history of colorectal carcinoma in adolescents. Cancer 1982;49:1716–20.

16. Hoerner MT. Carcinoma of the colon and rectum in persons under 20 years of age. Am J Surg 1958;96:47–53.

17. Kazama Y, Watanabe T, Kanazawa T, et al. Mucinous carcinomas of the colon and rectum show higher rates of microsatellite instability and lower rates of chromosomal instability: A study matched for T classification and tumor location. Cancer 2005;103:2023–9.

18. Alexander J, Watanabe T, Wu TT, et al. Histopathological identification of colon cancer with microsatellite instability. Am J Pathol 2001;158:527–35.

19. Messerini L, Vitelli F, De Vitis LR, et al. Microsatellite instability in sporadic mucinous colorectal carcinomas: Relationship to clinico-pathological variables. J Pathol 1997;182:380–4.

20. Lynch HT, de la Chapelle A. Hereditary colorectal cancer. N Engl J Med 2003;348:919–32.

21. Vasen HF, Watson P, Mecklin JP, Lynch HT. New clinical criteria for hereditary nonpolyposis colorectal cancer (HNPCC, Lynch syndrome) proposed by the International Collaborative group on HNPCC. Gastroenterology 1999;116:1453–6.

22. Syngal S, Fox EA, Eng C, et al. Sensitivity and specificity of clinical criteria for hereditary non-polyposis colorectal cancer associated mutations in MSH2 and MLH1. J Med Genet 2000;37:641–5.

23. Hampel H, Frankel WL, Martin E, et al. Screening for the Lynch syndrome (hereditary nonpolyposis colorectal cancer). N Engl J Med 2005;352:1851–60.

24. Barnetson RA, Tenesa A, Farrington SM, et al. Identification and survival of carriers of mutations in DNA mismatch-repair genes in colon cancer. N Engl J Med 2006;354:2751–63.

25. Ribic CM, Sargent DJ, Moore MJ, et al. Tumor microsatellite-instability status as a predictor of benefit from fluorouracil-based adjuvant chemotherapy for colon cancer. N Engl J Med 2003;349:247–57.

26. Carethers JM, Smith EJ, Behling CA, et al. Use of 5-fluorouracil and survival in patients with microsatellite-unstable colorectal cancer. Gastroenterology 2004;126:394–401.

27. Iannaccone R, Laghi A, Passariello R. Colorectal carcinoma: Detection and staging with multislice CT (MSCT) colonography. Abdom Imaging 2005;30:13–9.

28. Low RN, McCue M, Barone R, et al. MR staging of primary colorectal carcinoma: Comparison with surgical and histopathologic findings. Abdom Imaging 2003;28:784–93.

29. Sahani DV, Kalva SP, Fischman AJ, et al. Detection of liver metastases from adenocarcinoma of the colon and pancreas: Comparison of mangafodipir trisodium-enhanced liver MRI and whole-body FDG PET. AJR Am J Roentgenol 2005;185:239–46.

30. COSTSG A comparison of laparoscopically assisted and open colectomy for colon cancer. N Engl J Med 2004;350:2050–9.

31. Weeks JC, Nelson H, Gelber S, et al. Short-term quality-of-life outcomes following laparoscopic-assisted colectomy vs open colectomy for colon cancer: A randomized trial. JAMA 2002;287:321–8.

32. Astler VB, Coller FA. The prognostic significance of direct extension of carcinoma of the colon and rectum. Ann Surg 1954;139:846–52.

33. Greene FL. AJCC Cancer Staging Manual, American Joint Committee on Cancer, American Cancer Society, 6th edition. New York: Springer-Verlag; 2002.

34. Benson AB, III Schrag D, Somerfield MR, et al. American Society of Clinical Oncology recommendations on adjuvant chemotherapy for stage II colon cancer. J Clin Oncol 2004;22:3408–19.

35. Swanson RS, Compton CC, Stewart AK, Bland KI. The prognosis of T3N0 colon cancer is dependent on the number of lymph nodes examined. Ann Surg Oncol 2003; 10:65–71.

36. Cancer Care Ontario: Gastrointestinal Cancer Evidence-based Series and Practice Guidelines. http://wwwcancer careonca/index_gastrointestinalCancerguidelineshtm; Accessed July 30, 2006.

37. Cancer Care Ontario Practice Guideline Initiative: Postoperative Adjuvant Radiotherapy and/or Chemotherapy for Resected Stage II or III Rectal Cancer. Vol. Report #2–3. Toronto, ON: Cancer Care Ontario; 2001.

38. Kim DW, Lim SB, Kim DY, et al. Preoperative chemo-radiotherapy improves the sphincter preservation rate in patients with rectal cancer located within 3 cm of the anal verge. Eur J Surg Oncol 2006;32:162–7.

39. Goethals L, Haustermans K, Perneel C, et al. Chemo-radiotherapy versus radiotherapy alone in the preoperative treatment of resectable rectal cancer. Eur J Surg Oncol 2005;31:969–76.

40. Cordts AE, Chabot JR. Jejunal carcinoma in a child. J Pediatr Surg 1983;18:180–1.

41. Kabra SK, Kumar CL, Mathur M, Choudhry VP. Adenocarcinoma of small bowel. Indian Pediatr 1990;27:987–9.

42. Tankel JW, Galasko CS. Adenocarcinoma of small bowel in 12-year-old girl. J R Soc Med 1984;77:693–4.

43. Dunsmore KP, Lovell MA. Small bowel adenocarcinoma metastatic to the ovaries in a 12-year-old girl. J Pediatr Hematol Oncol 1998;20:498–501.

44. Busing CM, Haag D, Geiger H, Tschahargane C. Microscopic and pulse cytophotometric investigation of a carcinoma of the jejunum in a seven year old child. Virchows Arch A Pathol Anat Histol 1977;375:115–22.

45. Goldman LI, Bralow SP, Cox W, Peale AR. Adenocarcinoma of the small bowel complicating Crohn's disease. Cancer 1970;26:1119–25.

46. Cobrin GM, Pittman RH, Lewis BS. Increased diagnostic yield of small bowel tumors with capsule endoscopy. Cancer 2006;107:22–7.

47. Modlin IM, Lye KD, Kidd M. A 5-decade analysis of 13,715 carcinoid tumors. Cancer 2003;97:934–59.

48. Crocetti E, Paci E. Malignant carcinoids in the USA, SEER 1992–1999. An epidemiological study with 6830 cases. Eur J Cancer Prev 2003;12:191–4.

49. Godwin JD, 2nd. Carcinoid tumors. An analysis of 2,837 cases. Cancer 1975;36:560–9.

50. Dymock RB. Pathological changes in the appendix: A review of 1000 cases. Pathology 1977;9:331–9.

51. Dall'Igna P, Ferrari A, Luzzatto C, et al. Carcinoid tumor of the appendix in childhood: The experience of two Italian institutions. J Pediatr Gastroenterol Nutr 2005;40:216–9.

52. Doede T, Foss HD, Waldschmidt J. Carcinoid tumors of the appendix in children—epidemiology, clinical aspects and procedure. Eur J Pediatr Surg 2000;10:372–7.

53. Chow CW, Sane S, Campbell PE, Carter RF. Malignant carcinoid tumors in children. Cancer 1982;49:802–11.

54. Weitzner S. Carcinoid of Meckel's diverticulum. Report of a case and review of the literature. Cancer 1969;23:1436–40.

55. Rubin SZ, Mancer JF, Stephens CA. Carcinoid in a rectal duplication: A unique pediatric surgical problem. Can J Surg 1981;24:351–2.

56. Volpe A, Willert J, Ihnken K, et al. Metastatic appendiceal carcinoid tumor in a child. Med Pediatr Oncol 2000;34:218–20.

57. Spunt SL, Pratt CB, Rao BN, et al. Childhood carcinoid tumors: The St Jude Children's Research Hospital experience. J Pediatr Surg 2000;35:1282–6.

58. Pelizzo G, La Riccia A, Bouvier R, et al. Carcinoid tumors of the appendix in children. Pediatr Surg Int 2001;17:399–402.

59. Parkes SE, Muir KR, al Sheyyab M, et al. Carcinoid tumours of the appendix in children 1957–1986: Incidence, treatment and outcome. Br J Surg 1993;80:502–4.

60. Mihaljevic B, Nedeljkov-Jancic R, Vujicic V, et al. Primary extranodal lymphomas of gastrointestinal localizations: A single institution 5-yr experience. Med Oncol 2006;23:225–35.

61. Koh PK, Horsman JM, Radstone CR, et al. Localised extranodal non-Hodgkin's lymphoma of the gastrointestinal tract: Sheffield Lymphoma Group experience (1989–1998). Int J Oncol 2001;18:743–8.

62. Krugmann J, Dirnhofer S, Gschwendtner A, et al. Primary gastrointestinal B-cell lymphoma. A clincopathological and immunohistochemical study of 61 cases with an evaluation of prognostic parameters. Pathol Res Pract 2001;197:385–93.

63. Haselkorn T, Whittemore AS, Lilienfeld DE. Incidence of small bowel cancer in the United States and worldwide: Geographic, temporal, and racial differences. Cancer Causes Control 2005;16:781–7.

64. Hameed R, Parkes S, Davies P, Morland BJ. Paediatric malignant tumours of the gastrointestinal tract in the West Midlands, UK, 1957–2000: A large population based survey. Pediatr Blood Cancer 2004;43:257–60.

65. Skinner MA, Plumley DA, Grosfeld JL, et al. Gastrointestinal tumors in children: An analysis of 39 cases. Ann Surg Oncol 1994;1:283–9.

66. Temmim L, Baker H, Amanguno H, et al. Clinicopathological features of extranodal lymphomas: Kuwait experience. Oncology 2004;67:382–9.

67. Magrath IT. African Burkitt's lymphoma. History, biology, clinical features, and treatment. Am J Pediatr Hematol Oncol 1991;13:222–46.

68. Rochford R, Cannon MJ, Moormann AM. Endemic Burkitt's lymphoma: A polymicrobial disease? Nat Rev Microbiol 2005;3:182–7.

69. Lecuit M, Abachin E, Martin A, et al. Immunoproliferative small intestinal disease associated with Campylobacter jejuni. N Engl J Med 2004;350:239–48.

70. Salem PA, Estephan FF. Immunoproliferative small intestinal disease: Current concepts. Cancer J 2005;11:374–82.

71. Magrath IT, Sariban E. Clinical features of Burkitt's lymphoma in the USA. IARC Sci Publ 1985:119–127.

72. Wright D, McKeever P, Carter R. Childhood non-Hodgkin lymphomas in the United Kingdom: Findings from the UK Children's Cancer Study Group. J Clin Pathol 1997; 50:128–34.

73. Levine PH, Kamaraju LS, Connelly RR, et al. The American Burkitt's Lymphoma Registry: Eight years' experience. Cancer 1982;49:1016–22.

74. Divine M, Casassus P, Koscielny S, et al. Burkitt lymphoma in adults: A prospective study of 72 patients treated with an adapted pediatric LMB protocol. Ann Oncol 2005;16:1928–35.

75. Azar HA. Cancer in Lebanon and the Near East. Cancer 1962;15:66–78.

76. Ramot B, Shahin N, Bubis JJ. Malabsorption syndrome in lymphoma of small intestine. A study of 13 cases. Isr Med J 1965;47:221–6.

77. Seijffers MJ, Levy M, Hermann G. Intractable watery diarrhea, hypokalemia, and malabsorption in a patient with Mediterranean type of abdominal lymphoma. Gastroenterology 1968;55:118–24.

78. Rambaud JC, Bognel C, Prost A, et al. Clinico-pathological study of a patient with "Mediterranean" type of abdominal lymphoma and a new type of IgA abnormality ("alpha chain disease"). Digestion 1968;1:321–36.

79. Seligmann M, Danon F, Hurez D, et al. Alpha-chain disease: A new immunoglobulin abnormality. Science 1968;162:1396–7.

80. Isaacson PG, Muller-Hermelink HK, Piris MA, et al. Extranodal marginal zone B-cell lymphoma of mucosa-assciated lymphoid tissue (MALT lymphoma). In: Jaffe ES, Harris NL, Stein H, Vardiman JW, editors. World Health Organization Classification of Tumours: Pathology and Genetics of Tumours of Haematopoietic and Lymphoid Tissues. Lyon, France: IARC Press; 2001. p. 157–60.

81. Al-Saleem T, Al-Mondhiry H. Immunoproliferative small intestinal disease (IPSID): A model for mature B-cell neoplasms. Blood 2005;105:2274–80.

82. Khojasteh A, Haghighi P. Immunoproliferative small intestinal disease: Portrait of a potentially preventable cancer from the Third World. Am J Med 1990;89:483–90.

83. Khojasteh A, Haghshenass M, Haghighi P. Current concepts immunoproliferative small intestinal disease. A "Third-World lesion." N Engl J Med 1983;308:1401–5.

84. Crow J, Asselah F. Immunoproliferative small intestinal disease in Algerians. II. Ultrastructural studies in alpha-chain disease. Cancer 1984;54:1908–13.

85. Nikbin B, Banisadre M, Ala F, Mojtabai A. HLA AW19, B12 in immunoproliferative small intestinal disease. Gut 1979;20:226–8.

86. Ben-Ayed F, Halphen M, Najjar T, et al. Treatment of alpha chain disease. Results of a prospective study in 21 Tunisian patients by the Tunisian-French intestinal Lymphoma Study Group. Cancer 1989;63:1251–6.

87. Akbulut H, Soykan I, Yakaryilmaz F, et al. Five-year results of the treatment of 23 patients with immunoproliferative small intestinal disease: A Turkish experience. Cancer 1997; 80:8–14.

88. Catassi C, Bearzi I, Holmes GK. Association of celiac disease and intestinal lymphomas and other cancers. Gastroenterology 2005;128:S79–86.

89. Arnaud-Battandier F, Schmitz J, Ricour C, Rey J. Intestinal malignant lymphoma in a child with familial celiac disease. J Pediatr Gastroenterol Nutr 1983;2:320–3.

90. Schweizer JJ, Oren A, Mearin ML. Cancer in children with celiac disease: A survey of the European Society of Paediatric Gastroenterology, Hepatology and Nutrition. J Pediatr Gastroenterol Nutr 2001;33:97–100.

91. Askling J, Linet M, Gridley G, et al. Cancer incidence in a population-based cohort of individuals hospitalized with celiac disease or dermatitis herpetiformis. Gastroenterology 2002;123:1428–35.

92. Takahashi H, Hansmann ML. Primary gastrointestinal lymphoma in childhood (up to 18 years of age). A morphological, immunohistochemical and clinical study. J Cancer Res Clin Oncol 1990;116:190–6.

93. Bollen P, Bourgain C, Van Berlaer G, et al. Non-Hodgkin lymphoma presenting as a solitary rectal polyp. J Pediatr Gastroenterol Nutr 2000;31:193–4.

94. Harris NL, Horning SJ. Burkitt's lymphoma—the message from microarrays. N Engl J Med 2006;354:2495–8.

95. Dave SS, Fu K, Wright GW, et al. Molecular diagnosis of Burkitt's lymphoma. N Engl J Med 2006;354:2431–42.

96. Hummel M, Bentink S, Berger H, et al. A biologic definition of Burkitt's lymphoma from transcriptional and genomic profiling. N Engl J Med 2006;354:2419–30.

97. Miettinen M, Makhlouf H, Sobin LH, Lasota J. Gastrointestinal stromal tumors of the jejunum and ileum: A clinicopathologic, immunohistochemical, and molecular genetic study of 906 cases before imatinib with long-term follow-up. Am J Surg Pathol 2006;30:477–89.

98. Miettinen M, Sobin LH, Lasota J. Gastrointestinal stromal tumors of the stomach: A clinicopathologic, immunohistochemical, and molecular genetic study of 1765 cases with long-term follow-up. Am J Surg Pathol 2005;29:52–68.

99. Prakash S, Sarran L, Socci N, et al. Gastrointestinal stromal tumors in children and young adults: A clinicopathologic, molecular, and genomic study of 15 cases and review of the literature. J Pediatr Hematol Oncol 2005;27:179–87.

100. Miettinen M, Lasota J, Sobin LH. Gastrointestinal stromal tumors of the stomach in children and young adults: A clinicopathologic, immunohistochemical, and molecular genetic study of 44 cases with long-term follow-up and review of the literature. Am J Surg Pathol 2005;29:1373–81.

101. Cypriano MS, Jenkins JJ, Pappo AS, et al. Pediatric gastrointestinal stromal tumors and leiomyosarcoma. Cancer 2004;101:39–50.

102. Fletcher CD, Berman JJ, Corless C, et al. Diagnosis of gastrointestinal stromal tumors: A consensus approach. Hum Pathol 2002;33:459–65.

103. Yantiss RK, Rosenberg AE, Selig MK, Nielsen GP. Gastrointestinal stromal tumors: An ultrastructural study. Int J Surg Pathol 2002;10:101–13.

104. Furuzono S, Ohya S, Inoue S, et al. Inherent pacemaker function of duodenal GIST. Eur J Cancer 2006;42:243–8.

105. Min KW, Sook Seo I. Intestitial cells of Cajal in the human small intestine: Immunochemical and ultrastructural study. Ultrastruct Pathol 2003;27:67–78.

106. Hirota S, Isozaki K, Moriyama Y, et al. Gain-of-function mutations of c-kit in human gastrointestinal stromal tumors. Science 1998;279:577–80.

107. Heinrich MC, Corless CL, Duensing A, et al. PDGFRA activating mutations in gastrointestinal stromal tumors. Science 2003;299:708–10.

108. Kubota T. Gastrointestinal stromal tumor (GIST) and imatinib. Int J Clin Oncol 2006;11:184–9.

109. Miettinen M, Lasota J. Gastrointestinal stromal tumors–definition, clinical, histological, immunohistochemical, and molecular genetic features and differential diagnosis. Virchows Arch 2001;438:1–12.

110. Loughrey MB, Trivett M, Beshay V, et al. KIT immunohistochemistry and mutation status in gastrointestinal stromal tumours (GISTs) evaluated for treatment with imatinib. Histopathology 2006;49:52–65.

111. Tzen CY, Mau BL. Analysis of CD117-negative gastrointestinal stromal tumors. World J Gastroenterol 2005;11:1052–5.

112. Hirota S, Isozaki K. Pathology of gastrointestinal stromal tumors. Pathol Int 2006;56:1–9.

113. Hirota S, Okazaki T, Kitamura Y, et al. Cause of familial and multiple gastrointestinal autonomic nerve tumors with hyperplasia of interstitial cells of Cajal is germline mutation of the c-kit gene. Am J Surg Pathol 2000;24:326–7.

114. Chompret A, Kannengiesser C, Barrois M, et al. PDGFRA germline mutation in a family with multiple cases of gastrointestinal stromal tumor. Gastroenterology 2004;126:318–21.

115. Hirota S, Isozaki K, Nishida T, Kitamura Y. Effects of loss-of-function and gain-of-function mutations of c-kit on the gastrointestinal tract. J Gastroenterol 2000;35:75–9.

116. Carney JA, Sheps SG, Go VL, Gordon H. The triad of gastric leiomyosarcoma, functioning extra-adrenal paraganglioma and pulmonary chondroma. N Engl J Med 1977;296:1517–8.

117. Carney JA, Stratakis CA. Familial paraganglioma and gastric stromal sarcoma: A new syndrome distinct from the Carney triad. Am J Med Genet 2002;108:132–9.

118. Boccon-Gibod L, Boman F, Boudjemaa S, et al. Separate occurrence of extra-adrenal paraganglioma and gastrointestinal stromal tumor in monozygotic twins: Probable familial Carney syndrome. Pediatr Dev Pathol 2004;7:380–4.

119. Perez-Atayde AR, Shamberger RC, Kozakewich HW. Neuroectodermal differentiation of the gastrointestinal tumors in the Carney triad. An ultrastructural and immunohistochemical study. Am J Surg Pathol 1993;17:706–14.

120. Kerr JZ, Hicks MJ, Nuchtern JG, et al. Gastrointestinal autonomic nerve tumors in the pediatric population: A report of four cases and a review of the literature. Cancer 1999;85:220–30.

121. Kinoshita K, Hirota S, Isozaki K, et al. Absence of c-kit gene mutations in gastrointestinal stromal tumours from neurofibromatosis type 1 patients. J Pathol 2004;202:80–5.

122. Miettinen M, Fetsch JF, Sobin LH, Lasota J. Gastrointestinal stromal tumors in patients with neurofibromatosis 1: A clinicopathologic and molecular genetic study of 45 cases. Am J Surg Pathol 2006;30:90–6.

123. Andersson J, Sihto H, Meis-Kindblom JM, et al. NF1-associated gastrointestinal stromal tumors have unique clinical, phenotypic, and genotypic characteristics. Am J Surg Pathol 2005;29:1170–6.

124. Maertens O, Prenen H, Debiec-Rychter M, et al. Molecular pathogenesis of multiple gastrointestinal stromal tumors in NF1 patients. Hum Mol Genet 2006;15:1015–23.

125. Cummings SP, Lally KP, Pineiro-Carrero V, Beck DE. Colonic leiomyoma—an unusual cause of gastrointestinal hemorrhage in childhood. Report of a case. Dis Colon Rectum 1990;33:511–4.

126. Tervit GJ, Forster AL. Leiomyoma of the small intestine in an 11-year-old boy. Eur J Pediatr Surg 1997;7:44.

127. Ameh EA, Shehu SM, Rafindadi AH, Nmadu PT. Small intestinal leiomyoma in childhood: A case report. West Afr J Med 2002;21:157–8.

128. Riggle KP, Boeckman CR. Duodenal leiomyoma: A case report of hematemesis in a teenager. J Pediatr Surg 1988;23:850–1.

129. Chu MH, Lee HC, Shen EY, et al. Gastrointestinal bleeding caused by leiomyoma of the small intestine in a child with neurofibromatosis. Eur J Pediatr 1999;158:460–2.

130. Gupta AK, Berry M, Mitra DK. Gastrointestinal smooth muscle tumors in children: Report of three cases. Pediatr Radiol 1994;24:498–9.

131. Miser JS, Pizzo PA. Soft tissue sarcomas in childhood. Pediatr Clin North Am 1985;32:779–800.

132. Kennedy AP, Jr, Cameron B, Dorion RP, McGill C. Pediatric intestinal leiomyosarcomas: Case report and review of the literature. J Pediatr Surg 1997;32:1234–6.

133. McGrath PC, Neifeld JP, Kay S, Salzberg AM. Principles in the management of pediatric intestinal leiomyosarcomas. J Pediatr Surg 1988;23:939–41.

134. Furuta GT, Bross DA, Doody D, Kleinman RE. Intussusception and leiomyosarcoma of the gastrointestinal tract in a pediatric patient. Case report and review of the literature. Dig Dis Sci 1993;38:1933–7.

135. Yamamoto H, Tsuchiya T, Ishimaru Y, et al. Infantile intestinal leiomyosarcoma is prognostically favorable despite histologic aggressiveness: Case report and literature review. J Pediatr Surg 2004;39:1257–60.

136. Kusumoto H, Takahashi I, Yoshida M, et al. Primary malignant tumors of the small intestine: Analysis of 40 Japanese patients. J Surg Oncol 1992;50:139–43.

137. Simpson BB, Reynolds EM, Kim SH, et al. Infantile intestinal leiomyosarcoma: Surgical resection (without adjuvant therapy) for cure. J Pediatr Surg 1996;31:1577–80.

138. Granovsky MO, Mueller BU, Nicholson HS, et al. Cancer in human immunodeficiency virus-infected children: A case series from the Children's Cancer Group and the National Cancer Institute. J Clin Oncol 1998;16:1729–35.

139. Molle ZL, Bornemann P, Desai N, et al. Endoscopic features of intestinal smooth muscle tumor in a child with AIDS. Dig Dis Sci 1999;44:910–5.

140. Chadwick EG, Connor EJ, Hanson IC, et al. Tumors of smooth-muscle origin in HIV-infected children. JAMA 1990;263:3182–4.

141. Suankratay C, Shuangshoti S, Mutirangura A, et al. Epstein-Barr virus infection-associated smooth-muscle tumors in patients with AIDS. Clin Infect Dis 2005;40:1521–8.

142. Jenson HB, Leach CT, McClain KL, et al. Benign and malignant smooth muscle tumors containing Epstein-Barr virus in children with AIDS. Leuk Lymphoma 1997;27:303–14.

143. Tulbah A, Al-Dayel F, Fawaz I, Rosai J. Epstein-Barr virus-associated leiomyosarcoma of the thyroid in a child with congenital immunodeficiency: A case report. Am J Surg Pathol 1999;23:473–6.

144. Timmons CF, Dawson DB, Richards CS, et al. Epstein-Barr virus-associated leiomyosarcomas in liver transplantation recipients. Origin from either donor or recipient tissue. Cancer 1995;76:1481–9.

145. Wu TT, Swerdlow SH, Locker J, et al. Recurrent Epstein-Barr virus-associated lesions in organ transplant recipients. Hum Pathol 1996;27:157–64.

146. Boudjemaa S, Boman F, Guigonis V, Boccon-Gibod L. Brain involvement in multicentric Epstein-Barr virus-associated smooth muscle tumours in a child after kidney transplantation. Virchows Arch 2004;444:387–91.

147. Brichard B, Smets F, Sokal E, et al. Unusual evolution of an Epstein-Barr virus-associated leiomyosarcoma occurring after liver transplantation. Pediatr Transplant 2001;5:365–9.

148. Rogatsch H, Bonatti H, Menet A, et al. Epstein-Barr virus-associated multicentric leiomyosarcoma in an adult patient after heart transplantation: Case report and review of the literature. Am J Surg Pathol 2000;24:614–21.

149. Sadahira Y, Moriya T, Shirabe T, et al. Epstein-Barr virus-associated post-transplant primary smooth muscle tumor of the liver: Report of an autopsy case. Pathol Int 1996; 46:601–4.

150. Shekitka KM, Sobin LH. Ganglioneuromas of the gastrointestinal tract. Relation to Von Recklinghausen disease and other multiple tumor syndromes. Am J Surg Pathol 1994;18:250–7.

151. Donnelly WH, Sieber WK, Yunis EJ. Polypoid ganglioneurofibromatosis of the large bowel. Arch Pathol 1969;87:537–41.

152. Grobmyer SR, Guillem JG, O'Riordain DS, et al. Colonic manifestations of multiple endocrine neoplasia type 2B: Report of four cases. Dis Colon Rectum 1999;42:1216–9.

153. Carney JA, Go VL, Sizemore GW, Hayles AB. Alimentary-tract ganglioneuromatosis. A major component of the syndrome of multiple endocrine neoplasia, type 2b. N Engl J Med 1976;295:1287–91.

154. Pham BN, Villanueva RP. Ganglioneuromatous proliferation associated with juvenile polyposis coli. Arch Pathol Lab Med 1989;113:91–4.

155. Mendelsohn G, Diamond MP. Familial ganglioneuromatous polyposis of the large bowel. Report of a family with associated juvenile polyposis. Am J Surg Pathol 1984;8:515–20.

156. Schreibman IR, Baker M, Amos C, McGarrity TJ. The hamartomatous polyposis syndromes: A clinical and molecular review. Am J Gastroenterol 2005;100:476–90.

157. Losty P, Hu C, Quinn F, Fitzgerald RJ. Gastrointestinal manifestations of neurofibromatosis in childhood. Eur J Pediatr Surg 1993;3:57–8.

158. Kataria R, Bhatnagar V, Gupta SD, Mitra DK. Mesenteric neurofibroma in von Recklinghausen's disease. J Pediatr Surg 1997;32:128–9.

159. Buntin PT, Fitzgerald JF. Gastrointestinal neurofibromatosis. A rare cause of chronic anemia. Am J Dis Child 1970;119:521–3.

160. Ghrist TD. Gastrointestinal involvement in neurofibromatosis. Arch Intern Med 1963;112:357–62.

161. Rangiah DS, Cox M, Richardson M, et al. Small bowel tumours: A 10 year experience in four Sydney teaching hospitals. ANZ J Surg 2004;74:788–92.

162. Miettinen M, Shekitka KM, Sobin LH. Schwannomas in the colon and rectum: A clinicopathologic and immunohistochemical study of 20 cases. Am J Surg Pathol 2001;25:846–55.

163. Coffin CM, Dehner LP. Vascular tumors in children and adolescents: A clinicopathologic study of 228 tumors in 222 patients. Pathol Annu 1993;28:97–120.

164. Phung TL, Hochman M, Mihm MC. Current knowledge of the pathogenesis of infantile hemangiomas. Arch Facial Plast Surg 2005;7:319–21.

165. Smolinski KN, Yan AC. Hemangiomas of infancy: Clinical and biological characteristics. Clin Pediatr (Phila) 2005;44:747–66.

166. Boyle L, Lack EE. Solitary cavernous hemangioma of small intestine. Case report and literature review. Arch Pathol Lab Med 1993;117:939–41.

167. Sakaguchi M, Sue K, Etoh G, et al. A case of solitary cavernous hemangioma of the small intestine with recurrent clinical anemic attacks in childhood. J Pediatr Gastroenterol Nutr 1998;27:342–3.

168. Andiran F, Tanyel FC. Hemangioma of the cecum: An overlooked cause of rectal bleeding. J Pediatr Gastroenterol Nutr 2000;30:330–1.

169. Basaklar AC. Haemangiomas of the gastrointestinal tract in children. Z Kinderchir 1990;45:114–6.

170. Gandhi RK, Udwadia TE, Kinare SG, Shah DD. Intussuscepting haemangio-lymphangioma of the intestine in a child. J Postgrad Med 1968;14:136–8.

171. Condon RE, Loyd RD. Hemangioma of the colon. Am J Surg 1968;115:720–3.

172. Copple PJ, Kingsbury RA. Hemangiomas of the small bowel in children. Report of a case and review of the literature. J Pediatr 1961;59:243–7.

173. Aziz A, Kane TD, Meza MP, et al. An unusual cause of rectal bleeding and intestinal obstruction in a child with peripheral vascular malformations. Pediatr Surg Int 2005;21:491–3.

174. Fishman SJ, Smithers CJ, Folkman J, et al. Blue rubber bleb nevus syndrome: Surgical eradication of gastrointestinal bleeding. Ann Surg 2005;241:523–8.

175. Ghahremani GG, Kangarloo H, Volberg F, Meyers MA. Diffuse cavernous hemangioma of the colon in the Klippel-Trenaunay syndrome. Radiology 1976;118:673–8.

176. Byard RW, Burrows PE, Izakawa T, Silver MM. Diffuse infantile haemangiomatosis: Clinicopathological features and management problems in five fatal cases. Eur J Pediatr 1991;150:224–7.

177. Browne AF, Katz S, Miser J, Boles ET, Jr. Blue Rubber Bleb Nevi as a cause of intussusception. J Pediatr Surg 1983;18:7–9.

178. Buckmiller LM. Update on hemangiomas and vascular malformations. Curr Opin Otolaryngol Head Neck Surg 2004;12:476–87.

179. Miller T, Frieden IJ. Hemangiomas: New insights and classification. Pediatr Ann 2005;34:179–87.

180. Smith JA, Bhathal PS, Cuthbertson AM. Angiosarcoma of the colon. Report of a case with long-term survival. Dis Colon Rectum 1990;33:330–3.

181. Hanid MA, Suleiman M, Haleem A, et al. Gastrointestinal Kaposi's sarcoma in renal transplant patients. Q J Med 1989;73:1143–9.

182. Abhyankar SH, Burns RG, Godder KT, et al. Kaposi's sarcoma of the intestine in an HIV-negative patient associated with immunosuppressive therapy for severe aplastic anemia. J Pediatr Hematol Oncol 1997;19:86–8.

183. Moosa MR. Kaposi's sarcoma in kidney transplant recipients: A 23-year experience. Q J Med 2005;98:205–14.

184. de Perrot M, Rostan O, Morel P, Le Coultre C. Abdominal lymphangioma in adults and children. Br J Surg 1998;85:395–7.

185. Hornick JL, Fletcher CD. Intra-abdominal cystic lymphangiomas obscured by marked superimposed reactive changes: Clinicopathological analysis of a series. Hum Pathol 2005;36:426–32.

186. Luo CC, Huang CS, Chao HC, et al. Intra-abdominal cystic lymphangiomas in infancy and childhood. Chang Gung Med J 2004;27:509–14.

Intestinal Motility

24.1. Normal Motility and Development of the Intestinal Neuroenteric System

Gabriella Boccia, MD
Annamaria Staiano, MD

NORMAL ASPECTS OF SMALL INTESTINAL MOTILITY

Gastrointestinal motility is a complex process deriving from the integration of several mechanisms including myoelectrical activity and contractile activities, tone, compliance, and transit. Initiation and coordination of muscle contraction is regulated by neural and hormonal input. Under physiologic conditions, in the postprandial and fasting period, two basic organized motor patterns characterize the small intestine contractility.

In the fasted state, motor activity is highly organized into distinct and cyclically recurrent events known as the *interdigestive cycle*.[1,2] The interdigestive cycle consists of at least three distinct phases that occur in sequence, with a combined total average duration of about 60 to 90 minutes (Figure 1). At first, the gut is relatively quiet and exhibits very few contractions. This absence of motor contraction lasts for approximately 60% of the total cycle and is called *motor quiescence*, or phase I. Phase I is gradually replaced by a pattern characterized by increasing but irregular contractions, phase II. Phase III represents the hallmark of the fasting condition and reflects the neuromuscular function. This final pattern is called the *migrating motor complex* (MMC) and consists of a series of intense phasic contractions that are sustained for approximately 5 to 10 minutes and sweep distally throughout the intestine from the distal stomach to the ileum. The propagation velocity also varies, with about 10 cm/min in the duodenum, 7 cm/min in the proximal jejunum, and about 1 cm/min in the distal ileum.

Most phase III complexes originate in the gastroduodenal region, but about one-third of them begin distal to the ligament of Treitz. It has been reported that the terminal pressure waves of phase III in the proximal duodenum are mainly retroperistaltic.[3] The MMC develops before birth and persists in a stable fashion throughout life; it is responsible for the aboral movement of intraluminal contents and has such been termed the gut "housekeeper."

An additional brief period of transitional motor activity from the intense phase III to the quiescence of phase I (the phase IV) has been observed.

When nutrients are ingested, the cycling activity of the interdigestive cycle is interrupted by a second motor pattern. The postprandial pattern is induced 5 to 10 minutes after ingestion of a meal, peaks after 10 to 20 minutes and persists as long as food remains in the stomach. The myoelectric pattern of a meal consists of random bursts of spike potentials with the motor findings of continuous sustained contraction of variable amplitude superimposed on small changes of tone (Figure 2). This pattern of muscle contractions results in the mixing and churning of nutrients so that they may be mixed with gastrointestinal secretions and peptides and than exposed to the mucosal surface for absorption. The length of the fed motor period is dependent upon the type of nutrients ingested and the number of calories consumed, with fats inducing a more prolonged fed pattern than proteins or carbohydrates.[4]

The type of nutrients ingested together with the manner in which babies are fed and the timings of enteral feeding have been shown to be crucial factors in the development of intestinal motor activity in children. Recent advances in biomedical engineering have allowed the study of gastrointestinal motility even in very premature infants. By using miniaturized feeding catheters with an outer diameter of less than 2 mm, multiple recording sites and sleeve sensors, and with rates of water infusion ranging between 0.005 and 0.04 mL/min, we have learned a great deal about the functional ontogeny of esophageal and antroduodenal motility in humans.

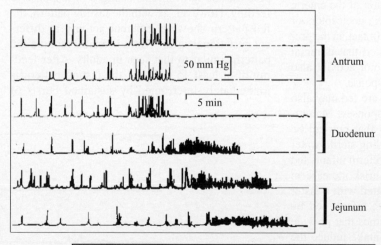

Figure 1 Fasting antroduodenal motor activity. The manometric tracing shows the sequence of phase I, phase II, and the migrating motor complex (MMC).

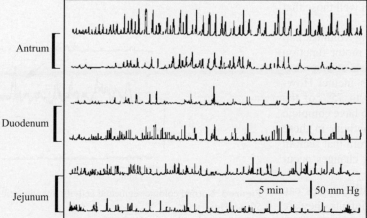

Figure 2 Postprandial small intestinal motor activity. The manometric tracing shows random bursts of contractions.

Development of Small Intestinal Motility in Children

There is convincing evidence that acute response of motor activity and peptide release are present with the first enteral feeding and that the provision of early enteral feedings facilitates functional maturation of the human intestine. Babies can respond to enteral nutrition as early as 25 weeks of gestational age.[5,6] The evidence also suggests that the small intestinal fed response is a more primitive form of motor activity than is the fasting motor activity. For this reason the practice of delaying the use of enteral nutrition in the very low birth weight infant may not coincide with preterm intestinal motor physiology. Several studies have shown that gut function and subsequent milk tolerance is improved by trophic feeding.[7–12]

Trophic feeding (minimal enteral feeding, gut priming, early hypocaloric feeding) is a practice that involves feeding small volumes of milk, nutritionally insignificant but beneficial to the developing gut. Typical volumes are from 1 to 24 mL daily/kg/body weight.[7,8] Several studies have reported that this practice accelerates the whole gut transit probably by enhancing the MMC. The mechanism by which trophic feeding exerts its influence is unknown. It is responsible for surges in the plasma concentration of several enteric hormones, neurotransmitters, and other peptides that alter gut motility (motilin, gastrin, neurotensin, and peptide YY). For example, infants who are given small enteral feedings have more mature small intestinal pattern and higher plasma gastrin and motilin concentration than do infants who have been given no feeding.[9] Furthermore, trophic feeding may cause stimulation of the enteric nervous system (ENS) directly via nociceptors or indirectly via hormone release.[10] In fact, in the preterm intestine it has been reported that minimal enteral feeding can stimulate motor activity also independently from hormonal response.

The manner in which babies are fed may also trigger differences in motor responses. Maturation of motor function requires that nutrient be fed to the neonates because feeding sterile water does not produce this effect.[11] Preterm infants fed by a 2-hour infusion display a brisk increase in motor contraction that is associated with a faster gastric emptying compared with infants fed by 15-minute bolus. Feedings volumes that provide as little as 10% of daily fluid intake induce the premature appearance of MMC as well those that provide 30 or 100%.[12]

In conclusion minimal feeding volumes can be used to trigger maturation of motor function avoiding at the same time the risk of enterocolitis that larger feeding volumes incute. However, since clusters represent 60 to 75% of the motor activity in term infants who have complete interdigestive cycle, the motor activity in these neonates is still very dissimilar from that seen in the adult, suggesting that further changes occur throughout infancy.

Although complete interdigestive cycles can be observed occasionally in term infants, they are very rarely seen in preterm infants. Approximately 75% of the neonatal intestinal motor activity is occupied by a motor pattern that is not typically seen in adults: the nonpropagating cluster of contractions. This pattern consists of bursts of 11 to 13/min contractions last 1 to 3 minutes, which do not migrate distally from the stomach to the distal gut and is prominent in both term and preterm infants.[13,14] With increasing gestational age, motor contractions become more organized, the duration of a single cluster becomes longer as does the duration of the motor quiescence separating clusters.

Preterm neonates of 27 to 28 weeks' gestational age have short clusters of activity, with a duration of less than 1.5 minutes, which are separated by brief periods (0.25 to 0.5 minutes) of motor quiescence. Compared with older children and adults, the clusters occur more frequently, with a rate of 12 to 14 times per minute. With increasing gestational age, the duration of a single cluster and motor quiescence periods become longer, with period of activity of 2 to 3 minutes occurring 8 to 10 times per minute at 32 weeks of gestation.[15] As a result, in term neonates this dominant pattern still occupies 75% of the recordings, but clusters last 3 to 4 minutes and their occurrence is lower with a frequency of 6 to 8 times per minute.

The migrating motor complexes (MMCs) appear between 32 and 35 weeks' postconception, as the overall occurrence of clusters decreases.[16] Some of these MMCs are poorly organized with slower propagation velocities.

In spite of an apparent immaturity of fasting activity, the intestinal motor activity pattern in preterm and term infants changes in response to feeding. However, as with the fasting pattern, the fed pattern shows a different activity at different gestational ages.[17] Term neonates report a fed pattern similar to that seen in adults. After feeding of at least 15 minutes, the fasting pattern is immediately interrupted by sustained bursts of motor contractions. In contrasts to term infants, only 25% of preterms display a mature type of fed pattern. About 75% of preterm neonates display a prompt cessation of motor contraction after feeding that lasts for approximately 15 to 20 minutes. This pattern of sustained motor quiescence, associated with a delay in gastric emptying, is probably due to immaturity of vagal regulation.

COLON MOTILITY: NORMAL FEATURES AND DEVELOPMENT

The physiology of the human colon requires motor activities that are different from those of the upper gut, to propel intraluminal contents distally, to mix them in a continuous manner and to store and eventually expel the residuals.

Colonic motility may be divided into two main patterns of contraction: the segmental activity and the propagated activity.[18] The segmental activity is represented by single contractions or bursts that appear usually arrhythmical and constitute most of the overall colonic motility (Figure 3). Only in a small percentage of time (<6% of the overall contractile daily activity) will these contractions assume a rhythmic frequency with ranges of 3 cycles/min. This motor pattern has the function of moving the fecal matter distally toward the rectum, allowing absorption of water, electrolytes, short-chain fatty acids, and bacterial metabolites.[19]

The propagated activity could be classified, on the basis of the contraction wave amplitude, as low-amplitude propagated contractions (LAPCs) and high-amplitude propagated contractions (HAPCs) (Figures 4 and 5). LAPCs appear with an amplitude of less than 50 mm Hg and a high frequency (more than 100 event/die). They allow the transport of fluid contents within the colon, the passage of flatus and the distention of lumen. HAPCs are powerful contractions with an amplitude of more than

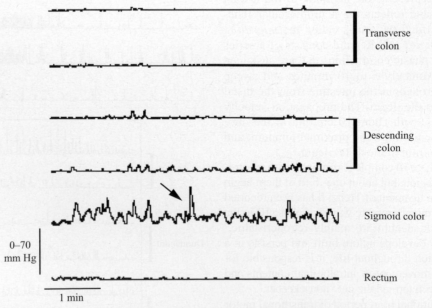

Figure 3 Normal colonic segmental activity: manometric tracing. The arrow points out sporadic contractions exceeding 50 mm Hg.

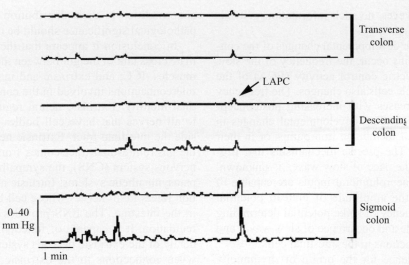

Figure 4 Manometric tracing of colonic propagated activity. The arrow points out a low-amplitude propagated contraction (LAPC).

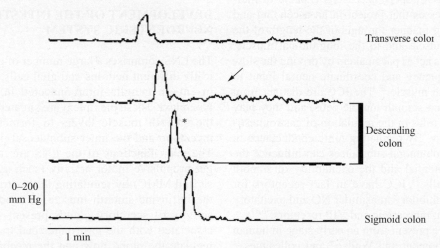

Figure 5 Normal colonic propagated activity. The manometric tracing shows high-amplitude propagated contractions (*asterisk*). Note the background arrhythmic segmental activity (*arrow*).

100 mm Hg that occur about 6 times/d. These contractions play a key role in the defecatory mechanism, as they precede the expulsion of stools.[20]

Periodic motor phenomena, the "rectal motor complex" and the "periodic colonic motor activity" have been documented in the rectum and in the more distal colonic segments, respectively.[21] No cyclic or periodic motor activity has been documented in the anal canal. Furthermore, a circadian trend is recognizable with a peak of activity after awaking in the morning and after meals and a deep inhibition during sleep. However, the major stimulus for colonic motor activity is represented by ingestion of food with an increase in smooth muscle tone and in segmental contractions. The type of nutrients influences the motor response with fatty meals eliciting a more sustained motor response than carbohydrates.[22]

In contrast to the upper gastrointestinal tract, very little is known about the development of colonic motility in infants and children. Placement of manometric or barostat catheters in the colon requires endoscopy and cannot be justified in healthy infants while noninvasive techniques such as scintigraphic transit studies or ultrasonographic evaluations have not been standardized yet in children.

Enteral nutrition represents a major factor in the ontogeny of colon motility. It seems that colon motilty matures late in gestation and has different characteristics in infants compared to older children and adults. Meconium can be found in the fetal rectum after the 21 weeks of gestation and as much as 10 to 20% of total amniotic fluid proteins derive from the fetal gut. These data suggest that defecation in utero occurs physiologically during the late stages of pregnancy and it is now believed that the detection of meconium in the amniotic fluid might reflect impaired clearance of meconium rather than excessive or inappropriate elimination in the amniotic fluid. Term newborn infants average 4 bowel movements/day for the first week of life. The frequency of defecation decreases with age, so that 85% of children 1 to 4 years old defecate once or twice daily.

As described previously, HAPCs (> 60 mm Hg) are the manometric correlate of the radiologic "mass movements" and are responsible for the rapid movement of feces in the aboral direction. The presence of HAPCs together with an increase in colonic motility after a meal, are markers for neuromuscular integrity of the colon in toddlers and children.[23] HAPCs decrease in frequency from several per hour after a meal in

awake toddlers to just a few per day in adults.[24] The gastrocolonic response seems also more prominent in younger compared to older children. Nevertheless the colon in toddlers seems to have fewer tonic and phasic non-HAPCs contractions compared to the colon of older subjects. Information about age related changes in colonic tone is absent

The ongoing developmental maturation of bowel function results in intestinal hypomotility with consequent postponement of meconium passage. The first studies to measure intestinal transit in humans used amniography and aboral transport of contrast did not occur in the intestinal tract of fetuses younger than 30 weeks' gestation. Using amniography, McLain observed that gastrointestinal motility increased with advancement of gestational age. Progression of contrast material from the oral cavity to the colon took as long as 9 hours at 32 weeks of gestational age, but only half as long by the time of labor.[25] Intestinal transit is approximately three times slower in preterm infants compared with that seen in the adults.

It has been noted that more than 90% of fullterm infants and 100% of postterm infants passed their meconium within the 24 hours. It is generally believed that the passage of meconium into the amniotic fluid is an indicator of fetal distress. Nevertheless, meconium-stained amniotic fluid is found up to 30% of all deliveries, and no cause of fetal distress is found in up to 25% of all occurrences of meconium stained amniotic fluid.[26]

In premature infants with a birth weight of 1,000 g or less the first stool is passed at a median age of 3 days and 90% have their first stool by 12 days after birth.[27] Meetze and colleagues[28] found a median age of 43 hours for passage of the first stool in 47 patients with birth weights 1,259 grams or less. One-fourth of these infants had not passed stool by 10 days of age. Weaver and Lucas[29] reported 32% delay in passing meconium greater than 48 hours with an inverse relation between gestational age and the time of first bowel movement. Extreme prematurity and delayed enteral feeding were significantly associated with delayed passage of the first stool in several studies.[30,31]

There is a well demonstrated correlation between early enteral feeding, passage of the first stool, and stool frequency and consistency. Coordinated sucking and swallowing, required for the independent utilization of milk feeds, is not achieved until 32 to 34 weeks' gestation, after which time most preterm infants are capable of taking feeds by mouth. This gestational age coincides with a significant increase in defecation rate and a surge in circulating concentrations of intestinal regulatory polypeptides (gastrin, motilin, and neurotensin) in response to milk feeds.

In newborn infants, who do not have voluntary control, evacuation probably occurs in response to an increasing volume of stool in the rectum. In a large study of bowel habits in 844 preterm infants, a direct relation between the volume of milk ingested and stool frequency throughout the first eight weeks after birth was reported.[29] Infants who received no milk had a modal frequency of one stool each day whereas those receiving greater than 150 mL/kg/d passed between three and four stools each day. Infants receiving human milk had consistently higher defecation rate, and passed softer stools, than those receiving formula milk, irrespective of gestational age and feed volume.

The finding of a modal frequency of one stool each day in the unfed neonate suggests that there is an intrinsic pattern of large bowel motor activity present as early as 25 weeks of gestation. This daily passage of stool may perform the "housekeeping" function of clearing the colon of intestinal secretions and other unwanted material. Probably milk feeds override the intrinsic fasting.

Motor activity of the colon and induce regular defecation at a frequency determined directly by the volume of the products of digestion that reach the rectum: the more feeds, the more stools.

In full term and preterm infants, the peak stool frequency occurs during the first week after birth, after which there is a decrease, in spite of increasing milk intake, indicating a maturation of the water conserving ability of the gut. It is not known, however, whether this is due to the increasing efficiency of small intestinal absorption or colonic water retention.

REGULATION OF GUT MOTILITY

The fetal development of the structure and function of the gastrointestinal tract is a complex process. Normal intestinal motility requires the coordinated development of the smooth muscle layers, nerve plexi, and interstitial cells of Cajal (ICC) in the gut wall. These structures allow all the integrated intestinal functions, such as myoelectrical activity, contractile activity, tone, compliance, and transit by generation and modulation of local and circulating neurohumoral substances.

Throughout the intestine, three layers of muscle contract in a coordinated fashion: the muscularis mucosa, a thin layer that lies beneath the villi; the circular muscle, which lies outside of the muscularis mucosa and serves as the pacemaker for gut muscle contraction; and the longitudinal muscle, the outer most layer of the three muscles. These muscles have oscillatory membrane potentials and their contraction rate is reflective of the electrical slow waves. The slow wave has a different frequency at each level of the gut (ie, 9 to 11 times per minute in the duodenum, 8 to 10 times per minute in the jejunum, and so forth). Thus, at each level of the gut, there is an intrinsic phasic contraction rate.

The muscular layers differentiate from the mesenchymal tissue in the gut by the 4th to the 6th week of gestation in a rostral to caudal fashion. The circular muscle layer appears first, and is presenting the small intestine and colon by week 8, followed, after 2 to 3 weeks, by the longitudinal muscle coat, while the muscularis mucosa is formed later, by 22 to 23 weeks' gestation.[32,33] Similarly, the contractile proteins of smooth muscle cells in animal models appear in a hierarchic

manner; however, no such information is available in humans.

Just as the developmental changes of the contractile proteins occur, the frequency of the slow waves or electric control activity (ECA) of the smooth muscle cells also changes. The frequency of ECA increases with increasing postconceptional age, reflecting developmental changes in the activity of membrane iron pumps or in their modulation. The precise mechanisms that trigger and set the pace of slow waves is unknown. Only a few neurohumoral inputs are capable of influencing the amplitude of plateau potential and the frequency of spike potential determining the magnitude and occurrence of slow waves and phasic contractions in the intestinal cells.[34]

The evidence for the origin of rhythmicity in intestinal contraction suggests that groups of mesenchymal progenitor cells differentiate to form the ICC, specialized cells capable of multiple processes that project in an ascending and descending manner throughout the length of the circular muscle and to the longitudinal muscle. These cells act as pacemakers by driving the slow wave frequency and coordinate neural input to gut smooth muscle.[32] The ICC are distinct from neurons and smooth muscle cells, and they play important roles in the regulation of gastrointestinal motility. By regulating ionic conductance in ICC, neurohumoral substances can influence the resting potential and the excitability of smooth muscle cells.[35] ICC have in fact receptors for both the inhibitory transmitter NO and excitatory tachykinin; muscarinic and VIP receptors.[36,37]

ICC are present from an early stage in human gut development and Wallace and colleagues.[33] identified Kit-positive ICC in the human intestine by week 9, after the colonization of the gut by neural crest cells and following the differentiation of the circular muscle layer. The finding that c-Kit positive ICC are present when neural crest colonization of the gut is approaching completion, is consistent with a modulating effect of the fetal ENS on ICC development.

Anatomic studies characterizing the distribution of ICC have measured the immunoreactivity to c-Kit, a protooncogene coding for a receptor tyrosine kinase. Six distinct ICC populations were identified in the gut, including intramuscular ICC, ICC within the myenteric plexus, submucosal ICC in the colon, and ICC in the deep muscular plexus of the small intestine. A regional variability has been reported in colonic ICC with the highest density observed in the transverse colon.[38]

Intrauterine maturation of ICC correlates with the initiation of electrical rhythmicity. In fact, in mutant mice lacking ICC, no spontaneous pacemaker activity is seen.[39] Such loss of pacemaker function leads to disruption of organized luminal propagation. Recent studies have reported that a delayed maturation of ICC could be involved in the pathophysiology of gastrointestinal dysmotility seen in some neonates and children.[40,41] However, since ICC development continues well into postnatal life, interpretation of apparent

abnormalities in their distribution as being of pathological significance should be tempered.

In conclusion it appears that there is an intimate cross talk in the gut between the developing muscles, ICC, and extrinsic and intrinsic neural interconnections involved in the control of intestinal motility. Extrinsic neural regulation refers to all nerves that have cell bodies located outside the intestinal tract. Extrinsic neural input to the gastrointestinal tract comes from the central nervous system (CNS), the sympathetic, and the parasympathetic systems. Intrinsic neural regulation refers to all nerves whose cell bodies reside in the intestine. The ENS provides most of this regulation. It is capable of functioning independently of the extrinsic nervous system in animals when connections to the extrinsic nerves have been severed.

DEVELOPMENT OF THE INTESTINAL NEUROENTERIC SYSTEM

The ENS comprises a large number of phenotypically different neurons and glial cells, arranged in enteric ganglia interconnected in complex plexiplexi. These plexiplexi are situated between the smooth muscle layers to form the outer myenteric and the inner submucosal plexiplexi. The main functions of the ENS are: to control gut propulsive motor activity (such as peristalsis and MMC) by regulating the contractility of the intrinsinc smooth muscle; to modulate the activity of secretory glands present within or associated with the gastrointestinal tract and to regulate the blood flow and the mechanisms of secretion/absorption.

In many aspects, the ENS of vertebrates is similar to the CNS, which has led to its characterization as the "second brain." In fact, unlike the innervation of other organs, the ENS is capable of mediating reflex activity in the absence of input from the brain or spinal cord, due to the presence of motor circuits including sensory neurons, intrinsic primary afferent neurons, interneurons, and excitatory and inhibitory motor neurons.

During the development of the gastrointestinal tract, neuroectoderm-derived neuronal precursors colonize the lengthening gut and become distributed in concentric plexi within the gut wall to form the ENS. All neurons and glial cells of the ENS are derived from the neural crest. Neural crest cells (NCCs) ablation studies,[42] quail-chicks interspecies grafting,[43] and other cell-tracing experiments[44] have allowed the origin of ENS cells to be assigned to the vagal region of the neural crest, adjacent to somites 1 to 7, which populates the entire length of the gut. A second region of the neuraxis, the sacral neural crest, posterior to somite 28, was also shown to provide cells to the hindgut.[45]

Vagal derived ENS progenitors, which give rise to the majority of neurons and glia of the enteric ganglia, enter the foregut mesenchyme and migrate in an anteroposterior direction colonising the entire length of the gut (primary migration wave). Lineage and genetic studies in mouse embryos have suggested that the enteric component of the vagal neural crest generates two distinct lineages: the sympathoenteric lineage which is derived from neural tube at the level of somites 1 to 5 and contributes to the formation of the enteric ganglia and the superior cervical ganglia of the sympathetic chain, and the second, the sympathoadrenal lineage, which generates progeny that colonizes primarily the enteric ganglia of the foregut (esophagus and stomach).[46] A secondary migration wave of NCCs takes place across the radius of the developing gut in mice and chicks.[45,47] In the small and large intestine of mice and small intestine of chicks, neurons and glia initially coalesce into ganglion plexiplexi in the myenteric region, while the submucosal plexus develops later.[48,49] However, the submucosal plexus develops before the myenteric plexus in the large intestine of chicks. In contrast to the vagal derived NCCs, the vast majority of the sacral-derived neural crest progeny is restricted to the colorectum, whereas, far fewer cells are also present in the ceca and in the postumbilical intestine.[50]

Numerous studies have investigated the phases of NCCs spatiotemporal migration within the gut, the possible prespecification of NCCs as ENS precursors and the possible factors implicated in the coordinated migration, proliferation, differentiation, and survival of NCCs within the developing gut. The combination of quail-chicks interspecies grafting to selectively label subpopulations of NCCs, together with antibody double-labeling to identify quail cells and neuronal and glial phenotypes within chick enteric ganglia, has allowed the identification of the subsequent phenotypes of crest-derived cells within the gut and consequently the vagal and sacral NCCs spatiotemporal migration pathways.[43,45,50] Vagal NCCs initially accumulate in the caudal branchial arches, then enter the foregut mesenchime at E3 and migrate in a single rostrocaudal wave reaching the level of umbilicus in the chicken at E5, the cecal region at E6 and the colorectum at E7.5. The entire length of the chick gut is colonized by E8.5. Sacral NCCs colonize the gut in an opposing caudorostral direction. They were found to initially congregate in the dorsal wall of the hindgut where they form the nerve of Remak until E7, when nerve fibres project into the hindgut, than migrate into the gut along these nerve fibres colonising the hindgut in large numbers from E10. From these findings, the sacral NCCs appear to colonize the hindgut 2 to 3 days after it had been colonized by vagal NCCs, supporting the idea that sacral crest derived cells require the presence of signaling molecules released by vagal-derived cells in order to colonize the hindgut.

The same authors demonstrated that unlike the colorectum in avians and mammals, where NCCs initially colonize the myenteric plexus while the submucosal plexus arises from the secondary migration of cells throughout the myenteric region, in chicks vagal NCCs colonize the submucosal region first, before migrating outward

through the circular muscle layer to populate the myenteric plexus region in a second movement.[45] Furthermore, these experiments revealed differences in the migration pathways of vagal NCCs within different regions of the chick gut. In fact, migrating crest cells appear randomly distributed within the mesenchyme in the colonization of preumbilical intestine, being muscle layers undeveloped. In the postumbilical intestine the vagal NCCs migration front is initially located in the outermost layers of the mesenchyme, adjacent to the serosal ephitelium. As the circular muscle layer begins to develop, while the crest cells progress along the gut to reach the cecum, they become orientated on either side of the circular muscle layers to form the presumptive myenteric and submucosal ganglia.[45]

The topographical pattern of differentiation of human NCCs and gut mesenchyme has been recently studied (Fu and colleagues 2004).[32] Previous studies reported that vagal NCCs migrate from the foregut to the hindgut of human embryos between gestational age week 4 and week 7 and that the NCCs at level of the colon differentiate into neurons and glia by week 7 without coalescing into ganglion plexus.[51]

Fu and colleagues[32] reported that rostral to caudal colonization of the entire gut by the NCC is completed by week 7 of gestation. The formation of the myenteric plexus follows a rostral to caudal pattern. Coalescence of neurons and glia into the myenteric plexus coincides with the differentiation of the longitudinal and circular muscles between gestational weeks 7 and 14. The submucosal plexus develops after the appearance of the myenteric plexus and before the differentiation of the muscularis mucosae. A discernable myenteric plexus first appears at the foregut in week 7 when the mesenchyme surrounding the ganglion has started to differentiate into muscle. At week 7, neurons and glia are localized at the hindgut mesenchyme but are randomly distributed and have not coalesced into recognizable ganglion plexus. Neurons and glia coalesce into plexi in the myenteric region at the hindgut by week 9, 2 weeks after the appearance of myenteric plexus at the foregut. The myenteric plexus is small and consists of a few, closely packed neurons and glia at week 7. From week 12 to week 20 plexus increases in size and neurons and glia become less packed. Intraplexus nerve fascicles become clearly visible from week 14 to week 20. The submucosal plexus develops after the appearance of the myenteric plexus and before the differentiation of muscularis mucosae. Scattered NNCs and glia are first seen at the presumptive submucosa of the foregut and mid gut at week 9 and coalesce into small ganglion plexi in the submucosa inner to the nascent circular muscle layer in these sites. By week 12 the submucosal plexus at the foregut increases in size, remaining relatively small in the midgut. By week 14 intercellular spaces and intraplexus nerve fascicles are visible at the foregut and midgut. At the same gestational age the submucosal plexus is seen at the hindgut, firstly localized at the submucosa inner to the

circular muscle. By week 20 it is also localized in the inner submucosa further away from the circular muscle layer at the foregut and the midgut and intraplexus nerve fascicles are evident in the hindgut submucosal plexus. The observation that in the human fetal gut neurons and glia initially coalesce into ganglion plexi at the myenteric region, and that the submucosal plexus develops later, argues for a secondary migration of NCCs from the myenteric region to the submucosa.

The temporal development of ganglion plexi in the human fetal gut is in line with that reported in mice and the small intestine of chicks, but differs from the large intestine of chicks.[45,47] The molecular mechanisms that control the spatiotemporal development of the ENS in the gut are multiple and represent a field of research in continuous evolution.

Signals and Molecules that Control the Development of ENS

Crest derived cells probably do not migrate as an uniform array of committed and uncommitted precursors, but appear to constitute a heterogeneous population that changes progressively as a function of developmental stage, both as the cells migrate and after they arrive in the target bowel.

Several studies, performed over the past several decades, have clarified that since vagal and sacral NCCs differentiate into specific neuronal phenotypes when transplanted elsewhere along the neuraxis, it is possible that NCC precursors may have some level of prespecification or some special migratory properties that, together with a particular favorable and permissive environment, allow and regulate their spatiotemporal migration within the gut.[52–54] Another important concept is that vagal and sacral populations seem to present differences in the migratory properties, the rostral vagal NCCs being endowed with a higher invasive and proliferative capacity than sacral cells.[54,55] In fact by transplanting sacral crest to the trunk region and vice versa, Erickson and colleagues[55] found that crest cells behaved according to their new position, rather than their site of origin, concluding that sacral NCCs have no cell autonomous properties that allow them to colonize the gut and that at the sacral level the environment is sufficient to allow crest cells from other axial levels to enter the gut mesenchyme.

Along their route of travel the crest derived precursors have ample opportunity to interact with microenvironmental signaling factors, which include growth factors and elements of extracellular matrix (ECM) that irreversibly influence the precursors and contribute to the determination of their fate. The migration, proliferation, survival, and differentiation of enteric NCCs are primarily regulated by interactions between diffusible chemoattractive molecules that originate in the gut mesenchyme and their specific receptors expressed on the enteric NCCs. These essential factors include: glial cell line-derived neurotrophic factor (GDNF) and its receptor tyrosine kinase RET and Gfra1[56,57] neurotrophin-3 (NT-3) and TrkC receptor,[58] endothelin-3(EDN-3) and endothelin receptor-B (EDNRB),[59] netrin (NTN) and deleted in colorectal cancer (DCC),[60] bone morphogenetic proteins 2 and 4 (BPM2, BPM4) and the BPM receptors,[61] sonic hedgehog.[62]

Two intercellular signaling pathways are absolutely necessary for complete colonization of the gut by neural precursors: those mediated by RET and EDNRB.

GDNF GFRα-RET Mediated Pathway

RET is a transmembrane tyrosine kinase and represents the signaling component of multisubunit receptor complexes for the GDNF family ligands (GFLs). There are four distant members of the transforming growth factors TGF-β superfamily: GDNF, neurturin (NRTN), artemin(ARTN), and persephin (PSPN).[63] RET activation requires a glycosylphosphatidilinositol (GPI)-linked coreceptor (Gfrα1-4) that determines RET ligand specificity. Gfrα1 interacts preferentially with GDNF; Gfrα2 with NRTN; Gfrα3 with ARTN, and GRFα4 with PSPN.[64]

The role of RET in ENS development is well documented and several studies have demonstrated the role of RET-positive NCCs as multipotential ENS progenitors. Taraviras and colleagues[46] studied the response to GDNF and NTN of primary neuronal cultures (peripheral sensory and central dopaminergic neurons) derived from wild-type and RET-deficient mice and showed that the absence of functional RET receptors abrogates the biological responses of neuronal cells to both GDNF and NTN. Furthermore, cultures of Ret+-NCCs, isolated from the gut of rat embryos failed to survive or differentiate in the absence of neurotrophic factors. These findings suggest that GDNF and NRTN promote the survival, proliferation, and differentiation of multipotential ENS progenitors present in the gut rat embryos at relatively early stage of embryogenesis (E12.5 to 13.5). These effects seem to be stage specific, since similar ENS cultures established from later stage embryos (E14.5 to 15.5) had a drastically reduced response to both neurotrophic factors. On the contrary another neurotrophic factor, NT-3, has no effect on early Ret+-NCCs progenitors while it promotes the generation of neurons and glia in late NCC derived cultures (E14.5).[46,65–66]

Despite the comparable ability of GDNF and NRTN to promote ENS precursors proliferation and axonal extension in vitro, the phenotype of Gdnf−/− and Nrtn−/− mice is very different. Gdnf−/− mice have hypoganglionosis in the stomach and ganglionosis of the small bowel and colon.[67] Nrtn−/− mice have a normal number of myenteric neurons but a reduced neuronal fiber density and abnormal intestinal contractility.[68] Gianino and colleagues[64] have examined the ENS in mice deficient in both GDNF and NRTN (Gdnf −/−/Ntrn−/−) and in mice heterozygous for GDNF (Gdnf+/−) as well as Gdnf +/−/ Nrtn−/−, Ret+/−, and Gfra1+/−. They confirmed that Gdnf+/− mice have enteric hypoganglionosis

that occurs because GDNF availability determines the rate of ENS precursor proliferation.

Unlike most other parts of the nervous system, neuron number in the wild-type ENS appears to be largely determined by controlling ENS precursor proliferation rather than by programmed cell death. By contrast, NRTN availability determines acetylcholinesterase-stained neuronal fiber density in the mature ENS, but does not influence myenteric neuron number; it may play a minor role in determining submucosal neuron number. Heterozygous mutation produces motility defects, but no major neuron-anatomical changes within the ENS. The hypoganglionosis in Gdnf+/− mice and the reduction in neural cell size and acetylchilinesterase-stained myenteric fiber density in Ntrn−/− mice provides strong evidence that mature enteric neurons and their precursors are trophic factor dependent. This dependence appears to switch during development. In the early stages of cell migration and proliferation, GDNF activation of Ret via GRFα1 is absolutely required for both survival and proliferation of all ENS precursors in the small bowel and colon. As development proceeds, many enteric neurons become dependent on NTRN and GFRα2 for trophic support. However, because of the complexity of the ENS, it seems likely that subpopulations of enteric neurons will be supported by distinct neurotrophic factors and neuropoietic cytokines.

Yang and colleagues[69] demonstrated that mesenchymally derived GDNF in addition to its role in survival, proliferation, and neuronal differentiation, plays a role in retaining vagal NCCs within the gut mesenchyme so that they do not migrate into the neighboring tissues via mesentery and promote the migration of NCCs along the gut. The authors postulated that GDNF protein levels could be higher in more caudal uncolonized areas that could act as GDNF "sinks." So the net direction of neuronal precursor cell migration, and the direction of axon projection pattern of the first enteric neurons, could be attracted towards these areas with higher levels of untapped GDNF protein in a gradient-dependent manner. Further supporting this evidence is the study from Natarajan and colleagues.[57] The authors found that NCCs present within fetal small intestine explants migrate towards an exogenous source of GDNF in a RET-dependent fashion. The chemoattractant role of GDNF is likely to depend on the spatial and temporal regulation of GDNF expression along the developing bowel. When vagal cells colonized the foregut, GDNF expression was high in the stomach and when present in the midgut, GDNF expression was upregulated in a more posterior region, the cecum.

The progressive wave front of the NCCs following the areas with GDNF upregulation has not been described in the hindgut. It appears that during hindgut colonization by ENS progenitors, the cecal domain of GDNF expression extends posteriorly alongside the front of migration cells. This suggests a permissive, rather than an instructive role for GDNF in the postcecal region with distinct mechanisms directing hindgut colonization.

The role of GDNF in promoting proliferation and survival of ENS precursors seem to be modulated by EDN3 which had been shown to inhibit the differentiation of migrating NCCs ensuring that sufficient ENS precursors are available to colonize the entire gut. In fact, in the absence of EDN3, enteric precursors differentiate prematurely and fail to colonize the entire length of the gut.

EDN3/EDNRB-Mediated Pathway

Endothelins -1, -2, and -3 (EDN1-3) constitute a small family of 21 amino acid peptides which activate heptahelical G-protein-coupled receptors. Only EDN3 is known to be required for normal enteric neurodevelopment. EDN3 is produced by mesenchymal cells adjacent to NCCs as they colonize the gut and the skin, and is expressed at particularly high levels in the ileocecum.[70] Mature endothelins are produced from large precursor molecules, called pre-proendothelins that are cleaved enzymatically to produce 38-41 amino acid long biologically inactive intermediates, the "big endothelins." The big endothelins are than cleaved by endothelin converting enzyme 1 (ECE-1) to the biologically active 21 amino acid long endothelins.

Mice deficient in ECE-1 exhibit craniofacial and cardiac abnormalities and fail to generate enteric neurons and melanocytes, reproducing the phenotype observed in EDN3 and EDNB-deficient animals.[71] These findings confirm that ECE-1 is the protease responsible for the in vivo formation of active EDN-1 and EDN3. In vitro studies of cell cultures of ENS precursors suggest that EDNRB activation inhibits differentiation.[72] A similar phenomenon is believed to occur in vivo to maintain a critical mass of mitotically active crest cell precursors, which are required to colonize the entire length of the large intestine. In the absence of EDNRB or EDN3, colonization of the small intestine is slightly retarded and spread of neuronal precursors from the distal ileum to the cecum is severely impaired. The most commonly held hypothesis is that EDN3 activity maintains the pool of enteric NCC precursors by promoting their proliferation and inhibiting their differentiation into neurons. While several studies have confirmed the capacity of EDN3 to inhibit neurogenesis in cultured NCCs, it has been recently reported that the absence of EDNRB in enteric neural steam cells, does not increase neurogenesis.[73]

Recently Nagy and colleagues[62] have studied the role of EDN3 during formation of the avian hindgut ENS. They created chick-quail intestinal chimeras by transplanting preganglionic quail hindguts into the coelomic cavity of chick embryos. The quail grafts develop two ganglionated plexi of differentiated neurons and glial cells originating entirely from the host neural crest. The presence of excess of EDN3 in the graft results in a significant increase in ganglion cell number, while inhibition of EDNRB signaling in the hindgut leads to severe hypoganglionosis. This hypoganglionosis does not derive by increased apoptotic cell death. The EDN3-induced hyperganglionosis can result from effects on NCCs proliferation, survival, and/or differentiation. This result is consistent with previous in vitro works where EDN3 promoted proliferation of cultured NCC and of undifferentiated enteric crest-derived cells.[74] In the absence of EDN3 signaling there are only enough NCCs precursor to populate the intestine to the level of the cecum.

The cecum seems to occupy a very central role in EDN3 function. The cecal expression of EDN3 and GDNF in avians appears just prior to the arrival of crest-derived cells at E5.5, suggesting that these factors may locally influence, directly or indirectly, enteric NCCs and the migratory wavefront. Inhibition of EDNRB activity in the avian gut leads to arrested migration precisely at the level of the cecum,[62] while EDN3 signaling is only required between E10.5 and E12.5 in mice, just when migrating crest cells are crossing the ileocecal junction. Furthermore, NCC migration appears normal in EDN3 and EDNRB mutant mice until those cells reach the cecum, at which time there is a transient migratory arrest.[75] These observations suggest that EDN3 may have a specific effect on migrating crest-derived cells as they reach the cecum, serving to expand the population precursors at that point so that they can populate the remaining intestine.

While several studies have supported the capacity of EDN3 to promote NCCs proliferation, it has been reported that the absence of EDNRB in enteric neural stem cells does not increase neurogenesis and that EDN3 also inhibits neuronal differentiation in the ENS, as demonstrated by the absence of nNos-expressing cells in EDN-3 treated hindgut.[62,73] In contrast, terminally differentiated crest-derived cells are present in the cecum reflecting their premature differentiation and inability to migrate further along the gut and confirming the role of EDN3 in expanding the population of precursors in the cecum to allow migration in the remaining intestine where they mature. The role of EDN3-EDNBR signaling is relevant not only in the cecum but also in the hindgut, where EDN3 becomes expressed as NCCs are arriving; in this way, deficient EDN3 activity may create a hindgut environment that does not allow normal colonization by enteric crest derived cells.[62]

One of the most exciting areas of investigation concerns potential genetic and molecular interactions between the GDNF/RET/GFRα1 and EDN3/ENDRB pathways.

Coexistent alterations in genes from both pathways confer a significantly greater risk of enteric aganglionosis than the same genetic alterations in isolation. In contrast with homozygotes, Ret[+/−] heterozygotes do not exhibit aganglionosis. Similarly, Ednrb[sl/sl] mice, have ganglion cells throughout their gastrointestinal tracts. On the contrary, aganglionosis is observed in 100% of Ret[+/−]:Ednrb[sl/sl], indicating that mutations at one locus will modify the phenotype associated with mutations at the other locus.

The restriction of aganglionosis in EDNRB and EDN3 deficient mouse to the distal colon initially suggested that this pathway could play a role only during late stages of gut colonization such as E11.5 to E12.5, during which time enteric NCCs cross the cecum and colonize the proximal colon.[76,78] Recent studies in humans and mice have demonstrated that an interaction between the RET and EDNBR loci regulates ENS development not only in the distal colon,[76,77] but also into prececal segment.[74] Barlow and colleagues[74] studying double mutant embryos, reported that EDN3 specifically cooperates with GDNF to promote the proliferation of the uncommitted ENS progenitors; this function in addition to its antagonistic effects on neuronal differentiation, suggests that endothelins represent a class of extracellular signals that regulate the number of undifferentiated neuroectodermal precursors. At the same time, activation of the EDNRB inhibits the chemoattractive effect of GDNF on ENS progenitors. In fact, EDN3 is expressed at highest levels just near and ahead of the front of migration of enteric NCC, probably regulating the orderly colonization of the gut. In this respect, it is interesting that in EDN3 deficient mice, ectopic ganglia have been identified in the pelvic region outside the enteric musculature in the adventitia of the colon[79] indicating a possible derivation from ENS progenitors that fail to follow the correct migratory pathways established by GDNF. The mechanism by which EDN3 blocks GDNF-induced chemoattraction wavefront seems to be related to the inhibition of a protein Kinase A (PKA).[74]

Finally, EDN3 may also affect the environment through which NCCs migrate, in fact in vivo and in vitro studies have shown that EDNRB-mRNA is expressed by non-NCCs in the gut wall; these cells produce high levels of laminin when EDN3 is deficient.[72,80] These findings support the hypothesis that a nonneural crest, ECM mediated, indirect effect of EDN3/EDNRB signaling promotes premature differentiation of neural precursors.

Extracellular matrix molecules could contribute in several ways to ENS development. They provide the matrices for navigation during cell migration, promote neronal overgrowth, neuronal differentiation, and cell survival. Alterations in ECM molecules including laminin, collagen type IV, tenascin, fibronectin, and nidogen have been documented in patients with Hirschsprung's disease, thus implicating ECM molecules in enteric neurogenesis.[80–83] The production and deposition of the neurotrophic factors and ECM molecules changes as the gut mesenchyme differentiates. The migratory NCCs may recognize the differentiation state of the mesenchyme by the interpretation of the repertoire of neurotrophic factors and ECM molecules as microenvironmental cues.

Netrin/DCC Mediated Pathway

Netrins are members of a family of laminin-related proteins which include the UNC-6 gene product of nematodes, netrin A and B of Drosophila, netrins 1 and 2 of chicks, netrin 3 of mice, and NTN2L of humans. They attract or repel sets of axons; the chemoattractant effects are mediated by the DCC family of plasmalemmal receptors. The adenosine A2b receptor also binds netrins probably acting as a DCC coreceptor.[84] Whether effects of netrins are attractive or repulsive depends on coreceptors.[85]

Unlike the colorectum in birds, in the intestine of mammals including humans, NCC initially colonize the myenteric plexus. Then cells migrate from the outmoster layers of gut mesenchyme taking a critical perpendicular turn and entering the submucosa to give rise to the submucosal plexus.[45,47] Recent studies have implicated netrins in the guidance of this secondary migration to the submucosa and pancreas respectively.[60] These authors demonstrated that netrins and netrins receptor DCC, neogenin and the adenosin A2b receptor are expressed in the fetal mucosa and pancreas at early stages in development. DCC expression quantified in the murine gut, was detectable as early as E11 when crest-derived cells are known to be present in the small intestine.[47] By E13 DCC expression reaches a peak; this is the period in which the hindgut is colonized (E12.3 to E14.5) and coincides with the secondary migration of the NCCs in the small intestine from the outer gut mesenchyme to the submucosa.

A subset of enteric crest derived cells thus expresses DCC. These cells migrate towards endogenous sources of netrin within the gut, inwardly through the developing circular muscle and give rise to the submucosal plexus. Expression of DCC by enteric NCCs is maximal when they make their turn to colonize the submucosal plexus and when others enter the pancreas. Transgenic mice that lack DCC lack both the submucosal plexus in the bowel and ganglia in the pancreas, confirming that netrins interact with DCC expressed by crest-derived precursors to guide these cells to the submucosa and pancreas.

A repulsive signal, which prevents crest-derived cells from migrating any further than the submucosa is laminin. Laminin, secreted in abundance by the developing enteric mucosa, converts the attractive effect of netrin to repulsion,[86] preventing NCC from entering the mucosa and encouraging these precursors to differentiate only in the submucosa.

The presence of netrin in the outer gut mesenchyme may be important also in preventing premature apoptosis among the migrating crest derived cells; in fact, in the absence of ligands, DCC mediates apoptosis.[87,88]

It can be concluded that the netrin/DCC signaling pathway play a critical role in the development of the ENS for the formation of the submucosal and pancreatic plexi. However, this pathway may also play a role in the establishment of the extrinsic vagal innervation of the intestinal ganglia, the development of intraenteric connections and the regulation of cellular apoptosis.

Role of Sonic Hedgehog (Shh) and the Bone Morphogenetic Proteins (BMP)

The molecular mechanism that controls the secondary migration of NCCs together with the spatiotemporal development of the annular structures of the gut wall are poorly understood. The development of the annular structure of the gut wall seems to be regulated by the mucosal secretion of the Sonic hedgehog (Shh) into the underlying mesenchyme. In response to Shh induction, mesenchyme produces and secretes bone morphogenetics proteins (BMPs) into the ECM.[89,90]

In developing gut it has been shown that Shh is expressed in the endodermal epithelium and induces patched and BMP4 expression in the mesenchyme of gut.[90,91] Sukegawa and colleagues[89] have investigated the expression and function of the genes that regulate the molecular mechanisms involved in concentric differentiation of chicken gut mesenchyme. They reported that all gut mesenchymal cells have the potency of differentiating into smooth muscle cells and that epithelium inhibits this differentiation. Epithelium seems to inhibit also proliferation of enteric neurons and controls their distribution within the gut mesenchyme. The authors demonstrated that Shh could mimic the effect of epithelium on the topographical differentiation of the gut.

Shh secretion is first detected in the endodermal epithelium just after the establishment of the digestive tube and continue throughout development.[91] Later in development Shh is involved in the region-specific differentiation of both epithelium and mesenchyme. Shh-mediated signaling inhibits differentiation of smooth muscle resulting in differentiation of nonmuscle layers such as the lamina propria and submucosa. The influence of this molecule on the mesenchyme can be monitored by the expression of Shh-responsive genes such as patched and BMP4. These genes are expressed in cells in close proximity of epithelium that are the main sources of Shh.

Shh also inhibit the differentiation of enteric neuronal cells which appear restricted to regions distant from the sources of Shh. It has been reported that Shh-knockout mouse shows an alteration in smooth muscle differentiation and in the increase of the number of enteric neuronal cells that appear abnormally distributed in the mesenchyme. The gradient of Shh concentration across the radius of the gut may regulate the second migration and differentiation of NCC by the modulation of competence of NCCs towards special microenvironmental "cues" such as GDNF and EDN3 from the differentiated mesenchyme.

Shh has been shown to inhibit neuron differentiation of NCC in the gut by inducing BMP4,[89,90] while it controls smooth muscle differentiation directly or via induction of factors other that BMP4. However, studies in the rat gut in vivo have demonstrated that BMP2 induces neuron differentiation of NCC due to the addition of mesenchyme derived factors.[92] In response to Shh induction, mesenchyme produces and secretes BMPs.

Bone morphogenetic proteins comprise a subgroup of the TGF-β family of secreted signaling molecules. BMP2, 4, and 7 transduce their signal by binding to a heterodimer consisting of a type I receptor, BMPRIA, or BMPRIB or, in case of BMP7, activin receptor like kinase (Alk-2) and type II (BMPRII) receptor. Receptor activation leads to phosphorylation and activation of the Smad-signaling cascade.[90,91] BMP regulates multiple critical functions during organogenesis including the epithelial-mesenchymal interactions that underlie specification, regionalization, and differentiation within the developing gut. In the early embryo BMP directs the formation of NCCs in the dorsal neural tube. During the neural crest migration they continue to act as local environmental cues to promote the development of autonomic neurons. Later in development, exposure to BPM promotes dendrite specific process outgrowth, promoting differentiation to an autonomic neuronal fate and modulating trophic factor responsiveness in primary sympathetic cultures in cell lines.[93–95]

The role of BMP signaling in enteric neuronal differentiation is controversial. BMP4 has been to shown to either promote or inhibit enteric neuronal differentiation while BMP2 promotes neuronal differentiation of postmigratory enteric crest cells.[91]

Pisano and colleagues[92] reported that BMP2 influences the number of neurones that develop from sympathetic and enteric precursors cells, acting through multiple mechanisms that include regulation of differentiation, proliferation, and survival. The acquisition of trophic factor responsiveness and the increase in expression of neurofilament proteins, in conjunction with studies showing BMP-dependent regulation of neuropeptide expression and dendritic development, argue that BMP promotes neuronal maturation in neural crest derived lineages. The final phenotype of these neurons is determined by BMP signal in the context of other signals expressed in the local environment. This model of multiple interacting signals is supported by studies demonstrating that BMP act in conjunction with retinoic acid to induce expression of a GDNF receptor and to enhance the acquisition of GDNF and NT-3 responsiveness.[96,97]

Recently Goldstein and colleagues.[59] reported that targeted inhibition of intestinal BMP activity using the BMP inhibitor *noggin*, leads to impaired migration of enteric crest cells by interfering with their responsiveness to GDNF. Enteric crest cells underwent a significant delay in their migration and failed to reach the distal hindgut until well beyond the stage at which this normally occurs. Multiple factors can contribute to delay in migration: increased cell death, premature neuronal differentiation or direct effect on migration. The authors found that there was no change in the rate of cell death or in the timing of neuronal and glial differentiation. Since BMP4 alone is not sufficient to promote migration of crest-derived cells from the gut, they demonstrated that BMP4 can modulate the effect of a known migratory factor: the GDNF.

This observation extend the previously reported data that an interaction between GDNF and BMP4 synergystically enhances enteric neuronal development[59,98] The migratory response of ENS cells to GDNF is known to be mediated by several factors, the activation of RET signaling pathways and the interaction with neuronal cell adhesion molecule (NCAM). In addition, both the EDN3 and Shh pathways appear to be involved, inhibiting the migration of crest-derived cells in response to GDNF.[57,61,63,64,99] Since BMP4 is expressed both in crest and noncrest derived cells within the gut, its influence on migration may be either a direct effect on the crest cells itself or an indirect one through other molecules produced by the intestinal microenvironment.

Secondly, in the absence of BMP activity, fewer numbers of NCC reach the hindgut and subsequently fail to aggregate normally into clusters to form ganglia. Studies in vitro and in vivo show that BMP2 and BMP4 are required to promote aggregation of isolated enteric neurons to form clusters of cells simulating the appearance of enteric ganglia. This mechanism also requires activation of GDNF which increases the number of neurons per clusters and the ganglion size.[59,65]

In conclusion, development of the ENS is a complex process during all of embryogenesis and continues in fetal and early postnatal life. Its spatiotemporal determination is dictated by innumerable and complex interactions between different intercellular signaling systems. Alterations in this subtle equilibrium could induce anatomic and physiologic defects in the gut wall, some of which are recognized as specific forms of intestinal dysmotility patterns in humans. Further studies of ENS development and all of the molecules involved in its complex mechanisms of control will improve the understanding of these conditions, leading to better diagnosis and treatment of affected individuals.

REFERENCES

1. Kellow JE, Borody TJ, Phillips SF, et al. Human interdigestive motility: Variations in patterns from esophagus to colon. Gastroenterology 1986;91:386.
2. Sarna SK. Cyclic motor activity: Migrating motor complex. Gastoenterology 1985;89:894.
3. Castedal M, Abrahamsson H. High-resolution analysis of the duodenal interdigestive phase III in humans. Neurogastroenterol Motil 2001;13:437–481.
4. Feinle C, O'Donovan D, Doran S, et al. Effects of fat digestion on appetite, APD motility, and gut hormones in response to duodenal fat infusion in humans. Am J Physiol Gastrointest Liver Physiol 2003;284:G798–807.
5. Berseth CL. Neonatal small intestinal motility: Motor responses to feeding in term and preterm infants. J Pediatr 1990;117:777–82.
6. Al Tawil Y, Berseth C. Gestational and postnatal maturation of duodenal motor responses to intragastric feeding. J Pediatr 1996;129:374–81.
7. Troche B, Harvey-Wilkes K, Engle WD, et al. Early minimal feedings promote growth in critically ill premature infants. Biol Neonate 1995;67:172–81.
8. Berseth CL. Effect of early feeding on maturation of the preterm infant's samll intestine. J Pediatr 1992;120:947–53.
9. Shulman DI, Konterek K. Gastrin, motilin, insulin, and insulin-likegrowth factor-1 concentrations in very low birth weight infants receving enteral or parenteral nutrition. J Parenter Enteral Nutr 1993;17:130–5.
10. McClure RJ, Newell SJ. Randomised controlled trial of trophic feeding and gut motility. Arch Dis Child Fetal Neonatal 1999;80:F54–8.
11. Berseth CL, Nordyke C. Enteral nutrients promote postnatal maturation of intestinal motor activity in preterm infants. Am J Pyisiol 1993;27:G1046–51.
12. Owens L, Burrin DG, Berseth CL. Minimal enteral feeding induces maturation of intestinal motor function but not mucosal growth in neonatal dogs. J Nutr 2002;132:2717–22.

13. Bisset WM, Watt JB, Rivers RPA, et al. Ontogeny of fasting small intestinal motor activity in human infants. Gut 1988;29:483.
14. Owens L, Burrin D, Berseth CL. Enteral nutrition has a dose-response effect on maturation of neonatal canine motor activity. Gastroenterology 1996;110:828.
15. Berseth CL. Assessment in intestinal motility as a guide in the feeding management of the newborn. Clin in Perinatol 1999;26:1007–15.
16. Ittman PI, Amarnath R, Berseth CL. Maturation of antroduodenal motor activity in preterm and term infants. Dig Dis Sci 1992;37:14–9.
17. Al-Tawil Y, Berseth CL. Gestational and postnatal maturation of duodenal motor responses to intragastric feeding. J Pediatr 1996;129:374.
18. Bassotti G, de Roberto G, Castellani D, et al. Normal aspects of colorectal motility and abnormalities in slow trasit constipation. World J Gastroenterol 2005;11:2691–6.
19. Cook IJ, Furukawa Y, Panagopoulus V, et al. Relationships between spatial patterns of colonic pressure and individual movements of content. Am J Physiol Gastrointest Liver Physiol 2000;278:G329–41.
20. Bampton PA, Dinning PG, Kennedy ML, et al. Spatial and temporal organization of pressure patterns throughout the unprepared colon during spontaneous defecation. Am J gastroenterol 2000;95:1027–35.
21. Hagger R, Kumar D, Benson M, et al. Periodic colonic motor activity identified by 24-h pancolonic ambulatory manometry in humans. Neurogastroenterol Mot 2002;14:271–8.
22. Rao SS, Kaveloc R, Beaty J, et al. Effects of fat and carbohydrate meals on colonic motor response. Gut 2000;46:205–11.
23. Di Lorenzo C, Hyman PE. Gastrointestinal motility in neonatal and pediatric practice. Gastroenterol Clin North Am 1996;25:203–23.
24. Di Lorenzo C, Flores AF, Hyman PE. Age related changes in colon motility. J Pediatr 1995;127:593–6.
25. McLain CR. Amniography studies of the gastrointestinal motility of the human fetus. Am J Obstet Gynecol 1963;86:1079–87.
26. Ciftci AO, Tanyel FC, Bingol-Kologlu M, et al. Fetal di stress does not affect in utero defecation but does impari the clearance of amniotic fluid. J Pediatr Surg 1999;34:246–50.
27. Verma A, Ramasubbareddy D. Time of first stool in extremely low birth weight ($\leq$ 1000 grams) infants. J Pediatr 1993;122:626–9.
28. Meetze WH, Palazzolo VL, Dowling D, et al. Meconium passage in very low birth weight infants. JPEN 1993;17:537–40.
29. Weaver LT, Lucas A. Development of bowel habit in preterm infants. Arch Dis Child 1993;68:317–20.
30. Wang PA, Huang FY. Time of the first defecation and urination in very low birth weight infants. Eur J Pediatr 1994;153:279–83.
31. Jhaveri MK, Kumar SP. Passage of the first stool in very low birth weight infants. Pediatrics 1987;79:1005–7.
32. Fu M, Tam PKH, Sham MH, et al. Embryonic development of the ganglionic plexi and the concentric layer struture of human gut: A topographyc study. Anat Embryol 2004;208:33–41.
33. Wallace AS, Burns AJ. Development of the enteric nervous system, smooth muscle and interstitial cells of Cajal in the human gastrointestinal tract. Cell Tissue Res 2005; 319:367–82.
34. Hansen MB. Neurohumoral control of gastrointestinal motility. Physiol Res 2003;52:1–30.
35. Ward SM, Beckett EA, Wang X, et al. Interstitial cells of Cajal mediate cholinergic neurotransmssion from enteric motor neurons. J Neurosci 2000;20:1393–403.
36. Camilleri M. Enteric nervous system disorders: Genetic and molecular insights for the neurogastroenterologist. Neurogastroenterol Motil 2001;13:277–95.
37. Keef KD, Anderson U, O'DriscollK, et al. Electical activity induced by nitric oxide in canine colonic circular muscle. Am J Physiol 2002;282:G123–9.
38. Hagger R, Gharaie S, FinlaysonC, et al. Regional and transmural density of interstitial cells of Cajal in human colon and rectum. Am J Physiol 1998;275:G1309–16.
39. Der-Silaphet T, Malysz J, Hagel S, et al. Interstitial cells of Cajal direct normal propulsive contractile activity in the mouse small intestine. Gastroenterology 1998;114:724–36.
40. Kenny SE, Vanderwiden JM, Rintala RJ, et al. Delayed maturation of the interstitial cells of Cajal: A new diagnosis for transient neonatal pseudoobstruction. Report of two cases. J Pediatr Surg 1998;33:94–8.
41. Sabri M, Barksdale E, Di Lorenzo C. Constipation and lack of colonic interstitial cells of Cajal. Dig Dis Sci 2003; 48:849–53.
42. Peters-van der Sanden MJ, Krby ML, Gittenberger-de Groot A, et al. Ablation of various regions within the avian vagal neural crest has differential effects on ganglion formation in the fore-, mid-and hindgut. Dev Dyn 1993;196:183–94.
43. Burns AJ, Le Dourain NM. Enteric nervous system development: Analysis of the selective developmental potentialities of vagal and sacral neural crest cells using quail-chick chimeras. Anat Rec 2001;262:16–28.
44. Epstain ML, Mikawa T, Brown AM, et al. Mapping the origin of avian enteric nervous system with a retroviral marker. Dev Dyn 1994;201:236–44.
45. Burns AJ, Le Dourain NM. The sacral neural crest contributes neurons and glia to the postumbilical gut: Spatiotemporal analysis of the development of the enteric nervous system. Development 1998;125:4335–47.
46. Taraviras S, Pachnis V. Development of the mammalian enteric nervous system. Curr Opin Genet Dev 1999;9:321–7.
47. McKewon SJ, Chow CW, Young HM. Development of the submucous plexus in the large intestine of the mouse. Cell Tissue Res 2001;303:301–5.
48. Conner PJ, Focke PJ, Noden DM, et al. Appearance of neurons and glia with respect to the wavefront during colonization of the avian gut by neural crest cells. Dev Dyn 2003;226:91–8.
49. Young HM, Bergner AJ, Muller T. Acquisition of neuronal and glial markers by neural crest-derived cells in the mouse intestine. J Comp Neurol 2003;456:1–11.
50. Burns AJ, Champeval D, Le Durain NM. Sacral neural crest cells colonise aganglionic hindgut in vivo but fail to compensate for lack of enteric ganglia. Dev Biol 2000;219:30–43.
51. Fu M, Lui VCH, Sham MH, et al. HOXB5 expression is spatially and temporally regulated in human embryonic gut during neural crest cell colonization and differentiation of enteric neuroblasts. Dev Dyn 2003;228:1–10.
52. Le Durain NM, Teillet MA. Experimental analysis of the migration and differentiation of neuroblasts of the autonomic nervous system and of neuroectodermal mesenchymal derivatives, using a biological cell marking tecnique. Dev Biol 1974;41:162–84.
53. Rothman TP, Sherman D, Cochard P, et al. Development of the monoaminergic innervation of the avian gut: Transient and permanent expression of phenotypic markers. Dev Biol 1986;116:357–80.
54. Burns AJ, Delande JM, Le Duraine NM. In ovo transplantation of enteric nervous system precursors from vagal to sacral neural crest results in extensive hindgut colonization. Development 2002;129:2785–96.
55. Erickson CA, Goins TL. Sacral neural crest cell migration to the gut is dependent upon the migratory environment and not cell-autonomous migratory properties. Dev Biol 2000;219:79–97.
56. Homma S, Oppenheim RW, Yaginuma H, et al. Expression pattern o GDNF, c-ret, and GFRalphas suggests novel roles for GDNF ligands during early organogenesis in the chick embryio. Dev Biol 2000;217:121–37.
57. Natarajan D, Marcos-Gutierres C, Pachnis V, et al. Requirement of signalling by receptor tirosine kinase RET for the directed migration of enteric nervous system progenitor cells during mammalian embryogenesis. Development 2002;129:5151–60.
58. Chalazonitis A, Rothman TP, Chen J, et al. Neurotrophin-3 induces neuralcrest derived cells from fetal gut develop in vitro as neurons or glia. J Neurosci 1994;14:6571–84.
59. Goldstain AM, Brewer KC, Doyle AM, et al. BMP signalling is necessary for neural crest cells migration and ganglion formation in the enteric nervous system. Mech Dev 2005;122:821–33.
60. Jiang Y, Liu MT, Grshon MD. Netrins and DCC in the guidance of migrating neural crest-derived cells in the developing bowel and pancreas. Dev Biol 2003;258:364–84.
61. Fu M, Lui VC, Sham MH, et al. Sonic hedgehog regulates the proliferation, differentiation, and migration of enteral neural crest cells in gut. J Cell Biol 2004;166:673–84.
62. Nagy N, Goldstein AM. Endothelin-3 regulates neural crest cell proliferation and differentiation in the hindgut enteric nervous system. Dev Biol 2006;293:203–17.
63. Manic S, Santoro M, Fusco A, et al. RET receptor: Function in development and dysfunction in congenital marformation. Trends Genet 2001;17:580–9.
64. Gianino S, Grider J R, Cresswell J, et al. GDNF availability determines enteric neuron number by controlling precursor proliferation. Development 2003;130:2187–98.
65. Chalazonitis A, Rothman TP, Chen J, et al. Age dependent differences in the effects of GDNF and NT-3 on the development of neurons and glia from neural crest-derived precursors immunoselcted from the fetal rat gut: Expression of GRFalpha-1 in vitro and in vivo. Dev Biol 1998;204:385–406.
66. Natarajan D, Grigoriou M, Marcos-Gutierrez CV, et al. Multipotential progenitors of the mammalian enteric nervous system capable of colonising aganglionic bowel in organ culture. Develpement 1999;126:157–68.
67. Moore MW, Klein RD, Farinas I, et al. Renal and neuronal abnormalities in mice lacking GDNF. Nature 1996;382:76–9.
68. Heuckeroth RO, Enomoto H, Grider JR, et al. Gene targeting reveals a critical roles for neurturin in the development and maintenance of enetric, sensory, and parasympathetic neurons. Neuron 1999;22:253–63.
69. Young HM, Hearn CJ, Farlie PG, et al. GDNF is a chemoattractant for enteric neural cells. Dev Biol 2001;229:503–16.
70. Leibl MA, Ota T, Woodward MN, et al. Expression of endothelin 3 by mesenchymal cells of embryonic mouse caecum. Gut 1999;44:246–52.
71. Yanagisawa H, Yanagisawa M, Kapur RP. Dual genetic pathways of endothelin-mediated intracellular signalling revealed by targetd distruption of ndothlin converting ezyme-1 gene. Development 1998;125:825–36.
72. Wu JJ, Chen JX, Rothman TP, et al. Inhibition of in vitro enteric neuronal development by endothelin-3: Mediation by endothelin B rceptors. Development 1999;126:1161–73.
73. Kruger GM, Mosher JT, Tsai YH, et al. Temporally distinct requirements for endothelin receptor B in the generation and migration of gut neural crest stem cells. Neuron 2003;40:917–29.
74. Barlow A, degraaff E, Pachnis V. Enteric nervous system progenitoers are coordinately controlled by the G-protein-coupled receptor EDNRB and the receptor tyrosine kinase RET. Neuron 2003;40:905–16.
75. Lee HO, Levorse JM, Shin MK. The endothelin receptod B is required for the migration of neural crest-derived melanocyte and enteric neurons precursors. Dev Biol 2003;259:246–52.
76. Carrasquillo MM, McCallion AS, Puffenberger, et al. Genome-wide association study and mouse model identify interaction between RET and ENDRB pathways in hirschsprung's disease. Nature Genet 2002;32:237–44.
77. McCallion AS, Stames E, Conlon RA, et al. Phenotypic variation in two-locus mouse models od Hirschprung disease: Tissue specific interaction between Ret and ENDRB. Proc Natl Acad Sci U S A 2003;100:1826–31.
78. Sidebotham EL, Woodward MN, Kenny SE, et al. Localization and endhotelin-3 dependence of stem cells of the enteric nervous system in the embryonic colon. J Oediatr Surg 2002;37:145–50.
79. Payette RF, Tennyson VM, Gershon MD. Origin and morphology of nerve fibers in the aganglionic colon of the lethal spotted(IsIIs) mutant mouse. J Comp Neurol 1987;257: 237–52.
80. Rothman TP, Chen J, Howard MJ, et al. Increased expression of laminin-1 and collagen (IV) subunits in the aganglionic bowel of Is/Is, but not c-ret$^{-/-}$ mice. Dev Biol 1996;178:498–513.
81. Parikh DH, Tam PK, Van Velzen. The extracellular matrix components, tenascin and fibronectin, in Hirschsprung's disease and immunohistochemical study. J Pediatr Surg 1994;29:1302–6.
82. Parikh DH, Leibl M, Tam PK, et al. Abnormal expression and distribution of nidogen in Hirschprung's disease. J Pediar Surg 1995;30:1687–93.
83. Rauch U, Schafer KH. The extracellular matrix and its role in cell migration and development of enteric nervous system. Eur J Pediatr Surg 2003;13:158–62.
84. Corset W, Nguyen-Ba-Chrvet KT, Forcet T, et al. Netrin-1 mediated axon outhgrowth and cAMP production requires interactions with adenosisne Ab2 receptors. Nature 2000;407:747–50.
85. Barret C, Guthrie S. Expression patterns of the netrin receptor UNC5H1 among developing motor neurons in the embryonic rat hindbrain. Mech Dev 2001;106:163–6.
86. Hopker V, Shewan D, Tessier-Lavigne M, et al. Growth-cone attraction to netrin-1 is converted to repulsion by laminin-1. Nature 1999;401:69–73.
87. Forcet C, Ye X, Granger L, et al. The dependence receptor DCC (deleted in colorectal cancer) defines an alternative mechanism for caspase activation. Proc Natl Acad Sci U S A 2001;98:3416–21.
88. Llambi F, Causeret F, Bloch-Gallego E, et al. Netrin-1 acts as survival factor via receptors UNC5H and DCC. EMBO J 2001;20:2715–22.
89. Sukegawa A, Narita T, Kameda T, et al. The concentric structure of the developing gut is regulated by Sonic hedgehog derived from endodermal epithelium. Development 2000;127:1971–80.
90. Roberts DJ, Johnson RL, Burke AC, et al. Sonic hedgehoog is an endodermal signal inducing Bpm-4 and Hox genes during induction and regionalization of the chick hindgut. Development 1995;121:3163–74.
91. Narita T, Ishii Y, Nohno T, et al. Sonic hedgehog expression in developing chicken digestive organs is regulated by epithelial–mesenchymal interactions. Dev Growth Differ 1998;40:67–74.
92. Pisano JM, Colon-Hasting F, Birren SJ. Postmigratory enteric and symapthetic neural precursors share common

developmentally regulated responses to BPM2. Dev Biol 2000;227:1–11.

93. Guo X, Rueger D, Higgins D. Osteogenic protein-1 and related bone morphogenetic proteins regulate dendritic growth and the expression of microtubule-associated protein-2 in rat sympathetic neurons. Neurosci Lett 1998;245;131–4.

94. Song Q, Mehler MF, Kessler JA. Bone morphogenetic proteins induce apoptosis and growth factor dependence of cultured sympathoadrenal progenitor cells. Dev Biol 1998;196:119–27.

95. Zhang D, Meheler MF, Song Q, et al. Development of bone morphogenetic protein receptors in the nervous system and possible roles in regulationg trkC expression. J Neurosci 1998;18:3314–26.

96. Kobayashi M, Fuji M, Kurihara K, et al. Bone morphogenetic protein-2 and retinoic acid induce neurothrophin-3 responsiveness in developing rat sympathetic Neurons. Brain Res Mol Brain Res 1998;53:206–17.

97. Thang SH, Kobayashi M, Matsuoka I. Regulation of glial cell line-derived neurotrophic factor responsiveness in developing rat sympathetic neurons by retinoic acid and bone morphogenetic protein-2. J Neurosci 2000;20:2917–25.

98. Chalazonitis A, D'Autreaux F, Gutha U, et al. Bone morphogenetic protein-2 and-4 limit the number of enteric neurons bur promote development of a TrkC-expressing neuro-trophin-3-dependent subset. J Neurosci 2004;24:4266–82.

99. Paratcha G, Ledda F, Ibanez CF. The neural cell adhesion molrculr NCAM is an alternative signalling receptor for GDNF family ligands. Cell 2003;113:867–79.

24.2 Motility Disorders
24.2a. Functional Constipation

Riad Rahhal, MD
Aliye Uc, MD

Constipation is one of the most common reasons a child is referred to a pediatric gastroenterologist. In the vast majority, no structural, endocrine, or metabolic etiology is identified and the constipation is called "idiopathic" or "functional." Despite its common and benign nature, constipation creates a significant amount of distress and anxiety for the families. Constipation does not usually present a diagnostic challenge for the health care professionals. Diagnosis can be easily made and organic conditions can be ruled out by a detailed history and physical examination. However, 30 to 50% of children with functional constipation will continue to have prolonged symptoms despite initial intensive medical management. The treatment is long-lasting and relapses are common. Pediatricians and pediatric gastroenterologists who treat children with constipation will have to work closely with the families, continue to educate the child and the parents, be available to answer questions, adjust medications as needed, and do further work-up if the child does not respond to routine management. In this chapter, we will focus on the diagnostic approach to functional constipation, the work-up necessary to rule out organic causes and the treatment regimens that have proven to work in children.

DEFINITION

The term constipation is derived from the Latin word "constipare," meaning to crowd together. In general, there is not a uniform definition of constipation among physicians and the term is often interpreted differently by parents and doctors. Constipation may be characterized by infrequent bowel movements, firm consistency, large stool size, pain or discomfort with defecation, delayed intestinal transit time, increased weight of evacuated stools, and accompanied retentive posturing.[1-3] Retentive posturing or stool withholding behavior may manifest as tip toeing, holding onto furniture, leg stiffening or crossing, and hiding in a corner (Figure 1). These maneuvers contract the pelvic floor muscles, move the stool upwards and help the child to get rid of the urge to have a bowel movement.[4]

Infrequent defecation, usually less than three stools per week, is among the commonly used measures to define constipation.[2,5] Stool frequency changes in children with age. Defecation does not typically occur in fetal life and it is a sign of fetal distress if noted in utero. The first stool is typically passed within 48 hours after birth in more than 99% of term neonates.[6] Passage of meconium may be delayed in preterm babies.[7,8] Breast-fed infants have a different defecation pattern compared to formula fed infants; the frequency of their bowel movements may vary between multiple stools per day to one stool per week.[7-10] The stool frequency gradually declines from more than 4 stools/d during the first week of life to 1 to 2 stools/d by the age of 4 years. An adult defecation pattern is achieved after 4 years. The decline in stool frequency is accompanied with an increase in stool size and prolonged gastrointestinal transit time.[11-15] Mean intestinal transit time is approximately 8.5 hours in young infants. After puberty, intestinal transit time ranges between 30 and 48 hours.[16,17]

There has been an effort to standardize the childhood constipation terminology and create a consensus on the definition of pediatric defecatory disorders. Initial work was done by a pediatric working team to characterize different functional gastrointestinal disorders, including

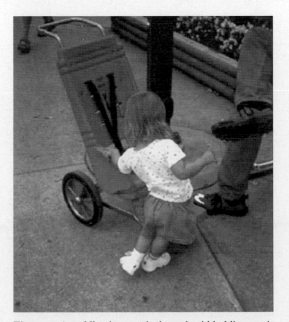
Figure 1 A toddler in a typical stool withholding position, contracting the pelvic and gluteal muscles to avoid stooling.

functional constipation (1999 Rome II criteria)[18] These criteria were found as too restrictive by others.[19,20] A group of pediatric gastroenterologists and pediatricians with an interest in gastrointestinal motility, gathered at the 2nd World Congress of Pediatric Gastroenterology, Hepatology and Nutrition in Paris in July 2004 to seek a consensus on childhood constipation terminology (PACCT).[21] Functional constipation definition described by PACCT was used as a basis for the 2006 Rome III Diagnostic Criteria for Childhood Functional Gastrointestinal Disorders.[22,23] These criteria included a separate but somewhat similar symptom-based diagnostic criteria for functional constipation in two age groups: neonates/toddlers and young children/adolescents (Table 1).[22,23] PACCT and Rome III criteria aim to unify the commonly used definitions and encourage researchers to further study the basis, treatment, and outcome of constipation. PACCT also recommended that the usage of terms *"soiling" and "encopresis"* should be discontinued and replaced by a more specific term *"fecal incontinence."*

Two other pediatric functional defecatory disorders are important in the differential diagnosis of functional constipation: infant dyschezia and nonretentive fecal incontinence. *Infant dyschezia* is described in young infants who experience at least 10 minutes of straining and crying before successful defecation in the absence of any underlying health problems. The complex defecation process is a learned practice and may be still immature in this age group. This may result in failure to coordinate abdominal muscle contraction with pelvic floor relaxation.[22] In other terms, these babies are still trying to learn "how to poop." We recommend no treatment for these babies. Physicians should reassure the parents that the infants will soon be able to master these important skills. *Nonretentive fecal incontinence* is characterized by repeated socially inappropriate stool passage in the absence of fecal retention or any other predisposing medical condition.[23] These children are older than 4 years and have no evidence of constipation. Treatment of these patients differs from those with functional constipation. We recommend educating the family, a rigorous toilet training program and caution against an intensive use of stool softeners.[24,25]

Table 1 Functional Constipation-Rome III Criteria

In infants/toddlers (<4 yr of age)

One month of at least 2 of the following[22]:

- ≤2 defecations per wk
- ≥1 episode per wk of incontinence after the acquisition of toileting skills
- History of excessive stool retention or history of painful or hard bowel movements
- Presence of a large fecal mass in the rectum
- History of large-diameter stools that may obstruct the toilet

Accompanying symptoms may include irritability, decreased appetite and/or early satiety. The accompanying symptoms disappear immediately following passage of a large stool.

In older children/adolescents (>4 yr of age)

Two months of at least 2 or more of the following[23]:

- ≤2 defecations in the toilet per wk
- ≥1 episode of fecal incontinence per wk
- History of retentive posturing or excessive volitional stool retention.
- History of painful or hard bowel movements
- Presence of a large fecal mass in the rectum
- History of large diameter stools that may obstruct the toilet

EPIDEMIOLOGY

Constipation is a common symptom in children accounting for 3% of general pediatric outpatient visits and up to 25% of visits to pediatric gastroenterologists.[26,27] Estimates of the worldwide prevalence of childhood constipation vary from 0.3% to 28%.[28–31] The lack of consensus in diagnostic criteria may have contributed to the wide variation of the prevalence in the literature.

The incidence of functional constipation in children seems to be rising over the last few decades. The number of physician visits for constipation has doubled in children less than 9 years of age between 1958 and 1986. Most of the increase was in children younger than 2 years of age.[29] The reason for this increase is not well known, but may be due to changing patterns in toilet training, diminished dietary fiber intake, or more access to health care services.[32,33]

Constipation may occur at any age but children appear most vulnerable in one of three phases: (1) infants with the introduction of cereals and other solids and weaning of breast milk; (2) toddlers at the time of toilet training, which is the peak incidence; and (3) older children who avoid bathrooms at school.[7] The prevalence of constipation in prepubertal males is noted to be higher than females in some[34,35] but not all studies.[17] In adulthood, constipation is three times more common in women than men.[36] Constipation also seems to be more prevalent in families with lesser education and lower socioeconomic status[36,37]

DEFECATION PHYSIOLOGY

Normal defecation is a complex process involving the coordinated activity of the abdominal, pelvic, and anal sphincter musculature and the autonomic and somatic nervous systems. When the rectum is empty and the internal anal sphincter is closed, there is no urge to defecate (Figure 2A–D). The entry of the stool into the rectum and the distension of the rectal wall cause a sudden drop in the internal anal sphincter tone, a phenomenon also known as the rectoanal inhibitory reflex (involuntary phase). The relaxation of the internal anal sphincter allows the stool to descend further and get in contact with the anal canal. This creates awareness that passage of a bowel movement is imminent. Rectal distension leads to rectal contractions and evacuation may be completed by the voluntary increase in intra-abdominal pressure, relaxation of the puborectalis, and levator ani muscles of the external sphincter (voluntary phase). If it is not socially acceptable to have a bowel movement, defecation can be inhibited by voluntary contraction of the pelvic floor muscles. A child who has had previous painful bowel movements may go into a withholding posture in order to prevent another painful experience (Figure 2E–H). The child will contract the pelvic floor muscles, prevent the passage of the stool, and push the stool to a level that is no longer in contact with the anal canal. If the external sphincter complex remains contracted, the rectal wall will distend and adapt to the increased rectal volume. With repeated attempts, the rectal fecal mass will develop and more liquidy stools will seep around this mass, causing fecal incontinence.

Many children achieve at least partial stool continence by 18 months of age but the age of complete bowel control is variable. Around 98% of healthy children are toilet trained by the age of 4 years.[38,39] Boys take slightly longer to toilet train than girls. Acquisition of bowel and bladder control is a maturational process, which cannot be accelerated by early and high intensity pottytraining.[38,40]

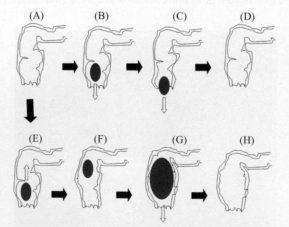

Figure 2 (A–D) Normally, defecation is triggered by stool stretching the walls of rectum. Internal anal sphincter relaxes and stool is evacuated by the relaxation of the pelvic floor muscles and contraction of the abdominal muscles. (E, F) Voluntary stool withholding pushes the stool higher in rectum; the urge to defecate disappears. (G, H) Rectum gets distended with impacted stool and large fecal mass becomes more difficult to pass. Internal anal sphincter remains open due to rectal distension and more liquidy stool seep around the fecal mass. (Adapted from reference 130.)

PATHOGENESIS

The pathophysiology of constipation is most likely multifactorial involving a dysfunction at any step of the normal defection process. In the overwhelming majority, the constipation is "idiopathic" or "functional," so an underlying structural, endocrine, or metabolic cause cannot be identified. Constipation seems to cluster in families: a positive family history is reported in 28% to 50% of constipated children with a higher incidence noted in monozygotic than dizygotic twins.[41,42] These findings suggest a genetic predisposition for functional constipation, but the contribution of physical, environmental, and social factors cannot be entirely ruled out. Most childhood constipation results from purposeful or subconscious stool withholding after an unpleasant experience with passing a bowel movement.

In neonates and infants, changing stool characteristics may occur after dietary modifications. The introduction of a new formula or solid foods may firm up the stools and lead to a different and perhaps frightening defecation experience.[7] Passage of large and hard stools may cause anal irritation and/or fissures which will in turn frighten the child each time he/she has an urge to have a bowel movement. After experiencing pain with stooling, toddlers may decide to avoid defecation. This often leads to stool withholding behavior as the child forcefully contracts the pelvic and gluteal muscles in an effort to inhibit evacuation (Figure 1). A child may also refuse defecation as part of control and independence struggle with parents during toilet training. Toilet mastery is truly a developmental milestone in children's lives, as they enhance their physical abilities, react to external pressures and develop self-esteem. Toilet training can be an extremely difficult phase for children and parents, because pressure on the child to conform to parental expectations will clash with the child's pursuit for independence. The American Academy of Pediatrics strongly recommends that parents avoid pushing their child into toilet training. The toilet training process should begin only when the child shows signs of readiness.[43]

A significant number of school-aged children refuse to use school toilets, often citing poorly maintained and unhygienic facilities. Students may also have restricted toilet access during classroom hours. Bullying while using toilet facilities may also deter some children.[44]

There is a general belief that cow's milk can be constipating in children. There are only a few reports linking cow's milk consumption to constipation.[45–48]

Colon absorbs fluid and electrolytes from the retained stool, leading to progressively larger stool volume and harder stool consistency. This makes the defecation even more difficult and painful. The rectal vault stretches and the anal canal shortens over time.[49] Chronic rectal distension eventually overcomes the ability of the external anal sphincter to maintain continence, followed by overflow soiling, which is also known as fecal incontinence. Rectal distension is accompanied by diminished rectal sensitivity and loss of normal defecation urge.

CLINICAL PRESENTATION

In most cases, the diagnosis of functional constipation can be easily made with a typical history and physical examination. In the absence of "red flag" symptoms (Table 2), no further testing is needed.

The medical history of children with constipation should include questions about the time of the first bowel movement after birth. Failure to pass the meconium within the first 24 hours of life raises the suspicion for Hirschsprung's disease. The interviewer should inquire about the age of onset, the stool frequency, stool consistency and size, painful defecation, presence of blood in the stool/on the toilet paper, and retentive posturing[50,51] Information about the soiling frequency, day and/or nighttime soiling, role of social and emotional factors are also important. The patient with functional constipation is typically an infant after the introduction of solids and weaning the breast milk; a toddler at the time of toilet training or a school-age child refusing to use the bathrooms at school. The child has hard, large, and infrequent stools that are painful to pass. The stools may be large enough to clog the toilet. Large-size stools may cause anal fissures commonly manifested as blood on the toilet paper with wiping.

Fecal incontinence may occur intermittently or several times a day, with passage of small smears to a full bowel movement into the underwear.[52] It can be mistaken as diarrhea by some parents. Passage of large stools may be followed by a short interval of decreased soiling and abdominal pain until a new rectal fecal mass accumulates. Fecal incontinence can be a source of considerable social embarrassment for children.[53] Low self-esteem, depression, shame, social withdrawal, and fear of discovery may lead the child to hide the soiled underwear.[53] Parents may accuse encopretic children with laziness, carelessness, or reluctance to use the toilet, occasionally leading to punishment or negative reinforcement.

Table 2 Red Flags for Childhood Constipation[7]
Onset <12 mo
Delayed passage of meconium
No stool withholding
No soiling
Intermittent diarrhea and explosive stools
Failure to thrive
Empty rectal ampulla
Tight anal sphincter
Gushing of the stool with the rectal exam
Abnormal neurological exam
Pigmentary abnormalities
Heme positive stools
Presence of extraintestinal symptoms
Bladder disease
No response to conventional treatment

The examiner should ask about the presence of abdominal pain, abdominal distension, urinary tract symptoms, fever, nausea, vomiting, change in appetite, weight loss or poor weight gain, and abnormal neuromuscular development. Abdominal pain associated with functional constipation is usually nonspecific and not well-localized.[34] Pain may be precipitated by eating and waking up from sleep, as a response to increased colonic motility. Enuresis and urinary tract infection are reported in a significant subset of constipated children.[54–56] This results from reduced bladder capacity or urinary stasis from the large rectal stool volume that compresses the bladder. Failure to thrive, developmental delay, presence of extraintestinal symptoms, and bladder disease are "red flags" (Table 2) and necessitate further testing.

Inquiry about psychological and behavioral problems should also be performed. Prognosis may be worse in children with behavioral disorders and poor social situation.[57] The examiner should also inquire about the dietary history, the volume of fluids and the amount of fiber in the diet. The history of previous treatments with medication names, doses, and the duration or treatment should be obtained. A stool diary may be helpful to learn about the stooling habits of the child, but the reliability of the recall of bowel habits is still under debate.[58]

PHYSICAL EXAMINATION

A thorough physical examination with particular attention to neurological assessment should be performed in all children with constipation. Abdominal examination will help detect fecal masses and signs of intestinal obstruction. Abdominal distension is seen in functional constipation only if large volumes of stool are retained. Evaluation of the perianal region provides valuable information about the position of the anus, evidence of fecal soiling, skin irritation, fissures, hemorrhoids, and signs of possible sexual abuse. A digital rectal examination is recommended in all patients at least during the initial assessment, except in very few scenarios: an uncooperative child, presence of neutropenia or history of sexual abuse. The digital rectal examination assesses the perianal sensation, anal wink, anal tone, size of the rectal vault, volume and consistency of the stool in the rectum, and the voluntary contraction and relaxation of the anal sphincter. The lumbosacral area should be inspected for sacral dimple or a tuft of hair.

DIFFERENTIAL DIAGNOSIS

Constipation may be the result of a wide variety of disorders or secondary to various medications. Presence of "red flags" (Table 2) raises the suspicion for an organic disorder and necessitates further workup. A list of such organic etiologies is provided in Table 3. Onset at a young age, delayed passage of meconium, abdominal distension, intermittent diarrhea, and explosive stools, a tight anal sphincter on rectal exam with

Table 3 Organic Causes of Constipation[75]
Abnormalities of colon and rectum
Anal or colonic stenosis
Imperforate anus
Anteriorly displaced or ectopic anus
Chronic intestinal pseudo-obstruction
Spinal cord abnormalities
Meningomyelocele
Spinal cord tumor
Sacral agenesis
Diastematomyelia
Neuropathic gastrointestinal disorders
Hirschsprung's disease
Intestinal neuronal dysplasia
Chaga's disease
Systemic disorders
Hypothyroidism
Hypercalcemia
Hypocalcemia
Diabetes mellitus
Diabetes insipidus
Panhypopituitarism
Cerebral palsy
Amyotonia congenita
Scleroderma
Amyloidosis
Mixed connective tissue disease
Myotonic dystrophy
Multiple sclerosis
Abnormal abdominal musculature
Prune belly syndrome
Gastroschisis
Drugs
Opiates
Anticholinergics
Antiacids
Antihypertensives
Antimotility agents
Cholestyramine
Psychotropics
Diuretics
Others
Cystic fibrosis
Celiac disease
Heavy metal ingestion (lead, mercury)

no evidence of rectal impaction, gushing of stool upon removal of the finger raise the suspicion for Hirschsprung's disease. A complete neurological exam may reveal abnormal deep tendon reflexes, absent cremasteric reflex and anal wink, a lumbosacral dimple, and tuft of hair, all pointing to a spinal cord anomaly as the cause of constipation. In rare patients with intractable constipation, neurological exam may be normal and spinal cord lesions can only be detected by an MRI.[59]

DIAGNOSTIC TESTS

A complete medical history and a thorough physical examination are usually sufficient to confirm the diagnosis of functional constipation in most children. Obtaining symptom diaries about defecation and soiling characteristics may help establish the diagnosis and aid with the follow-up monitoring. In a small subset of children, clinical evaluation is not adequate and further diagnostic interventions are warranted to establish or refute organic etiologies.

These may include plain abdominal radiographs, colon transit studies, anorectal manometry, contrast studies, or rectal suction biopsies.

Abdominal X-ray

The diagnosis of functional constipation may be difficult if the typical symptoms are not present or when the physical examination is limited. In these cases, a plain abdominal radiograph can be useful in the assessment of fecal retention. The North American Society for Pediatric Gastroenterology and Nutrition (NASPGHAN) clinical practice guidelines recommends taking a plain abdominal radiograph in case of doubt about the presence of constipation, such as: a child refusing a rectal examination; or rectal examination considered to be traumatic.[26] On the other hand, there is no clear correlation between clinical symptoms and radiological features of childhood constipation. We would expect to see some stool collection on X-ray, because one of the key functions of the colon is to store the stool before evacuation. Different scoring systems have been developed to determine the amount of stool loading on abdominal radiographs,[60–62] but a great deal of interobserver and intraobserver variation exists in quantifying the amount of stool with this technique.[63–65] We use abdominal radiograph only in limited clinical settings such as poor or unreliable history, difficult examinations (ie, obese or uncooperative patients), or when rectal examination is deemed traumatic (ie, children with a history of sexual abuse).[24]

Colon Transit Studies

Colonic transit time (CTT) measurement with radiopaque markers is a simple and noninvasive tool to assess defecation disorders. A variety of markers have been employed, including commercially available Sitzmarks or 1 cm cut segments of a size 10 radiopaque nasogastric tube. There is not a consensus on the amount of markers to ingest and the number and timing of X-rays to follow the progression of the markers. Some use Bouchoucha method, in which segmental and total CTT is calculated from a single X-ray obtained on the seventh day, after the child ingests the markers for 6 consecutive days.[66] Others use Metcalf method that recommends the intake of markers for 3 consecutive days, followed by an X-ray on the fourth day.[67] Some investigators recommend cleaning the colon before a transit study as the markers may get "stuck" in an impacted colon, others advocate against any laxatives that would affect the bowel function.[68] Slow marker propagation as assessed by plain radiographic images at one or multiple time points after ingestion can point to dysfunction in distinctive colonic segments. There is a great variation between total colonic transit times in healthy children, ranging between 25 and 84 hours.[17,69,70] Three different patterns of colonic transit time can be described based on colonic transit studies. These include *normal colonic transit, colonic inertia* (also known as slow-transit constipation with slow propagation throughout all colonic segments), and *outlet obstruction* (delay is mainly in the rectosigmoidal region). Outlet obstruction is the most commonly encountered form in functional constipation.[17,66,71] CTT may be normal in up to 50% of children with constipation.[64,72] Slow transit constipation has been reported in children, but it seems to be more common in adults. The marker test may be useful in differentiating between children with constipation and children with nonretentive fecal incontinence.[18] Those with nonretentive fecal incontinence usually have normal colonic transit values and no rectal mass on physical examination.[24] These children should be treated with intensive toilet training; laxatives will increase the frequency of soiling.[25]

Manometry

Colonic manometry is a valuable diagnostic tool in children with defecation disorders to differentiate normal colonic motor function from colonic neuromuscular disorders.[26,73] In children with functional constipation, one would expect the presence of high amplitude propagating contractions (HAPCs) and an increased motility following a meal. Colonic manometry may be useful in children with long-standing and intractable constipation if a gastrointestinal motility disorder is suspected. Colonic manometry tracings have to be carefully interpreted because the findings may not be due to a primary colonic motility disorder but secondary to the dilatation of the bowel. In one study, treatment recommendations were changed in 93% of patients with intractable constipation; in 68% of patients surgical therapy was suggested, leading to a clinical improvement in 88% of patients.[74] The role of colonic manometry in identifying abnormal segments of colon requiring surgical removal needs to be further explored.

Anorectal manometry is most useful in determining the presence of the rectoanal inhibitory reflex and therefore excluding Hirschsprung's disease. It may have a role in predicting the outcome and response to treatment in some patients.[51]

TREATMENT

General Considerations

The goals of treatment of childhood constipation are: to restore a regular defecation pattern (soft and painless stools, no fecal incontinence) and to prevent relapses. Oral laxatives and structured toilet training are the main pillars of a successful treatment. In a position paper published by the NASPGHAN, the following four important steps were recommended for the evaluation and treatment of childhood constipation: (1) education, (2) disimpaction, if present, (3) prevention of rectal reimpaction, and (4) regular follow up.[26,75] The treatment starts with explaining the problem to the child and family, including the purpose of each intervention and the potential difficulties to be encountered. The plan should be communicated with the child in simple terms whenever possible. Clarifying to the family that fecal incontinence is due to the rectal impaction and beyond the child's control usually eliminates parental negative attributions and relieves tensions between children and their parents.[76] Some younger children and toddlers may still continue to withhold the stools after laxatives are started. It will be helpful to explain that the child may still continue the withholding behavior until he/she trusts that the bowel movements will no longer be painful. Information regarding the long duration of therapy from 6 to 24 months and periods of setbacks should be relayed early to the family. It may be necessary to repeat the education several times during treatment.[76,77]

Dietary Modifications

Dietary measures are commonly recommended for constipated children. This may include increasing fluid, carbohydrate, or fiber intake. Few small studies have evaluated the efficacy of increased fluid intake and nonabsorbable carbohydrates for the treatment of constipation. These studies do not support such interventions for childhood constipation; they report increased urine production only and no change in stool consistency or frequency.[78,79] The role of dietary changes in functional constipation is not well established. Extreme dietary interventions (ie, substituting milk with other liquids), especially in young infants, may lead to nutritional deficiencies and negatively impact growth.

The relationship between constipation and low fiber intake is not well known. Some studies demonstrated low fiber intake in constipated children compared to healthy controls[80,81] but others did not support this finding.[82,83] The recommended dietary fiber intake in children older than 2 years of age is equivalent to age (in years) plus 5 g/d, with a safe range between age plus 5 and age plus 10 g/d.[84] Fiber supplements, such as Metamucil and Citrucel are gritty, thicken quickly and not preferred by children. On the other hand, water soluble fiber supplements, such as glucomannan do not have the unpleasant taste and may have a role in the treatment of childhood constipation. Loening-Baucke and colleagues showed in a randomized controlled trial that *glucomannan*, a fiber gel polysaccharide from the tubers of the Japanese Konjac plant, at 100 mg/kg daily (maximal 5 g/d) improved constipation better than placebo, especially in children with encopresis.[83] Similar results were found in another study conducted by Staiano and colleagues,[85] glucomannan at 100 mg/kg twice daily improved stool frequency in neurologically impaired children with no effect on colonic motility.[85]

There is a general belief that milk can cause constipation in children. The clinical practice guidelines from NASPGHAN only recommends a time limited trial of cow's milk free diet in children unresponsive to conventional medical and behavioral treatment.[75] One double-blind crossover study in 65 infants found that constipation might be a manifestation of cow's milk intolerance.[48] In that study, two-thirds of patients with constipation improved after switching to a soy-based milk. This has not been confirmed by larger studies.

The practice of using infant formulas without iron fortification to treat or prevent constipation has no scientific basis and places infants at risk for iron deficiency anemia. A randomized controlled trial in 93 term infants showed no difference in gastrointestinal symptoms, stool frequency, or consistency in babies taking formula with or without iron fortification.[86]

Medical Treatment

Fecal disimpaction prior to maintenance therapy is recommended to ensure success, reduce the amount of overflow incontinence and abdominal pain. Children treated with some form of disimpaction followed by daily laxatives respond better to treatment after 2 months compared with children treated with less aggressive measures.[87] Various disimpaction protocols using oral and/or rectal routes have been published.[88–90] Youssef and colleagues reported successful treatment of fecal impaction with polyethylene glycol (PEG) 3350 (MiraLax; Braintree Laboratories, Braintree, or Glycolax, Schwarz Pharma Inc.) at a dose of 1 to 1.5 g/kg/d for 3 days.[88] Rectal disimpaction can also be performed with phosphate soda enemas (Fleet), saline, or mineral oil enemas followed by a phosphate enema. When using enema therapy for disimpaction, low-volume enemas with short retention times may reduce the risk of potential complications. Intravascular volume status should be evaluated before using enemas involving hypertonic solutions. Infrequent but important complications including metabolic derangements in serum phosphate, magnesium, sodium, calcium, and potassium have been described with the use of phosphate enemas.[91–93] The use of soapsuds, tap water, and magnesium enemas is not recommended because of their potential toxicity.[94–95] Milk and molasses enemas have been linked to severe and occasionally fatal acute respiratory and hemodynamic decompensation in pediatrics.[96] In infants, rectal disimpaction can be effectively performed with glycerin suppositories.[97] Doses of commonly used oral laxatives for disimpaction are listed in Table 4.

Oral daily laxative therapy should be started immediately after disimpaction. The aim of maintenance therapy is to produce soft and painless stools, prevent stool reaccumulation and recurrence of stool withholding behavior. The laxative dose should be adjusted as needed to reach the desired stool consistency and frequency. Based on the mode of action, laxatives have been traditionally divided into bulking agents, osmotic laxatives, stimulant laxatives, lubricating laxatives, and prokinetics. Doses of commonly used oral laxatives for maintenance treatment are listed in Table 5.

Bulking Agents. Bulking agents include dietary or processed natural fibers, chemically modified cellulose and synthetic polymers. These agents are subjected to bacterial fermentation in the colon with the production of short chain fatty acids (SCFA). SCFA may increase the stool osmolality and volume, and produce softer, bulkier stools.[98] Efficacy of bulking agents has not been established in children.

Osmotic Laxatives. Osmotic laxatives are a heterogenous group that include poorly absorbable ions (magnesium, phosphate, and sulfate salts), agents that are not absorbed in the small bowel but metabolized in the colon (lactulose and sorbitol), and metabolically inert compounds (PEG). Osmotic laxatives soften the stools by retaining water within the colon through osmosis.

Lactulose is a semisynthetic nonabsorbable disaccharide, consisting of galactose and fructose. It is not digested in the small intestine, but broken down by colonic bacteria into low molecular weight compounds that can acidify the colonic contents. Pediatric dosages have not been well established. In infants, commonly used dosing is 2.5 to 10 mL per day divided into 2 to 4 dosages. The usual dose for older children and adolescents is 40 to 90 mL per day in divided doses. Common side effects are due to colonic bacterial digestion causing flatulence, abdominal cramps, and bloating.

Magnesium hydroxide (Milk of magnesia). It is the most commonly used magnesium salt that acts by osmosis but it may also enhance colonic motility by affecting enteric hormones.[99] The recommended dose ranges from 1 to 4 mL/kg/d. Partial absorption of the ion may occur but hypermagnesemia is extremely rare.[100] The use of magnesium salts should be avoided in patients with renal insufficiency. Overall, magnesium hydroxide is safe and effective, but not well accepted by children due to its taste.

Polyethylene glycols (PEG) are nonabsorbable compounds with high molecular masses that are not metabolized by colonic bacteria. PEG 3350 without electrolytes is available as a powder. It is a tasteless, colorless molecule that can be dissolved in a beverage such as water or juice. Because of its palatability, it is well accepted by children and widely used to treat childhood constipation. The lack of colonic metabolism offers an advantage compared with fermentable laxatives. Several studies have assessed the safety and efficacy of PEG 3350 in the treatment of childhood constipation.[101–103] Pashankar and colleagues reported a mean effective dose of 0.84 g/kg/d with a range of 0.27 to 1.42 g/kg/d.[103] We generally recommend an initial dose of 1 g/kg/d with adjustments every 3 days to achieve 1 to 2 soft bowel movements per day. Long-term therapy with a mean duration of 8.4 months and a range of 3 to 30 months, was reported to be effective in the treatment of chronic childhood constipation with and without encopresis.[103] In one study, milk of magnesia was as effective as PEG in children with constipation and encopresis; however, 33% of children refused to take milk of magnesia, whereas none refused PEG.[101] In a crossover study, PEG was as effective as lactulose for the treatment of constipation in children in a 2-week trial, but PEG was preferred by children over lactulose.[104]

Lubricating Laxatives. Mineral oil or liquid paraffin is the most commonly used lubricant laxative. It is composed of saturated hydrocarbons obtained from petroleum. Mineral oil acts by coating and lubricating stools, reducing colonic absorption of fecal water and facilitating the evacuation of the stools. Mineral oil is not chemically active, and serious adverse effects are uncommon. Anal seepage of oily material is the most common problem. Lipoid pneumonia may occur as a result of mineral oil aspiration.[105] Mineral oil should not be used in patients with a tendency for regurgitation or pulmonary aspiration. In general, mineral oil does not interfere with the absorption of fat soluble vitamins.[106]

Stimulant Laxatives. Stimulant laxatives increase intestinal motility and interfere with the epithelial transport of water and electrolytes. This class of agents includes diphenylmethane derivatives (phenolphthalein, bisacodyl, and sodium picosulfate), anthranoids (senna), ricinoleic acid (castor oil), and surface-acting agents (docusates). *Phenolphthalein* was commonly used in the United States but has been banned because of its potential carcinogenic effects. *Castor oil* is hydrolyzed in the small intestine to ricinoleic acid, which alters the intestinal absorption of water and electrolytes and increases colonic motility. Abdominal cramping is the most common side effect. *Docusates* have emulsifying and detergent properties that allow water to seep more effectively into the feces, producing looser stools. They have relatively subtle stimulatory effects on the gut mucosa. They may enhance the gastrointestinal or hepatic uptake of other drugs and increase

Table 5 Commonly Used Oral Laxatives for Maintenance Therapy[75]	
Lactulose	1–3 cc/kg/d in divided doses
Mineral oil	Not recommended <1 year 1–3 cc/kg/d in divided doses*
Magnesium hydroxide	1–3 cc/kg/d in divided doses
PEG 3350 with-out electrolytes	1 g/kg/d
Sorbitol	1–3 cc/kg/d in divided doses
Senna	55–436 mg once or twice daily*
Docusate	10–400 mg in divided doses

*Variable dose based on patient's age.

Table 4 Commonly Used Oral Laxatives for Disimpaction	
Mineral oil[68]	15–30 cc/yr of age per day (max 240 cc) for 3–4 d
PEG 3350 without electrolytes[88]	1–1.5 g/kg/d for 3 d
PEG with electrolytes[75]	20–25 cc/kg/h for 4 h (max 4 L)

their potential toxicities. Docusates may damage ganglion cells in the myenteric plexus and produce structural changes in the gut mucosa.[107,108] The clinical significance of this finding is not known. Overall, infrequent and small doses of stimulant laxatives are unlikely to cause significant harm, but long-term use should be avoided.

Others. Cisapride has been shown be effective in the treatment of childhood constipation at 0.2 mg/kg/dose, given three times daily. Twenty-seven children completed a 12-week study, with 76% success rate with cisapride compared to 37% with placebo. Cisapride is no longer available in the United Sates because of its effect on QTc interval and cardiac arrhythmias. The clinical practice guideline from NASPGHAN does not recommend its use, as the benefits do not outweigh the risks.[75]

Toilet training along with the use of age specific reward systems is an integral part of the treatment of childhood constipation. The aim is to overcome the fear of using the toilet and restore normal bowel habits by positive reinforcement and encouragement. The child is instructed to sit on the toilet after waking up from sleep and following meals when colonic motor activity is at its highest. The child usually does the toilet sitting for 5 to 10 minutes with proper foot support for leverage. A high level of motivation and perseverance are necessary on the parents' part for these measures to be successful. Psychological referral is indicated in children with severe emotional problems who fail intensive medical treatment.

Biofeedback Training

Biofeedback or pelvic floor retraining has been employed for decades as a treatment of defecation disorders. Biofeedback is based on the principle of learning through reinforcement and it is used to emphasize normal coordination and function of the anal-sphincter and pelvic-floor muscles. Patients receive visual and auditory feedback by simulating an evacuation with a rectal balloon of adjustable volume. In patients with constipation, biofeedback is believed to enhance rectal sensation, improve muscle control, and coordination, leading to normal defecation and continence. In a significant portion of children with defecation disorders, external anal sphincter and puborectalis muscle do not relax during stooling.[34,109] Lack of sphincter relaxation is sometimes seen as an abnormal contraction. This condition is usually called *pelvic floor dyssynergia*.[21] Biofeedback training may be helpful in patients with constipation who have pelvic floor dyssynergia.[110,111]

There is a wide range of success rates (50 to 100%) reported with biofeedback training in constipated children. Nolan and colleagues showed no association between achievement of normal defecation dynamics and clinical outcome in 194 constipated children randomized to conventional treatment alone *vs.* conventional treatment plus biofeedback training.[109] In this study, biofeedback training did not result in higher success rates in chronically constipated children compared to conventional therapy alone.[109] A meta-analysis by Heymen and colleagues compared the various biofeedback treatment protocols and outcomes in children and adults treated for constipation.[112] Thirty-eight studies were included and ten studies were reviewed in detail. Mean success rate of studies using pressure biofeedback was superior to studies using electromyography biofeedback (78% vs 70%). There were significant inconsistencies in regards to the etiology and severity of symptoms, patient selection, and the definition of a successful outcome. Anatomical, physiological, or demographic variables were not predictive of a treatment response.[112] Biofeedback studies in children have small patient groups, lack long-term follow-up and do not share common outcome measures. Therefore, we cannot make any comments on the usefulness of such intervention. Biofeedback treatment may be beneficial in a small subgroup of patients with intractable constipation.[75]

Surgery

Although functional constipation usually improves or resolves with conventional therapy, a small minority continues to have intractable symptoms. Surgery has been occasionally offered as an alternative treatment in this population. A number of surgical procedures have been described, including anorectal myectomy, antegrade continence enema (ACE), sigmoid irrigation tube placement, colostomy, total and subtotal colectomies with ileorectal resection, and segmental colonic resection. Improved stool frequency and quality of life were reported postoperatively, but diarrhea and incontinence were common complications.[113,114]

There are only a few studies reporting surgical treatment in children with intractable constipation. In a retrospective study, Youssef and colleagues described almost 90% success rate with subtotal colectomy in 19 neurologically normal children with intractable constipation and abnormal colonic motility.[115]

ACE has been offered as a therapeutic option for defecation disorders that failed maximal medical therapy. Antegrade delivery of an enema for colonic cleansing at regular intervals prevents fecal accumulation and reduces soiling episodes. ACE can be achieved by creating an appendicocecostomy or by percutaneous endoscopic cecostomy.[116,117] A wide variety of irrigation solutions can be used as antegrade enemas including PEG, saline and glycerin solutions, and phosphate enemas. Adverse events include skin lacerations, stomal stenosis, granulation tissue formation, leakage of irrigation solution, and tube dislodgement. Several small studies documented a significant increase in frequency of stooling, decrease in soiling and improved quality of life in children with functional constipation following ACE.[118,119] Curry and colleagues reported follow-up data on 273 of 300 ACE procedures performed in the United Kingdom, with a mean follow-up of 2.4 years. They had full or partial success in 79% of cases. However, when the results were analyzed by underlying disease category, success was only reported in 12 of 23 (52%) patients with functional constipation. The overall complication rate was 40%, with 30% stomal stenosis reported.[120]

Koszutski and colleagues described 19 constipated children who underwent anal divulsion with almost 85% reporting symptom improvement. Sphincter myectomy were performed in 2 patients with good outcome.[121] Early reports using anorectal myectomy in constipation were encouraging,[122] but long-term data have shown only 70% improvement.[123]

Woodward and colleagues reported the results of the Hartmann procedure in 10 constipated children, mostly with neurodevelopmental impairment. These patients had proximal sigmoid colostomy, limited anterior resection of hypertrophic proximal rectosigmoid, with oversewing of the rectal stump. Four patients had complications and two patients failed reversal surgery.[124]

Larger studies are needed to analyze the usefulness of surgical intervention in children with idiopathic constipation. In a highly selected subset of patients surgery may be considered.

PROGNOSIS

Many studies have estimated constipation remission rates to range between 60 and 90% after 1 year of treatment.[51,65,125] Van Ginkel and colleagues followed 418 constipated patients for a median duration of 5 years (range 1 to 8 years). Successful treatment was reported in 60% of patients by 1 year and 80% by 8 years of treatment. Successful rate was higher if fecal incontinence was absent and constipation started after 4 years of age. Half of the successfully treated patients had at least one relapse and boys experienced more relapses than girls. One-third of the children followed up beyond puberty continued to have severe complaints of constipation.[126] Other studies reported higher failure rates. Staiano and colleagues described that 52% of 62 constipated children remained symptomatic at 5 years after diagnosis despite intensive initial medical and behavioral therapy. Early onset constipation (<1 year of age) and a positive family history were predictive of persistent symptoms.[101,127–129]

SUMMARY

Functional constipation is a common and challenging problem in pediatrics with a significant psychological and social impact on children and their families. Careful evaluation is necessary to determine potential underlying causes. Most children can be successfully managed with a combination of medical and behavioral therapies. Treatment is often lengthy and a significant proportion of children will have persistent symptoms beyond puberty. Regular follow-up and adjustment of therapy are keys to successful outcome. Future research should focus on further understanding the pathophysiology of functional constipation, comparing safety and efficacy of the various treatments available and determining long-term outcome.

REFERENCES

1. Lewis G, Rudolph CD. Practical approach to defecation disorders in children. Pediatr Ann 1997;26:260–8.
2. Seth R, Heyman MB. Management of constipation and encopresis in infants and children. Gastroenterol Clin North Am 1994;23:621–36.
3. Castiglia PT. Constipation in children. J Pediatr Health Care 2001;15:200–2.
4. Taubman B, Blum NJ, Nemeth N. Children who hide while defecating before they have completed toilet training: A prospective study. Arch Pediatr Adolesc Med 2003;157:1190–2.
5. Loening-Baucke V. Chronic constipation in children. Gastroenterology 1993;105:1557–64.
6. Clark DA. Times of first void and first stool in 500 newborns. Pediatrics 1977;60:457–9.
7. Di Lorenzo C. Pediatric anorectal disorders. Gastroenterol Clin North Am 2001;30:269–87, ix.
8. Weaver LT, Lucas A. Development of bowel habit in preterm infants. Arch Dis Child 1993;68:317–20.
9. Hyams JS, Treem WR, Etienne NL, et al. Effect of infant formula on stool characteristics of young infants. Pediatrics 1995;95:50–4.
10. Weaver LT, Ewing G, Taylor LC. The bowel habit of milk-fed infants. J Pediatr Gastroenterol Nutr 1988;7:568–71.
11. Nyhan WL. Stool frequency of normal infants in the first week of life. Pediatrics 1952;10:414–25.
12. Lemoh JN, Brooke OG. Frequency and weight of normal stools in infancy. Arch Dis Child 1979;54:719–20.
13. Weaver LT, Steiner H. The bowel habit of young children. Arch Dis Child 1984;59:649–52.
14. Fontana M, Bianchi C, Cataldo F, et al. Bowel frequency in healthy children. Acta Paediatr Scand 1989;78:682–4.
15. Tham EB, Nathan R, Davidson GP, et al. Bowel habits of healthy Australian children aged 0–2 years. J Paediatr Child Health 1996;32:504–7.
16. Dimson SB. Carmine as an index of transit time in children with simple constipation. Arch Dis Child 1970;45:232–5.
17. Corazziari E, Cucchiara S, Staiano A, et al. Gastrointestinal transit time, frequency of defecation, and anorectal manometry in healthy and constipated children. J Pediatr 1985;106:379–82.
18. Rasquin-Weber A, Hyman PE, Cucchiara S, et al. Childhood functional gastrointestinal disorders. Gut 1999;45:II60–8.
19. Loening-Baucke V. Functional fecal retention with encopresis in childhood. J Pediatr Gastroenterol Nutr 2004;38: 79–84.
20. Voskuijl WP, Heijmans J, Heijmans HS, et al. Use of Rome II criteria in childhood defecation disorders: Applicability in clinical and research practice. J Pediatr 2004;145:213–7.
21. Benninga M, Candy DC, Catto-Smith AG, et al. The Paris Consensus on Childhood Constipation Terminology (PACCT) Group. J Pediatr Gastroenterol Nutr 2005;40: 273–5.
22. Hyman PE, Milla PJ, Benninga MA, et al. Childhood functional gastrointestinal disorders: Neonate/toddler. Gastroenterology 2006;130:1519–26.
23. Rasquin A, Di Lorenzo C, Forbes D, et al. Childhood functional gastrointestinal disorders: Child/adolescent. Gastroenterology 2006;130: 1527–37.
24. Benninga MA, Büller HA, Heymans HS, et al. Is encopresis always the result of constipation? Arch Dis Child 1994;71:186–93.
25. van Ginkel R, Benninga MA, Blommaart PJ, et al. Lack of benefit of laxatives as adjunctive therapy for functional nonretentive fecal soiling in children. J Pediatr 2000;137: 808–13.
26. Baker SS, Liptak GS, Colletti RB, et al. Constipation in infants and children: Evaluation and treatment. A medical position statement of the North American Society for Pediatric Gastroenterology and Nutrition. J Pediatr Gastroenterol Nutr 1999;29:612–26.
27. Molnar D, Taitz LS, Urwin OM, Wales JK. Anorectal manometry results in defecation disorders. Arch Dis Child 1983;58:257–61.
28. Loening-Baucke V. Constipation in early childhood: Patient characteristics, treatment, and longterm follow up. Gut 1993;34:1400–4.
29. Sonnenberg A, Koch TR. Physician visits in the United States for constipation: 1958 to 1986. Dig Dis Sci 1989;34:606–11.
30. de Araujo Sant'Anna AM, Calcado AC. Constipation in school-aged children at public schools in Rio de Janeiro, Brazil. J Pediatr Gastroenterol Nutr 1999;29:190–3.
31. Uc A, Hyman PE, Walker LS. Functional gastrointestinal disorders in African American children in primary care. J Pediatr Gastroenterol Nutr 2006;42:270–4.
32. Burkitt DP, Walker AR, Painter NS. Dietary fiber and disease. JAMA 1974;229:1068–74.
33. Borowitz SM, Cox DJ, Tam A, et al. Precipitants of constipation during early childhood. J Am Board Fam Pract 2003;16:213–8.
34. van der Plas RN, Benninga MA, Büller HA, et al. Biofeedback training in treatment of childhood constipation: A randomised controlled study. Lancet 1996;348:776–80.
35. van Ginkel R, Büller HA, Boeckxstaens GE, et al. The effect of anorectal manometry on the outcome of treatment in severe childhood constipation: A randomized, controlled trial. Pediatrics 2001;108: E9.
36. Sonnenberg A, Koch TR. Epidemiology of constipation in the United States. Dis Colon Rectum 1989;32:1–8.
37. Bytzer P, Howell S, Leemon M, et al. Low socioeconomic class is a risk factor for upper and lower gastrointestinal symptoms: A population based study in 15,000 Australian adults. Gut 2001;49:66–72.
38. Largo RH, Stutzle W. Longitudinal study of bowel and bladder control by day and at night in the first six years of life. II: The role of potty training and the child's initiative. Dev Med Child Neurol 1977;19:607–13.
39. Blum NJ, Taubman B, Nemeth N. During toilet training, constipation occurs before stool toileting refusal. Pediatrics 2004;113:e520–2.
40. Largo RH, Molinari L, von Siebenthal K, Wolfensberger U. Does a profound change in toilet-training affect development of bowel and bladder control? Dev Med Child Neurol 1996;38:1106–16.
41. Morris-Yates A, Talley NJ, Boyce PM, et al. Evidence of a genetic contribution to functional bowel disorder. Am J Gastroenterol 1998;93:1311–7.
42. Bakwin H, Davidson M. Constipation in twins. Am J Dis Child 1971;121:179–81.
43. Stadtler AC, Gorski PA, Brazelton TB. Toilet training methods, clinical interventions, and recommendations. American Academy of Pediatrics 1999;103:1359–68.
44. Barnes PM, Maddocks A. Standards in school toilets—a questionnaire survey. J Public Health Med 2002;24:85–7.
45. Andiran F, Dayi S, Mete E. Cow's milk consumption in constipation and anal fissure in infants and young children. J Paediatr Child Health 2003;39:329–31.
46. Carroccio A, Montalto G, Custro N, et al. Evidence of very delayed clinical reactions to cow's milk in cow's milk-intolerant patients. Allergy 2000;55:574–9.
47. Daher S, Tahan S, Solé D, et al. Cow's milk protein intolerance and chronic constipation in children. Pediatr Allergy Immunol 2001;12:339–42.
48. Iacono G, Cavataio F, Montalto G, et al. Intolerance of cow's milk and chronic constipation in children. N Engl J Med 1998;339:1100–4.
49. Loening-Baucke VA, Younoszai MK. Abnormal and sphincter response in chronically constipated children. J Pediatr 1982;100:213–8.
50. Partin JC, Hamill SK, Fischel JE, Partin JS. Painful defecation and fecal soiling in children. Pediatrics 1992;89:1007–9.
51. Loening-Baucke V. Factors determining outcome in children with chronic constipation and faecal soiling. Gut 1989;30:999–1006.
52. Benninga MA, Büller HA, Tytgat GN, et al. Colonic transit time in constipated children: Does pediatric slow-transit constipation exist? J Pediatr Gastroenterol Nutr 1996;23:241–51.
53. Fishman L, Rappaport L, Schonwald A, Nurko S. Trends in referral to a single encopresis clinic over 20 years. Pediatrics 2003;111:e604–7.
54. Hellerstein S, Linebarger JS. Voiding dysfunction in pediatric patients. Clin Pediatr (Phila) 2003;42:43–9.
55. Romanczuk W, Korczawski R. Chronic constipation: A cause of recurrent urinary tract infections. Turk J Pediatr 1993;35:181–8.
56. O'Regan S, Yazbeck S. Constipation: A cause of enuresis, urinary tract infection and vesico-ureteral reflux in children. Med Hypotheses 1985;17:409–13.
57. Sutphen JL, Borowitz SM, Hutchison RL, Cox DJ. Long-term follow-up of medically treated childhood constipation. Clin Pediatr (Phila) 1995;34:576–80.
58. Pless CE, Pless IB. How well they remember. The accuracy of parent reports. Arch Pediatr Adolesc Med 1995;149:553–8.
59. Rosen R, Buonomo C, Andrade R, Nurko S. Incidence of spinal cord lesions in patients with intractable constipation. J Pediatr 2004;145:409–11.
60. Leech SC, McHugh K, Sullivan PB. Evaluation of a method of assessing faecal loading on plain abdominal radiographs in children. Pediatr Radiol 1999;29:255–8.
61. Blethyn AJ, Verrier Jones K, Newcombe R, et al. Radiological assessment of constipation. Arch Dis Child 1995;73: 532–3.
62. Barr RG, Levine MD, Wilkinson RH, Mulvihill D. Chronic and occult stool retention: A clinical tool for its evaluation in school-aged children. Clin Pediatr (Phila) 1979;18:674, 676, 677–9, passim.
63. de Lorijn F, van Rijn RR, Heijmans J, et al. The Leech method for diagnosing constipation: intra- and interobserver variability and accuracy. Pediatr Radiol 2006;36:43–9.
64. Benninga MA, Büller HA, Staalman CR, et al. Defecation disorders in children, colonic transit time versus the Barr-score. Eur J Pediatr 1995;154:277–84.
65. Abrahamian FP, Lloyd-Still JD. Chronic constipation in childhood: A longitudinal study of 186 patients. J Pediatr Gastroenterol Nutr 1984;3:460–7.
66. Bouchoucha M, Devroede G, Arhan P, et al. What is the meaning of colorectal transit time measurement? Dis Colon Rectum 1992;35: 773–82.
67. Metcalf AM, Phillips SF, Zinsmeister AR, et al. Simplified assessment of segmental colonic transit. Gastroenterology 1987;92:40–7.
68. Benninga MA, Voskuijl WP, Taminiau JA. Childhood constipation: Is there new light in the tunnel? J Pediatr Gastroenterol Nutr 2004;39:448–64.
69. Tota G, Messina M, Meucci D, et al. Use of radionuclides in the evaluation of intestinal transit time in children with idiopathic constipation. Pediatr Med Chir 1998;20:63–6.
70. Wagener S, Shankar KR, Turnock RR, et al. Colonic transit time—what is normal? J Pediatr Surg 2004;39:166–9; discussion 166–9.
71. Maurer AH, Krevsky B. Whole-gut transit scintigraphy in the evaluation of small-bowel and colon transit disorders. Semin Nucl Med 1995;25:326–38.
72. Gutierrez C, Marco A, Nogales A, Tebar R. Total and segmental colonic transit time and anorectal manometry in children with chronic idiopathic constipation. J Pediatr Gastroenterol Nutr 2002;35:31–8.
73. Di Lorenzo C, Hillemeier C, Hyman P, et al. Manometry studies in children: Minimum standards for procedures. Neurogastroenterol Motil 2002;14:411–20.
74. Pensabene L, Youssef NN, Griffiths JM, Di Lorenzo C. Colonic manometry in children with defecatory disorders. role in diagnosis and management. Am J Gastroenterol 2003;98:1052–7.
75. Evaluation and treatment of constipation in infants and children: Recommendations of the North American Society for Pediatric Gastroenterology, Hepatology, and Nutrition. J Pediatr Gastroenterol Nutr 2006;43:e1–13.
76. Rappaport LA, Levine MD. The prevention of constipation and encopresis: A developmental model and approach. Pediatr Clin North Am 1986;33:859–69.
77. Felt B, Wise CG, Olson A, et al. Guideline for the management of pediatric idiopathic constipation and soiling. Multidisciplinary team from the University of Michigan Medical Center in Ann Arbor. Arch Pediatr Adolesc Med 1999;153:380–5.
78. Ziegenhagen DJ, Tewinkel G, Kruis W, Herrmann F. Adding more fluid to wheat bran has no significant effects on intestinal functions of healthy subjects. J Clin Gastroenterol 1991;13:525–30.
79. Chung BD, Parekh U, Sellin JH. Effect of increased fluid intake on stool output in normal healthy volunteers. J Clin Gastroenterol 1999;28:29–32.
80. Morais MB, Vítolo MR, Aguirre AN, Fagundes-Neto U. Measurement of low dietary fiber intake as a risk factor for chronic constipation in children. J Pediatr Gastroenterol Nutr 1999;29:132–5.
81. Roma E, Adamidis D, Nikolara R, et al. Diet and chronic constipation in children: The role of fiber. J Pediatr Gastroenterol Nutr 1999;28:169–74.
82. McClung HJ, Boyne L, Heitlinger L. Constipation and dietary fiber intake in children. Pediatrics 1995;96:999–1000.
83. Loening-Baucke V, Miele E, Staiano A. Fiber (glucomannan) is beneficial in the treatment of childhood constipation. Pediatrics 2004;113:e259–64.
84. Williams CL, Bollella M, Wynder EL. A new recommendation for dietary fiber in childhood. Pediatrics 1995;96: 985–8.
85. Staiano A, Simeone D, Del Giudice E, et al. Effect of the dietary fiber glucomannan on chronic constipation in neurologically impaired children. J Pediatr 2000;136:41–5.
86. Iron-fortified formulas and gastrointestinal symptoms in infants: A controlled study, With the cooperation of The Syracuse Consortium for Pediatric Clinical Studies. Pediatrics 1980;66:168–70.
87. Borowitz SM, Cox DJ, Kovatchev B, et al. Treatment of childhood constipation by primary care physicians: Efficacy and predictors of outcome. Pediatrics 2005;115:873–7.
88. Youssef NN, Peters JM, Henderson W, et al. Dose response of PEG 3350 for the treatment of childhood fecal impaction. J Pediatr 2002;141:410–4.
89. Tolia V, Use of a balanced lavage solution in the treatment of fecal impaction. J Pediatr Gastroenterol Nutr 1988;7: 299–301.

90. Tolia V, Lin CH, Elitsur Y. A prospective randomized study with mineral oil and oral lavage solution for treatment of faecal impaction in children. Aliment Pharmacol Ther 1993;7:523–9.

91. Craig JC, Hodson EM, Martin HC. Phosphate enema poisoning in children. Med J Aust 1994;160:347–51.

92. Davis RF, Eichner JM, Bleyer WA, Okamoto G. Hypocalcemia, hyperphosphatemia, and dehydration following a single hypertonic phosphate enema. J Pediatr 1977;90: 484–5.

93. Grosskopf I, Graff E, Charach G, et al. Hyperphosphataemia and hypocalcaemia induced by hypertonic phosphate enema–an experimental study and review of the literature. Hum Exp Toxicol 1991;10:351–5.

94. Chertow GM, Brady HR. Hyponatraemia from tap-water enema. Lancet 1994;344:748.

95. Ashton MR, Sutton D, Nielsen M. Severe magnesium toxicity after magnesium sulphate enema in a chronically constipated child. BMJ 1990;300:541.

96. Walker M, Warner BW, Brilli RJ, Jacobs BR. Cardiopulmonary compromise associated with milk and molasses enema use in children. J Pediatr Gastroenterol Nutr 2003;36:144–8.

97. Weisman LE, Merenstein GB, Digirol M, et al. The effect of early meconium evacuation on early-onset hyperbilirubinemia. Am J Dis Child 1983;137:666–8.

98. Schiller LR. Clinical pharmacology and use of laxatives and lavage solutions. J Clin Gastroenterol 1999;28:11–8.

99. Gattuso JM, Kamm MA. Adverse effects of drugs used in the management of constipation and diarrhoea. Drug Saf 1994;10:47–65.

100. Alison LH, Bulugahapitiya D. Laxative induced magnesium poisoning in a 6-week old infant. BMJ 1990;300:125.

101. Loening-Baucke V. Polyethylene glycol without electrolytes for children with constipation and encopresis. J Pediatr Gastroenterol Nutr 2002;34:372–7.

102. Pashankar DS, Loening-Baucke V, Bishop WP. Safety of polyethylene glycol 3350 for the treatment of chronic constipation in children. Arch Pediatr Adolesc Med 2003;157:661–4.

103. Pashankar DS, Bishop WP. Efficacy and optimal dose of daily polyethylene glycol 3350 for treatment of constipation and encopresis in children. J Pediatr 2001;139:428–32.

104. Gremse DA, Hixon J, Crutchfield A. Comparison of polyethylene glycol 3350 and lactulose for treatment of chronic constipation in children. Clin Pediatr (Phila) 2002;41:225–9.

105. Bandla HP, Davis SH, Hopkins NE. Lipoid pneumonia: A silent complication of mineral oil aspiration. Pediatrics 1999;103:E19.

106. Sharif F, Crushell E, O'Driscoll K, Bourke B. Liquid paraffin: A reappraisal of its role in the treatment of constipation. Arch Dis Child 2001;85:121–4.

107. Fox DA, Epstein ML, Bass P. Surfactants selectively ablate enteric neurons of the rat jejunum. J Pharmacol Exp Ther 1983;227:538–44.

108. Saunders DR, Sillery J, Rachmilewitz D. Effect of dioctyl sodium sulfosuccinate on structure and function of rodent and human intestine. Gastroenterology 1975;69:380–6.

109. Nolan T, Catto-Smith T, Coffey C, Wells J. Randomised controlled trial of biofeedback training in persistent encopresis with anismus. Arch Dis Child 1998;79:131–5.

110. Loening-Baucke V. Persistence of chronic constipation in children after biofeedback treatment. Dig Dis Sci 1991;36:153–60.

111. Keren S, Wagner Y, Heldenberg D, Golan M. Studies of manometric abnormalities of the rectoanal region during defecation in constipated and soiling children: Modification through biofeedback therapy. Am J Gastroenterol 1988; 83:827–31.

112. Heymen S, Jones KR, Scarlett Y, Whitehead WE. Biofeedback treatment of constipation: A critical review. Dis Colon Rectum 2003;46:1208–17.

113. FitzHarris GP, Garcia-Aguilar J, Parkere SC, et al. Quality of life after subtotal colectomy for slow-transit constipation: Both quality and quantity count. Dis Colon Rectum 2003;46:433–40.

114. Lundin E, Karlbom U, Påhlman L, Graf W. Outcome of segmental colonic resection for slow-transit constipation. Br J Surg 2002;89:1270–4.

115. Youssef NN, Pensabene L, Barksdale E, Jr, Di Lorenzo C. Is there a role for surgery beyond colonic aganglionosis and anorectal malformations in children with intractable constipation? J Pediatr Surg 2004;39:73–7.

116. Malone PS, Ransley PG, Kiely EM. Preliminary report: The antegrade continence enema. Lancet 1990;336:1217–8.

117. Cascio S, Flett ME, De la Hunt M, et al. MACE or caecostomy button for idiopathic constipation in children: A comparison of complications and outcomes. Pediatr Surg Int 2004;20:484–7.

118. Youssef NN, Barksdale E, Jr, Griffiths JM, et al. Management of intractable constipation with antegrade enemas in neurologically intact children. J Pediatr Gastroenterol Nutr 2002;34:402–5.

119. Mousa HM, van den Berg MM, Caniano DA, et al. Cecostomy in children with defecation disorders. Dig Dis Sci 2006; 51:154–60.

120. Curry JI, Osborne A, Malone PS. The MACE procedure: Experience in the United Kingdom. J Pediatr Surg 1999;34: 338–40.

121. Koszutski T, Bohosiewicz J, Kudela G, Owczarek K. Diagnostics and treatment of chronic constipation in children–the experience of the department of paediatric surgery. Wiad Lek 2004;57:193–6.

122. Yoshioka K, Keighley MR. Randomized trial comparing anorectal myectomy and controlled anal dilatation for outlet obstruction. Br J Surg 1987;74:1125–9.

123. Pinho M, Yoshioka K, Keighley MR. Long-term results of anorectal myectomy for chronic constipation. Dis Colon Rectum 1990;33:795–7.

124. Woodward MN, Foley P, Cusick EL. Colostomy for treatment of functional constipation in children: A preliminary report. J Pediatr Gastroenterol Nutr 2004;38:75–8.

125. Levine MD, Bakow H. Children with encopresis: A study of treatment outcome. Pediatrics 1976;58:845–52.

126. van Ginkel R, Reitsma JB, Büller HA, et al. Childhood constipation: longitudinal follow-up beyond puberty. Gastroenterology 2003;125:357–63.

127. Staiano A, Andreotti MR, Greco L, et al. Long-term follow-up of children with chronic idiopathic constipation. Dig Dis Sci 1994;39:561–4.

128. Borowitz SM, Cox DJ, Sutphen JL, Kovatchev B. Treatment of childhood encopresis: A randomized trial comparing three treatment protocols. J Pediatr Gastroenterol Nutr 2002;34:378–84.

129. Loening-Baucke V. Encopresis. Curr Opin Pediatr 2002; 14:570–5.

130. Fleisher DR. Diagnosis and treatment of disorders of defecation in children. Pediatr Ann 1976;5:700–22.

24.2b. Hirschsprung's Disease

Essam Imseis, MD

Cheryl E. Gariepy, MD

Hirschsprung's disease is the congenital absence of the enteric nervous system (ENS) extending continuously for a variable distance to the internal anal sphincter. The ENS consists of ganglion cells in the myenteric and submucosal plexuses and associated connecting nerves within the wall of the intestine. Short-segment Hirschsprung's disease is restricted to the rectum and sigmoid colon and accounts for nearly 90% of cases. Long-segment Hirschsprung's disease generally describes disease that begins proximal to the sigmoid colon. Long-segment disease accounts for approximately 10% of cases. This includes disease that involves the entire colon (total colonic aganglionosis, approximately 5% of cases) and portions of the small bowel.[1] Rarely, aganglionosis includes most or all of the small intestine.[1–4] The existence (and definition) of an "ultrashort" form of the disease is debated.

In recent years, great progress has been made in our understanding of the molecular genetics of this disorder, which appear to be quite complicated. Hirschsprung's disease has become a paradigm for multigene disorders because the same basic phenotype is associated with mutations in at least 11 distinct genes. This chapter will discuss the history, diagnosis, and treatment of the disorder as well as the current understanding of the pathogenesis and genetics of Hirschsprung's disease and the potential practical applications of this information.

HISTORY

In 1886, Harald Hirschsprung provided the first detailed description of the disease that bears his name when he reported the autopsy of two infants, age 8 months and 11 months, who presented with constipation and megacolon.[5]

After Hirschsprung's description, great debate ensued regarding the etiology of this disease. It was not until 1948 when Whitehouse and Zuelzer independently confirmed an absence of ganglion cells in the distal colon of affected individuals that this abnormality was widely accepted as the cause of Hirschsprung's disease.[6,7] At roughly the same time, Orvar Swenson performed the first successful operation for the disease, involving resection of the aganglionic bowel with anastomosis of ganglionic bowel near the internal anal sphincter.[8]

EPIDEMIOLOGY

The general incidence of Hirschsprung's disease is approximately 1/5,000 live births.[9–11] Recent studies suggest that incidence rates varies among different ethnicities with incidence rates in Caucasians, African Americans, Asians, and Pacific Islanders of 1/7,000, 1/5,000, 1/3,600, and 1/1,300 respectively.[12,13] The ratio of short-segment to long-segment disease may also vary between ethnic groups, with long-segment disease being relatively more common in those of African ancestry and short-segment disease being relatively more common in those of Asian ancestry. The male-female ratio for Hirschsprung's disease is 4:1 for short-segment disease and approaches 1:1 as the length of involved segment increases. Overall, 7% of cases have a family history of the disorder. However, the family prevalence is 21% in individuals with total colonic disease.[14]

Approximately 15% of individuals with Hirschsprung's disease present with at least one other congenital anomaly.[15,16] Excluding individuals with Down's syndrome, cardiac anomalies are found in 4.5%, CNS anomalies are found in 3.9%, genitourinary anomalies are found in 5.6%, and other gastrointestinal anomalies are found in 3.9% of individuals with Hirschsprung's disease.[15] In some instances, these anomalies may constitute part of a known syndromic disorder (Table 1).

Chromosomal anomalies are seen in 12% of individuals with Hirschsprung's disease. Trisomy 21 is the most commonly associated chromosomal abnormality and is found in 2 to 8% of individuals with Hirschsprung's disease.[1,10,15,17]

PATHOPHYSIOLOGY AND MOLECULAR GENETICS

ENS precursors are derived from the neural crest and colonize the gut in a cranial-to-caudal progression between weeks 5 and 12 of embryogenesis. Hirschsprung's disease is caused by failure of the ENS precursors to colonize the distal intestine.[18] ENS precursors are identified in the proximal gut of animal models of Hirschsprung's disease suggesting that the colonization failure results from migration or proliferation defects.[19,20] Absence of the myenteric and submucosal nerve plexus in the affected bowel results in inadequate relaxation of the bowel and bowel wall hyperto-

nicity (see Chapter 24.1, "Normal Motility and Development of the Intestinal Neuroenteric System" for further details). The hypertonic bowel causes intestinal obstruction, which can lead to bacterial overgrowth and enterocolitis.

The inheritance pattern of Hirschsprung's disease can be autosomal dominant or recessive. The genetics of Hirschsprung's disease displays three characteristics: (1) the penetrance of mutations is generally low, (2) there is a sex difference in the penetrance and expression of mutations, and (3) the penetrance of a gene mutation depends upon the extent of aganglionosis in affected family members. Most identified gene mutations associated with Hirschsprung's disease are best thought of as susceptibility genes. That is, the mutation increases the individual's odds of having Hirschsprung's disease, but is not predictive of the abnormality.

Multiple Hirschsprung's disease susceptibility genes are identified, primarily through studies of animal models (Table 2). Among the identified gene mutations are two signaling pathways, one involving the RET receptor and the other involving the endothelin-B receptor.

The *RET* gene encodes a transmembrane receptor tyrosine kinase and is the major Hirschsprung susceptibility gene. Coding sequence mutations of *RET* were the first gene mutations identified in Hirschsprung's disease.[21,22] *RET* loss-of-function (resulting in an absence of RET protein function) or dominant negative (in which the abnormal gene product interferes with functioning of the normal gene product) mutations are associated with up to 50% of familial Hirschsprung cases.[21–25] *RET* coding sequence mutations are more common in long-segment Hirschsprung's disease where they can be identified in up to 75% of individuals.[26] In addition, Emison and colleagues identified a noncoding *RET* variant that is quite common in many parts of the world and is associated with Hirschsprung's disease.[27] This sequence was subsequently demonstrated to encode an enhancer element that drives *RET* expression in the digestive tract during embryogenesis.[28] The enhancer mutation is present in 25% of Europeans, 45% of Asians, and less than 1% of Africans. The presence of this enhancer mutation appears to correlate with the incidence of short-segment disease since it is twice a common in Asia compared to Europe.[27] The relatively low prevalence of this enhancer mutation in Africans may also explain the lower incidence of short-segment disease

Table 1 Anomalies Associated with Hirschsprung's Disease

Syndromes	Key Features
*Chromosomal**	
Down's syndrome	Mental retardation with characteristic features
Syndromes requiring Hirschsprung's disease	
Goldberg-Shprintzen syndrome	Cleft palate, hypotonia, mental retardation, and facial dysmorphism
Shah-Waardenburg†	Pigmentary abnormalities (white forelock, depigmentation of skin, premature greying, heterochromic irides), and sensorineural deafness
Hirschsprung's disease w/ distal limb anomalies(several syndromes)	Polydactyly, brachydactyly, or nail hypoplasia with other assorted anomalies
BRESHEK	Brain abnormalities, mental retardation, ectodermal dysplasia, skeletal malformation, ear/eye anomalies, kidney dysplasia
Syndromes w/ Hirschsprung's disease as an occasional finding	
Mowat-Wilson	Facial dysmorphic features, mental retardation
Congenital central hypoventilation	Abnormal autonomic control of respiration
Bardet-Biedl	Pigmentary retinopathy, obesity, hypogonadism, mild mental retardation postaxial polydactyly
MEN2A	Medullary thyroid carcinoma, pheochromocytoma, parathyroid hyperplasia heart defect
Kauffman-McKusick	Hydrometrocolpos, postaxial polydactyly, congenital
Smith-Lemli-Opitz	Growth retardation, microcephaly, mental retardation, hypospadias, syndactyly of second, and third toes, dymorphic features
Cartilage–Hair Hypoplasia	Short-limb dwarfism, metaphyseal dysplasia, transient macrocytic anemia, immunodeficiency, fine, and sparse blond hair
Syndromes w/ a possible association with Hirschsprung‡	
Fukuyama congenital muscular dystrophy	Muscular dystrophy, polymicrogyria, hydrocephalus, mental retardation, seizures
Clayton-Smith	Dysmorphic features, hypoplastic toes and nails, deafness, ichthyosis
Kaplan	Agenesis of the corpus callosum, adducted thumbs, ptosis, muscle weakness
Dermotrichic	Alopecia, ichthyosis, mental retardation, seizures
Okamoto	Hydrocephalus, cleft palate, agenesis of the corpus callosum, familial dyautonomia

Adapted from Chakravarti, Lyonnet.[29]

*Hirschsprung's disease is also seen in association with the following chromosomal disorders: chromosome 2p deletion syndrome, chromosome 22q11.2 deletion, cat-eye syndrome (supernumerary dicentric chromosome 22q), 20p deletion, and deletions/duplications of chromosme 17q21–q23.

†Other neurocristopathies are reported in association with Hirschsprung's disease that likely share a molecular basis with Shah-Waardenburg. These include Yemenite deaf-blind hypopigmentation (OMIM #601706), ABCD syndrome (OMIM #600501), familial piebaldism (OMIM #172800), and congenital deafness.

‡Hirschsprung's disease is also reported in association with the following syndromes: Pallister-Hall, Fryns, Jeune asphyxiating thoracic, Frontonasal dysplasia, osteopetrosis, Goldenhar, Lesch-Nyhan, Rubinstein-Taybi, Toriello-Carey, and spondyloepimetaphyseal dysplasia with joint laxity.[29]

noted in African Americans versus non-African Americans.[29] *RET* mutations, coding and/or noncoding, are probably present in the vast majority of individuals with Hirschsprung's disease. However, these mutations are not sufficient to cause Hirschsprung's disease since penetrance of the phenotype requires mutations in additional genes.[27] The enhancer mutation may also account for the sex difference in the observed incidence of Hirschsprung's disease. For reasons that are unclear, this mutation is more likely to be transmitted to male offspring and the mutation is more likely to be penetrant in males.[27]

Mutations in the gene encoding the RET ligand, glial-cell line derived neurotrophic factor (GDNF), are also associated with Hirschsprung's disease, and loss-of-function mutations in its coreceptor, GFR$_\alpha$-1, cause a similar disease in mice.[30–32]

RET and GFR$_\alpha$-1 are expressed in multipotent progenitors of the mammalian ENS as they migrate through and colonize the gut during embryogenesis.[30,33,34] GDNF is expressed by the mesenchyme of the developing gut.[35,36] Mice deficient in ret signaling display an absence of ENS development distal to the stomach along with renal anomalies.[30,31,37–39] In mice, RET-deficient ENS precursors fail to colonize the gut beyond the gastric cardia and a reduced population of neurons and glia survive in the esophagus.[40] RET–GDNF interaction is implicated in proliferation, survival, and migration of ENS precursors in the developing gut.[41,42] RET may be a "dependence receptor" that induces survival signals in the presence of ligand and cell death signals in the absence of ligand.[43] GDNF appears to act as a chemoattractant for RET-expressing neural crest cells, driving migration of the cells through the small bowel to cecum.

In addition to Hirschsprung's disease, germline *RET* mutations also cause the multiple endocrine neoplasia syndromes MEN2A and MEN2B as well as familial/sporadic cases of medullary thyroid carcinoma.[44–48] These mutations are activating mutations, leading to dimerization of the receptor and ligand-independent activation of its tyrosine kinase domain. Interestingly, some of the same *RET* mutations that cause Hirschsprung's disease cause MEN2A.[49] Several studies suggest that a subset of mutations promoting high cell proliferation may also impaired cell migration in response to GDNF.[50–52] Thus, while the neoplastic phenotype may result from a high level of *RET* signaling within the cell, the aganglionosis phenotype may result from a lack of ligand responsiveness. This phenotypic overlap suggests that some individuals with Hirschsprung's disease and their family members are at risk for neuroendocrine tumors (see "Genetic Counseling" below).[32,53]

Endothelins are 21 amino acid peptides that interact with G-protein coupled receptors and play a number of roles in mammalian physiology and development. Mutations in the endothelin-B receptor and its ligand, endothelin-3, cause Hirschsprung's disease that may be associated with pigmentary abnormalities (regional hypopigmentation, white forelock, bicolored irides) and sensorineural deafness.[54–56] This combination of defects is known as Waardenburg syndrome type 4, or Shah-Waardenburg syndrome. Patients homozygous for mutations in the endothelin-B or endothelin-3 gene express the complete Shah-Waardenburg syndrome, whereas patients heterozygous for mutations in these genes may have isolated Hirschsprung's disease or Waardenburg syndrome.[29] Mutations in endothelin-B are found in approximately 5% of individuals with isolated Hirschsprung's disease, as are mutations in endothelin-3.[55–59] Unlike *RET* mutations, endothelin-B mutations are often associated with short-segment Hirschsprung's disease. Hirschsprung's disease is reported in one patient with a large deletion near, but not including, the endothelin-B gene. This suggests that nearby genomic rearrangements may affect endothelin-B expression and may explain why mutations within the gene are not found more commonly in individuals with Hirschsprung's disease.[60]

Mutations in the gene encoding endothelin-converting-enzyme-1, a protease responsible for the biological activation of endothelin-3, may also be associated with Hirschsprung's disease. An endothelin-converting-enzyme-1 mutation is reported in a single individual with Hirschsprung's disease associated with cardiac, craniofacial, and other abnormalities.[61]

Endothelin-B is expressed by early ENS precursors and endothelin-3 is expressed by the surrounding mesenchyme.[62] Studies in the mouse demonstrate that, in the absence of endothelin-B activation, ENS precursors show abnormalities in gut colonization beginning in the region of the cecum. Several lines of evidence suggest that endothelin-B activation during this phase of intestinal colonization is critical for complete colonization of the distal gut.[63–66] In vitro evidence indicates that endothelin-3/endothelin-B signaling inhibits neuronal differentiation.[67,68] It

Table 2 Selected Gene Mutations Associated with Hirschsprung's Disease

Gene	Gene Product	Human Locus	% of Hirschsprung's Disease	Human Homozygote Phenotype	Human Heterozygote Phenotype	Penetrance of Hirschsprung Phenotype	Animal Model
RET	Receptor tyrosine kinase	10q11.2	Familial-50% Sporadic - 15–35%	Long-segment Hirschsprung's disease (1 case reported)	Hirschsprung's disease	51–72%	Mouse
GDNF	Glial-cell line derived neurotrophic factor (RET ligand)	5p12–13.1	<1%	None reported	Hirschsprung's disease	Unknown	Mouse
GFRα1	GDNF family receptor alpha-1	10q26	None reported	None reported	None reported	Unknown	Mouse
EDNRB	Endothelin-B receptor	13q22	5%	Shah-Waardenburg syndrome (often with total intestinal aganglionos)	Hirschsprung's disease (with or without features of Waardenburg syndrome)	30–85%	Mouse, rat, horse
EDN3	Endothelin-3	20q13.2–13.3	<5%	Long-segment Shah-Waardenburg syndrome	Shah-Waardenburg syndrome (1 case reported)	Unknown	Mouse
ECE1	Endothelin converting enzyme-1	1p36.1	<1%	None noted	Hirschsprung's disease with cardiac defects, craniofacial defects, and autonomic dysfunction (1 case reported)	Unknown	Mouse
SOX10	SRY-related HMG box gene 10, transcription factor	22q13.1	<1%	None noted	Shah-Waardenburg syndrome often with other neurologic deficits	>80%	Mouse
ZFHX1B (SIP1)	Zinc finger homeobox 1B (SMAD interacting protein-1), transcription factor	2q22	<1%	Hirschsprung's disease with microcephaly, mental retardation, epilepsy, and characteristic facial features	Hirschsprung's disease with microcephaly, mental retardation, epilepsy, and characteristic facial features	Unknown	Mouse
Phox2b	Paired-like homeobox transcription factor	4p12	<1%	None reported	Congenital central hypoventilation syndrome (when Hirschsprung is present known as Haddad syndrome)	15–20%	Mouse
L1CAM	Immunoglobulin gene supperfamily of neural-cell adhesion molecules	Xq28	<1%	Homozygous female not reported	Hydrocephalus, adducted thumbs and Hirschsprung's disease in hemizygous males	3% (males)	Mice have developmental abnormalities of ENS, but not aganglionosis

is hypothesized that, by inhibiting differentiation, endothelin-B signaling maintains the ENS precursors in a colonization-competent state. Mice and rats with mutations affecting endothelin-B signaling are reported to exhibit abnormalities in the ganglia of ENS-containing bowel. These abnormalities are hypothesized to play a role in the prolonged dysmotility observed in some Hirschsprung patients after surgical resection of aganglionic bowel.[69–71] Reduced expression of endothelin-3 and endothelin converting enzyme-1 in males may contribute to the increased incidence of Hirschsprung's disease in males.[72]

Mutations in *SOX10* also cause Shah-Waardenburg syndrome.[73] Most *SOX10* mutations are dominant and frequently occur de novo. While the penetrance of the identified mutations is high, some individuals with *SOX10* mutations may have only some of the features of Shah-Waardenburg syndrome.[74] They tend to have short-segment aganglionosis or even hypoganglionosis of the colon. Some of these individuals show other abnormalities involving the central or peripheral nervous systems.[74–76] Not all patients with Shah-Waardenburg syndrome have identified mutations in the genes encoding endothelin-B, endothelin-3, or *SOX10*.

SOX10 is a transcription factor that is expressed in early ENS precursors and appears to support their survival. In mice homozygous for *SOX10* mutations, ENS precursors undergo apoptosis before they reach the foregut. Mice heterozygous for *SOX10* mutations exhibit early delays in ENS precursor migration, though final gut colonization may be complete. This observation has led to the hypothesis that haploinsufficiency for *SOX10* selectively affects an early subset of ENS precursors.[77,78] Zhu and colleagues[79] identified binding sites for *SOX10* in an Ednrb enhancer activated as the ENS precursors approach the colon, Owens and colleagues performed a genome wide scan to identify genes that modify the ENS phenotype of *SOX10* heterozygous mutant mice. They identified both Ednrb and Phox2b as likely modifying alleles.[80]

Inactivating mutations in the gene encoding the zinc finger homeobox 1B gene, *ZFHX1B* (formerly *SIP1*), cause Mowat-Wilson syndrome (characteristic facial features, microcephaly, mental retardation) with or without Hirschsprung's disease.[81] Individuals with Mowat-Wilson syndrome carry dominant, de novo mutations in this gene.[81,82] *ZFHX1B* is believed to be a transcriptional repressor that directly binds promoters and interacts with Smad proteins.[81–83]

Individuals with Goldberg-Shprintzer syndrome have distinct facial and CNS features from Mowat-Wilson syndrome, though they also suffer from microcephaly and metal retardation associated with Hirschsprung's disease. Brooks and colleagues have recently described mutations in a novel, evolutionarily conserved, widely expressed gene, *KIAA1279* in this syndrome. Little is yet known regarding the function of this gene product.[84]

Phox2B is a paired-like homeobox transcription factor that modulates RET expression. Inactivating mutations in this gene are linked to congenital central hypoventilation syndrome (CCHS) and automonic system abnormalities (including Hirschsprung's disease) in humans and a similar syndrome in mice. Ninety-eight percent of individuals with CCHS have Phox2b mutations and 15 to 20% of these individuals have Hirschsprung's disease (usually long segment).[85–87]

Finally, several factors are thought to contribute to the pathophysiology of Hirschsprung associated enterocolitis. The major problem is likely bowel stasis. In addition, defects in intestinal epithelial defense mechanisms are identified in Hirschsprung's disease. These include luminal IgA deficiency and altered mucin composition.[88,89] How these defects relate to the identified gene mutations in Hirschsprung's disease is unclear.

CLINICAL MANIFESTATIONS

The clinical manifestations of Hirschsprung's disease depend upon the age of presentation and the length of aganglionic bowel. Kleinhaus and colleagues reported that 40% of individuals with Hirschsprung's disease are diagnosed in the first 3 months of life and 60% are diagnosed in the first year of life.[14] Over the past few decades, the mean age at diagnosis has decreased so that the majority of patients are now diagnosed in the first 3 months of life. Individuals with total colonic disease tend to be diagnosed earlier than individuals with short-segment disease.[90] Breast-fed infants may present later than formula-fed infants.[91]

The neonate with Hirschsprung's disease is usually full term and with normal birth weight. Failure to pass meconium on the first day of life in a term infant should raise the suspicion of Hirschsprung's disease, but 30 to 40% of infants with Hirschsprung's disease are reported to pass meconium in the first 24 hours. Only approximately half of term infants with Hirschsprung's disease fail to pass meconium in the first 48 hours of life.[92,93] Delayed passage of meconium is a common finding in premature infants, particularly very low birth weight and sicker premature infants, and is not a useful indicator of Hirschsprung's disease.[94–96] Abdominal distention, vomiting, constipation, and poor feeding are also commonly seen in neonates with Hirschsprung's disease. Diarrhea is seen in approximately one in four neonates with Hirschsprung's disease[97] and generally indicates the presence of enterocolitis, the most common cause of morbidity and mortality in Hirschsprung's disease.

Bowel perforation is an uncommon presentation in infants with Hirschsprung's disease, noted in about 3 to 5% of patients, almost exclusively in infants less than 2 months of age.[97–101] Perforations tend to occur in the appendix and proximal colon and are more common in long-segment or total colonic Hirschsprung's disease.

The infant or child with Hirschsprung's disease usually presents with constipation that begins in infancy and responds poorly to medical management. Fecal urgency, stool holding behaviors, and fecal soiling are usually not noted. Poor weight gain, anemia, hypoalbuminemia, and bouts of diarrhea (associated with enterocolitis) are common. Urinary stasis due to mechanical factors associated with fecal retention rarely results in recurrent urinary tract infections, urothithiasis, and hydronephrosis.[97,102–104]

Physical examination may reveal a tympanitic distended abdomen with palpable fecal masses, particularly in the older infant and child. A rectal examination is essential to evaluate for imperforate anus, an anteriorly displaced anus, and anal stenosis. The digital rectal examination in Hirschsprung's disease will demonstrate a normally placed anus that will easily admit the finger but may remain somewhat tight. Stool is generally not found in the distal rectum, and the rectal mucosa remains snug to the examiner's finger (the "finger in glove" sensation). Often there is an explosive release of air and liquid stool as the examiner's finger is removed due to temporary relief of the obstruction in the distal bowel. The patient with enterocolitis will have diarrhea and appear ill, usually with fever and lethargy.

DIFFERENTIAL DIAGNOSIS

The clinical history and physical findings are very valuable in differentiating Hirschsprung's disease from other disorders. Hirschsprung's disease should be considered in any child who has a history of constipation dating back to the newborn period. Suspicion should increase in any child with associated abdominal distension, vomiting, and/or poor growth. Suspicion should also increase in a child with a family history of Hirschsprung's disease.

It is important to differentiate Hirschsprung's disease from functional constipation (Table 3). The patient with Hirschsprung's disease often has problems that begin in the neonatal period with delayed passage of meconium and poor growth. Stool caliber in Hirschsprung's disease is often small and ribbon-like while children with functional constipation occasionally pass large stools. Rectal examination in Hirschsprung's disease generally fails to detect stool in the rectal vault.

In addition to functional constipation, the clinical findings associated with Hirschsprung's disease can mimic several other clinical entities. Anatomic causes of intestinal obstruction, endocrine disorders, electrolyte imbalances, sepsis, and drug side effects should all be included in the differential (see Chapter 24.2a, "Functional Constipation").

INVESTIGATIONS

Radiographic Studies

Abdominal radiographs frequently show loops of distended intestine and may show a paucity of air in the rectum. Prone films are particularly helpful as this position facilitates the movement of air into the rectum of individuals without an obstruction. The presence of free air indicates a perforation and is more frequently seen in infants.[105]

Because the proximal, ganglionic intestine may not be significantly dilated in the first few weeks of life, an unprepared contrast enema is most likely to aid in the diagnosis of Hirschsprung's disease in children greater than 1 month of age. Similar difficulties arise in interpreting contrast studies in individuals with total colonic aganglionosis (Figure 1C). Classic findings include a contracted distal colon with an abrupt transition to a widely dilated proximal colon (Figure 1B). In the absence of this finding, it is important to compare the diameter of the rectum to that of the sigmoid colon. A rectal diameter that is the same as or smaller than the diameter of the sigmoid colon is suggestive of Hirschsprung's disease (Figure 1A). A radiograph taken 24 hours after the study may also be helpful in showing retained contrast in individuals with Hirschsprung's disease.[106]

The transition zone demonstrated by the contrast study (and by gross inspection of the intestine) does not necessarily provide reliable evidence regarding the length of aganglionosis.[107] Only histologic analysis can determine how much bowel will need to be resected. Finally, a contrast enema should not be undertaken in a patient with clinical enterocolitis or recent rectal biopsy because the risk of perforation is increased.

Anorectal Manometry

Anorectal manometry is a measure of ENS function. Distension of a proximal colonic segment normally leads to relaxation of the neighboring distal segment. The technique looks for relaxation of the internal anal sphincter in response to distension of the rectum with a balloon (Figure 2). The reported sensitivity and specificity of the test vary widely.[108–110] In experienced hands, the technique can be quite sensitive.[111,112] However, the procedure generally requires some patient cooperation and can be difficult to perform on young children in the absence of sedation. In addition, the anorectal reflex may not be completely developed in premature or full-term

Table 3 Clinical Features Differentiating Hirschsprung's Disease and Functional Constipation

	Hirschsprung's Disease	Functional Constipation
Age at onset	Under 1 yr of age	Over 1 yr of age
Passage of meconium	Delayed	Normal
Encopresis	Absent	Present
Growth	Poor	Normal
Abdominal pain	Rare	Frequent and colicky
Stool size	Small ribbon-like or pebble-like	Large
Stool withholding behavior	Absent	Present
Abdominal examination	Distended	Not distended
Rectum	Empty	Filled with stool
Rectal examination	Explosive passage of stool	Stool in rectum

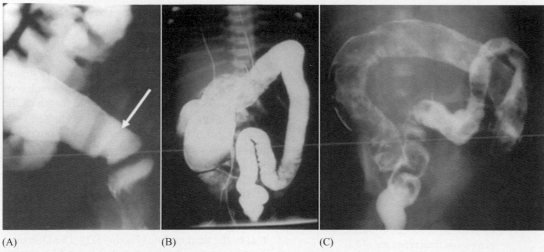

(A)   (B)   (C)

Figure 1 Contrast enema in Hirschsprung's disease. (A) Contrast enema of an infant with short-segment Hirschsprung's disease. Arrow indicates rectum. Note that although the distal sigmoid is not dilated, the rectal diameter is smaller than that of the sigmoid colon. (Provided by Peter Strouse, Department of Pediatric Radiology, University of Michigan, Ann Arbor.) (B) Typical contrast enema appearance in long-segment Hirschsprung's disease. The transition zone is in the ascending colon. (Provided by Daniel Teitelbaum, Department of Pediatric Surgery, University of Michigan, Ann Arbor.) (C) Contrast enema in an infant with total colonic aganglionosis. Note the consistent small caliber of the colon and the lack of an identifiable transition zone. (Reprinted with permission from reference 118.)

infants less that 12 days of age[113] and the technique can be technically difficult in very young infants. Anorectal manometry is best done by a very experienced operator.

Rectal Biopsy

Rectal biopsy is the gold standard for diagnosing Hirschsprung's disease. The diagnosis is usually established by a rectal suction biopsy, which can be performed at the bedside or in an outpatient setting. Two difficulties most commonly arise with the technique. The first is in obtaining an adequate amount of submucosa to adequately evaluate the ganglion cells. The other difficulty is in getting biopsies from the appropriate location. A segment of hypoganglionosis exists normally in the submucosal plexus just above the dentate line. This ranges from 3 to 17 mm in length.[114] In order to avoid taking biopsies in this area, the general practice is to obtain suction rectal biopsies no closer that 2 cm above the dentate line. If an adequate specimen is obtained from the correct location, the test is highly accurate. The technique is also quite safe, though perforations and significant hemorrhages are reported.[115] Because the length of normal hypoganglionosis above the dentate line is shorter in the myenteric plexus, full thickness biopsies can be obtained more distally than rectal suction biopsies. They are generally reserved for difficult cases in which rectal suction biopsies have failed to resolve the clinical question.

In experienced hands, examination of hematoxylin and eosin stained sections from an adequate biopsy is sufficient to establish a diagnosis of Hirschsprung's disease (Figure 3).[116] Acetylcholinesterase staining on unfixed specimens can aid the diagnosis. Hypertrophied extrinsic nerve fibers in the lamina propria and muscularis mucosa are often, but not always, identified in the aganglionic bowel in Hirschsprung's disease (Figure 4). Acetylcholinesterase staining is most useful if the biopsy contains limited submucosa and no ganglion cells are identified. In this case, acetylcholinesterase staining typical for Hirschsprung's disease can be diagnostic.[117]

Ultrashort segment Hirschsprung's disease is also referred to as anorectal achalasia and may represent a different pathophysiologic process. The major controversy with this disease entity is that the gold standard for diagnosing Hirschsprung's disease (a rectal biopsy 3 to 5 cm above the dentate line) is normal. In addition, the clinical history is generally consistent with functional constipation (often with encopresis). Only anorectal manometry demonstrates the characteristic abnormality of Hirschsprung's disease—failure of reflex relaxation of the internal anal sphincter upon distension of the rectum. This disorder may go undiagnosed because many centers do not routinely perform anorectal manometry on patients with this presentation.

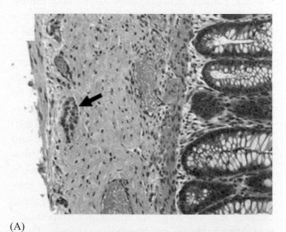

(A)

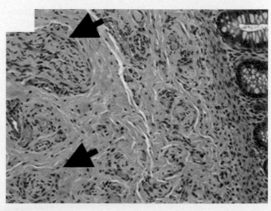

(B)

Figure 3 Hematoxylin and eosin stained sections of a surgically resected specimen from a patient with Hirschsprung's disease (magnification 200×). (A) Proximal section demonstrating normal myenteric ganglia (small arrow). (B) Distal (rectal) section showing numerous hypertrophic peripheral nerves (large arrows). Ganglion cells are not identified. (Photo provided by Robert Ruiz, Department of Pathology, University of Michigan, Ann Arbor.)

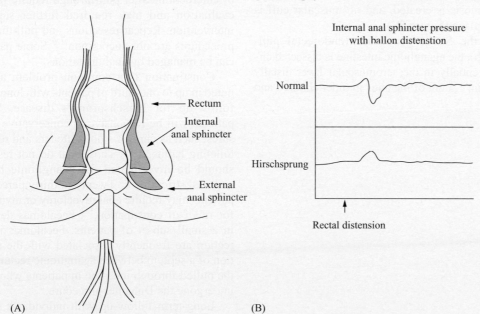

(A)   (B)

Figure 2 Anorectal manometry. (A) Illustration of placement of a triple balloon anorectal manometry catheter. (B) Anorectal manometric tracing demonstrating the response to rectal distension. Normal relaxation of the internal anal sphincter is illustrated in the top tracing and the absence of relaxation of the internal anal sphincter in a patient with Hirschsprung's disease is illustrated in the bottom tracing.

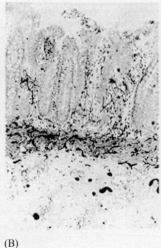

(A)   (B)

Figure 4 Acetylcholinesterase staining of rectal suction biopsy frozen sections. (A) In an individual without Hirschsprung's disease, staining is limited to a few nerve twigs in the muscularis mucosa. (B) In Hirschsprung's disease, staining reveals more and thicker nerve fibers in the muscularis mucosa and the lamina propria than in normal tissue. (Reprinted with permission from reference 116.)

TREATMENT

Definitive treatment for Hirschsprung's disease is surgical. Medical management is important in stabilizing the patient, especially if the patient has enterocolitis, and to adequately prepare the bowel for surgery.

The treatment of Hirschsprung-associated enterocolitis involves the placement of a soft rectal tube to decompress the colon and to allow saline washes. Patients generally need intravenous antibiotics. Rectal tube decompression and washes may not be effective in long segment disease, in which case a decompressing ostomy may be required.

The bowel should be prepared for surgery with warm saline enemas (10 mL/kg) through a rectal tube. In addition, the patient should be given a clear liquid diet for 2 to 3 days or a polyethylene glycol electrolyte solution (25 mL/kg/h) for 8 hours on the day prior to the procedure and monitored closely for worsening abdominal distention.[118] Hypertonic phosphate enemas should never be given to a patient with proven or suspected Hirschsprung's disease. Retention of these enemas leads to hyperphosphatemia, hypocalcemia, hypokalemia, and metabolic acidosis. These abnormalities may result in tetany, dehydration, acute renal failure, cardiac arrest, and death.[119]

Four surgical pull-through approaches are commonly used in the treatment of Hirschsprung's disease: the Rehbein, Swenson, Soave, and Duhamel procedures. Historically, obstruction was relieved in all infants with the creation of a stoma proximal to the aganglionic segment. Definitive surgery was delayed until the child weighed 9 to 10 kg (20 lbs) or until the dilated proximal segment regained a normal caliber. Currently, many infants undergo a primary pull-through procedure, often done laparoscopically. Results with the primary pull-through appear comparable to those with the staged procedure.[120–123]

In the Rehbein procedure (which is more frequently used in Europe than the United States), an anterior approach is used to remove the defective aganglionic tissue. The procedure leaves 3 to 5 cm of aganglionic colon above the dentate line (Figure 5A).

The Swenson procedure consists of dissection of the rectal wall distally to the level of the internal anal sphincter. The ganglion-containing bowel is pulled through the pelvis and anastomosed end to end to the rectum within 2 cm of the dentate line. Both a muscular and mucosal anastomosis is created, and no muscular cuff is left in place (Figure 5B).

In the Soave procedure (endorectal pull-through), the aganglionic intestine is dissected circumferentially in the seromuscular layer distally to within 1.5 cm of the anus in older children and less than 1 cm in newborns. The ganglionic intestine is incised, pulled through the muscular cuff, and an anastomosis is created to the submucosal–mucosal tube close to the anus (Figure 5C).[118] The Soave procedure has been associated with a higher incidence of postoperative enterocolitis and constipation. This may be related to the length of the muscular cuff. Because of this concern, a muscular cuff that extends no more than 1 to 2 cm above the levator muscle complex is advocated.[118]

The Duhamel procedure involves positioning the proximal ganglionic intestine posterior to the rectum. The ganglionic bowel is anastomosed side-to-side to the posterior wall of the aganglionic rectum through an incision 1 to 2 cm proximal to the dentate line (Figure 5D). The Duhamel procedure has been modified by Martin. The Martin-Duhamel procedure involves an extended side-to-side anastomosis of the small intestine to the aganglionic left colon.

LONG-TERM COMPLICATIONS AND RESULTS

Hirschsprung-associated enterocolitis remains the major cause of morbidity and mortality in the disease. Enterocolitis may be a presenting complaint in Hirschsprung's disease but it also frequently occurs after pull-through. The published mortality rates range from 6 to 30%[14,124,125] and appear to be decreasing.[126] Individuals with Down's syndrome are at increased risk for enterocolitis.[123,127] The risk of postoperative enterocolitis may also be increased in individuals with a history of an anastomotic leak, those with an anastomotic stricture, anal stenosis, and individuals with intestinal obstruction secondary to adhesions. This increased risk is likely related to intestinal stasis with subsequent bacterial overgrowth and mucosal invasion.[128] Patients with repeated episodes of enterocolitis after pull-through require further evaluation and may required further surgical intervention. Repeat resections and pull-through procedures are not uncommon.[129] Some patients can be managed by anal dilatations.

Constipation is a common problem and is noted in up to one-third of patients with long-term follow-up for Hirschsprung's disease. Some patients will be responsive to conservative measures, such as chronic stool softeners and regular toileting habits.[130,131] Those that do not respond should be investigated for aganglionic bowel and anal strictures.[132] Twenty to thirty percent of patients may require anal myectomy or myotomy for relief of constipation.[133] Fecalomas develop in a small subset of patients. Fecalomas in the rectum are frequently associated with the retention of a septum between aganglionic rectum and the pulled-through intestine in patients who have undergone the Duhamel procedure.

Long-term follow-up with individuals surgically treated for Hirschsprung's disease reveals that ongoing difficulties with fecal incontinence and weight gain are not uncommon. Ludman and colleagues found that 7 to 17 years after definitive

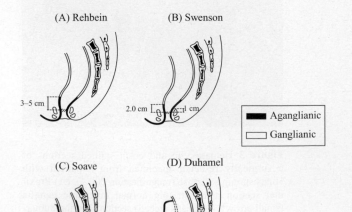

(A) Rehbein   (B) Swenson

3–5 cm   2.0 cm

■ Aganglianic
□ Ganglianic

(C) Soave   (D) Duhamel

Figure 5 Summary of anorectal anatomy following the more commonly performed pull-through procedures for Hirschsprung's disease. (Reprinted with permission from reference 118.)

operation, 60% of patients treated for rectosigmoid aganglionosis were incontinent while 86% of patients treated for total colonic aganglionosis were incontinent.[134] Similarly, Tsuji and colleagues[135] found that, in patients with total colonic disease, the fecal incontinence rates were 82% at 5 years, 57% at 10 years, and 33% at 15 years. With time, most individuals have improved fecal continence, but this may not occur until late adolescence. Yanchar and colleagues surveyed teenage patients who underwent definitive surgical treatment in the first year of life and their parents. They concluded that incontinence significantly impacted the patients' social and family life. Despite this, most parents were satisfied with their child's outcome.[136] Individuals with Down's syndrome appear to have prolonged difficulties with continence, particularly at night.

Di Lorenzo and colleagues performed colonic manometry on 46 symptomatic individuals who were more than 10 months status-post surgical resection of aganglionic bowel. Almost 40% of these individuals were found to have high-amplitude propagating contractions migrating through the neorectum and to the anal sphincter. This type of contraction does not propate beyond the sigmoid colon in healthy children and may play a significant role in incontinence after distal colonic resection for Hirschsprung's disease. Low dose amitriptyline at bedtime may improve continence in these individuals.[137] Over 30% of individuals exhibited an absence of high-amplitude propagating contractions or they had persistent simultaneous contractions, suggesting a neuropathic motility disorder proximal to the aganglionic colon. About 9% of children studied had normal colonic manometry but a hypertensive internal anal sphincter. Finally, 20% of children with symptoms after resection had normal manometry studies and were felt to have primarily behavioral issues related to defecation.[138]

Little data exist regarding possible damage to pelvic neuronal structures in the process of the pull-through procedure. Most reports fail to mention the subject. Sherman and colleagues found no abnormalities in urinary or sexual function in his review of a large number of adult postoperative patients.[105]

After resection of aganglionic bowel, some patients are unable to absorb adequate nutrients and are dependent upon parenteral nutrition. This includes patients with extensive aganglionosis involving the small bowel and patients with dysmotility in the remaining bowel. Dysmotility may improve with time and often no histologic abnormality in the remaining bowel can be identified. Rarely individuals with Hirschsprung's disease also exhibit intestinal neuronal dysplasia (IND B), characterized by hyperplastic submucosal ganglia (see Chapter 24.2c, "Other Dysmotilities Including Chronic Intestinal Pseudo-Obstruction Syndrome").[139] In addition, Hirschsprung's disease is identified in up to 20% of individuals diagnosed with IND B in the proximal intestine.[140] While specific histologic features of IND B are defined, a recent study demonstrated high interobserver variation in making the diagnosis.[141] No genetic link is established between Hirschsprung's disease and IND.[142] Finally, abnormalities in the network of interstitial cells of Cajal in the ganglion-containing bowel of patients with Hirschsprung's disease are reported and may contribute to dysmotility.[143]

GENETIC COUNSELING

Hirschsprung's disease is a sex-modified multifactorial disorder. The generalized risk to siblings is 4% and increases as the length of involved segment increases.[1,17] In Hirschsprung's disease associated with known syndromes, genetic counseling may focus more on the prognosis related to the syndrome and testing can be undertaken when a causative gene is known. In isolated Hirschsprung's disease, there is a general recurrence risk table (Table 4). Prenatal diagnosis is possible if the mutation within the family is known. However, because the penetrance of single gene mutations is low (except for *SOX10* mutations), the clinical usefulness of genetic testing is limited.

In addition to prenatal evaluation and assessments of recurrence risks, genetic testing in Hirschsprung's disease has the potential to identify significant risks for other diseases in the individual with Hirschsprung's disease or their family members. Currently, this is most clearly illustrated in Hirschsprung patients with *RET* mutations identical to those observed in individuals with MEN2A. Mutations of *RET* codons 609, 618, and 620 (within exon 10) are associated with MEN2A and Hirschsprung's disease. In addition, there have been rare cases of Hirschsprung's disease with exon 10 mutations identical to those found in hereditary medullary thyroid carcinoma.[50] A family history of thyroid, parathyroid, or adrenal cancer should be sought in all patients with Hirschsprung's disease. There is a growing trend to recommend mutation screening for those *RET* mutations common between Hirschsprung's disease and MEN2A in both nonsyndromic sporadic and familial Hirschsprung cases. However, before mutational analysis is undertaken, genetic counseling should address the follow-up when a MEN2A-related *RET* mutation is identified. While the vast majority of these tests will be negative, the significance of identifying a MEN2A mutation carrier to that individual and family justifies such testing.[144]

Newby and colleagues assessed the in vivo vasomotor responses to endothelin-B stimulation in a group of healthy adults with a history of nonsyndromic Hirschsprung's disease, without regard to the length of aganglionosis or genetic mutation. They reported that the individuals with a history of Hirschsprung's disease exhibited an abnormal vascular response to the injection of the endothelin-B selective agonist and that the pattern of abnormality suggested a defect in endothelin-B signaling.[145] This result raises the possibility that children treated for Hirschsprung's disease may be at increased risk for cardiovascular disease in adulthood. Endothelin-B is normally expressed on the vascular endothelium and smooth muscle where it appears to be involved in the maintenance of basal vascular tone. Rats genetically deficient in endothelin-B exhibit salt-sensitive hypertension.[146] However, no association has yet been made between Hirschsprung's disease and noncongenital cardiovascular disease.

FUTURE DIRECTIONS

Theoretically, Hirschsprung's disease and other congenital or acquired enteric neuromuscular disorders could be truly cured by restoration or replacement of missing or dysfunctional ganglia with healthy ganglia. Hopes for the development of such a treatment for Hirschsprung's disease have increased recently with advances related to CNS neural stem cell transplantation as well as the identification and successful in vitro transplantation of enteric neural crest stem cells.

CNS-derived neural stem cells have been transplanted to the gut where they formed neurons and improved gastrointestinal function. Mucci and colleagues transplanted CNS-derived neural stem cells into the pyloric region of a transgenic model of pyloric stenosis (the nNOS "knockout" mouse in which the pylorus is unable to relax and open appropriately). Some of these cells survived and differentiated into neurons expressing nNOS. Most importantly, the graft resulted in significantly improved gastric emptying, at least in the short term (1 week after transplantation). The long-term survival of the grafted cells was not assessed in this study.[147]

Because they may respond more appropriately to the intestinal microenvironment, gut-specific neural stem cells may be better suited to building or repairing the ENS. Neural crest-derived stem cells can be isolated from the fetal as well as adult ENS[66,148–151] and they appear to be somewhat restricted to gut phenotypes. Endothelin-3

Table 4 Percent Recurrence Risk of Hirschsprung's Disease by Profound and Consult and Gender						
Consult and Gender	Aganglionosis Proximal to Splenic Flexure		Aganglionosis Beginning in the Descending Colon		Aganglionosis of Rectum and/ or Sigmoid only	
	Male	Female	Male	Female	Male	Female
Sib of affected male	11	8	10	7	4	1
Sib of affected female	23	18	13	10	6	2
Offspring of affected male	18	13	11	9	~0	~0
Offspring of affected female	28	22	15	11	~0	~0
Reprinted with permission from Chakravarti, Lyonnet.[29]						

and *SOX10* help maintain these cells in an uncommitted state[152] and GDNF promotes their survival through PI-3 kinase.[153]

Most importantly from the standpoint of a potential treatment of Hirschsprung's disease is the finding that ENS precursors can be isolated from the unaffected segments of gut in two animal models of Hirschsprung's disease; RET mutant mice and endothelin-B mutant rats.[19,154] Transplantation of human ENS precursors isolated from biopsy specimens from infants up to 5 months of age into aganglionic bowel in organ culture has also recently been reported.[155] Despite these advances, several significant hurdles remain to be overcome before transplantation strategies can reach the clinic. Posttransplant survival of the ENS precursors remains a critical limiting factor and successful treatment of Hirschsprung's disease will required the transplanted cells to form a highly complex network of ganglia expressing a wide range of neurotransmitters. Successful engraftment will depend not only on isolation and expansion of a population of stem cells, but will depend critically on the cellular and extracellular environment of the gut receiving the graft. For example, inflammation has a profound effect on survival and differentiation of transplanted neural stem cells.[156,157]And, while fetal gut provides important survival and differentiation cues to stem cells, many of these signals are downregulated in postnatal life. While the preliminary experimental results are exciting, it will take the continued significant research efforts of many individuals before we are able to manipulate precursor cells and the gut environment to build a functional distal ENS for individuals with Hirschsprung's disease and minimize the need for surgical resection.

REFERENCES

1. Russell MB, Russell CA, Niebuhr E. An epidemiological study of Hirschsprung's disease and additional anomalies. Acta Paediatr 1994;83:68–71.
2. Descos B, Lachaux A, Louis D, et al. Extended intestinal aganglionosis in siblings. J Pediatr Gastroenterol Nur 1984;3:641–3.
3. Ward J, Sierra IA, D'Croz E. Cat eye syndrome associated with aganglionosis of the small and large intestine. J Med Genet 1989;26:647–8.
4. Inoue K, Shimotake T, Iwai N. Mutational analysis of RET/GDNF/NTN genes in children with total colonic aganglionosis with small bowel involvement. Am J Med Genet 2000;93:278–84.
5. Hirschsprung H. Stuhltragheit neugeborener in folge von delitation und hypertrophie des colons. Jahrb Kinderheilk 1888;27:1–7.
6. Whitehouse ER, Kernohan JW. The myenteric plexus in congenital megacolon. Arch Intern Med 1948;82:75.
7. Zuelzer WW, Wilson JL. Functional intestinal obstruction on a congenital neurogenic basis in infancy. Am J Dis Child 1948;75:40–64.
8. Swenson O, Rheinlander HF, Diamond I. Hirschsprung's disease: A new concept of the operative results in 34 patients. N Engl J Med 1949;241:551.
9. Passarge E. The genetics of Hirschsprung's disease. Evidence for heterogeneous etiology and a study of sixty-three families. N Engl J Med 1967;276:138–43.
10. Spouge D, Baird PA. Hirschsprung's disease in a large birth cohort. Teratology 1985;32:171–7.
11. Goldberg EL. An epidemiological study of Hirschsprung's disease. Int J Epidemiol 1984;13:479–85.
12. Torfs CP. An epidemiologic study of Hirschsprung's disease in a large multiracial California population. The second international meeting: Hirschsprung's disease and related neurocristopathies. Cleveland, OH, USA, 1995.
13. Meza-Valencia B, de Lorimier A, Person DA. Hirschsprung's disease in the United States associated Pacific Islands (USAPI): More common than expected. J Pediatr Gastroenterol Nur 2002;35:431.
14. Kleinhaus S, Boley SJ, Sheran M, Sieber WK. Hirschsprung's disease—a survey of the members of the surgical section of the American Academy of Pediatrics. J Pediatr Surg 1979;14:588–97.
15. Ryan ET, Ecker JL, Christakis NA, Folkman J. Hirschsprung's disease: Associated abnormalities and demography. J Pediatr Surg 1992;27:76–81.
16. Brown RA, Cywes S. Disorders and congenital malformations associated with Hirschsprung's disease. In: Holschneider AM, Puri P, editors. Hirschsprung's Disease and Allied Disorders, 2nd edition. Amsterdam: Harwood Academic Publishers; 2000. p. 137–45.
17. Badner JA, Sieber WK, Garver KL, Chakravarti A. A genetic study of Hirschsprung's disease. Am J Hum Genet 1990;46:568–80.
18. Le Douarin NM, Teillet MA. The migration of neural crest cells to the wall of the digestive tract in avian embryo. J Embryol Exp Morphol 1973;30:31–48.
19. Bondurand N, Natarajan D, Thapar N, et al. Neuron and glia generating progenitors of the mammalian enteric nervous system isolated from foetal and postnatal gut cultures. Dev 2003;130:6387–400.
20. Kruger GM, Mosher JT, Tsai YH, et al. Temporally distinct requirements for endothelin receptor B in the generation and migration of gut neural crest stem cells. Neuron 2003;40:917–29.
21. Romeo G, Ronchetto P, Luo Y, et al. Point mutations affecting the tyrosine kinase domain of the RET proto-oncogene in Hirschsprung's disease. Nature 1994;367:377–8.
22. Edery P, Lyonnet S, Mulligan LM, et al. Mutations of the RET proto-oncogene in Hirschsprung's disease. Nature 1994;367:378–80.
23. Attie T, Pelet A, Edery P, et al. Diversity of RET proto-oncogene mutations in familial and sporadic Hirschsprung's disease. Hum Mol Genet 1995;4:1381–6.
24. Hofstra RM, Wu Y, Stulp RP, et al. RET and GDNF gene scanning in Hirschsprung patients using two dual denaturing gel systems. Hum. Mutat 2000;15:418–29.
25. Lantieri F, Griseri P, Ceccherini I. Molecular mechanisms of RET-induced Hirschsprung pathogenesis. Ann Med 2006;38:11–9.
26. Seri M, Yin L, Barone V, et al. Frequency of RET mutations in long- and short-segment Hirschsprung's disease. Hum Mutat 1997;9:243–9.
27. Emison ES, McCallion AS, Kashuk CS, et al. A common sex-dependent mutation in a RET enhancer underlies Hirschsprung's disease risk. Nature 2005;434:857–63.
28. Grice EA, Rochelle ES, Green ED, et al. Evaluation of the RET regulatory landscape reveals the biological relevance of a HSCR-implicated enhancer. Hum Mol Genet 2005;14:3837–45.
29. Chakravarti A, Lyonnet S. Hirschsprung's disease. In: Scriver CR, Beaudet AL, Sly WS, Valle D, editors. The Metabolic and Molecular Basis of Inherited Disease, 8th edition. New York: McGraw Hill; 2001. p. 931–42.
30. Enomoto H, Araki T, Jackman A, et al. GFR alpha1-deficient mice have deficits in the enteric nervous system and kidneys. Neuron 1998;21:317–24.
31. Cacalano G, Farinas I, Wang LC, et al. GFRalpha1 is an essential receptor component for GDNF in the developing nervous system and kidney. Neuron 1998;21:53–62.
32. Angrist M, Bolk S, Halushka M, et al. Germline mutations in glial cell line-derived neurotrophic factor (GDNF) and RET in a Hirschsprung's disease patient. Nat Genet 1996;14:341–4.
33. Pachnis V, Mankoo B, Costantini F. Expression of the c-ret proto-oncogene during mouse embryogenesis. Dev 1993;119:1005–17.
34. Natarajan D, Grigoriou M, Marcos-Gutierrez CV, et al. Multipotential progenitors of the mammalian enteric nervous system capable of colonising aganglionic bowel in organ culture. Dev Suppl 1999;126:157–68.
35. Trupp M, Ryden M, Jornvall H, et al. Peripheral expression and biological activities of GDNF, a new neurotrophic factor for avian and mammalian peripheral neurons. J Cell Biol 1995;130:137–48.
36. Treanor JJ, Goodman L, de Sauvage F, et al. Characterization of a multicomponent receptor for GDNF. Nature 1996;382:80–3.
37. Schuchardt A, D'Agati V, Larsson-Blomberg L, et al. Defects in the kidney and enteric nervous system of mice lacking the tyrosine kinase receptor Ret. Nature 1994;367:380–3.
38. Moore MW, Klein RD, Farinas I, et al. Renal and neuronal abnormalities in mice lacking GDNF. Nature 1996;382:76–9.
39. Tomac AC, Grinberg A, Huang SP, et al. Glial cell line-derived neurotrophic factor receptor alpha1 availability regulates glial cell line-derived neurotrophic factor signaling: Evidence from mice carrying one or two mutated alleles. Neuroscience 2000;95:1011–23.
40. Taraviras S, Marcos-Gutierrez CV, Durbec P, et al. Signalling by the RET receptor tyrosine kinase and its role in the development of the mammalian enteric nervous system. Dev Suppl 1999;126:2785–97.
41. Chalazonitis A, Rothman TP, Chen J, Gershon MD. Age-dependent differences in the effects of GDNF and NT-3 on the development of neurons and glia from neural crest-derived precursors immunoselected from the fetal rat gut: Expression of GFRa-1 in vitro and in vivo. Dev Biol 1998;204:385–406.
42. Heuckeroth RO, Lampe PA, Johnson EM, Milbrandt J. Neurturin and GDNF promote proliferation and survival of enteric neuron and glial progenitors in vitro. Dev Biol 1998;200:116–29.
43. Bordeaux MC, Forcet C, Granger L, et al. The RET proto-oncogene induces apoptosis: A novel mechanism for Hirschsprung's disease. EMBO J 2000;19:4056–63.
44. Hofstra RM, Landsvater RM, Ceccherini I, et al. A mutation in the RET proto-oncogene associated with multiple endocrine neoplasia type 2B and sporadic medullary thyroid carcinoma. Nature 1994;367:375–6.
45. Carlson KM, Dou S, Chi D, et al. Single missense mutation in the tyrosine kinase catalytic domain of the RET protooncogene is associated with multiple endocrine neoplasia type 2B. Proc Natl Acad Sci U S A 1994;91:1579–83.
46. Mulligan LM, Eng C, Attie T, et al. Diverse phenotypes associated with exon 10 mutations of the RET proto-oncogene. Hum Mol Genet 1994;3:2163–7.
47. Mulligan LM, Eng C, Healey CS, et al. Specific mutations of the RET proto-oncogene are related to disease phenotype in MEN 2A and FMTC. Nat Genet 1994;6:70–4.
48. Eng C, Smith DP, Mulligan LM, et al. Point mutation within the tyrosine kinase domain of the RET proto-oncogene in multiple endocrine neoplasia type 2B and related sporadic tumours. Hum Mol Genet 1994;3:237–41.
49. Verdy M, Weber AM, Roy CC, et al. Hirschsprung's disease in a family with multiple endocrine neoplasia type 2. J Pediatr Gastroenterol Nur 1982;1:603–7.
50. Takahashi M, HIwashita T, Santoro M, et al. Cosegregation of MEN2 and Hirschsprung's disease: The same mutation of RET with both gain and loss-of-function. Hum Mutat 1999;13:331–6.
51. Mograbi B, Bocciardi R, Bourget I, et al. The sensitivity of activated Cys Ret mutants to glial cell line-derived neurotrophic factor is mandatory to rescue neuroectodermic cells from apoptosis. Mol Cell Biol 2001;21:6719–30.
52. Arighi E, Popsueva A, Degl'Innocenti D, et al. Biological effects of the dual phenotypic Janus mutation of ret cosegregating with both multiple endocrine neoplasia type 2 and Hirschsprung's disease. Mol Endocrinol 2004;18:1004–17.
53. Sijmons RH, Hofstra RM, Wijburg FA, et al. Oncological implications of *RET* gene mutations in Hirschsprung's disease. Gut 1998;43:542–7.
54. Puffenberger EG, Hosoda K, Washington SS, et al. A missense mutation of the endothelin-B receptor gene in multigenic Hirschsprung's disease. Cell 1994;79:1257–66.
55. Hofstra RM, Osinga J, Tan-Sindhunata G, et al. A homozygous mutation in the endothelin-3 gene associated with a combined Waardenburg type 2 and Hirschsprung phenotype (Shah-Waardenburg syndrome). Nat Genet 1996;12:445–7.
56. Edery P, Attie T, Amiel J, et al. Mutation of the endothelin-3 gene in the Waardenburg-Hirschsprung's disease (Shah-Waardenburg syndrome). Nat Genet 1996;12:442–4.
57. Attie T, Till M, Pelet A, et al. Mutation of the endothelin-receptor B gene in Waardenberg-Hirschsprung's disease. Hum Molec Genet 1995;4:2407–9.
58. Amiel J, Attie T, Jan D, et al. Heterozygous endothelin receptor B (EDNRB) mutations in isolated Hirschsprung's disease. Hum Mol Genet 1996;5:355–7.
59. Auricchio A, Casari G, Staiano A, Ballabio A. Endothelin-B receptor mutations in patients with isolated Hirschsprung's disease from a non-inbred population. Hum Mol Genet 1996;5:351–4.
60. Chakravarti A. Endothelin receptor-mediated signaling in Hirschsprung's disease. Hum Molec Genet 1996;5:303–7.
61. Hofstra RM, Valdenaire O, Arch E, et al. A loss-of-function mutation in the endothelin-converting enzyme 1 (ECE-1) associated with Hirschsprung's disease, cardiac defects, and autonomic dysfunction. Am J Hum Genet 1999;64:304–8.
62. Brand M, Le moullec JM, Corvol P, Gase JM. Ontogeny of endothelins-1 and -3, their receptors, and endothelin converting enzyme-1 in the early human embryo. J Clin Invest 1998;101:549–59.
63. Coventry S, Yost C, Palmiter RD, Kapur RP. Migration of ganglion cell precursors in the ileoceca of normal and

lethal spotted embryos, a murine model for Hirschsprung's disease. Lab. Invest 1994;71:82–93.
64. Shin MK, Levorse JM, Ingram RS, Tilghman SM. The temporal requirement for endothelin receptor-B signalling during neural crest development. Nature 1999;402:496–501.
65. Woodward MN, Kenny SE, Vaillant C, et al. Time-dependent effects of endothelin-3 on enteric nervous system development in an organ culture model of Hirschsprung's disease. J Pediatr Surg 2000;35:25–9.
66. Sidebotham EL, Woodward MN, Kenny SE, et al. Localization and endothelin-3 dependence of stem cells of the enteric nervous system in the embryonic colon. J Pediatr Surg 2002;37:145–50.
67. Hearn CJ, Murphy M, Newgreen D. GDNF and ET-3 differentially modulate the numbers of avian enteric neural crest cells and enteric neurons in vitro. Dev Biol 1998;197:93–105.
68. Wu JJ, Chen JX, Rothman TP, Gershon MD. Inhibition of in vitro enteric neuronal development by endothelin-3: Mediation by endothelin-B receptors. Dev 1999;126:1161–73.
69. Sandgren K, Larsson LT, Ekblad E. Widespread changes in neurotransmitter expression and number of enteric neurons and interstitial cells of Cajal in lethal spotted mice: An explanation for persisting dysmotility after operation for Hirschsprung's disease? Dig Dis Sci 2002;47:1049–64.
70. Nagahama M, Tsutsui Y, Ozaki T, Hama K. Myenteric and submucosal plexuses of the congenital aganglionosis rat (spotting lethal) as revealed by scanning electron microscopy. Biol Signals 1993;2:136–45.
71. Von Boyen GB, Krammer HJ, Suss A, et al. Abnormalities of the enteric nervous system in heterozygous endothelin B receptor deficient (spotting lethal) rats resembling intestinal neuronal dysplasia. Gut 2002;51:414–9.
72. Vohra BP, Planer W, Armon J, et al. Reduced endothelin converting enzyme-1 and endothelin-3 mRNA in the developing bowel of male mice may increase expressivity and penetrance of Hirschsprung disease-like distal intestinal aganglionosis. Dev Dyn 2007;236:106–17.
73. Pingault V, Bondurand N, Kuhlbrodt K, et al. *SOX10* mutations in patients with Waardenburg-Hirschsprung's disease. Nat Genet 1998;18:171–3.
74. Southard-Smith EM, Angrist M, Ellison JS, et al. The *SOX10*(Dom) mouse: Modeling the genetic variation of Waardenburg–Shah (WS4) syndrome. Genome Res 1999;9:215–25.
75. Touraine RL, Attie-Bitach T, Manceau E, et al. Neurological phenotype in Waardenburgh syndrome type 4 correlates with novel *SOX10* truncating mutations and expression in developing brain. Am J Hum Genet 2000;66:1496–503.
76. Inoue K, Tanabe Y, Lupski JR. Myelin deficiencies in both the central and the peripheral nervous systems associated with a *SOX10* mutation. Ann Neurol 1999;46:313–8.
77. Kapur RP. Early death of neural crest cells is responsible for total enteric aganglionosis in *SOX10*Dom/*SOX10*Dom mouse embryos. Pediatr Dev Pathol 1999;2:559–69.
78. Southard-Smith EM, Kos L, Pavan WJ. *SOX10* mutation disrupts neural crest development in Dom Hirschsprung mouse model. Nat Genet 1998;18:60–4.
79. Zhu L, Lee HO, Jordan CS, et al. Spatiotemporal regulation of endothelin receptor-B by *SOX10* in neural crest-derived enteric neuron precursors. Nat Genet 2004;36:732–7.
80. Owens SE, Broman KW, Wiltshire T, et al. Genome-wide linkage identifies novel modifier loci of aganglionosis in the *SOX10*Dom model of Hirschsprung's disease. Hum Mol Genet 2005;14:1549–58.
81. Wakamatsu N, Yamada Y, Yamada K, et al. Mutations in SIP1, encoding Smad interacting protein-1, cause a form of Hirschsprung's disease. Nat Genet 2001;27:369–70.
82. Yamada K, Yamada Y, Nomura N, et al. Nonsense and frameshift mutations in *ZFHX1B*, encoding Smad-interacting protein 1, cause a complex developmental disorder with a great variety of clinical features. Am J Hum Genet 2001;69:1178–85.
83. Verschueren K, Remacle JE, Collart C, et al. SIP1, a novel zinc finger/homeodomain repressor, interacts with Smad proteins and binds to 5′-CACCT sequences in candidate target genes. J Biol Chem 1999;274:20489–98.
84. Brooks AS, Bertoli-Avella AM, Burzynski GM, et al. Homozygous nonsense mutations in *KIAA1279* are associated with malformations of the central and enteric nervous systems. Am J Hum Genet 2005;77:120–6.
85. Trang H, Dehan M, Beaufils F, et al. The French Congenital Central Hypoventilation Syndrome Registry: General data, phenotype, and genotype. Chest 2005;127:72–9.
86. Vanderlaan M, Holbrook CR, Wang M, et al. Epidemiologic survey of 196 patients with congenital central hypoventilation syndrome. Pediatr Pulmonol 2004;37:217–29.
87. Pattyn A, Morin X, Cremer H, et al. The homeobox gene Phox2b is essential for the development of autonomic neural crest derivatives. Nature 1999;399:366–70.
88. Teitelbaum DH, Caniano DA, Qualman SJ. The pathophysiology of Hirschsprung's-associated enterocolitis: Importance of histologic correlates. J Pediatr Surg 1989;24:1271–7.
89. Akkary S, Sahwy E, Kandil W, Hamdy MH. A histochemical study of the mucosubstances of the colon in cases of Hirschsprung's disease with and without enterocolitis. J Pediatr Surg 1981;16:664–8.
90. Klein MD, Philippart AI. Hirschsprung's disease: Three decades' experience at a single institution. J Pediatr Surg 1993;28:1291–3; discussion 3–4.
91. Harrison MW, Deitz DM, Campbell JR, Campbell TJ. Diagnosis and management of Hirschsprung's disease. A 25-year perspective. Am J Surg 1986;152:49–56.
92. Reding R, de Ville de Goyet J, Gosseye S, et al. Hirschsprung's disease: A 20-year experience. J Pediatr Surg 1997;32:1221–5.
93. Klein MD, Coran AG, Wesley, JR, Drongowski RA. Hirschsprung's disease in the newborn. J Pediatr Surg 1984; 19:370–4.
94. Jhaveri MK, Kumar SP. Passage of the first stool in very low birth weight infants. Pediatr 1987;79:1005–7.
95. Kumar SL, Dhanireddy R. Time of first stool in premature infants: Effect of gestational age and illness severity. J Pediatr 1995;127:971–4.
96. Meetze WH, Palazzolo VL, Bowling D, et al. Meconium passage in very-low-birth-weight infants. JPEN J Parenter Enteral Nutr 1993;17:537–40.
97. Swenson O, Sherman JO, Fisher JH. Diagnosis of congenital megacolon: An analysis of 501 patients. J Pediatr Surg 1973;8:587–94.
98. Sarioglu A, Tanyel FC, Buyukpamukcu N, Hicsonmez A. Appendiceal perforation: A potentially lethal initial mode of presentation of Hirschsprung's disease. J Pediatr Surg 1997;32:123–4.
99. Arliss J, Holgersen LO. Neonatal appendiceal perforation and Hirschsprung's disease. J Pediatr Surg 1990;25:694–5.
100. Newman B, Nussbaum A, Kirkpatrick JA, Jr, Colodny A. Appendiceal perforation, pneumoperitoneum, and Hirschsprung's disease. J Pediatr Surg 1988;23:854–6.
101. Newman B, Nussbaum A, Kirkpatrick JA, Jr. Bowel perforation in Hirschsprung's disease. AJR Am J Roentgenol 1987;148:1195–7.
102. Sarioglu A, Tanyel FC, Buyukpamukcu N, Hicsonmez A. Urolithiasis in patients with Hirschsprung's disease. Eur J Pediatr Surg 1997;7:149–51.
103. Dierks SM, Colberg JW. Urinary retention in a child secondary to Hirschsprung's disease. Br J Urol 1997;79:806.
104. Yazbeck S, O'Regan S. Hirschsprung's disease and urinary tract infection: Unrecognized association. Nephron 1986;43:211–3.
105. Sherman JO, Snyder ME, Weitzman JJ, et al. A 40-year multinational retrospective study of 880 Swenson procedures. J Pediatr Surg 1989;24:833–8.
106. Rosenfield NS, Ablow RC, Markowitz RI, et al. Hirschsprung disease: Accuracy of the barium enema examination. Radiol 1984;150:393–400.
107. Smith GH, Cass DT. Infantile Hirschsprung's disease is a barium enema useful? Pediatr Surg Int 1991;6:318.
108. Mishalany HG, Woolley MG. Chronic constipation. Manometric patterns and surgical considerations. Arch Surg 1984;119:1257–9.
109. Meunier P, Marechal JM, Mollard P. Accuracy of the manometric diagnosis of Hirschsprung's disease. J Pediatr Surg 1978;13:411–5.
110. Loening-Baucke VA. Anorectal manometry: Experience with strain gauge pressure transducers for the diagnosis of Hirschsprung's disease. J Pediatr Surg 1983;18:595–600.
111. Tamate S, Shiokawa C, Yamada C, et al. Manometric diagnosis of Hirschsprung's disease in the neonatal period. J Pediatr Surg 1984;19:285–8.
112. Yokoyama J, Namba S, Ihara N, et al. Studies on the rectoanal reflex in children and in experimental animals: An evaluation of neuronal control of the rectoanal reflex. Prog Pediatr Surg 1989;24:5–20.
113. Holschneider AM, Kellner E, Streibl P, Sippell WG. The development of anorectal continence and its significance in the diagnosis of Hirschsprung's disease. J Pediatr Surg 1976;11:151–6.
114. Aldridge RT, Campbell PE. Ganglion cell distribution in the normal rectum and anal canal. A basis for the diagnosis of Hirschsprung's disease by anorectal biopsy. J Pediatr Surg 1968;3:475–90.
115. Rees BI, Azmy A, Nigam M, Lake BD. Complications of rectal suction biopsy. J Pediatr Surg 1983;18:273–5.
116. Dahms B. The gastrointestinal tract. In: Stocker J, and Dehner L, editors. Pediatric Pathology, 2nd edition. Philadelphia: Lippincott Williams and Wilkins, 2001. p 631–704.
117. Kapur RP. Hirschsprung's disease and other enteric dysganglionoses. Crit Rev Clin Lab Sci 1999;36:225–73.
118. Teitelbaum D, Coran AG, Weitzman J, et al. Hirschsprung's disease and related neuromuscular disorders of the intestine. In: James A. O'Neill J, Rowe MI, Gosfeld JL, et al, editors. Pediatric Surgery, 5th edition. St. Louis: Mosby-Year Book, Inc; 1998.
119. Harris P, Zhuo J, Mendelsohn F, Skinner S. Haemodynamic and renal tubular effects of low doses of endothelin in anaesthetized rats. J Physiol 1991;422:25–39.
120. Cilley RE, Statter MB, Hirschl RB, Coran AG. Definitive treatment of Hirschsprung's disease in the newborn with a one-stage procedure. Surgery 1994;115:551–6.
121. Curran TJ, Raffensperger JG. Laparoscopic Swenson pull-through: A comparison with the open procedure. J Pediatr Surg 1996;31:1155–6; discussion 6–7.
122. De La Torre-Mondragon L, Ortega-Salgado JA. Transanal endorectal pull-through for Hirschsprung's disease. J Pediatr Surg 1998;33:1283–6.
123. Teitelbaum DH, Cilley RE, Sherman NJ, et al. A decade of experience with the primary pull-through for Hirschsprung's disease in the newborn period: A multicenter analysis of outcomes. Ann Surg 2000;232:372–80.
124. Bill JAH, Chapman ND. The enterocolitis of Hirschsprung's disease: Its natural history and treatment. Am J Surg 1962;103:70.
125. Ikeda K, Goto S. Diagnosis and treatment of Hirschsprung's disease in Japan. An analysis of 1628 patients. Ann Surg 1984;199:400–5.
126. Coran AG, Teitelbaum DH. Recent advances in the management of Hirschsprung's disease. Am J Surg 2000;180:382–7.
127. Caniano DA, Teitelbaum DH, Qualman SJ. Management of Hirschsprung's disease in children with trisomy 21. Am J Surg 1990;159:402–4.
128. Hackam DJ, Filler RM, Pearl RH. Enterocolitis after the surgical treatment of Hirschsprung's disease: Risk factors and financial impact. J Pediatr Surg 1998;33:830–3.
129. Van Leeuwen K, Teitelbaum DH, Elhalaby EA, Coran AG. Long-term follow-up of redo pull-through procedures for Hirschsprung's disease: Efficacy of the endorectal pull-through. J Pediatr Surg 2000;35:829–33; discussion 33–4.
130. Marty TL, Seo T, Matlak ME, et al. Gastrointestinal function after surgical correction of Hirschsprung's disease: Long-term follow-up in 135 patients. J Pediatr Surg 1995;30:655–8.
131. Holschneider AM, Puri P. Hirschsprung's Disease and Allied Disorders, 2nd edition. In: Holschneider AM, Puri P, editors. Amsterdam: Hardwood Academic Publishers; 2000. p. 457–66.
132. Teitelbaum DH, Coran AG. Reoperative surgery for Hirschsprung's disease. Semin Pediatr Surg 2003;12:124–31.
133. Abbas Banani S, Forootan H. Role of anorectal myectomy after failed endorectal pull-through in Hirschsprung's disease. J Pediatr Surg 1994;29:1307–9.
134. Ludman L, Spitz L, Tsuji H, Pierro A. Hirschsprung's disease: Functional and psychological follow up comparing total colonic and rectosigmoid aganglionosis. Arch Dis Child 2002;86:348–51.
135. Tsuji H, Spitz L, Kiely EM, et al. Management and long-term follow-up of infants with total colonic aganglionosis. J Pediatr Surg 1999;34:158–61; discussion 62.
136. Yanchar NL, Soucy P. Long-term outcome after Hirschsprung's disease: Patients' perspectives. J Pediatr Surg 1999;34:1152–60.
137. Hyman PE. Defecation disorders after surgery for Hirschsprung's disease. J Pediatr Gastroenterol Nur 2005;41:S62–3.
138. Di Lorenzo C, Solzi GF, Flores AF, et al. Colonic motility after surgery for Hirschsprung's disease. Am J Gastroenterol 2000;95:1759–64.
139. Kobayashi H, Hirakawa H, Surana R, et al. Intestinal neuronal dysplasia is a possible cause of persistent bowel symptoms after pull-through operation for Hirschsprung's disease. J Pediatr Surg 1995;30:253–7; discussion 7–9.
140. Fadda B, Maier WA, Meier-Ruge W, et al. Neuronal intestinal dysplasia. Critical 10 years' analysis of clinical and biopsy diagnosis. Zeitschrift fur Kinderchirurgie 1983;38:305–11.
141. Koletzko S, Jesch I, Faus-Kebetaler T, et al. Rectal biopsy for diagnosis of intestinal neuronal dysplasia in children: A prospective multicentre study on interobserver variation and clinical outcome. Gut 1999;44:853–61.
142. Gath R, Goessling A, Keller KM, et al. Analysis of the RET, GDNF, EDN3, and EDNRB genes in patients with intestinal neuronal dysplasia and Hirschsprung's disease. Gut 2001;48:671–5.
143. Rolle U, Piotrowska AP, Nemeth L, Puri P. Altered distribution of interstitial cells of Cajal in Hirschsprung's disease. Archives of Pathology & Laboratory Medicine 2002;126:928–33.
144. Brandi ML, Gagel RF, Angeli A, et al. Guidelines for diagnosis and therapy of MEN type 1 and type 2. J Clin Endocrinol Metab 2001;86:5658–71.

145. Newby DE, Strachan FE, Webb DJ. Abnormal endothelin B receptor vasomotor responses in patients with Hirschsprung's disease. Q J Med 2002;95:159–63.

146. Gariepy CE, Ohuchi T, Williams SC, et al. Salt-sensitive hypertension in endothelin-B receptor-deficient rats. J Clin Invest 2000;105:925–33.

147. Micci MA, Kahrig KM, Simmons RS, et al. Neural stem cell transplantation in the stomach rescues gastric function in neuronal nitric oxide synthase-deficient mice. Gastroenterology 2005;129:1817–24.

148. Kruger GM, Mosher JT, Bixby S, et al. Neural crest stem cells persist in the adult gut but undergo changes in self-renewal, neuronal subtype potential, and factor responsiveness. Neuron 2002;35:657–69.

149. Bixby S, Kruger GM, Mosher JT, et al. Cell-intrinsic differences between stem cells from different regions of the peripheral nervous system regulate the generation of neural diversity. Neuron 2002;35:643–56.

150. Suarez-Rodriguez R, Belkind-Gerson J. Cultured nestin-positive cells from postnatal mouse small bowel differentiate ex vivo into neurons, glia, and smooth muscle. Stem Cells 2004;22:1373–85.

151. Burns AJ. Migration of neural crest-derived enteric nervous system precursor cells to and within the gastrointestinal tract. Int J Dev Biol 2005;49:143–50.

152. Bondurand N, Natarajan D, Barlow A, et al. Maintenance of mammalian enteric nervous system progenitors by *SOX10* and endothelin 3 signalling. Dev 2006;133:2075–86.

153. Srinivasan S, Anitha M, Mwangi S, Heuckeroth RO. Enteric neuroblasts require the phosphatidylinositol 3-kinase/Akt/Forkhead pathway for GDNF-stimulated survival. Mol Cell Neurosci 2005;29:107–19.

154. Kruger GM, Mosher JT, Tsai YH, et al. Temporally distinct requirements for endothelin receptor B in the generation and migration of gut neural crest stem cells. Neuron 2003;40:917–29.

155. Rauch U, Hansgen A, Hagl C, et al. Isolation and cultivation of neuronal precursor cells from the developing human enteric nervous system as a tool for cell therapy in dysganglionosis. Int J Colorectal Dis 2006;21:554–9.

156. Butovsky O, Ziv Y, Schwartz A, et al. Microglia activated by IL-4 or IFN-gamma differentially induce neurogenesis and oligodendrogenesis from adult stem/progenitor cells. Mol Cell Neurosci 2006;31:149–60.

157. Sheng WS, Hu S, Ni HT, et al. TNF–induced chemokine production and apoptosis in human neural precursor cells. J Leukocyte Biol 2005;78:1233–41.

24.2c. Other Dysmotilities Including Chronic Intestinal Pseudo-Obstruction Syndrome

Sibylle Koletzko, MD
Andrea Schwarzer, MD

The motility of the small and large intestine is a function of the intestinal smooth muscle, which is controlled by the enteric nervous system (ENS) and the interstitial cells of Cajal (ICC). Gastrointestinal (GI) motility is modulated by the extrinsic input from the autonomic (parasympathetic vagal and sacral and thoracolumbar sympathetic) and central nervous system (CNS), from GI hormones, and the immune system. Any disturbances of one or more of these systems may lead to dysmotility, which may be restricted to a particular bowel segment or may involve the entire gut, with or without the esophagus and stomach. The first-half of this chapter is a systematic review of intestinal motility disorders excluding functional disorders and Hirschsprung's disease in its isolated or syndromatic form. Some of these entities have only been described in a few patients. A particular pattern of intestinal and extraintestinal manifestation may be the hint for further classification, if a complete histopathology is not available. Most enteric neuropathies and myopathies show a wide spectrum of clinical manifestations and many of them may present as chronic intestinal pseudo-obstruction (CIP). Therefore, CIP is not a diagnosis, but a symptom of different dysmotility disorders and the most severe form of manifestation. The diagnostic and therapeutic approach of a child presenting with CIP is one of the most challenging tasks for a pediatric gastroenterologist. After the description of the different disease entities, the reader may find at the end of this chapter some practical help how to approach a child with CIP. Although the therapeutic options are limited and often not specific to the underlying etiopathology, the aim should always be to classify as good as possible. Only the assignment to a certain diagnosis enables the physician to give a more precise prognosis and for genetic counseling.

Dysmotility diseases are classified into primary visceral myopathies, primary visceral neuropathies, and secondary to toxic, metabolic, infectious, or other systemic disorders affecting the smooth muscle or the enteric or extrinsic nervous system. Some diseases do not fit into this rough classification because both the muscle layer and the enteric nervous plexuses are involved either primarily, as in some of the mitochondrial disorders, or secondarily, as in

fibrosis or ischemia. The term "idiopathic" is applied if the disorder does not fulfill the criteria of a recognizable genetic syndrome, if there is no apparent underlying disease, and if affected tissue is unavailable for investigation or appears normal under histologic examination.

The classification of dysmotility disorders has been changed over the years, because new techniques or molecular genetics identified new disorders that have been only described by clinical symptoms or histopathology. More sophisticated techniques have been applied, including imaging techniques, different types of fixation, cutting, and staining of the tissue, light and transmission electron microscopy, and several enzyme histochemical and immunohistochemical methods using a wide variety of markers. Applying these new techniques identified abnormalities of the intestinal muscle layers in enteric neuropathies like aganglionosis or hypoganglionosis with deficiency of ICCs and enteric glial cells (EGC).[1-3] Secondary involvement of the smooth muscle in neuropathies and vice versa seems to be a common phenomenon, which makes the classification into neuropathies and myopathies even more difficult.

Another problem of classifying the motility disorders by histopathologic findings is the fact that interpretation of morphologic features for histologic diagnosis is a subjective integrating process that is influenced by an individual's expertise and subject to marked interobserver variation.[4] Comparisons of morphologic findings between single case reports or series of patients are therefore difficult to interpret. Secondary phenomena owing to severe chronic bowel dilatation or therapeutic interventions (ie, drugs or surgery interrupting the flow of the chyme) need to be distinguished from primary pathology. More data are now available on the normal postnatal maturation and appearance of the ENS in premature infants and during early childhood. These data indicate that not all enteric nerve cells are morphologically mature at birth, and maturation continues for at least the first 2 to 4 years of life.[5-7] With the new knowledge, it became clear that findings are now considered a variation of normal, which have been previously identified as a pathologic entity.[7] In clinical practice, histologic classification of neuromuscular disorders of the gut is also

hampered by the fact that full-thickness biopsies are usually required for the pathomorphologic diagnosis. Exceptions are Hirschsprung's disease and a few other neuropathies in which a definite histopathologic diagnosis can be made from rectal suction or deep forceps biopsies. After exclusion of aganglionosis, the knowledge of the exact neuromuscular classification hardly alters therapeutic management in most affected children with primary dysmotility disorders. Therefore, full-thickness bowel biopsies are usually not justified unless an operation is necessary for other clinical indications (ie, ileostomy and resection).

Beside, histopathology, classification has also been attempted based on clinical phenotypes such as age at onset, bowel and bladder involvement, or mode of inheritance. This approach can be very misleading, but it is helpful in a few cases with distinguished concurrent extraintestinal features. For example, the megacystis-microcolon-intestinal hypoperistalsis syndrome (MMIHS) describes a certain phenotype, but histopathologic investigations reveal myopathic changes in most children, myopathic and neuropathic changes in other children, or both. In some children, no histologic abnormalities are found. Progress in molecular genetics has been proven to be very helpful to define additional familial forms of GI motility disorders.

CLINICAL MANIFESTATIONS OF GI DYSMOTILITY

Clinical symptoms are variable and often nonspecific. The location of the affected bowel (diffuse or segmental) seems a more important determinant of clinical manifestation than the underlying cause. Within the same family with a defined genetic disorder, a spectrum of symptoms may occur, ranging from none to CIP, which represents the extreme end of the clinical manifestation. Primary and secondary neuromuscular disorders of the intestine may present at any age, but most children become symptomatic during the neonatal period or early infancy. In congenital disorders, antenatal ultrasonography may show dilated bladder and/or bowel loops with or without polyhydramnios.[8-11] After birth, the main symptoms are bilious vomiting, failure to pass meconium, severe constipation, and a distended abdomen. Differentiation from mechanical obstruction is often very difficult, and many of these infants undergo exploratory laparotomy. If the bladder is involved, failure to void and urinary infection owing to incomplete emptying may be the initial symptoms. Megacystis associated with motility disorders make the diagnosis easier and may avoid unjustified exploratory laparotomy. Common symptoms reported in children with an acquired dysmotility disorder include abdominal distention, constipation, vomiting, failure to thrive, dyspepsia, and abdominal pain. Intermittent diarrhea occurs in some children as a result of bacterial overgrowth and malabsorption. CIP is the most severe form of manifestation of gut dysmotility, but not a specific disease. CIP can occur in most intestinal neuromuscular diseases. The diagnostic and therapeutic approach of this disabling condition is discussed below.

DISORDERS OF THE INTESTINAL SMOOTH MUSCLE

Intestinal dysmotilities are less frequently caused by smooth muscle than by neural disorders. In general, symptoms are more severe, and the prognosis is worse in primary myopathies compared with primary neuropathies. Most affected children develop symptoms at birth or shortly thereafter. Definite diagnosis requires careful study of the full thickness of the GI wall with sectioning across muscle fibers. In addition to conventional staining with hematoxylin/eosin and Masson's trichrome, antibodies against smooth muscle α-actin (α-SMA), smooth muscle myosin heavy chain, novel markers smoothelin, and histone deacetylase 8 (HDAC8) may be helpful to reveal abnormalities of the intestinal musculature in both myopathies and neuropathies.[2,12]

In cases in which no tissue is available for investigation, characteristic myopathic pattern on antroduodenal manometry may support the diagnosis. The term "hollow visceral myopathy" is used when smooth muscle of both the GI and the urinary tract is affected.

Primary Visceral Myopathies (Familial Visceral Myopathy)

Primary disorders of the intestinal smooth muscle represent abnormalities in morphogenesis, resulting in alterations in intestinal muscle layering (additional muscle coat or an absence of a muscle layer) or intrinsic myocyte defects comprising varying degrees of fibrosis, myocyte atrophy, vacuolation, or an altered contractile protein. Smith and Milla identified five histologic phenotypes of smooth muscle disease in full-thickness biopsies from children with functional obstruction using routine microscopy, histochemistry, immunohistochemistry with monoclonal antibodies against different neural and smooth muscle markers, and electron microscopy.[13] Routine microscopy on paraffin sections of the smooth muscle was

abnormal in only 15 of 27 patients. In the remaining patients, myopathic changes would have been missed without application of other techniques. Twenty-five of the children had a primary myopathy, and two had an acquired enteric myopathic disorder.

Clinically, primary visceral myopathies occur as familial genetic diseases with a defined mode of inheritance or as sporadic cases. Four types of familial visceral myopathies (FVMs) have been described so far. They may begin at any age, but particularly in the second decade; therefore, they should be considered when symptoms begin in school-age children. A few families with probable hereditary forms of infantile or childhood visceral myopathies have been reported; all affected children presented at birth, during infancy, or during early childhood.[14]

Familiar Visceral Myopathy Type 1. Familial occurrence of megaduodenum resembling type 1 FVM was first described in 1938 in a German family.[15] Since then, several families have been reported and confirmed that type 1 FVM is transmitted by an autosomal dominant inheritance, although there is female predominance in frequency and severity.[14,15] The disease is characterized by esophageal dilatation, megaduodenum, and an elongated, redundant, usually dilated colon.[16] Barium studies show an aperistaltic esophagus and often normal gastric emptying but a flaccid and dilated duodenum with prolonged retention of barium (up to 19 days in one case).[17] The small intestinal caliber is normal, except the proximal jejunum, which may be dilated. The bladder is affected in about half of the cases, but megacystis is often asymptomatic.

Most patients, especially females, become symptomatic around puberty with recurrent abdominal pain, nausea, vomiting, heartburn, and severe constipation or, occasionally, diarrhea. Some affected family members remain asymptomatic despite abnormal barium studies. Mydriasis is common in type 1 FVM.

Schuffler and Pope investigated full-thickness intestinal biopsies of a 15-year-old girl with type 1 FVM by using different staining methods, including Masson's trichrome in addition to electron microscopy. They observed marked thinning and degeneration and vacuolation of smooth muscle with replacement by fibrous tissue.[14]

Treatment that depends on the severity of symptoms includes dietary modification with a diet low in fat, fiber, and lactose and intermittent use of antibiotics to treat bacterial overgrowth. Neostigmine was helpful in one patient to improve severe constipation, although systemic side effects limit the use of the drug.[16] Surgical treatment is indicated in patients which are refractory to dietary and medical management and in cases with pseudo-obstruction. Side-to-side duodenojejunostomy to drain the duodenum or partial duodenal resection below the papilla of Vater and anastomosis with the jejunum have benefited in carefully selected patients.[17,18]

Mitochondrial Neurogastrointestinal Encephalomyopathy (Familiar Visceral Myopathy Type 2). Mitochondrial neurogastrointestinal encephalomyopathy (MNGIE) forms part of a heterogeneous group of disorders that result from structural, biochemical, or genetic derangements of mitochondria. First reported as oculogastrointestinal muscular dystrophy or polyneuropathy-ophthalmoplegia-leukoencephalopathy-intestinal-pseudo-obstruction syndrome (POLIP syndrome), this was renamed MNGIE. MNGIE is an autosomal recessive multisystem disorder caused by thymidine phosphorylase (TP) deficiency, resulting in severe GI dysmotiltiy and skeletal muscles abnormalities.[19] A total of 72 cases have been reported.[20] Phenotypic features include external ophthalmoplegia with ptosis and diplopia (91%), hearing loss (55%), leucencephalopathy (96%), cardiac conduction defect, mild muscular atrophy, and dilatation of the entire GI tract with scattered small-bowel diverticula on the mesenteric border.[21] They may be responsible for life-threatening complications such as perforation or abscesses.[20] GI symptoms of this progressive and potentially lethal disorder may develop during teenage years with dysphagia, dyspepsia due to gastroparesis, heartburn, abdominal pain, chronic diarrhea, and weight loss. Skeletal muscle biopsy specimens (Gomori trichrome stain) show megamitochondria at a subsacolemmal location giving the appearance of "ragged" red fibers that are typical of mitochondrial myopathies.[22] Different mutations mapped to locus 22q13.32qter of the TP gene have been reported, including missense, splice site, microdeletions, and nucleotide insertion.[23-26] TP is a nuclear encoded enzyme catalyzing phosphorolysis of thymidine to thymine and deoxyribose 1-phosphate. Lack of TP activity leads to accumulation of thymidine and deoxyuridine. This results in mitochondrial DNA (mtDNA) alterations with deletion, depletion, and somatic point mutations. Biochemical assays with the determination of plasma nucleosides thymidine and deoxyuridine in plasma or TP enzyme activity in the buffy coat have been suggested to confirm the diagnosis of patients with the clinical suspicion of MNGIE.[26]

Diagnostic criteria include GI dysmotility, cachexia, ptosis, external ophthalmoparesis, peripheral neuropathy, and leucoencephalopathy. Lactate and thymidine levels are elevated in about three-quarters of the patients.[20] A deficiency of cytochrome c oxidase in the muscle fibers has been demonstrated. The histologic features of the GI smooth muscle are similar to those of type 1 FVM; however, some patients also showed signs of intestinal neuropathy or a mixed myopathic–neuropathic pattern.[22] The mitochondrial abnormalities in the gut are seen by electron microscopy, both in the muscle cell and in the ganglion cells and are similar to those observed in skeletal muscle of patients affected by mtDNA depletion, which was confined to the external layer of muscularis propria in one patient.[27] A single case of MNGIE with a homozygous splice site mutation in TP; but with lack of skeletal muscle involvement has been reported.[24]

The prognosis is poor with CIP in the majority of cases. Most patients require total parenteral nutrition (TPN) because neither medical nor surgical treatment is effective.[28,29]

Other disorders of oxidative phosphorylation may also show GI dysmotility, this includes Leigh syndrome (subacute necrotizing encephalomyelopathy), Kearns-Sayre syndrome (chronic progressive external ophthalmogplegia, atypical pigmentary retinopathy, ataxia, and heart block), Pearson's marrow-pancreas syndrome (pancreatic exocrine insufficiency, Fanconi anemia, and hepatic dysfunction) and mitochondrial encephalopathy, lactic acidosis and stroke-like episodes (MELAS syndrome).[30]

Familiar Visceral Myopathy Type 3. Anuras and colleagues reported four siblings with dilatation of the entire GI tract but no extraintestinal manifestations.[31] One of the siblings died at the age of 7 years with intestinal obstruction; the others became symptomatic during adulthood. The prognosis of this autosomal recessive disorder is poor.

Familiar Visceral Myopathy Type 4. Two families have been described with this type 4 FVM, which is characterized by gastroparesis, a tubular narrow small intestine, and a normal esophagus and colon.[32,33] Symptoms, including vomiting, abdominal pain and distention, and diarrhea, occurred as early as 2 years of age. The hypertrophy of circular muscle layer produces the tubular narrowing of the small intestine. An autosomal recessive trait is assumed because in one family two siblings and in the other family three siblings were affected.

Familial Childhood Visceral Myopathy with Diffuse Abnormal Muscle Layering, Short Gut, and Malrotation. Three related males have been described with this disorder: the index case, his half-brother from the same mother, and his maternal uncle, suggesting an X-linked inheritance.[13] All presented during the neonatal period with vomiting and abdominal distention. All had short gut and malrotation. The most striking histologic finding was an extracircular muscle coat between the outer and inner layer of the muscularis propria; the myenteric plexus appeared to be embedded within them.

Sporadic Infantile or Childhood Visceral Myopathy. Most cases occur sporadically, but new dominant mutations may be responsible for some.[11] In families with several members affected, a dominant gene with variable expressivity and incomplete penetrance, or an autosomal recessive inheritance, is possible.[11,34] Most affected children develop symptoms at birth or within the first year, including severe constipation, bowel dilatation, and abdominal distention (Figure 1). Failure to thrive and malnutrition are common. When the disease progresses to CIP, most patients depend on long-term parenteral nutrition (PN) or require bowel transplant. Distal to the esophagus, the entire GI tract is affected and markedly dilated.

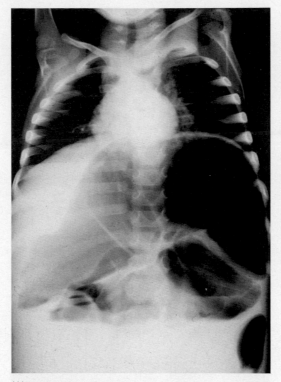 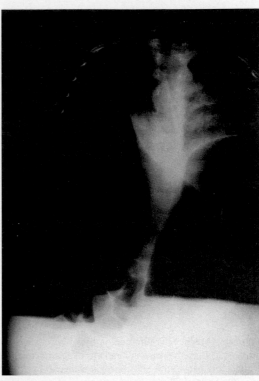

(A) (B)

Figure 1 Sporadic form of visceral myopathy of the entire bowel and urinary tract involvement. The boy presented at birth with a distended abdomen and chronic intestinal pseudo-obstruction. Abdominal radiographs at 2 years (A) and 3.5 years of age (B).

Almost all patients have involvement of the urinary tract system with megaureters and megacystis (hollow visceral myopathy).[11,35] Microscopic findings from the small and large bowel reveal gross fibrosis of the muscularis propria identified with the Masson trichrome staining and profound atrophy of the smooth muscle cells,[36] similar to those from adults with familial and sporadic forms of visceral myopathy.[37,38] In some sporadic cases, α-actin deficiency could be shown.[39] Smith and Milla related these changes to an intrinsic myocyte defect and/or changes in the extracellular matrix. Using different staining techniques, they distinguished two subtypes: a myopathy with autophagic activity and a pink blush myopathy with nuclear crowding.[13] The prognosis is poor in patients with diffuse disease; many die during childhood owing to complications of malnutrition or long-term TPN.[11,35] Some patients tolerate oral feeding and survive into adulthood.

African Degenerative Leiomyopathy. This disease is now recognized as a distinctive, nonfamilial form of degenerative visceral myopathy of uncertain etiology that occurs largely in Africa (particularly southern, eastern, and central Africa). Histologic features include atrophy of myocytes with vacuolated cytoplasm, extracellular edema, and gross fibrous replacement in the circular muscle layer.[36,40] Neuronal loss was absent, but hyperplasia of the myenteric plexus was observed in some cases. Bowel dilatation with severe constipation and pseudo-obstruction developed after the age of 6 months, with a mean age of presentation of 9.5 years.[36] The bladder was affected in about 10% of the patients.

Therapy included neostigmine, a low-residue diet, laxatives, enemas, and surgical intervention. Steroids or another immunosuppressive treatment has not been tried.

Megacystis-Microcolon-Intestinal Hypoperistalsis Syndrome. This most severe form of pseudo-obstruction was first described in 1976 by Berdon and colleagues[41] and more than 90 cases have been reported to date. MMIHS affects female infants four times more often than males.[10] In some cases, the syndrome can be detected by prenatal ultrasound scans showing megacystis, hydronephrosis with hydroureter, and/or bowel abnormalities or gastric distention.[10] Increased concentrations of digestive enzymes in the amniotic fluid have been reported in 8/10 cases with MMIHS compared to only 7 of 63 controls with megabladder of another origin.[42]

The syndrome is identified by a marked, nonobstructive bladder enlargement, a dilated aperistaltic proximal small bowel, a narrowed distal small bowel, and a malrotated microcolon located entirely on the left side of the abdomen[41] (Figure 2A to C). Occasionally, a megaesophagus is associated.[43] The intestinal length is shortened to up to one-third of normal. MMIHS is usually caused by a myopathy with vacuolar degenerative changes of the smooth muscle cells.[44] However, the phenotype can also be a manifestation of a neuropathy with hypo- or hyperganglionosis and giant ganglia, indicating genetic heterogeneity. Based on findings from affected siblings, an autosomal recessive pattern of inheritance has been suggested in some families.[45,46] However, most cases are sporadic.

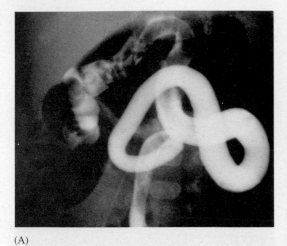

(A)

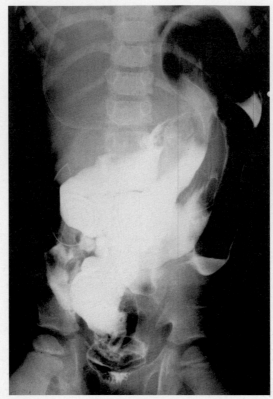

(B)

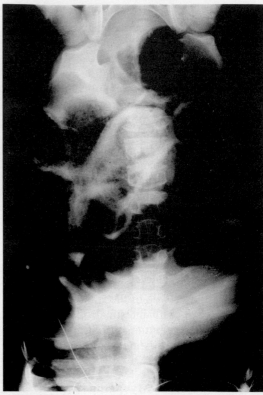

(C)

Figure 2 Megacystis-microcolon-hypoperistalsis syndrome. (A) Barium enema at 2 months of age: microcolon without any haustration. (B) Barium enema at 3 years of age. (C) Abdominal radiograph at 6 years of age. By that time girl had developed a megacolon. She died at 10 years of age. (With courtesy Prof. Dr Karl Schneider.)

There is now some indication that the absence of the α3 subunit containing nicotinic acetylcholine receptor plays a role in this congenital disorder. The neuronal nicotinic acetylcholine receptor subunits are widely expressed throughout the central, peripheral, and autonomous nervous systems. They are pentamers made up by at least eight α subunits (α2 to α9) and three β subunits (β2 to β4) encoded by 11 distinct genes. Transgenic mice lacking the α3 or both β2 and β4 subunits show some of the phenotypic features of MMIHS. Richardson and colleagues used in situ hybridization and immunocytochemistry to study the expression of this subunit in tissue from 10 patients with MMIHS and 12 control children.[47] They found a wide distribution of α3 messenger ribonucleic acid in the enteric ganglion cells, smooth muscle, and epithelium of normal small bowel but not in MMIHS patients.[47] However, in affected individuals with MMIHS and/or their parents, no loss of function mutations have been identified to date within the genes encoding for α3 or β3 subunit.[48]

After birth, the children develop massive abdominal distention, which is often relieved when a huge bladder, which may contain several hundred milliliters of urine, is catheterized. Most patients require several operations on the GI and urinary tract and continue to remain dependent on PN. The prognosis is poor because there is no effective medical treatment. Most children die within the first year of life owing to renal insufficiency, postoperative complications, or sepsis.[45] No patient has reached adulthood. Bowel transplant may be an option for some children.[49,50]

The MMIHS must be differentiated from the prune-belly sequence owing to early intrauterine urethral obstruction. This disorder affects predominantly male infants, who present with a dilated abdomen, constipation, hydronephrosis, megacystis, and often intestinal malrotation, but no intestinal hypoperistalsis or microcolon.

Systemic Disorders Involving the Intestinal Smooth Muscle (Secondary Myopathies)

Most secondary myopathies have been described in adults because it may take several years of a disease process such as a connective tissue disorder until the intestinal smooth muscle layer is damaged. An exception is the autoimmune enteric leiomyositis, which may occur in any age, even young children.[51] With modern histologic techniques and the availability of intestinal manometry, secondary myopathies are recognized even in young children. It is important to identify these entities because sometimes medical treatment can achieve symptomatic improvement and prevent secondary complications or progression of the disease process.

Connective Tissue Disorders. Scleroderma or progressive systemic sclerosis is a systemic disease characterized by excessive deposition of collagen and other matrix elements by fibroblasts in the skin and, in the systemic form, in multiple internal organs. It is associated with prominent and often severe alterations of the microvasculature, the autonomic nervous system, and the immune system. GI dysmotility is prevalent in 90% with symptoms of clinical relevance and in at least 50% of all patients with systemic sclerosis.[52] It affects less often and later in patients with the limited cutaneous systemic sclerosis, the CREST variant (calcinosis, Raynaud's phenomenon, esophageal dysmotility, sclerodactyly, and telangiectasias). The esophagus is the most commonly affected organ, with 75 to 90% of all patients showing abnormalities on esophageal motility testing. Gastroesophageal reflux disease (GERD) is a problem in children and adolescents with scleroderma and CREST syndrome.[53] Involvement of the anorectum is the next most frequent manifestation (50 to 70%), followed by small-bowel hypomotility in 40%. In spite of severe dysmotilities, clinical symptoms may be mild or absent owing to a concurrent visceral sensory neuropathy.

The lesions of scleroderma are similar throughout the GI tract, with atrophy and fragmentation of the muscularis propria, collagen infiltration, and fibrosis in the late stage of the disease. The findings are more marked in the circular than in the longitudinal layer. The same histologic findings have been reported in adults and even in a child with intestinal myopathy, who did not have any cutaneous manifestations of scleroderma.[54]

Symptoms of small-bowel involvement of scleroderma include nausea, vomiting, distention, abdominal cramps, diarrhea with malabsorption, or severe slow-transit constipation if the colon is markedly affected. Fecal incontinence is the most common colonic presentation of systemic sclerosis. Episodes of pseudo-obstruction occur only in patients with advanced systemic sclerosis. Manometric studies in patients with gastric and intestinal involvement of scleroderma may show a complete absence of the migrating motor complex (MMC), which predisposes the patient to bacterial overgrowth and bezoars formation.

Therapy includes dietary recommendations (avoidance of fatty and large meals, high residue diet) and lifestyle changes (no smoking and raise the head of bed) and medications, rarely surgery. High-dose PPIs is essential for treatment of GERD. Prokinetics are helpful for gastroparesis (erythromycin and domperidone) or delayed bowel transit (metoclopramide and tegaserod).[52] In the early stage of the disease with predominant neuropathic impairment, MMCs can be generated by the long-acting somatostatin analog octreotide, the cholinergic agonist cisapride, or the motilin agonist erythromycin.[55] Antibiotics (metronidazole) against bacterial overgrowth, loperamide in cases of diarrhea, and macrogol (polyethylenglycol 3300) with sufficient fluid in constipated patients are other supportive measures.

GI dysmotilities, including CIP owing to progressive atrophy and fibrosis of the intestinal smooth muscle, have occasionally been reported in patients with collagen vascular diseases such as dermatomyositis, polymyositis, or mixed connective tissue disease,[56,57] and in Ehlers-Danlos syndrome. Smooth muscle dysfunction with bowel dilatation can also result from systemic lupus erythematosus–induced vasculitis.[58]

Chronic Enteric Myositis and Autoimmune Myopathy. Infiltration of intestinal smooth muscle layer by lymphocytes is found in Crohn's disease and other forms of chronic intestinal inflammation associated with altered motility.

Acquired myositis of the muscularis propria was reported in a total of six young children between 0.5 and 5 years of age[13,51,59–61] and a 16-year-old girl[62] who presented with functional intestinal obstruction. Antibodies against smooth muscle were detected in three of the patients, indicating an autoimmune process. Dense lymphocytic infiltrates, mainly of CD8[+] T cells, were found in the muscular layers along the large and small intestine on full-thickness biopsies. With progress of the disease, an increasing fibrosis and atrophy of the muscularis propria with diminution of the myenteric plexus were noted in some cases. Three cases developed the disease after an acute gastroenteritis. One of the cases, a 5-year-old girl developed the myositis with signs of intestinal pseudo-obstruction 3 years after autoimmune hepatitis type 1 had been diagnosed.[51] A rapid diagnosis with laparoscopic-assisted full-thickness biopsies is crucial for successful treatment, because combined immunosuppressive therapy including different combinations of prednisolone, budesonide, azathioprine, and tacrolimus were successful in most cases and allowed weaning off PN.

Myotonic Muscular Dystrophy. Myotonic muscular dystrophy is a progressive systemic disease characterized by myotonia and wasting of skeletal muscle. The major features of the congenital form of the disease are reduced fetal movements and polyhydramnios, severe muscular hypotonia, facial diplegia, respiratory insufficiency, difficulties in sucking and swallowing, and skeletal anomalies such as talipes equinovarus. Cataracts and endocrine disturbances, which are typical for the adult form of the disease, are not found in infants and young children. Involvement of the smooth muscle of various organs, including the GI tract and the bladder, is well documented.

Histologic studies of small intestinal and colonic smooth muscle have shown similar changes to those described in dystrophic skeletal muscle, with swollen, partially destroyed smooth muscle cells that are progressively replaced by fat. Motor abnormalities are found in the entire GI tract, from the esophagus to the anal sphincter. GI symptoms with dysphagia, abdominal cramping, diarrhea, malabsorption, or severe constipation are frequent and may precede other clinical manifestations of the disease for years. Lenard and colleagues reported on two brothers whose mother and maternal grandmother were affected by the adult form of the disease.[63] The younger brother, who presented with typical features of congenital myotonic dystrophy at birth, developed severe constipation and megacolon during the second year of life. The presenting symptoms of the older brother were repeated episodes of pseudo-obstruction in the neonatal period and diarrhea, vomiting, and abdominal distention during the first 2 years of life. Thereafter, he suffered from severe constipation with encopresis owing to megacolon. Repeated electromyographic examinations between 2 and 6 years of age were normal, and the first myotonic tracing was obtained when he was 8 years of age.

Duchenne's Muscular Dystrophy. Duchenne's muscular dystrophy is an X-linked disorder that causes skeletal and cardiac muscle degeneration leading to progressive weakness and death, usually from respiratory failure. Histologic studies of skeletal muscle show myofiber degeneration accompanied by necrosis and accumulation of fat and connective tissue and hypertrophy of the remaining muscle fibers. The cause of the disease is a deficiency of dystrophin, which has also been identified in the heart and in smooth muscle. Visceral smooth muscle involvement of the GI tract can be detected by manometry with a typical myopathic pattern in many children, even in those who have only minimal skeletal muscle symptoms and an absence of GI dysfunction. Symptoms such as diarrhea, constipation, and abdominal cramping may be related to dysmotility of the small and large intestine. CIP as a complication of Duchenne's muscular dystrophy is rare.[64]

DISORDERS OF THE ENTERIC AND AUTONOMOUS NERVOUS SYSTEM

The ENS is a collection of neurons in the GI tract, which has been referred to as the "brain of the gut." It can function independently of the CNS. The cell bodies of the ENS are grouped into small ganglia that are connected by bundles of nerve processes forming two major plexus. The myenteric (or Auerbach's) plexus is located between the longitudinal and circular muscle layers and primarily provide them with motor innervation. The submucous (or Meissner's) plexus, which lies in the submucosa between the circular muscle layer and the muscularis mucosae, is important in regulating secretory control. The ganglia of the plexus consist of tightly packed nerve cell bodies,

terminal bundles of nerve fibers, and glial cells, which even outnumber enteric neurons. There are numerous projections between the two plexuses, and both are connected to the central autonomic neural network in the CNS by parasympathetic and sympathetic nerves.[65] Based on histochemical and electrophysiological properties, the neurons of the ENS can be classified into functionally distinct subpopulations, including intrinsic primary afferent neurons, interneurons, motor neurons, and secretomotor and vasomotor neurons.

The ENS controls the segmental and forward propagating contractions, the exocrine and the endocrine secretions, the microcirculation, and the immune and inflammatory processes in the GI tract. Both quantitative (eg, hypo- or hyperganglionosis or aganglionosis) and qualitative abnormalities (ie, degeneration, immaturity, and intranuclear inclusions) of the ENS have been identified using different staining methods. In children, the results should be interpreted with respect to age because there are notable postnatal alterations in the myenteric plexus with a steep decline of nerve cell density.[6,7,66]

Staining for the different neurotransmitters identified different disorders, in which the loss of intrinsic inhibitory neurons, such as NO, VIP, or somatostatin, have been described. These disorders may be primary and confined to dysfunction of sphincteric regions like achalasia or infantile hypertrophy of the pylorus, or acquired neurotransmitter disorders. This has been particularly discussed for adults[67] and partly also in children[68] with slow-transit constipation. However, it remains uncertain whether the dysmotility disorder is related to the decreased neuron transmitters.[67]

Specific neuronal abnormalities have not been linked to specific clinical symptoms, making it difficult for a patient to be classified into any specific category. Combined clinical and histopathologic studies may enable a more precise classification. Most patients have disturbances in GI transit and functional obstruction from infancy. Excessive intestinal secretion or other features of ENS dysfunction often remain clinically unrecognized. Visceral neuropathies are called diffuse if the entire small and large intestine is affected or segmental with only certain parts of the bowel being involved. Apart from aganglionosis only a few visceral neuropathies (ie, ganglioneuromatosis)[69] or neuronal intranuclear inclusion neuropathy[70] can be classified by investigating only the submucous plexus in specimens obtained from rectal suction or deep forceps biopsies.[9]

Intestinal Neuronal Dysplasia

Intestinal neuronal dysplasia (IND) is a term that has been used over the last decades to describe different quantitative (ie, hypo- and hyperganglionosis) and qualitative (ie, immature or heterotopic ganglion cells) abnormalities of the myenteric or submucous plexus or both. The term has raised confusion and controversy among clinicians and pathologists. IND has been observed in an isolated form and proximal to an aganglionic segment. It has been reported in all age groups, mostly infants, but also in adults with chronic constipation not dating back into childhood.[71] It was first considered to be a developmental defect of the submucous plexus,[72] but others suggested that some of the histologic features may be secondary to functional or mechanical obstruction.[73] Other intra- and extraintestinal anomalies are found in a high percentage of children diagnosed to have IND.[74] Diagnosed often in Switzerland and Germany[4,75] IND was rarely reported in British or North American series.[76–78] One of the main criteria of IND, the presence of giant ganglia in the submucous plexus defined as more than eight ganglion cells per ganglion[79] has been considered a normal finding of the enteric plexus in patients without any gut dysmotility.[7,80] The confusion was complete when IND was used not only as a histologic description, but also as a clinical diagnosis. Although neither retrospective nor prospective studies showed a correlation between the morphologic features of IND and symptoms or long-term outcome, surgical procedures were recommended. Sphinctermyectomies and bowel resections have been performed in both children and adults with uncomplicated constipation who were found to have IND on intestinal biopsies. The histologic definitions of IND have changed considerably over time, and this may be responsible for some of the discrepancies. However, even when the same criteria for the diagnosis of IND were applied to a prospective study of rectal biopsies, the interobserver variation was enormous and close to chance agreement.[4] In this study, 377 coded specimens from 108 children, aged 4 days to 15 years with intestinal dysmotilities, were judged for 20 histologic features and a final diagnosis by three pathologists, who had previously participated in a consensus meeting on diagnostic guidelines. There was complete agreement for the diagnosis of Hirschsprung's disease, but in only 14% of the remaining children was there a concordant diagnosis by the pathologists. The criteria were significantly more often fulfilled in infants compared with older children. Furthermore, the diagnosis of IND had no prognostic value for the outcome in constipated children, as assessed by clinical symptoms 1 year after the biopsies.[4] Most recently, Meier-Ruge suggested more strict criteria for the diagnosis of IND with more than 20% of submucosal ganglia containing more than 8 nerve cells (giant ganglia) and that at least 30 sections should be viewed.[81] In his most recent paper, he concluded that the diagnosis should not be made prior to 1 year of age. He now considers IND type B as a mild form of gut dysmotility and that the morphologic abnormalities in isolated cases usually disappear spontaneously by 4 years of age.[82]

Genetic studies in children with histologic features of IND could not identify any mutations in the coding regions of the *RET, GDNF, EDNRB*, and *EDN3* genes.[83] Mice with mutations of Hox11L1, a homeobox gene involved in nervous system development, show a megacolon with ENS pathology with increased neuron numbers in the colon.[84] The human homolog of this gene has been found on chromosome 2p13.1 but, to date, no patients with GI motility disorder and proposed histologic features of IND have been found to have a mutation of this possible candidate gene.[85]

Because the term IND type B describes neither a specific histologic nor a clinical entity in infants and children, the term should not be used until better defined. IND type A has not been reported since the first descriptions and is even less classified. For these reasons, IND has not been included in Table 2 and is not further discussed in this chapter.

Primary Visceral Neuropathies

Primary visceral neuropathies can be subdivided into familial visceral neuropathies, which follow a certain trait of inheritance, and sporadic cases characterized by distinct morphologic and clinical findings. In clinical practice, many neuropathic motility disorders remain unclassified (idiopathic).

Familial Visceral Neuropathy

Familial Visceral Neuropathy without Extraintestinal Manifestations. This is an autosomal dominant disorder that affects mainly the large and distal part of the small bowel.[86] Age at onset differs within the same family, but symptoms develop after infancy. Severe slow-transit constipation, with or without intermittent diarrhea, nausea, abdominal distention, and cramping, is the main complaint. Pseudo-obstructive episodes with severe intestinal dilatation occur in approximately half of the patients and may require colonoscopic decompression. There is no evidence of extrinsic autonomic dysfunction. Histologic findings include a markedly reduced number and degeneration of argyrophilic neurons and nerve fibers of the myenteric plexus, with hypertrophy of the smooth muscle. No Schwann's cell proliferation, intranuclear inclusions, or inflammatory cells are observed. Subtotal colectomy may give transient relief but may accelerate small-bowel disease; therefore, it is contraindicated. Camilleri reported an intestinal pseudo-obstruction without evidence of autonomic or extraintestinal manifestations in mother and daughter.[87] Both patients underwent subtotal small-bowel resection with recurrence of symptoms. Histology revealed reduced numbers of ganglion cells with degeneration of neurons and axons.

Familial Visceral Neuropathy with Neuronal Intranuclear Inclusions and Apoptosis. This neuropathy is an autosomal dominant disorder because it was described in three siblings (2 females and 1 male) and their father[70] and in 10 members of a family in 4 generations.[88] Most patients develop symptoms during childhood. GI symptoms included dysphagia, diarrhea, constipation, and intestinal pseudo-obstruction. Autonomic dysfunction, achalasia or diffuse esophageal spasm, irregular and unresponsive pupils, ataxia, dysarthria, mental retardation, and dementia are part of this neuropathic disease in some but not all of the affected persons indicating marked variation in expression. Characteristic eosinophilic intranuclear inclusions have been identified in the neurons of the degenerated myenteric plexus all along the GI tract.[9,88] The same inclusions are found postmortem in nerve cells of the central and peripheral nervous systems.[89] In some patients, the intranuclear inclusions could be detected within the ganglion cells of the plexus mucous on rectal biopsies. Electron microscopy and histochemistry identified the inclusions as nonviral proteinaceous material without evidence of DNA, RNA, or carbohydrates. Manometric studies showed a typical neuropathic pattern with lack of phase III of the MMC and irregular, nonpropagated contractions in the small intestine. There is no treatment; some patients survive into mid- or late adulthood.[90]

Familial Visceral Neuropathy with Short Bowel, Malrotation, and Pyloric Hypertrophy. This sequence has been described in several families.[91] Symptoms of functional obstruction occur in the neonatal period, and most patients die during the first year of life. Morphologic studies of the bowel showed abnormalities of the myenteric plexus, with shrunken, degenerated neurons, clumped chromatin within the nuclei, and lack of argyrophilic neurons. This syndrome may be inherited in an autosomal recessive pattern because it occurred in siblings of both genders and in families with consanguineous marriages.[91,92] An autosomal dominant pattern was likely in one family with an infected 2-year-old girl, her mother, and her maternal grandfather (personal observation). In addition to malrotation, short bowel, and pyloric hypertrophy, an abnormal ileocecal connection with an absent appendix was noted during laparoscopy in all three. Auricchio and colleagues performed linkage analysis in a family in which, over four generations, only the male members related through female members were affected. The authors assigned the defect to a gene locus on the chromosome Xq28 region, but suggested that the same clinical entity may be associated with different loci.[93] Recently the same group described a 2 bp deletion in exon 2 of the filamin A gene in an affected male who suffered also from CNS involvement.[94] The FLNA mutation was present at the heterozygous state in the carrier females of the family. Interestingly, mutations of the filamin A gene with a loss of function have been associated with X-linked dominant nodular ventricular heterotopia (PVNH), a CNS migration defect that presents with seizures in females and lethality in males. The frameshift mutation is located between two close methionines at the filamin N-terminus and codes for a protein truncated shortly after the first predicted methionine. The authors conclude that the filamin N-terminal region between the initial two methionines is crucial for proper enteric neuron development.

Familial Visceral Neuropathy with Neurologic Involvement. Several families with at least two affected siblings have been reported. Symptoms occurred during early childhood with neuropathic GI dysmotilities and involvement of the peripheral or CNS. The trait of inheritance remains unclear. Faber and colleagues reported two Jewish families of Iranian origin with a progressive sensory and motor peripheral neuropathy, ophthalmoplegia, and hearing loss but no evidence of CNS involvement.[95] The description and combination of the pathologic findings make a mitochondrial disorder likely. Cockel and colleagues described a familial disorder defined by megaduodenum, dilatation of the small bowel, steatorrhea, mental retardation, and calcification in the subcortical white matter of the brain and basal ganglia.[96] The age at onset was during childhood. The myenteric plexus appeared normal on conventional light microscopy, but silver staining revealed a degeneration of argyrophobic cells. A similar case was reported by Navarro and colleagues.[9]

A de novo mutation of the *SOX10* gene with a heterozygous deletion of 1 bp (795delG) in the last coding exon with CIP, peripheral neuropathy with unusual multiplication of nerve fascicles, and deafness since early infancy has been described in an 8-year-old girl.[97]

Familial Visceral Neuropathy (Ganglioneuromatosis) Associated with Multiple Endocrine Neoplasia Type IIB. Of the three different multiple endocrine neoplasia (MEN) type II syndromes (MEN IIA, MEN IIB, and isolated medullary thyroid carcinoma), MEN IIB is the only form that involves the GI tract. The susceptibility gene for these autosomal dominant inherited disorders is the RET proto-oncogene located on chromosome 10q11.2, which encodes a plasma membrane-bound tyrosine kinase enzyme, the RET receptor, which is expressed by neuroendocrine and neural cells, including thyroid C cells, adrenal medullary cells, parasympathetic, sympathetic, and colonic ganglia, cells of the urogenital tract, and parathyroid cells derived from branchial arches. The RET plays an important role in the development, function, and migration of cells of neural crest origin. MEN II is transmitted in an autosomal dominant pattern, and affects approximately 1 in 30,000 individuals; however, only ~5% account for MEN II cases. In MEN IIB, 94% of cases are due to a single identical germline point mutation at codon 918 in exon 16. In the remaining patients, a mutation at codon 883 in exon 15, or compound heterozygous mutations of V804M with Y806C and V804M with S904 C or no RET mutation were found.[98] Approximately 50% of diagnosed cases seem to be due to de novo mutations. In most affected patients, GI dysmotility is the first manifestation of the disease. It is important to be aware of possible other symptoms in combination with the typical features of MEN IIB (Table 1).

The characteristic pathologic finding of intestinal ganglioneuromatosis is an increased density of ganglion cells in the submucous and myenteric plexus, with penetration of hyperplastic nerves into the mucosal zone. Hyperplasia of the ner-

---

Table 1 Features of Multiple Endocrine Neoplasia Type IIB

Gastrointestinal manifestations
  Abdominal distension
  Feeding problems
  Dysphagia
  Vomiting
  Chronic constipation
  Paradoxal diarrhea
  Megacolon
  Intestinal pseudo-obstruction
  Ganglioneuromatosis

Facial abnormalities
  Elongated face
  Thickened and everted upper eyelids
  Prominent eyebrows
  Neuromas on eyelids and conjunctiva
  Thickened corneal nerves
  Thickened lips
  Neuromas of buccal mucosa, tongue, and palate
  High-arched palate

Extraintestinal manifestations
  Marfanoid habitus/musculoskeletal manifestations
  Tall stature
  Long extremities
  Kyphoscoliosis or lordosis
  Joint laxity
  Pes cavus
  Pectus excavatum
  Slipped capital femoral epiphysis
  Dental abnormalities

Tumors and endocrine manifestations
  C-cell hyperplasia/medullary thyroid carcinoma
  Pheochromocytoma
  Parathyroid hyperplasia

---

vous tissue is characterized by large ganglionic nodes with numerous glial cells. Acetylcholinesterase staining reveals increased activity along the hypertrophic myenteric plexus and within the lamina propria, but less than that observed in Hirschsprung's disease. These abnormalities are present along the entire GI tract, from the mouth to the anus, including the appendix. Ganglioneuromatosis may be confused with isolated, diffuse, or segmental hyperganglionosis, characterized by an excess of intestinal neurons only or, preferentially, in the myenteric plexus (see below).

Colonic dysfunction with chronic constipation and bowel dilatation are the prominent clinical features. If it presents at birth, this disorder may be confused with Hirschsprung's disease. Serious complications of ganglioneuromatosis are failure to thrive, CIP, severe colonic diverticulosis, and bowel perforation. Defunctioning ileostomy or elective subtotal colectomy for chronic constipation may be required. GI symptoms often develop years before other features of the syndrome are recognized and MEN IIB is diagnosed.[99] Searching for a RET mutation is recommended in patients with apparently isolated intestinal ganglioneuromatosis or hyperganglionosis proven by rectal suction biopsy or a resected bowel segment.[69] Medullary thyroid carcinoma in MEN IIb has the most aggressive malignant potential with a very high risk for early manifestation.[98] Early diagnosis of

---

MEN IIB is essential to perform prophylactic thyroidectomy by the age of 6 months before medullary thyroid carcinoma develops. In patients who are diagnosed later in life lymph node metastases are usually present and require dissection of the central and both lateral compartments. In addition, screening for development of pheochromocytoma should be performed. In contrast to medullary thyroid carcinoma, pheochromocytoma is rarely malignant and extra-adrenal. The absence of metastatic pheochromaocytoma in patients with MEN II and the risk of morbidity and death from adrenal insufficiency after bilateral total adrenalectomy support the surgical practice of cortex-sparing adrenalectomy. Prophylactic adrenalectomy is not recommended.[98]

Visceral Neuropathy Associated with Neurofibromatosis (von Recklinghausen's Disease). Single or multiple neurofibromas in the small intestine occur in about 10% of patients with this autosomal dominant disorder. Intestinal neuromas may cause both functional and mechanical obstruction.[100,101]

Nonfamilial or Sporadic Visceral Neuropathies

Hypoganglionosis. Hypoganglionosis is defined by a reduced number of ganglion cells in the myenteric plexus and in the submucous plexus in some cases. The location of the sample within the bowel is important for comparison with age-matched controls, and the same methods of tissue preparation (cutting, staining, and counting) need to be applied to both. Whereas, aganglionosis is easily recognized on rectal suction biopsies, hypoganglionosis of the myenteric plexus requires a full-thickness sample of adequate size (>1 cm length). Because the subjective impression of hypoganglionosis can be very misleading, morphometric measurements are required using standardized neuron counts in a sufficient number of sections. The few published studies on neuronal density in control subjects gave very conflicting results, perhaps because of the different methods applied or the different selection criteria used for controls. Neuronal density is affected by the age of the patient, tissue freshness, different diseases, and intestinal dilatation, especially when the specimen is cut transversely to the long axis of the bowel. Sections should be at least 30 m apart to avoid counting each neuron more than once. In postmortem specimens from non-gut-diseased children of different ages, Smith reported a mean neuronal density of 3.6/mm for the jejunum, 4.3/mm for the ileum, and 7.7/mm for the colon, with no major differences between transversal and longitudinal sections.[66] Depending on the section thickness and various techniques used, neuronal density may differ by a factor up to 200.[6]

Hypoganglionosis can always be detected in a short segment, called the transitional zone, proximal to the aganglionic bowel in Hirschsprung's disease. An extensively long hypoganglionic segment may cause symptoms of dysmotility after the pull-through operation. Non-Hirschsprung's disease-related hypoganglionosis, with a morphologic picture similar to the histology of the transition zone, has been reported in many children with severe chronic constipation. It was the most frequent diagnosis in two large series reported on children with CIP owing to visceral neuropathy.[9,102] Navarro and colleagues reported hypoganglionosis of the myenteric plexus in 13 of their 26 patients.[9] Ganglions were smaller than normal and often infiltrated with collagen fibers. Ganglion cells were sparse and sometimes difficult to identify with conventional staining techniques. Immunostaining with different neuronal markers confirmed the paucity of the nervous tissue. Between the ganglion nodes, there were numerous and thickened Schwann's nerve fibers that stained strongly with acetylcholinesterase. In the majority of their patients, hypoganglionosis was confined to the distal segment of the colon. Diffuse disease was reported in only two patients, one of whom presented with intestinal obstruction on the second day of life, had a severe course of the disease, and died of sepsis 1 year later. The second patient with diffuse hypoganglionosis presented at the age of 1 month with pseudo-obstructive episodes. She was the only patient in this series who developed extraintestinal symptoms with severe progressive peripheral neuropathy, absent deep tendon reflexes, ataxia, and tetraplegia. In addition to hypoganglionosis and Schwann's cell hypertrophy, she had intranuclear inclusions within the enteric neurons and in peripheral nerve cells. Her disease fit the pattern of familial visceral neuropathy with intranuclear inclusions described above. This case illustrated that visceral hypoganglionosis (like hyperganglionosis; see below) is not confined to a certain disease entity. The second series of children with intestinal pseudo-obstruction owing to visceral neuropathies was reported by Krishnamurthy and colleagues.[102] They performed hematoxylin–eosin and silver staining on biopsies from 26 children aged 2 months to 10 years and 14 control infants who died of several non-gut-related causes. They distinguished three groups of patients by different morphologic criteria. Group 1 consisted of three children with absence of the myenteric plexus by hematoxylin–eosin and silver staining but the presence of submucosal neurons. Group 2 included four patients with hypoganglionosis of the myenteric plexus by hematoxylin–eosin staining but no nerve tracts and mesh-like structures of the myenteric plexus by silver staining. Group 3 consisted of 19 patients with normal or slightly abnormal neuron density but deficiency of argyrophilic neurons by silver staining. The latter finding has to be interpreted with caution in infants because argyrophilic neurons were found to be absent in preterm babies and could be detected in only some non-gut-diseased infants until the age of 1 year.[103] Many neurons in these patients were abnormal, with scant cytoplasm, enlarged nuclei, and prominent chromatin. Argyrophilic neurons, when present, were small and had few processes. The authors speculated that a maturational arrest at different stages of development could be responsible for the findings. In the

first two groups, migration of the neurons may have been arrested or hampered, whereas in the third group, the maturation process of normally migrated neurons was disturbed. Maturation of enteric neuronal structures continue after birth. This postnatal maturation process may explain why some of the patients with pseudo-obstructive symptoms at birth show improvement or complete resolution of their GI dysmotility during the first years of life (Figure 3).

The clinical course of patients with hypoganglionosis varies markedly. Most cases present in the newborn period with symptoms of Hirschsprung's disease, but some become symptomatic as late as 4 years of age. Most undergo operation (ileostomy, colonic resection, and pull-through procedure), which relieves symptoms in only a few; many children remain dependent on PN or die. This diverse outcome emphasizes that clinical decisions should not be based on the morphologic finding of enteric hypoganglionosis.

Hyperganglionosis. Hyperganglionosis is characterized by an excess of intestinal neurons in the myenteric plexus with or without involvement of the submucous plexus. Knowledge of normal neuronal density is a *conditio sine qua non* for this diagnosis. Because hyperplasia of the submucosal plexus with large ganglia containing more than seven ganglion cells (giant ganglia) was one of the main criteria of IND, the age dependency of neuronal density is relevant to the accuracy of diagnosis. Several authors reported a significantly higher proportion of infants, especially newborn babies, fulfilling these criteria compared with older children.[4,7,66] In non-gut-diseased children, a higher neuronal density in the submucosal plexus is found in infants than in older children.[6,66] Using whole-mount preparations stained with reduced nicotinamide adenine dinucleotide phosphate diaphorase histochemistry (identical to nitric oxide synthetase) and cuprolinic blue (a general neuronal marker), Wester and colleagues described an exponential decrease of ganglion cells within the myenteric plexus meshwork during the first 4 years of life.[6] Therefore, the finding of hyperganglionosis in a young infant with dysmotility needs to be interpreted with caution.

Severe hyperganglionosis is the hallmark of the visceral neuropathy (ganglioneuromatosis) occurring in patients with MEN IIB (see above). In fact, many of the young children reported to have severe hyperganglionosis later developed medullary thyroid carcinoma; some of them were initially labeled as having neuronal intestinal dysplasia. Severe myenteric and submucous plexus hyperplasia with signs of penetration of hyperplastic nerves into the mucosal were typical findings in children with MEN IIB, reported by Navarro and colleagues.[9] In contrast, four patients with no signs of MEN IIB on follow-up showed only mild-to-moderate hyperganglionosis. Their findings were much more pronounced in the myenteric than in the submucosal plexus. Three patients presented with

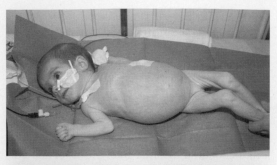

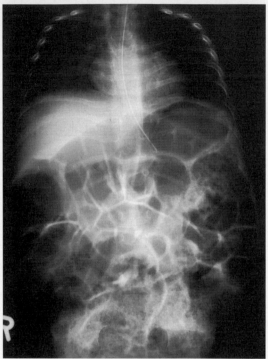

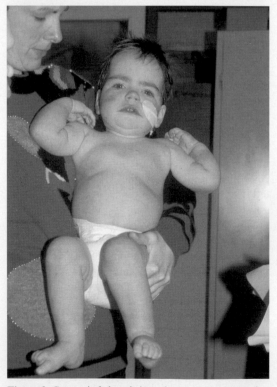

Figure 3 Congenital chronic intestinal pseudo-obstruction of unknown cause: enteral feeding was possible during the first 10 months of life, but she completely recovered by 2 years of age except for some behavioral feeding problems and developmental delay. (A) Severe malnutrition at 7 months of age, (B) abdominal X-ray at 7 months: dilated bowel loops, and (C) enteral feeding via mouths and nasogastric tube at 21 months of age.

obstructive symptoms and one with enterocolitis during the neonatal period. Two of these children became asymptomatic after ileostomy, and the other two recovered without surgical treatment.

These observations underline the quantitative and qualitative differences between isolated hyperganglionosis and ganglioneuromatosis associated with MEN IIB. Infants and children with severe hyperganglionosis, especially when the submucous plexus is involved, should be investigated for a mutation within the *RET* gene, regardless of a negative family history for MEN IIB. In contrast, mild hyperganglionosis in a young infant seems to have a much better prognosis and may be an age-related variation of the normal enteric maturation process.[6,7] Further work is needed, using more sophisticated techniques, to clarify whether isolated mild or moderate segmental hyperganglionosis is a distinct entity that causes long-term motility problems.

Hyperplasia of the myenteric and submucous plexus proximal to the transition zone has been reported in patients with Hirschsprung's disease.[4] Most of them had increased acetylcholinesterase activity in the lamina propria of the affected bowel segment. The significance of these findings for motility problems after the pull-through procedure remains controversial. Nevertheless, patients with disabling motility disturbances after a pull-through procedure or after colostomy, who have proven hyperganglionosis in both plexuses, may benefit from resection of the affected part of the colon. Interestingly, mucosal neuromas or extraintestinal features of MEN IIB have not been reported in patients with Hirschsprung's disease–associated hyperganglionosis. The RET mutation found in aganglionosis results in a loss of function effect, whereas in MEN IIB mutations, a common gain of function has been shown.[98] It is unknown whether patients with Hirschsprung's disease–associated effect has hyperganglionosis have more mutations in the *RET* gene than patients without these morphologic findings in the bowel proximal to the aganglionic segment.

Secondary or Acquired Visceral Neuropathies

In secondary or acquired neuropathies, the damage of the ENS is due to a known agent (ie, toxic and infectious) or secondary to a systemic disease (ie, endocrine or metabolic disorder and chronic inflammation). Secondary visceral neuropathies may manifest at any age, even after birth if the damaging agent was present in utero. They occur less often in children compared with adults because it may take many years to cause neuronal damage severe enough to cause dysmotility.

Infectious Agents. Enteric ganglionitis can occur in the course of infectious disease and may cause gut dysmotility.[104] Chagas' disease, an endemic disorder of South America, is caused by infection with *Trypanosoma cruzi* and a well-known example of ENS destruction. The neuronal degeneration is not caused by the parasite itself but is due to an immune response elicited by the infection. The neuropathy is the result

of a molecular mimicry that leads to immune crossreactivity between the parasite end enteric neurons. The *T. cruzi* flagellar antigen Fl-160 mimics a 48-kDa protein expressed by mammalian axons and myenteric neurons. The immune-mediated damage contributes to the complete loss of enteric neurons. Patient with Chagas' disease show high titers of circulating antibodies directed against the type 2 muscarinic acetylcholine receptor. These autoantibodies have smooth muscle cells as a target, not the neurons, and act as agonist resulting in muscle contraction. The most common clinical presentation is achalasia, followed by dysfunction of the large intestine (megacolon) and small intestine (megaduodenum), including episodes of CIP.

A viral etiology was suspected in patients infected with neurotropic viruses including cytomegalovirus, varicella-zoster virus, Epstein–Barr virus (EBV), herpes simplex virus type 1, and human immunodeficiency virus.[8,105] Debinski and colleagues provided the first proof for a viral etiology by identifying EBV in the myenteric plexus of a patient with chronic pseudo-obstruction.[106] Full-thickness biopsies of the patient showed myenteric inflammatory infiltrates but no evidence for a myopathy. Because the authors did not identify virus material in the tissue of 12 other patients with chronic pseudo-obstruction, they concluded that viral infection is a rare cause of severe intestinal dysmotility. Besnard and colleagues reported a 13-year-old boy with intestinal pseudo-obstruction, acquired hypoganglionosis, and severe acute dysautonomia related to EBV reactivation.[107] Cytomegalovius (CMV) was found to be the cause in at least two infants presenting with CIP.[108,109] Both cases presented at 2 months of age with severe CIP and were positive for both IgG- and IgM-specific CMV antibodies. The virus was identified in intestinal biopsies in the case of Ategbo and colleagues. This child had also respiratory distress due to diffuse interstitial pneumonia. Inspite of total PN, an ilostomy was necessary because of severe distention. No MMC was observed on antroduodenal manometry tracing. The child spontaneously improved at the age of 6 months and could be weaned from parenteral nutrition 2 months later. The child completely recovered without relapse during the following years.[109] An undiscovered viral agent may therefore be the cause in infants with severe dysmotility and spontaneous recovery that may be falsely attributed to a delay in the maturation process of the ENS.

Following an acute bout of enteric infection, a significant proportion of both adults and children develop symptoms of irritable bowel syndrome, such as abdominal pain, fullness, or nausea.[110] In children, symptoms are often transient and resolve over weeks or months, but may be the beginning of IBS depending also in the presence of psychological and other biological factors.

Toxic Agents. Abnormal antroduodenal manometry suggestive of enteric neuropathy was reported in five children with fetal alcohol syndrome.[111]

All patients presented during infancy with disabling symptoms of GI dysmotility, including vomiting, abdominal pain and distention, constipation, and intermittent diarrhea, resulting in failure to thrive. However, prior to referral between the ages of 20 months and 9 years, all patients had undergone multiple operations. Nissen fundoplication, with pyloric emptying procedures, was performed in four children and bowel resection in one. Because no tissue was available from these patients, it remains undetermined whether the observed manometric motility pattern was the direct result of in utero alcohol neurotoxicity on the enteric nerves

Drugs. Drugs may affect GI motility as a main target organ by intent (eg, various prokinetics or loperamide) or as unwarranted side effects (ie, opiate analgesics, macrolides, or anticonvulsive drugs). Symptoms such as diarrhea, abdominal cramping, or constipation resolve as soon as the drugs are stopped. Two infants with hypoperistalsis and idiopathic intestinal pseudo-obstruction have been reported, who were treated during the perinatal period with zidovudine.[112] In both, symptoms resolved when the drug was discontinued. Nonreversible visceral neuropathy owing to long-term intake of cathartics or chemotherapeutic agents has been reported in adults.

Radiation. Radiation damages all structures of the small and large bowel, including the mucosa, blood vessels, connective tissue, nerves, and smooth muscle. Acute manifestations usually subside within weeks, whereas late complications may appear months to decades after radiotherapy. Most affected patients are adults. Symptoms of the late radiation enteropathy include diarrhea, urge defecation, abdominal pain, nausea, vomiting, bloating, and pseudo-obstructive episodes. Late radiation injury is characterized by vascular degeneration and intestinal wall fibrosis evident in all layers of the gut wall. Both neuronal and muscular structures of the bowel are affected and contribute to the motility disorder. Contrast studies may show dilated loops, hypoperistalsis, and a thickened wall. Antroduodenal manometry showed a wide variety of abnormalities, preferentially in patients with more severe symptoms and malnutrition.[113] Major features were an attenuated postprandial motor response and a reduced intensity of the MMC during the night.

Chronic Inflammation and Autoimmune Disease. Gut dysmotility has been reported in patients with different noninfectious inflammatory diseases. Enteric ganglionitis is characterized by a dense infiltrate of lymphocytes with a predominant T-cytotoxic activity and plasma cells involving either the two major ganglionated plexus and related axonal processes of the ENS, or more commonly, only the myenteric plexus (myenteric ganglionitis). Eosionophilic and neutrophils may also be involved. Dense eosiophilic infiltrates and neuronal expression of IL-5 has been described in three children with CIP.[114] Besides the cellular response, a wide spectrum of circulating antineuronal antibodies indicate humoral mechanisms. Detection of antibodies is helpful for the diagnosis of myenteric ganglionitis as a cause of gut motility disorders. These antibodies can be found in idiopathic forms of ganglionitis or associated with an underlying disease. In adults, antineuronal autoantibodies like ANNA (or anti-Hu antibodies), antivoltage-gated Ca^{2+} channels or anit-Yo (Cdr2) antibodies should initiate a search for tumors, because they are part of a paraneoplastic syndrome of different underlying tumors.[67]

Chronic and acute transmural inflammation as in Crohn's disease or postnecrotizing enterocolitis causes fibrosis and ischemia and may damage enteric nerves and glial cells and muscular structures of the bowel. Dysmotility in untreated celiac disease is probably due to mucosal atrophy, resulting in disturbed secretion of several GI hormones. Neuropathic changes have not been reported. Common complaints are symptoms of delayed gastric emptying, abdominal distention, and bloating. Hypoperistalsis of the small and large bowel results in constipation in about 10 to 15% of untreated celiac patients in spite of malabsorption. A few celiac patients with intestinal pseudo-obstruction have been described. Symptoms of dysmotility resolve on a strict gluten-free diet.

Several patients have been reported with an idiopathic autoimmune visceral neuropathy (ganglionitis) and acquired progressive aganglionosis as a result of a severe T-cell–mediated inflammatory ganglionitis of both enteric plexuses.[115] Both patients became symptomatic during childhood, with severe constipation, anorexia, abdominal distention, and abdominal pain, and later developed pseudo-obstructive episodes. No extraintestinal involvement or autonomic dysfunction was observed. High titers of immunoglobulin G class autoantibody directed against enteric neurons were found in both patients. There was no evidence of a paraneoplastic syndrome because no tumor was found during a period of up to 8 years. The autoimmune inflammatory nature of this acquired severe neuropathy with secondary aganglionosis is supported by the improvement of symptoms during treatment with prednisone and relapse after withdrawal of steroids.

Severe constipation and abdominal pain and occasionally intestinal pseudo-obstruction in patients with recurrent fever (>38°C) and myalgia and/or a migratory erythematous rash may be the manifestation of the period fever syndrome, tumor necrosis factor receptor–associated periodic syndrome.[116] This autosomal dominantly inherited disease is related to mutations in the tumor necrosis factor receptor soluble form 1A on chromosome 12p13. The symptoms start during childhood, but in almost half of the cases intra-abdominal surgery is performed before the diagnosis is made. This autoinflammatory disease with high levels of TNF-α and increased inflammatory signs (ESR and CRP) is successfully treated with corticosteroids, or with TNF-α–blocking agents like infliximab or etanercept.

Autonomic Neuropathy. The autonomic nervous system constitutes one of the three levels of control of GI motor function and interacts with the ENS and the excitable smooth muscle cells. Therefore, disorders affecting the extrinsic nervous system of the gut may cause intestinal dysmotility, even in the absence of morphologic abnormalities of the ENS.[117] Children with autonomic dysfunction may have very unspecific symptoms like feeding problems with poor sucking due to oropharyngeal dysmotility, dysphagia due to esophageal spasm and achalasia, and finally bowel dysmotility causing recurrent vomiting or profound constipation or diarrhea.

About half of the children with the autosomal recessive inherited familial dysautonomia (Riley-Day syndrome) develop GI problems.[118] Attacks of severe vomiting affect children after the age of 3 years and are one of the most disturbing afflictions of the disorder. The crises usually last less than 24 to 72 hours and are associated with hypertension, sweating, and erythematous blotching of the skin. Severe gastric distention and abdominal pain may accompany the attacks. The children are at high risk for profound dehydration and aspiration. Children with triple A syndrome (achalasia-addisonian-alacrimia syndrome or Allgrove's syndrome), an autosomal recessive disorder, often suffer from a variety of neurologic features with autonomic dysfunction, including GI dysmotility with vomiting, retching, diarrhea, or constipation. The AAAS gene has been mapped on chromosome 12q13 and encodes a protein, which is involved in signal transduction, ribonucleic acid processing, and transcription.[119,120]

An acquired idiopathic autonomic neuropathy was described in 27 patients aged 7 to 75 years from the Mayo Clinic, most of whom had an acute or subacute onset of symptoms.[121] In 16 cases, a presumed viral infection preceded symptoms. GI symptoms, reported in 19 patients, consisted of various combinations of nausea, vomiting, diarrhea, and severe constipation. Most of the patients had a partial recovery without relapse. An immune-mediated mechanism comparable to Guillain-Barré syndrome was considered a possible cause by the authors.

Autonomic neuropathy owing to poorly controlled diabetes mellitus is common in adults but rarely reaches clinical significance in childhood. Gastroparesis and diarrhea are the main manifestations. Celiac disease needs to be excluded because it affects 3 to 5% of children with insulin-dependent diabetes mellitus.

Endocrine Disorders. Several endocrine disorders with decreased or excessive hormone release may manifest with symptoms of GI dysmotility. Severe slow-transit constipation or even pseudo-obstructive episodes may be the presenting symptom of hypothyroidism, whereas diarrhea with or without steatorrhea owing to rapid intestinal transit occurs in hyperthyroidism. Impaired gut contractile activity with small-bowel dysmotility and steatorrhea has been observed in children

with hypoparathyroidism, especially when it is part of a polyendocrine deficiency syndrome. Tumors producing catecholamines or vasoactive peptides, that is, neuroblastoma, pheochromocytoma, carcinoid, ganglioneuroblastoma, VIPoma, and gastrinoma, may present with dilated small-bowel loops and dysmotility in addition to watery diarrhea.[122]

Metabolic Disorders. Several metabolic disorders, with or without electrolyte disturbances, may result in acute or chronic GI dysmotility (eg, organic aciduria, end-stage liver disease, or renal disease). In some disorders, material stored within the bowel wall may result in permanent damage of the neuromuscular structures (ie, Fabry's disease and amyloidosis).

Anorexia Nervosa and Bulimia. Patients with eating disorders frequently complain of bloating, early satiety, fullness, and constipation. Delayed gastric emptying and slow bowel transit have been documented. Symptoms improve or resolve when the behavioral problem is successfully treated.

Degenerative Neuropathy due to Intestinal Obstruction. Degeneration of the ENS can be secondary to long-standing bowel dilatation as a consequence of unrecognized obstruction. A 14-year-old girl was reported with obstruction of the upper small bowel due to Ladd's band and malrotation that had been overlooked at two previous operations.[123] Based on symptoms with pain and bilious vomiting dating back to infancy, a histology with signs of "hyperganglionosis" and manometric pattern suggestive of neuropathy, she had previously been diagnosed to have chronic intestinal pseudo-obstruction. The histology at the time of final operation showed degenerative changes in the massively dilated duodenum proximal to the obstruction with normal histology beyond the obstruction. This case report illustrates that an enteric neuropathology may occur secondary to untreated long-lasting bowel obstruction and that the results of antroduodenal manometry and histology from full-thickness biopsies can be very misleading.

Acute Colonic Pseudo-obstruction (Ogilvie's Syndrome). This is a severe form of adynamic ileus with massive dilatation of the colon in the absence of mechanical obstruction.[124] It occurs in hospitalized patients with a wide variety of medical and surgical conditions. The pathogenesis is not well understood, but it is thought to be due to imbalance in the autonomic regulation of the colon with either excessive parasympathetic suppression or sympathetic stimulation. The severe dilatation of the colon has a high risk of ischemia and perforation. Most cases respond to supportive therapy with nothing by mouth, correction of fluid and electrolyte imbalances, nasogastric tube suction and rectal tube drainage. If there is no response within 24 hours of conservative treatment, intravenous neostigmine (in adults: 2 mg given over 5 minutes) was very effective to decompress the colon in one randomized placebo controlled trial and several open studies in adults.[124,125] It seems to be much safer compared to colonoscopic decompression, which should be reserved to patients who do not respond to neostigmine or where it is contraindicated.

Interstitial Cells of Cajal

Throughout the GI tract, there are nonneural cells derived from mesenchymal precursors, the ICC, which generate and propagate slow waves. These cells form extensive networks of electrically coupled cells and are very important modulators of communication between nerves and muscle, and loss or defects of ICC significantly compromise neuronal regulation of GI motility.[126,127] ICC can be identified in normal tissue by their immunoreactivity for the tyrosine kinase receptor Kit and by ultrastructural criteria in transmission electron microscopy. There are at least two populations of ICC in the GI tract.[128] Some cells lie between or at the edge of the muscles layers and generate and propagate electrical slow-wave activity, and others lie within muscle bundles in close apposition with enteric neurons.[129] However, some limitations and pitfalls are reported with respect to identification of ICC in disease states: The ultrastructural criteria for ICC may not apply to pathologic conditions, and absence of detectable Kit-positive cells may not only indicate loss of ICC but may also be due to artifactual loss of Kit positivity by ICC. For example, Kit positivity is impaired by paraffin embedding, and certain antigen retrieval procedures are mandatory to detect Kit positivity on such material.[126] In addition, long-standing dilatation of the intestine or hypertrophy makes it difficult to quantify the number of both neuronal cells and ICC, and may result in an underestimation or overestimation of the cell density. Most important, any changes with respect to ICC observed in tissue from patients with advanced intestinal motility problems may be the cause of the disease or be secondary to the disease process. In animal models, it could be demonstrated that chronic bowel obstruction or chronic inflammation results in defects in ICC networks.[130] However, ICC display a high degree of plasticity, and loss of these cell in pathologic conditions does not necessarily mean permanent loss. For example, removal of the obstruction or healing after surgery caused restoration of functional ICC.[131] At this point we can only summarize the recent knowledge of the role of ICC in human GI motility disorders.

Delayed Maturation of ICC

Two infants, one of whom was born prematurely, with neonatal intestinal pseudo-obstruction, have been reported who showed lack of ICC in the intestine at the side of ileostomy.[132] The intestinal motility normalized over the first months of life, and at the time of closure of the stoma, a normal distribution of Kit-positive ICC was documented. The authors speculated that a developmental delay of Kit-positive ICC may have been the underlying mechanism. Their finding was confirmed

in six other children with meconium ileus who required ileostomy during the neonatal period. No Kit-positive ICC were detected in the colonic biopsies of two children, and there was a scanty distribution in the remaining four compared with controls. All children showed a normal pattern of ICC when the ileostomies were closed between 39 and 104 days of age.[133]

Reduced Density or an Abnormal Distribution of Kit-Positve ICC

This has been described in patients with children with hypoganglionosis,[134] in a woman with intestinal pseudo-obstruction and megaduodenum owing to myopathy,[135] and in the colon of adults with slow-transit constipation.[136,137] A decreased density of ICC around the myenteric plexus has been described in a 5-year-old girl with congenital generalized myopathy and gut dysmotility.[138] However, the relationship between cause and consequence in these cases remain unresolved.

Enteric Glial Cells

EGCs have been recently recognized as important components of mucosal protection, inflammatory responses, and signaling.[3] EGCs resemble in many aspects the astroglia in the CNS and are more than passive scaffolding the support the neurons in the ENS. In transgenic mice lacking their EGCs, severe-to-fatal gut inflammation occurs, which is not related to bacterial overgrowth. EGCs seem to play a major role for the epithelial barrier function to provide protection against transepithelial invasion by pathogens, but possibly also the normal gut flora. The number of EGCs is increased in patients with inflammatory bowel diseases such as Crohn's disease and ulcerative colitis with and enhanced expression of the major histocompatibility complex class II antigen on their surface. This may indicate that these cells are involved in antigen presentation and immune response in IBD. So far, no specific disease has been identified in humans caused by an increase, decrease, or dysfunction of EGCs. However, there are no doubts on their active role in the functioning of the ENS and the whole bowel.[139]

Chronic Intestinal Pseudo-Obstruction Syndrome

CIP describes a rare and severe GI dysmotility leading to signs and symptoms of bowel obstruction in the absence of a mechanical obstructive lesion. It was defined by pediatric and adult gastroenterologists as "a rare, severe, disabling disorder characterized by repetitive episodes or continuous symptoms and signs of bowel obstruction, including radiographic documentation of dilated bowel with air–fluid levels, in the absence of a fixed, lumen-occluding lesion."[140] The rather strict definition that makes radiological signs obligatory has been criticized because in some patients with severe disabling symptoms, bowel dilatation and air–fluid levels are found only intermittently. In addition, dilated bowel loops with air–fluid levels can be observed in newborns

with severe diarrhea owing to congenital transport defects, that is, chloride diarrhea, imitating a severe GI motility disease. CIP may be congenital or acquired, primary or secondary.[140] Congenital pseudo-obstruction lasting for the first 2 months of life or the acquired disorder persisting for more than 6 months is considered chronic. Based on histopathology and patterns of motility abnormalities, patients with CIP can be subdivided into neuropathic type, myopathic type, and unclassified forms.[141–143] Although familial forms with autosomal dominant or recessive modes of inheritance have been reported,[141,144–146] most cases of CIP appear to be unrelated to familial clusters and therefore are referred to as sporadic forms. Mitochondrial disorders also may be complicated by neuropathic pseudo-obstruction such as mitochondrial neurogastroencephalopathy.[28] In addition deficiency of the GI pacemaker cells, the ICC, has been recently described with motility disorders.[132,147–149] Although research has improved the understanding and management of dysmotility disorders,[150] CIP is one of the most severe intractable problems in pediatric gastroenterology: almost half of the children never tolerate enteral feeding.[8,142]

Pathophysiology

The pathophysiology depends on the underlying condition causing CIP (Table 1). Most of the primary or secondary neuropathic or myopathic disorders may cause CIP. The histology and pathophysiological mechanisms of the different diseases, if known, are discussed in the first part of this chapter.

Clinical Features

In most pediatric cases, symptoms are present from birth or early infancy.[143] The exact prevalence of CIP is not known, but it has been estimated that approximately 100 infants with congenital CIP are born in the United States each year[141] and many more develop acquired forms of the disease. Two-thirds of patients present within the first month of life and 80% by 1 year of age.[8,143,151] The male-to-female ratio in CIP is thought to be 1:1. Girls are more frequently affected with the neonatal forms.[8,46,143]

Clinical Presentation

In ~20% of cases CIP is detected prenatally. In MMIHS, signs of an obstructed urinary system leading to an abdominal distension may be the presenting feature, with symptoms of intestinal obstruction appearing within days to 12 month later (see above). Some reports have described the detection of these sign by ultrasonography as early as 16 weeks. But most times the abnormalities are noted very late in gestation.

The neonatal presentation of CIP includes intestinal occlusion, severe abdominal distension, and bilious vomiting. Abdominal distension and diarrhea may also be secondary to bacterial overgrowth. The diagnosis of CIP in neonates and particularly preterm infants should be made with caution. The MMC does not appear in its mature form until a gestational age of 34 to 35 weeks, and CIP may be mimicked by the immaturity of intestinal motility.

Manifestations later in infancy and childhood include abdominal bloating, severe constipation, failure to thrive, and bilious vomiting with an initially normal intestinal transit.[152] The symptoms depend on the regions of the GI tract involved and may be acute or insidious or chronic persistent or intermittent. Diarrhea owing to bacterial overgrowth is frequent and may alternate with constipation or episodes of partial obstruction. Severe abdominal pain often results in feeding difficulties and malnutrition. Involvement of the esophagus is rarely reported.[153] The colonic form of CIP (colonic inertia) may result in severe intractable constipation without upper digestive tract involvement.[8]

Urological involvement is reported in 33 to 92% of children with CIP in both, neuropathic and myopathic forms, and includes megacystis, hydronephrosis, urinary retention, and urinary tract infections.[8,154,155] In myopathic forms of CIP without megacystis, urinary tract infection remains a frequent problem.[143] Providing a good and careful management of the adynamic bladder for preventing urinary tract infections, the renal prognosis is generally good.[154] The histology from biopsies of the bladder reveals nonspecific fibrotic changes which are not useful for subtype classification of CIP.

Diagnosis. Due to the different etiologies for CIP and a wide variety of clinical presentations, the diagnosis of CIP is difficult. Specific diagnostic tests are not available. The diagnosis should be considered in children with symptoms of intestinal obstruction without mechanical obstructive lesions, persistent GI symptoms after surgery for malrotation,[156] intestinal obstruction associated with bladder dysmotility, or persistent symptoms after exclusion of Hirschsprung's disease and hypothyroidism. Although children are affected predominantly by primary disorders of the enteric neuromusculature structures, a secondary cause of CIP should always be considered (see Table 2). This is of great importance because the specific treatment of the condition may lead to cure of the dysmotility.

The following three steps are important in the diagnostic work up of patients with suspected "pseudo-"obstruction:

1. To rule out a fixed, occluding lesion.
2. To confirm an abnormal motility of the GI tract.
3. To find or exclude a treatable systemic cause of secondary CIP

An algorithm for the diagnostic work up of CIP is shown in Figure 4.

History

A review of symptoms may identify disturbance of neuromuscular function or collagen vascular disease that can be associated with GI

Table 2 Causes of Intestinal Pseudo-Obstruction in Infants and Children

Primary visceral myopathies
  Familial myopathy with megaduodenum
  MNGIE
  Familial myopathy with short gut, malrotation, and abnormal muscle layering
  Megacystis-microcolon-intestinal hypoperistalsis syndrome
  African degenerative leiomyopathy

Systemic disorders affecting primarily the gastrointestinal smooth muscle
  Connective tissue disorders
    Dermatomyositis/polymyositis
    Systemic lupus erythematosus
    Mixed connective tissue diseases
    Scleroderma
    Ehlers-Danlos syndrome type IV
  Myopathies affecting also the striated muscles
    Myotonic dystrophy
    Duchenne's muscular dystrophy
    Desmin myopathy
    Mitochondrial myopathy with or without liver involvement
  Infiltrative and inflammatory diseases
    Amyloidosis
    Ceroidosis (Brown bowel syndrome)
    Leiomyositis (autoimmune)

Primary neuropathies of the ENS
  Autosomal dominant familial visceral neuropathy without extraintestinal manifestation
  Autosomal dominant visceral neuropathy with neuronal intranuclear inclusions and autonomic dysfunction
  Familial visceral neurophathy with peripheral and central neuropathy
  Ganglioneuromatosis with MEN type IIB (autosomal dominant)
  Sporadic and familial forms of aganglionosis
  Unclassified enteric neuropathies (normal histology, hypoganglionosis, transmitter deficiency, etc)
  Disorders of the interstitial cells of Cajal (reduced density, delayed maturation)

Systemic disorders affecting primarily the enteric nervous system
  Central or peripheral generalized neural diseases
    Familial dysautonomia (Riley–Day syndrome)
    Acquired cholinergic dysautonomia or pandysautonomia
    Diabetic polyneuropathy
    Mitochondrial neurogastrointestinal encephalopathy
  Infectious/postinfectious
    Postviral (CMV, EBV, HZV, rotavirus, and others)
    Trypanosoma cruzi
    Lyme's disease
    Chagas' disease
    Kawasaki's disease
    Guillan-Barré syndrome
  Immune/autoimmune
    Celiac disease
    Autoimmune enteric ganglionitis (with positive antibodies)
    Eosinophilic gastroenteritis
  Endocrine/metabolic
    Electrolyte imbalance (K^+, Mg^{2+}, Ca^{2+})
    Uremia
    Porphyria
    Hypothyroidism
    Hypoparathyroidism
    Carnitine deficiency
    Vitamin E deficiency
  Tumor-associated
    Chemotherapy and/or bone marrow/stem cell transplant
    Thymoma (with antiacetylcholine receptor antibodies)
    Neural crest cell tumor: neuroblastoma, ganglioneuroblastoma, pheochromocytoma
    Paraneoplastic syndrome (with different tumors and positive antibodies)
  Toxic
    Drugs: ketamine, carbamazepine, clonidine, atro-pine, anticholinergics, theophylline, fludarabine
    Vinblastine/other vinca alkaloids, neuroleptics, antidepressants, phenothiazine, opiates, calcium channel blockers
    Fetal alcohol syndrome
    Jellyfish envenomation
  Miscellaneous
    Angioedema
    Postradiation enteropathy
    Crohn's disease
    Acute colonic pseudo-obstruction (Ogilvie's syndrome) postsurgery, post-trauma, and others

manifestations.[157] A past history of other neurologic disorders or diabetes mellitus, concomitant use of medications that cause neurologic dysfunction of the intestine (such as anticholinergics, phenothiazines, antihypertensives, tricyclic antidepressants, serotoninergic agents, dopaminergic drugs, opiates, and calcium channel blockers), or any prior exposure to radiation or recent travel to tropical countries are also important clues from the patient's history. The possibility of a viral infection such as CMV or EBV should be considered. Even rotavirus has been described as a cause of both severe and prolonged gastroparesis.[158] For any neurologic, myopathic, and autoimmune disease, the family history should be exactly explored.

The main physical findings are abdominal distension and a succession splash. But the physical examination should also encompass thorough neuromuscular assessment to identify conditions associated with autonomic neuropathy or mitochondrial diseases. Dermatologic examination should note signs of connective tissue diseases (systemic sclerosis and lupus) including Raynaud phenomenon, skin eruption, palmar erythema, teleangiectasia, nodules, and scleroderma of the hands, feet, face, and forearms. Typical facial finding with an elongated shape, thickened and everted upper eyelids, prominent eyebrows, and a marphanoid habitus points to the diagnosis of MEN (see above). Audiologic assessment is important to rule out deafness associated with a *SOX10* gene mutation.[97] External ophthalmoplegia associated with deafness suggests a MNGIE defect.[28] Cardiac function should be evaluated to rule out a suspected muscular disease such as desmin myopathies.[159] Neural crest-derived tumors and pheochromocytoma should be suspected and ruled out in children and infants with CIP by appropriate computed tomography and ultrasonographic studies.[160] In atypical cases, and with normal manometry, Munchausen syndrome by proxy should be considered[161] (see below).

Blood Testing and Assessment of Nutritional Status

At an early stage, it is important to assess the nutritional and metabolic consequences of the motility disorder, especially the measurement of serum electrolytes and albumin. Hypokalemia and metabolic acidosis may occur in the case of prominent diarrhea, or hypokalemia and metabolic alkalosis in prominent vomiting. Hypoalbuminemia is a sign of malnutrition, but may also indicate protein loss into the gut lumen or ascitic fluid. Due to bacterial overgrowth, serum vitamin B12 concentrations can be low. Carnitine and vitamin E levels should be checked in cases with possible fat maldigestion or malabsorption. Severe deficiencies may cause by itself a neuropathy, but also have been reported in enteric myopathic disorders with deposition of lipofuscin in smooth muscle cells.[162–164] Laboratory testing should also include thyroid-stimulating hormone, free thyroxine, antitransglutaminase antibodies for celiac disease, urinary catecholamines, plasma vasoactive intestinal peptides, erythrocyte sedimentation rate, fraction of complements 3 and 4, and antinuclear antibodies. The results of hemagglutination testing and complement fixation for Chagas' disease may be positive in patients who have lived in South America. Determinations of blood lactate, pyruvate, CPK, ALT, and leukocyte TP are used to screen for mitochondrial cytopathies.[165] Anti-HU (antineuronal nuclear and ANNA-1) antibodies appear to be a useful serological marker in cases of CIP caused by autoimmune gangliositis.[104,115,166]

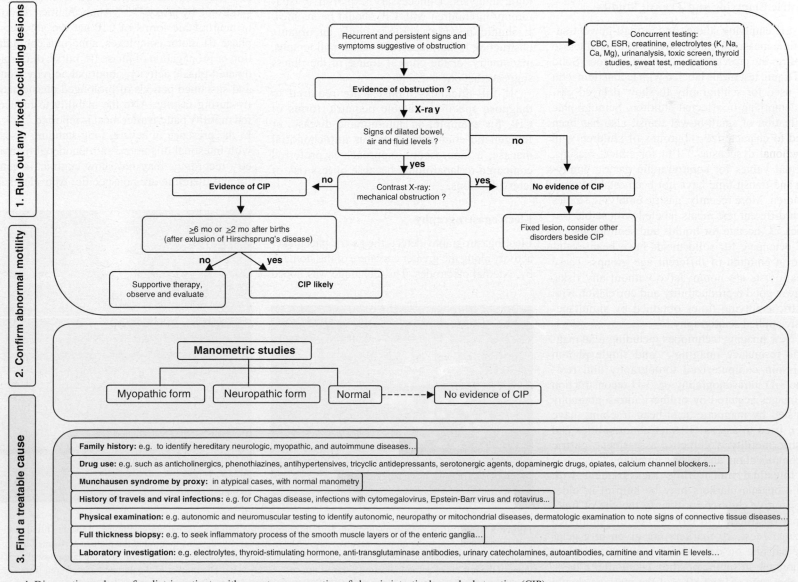

Figure 4 Diagnostic work up of pediatric patients with symptoms suggestive of chronic intestinal pseudoobstruction (CIP)

Radiological and Other Imaging Studies

Radiographic studies do not usually provide an etiologic diagnosis but are helpful in localizing the site of GI tract involvement. Radiological testing including plain films of the abdomen on left lateral position and an upper GI series may show typical signs of intestinal obstruction with dilated stomach, loops of small bowel and/or colon with air–fluid levels, except in patients who are not being fed and have venting entero-ostomies. Contrast studies should be performed to exclude any intraluminal or extrinsic lesion, using water-soluble, nontoxic isotonic material. Progression of the contrast medium may be slow, impaired, and retrograde peristalsis may occur. To rule out a partial mechanical obstruction, enteroclysis may be necessary. Sometimes normal results of a contrast enema can be found if only the upper digestive tract is involved. A microcolon can be found in neonates. Malrotation is frequent, especially in neonates, and was reported in cases of myopathy, neuropathy, and as part of a familial syndrome with associated CIP and pyloric stenosis.[93,167] Diverticulosis of the small bowel or colon has been reported as severe form of radiation-induced dysmotility.[107,168,169]

Gastric Emptying and Transit Studies

Gastric emptying studies and a small-bowel transit time measurement are useful additional test to confirm the presence of a motility disorder. Solid and liquid test meals labeled with technetium 99m are used for scintigraphy to show delayed gastric emptying in affected children. Scintigraphic evaluation of small-bowel transit also has been used to characterize subgroups of children with functional dyspepsia.[170] But for ethical reasons, normal values for scintigraphic gastric emptying and transit time have not been established in children. More recently, gastric emptying studies with different test meals labeled with stable isotopes ^{13}C-acetate for liquids and semiliquids and ^{13}C-octanoate for solid meals have been evaluated in children of different age groups. These breath tests are noninvasive without any risks, show a good reproducibility and correlation with gastric emptying times obtained by simultaneously applied scintigraphy.[171]

New imaging techniques including fetal magnetic resonance imaging[172] and single photon emission–computerized tomography and real-time 3-D ultrasonography or, 3-D reconstruction of images acquired by ordinary ultrasonography assisted by magnetic scan-head tracking, have been tried to assess GI tract abnormalities and gastric motility, volumetric assessment, gastric accommodation, and gastric emptying.[173]

Intestinal transit time measurement with radio-opaque markers may be helpful in older cooperative children to identify the site of functional obstruction in CIP.[174] For the simplified Sitzmark test, 20 markers are given in a gelatine capsule on day 0 with a abdominal plain radiograph in supine position taken after 5 days. By that time at least 80% of the markers should

be excreted. For measurement of total and segmental colonic transit times the markers should be swallowed on 6 consecutive days with a radiograph on day 7. From the number and the location of the retained markers, the transit time can be calculated[175] (Figure 5). For interpretation of transit time tests, an evacuation disorder needs to be excluded be anorectal manometry and balloon expulsion maneuver—because this may mimic colonic inertia with a hold up of the markers in the right-sided colon.

H_2-breath testing using substrates such as lactulose are inaccurate in intestinal pseudo-obstruction since the substrate can be metabolized by bacteria overgrowing in the small intestine.

Laparotomy and Laparoscopy

Variable clinical presentation and lack of specific diagnostic test may lead to exploratory surgery for diagnosis. Especially children and adolescents with an acute presentation usually undergo exploratory laparotomy. For these reasons, the prevalence of surgery at diagnosis of pediatric CIP approaches 50%.[8,102,143,176] If the diagnosis of CIP is strongly suggested from the surgical exploration, intestinal full-thickness biopsies should be taken at different levels for histopathologic analysis. Unnecessary explorative laparotomy in children with CIP should be avoided. It should be reserved to exclude an organic obstructing lesion in cases in which radiographs, manometry, or the clinical course of the illness suggests that one is likely.

If full-thickness biopsies are required to diagnose specific treatable pediatric forms of CIP, for example, an autoimmune disease, or for genetic counseling, such as mitochondrial disease, a laparoscopic approach is preferred compared to laparotomy because of less risk of later adhesions.

Electrogastrography

Electrogastrography detects the gastric pacemaker activity along the greater curvature of the stomach by external electrodes. The technique was hoped

to identify gastric dysrhythmia and dysmotility and to screen in a noninvasive matter for motility disorders. Unfortunately, the technique is prone to artifacts, the finding of bradygastric or tachygastric episodes is nonspecific and also found in normal individuals, the pattern correlate poorly with symptoms, and do not differentiate CIP from other forms of intestinal dysmotility. Therefore, further validation of this technique is needed and manometry is now considered a more definitive investigation for pseudo-obstruction.[177]

Manometry

Antroduodenal manometry provides important information to determine the pathophysiology of symptoms in CIP. Manometry can be useful to rule out a mechanical obstruction of the intestine, which typically shows simultaneous, prolonged contractions at the level of small intestine.[178] Dysmotilities of the upper digestive tract are almost always seen in children with CIP.[179] A normal antroduodenal manometry essentially rules out the diagnosis of CIP.[177] In patients presented with symptoms of intestinal pseudo-obstruction, the present normal manometry studies should alert the physician to the possibility of psychological or behavioral disorders, as well as Munchausen syndrome by proxy.[161,180] Abnormalities reported in neuropathic forms of CIP are the absence of phase III motor complexes, abnormal configuration or propagation of phase III, bursts of uncoordinated phasic activity, abnormal activity fronts, and sustained periods of prolonged phasic activity during fasting. Also the inability to induce a fed motility pattern after meal is reported.[153,181,182] In the presence of severe, long-standing disease with intestinal dilatation, antroduodenal manometry recordings may not show contractile activity and therefore are nonspecific. Antroduodenal

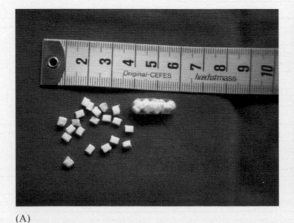

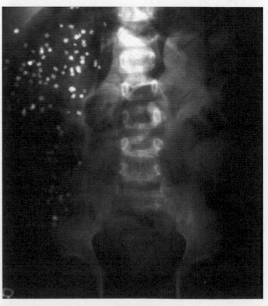

(A)   (B)

Figure 5 Transit time measurements with barium impregnated pellets. The patient swallows 2 capsules filled with 10 pellets each in the morning on 6 consecutive days (A). On the seventh day, an abdominal flat plate is performed in supine position. In this 5-year-old boy with severe dysmotility of the colon, all 120 pellets remained in the large bowel, most of them in the left-sided colon indicating a transit time of >7 days (B). The mother of the patient had suffered from severe constipation and episodes of neuropathic CIP. Both patients improved after colectomy and ileorectal anastomosis.

manomety may also be of value for prognosis[182] and likely response to prokinetic treatment.[183] Tolerating enteral feeding is more likely in the presence of phase III of MMC or organized and propagated clusters of contractions in the duodenum–jejunum.[184] The severity of motility dysfunction varies throughout the GI tract. Motility studies of the rest of the gut may identify areas with preserved motility and different feeding strategies then may be devised, bypassing the affected segments.

Esophageal manometry has been found abnormal in 50 to 90% of patients with both forms of CIP, independent of esophageal symptoms.[185] Anorectal manometry is extremely useful to rule out Hischsprung's disease, but the rectoanal inhibitory reflex is found in almost all patients with CIP not due to aganglionosis.[153] Colonic manometry may show distal motility impairment in patients with visceral neuropathy, with a weak basal activity and an absence of gastrocolic response during fasting and after stimulation with a meal, a laxative, or prokinetic drugs.[184]

Autonomic Testing

Autonomic tests are available to evaluate sympathetic adrenergic, sympathetic cholinergic, and vagal innervation of the viscera. They might be helpful in patients with the evidence of neuropathic dysmotility on previous testing but without a known underlying neurologic disorder. All systems can be involved such as the vasomotor/cardiovascular, ophthalmologic, respiratory, sudomotor, neurologic, and urologic system. Peripheral dysautonomia requires further screening for a toxic, metabolic, or paraneoplastic process. In some cases where a central lesion is suggested, a brain and spinal cord magnetic resonance imaging is essential. Dysautonomia may be familial or acquired.[117,186] In familial cases, reported in Ashkenazi Jewish families, the clinical diagnosis is based on the presence of five signs: lack of axon flare after intradermal injection of histamine, absence of fungiform papillae in the tongue, myosis of the pupil after conjunctival instillation of methacholine, absent deep tendon reflexes, and diminished tear flow.[118] Chronic vomiting and retching is the main GI symptom in these cases.[187]

Histology

Histopathologic finding on full-thickness biopsy specimen are essential to make a specific pathologic diagnosis. Descriptions and classifications of the various types of visceral myopathies and neuropathies are provided above. Unnecessary explorative laparotomy in children with CIP for histopathologic analysis should be avoided. Full-thickness intestinal wall specimens should only be taken during surgery when an ostomy is needed and performed or if an inflammatory process is suspected (leiomyositis and enteric gangliositis) via laparoscopy. Large samples of at least 1.5 cm should be obtained and be divided to send some tissue for routine light microscopy, for electron

microscopy, and snap-frozen samples for immunohistochemistry and enzyme histochemistry to a pathologist who is experienced with enteric myopathies and neuropathies. To show abnormalities in ICC distribution in children with CIP, immunoreactivity for c-Kit as a marker for ICC has been used.[188] If a mitochondrial disorder is suspected, tissue should also be taken from a striated muscle, and in case of abnormal liver function test, of the liver. Investigations such as in situ hybridization for specific abnormalities may be diagnostic. For example, abnormalities of the nicotinic acetylcholine receptor can be found in some patients with megacystis-microcolon hypoperistalsis syndrome.[47]

Treatment

Patients with CIP require a multidisciplinary approach with participations of different specialties based on the presence of comorbidities. Treatment options for CIP are still limited, and mainly focus on support of hydration, correcting nutritional deficiencies and preventing weight loss and malnutrition, minimizing symptoms, suppression of bacterial overgrowth, stimulation of motility with prokinetics or to counteract dumping, and rapid transit by somatostatin analogs. Venting enterostomy or localized resections are required to provide decompression for symptom relief.

Symptomatic Support

Abdominal pain, bloating, nausea, and vomiting in patients with small intestinal dysmotility are often related to eating. Bowel decompression by nasogastric suction is useful during acute exacerbations in patients with cyclical symptoms. Venting ostomies should early be performed in patients with frequent exacerbations or chronic distension to decrease bowel dilatation, to improve intestinal transit, and to provide symptomatic relief from vomiting and pain.[50,141] However, the management of intestinal or visceral pain in patients with CIP is very difficult. Although the parenteral administration of narcotics may be required during episodes of obstruction, long-term narcotic use should be avoided because narcotics can further disturb GI motility, and the risk of addiction is very high. The use of nonopioid analgesia with full psychological and psychiatric support, including behavioral or relaxation therapy, is the best way to help these children.[189]

Due to the increased understanding of the pathophysiologic disturbance responsible for many functional bowel disorders, many putative therapeutic targets for treatment of visceral pain are now available, although most of them are not released for children and only a few for adults. These include cholecystokinin A antagonists, serotonergic agonists and antagonists, selective agonist, tachykinin receptor antagonists, somatostatin analogs, cannabinoids γ, and amino butyric acid receptor modulators.[190] Gabapentin and tricyclic antidepressants also may be beneficial.[191,192]

Nutritional Support

An early nutritional support is important, particularly for patients with recurrent vomiting, reduced oral intake, or malnutrition in the course of the disease. Optimal nutrition by enteral or parenteral routes is of most importance for both supporting normal growth and development, and to avoid further gut dysfunction due to specific deficiencies like potassium, different vitamins, or carnitin. Normalization of the nutritional status may also lead to improvement of intestinal dysmotility. Enteral feeding should always be preferred to using PN. Even when parenteral feeding are required, at least small volumes of enteral feeding are desirable to prevent cholestatic liver disease and to maintain bowel mucosal integrity. Therefore gastrostomies and jejunostomies may also be used for slow administration of enteral formulas.[193] In neuropathic disorders, enteral nutrition is typically used, while PN may be necessary for patients with severe myopathies. About two-thirds of pediatric patients with CIP require more or less prolonged PN during the course of their disease.

Antibiotics

Abnormal motility is associated with bacterial overgrowth,[194,195] which by itself causes mucosal inflammation and maldigestion, further impairing GI motility and creating a vicious cycle.[196] Bacterial overgrowth is a frequent complication of CIP and often causes villous atrophy and malabsorption and may be associated with increased mucosal permeability of macromolecules and bacterial translocation across the bowel.[197–199] Treatment with 1- to 2-week cycles of broad-spectrum antibiotics such as metronidazole, amoxicillin and clavulanic acid, cotrimoxazole, or neomycin may decrease the risk of hepatic complication of TPN and sepsis, improve digestion and motility.[200] However, protracted and/or repeated antibiotic administration may be responsible for selection of highly resistant gram-negative bacteria. Antibiotic therapy should be monitored carefully with the support of an outstanding microbiology laboratory. There is no evidence-based study demonstrating the benefits of antibiotic in CIP.

Prokinetic Agents

Prokinetic agents, particularly erythromycin, cisapride, octreotide, and tegaserod may be useful for acute and chronic therapy of intestinal pseudo-obstruction. Combining a prokinetic agent with an antiemetic medication it is appropriate for symptoms relief. The 5-HT4 agonist cisapride increases the antroduodenal motility index and may improve tolerance of enteral feeds.[183,201] Unfortunately, cisapride has been associated with a number of drug interactions and fatal cardiac arrhythmias including tordade des Points, leading to its withdrawal from the market in most countries. Tegaserod is a new prokinetic agent with a similar mode of action to cisapride, a partial 5-HT4 agonist, but without causing cardiac dysrhythmia. It may be helpful particularly in patients with colonic involvement.[50] However, its release has been suspended due to an increased occurrence of cardiovascular insults in adults. 5-HT4 receptors are transmembrane domain receptors coupled to G proteins. They are responsible for eliciting the depolarizing action of serotonin that results in acetylcholine release from the enteric neurons. Another potent prokinetic from this class is prucalopride, which accelerated GI and colonic transit in patients with severe constipation.

Erythromycin is a motilin receptor agonist, mimicking the prokinetic hormone, motilin, which induces phase III of the MMC. It has been used in subantibiotic doses (3 mg/kg bodyweight per dose) with benefit in CIP.[202] Erythromycin in combination with octreotide that induces duodenal phase III-like contractions has been tested with success in adults with systemic sclerosis and pseudo-obstruction.[55] Octreotide is the most potent enterokinetic medication currently available and has been found to be beneficial in adult patients with CIP and bacterial overgrowth. Since it decreases gastric emptying and gall bladder contractibility, the combination with erythromycin seems useful.[203]

Neostigmine, an acetylcholinesterase inhibitor, was repeated reported to be successful in the therapy of acute pseudo-obstruction in adults and in children.[204] There are no comparable data for treatment of children with chronic pseudo-obstruction, although successful use in an adult with chronic symptoms was reported.[205] Metoclopramide, domperidone, misoprostol, trimebutine, leuprolide, and naloxone have been sporadically tried and may be useful in selected cases.

Immunmodulatory Therapy

The rare forms of CIP due to primary myenteric ganglionitis[104,206] or enteric leiomyositis[51,62] should be treated with immunosuppression including high-dose corticosteroids (see above). Due to the rarity of these conditions, there are no controlled data to guide therapy.

Surgery

Surgical options must be evaluated carefully.[207] Unnecessary abdominal surgery in children with CIP should be avoided because they bear the risk of prolonged postoperative ileus and developing adhesions, creating a diagnostic problem each time there is a new obstructive episode.

Gastrostomy Tubing. Repeated acute episodes of bowel obstruction as well as chronic intestinal distension require bowel decompression by using nasogastric suction. The placement of venting gastrostomy is of great benefit in avoiding the recurrent placement of nasogastric tubes. Percutaneous endoscopic gastrostomy tube placement is easily achieved in these children. When surgery is required, a gastrostomy may be performed during the same surgical procedure. Since enteral feeding should always be preferred to using PN, intragastric administration of feeding may

be achieved by the gastric tube as continuous or bolus enteral feeding.

Enterostomy. In neonates and young infants, intestinal obstruction may last several weeks or months requiring TPN with subsequent complications including catheter-related sepsis and liver disease. Enterostomy may offer the chance to restart intestinal transit allowing feeding and reducing PN.

In some patients, attacks of intestinal obstruction are frequent or life threatening. Chronic bowel dilatation impairs intestinal motility creating a vicious circle that increases intraluminal bacterial overgrowth with the subsequent risk of intestinal translocation. Enterostomy should be performed to bypass the functional obstruction and obtain digestive decompression. The location of enterostomy is a matter of debate. In case of obvious megacystis-microcolon syndrome and in most other forms of CIP a terminal ileostomy is the preferred stoma, because a colostomy is in most instances not sufficient. Terminal ileostomy usually enables transit to resume and leads to a major long-term reduction in obstructive episodes. However, less than 50% of patients improve after ileostomy by being weaned from PN. If the decompression ileostomy has produced relief, but there is diffuse disease, the urge to re-establish connection with the defunctioned limb of the bowel should be resisted as this will only result in further episodes of obstruction. In other words, performing an ileostomy and closing it because of clinical improvement results in the patient undergoing two surgical without resolution of the primary issues. This should be avoided. Conversely, in patients in which clear improvement from ileostomy is observed, with PN weaning and at least 2 years follow-up on enteral/oral feeding without exacerbations, total colectomy, and ileorectal anastomosis may be considered.

Cecostomies or even sigmoidostomies have been used to administer antegrade enemas when intractable constipation appears to be the prominent symptom.[208]

Recurrent Laparotomies. Patients with an enterostomy who continue to present with exacerbation of bowel obstruction are thought to have a mechanical obstruction. In the past, many children underwent multiple surgical procedures resulting in dense adhesions further aggravating obstruction. An excessive number of surgical procedures should be avoided. In the largest study involving 105 pediatric infants and children with CIP, 71 patients underwent surgery during their illness, and 217 surgical procedures, a mean of 3 per patient, were performed.[8] Ostomy was the most performed procedure. Surgery may cause adhesions, so interpretations of subsequent obstructive episodes are difficult. Exploratory laparotomy for obstruction should be performed only when a clear mechanical obstruction has been demonstrated. Signs of peritonitis, extreme dilatation, and pain in association with specific episode of obstruction points more toward a mechanical

obstruction than functional obstruction and laparotomy may be required to relieve it.

Some patients, in whom there was no evidence of mechanical obstruction but segmented bowel dilatation, had improvement by placing a jejunostomy tube within a dilated loop. The use of this jejunostomy button device for daily intermittent bowel decompression may improve bowel function allowing decreased PN intake. For some children this means three tubes: gastrostomy, jejunostomy, and terminal ileostomy.

Gastric and Intestinal Pacemaker

The implantation of gastric or intestinal pacemaker aimed at improving motility constitutes a promising investigational approach in patients with severe motility disorders. The use of gastric electrical stimulation has been shown a significant improvement in nausea and vomiting not only in patients with diabetic gastroparesis, but more recently also in three adult patients with familial and one with postsurgical CIP and disabling nausea and vomiting.[209] The weekly vomiting frequency decreased from 24 before implantation of the gastric pacemaker to 6.9 after 12 months. The clinical response was unrelated to the presence or improvement of delayed gastric emptying in these patients. Although placements of the electrodes along the anterolateral surface of the stomach was successful in most patients by laparoscopic implantation, the procedure is not without risk since the electrodes caused ileus, which made explantation and a short intestinal resection necessary.[209]

Intestinal Transplantation

In many cases of CIP, outcome is poor, with a constant risk of sepsis from intestinal bacterial overgrowth, and water-electrolyte disorders related to intraluminal fluid retention. Intestinal transplantation with liver transplantation in case of progressive cholestatic liver disease represents the only definitive cure for patients with permanent intestinal failure due to chronic intestinal pseudo-obstruction at the present time. Graft rejection, graft-versus-host diseases, and immunosuppression-related lymphoproliferative disorders are more common than other organ transplants.[210] The risk–benefit ratio in children with CIP is less clear than for other indication of intestinal failure like short-gut syndrome, total aganglionosis, microvillous inclusion disease, or epithelial dysplasia. Complications seem to be more common due to multiple previous abdominal surgeries, dysmotility of the stomach and esophagus, and extraintestinal manifestations including dysfunction of the urinary tract, the immune, and the neurologic system.[49]

Transplant procedures vary according to indication for liver transplant and based on the experience of the transplant surgical team. Combined small-bowel–liver transplantations or multivisceral transplantations (MVTxs), including the stomach, have been performed in refractory form of CIP associated with end-stage liver disease. MVTx was reported in 16 children at median age of 4 years.[211,212] Indications for MVTx were liver failure ($n = 10$), loss of venous access ($n = 3$), or sepsis ($n = 3$). Modified MVTx without the liver was performed in six patients. Actual patient survival for 1 year/2 years for the period before 2001 and the period from 2001-2004, were 57.1/42.9% and 88.9/77.8%. None of the long-term survivors are on PN and all tolerate enteral feedings. Gastric emptying was substantially affected in one case. Bladder function did not improve in those with urinary retention problems. MVTx for CIP offers a lifesaving option with excellent function of the transplanted pancreas and stomach among survivors. It is unclear which method offers the best chance for restoration of normal gut function.

Ethical dilemmas may arise with children who will never be able to tolerate full enteral feeding. Some patients with severe CIP may be disabled because of chronic, massive GI dilatation refractory to stomal decompression, or partial enterectomy. The poor quality of life might serve as indication for intestinal transplantation, although usual criteria include progressive liver disease, the loss of vascular access, and absence recurring life-threatening sepsis. In any case, parents must be extensively informed about the risks of the procedure and about the outcomes of all decisions. Extensive workup and careful consideration is required before transplantation is undertaken. However, early referral is essential on initial presentation of complications for these patients to be provided optimal medical care ensuring transplantation an option.[213]

Others

Botulinum toxin injection in the pylorus and anal sphincter has been used to improve gastric emptying and defecation, respectively, in case of obstruction, but in the absence of stenosis.[214] The use of hyperbaric oxygenation in a child with myopathic CIP has been reported.[215]

Outcome and Prognosis

The outcome of children with CIP is variable.[8,176,216,217] In secondary and acquired forms of CIP the outcome depends on the underlying responsible disease. Some causes of secondary pseudo-obstruction that have been described are treatable and may lead to the total cure of the disease.[61,140] In primary forms of CIP, the prognosis is poor, with the exception of some neonatal forms due to delayed maturation of the ENS or ICCs. In a large multicenter study of 105 pediatric patients, two-thirds required PN; and 41% did not tolerate enteral feeding.[8] Surgery was required as a treatment in 71 patients. Only 24 of 58 patients who underwent bypass surgery were able to eat normally. If TPN is required for more than 6 months, the child will probably be TPN dependent for at least 4 years.[143]

A poor prognosis was associated with neonatal onset, urinary tract involvement, requirement for surgery during the course of the disease, and myopathic disorders.[8,142,143] Prognostic factors for a better outcome and for tolerance of enteral feeding are the presence of phase III of the MMC on antroduodenal manometry.

Despite ongoing progress in our understanding and management of PN, medical, and surgical therapies, children suffering from CIP have a high morbidity and mortality. In recent pediatric studies, mortality varied from 10% to up to 25% at a median follow-up time of 2 years.[142] Most common causes of death are complications of long-term PN-related, including cholestatic liver disease, central venous catheter-associated sepsis, thrombembolic complications, and post-transplant death.[8,49,142,143] With an early recognition, avoidance of unnecessary surgery and a good nutritional support, psychological coping strategies, pain management and new drugs, survival, and quality of life are improving for patients with CIP.

MUNCHAUSEN SYNDROME BY PROXY

Munchausen syndrome by proxy is a form of child abuse characterized by a caretaker secretly causing illness with the inadvertent collusion of medical professionals. It commonly involves GI symptoms, and may mimic CIP. It may affect previously healthy children or children with an underlying organic disease and has been described even in a child after small-bowel transplantation.[218] The most frequent complaints reported by caregivers who falsify illness in their children included the GI-related symptoms of anorexia/feeding problems (24.6%), diarrhea (20.0%), and pain (8.0%).[219] In a series of 117 cases, the mortality rate was 9%.[220] Apnea, cyanosis, and vomiting were the most frequently reported symptoms among victims who had died. A previous review also found high rates of vomiting (10%) among suspected abusers.[220]

Sheridan recently reviewed the literature and analyzed 451 cases.[219] There is no gender preference. The average age at diagnosis was 48 months (range >1 to 204 months) with an average length of history of almost 22 months (range 0 to 195 months). In the review by Sheridan, 25% of siblings of victims were known to be dead and 61% of the siblings had symptoms that were similar to those of the victims. In 76% of the cases, the mother was the perpetrator, and in only 6.7% of the cases the father was identified fabricating the symptoms. Perpetrators are frequently characterized as having Munchausen syndrome, and more than 20% had or claimed a personal history of abuse during childhood or partner relationship.

While insufficient for diagnosis, warning signs *related to the illness* include that the illness (or test result) does not make medical sense, is oddly difficult to effectively treat, is exceedingly rare, or does not follow a normal illness or recovery trajectory. Warning signs in cases of falsified CIP include: (a) daily abdominal pain, (b) illness involving three or more organ systems, (c) an accelerating disease trajectory, (d) a reported history of preterm birth, (e) absence of dilated bowel on X-ray, (f) normal antroduodenal manometry, and (g) no urinary neuromuscular disease.[161] While these findings are not presented as diagnostic criteria, the index of illness falsification suspicion should rise with the number of warning signs. General warning signs *of a suspected abuser* include: symptoms only occur in the caregiver's presence or after the caregiver has been present; the caregiver is unusually attentive to medical issues; the caregiver appears less or more worried about child's illness than medical staff (does not take cues related to level of alarm from clinicians); the caregiver is medically knowledgeable or attempts to appear so; the caregiver requests unnecessary or dangerous medical procedures; or the caregiver has a pattern of lying. *Family history warning signs* include: caregiver reports medical interests or experience; or the caregiver or the family has an extensive history of illness.

A team approach is recommended for a scientific, systematic, safe, thorough, and objective assessment without unnecessarily alarming the family or creating undo conflict among team members. Team members might include attending physicians and residents, nursing, the hospital child protection team, social work, psychiatry/psychology, child life, security, and other consultants involved (such as nutrition services, medical consultants, and physical therapy).

A written protocol may be helpful and suggest which team members are best suited to interviews and may clarify procedures, including frequent communication with the family and among team members; obtaining and reviewing past records; collateral contacts with past clinicians and other caregivers; guidelines for documentation and for the collection of physical specimens that could be evidence; planning for family, child, and team emotional support; developing an assessment and treatment plan; discussing and arranging safety parameters for the child and family members; and deciding when/if contact with outside authorities is required. Safety issues to consider for inpatients include location of the child (intensive care unit, private room, near nurses station, etc); level of monitoring (telemetry, sitter, visitation, hours, covert videotape surveillance, etc)[221]; and emergency response plans (in case of acute medical event or attempted discharge by caregiver and legal issues). Details for assignments are reached by consensus, and once team members leave the team meeting, there is no discord among team members.

Clinical Evaluation

The issue of definitive proof is very important. A high degree of accuracy is important to finally protect the child from abuse and caretakers from false allegations.[219] In order to conduct an objective evaluation, one must discount the parental report of symptoms and rely on direct observations and on closely monitored medical tests. For legal issues every observation should be recorded and possibly testified by two persons. It is important to think about how one could simulate or induce a particular symptom and then assess for evidence of such behavior. For example, abnormal results of a pH probe might be discounted if a suspicious parent was alone with the child during the procedure. Tap water or blood can be added to stools to simulate bloody diarrhea. The history provided by the parent will enable the clinician to challenge claims. Therefore, all diagnostic tests should be performed under complete observation. A bedside commode and a sitter will stop false claims of diarrhea. Medications should be systematically removed if it is suspected that they are not needed. Physical therapy or other interventions can be recommended to optimize functioning. Because it is not the normal process for determining a differential diagnosis, and because it can be highly stressful, it is helpful to discuss the assessment plan with an experienced psychologist.

At admission and during increases in observed symptoms, obtain lab specimens for toxicology (urine, stool, blood or even hair, depending on suspected drugs or toxins). The specimens should be obtained under supervision of two health professionals. An emetine screen may be indicated for persistent vomiting. The chain of evidence must be preserved to establish that specimens were not contaminated or exchanged.

There is no consistent psychological profile of someone who has engaged in illness falsification.[222] Many abusers appear "normal" as parents. Therefore, a psychiatric interview and/or psychological testing of the suspected caretaker may not indicate any psychopathology. However, children are adversely impacted by this form of abuse and may become distressed during the hospitalization.[223] Psychiatric and developmental evaluations of the child are indicated as part of the initial evaluation. Additionally, ongoing support to the child, family and team, and assistance with rehabilitation treatment planning can be helpful contributions by mental health professionals.

Separation of the child from the suspected abuser can be a powerful way to determine if illness falsification has occurred. However, persistent symptoms do not rule out past illness falsification. Continued symptoms suggest that some or all of the symptoms are legitimate, that the child has been permanently injured, or that the child is not being sufficiently protected. Additionally, if medical treatment is altered at the time that separation occurs, it can be difficult to discern the cause for a change in health.

Long-Term Outcome and Prognosis. After proving this form of child abuse, many children need to be separated from their families in order to protect them from further damage.[224] If the child remains with their biological mother, the risk of further fabrications of illness is 30 to 50%.[225] Besides permanent organic health problems, conduct and emotional disorders and school problems were very common and found in half of the victims on long-term follow-up.[223,225]

REFERENCES

1. Iantorno G, Bassotti G, Kogan Z, et al. The enteric nervous system in chagasic and idiopathic megacolon. Am J Surg Pathol 2007;31:460–8.
2. Wedel T, Van Eys GJ, Waltregny D, et al. Novel smooth muscle markers reveal abnormalities of the intestinal musculature in severe colorectal motility disorders. Neurogastroenterol Motil 2006;18:526–38.
3. Rühl A. Glial cells in the gut. Neurogastroenterol Motil 2005;17:777-90.
4. Koletzko S, Jesch I, Faus-Keßler T, et al. Rectal biopsy for diagnosis of intestinal neuronal dysplasia in children: A prospective multicentre study on interobserver variation and clinical outcome. Gut 1999;44:853–61.
5. Smith B. Pre- and postnatal development of the ganglion cells of the rectum and its surgical implications. J Pediatr Surg 1968;3:386–91.
6. Wester T, O'briain DS, Puri P. Notable Postnatal Alterations In The Myenteric Plexus Of Normal Human Bowel. Gut 1999;44:666–74.
7. Coerdt W, Michel JS, Rippin G, et al. Quantitative morphometric analysis of the submucous plexus in age-related control groups. Virchows Arch 2004;444:239–46.
8. Faure C, Goulet O, Ategbo S, et al. Chronic intestinal pseudoobstruction syndrome: Clinical analysis, outcome, and prognosis in 105 children. French-speaking group of pediatric gastroenterology. Dig Dis Sci 1999;44:953–9.
9. Navarro J, Sonsino E, Boige N, et al. Visceral neuropathies responsible for chronic intestinal pseudo-obstruction syndrome in pediatric practice: Analysis of 26 cases. J Pediatr Gastroenterol Nutr 1990;11:179–95.
10. White SM, Chamberlain P, Hitchcock R, et al. Megacystis-microcolon-intestinal hypoperistalsis syndrome: The difficulties with antenatal diagnosis. case report and review of the literature. Prenat Diagn 2000;20:697–700.
11. Guze CD, Hyman PE, Payne VJ. Family studies of infantile visceral myopathy: A congenital myopathic pseudo-obstruction syndrome. Am J Med Genet 1999;82:114–22.
12. Knowles CH, Silk DB, Darzi A, et al. Deranged smooth muscle alpha-actin as a bio-marker of intestinal pseudo-obstruction: A controlled multinational case series. Gut 2004;53:1583–9.
13. Smith VV, Milla PJ. Histological phenotypes of enteric smooth muscle disease causing functional intestinal obstruction in childhood. Histopathology 1997;31:112–22.
14. Schuffler MD, Pope CE. Studies of idiopathic intestinal pseudoobstruction. II. hereditary hollow visceral myopathy: Family studies. Gastroenterology 1977;73:339–44.
15. Faulk DL, Anuras S, Gardner GD, et al. A familial visceral myopathy. Ann Intern Med 1978;89:600–6.
16. Shaw A, Shaffer HA, Anuras S. Familial visceral myopathy: The role of surgery. Am J Surg 1985;150:102–8.
17. Schuffler MD, Lowe MC, Bill AH. Studies of idiopathic intestinal pseudoobstruction. I. Hereditary hollow visceral myopathy: Clinical and pathological studies. Gastroenterology 1977;73:327–38.
18. Schuffler MD, Deitch EA. Chronic idiopathic intestinal pseudo-obstruction. A surgical approach. Ann Surg 1980;192:752–61.
19. Mueller LA, Camilleri M, Emslie SA. Mitochondrial neurogastrointestinal encephalomyopathy: Manometric and diagnostic features. Gastroenterology 1999;116:959–63.
20. Blondon H, Polivka M, Joly F, et al. Digestive smooth muscle mitochondrial myopathy in patients with mitochondrial-neurogastrointestinal encephalomyopathy (MNGIE). Gastroenterol Clin Biol 2005;29:773–8.
21. Anuras S, Mitros FA, Nowak TV, et al. A familial visceral myopathy with external ophthalmoplegia and autosomal recessive transmission. Gastroenterology 1983;84:346–53.
22. Perez AA, Fox V, Teitelbaum JE, et al. Mitochondrial neurogastrointestinal encephalomyopathy: Diagnosis by rectal biopsy. Am J Surg Pathol 1998;22:1141–7.
23. Nishino I, Spinazzola A, Papadimitriou A, et al. Mitochondrial neurogastrointestinal encephalomyopathy: An autosomal recessive disorder due to thymidine phosphorylase mutations. Ann Neurol 2000;47:792–800.
24. Szigeti K, Wong LJ, Perng CL, et al. MNGIE with lack of skeletal muscle involvement and a novel Tp splice site mutation. J Med Genet 2004;41:125–9.
25. Gamez J, Ferreiro C, Accarino ML, et al. Phenotypic variability in a Spanish family with MNGIE. Neurology 2002; 59:455–7.
26. Marti R, Spinazzola A, Tadesse S, et al. Definitive diagnosis of mitochondrial neurogastrointestinal encephalomyopathy by biochemical assays. Clin Chem 2004;50:120–4.
27. Giordano C, Sebastiani M, Plazzi G, et al. Mitochondrial neurogastrointestinal encephalomyopathy: Evidence of mitochondrial DNA depletion in the small intestine. Gastroenterology 2006;130:893–901.
28. Teitelbaum JE, Berde CB, Nurko S, et al. Diagnosis and management of MNGIE syndrome in children: Case report and review of the literature. J Pediatr Gastroenterol Nutr 2002;35:377–83.
29. Chitkara DK, Nurko S, Shoffner JM, et al. Abnormalities in gastrointestinal motility are associated with diseases of oxidative phosphorylation in children. Am J Gastroenterol 2003;98:871–7.
30. Hom XB, Lavine JE. Gastrointestinal complication of mitochondrial disease. Mitochondrion 2004;4:601–7.
31. Anuras S, Mitros FA, Milano A, et al. A familial visceral myopathy with dilatation of the entire gastrointestinal tract. Gastroenterology 1986;90:385–90.
32. Kansu A, Ensari A, Kalayci AG, Girgin N. A very rare cause of intestinal pseudo-obstruction: Familial visceral myopathy type IV. Acta Paediatr 2000;89:733–6.
33. Jacops E, Ardichvilli D, Perissino A, et al. A case of familial visceral myopathy with atrophy and fibrosis of the longitudinal muscle layer of the entire small bowel. Gastroenterology 1979;77:745–50.
34. Nonaka M, Goulet O, Arahan P, et al. Primary intestinal myopathy, a cause of chronic idiopathic intestinal pseudoobstruction syndrome (CIPS): Clinicopathological studies of seven cases in children. Pediatr Pathol 1989;9:409–24.
35. Ghavamian R, Wilcox DT, Duffy PG, Milla PJ. The urological manifestations of hollow visceral myopathy in children. J Urol 1997;158:1286–90.
36. Moore SW, Schneider JW, Kaschula RO. Unusual variations of gastrointestinal smooth muscle abnormalities associated with chronic intestinal pseudo-obstruction. Pediatr Surg Int 2002;18:13–20.
37. Moore SW, Schneider JW, Kaschula RD. Nonfamilial visceral myopathy: Clinical and pathologic features of degenerative leiomyopathy. Pediatr Surg Int 2002;18:6–12.
38. Munoz-Yague MT, Marin JC, Colina F, et al. Chronic primary intestinal pseudo-obstruction from visceral myopathy. Rev Esp Enferm Dig 2006;98:292–302.
39. Smith VV, Lake BD, Kamm MA, Nicholls RJ. Intestinal pseudo-obstruction with deficient smooth muscle alpha-actin. Histopathology 1992;21:535–42.
40. Kaschula ROC, Cywes S, Katz A, Louw JH. Degenerative leiomyopathy with massive megacolon. Myopathic form of chronic intestinal pseudo-obstruction occurring in indigenous Africans. Perspect Pediatr Pathol 1987;11:193–213.
41. Berdon WE, Baker DH, Blane WA, et al. Megacystismicrocolon-intestinal hypoperistalsis syndrome. A new cause of intestinal obstruction in the newborn. Report of radiological findings in five newborn girls. Am J Roentgenol 1976;126:957–64.
42. Muller F, Dreux S, Vaast P, et al. Prenatal diagnosis of megacystis-microcolon-intestinal hypoperistalsis syndrome: Contribution of amniotic fluid digestive enzyme assay and fetal urinalysis. Prenat Diagn 2005;25:203–9.
43. Al Harbi A, Tawil K, Crankson SJ. Megacystis-microcolon-intestinal hypoperistalsis syndrome associated with megaesophagus. Pediatr Surg Int 1999;15:272–4.
44. Rolle U, O'briain S, Pearl RH, Puri P. Megacystis-microcolon-intestinal hypoperistalsis syndrome: Evidence of intestinal myopathy. Pediatr Surg Int 2002;18:2–5.
45. Anneren G, Meurling S, Ohlsen L. Megacystis-microcolon-intestinal hypoperistalsis syndrome (MMIHS), an autosomal recessive disorder: Clinical reports and review of the literature. Am J Med Genet 1991;41:251–4.
46. Granata C, Puri P. Megacystis-microcolon-intestinal hypoperistalsis syndrome. J Pediatr Gastroenterol Nutr 1997;25:12–9.
47. Richardson CE, Morgan JM, Jasani B, et al. Megacystis-microcolon-intestinal hypoperistalsis syndrome and the absence of the alpha3 nicotinic acetylcholine receptor subunit. Gastroenterology 2001;121:350–7.
48. Lev-Lehman E, Bercovich D, Xu W, et al. Characterization of the human beta4 NACHR gene and polymorphisms in CHRNA3 and CHRNB4. J Hum.Genet. 2001;46:362–6.
49. Goulet O, Ruemmele F. Causes and management of intestinal failure in children. Gastroenterology 2006;130: S16–S28.
50. Connor FL, Di Lorenzo C. Chronic intestinal pseudo-obstruction: Assessment and management. Gastroenterology 2006;130:S29–S36.
51. Haas S, Bindl L, Fischer HP. Autoimmune enteric leiomyositis: A rare cause of chronic intestinal pseudo-obstruction with specific morphological features. Hum Pathol 2005;36:576–80.
52. Sallam H, Mcnearney TA, Chen JD. Systematic review: Pathophysiology and management of gastrointestinal dysmotility in systemic sclerosis (scleroderma). Aliment Pharmacol Ther 2006;23:691–712.

53. Weber P, Ganser G, Frosch M, et al. Twenty-four hour intraesophageal pH monitoring in children and adolescents with scleroderma and mixed connective tissue disease. J Rheumatol 2000;27:2692–5.
54. Jayachandar J, Frank JL, Jonas MM. Isolated intestinal myopathy resembling progressive systemic sclerosis in a child. Gastroenterology 1988;95:1114–8.
55. Verne GN, Eaker EY, Hardy E, Sninsky CA. Effect of octreotide and erythromycin on idiopathic and scleroderma-associated intestinal pseudoobstruction. Dig Dis Sci 1995;40:1892–901.
56. Weston S, Thumshirn M, Wiste J, Camilleri M. Clinical And upper gastrointestinal motility features in systemic sclerosis and related disorders. Am J Gastroenterol 1998;93:1085–9.
57. Alva S, Abir F, Longo WE. Colorectal manifestations of collagen vascular disease. Am J Surg 2005;189:685–93.
58. Cacoub P, Benhamou Y, Barbet P, et al. Systemic lupus erythematosus and chronic intestinal pseudoobstruction. J Rheumatol 1993;20:377–81.
59. Ruuska TH, Karikoski R, Smith VV, Milla PJ. Acquired myopathic intestinal pseudo-obstruction may be due to autoimmune enteric leiomyositis. Gastroenterology 2002;122:1133–9.
60. Nezelof C, Vivien E, Bigel P, et al. Idiopathic myositis of the small intestine. an unusual cause of chronic intestinal pseudo-obstruction in children. Arch Fr Pediatr 1985;42:823–8.
61. Ginies JL, Francois H, Joseph MG, et al. A curable cause of chronic idiopathic intestinal pseudo-obstruction in children: Idiopathic myositis of the small intestine. J Pediatr Gastroenterol Nutr 1996;23:426–9.
62. Oton E, Moreira V, Redondo C, et al. Chronic intestinal pseudo-obstruction due to lymphocytic leiomyositis: Is there a place for immunomodulatory therapy? Gut 2005;54:1343–4.
63. Lenard HG, Goebel HH, Weigel W. Smooth muscle involvement in congenital myotonic dystrophy. Neuropädiatrie 1976;8:42–52.
64. Leon SH, Schuffler MD, Kettler M, Rohrmann CA. Chronic intestinal pseudo-obstruction as a complication of Duchenne's muscular dystrophy. Gastroenterology 1986;90:455–9.
65. Goyal RK, Hirano I. The enteric nervous system. N Engl J Med 1996;334:1106–15.
66. Smith VV. Intestinal neuronal density in childhood: A baseline for the objective assessment of hypo- and hyperganglionosis. Pediatr Pathol 1993;13:225–37.
67. De Giorgio R, Camilleri M. Human enteric neuropathies: Morphology and molecular pathology. Neurogastroenterol Motil 2004;16:515–31.
68. Hutson JM, Chow CW, Borg J. Intractable constipation with a decrease in substance P-immunoreactive fibres: Is it a variant of intestinal neuronal dysplasia? J Pediatr Surg 1996;31:580–3.
69. Eng C, Marsh DJ, Robinson BG, et al. Germline RET codon 918 mutation in apparently isolated intestinal ganglioneuromatosis. J Clin Endocrinol Metab 1998;83:4191–4.
70. Barnett JL, Mcdonnell M, Appelman HD, Dobbins WO. Familial visceral neuropathy with neuronal intranuclear inclusions: Diagnosis by rectal biopsy. Gastroenterology 1992;102:684–91.
71. Stoss F, Meier-Ruge WA. Experience with neuronal intestinal dysplasia (NID) in adults. Eur J Pediatr Surg 1994;4: 289–302.
72. Meier-Ruge WA. Epidemiology of congenital innervation defects of the distal colon. Virchows Arch A Pathol Anat 1992;420:171–7.
73. Sacher P, Briner J, Hanimann B. Is intestinal neuronal dysplasia (NID) a primary disease or a secondary phenomenon? Eur J Pediatr Surg 1993;3:228–30.
74. Martucciello G, Torre M, Pini-Prato A, et al. Associated anomalies in intestinal neuronal dysplasia. J Pediatr Surg 2002;37:219–23.
75. Meier-Ruge WA, Gambazzi F, Käufeler RE, et al. The neuropathological diagnosis of neuronal intestinal dysplasia (NID B). Eur J Pediatr Surg 1993;4:267–73.
76. Schofield DE, Yunis EJ. Intestinal neuronal dysplasia. J Pediatr Gastroenterol Nutr 1991;12:182–9.
77. Smith VV. Isolated intestinal neuronal dysplasia: A descriptive histological pattern or a distinct clinicopathological entity. In: Hadziselimovic F, Herzog B, editors. Inflammatory Bowel Disease and Morbus Hirschsprung. Dordrecht, Boston, London: Kluwer Academic Publishers; 1992. p. 203–14.
78. Lake BD. Intestinal neuronal dysplasia—why does it only occur in parts of Europe? Virchows Arch 1995;426:537–9.
79. Borchard F, Meier-Ruge WA, Wiebecke B, et al. Innervationsstörungen Des Dick-darms: Klassifikation Und Diagnostik. Pathologe 1991;12:171–4.
80. Lumb PD, Moore L. Are giant ganglia a reliable marker of intestinal neuronal dysplasia type B (IND B)? Virchows Arch. 1998;432:103–6.
81. Meier-Ruge WA, Ammann K, Bruder E, et al. Updated results on intestinal neuronal dysplasia (IND B). Eur J Pediatr Surg 2004;14:384–91.
82. Meier-Ruge WA, Bruder E, Kapur RP. Intestinal neuronal dysplasia type B: One giant ganglion is not good enough. Pediatr Dev Pathol 2006;9:444–52.
83. Gath R, Goessling A, Keller KM, et al. Analysis of the RET, GDNF, EDN3, and EDNRB genes in patients with intestinal neuronal dysplasia and Hirschsprung disease. Gut 2001;48:671–5.
84. Puliti A, Cinti R, Betsos N, et al. Hox1111, A gene involved in peripheral nervous system development, maps to human chromosome 2p13.1→P12 and mouse chromosome 6c3-D1. Cytogenet Cell Genet 1999;84:115–7.
85. Newgreen D, Young HM. Enteric nervous system: Development and developmental disturbances—Part 1. Pediatr Dev Pathol 2002;5:224–47.
86. Mayer EA, Schuffler MD, Rotter JI, et al. Familial visceral neuropathy with autosomal dominant transmission. Gastroenterology 1986;91:1528–35.
87. Camilleri M, Carbone LD, Schuffler MD. Familial enteric neuropathy with pseudo-obstruction. Dig Dis Sci 1991;36: 1168–71.
88. Roper EC, Gibson A, Mcalindon ME, et al. Familial visceral neuropathy: A defined entity? Am J Med Genet 2005; 137a:249–54.
89. Zannolli R, Gilman S, Rossi S, et al. Hereditary neuronal intranuclear inclusion disease with autonomic failure and cerebellar degeneration. Arch Neurol 2002;59:1319–26.
90. Bird TD, Sumi SM, Schuffler MD. Neuronal intranuclear inclusion disease in two adult siblings. Ann Neurol 1985;17:212–3 [Letter].
91. Erez I, Reish O, Kovalivker M, et al. Congenital short-bowel and malrotation: Clinical presentation and outcome of six affected offspring in three related families. Eur J Pe-diatr Surg 2001;11:331–4.
92. Tanner MS, Smith B, Lloyd JK. Functional intestinal obstruction due to deficiency of argyrophil neurones in the myenteric plexus. Familial syndrome presenting with short small bowel, malrotation, and pyloric hypertrophy. Arch Dis Child 1976;51:837–41.
93. Auricchio A, Brancolini V, Casari G, et al. The locus for a novel syndromic form of neuronal intestinal pseudoobstruction maps to Xq28. Am J Hum.Genet. 1996;58:743–8.
94. Gargiulo A, Auricchio R, Barone MV, et al. Filamin A is mutated in X-linked chronic idiopathic intestinal pseudo-obstruction with central nervous system involvement. Am.J Hum.Genet. 2007;80:751–8.
95. Faber J, Fich A, Steinberg A, et al. Familial intestinal pseudoobstruction dominated by a progressive neurologic disease at a young age. Gastroenterology 1987;92:786–90.
96. Cockel R, Hill EE, Rushton DI, et al. Familial steatorrhea with calcification of the basal ganglia and mental retardation. Q J Med 1973;42:771–83.
97. Pingault V, Guiochon-Mantel A, Bondurand N, et al. Peripheral neuropathy with hypomyelination, chronic intestinal pseudo-obstruction and deafness: A developmental "Neural Crest Syndrome" related to A Sox10 mutation. Ann Neurol 2000;48:671–6.
98. Kouvaraki MA, Shapiro SE, Perrier ND, et al. RET proto-oncogene: A review and update of genotype-phenotype correlations in hereditary medullary thyroid cancer and associated endocrine tumors. Thyroid 2005;15:531–44.
99. De Krijger RR, Brooks A, Van-Der HE, et al. Constipation as the presenting symptom in de novo multiple endocrine neoplasia type 2b. Pediatrics 1998;102:405–8.
100. Bahuau M, Laurendeau I, Pelet A, et al. Tandem duplication within the neurofibromatosis type 1 gene (NF1) and reciprocal T(15;16)(Q26.3;Q12.1) Translocation in famil-ial association of NF1 with intestinal neuronal dysplasia type B (IND B). J Med Genet 2000;37:146–50.
101. Sinha Sk, Kochhar R, Rana S, et al. Intestinal pseudo-obstruction due to neurofibromatosis responding to cisapride. Ind J Gastroenterol 2000;19:83–4.
102. Krishnamurthy S, Heng Y, Schuffler MD. Chronic intestinal pseudo-obstruction in infants and children caused by diverse abnormalities of the myenteric plexus. Gastroenterology 1993;104:1398–408.
103. Smith VV, Milla PJ. Argyrophilia in the developing human myenteric plexus. Br J Biomed Sci 1996;53:278–83.
104. De Giorgio R, Guerrini S, Barbara G, et al. Inflammatory neuropathies of the enteric nervous system. Gastroenterology 2004;126:1872–83.
105. Sonsino E, Mouy R, Foucaud P, et al. Intestinal pseudoobstruction related to cytomegalovirus infection of myenteric plexus. N Engl J Med 1984;311:196–7 [Letter].
106. Debinski HS, Kamm MA, Talbot IC, et al. DNA viruses in the pathogenesis of sporadic chronic idiopathic intestinal pseudo-obstuction. Gut 1997;41:100–6.
107. Besnard M, Faure C, Fromont-Hankard G, et al. Intestinal pseudo-obstruction and acute pandysautonomia associated with Epstein–Barr virus infection. Am J Gastroenterol 2000;95:280–4.
108. Foucaud P, Sonsino E, Mouy R, et al. Pseudo-Obstruction Intestinale Et Infection A Cytomegalovirus Des Plexus Myenteriques. [Intestinal pseudo-obstruction and cytomegalovirus infection of myenteric plexuses]. Arch Fr Pediatr 1985;42:713–5.
109. Ategbo S, Turck D, Gottrand F, et al. Chronic intestinal pseudo-obstruction associated with cytomegalovirus infection in an infant. J Pediatr Gastroenterol Nutr 1996;23:457–60.
110. Spiller RC. Postinfectious irritable bowel syndrome. Gastroenterology 2003;124:1662–71.
111. Uc A, Vasiliauskas E, Piccoli DA, et al. Chronic intestinal pseudoobstruction associated with fetal alcohol syndrome. Dig Dis Sci 1997;42:1163–7.
112. Neuman MI, Molle Z, Handelsman EL, et al. Neonatal hypoperistalsis associated with perinatal zidovudine administration. J Perinatol 1998;18:20–3.
113. Husebye E, Hauer JM, Kjorstad K, Skar V. Severe late radiation enteropathy is characterized by impaired motility of proximal small intestine. Dig Dis Sci 1994;39:2341–9.
114. Schappi MG, Smith VV, Milla PJ, Lindley KJ. Eosinophilic myenteric ganglionitis is associated with functional intestinal obstruction. Gut 2003;52:752–5.
115. Smith VV, Gregson N, Foggensteiner L, et al. Acquired intestinal aganglionosis and circulating autoantibodies without neoplasia or other neural involvement. Gastroenterology 1997;112:1366-71 [see comments].
116. Marie I, Herve F, Dode C, et al. Intestinal pseudo-obstruction as a manifestation of tumor necrosis factor receptor-associated periodic syndrome. Dig Dis Sci 2006;51:1061–2.
117. Axelrod FB, Chelimsky GG, Weese-Mayer DE. Pediatric autonomic disorders. Pediatrics 2006;118:309–21.
118. Axelrod FB. Familial dysautonomia. Muscle Nerve 2004;29:352–63.
119. Prpic I, Huebner A, Persic M, et al. Triple A syndrome: Genotype–phenotype assessment. Clin Genet 2003;63:415–7.
120. Huebner A, Yoon SJ, Ozkinay F, et al. Triple A syndrome—clinical aspects and molecular genetics. Endocr Res 2000;26:751–9.
121. Suarez GA, Fealey RD, Camilleri M, Low PA. Idiopathic autonomic neuropathy: Clinical, neurophysiologic, and follow-up studies on 27 patients. Neurology 1994;44:1675–82.
122. Malik M, Connors R, Schwarz KB, O'dorisio TM. Hormone-producing ganglioneuroblastoma simulating intestinal pseudoobstruction. J Pediatr 1990;116:406–8.
123. Di Nardo G, Stanghellini V, Cucchiara S, et al. Enteric neuropathology of congenital intestinal obstruction: A case report. World J Gastroenterol 2006;12:5229–33.
124. Saunders MD, Kimmey MB. Systematic review: Acute colonic pseudo-obstruction. Aliment Pharmacol Ther 2005;22:917–25.
125. Borgaonkar MR, Lumb B. Acute on chronic intestinal pseudoobstruction responds to neostigmine. Dig Dis Sci 2000;45:1644–7.
126. Vanderwinden JM, Rumessen JJ. Interstitial cells of Cajal in human gut and gastrointestinal disease. Microsc Res Tech 1999;47:344–60.
127. Ward SM, Sanders KM. Physiology and pathophysiology of the interstitial cell of Cajal: From bench to bedside. I. Functional development and plasticity of interstitial cells of Cajal networks. Am J Physiol Gastrointest Liver Physiol 2001;281:G602–G611.
128. Sanders KM, Ward SM. Interstitial cells of Cajal: A new perspective on smooth muscle function. J Physiol 2006;576: 721–6.
129. Sanders KM, Koh SD, Ward SM. Interstitial cells of Cajal as pacemakers in the gastrointestinal tract. Annu Rev Physiol 2006;68:307–43.
130. Sanders KM, Ordog T, Ward SM. Physiology and pathophysiology of the interstitial cells of Cajal: From bench to bedside. IV. Genetic and animal models of GI motility disorders caused by loss of interstitial cells of Cajal. Am J Physiol Gastrointest Liver Physiol 2002;282:G747–56.
131. Chang IY, Glasgow NJ, Takayama I, et al. Loss of interstitial cells of Cajal and development of electrical dysfunction in murine small bowel obstruction. J Physiol 2001;536:555–68.
132. Kenny SE, Vanderwinden JM, Rintala RJ, et al. Delayed maturation of the interstitial cells of Cajal: A new diagnosis for transient neonatal pseudoobstruction. report of two cases. J Pediatr Surg 1998;33:94–8.
133. Yoo SY, Jung SH, Eom M, et al. Delayed maturation of interstitial cells of Cajal in meconium obstruction. J Pediatr Surg 2002;37:1758–61.
134. Rolle U, Yoneda A, Solari V, et al. Abnormalities of C-Kit-positive cellular network in isolated hypoganglionosis. J Pediatr Surg 2002;37:709–14.

135. Boeckxstaens GE, Rumessen JJ, De Wit L, et al. Abnormal distribution of the interstitial cells of Cajal in an adult patient with pseudo-obstruction and megaduodenum. Am J Gastroenterol 2002;97:2120–6.
136. He CL, Burgart L, Wang L, et al. Decreased interstitial cell of Cajal volume in patients with slow-transit constipation. Gastroenterology 2000;118:14–21.
137. Wedel T, Spiegler J, Soellner S, et al. Enteric nerves and interstitial cells of Cajal are altered in patients with slow-transit constipation and megacolon. Gastroenterology 2002; 123:1459–67.
138. Kubota M, Kanda E, Ida K, et al. Severe gastrointestinal dysmotility in a patient with congenital myopathy: Causal relationship to decrease of interstitial cells of Cajal. Brain Dev 2005;27:447–50.
139. Grundy D, Al-Chaer ED, Aziz Q, et al. Fundamentals of neurogastroenterology: Basic science. Gastroenterology 2006;130:1391–411.
140. Rudolph CD, Hyman PE, Altschuler SM, et al. Diagnosis and treatment of chronic intestinal pseudo-obstruction in children: Report of consensus workshop. J Pediatr Gastroenterol Nutr 1997;24:102–12 [see comments].
141. Di Lorenzo C. Pseudo-obstruction: Current approaches. Gastroenterology 1999;116:980–7.
142. Mousa H, Hyman PE, Cocjin J, et al. Longterm outcome of congenital intestinal pseudoobstruction. Dig Dis Sci 2002;47:2298–305.
143. Heneyke S, Smith VV, Spitz L, Milla PJ. Chronic intestinal pseudo-obstruction: Treatment and long term follow up of 44 patients. Arch Dis Child 1999;81:21–7.
144. Stanghellini V, Camilleri M, Malagelada JR. Chronic idiopathic intestinal pseudo-obstruction: Clinical and intestinal manometric findings. Gut 1987;28:5–12.
145. De GR, Sarnelli G, Corinaldesi R, Stanghellini V. Advances in our understanding of the pathology of chronic intestinal pseudo-obstruction. Gut 2004;53:1549–52.
146. Coulie B, Camilleri M. Intestinal pseudo-obstruction. Annu Rev Med 1999;50:37–55.
147. Streutker CJ, Huizinga JD, Campbell F, et al. Loss of Cd117 (C-Kit)- and CD34-positive ICC and associated CD34-positive fibroblasts defines a subpopulation of chronic intestinal pseudo-obstruction. Am J Surg Pathol 2003;27: 228–35.
148. Jain D, Moussa K, Tandon M, et al. Role of interstitial cells of Cajal in motility disorders of the bowel. Am J Gastroenterol 2003;98:618–24.
149. Isozaki K, Hirota S, Miyagawa J, et al. Deficiency of C-Kit+ cells in patients with a myopathic form of chronic idiopathic intestinal pseudo-obstruction. Am J Gastroenterol 1997;92:332–4.
150. Chitkara DK, Di Lorenzo C. From the bench to the 'Crib'-side: Implications of scientific advances to paediatric neurogastroenterology and motility. Neurogastroenterol Motil 2006;18:251–62.
151. Mousa H, Bueno J, Griffiths J, et al. Intestinal motility after small bowel transplantation. Transplant Proc 1998;30: 2535–6.
152. Goulet O, Jobert-Giraud A, Michel JL, et al. Chronic Intestinal pseudo-obstruction syndrome in pediatric patients. Eur J Pediatr Surg 1999;9:83–9.
153. Boige N, Faure C, Cargill G, et al. Manometrical evaluation in visceral neuropathies in children. J Pediatr Gastroenterol Nutr 1994;19:71–7.
154. Lapointe SP, Rivet C, Goulet O, et al. Urological manifestations associated with chronic intestinal pseudo-obstructions in children. J Urol 2002;168:1768–70.
155. Higman D, Peters P, Stewart M. Familial hollow visceral myopathy with varying urological manifestations. Br J Urol 1992;70:435–8.
156. Devane SP, Coombes R, Smith VV, et al. Persistent gastrointestinal symptoms after correction of malrotation. Arch Dis Child 1992;67:218–21.
157. Camilleri M. Disorders of gastrointestinal motility in neurologic diseases. Mayo Clin Proc 1990;65:825–46.
158. Sigurdsson L, Flores A, Putnam PE, et al. Postviral gastroparesis: Presentation, treatment, and outcome. J Pediatr 1997;131:751–4.
159. Ariza A, Coll J, Fernandez-Figueras MT, et al. Desmin myopathy: A multisystem disorder involving skeletal, cardiac, and smooth muscle. Hum Pathol 1995;26:1032–7.
160. Gohil A, Croffie JM, Fitzgerald JF, et al. Reversible intestinal pseudoobstruction associated with neural crest tumors. J Pediatr Gastroenterol Nutr 2001;33:86–8.
161. Hyman PE, Bursch B, Beck D, et al. Discriminating pediatric condition falsification from chronic intestinal pseudo-obstruction in toddlers. Child Maltreat 2002;7:132–7.
162. Weaver LT, Rosenthal SR, Gladstone W, Winter HS. Carnitine deficiency: A possible cause of gastrointestinal dysmotility. Acta Paediatr 1992;81:79–81.
163. Ward Hc, Leake J, Milla PJ, Spitz L. Brown bowel syndrome: A late complication of intestinal atresia. J Pediatr Surg 1992;27:1593–5.
164. Horn T, Svendsen LB, Nielsen R. Brown-bowel syndrome. Review of the literature and presentation of cases. Scand J Gastroenterol 1990;25:66–72.
165. Haftel LT, Lev D, Barash V, et al. Familial mitochondrial intestinal pseudo-obstruction and neurogenic bladder. J Child Neurol 2000;15:386–9.
166. De Gr, Barbara G, Stanghellini V, et al. Clinical and morphofunctional features of idiopathic myenteric ganglionitis underlying severe intestinal motor dysfunction: A study of three cases. Am J Gastroenterol 2002;97:2454–9.
167. Royer P, Ricour C, Nihoul-Fekete C, Pellerin D. The familial syndrome of short small intestine with intestinal malrotation and hypertrophic stenosis of the pylorus in infants. Arch Fr Pediatr 1974;31:223–9.
168. Simon LT, Horoupian DS, Dorfman LJ, et al. Polyneuropathy, ophthalmoplegia, leukoencephalopathy, and intestinal pseudo-obstruction: Polip syndrome. Ann Neurol 1990;28:349–60.
169. Krishnamurthy S, Schuffler MD. Pathology of neuromuscular disorders of the small intestine and colon. Gastroenterology 1987;93:610–39.
170. Chitkara DK, Gado-Aros S, Bredenoord AJ, et al. Functional dyspepsia, upper gastrointestinal symptoms, and transit in children. J Pediatr 2003;143:609–13.
171. Braden B, Peterknecht A, Piepho T, et al. Measuring gastric emptying of semisolids in children using the 13c-acetate breath test: A validation study 2004. Dig Liver Dis 2004;36:260–4.
172. Garel C, Dreux S, Philippe-Chomette P, et al. Contribution of fetal magnetic resonance imaging and amniotic fluid digestive enzyme assays to the evaluation of gastrointestinal tract abnormalities. Ultrasound Obstet Gynecol 2006;28:282–91.
173. Camilleri M. New imaging in neurogastroenterology: An overview. Neurogastroenterol Motil 2006;18:805–12.
174. Hase T, Kodama M, Kishida A, et al. The application of radioopaque markers prior to ileostomy in an infant with chronic intestinal pseudo-obstruction: Report of a case. Surg Today 1998;28:83–6.
175. Metcalf AM, Phillips SF, Zinsmeister AR, et al. Simplified assessment of segmental colonic transit. Gastroenterology 1987;92:40–7.
176. Vargas J, Sachs P, Ament ME. Chronic intestinal pseudo-obstruction syndrome in pediatrics. Results of a national survey by members of the North American Society Of Pediatric Gastroenterology and Nutrition. J Pedtr Gastroenterol Nutr 1988;7:323–32.
177. Cucchiara S, Borrelli O, Salvia G, et al. A normal gastrointestinal motility excludes chronic intestinal pseudoobstruction in children. Dig Dis Sci 2000;45:258–64.
178. Camilleri M. Jejunal manometry in distal subacute mechanical obstruction: Significance of prolonged simultaneous contractions. Gut 1989;30:468–75.
179. Cucchiara S, Annese V, Minella R, et al. Antroduodenojejunal manometry in the diagnosis of chronic idiopathic intestinal pseudoobstruction in children. J Pediatr Gastroenterol Nutr 1994;18:294–305.
180. Hyman PE, Napolitano JA, Diego A, et al. Antroduodenal manometry in the evaluation of chronic functional gastrointestinal symptoms. Pediatrics 1990;86:39–44.
181. Hyman PE, Mcdiarmid SV, Napolitano J, et al. Antroduodenal motility in children with chronic intestinal pseudo-obstruction. J Pediatr 1988;112:899–905.
182. Fell JM, Smith VV, Milla PJ. Infantile chronic idiopathic intestinal pseudo-obstruction: The role of small intestinal manometry as a diagnostic tool and prognostic indicator. Gut 1996;39:306–11.
183. Hyman PE, Di LC, Mcadams L, et al. Predicting the clinical response to cisapride in children with chronic intestinal pseudo-obstruction. Am J Gastroenterol 1993;88: 832–6.
184. Di Lorenzo C, Flores AF, Reddy SN, et al. Colonic manometry in children with chronic intestinal pseudo-obstruction. Gut 1993;34:803–7.
185. Schuffler MD, Pope CE. Esophageal motor dysfunction in idiopathic intestinal pseudo-obstruction. Gastroenterology 1976;70:677–82.
186. Slaugenhaupt SA, Gusella JF. Familial dysautonomia. Curr Opin Genet Dev 2002;12:307–11.
187. Gold-Von-Simson G, Axelrod FB. Familial dysautonomia: Update and recent advances. Curr Probl Pediatr Adolesc Health Care 2006;36:218–37.
188. Feldstein AE, Miller SM, El Youssef M, et al. Chronic intestinal pseudoobstruction associated with altered interstitial cells of Cajal networks. J Pediatr Gastroenterol Nutr 2003;36:492–7.
189. Hyman PE, Di LC, Rehm D. Chronic intestinal pseudo-obstruction: A cause of intestinal failure. Transplant Proc 1994;26:1440.
190. Hunt RH, Tougas G. Evolving concepts in functional gastrointestinal disorders: Promising directions for novel pharmaceutical treatments. Best Pract Res Clin Gastroenterol 2002;16:869–83.
191. Heughan CE, Sawynok J. The interaction between gabapentin and amitriptyline in the rat formalin test after systemic administration. Anesth Analg 2002;94:975–80 (Table).
192. Gottrup H, Juhl G, Kristensen Ad, et al. Chronic oral gabapentin reduces elements of central sensitization in human experimental hyperalgesia. Anesthesiology 2004;101: 1400–8.
193. Di Lorenzo C, Flores AF, Buie T, Hyman Pe. Intestinal motility and jejunal feeding in children with chronic intestinal pseudo-obstruction. Gastroenterology 1995;108: 1379–85.
194. Nieuwenhuijs VB, Verheem A, Van Duijvenbode-Beumer H, et al. The role of interdigestive small bowel motility in the regulation of gut microflora, bacterial over-growth, and bacterial translocation in rats. Ann Surg 1998;228: 188–93.
195. Stotzer PO, Bjornsson ES, Abrahamsson H. Interdigestive and postprandial motility in smallintestinal bacterial overgrowth. Scand J Gastroenterol 1996;31:875–80.
196. Husebye E. Gastrointestinal motility disorders and bacterial overgrowth. J Intern Med 1995;237:419–27.
197. Pignata C, Budillon G, Monaco G, et al. Jejunal bacterial overgrowth and intestinal permeability in children with immunodeficiency syndromes. Gut 1990;31:879–82.
198. Van Leeuwen PA, Boermeester MA, Houdijk AP, et al. Clinical significance of translocation. Gut 1994;35: S28–34.
199. Berg Rd. Bacterial translocation from the gastrointestinal tract. J Med 1992;23:217–44.
200. Madrid AM, Hurtado C, Venegas M, et al. Longterm treatment with cisapride and antibiotics in liver cirrhosis: Effect on small intestinal motility, bacterial overgrowth, and liver function. Am J Gastroenterol 2001;96:1251–5.
201. Di LC, Reddy SN, Villanueva-Meyer J, et al. Cisapride in children with chronic intestinal pseudoobstruction. An acute, double-blind, crossover, placebo-controlled trial. Gastroenterology 1991;101:1564–70.
202. Minami T, Nishibayashi H, Shinomura Y, Matsuzawa Y. Effects of erythromycin in chronic idiopathic intestinal pseudo-obstruction. J Gastroenterol 1996;31:855–9.
203. Di Lorenzo C, Lucanto C, Flores AF, et al. Effect of sequential erythromycin and octreotide on antroduodenal manometry. J Pediatr Gastroenterol Nutr 1999;29:293–6.
204. Gmora S, Poenaru D, Tsai E. Neostigmine for the treatment of pediatric acute colonic pseudo-obstruction. J Pediatr Surg 2002;37:E28.
205. Calvet X, Martinez JM, Martinez M. Repeated neostigmine dosage as palliative treatment for chronic colonic pseudo-obstruction in a patient with autonomic paraneoplastic neuropathy. Am J Gastroenterol 2003;98:708–9.
206. Ghirardo S, Sauter B, Levy G, et al. Primary intestinal autoimmune disease as a cause of chronic intestinal pseudo-obstruction. Gut 2005;54:1206–7.
207. Goulet O, Sauvat F, Jan D. Surgery for pediatric patients with chronic intestinal pseudo-obstruction syndrome. J Pediatr Gastroenterol Nutr 2005;41:S66–8.
208. Di Lorenzo C. Surgery in intestinal pseudo-obstruction. Pro J Pediatr Gastroenterol Nutr 2005;41:S64–5.
209. Andersson S, Lonroth H, Simren M, et al. Gastric electrical stimulation for intractable vomiting in patients with chronic intestinal pseudoobstruction. Neurogastroenterol Motil 2006;18:823–30.
210. Lee RG, Nakamura K, Tsamandas AC, et al. Pathology of human intestinal transplantation. Gastroenterology 1996;110:1820–34.
211. Loinaz C, Rodriguez MM, Kato T, et al. Intestinal and multivisceral transplantation in children with severe gastrointestinal dysmotility. J Pediatr Surg 2005;40:1598–604.
212. Loinaz C, Mittal N, Kato T, et al. Multivisceral Transplantation for pediatric intestinal pseudo-obstruction: Single center's experience of 16 cases. Transplant Proc 2004;36: 312–3.
213. Sauvat F, Dupic L, Caldari D, et al. Factors influencing outcome after intestinal transplantation in children. Transplant Proc 2006;38:1689–91.
214. Friedenberg F, Gollamudi S, Parkman HP. The use of botulinum toxin for the treatment of gastrointestinal motility disorders. Dig Dis Sci 2004;49:165–75.
215. Yokota T, Suda T, Tsukioka S, et al. The striking effect of hyperbaric oxygenation therapy in the management of chronic idiopathic intestinal pseudo-obstruction. Am J Gastroenterol 2000;95:285–8.

216. Lopez-Santamaria M, Gamez M, Murcia M, et al. Pediatric Intestinal Transplantation. Transplant.Proc. 2003;35:1927–8.

217. Grant D. Intestinal transplantation: 1997 Report of the international registry. Intestinal Transplant Registry. Transplantation 1999;67:1061–4.

218. Kosmach B, Tarbell S, Reyes J, Todo S. "Munchausen by proxy" syndrome in a small bowel transplant recipient. Transplant Proc 1996;28:2790–1.

219. Sheridan Ms. The Deceit Continues: An Updated Literature Review Of Munchausen Syndrome By Proxy. Child Abuse Negl 2003;27:431–51.

220. Rosenberg DA. Web of deceit: A literature review of munchausen syndrome by proxy. Child Abuse Negl 1987;11:547–63.

221. Hall DE, Eubanks L, Meyyazhagan LS, et al. Evaluation of covert video surveillance in the diagnosis of Munchausen syndrome by proxy: Lessons from 41 cases. Pediatrics 2000;105:1305–12.

222. Parnell TF, Day DO. Munchausen By Proxy Syndrome: Misunderstood Child Abuse. Thousand Oaks, CA: Sage Publications; 1998. p. 8.

223. Ayoub CC. Emotional impact of Munchausen by proxy on the child victims: A five-year follow-up study. Symposium Meeting Of The American Academy Of Child & Adolescent Psychiatry, Chicago; 1999.

224. Sanders MJ, Bursch B. Forensic assessment of illness falsification, Munchausen by proxy, and factitious disorder, nos. Child Maltreat 2002;7:112–4.

225. Bools CN, Neale BA, Meadow SR. Follow up of victims of fabricated illness (Munchausen syndrome by proxy). Arch Dis Child 1993;69:625–30.

24.3. Chronic Abdominal Pain Including Functional Abdominal Pain, Irritable Bowel Syndrome, and Abdominal Migraine

Arine M. Vlieger, MD
Marc A. Benninga, MD, PhD

Chronic abdominal pain is one of the most commonly encountered symptoms in childhood and adolescence with reported prevalences of 1 to 19% and accounting for 2 to 4% of pediatric office visits.[1,2] It is characterized by chronic, recurrent, or continuous abdominal pain not well localized. The pain may wax and wane, with asymptomatic episodes interposed with painful periods and can profoundly affect daily activities. Children often have feelings of anxiety and distress leading to significant school absence and their parents tend to be very worried. Studies of these children revealed self-reported quality-of-life scores comparable to children with inflammatory bowel diseases, highlighting the clinical significance of this problem.[3]

Many pathologic conditions such as infectious, inflammatory, metabolic, or anatomic disorders can cause recurrent abdominal pain (RAP); however, in the vast majority of these children the pain is functional, that is, without objective evidence of an underlying disorder. In the last years chronic or RAP is classified according to the revised Rome criteria into five different abdominal pain-related functional gastrointestinal disorders (FGIDs).[4] The etiology and pathogenesis of these disorders are still largely unknown, but a growing body of evidence suggests that the pain is a result of disordered brain-gut communication. Visceral hypersensitivity, altered conscious awareness of gastrointestinal sensory input, and gastrointestinal dysmotility play a role. This chapter places particular emphasis on new insights in the pathophysiology of chronic, functional abdominal pain (FAP), and abnormalities found at the level of the gut and the brain are discussed.

Children with chronic abdominal pain may present a sometimes frustrating challenge to their treating physicians since they have to determine which children might have an organic disorder and need further diagnostic tests. This chapter tries to provide guidance for the clinician in the diagnostic evaluation of the child with chronic abdominal pain. The importance of the recognition of the so-called alarm symptoms and "red flag" signs is discussed. Finally, evidence-based treatment options for children with FAP are discussed including medications, dietary interventions, and psychological and complementary therapies. For the treatment of organic causes of chronic abdominal pain, readers are referred to the specific chapters on those diseases.

DEFINITIONS

In 1958, Apley and Naish defined RAP as three or more episodes of abdominal pain, severe enough to affect daily activities, occurring over a period of at least 3 months.[5] For decades these criteria have been widely used, although often the o)riginal term *recurrent* abdominal pain was replaced by *chronic* or *functional* abdominal pain. Nowadays, the terms recurrent and chronic abdominal pain are abandoned and replaced by "pain-related functional gastrointestinal disorders." FGIDs are defined as a variable combination of chronic or recurrent gastrointestinal symptoms not explained by structural or biochemical abnormalities. In 1999 in Rome, a group of experts in the field of pediatric gastroenterology made an attempt to set criteria for FGIDs in childhood, the so-called Rome II criteria.[6] These criteria have provided clinicians for the first time with a method for standardizing their definition of clinical disorders and have allowed researchers from various fields to study the pathophysiology and treatment of the same disorders from different points of view. At that time, however, no evidence was available to support a classification for RAP in children in four pain-related FGIDs; that is, functional dyspepsia (FD), irritable bowel syndrome (IBS), functional abdominal pain, and abdominal migraine. Furthermore, the interobserver reliability in diagnosis while using the pediatric Rome II criteria among pediatric gastroenterologists and fellows was low.[7] In recent years, however, a preliminary validation of a questionnaire on pediatric gastrointestinal symptoms and features related to FGIDs, as defined by the Rome II criteria was reported.[8] Since then three publications using the same questionnaire documented the prevalence of FGIDs in tertiary care clinics and in African American children in primary care in the United States.[9–11] In Europe a study reported the prevalence of FGIDs in Italian children consulting primary care pediatricians.[12]

These publications have offered valid criticism of some disorders and provided preliminary validation of others.

Based on these latter studies, clinical experience and consensus between the members of the Rome III committee, the revised and updated Rome III pediatric criteria appeared in 2006.[4] Because of the great variability in the severity and phenotypic presentation of children with abdominal pain–related FGIDs, the previously inclusive category of FAP was divided into two separate disorders, childhood functional abdominal pain and childhood functional abdominal pain syndrome (FAPS). Furthermore, the required duration of symptoms was changed from to 3 to 2 months. More importantly, and in contrast to the Rome II criteria, the Rome III criteria for FAP in childhood now differs from the criteria in adults. The new classifications for FAP in children are listed in Table 1. These new Rome III pediatric criteria need to be validated in prospective studies on children with FAP. Furthermore, their relevance in terms of therapeutic interventions or predicting prognosis must be evaluated in long-term follow-up studies.

EPIDEMIOLOGY

Chronic or RAP is one of the most common pediatric complaints with reported prevalences in western countries of 0.3 to 19% and a median of 8.4% (reviewed by Chitkara and colleagues[1]). This very wide range is caused by different methodologies used to assess the diagnosis such as personal interviews versus questionnaires and different criteria used to make the diagnosis of RAP. There is evidence to suggest a bimodal age peak in which the symptoms of RAP are more prevalent. Apley and Naish observed already in their original study a steady rise in children below 5 years of age and then another rise between 8 and 10 years of age.[5] This observation has been supported by many others studies evaluating the prevalence of RAP (reviewed by Chitkara and colleagues[1]). Females seem to have a higher prevalence of RAP compared to males, but this difference manifests not earlier than around puberty.[13] Other factors associated with a higher RAP prevalence are familial and socioeconomic factors. Bode and colleagues

Table 1 Classifications of Pediatric Functional Abdominal Pain Disorders According to the Rome III Criteria[4]

Functional dyspepsia
- Persistent or recurrent pain or discomfort centered in the upper abdomen (above the umbilicus)
- Not relieved by defecation or associated with the onset of a change in stool frequency or stool form (ie, not IBS)
- Criteria fulfilled at least once per week for at least 2 months before diagnosis

Irritable bowel syndrome
- Abdominal discomfort (an uncomfortable sensation not described as pain) or pain associated with 2 *or more* of the following at least 25% of the time:
  a) Improved with defecation
  b) Onset associated with a change in frequency of stool
  c) Onset associated with a change in form (appearance) of stool
- Criteria fulfilled at least once per week for at least 2 months before diagnosis

Symptoms that cumulatively support the diagnosis of IBS are (1) abnormal stool frequency (four or more stools per day and two or less stools per week), (2) abnormal stool form (lumpy/hard or loose/watery stool), (3) abnormal stool passage (straining, urgency, or feeling of incomplete evacuation), (4) passage of mucus, and (5) bloating or feeling of abdominal distension.

Abdominal migraine
- Paroxysmal episodes of intense, acute periumbilical pain that lasts for 1 h or more
- Intervening periods of usual health lasting weeks to months
- The pain interferes with normal activities
- The pain is associated with two or more of the following:
  a) Anorexia
  b) Nausea
  c) Vomiting
  d) Headache
  e) Photophobia
  f) Pallor
- All above criteria must be included and fulfilled >2 times in the preceding 12 months

Childhood functional abdominal pain
- Episodic or continuous abdominal pain
- Insufficient criteria for other FGIDs
- Criteria fulfilled at least once per week for at least 2 months before diagnosis

Childhood functional abdominal pain syndrome
- Must include functional abdominal pain at least 25% of the time and 1 or more of the following:
  1. Some loss of daily functioning
  2. Additional somatic symptoms such as headache, limb pain, or difficulty sleeping
- Criteria fulfilled at least once per week for at least 2 months before diagnosis

In all subgroups no evidence is found of an inflammatory, anatomic, metabolic, or neoplastic process that explains the subject's symptoms.
FGIDs = functional gastrointestinal disorders; IBS = irritable bowel syndrome.

demonstrated that a single parent household [odds ratio (OR) 2.9] and having a parent with gastrointestinal complaints (OR: 5.3) were significantly associated with having a child with RAP.[14] Furthermore, a lower socioeconomic environment has been associated with RAP and in addition, children of immigrants reported RAP in a significantly higher proportion compared to the indigenous population.[1] No population-based study has prospectively evaluated the incidence of RAP in children over time.

Several studies have investigated the relative frequency of the different pain-related FGIDs, defined by the pediatric Rome II criteria as described in the section above.[9,10,12,15–17] IBS was diagnosed in 0.2% of children seen by primary care pediatricians, in 13 to 20% of Chinese and Russian adolescents, and in 22 to 45% of children aged 4 to 18 years presenting to tertiary care clinics for a FGID. The prevalence of FD was 0.3% in primary care, 22% in Russian adolescents, and between 12.5 and 15.9% in tertiary care settings. Abdominal migraine and FAP are less prevalent; in pediatric gastroenterology clinics, abdominal migraine was diagnosed in 2.2 to 5% of the children and FAP in 0 to 7.5%.

The figures from tertiary care clinics in North America with a predominance of IBS and FD are in contrast to the findings of Rowland and colleagues: in a group of 125 Irish children with RAP only 3% fulfilled the Rome II criteria for IBS and 5% for FD.[18] Whether this remarkable difference is caused by geographical factors or a different interpretation of the Rome criteria is unknown.

Of the patients with RAP, 11 to 24% did not meet the Rome II criteria for any FGID.[9,15] Most common reasons were: (1) having too few symptoms to meet the criteria for IBS or abdominal migraine but too many for FAP and (2) the pain episodes were less frequent than the 12 weeks required by the Rome II criteria for FAP. Since in the Rome III criteria the required duration of symptoms has changed from 3 to 2 months, the number of patients not meeting the criteria will probably decrease. It may be clear that large studies, using the recently revised Rome III criteria, need to be performed, not only among referred patients, but also in unselected populations to validate the new criteria and to assess epidemiology of the different subtypes of painrelated FGIDs.

PATHOPHYSIOLOGY OF FUNCTIONAL ABDOMINAL PAIN

There is general agreement that functional pain is genuine and not simply social modeling, imitation of parental pain, or a means to avoid an unwanted experience. The exact etiology and pathogenesis of the pain are unknown. Yet, there is a growing body of evidence that the pain is the result of disordered brain-gut communication involving both the efferent and the afferent pathways by which the enteric and central nervous system (CNS) communicate. It is not clear whether the different subcategories of functional pain result from a heterogeneous group of disorders with different pathophysiological mechanisms or represent variable expressions of the same disorder. The frequent occurrence of upper and lower symptoms in the same patient, for example, dyspepsia and IBS suggest that the latter scenario may indeed be the case. Most of the studies evaluating the pathophysiological mechanisms in functional pain disorders have been performed in adults with IBS. Since it has been shown that RAP in children can progress to IBS in adults,[19,20] it seems logical to assume that the etiology of functional pain disorders in children does not differ much from functional pain disorders in adults and nowadays RAP is seen as a possible precursor of IBS. The higher rate of spontaneous remission in children (30 to 70%), however, suggests that self-limiting developmental factors may also be involved in the pathophysiology of abdominal pain in children.

The prevailing viewpoint is that the pathogenesis of functional pain disorders involves the interrelationship between altered gastrointestinal motility and changes in visceral sensation, the so-called visceral hyperalgesia or hypersensitivity. The symptoms of altered motility can be diarrhea, constipation, bloating, and distension, whereas the symptoms of hypersensitivity are pain and discomfort. Hypersensitivity and dysmotility are probably strongly related. Altered sensitivity may exacerbate motility disturbances by upregulating sensory-motor reflex loops in the gut and disordered motility may exacerbate hypersensitivity by creating excess stimuli through distension due to poor transit or high pressures due to spasms. Several hypotheses have been put forward to explain the altered motility and hypersensitivity and they will be discussed in the following sections.

Visceral Hypersensitivity

In the last decade, visceral hyperalgesia has been recognized as playing an important role in symptom generation in FAPSs not only in adults, but also in children. In one study rectal sensitivity was measured by electric barostat in children with IBS and healthy controls. Children with IBS had a lower threshold for rectal sensations than controls.[21] This finding was confirmed in another study where gastric and rectal sensitivity was measured in children with FGIDs. The group of children with FAP was hypersensitive in both upper and lower gastrointestinal tract compared to healthy controls; those with IBS displayed only visceral hypersensitivity in the rectum. In most of the patients, their typical abdominal pain was reproduced by the barostat procedure.[22] Finally, meal-related visceral sensation was evaluated in adolescents with FD and they experienced an increased postprandial nausea and bloating compared to healthy controls.[23] In conclusion, visceral hypersensitivity appears to be a reproducible observation in children with FAP disorders. Interesting is the finding of differences in the predominant site of hyperalgesia in children with distinct FGIDs. It is hypothesized that the specific site of the hyperalgesia is important for the phenotypic presentation of these children, with the more severe rectal hyperalgesia being associated with IBS symptoms and more generalized (but not as severe in the rectum) hyperalgesia with FAP. The mechanism of hypersensitivity, whether generalized or rectal, is not fully understood yet and can be through changes peripheral in the gut and the enteric nervous system (ENS) or central in the spinal cord or brain. Several factors (ie, changes in serotonin signaling, genetic, inflammatory, stress, and psychiatric factors) have been proposed as contributing to alterations in enteric and spinal neural function and in CNS modulation of pain perception.

Altered Central Modulation of Sensation

Central processing of pain is complex and occurs through different pathways. Pain is thought to have two dimensions: a sensory-discriminative component and an affective-motivational component.[24] The discriminative component of gastrointestinal pain encodes location, intensity, and nature of pain and follows a route from the gut, via the dorsal horn of the spinal cord, the ventral posterior portions of the thalamus to the insula, an infolding of the temporal lobe. The affective-motivational component is thought to encode pain affect and suffering and runs through the spinal cord, the reticular formation of the brainstem, via the medial portions of the thalamus to the limbic system, particularly the part called the anterior cingulated cortex (ACC) (Figure 1). The ACC is

a critical center involved in the "unpleasantness" of the pain. Patients with ACC surgical lesions have an impaired pain interpretation and they report they can still feel the pain, but it is not bothersome to them.

Advances in functional brain imaging with either positron emission tomography or functional MRI have recently allowed study of these processes in healthy controls and IBS patients. Several studies demonstrated an increased activation of the ACC in IBS patients compared to healthy controls. This activation occurred both during actual painful stimuli applied to the colon and anticipation of such painful stimuli.[25,26] The clinical relevance of these altered patterns of activation is supported by several different findings. First, successful pharmacological interventions in IBS patients with either alosetron, a 5-HT3 antagonist or amitriptyline, a tricyclic antidepressant are associated with reduced activation of the ACC.[27,28] Second, gut-directed hypnotherapy has been proven to be a successful therapy for IBS patients (see section on "Therapy"). Several investigators have shown that hypnotic modulation of painful stimuli leads to significant changes within the ACC, suggesting that gut-directed hypnotherapy might have its effect through modulation of the affective-motivational component of pain.[29,30] The exact mechanism leading to an increased activation of the limbic system is unclear. It is hypothesized that emotional processes like anxiety and cortical factors like previous experience of pain, coping mechanisms, and psychosocial stressors could interact with limbic circuits to amplify the pain experience.[31]

Genetics

Familial clustering of FGIDs has been described and suggests a genetic transmittance of these disorders. Studies completed in adults, for example, have demonstrated that IBS is more common in first-degree relatives of individuals with IBS.[32,33] Furthermore, children with RAP are more likely to have a parent with functional gastrointestinal complaints.[14] A twin study, performed by Levy and colleagues, showed a 17% concor-

dance for IBS in monozygotic patients with only 8% concordance in dizygotic twins, supporting a genetic contribution to IBS.[34] This study however, also showed that a parental history of IBS was a stronger predictor of IBS than having a twin with IBS, suggesting that social learning is much more important than genetic factors. Recently, this was confirmed by Mohammed and colleagues, who found almost similar prevalences of IBS in monozygotic (17%) and dizygotic (16%) twins, showing that genetic factors are probably of little or no influence on IBS.[35] It is therefore more likely that familial clustering is a reflection of a shared exposure to environmental factors including learned responses to abdominal complaints than of a genetic predisposition. Finally, studies, that examined possible associations between polymorphisms in the human serotonin transporter gene and IBS, have offered little evidence to suggest a genetic transmittance of FGIDs.[36]

Role of Serotonin

Serotonin (5-HT) is a neurotransmitter found both in the enteric and in the CNS. It has emerged as a key mediator in modulating visceral sensitivity and motility.[37] 5-HT is synthesized and stored in the gut in a subset of epithelial cells, the so-called enterochromafin cells (EC-cells) from where it is released in response to luminal stimuli. This leads to activation of local secretory and motor reflexes as well as stimulation of afferent sensory nerves to the CNS. Serotonin uses different receptor types such as $5-HT_{1a-e}$, $5-HT_{2a-c}$, $5-HT_3$, $5-HT_4$, $5-HT_5$, $5-HT_6$, and $5-HT_7$. Some of these receptors have been identified only in the gut, while others are being located in the nervous system.[38] Activation can lead to different effects, for example, some receptors will inhibit and others will stimulate the peristaltic reflex. The signal of 5-HT is terminated mainly through a serotonin-selective reuptake transporter (SERT), that is expressed on gut epithelial cells, nerve endings, and platelets. The different effects of 5-HT can be augmented by selective serotonin reuptake inhibitors (SSRIs) as well as 5-HT receptor agonists or partial antagonists (see section on "Therapy").

It is becoming increasingly clear that changes in serotonin signaling occur in patients with IBS. Various elements of 5-HT signaling that have been reported to be different in IBS patients are the number of EC-cells, 5-HT content in EC-cells, expression of SERT, and free serum 5-HT levels (studies reviewed by Mawe and colleagues[39]). The results of the studies performed so far are, however, not entirely in harmony, so the exact role of serotonin in the pathophysiology of IBS remains unclear. It is also not fully understood yet whether the changes in 5-HT signaling contribute to the alterations in motility and sensitivity or are just a response to altered gut function. In other words, what is cause and what is effect? Further studies are required to answer this question and also to gain a more complete picture of the changes that are occurring, not only in

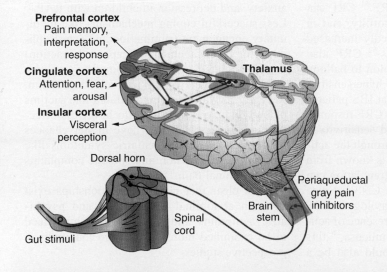

Figure 1 Uncomfortable sensations from the gut are relayed to the dorsal horn of the spinal cord and are then send to the brainstem and the thalamus. From these two areas afferent messages are relayed to the insula for discriminative processing and to the anterior cingulate cortex for affective (emotional) coding. Ultimately messages from both sources reach the frontal cortex where cognitive processing of the discomfort occurs.

5-HT signaling in patients with IBS, but also in patients with other pain-related FGIDs.

Inflammation

Evidence exists that a low-grade mucosal inflammatory process may play a role in IBS pathogenesis. First, it is well known that a proportion of patients with IBS describe that their symptoms have begun after an acute enteric infection. This observation was confirmed by Gwee and colleagues who reported that 20 to 25% of adult patients admitted to the hospital for bacterial gastroenteritis developed symptoms consistent with IBS in the first three months.[40] Postinfectious irritable bowel syndrome (PI-IBS) seems to occur particularly after Campylobacter and Shigella enteritis and it has been suggested that the severity of tissue damage and ulceration, which is a marked feature of these two infections, is a key factor in developing PI-IBS. Both in animal studies and in patients with PI-IBS elevations of the number of EC-cells and 5-HT levels are found. These observations suggest that transient inflammation may result in persistent changes in the neuromuscular apparatus of the gut.

Second, an increased number of inflammatory cells (eg, mast cells, T lymphocytes, macrophages) has been detected in the colonic and ileal mucosa as well as in the muscularis externa of the jejunum of patients with IBS (summarized by Barbara and colleagues).[41] These activated inflammatory cells can release many different mediators, including interleukins, nitric oxide, histamine, and proteases. These mediators are capable of affecting the ENS leading to altered bowel function and an increased visceral sensory input generating feelings of abdominal discomfort and pain. So far, one has not been successful yet to influence the inflammatory process in IBS. An attempt to reduce intestinal inflammation with steroids in PI-IBS failed to demonstrate any symptomatic improvement, but further studies are now awaited.[42]

Stressful Events

Early stressful childhood events, both physical and psychological, have been theorized to be a contributory factor toward sensitization of visceral afferents, with possible life-long consequences. In an animal study it has been demonstrated that rats subjected to maternal separation were more likely to develop visceral hyperalgesia and increased colonic motility later in life.[43] Furthermore, neonatal rats subjected to colonic, mechanical, or chemical irritation developed visceral hypersensitivity as adults.[44] Clinical observations have also supported the theory that stress factors during early childhood may be influential toward the development of visceral hyperalgesia. Loss and separation during childhood, conflicting maternal relationships, and an environment of physical, sexual, or emotional abuse are all associated with the development of IBS. Much attention has been given to the role of abuse. Population- and clinic-based studies have consistently suggested that a considerable number of individuals with IBS report histories of physical, emotional, and sexual abuse. Prevalences of physical abuse range from 6.2 to 26%, significantly higher than the prevalence rates observed in the general population. Sexual abuse is the most common type of abuse reported by people with IBS and the rates range from 13 to 54%, depending on the methods of assessment and definitions of abuse used (reviewed by Koloski and Talley[45]).

Also in children with RAP a clear association with stressful events has been found. Two studies in the 1980s demonstrated that children with RAP had experienced significantly more traumatic events such as illness, hospitalization, and death, and had more stress associated with these events than did healthy children.[46,47] These results were confirmed by two other studies reporting stressful life events to be important predictors of RAP in children.[48,49] Every pediatrician is also aware of the association of RAP with frequently occurring social and behavioral factors like marital turmoil, pestering by peers, and tendency to perfectionism.[50] There are no data yet on the incidence of physical or sexual abuse in children with RAP. However, the high incidence of abuse among adult patients with IBS and the fact that RAP is seen as a precursor of IBS suggest that abuse can be an important factor in the etiology of RAP in childhood and that pediatricians should be well aware of this possibility.

Stressful events later in life also play a role in IBS. Adult patients often describe a correlation between stress and the onset or exacerbation of their symptoms. Moreover, patients who develop an intercurrent bacterial enteritis are more likely to develop a PI-IBS if the infection occurs at the time when there are more stressful life events in the individual's life.[40]

One of proposed mechanisms in which stress, both early and later in life could modulate symptoms in functional pain disorders is through the corticotrophin-releasing factor (CRF), one of the important hormones involved in the stress response. Studies have shown that stress early in life results in both acute and chronic changes in the activity and regulation of the hypothalamo-pituitary-adrenal (HPA) axis, particularly in the form of hypersecretion of CRF.[51] CRF can induce an increase in colonic motility, and in IBS this motility effect is markedly increased compared to normal individuals.[52] CRF also increases the sensitivity of the colon to balloon distension, analogous to visceral hypersensitivity in IBS.[53] It is thus possible that IBS patients have a perturbation in their stress CRF response leading to increased motility and sensitivity.[54] Another possible mechanism is through the activation of mast cells in the gut. It is known from animal studies that mast cell degranulation can be evoked by stimulation of the CNS.[55] Since it has been shown that symptomatology in IBS patients was correlated with the presence of activated mast cells in the colonic mucosa,[56] this brain-to-mast cell connection could also be a good candidate to link psychoemotional status like stress to gastrointestinal symptomatology. More research is needed in this area, preferably also in pediatric patients, since early modulation of the stress response could be an interesting therapeutic target.

Psychiatric Factors

Several investigators have addressed the issue of psychiatric symptoms in children with RAP. An anxiety disorder is found in approximately 80% of the children and almost 40% meets the criteria for a depressive disorder.[57–59] These percentages may seem high, but are not surprising since decades of similar cross-sectional surveys already have shown that chronic pain, depression, and anxiety often coexist. Potential explanations for the observed associations are: (1) pain causes mood and anxiety disorders; (2) affective disorders cause or increase pain; (3) a common biological predisposition underlies both pain and affective disorders; or (4) pain or affective disorders do not directly cause the other but frequently associate with a true causal variable such as somatization, social stress, or ineffective coping style.[60] In primary care settings it has been shown that a persistent pain disorder at baseline predicted the onset of mood or anxiety disorders to the same degree that a baseline psychiatric disorder predicted the subsequent onset of chronic pain.[61] So, evidence exists for bidirectional causal links between pain and mood.

It is also possible that pain and mood are both the result of a biological factor, for example, an aberrant functioning HPA -axis due to stress as stated above. Apart from increasing colonic motility and hypersensitivity of the gut,[52,53] changes in the HPA axis also induce alteration in the serotonergic system, which in turn may contribute to the onset of depression and anxiety.[51]

Finally there is also evidence for the fourth proposed mechanism, that is, both pain and symptoms of depression and anxiety are the result of ineffective mechanisms of coping with stress. A study performed by Thomsen and colleagues. showed that successful coping mechanisms like problem solving, acceptance, and positive thinking were associated with less pain, anxiety, and depression in children with RAP.[62] Less successful coping mechanisms like involuntary engagement (rumination and catastrophizing) or disengagement (escape and inaction) were associated with more somatic symptoms and higher levels of anxiety and depression. Recently, it was also demonstrated that victims of bullying, who are likely to have less effective coping mechanisms, have higher chances of developing new psychiatric symptoms like anxiety and depression and somatic complaints like abdominal pain.[63]

It is clear that complex relationships exist between abdominal pain, stress, and psychiatric symptoms and these relationships need to be examined more carefully in longitudinal, prospective studies.

Parental Factors

Chronic abdominal pain is more common in families with higher rates of reported physical illness and psychological symptoms like anxiety.[14,19,64,65] The relation between abdominal pain in childhood and these parental factors suggests that parental anxiety and preoccupation with physical health may reinforce the child's own concerns about physiological and minor medical bodily sensations. The children may adopt the pain behavior of their parents and one could hypothesize that this pain behavior might attribute to visceral hyperalgesia.[64]

Several studies have also demonstrated the importance of the acceptance by parents of the role of psychological factors like stress for the resolution of RAP in children.[66,67] This suggests that these children may have learned to complain of pain or adopt the sick role model rather than to deal with stress or other emotional problems.

Another parental factor that has considerable impact on symptom severity in children with FAP is the parents' direct response to their child's symptoms. When children express pain, parents are faced with a variety of choices like ignoring the pain behavior, distracting the child, or expressing sympathy. Parents often believe that attention to somatic complaints is a good thing and distraction is potentially harmful.[68] The opposite however, seems true. In a randomized, controlled trial Walker and colleagues. compared the effect of parent's attention versus distraction or no instruction following induction of visceral discomfort in their child. Compared to the "no instruction" group, symptom complaints nearly doubled in the attention group and were reduced by half in the distraction group. The children in the distraction group rated parents as making them feel better compared to the attention group.[68] Although more research is needed, this study demonstrates the importance of parents' response to their child's pain, which potentially has therapeutic consequences.

Dysmotility

In addition to a greater intestinal sensitivity, patients with functional bowel disorders may display abnormal gut motility. Exaggerated intestinal motor responses have been shown in adults with IBS after meal ingestion, stress, or mechanical stimulation.[69] Furthermore, there is evidence that gas may be propelled abnormally through the gut: in normal subjects, gas experimentally infused in the small bowel was propelled rapidly through the bowel and consequently expelled. Conversely, a high proportion of IBS patients retained a significant amount of gas resulting in complaints of abdominal pain and bloating.[70] Motility studies have been performed also in pediatric patients with FGIDs. Heterogeneous abnormalities in antroduodenal motility have been described in small groups of children with RAP (reviewed by Dilorenzo).[71] Furthermore, children with IBS have been shown to have altered contractile responses in the rectum to a meal.[21]

The relevance of these findings remains elusive for several reasons. First, in most studies an association between motor abnormalities and patient's symptoms perception could not be found. Second, these motility changes are not found in all patient with IBS or FAP. Third, drugs that have targeted gut motility such as antispasmodics or prokinetics have traditionally provided disappointing results.[72] It is therefore now believed that motility disorders are more likely to be the result of other disturbances, rather than being a primary causal factor.

Role of Intestinal Gas and Aerophagia

The so-called gas-related symptoms such as flatulence, bloating, and distension are common among patients with FAP and especially IBS. The origin of these symptoms seems to be a combination of impaired gas clearance, hypersensitivity to normal amounts of gas, and an excessive gas production. The gut in healthy subjects is able to transport and evacuate large gas loads, virtually up to any demand, without discomfort.[73] IBS subjects, however, have an impaired capability to propel intestinal gas infused in the jejunum, leading to symptoms.[70] Furthermore, this impaired propulsion is coupled to a visceral hypersensitivity to normal amounts of gas and gas retention in response to physiological concentrations of intestinal lipids.[74] Moreover, it has been suggested that gas production could be increased due to small intestinal bacterial overgrowth. The changes in the intestinal microflora may only be subtle with local increases in gas production, sufficient enough to be sensed as bloating or distension in patients with hypersensitivity, but too low to lead to a detectable elevation in breath hydrogen excretion. The fact that some patients benefit from manipulation of the intestinal flora by either antibiotics or probiotics adds prove to this hypothesis.[75]

The role of gas in children with abdominal pain is less well studied and most attention has been on infantile colic and aerophagia. Pathologic childhood aerophagia (PCA), that is, the swallowing of excessive volumes of air, can cause burping, abdominal cramps, bloating, flatulence, and even chronic diarrhea. Therefore, it is not surprising that PCA frequently is diagnosed as FD, RAP, or IBS. PCA, however, is seen as a distinct clinical entity and should be distinguished from other functional gastrointestinal disorders. Essential diagnostic criteria are an abdominal distension that increases progressively during the day, increased flatus on sleep, visible, or audible air swallowing and an esophageal air sign in a chest radiograph.[76]

Concluding Remarks on Pathophysiology

The very different findings described above support the concept that a simple universal etiology for IBS does not exist. It is likely that there is a complex interaction of biopsychosocial factors that generate the symptoms we know as IBS (Figure 2). Genetic influences and early social learning may result in a predisposition that is

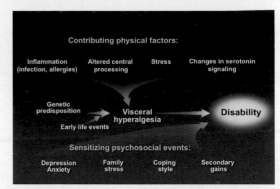

Figure 2 Contributing physical and psychosocial factors in the etiology of pain-related functional gastrointestinal disorders.

influenced by later psychological experiences and physiological factors. The relative contribution of each of these factors may vary among patients. Whether this pathophysiological concept is also applicable to all Rome III subtypes of FAP in childhood is far from clear and more research has to be done to elucidate this.

DIAGNOSIS OF FUNCTIONAL ABDOMINAL PAIN

Because the exact etiology and pathogenesis of abdominal pain-related FGIDs are unknown and no specific diagnostic markers exist for any of them, FAP (syndrome), IBS, FD, and abdominal migraine are often perceived as diagnosis of exclusion. Physicians are tempted to perform multiple tests to rule out an organic disease at all costs, before they are willing to make the diagnosis of FAP. This is often traumatic for the child and expensive for the health service system. Negative test results generally do not reassure the patient,[77] but rather reinforce a medical model of disease, making it more difficult to introduce the diagnosis of a functional disorder. It is therefore important to keep diagnostic investigations to a minimum. It is the clinical presentation, together with a well-structured medical history and physical examination, that usually indicates that a functional gastrointestinal disorder is the likely diagnosis in an individual child presenting with chronic abdominal pain (see Figure 3).

History and Physical Examination

Many pathologic conditions such as infectious, inflammatory, metabolic, or anatomic disorders can cause chronic or RAP; however, in the majority of pediatric patients the pain is functional, that is without objective evidence of an underlying organic disorder. In his original study, Apley and Naish reported an organic disorder in only 8% of the studied patients.[5] Others found an identifiable cause up to 27%; these higher percentages may be due to selection bias in tertiary centers or reflect improved diagnostic abilities.[78] Differential diagnosis is presented in Table 2.

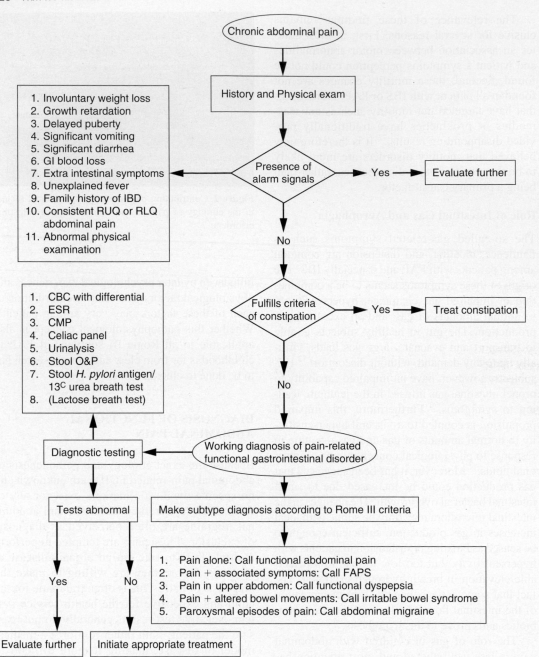

Figure 3 The authors' algorithm for the evaluation of children with chronic abdominal pain. CBC = complete blood count; CMP = comprehensive metabolic panel; ESR = erythrocyte sedimentation rate; FAPS = functional abdominal pain syndrome; GI = gastrointestinal; *H. pylori* = *Helicobacter pylori*; IBD = inflammatory bowel disease; O&P = ovum parasite examination; RLQ = right lower quadrant; RUQ = right upper quadrant.

Table 2 Differential Diagnosis of Chronic or Recurrent Abdominal Pain

Functional disorders
   Functional abdominal pain
   Functional abdominal pain syndrome
   Irritable bowel syndrome
   Functional dyspepsia
   Abdominal migraine
   Aerophagia

GI tract
   Gastroesophageal reflux disease
   Helicobacter pylori gastritis
   Peptic ulcer
   Esophagitis
   Lactose intolerance
   Celiac disease
   Parasitic infection (*Giardia, Blastocystis hominis*)
   Inflammatory bowel disease
   Meckel diverticulum
   Malrotation with intermittent volvulus
   Chronic appendicitis

Galbladder, liver, and pancreas
   Cholelithiasis
   Choledochal cyst
   Hepatitis
   Liver abcess
   Recurrent pancreatitis

Genitourinary tract
   Urinary tract infection
   Hydronephrosis
   Urolithiasis
   Dysmenorrhea
   Pelvic inflammatory disease

Miscellaneous causes
   Gilbert's syndrome
   Familial Mediterranean fever
   Malignancies
   Sickle cell crisis
   Lead poisoning
   Vasculitis (especially Henoch Schönlein Purpura)
   Angioneurotic edema
   Acute intermittent porphyria

Only few items from medical history and physical examination provide clues for the possibility of an organic disease. Several studies, evaluating histories of children with chronic abdominal pain, have provided some evidence that frequency, severity, location, and timing (postprandial and waking during the night) of abdominal pain do not help distinguishing between organic and FAP.[79] The same can be said for the so-called associated symptoms: children with chronic abdominal pain are very likely to have associated symptoms like anorexia, nausea, episodic vomiting, altered bowel movements, headache, back pain, arthralgia, or eye problems. Yet, none of these symptoms have been reported to help to distinguish between organic and FAP.[80] RAP can result in interference with normal school attendance and performance, peer relationships, participation in

organizations and sports, and other personal and family activities. Liebman found that only 1 of 10 children with FAP attended school regularly and that absenteeism was greater than 1 day in 10 in 28% of patients.[50] Again, inability to attend school is not associated with organic disease; only with the decision to consult a physician.[80]

As described in the section on pathophysiology, stressful life events, emotional symptoms like anxiety and depression, and family factors play a role in FAP. Several studies have evaluated whether the psychosocial history of the patient is relevant in the differential diagnosis of chronic abdominal pain and can be of value in predicting the existence of a functional disorder. Two small trials found no difference in significant recent life events between children with RAP and minor organic disease.[81,82] However, a diary study found that children with

RAP report significantly more daily stressors than healthy children; moreover, the relation between daily stressors and somatic complaints was significantly stronger for patients with abdominal pain than for healthy school children.[83] Thus, although there is no evidence that life stress helps to distinguish between FAP and organic disease, attention must be paid to this part of the history especially with respect to treatment options. It is also known that children with chronic abdominal pain are more often anxious or depressed than healthy children, but again this aspect cannot be used to differentiate from children with organic disease, since no studies have found a significant difference between patients with abdominal pain that is functional or organic in etiology with respect to their emotional and behavioral symptoms.[82,84] Finally, also family characteristics have not proven useful in distinguishing between functional and organic abdominal pain.[79]

Physical examination of children with FAP has been described rarely. The presence of tenderness on abdominal palpitation has been reported to be characteristic of children with FAP when compared to control children.[85] Furthermore, since almost 50% of the children with functional constipation present with chronic abdominal pain,[86] one should carefully look for signs of constipation in this phase of establishing a working diagnosis. In children with functional constipation, a fecal mass is commonly found upon abdominal examination. External examination of the perineum and rectal area may show visible fecal incontinence. Although controversy exists, it is recommended that digital rectal examination be performed at least once.[87]

According to experts, only the presence of the so-called alarm symptoms or "red flags" suggests a higher prevalence of organic disease and definitely indicate the performance of diagnostic tests, but so far, no studies have evaluated the value of these red flags in discriminating organic from FAP.[79] Alarm signals in the history include: involuntary weight loss, growth retardation, delayed puberty, significant vomiting, significant diarrhea, gastrointestinal blood loss, unexplained fever, rash, arthritis, or a family history of inflammatory bowel disease. Red flags in the physical examination are localized tenderness in the right upper or lower quadrant, localized fullness or mass effect, hepatomegaly, splenomegaly, spine or costovertebral angle tenderness, oral ulcers, and perianal fissure or fistula.

In conclusion, the key variables that point toward a functional diagnosis are the absence of alarm symptoms for an organic disorder and a normal physical examination, other than abdominal pressure tenderness.

Laboratory Tests

There are no studies that have evaluated the usefulness of common laboratory tests (complete blood count, comprehensive metabolic panel that screens for liver, kidney and pancreatic dysfunction, erythrocyte sedimentation rate, urinalysis, and stool analysis of ova and parasites (eg, *Giardia lambliae or Dientamoeba fragilis*) to distinguish between organic and FAP. Since these tests are neither very invasive nor expensive, most clinicians will order for these tests, even in the absence of alarm signals. One should however realize that performing multiple tests may provide results that are unrelated to the presenting symptom or have no clinical relevance (such as a mildly elevated sedimentation rate). Repeating these tests to confirm the serendipitous findings may further increase anxiety in patients and parents and undermine the clinical diagnosis of a functional disorder. The value of testing for food allergies by IgE and IgG antibodies is debatable, although many clinicians will still include this in their initial workup.[88,89]

Apart from the above-mentioned tests, the diagnostic workup can include several other investigations, that is, a celiac panel, screening for *Helicobacter pylori* and a lactose breathing test. Several studies have evaluated the usefulness of screening for celiac disease in children with RAP and the results are conflicting.[89,90] Because of the high frequency of celiac disease in the general population and the possible long-term

consequences, most clinicians do include a celiac panel in their diagnostic workup. *H. pylori* infection can be found in a small percentage of children with RAP.[89] This does, however, not necessarily indicate a causal relationship between the two, since children with *H. pylori* infection are not more likely to have abdominal pain than children without *H. pylori*.[14] Lactose malabsorption can also be found in a subset of children. However, treatment of lactose malabsorption often does not result in resolution of abdominal pain, again questioning the causal relationship and the usefulness of performing this test in children with chronic abdominal pain.[91,92]

Other Diagnostic Tests

The usefulness of abdominal ultrasonography has been examined in children with recurrent episodes of abdominal pain without alarm symptoms; abnormalities were found in fewer than 1%. When atypical symptoms were present, such as jaundice, urinary symptoms, back or flank pain, vomiting, or abnormal findings on physical examination, the percentage increased to 11%. It was concluded in this study that ultrasonography should be used in children with RAP and atypical clinical features.[93] In children without alarm symptoms, ultrasonographic examination might be done as a reassurance to parents and patient.

Studies of endoscopy, biopsy, and/or esophageal pH monitoring performed in children with RAP have demonstrated abnormalities in 25 to 56%, but reports have been limited by small sample size, sample bias, variability of findings, and questionable specificity and generalizability.[79] Since there is little evidence so far to suggest that the use of these diagnostic tests in the absence of alarm symptoms has a significant yield of organic disease, the inconvenience associated with these tests and their costs preclude its use in the initial evaluation of children with chronic abdominal pain. However, the reassuring effect of a normal endoscopy can have value in certain cases. Decisions regarding extensive diagnostic testing to rule out organic disease should be individualized, based on the child's predominant symptoms, degree of impairment, and parental anxiety.

Gastric and rectal barostat are increasingly used in scientific studies to detect visceral hyperalgesia (see section on "Pathophysiology"). Since not every patient has an abnormal barostat, these tests cannot be used to distinguish functional from organic abdominal pain. Furthermore, gastric barostat is very invasive and to our opinion should thus only be used in the context of research. Rectal barostat is less invasive and can sometimes have an educational value for the patient by demonstrating rectal hypersensitivity.

Establishing a Working Diagnosis According to Rome III

When history, physical exam, and limited screening tests reveal no abnormalities, the diagnosis of an abdominal pain-related functional gastrointestinal disorder can be made. The next step is to clas-

sify according to the Rome III criteria as described earlier. Some remarks about this classification need to be made. First, it is not rare that children fulfill criteria of more than one FGID (especially the combination of FD and IBS can be found) or change from one FGID to another over time.[15] Second, a small percentage of children, who initially have received a diagnosis of FGID can have a change in diagnosis to an organic disease and therefore clinical follow-up to monitor for change in symptoms is mandatory.[12] Finally, the value of subclassifying chronic FAP in different conditions is questioned by some clinicians. So far it is unknown whether RAP indeed represents a group of heterogeneous conditions, and furthermore, if subclassifying RAP in separate FGIDs benefits the children in terms of treatment or predicting prognosis.[94] Furthur research is needed to answer these questions.

THERAPY

Only few studies exist on the pharmacological and behavioral therapy of functional RAP in children. Moreover no placebo-controlled trials have been performed with adequate sample size and adequate duration of medications or psychological interventions in the treatment of any of the specific Rome-defined subtypes of pain-related FGIDs, that is, pediatric IBS, FD, abdominal migraine, or FAP (syndrome). Consequently, this section on therapy will focus on FAP broadly, defined to mean a FGID where abdominal pain is the predominant symptom. When appropriate, the treatment of the different subtypes will be discussed separately. Relevant studies on adults will be mentioned where pediatric data are missing. Furthermore, one should keep in mind that the evaluation of any therapeutic intervention for the pain-related FGIDs is complicated by an important observation. A very high placebo response rate exists in virtually all clinical trials involving FGIDs in adults, and no reason to believe that this is different in children. The placebo rate ranges from 20 to 50%, so evaluation of any intervention needs to be compared to this high baseline therapeutic effect of placebo.[95] The high placebo response embraces not only the nonspecific response to placebo, but also the natural history of the disease. Although the natural history of pain-related FGIDs in children is not well characterized, it is well appreciated that there is a significant variability in severity over time.

The current practice of many pediatricians in treating children with FAP and IBS is that of support and empathy for the family with the assurance that no serious disease is present and that children will likely outgrow it. With this approach approximately 40 to 70% of the children have resolution of their complaints (see section on prognosis). However, the remainder continues to exhibit symptoms and goes on to be adults with abdominal pain. In this group specific treatment including education, identification, and modification of physical and psychological stress factors, dietary interventions, drug therapy, and

Table 3 Therapeutic Options

Treatment	Evidence	Costs and Restraints	Comments
Dietary interventions			
Fibers enriched	Two RCTs (n = 92) in children with RAP are inconclusive[99,100]	Simple and inexpensive	A short trial of 2 mo might benefit some children
Lactose free	Two RCTs (n = 77) show no effect of a lactose-free diet[91, 92]		Not recommended
Food antigens	No RCTs with elimination and placebo-controlled food –challenges	Food restriction can have significant impact on daily life	Elimination diet only recommended when a food allergy is strongly suspected
Probiotics	Two RCTs with LGG (n = 154) in children with FGID's[110,111]	Simple, but sometimes expensive	Inconsistent data, might be helpful in children with IBS
Pharmacological treatment			
H2 blockers	Small RCT (n = 25) in children with functional dyspepsia[114]		Short trial of 4 weeks might benefit some children
Serotoninergic agents	One RCT (n = 14) shows effect of pizotifen in children with abdominal migraine[115]		Larger studies are necessary
	Citalopram effective in open-label trial (n = 25)[116]		RCT's are needed
Tricyclic antidepressants	One RCT (n = 33) shows effect in adolescents with IBS[119]		Not recommended as first-line therapy
Psychological approaches			
Cognitive-behavorial therapy	Three RCTs (n = 129) in children with RAP show CBT to be effective[120–122]	Time consuming	Recommended
Gut-directed hypnotherapy	One RCT (n = 52) shows effect in children with FAP or IBS [130]	Time consuming	Recommended
Complementary therapies			
Peppermint oil capsules	One RCT (n = 42) shows decrease in symptom severity[136]	Not expensive, over the counter	2-wk trial might benefit some children
Ginger	Proven to be effective in nausea, no RCTs in FGID		Not recommended
Acupuncture	No RCTs in children, no effect in adults		Not recommended
Massage therapy	No RCTs in children		Studies are necessary

CBT = cognitive behavioral therapy; FAPS = functional abdominal pain; FGIDs = functional gastrointestinal disorders; IBS = irritable bowel syndrome; RAP = recurrent abdominal pain.

psychological therapies may be needed (Table 3). Hospitalization is rarely indicated for children with FAP.

Education and Goals of Therapy

Education of the family and the patient is an important part of the treatment of the child with chronic FAP. One need to emphasize that although the pain is real, there is no underlying serious or chronic disease and that this so-called functional pain is the most common etiology of chronic abdominal pain in children. Reassurance that FAP will not affect future health can have positive effects. It may also be helpful to explain what is known so far on the pathogenesis (ie, visceral hyperalgesia and an altered brain–gut communication) in simple and age-appropriate language. Furthermore, parents and child should

be encouraged to ask questions and share their concerns, which must be addressed in depth to avoid fears and misconceptions.

The primary goal of the therapy is not complete eradication of pain, but resumption of a normal lifestyle with regular school attendance, school performance to the child's ability, participation in desired extracurricular activities, and a normal sleep pattern. An important factor in resumption of a normal lifestyle is the parents' response to the complaints of the child. Parental over involvement in pain behavior and parent reinforcement of sick role behavior are thought to be associated with ineffective coping with chronic pain and a perseverance of the complaints. Therefore, the family should be discouraged from reinforcing the symptoms by allowing the child to miss school and leisure activities and from paying too much positive attention to the

symptoms. On the other hand, negative attention to pain in children with low self-esteem has also been associated with increased pain behavior, possibly by creating affective distress that may further contribute to somatic symptoms.[96] Thus, the parents' attitude toward the pain should be balanced, showing enough support and understanding, but being aware that excessive attention and irregular attendance at school may provide the child with secondary gain.

Identification and Modification of Stress Factors

An important goal in the therapeutic phase is to identify, clarify, and possibly reverse physical and psychological stress factors that may have an important role in the onset, exacerbation, or maintenance of pain. In some cases, painful sensations may be provoked by physiological phenomena, including postprandial gastric or intestinal distension, intestinal contractions, intestinal gas, or gastroesophageal reflux. In these cases pharmacological interventions like antispasmodics or antireflux therapy might be useful. Psychological stressful life events that may exacerbate abdominal pain include death or separation of a significant family member, school problems, altered peer relationships, and family marital or financial problems. Many parents find it difficult to accept that these kinds of psychological factors can influence or even cause the abdominal pain of their child and may be unwilling to discuss this. Nevertheless, it is important to pay attention to these factors since it has been shown that acceptance by parents of a psychological factor in the etiology of their child's complaint is important in the resolution of symptoms (see also section on "Prognosis").[66,67]

Identification of a child's physical and psychological stressors can be done by means of a simple pain diary. In this diary frequency, duration and intensity of pain must be noted as well as accompanying symptoms like headaches, defecation, bloating, and nausea. Furthermore, patients are encouraged to look for a relation between pain and stress factors like those mentioned above or a relation with eating and food substances.

Dietary Interventions

Parents frequently believe that food intolerances are to blame for many of the abdominal symptoms of their child as they have noticed that pain episodes often worsen in the postprandial period. Not uncommonly however, this is caused by a nonspecific increase in gut and colonic motility that occurs with food ingestion. Given that increased colonic motor activity has been shown to be associated strongly with abdominal pain in patients with IBS,[97] it is important for parents and patients to realize that the process of eating, irrespective of what is eaten, may exacerbate the symptoms. Nevertheless, dietary manipulation may result in substantial improvement in symptomatology in patients, provided it is individualized. Below, several options for dietary interventions are discussed.

FIBERS

The most common form of dietary advice offered to patients with RAP has been to increase their intake of fiber. As fibers decrease the whole-gut transit time, fiber-enriched diets may be more useful in the subgroup of patients with constipation.[98] In children with RAP two randomized, controlled studies have evaluated the effect of adding fiber to the diet.[99,100] In the first study, the addition of 10 g of insoluble dietary corn fiber in a cookie was tested during 6 weeks and in the second study the children received fibers in the form of cereals (165 g) for a period of 7 weeks. The primary outcomes in both studies were the number of pain episodes. Analyzing the results of both studies it was concluded that the evidence supporting the use of fiber is, at best, weak and, at worse, inconclusive.[101] However, the addition of fiber each day is a simple and inexpensive intervention that might benefit some children with pain-related FGIDs.

LACTOSE AVOIDANCE

The role of lactose intolerance in chronic abdominal pain has been addressed by several investigators. Two studies have examined the effect of a trial of lactose avoidance in children with chronic abdominal pain.[91,92] In both studies all children were tested for lactose malabsorption. During the diet trials, there were no differences in the number of children who claimed relief, whether they were lactose intolerant or tolerant or whether they received lactose or lactose-free milk. Thus, there seems to be no association between RAP in children and lactose intolerance and a lactose-free diet is unlikely to improve the symptoms of RAP.

FOOD ALLERGIES

Many parents are convinced that food allergies play a role in the symptoms of their child, leading to the initiation of a strict dietary regime without first consulting health care professionals.[102] The role of food allergies and especially cow's milk allergy in RAP and the best ways of diagnosing these allergies are still under debate, but adverse reactions to food probably are a causative factor in less than 5% of the children with RAP.[89] Until new and more reliable tests to diagnose food allergy have been developed and implemented in clinical settings, an elimination diet followed by a double-blind placebo-controlled food challenge should be performed when a food allergy is considered. This food challenge should take at least a week considering the suspected immunological delayed-type reactions. When the challenge is considered positive, patients are advised to follow an elimination diet, supervised by a dietician to prevent nutritional deficiencies. In some patients, however, compliance with the dietetic regimen is poor and in others it may be difficult to remove all traces of the offending food from the diet. To overcome these problems one might

prescribe sodium cromoglycate. In adult patients with IBS and suspected food allergies, symptoms improved in 60% of patients treated with an elimination diet compared to 67% of those treated with oral cromolyn sodium.[103] Also, in an Italian study among 153 children with abdominal pain and diarrhea treatment with oral sodium cromoglycate (mean 63 mg/kg/d) appeared to be superior to an elimination diet in reducing intestinal symptoms.[104]

PROBIOTICS

A probiotic can be defined as a beneficial species of bacteria that colonizes and replicates in the human intestinal tract and provides a positive benefit to the host.[105] Probiotics play a role in preventing overgrowth of potentially pathogenic bacteria and maintaining the integrity of the gut mucosal barrier. The effects of probiotics have been studied in adults with IBS,[106–108] but so far the evidence of benefit is not compelling. Improvement of bloating, flatulence, and abdominal pain in some studies has been reported, but the studies are difficult to compare because of differences in study design, probiotic dose, and strain. Recently O'Mahony and colleagues examined the effect of two probiotics (*Lactobacillus salivarius* and *Bifidobacterium infantis*) compared to placebo in 60 adults with IBS.[109] Only *B. infantis* alleviated significantly symptoms like pain, abdominal distension, and bowel movement difficulty. Since, however, an effect on quality of life was not seen, it is questionable if this symptom reduction was relevant. Interestingly, the symptomatic response was associated with normalization of the ratio of an anti-inflammatory cytokine (IL-10) to a proinflammatory cytokine (IL-12), suggesting an immunomodulating role for this organism.

In children with abdominal pain disorders two randomized, controlled trials have been performed, both with capsules containing *Lactobacillus* GG or placebo.[110,111] In the first trial ($n = 50$) no difference in gastrointestinal symptoms was found except for a lower incidence of perceived abdominal distension. In the second study ($n = 104$) an improvement in pain severity was found in IBS patients, but no effect of probiotics was seen in FAP patients nor in FD patients. Clearly further studies are indicated to determine the role of the different strains of probiotics in patients with IBS or FAPS. In these studies, the focus should not only be on symptomatology and quality of life but also on inflammatory and immunological markers to learn more about pathophysiology.[112]

Pharmacological Treatment

Drug therapy for pain-related FGIDs has generally been directed at symptom alleviation, rather than at precise pathophysiological abnormalities. However, with an increased understanding on the etiology of visceral hypersensitivity and dysmotility, new therapeutic strategies are being developed aiming at modulation of

gastrointestinal motor function, neurohormonal stress responses, cytokines involved in inflammation and central processing of pain information.[113]

While awaiting these new strategies, medications for FAP in children are best described judiciously as part of a multifaceted, individualized approach to relieve symptoms and disability.[79] This recommendation is based on the fact that in contrast to adults with IBS there is only a paucity of studies examining pharmacological interventions in children with RAP and the evidence for these interventions is often inconclusive. The decision to medicate a child must therefore be considered in the context of this limited knowledge and must balance the potential risks and benefits of the intervention.

H2 BLOCKERS

One double-blind, placebo-controlled trial examined the effect of famotidine, an H2-receptor antagonist, in 25 children with abdominal pain. The global evaluation suggested that there was only a small benefit of famotidine over placebo, but the study population was heterogeneous. A subset of patients with dyspeptic symptoms did however show a significant improvement in symptoms. It seems therefore that H2-receptor antagonists might be prescribed to patients with FD.[114]

SEROTONERGIC AGENTS

In the section on "Pathophysiology", the role of serotonin as a key mediator in modulating visceral sensitivity and motility has been discussed. Serotonin can be modulated by (partial) antagonists as well as SSRIs. Both type of medications can indeed provide symptom relief in patients with functional abdominal complaints, but most studies have been performed in adults. Only pizotifen, a potent antagonist of the serotonin 2A (5-HT2A) receptor and citalopram, a selective serotonin reuptake inhibitor have been studied in children. Pizotifen was compared to placebo in 14 children with abdominal migraine; it was well tolerated and resulted in a decrease in the number of days with abdominal pain.[115] However, this drug is not approved in the United States and its use is thus limited. The efficacy, tolerability, and safety of citalopram in the treatment of functional pediatric abdominal pain was studied in 25 children in a 12-week, open-label trial.[116] Twenty-one subjects (84%) were classified as responders and ratings of abdominal pain, anxiety, depression, and other somatic symptoms improved significantly over time. The medication was generally well tolerated. It was concluded that citalopram is a promising treatment, but randomized, controlled studies are needed.

Novel pharmacological approaches in adults with IBS include serotonergic type 3 (5-HT3) antagonists such as alosetron and cilansetron, and tegaserod, a serotonergic type 4 (5-HT4) partial agonist. They all provide a modest symptom improvement, but due to severe side effects (drug-related ischemic colitis and an unexpected high number of ischemic cardiocvascular events) these drugs have been withdrawn from the market. Several other serotonin neuromodulators are in the pipeline, it is unclear however whether they will be more safe and effective.

TRICYCLIC ANTIDEPRESSANTS

The recommendation in the past for use of tricyclic antidepressants (TCAs) to treat FAP in children had been based primarily on anecdotal experience[117] and positive results in adults with IBS. Potential mechanisms of action of TCAs include reduction of central pain perception, alternations in gastrointestinal physiology, and a psychopharmacological affect. A meta-analysis of 12 studies among adults with IBS suggested efficacy, with three to four patients needed to treat to demonstrate benefit over placebo.[118] However, many of the studies included in this report have been criticized as methodologically flawed. A later conducted, well-controlled trial of desipramine versus placebo in 216 adult patients with IBS did not show a significant difference in pain relief. Recently, a small RCT in 33 adolescents with IBS showed improvement in quality of life and reduction of abdominal pain, although the effects decreased after cessation of the drug.[119] The potential side effects of TCAs, including the reports of sudden death in young children, a very low therapeutic index and a lack of efficacy in comorbid depression prevent recommendation as a first-line treatment option in children with FAP.

PSYCHOLOGICAL APPROACHES

Since children with RAP are significantly more likely to have high levels of anxiety and depression symptoms,[57–59] therapies that are capable of addressing these symptoms seem ideal for treating this group of patients. Cognitive behavioral therapy (CBT) has been proven efficacious in the treatment of anxiety and depression disorders in children. Therefore, a strong rationale exists for using CBT in this group of patients. Two Australian and one American randomized, controlled trials have examined the effect of CBT on children with RAP.[120–122] Treatment programs in the three studies differed slightly and consisted of increasing the understanding of pain and pain management, reinforcement of well behavior, and teaching cognitive coping skills. The first study showed decreased levels of pain in both the experimental and the control group. However, the CBT group improved more quickly, the effects generalized to the school setting and a larger proportion of subjects were completely pain free by 3 months follow-up.[120] In the second study, the CBT group had a higher rate of complete elimination of pain, lower levels of relapse at 6 and 12 months follow-up, and lower levels of interference with their activities as a result of pain.

After controlling for pretreatment levels of pain, children's active self-coping and mothers' caregiving strategies were significant independent predictors of pain behavior after treatment.[121] Finally in the third study, children and parents participating in the CBT intervention reported significantly less pain immediately following the intervention and up to 1 year after study entry, as well as significantly fewer school absences.[122] However, this last study suffered from methodological limitations such as significant differences at baseline and inadequate randomization procedures. Nevertheless, it can be concluded that there is evidence that CBT can be useful in improving pain and disability in children with FAP. More studies are needed to asses the cost-benefit of CBT in comparison to standard medical care, the effect on comorbid internalizing psychopathology, and the long-term follow-up.

Another psychological approach that might be useful in the treatment of children with FAP and IBS is gut-directed hypnotherapy. In this therapy a hypnotic trance is induced in which patients are given suggestions, directed toward control and normalization of gut function in addition to relevant ego-strengthening interventions. The first RCT with gut-directed hypnotherapy was performed in 1984 and involved 30 adult patients with IBS; the hypnotherapy group showed a dramatic improvement in abdominal pain and general well being.[123] A follow-up study among more than 200 patients with IBS who were refractory to conventional treatments showed that 71% of the patients initially responded to therapy. Of these, 81% maintained their improvement over time, while the majority of the remaining 19% claimed that deterioration of symptoms had only been slight.[124] Not only symptom scores improved, but also quality of life and anxiety and depression scores. Similar findings have also independently been reported by others (reviewed by Tan and colleagues)[125]. The mechanism of action is not well understood yet. Relief of pain could occur at the level of the gut or through modification of CNS processes. It has been shown that hypnosis reduces colonic motility and normalizes disordered rectal sensitivity. At the same time, brain imaging studies have demonstrated that hypnosis can modify cerebral processing of pain signals in the anterior cingulate cortex.[126] In children with RAP three uncontrolled studies have shown the feasibility of the use of (self-)hypnosis and guided imagery: 29 out of 33 children showed significant improvement with a decrease in weekly pain episodes.[127–129] Recently, a RCT in 52 children with either FAP or IBS demonstrated that gut-directed hypnotherapy was highly superior to standard medical therapy with 85 versus 25% of the children in clinical remission one year after treatment.[130]

COMPLEMENTARY THERAPIES

Despite all the above-described therapeutic interventions, there is still a considerable amount of patients with persisting complaints for whom effective therapies are lacking. A lot of patients

with functional bowel disorders have therefore prompted an interest in complementary and alternative therapies such as herbal remedies, acupuncture, or massage.[131,132] It might be useful for pediatricians and gastroenterologists to become familiar with these therapies; it is likely their patients already are. Furthermore, especially herbal medications are not without adverse effects and patients should not take these products without medical supervision.

Different herbal medicines have been tried in patients with IBS and RAP with mixed results. Most studies have been performed in adults. An Australian randomized-placebo-controlled trial demonstrated that Chinese herbal medicine, both standard and individualized formulations, may offer improvement in adults.[133] Peppermint is commonly found in over-the counter preparations for IBS and has been found effective.[134] The mechanism of action is thought to be from the menthol component of peppermint that relaxes gastrointestinal smooth muscle by blocking calcium channels.[135] Also in children with IBS the use of peppermint oil seems to be beneficial. In a small randomized, double-blind, controlled "only" 2-week trial 76% of the patients receiving enteric-coated peppermint oil capsules reported a decrease in symptom severity versus only 19% in the placebo group.[136] Curcuma and fumitory, two other over-the counter remedies, did not show any therapeutic benefit over placebo in adult patients with IBS. Finally, ginger (*Zingiber officinale*) is used by some patients, especially those with nausea, dyspepsia, or diarrhea as one of the main complaints. It has a prokinetic action, probably mediated by spasmolytic constituents of the calcium antagonist type.[137] Ginger has been proven effective for reducing postoperative nausea and vomiting[138] and nausea in early pregnancy.[139] It seems to be relatively safe, although abdominal discomfort has been noted in some patients. No RCTs in pediatric FGIDs have been performed so far.

Massage therapy is a commonly used complementary medicine modality in patients with chronic pain. Its use is based amongst others on the assumption that massage may reduce excitation of visceral afferent fibers and possibly affect central pain perception and processing. Recently, it was shown that massage can increase vagal tone and gastric motility.[140] In adults with IBS a small, single-blind trial did not show any benefit of reflexology foot massage on abdominal pain, defecation frequency, and abdominal distension.[141] In children one study examined the effect of massage in infants with colicky symptoms.[142] The authors concluded that the decrease of total and colicky crying hours reflected more the natural course of early infant crying and colic than a specific effect of the intervention. Studies with massage among children with IBS or FAP have not yet been performed.

Acupuncture is part of the traditional Chinese medicine and has become very popular in western countries in the last decades. Acupuncture and acupressure appear to ameliorate postoperative nausea and vomiting and thus might be useful in functional gastrointestinal complaints.[143] It is claimed that acupuncture is effective for IBS, but there are no data to support this. A recent prospective, blinded and sham/acupuncture-controlled study in 59 adult patients with IBS found a small but nonsignificant difference in response rate (40.7 vs 31.2% relief).[144] A second similar study among 43 patients found no differences and it was concluded that acupuncture in IBS is primarily a placebo response.[145] No good studies have been performed examining the benefits of acupuncture in children with FGIDs.

CONCLUDING REMARKS ON THERAPY

Because the pain-related FGIDs tend to be chronic, waxing and waning, a quick cure in every patient by any therapy is unlikely. Because of the high spontaneous remission of 30 to 70%, a stepwise approach is reasonable with the first step being education, identification, and modification of stress factors and dietary interventions if necessary. When symptoms persist or reoccur, the next step could be a trial of one of the psychological treatments like CBT, (self-)hypnosis, or guided imagery. It seems reasonable to reserve pharmacological interventions for patients who fail the above-mentioned therapies or are unwilling to consider it. There is no doubt that additional research is needed; randomized, double-blind, placebo-controlled trial are required for new drugs that are currently tested in adults with FGIDs.

FOLLOW-UP AND PROGNOSIS

Scarce data exist on the natural history of abdominal pain in children with only a limited number of longitudinal studies following children with RAP into adolescence and adult life. In the 1970s and 1980s several authors regarded pediatric RAP a short-term phenomenon.[50,146] However, later studies, studying the long-term follow-up (5 to 30 years) of RAP in childhood, showed that a significant proportion of 25 to 66% either continues to experience abdominal pain symptoms or develops other symptoms such as chronic headache, back pain, fibromyalgia, anxiety, and sleep disturbances throughout adolescence and adulthood.[19,64,147–151]

Some studies have evaluated the natural history of childhood abdominal pain and its suggested association with adult IBS. In an English study, following a cohort of 5,362 subjects from birth until the age of 43 years,[64] the presence of RAP was evaluated at three time points in childhood (at age 7, 11, and 15 years) and at adulthood. The prevalence of childhood abdominal pain was more or less 20% on each occasion. Only 2% experienced RAP on all three time points, suggesting that around 10% of the children with RAP in the general population continue to exhibit symptoms into adolescence. Persistent abdominal pain in childhood was modestly associated with other common physical symptoms in adulthood

and was a strong predictor of adult psychiatric disorders. It did not predict, however, abdominal pain in adulthood. This is in contrast to a birth cohort study from New Zealand, where 1,037 children were followed until the age of 26 years.[20] IBS at the of age 26 years was significantly more common among individuals with a history of RAP between the age of 7 and 9 years compared to those with no history of RAP. It is unclear why adult IBS was specifically linked to RAP reported at 9 years, but not at other time reports.

Walker and colleagues showed that 5 years after the initial evaluation, 45% of the 76 children with a history of RAP still had frequent abdominal pain compared to 20% of the control subjects.[19] Furthermore, female patients with a history of RAP appeared to be at an increased risk of IBS during adolescence and young adulthood. A recent study by Pace and colleagues confirms these observations indicating that pediatric RAP can predict later development of IBS. A cohort of 52 patients with RAP was followed up between 5 to 13 years; IBS was present in 29% of the patients at follow-up. Subjects who had developed IBS-like symptoms were almost three times more likely to present at least one sibling with similar symptoms. This suggests that a positive family history on RAP or IBS is an important determinant of persistent abdominal pain in adulthood, possibly through the learning of specific illness behavior (see also section on "Pathophysiology").[150]

Two studies examined adverse prognostic factors in children with RAP.[66,67] In the first study, 28 children with RAP of sufficient severity to necessitate hospitalization were evaluated; 14 continued to complain of pain. Only 1 of 14 parents of children with ongoing pain believed that there was a psychological cause for their child's pain, whereas 11 of 14 parents of the recovered children believed that the cause was attributable to psychological factors. It was concluded that acceptance by parents of a biopsychosocial model

of illness is important for the resolution of RAP in children.[66] These findings were confirmed by Lindley and colleagues who carried out a retrospective analysis in a cohort of 23 children aged <16 years with FAP. Poor outcome, defined as continued pain and failure to return to normal functioning >12 months after onset, was associated with refusal to engage with psychological services and lack of development of insight into psychosocial influences on symptoms. Moreover, involvement of more than three consultants and lodging of a manipulative complaint with hospital management by the child's family were adverse prognostic factors.[67]

In conclusion, 25 to 66% of children seeking medical help for RAP continue to experience similar symptoms in adulthood. They are at increased risk of developing other physical symptoms or psychiatric problems like anxiety. A family history of IBS, parental refusal to acknowledge the role of psychological factors in the genesis and maintenance of abdominal pain and an increased health-care consumerism are associated with persistence of symptoms.

REFERENCES

1. Chitkara DK, Rawat DJ, Talley NJ. The epidemiology of childhood recurrent abdominal pain in western countries: A systematic review. Am J Gastroenterol 2005;100:1868–75.
2. Starfield B, Gross E, Wood M, et al. Psychosocial and psychosomatic diagnoses in primary care of children. Pediatrics 1980;66:159–67.
3. Youssef NN, Murphy TG, Langseder AL, Rosh JR. Quality of life for children with functional abdominal pain: A comparison study of patients' and parents' perceptions. Pediatrics 2006;117:54–9.
4. Rasquin A, Di LC, Forbes D, et al. Childhood functional gastrointestinal disorders: Child/adolescent. Gastroenterology 2006;130:1527–37.
5. Apley J, Naish N. Recurrent abdominal pains: A field survey of 1,000 school children. Arch Dis Child 1958;33:165–70.
6. Rasquin-Weber A, Hyman PE, Cucchiara S, et al. Childhood functional gastrointestinal disorders. Gut 1999;45: ii60–ii68.
7. Saps M, Di LC. Interobserver and intraobserver reliability of the Rome II criteria in children. Am J Gastroenterol 2005;100:2079–82.

Table 4 Summary with Main Recommendations

1. Many pathologic conditions such as infectious, inflammatory, metabolic, or anatomic disorders can cause chronic or recurrent abdominal pain. However, in the majority of pediatric patients the pain is functional, that is without objective evidence of an underlying organic disorder.
2. Pain-related functional gastrointestinal disorders like IBS, FAP, and abdominal migraine are highly prevalent with significant clinical impact often resulting in interference with normal school attendance and performance, peer relationships, participation in organizations and sports, and other personal and family activities.
3. There is a growing body of evidence that functional abdominal pain is the result of visceral hypersensitivity due to a disordered brain–gut communication. Symptoms are generated by a complex interaction of biopsychosocial factors like genetic influences, early social learning, stressful life events, changes in serotonin signaling and emotional symptoms like anxiety and depression.
4. The key variables that point toward the diagnosis of a functional gastrointestinal disorder are the absence of alarm symptoms for an organic disorder and a normal physical examination, other than abdominal pressure tenderness.
5. Diagnostic tests should be kept to a minimum and one should realize that performing multiple tests may provide results that are unrelated to the presenting symptom or have no clinical relevance.
6. Because of the high spontaneous remission of 30 to 70%, a step-wise approach is reasonable with the first step being education, identification, and modification of stress factors and dietary interventions if necessary.
7. When symptoms persist or reoccur, the next step could be a trial of one of the psychological treatments like cognitive behavioral therapy or (self-)hypnosis. Pharmacological interventions need to be reserved for patients who fail the above-mentioned therapies or are unwilling to consider it.

FAP = functional abdominal pain; IBS = irritable bowel syndrome.

8. Caplan A, Walker L, Rasquin A. Development and preliminary validation of the questionnaire on pediatric gastrointestinal symptoms to assess functional gastrointestinal disorders in children and adolescents. J Pediatr Gastroenterol Nutr 2005;41:296–304.
9. Walker LS, Lipani TA, Greene JW, et al. Recurrent abdominal pain: Symptom subtypes based on the Rome II criteria for pediatric functional gastrointestinal disorders. J Pediatr Gastroenterol Nutr 2004;38:187–91.
10. Caplan A, Walker L, Rasquin A. Validation of the pediatric Rome II criteria for functional gastrointestinal disorders using the questionnaire on pediatric gastrointestinal symptoms. J Pediatr Gastroenterol Nutr 2005;41:305–16.
11. Uc A, Hyman PE, Walker LS. Functional gastrointestinal disorders in African American children in primary care. J Pediatr Gastroenterol Nutr 2006;42:270–4.
12. Miele E, Simeone D, Marino A, et al. Functional gastrointestinal disorders in children: An Italian prospective survey. Pediatrics 2004;114:73–8.
13. Perquin CW, Hazebroek-Kampschreur AA, Hunfeld JA, et al. Pain in children and adolescents: A common experience. Pain 2000;87:51–8.
14. Bode G, Brenner H, Adler G, Rothenbacher D. Recurrent abdominal pain in children: Evidence from a population-based study that social and familial factors play a major role but not *Helicobacter pylori* infection. J Psychosom Res 2003;54:417–21.
15. Schurman JV, Friesen Ca, Danda CE, et al. Diagnosing functional abdominal pain with the Rome II criteria: Parent, child, and clinician agreement. J Pediatr Gastroenterol Nutr 2005;41:291–5.
16. Reshetnikov OV, Kurilovich SA, Denisova DV, et al. Prevalence of dyspepsia and irritable bowel syndrome among adolescents of Novosibirsk, Western Siberia. Int J Circumpolar Health 2001;60:253–7.
17. Dong L, Dingguo L, Xiaoxing X, Hanming L. An epidemiologic study of irritable bowel syndrome in adolescents and children in China: A school-based study. Pediatrics 2005;116:E393–6.
18. Rowland M, Gormally SM, Daly LE, et al. Clinical relevance of the paediatric Rome criteria for the diagnosis of recurrent abdominal pain in children. Gut 2001;A2324.
19. Walker LS, Guite JW, Duke M, et al. Recurrent abdominal pain: A potential precursor of irritable bowel syndrome in adolescents and young adults. J Pediatr 1998;132: 1010–5.
20. Howell S, Poulton R, Talley NJ. The natural history of childhood abdominal pain and its association with adult irritable bowel syndrome: Birth-cohort study. Am J Gastroenterol 2005;100:2071–8.
21. Van Ginkel R, Voskuijl WP, Benninga MA, et al. Alterations in rectal sensitivity and motility in childhood irritable bowel syndrome. Gastroenterology 2001;120:31–8.
22. Di Lorenzo C, Youssef NN, Sigurdsson L, et al. Visceral hyperalgesia in children with functional abdominal pain. J Pediatr 2001;139:838–43.
23. Chitkara DK, Camilleri M, Zinsmeister AR, et al. Gastric sensory and motor dysfunction in adolescents with functional dyspepsia. J Pediatr 2005;146:500–5.
24. Treede RD, Kenshalo DR, Gracely RH, Jones Ak. The cortical representation of pain. Pain 1999;79:105–11.
25. Mertz H, Morgan V, Tanner G, et al. Regional cerebral activation in irritable bowel syndrome and control subjects with painful and nonpainful rectal distention. Gastroenterology 2000;118:842–8.
26. Naliboff BD, Derbyshire SW, Munakata J, et al. Cerebral activation in patients with irritable bowel syndrome and control subjects during rectosigmoid stimulation. Psychosom Med 2001;63:365–75.
27. Berman SM, Chang L, Suyenobu B, et al. Condition-specific deactivation of brain regions by 5-HT3 receptor antagonist alosetron. Gastroenterology 2002;123:969–77.
28. Morgan V, Pickens D, Gautam S, et al. Amitriptyline reduces rectal pain related activation of the anterior cingulate cortex in patients with irritable bowel syndrome. Gut 2005;54:601–7.
29. Rainville P, Duncan GH, Price DD, et al. Pain affect encoded in human anterior cingulate but not somatosensory cortex. Science 1997;277:968–71.
30. Hofbauer RK, Rainville P, Duncan GH, et al. Cortical representation of the sensory dimension of pain. J Neurophysiol 2001;86:402–11.
31. Mertz H. Altered CNS processing of visceral pain in IBS. In: Camilleri M, Spiller RC, editors. Irritable Bowel Syndrome. Diagnosis And Treatment, 1st edition. Philadelphia: WB Saunders; 2002. p. 55–68.
32. Kalantar JS, Locke Gr, III, Zinsmeister AR, et al. Familial aggregation of irritable bowel syndrome: A prospective study. Gut 2003;52:1703–7.
33. Locke Gr, III, Zinsmeister AR, Talley NJ, et al. Familial association in adults with functional gastrointestinal disorders. Mayo Clin Proc 2000;75:907–12.
34. Levy RL, Jones KR, Whitehead WE, et al. Irritable bowel syndrome in twins: Heredity and social learning both contribute to etiology. Gastroenterology 2001;121:799–804.
35. Mohammed I, Cherkas Lf, Riley SA, et al. Genetic influences in irritable bowel syndrome: A twin study. Am J Gastroenterol 2005;100:1340–4.
36. Chitkara DK, Di Lorenzo C. From The bench to the "crib"-side: Implications of scientific advances to paediatric neurogastroenterology and motility. Neurogastroenterol Motil 2006;18:251–62.
37. Read NW, Gwee KA. The importance of 5-hydroxytryptamine receptors in the gut. Pharmacol Ther 1994;62:159–73.
38. Gershon MD. Review article: Serotonin receptors and transporters—roles in normal and abnormal gastrointestinal motility. Aliment Pharmacol Ther 2004;20:3–14.
39. Mawe GM, Coates MD, Moses PL. Review article: Intestinal serotonin signalling in irritable bowel syndrome. Aliment Pharmacol Ther 2006;23:1067–76.
40. Gwee KA, Leong YL, Graham C, et al. The role of psychological and biological factors in postinfective gut dysfunction. Gut 1999;44:400–6.
41. Barbara G, De GR, Stanghellini V, et al. New pathophysiological mechanisms in irritable bowel syndrome. Aliment Pharmacol Ther 2004;20:1–9.
42. Dunlop SP, Jenkins D, Neal KR, et al. Randomized, double-blind, placebo-controlled trial of prednisolone in post-infectious irritable bowel syndrome. Aliment Pharmacol Ther 2003;18:77–84.
43. Coutinho SV, Plotsky PM, Sablad M, et al. Neonatal maternal separation alters stress-induced responses to viscerosomatic nociceptive stimuli in rat. Am J Physiol Gastrointest Liver Physiol 2002;282:G307–16.
44. Al-Chaer ED, Kawasaki M, Pasricha PJ. A new model of chronic visceral hypersensitivity in adult rats induced by colon irritation during postnatal development. Gastroenterology 2000;119:1276–85.
45. Koloski NA, Talley NJ. Role of sexual or physical abuse in IBS. In: Camilleri M, Spiller RC, editors. Irritable Bowel Syndrome. Diagnosis And Treatment, 1st edition. Philadelphia WB Saunders; 2002. p. 37–43.
46. Hodges K, Kline JJ, Barbero G, Flanery R. Life events occurring in families of children with recurrent abdominal pain. J Psychosom Res 1984;28:185–8.
47. Wasserman AL, Whitington PF, Rivara FP. Psychogenic basis for abdominal pain in children and adolescents. J Am Acad Child Adolesc Psychiatr 1988;27:179–84.
48. Robinson JO, Alverez JH, Dodge JA. Life events and family history in children with recurrent abdominal pain. J Psychosom Res 1990;34:171–81.
49. Boey CC, Goh KL. The significance of life-events as contributing factors in childhood recurrent abdominal pain in an urban community in Malaysia. J Psychosom Res 2001;51:559–62.
50. Liebman WM. Recurrent abdominal pain in children: A retrospective survey of 119 patients. Clin Pediatr (Phila) 1978;17:149–53.
51. Leonard BE. The HPA and immune axes in stress: The involvement of the serotonergic system. Eur Psychiatr 2005;20:S302–6.
52. Fukudo S, Nomura T, Hongo M. Impact of corticotropin-releasing hormone on gastrointestinal motility and adrenocorticotropic hormone in normal controls and patients with irritable bowel syndrome. Gut 1998;42:845–9.
53. Lembo T, Plourde V, Shui Z, et al. Effects of the corticotropin-releasing factor (CRF) on rectal afferent nerves in humans. Neurogastroenterol Motil 1996;8:9–18.
54. Posserud I, Agerforz P, Ekman R, et al. Altered visceral perceptual and neuroendocrine response in patients with irritable bowel syndrome during mental stress. Gut 2004;53:1102–8.
55. Santos J, Saperas E, Mourelle M, et al. Regulation of intestinal mast cells and luminal protein release by cerebral thyrotropin-releasing hormone in rats. Gastroenterology 1996;111:1465–73.
56. Barbara G, Stanghellini V, De Giorgio R, et al. Activated mast cells in proximity to colonic nerves correlate with abdominal pain in irritable bowel syndrome. Gastroenterology 2004;126:693–02.
57. Campo JV, Bridge J, Ehmann M, et al. Recurrent abdominal pain, anxiety, and depression in primary care. Pediatrics 2004;113:817–24.
58. Garber J, Zeman J, Walker LS. Recurrent abdominal pain in children: Psychiatric diagnoses and parental psychopathology. J Am Acad Child Adolesc Psychiatr 1990;29:648–56.
59. Liakopoulou-Kairis M, Alifieraki T, Protagora D, et al. Recurrent abdominal pain and headache—psychopathology, life events and family functioning. Eur Child Adolesc Psychiatr 2002;11:115–22.
60. Robinson ME, Riley JL. The role of emotion in pain. In: Gatchel RJ, Turk DC, editors. Psychosocial Factors In Pain: Critical Perspectives. New York: Guilford Press; 1999. p. 74–88.
61. Gureje O, Simon GE, Von Korff M. A cross-national study of the course of persistent pain in primary care. Pain 2001;92: 195–200.
62. Thomsen AH, Compas BE, Colletti RB, et al. Parent reports of coping and stress responses in children with recurrent abdominal pain. J Pediatr Psychol 2002;27:215–26.
63. Fekkes M, Pijpers FI, Fredriks AM, et al. Do bullied children get ill, or do ill children get bullied? A prospective cohort study on the relationship between bullying and health-related symptoms. Pediatrics 2006;117:1568–74.
64. Hotopf M, Carr S, Mayou R, et al. Why do children have chronic abdominal pain, and what happens to them when they grow up? Population based cohort study. BMJ 1998;316:1196–200.
65. Ramchandani PG, Stein A, Hotopf M, Wiles NJ. Early parental and child predictors of recurrent abdominal pain at school age: results of a large population-based study. J Am Acad Child Adolesc Psychiatr 2006;45:729–36.
66. Crushell E, Rowland M, Doherty M, et al. Importance of parental conceptual model of illness in severe recurrent abdominal pain. Pediatrics 2003;112:1368–72.
67. Lindley KJ, Glaser D, Milla PJ. Consumerism in healthcare can be detrimental to child health: Lessons from children with functional abdominal pain. Arch Dis Child 2005;90:335–7.
68. Walker LS, Williams SE, Smith CA, et al. Parent attention versus distraction: impact on symptom complaints by children with and without chronic functional abdominal pain. Pain 2006;122:43–52.
69. Camilleri M, Ford MJ. Review article: Colonic sensorimotor physiology in health, and its alteration in constipation and diarrhoeal disorders. Aliment Pharmacol Ther 1998;12:287–302.
70. Serra J, Azpiroz F, Malagelada JR. Impaired transit and tolerance of intestinal gas in the irritable bowel syndrome. Gut 2001;48:14–9.
71. Di Lorenzo C. Abdominal pain: Is it in the gut or in the head? J Pediatr Gastroenterol Nutr 2005;41:S44–6.
72. Cremonini F, Talley NJ. Diagnostic and therapeutic strategies in the irritable bowel syndrome. Minerva Med 2004;95:427–41.
73. Serra J, Azpiroz F, Malagelada JR. Intestinal gas dynamics and tolerance in humans. Gastroenterology 1998;115:542–50.
74. Serra J, Salvioli B, Azpiroz F, Malagelada JR. Lipid-induced intestinal gas retention in irritable bowel syndrome. Gastroenterology 2002;123:700–6.
75. Lin HC. Small intestinal bacterial overgrowth: A framework for understanding irritable bowel syndrome. JAMA 2004;292:852–8.
76. Hwang JB, Choi WJ, Kim JS, et al. Clinical features of pathologic childhood aerophagia: Early recognition and essential diagnostic criteria. J Pediatr Gastroenterol Nutr 2005;41:612–6.
77. Heaton KW. Diagnosis of acute non-specific abdominal pain. Lancet 2000;355:1644.
78. Croffie JM, Fitzgerald JF, Chong SK. Recurrent abdominal pain in children—a retrospective study of outcome in a group referred to a pediatric gastroenterology practice. Clin Pediatr (Phila) 2000;39:267–74.
79. Di Lorenzo C, Colletti RB, Lehmann HP, et al. Chronic abdominal pain in children: A technical report of the american academy of pediatrics and the North American Society For Pediatric Gastroenterology, Hepatology And Nutrition. J Pediatr Gastroenterol Nutr 2005;40:249–61.
80. Alfven G. The covariation of common psychosomatic symptoms among children from socio-economically differing residential areas. An epidemiological study. Acta Paediatr 1993;82:484–7.
81. Mcgrath PJ, Goodman JT, Firestone P, et al. Recurrent abdominal pain: a psychogenic disorder? Arch Dis Child 1983;58:888–90.
82. Walker LS, Garber J, Greene JW. Psychosocial correlates of recurrent childhood pain: A comparison of pediatric patients with recurrent abdominal pain, organic illness, and psychiatric disorders. J Abnorm Psychol 1993;102:248–58.
83. Walker LS, Garber J, Smith CA, et al. The relation of daily stressors to somatic and emotional symptoms in children with and without recurrent abdominal pain. J Consult Clin Psychol 2001;69:85–91.
84. Walker LS, Greene JW. Children with recurrent abdominal pain and their parents: More somatic complaints, anxiety, and depression than other patient families? J Pediatr Psychol 1989;14:231–3.

85. Alfven G. The pressure pain threshold (PPT) of certain muscles in children suffering from recurrent abdominal pain of non-organic origin. An algometric study. Acta Paediatr 1993;82:481–3.

86. Van Der Plas RN, Benninga MA, Buller HA, et al. Biofeedback training in treatment of childhood constipation: A randomised controlled study. Lancet 1996;348:776–80.

87. Baker SS, Liptak GS, Colletti RB, et al. Constipation in infants and children: Evaluation and treatment. A medical position statement of The North American Society For Pediatric Gastroenterology And Nutrition. J Pediatr Gastroenterol Nutr 1999;29:612–26.

88. Liebman WM. Serum IGE levels and recurrent abdominal pain in children. South Med J 1978;71:1485–6.

89. Kokkonen J, Haapalahti M, Tikkanen S, et al. Gastrointestinal complaints and diagnosis in children: A population-based study. Acta Paediatr 2004;93:880–6.

90. Fitzpatrick KP, Sherman PM, Ipp M, et al. Screening for celiac disease in children with recurrent abdominal pain. J Pediatr Gastroenterol Nutr 2001;33:250–2.

91. Lebenthal E, Rossi TM, Nord KS, Branski D. Recurrent abdominal pain and lactose absorption in children. Pediatrics 1981;67:828–32.

92. Dearlove J, Dearlove B, Pearl K, Primavesi R. Dietary lactose and the child with abdominal pain. Br Med J (Clin Res Ed) 1983;286:1936.

93. Yip WC, Ho TF, Yip YY, Chan KY. Value of abdominal sonography in the assessment of children with abdominal pain. J Clin Ultrasound 1998;26:397–400.

94. Rowland M, Bourke B, Drumm B. Do the Rome criteria help the doctor or the patient? J Pediatr Gastroenterol Nutr 2005;41:S32–3.

95. Pitz M, Cheang M, Bernstein CN. Defining the predictors of the placebo response in irritable bowel syndrome. Clin Gastroenterol Hepatol 2005;3:237–47.

96. Walker LS, Claar RL, Garber J. Social consequences of children's pain: When do they encourage symptom maintenance? J Pediatr Psychol 2002;27:689–98.

97. Chey WY, Jin HO, Lee MH, et al. Colonic motility abnormality in patients with irritable bowel syndrome exhibiting abdominal pain and diarrhea. Am J Gastroenterol 2001;96:1499–506.

98. Hillemeier C. An overview of the effects of dietary fiber on gastrointestinal transit. Pediatrics 1995;96:997–99.

99. Feldman W, Mcgrath P, Hodgson C, et al. The use of dietary fiber in the management of simple, childhood, idiopathic, recurrent, abdominal pain. Results in a prospective, double-blind, randomized, controlled trial. Am J Dis Child 1985;139:1216–8.

100. Christensen MF. Recurrent abdominal pain and dietary fiber. Am J Dis Child 1986;140:738–9.

101. Weydert JA, Ball TM, Davis MF. Systematic review of treatments for recurrent abdominal pain. Pediatrics 2003; 111:E1–11.

102. Stordal K, Bentsen BS. Recurrent abdominal pain in school children revisited: Fitting adverse food reactions into the puzzle. Acta Paediatr 2004;93:869–71.

103. Stefanini GF, Saggioro A, Alvisi V, et al. Oral cromolyn sodium in comparison with elimination diet in the irritable bowel syndrome, diarrheic type. Multicenter study of 428 patients. Scand J Gastroenterol 1995;30:535–41.

104. Grazioli I, Melzi G, Balsamo V, et al. Food intolerance and irritable bowel syndrome of childhood: Clinical efficacy of oral sodium cromoglycate and elimination diet. Minerva Pediatr 1993;45:253–8.

105. Vanderhoof JA, Young RJ. Pediatric applications of probiotics. Gastroenterol Clin North Am 2005;34:45i–ix.

106. Kajander K, Hatakka K, Poussa T, et al. A probiotic mixture alleviates symptoms in irritable bowel syndrome patients: A controlled 6-month intervention. Aliment Pharmacol Ther 2005;22:387–394.

107. Kim HJ, Vazquez Roque MI, Camilleri M, et al. A randomized controlled trial of a probiotic combination Vsl# 3 and placebo in irritable bowel syndrome with bloating. Neurogastroenterol Motil 2005;17:687–96.

108. Nobaek S, Johansson ML, Molin G, et al. Alteration of intestinal microflora is associated with reduction in abdominal bloating and pain in patients with irritable bowel syndrome. Am J Gastroenterol 2000;95:1231–8.

109. O'mahony L, Mccarthy J, Kelly P, et al. Lactobacillus and bifidobacterium in irritable bowel syndrome: Symptom responses and relationship to cytokine profiles. Gastroenterology 2005;128:541–51.

110. Bausserman M, Michail S. The use of lactobacillus Gg in irritable bowel syndrome in children: A double-blind randomized control trial. J Pediatr 2005;147:197–201.

111. Gawronska A, Dziechciarz P, Horvath A, Szajewska H. A randomized double-blind placebo-controlled trial of lactobacillus Gg for abdominal pain disorders in children 1. Aliment Pharmacol Ther 2007;25:177–84.

112. Spiller R. Probiotics: An ideal anti-inflammatory treatment for IBS? Gastroenterology 2005;128:783–5.

113. Cremonini F, Talley NJ. Treatments targeting putative mechanisms in irritable bowel syndrome. Nat Clin Pract Gastroenterol Hepatol 2005;2:82–8.

114. See MC, Birnbaum AH, Schechter CB, et al. Double-blind, placebo-controlled trial of famotidine in children with abdominal pain and dyspepsia: Global and quantitative assessment. Dig Dis Sci 2001;46:985–92.

115. Symon DN, Russell G. Double blind placebo controlled trial of pizotifen syrup in the treatment of abdominal migraine. Arch Dis Child 1995;72:48–50.

116. Campo Jv, Perel J, Lucas A, et al. Citalopram treatment of pediatric recurrent abdominal pain and comorbid internalizing disorders: An exploratory study. J Am Acad Child Adolesc Psychiatry 2004;43:1234–42.

117. Hyams JS, Hyman PE. Recurrent abdominal pain and the biopsychosocial model of medical practice. J Pediatr 1998;133:473–8.

118. Jackson JL, O'malley PG, Tomkins G, et al. Treatment of functional gastrointestinal disorders with antidepressant medications: A meta-analysis. Am J Med 2000;108: 65–72.

119. Collins BS, Bahar RJ, Steinmetz BA, Ament ME. Double-blind placebo-controlled trial of low-dose amitriptyline for the treatment of irritable bowel syndrome in adolescents. Gastroenterology 2007;132:A T1343.

120. Sanders MR, Rebgetz M, Morrison M, et al. Cognitive-behavioral treatment of recurrent nonspecific abdominal pain in children: An analysis of generalization, maintenance, and side effects. J Consult Clin Psychol 1989;57: 294–300.

121. Sanders MR, Shepherd RW, Cleghorn G, Woolford H. The treatment of recurrent abdominal pain in children: A controlled comparison of cognitive-behavioral family intervention and standard pediatric care. J Consult Clin Psychol 1994;62:306–14.

122. Robins PM, Smith SM, Glutting JJ, Bishop CT. A randomized controlled trial of a cognitive-behavioral family intervention for pediatric recurrent abdominal pain. J Pediatr Psychol 2005;30:397–408.

123. Whorwell PJ, Prior A, Faragher EB. Controlled trial of hypnotherapy in the treatment of severe refractory irritable-bowel syndrome. Lancet 1984;2:1232–4.

124. Gonsalkorale WM, Miller V, Afzal A, Whorwell PJ. Long term benefits of hypnotherapy for irritable bowel syndrome. Gut 2003;52:1623–9.

125. Tan G, Hammond DC, Joseph G. Hypnosis and irritable bowel syndrome: A review of efficacy and mechanism of action. Am J Clin Hypn 2005;47:161–78.

126. Gonsalkorale WM, Whorwell PJ. Hypnotherapy in the treatment of irritable bowel syndrome. Eur J Gastroenterol Hepatol 2005;17:15–20.

127. Anbar RD. Self-hypnosis for the treatment of functional abdominal pain in childhood. Clin Pediatr (Phila) 2001;40:447–51.

128. Ball TM, Shapiro DE, Monheim CJ, Weydert JA. A pilot study of the use of guided imagery for the treatment of recurrent abdominal pain in children. Clin Pediatr (Phila) 2003;42:527–32.

129. Youssef NN, Rosh JR, Loughran M, et al. Treatment of functional abdominal pain in childhood with cognitive behavioral strategies. J Pediatr Gastroenterol Nutr 2004;39:192–6.

130. Vlieger AM, Menko-Frankenhuis C, Wolfkamp SC, et al. Hypnotherapy for children with functional abdominal pain or irritable bowel syndrome: A randomized controlled trial. Gastroenterology (in press).

131. Day AS. Use of complementary and alternative therapies and probiotic agents by children attending gastroenterology outpatient clinics. J Paediatr Child Health 2002;38:343–6.

132. Kong SC, Hurlstone DP, Pocock CY, et al. The incidence of self-prescribed oral complementary and alternative medicine use by patients with gastrointestinal diseases. J Clin Gastroenterol 2005;39:138–41.

133. Bensoussan A, Talley NJ, Hing M, et al. Treatment of irritable bowel syndrome with Chinese herbal medicine: A randomized controlled trial. JAMA 1998;280:1585–9.

134. Pittler MH, Ernst E. Peppermint oil for irritable bowel syndrome: A critical review and metaanalysis. Am J Gastroenterol 1998;93:1131–5.

135. Hills JM, Aaronson PI. The mechanism of action of peppermint oil on gastrointestinal smooth muscle. An analysis using patch clamp electrophysiology and isolated tissue pharmacology in rabbit and guinea pig. Gastroenterology 1991;101:55–65.

136. Kline RM, Kline JJ, Di PJ, Barbero GJ. Enteric-coated, pH-dependent peppermint oil capsules for the treatment of irritable bowel syndrome in children. J Pediatr 2001;138:125–8.

137. Ghayur MN, Gilani AH. Pharmacological basis for the medicinal use of ginger in gastrointestinal disorders. Dig Dis Sci 2005;50:1889–97.

138. Chaiyakunapruk N, Kitikannakorn N, Nathisuwan S, et al. The efficacy of ginger for the prevention of postoperative nausea and vomiting: A meta-analysis. Am J Obstet Gynecol 2006;194:95–9.

139. Borrelli F, Capasso R, Aviello G, et al. Effectiveness and safety of ginger in the treatment of pregnancy-induced nausea and vomiting. Obstet Gynecol 2005;105:849–56.

140. Diego MA, Field T, Hernandez-Reif M. Vagal activity, gastric motility, and weight gain in massaged preterm neonates. J Pediatr 2005;147:50–5.

141. Tovey P. A single-blind trial of reflexology for irritable bowel syndrome. Br J Gen Pract 2002;52:19–23.

142. Huhtala V, Lehtonen L, Heinonen R, Korvenranta H. Infant massage compared with crib vibrator in the treatment of colicky infants. Pediatrics 2000;105:E84.

143. Stern RM, Jokerst MD, Muth ER, Hollis C. Acupressure relieves the symptoms of motion sickness and reduces abnormal gastric activity. Altern Ther Health Med 2001;7:91–4.

144. Forbes A, Jackson S, Walter C, et al. Acupuncture for irritable bowel syndrome: A blinded placebo-controlled trial. World J Gastroenterol 2005;11:4040–4.

145. Schneider A, Enck P, Streitberger K, et al. Acupuncture treatment in irritable bowel syndrome. Gut 2006;55:649–54.

146. Levine MD, Rappaport LA. Recurrent abdominal pain in school children: The loneliness of the long-distance physician. Pediatr Clin North Am 1984;31:969–91.

147. Hyams JS, Burke G, Davis PM, et al. Abdominal pain and irritable bowel syndrome in adolescents: A community-based study. J Pediatr 1996;129:220–6.

148. Walker LS, Garber J, Van Slyke DA, Greene JW. Long-term health outcomes in patients with recurrent abdominal pain. J Pediatr Psychol 1995;20:233–45.

149. Magni G, Pierri M, Donzelli F. Recurrent abdominal pain in children: A long term follow-up. Eur J Pediatr 1987;146:72–4.

150. Pace F, Zuin G, Di GS, et al. Family history of irritable bowel syndrome is the major determinant of persistent abdominal complaints in young adults with a history of pediatric recurrent abdominal pain. World J Gastroenterol 2006;12:3874–7.

151. Campo JV, Di LC, Chiappetta L, et al. Adult outcomes of pediatric recurrent abdominal pain: Do they just grow out of it? Pediatrics 2001;108:E1.

25

Gastrointestinal System in Systemic Endocrinopathies

Jonathan E. Teitelbaum, MD

Systemic endocrinopathies have effects on multiple organ systems including the gastrointestinal (GI) tract. Effects on the gastrointestinal system are secondary to shared genetic susceptibilities (eg, diabetes and celiac disease) as well as altered homeostatic and metabolic functions (eg, hyperthyroidism and diarrhea). The pathophysiologic basis for these alterations is often poorly understood. In part, the effects can be meditated through the effects of the endocrinopathies on other organ systems, such as the enteric nervous system. Finally, since the endocrine system plays a vital role in organ development and growth, endocrinopathies have effects on both the developing gut as well as the mature intestine.

DIABETES MELLITUS

Type 1 diabetes mellitus (DM) is a common, serious disease of childhood and adolescence. Previously called juvenile-onset diabetes, these patients are insulinopenic and require exogenous insulin to prevent ketosis and preserve life. The prevalence of type 1 diabetes in the United States among children and adolescence is between 1.2 and 1.9 cases per 1,000 members of this age group.[1]

Type 2 diabetes is most commonly found among adults and obese persons. Previously called adult-onset diabetes, this type of diabetes is the result of insulin resistance without adequate compensatory insulin secretion. Thus a relative, not absolute, insulin deficiency occurs. Affected patients are not dependent on insulin for survival, but may require exogenous insulin for metabolic control.

The diagnosis of diabetes in a child is rarely subtle. Most children present with classic symptoms of polyuria, polydipsia, polyphagia, weight loss, and lethargy. Gastrointestinal manifestations are well described (Table 1), although many adult studies will combine the data obtained from both type 1 and type 2 patients. Thus one must be cautious in applying these findings to pediatric patients where type 1 disease is the most prevalent.

Mechanisms leading to these gastrointestinal disturbances include autonomic neuropathy, microangiopathy, hyperglycemia, electrolyte disturbances, and abnormalities in plasma insulin, glucagon, and other hormones such as motilin and gastric inhibitory polypeptide.[2]

Infants of Diabetic Mothers

Gestational diabetes is defined as carbohydrate intolerance resulting in hyperglycemia of variable severity with onset during pregnancy irrespective of whether or not insulin is used for the treatment or if the condition persists after pregnancy. The frequency of gestational diabetes is variable, and mirrors the frequency of type 2 diabetes in the population. In China and South India the rate is 0.6%, in Australia 15%, in the USA 4%.[3] A normal glucose tolerance test early in pregnancy does not exclude the development of this condition later in gestation. There are significant morbidities and mortality associated with children born to diabetic mothers. Indeed, early descriptions of these parents read "they gave birth astride a grave, with a grave awaiting both the mother and fetus."[3] The mother is also at risk for preterm labor, pyelonephritis, and hypertension.

Infants of diabetic mothers (IDM) have been documented to have a large number of associated anomalies. The fetus carries an increased risk of abortion, congenital malformations, macrosomia, intrauterine growth retardation, trauma, asphyxia, respiratory distress syndrome, hypoglycemia, hypocalcemia, jaundice, and cardiomyopathy. Most important among these is the marked increase in perinatal mortality, with an incidence of up to 30% in those who have poorly controlled diabetes. This can be decreased to 2 to 4% with strict glycemic control throughout the pregnancy.[4] Thirty to forty percent of these deaths are associated with congenital malformations. Overall, the incidence of such malformations is 6 to 13%, which is 2 to 4 times that seen in the general population.[4] In the Diabetes Control and Complication trial, 1,441 type 1 diabetics had 270 births. If there was excellent glucose control (HgA1c 4.7 standard deviations above the mean) during pregnancy then the rate of congenital malformations and abortions was similar to the general population (0.7%).[3] Also in this group the incidence of SGA babies was 20% vs 11% in healthy controls.[5] However, conventional control (HgA1c 6.3 standard deviations above the mean) had a rate of malformations at 5.9%. These results suggested that the goal should be to maintain a HgA1c less than 5 standard deviations above the mean.[3] The exact teratogen remains unknown with the major candidates being hyperglycemia, hypoglycemia, increased ketones, effects of increased glycosylation products, changes in amino acid or prostaglandin profiles, and increased free radical production. A study of placental pathology in children born to diabetic mothers revealed greater numbers of histological abnormalities such as the presence of nucleated fetal red blood cells, fibrinoid necrosis, villous immaturity, and chorangiosis as compared to normal controls.[6]

The children of diabetic mothers can demonstrate an increase in organ size, specifically the heart and liver, while the brain and kidney do not demonstrate visceromegaly. The etiology of hepatomegaly is based on the increase in maternal blood glucose. This increase causes a similar rise in fetal blood glucose. The fetus, therefore, has an appropriate increase in insulin production to obtain euglycemia. Insulin is the primary anabolic hormone in the growing fetus and results in visceromegaly. Macrosomia is the result of

Table 1 Effects of Diabetes Mellitus on the Gastrointestinal System	
Abnormality/Association	Gastrointestinal Manifestation
Diabetic ketoacidosis (DKA)	Nausea, anorexia, vomiting
Esophageal dysmotility	Dysphagia, reflux esophagitis
Esophageal candidiasis	Odynophagia, dysphagia
Gastroparesis/gastritis	Nausea, vomiting, gastric outlet obstruction
Small intestine dysmotility	Malabsorption, diarrhea, bacterial overgrowth
Impaired intestinal fluid reabsorption	Diabetic diarrhea
Celiac disease	Diarrhea, steatorrhea
Steatohepatitis	Abnormal transaminases, hepatic fibrosis
Hepatocellular carcinoma	Twofold increase risk
Cholelithiasis	Biliary sepsis
Adapted from Weber, Ryan.[113]	

increased adipose tissue and birth weight correlates with blood insulin levels[7] as well as cord blood leptin levels.[8] Ultrasound monitoring of the fetus can be helpful in predicting fetal well being. Measurements of fetal abdominal circumference (AC) between 29 to 33 weeks' gestation can identify those infants with an AC greater than the 75 percentile. If these women are then treated with insulin the rate of macrosomia is decreased from 45% to 13%. Those children who have a greater than 1.1cm increase in their AC per week appear to be at risk for macrosomia. A nationwide study in the Netherlands including 289 children born to insulin dependent diabetic mothers reported an incidence of macrosomia of 48.8% despite good diabetic control (HgA1c ≤7%) in 84% of mothers. Third trimester HgA1C was the most powerful predictor of macrosomia but its predictive capacity was weak, accounting for less than 5% of the variance.[9] Vohr reported that previously macrosomic infants who were followed up at ages of 4 and 7 years had increased body size and adiposity as compared to controls and those infants born to gestational diabetics who were born at appropriate weight.[10]

Infants of diabetics are also noted to have increased levels of bilirubin, which in one study affected 35.7%.[11] While some suggest that prematurity, ABO incompatibility, red blood cell life span, or osmotic fragility accounted for this increase; other studies do not support a difference in these parameters between IDM and normals.[4] Stevenson suggested that the delayed clearance of bilirubin was a factor.[12] However, polycythemia is felt to be the most important factor accounting for elevated levels of indirect bilirubin in this population.[4]

Neonatal small-left colon was first described by Davis and colleagues in 1974. It results in a low obstruction of the large bowel which clinically is manifested by failure to pass meconium in a timely fashion, tympanic abdominal distention, or bilious vomiting. Barium enema reveals smooth narrowing of the sigmoid and descending colon with proximal dilatation (Figure 1). An early series of 20 patients revealed that 17 did well after diagnostic/therapeutic enema.[13] Eight of the twenty (40%) had diabetic mothers. Perforation, typically of the cecum also has been reported. The etiology is still unclear and theories include disorders of fetal colonic motility perhaps secondary to temporary ganglionic dysfunction[14] or to the effects of glucagons and hypoglycemia on intestinal motility.[15] Treatment is typically conservative with initial parenteral nutrition and nasogastric decompression. At times, the barium enema has been therapeutic and allowed for a graded approach to feeding. The condition commonly resolves within the first 1 to 2 weeks of life. Differentiation between infants with small left colons and Hirschprung's disease can be difficult as they share similar features.[16] However, the caliber of the colons in infants with small left colons is significantly reduced (typically less than 1 cm) as compared to the normal caliber of the aganglionic colon.

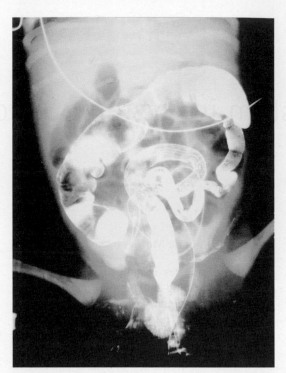

Figure 1 Barium enema of a newborn with small left colon syndrome. (Courtesy of Thomas J. Kelly, MD. Monmouth Medical Center, NJ.)

Diabetic Ketoacidosis and GI Tract

Diabetic ketoacidosis (DKA) is commonly associated with gastrointestinal symptoms such as nausea, anorexia, and vomiting. At times, the abdominal presentations are severe and raise concerns about coexistent appendicitis or other causes of an acute abdomen. While surgical emergencies such as intestinal ischemia can rarely occur with the onset of diabetes mellitus,[17] clinicians should recognize that the symptoms can be solely due to the associated metabolic derangements, and they will resolve with correction of the acidosis.[18] The patient should be closely observed and correction of the metabolic disturbances undertaken prior to any invasive interventions.

Elevations of amylase may be present and raise concerns about pancreatitis. However, isoenzyme analysis often shows that the amylase is of salivary origin.[19] Marked dilatation of the stomach during DKA has been reported and resolves with nasogastric tube decompression.[20] Acute hypermagnesemia can also contribute to the dysmotility seen with DKA.[20] Upper gastrointestinal hemorrhage has also been reported, typically secondary to erosive esophagitis,[21] and responds to acid blockade therapy.

Diabetes and GI Neuropathy

Since the motility of the GI tract is dependent on the enteric nervous system, neuropathic changes can adversely affect function. Neuropathic changes within the GI tract of diabetics are typically thought to occur over prolonged periods of time with poor diabetic control. Accordingly, diabetic neuropathy among diabetic children is a rare event. However, studies of neuropathic changes, as documented by alteration in nerve conduction and parasympathetic nerve function

(R–R variations), have shown that 25% of children have evidence of low sensory nerve conduction and autonomic dysfunction at the time of diagnosis prior to achieving remission.[22] After 2 years of disease, deterioration in function was common with a correlation between nerve conduction and glycemic control.[22]

Studies in adults suggest that over 75% of diabetics have gastrointestinal symptoms related to neuropathy. Among this population many have documented motility abnormalities although such abnormalities correlate poorly with symptoms. Many explain this discordance as a possible underreporting of complaints, such as dysphagia or fullness.

The neuropathy associated with DM appears to be the result of altered sympathetic function and cholinergic denervation. Although there is damage to the vagus nerve resulting in vagal nerve dysfunction, most alterations are thought to be in the postganglionic nerves, sympathetic ganglia, and intramural adrenergic plexus. The sympathetic nerve dysfunction is particularly implicated in anal sphincter dysfunction. Others suggest that neurotransmitters (ie, an increase in vasoactive intestinal polypeptide [VIP]) are the etiology of such dysfunction.[20] One must also consider the effects of polypharmacy and electrolyte disturbances on nerve function.

Histologically nerves in patients with diabetic neuropathy can appear swollen with irregular processes, vacuolization, and there can be fragmentation of dendrites or Schwan cells.[23]

Diabetes and Nonspecific Abdominal Pain

Due to the altered intestinal motility associated with the autonomic neuropathy of longstanding diabetes, there has been an assumption that nonspecific abdominal pain is more common among patients with diabetes. Studies evaluating the prevalence of chronic dyspepsia and chronic constipation among diabetics are somewhat conflicting. Among children with diabetes one uncontrolled study indicated that the prevalence of gastroesophageal reflux disease (GERD) was 7%.[24] Those affected had poor linear growth, and more frequent hospital admissions. By contrast a larger study[25] of 118 children and adolescents with type 1 diabetes was unable to demonstrate a significant difference in the frequency of recurrent abdominal pain, chronic constipation, or chronic dyspepsia between those with diabetes and controls.

A study[26] of adult diabetics found no significant difference in the presence of upper and lower GI tract symptoms among 75 patients with type 1 diabetes compared to controls. However, among 68 patients with type 2 diabetes there is more constipation (22.1% vs 10.3%, $p < .05$) as well as nausea (11.8% vs 2.9%, $p < .5$). The difference among those with type 2 diabetes is not likely to be due to autonomic neuropathy as diabetes duration and glycemic control did not influence the frequency of symptoms. It seems more likely that these changes are due to an altered pathophysiology in obese patients, since obesity has been reported to result in increased amounts of GERD [27,28] and constipation.[29] A larger study by Xia and colleagues surveyed 429 diabetic patients (both type 1 [$n = 49$] and type 2 [$n = 380$]) and compared them to 170 controls. There was no difference in the percentage of patients with gastrointestinal complaints such as epigastric pain, bloating, distention, early satiety, heartburn, nausea, or vomiting between diabetics and the controls (51% vs 44.7%).[30]

It is unclear if pancreatic transplant can reverse preexisting intestinal damage. However in a study of 32 patients who underwent transplant, 24 of whom had gastrointestinal symptoms, almost all (96%) had fewer gastrointestinal complaints after transplant. One must be aware that with the transplant the patients had correction of multiple metabolic derangements so that the underlying etiology of the improvement is unclear.[31]

Diabetes and the Esophagus

Alterations in esophageal function in children with diabetes are rare. The majority of reported abnormalities described are limited to case reports including that of one child with a 4-year history of DM who presented with dysphagia and was found to have manometric features of a nutcracker esophagus.[32]

Although many adult patients with peripheral neuropathy secondary to DM have documented alterations in esophageal motility or gastric emptying, only 30% have clinical symptoms of chest pain, heartburn, or dysphagia. Motility disturbances documented by esophageal manometry reveal few alterations in upper esophageal sphincter function. However, the length of the esophagus can demonstrate a decrease in the amplitude of contractions, aperistaltic contractions, and prolonged contractions, as well as decreased lower esophageal sphincter tone.[20] A study of adults with type 2 diabetes showed that an aldose reductase inhibitor (which is effective in helping diabetic peripheral neuropathy) improved parameters related to GERD and esophageal motility.[33] Peristaltic alterations can result in a prolonged esophageal transit time. This, along with possible alterations in the immune system[34] can result in candida esophagitis in this population with resulting odynophagia.[35]

Adult patients with type 2 diabetes appear to be at risk for symptomatic GERD. Here there appears to be an association with body mass index, disease duration, and quality of diabetic control.[36] Studies suggesting similar associations in children are lacking.

Diabetes and the Stomach

Gastroparesis in DM was first described in 1945. Alterations in gastric emptying among pediatric diabetics are uncommon and mainly limited to case reports and small case series. Reid described 3 children, 1 to 7 years after the onset of diabetes with delayed gastric emptying and postprandial antral hypomotility.[37] Oduwole described an adolescent with severe gastroparesis that developed despite good glycemic control and a HbA1c of 7.4%, which normalized after 2 months of treatment with metoclopromide.[38]

Studies have documented delays in gastric emptying in up to 58% of adult diabetics. The onset of symptoms is typically insidious with early satiety, decreased weight, anorexia, postprandial nausea and vomiting, and epigastric distress. A sense of fullness or bloating correlate with a delay in gastric emptying, where as nausea and vomiting do not.[39] Physical examination may reveal a succession splash and gastric distention.

The gold standard of diagnosis is scintigraphy. The study should be done during a period of euglycemia, and preferably using solids. The development of scintigraphic breath tests[39] and the use of ultrasonographic measurements of gastric emptying[40] will likely be useful screening tools in the future. Alterations can be documented with a gastric emptying scan, and endoscopy or contrast radiography can rule out pathologic narrowing or obstruction.

The etiology of delayed gastric emptying appears to be due to vagal dysfunction. This dysfunction can be documented by a rise in serum gastrin and fall in acid secretion during sham feeding.[41] Nerve dysfunction may be related to the direct effect of hyperglycemia on nerves. For instance, experimentally neurons in the small intestines of rats have been proven to be responsive to glucose concentration.[42] In diabetics, as well as normal subjects who experience acute hyperglycemia with serum glucose concentrations above 200 mg/dL, one can observe a marked delay in gastric emptying.[43,44] Motility studies reveal a decrease in the frequency of migrating motor complexes in patients with gastroparesis. This may account for the observed increase in motilin in these patients, perhaps as a compensatory change. These changes are reversed with the use of prokinetics.[45] In diabetic mice interstitial cells of Cajal, which provide pacemaker activity for the stomach, are greatly depleted in the antrum. Accordingly, these mice have delayed gastric emptying.[46] However, such histologic changes have not been reported in humans. Animal studies have also implicated defects in nitric oxide mediated endothethium-dependent relaxation of blood vessels and subsequent free radical species formation resulting in defective nonadrenergic noncholinergic neurotransmission within the gastric fundus.[47]

Alteration in the fasting and fed pattern of these patients reveals that there are postcibal alterations in antral rhythm and poor receptive relaxation. Electrogastrography reveals alterations in the normal 3 cpm electrical pace of the stomach such that one sees bradyrhythmias (1 to 2.5 cpm) and tachyrhythmias (3.7 to 10 cpm). Also, the perception of normal patients with nausea, fullness, and distention is more intense with increased levels of serum glucose.[39] Delaying emptying of a solid in the fasting state can contribute to bezoar formation.[20] In the postprandial state, antral contractions are decreased in number and amplitude. In addition, the pylorus exhibits prolonged high-amplitude contractions.[20] Delayed gastric emptying in the postprandial state may result in hypoglycemia in insulin treated patients.[48]

Treatment of these motor disorders begins with better glycemic control. Dietary changes, with the introduction of smaller more frequent meals and liquid supplements can be beneficial. In addition, patients should be advised to consume diets with low amounts of residue so as to avoid bezoar formation.[20] Alternative treatments include gastric pacemakers and *Clostidium botulinum* toxin injection into the pylorus to improve gastric emptying.[49]

Pharmacotherapy is also helpful as adjunctive therapy. Antiemetics do not appear to help to any great degree. Prokinetics coordinate pyloric relaxation and duodenal peristalsis with smooth muscle contraction in the stomach thus promoting improved gastric emptying.[50,51] Erythromycin which stimulates the motilin receptor,[52] has had some effect although some patients develop tachyphylaxis to the drug. A study in DM children with dyspepsia and delayed gastric emptying revealed that domperidone is superior to cisapride in reversing delayed gastric emptying and relieving clinical symptoms.[53] In diabetic mice tegaserod, a 5-HT receptor agonist, improved gastric emptying.[54] Intravenous ghrelin has also been shown to enhance gastric emptying in insulin dependant diabetic humans,[55] which may relate to histologic evidence of decreased numbers of ghrelin cell density in the GI tracts of animal models of diabetes.[56] Rarely, recalcitrant patients require parenteral nutrition or transpyloric enteral tube feeding.

Other gastric alterations that have been described in DM include hemorrhagic gastritis, acute and chronic gastritis, atrophic gastritis, and pernicious anemia. The incidence of pernicious anemia among diabetics is 10.5/1,000 vs 2/1,000 in the general population.[20] Peptic ulcers among diabetics appear to occur at a lower rate compared to the general population. It is hypothesized that this is due to the increase in glucagon in response to the hyperglycemia, which subsequently decreases the production of gastric acid.[20]

Diabetes and *Helicobacter pylori*

Simon and colleagues were the first to suggest that *Helicobacter pylori* infection is more prevalent among patients with DM.[57] Some have hypothesized that the immune dysregulation associated with DM, coupled with the autonomic neuropathy that can lead to gastroparesis, place diabetics at increased risk for *H. pylori* infection. However, a large study by Xia, including 429 patients with DM, found no difference in the incidence of *H. pylori* infection between the diabetic patients and controls (32.9% vs 31.7%).[30] Smaller studies of children with diabetes also found no difference in the overall rate of infection between the diabetics and controls.[58]

A study by Jones and colleagues[59] comparing diabetic adults with *H. pylori* infection and those without found no difference in the number with gastrointestinal symptoms, rate of gastric emptying, glycemic control, or autonomic function. Indeed, the overall rate of infection with *H. pylori* was identical to the population without diabetes indicating that DM is not a risk factor for infection. A study in Bangladesh of 520 DM patients came to the same conclusion.[60] This is in contrast to other studies, which report that DM patients with *H. pylori* have slower gastric emptying [61] or increased numbers of upper gastrointestinal symptoms and subsequent improvement after eradication of the infection.[62,63]

It has been suggested that eradication of *H. pylori* among those with diabetes can result in better glycemic control; however, the evidence for such a change is weak. The proposed mechanism of this improvement is based on the ability of *H. pylori* to cause an increase in the production of various cytokines including tumor necrosis factor alpha, interferon gamma, and interleukins 1, 6, and 8, respectively.[64] In such studies Begue found no change in insulin requirements over the 2 years after eradication of *H. pylori*, but there was a modest decrease (2%) in the children's hemoglobin A1c levels .[65] This is similar to other pediatric studies, which found no difference in glycemic control after *H. pylori* eradication.[25,66]

Diabetes and Autoimmune Gastritis

Fifteen to twenty percent of DM patients have parietal cell antibodies (PCA) compared to 2 to 10% of nondiabetic patients.[67,68] Thus, diabetic patients account for 20 to 40% of all PCA-positive patients. Such antibodies target the gastric proton pump (H/K ATPase) and are a serologic marker for autoimmune atrophic gastritis. This, in turn, is associated with iron deficiency anemia, pernicious anemia, and may predispose to gastric cancer and carcinoid tumors. A study of 229 diabetic patients[69] found 69 to be PCA-positive. The presence of PCA was associated with HLA-DQA1*0501-B1*0301. In those patients with PCA there is a higher prevalence of iron deficiency anemia, pernicious anemia, autoimmune gastritis, and hypochlorhydria. Signs of preatrophic gastritis are also more common and documented by histologic features including pronounced lymphocytic infiltration in the corpus mucosa and parietal atrophy of oxyntic glands. The presence of concomitant *H. pylori* infection does not represent a separate risk factor for these findings.[69] Similar studies in pediatric patients with DM are lacking.

Diabetes and Small Bowel Motility

Like other portions of the gut, small intestinal motility can be affected by the neuropathic changes of long-standing DM. Delayed intestinal transit can be seen in up to 33% of diabetics, as demonstrated by breath hydrogen test.[70] This is due to decreases in the amplitude of contractions as well as alterations in migrating motor complexes. Limited evidence suggests that in a select group of patients with delayed small bowel transit and bacterial overgrowth, eradication of the bacterial overgrowth can improve orocecal transit time.[71]

Diabetes and Celiac Disease

In 1969, Walker-Smith described an 8-year-old with DM who developed celiac disease (CD).[72] Celiac disease is associated with HLA DQ2 and DQ8, while diabetes is also linked to the same DQ2 molecule.[73] In diabetes it is the DQ molecule that influences the selection and binding to autoantigenic peptides.[73] The prevalence of CD in DM is 10 to 30 times the general population, with an incidence of 2 to 8.5%. The wide variation is based on how CD is defined, where using clinical symptoms and histology the incidence is at the lower end, 2%. If, however, seropositivity is the defining characteristic then the incidence is 8 to 9%.[74] Among children of type 1 diabetics, 3.5% have CD.[75] CD does not appear to be increased among patients with type 2 diabetes.[75]

A meta-analysis of 20 studies evaluating the incidence of a dual diagnosis of CD and DM found rates in children between 1 in 6 (16.4%) and 1 in 103 (0.97%).[74] If one excludes the study from Algeria, which accounted for the highest prevalence, the remainder of the studies reported prevalence between 0.97 and 6.2%. In adults, a meta-analysis of 10 studies revealed rates ranging from 1 in 16 (6.4%) to 1 in 76 (1.3%)[74]

A large study by Pocecco and Ventura[73] evaluated 4,500 type I diabetics and found two subgroups of patients. The first group included those with type I DM who were later found to have "silent CD," this represented 88% of the dual-diagnosis cases. The second group was those with prediagnosed CD who were later found to have type I DM, representing 12% of the cases. Group 1 had minimal gastrointestinal symptoms and was diagnosed with CD between 11 and 17 years of age. Group 2, however, experienced numerous gastrointestinal symptoms and was diagnosed with CD at younger ages (between 6 and 10 years). It is thought that the later age in which CD was diagnosed among the group 1 patients was due to the minimal gastrointestinal symptoms they exhibited. Indeed in some studies short stature is the only sign, accounting for up to 33% of the patients.[74] Maki[76] screened 238 DM patients with IgA antireticulin antibodies (ARA) and 16 were positive. However, of these 11 were negative at first screening. CD was confirmed in nine with typical changes on small bowel histology. Of note, two children had negative ARA and normal small intestinal biopsy at the time of DM diagnosis. One then developed rising ARA titers and after 2 years had flat villi on biopsy. The other child had a positive ARA, but after 8 years villi were still normal even though there were increased numbers of intraepithelial lymphocytes.[76] The North American Society for Pediatric Gastroenterology, Hepatology and Nutrition suggests screening all children with type I diabetes using antitissue transglutaminases IgA antibodies.[77] Others have suggesting using serum testing for both serum antiendomysial IgA antibodies and antiendomysial IgG1 antibodies to improve the screening sensitivity among diabetic patients.[78]

If the patient had clinical symptoms of CD then the gluten free diet typically results in improved diabetic control.[74] However, in those patients that were diagnosed by routine screening alone studies are varied with some revealing no improvement in glycemic control, while others show better control or fewer hypoglycemic events.[74]

Similarities in peptide sequences can result in a cross-reaction of epitopes at the T-cell level. However, it is unclear whether such similarities exist between gliadin and tissue transglutaminase (tTG) and glutamic acid decarboxylase (GAD) or insulin. If such cross-reactivity does exist then the coexistence of DM and CD can be explained by "molecular mimicry."[73] A study of nonobese diabetic rats provided regular chow versus a gluten-free diet for 320 days decreased the incidence of type 1 diabetes from 64 to 15%.[79]

Diabetes and the Liver

The most common cause of elevated transaminase levels or hepatomegaly among patients with diabetes is steatosis. This is the result of deposition of large, macronodular fat droplets within the parenchyma of the liver. When the fat deposition is associated with an inflammatory infiltrate one can make a histologic diagnosis of nonalcoholic steatohepatitis (NASH) which in some instances can progress to fibrosis and cirrhosis.[80] The predominant lipid deposited is the triglyceride, but fatty acids also contribute to the toxic effects. The accumulation is the result of fatty acids brought to the liver at a rate greater than the liver can either metabolize the fatty acid or secrete VLDL. Furthermore the increase in liver size can be secondary to increased glycogen stores.[81] Overall, fatty liver is diagnosed in 4.5 to 17% of type 1 diabetics. It typically reflects poor glycemic control, and resolves with better control of the diabetes. In type 2 diabetics the incidence of fatty liver is 45%. This suggests that the increase in incidence among type 2 diabetics is likely secondary to obesity rather than the diabetes itself. However, some studies suggest that histologic evidence of steatosis is even more common than appreciated by transaminase elevation or imaging alone. For example, one study of 68 insulin treated children found evidence of increased glycogen in the cytoplasm and nucleus of hepatocytes in 58%.[82]

A distinct entity of glycogenic hepatopathy has also been reported in diabetics. This is characterized by a pathologic overloading of hepatocytes with glycogen and is associated with poorly controlled diabetes. Clinically patients have hepatomegaly, abdominal pain, and elevated transaminases (range 50 to 1,600 IU/L). Histologically steatosis and fibrosis are typically absent.[83]

Imaging of the liver with CT or ultrasound can be helpful in identifying the respective enhancement or echogenicity associated with fatty liver. The degree of transaminase elevation does not correlate to the degree of liver injury. Treatments include weight loss, better glycemic control, and, possibly, vitamin E supplementation.[84] Rapid weight loss can be detrimental and it is, therefore, suggested that the loss be no faster than 1.6kg/wk.

Mauriac syndrome refers to hepatomegaly associated with increased glycogen stores, hypoglycemia, dwarfism, and a Cushingoid appearance.[85] Previously, it was described in patients classified as brittle diabetics. This is less frequently seen due to advances in insulin preparations and glucose monitoring. The disease results from increased serum glucose leading to moderate hepatic glycogen accumulation, which subsequently inactivates glycogen phosphorylase. This inactivation leads to an inhibition of glycogenolysis and increased glycogen synthase and subsequent increase in glycogen stores. Treatment with insulin results in continued activation of glycogen synthase and further glycogen accumulation. Hypercortisolism is thought to be responsible for the growth retardation and delayed puberty. Better glycemic control results in resolution of the syndrome.

Among diabetics receiving peritoneal dialysis with added insulin there is a risk of developing subcapsular fatty changes.[81] Also, hepatocellular carcinoma is twice as prevalent in diabetic patients.[20] It has also been suggested that Hepatitis C infection is more common in diabetic patients, and that this may be unrelated to the use of needles.[86]

Diabetes and Biliary Function

An increase in the frequency of cholecystitis and cholelithiasis is seen in adult diabetics with the risk of cholelithiasis being twice that of the general population.[20] These increases in prevalence are thought to be secondary to decreased motility and a lithogenic bile composition.[20] Evidence suggests that diabetics with stones may have decreased gene expression of CCK-A receptor within the smooth muscle of the gallbladder accounting for the hypomotility.[87] Despite these increases in risk, the routine practice of cholecystectomy among diabetics has fallen out of favor.

A study of 20 diabetic children found that the fasting gallbladder volume in these children was greater than in controls. However, there was no difference in ejection fraction or maximal contraction between the two groups.[88] It is questioned whether the dilation of the gallbladder heralds future autonomic neuropathy and an increased risk for gallstone formation. In addition, there is an increased risk of ascending cholangitis. Reports of organisms, such as Yersinea enterocolitica,[89] have been found to rarely be causative.

Diabetes and the Exocrine Pancreas

Thirty percent of adult diabetics have decreased exocrine pancreatic secretion although this is typically not associated with clinical symptoms. The decrease is likely due to glucagon excess, malnutrition, vagal nerve dysfunction, and a decrease in insulin effects. A study of 94 children and adolescents with type 1 diabetes found 35% to have mild exocrine pancreatic insufficiency, while 10% had severe pancreatic insufficiency as determined by stool elastase and fecal fat excretion.

No significant affect of pancreatic insufficiency was seen on patient's height, weight, or diabetes status.[90] Among those diabetics who consume alcohol, there is a two-to-four-fold risk of adenocarcinoma of the pancreas compared with the general adult population.[20]

Diabetic Diarrhea

Diabetic associated diarrhea can occur in up to 20% of patients with DM. It is typically worse at night and more common among males. The etiology is likely multifactorial and can be associated with rapid intestinal transit or a defect in adrenergic stimulation of colonic water reabsorption. One should consider confounding causes such as drugs, including sorbitol found in sugar free foods,[91] and small bowel bacterial overgrowth.[92] Some studies suggest that clonidine can aid in increasing water reabsorption. Octreotide has also been used to decrease the diarrhea.[23] Among those with diarrhea 40% suffer from fecal incontinence. This is hypothesized to be secondary to decreased anal sphincter tone and decreased sensation to rectal distention. Although diarrhea is a relatively common complaint among young diabetics, the disabling form of autonomic diabetic diarrhea rarely begins before middle age. One should thus consider other causes, including those confounders mentioned above, routine enteric infections and celiac disease in DM children with persistent diarrhea.

Maternally Inherited Diabetes and Deafness

First described in 1992 by Ballinger and colleagues maternally inherited diabetes and deafness (MIDD, MIM # 520000) appears to be the result of a mutation in the mitochondrial tRNA (Leu-UUR) gene. Gastrointestinal symptoms in these patients appear to be common, especially among those with the 3,243 mutations. Narbonne and colleagues[93] studied 10 patients with MIDD 88% had constipation, diarrhea, or both, as compared to 28% of matched controls with diabetes type 1. Among those studied one patient had fatal intestinal pseudo-obstruction.

Neonatal Diabetes with Hypoplastic Pancreas, Intestinal Atresia, and Gallbladder Hypoplasia

Five infants have been described with neonatal diabetes, hypoplastic or annular pancreas, jejunal atresia, duodenal atresia, and gallbladder aplasia or hypoplasia. One patient with a mild form is surviving free of insulin, while the other died in the first year of life. Pancreatic immunohistochemistry revealed complete absence of insulin, glucagons, and somatostatin. Exocrine histology was variable. The inheritance appears to be autosomal recessive.[94]

AUTOIMMUNE POLYGLANDULAR SYNDROME

Autoimmune polyglandular syndrome type I (MIM #240300), also known as autoimmune polyendocrinopathy-candidiasis-ectodermal

dystrophy (APECED) is typically an autosomal recessive disease. The disease is characterized by the combination of:

1. failure of parathyroid, adrenal cortex, gonads, beta cells, parietal cells, thyroid, and/or hepatitis
2. chronic mucocutaneous candidiasis
3. dystrophy of dental enamel, nails, alopecia, vitiligo, and/or keratopathy[95]

Patients are typically of Iranian, Jewish, Finnish, or Scandinavian descent.[96] A multicenter review of patients with chronic mucocutaneous candidiasis demonstrated that 50% later developed disease components typical of autoimmune polyglandular syndrome.[97] Finland has published the largest cohort of these patients[95] encompassing a group of 68 patients, with a mean follow up of 11.2 years between 1910 and 1988. Due to a founder effect, one major mutation accounts for approximately 90% of these cases. Linkage studies identified a gene at 21q22.3. This gene, likely a transcription regulator, has been cloned and named autoimmune regulator 1 (AIRE-1).[96,98] The AIRE protein has been found in numerous tissues including thymus, ovary, lung, testis, kidney, adrenal gland, spleen, lymph nodes, and bone marrow.[98]

Within the Finnish group,[95] the number of endocrine organs involved varied between one and eight, with most having four. Hypoparathyroidism is the most common (79%) and was diagnosed between 19 months and 44 years of age. Adrenocortical failure is second at 72%, being diagnosed between 4.2 and 41 years. Cortisol and aldosterone deficiency occur at the same time in 38/49 patients. Gonadal failure occurs in 60% of the females and 14% of males, all by age 30 years. Diabetes is diagnosed in 12% and vitamin B12 deficiency in 13%. Rarely patients have been documented to have coexistent celiac disease,[99] or intestinal lymphangiectasia.[100]

The majority of patients (78%) have documented nonendocrine manifestations prior to the first endocrinopathy. In 60% of cases this includes oral candidiasis, 9% malabsorption, 4% keratopathy, and 1 case of hepatitis. Endocrine problems arose at mean ages of 8.7 years for the first, 13.3 years for the second, and 16 years for the third. In those patients with adrenal failure as their first endocrinopathy, they had fewer additional organs involved. However, those patients with malabsorption or keratopathy as their first manifestation often had five subsequent organs involved.

All patients have oral candidiasis, the onset of which varied between 1 month and 21 years. Nail involvement is seen in 71% and dermal involvement, typically the hands and face, in 9%. Four patients have had documented esophageal candidiasis, one with a stricture. However, an additional 11 patients had retrosternal pain that resolved with antifungal treatment. Malabsorption was documented in 18% at a time 4 months to 21 years from onset of disease. All but one of these patients had decreased parathyroid function, and decreased serum calcium appeared to correlate with the malabsorption. Of the 43 patients evaluated 33 had evidence of dental enamel hypoplasia, unrelated to hypoparathyroid status. Patients also appear to be at a greater risk for developing carcinoma of the oral mucosa, likely due to the chronic candidiasis.

Overall, autoimmune hepatitis appears to a component of the disease in 10 to 18%.[95] Indeed, there are reports in which a sudden onset of hepatitis resulted in death. The first hepatic autoantigen in these patients was identified as cytochrome P450 1A2.[101] A second autoantigen was identified as aromatic-L-amino acid decarboxylase (AADC).[102] This enzyme, active in the biosynthesis of neurotransmitters, is expressed in the cytosol and was originally described as a beta-cell autoantigen. Among the Finnish cohort 50% of those tested had AADC autoantibodies. However, up to 92% of autoimmune polyglandular syndrome type I patients with vitiligo and autoimmune hepatitis had such antibodies.[96]

HYPERPARATHYROIDISM

Primary hyperparathyroidism (PHPT) is a rare condition in childhood, and often goes undiagnosed. The disease is identified in those patients with hypercalcemia, low-normal phosphate level, and elevated parathyroid hormone (PTH). Since its initial description in 1939, approximately 100 cases have been reported among children and adolescents less than 16 years. The etiology of the disease is similar to the adults, with sporadic adenomas being causative. Rarely the hyperparathyroidism is a manifestation of a systemic disease such as MEN types 1 or 2. Fewer than 40 neonatal cases have been reported. Here the etiology involves hyperplasia of the parathyroid chief cells. The clinical manifestations of hypercalcemia include muscle weakness, paralysis, and hyporeflexia. Gastrointestinal symptoms (Table 2) may be absent or nonspecific including fatigue, poor appetite, weight loss, abdominal pain, nausea, constipation, peptic ulcer disease, and vomiting.[103] A case report of an adolescent with hyperparathyroidism revealed that hypercalcemia was the etiology of his acute pancreatitis.[104] Abdominal symptoms appear to be seen more frequently among children affected by PHPT than adults, 8% vs 1% respectively.[105] Nephrocalcinosis has been described in 30 to 70% of PHPT children. Severe pancreatitis immediately following parathyroidectomy for PHPT may occur in as many as 3% of patients.[10]

Table 3 Effects of Hypothyroidism on the Gastrointestinal System

Abnormality/Association	Gastrointestinal Manifestation
Altered colonic function/transit	Constipation, pseudo-obstruction
Impaired esophageal motility	Reflux esophagitis
Liver test abnormalities	Normal histology, prolonged neonatal jaundice
Celiac disease	Diarrhea, steatorrhea

Adapted from Weber, Ryan.[113]

HYPOPARATHYROIDISM

Hypoparathyroidism among children is rare, although it can be a part of other systemic syndromes such as autoimmune polyglandular syndrome, Pearson marrow pancreas syndrome, and DiGeorge syndrome. Biochemically there is hypocalcemia, hyperphosphatemia, and decreased parathyroid hormone levels. The clinical manifestations of hypocalcemia predominate and result in neuromuscular instability with seizure, tetany, paraesthesias, laryngospasm, bronchospasm, or prolonged QTc. Idiopathic hypoparathyroidism is also associated with malabsorption, pernicious anemia, and Addison's disease. Indeed, approximately 11% of those with decreased parathyroid function have chronic diarrhea or steatorrhea.[107]

The mechanisms by which parathormone is involved in intestinal absorption is unknown, but symptoms of malabsorption may be the earliest sign of hypoparathyroidism. The diarrhea typically ceases with vitamin D therapy.[107] It has been noted that magnesium deficiency must be ruled out in patients who present with malabsorption and findings of hypoparathyroidism as functional hypoparathyroidism occurs in patients with severe and prolonged hypomagnesemia.[108] Intestinal lymphangiectasia with protein-losing enteropathy also has been reported in association with malabsorption and hypoparathyroidism.[109]

Gastrointestinal problems similar to, but less severe than those found in hypoparathyroidism, are found in pseudohypoparathyroidism, but plasma parathyroid hormone levels are high.

HYPOTHYROIDISM

Hypothyroidism is defined as a state in which the thyroid gland fails to secrete sufficient quantities of thyroid hormone. Congenital hypothyroidism has been associated with gastrointestinal manifestations (Table 3) including constipation, feeding difficulties, and prolonged neonatal jaundice. The frequency of celiac disease in patients with

autoimmune thyroid disease is 4.3% compared to nonautoimmune hypothyroid controls of 0.4%.[73] The association is likely due to a common genetic predisposition, namely the DQ2 allele.

Among hypothyroid adults studies show that affected patients have an average of 3 bowel movements a week (range of 1 to 7/wk).[110] Studies to determine the pathophysiologic basis of the constipation include anorectal manometry studies, which reveal that hypothyroid individuals have normal maximal resting and squeeze pressures. However, sensation threshold for impending evacuation greater than controls. There is no change in whole gut transit time.[110] Gastric myoelectrical activity in hypothyroid individuals has been measured by EGG and abnormal slow wave activity correlates with clinical complaints of dyspepsia.[111] Although there is evidence of increased VIP expression from the anterior pituitary of hypothyroid rats, it is unlikely these changes play a pathophysiological role in gastrointestinal disorders seen with hypothyroidism.[112]

Myxedema has also been associated with decreased esophageal peristalsis and impaired lower esophageal sphincter function resulting in reflux esophagitis. Hypothyroidism can also cause severe gastric hypomotility and secondary pseudo-obstruction.[113]

Studies of hypothyroid murine models reveal that hypothyroidism decreases the DNA and protein content of the intestinal mucosa. Villi in the jejunum appear shorter as does crypt depth. In addition, hypothyroidism decreases the rates of glucose and glutamine utilization by epithelial cells of the small intestine and colon.[114]

Liver transaminases are mildly abnormal in 50% of hypothyroid patients, however liver histology is typically normal.[115] Hypothyroidism can cause exudative ascites in the absence of overt liver disease.[113] Rarely, one can have associated chronic active hepatitis, diabetes mellitus, or Cronkhite–Canada syndrome. Hashimoto's thyroiditis has also been associated with ulcerative colitis.[113]

HYPERTHYROIDISM

Hyperthyroidism occurs when excessive amounts of circulating thyroid hormone are present. Hyperthyroidism (Table 4) has been associated with diarrhea, with some studies showing that such individuals pass an average of 14 bowel movements per week (range 7 to 21/wk).[24] Attempts at discerning the etiology of the diarrhea include anorectal manometry studies which reveal that hyperthyroid individuals have a lower maximal

Table 2 Effects of Hyperparathyroidism on the Gastrointestinal System

Abnormality/Association	Gastrointestinal Manifestation
Increased serum calcium	Constipation, nausea, vomiting
Peptic ulceration	Bleeding, abdominal pain, perforation
Pancreatitis	Acute pancreatitis
MEN-1	Gastrinoma, VIPoma

Adapted from Weber, Ryan.[113]

Table 4 Effects of Hyperthyroidism on the Gastrointestinal System

Abnormality/Association	Gastrointestinal Manifestation
Accelerated intestinal transit	Diarrhea
Myopathy of the upper esophagus	Dysphagia
Liver test abnormalities	Minor histologic changes
Ulcerative colitis	Bloody diarrhea

Adapted from Weber, Ryan.[113]

resting pressure and maximal squeeze pressure compared to controls.[110] In addition, they have a lower threshold sensation for impending evacuation.[110]

Studies of intestinal motility reveal no difference in gastric emptying between controls and hyperthyroid adults. However, hyperthyroid individuals have accelerated small bowel and colonic transit. Small bowel transit time appears to be inversely related to T3 concentrations.[116] Gastric myoelectrical activity in hyperthyroid individuals has been measured by EGG a high percentage of postprandial tachygastria was demonstrate.[111] Furthermore, increased small intestinal myoelectric activity has been reported.[117] This presumably accounts for the gastrointestinal symptoms and diarrhea exhibited by hyperthyroid individuals. However, there is also evidence for a secretory component to the diarrhea as thyroid hormone can cause increased intestinal secretion via an increase in intracellular levels of cyclic AMP.[113] Changes in intestinal transit appear to normalize once patients are rendered euthyroid.[118]

Hyperthyroidism may cause myopathy, resulting in dysfunction of the striated muscles of the pharynx and proximal esophagus. Decreased propulsive force of the muscles and abnormal closure of the upper esophageal sphincter can result in dysphagia and aspiration. Esophageal peristalsis in increased in thyrotoxic patients.[113]

Appreciation of the gastrointestinal disturbances in thyroid disease is often overshadowed by other organ dysfunction including cardiovascular, neuromuscular, and ocular systems. Of note, Grave's disease is associated with ulcerative colitis.[113] Also, hyperthyroidism is associated with minor histologic changes in the liver. One can detect mildly elevated transaminases in approximately 33% of patients, and 5% have an unconjugated hyperbilirubinemia.[113]

PITUITARY HORMONES

Pituitary hormones have important effects on the gut. Adrenocorticotropic hormone stimulates cortisol secretion and enhances brush–border enzyme activity, and thyrotropin stimulating hormone causes thyroxin secretion with major effects on gut motility.[119] Growth hormone causes intestinal villus growth and enhances absorption.[120] Infants with intrauterine hypopituitarism may present at birth with hypoglycemia, prolonged jaundice,[121] and in males, micropenis and undescended testes. Excessive secretion of pituitary growth hormone results in acromegaly,

which is associated with an increased incidence of adenomatous colonic polyps and cancers of the colon and stomach.[113]

An association between liver disease and hypopituitarism in children and adults has been described.[122–124] Patients with hypopituitarism develop a phenotype similar to metabolic syndrome with central obesity and diabetes. Adams and colleagues[122] described 21 such patients with associated nonalcoholic fatty liver disease (NAFLD). The NAFLD was diagnosed and average of 6.4 years after pituitary dysfunction. The majority had associated dyslipidemia and elevated glucose levels. Of the ten that underwent liver biopsy six had cirrhosis, two had nonalcoholic steatohepatitis with fibrosis, and two had simple steatosis. Long-term follow-up revealed two undergoing liver transplant, and six liver related deaths. One teenager had rapid recurrence of the NAFLD after successful transplantation.[124]

HYPOADRENOCORTICISM

The adrenal cortex secretes glucocorticoids and mineralocorticoids. Glucocorticoids bind to specific cytoplasmic receptors on the enterocyte, and the activated receptor-steroid complex is translocated to the nucleus where it triggers the synthesis of mRNA. The net effect is to increase the absorptive capacity of the small intestine and enhance brush–border membrane digestive capacity without increasing the number of cells.[125] The dominant gastrointestinal effect of adrenal gland disorders is related to abnormalities of aldosterone metabolism. Although the effect of increased aldosterone production in increasing sodium absorption in the colon is overshadowed by its effect on the kidney, lack of aldosterone production and end-organ failure to respond to aldosterone are often associated with marked intestinal salt wasting in addition to urinary losses.[126] Thus, in salt-losing states associated with hyperadrenocorticism, the intestinal losses contribute to dehydration.

Some patients with Addison's disease have steatorrhea with normal jejunal histology,[127] which resolves with hormone replacement. Gastrointestinal symptoms can include anorexia, weight loss, vomiting, and abdominal pain. There is a high incidence of associated anomalies in children with Addison's disease including autoimmune polyglandular syndrome, adrenoleukodystrophy, and AAA syndrome (Addison's, achalasia, and alacrimation).

DIENCEPHALIC SYNDROME

Diencephalic syndrome is a complex of signs and symptoms related to hypothalamic dysfunction. The association between brain tumors of the anterior hypothalamus and severe failure to thrive is almost exclusively seen in infants and young children, with 85% occurring at ages less than 2 years.[128] Most patients have space occupying lesions in the region of the optic chiasm, typically a low grade, slow growing, glioma, or a juvenile pilocytic astrocytoma.

Three major features include failure to thrive in spite of normal energy intake, motor hyperactivity, and apparent euphoria. Autonomic disturbances include skin pallor, profuse sweating, and erratic temperature control. Rotary nystagmus may be the only neurologic sign.[128]

At the time of diagnosis, length is typically maintained and head circumference is normal, except in the 33 to 58% with hydrocephalus. Classically vomiting occurs in 68% of affected patients [128] although one series reports an incidence of only 36%.[129] The etiology of the extreme loss of subcutaneous fatty tissue is unclear. Some suspect increased lipolysis secondary to elevated growth hormone excretion, while others feel it is the effect of the tumor on the satiety center.[128,129] There is some evidence that these patients have a 30 to 50% increase in resting energy expenditure.[130] Optimal treatment involves complete tumor resection, although this is not always possible. Chemotherapy and radiation have also proven effective.

REFERENCES

1. Plotnick LP. Type 1 (insulin-dependent) diabetes mellitus. In: McMillan JA, DeAngelis CD, Feigin RD, Warshaw JB, editors. Oski's Pediatrics: Principles and Practice. New York: Lippincott, Williams &Wilkins; 1999. p. 1793–1803.
2. Falchuk KR, Conlin D. The intestinal and liver complications of diabetes mellitus. Adv Intern Med 1993;38:269–86.
3. Coetzee EJ, Levitt NS. Maternal diabetes and neonatal outcome. Semin Neonatol 2000;5:221–9.
4. Schwartz R, Teramo KA. Effects of diabetic pregnancy on the fetus and newborn. Semin Perinatol 2000;24:120–35.
5. Langer O, Levy J, Brustman L, et al. Glycemic control in gestational diabetes. How tight is tight enough? Small for gestational age versus large for gestational age? Am J Obstet Gynecol 1989;161:646–53.
6. Evers I, Nikkels P, Sikkema J, Visser G. Placental pathology in women with type 1 diabetes and in a control group with normal and large-for-gestational-age infants. Placenta 2003;24:819–25.
7. Schwartz R, Gruppuso PA, Petzold K, et al. Hyperinsulinemia and microsomia in the fetus of the diabetic mother. Diabetes Care 1994;17:640–8.
8. Tapanainen P, Leinonen E, Ruokonen A, Knip M. Leptin concentrations are elevated in newborn infants of diabetic mothers. Horm Res 2001;55:185–90.
9. Evers I, Valk Hd, Mol B, et al. Macrosomia despite good glycaemic control in Type I diabetic pregnancy; results of a nationwide study in The Netherlands. Diabetologia 2002;45:1484–9.
10. Vohr BR, McGarvey ST, Tucker R. Effects of maternal gestational diabetes on offspring adiposity at 4–7 years of age. Diabetes Care 1999;22:1284–91.
11. Tanir H, Sener T, Gurer H, Kaya M. A ten-year gestational diabetes mellitus cohort at a university clinic of the mid-Anatolian region of Turkey. Clin Exp Obstet Gynecol 2005;32:241–4.
12. Stevenson DK. Bilirubin metabolism in the infant of the diabetic mother: An overview. In: Gabbe SG, Oh W, editors. Report of the 93rd Ross Conference on Pediatric Research. Columbus, 1987:109–117.

13. Davis WS, Allen RP, Favara BE, Slovis TL. Neonatal small left colon syndrome. Am J Roentgenol Radium Ther Nucl Med 1974;120:322–9.
14. Rangecroft L. Neonatal small left colon syndrome. Arch Dis Childhood 1979;54:635–47.
15. Cohen M. Infants of diabetic mothers and neonatal small left colon. Am J Med Genet A 2003;122:301–2.
16. Berdon W, Slovis T, Campbell J, et al. Neonatal small left colon syndrome: Its relationship to aganglionosis and meconium plug syndrome. Radiology 1977;125:457–62.
17. DiMeglio L, Chaet M, Quigley C, Grosfeld J. Massive ischemic intestinal necrosis at the onset of diabetes mellitus with ketoacidosis in a three-year-old girl. J Pediatr Surg 2003;38:1537–9.
18. Umpierrez G, Freire A. Abdominal pain in patients with hyperglycemic crises. J Crit Care 2002;17:63–7.
19. Kwarshaw AL, Feller ER, Lee KH. On the cause of raised serum amylase in diabetic ketoacidosis. Lancet 1977:929–30.
20. Verne GN, Sninsky CA. Diabetes and the gastrointestinal tract. Gastroenterol Clin North Amer 1998;27:861–74.
21. Faigel DO, Metz DC. Prevelence, etiology, and prognostic significance of upper gastrointestinal hemorrhage in diabetic ketoacidosis. Dig Dis Sci 1996;41:1–8.
22. Solders G, Thalme B, Aguirre-Aquino M, et al. Nerve conduction and autonomic nerve function in diabteic children. A 10-year follow-up study. Acta Paediatr 1997;86:361–6.
23. Camilleri M. Gastrointestinal problems in diabetes. Endocr Metab Clinics North Amer 1996;25:361–78.
24. Burghen GA, Murrell LR, Whitington GL, et al. Acid peptic disease in children with type 1 diabetes mellitus. A complicating relationship. Am J Dis Child 1992;146:718–22.
25. Vazeou A, Papadopoulou A, Booth IW, Bartsocas CS. Prevalence of gastrointestinal symptoms in children and adolescents with type 1 diabetes. Diabetes Care 2001;24:962–4.
26. Enck P, Rathmann W., Spiekermann M, et al. Prevalence of gastrointestinal symptoms in diabetic patients and non-diabetic patients. Z Gastroenterol 1994;32:637–41.
27. Fisher BL, Pennathur A, Mutnick JL, Little AG. Obesity correlates with gastroesophageal reflux. Dig Dis Sci 1999;44:2290–4.
28. Ruhl CE, Everhart JE. Overweight, but not high dietary fat intake, increases risk of gastroesophageal reflux disease hospitalization: The NHANES I Epidemilogic Follow-Up Study. First National Health and Nutrition Examination Survey. Ann Epidemiol 1999;9:424–35.
29. Pecora P, Suraci C, Antonelli M, et al. Constipation and obesity: A statistical analysis. Boll Soc Biol Sper 1981;57:2384–8.
30. Xia HHX, Talley NJ, Kam EPY, et al. *Helicobacter pylori* infection is not associated with diabetes mellitus, nor with upper gastrointestinal symptoms in diabetes mellitus. Am J Gastroenterol 2001;96:1039–46.
31. Zehr PS, Milde FK, Hart LK, Corry RJ. Pancreas transplantation: Assessing secondary complications and life quality. Diabetologia 1991;34: S138–40.
32. Solzi GF, DiLorenzo C. Nutcracker esophagus in a child with insulin-dependent diabetes mellitus. J Pediatr Gastroenterol Nutr 1999;29:482–484.
33. Kinekawa F, Kubo F, Matsuda K, et al. Effect of an aldose reductase inhibitor on esophageal dysfunction in diabetic patients. Hepatogastroenterology 2005;52:471–4.
34. Moutschen MP, Scheen AJ, Lefebvre PJ. Impaired immune responses in diabetes mellitus: Analysis of the factors and mechanisms involved. Relevance to the increased susceptibility of diabetic patients to specific infections. Diabetes Metab 1992;18:187–201.
35. Parkman HP, Schwartz SS. Esophagitis and gastroduodenal disorders associated with diabetic gastroparesis. Arch Intern Med 1987;147:1477–80.
36. Nishida T, Tsuji S, Tsujii M, et al. Gastroesophageal reflux disease related to diabetes: Analysis of 241 cases with type 2 diabetes mellitus. J Gastroenterol Hepatol 2004;19:258–65.
37. Reid B, DiLorenzo C, Travis L, et al. Diabetic gastroparesis due to postprandial antral hypomotility in childhood. Pediatrics 1992;90:43–6.
38. Oduwole A, Marcon M, Bril V, Ehrlich RM. Transient autonomic neuropathy in an adolescent with insulin dependent diabetes mellitus. J Pediatr Endocrinol Metab 1995;8:195–7.
39. Horowitz M, O'Donovan D, Jones KL, et al. Gastric emptying in diabetes: Clinical significance and treatment. Diabetic Medicine 2002;19:177–94.
40. Darwiche G, Bjorgell O, Thorsson O, Almer L. Correlation between simultaneous scintigraphic and ultrasonographic measurement of gastric emptying in patients with type 1 diabetes mellitus. J Ultrasound Med 2003;22:459–66.
41. Dooley CP, Newihi HM, Zeider A, et al. Abnormalities of the migrating motor complex in diabetics with autonomic neuropathy and diarrhea. Scand J Gastroenterol 1988;23:217–23.
42. Liu M, Seino S, Kirchgessner AL. Identification and characterization of glucoresponsive neurons in the enteric nervous system. J Neurosci 1999;19:10305–17.
43. Fraser RJ, Horowitz M, Maddox AF, et al. Hyperglycaemia slows gastric emptying in type I (insulin-dependent) diabetes mellitus. Diabetologia 1990;33:675–80.
44. MacGrgor IL, Gueller R, Watts HD, et al. The effect of acute hyperglycemia on gastric emptying in man. Gastroenterol 1976;70:190–6.
45. Achem-Karam SR, Funakoshi A, Vinik AI, et al. Plasma motilin concentration and interdigestive migrating motor complex in diabetic gastroparesis: Effect of metoclopramide. Gastroenterology 1985;88:492–5.
46. Ordog T, Takayama I, Cheung WKT, et al. Remodeling of networks of interstitial cells of Cajal in a murine model of diabetic gastroparesis. Diabetes 2000;49:1731–9.
47. Gibson T, Cotter M, Cameron N. Effects of poly(ADP-ribose) polymerase inhibition on dysfunction of nonadrenergic noncholinergic neurotransmission in gastric fundus in diabetic rats. Nitric Oxide 2006;15:34–50.
48. Lysy J, Israeli E, Strauss-Liviatan N, Goldin E. Relationships between hypoglycaemia and gastric emptying abnormalities in insulin-treated diabetic patients. Neurogastroenterol Motil 2006;18:433–40.
49. Koch K. Electrogastrography: Physiological basis and clinical application in diabetic gastropathy. Diabetes Technol Therap 2001;3:51–62.
50. Brown CK, Khanderia U. Use of metoclopramide, domperidone, and cisapride in the management of diabetic gastroparesis. Clin Pharmacol 1990;9:357–65.
51. Feldman M, Smith HJ. Effect of cisapride on gastric emptying of indigestible solids in patients with gastroparesis diabeticorum: A comparison with metoclopramide and placebo. Gastroenterology 1987;92:171–4.
52. Steinmetz WE, Shapiro BL, Roberts JJ. The structure of erythromycin enol ether as a model for its activity as a motilide. J Med Chem 2002;45:4899–902.
53. Franzese A, Borrelli O, Corrado G, et al. Domperidone is more effective than cisapride in children with diabetic gastroparesis. Aliment Pharmacol Ther 2002;16:951–7.
54. Crowell M, Mathis C, Schettler V, et al. The effects of tegaserod, a 5-HT receptor agonist, on gastric emptying in a murine model of diabetes mellitus. Neurogastroenterol Motil 2005;17:738–43.
55. Murray C, Martin N, Patterson M, et al. Ghrelin enhances gastric emptying in diabetic gastroparesis: A double blind, placebo controlled, crossover study. Gut 2005;54:1693–8.
56. Rauma J, Spangeus A, El-Salhy M. Ghrelin cell density in the gastrointestinal tracts of animal models of human diabetes. Histol Histopathol 2006;21:1–5.
57. Simon L, Tornoczky J, Toth M, et al. The significance of Campylobacter pylori in gastroenterologic and diabetic practice. Orv Hetil 1989;130:1325–9.
58. Salardi S, Cacciari E, Menegatti M, et al. *Helicobacter pylori* and type 1 diabetes in children. J Pediatr Gastroenterol Nutr 1999;28:307–9.
59. Jones KL, Wishart JM, Berry M, et al. *Helicobacter pylori* infection is not associated with delayed gastric emptying or upper gastrointestinal symptoms in diabetes mellitus. Dig Dis Sci 2002;47:704–9.
60. Miah MAR, Rahman MT, Hasan M, Khan AKA. Seroprevalence of *Helicobacter pylori* among the diabetic population in Bangladesh: A comparative serological study on the newly diagnosed and older diabetics. Bangladesh Med Res Counc Bull 2001;27:9–18.
61. Fock KM, Khoo TK, Chia KS, Sim CS. *Helicobacter pylori* infection and gastric emptying of indigestible solids in patients with dysmotility-like dyspepsia. Scand J Gastroenterol 1997;32:676–80.
62. Gasbarrini A, Ojetti V, Pitocco D, et al. Insulin-dependant diabetes mellitus affects eradication rate of *Helicobacter pylori* infection. Eur J Gastroenterol Hepatol 1999;11: 713–6.
63. Gasbarrini A, Ojetti V, Pitocco D, et al. Efficacy of different *Helicobacter pylori* eradication regiments in patients affected by insulin-dependant diabetes mellitus. Scand J Gastroenterol 2000;35:260–3.
64. Genta RM. The immunobiology of *Helicobacter pylori* gastritis. Semin Gastrointest Dis 1997;8:2–11.
65. Begue RE, Gomez R, Compton T, Vargas A. Effect of *Helicobacter pylori* eradication in the glycemia of children with type 1 diabetes: A preliminary study. Southern Med J 2002;95:842–5.
66. Gulcelik N, Kaya E, Demirbas B, et al. *Helicobacter pylori* prevalence in diabetic patients and its relationship with dyspepsia and autonomic neuropathy. J Pediatr Gastroenterol Nutr 2004;38:422–5.
67. Riley WJ, Toskes PP, Maclaren NK, Silverstein J. Predictive value of gastric parietal cell autoantibodies as a marker for gastric and hematologic abnormalities associated with insulin dependant diabetes. Diabetes 1982;31:1051–5.
68. DeBlock CEM, VanGaal LF, Leeuw IH. High prevalence of manifestations of gastric autoimmunity in parietal cell-antibody positive type 1 (insulin dependent) diabetic patients. J Clin Endocrinol Metab 1999;84:4062–7.
69. DeBlock CEM, DeLeeuw IH, Bogers JJPM, et al. *Helicobacter pylori*, parietal cell antibodies and autoimmune gastropathy in type 1 diabetes mellitus. Aliment Pharmacol Ther 2002;16:281–9.
70. Keshavarzian A, Iber FL. Intestinal transit in insulin-requiring diabetics. Am J Gastroenterol 1986;81:257–60.
71. Cuoco L, MMontalto, Jorizzo R, et al. Eradication of small intestinal bacterial overgrowth and oro-cecal transit in diabetics. Hepatogastroenterology 2002;49:1582–6.
72. Walker-Smith JA, Grigor W. Coeliac disease is a diabetic child. Lancet 1969;1:1021.
73. Kumar V, Rajadhyaksha M, Wortsman J. Celiac disease-associated autoimmune endocrinopathies. Clin Diagn Lab Immunol 2001;8:678–85.
74. Holmes GK. Coeliac disease and type 1 diabetes mellitus-the case for screening. Diabet Med 2001;18:169–77.
75. Schuppan D, Hahn EG. Celiac disease and its link to type 1 diabetes mellitus. J Pediatr Endocrinol Metab 2001;14:597–605.
76. Maki M, Huupponen T, Holm K, Hallstrom O. Seroconversion of reticulin autoantibodies predicts coeliac disease in insulin dependent diabetes mellitus. Gut 1995;36:239–42.
77. Hill I, Dirks M, Liptak G, et al. Guideline for the diagnosis and treatment of celiac disease in children: Recommendations of the North American Society for Pediatric Gastroenterology, Hepatology and Nutrition. J Pediatr Gastroenterol Nutr 2005;40:1–19.
78. Picarelli A, Sabbatella L, Tola MD, et al. Antiendomysial antibody of IgG1 isotype detection strongly increases the prevalence of coeliac disease in patients affected by type I diabetes mellitus. Clin Exp Immunol 2005;142:111–5.
79. Funda DP, Kaas A, Bock T, et al. Gluten-free diet prevents diabetes in NOD mice. Diabetes Metab Res Rev 1999;15:323–7.
80. American Gastroenterological Association Medical Position Statement: Nonalcoholic fatty liver disease. Gastroenterology 2002;123:1702–4.
81. VanSteenbergen WV, Lanckmans S. Liver disturbances in obesity and diabetes mellitus. Intern J Obesity 1995;19: S27–36.
82. Lorenz G, Barenwald G. Histologic and electron-microscopic changes in diabetic children. Acta Hepatogastroenterol 1979;26:435–8.
83. Torbenson M, Chen Y, Brunt E, et al. Glycogenic hepatopathy: An underrecognized hepatic complication of diabetes mellitus. Am J Surg Pathol 2006;30:508–13.
84. Lavine JE. Vitamin E treatment of nonalcoholic steatohepatitis in children: A pilot study. J Pediatr 2000;136:734–8.
85. Franzese A, Iorio R, Buono P, et al. Mauriac syndrome still exists. Diabetes Res Clin Pract 2001;54:219–21.
86. Banerjee S, Banerjee M. Hepatitis C and diabetes mellitus. J Indian Med Assoc 2006;104:86–9.
87. Ding X, Lu C, Mei Y, et al. Correlation between gene expression of CCK-A receptor and emptying dysfunction of the gallbladder in patients with gallstones and diabetes mellitus. Hepatobiliary Pancreat Dis Int 2005;4:295–8.
88. Arslanoglu I, Unal F, Sagin F, et al. Real-time sonography for screening gallbladder dysfunction in children with type 1 diabetes mellitus. J Pediatr Endocrinol Metab 2001; 14:61–9.
89. Watson JA, Windsor JA, Wynne-Jones G. Conservative management of a yersinea entercolitica hepatic abscess. Aust NZ J Surg 1989;59:353–4.
90. Laass M, Henker J, Thamm K, et al. Exocrine pancreatic insufficiency and its consequences on physical development and metabolism in children and adolescents with type 1 diabetes mellitus. Eur J Pediatr 2004;163:681–2.
91. Badiga MS, Jain NK, Casanova C, Pitchumoni CS. Diarrhea in diabetes: The role of sorbitol. J Am Coll Nutr 1990;9:578–82.
92. Virally-Monod M, Tielmans D, Kevorkian JP, et al. Chronic diarrhoea and diabetes mellitus: Prevalence of small intestinal bacterial overgrowth. Diabetes Metab 1998;24:530–6.
93. Narbonne H, Paquis-Fluckinger V, Valero R, et al. Gastrointestinal tract symptoms in maternally inherited diabetes and deafness (MIDD). Diabetes Metab 2004;30:61–6.
94. Mitchell J, Punthakee Z, Lo B, et al. Neonatal diabetes, with hypoplastic pancreas, intestinal atresia and gall bladder hypoplasia: Search for the aetiology of a new autosomal recessive syndrome. Diabetologia 2004;47:2160–7.
95. Ahonen P, Myllarniemi S, Sipila I, Perheentupa J. Clinical variation of autoimmune polyendocrinopathy-candidiasis ectodermal dystrophy (APECED) in a series of 68 patients. N Engl J Med 1990;322:1829–36.

96. Obermayer-Straub P, Manns M. Autoimmune polyglandular syndromes. Baillieres Clin Gastroenterol 1998;12: 293–315.

97. Herrod HG. Chronic mucocutaneous candidiasis and complications of noncandida infection. A report of the Pediatric Immunodeficiency Collaborative Study Group. J Pediatr 1990;116:377–82.

98. Ruan QG, She JX. Autoimmune polyglandular syndrome type 1 and the autoimmune regulator. Clin Lab Med 2004;24:305–17.

99. Valentino R, Savastano S, Tommaselli AP, et al. Unusual association of thyroiditis, Addison's disease, ovarian failure and celiac disease. J Endocrinol Invest 1999;22:390–4.

100. Bereket A, Lowenheim M, Blethen SL, et al. Intestinal lymphangiectasia in a patient with autoimmune polyglandular disease type I and steatorrhea. J Clin Endocrinol Metab 1995;80:933–5.

101. Clemente MG, Obermayer-Straub P, Meloni A, et al. Cytochrome P450 1A2 is a hepatic autoantigen in autoimmune polyglandular syndrome type 1. J Clin Endocrinol Metab 1997;82:1353–61.

102. Rorsman F, Husebye ES, Winqvist O, et al. Aromatic-L-amino-acid decarboxylase, a pyridoxal phosphate-dependent enzyme, is a beta-cell autoantigen. Proc Natl Acad Sci USA 1995;92:8626–9.

103. Damiani D, Aguiar CH, Bueno VS, et al. Primary hyperparathyroidism in children: Patient report and review of the literature. J Pediatr Endocrinol Metab 1998;11:83–6.

104. Nieves-Rivera F, Gonzalez-Pijem L. Primary hyperparathyroidism: An unusual cause of pancreatitis in adolescence. PRHSJ 1995;14:233–6.

105. Cronin CS, Reeve TS, Robinson B, et al. Primary hypoparathyroidism in childhood and adolescence. J Paediatr Child Health 1996;32:397–9.

106. Willems D, Hooghe L, Kinnaert P, AVanGeertruyden J. Postoperative pancreatitis, hyperamylasemia and amylase isoenzymes after parathyroidectomy for primary hyperparathyroidism. Gastroenterol Clin Biol 1988;12:347–53.

107. Gay JD, Grimes JD. Idiopathic hypoparathyroidism with impaired vitamin B12 absorption and neuropathy. CMA Journal 1972;107:54–8.

108. Root AW, Diamond FB. Disorders of calcium and phosphorus metabolism in adolescent. Pediatr Clin North Am 1993;22:573–92.

109. O'Donnell P, Myers AM. Intestinal lymphangectasia and protein-losing enteropathy, toxic copper accumulation and hypoparathyroidism. Aust NZ J Med 1990;20: 167–9.

110. Deen KI, Sen!viratne SL, DeSilva HJ. Anorectal physiology and transit in patients with disorders of thyroid metabolism. J Gastroenterol Hepatol 1999;14:384–87.

111. Gunsar F, Yilmaz S, Bor S, et al. Effect of hypo- and hyperthyroidism on gastric myoelectrical activity. Dig Dis Sci 2003;48:706–12.

112. Buhl T, Nilsson C, Ekblad E, et al. Expression of prepro-VIP derived peptides in the gastrointestinal tract of normal, hypothyroid and hyperthyroid rats. Neuropeptides 1996;30:237–47.

113. Weber JR, Ryan JC. Effects on the gut of systemic disease and other extraintestinal conditions. In: Feldman M, Scharschmidt BF, Sleisenger M, editors. Sleisenger and Fodtran's Gastrointestinal and Liver Disease: Pathophysiology, Diagnosis, and Management, Volume 6. Philadelphia: WB Saunders Company; 1998. p. 411–38.

114. Ardawi MSM, Jalalah SM. Effects of hypothyroidism on glucose and glutamine metabolism by the gut of the rat. Clin Sci 1991;81:347–55.

115. Tajri J, Shimada T, Naomi S, et al. Hepatic dysfunction in primary hypothyroidism. Endocrinol Jpn 1984;31:83.

116. Wegener M, Wedmann B, Langhoff T, et al. Effect of hyperthyroidism on the transit of a caloric solid–liquid meal through the stomach, the small intestine, and the colon in man. J Clin Endocrinol Metab 1992;75:745–9.

117. Christensen J, Schedl HP, Clifton JA. The basic electric rhythm of the duodenum in normal subjects and in patients with thyroid disease. J Clin Invest 1964;43:1659–67.

118. Tobin MV, Fisken RA, Diggory RT, et al. Orocaecal transit time in health and in thyroid disease. Gut 1989;30:26–9.

119. Rahman Q, Haboubi NY, Hudson PR, et al. The effect of thyroxin on small intestinal motility in the elderly. Clin Endocrinol (Oxf) 1991;35:443–6.

120. Gu Y, Wu ZH. The anabolic effects of recombinant human growth hormone and glutamine on parenterally fed, short bowel rats. World J Gastroenterol 2002;8:752–7.

121. Ellaway CJ, Silink M, Cowell CT, et al. Cholestatic jaundice and congenital hypopituitarism. J Paediatr Child Health 1995;31:51–3.

122. Adams L, Feldstein A, Lindor K, Angulo P. Nonalcoholic fatty liver disease among patients with hypothalamic and pituitary dysfunction. Hepatology 2004;39:909–14.

123. Nakajima K, Kaneda H, Tokushige K, et al. Pediatric nonalcoholic steatohepatitis associated with hypopituitarism. J Gastroenterol 2005;40:312–5.

124. Jonas M, Krawczuk L, Kim H, et al. Rapid recurrence of nonalcoholic fatty liver disease after transplantation in a child with hypopituitarism and hepatopulmonary syndrome. Liver Transpl 2005;11:108–10.

125. Scott J, Batt RM, Peters TJ. Enhancement of ileal adaptation by prednisolone after proximal small bowel resection in the rat. Gut 1979;20:858–64.

126. Oberfield SE, et al. Pseudohypoaldosteronism: Multiple target unresponsiveness to mineralocorticoid hormone. J Clin Endocrinol 1979;48:228–34.

127. McBrien DJ, Jones RV, Creamer B. Steatorrhea in Addison's disease. Lancet 1963;i:25–6.

128. Ertem D, Acar Y, Alper G, et al. An uncommon and often overlooked cause of failure to thrive: Diencephalic syndrome. J Pediatr Gastroenterol Nutr 2000;30:453–7.

129. Fleischman A, Brue C, Poussaint T, et al. Diencephalic syndrome: A cause of failure to thrive and a model of partial growth hormone resistance. Pediatrics 2005;115:e742–8.

130. Vlachopapadopoulou E, Tracey KJ, Capella M, et al. Increased energy expenditure in a patient with diencephalic syndrome. J Pediatr 1993;122:922–4.

Gastrointestinal Injury

26.1a. Drug-Induced Bowel Injury

Miho Inoue, MD

Shinya Ito, MD, FRCPC

Pharmacotherapy is often associated with adverse effects in the gastrointestinal tract. Oral administration of drugs exposes gastrointestinal mucosa to relatively high concentrations of the drug. Even parenteral use of drugs may cause adverse reactions, which are specific to the gastrointestinal system. The classification system of adverse drug reactions (ADRs) proposed by Patterson and colleagues categorizes them as predictable or unpredictable (idiosyncratic effects), providing a practical framework for risk assessment and communication.[1] ADRs that target the gastrointestinal tract are numerous, ranging from nausea and vomiting without significant pathology to severe colitis. This chapter describes drug-induced bowel injury defined as gastrointestinal ADRs with pathologic changes. Although nausea and vomiting without gastrointestinal pathology are commonly encountered, they are not discussed. Similarly, overdoses and poisonings with corrosive nonmedicinal agents are beyond the scope of the chapter. The ADRs are discussed in a section of each major target anatomic site, but it is important to note that multiple sites may be involved. Because the field of pediatrics encompasses premature infants to young adults, the chapter covers both pediatric-specific ADRs and those commonly reported in adults.

THE ESOPHAGUS

Pill Esophagitis

Tablets and capsules are common drug formulations for older children, adolescents, and adults. These drug formulations are designed for optimal dissolution in an appropriate gastrointestinal environment for absorption. As a conduit for ingested substances, the esophagus is not directly involved in drug absorption. However, a swallowed tablet or capsule may lodge itself in the esophagus, releasing its contents onto the esophageal mucosa. If a pill is dissolved in such a confined small area, concentrations of active ingredients in the local milieu may become extremely high. If exposed to the drug at a high concentration for a prolonged period of time, the esophageal mucosa may be damaged. Hence, lodged and immobilized pills become a cause of esophageal mucosal injury. This condition is called pill esophagitis or pill-induced esophageal injury. Although the risks of developing pill esophagitis may be small, it is estimated that 10,000 cases occur per year in the United States.[2]

The patients with pill esophagisits vary in age, ranging from 3 to 98 years in the published reports.[2] Majority of them have no apparent predisposing conditions, such as esophageal or neuromuscular disorders. However, delayed transit of esophageal content for pathological anatomical and/or functional conditions causes prolonged exposure of esophageal mucosa to pills and can predispose patients for pill esophagitis. Ingestion of pills without sufficient fluid, supine positioning, certain formulations (eg, larger pills, gelatinous capsules, sustained-release formulations), and chemical characteristics of pills are considered to be risk factors for developing the condition.[3]

Drugs reported to cause pill esophagitis are numerous (Table 1), but the most frequently quoted medications include antibiotics, potassium chloride, nonsteroidal anti-inflammatory drugs (NSAIDs), and quinidine, comprising

Table 1 Drugs Frequently Implicated for Esophageal Mucosal Injury

Antimicrobials
 Ampicillin
 Doxycycline
 Minocycline
 Oxytetracycline
 Penicillin
 Tetracycline
 Zidovudine

NSAIDs
 Aspirin
 Ibuprofen
 Indomethacin
 Naproxen
 Piroxicam

Others
 Bisphosphonates (alendronate, pamidronate)
 Potassium chloride
 Ferrous sulfate/succinate
 Quinidine
 Theophylline
 Corticosteroids

Adapted and modified from Kikendall.[2]
NSAID = nonsteroidal anti-inflammatory drug.

nearly 90% of all reported cases.[2] Despite the recent introduction into clinical practice, case reports of esophageal injury by bisphosphonates such as alendronate and pamidronate are relatively common and severe in nature. However, drug-specific incidences of pill esophagitis are unknown. The mechanisms of injury to esophageal mucosa may differ among these offending drugs and are not fully understood. Postulated mechanisms include acidity (eg, tetracycline, doxycycline, ascorbic acid, and ferrous sulfate), high osmolarity of drug formulations, accumulation of toxic concentration of the drugs in mucosa, and induction of reflux by decreasing lower esophageal sphincter tone (eg, theophylline).[2,4] The common symptoms are acute-onset retrosternal pain that is continuous or worsened by swallowing (ie, odynophagia), chest pain, vomiting, dysphagia, and hematemesis.[2,4,5] A long-standing injury may lead to a stricture. Esophageal hemorrhage, perforation, penetration, strictures, and mediastinitis have been reported in those receiving drugs such as NSAIDs,[6,7] potassium chloride,[8] alendronate,[9] sustained-release ferrous sulfate, and sustained-release valproate.[10] Endoscopic examinations usually confirm the diagnosis. Symptoms of pill esophagitis improve in a few days to weeks in most patients on discontinuation of the offending drug. The best treatment is removal of the offending drugs, followed by supportive care. Antiacids are commonly prescribed. In severe cases, patients may require parenteral nutrition, therapeutic endoscopy for hemorrhage and chronic stricture, or surgery for massive esophageal hemorrhage or perforation.

Oral and Esophageal Mucositis Induced by Cancer Chemotherapy

Anticancer drugs affect tissue turnover and remodeling maintained by rapidly proliferating epithelial cells in the gastrointestinal tract. Consequently, ulceration and inflammation may occur following systemic administration of cancer chemotherapy agents throughout the gastrointestinal system, including oral cavity mucosa, the esophagus, and other parts of the gastrointestinal tract. Usually, oral lesions accompany the esophageal changes. Methotrexate, vinca alkaloids (such as vincristine and vinblastine), dactinomycin, doxorubicin, bleomycin, cytosine arabinoside, and 5-fluorouracil are often implicated as causative agents.[11] Treatment is supportive, and uncomplicated lesions usually heal in 2 weeks. A well-known example of effective prevention of toxicities caused by high-dose methotrexate regimens is folinic acid (leucovorin) rescue.

STOMACH AND DUODENUM

NSAID-Induced Gastroduodenal Ulcer

NSAIDs (in this chapter, NSAIDs indicate salicylates and traditional nonselective cyclooxygenase [COX] inhibitors and do not include selective COX-2 inhibitors, unless otherwise stated) are the most common medications taken for pain, inflammation and fever. Aspirin in a low dose is also widely used as an antiplatelet agent. Although NSAIDs are generally well tolerated, mucosal injury of the stomach and duodenum induced by NSAIDs has been one of the major clinical issues.

Mechanism. The mechanisms of mucosal damage are considered to be multifactorial, which include inhibition of gastric prostaglandin synthesis, reduction in gastric mucosal blood flow, topical irritant effects, and impairment of healing process of mucosal damage.[12] NSAIDs inhibit COX-1, a constitutive enzyme in gastric mucosa responsible for production of protective prostaglandins such as PGE2.[12,13] Decrease in prostaglandin synthesis in gastric mucosa leads to decreases in epithelial mucus, bicarbonate secretion, mucosal blood flow, epithelial proliferation, and mucosal barrier function. The impaired mucosal barrier permits gastric injury by irritants such as acid, pepsin, and medications. This pathologic process develops not only through topical mucosal contact with the offending agents but, more importantly, via the systemic effects of the drugs.[13]

Epidemiology. Dyspepsia is the most common cause of discontinuation of traditional NSAIDs. At least 15 to 25% of adult patients receiving NSAIDs on a regular basis have dyspeptic symptoms.[14] However, there is no clear correlation between severity of symptoms and endoscopic findings.[15] In an adult study, dyspeptic symptoms were present in 19% of those with completely normal endoscopy and in only 9% of those with abnormal endoscopic findings.[16] Another study reported that 55% of the patients with ulcers were asymptomatic.[17] Risk factors for developing NSAID-induced gastroduodenal ulcers include advanced age, past history of ulcer, use of concurrent corticosteroids, higher NSAID doses, multiple NSAID use, anticoagulant use, and serious systemic disorder.[13,18] In adults, the risk of NSAID-induced upper gastrointestinal mucosal damage is highest within the first month of its use, although the risk seems to accumulate during the first 6 months.[19]

In a large prospective study of more than 8,000 adult patients with rheumatoid arthritis,

the rate of serious gastrointestinal complications, such as bleeding, perforation, and gastric outlet obstruction, was found to be about 0.8% per 6 months,[19] approaching an annual incidence of 2%. In patients without risk factors such as old age (75 years or older) and previous peptic ulcer and bleeding, they reported that the logistic regression model predicted a risk for developing gastrointestinal complications such as bleeding and endoscopically proven mucosal lesions of 0.4%.[17] Users of NSAIDs are about 3 times as likely as nonusers to develop serious adverse gastrointestinal events.[18] The risk in pediatric patients is probably close to this estimate, although there are no explicit data. In a retrospective study of 702 pediatric patients with juvenile rheumatoid arthritis, 5 children had a total of 10 events of symptomatic "gastropathy," defined as esophagitis, gastritis, or peptic ulcer disease, which were associated with NSAIDs, including tolmetin, diclofenac, aspirin, and indomethacin.[20] In premature infants receiving corticosteroids or NSAIDs for lung maturation or closure of patent ductus arteriosus, severe gastrointestinal complications such as perforation have been well recognized (see dexamethasone-induced gastrointestinal perforation and NSAID-induced intestinal injury in the section on the small intestine and colon).

Although there is an apparent rank order of ulcer bleeding and perforation risks of NSAIDs (eg, low risk: ibuprofen and diclofenac; medium risk: naproxen, indomethacin, and piroxicam; high risk: ketoprofen and azapropazone),[21] caution should be exercised in interpreting it because the data are not available for risks standardized by equivalent doses. Given the dose-response relationship between NSAID use and the risk of gastrointestinal complications, this aspect cannot be ignored.

Children with the acute phase of Kawasaki disease are treated with immunoglobulin and high-dose aspirin, followed by low-dose aspirin therapy during the convalescent phase. Surprisingly, there has been no systematic study on aspirin-induced gastrointestinal damages in children with Kawasaki disease. A report in 1996 described two children with overt gastrointestinal hemorrhage during aspirin therapy for Kawasaki disease in the convalescent phase.[22]

COX-2 Inhibitors. A new subclass of NSAIDs (eg, celecoxib and lumiracoxib) has more selective inhibitory effects on COX-2 than traditional NSAIDs. They are called coxibs, COX-2 inhibitors, or COX-1–sparing NSAIDs. COX-2 is an inducible form associated with inflammation, which has been established as an effective therapeutic target. The gastrointestinal tract constitutively expresses COX-1, which plays a key role in protecting and maintaining the integrity of the gastrointestinal mucosa by producing mucosa-protective prostaglandins.[16] Therefore, by sparing COX-1, these COX-2 inhibitors appear to be beneficial in minimizing the risk of the mucosal damages.

Clinical trials in adults suggest that the COX-2 inhibitors are better tolerated than

nonselective NSAIDs such as ibuprofen, diclofenac, or naproxen.[23–25] In patients receiving no aspirin, the annualized occurrence rate of gastroduodenal ulcers and their complications was 0.44% for celecoxib and 1.27% for the nonselective NSAIDs.[24] Similarly, in adults with rheumatoid arthritis, rofecoxib (removed from market in 2004) was associated with fewer gastrointestinal ulcers and complications (2.1% per year) than naproxen (4.5% per year); the difference was most pronounced in the frequency of gastric ulcer.[23] In the study comparing lumiracoxib with two NSAIDs, naproxen and ibuprofen, in osteoarthritis patients, the cumulative 1-year incidence of ulcer complications with lumiracoxib was lower than with NSAIDs (0.25% vs 1.09%).[25] Together with other studies,[26–28] these data suggest an improved adverse effect profile of the COX-2 inhibitors, especially for complicated ulcer. However, increase in the risk of cardiovascular events in adults on rofecoxib and celecoxib was reported in large clinical trials[23,29,30] and case-control studies.[31,32] These findings led to the product recall of rofecoxib and the boxed warning highlighting the potential for increased risk of cardiovascular events with celecoxib. Considering the relatively low risk of gastrointestinal complications and cardiac events in children, the benefit of the relatively expensive COX-2–selective inhibitors over inexpensive traditional NSAIDs in pediatric populations is not clear and remains to be demonstrated.

***Helicobacter pylori* and NSAID-Induced Ulcer.** *Helicobacter pylori* infection and NSAID use are major and independent risk factors for gastroduodenal mucosal injury. Although the prevalence of *H. pylori* infection is lower in the pediatric population than in adults, it remains an etiologically important risk factor for gastroduodenal lesions. When endoscopically confirmed mucosal damages caused by NSAIDs are used as an end point, *H. pylori* infection does not seem to substantially increase the frequency and severity of the NSAID-induced mucosal damages for both short and long-term (more than 4 weeks) use of the drug.[33] However, it is recommended that *H. pylori* be eradicated in those NSAID-receiving patients with *H. pylori*-associated ulcers because the two conditions are clinically indistinguishable.[34] Currently, no evidence exists to clearly support or refute *H. pylori* eradication before NSAID use in adult patients with no preexisting mucosal lesions.

Prophylaxis and Treatment. Pharmacologic approaches (Table 2) to counteract ulcerogenic effects of NSAIDs include the use of misoprostol,[19,35–37] proton pump inhibitors (PIPs),[38–40] histamine 2 (H2) receptor antagonists,[41–43] and nitric oxide. In adults, misoprostol, PPIs, and high-dose H2 receptor antagonists (double the standard dose) were all shown to reduce the risk of endoscopic gastric and duodenal ulcers induced by NSAIDs, but misoprostol is the only prophylactic drug directly shown to decrease

Table 2 Main Pharmacological Approaches for NSAID-Induced Gastroduodenal Injury

Drug/Drug Group	Indications
Misoprostol	Ulcer prophylaxis
Proton pump inhibitors	Ulcer prophylaxis
	Dyspepsia treatment
	Ulcer treatment*
H2 receptor antagonists	Dyspepsia treatment
	Ulcer treatment†

*In patients who continue nonsteroidal anti-inflammatory drug (NSAID) treatment.
†For those who discontinued NSAIDs.

the risk of severe complications of NSAID-induced ulcers.[44] Misoprostol, a prostaglandin E analogue, is expected to replace cytoprotective prostaglandins depleted by NSAIDs. Misoprostol 800 µg per day for 6 months is effective in reducing the risk of NSAID-induced serious gastrointestinal complications (bleeding, perforation and gastric outlet obstruction) from 0.95 to 0.38% in patients with chronic rheumatoid arthritis.[19] The meta-analysis showed that misoprostol significantly reduces the relative risk of endoscopic gastric and duodenal ulcers by 74% and 53%.[44] However, 27% of the adult patients receiving this standard dose of misoprostol experiences adverse effects including nausea, diarrhea and abdominal discomfort. Misoprostol 400 µg per day is associated with lower risk of the adverse events but is not as effective as 800 µg per day for ulcer prevention.

Overall, PPIs and high-dose H2 receptor antagonists (about twofold higher than the standard dose: eg, 80 mg/d famotidine or 600 mg/d ranitidine) are effective for preventing NSAID-related endoscopic gastric and duodenal ulcers, and also better tolerated than misoprostol. However, H2 receptor antagonists in a standard dose are effective for reducing dyspepsic symptoms and the risk of NSAID-induced duodenal ulcers, but ineffective in preventing gastric ulcers. Relative efficacy of misoprostol and PPIs at their effective doses in reducing NSAID-induced gastric and duodenal ulcers has yet to be defined.[45,46]

Nitric oxide shares multiple antiulcerogenic effects with mucosa-protective prostaglandins. A case-control study showed that the use of nitric oxide-releasing nitrovasodilators is associated with a reduced risk of upper gastrointestinal bleeding in adults receiving NSAIDs or low-dose aspirin.[47] Nitric oxide-releasing NSAIDs are currently under investigation for clinical use.[48,49]

In children, a case series suggested that misoprostol alleviates gastrointestinal symptoms associated with NSAIDs.[35] In that series, only 1 of the 25 children receiving an NSAID and misoprostol had diarrhea, which is in sharp contrast to the adult study.[36] The case series included 22 pediatric rheumatology patients on misoprostol for gastrointestinal tract symptoms, and more than 90% of the patients had improvement in the symptoms. Only adverse effect was self-limited diarrhea in one patient.

Omeprazole-Associated Gastric Polyps

Omeprazole, a proton pump inhibitor (PPI), has been widely used to suppress gastric acid for the treatment of gastroesophageal reflux disease, gastritis and gastroduodenal ulcer in children. There have been reports of the development of gastric polyps in adults,[50] and children,[51] receiving long-term omeprazole therapy. No dysplastic changes in polyps are reported in these studies. Large retrospective studies in adults have shown conflicting results regarding the association between fundic gland polyps and PPI use.[52–54] The exact mechanism of polyp formation is not clear. Hypergastrinemia is known to occur with long-term omeprazole therapy,[55,56] but no association between polyps and gastrin concentration was shown in a small pediatric study.[51]

Prostaglandin E1-Induced Antral Hyperplasia

Antral mucosal hyperplasia, with no evidence of pyloric stenosis, causing gastric outlet obstruction has been reported in neonates who were receiving prostaglandin E1 infusion to sustain the ductus arteriosus for congenital heart disease such as transposition of great arteries and hypoplastic left heart syndrome.[57] The condition is distinct from infantile hypertrophic pyloric stenosis because there is significant hyperplasia of the antral mucosal glands with no muscular thickening at the pyloric sphincter. Five of seventy-four neonates who received prostaglandin E1 in the case series had clinical, radiologic, and pathologic evidence of the gastric outlet obstruction with no evidence of hypertrophic pyloric stenosis. These five patients received the drug for a significantly longer period (mean 569 hours) at significantly higher cumulative doses than the remaining neonates. On withdrawal of the drug in two patients, the condition improved clinically and ultrasonographically. Close monitoring of the gastric out-let functioning is warranted in neonates receiving prostaglandin E1 for more than 120 hours.

Erythromycin-Induced Infantile Hypertrophic Pyloric Stenosis

The association between exposures to erythromycin in infants and development of infantile hypertrophic pyloric stenosis has been suggested since 1976.[58] Infantile hypertrophic pyloric stenosis (IHPS) is a condition of infancy in which hypertrophy of the pylorus results in the obstruction of gastric outlet. IHPS is seen in 1.5 to 4 per 1,000 live births with a male-to-female ratio of 4 to 6:1.[59–61] The epidemiological investigations of the link were prompted by seven cases of IHPS among infants who received systemic erythromycin for prophylaxis after a cluster of neonatal perutssis cases in 1999.[62] Retrospective cohort studies showed that systemic use of erythromycin in the first 2 weeks of life is associated with 7- to 10-fold increase in the risk of pyloric stenosis.[59,60,63] The role of erythromycin in pathogenesis of IHPS is not fully understood.

Erythromycin is a potent motilin receptor agonist and induces large amplitude contractions in the stomach called migrating motor complexes. It specifically increases motility of gastric antrum and contraction of pyloric muscles. These effects of erythromycin are hypothesized to cause hypertrophy of pyloric bulb.[63]

The epidemiologic link between erythromycin use in newborns and IHPS raised a concern about erythromycin use in pregnant women. Erythromycin is a treatment of choice for genital infection by chlamydia, mycoplasma, and ureaplasma during pregnancy. Transplacental transfer of erythromycin is limited and the serum concentration of the drug in fetus may not reach a therapeutic level.[64] Three retrospective studies did not find increase in the risk of IHPS in infants with prenatal exposure to erythromycin either in late pregnancy or at any time during pregnancy.[60,65,66]

Erythromycin is also commonly used in preterm neonates as a prokinetic agent. It often takes several days and even weeks for preterm neonates to establish full enteral feeding because of functional immaturity of gastrointestinal motility. To enhance this process and to avoid adverse effects of prolonged parenteral nutrition, low-dose erythromycin (3–12 mg/kg/d) has been used in some neonatal intensive care units. In studies evaluating the efficacy of erythromycin in improving feeding, no increase in IHPS is reported.[67,68]

Erythromycin is excreted into breast milk. The level of erythromycin in breast milk of women receiving the drug at daily doses of 1.2 to 2 g was reported to range from 0.4 mg/L to 3.2 mg/L.[69] Assuming an average milk intake of 150 mL/kg/d, an estimated infant dose is less than 0.5 mg/kg/d. Although a retrospective study suggested the epidemiological link between exposure to erythromycin through breast milk and the development of IHPS,[70] it seems unlikely that such a low level exposure exerts a clinically meaningful effect.

There are paucity of data for other macrolides, such as clarithromycin and azithromycin. It is not clear whether the findings with erythromycin can be extrapolated to other macrolides. Continued surveillance of the incidence of IHPS in those infants who have prenatal or postnatal exposure to macrolide antibiotics is warranted.

SMALL INTESTINE AND COLON

Neutropenic Enterocolitis (Typhlitis, Necrotizing Enterocolitis, Ileocecal Syndrome)

Severe inflammation leading to bowel necrosis may be seen in the cecum, ascending colon, and terminal ileum of leukemic patients receiving chemotherapy.[71] The condition is also seen in noncancer patients, such as those with drug-induced neutropenia, acquired immune deficiency syndrome (AIDS), or organ transplants.[72–74] The patient usually has severe granulocytopenia (<500–1,000 cells/mm³), and mortality may be as high as 50%.[75] Although the etiology is likely to be multiple and the pathophysiology poorly understood, cytotoxic drugs apparently play a key role in some patients. Vinca alkaloid-induced myenteric nerve damages may contribute to paralytic ileus and cecal distention that further enhances intestinal ischemia.

Pain in the right lower quadrant of the abdomen, fever, diarrhea with or without blood, and nausea and vomiting are usually seen. As the disease progresses, clinical signs of intestinal perforation, peritonitis, and sepsis may become apparent. Abdominal computed tomography, ultrasonography, and radiography provide diagnostic clues, including a fluid-filled dilated lumen, pneumatosis, and cecal wall thickening.

Treatment for the drug-induced neutropenic enterocolitis is no different from treatments for other forms of necrotizing enterocolitis. Namely, the therapy includes antibiotics covering intestinal bacteria, antifungal agents, supportive measures, and surgical resection.

Intestinal Mucositis Induced by Cancer Chemotherapy

Cancer chemotherapeutic agents affect intestinal cells with rapid cell turnover, disrupting the integrity of the epithelia (see "Esophagus"). Methotrexate is one of the most commonly cited offending agents. The affected patients have abdominal pain, diarrhea, vomiting, and occasionally, melena. Protein-losing enteropathy has also been reported.

Drug-Induced Intestinal Hypomotility

Intestinal motility is reduced by drugs with anticholinergic properties (eg, anticholinergics, tricyclic antidepressants, and opioids). These are consequences of their pharmacologic actions of functional cholinergic inhibition. In contrast, vincristine damages nerve tissues, including the myenteric plexus, which may lead to paralytic ileus.[11] The condition develops within 2 to 3 days of the therapy.[11] Conservative treatment usually brings complete recovery in 2 weeks unless other complications, such as neutropenic enterocolitis (above), develop. If patients concomitantly receive itraconazole, vincristine neurotoxicity, including paralytic ileus, may become more severe.[76] This vincristine-itraconazole interaction may be due to itraconazole inhibition of a drug-metabolizing enzyme (eg, cytochrome P-450 3A4) and a drug transporter (eg, P-glycoprotein), which handle vincristine as a substrate.

Dexamethasone-Induced Intestinal Perforation in Premature Infants

A clinical trial of early use of high-dose dexamethasone in extremely low birth weight infants to prevent chronic lung disease was terminated before completion owing to a high incidence of spontaneous gastrointestinal perforation.[77] The rate of gastrointestinal perforation without necrotizing enterocolitis during the first 2 weeks of life was 13% (14 of 111) in the dexamethasone group that received a 10-day tapered course of the drug starting at 0.15 mg/kg/d within 24 hours after birth. The incidence in the placebo group was 4% (4 of 109). The sites of perforation were the small bowel (13 infants), the stomach (1), and unknown (4). A concurrent use of indomethacin appeared to contribute to development of the adverse event in both groups. Trends toward higher rates of spontaneous perforation associated with dexamethasone or indomethacin were also reported in other studies.[78–82] Given the established inhibitory effects of corticosteroids and NSAIDs on gastrointestinal prostaglandin synthesis, it is not surprising to see an increased incidence of spontaneous gastrointestinal perforation in this vulnerable patient population.

Antibiotic-Associated Diarrhea

Antibiotics are responsible for about one-fourth of the cases of drug-induced diarrhea.[83] About 70 to 80% of the cases of diarrhea associated with antibiotics use are nonspecific, self-limited, and unrelated to *Clostridium difficile*.[84,85] Some of these patients may develop the condition as a result of altered carbohydrate metabolism induced by changes in intestinal bacterial flora. Erythromycin may cause diarrhea owing to its prokinetic property. The nonspecific diarrhea subsides on discontinuation of the antibiotics.

C. difficile infection is a nosocomial illness, comprising about 20% of antibiotic-associated diarrhea.[84] *C. difficile* produces toxins, causing intestinal damage with a wide spectrum of severity. *C. difficile* disease occurs 4 to 18 days after a first dose of the offending agent[86] and usually requires a cascade of events: Changes in normal gut flora, acquisition and colonization of the bacteria, and toxin production. Clearly, loss of colonization resistance against *C. difficile* as a result of disruption of the normal intestinal microflora by antibiotics is an important etiologic process, although *C. difficile* disease in pediatric patients may be less dependent on prior exposures to antibiotics than in adults.[85] The most commonly implicated antibiotics are ampicillin, amoxicillin, cephalosporins (second and third generations), lincomycin, and clindamycin, but use of virtually any antibiotic can be a predisposing factor.[87–89] Notably, as many as 60% of neonates and infants are asymptomatically colonized by *C. difficile*, the mechanism of which is not fully understood.[84,90,91] Compared with neonates, the isolation rates of the bacteria decrease to 0 to 3% in older asymptomatic children, similar to those seen in asymptomatic healthy adults.[85] Clinical pictures of *C. difficile* infections range from asymptomatic carriers, mild diarrhea, and uncomplicated colitis to pseudomembranous colitis and fulminant colitis.

Pseudomembranous enterocolitis affects mainly the large intestine and rarely the small intestine. *C. difficile* has been the most common cause, often induced by preceding antibiotic therapy. Other causes of pseudomembranous colitis include ischemia, verotoxin-producing *Escherichia coli*, and drugs such as chlorpropamide, gold, and NSAIDs.[84]

C. difficile infections usually present with profuse watery or mucoid diarrhea with or without blood, abdominal pain, and fever. Supportive care and discontinuation of the offending antibiotics, if any, may be sufficient for those with mild symptoms. Symptomatic therapy with antidiarrheal agents should be avoided. Patients with severe symptoms, for whom supportive therapy has failed, may be treated with oral metronidazole or vancomycin for 1 to 2 weeks. Of those who underwent the therapy for the first time, as high as 40 to 60% may relapse.[92–94] Currently, a new strategy to neutralize the toxin by a synthetic oligosaccharide mimicking toxin receptors is being tested for treating recurrent *C. difficile* infections.[85]

NSAID-Induced Intestinal Injury

NSAIDs can cause a variety of side effects in small intestine including increased intestinal permeability, inflammation, ulcer, strictures, obstructions, bleeding, and perforations. These conditions may lead to iron deficiency anemia owing to chronic blood loss, a protein-losing enteropathy, and mild lipid malabsorption. Small intestinal perforation associated with slow-release NSAIDs is well documented in adults,[95] suggesting that slow-release formulations simply shift a target site of NSAID-induced mucosal injury from the stomach to the more distal intestinal tract.

NSAIDs can also lead to colitis resembling inflammatory bowel disease (IBD).[96] Lesions in colon are less commonly reported than those in small intestine. This may be due to a progressively small amount of orally ingested NSAIDs reaching the colon in most patients as a result of nearly complete absorption in the proximal intestinal tract. Indeed, ulcers and strictures are seen, if at all, mostly in the right side of the colon.[97] Inhibition of prostaglandin synthesis, decrease in blood flow, and increased permeability of intestinal mucosa are postulated to mechanisms of NSAID-induced intestinal injury.

Incidence of NSAID-induced small bowel injury has been evaluated in a number of studies using different diagnostic methods. A study using video capsule endoscopy found that 71% of chronic NSAID users (>3 months' duration) compared with 10% of controls had small bowel injury including red spots, small erosions, large erosions, or ulcers.[98] In another randomized study with video capsule endoscopy, celecoxib was associated with fewer small bowel lesions than naproxen plus omeprazole.[99] An autopsy study including 249 adult patients on NSAIDs found the prevalence of small intestinal ulcers to be 8.4% compared with 0.6% in the control group.[100] Although gastric and duodenal ulcers were also seen in the NSAID users, no correlation was found between the gastric or duodenal lesions and the small intestinal ulcers,[100] implying that prediction of the small intestinal ulcers from the upper gastrointestinal damages may not be valid.

In children, data are scarce, but preterm neonates appear to be more susceptible to the adverse effects of NSAIDs. For example, 1 in 10 premature infants with a patent ductus arteriosus, who received indomethacin, were found to have intestinal perforation compared with none in surgically treated babies.[101] Overall, perforation has been reported to occur throughout the gastrointestinal tract in premature neonates receiving NSAIDs.[78,80–82,101]

NSAID-induced colitis is clinically characterized by acute diarrhea with or without mucus or blood. In addition to the de novo colitis, NSAIDs may exacerbate preexisting IBD.[102,103] Patients with ulcerative colitis on short-term treatment with celecoxib up to 14 days did not have increased risk for exacerbation compared to those on placebo,[104] but the effect of long-term COX-2 inhibitor therapy on the activity of IBD remains to be studied.

Most of NSAID-induced mucosal lesions improve upon discontinuation of offending drugs. Stricture may require endoscopic dilatation or surgical resection. Surgery is also indicated for major bleeding and perforations.

Enterocolitis by Mycophenolic Acid

Mycophenolate mofetil (MMF) is one of the standard immunosuppressive drugs used in combination with corticosteroids and calcineurin inhibitors for the prophylaxis of rejection after solid organ transplants. In addition, it has been used in patients with inflammatory bowel disease and lupus nephritis. MMF is rapidly hydrolyzed in liver to an active metabolite, mycophenolic acid (MPA). Gastrointestinal side effects including nausea, vomiting, diarrhea, gastritis, ulcers, enterocolitis, bleeding, and intestinal perforation have been reported in patients on MMF.[105,106] The incidence of gastrointestinal side effects in renal transplant patients receiving MMF as a part of combination therapy ranges from 12 to 50% in adults,[38,106–110] and children.[111,112] The mechanism of gastrointestinal toxicities of MMF is not clear. Renal transplant recipients with MMF-associated chronic diarrhea show histological findings such as Crohn's disease-like enterocolitis,[113,114] duodenal villous atrophy,[115] and a graft-versus-host disease-like pattern.[116] Diarrhea resolves in most of patients after reducing or discontinuing MMF.[113,115] However, patients with dose reduction or discontinuation of MMF had two to threefold increase in the risk of graft failure.[117]

REFERENCES

1. Patterson R, DeSwarte RD, Greenberger PA, et al. Drug allergy and protocols for management of drug allergies. Allergy Proc 1994;15:239–64.
2. Kikendall JW. Pill esophagitis. J Clin Gastroenterol 1999;28:298–305.
3. Bonavina L, DeMeester TR, McChesney L, et al. Drug-induced esophageal strictures. Ann Surg 1987;206:173–83.
4. Jaspersen D. Drug-induced oesophageal disorders: Pathogenesis, incidence, prevention and management. Drug Saf 2000;22:237–49.
5. Abid S, Mumtaz K, Jafri W, et al. Pill-induced esophageal injury: Endoscopic features and clinical outcomes. Endoscopy 2005;37:740–4.
6. Sacca N, Rodino S, De Medici A, et al. NSAIDs-induced digestive hemorrhage and esophageal pseudotumor: A case report. Endoscopy 1995;27:632.
7. Kahn LH, Chen M, Eaton R. Over-the-counter naproxen sodium and esophageal injury. Ann Intern Med 1997;126:1006.
8. Henry JG, Shinner JJ, Martino JH, Cimino LE. Fatal esophageal and bronchial artery ulceration caused by solid potassium chloride. Pediatr Cardiol 1983;4:251–2.
9. de Groen PC, Lubbe DF, Hirsch LJ, et al. Esophagitis associated with the use of alendronate. N Engl J Med 1996;335:1016–21.
10. Yamaoka K, Takenawa H, Tajiri K, et al. A case of esophageal perforation due to a pill-induced ulcer successfully treated with conservative measures. Am J Gastroenterol 1996;91:1044–5.
11. Mitchell EP. Gastrointestinal toxicity of chemotherapeutic agents. Semin Oncol 1992;19:566–79.
12. Wallace JL. Pathogenesis of NSAID-induced gastroduodenal mucosal injury. Best Pract Res Clin Gastroenterol 2001;15:691–703.
13. Wolfe MM, Lichtenstein DR, Singh G. Gastrointestinal toxicity of nonsteroidal antiinflammatory drugs. N Engl J Med 1999;340:1888–99.
14. Scheiman JM. Unmet needs in non-steroidal anti-inflammatory drug-induced upper gastrointestinal diseases. Drugs 2006;66:15–21; discussion 29–33.
15. McCarthy D. Nonsteroidal anti-inflammatory drug-related gastrointestinal toxicity: Definitions and epidemiology. Am J Med 1998;105:3S–9S.
16. Larkai EN, Smith JL, Lidsky MD, Graham DY. Gastroduodenal mucosa and dyspeptic symptoms in arthritic patients during chronic nonsteroidal anti-inflammatory drug use. Am J Gastroenterol 1987;82:1153–8.
17. Taha AS, Dahill S, Sturrock RD, et al. Predicting NSAID related ulcers–assessment of clinical and pathological risk factors and importance of differences in NSAID. Gut 1994;35:891–5.
18. Gabriel SE, Jaakkimainen L, Bombardier C. Risk for serious gastrointestinal complications related to use of nonsteroidal anti-inflammatory drugs. A meta-analysis. Ann Intern Med 1991;115:787–96.
19. Silverstein FE, Graham DY, Senior JR, et al. Misoprostol reduces serious gastrointestinal complications in patients with rheumatoid arthritis receiving nonsteroidal anti-inflammatory drugs. A randomized, double-blind, placebo-controlled trial [see comment]. Ann Intern Med 1995;123:241–9.
20. Keenan GF, Giannini EH, Athreya BH. Clinically significant gastropathy associated with nonsteroidal antiinflammatory drug use in children with juvenile rheumatoid arthritis. J Rheumatol 1995;22:1149–51.
21. Langman MJ, Weil J, Wainwright P, et al. Risks of bleeding peptic ulcer associated with individual non-steroidal anti-inflammatory drugs. Lancet 1994;343:1075–8.
22. Matsubara T, Mason W, Kashani IA, et al. Gastrointestinal hemorrhage complicating aspirin therapy in acute Kawasaki disease. J Pediatr 1996;128:701–3.
23. Bombardier C, Laine L, Reicin A, et al. Comparison of upper gastrointestinal toxicity of rofecoxib and naproxen in patients with rheumatoid arthritis. VIGOR Study Group. N Engl J Med 2000;343:1520–8.
24. Silverstein FE, Faich G, Goldstein JL, et al. Gastrointestinal toxicity with celecoxib vs nonsteroidal anti-inflammatory drugs for osteoarthritis and rheumatoid arthritis: The CLASS study: A randomized controlled trial. Celecoxib Long-term Arthritis Safety Study [see comment]. JAMA 2000;284:1247–55.
25. Schnitzer TJ, Burmester GR, Mysler E, et al. Comparison of lumiracoxib with naproxen and ibuprofen in the Therapeutic Arthritis Research and Gastrointestinal Event Trial (TARGET), reduction in ulcer complications: Randomised controlled trial. Lancet 2004;364:665–674.
26. Simon LS, Weaver AL, Graham DY, et al. Anti-inflammatory and upper gastrointestinal effects of celecoxib in rheumatoid arthritis: A randomized controlled trial. JAMA 1999;282:1921–8.
27. Chan FK, Hung LC, Suen BY, et al. Celecoxib versus diclofenac and omeprazole in reducing the risk of recurrent ulcer bleeding in patients with arthritis. N Engl J Med 2002;347:2104–10.
28. Langman MJ, Jensen DM, Watson DJ, et al. Adverse upper gastrointestinal effects of rofecoxib compared with NSAIDs. JAMA 1999;282:1929–33.
29. Bresalier RS, Sandler RS, Quan H, et al. Cardiovascular events associated with rofecoxib in a colorectal adenoma chemoprevention trial. N Engl J Med 2005;352:1092–102.
30. Solomon SD, McMurray JJV, Pfeffer MA, et al. Cardiovascular risk associated with celecoxib in a clinical trial for colorectal adenoma prevention. N Engl J Med 2005;352:1071–80.
31. Solomon DH, Schneeweiss S, Glynn RJ, et al. Relationship between selective cyclooxygenase-2 inhibitors and acute myocardial infarction in older adults. Circulation 2004;109:2068–73.
32. Graham DJ, Campen D, Hui R, et al. Risk of acute myocardial infarction and sudden cardiac death in patients treated with cyclo-oxygenase 2 selective and non-selective non-steroidal anti-inflammatory drugs: Nested case-control study. Lancet 2005;365:475–81.
33. Lazzaroni M, Bianchi Porro G. Nonsteroidal anti-inflammatory drug gastropathy and Helicobacter pylori: The search for an improbable consensus. Am J Med 2001;110:50S–54S.
34. Hawkey CJ, Lanas AI. Doubt and certainty about nonsteroidal anti-inflammatory drugs in the year 2000: A multidisciplinary expert statement. Am J Med 2001;110:79S–100S.
35. Gazarian M, Berkovitch M, Koren G, et al. Experience with misoprostol therapy for NSAID gastropathy in children. Ann Rheum Dis 1995;54:277–80.
36. Graham DY, Agrawal NM, Roth SH. Prevention of NSAID-induced gastric ulcer with misoprostol: Multicentre, double-blind, placebo-controlled trial. Lancet 1988;2:1277–80.
37. Walt RP. Misoprostol for the treatment of peptic ulcer and antiinflammatory-drug-induced gastroduodenal ulceration. N Engl J Med 1992;327:1575–80.
38. Yeomans ND, Tulassay Z, Juhasz L, et al. A comparison of omeprazole with ranitidine for ulcers associated with nonsteroidal antiinflammatory drugs. Acid Suppression Trial: Ranitidine versus Omeprazole for NSAID-associated Ulcer Treatment (ASTRONAUT) Study Group. N Engl J Med 1998;338:719–26.
39. Hawkey CJ, Karrasch JA, Szczepanski L, et al. Omeprazole compared with misoprostol for ulcers associated with nonsteroidal antiinflammatory drugs. Omeprazole versus Misoprostol for NSAID-induced Ulcer Management (OMNIUM) Study Group. N Engl J Med 1998;338:727–34.
40. Lai KC, Lam SK, Chu KM, et al. Lansoprazole for the prevention of recurrences of ulcer complications from long-term low-dose aspirin use. N Engl J Med 2002;346:2033–8.
41. Ehsanullah RS, Page MC, Tildesley G, Wood JR. Prevention of gastroduodenal damage induced by non-steroidal anti-inflammatory drugs: Controlled trial of ranitidine. BMJ 1988;297:1017–21.
42. Robinson MG, Griffin JW, Jr, Bowers J, et al. Effect of ranitidine on gastroduodenal mucosal damage induced by nonsteroidal antiinflammatory drugs. Dig Dis Sci 1989;34:424–8.
43. Lancaster-Smith MJ, Jaderberg ME, Jackson DA. Ranitidine in the treatment of non-steroidal anti-inflammatory drug associated gastric and duodenal ulcers. Gut 1991;32:252–5.
44. Rostom A, Dube C, Wells G, et al. Prevention of NSAID-induced gastroduodenal ulcers. Cochrane Database Syst Rev 2002;Issue 4 Art No:CD002296.
45. Hawkey C, Kahan A, Steinbruck K, et al. Gastrointestinal tolerability of meloxicam compared to diclofenac in osteoarthritis patients. International MELISSA Study Group. Meloxicam Large-Scale International Study Safety Assessment. Br J Rheumatol 1998;37:937–45.
46. Graham DY, Agrawal NM, Campbell DR, et al. Ulcer prevention in long-term users of nonsteroidal anti-inflammatory drugs: Results of a double-blind, randomized, multicenter, active- and placebo-controlled study of misoprostol vs lansoprazole. Arch Intern Med 2002;162:169–75.
47. Lanas A, Bajador E, Serrano P, et al. Nitrovasodilators, low-dose aspirin, other nonsteroidal antiinflammatory drugs, and the risk of upper gastrointestinal bleeding. N Engl J Med 2000;343:834–9.
48. Bandarage UK, Chen L, Fang X, et al. Nitrosothiol esters of diclofenac: Synthesis and pharmacological characterization as gastrointestinal-sparing prodrugs. J Med Chem 2000;43:4005–16.
49. Low SY. Application of pharmaceuticals to nitric oxide. Mol Aspects Med 2005;26:97–138.
50. el-Zimaity HM, Jackson FW, Graham DY. Fundic gland polyps developing during omeprazole therapy. Am J Gastroenterol 1997;92:1858–60.
51. Pashankar DS, Israel DM. Gastric polyps and nodules in children receiving long-term omeprazole therapy. J Pediatr Gastroenterol Nutr 2002;35:658–62.
52. Vieth M, Stolte M. Fundic gland polyps are not induced by proton pump inhibitor therapy. Am J Clin Pathol 2001;116:716–20.
53. Choudhry U, Boyce HW, Jr, Coppola D. Proton pump inhibitor-associated gastric polyps: A retrospective analysis of their frequency, and endoscopic, histologic, and ultrastructural characteristics [see comment]. Am J Clin Pathol 1998;110:615–21.

54. Jalving M, Koornstra JJ, Wesseling J, et al. Increased risk of fundic gland polyps during long-term proton pump inhibitor therapy. Aliment Pharmacol Ther 2006;24:1341–8.

55. Schenk BE, Kuipers EJ, Klinkenberg-Knol EC, et al. Hypergastrinaemia during long-term omeprazole therapy: Influences of vagal nerve function, gastric emptying and *Helicobacter pylori* infection. Aliment Pharmacol Ther 1998;12:605–12.

56. Klinkenberg-Knol EC, Nelis F, Dent J, et al. Long-term omeprazole treatment in resistant gastroesophageal reflux disease: Efficacy, safety, and influence on gastric mucosa. Gastroenterology 2000;118:661–9.

57. Peled N, Dagan O, Babyn P, et al. Gastric-outlet obstruction induced by prostaglandin therapy in neonates. N Engl J Med 1992;327:505–10.

58. SanFilippo A. Infantile hypertrophic pyloric stenosis related to ingestion of erythromycine estolate: A report of five cases. J Pediatr Surg 1976;11:177–80.

59. Cooper WO, Griffin MR, Arbogast P, et al. Very early exposure to erythromycin and infantile hypertrophic pyloric stenosis. Arch Pediatr Adolesc Med 2002;156:647–50.

60. Mahon BE, Rosenman MB, Kleiman MB. Maternal and infant use of erythromycin and other macrolide antibiotics as risk factors for infantile hypertrophic pyloric stenosis. J Pediatr 2001;139:380–4.

61. Applegate MS, Druschel CM. The epidemiology of infantile hypertrophic pyloric stenosis in New York State, 1983 to 1990. Arch Pediatr Adolesc Med 1995;149:1123–9.

62. Centers for Disease Control and Prevention. Hypertrophic pyloric stenosis in infants following pertussis prophylaxis with erythromycin–Knoxville, Tennessee, 1999. MMWR Morb Mortal Wkly Rep 1999;48:1117–20.

63. Honein MA, Paulozzi LJ, Himelright IM, et al. Infantile hypertrophic pyloric stenosis after pertussis prophylaxis with erythromcyin: A case review and cohort study. Lancet 1999;354:2101–5.

64. Heikkinen T, Laine K, Neuvonen PJ, Ekblad U. The transplacental transfer of the macrolide antibiotics erythromycin, roxithromycin and azithromycin. BJOG 2000;107:770–5.

65. Louik C, Werler MM, Mitchell AA. Erythromycin use during pregnancy in relation to pyloric stenosis. Am J Obstet Gynecol 2002;186:288–90.

66. Cooper WO, Ray WA, Griffin MR. Prenatal prescription of macrolide antibiotics and infantile hypertrophic pyloric stenosis. Obstet Gynecol 2002;100:101–6.

67. Ng PC, So KW, Fung KS, et al. Randomised controlled study of oral erythromycin for treatment of gastrointestinal dysmotility in preterm infants. Arch Dis Child Fetal Neonatal Ed 2001;84:F177–82.

68. Nuntnarumit P, Kiatchoosakun P, Tantiprapa W, Boonkasidecha S. Efficacy of oral erythromycin for treatment of feeding intolerance in preterm infants. J Pediatr 2006;148:600–5.

69. Stang H. Pyloric stenosis associated with erythromycin ingested through breastmilk. Minn Med 1986;69:669–70, 682.

70. Toft Sorensen HT, Vinther Skriver Mette MV, Pedersen L, et al. Risk of infantile hypertrophic pyloric stenosis after maternal postnatal use of macrolides. Scand J Infect Dis 2003;35:104–106.

71. Wade DS, Nava HR, Douglass HO, Jr. Neutropenic enterocolitis. Clinical diagnosis and treatment. Cancer 1992;69:17–23.

72. Till M, Lee N, Soper WD, Murphy RL. Typhlitis in patients with HIV-1 infection. Ann Intern Med 1992;116:998–1000.

73. Otaibi AA, Barker C, Anderson R, Sigalet DL. Neutropenic enterocolitis (typhlitis) after pediatric bone marrow transplant. J Pediatr Surg 2002;37:770–2.

74. Kurbegov AC, Sondheimer JM. Pneumatosis intestinalis in non-neonatal pediatric patients. Pediatrics 2001;108:402–6.

75. Katz JA, Wagner ML, Gresik MV, et al. Typhlitis. An 18-year experience and postmortem review. Cancer 1990;65:1041–7.

76. Bohme A, Ganser A, Hoelzer D. Aggravation of vincristine-induced neurotoxicity by itraconazole in the treatment of adult ALL. Ann Hematol 1995;71:311–2.

77. Stark AR, Carlo WA, Tyson JE, et al. Adverse effects of early dexamethasone in extremely-low-birth-weight infants. National Institute of Child Health and Human Development Neonatal Research Network. N Engl J Med 2001;344:95–101.

78. Aschner JL, Deluga KS, Metlay LA, et al. Spontaneous focal gastrointestinal perforation in very low birth weight infants. J Pediatr 1988;113:364–7.

79. Ng PC, Brownlee KG, Dear PR. Gastroduodenal perforation in preterm babies treated with dexamethasone for bronchopulmonary dysplasia. Arch Dis Child 1991;66:1164–6.

80. Buchheit JQ, Stewart DL. Clinical comparison of localized intestinal perforation and necrotizing enterocolitis in neonates. Pediatrics 1994;93:32–6.

81. Shorter NA, Liu JY, Mooney DP, Harmon BJ. Indomethacin-associated bowel perforations: A study of possible risk factors. J Pediatr Surg 1999;34:442–4.

82. Van Overmeire B, Smets K, Lecoutere D, et al. A comparison of ibuprofen and indomethacin for closure of patent ductus arteriosus. N Engl J Med 2000;343:674–81.

83. Bartlett JG. Antibiotic-associated diarrhea. Clin Infect Dis 1992;15:573–81.

84. Hurley BW, Nguyen CC. The spectrum of pseudomembranous enterocolitis and antibiotic-associated diarrhea. Arch Intern Med 2002;162:2177–84.

85. McFarland LV, Brandmarker SA, Guandalini S. Pediatric *Clostridium difficile*: A phantom menace or clinical reality? J Pediatr Gastroenterol Nutr 2000;31:220–31.

86. Ferroni A, Merckx J, Ancelle T, et al. Nosocomial outbreak of *Clostridium difficile* diarrhea in a pediatric service. Eur J Clin Microbiol Infect Dis 1997;16:928–33.

87. Fekety R. Guidelines for the diagnosis and management of *Clostridium difficile*-associated diarrhea and colitis. American College of Gastroenterology, Practice Parameters Committee. Am J Gastroenterol 1997;92:739–50.

88. McFarland LV, Surawicz CM, Stamm WE. Risk factors for *Clostridium difficile* carriage and C. difficile-associated diarrhea in a cohort of hospitalized patients. J Infect Dis 1990;162:678–84.

89. Kelly CP, Pothoulakis C, LaMont JT. *Clostridium difficile* colitis. N Engl J Med 1994;330:257–62.

90. Cerquetti M, Luzzi I, Caprioli A, et al. Role of *Clostridium difficile* in childhood diarrhea. Pediatr Infect Dis J 1995;14:598–603.

91. Delmee M, Verellen G, Avesani V, Francois G. *Clostridium difficile* in neonates: Serogrouping and epidemiology. Eur J Pediatr 1988;147:36–40.

92. Brunetto AL, Pearson AD, Craft AW, Pedler SJ. *Clostridium difficile* in an oncology unit. Arch Dis Child 1988;63:979–81.

93. Tvede M, Schiotz PO, Krasilnikoff PA. Incidence of *Clostridium difficile* in hospitalized children. A prospective study. Acta Paediatr Scand 1990;79:292–9.

94. Fekety R, McFarland LV, Surawicz CM, et al. Recurrent *Clostridium difficile* diarrhea: Characteristics of and risk factors for patients enrolled in a prospective, randomized, double-blinded trial. Clin Infect Dis 1997;24:324–33.

95. Deakin M. Small bowel perforation associated with an excessive dose of slow release diclofenac sodium. BMJ 1988;297:488–9.

96. Cryer B. Nonsteroidal anti-inflammatory drugs and gastrointestinal disease. In: Feldman M, Scharschmidt BF, Sleisenger MH, editors. Sleisenger and Fordtran's Gastrointestinal and Liver Disease: Pathophysiology, Diagnosis, and Management, Vol. 1, 6th edition. Philadelphia: WB Saunders Company; 1998. p. 343–57.

97. Gibson GR, Whitacre EB, Ricotti CA. Colitis induced by nonsteroidal anti-inflammatory drugs. Report of four cases and review of the literature. Arch Intern Med 1992;152:625–32.

98. Graham DY, Opekun AR, Willingham FF, Qureshi WA. Visible small-intestinal mucosal injury in chronic NSAID users. Clin Gastroenterol Hepatol 2005;3:55–9.

99. Goldstein JL, Eisen GM, Lewis B, et al. Video capsule endoscopy to prospectively assess small bowel injury with celecoxib, naproxen plus omeprazole, and placebo. Clin Gastroenterol Hepatol 2005;3:133–41.

100. Allison MC, Howatson AG, Torrance CJ, et al. Gastrointestinal damage associated with the use of nonsteroidal antiinflammatory drugs. N Engl J Med 1992;327:749–54.

101. Nagaraj HS, Sandhu AS, Cook LN, et al. Gastrointestinal perforation following indomethacin therapy in very low birth weight infants. J Pediatr Surg 1981;16:1003–7.

102. Kaufmann HJ, Taubin HL. Nonsteroidal anti-inflammatory drugs activate quiescent inflammatory bowel disease. Ann Intern Med 1987;107:513–6.

103. Felder JB, Korelitz BI, Rajapakse R, et al. Effects of nonsteroidal antiinflammatory drugs on inflammatory bowel disease: A case-control study. Am J Gastroenterol 2000;95:1949–54.

104. Sandborn WJ, Stenson WF, Brynskov J, et al. Safety of celecoxib in patients with ulcerative colitis in remission: A randomized, placebo-controlled, pilot study. Clin Gastroenterol Hepatol 2006;4:203–11.

105. Skelly MM, Logan RFA, Jenkins D, et al. Toxicity of mycophenolate mofetil in patients with inflammatory bowel disease. Inflamm Bowel Dis 2002;8:93–7.

106. Behrend M. Adverse gastrointestinal effects of mycophenolate mofetil: Aetiology, incidence and management. Drug Saf 2001;24:645–63.

107. The Tricontinental Mycophenolate Mofetil Renal Transplantation Study Group. A blinded, randomized clinical trial of mycophenolate mofetil for the prevention of acute rejection in cadaveric renal transplantation. Transplantation 1996;61:1029–37.

108. European Mycophenolate Mofetil Cooperative Study Group. Mycophenolate mofetil in renal transplantation: 3-year results from the placebo-controlled trial. Transplantation 1999;68:391–6.

109. Sollinger HW. Mycophenolate mofetil for the prevention of acute rejection in primary cadaveric renal allograft recipients. U.S. Renal Transplant Mycophenolate Mofetil Study Group. Transplantation 1995;60:225–32.

110. European Mycophenolate Mofetil Cooperative Study Group. Placebo-controlled study of mycophenolate mofetil combined with cyclosporin and corticosteroids for prevention of acute rejection. Lancet 1995;345:1321–5.

111. Butani L, Palmer J, Baluarte HJ, Polinsky MS. Adverse effects of mycophenolate mofetil in pediatric renal transplant recipients with presumed chronic rejection. Transplantation 1999;68:83–6.

112. Hocker B, Weber LT, Bunchman T, et al. Mycophenolate mofetil suspension in pediatric renal transplantation: Three-year data from the tricontinental trial. Pediatr Transplant 2005;9:504–11.

113. Maes BD, Dalle I, Geboes K, et al. Erosive enterocolitis in mycophenolate mofetil-treated renal-transplant recipients with persistent afebrile diarrhea. Transplantation 2003;75:665–72.

114. Dalle IJ, Maes BD, Geboes KP, et al. Crohn's-like changes in the colon due to mycophenolate? Colorectal Dis 2005;7:27–34.

115. Kamar N, Faure P, Dupuis E, et al. Villous atrophy induced by mycophenolate mofetil in renal-transplant patients. Transpl Int 2004;17:463–7.

116. Papadimitriou JC, Drachenberg CB, Beskow CO, et al. Graft-versus-host disease-like features in mycophenolate mofetil-related colitis. Transplant Proc 2001;33:2237–8.

117. Bunnapradist S, Lentine KL, Burroughs TE, et al. Mycophenolate mofetil dose reductions and discontinuations after gastrointestinal complications are associated with renal transplant graft failure. Transplantation 2006;82:102–7.

26.1b. Radiation-Induced Bowel Injury

Wallace K. MacNaughton, PhD

Biological Effects of Ionizing Radiation

The term "radiation" refers to the transfer of energy through space. The type of radiation commonly used for diagnostic and therapeutic purposes is *ionizing radiation*, which is comprised of energetic particles that generate ions when they interact with other atoms or molecules. The incident particle may be stopped, but generate another energetic particle, referred to as secondary or bremsstrahlung radiation, which may also have the ability to interact with other atoms or molecules to cause further ionization. The amount of energy transferred to material as an ionizing particle passes through it is referred to as the linear energy transfer (LET). Radiotherapy applications involve ionizing radiation with relatively high energy such as beta particles (high-energy electrons), gamma radiation, and X-rays (high-energy electromagnetic radiation). Quantification of radiation is expressed in different units, but most relevant to the clinical setting is the Gray (Gy). One Gy = 100 rad = 1 J/kg.

The biological effect of ionizing radiation, specifically cell death, has traditionally been thought to occur by direct interaction with DNA, causing a sufficient degree of double strand breakage to escape the cell's inherent repair capabilities. Double strand breaks will result in unbalanced amounts of DNA segregating into daughter cells during mitosis, causing cell death. Thus, this is often referred to as *mitotic cell death* and is the main reason why rapidly dividing cells, such as tumor cells, are susceptible to ionizing radiation. However, mitotic cell death also affects normal, rapidly dividing cells that might be within the irradiation field, such as those of the gastrointestinal epithelium. More recently, it has become recognized that ionizing radiation can impact other regions of the cell to cause cell death. For example, damaged mitochondria may trigger *apoptotic cell death*. In addition, injured cells may release free radicals or other mediators that alter the behavior of neighboring, unirradiated cells; the so-called *bystander effect*.[1] The different types of radiation-induced cell death are illustrated in Figure 1.

Epidemiology. The effects of ionizing radiation on the gastrointestinal tract were first observed by Walsh in 1897, where the "pain, tenderness on pressure, flatulency, colic, and diarrhea" associated with exposure of the abdomen to ionizing radiation for "2 hours daily" for "some weeks" was taken as evidence of "direct inflammation of the gastrointestinal mucous membranes."[2] Today, we recognize that treatment of abdominal and pelvic malignancies with radiation can result in inflammatory bowel injury or *radiation enteritis*. In children, the use of radiation therapy for neuroblastoma, rhabdomyosarcoma, or Wilms' tumor has diminished and is limited to the cases which have failed to respond to current conventional therapy. In addition, improvements in our understanding of dosing and fractionation, and the increased use of intensity-modulated radiotherapy (IMRT) have reduced the impact of abdominopelvic irradiation on the gut. Furthermore, the surgical use of tissue expanders and absorbable mesh slings to move the bowel out of the irradiation field has been useful in preventing radiation enteritis.[3,4] As a result, bowel injury secondary to abdominal

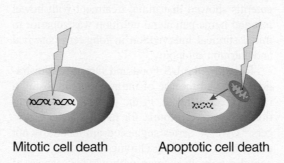

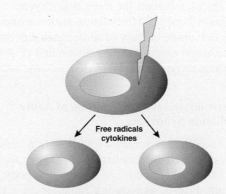

Figure 1 Ionizing radiation can induce cell death in a number of ways. First, the incident ionizing radiation can cause DNA double strand breaks that lead to *mitotic cell death* upon cell division. Second, ionizing radiation may damage organelles such as mitochondria, which could trigger *apoptotic cell* death. Finally, ionizing radiation may cause a cell to release free radicals, cytokines, or other mediators that could affect neighboring cells, the so-called *bystander effect*.

or pelvic radiation therapy is relatively uncommon in children, and most of recent literature about radiation enteritis is based on studies in adults.

Symptoms of radiation enteritis can present early during radiation therapy (*acute radiation enteritis*) or months to years after the completion of therapy (*chronic radiation enteritis*). The occurrence and severity of radiation enteritis are influenced by radiation dose, dose rate and dose per fraction, field size, volume of irradiated small bowel, concomitant chemotherapy, and previous abdominal or pelvic surgery.

In addition to radiation exposures in therapeutic settings, accidental radiation exposures are also well-known causes of bowel injury. In those cases of massive radiation exposure, gastrointestinal tissue damage is often part of multiorgan dysfunction, known as *acute radiation syndrome* (ARS).[5]

Clinical Effects of Abdominopelvic Irradiation

Acute Radiation Enteritis. The cytotoxic effects of radiotherapy are most pronounced in rapidly proliferating epithelial cells in the crypt region of the mucosa. Cell death in crypt cells is observed in the first 24 hours after exposure to radiation. While some of this damage is likely due to direct effects on the epithelial proliferative zone, there is also evidence that apoptotic damage to the endothelium in the mucosal microvasculature precedes crypt cell damage.[6] The severity of radiation enteritis may be related to commensal bacteria present in the gut, since mice raised in a germ-free environment are much more resistant to radiation-induced intestinal injury than mice having a normal intestinal microflora.[7] Regardless of the precipitating lesion, damage to crypt progenitor cells impairs normal replacement of surface epithelial cells with new crypt epithelial cells, which is associated with villous atrophy.[8] Ulceration may occur as the cumulative dose of radiation increases. The loss of absorptive surface leads to malabsorption of nutrients, electrolytes, and water. Nausea, vomiting, abdominal cramps, and diarrhea are common symptoms. Symptoms of acute radiation enteritis can develop within hours after the first dose of radiation, but usually begin during the first few weeks of radiotherapy and resolve 2 to 3 weeks after the completion of treatment. Diarrhea and other intestinal symptoms occur in up to 82% of adults undergoing abdominal or pelvic irradiation.[9–11] In children receiving radiotherapy with chemotherapy for abdominal solid tumor, 71% of patients have vomiting and diarrhea and 30% of patients require intravenous fluid therapy.[12]

The pathological changes that occur in the intestinal mucosa are usually reversible, and acute enteritis symptoms generally resolve 2 to 3 weeks after the completion of treatment. There is no specific diagnostic criterion, other than the temporal relationship between radiation and development of symptoms. An endoscopic examination is rarely warranted to make a diagnosis in the acute setting. Medical management includes treatment of diarrhea, dehydration, malabsorption, and abdominal discomfort. Diarrhea is usually managed with low-fiber diet and antidiarrheal drugs. For diarrhea secondary to bile malabsorption, cholestyramine is effective.[13] Inhibitors of one of the serotonin receptors, 5-hydroxytryptamine-3 (5-HT$_3$) receptor, are effective in reducing radiation-induced nausea and vomiting in randomized controlled trials.[14–17] Therefore, the prophylactic use of a 5-HT$_3$ antagonist is widely recommended.[18–20] Dexamethasone may also be useful when employed in addition to 5-HT$_3$ antagonists.[21] There are conflicting results about the efficacy of salicylates[11,22,23] and sucralfate[10,24,25] in preventing acute radiation enteritis and alleviating enteritis symptoms. The clinical value of these medications needs further evaluation.

Chronic Radiation Enteritis. Chronic radiation enteritis usually develops months to years following the completion of radiation therapy and is characterized by one or more of ulceration, stricture, obstruction, fistula, or perforation. Signs and symptoms include colicky abdominal pain, bloody diarrhea, tenesmus, steatorrhea, weight loss, nausea, and vomiting. It is estimated that 5 to 15% of adults treated with abdominal or pelvic radiation develop these chronic symptoms.[26] An older, retrospective study reported that 11% of children receiving whole abdominal radiation therapy have delayed signs and symptoms of small bowel obstruction.[12] A more recent study of children receiving adjunct radiotherapy for Wilms' tumor reported the frequency of small bowel obstruction of $9.5 \pm 4.5\%$, $13.0 \pm 5.5\%$, and $17.0 \pm 6.5\%$ at 5, 10, and 15-year follow-up, respectively.[27]

The pathogenesis of chronic radiation enteritis is not entirely clear, but is likely due to a combination of continuous signaling for connective tissue deposition and a downregulation of signals that normally turn off fibrogenesis. While several growth factors and cytokines have been implicated, there is strong evidence implicating transforming growth factor (TGF)-β. This cytokine stimulates fibrosis as part of the normal wound repair process, but is chronically upregulated following exposure to ionizing radiation.[28] In animal models, reduction of tissue levels of TGF-β is associated with a decrease in radiation-induced fibrosis.[29] In addition, the elevation of inducible nitric oxide synthase (iNOS) following irradiation of mice decreases the secretory component of epithelial barrier function.[30,31] Irradiation of mice infected with a bacterial pathogen results in a synergistic increase in bacterial transepithelial migration that is greater than that which is observed in mice receiving either radiation or pathogenic infection alone.[32]

The diagnosis of chronic radiation enteritis is established based on the history of radiation exposure, clinical symptoms, and radiographic findings. Plain abdominal radiographs are usually nonspecific, but may show signs of ileus. Radiocontrast studies of the small intestine and colon are useful to detect mucosal ulceration, strictures, and fistulae. CT scan of abdomen and pelvis may be helpful to identify abscesses and to distinguish strictures due to radiation enteritis from those by recurrent tumors. Colonoscopy is also used to evaluate lesions in the colon and terminal ileum. Hydrogen breath test has been used to diagnose small bowel bacterial overgrowth in patients with diarrhea, abdominal pain, nausea, or bloating due to bowel stricture.

Medical management includes control of diarrhea with antidiarrheal agents, nutritional support, and antibiotics for presumed bacterial overgrowth. Surgical intervention often leads to increased mortality and morbidity because of adhesions of the irradiated tissue, and should be reserved, therefore, for definite indications such as perforation, obstruction, abscess drainage, fistulae, and local wound infections. Even with a conservative approach to management, surgery will be required in one-third of patients with chronic radiation enteritis.[33] A recent retrospective study in patients with mechanical bowel obstruction due to chronic radiation enteritis showed that initial treatment with bowel rest and home parenteral nutrition was superior to initial surgical intervention in long-term survival and nutrition autonomy.[34]

Recently, the US Food and Drug Administration approved the use of intravenous amifostin, a radioprotectant agent, in the prevention of radiation-induced xerostomia for head and neck cancers.[35] A case series suggested amifostine is not effective in preventing chronic rectal and bladder complications in women with cervical cancer of the uterus followed for more than 5 years after radiation therapy.[36] More clinical studies are necessary to evaluate efficacy of amifostin in prevention of radiation enteritis during abdominal or pelvic radiation therapy, including in the pediatric setting.

Gastrointestinal Manifestation of Acute Radiation Syndrome

Acute radiation syndrome (ARS) is a serious illness caused by irradiation of greater than 1 Gy to the whole body, or most of the body, by a high dose of penetrating radiation in a very short period of time.[37] ARS is rare as it is usually observed in accidental, nonmedical settings. The median lethal dose of whole-body radiation at 60 days (LD$_{50/60}$) is 3.25 to 4 Gy in patients without access to medical care and 6 to 7 Gy in those under medical care.[38] Clinical components of ARS include the hematopoietic, gastrointestinal, cerebrovascular, and skin syndromes. ARS is characterized by four distinct phases: a prodromal period (0 to 2 days after exposure), a latent period (for a few hours to a few weeks), a period of illness (for weeks to months), and recovery or death. Gastrointestinal damage in the acute radiation syndrome is essentially a severe form of acute radiation enteritis in therapeutic settings. Severe nausea, vomiting, diarrhea, and abdominal cramps occur in a prodromal phase. The time to emesis is one indicator of radiation dose: most patients exposed to >3.5 Gy will vomit within 2 hours of exposure.[5,39] Then, a symptom-free, latent period lasts for a few hours or even up to a few weeks, depending on the size of the radiation dose. At doses greater than 6 to 8 Gy, the latent period is followed by an illness characterized with severe vomiting and bloody diarrhea. Life-threatening dehydration and electrolyte imbalance can result in circulatory collapse. Malabsorption and ileus are also common. Together with bone marrow suppression, depletion of circulating leukocytes, and decreased immune function, the disruption of intestinal epithelial barrier leads to bacterial translocation and sepsis. Aggressive fluid resuscitation, correction of electrolyte imbalance, control of emesis with serotonin receptor antagonists, prophylaxis of gastrointestinal ulcer, and nutritional support are crucial in patients with gastrointestinal symptoms arising from ARS.[37]

REFERENCES

1. Prise KM, Schettino G, Folkard M, Held KD. New insights on cell death from radiation exposure. Lancet Oncol 2005;6:520–8.
2. Walsh D. Deep tissue traumatism from roentgen ray exposure. BMJ 1897;2:272–3.
3. Meric F, Hirschl RB, Mahboudi S, et al. Prevention of radiation enteritis in children, using a pelvic mesh sling. J Pediatr Surg 1994;29:917–21.
4. Abhyankar A, Jenney M, Huddart SN, et al. Use of a tissue expander and a polyglactic acid (Vicryl) mesh to reduce radiation enteritis: Case report and literature review. Pediatr Surg Int 2005;21:755–7.
5. Berger ME, Christensen DM, Lowry PC, et al. Medical management of radiation injuries: Current approaches. Occupational Med (Oxf) 2006;56:162–72.
6. Paris F, Fuks Z, Kang A, et al. Endothelial apoptosis as the primary lesion initiating intestinal radiation damage in mice. Science 2001;293:293–7.
7. Crawford PA, JI Gordon. Microbial regulation of intestinal radiosensitivity. Proc Natl Acad Sci U S A 2005;102:13254–9.
8. Carr KE. Effects of radiation damage on intestinal morphology. Int Rev Cytol 2001;208:1–119.
9. Herbert SH, Curran WJ, Jr, Solin LJ, et al. Decreasing gastrointestinal morbidity with the use of small bowel contrast during treatment planning for pelvic irradiation. Int J Rad Oncol Biol Phys 1991;20:835–42.
10. Henriksson R, Franzen L, Littbrand B. Prevention and therapy of radiation-induced bowel discomfort. Scand J Gastroenterol Suppl 1992;27:7–11.
11. Resbeut M, Marteau P, Cowen D, et al. A randomized double blind placebo controlled multicenter study of mesalazine for the prevention of acute radiation enteritis. Radiother Oncol 1997;44:59–63.
12. Donaldson SS, Jundt S, Ricour C, et al. Radiation enteritis in children. A retrospective review, clinicopathologic correlation, and dietary management. Cancer 1975;35:1167–78.
13. Arlow FL, Dekovich AA, Priest RJ, Beher WT. Bile acids in radiation-induced diarrhea. South Med J 1987;80:1259–61.
14. Franzen L, Nyman J, Hagberg H, et al. A randomised placebo controlled study with ondansetron in patients undergoing fractionated radiotherapy. Ann Oncol 1996;7:587–92.
15. Prentice HG, Cunningham S, Gandhi L, et al. Granisetron in the prevention of irradiation-induced emesis. Bone Marrow Transplant 1995;15:445–8.

16. Priestman TJ, Roberts JT, Lucraft H, et al. Results of a randomized, double-blind comparative study of ondansetron and metoclopramide in the prevention of nausea and vomiting following high-dose upper abdominal irradiation. Clin Oncol (Royal College of Radiologists) 1990;2:71–5.

17. Spitzer TR, Bryson JC, Cirenza E, et al. Randomized double-blind, placebo-controlled evaluation of oral ondansetron in the prevention of nausea and vomiting associated with fractionated total-body irradiation. J Clin Oncol 1994;12:2432–8.

18. Kris MG, Hesketh PJ, Somerfield MR, et al. American Society of Clinical Oncology guideline for antiemetics in oncology: Update 2006. J Clin Oncol 2006;24:2932–47.

19. Maranzano E, Feyer P, Molassiotis A, et al. Evidence-based recommendations for the use of antiemetics in radiotherapy. Radiother Oncol 2005;76:227–33.

20. Feyer P, Maranzano E, Molassiotis A, et al. Radiotherapy-induced nausea and vomiting (RINV): Antiemetic guidelines. Support Care Cancer 2005;13:122–8.

21. Wong RK, Paul N, Ding K, et al. 5-Hydroxytryptamine-3 receptor antagonist with or without short-course dexamethasone in the prophylaxis of radiation induced emesis: A placebo-controlled randomized trial of the National Cancer Institute of Canada Clinical Trials Group (SC19). J Clin Oncol 2006;24:3458–64.

22. Kilic D, Egehan I, Ozenirler S, Dursun A. Double-blinded, randomized, placebo-controlled study to evaluate the effectiveness of sulphasalazine in preventing acute gastrointestinal complications due to radiotherapy. Radiother Oncol 2000;57:125–129.

23. Baughan CA, Canney PA, Buchanan RB, Pickering RM. A randomized trial to assess the efficacy of 5-Aminosalicylic acid for the prevention of radiation enteritis. Clin Oncol (Royal College of Radiologists) 1993;5:19–24.

24. Henriksson R, Franzen L, Littbrand B. Effects of sucralfate on acute and late bowel discomfort following radiotherapy of pelvic cancer. J Clin Oncol 1992;10:969–75.

25. Kneebone A, Mameghan H, Bolin T, et al. Effect of oral sucralfate on late rectal injury associated with radiotherapy for prostate cancer: A double-blind, randomized trial. Int J Radiat Oncol Biol Phys 2004;60:1088–97.

26. Waddell BE, Rodriguez-Bigas MA, Lee RJ, et al. Prevention of chronic radiation enteritis. J Am Coll Surg 1999;189:611–24.

27. Paulino AC, Wen BC, Brown CK, et al. Late effects in children treated with radiation therapy for Wilms' tumor. Int J Radiat Oncol Biol Phys 2000;46:1239–46.

28. Richter KK, Langberg CW, Sung CC, Hauer-Jensen M. Increased transforming growth factor β (TGF-β) immunoreactivity is independently associated with chronic injury in both consequential and primary radiation enteropathy. Int J Radiat Oncol Biol Phys 1997;39:187–95.

29. Denham JW, Hauer-Jensen M. The radiotherapeutic injury a complex "wound." Radiother Oncol 2002;63:129–45.

30. Freeman SL, MacNaughton WK. Ionizing radiation induces iNOS-mediated epithelial dysfunction in the absence of an inflammatory response. Am J Physiol Gastrointest Liver Physiol 2000;278:G243–50.

31. Freeman SL, MacNaughton WK. Nitric oxide inhibitable isoforms of adenylate cyclase mediate epithelial secretory dysfunction following exposure to ionising radiation. Gut 2004;53:214–21.

32. Skinn AC, Vergnolle N, Cellars L, et al. Combined challenge of mice with *Citrobacter rodentium* and ionizing radiation promotes bacterial translocation. Int J Radiat Biol 2007;83:375–82.

33. Regimbeau JM, Panis Y, Gouzi JL, Fagniez PL. Operative and long term results after surgery for chronic radiation enteritis. Am J Surg 2001;182:237–42.

34. Gavazzi C, Bhoori S, LoVullo S, et al. Role of home parenteral nutrition in chronic radiation enteritis. Am J Gastroenterol 2006;101:374–9.

35. Jellema AP, Slotman BJ, Muller MJ, et al. Radiotherapy alone, versus radiotherapy with amifostine 3 times weekly, versus radiotherapy with amifostine 5 times weekly: A prospective randomized study in squamous cell head and neck cancer. Cancer 2006;107:544–53.

36. Mitsuhashi N, Takahashi I, Takahashi M, et al. Clinical study of radioprotective effects of amifostine (YM-08310, WR- 2721) on long-term outcome for patients with cervical cancer. Int J Radiat Oncol Biol Phys 1993;26:407–11.

37. Waselenko JK, MacVittie TJ, Blakely WF, et al. Medical management of the acute radiation syndrome: Recommendations of the Strategic National Stockpile Radiation Working Group. Ann Int Med 2004;140:1037–51.

38. Anno GH, Young RW, Bloom RM, Mercier JR. Dose response relationships for acute ionizing-radiation lethality. Health Phys 2003;84:565–75.

39. Anno GH, Baum SJ, Withers HR, Young RW. Symptomatology of acute radiation effects in humans after exposure to doses of 0.5–30 Gy. Health Phys 1989;56:821–38.

INDEX